SAUNDERS

2004 ICD-9-CM,

Volumes 1, 2, and 3

AND

HCPCS Level II

SAUNDERS

2004 ICD-9-CM, Volumes 1, 2, and 3 AND HCPCS Level II

Includes Official Coding Guidelines!

Carol J. Buck, MS, CPC

Program Director (Ret.), Medical Secretary Programs
Northwest Technical College
East Grand Forks, Minnesota

Technical Collaborator:
Karla R. Lovaasen, RHIA, CCS
Director of Health Information Management
(Health Information and Business Office)
St. Francis Medical Center/Home
Breckenridge, Minnesota

SAUNDERS
An Imprint of Elsevier

SAUNDERS
An Imprint of Elsevier

11830 Westline Industrial Drive
St. Louis, Missouri 63146

DISCLAIMER

Every effort has been made to make this text complete and accurate, but no guarantee, warranty, or representation is made for its accuracy or completeness.

W.B. Saunders Company and Carol J. Buck are not providing any legal or professional service/advice in presenting these codes and bear no liability for how the codes are used.

THE PUBLISHER

Publishing Director: Andrew Allen
Executive Editor: Adrianne Cochran
Acquisitions Editor: Susan Cole
Developmental Editor: Beth LoGiudice
Publishing Services Manager: Linda McKinley
Project Manager: Ellen Kunkelmann
Designer: Mark Oberkrom

Saunders 2004 ICD-9-CM, Volumes 1, 2, and 3, and HCPCS Level II ISBN 1-4160-0046-1

Printed in the United States of America.

Last digit is the print number: 9 8 7 6 5 4 3 2 1

GUIDE TO USING THE SAUNDERS 2004 ICD-9-CM, Volumes 1, 2, and 3, AND HCPCS Level II

Medical coding has long been a part of the health care profession. Through the years medical coding systems have become more complex and extensive. Today, medical coding is an intricate and immense process that is present in every health care setting. The increased use of electronic submissions for health care services only increases the need for coders who understand the coding process.

Saunders 2004 ICD-9-CM Volumes 1, 2, & 3 and HCPCS Level II was developed to help meet the needs of students preparing for a career in medical coding by offering a comprehensive coding text at a reasonable price. This text combines the official coding guidelines, all three volumes of the ICD-9-CM, and HCPCS in one book—three books in one.

All material strictly adheres to the latest government versions available at the time of printing.

ILLUSTRATIONS AND ITEMS

The ICD-9-CM, Volume 1, Tabular List contains illustrations, pictures, and items to assist you in understanding difficult terminology, diseases/conditions, or coding in a specific category. Items are always printed in ▬ ink so the added material is not mistaken for official notations or instructions. Your ideas on what other descriptions or illustrations should be in future editions of this text are always appreciated.

Annotated

Throughout this text revisions and additions are indicated by the following symbols:

- ⬅ ➡ **Revised:** Revisions within the line or code from the previous edition are indicated by the black arrow.
- ◀ ▶ **New:** Additions to the previous edition are indicated by the color triangle.

The revision and addition symbols are the only symbols that appear in the ICD-9-CM indexes.

ICD-9-CM, Volume 1, Tabular List Symbols

- ● **Not a principal diagnosis:** These codes have a black dot before them. These codes give additional information or describe the circumstances affecting the health care encounter but are unacceptable as principal diagnosis codes.
- ● **Use additional digit(s):** The color dot cautions you that the code requires additional digit(s) to insure the greatest specificity.
- ❑ **Nonspecific code:** These have a square before the code. Although these codes are valid as a principal diagnosis, they are usually too general to be used as a principal diagnosis for Medicare, and you should continue to seek a code that is more specific.

ICD-9-CM, Volume 3, Tabular List Symbols

- ● **Use additional digit(s):** The color dot cautions you that the code requires additional digit(s) to insure the greatest specificity.
- ✖ **Valid O.R. procedure:** The color "x" is placed before a code that is a valid operating room (O.R.) procedure according to the DRG grouper.

In addition to the symbols, the official ICD-9-CM conventions appear throughout the text. Refer to the illustrations of conventions on the following pages and to the Introduction for further information on conventions.

HCPCS Symbols

- ◎ **Special coverage instructions** apply to these codes. Usually these special coverage instructions are included in the Medicare Carrier Manual (MCM) select references in Appendix A or in the Coverage Issues Manual (CIM) in Appendix B of this text.

- ◆ **Not covered by or valid for Medicare** is indicated by the diamond. Usually the reason for the exclusion is included in the Medicare Carrier Manual (MCM) select references in Appendix A or in the Coverage Issues Manual (CIM) in Appendix B of this text.

- * **Carrier discretion** is an indication that you must contact the individual third-party payors to find out the coverage available for codes identified by this symbol.

SAUNDERS
2004 ICD-9-CM, Volumes 1, 2, and 3, and HCPCS LEVEL II

Symbols Used in All Volumes of ICD-9-CM to Identify New or Revised Material

Volume 1, Tabular List

237.70 Neurofibromatosis, unspecified ◀ ← Indicates **new** information or a new code.

● **V01.1 Cholera** ⇐ ← Indicates a **revision** within the line or code.

Volume 2, Alphabetic Index

Illness—*see also* Disease
factitious 300.19 ⇐
with
combined physical and ◀
psychological symptoms 300.19
◀

Volume 3, Procedures, Index

Biopsy
peritoneum ⇐
closed 54.24 ◀

Volume 3, Procedures, Tabular List

37 **Other operations on heart and pericardium** ⇐
Code also any injection or infusion of platelet inhibitor (99.20)

92 **Stereotactic radiosurgery** ◀

Symbols for Volume 1, Tabular List

Use Additional Digit(s): The color dot cautions you that the code requires additional digit(s) to ensure the greatest specificity.

● **237.7 Neurofibromatosis**
von Recklinghausen's disease
❑ **237.70 Neurofibromatosis, unspecified**

Nonspecific code: These codes have a square before them. Although these codes are valid as a principal diagnosis, they are usually too general to be used as a principal diagnosis for Medicare, and you should continue to seek a code that is more specific.

Not a Principal Diagnosis: These codes have a black dot before them. These codes give additional information or describe the circumstances affecting the health care encounter but are unacceptable as principal diagnosis codes.

● **V01.1 Cholera**

Conventions for Volume 1, Tabular List

Notes define terms or give coding instructions.

2. NEOPLASMS (140–239)

Notes

1. Content

This chapter contains the following broad groups:

140–195 Malignant neoplasms, stated or presumed to be primary, of specified sites, except of lymphatic and hematopoietic tissue.

"Use additional digit(s)" directs you to use an additional code to give a more complete picture of the diagnosis.

510 Empyema
Use additional code to identify infectious organism (041.0–041.9)

"*Code first*" is used in those categories not intended as the principal diagnosis. In such cases, the code, title, and instructions appear in italics. The note requires that the underlying disease (etiology) be sequenced first.

366.4 Cataract associated with other disorders
366.41 Diabetic cataract
Code first diabetes (250.5)

A code with this note may be principal if no causal condition is applicable or known

428 Heart failure
Code, if applicable, heart failure due to hypertension first (402.0-402.9, with fifth-digit 1 or 404.0-404.9 with fifth-digit 1 or 3)

474 Chronic disease of tonsils and adenoids

"and" indicates a code that can be assigned if either of the conditions is present or if both of the conditions are present.

366.4 Cataract associated with other disorders

"with" indicates a code that can only be used if both conditions are present.

087 Relapsing fever
Includes: recurrent fever

The "Includes" note appears immediately under a code to further define, or give example of, the contents of the code.

420.0 ***Acute pericarditis in disease classified elsewhere***

Italicized type is used for all exclusion notes and to identify those codes that are not usually sequenced as the principal diagnosis.

150.2 Abdominal esophagus
Excludes: *recurrent fever*

Terms following the word "Excludes" are to be coded elsewhere. The term "Excludes" means "Do Not Code Here."

244.8 Other specified acquired hypothyroidism
Secondary hypothyroidism NEC

NEC means Not Elsewhere Classifiable and is to be used only when the information at hand specifies a condition but there is no more specific code for that condition.

Bold type is used for all codes and titles.

159.0 Intestinal tract, part unspecified
Intestine NOS

NOS means Not Otherwise Specified and is the equivalent of "unspecified."

426.89 Other
Dissociation:
atrioventricular [AV]

Brackets are used to enclose synonyms, alternative wording, or explanatory phrases.

158.8 Specified parts of peritoneum
Cul-de-sac (of Douglas)
Mesentery

Parentheses are used to enclose supplementary words that may be present or absent in the statement of a disease without affecting the code.

628.4 Of cervical or vaginal origin
Infertility associated with:
anomaly of cervical mucus
congenital structural anomaly

A colon is used after an incomplete term that needs one or more of the modifiers that follow in order to make it assignable to a given category.

Conventions for Volume 2, Alphabetic Index

Nonessential modifiers are enclosed in parentheses and are words that may be used to clarify the diagnosis but do not affect the code.

Ileus (adynamic) (bowel) (colon) (inhibitory) (intestine) (neurogenic) (paralytic)

Essential modifiers are NOT enclosed in parentheses and are subterms that DO affect the selection of the appropriate code.

Incoordination
esophageal-pharyngeal (newborn) 787.2

"see" is a cross reference directing you to look elsewhere.

Hereditary—*see* condition

Paralysis
embolic (current episode) (*see also* Embolism, brain) 434.1

"*see also*" is a cross reference directing you to look under another main term if all the information being searched for cannot be located under the first main term entry.

Delivery
completely normal case—*see* category 650

"*see* category" is a cross reference directing you to Volume 1, Tabular List for important information governing the use of the specific code.

Amputation
traumatic (complete) (partial)

"Notes" are used to define terms and give coding instructions

Note "Complicated" includes traumatic amputation with delayed healing, delayed treatment, foreign body, or major infection.

Adolescence NEC V21.2

NEC means Not Elsewhere Classifiable.

Conventions for Volume 3, Procedures Index

Arthrotomy 80.10
as operative approach—*omit code*

"*omit code*" identifies procedures or services that are included in another larger procedure or service. For example, an incision that is part of the main surgical procedure is not coded separately.

Ileal
bladder
closed 57.87 [*45.51*]

For some operative procedures it is necessary to record the individual components of the procedure. These procedures are termed **"synchronous procedures"** and are listed together in the Index. The codes are sequenced in the same order as displayed in the Index.

Operation
Thompson
cleft lip repair 27.54
correction of lymphedema 40.9
quadricepsplasty 83.86

Eponyms are operations named for people and are listed in the Index both under the eponym and under the term "Operation."

Thompson operation
cleft lip repair 27.54
correction of lymphedema 40.9
quadricepsplasty 83.86

Volume 3, Index to Procedures, also contains "*see*," "*see also*," "*see* category," "essential modifiers," "nonessential modifiers," "notes," NEC, and NOS as in Volume 2, Alphabetic Index.

Symbols for Volume 3, Procedures, Tabular List

Use additional digit(s): The color dot cautions you that the code requires additional digit(s) to ensure the greatest specificity.

● **31.9 Other operations on larynx and trachea**

✖ **31.91 Division of laryngeal nerve**

Valid O.R. procedure: The red X is placed before a code that is a valid operating room (O.R.) procedure according to the DRG grouper.

Conventions for Volume 3, Procedures, Tabular List

Bold type is used for all codes and titles.

88.4 Arteriography using contrast material

Includes: angiography of arteries
arterial puncture for injection of contrast material
radiography of arteries (by fluoroscopy)
retrograde arteriography

The "Includes" note appears to further define, or give example of, the contents of the code.

The fifth-digit subclassification identifies the site to be viewed, not the site of injection

Excludes: arteriography using:
radioisotopes or radionuclides (92.01–92.19)

Terms following the word "Excludes" are to be coded elsewhere. The term means "Do Not Code Here."

45.5 Isolation of intestinal segment

Code also any synchronous:
anastomosis other than end-to-end (45.90–45.94)
enterostomy (46.10–46.39)

For some operative procedures it is necessary to record the individual components of the procedure. These procedures are termed "synchronous procedures."

Symbols for HCPCS

Special coverage instructions apply to these codes. Usually these instructions are included in the Medicare Carrier Manual (MCM) select references in Appendix A or in the Coverage Issues Manual (CIM) in Appendix B of this text. → ✪

L3540 Miscellaneous shoe additions, sole, full
MCM 2079, CIM 70-3

Medicare Carrier Manual (MCM) and Coverage Issues Manual (CIM) give instructions regarding use of the code. MCM and CIM select references are located in the appendices of this text.

Not covered by or valid for Medicare is indicated by the diamond. Usually the reason for the exclusion is included in the Medicare Carrier Manual (MCM) references in Appendix A or in the Coverage Issues Manual (CIM) in Appendix B of this text. → ◆

A5074 Pouch, urinary; with faceplate attached; plastic or rubber
MCM 2130

Carrier discretion is an indication that you must contact the individual third-party payors to find out the coverage available for these codes. → ✻

A6154 Wound pouch, each

Indicates **new** information or a new code. → ▶

A4614 Peak expiratory flow rate meter, hand held

Indicates a **revision** within the line or code. → ➠

J0270 Injection alprostadil, per 1.25 mcg

GUIDE TO THE 2004 ICD-9-CM UPDATES and 2003 HCPCS Updates

VOLUME 1 CHANGES EFFECTIVE OCTOBER 1, 2003 AND CLASSIFICATION OF DISEASES AND E CODES

1. INFECTIOUS AND PARASITIC DISEASES (001–139)

038 Septicemia

Add Use additional code for systemic inflammatory response syndrome (SIRS), 995.91–995.92)

2. NEOPLASMS (140–239)

202 Other malignant neoplasms of lymphoid and histiocytic tissue

202.5 Letterer-Siwe disease

Revise **Excludes** *Hand-Schüller-Christian disease (277.89)*

Revise *histiocytosis (acute) (chronic) (277.89)*

Revise *histiocytosis X (chronic) (277.89)*

202.9 Other and unspecified malignant neoplasms of lymphoid and histiocytic tissue

Add Follicular dendritic cell sarcoma

Add Interdigitating dendritic cell sarcoma

Add Langerhans cell sarcoma

222 Benign neoplasm of male genital organs

222.2 Prostate

Revise **Excludes** *adenomatous hyperplasia of prostate (600.20–600.21)*

prostatic:

Revise *adenoma (600.20–600.21)*

Revise *enlargement (600.00–600.01)*

Revise *hypertrophy (600.00–600.01)*

238 Neoplasms of uncertain behavior of other and unspecified sites and tissues

238.7 Other lymphatic hematopoietic tissues

Revise **Excludes** *myelofibrosis (289.89)*

Revise *myelosclerosis NOS (289.89)*

3. ENDOCRINE, NUTRITIONAL AND METABOLIC DISEASES, AND IMMUNITY DISORDERS (240–279)

250 Diabetes mellitus

Revise **Excludes** *nonclinical diabetes (790.29)*

250.5 Diabetes with ophthalmic manifestations

Use additional code to identify manifestation as:

diabetic

Revise retinal edema (362.01)

254 Diseases of thymus gland

Revise **Excludes** *myasthenia gravis (358.00)*

255 Disorders of adrenal glands

255.1 Hyperaldosteronism

Delete ~~Aldosteronism (primary) (secondary)~~

~~Bartter's syndrome~~

~~Conn's syndrome~~

New code **255.10 Primary aldosteronism**

Aldosteronism NOS

Hyperaldosteronism, unspecified

New code **255.11 Glucocorticoid-remediable aldosteronism**

Familiar aldosteronism type I

New code **255.12 Conn's syndrome**

New code **255.13 Bartter's syndrome**

New code **255.14 Other secondary aldosteronism**

277 Other and unspecified disorders of metabolism

277.7 Dysmetabolic syndrome X

Use additional code for associated manifestation, such as:

Revise cardiovascular disease (414.00–414.07)

277.8 Other specified disorders of metabolism

Delete ~~Hand-Schuller-Christian disease~~

~~Histiocytosis (acute) (chronic)~~

~~Histiocytosis X (chronic)~~

Delete **Excludes** ~~histiocytosis~~

~~acute differentiated progressive (202.5)~~

~~X, acute (progressive) (202.5)~~

New code **277.81 Primary carnitine deficiency**

New code **277.82 Carnitine deficiency due to inborn errors of metabolism**

New code **277.83 Iatrogenic carnitine deficiency**

Carnitine deficiency due to:

Hemodialysis

Valproic acid therapy

New code **277.84 Other secondary carnitine deficiency**

New code **277.89 Other specified disorders of metabolism**

Hand-Schuller-Christian disease

Histiocytosis (acute) (chronic)

Histiocytosis (chronic)

Excludes *histiocytes:*

acute differentiated progressive (202.5)

X, acute (progressive) (202.5)

278 Obesity and other hyperalimentation

278.0 Obesity

278.01 Morbid obesity

Add Severe obesity

4. DISEASES OF THE BLOOD AND BLOOD-FORMING ORGANS (280–289)

280 Iron deficiency anemias

Revise **Excludes** *familial microcytic anemia (282.49)*

282 Hereditary hemolytic anemias

284.4 Thalassemias

Delete ~~Cooley's anemia~~

Delete ~~Hereditary leptocytosis~~

Delete ~~Mediterranean anemia (with other hemoglobinopathy)~~

Delete ~~Microdrepanocytosis~~

Delete ~~Sickle-cell thalassemia~~

Delete ~~Thalassemia (alpha) (beta) (intermedia) (major) (minima) (minor) (mixed) (trait) (with other hemoglobinopathy)~~

Delete ~~Thalassemia Hb-S disease~~

Revise **Excludes** *sickle cell:* ~~*anemia*~~ *disease (282.60–282.69)*

New code **282.41 Sickle-cell thalassemia without crisis**

Sickle-cell thalassemia NOS

Thalassemia Hb-S disease without crisis

New code **282.42 Sickle-cell thalasemia with crisis**

Sickle-cell thalassemia with vasoocculsive pain

Thalassemia Hb-S disease without crisis

Use additional code for types of crisis, such as:

Acute chest syndrome (517.3)

Splenic sequestration (289.52)

New code 282.49 **Other thalassemia**
Cooley's anemia
Hereditary leptocytosis
Mediterranean anemia (with other hemoglobinopathy)
Microdrepanocytosis
Thalassemia (alpha) (beta) (intermedia) (major) (minima) (minor) (mixed) (trait) (with other hemoglobinopathy)
Thalassemia NOS
282.5 **Sickle-cell trait**
Revise **Excludes** *that with thalassemia (282.490)*
Revise 282.6 **Sickle-cell ~~anemia~~ disease**
Add Sickle-cell anemia
Revise **Excludes** *sickle-cell thalassemia (282.41–283.42)*
Revise 282.60 **Sickle-cell ~~anemia~~ disease, unspecified**
Add Sickle-cell anemia NOS
Revise 282.61 **~~Hb-S~~ HB-SS, disease without ~~mention of~~ crisis**
Revise 282.62 **~~Hb-S~~ Hb-SS, disease with ~~mention of~~ crisis**
Add Hb-SS disease with vaso-occlusive pain
Add Use additional code for types of crisis, such as:
Add Acute chest syndrome (517.3)
Add Splenic sequestration (289.52)
Revise 282.63 **Sickle-cell/Hb-C disease without crisis**
Revise Hb-S/Hb-C disease without crisis
New code 282.64 **Sickle-cell/Hb-C disease with crisis**
Hb-S/Hb-C disease with crisis
Sickle-cell/Hb-C disease with vaso-occlusive pain
Use additional code for types of crisis, such as:
Add acute chest syndrome (517.3)
Add splenic sequestration (289.52)
New code 282.68 **Other sickle-cell disease without crisis**
Hb-S/Hb-D disease without crisis
Hb-S/Hb-E disease without crisis
Sickle-cell/Hb-D disease without crisis
Sickle-cell/Hb-E disease without crisis
Revise 282.69 **Other ~~hemoglobinopathies~~ sickle-cell disease with crisis ~~Disease~~**
Hb-S/Hb-D disease with crisis
Hb-S/Hb-E disease with crisis
Other sickle-cell disease with vaso-occlusive pain
Sickle-cell/Hb-D disease with crisis
Sickle-cell/Hb-E disease with crisis
Add Use additional code for types of crisis, such as:
Add acute chest syndrome (517.3)
Add splenic sequestration (289.52)
285 **Other and unspecified anemia**
285.2 **Anemia in chronic illness**
285.21 **Anemia in end-stage renal disease**
Add Erythropoieten-resistant (EPO resistant anemia)
289 **Other diseases of blood and blood-forming organs**
289.5 **Other disease of spleen**
New code 289.52 **Splenic sequestrian**
Add Code first sickle-cell disease in crisis (282.42, 282.62, 282.65, 282.69)
289.8 **Other specified diseases of blood and blood-forming organs**
Delete ~~Hypergammaglobulinemia~~
~~Myelofibrosis~~
~~Pseudocholinesteras deficiency~~

New code 289.81 **Primary hypercoagulable state**
Activated protein C resistance
Antithrombin III deficiency
Factor VI Leiden mutation
Lupus anticoagulant
Protein C deficiency
Protein S deficiency
Prothrombin gene mutation
New code 289.82 **Secondary hypercoagulable state**
New code 289.89 **Other specified disease of blood and blood-forming organs**
Hypergammaglobulinemia
Myelofibrosis
Pseudocholinesterase deficiency

5. MENTAL DISORDERS (290–319)
294 **Other organic psychotic conditons (chronic)**
294.1 **Dementia in conditions classified elsewhere**
Code first in any underlying physical conditions, as: dementia in:
Add Dementia with Lewy bodies (331.82)
Add Dementia with Parkinsonims (331.82)
Add Fontal dementia (331.19)
Add Frontotemporal dementia (331.19)
Revise Pick's disease of the brain (331.11)
302 **Sexual deviations and disorders**
302.7 **Psychosexual dysfunction**
302.71 **With inhibited sexual desire**
Add **Excludes** *decreased sexual desire NOS (799.81)*
310 **Specified nonpsychotic mental disorders due to organic brain damage**
310.1 **Organic personality syndrome**
Add **Excludes** *memory loss of unknown cause (780.93)*

6. DISEASES OF THE NERVOUS SYSTEM AND SENSE ORGANS (320–389)
331 **Other cerebral degeneration**
Revise 331.1 **~~Pick's disease~~ Frontotemporal dementia**
Add Use additional code for associated behavior disturbance (294.10–294.11)
New code 331.11 **Pick's disease**
New code 331.19 **Other frontotemporal dementia**
Frontal dementia
331.8 **Other cerebral degenerations**
New code 331.82 **Dementia with Lewy bodies**
Dementia with Parkinsonism
Lewy body dementia
Lewy body disease
Use additional code for associated behavioral disturbances (294.0–294.11)
332 **Parkinson's disease**
Add **Excludes** *dementia with Parkinsonism (331.82)*
348 **Other conditions of brain**
Revise 348.3 **Encephalopathy, ~~unspecified~~ not elsewhere classified**
New code 348.30 **Encephalopathy, unspecified**
New code 348.31 **Metabolic encephalopathy**
Septic encephalopathy
New code 348.39 **Other encephalopathy**
Excludes *encephalopathy:*
alcoholic (291.2)
hepatic (572.2)
hypertensive (347.2)
toxic (349.82)
358 **Myoneural disorders**
358.0 **Myasthenia gravis**
New code 385.00 **Myasthenia gravis not in (acute) exacerbation**
Myasthenia gravis NOS
New code 385.01 **Myasthenia gravis in (acute) exacerbation**
Myasthenia gravis in crisis

7. DISEASES OF THE CIRCULATORY SYSTEM (390–459)

411 Other acute and subacute forms of ischemic heart disease

411.8 Other

411.81 Acute coronary occlusion without myocardial infarction

Excludes *obstruction without infarction due to atherosclerosis (414.00–414.07)*
occlusion without infarction due to atherosclerosis (414.00–414.07)

414 Other forms of chronic ischemic heart disease

414.0 Coronary atherosclerosis

Revise **414.06 Of native coronary artery of transplanted heart**

New code **414.07 Of bypass graft (artery) (vein) of transplanted heart**

440 Artherosclerosis

440.8 Of other specified arteries

Revise **Excludes** *coronary (414.00–414.07)*

447 Other disorders of arteries and arterioles

447.6 Arteritis, unspecified

Revise **Excludes** coronary (414.00–414.07)

458 Hypotension

458.2 Iatrogenic hypotensions

Delete ~~Postoperative hypotension~~

New code **458.21 Hypotension of hemodialysis**
Intra-dialytic hypotension

New code **458.29 Other iatrogenic hypotension**
Postoperative hypotension

8. DISEASES OF THE RESPIRATORY SYSTEM (460–519)

466 Acute bronchitis and bronchiolitis

466.0 Acute bronchitis

Delete **Excludes** ~~acute bronchitis with:~~
Delete ~~bronchiectasis (494.1)~~
Delete ~~chronic obstructive pulmonary disease (491.21)~~

491 Chronic bronchitis

491.2 Obstructive chronic bronchitis

Revise **491.20 Without ~~mention of acute~~ exacerbation**

Revise **491.21 With (acute) exacerbation**
Delete ~~Acute bronchitis with chronic obstructive pulmonary disease [COPD]~~
Add Decompensated chronic obstructive pulmonary disease [COPD]
Add Decompensated chronic obstructive pulmonary disease [COPD] with exacerbation

492 Emphysema

492.8 Other emphysema

Delete **Excludes** emphysema:
Delete ~~with both acute and chronic bronchitis (491.21)~~
Delete with chronic bronchitis (491.20–491.21)

493 Asthma

Revise The following fifth-digit subclassification is for use with codes 493.0–493.2, 493.9:

Revise 0 ~~without mention of status asthmaticus or acute exacerbation or~~ unspecified

Revise 2 with (acute) exacerbation

New code **493.8 Other forms of asthma**

New code **493.81 Exercise induced bronchospasm**

New code **493.82 Cough variant asthma**

494 Bronchiectasis

494.1 Bronchietasis with acute exacerbation

Delete ~~Acute bronchitis with bronchiectasis~~

517 Lung involvement in conditions classified elsewhere

New code **517.3 Acute chest syndrome**
Code first sickle-cell disease in crisis (292.42, 282.62, 282.65, 282.69)

9. DISEASES OF THE DIGESTIVE SYSTEM (520–579)

530 Diseases of the esophagus

530.2 Ulcer of the esophagus

New code **530.20 Ulcer of esophagus without bleeding**
Ulcer of esophagus NOS

New code **530.21 Ulcer of esophagus with bleeding**

Excludes *bleeding esophageal varices (456.0, 456.20)*

530.8 Other specified disorders of the esophagus

New code **530.85 Barrett's esophagus**

558 Other and unspecified noninfectious gastroenteritis and colitis

558.3 Allergic gastroenteritis and colitis

Add Use additional code to identify type of food allergy (V15.01–V15.05)

593 Other disorders of kidney and ureter

593.9 Unspecified disorder of the kidney and ureter

Revise Renal disease (chronic) NOS

Add Renal insufficiency (acute) (chronic)

10. DISEASES OF THE GENITOURINARY SYSTEM (580–629)

600 Hyperplasia of prostate

600.0 Hypertrophy (benign) of prostate

New code **600.00 Hypertrophy (benign) of prostate without urinary obstruction**
Hypertrophy (benign) of prostate NOS

New code **600.01 Hypertrophy (benign) of prostate with urinary obstruction**
Hypertrophy (benign) of prostate with urinary retention

600.1 Nodular prostate

New code **600.10 Nodular prostate without urinary obstruction**
Nodular prostate NOS

New code **600.11 Nodular prostate with urinary obstruction**
Nodular prostate with urinary retention

600.2 Benign localized hyperplasia of prostate

Revise **Excludes** *hypertrophy of prostate (600.0–600.01)*

New code **600.20 Benign localized hyperplasia of prostate without urinary obstruction**
Benign localized hyperplasia of prostate NOS

New code **600.21 Benign localized hyperplasia of prostate with urinary obstruction**
Benign localized hyperplasia of prostate with urinary retention

600.9 Hyperplasia of prostate, unspecified

New code **600.90 Hyperplasia of prostate, unspecified, without urinary obstruction**
Hyperplasia of prostate NOS

New code **600.91 Hyperplasia of prostate, unspecified, with urinary obstruction**
Hyperplasia of prostate, unspecified, with urinary retention

607 Disorders of the penis

607.8 Other specified disorders of penis

New code **607.85 Peyronie's disease**

625 Pain and other symptoms associated with female genital organs

625.4 Premenstrual tension syndrome

Add Premenstrual dysphoric disorder

11. COMPLICATIONS OF PREGNANCY, CHILDBIRTH, AND THE PUERPERIUM (630–677)

674 Other and unspecified complications of the puerperium, not elsewhere classified

New code **674.5 Peripartum cardiomyopathy**
[0–4] Postpartum cardiomyopathy

674.8 Other
Postpartum:
Delete ~~cardiomyopathy~~

12. DISEASES OF THE SKIN AND SUBCUTANEOUS TISSUE (680–709)

13. DISEASES OF THE MUSCULOSKELETAL SYSTEM AND CONNECTIVE TISSUE (710–739)

710 Diffuse diseases of connective tissue

710.1 Systemic sclerosis

Use additional code to identify . . .

Revise lung involvement (517.2)

719 Other an unspecified disorder so joint

Revise The following fifth-digit subclassification is for use with codes 719.0–719.6, 719.8–718.9): valid digits are in [brackets] under each code. See list at beginning of chapter for definitions.

719.7 Difficulty walking

Delete ~~[0, 5–9]~~

728 Disorders of muscle, ligament, and fascia

Excludes *myoneural disorders (358.00–368.9)*

728.8 Other disorders of muscle ligament, and fascia

New code **728.87 Muscle weakness**

Excludes *generalized weakness (780.79)*

728.88 Rhabdomyolysis

14. CONGENITAL ANOMALIES (740–759)

752 Congenital anomalies of genital organs

752.8 Other specified anomalies of genital organs

Delete ~~Absence of:~~
~~prostate~~
~~spermatic cord~~
~~vas deferens~~
~~Anorchism~~
~~Aplasia (congenital) of:~~
~~prostate~~
~~round ligament~~
~~testicle~~
~~Atresia of:~~
~~ejaculatory duct~~
~~vas deferens~~
~~Fusion of testes~~
~~Hypoplasia of testes~~
~~Monorchism~~
~~Polyorchism~~

New code **752.81 Scrotal transposition**

New code **752.89 Other specified anomalies of genital organs**

Absence of:
prostate
spermatic cord
vas deferens
Anorchism
Aplasia (congenital) of:
prostate
round ligament
testicle
Atresia of:
ejaculatory duct
vas deferens
Fusion of testes
Hypoplasia of testes
Monorchism
Polyorchism

15. CERTAIN CONDITIONS ORIGINATING IN THE PERINATAL PERIOD (760–779)

766 Disorders relating to long gestation and high birth-weight

Revise **766.2** ~~**Post-term infant, not "heavy-for-dates" Late infant, not "heavy-for-dates"**~~

~~Fetus or infant with gestation period of 294 days or more [42 or more completed weeks], not "heavy" or "large for dates"~~
~~Postmaturity NOS"~~

New code **766.21 Post-term infant**

Infant with gestation period over 40 completed weeks to 42 completed weeks

New code **766.22 Prolonged gestation of infant**

Infant with gestation period over 42 completed weeks
Postmaturity NOS

767 Birth trauma

767.1 Injuries to scalp

Delete ~~Caput succedaneum~~
~~Cephalhematoma~~
~~Chignon (from vacuum extraction)~~
~~Massive epicranial subaponeurotic hemorrhage~~

New code **767.11 Epicranial subaponeurotic hemorrhage (massive)**

Subgaleal hemorrhage

New code **767.19 Other injuries to the scalp**

Caput succedaneum
Cephalhematoma
Chignon (from vacuum extraction)

779 Other and ill-defined conditions originating in the perinatal period

789.8 Other specified conditions originating in the perinatal period

New code **779.83 Delayed separation of umbilical cored**

16. SYMPTOMS, SIGNS, AND ILL-DEFINED CONDITIONS (780–799)

780 General symptoms

780.9 Other general symptoms

New code **780.93 Memory loss**

Amnesia (retrograde)
Memory loss NOS

Excludes *mild memory disturbance due to brain damage (310.1)*
transient global amnesia (437.7)

New code **780.94 Early satiety**

780.99 Other general symptoms

Delete ~~Amnesia (retrograde)~~

781 Symptoms involving nervous and musculoskeletal systems

781.9 Other symptoms involving nervous and musculoskeletal systems

New code **781.94 Facial weakness**

Facial droop

Excludes *facial weakness due to late effect of cerebrovascular accident (438.83)*

784 Symptoms involving head and neck

Revise **Excludes** *encephalopathy NOS (348.30)*

785 Symptoms involving cardiovascular system

785.5 Schock without mention of trauma

New code **785.52 Septic shock**

Code first systemic inflammtory response syndrome due to infectious process with organ dysfunction (995.92)

785.59 Other

Shock:

Delete ~~*septic*~~

788 Symptoms involving urinary system

788.6 Other abnormality of urination

New code **788.63 Urgency of urination**

Excludes *urge incontinenced (788.31–788.33)*

790 Nonspecific findings on examination of blood

Revise **790.2 Abnormal glucose** ~~**tolerance**~~ **test**

Add **Excludes** *diabetes mellitus (250.00–250.93)*
dysmetabolic syndrome X (277.7)
gestational diabetes (648.8)
glycosuria (791.5)
hypoglycomia (251.2)

New code **790.21 Impaired fasting glucose**
Elevated fasting glucose
New code **790.22 Impaired glucose tolerance test (oral)**
Elevated fasting glucose
New code **790.29 Other abnormal glucose**
Abnormal glucose NOS
Abnormal non-fasting glucose
Pre-diabetes NOS

799 Other ill-defined and unknown causes of morbidity and mortality
799.8 Other ill-defined conditions
New code **799.81 Decreased libido**
Decreased sexual desire
Excludes *psychosexual dysfunction with inhibited sexual desire (302.71)*
New code **799.89 Other ill-defined conditions**

17. INJURY AND POISONING (800–999)

850 Concussion
850.1 With brief loss of consciousness
New code **850.11 With loss of consciousness of 30 minutes or less**
New code **850.12 With loss of consciousness from 31–59 minutes**

CRUSHING INJURY (925–929)

Delete **Excludes** ~~*concussion (850.0–850.9)*~~
~~*fractures (800–829)*~~
~~*internal organs (860.0–869.1)*~~
~~*that incidental to:*~~
~~*internal injury (860.0–869.1)*~~
~~*intracranial injury (850.0–854.1)*~~
Add Use additional code to identify any associated injuries, such as:
fractures (800–829)
internal injuries (860.0–869.1)
intracranial injuries (850.0–854.1)

926 Crushing injury of trunk
Delete **Excludes** ~~*crush injury of internal organs (860.0–869.1)*~~
926.1 Other specified sites
926.19 Other
Delete **Excludes** ~~*crushing of chest (860.0–869.9)*~~

929 Crushing injury of multiple and unspecified sites
Delete **Excludes** ~~*multiple internal injury NOS (869.0–869.1)*~~

959 Injury, other and unspecified
959.1 Trunk
Delete ~~Abdominal wall~~
~~Back~~
~~Breast~~
~~Buttock~~
~~Chest wall~~
~~External genital organs~~
~~Flank~~
~~Groin~~
~~Interscapular region~~
~~Perineum~~
New code **959.11 Other injury of chest wall**
New code **959.12 Other injury of abdomen**
New code **959.13 Fracture of corpus cavernosum penis**
New code **959.14 Other injury of external genitals**
New code **959.19 Other injury of other sites of trunk**
Injury of trunk NOS

995 Certain adverse effects not elsewhere classified
995.9 Systemic inflammatory response syndrome (SIRS)
Add Code first underlying condition
995.91 Systemic inflammatory response syndrome due to infectious process without organ dysfunction
Add Sepsis
995.92 Systemic inflammatory response syndrome due to infectious process with organ dysfunction
Use additional code to specify organ dysfunction, such as:
Add acute renal failure (584.5–585.9)
Add acute respiratory failure (518.81)
Add critical illness myopathy (359.81)
Add critical illness polyneuropathy (357.82)
Revise encephalopathy (348.31)
Add hepatic failure (570)
Delete ~~heart failure (428.0–428.9)~~
Add septic shock (785.52)
New code **995.94 Systemic inflammatory response syndrome due to noninfectious process with organ dysfunction**
Use additional code to specify organ dysfunction, such as:
Add acute renal failure (584.5–585.9)
Add acute respiratory failure (518.81)
Add critical illness myopathy (359.81)
Add critical illness polyneuropathy (357.82)
Revise encephalopathy (348.31)
Add hepatic failure (570)
Delete ~~heart failure (428.0–428.9)~~
Add septic shock (785.52)

996 Complications peculiar to certain specified procedures
996.5 Mechanical complication of other specified prosthetic device, implant, and graft
New code **996.57 Due to insulin pump**

997 Complications affecting specified body systems, not elsewhere classified
997.4 Digestive system complication
Add **Excludes** *specified gastrointestinal complications classified elsewhere, such as:*
vomiting following gastrointestinal surgery (564.3)

V CODES

V04 Need for prophylactic vaccination and inoculation against certain viral diseases
Revise **V04.8 ~~Influenza~~ Other viral diseases**
New code **V04.81 Influenza**
New code **V04.82 Respiratory syncytial virus (RSV)**
New code **V04.89 other viral diseases**

V06 Need for prophylactic vaccination and inoculation against combinations of diseases
Revise **V06.1 Diphtheria-tetanus-pertussis, combined [DTP] [DTaP]**
Revise **V06.5 Tetanus-diphtheria [Td] [DT]**

V15 Other personal history presenting hazards to health
V15.8 Other specified personal history presenting hazards to health
New code **V15.87 History of Extracorporeal Membrane Oxygenation [ECMO]**

V25 Encounter for contraceptive management
V25.0 General counseling and advice
New code **V25.03 Encounter for emergency contraceptive counseling and prescription**
Encounter for postcoital contraceptive counseling and prescription

V43 Organ or tissue replaced by other means
Add Includes: organ or tissue assisted by other means
V43.2 Heart
New code **V43.21 Heart assist device**
New code **V43.22 Fully implantable artificial heart**

V45 Other ~~postsurgical~~ postprocedural states
V45.0 Cardiac device in situ
Add **Excludes** *artificial heart (V43.22)*
Add *heart assist device (V43.21)*
V45.8 Other ~~postsurgical~~ postprocedureal status
New code **V45.85 Insulin pump station**

V53 Fitting and adjustment of other device

V53.9 Other and unspecified diseases
New code V53.90 Unspecified device
New code V53.91 Fitting and adjustment of insulin pump
Insulin pump titration
New code V53.99 Other device
V54 Other orthopedic aftercare
Revise V54.0 Aftercare involving ~~removal of fracture plate or other~~ internal fixation
Delete ~~Removal of:~~
~~pins~~
~~plates~~
~~rods~~
~~screws~~
New code V54.01 Encounter for removal of internal fixation device
New code V54.02 Encounter for lengthening/adjustment of growth rod
New code V54.09 Other aftercare involving internal fixation device
V58 Encounter for other and unspecified procedures and aftercare
V58.6 Long-term (current) drug use
New code V58.63 Long-term (current) use of antiplatelet/antithrombotics
New code V58.64 Long-term (current) use of non-steroidal anti-inflammatories (NSAID)
V58.65 Long-term (current) use of steroids
V64 Person encountering health services for specific procedures, not carried out
Revise V64.4 ~~Laparoscopic~~ Closed surgical procedure converted to open procedure
New code V64.41 Laparoscopic surgical procedure converted to open procedure
New code V64.42 Thoracoscopic surgical procedure converted to open procedure
New code V64.41 Arthroscopic surgical procedure converted to open procedure
Revise V65 Other person seeking consultation ~~without complaint or sickness~~
V65.1 Person consulting on behalf of another person
New code V65.11 Pediatric pre-birth visit for expectant mother
New code V65.19 Other person consulting on behalf of another person
V65.4 Other counseling, not elsewhere classified
Revise **Excludes** *on behalf of third party (V65.11–V65.19)*
New code V65.46 Encounter for insulin pump training

E CODES

E928 Other and unspecified environmental and accidental causes
New code E928.4 External constriction caused by air
New code E928.5 External constriction caused by other object

VOLUME 3, PROCEDURE

00. PROCEDURE AND INTERVENTIONS, NOT ELSEWHERE CLASSIFIED (00)

00.1 Pharmaceuticals
New code 00.15 High-dose infusion interleukin-2 (IL-2)
Infusion (IV bolus, CIV) interleukin
Infusion aldesleukin
Excludes *low-dose infusion interleukin-2 (99.28)*
02.4 Revision, removal, and irrigation of ventricular shunt
New code 02.41 Irrigation and exploration of ventricular shunt
Re-programming of ventriculoperitoneal shunt

03 Operations on spiral cord and spinal cord canal structures
03.5 Plastic operations on spinal cord structures
03.53 Repair of vertebral fracture
Add **Excludes** *kyphoplasty (78.49)*
Add *vertebroplasty (78.49)*

1. OPERATIONS ON THE NERVOUS SYSTEM (01–05)

No changes

2. OPERATIONS ON THE ENDOCRINE SYSTEM (006–007)

No changes

3. OPERATIONS ON THE EYE (08–16)

No changes

4. OPERATIONS ON THE EAR (18–20)

No changes

5. OPERATIONS ON THE NOSE, MOUTH, AND PHARYNX (21–29)

No changes

6. OPERATIONS ON THE RESPIRATORY SYSTEM (30–34)

No changes

7. OPERATIONS ON THE CARDIOVASCULAR SYSTEM (35–39)

37 Other operations on heart and precardium
37.3 Pericardiectomy and excision of lesion of heart
Revise 37.33 Excision or destruction of other lesion or tissue of heart, open approach
Add Ablation of heart tissue (cryoablation) (electrocurrent) (laser) (microwave) (radiofrequency) (resection), open chest approach
Add Cox-maze procedure
Add Maze procedure
Add Modified maze procedure, trans-thoracic approach
Revise **Excludes** ~~*catheter*~~ *ablation, excision or destruction of lesion or tissues of heart, endovascular approach (37.34)*
Revise 37.34 ~~Catheter ablation~~ Excision or destruction of other lesion or tissue of heart, other approach
Add Ablation of heart tissue (cryoablation) (electrocurrent) (laser) (microwave) (radiofrequency) (resection), via peripherally inserted catheter
Delete ~~Cryoablation of lesion or tissues of heart~~
Delete ~~Electrocurrent of lesion or tissues of heart~~
Add Maze procedure, endovascular approach
Add Maze procedure, trans-thoracic approach
Delete ~~Resection of lesion or tissues of heart~~
Revise 37.5 Heart ~~transplantation~~ replacement procedures
New code 37.51 Heart transplant
Excludes *combined heart-lung transplantation (33.6)*
New code 37.52 Implantation of total replacement heart system
Artifical heart
Implantation of fully implantable total replacement heart system, including ventriculectomy
Excludes *implantation of heart assist system (37.62–37.65, 37.66)*
New code 37.53 Replacement or repair thoracic unit of total replacement heart system

Excludes *replacement and repair of heart assist system (37.63)*

New code **37.54 Replacement or repair of other implantatable component of total replacement heart system**

Implantable battery

Implantable controller

Transcutaneous energy transfer (TET) device

Excludes *replacement and repair of heart assist system (37.63)*

replacement or repair of thoracic unit of total replacement heart system (37.53)

Revise **37.6 Implantation of heart ~~assist~~ system**

37.62 Implant of other heart assist system

Add **Excludes** *implantation of total replacement heart system (37.52)*

37.63 Replacement and repair of heart assist system

Add **Excludes** *replacement or repair of other implantable component of total replacement heart system (37.54)*

replacement or repair of thoracic unit of total replacement heart system (37.53)

37.65 Implant of external, pulsatile heart assist system

Add **Excludes** *implantation of total replacement heart system (37.52)*

37.66 Implant of an implantable, pulsatile heart assist system

Add **Excludes** *implantation of total replacement heart system (37.52)*

37.9 Other operations on heart and pericardium

37.94 Implantation or replacement of automatic cardioverter/defibrillator, total system [AICD]

Revise Implantation of defibrillator with leads (epicardial patches), formation of pocket (abdominal fascia) (subcutaneous), any transvenous leads, intraoperative procedures for evaluation of lead signals, and obtaining defibrillator threshold measurements (electrophysiologic studies [EPS])

37.99 Other

Add **Excludes** *maze procedure (Cox-maze), open (37.33)*

maze procedure, endovascular approach (37.34)

39 Other operations on vessels

39.7 Endovascular repair of vessel

Revise **39.79 Other endovascular repair (of aneurysm) of other vessels**

8. OPERATIONS ON THE HEMIC AND LYMPHATIC SYSTEM (40–41)

No changes

9. OPERATIONS ON THE DIGESTIVE SYSTEM (42–54)

No changes

10. OPERATIONS ON THE URINARY SYSTEM (55–59)

No changes

11. OPERATIONS ON THE MALE GENITAL ORGANS (60–64)

No changes

12. OPERATIONS ON THE FEMALE GENITAL ORGANS (65–71)

67 Operations on cervix

67.5 Repair of internal cervical os

67.59 Other repair on internal cervical os

Add **Excludes** *laparoscopically assisted supracervical hysterectomy [LASH] (68.31)*

68 Other incision and excision of uterus

68.3 Subtotal abdominal hysterectomy

Delete ~~Supracervical hysterectomy~~

New code **68.31 Laparoscopic supracervical hysterectomy [LSH]**

Classic infrafascial SEMM hysterectomy [CISH]

Laparoscopically assisted supracervical hysterectomy [LASH]

New code **68.39 Other subtotal abdominal hysterectomy, NOS**

Supracervical hysterectomy

Excludes *classic infrafascial SEMM hysterectomy [CISH] (68.31)*

laparoscopic supracervical hysterectomy [LSH] (68.31)

68.9 Other and unspecified hysterectomy

Revise **Excludes** *abdominal hysterectomy, any approach (~~68.3~~, 68.31–68.39, 68.4, 68.6)*

13. OBSTETRICAL PROCEDURES (72–75)

No changes

14. OPERATIONS ON THE MUSCULOSKELETAL SYSTEM (76–84)

81 Repair and plastic operations on joint structures

81.0 Spinal fusion

Add Code also the total number of vertebrae fused (81.62–81.64)

81.3 Refusions of spine

Add Code also the total number of vertebrae fused (81.62–81.64)

81.6 Other procedures on spine

Add Note: Number of vertebrae

The vertebral spine consists of 25 vertebrae in the following order and number:

Cervical: C1 (atlas), C2 (axis), C3, C4, C5, C6, C7

Thoracic or Dorsal: T1, T2, T3, T4, T5, T6, T7, T8, T9, T10, T11, T12

Lumbar and Sacral: L1, L2, L3, L4, L5, S1

Coders should report only one code from the series 81.62, 81.63, 81.64 to show the total number of vertebrae fused on the patient.

Code also the level and approach of the fusion or refusion (81.00–81.08, 81.30–81.39).

81.61 360 degree spinal fusion, single incision approach

Add Code also the total number of vertebrae fused (81.62–81.64)

New code **81.62 Fusion or refusion of 2–3 vertebrae**

New code **81.63 Fusion or refusion of 4–8 vertebrae**

New code **81.64 Fusion or refusion of 9 or more vertebrae**

15. OPERATIONS ON THE INTEGUMENTARY SYSTEM (85–86)

No changes

16. MISCELLANEOUS DIAGNOSTIC AND THERAPEUTIC PROCEDURES (87–99)

92 Nuclear medicine

92.2 Therapeutic radiology and nuclear medicine

99.28 Injection or instillation of radioisotopes

Add Injection or infusion of radioimmunoconjugate

Add Iodine-131 [I-131] tositumomab

Add Radioimmunotherapy

Add Ytrium-90 [Y-90] ibritumomab tiuxetun

99 Other nonoperative procedures

99.2 Injection or infusion of other therapetuic or prophylactic substance

99.25 Injection or infusion of cancer chemotherapeutic substance

Revise **Excludes** *immunotherapy, antieoplastic (00.15, 99.28)*

99.28 Injection or infusion of biological response modifier [BRM] as an antineoplastic agent

Revise ~~High~~Low-dose interleukin-s [IL-2] therapy

Add **Excludes** *high-dose infusion interleukin-2 [IL-2] (00.15)*

HCPCS 2003 New/Revised/Deleted Codes and Modifiers

2004 HCPCS Updates are printed in Unit Three of this text and will also be posted on the companion website: http://evolve.elsevier.com/Buck/icd.

NEW CODES/MODIFIERS

A1	SQ	A4521	A6510	E0483	G0264	J0637	L0470	S0207
A2	ST	A4522	A6511	E0484	G0265	J0880	L0472	S0315
A3	SU	A4523	A6512	E0618	G0266	J1051	L0476	S0316
A4	SV	A4524	A7025	E0619	G0267	J1094	L0478	S0320
A5	TK	A4525	A7026	E0636	G0268	J1564	L0480	S0390
A6	TL	A4526	A7030	E0691	G0269	J1652	L0482	S1040
A7	TM	A4527	A7031	E0692	G0270	J1756	L0484	S2107
A8	TN	A4528	A7032	E0693	G0271	J1815	L0486	S2130
A9	TP	A4529	A7033	E0694	G0272	J1817	L0488	S2211
AU	TQ	A4530	A7034	E0701	G0273	J2324	L0490	S2262
AV	TR	A4531	A7035	E0761	G0274	J2501	L1652	S2265
AW	TS	A4532	A7036	E1011	G0275	J2675	L1836	S2266
AX	TS	A4533	A7037	E1012	G0278	J2788	L1901	S2267
BA	TT	A4534	A7038	E1013	G0279	J2916	L3651	S2405
BO	TU	A4535	A7039	E1014	G0280	J3315	L3652	S3655
CA	TV	A4536	A7042	E1015	G0281	J3487	L3701	S4005
CB	TW	A4537	A7043	E1016	G0282	J3590	L3762	S4013
EY	U1	A4538	A7044	E1017	G0283	J7317	L3909	S4014
H9	U2	A4606	A9512	E1018	G0288	J7342	L3911	S4017
HA	U3	A4609	A9513	E1020	G0289	J7350	L4386	S4023
HB	U4	A4610	A9514	E1025	G0290	J7633	L5781	S4035
HC	U5	A4632	A9515	E1026	G0291	J9010	L5782	S4036
HD	U6	A4633	A9516	E1027	G0292	K0556	L5848	S4037
HE	U7	A4634	A9517	E1037	G0293	K0557	L5995	S4040
HF	U8	A4639	A9518	E1038	G0294	K0558	L6025	S4993
HG	U9	A4653	A9519	E1161	G0295	K0559	L6638	S4995
HH	UA	A4930	A9520	E1231	H0031	K0581	L6646	S5100
HI	UB	A4931	A9521	E1232	H0032	K0582	L6647	S5101
HJ	UC	A4932	A9522	E1233	H0033	K0583	L6648	S5102
HK	UD	A6011	A9523	E1234	H0034	K0584	L7367	S5105
HL	A4266	A6410	A9524	E1235	H0035	K0585	L7368	S5110
HM	A4267	A6411	A9603	E1236	H0036	K0586	Q0144	S5111
HN	A4268	A6412	A9699	E1237	H0037	K0587	Q3000	S5115
HO	A4269	A6421	B4100	E1238	H0038	K0588	Q3019	S5116
HP	A4281	A6422	C1015	E1802	H0039	K0589	Q3020	S5120
HQ	A4282	A6424	C1020	G0245	H0040	K0590	Q3021	S5121
HR	A4283	A6426	C1021	G0246	H0041	K0591	Q3022	S5125
HS	A4284	A6428	C1022	G0247	H0042	K0592	Q3023	S5126
HT	A4285	A6430	C1775	G0248	H0043	K0593	Q3025	S5130
HU	A4286	A6432	C1783	G0249	H0044	K0594	Q3026	S5131
HV	A4405	A6434	C1888	G0250	H0045	K0595	S0104	S5135
HW	A4406	A6436	C1900	G0251	H0046	K0596	S0106	S5136
HX	A4407	A6438	C2614	G0252	H0047	K0597	S0108	S5140
HY	A4408	A6440	C2632	G0253	H0048	L0450	S0114	S5141
HZ	A4409	A6501	C9116	G0254	H1010	L0452	S0122	S5145
JW	A4410	A6502	C9119	G0255	H1011	L0454	S0124	S5146
KB	A4413	A6503	C9120	G0256	H2000	L0456	S0126	S5150
KX	A4414	A6504	C9121	G0257	H2001	L0458	S0128	S5151
QJ	A4415	A6505	E0117	G0259	J0287	L0460	S0130	S5160
SK	A4422	A6506	E0203	G0260	J0288	L0462	S0132	S5161
SL	A4450	A6507	E0445	G0261	J0289	L0464	S0135	S5162
SM	A4452	A6508	E0454	G0262	J0592	L0466	S0195	S5165
SN	A4458	A6509	E0461	G0263	J0636	L0468	S0201	S5170

NEW CODES/MODIFIERS — *Continued*

S5175	S8262	S9430	S9451	S9562	T1016	T1024	T1500	T2006
S5180	S8265	S9436	S9452	S9590	T1017	T1025	T1502	T2007
S5181	S8945	S9437	S9453	S9802	T1018	T1026	T1999	V5095
S5185	S9034	S9438	S9454	S9803	T1019	T1027	T2001	V5298
S5190	S9092	S9439	S9484	S9806	T1020	T1028	T2002	
S5199	S9145	S9444	S9490	S9900	T1021	T1029	T2003	
S8004	S9150	S9447	S9494	S9970	T1022	T1030	T2004	
S8042	S9401	S9449	S9546	S9975	T1023	T1031	T2005	

REVISED CODES/MODIFIERS

GN	A4389	A5054	E0443	G0214	G0230	J7340	L4360	S9330
GO	A4391	A5061	E0444	G0215	G0236	J7626	L4370	S9331
GP	A4462	A5062	E0574	G0216	G0239	K0082	L4380	S9338
K0	A4595	A5063	E0730	G0217	H0002	K0083	L7900	S9347
Q3	A4624	A5071	E0782	G0218	H0004	K0084	L7510	S9364
A0080	A4656	A5072	E1637	G0219	H0017	K0085	L9000	S9365
A0090	A4657	A5073	E1639	G0220	H0018	K0086	S0088	S9366
A0100	A4660	A6266	G0125	G0221	H0019	K0087	S0091	S9367
A0120	A4663	C1010	G0144	G0222	H0023	K0088	S0092	S9368
A0170	A4670	C1016	G0145	G0223	H0024	K0089	S0093	S9537
A0424	A4712	C1018	G0179	G0224	H0025	L0500	S0215	S9542
A4301	A4927	C1166	G0180	G0225	H0030	L0510	S2400	S9558
A4372	A4928	C1178	G0210	G0226	J1825	L1843	S4015	S9559
A4373	A5051	C1774	G0211	G0227	J2790	L1844	S9123	T1013
A4387	A5052	E0441	G0212	G0228	J3070	L3260	S9326	
A4388	A5053	E0442	G0213	G0229	J3240	L4350	S9327	

DELETED CODES/MODIFIERS

A4360	C1202	C1760	C1874	C2627	G0132	K0184	L0310	L5662
A4370	C1207	C1762	C1875	C2628	G0185	K0185	L0315	L5663
A4374	C1348	C1763	C1876	C2629	G0187	K0186	L0317	L5664
A4386	C1713	C1764	C1877	C2630	G0192	K0187	L0320	Q0184
A4454	C1714	C1766	C1878	C2631	G0193	K0188	L0321	Q3017
A4460	C1715	C1767	C1879	C9019	G0194	K0189	L0330	Q3030
A4464	C1717	C1768	C1880	C9020	G0195	K0548	L0331	S0085
A4572	C1721	C1769	C1881	C9100	G0196	K0551	L0340	S0087
A4801	C1722	C1770	C1882	C9108	G0197	K0561	L0350	S0112
A5123	C1724	C1771	C1883	C9110	G0198	K0562	L0360	S0206
A6263	C1725	C1772	C1885	C9114	G0199	K0563	L0370	S2180
A6264	C1726	C1773	C1887	C9115	G0200	K0564	L0380	S8002
A6265	C1727	C1776	C1891	C9117	G0201	K0565	L0390	S8003
A6405	C1728	C1777	C1892	C9118	G0240	K0566	L0391	S8105
A6406	C1729	C1778	C1893	C9708	G0241	K0567	L0400	S8200
C1012	C1730	C1779	C1894	E0608	J0286	K0568	L0410	S8205
C1013	C1731	C1780	C1895	E0690	J0635	K0569	L0420	S8401
C1014	C1732	C1781	C1896	E1091	J1050	K0570	L0430	S8403
C1058	C1733	C1782	C1897	E1638	J1095	K0571	L0440	S8404
C1064	C1750	C1784	C1898	G0002	J1561	K0572	L0900	S8405
C1065	C1751	C1785	C1899	G0004	J1755	K0573	L0910	S8433
C1066	C1752	C1786	C2615	G0005	J1820	K0574	L0920	S9216
C1087	C1753	C1787	C2617	G0006	J2500	K0575	L0930	S9217
C1094	C1754	C1788	C2619	G0007	J2915	K0576	L0940	S9218
C1096	C1755	C1789	C2620	G0015	J7316	K0577	L0950	S9543
C1097	C1756	C1813	C2621	G0026	K0021	K0578	L0986	S9800
C1098	C1757	C1815	C2622	G0027	K0034	K0579	L3218	
C1099	C1758	C1816	C2625	G0050	K0101	K0580	L3223	
C1188	C1759	C1817	C2626	G0131	K0183	L0300	L5660	

CONTENTS

Part IV Procedures, Volume 3 943

UNIT TWO HCPCS 2003: LEVEL II NATIONAL CODES 1139

UNIT THREE HCPCS 2004 UPDATES 1345

UNIT ONE

ICD-9-CM

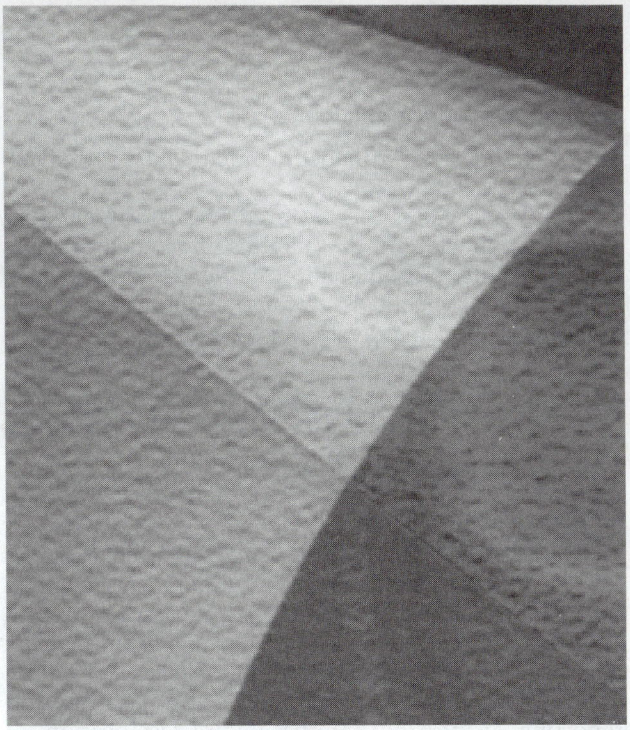

PART I

Introduction

ICD-9-CM BACKGROUND

The International Classification of Diseases, 9th Revision, Clinical Modification (ICD-9-CM) is based on the official version of the World Health Organization's 9th Revision, International Classification of Diseases (ICD-9). ICD-9 is designed for the classification of morbidity and mortality information for statistical purposes, and for the indexing of hospital records by disease and operations, for data storage and retrieval. The historical background of the International Classification of Diseases may be found in the Introduction to ICD-9 (Manual of the International Classification of Diseases, Injuries, and Causes of Death, World Health Organization, Geneva, Switzerland, 1977).

ICD-9-CM is a clinical modification of the World Health Organization's International Classification of Diseases, 9th Revision (ICD-9). The term "clinical" is used to emphasize the modification's intent: to serve as a useful tool in the area of classification of morbidity data for indexing of medical records, medical care review, and ambulatory and other medical care programs, as well as for basic health statistics. To describe the clinical picture of the patient, the codes must be more precise than those needed only for statistical groupings and trend analysis.

COORDINATION AND MAINTENANCE COMMITTEE

Annual modifications are made to the ICD-9-CM through the ICD-9-CM Coordination and Maintenance Committee (C&M). The Committee is made up of representatives from two Federal Government agencies, the National Center for Health Statistics and the Health Care Financing Administration. The Committee holds meetings twice a year which are open to the public. Modification proposals submitted to the Committee for consideration are presented at the meetings for public discussion. Those modification proposals which are approved are incorporated into the official government version of the ICD-9-CM and become effective for use October 1 of the year following their presentation. This CD-ROM contains the modifications approved from the 1995 C&M cycle.

This CD-ROM is the only official federal government version of the ICD-9-CM. It may be purchased through the Government Printing Office.

CHARACTERISTICS OF ICD-9-CM

ICD-9-CM far exceeds its predecessors in the number of codes provided. The disease classification has been expanded to include health-related conditions and to provide greater specificity at the fifth-digit level of detail. These fifth digits are not optional; they are intended for use in recording the information substantiated in the clinical record.

Volume I of ICD-9-CM contains five appendices:

Appendix A	Morphology of Neoplasms
Appendix B	Glossary of Mental Disorders
Appendix C	Classification of Drugs by American Hospital Formulary Service List Number and Their ICD-9-CM Equivalents
Appendix D	Classification of Industrial Accidents According to Agency
Appendix E	List of Three-Digit Categories

These appendices are included as a reference to the user in order to provide further information about the patient's clinical picture, to further define a diagnostic statement, to aid in classifying new drugs, or to reference three-digit categories.

Volume 2 of ICD-9-CM contains many diagnostic terms which do not appear in Volume 1 since the index includes most diagnostic terms currently in use.

The Disease Classification

ICD-9-CM is totally compatible with its parent system, ICD-9, thus meeting the need for comparability of morbidity and mortality statistics at the international level. A few fourth-digit codes were created in existing three-digit rubrics only when the necessary detail could not be accommodated by the use of a fifth-digit subclassification. To ensure that each rubric of ICD-9-CM collapses back to its ICD-9 counterpart the following specifications governed the ICD-9-CM disease classification:

Specifications for the Tabular List

1. Three-digit rubrics and their contents are unchanged from ICD-9.
2. The sequence of three-digit rubrics is unchanged from ICD-9.
3. Unsubdivided three-digit rubrics are subdivided where necessary to:
   a) Add clinical detail
   b) Isolate terms for clinical accuracy
4. The modification in ICD-9-CM is accomplished by the addition of a fifth digit to existing ICD-9 rubrics.
5. The optional dual classification in ICD-9 is modified.
   a) Duplicate rubrics are deleted:
      1) Four-digit manifestation categories duplicating etiology entries.
      2) Manifestation inclusion terms duplicating etiology entries.
   b) Manifestations of diseases are identified, to the extent possible, by creating five-digit codes in the etiology rubrics.
   c) When the manifestation of a disease cannot be included in the etiology rubrics, provision for its identification is made by retaining the ICD-9 rubrics used for classifying manifestations of disease.
6. The format of ICD-9-CM is revised from that used in ICD-9.
   a) American spelling of medical terms is used.
   b) Inclusion terms are indented beneath the titles of codes.
   c) Codes not to be used for principal tabulation of disease are printed with the notation, "Code first underlying disease."

Specifications for the Alphabetic Index

1. Format of the Alphabetic Index follows the format of ICD-9.
2. When two codes are required to indicate etiology and manifestation, the manifestation code appears in brackets, e.g., diabetic cataract 250.5X [366.41]. The etiology code is always sequenced first followed by the manifestation code.

ICD-9-CM Official Guidelines For Coding and Reporting

NOTE: Effective 10/1/02

The Centers for Medicare and Medicaid Services (CMS) formerly the Health Care Financing Administration (HCFA) and the National Center for Health Statistics (NCHS), two departments within the Department of Health and Human Services (DHHS) present the following guidelines for coding and reporting using the International Classification of Diseases, 9th Revision, Clinical Modification (ICD-9-CM). These guidelines should be used as a companion document to the official versions of the ICD-9-CM as published on CD-ROM.

These guidelines for coding and reporting have been developed and approved by the Cooperating Parties for ICD-9-CM: the American Hospital Association, the American Health Information Management Association, CMS, and the NCHS. These guidelines, published by the Department of Health and Human Services have also appeared in the Coding Clinic for ICD-9-CM, published by the American Hospital Association.

These guidelines have been developed to assist the user in coding and reporting in situations where the ICD-9-CM does not provide direction. Coding and sequencing instructions in volumes I, II, and III of ICD-9-CM take precedence over any guidelines. The conventions, general guidelines and chapter-specific guidelines apply to the proper use of ICD-9-CM, regardless of the health care setting. A joint effort between the attending physician and coder is essential to achieve complete and accurate documentation, code assignment, and reporting of diagnoses and procedures. These guidelines have been developed and approved by the Cooperating Parties to assist both the physician and the coder in identifying those diagnoses that are to be reported. The importance of consistent, complete documentation in the medical record cannot be overemphasized. Without such documentation the application of all coding guidelines is a difficult, if not impossible, task.

These guidelines are not exhaustive. The cooperating parties are continuing to conduct reviews of these guidelines and develop new guidelines as needed. Users of the ICD-9-CM should be aware that only guidelines approved by the cooperating parties are official. Revision of these guidelines and new guidelines will be published by the U.S. Department of Health and Human Services when they are approved by the cooperating parties. The term "admitted" is used generally to mean a health care encounter in any setting.

The guidelines have been reorganized into several new sections including an enhanced introduction that provides more detail about the structure and conventions of the classification usually found in the classification itself. The other new section, General Guidelines, brings together overarching guidelines that were previously found throughout the various sections of the guidelines. The new format of the guidelines also includes a resequencing of the disease-specific guidelines. They are sequenced in the same order as they appear in the tabular list chapters (Infectious and Parasitic Diseases, Neoplasms, etc.)

These changes will make it easier for coders, experienced and beginners, to more easily find the specific portion of the coding guideline information they seek.

Table of Contents

Section I Conventions, General Coding Guidelines and Chapter-Specific Guidelines

The conventions, general guidelines and chapter-specific guidelines are applicable to all health care settings unless otherwise indicated.

A. Conventions for the ICD-9-CM

The conventions for the ICD-9-CM are the general rules for use of the classification independent of the guidelines. These conventions are incorporated within the index and tabular of the ICD-9-CM as instructional notes. The conventions are as follows:

1. Format: The ICD-9-CM uses an indented format for ease in reference

2. Abbreviations

a. Index Abbreviations

NEC "Not elsewhere classifiable"

This abbreviation in the index represents "other specified" When a specific code is not available for a condition the index directs the coder to the "other specified" code in the tabular.

b. Tabular Abbreviations

NEC "Not elsewhere classifiable"

This abbreviation in the tabular represents "other specified" When a specific code is not available for a condition the tabular includes an NEC entry under a code to identify the code as the "other specified" code. (see "Other" codes)

NOS "Not otherwise specified" This abbreviation is the equivalent of unspecified. (see "Unspecified" codes)

3. Punctuation

[ ] Brackets are used in the tabular list to enclose synonyms, alternative wording or explanatory phrases. Brackets are used in the index to identify manifestation codes. (see etiology/manifestations)

( ) Parentheses are used in both the index and tabular to enclose supplementary words which may be present or absent in the statement of a disease or procedure without affecting the code number to which it is assigned. The terms within the parentheses are referred to as nonessential modifiers.

: Colons are used in the Tabular list after an incomplete term which needs one or more of the modifiers following the colon to make it assignable to a given category.

4. Includes and Excludes Notes and Inclusion terms

Includes: This note appears immediately under a three-digit code title to further define, or give examples of, the content of the category.

Excludes: An excludes note under a code indicate that the terms excluded from the code are to be coded elsewhere. In some cases the codes for the excluded terms should not be used in conjunction with the code from which it is excluded. An example of this is a congenital condition excluded from an acquired form of the same condition. The congenital and acquired codes should not be used together. In other cases, the excluded terms may be used together with an excluded code. An example of this is when fractures of different bones are coded to different codes. Both codes may be used together if both types of fractures are present.

Inclusion terms: List of terms are included under certain four and five digit codes. These terms are the conditions for which that code number is to be used. The terms may be synonyms of the code title, or, in the case of "other specified" codes, the terms are a list of the various conditions assigned to that code. The inclusion terms are not necessarily exhaustive. Additional terms found only in the index may also be assigned to a code.

5. Other and Unspecified codes

a. "Other" codes

Codes titled "other" or "other specified" (usually a code with a 4th digit 8 or fifth-digit 9 for diagnosis codes) are for use when the information in the medical record provides detail for which a specific code does not exist. Index entries with NEC in the line designate "other" codes in the tabular. These index entries represent specific disease entities for which no specific code exists so the term is included within an "other" code.

b. "Unspecified" codes

Codes (usually a code with a 4th digit 9 or 5th digit 0 for diagnosis codes) titled "unspecified" are for use when the information in the medical record is insufficient to assign a more specific code.

6. Etiology/manifestation convention ("code first", "use additional code" and "in diseases classified elsewhere" notes)

Certain conditions have both an underlying etiology and multiple body system manifestations due to the underlying etiology. For such conditions the ICD-9-CM has a coding convention that requires the underlying condition be sequenced first followed by the manifestation. Wherever such a combination exists there is a "use additional code" note at the etiology code, and a "code first" note at the manifestation code. These instructional notes indicate the proper sequencing order of the codes, etiology followed by manifestation.

In most cases the manifestation codes will have in the code title, "in diseases classified elsewhere." Codes with this title are a component of the etiology/ manifestation convention. The code title indicates that it is a manifestation code. "In diseases classified elsewhere" codes are never permitted to be used as first listed or principle diagnosis codes. They must be used in conjunction with an underlying condition code and they must be listed following the underlying condition.

There are manifestation codes that do not have "in diseases classified elsewhere" in the title. For such codes a "use additional code" note will still be present and the rules for sequencing apply.

In addition to the notes in the tabular, these conditions also have a specific index entry structure. In the index both conditions are listed together with the etiology code first followed by the manifestation codes in brackets. The code in brackets is always to be sequenced second.

The most commonly used etiology/manifestation combinations are the codes for Diabetes mellitus, category 250. For each code under category 250 there is a use additional code note for the manifestation that is specific for that particular diabetic manifestation. Should a patient have more than one manifestation of diabetes more than one code from category 250 may be used with as many manifestation codes as are needed to fully describe the patient's complete diabetic condition. The 250 diabetes codes should be sequenced first, followed by the manifestation codes.

"Code first" and "Use additional code" notes are also used as sequencing rules in the classification for certain codes that are not part of an etiology/ manifestation combination. See - Other multiple coding for a single condition in the General Guidelines section.

B. General Coding Guidelines

1. Use of Both Alphabetic Index and Tabular List

   Use both the Alphabetic Index and the Tabular List when locating and assigning a code. Reliance on only the Alphabetic Index or the Tabular List leads to errors in code assignments and less specificity in code selection.

2. Locate each term in the Alphabetic Index and verify the code selected in the Tabular List. Read and be guided by instructional notations that appear in both the Alphabetic Index and the Tabular List.

3. Level of Detail in Coding

   Diagnosis and procedure codes are to be used at their highest number of digits available.

   ICD-9-CM diagnosis codes are composed of codes with either 3, 4, or 5 digits. Codes with three digits are included in ICD-9-CM as the heading of a category of codes that may be further subdivided by the use of fourth and/or fifth digits, which provide greater detail.

   A three-digit code is to be used only if it is not further subdivided. Where fourth-digit subcategories and/or fifth-digit subclassifications are provided, they must be assigned. A code is invalid if it has not been coded to the full number of digits required for that code. For example, Acute myocardial infarction, code 410, has fourth digits that describe the location of the infarction (e.g., 410.2, Of inferolateral wall), and fifth digits that identify the episode of care. It would be incorrect to report a code in category 410 without a fourth and fifth digit.

   ICD-9-CM Volume 3 procedure codes are composed of codes with either 3 or 4 digits. Codes with two digits are included in ICD-9-CM as the heading of a category of codes that may be further subdivided by the use of third and/or fourth digits, which provide greater detail.

4. The appropriate code or codes from 001.0 through V83.89 must be used to identify diagnoses, symptoms, conditions, problems, complaints or other reason(s) for the encounter/visit.

5. The selection of codes 001.0 through 999.9 will frequently be used to describe the reason for the admission/encounter. These codes are from the section of ICD-9-CM for the classification of diseases and injuries (e.g., infectious and parasitic diseases; neoplasms; symptoms, signs, and ill-defined conditions, etc.).

6. Codes that describe symptoms and signs, as opposed to diagnoses, are acceptable for reporting purposes when a related definitive diagnosis has not been established (confirmed) by the physician. Chapter 16 of ICD-9-CM, Symptoms, Signs, and Ill-defined conditions (codes 780.0 - 799.9) contain many, but not all codes for symptoms.

7. Conditions that are an integral part of a disease process

   Signs and symptoms that are integral to the disease process should not be assigned as additional codes.

8. Conditions that are not an integral part of a disease process

   Additional signs and symptoms that may not be

associated routinely with a disease process should be coded when present.

9. Multiple coding for a single condition

In addition to the etiology/manifestation convention that requires two codes to fully describe a single condition that affects multiple body systems, there are other single conditions that also require more than one code. "Use additional code" notes are found in the tabular at codes that are not part of an etiology/manifestation pair where a secondary code is useful to fully describe a condition. The sequencing rule is the same, "use additional code" indicates that a secondary code should be added.

For example, for infections that are not included in chapter 1, a secondary code from category 041, Bacterial infection in conditions classified elsewhere and of unspecified site, may be required to identify the bacterial organism causing the infection. A "use additional code" note will normally be found at the infection code indicates a need for the organism code to be added as a secondary code.

"Code first" notes are also under certain codes that are not specifically manifestation codes but may be due to an underlying cause. When a "code first" note is present and an underlying condition is present the underlying condition should be sequenced first. "Code, if applicable, any causal condition first", notes indicate that this code may be assigned as a principal diagnosis when the causal condition is unknown or not applicable. If a causal condition is known, then the code for that condition should be sequenced as the principal or first-listed diagnosis.

Multiple codes may be needed for late effects, complication codes and obstetric codes to more fully describe a condition. See the specific guidelines for these conditions for further instruction.

10. Acute and Chronic Conditions

If the same condition is described as both acute (subacute) and chronic, and separate subentries exist in the Alphabetic Index at the same indentation level, code both and sequence the acute (subacute) code first.

11. Combination Code

A combination code is a single code used to classify:

two diagnoses, or

A diagnosis with an associated secondary process (manifestation)

A diagnosis with an associated complication

Combination codes are identified by referring to subterm entries in the Alphabetic Index and by reading the inclusion and exclusion notes in the Tabular List.

Assign only the combination code when that code fully identifies the diagnostic conditions involved or when the Alphabetic Index so directs. Multiple coding should not be used when the classification provides a combination code that clearly identifies all of the elements documented in the diagnosis. When the combination code lacks necessary specificity in describing the manifestation or complication, an additional code may be used as a secondary code.

12. Late Effects

A late effect is the residual effect (condition produced) after the acute phase of an illness or injury has terminated. There is no time limit on when a late effect code can be used. The residual may be apparent early, such as in cerebrovascular accident cases, or it may occur months or years later, such as that due to a previous injury. Coding of late effects generally requires two codes sequenced in the following order: The condition or nature of the late effect is sequenced first. The late effect code is sequenced second.

An exception to the above guidelines are those instances where the code for late effect is followed by a manifestation code identified in the Tabular List and title, or the late effect code has been expanded (at the fourth and fifth-digit levels) to include the manifestation(s). The code for the acute phase of an illness or injury that led to the late effect is never used with a code for the late effect.

13. Impending or Threatened Condition

Code any condition described at the time of discharge as "impending" or "threatened" as follows:

If it did occur, code as confirmed diagnosis.

If it did not occur, reference the Alphabetic Index to determine if the condition has a subentry term for "impending" or "threatened" and also reference main term entries for "Impending" and for "Threatened."

If the subterms are listed, assign the given code.

If the subterms are not listed, code the existing underlying condition(s) and not the condition described as impending or threatened.

C. Chapter-Specific Coding Guidelines

In addition to general coding guidelines, there are guidelines for specific diagnoses and/or conditions in the classification. Unless otherwise indicated, these guidelines apply to all health care settings.

C1. Infectious and Parasitic Diseases

A. Human Immunodeficiency Virus (HIV) Infections

1. Code only confirmed cases of HIV infection/illness. This is an exception to the hospital inpatient guideline Section II, H.

In this context, "confirmation" does not require documentation of positive serology or culture for HIV; the physician's diagnostic statement that the patient is HIV positive, or has an HIV-related illness is sufficient.

2. Selection and sequencing
   a. If a patient is admitted for an HIV-related condition, the principal diagnosis should be 042, followed by additional diagnosis codes for all reported HIV-related conditions.
   b. If a patient with HIV disease is admitted for an unrelated condition (such as a traumatic injury), the code for the unrelated condition (e.g., the nature of injury code) should be the principal diagnosis. Other diagnoses would be 042 followed by additional diagnosis codes for all reported HIV-related conditions.
   c. Whether the patient is newly diagnosed or has had previous admissions/encounters for HIV conditions (or has expired) is irrelevant to the sequencing decision.
   d. V08 Asymptomatic human immunodeficiency virus [HIV] infection, is to be applied when the patient without any documentation of symptoms is listed as being "HIV positive," "known HIV," "HIV test positive," or similar terminology. Do not use this code if the term "AIDS" is used or if the patient is treated for any HIV-related illness or is described as having any condition(s) resulting from his/her HIV positive status; use 042 in these cases.
   e. Patients with inconclusive HIV serology, but no definitive diagnosis or manifestations of the illness, may be assigned code 795.71, Inconclusive serologic test for Human Immunodeficiency Virus [HIV]
   f. Previously diagnosed HIV-related illness

      Patients with any known prior diagnosis of an HIV-related illness should be coded to 042. Once a patient had developed an HIV-related illness, the patient should always be assigned code 042 on every subsequent admission/encounter. Patients previously diagnosed with any HIV illness (042) should never be assigned to 795.71 or V08.
   g. HIV Infection in Pregnancy, Childbirth and the Puerperium

      During pregnancy, childbirth or the puerperium, a patient admitted (or presenting for a health care encounter) because of an HIV-related illness should receive a principal diagnosis of 647.6X, Other specified infectious and parasitic diseases in the mother classifiable elsewhere, but complicating the pregnancy, childbirth or the puerperium, followed by 042 and the code(s) for the HIV-related illness(es). Codes from Chapter 15 always take sequencing priority.

      Patients with asymptomatic HIV infection status admitted (or presenting for a health care encounter) during pregnancy, childbirth, or the puerperium should receive codes of 647.6X and V08.
   h. Encounters for Testing for HIV

      If a patient is being seen to determine his/her HIV status, use code V73.89, Screening for other specified viral disease. Use code V69.8, Other problems related to lifestyle, as a secondary code if an asymptomatic patient is in a known high risk group for HIV. Should a patient with signs or symptoms or illness, or a confirmed HIV related diagnosis be tested for HIV, code the signs and symptoms or the diagnosis. An additional counseling code V65.44 may be used if counseling is provided during the encounter for the test.

      When a patient returns to be informed of his/her HIV test results use code V65.44, HIV counseling, if the results of the test are negative.

      If the results are positive but the patient is asymptomatic use code V08, Asymptomatic HIV infection. If the results are positive and the patient is symptomatic use code 042, HIV infection, with codes for the HIV related symptoms or diagnosis. The HIV counseling code may also be used if counseling is provided for patients with positive test results.

B. Septicemia and Septic Shock
   1. When the diagnosis of septicemia with shock or the diagnosis of general sepsis with septic shock is documented, code

and list the septicemia first and report the septic shock code as a secondary condition. The septicemia code assignment should identify the type of bacteria if it is known.

2. Sepsis and septic shock associated with abortion, ectopic pregnancy, and molar pregnancy are classified to category codes in Chapter 11 (630-639).
3. Negative or inconclusive blood cultures do not preclude a diagnosis of septicemia in patients with clinical evidence of the condition.

C2. Neoplasms

Chapter 2 of the ICD-9-CM contains the code for most benign and all malignant neoplasms. Certain benign neoplasms, such as prostatic adenomas, may be found in the specific body system chapters. To properly code a neoplasm it is necessary to determine from the record if the neoplasm is benign, in-situ, malignant, or of uncertain histologic behavior. If malignant, any secondary (metastatic) sites should also be determined.

The neoplasm table in the Alphabetic Index should be referenced first. If the histological term is documented, that term should be referenced first, rather than going immediately to the Neoplasm Table, in order to determine which column in the Neoplasm Table is appropriate. For example, if the documentation indicates "adenoma," refer to the term in the Alphabetic Index to review the entries under this term and the instructional note to "see also neoplasm, by site, benign." The table provides the proper code based on the type of neoplasm and the site. It is important to select the proper column in the table that corresponds to the type of neoplasm. The tabular should then be referenced to verify that the correct code has been selected from the table and that a more specific site code does not exist.

A. If the treatment is directed at the malignancy, designate the malignancy as the principal diagnosis.

B. When a patient is admitted because of a primary neoplasm with metastasis and treatment is directed toward the secondary site only, the secondary neoplasm is designated as the principal diagnosis even though the primary malignancy is still present.

C. Coding and sequencing of complications associated with the malignant neoplasm or with the therapy thereof are subject to the following guidelines:

1. When admission/encounter is for management of an anemia associated with the malignancy, and the treatment is only for anemia, the anemia is designated at the principal diagnosis and is followed by the appropriate code(s) for the malignancy.
2. When the admission/encounter is for management of an anemia associated with chemotherapy or radiotherapy and the only treatment is for the anemia, the anemia is sequenced first followed by the appropriate code(s) for the malignancy.
3. When the admission/encounter is for management of dehydration due to the malignancy or the therapy, or a combination of both, and only the dehydration is being treated (intravenous rehydration), the dehydration is sequenced first, followed by the code(s) for the malignancy.
4. When the admission/encounter is for treatment of a complication resulting from a surgical procedure performed for the treatment of an intestinal malignancy, designate the complication as the principal or first-listed diagnosis if treatment is directed at resolving the complication.

D. When a primary malignancy has been previously excised or eradicated from its site and there is no further treatment directed to that site and there is no evidence of any existing primary malignancy, a code from category V10, Personal history of malignant neoplasm, should be used to indicate the former site of the malignancy. Any mention of extension, invasion, or metastasis to another site is coded as a secondary malignant neoplasm to that site. The secondary site may be the principal or first-listed with the V10 code used as a secondary code.

E. Admissions/Encounters involving chemotherapy and radiation therapy

1. When an episode of care involves the surgical removal of a neoplasm, primary or secondary site, followed by chemotherapy or radiation treatment, the neoplasm code should be assigned as principal or first-listed diagnosis. When an episode of inpatient care involves surgical removal of a primary site or secondary site malignancy followed by adjunct chemotherapy or radiotherapy, code the malignancy as the principal or first-listed diagnosis, using codes in the 140-198 series or where appropriate in the 200-203 series.
2. If a patient admission/encounter is

solely for the administration of chemotherapy or radiation therapy code V58.0, Encounter for radiation therapy, or V58.1, Encounter for chemotherapy, should be the first-listed or principal diagnosis. If a patient receives both chemotherapy and radiation therapy both codes should be listed, in either order of sequence.

3. When a patient is admitted for the purpose of radiotherapy or chemotherapy and develops complications such as uncontrolled nausea and vomiting or dehydration, the principal or first-listed diagnosis is V58.0, Encounter for radiotherapy, or V58.1, Encounter for chemotherapy.

F. When the reason for admission/encounter is to determine the extent of the malignancy, or for a procedure such as paracentesis or thoracentesis, the primary malignancy or appropriate metastatic site is designated as the principal or first-listed diagnosis, even though chemotherapy or radiotherapy is administered.

G. Symptoms, signs, and ill-defined conditions listed in Chapter 16 characteristic of, or associated with, an existing primary or secondary site malignancy cannot be used to replace the malignancy as principal or first-listed diagnosis, regardless of the number of admissions or encounters for treatment and care of the neoplasm.

C3. Endocrine, Nutritional, and Metabolic Diseases and Immunity Disorders

Reserved for future guideline expansion

C4. Diseases of Blood and Blood Forming Organs

Reserved for future guideline expansion

C5. Mental Disorders

Reserved for future guideline expansion

C6. Diseases of Nervous System and Sense Organs

Reserved for future guideline expansion

C7. Diseases of Circulatory System

A. Hypertension

The Hypertension Table, found under the main term, "Hypertension", in the Alphabetic Index, contains a complete listing of all conditions due to or associated with hypertension and classifies them according to malignant, benign, and unspecified.

1. Hypertension, Essential, or NOS Assign hypertension (arterial) (essential) (primary) (systemic) (NOS) to category code 401 with the appropriate fourth digit to indicate malignant (.0), benign (.1), or unspecified (.9). Do not use either .0 malignant or .1 benign unless medical record documentation supports such a designation.

2. Hypertension with Heart Disease

Heart conditions (425.8, 429.0-429.3, 429.8, 429.9) are assigned to a code from category 402 when a causal relationship is stated (due to hypertension) or implied (hypertensive). Use an additional code from category 428 to identify the type of heart failure in those patients with heart failure. More than one code from category 428 may be assigned if the patient has systolic or diastolic failure and congestive heart failure.

The same heart conditions (425.8, 428, 429.0-429.3, 429.8, 429.9) with hypertension, but without a stated casual relationship, are coded separately. Sequence according to the circumstances of the admission/encounter.

3. Hypertensive Renal Disease with Chronic Renal Failure

Assign codes from category 403, Hypertensive renal disease, when conditions classified to categories 585-587 are present. Unlike hypertension with heart disease, ICD-9-CM presumes a cause-and-effect relationship and classifies renal failure with hypertension as hypertensive renal disease.

4. Hypertensive Heart and Renal Disease

Assign codes from combination category 404, Hypertensive heart and renal disease, when both hypertensive renal disease and hypertensive heart disease are stated in the diagnosis. Assume a relationship between the hypertension and the renal disease, whether or not the condition is so designated. Assign an additional code from category 428, to identify the type of heart failure. More than one code from category 428 may be assigned if the patient has systolic or diastolic failure and congestive heart failure.

5. Hypertensive Cerebrovascular Disease

First assign codes from 430-438, Cerebrovascular disease, then the appropriate hypertension code from categories 401-405.

6. Hypertensive Retinopathy

Two codes are necessary to identify the condition. First assign the code from subcategory 362.11, Hypertensive retinopathy, then the appropriate code from categories 401-405 to indicate the type of hypertension.

7. Hypertension, Secondary

   Two codes are required: one to identify the underlying etiology and one from category 405 to identify the hypertension. Sequencing of codes is determined by the reason for admission/encounter.

8. Hypertension, Transient

   Assign code 796.2, Elevated blood pressure reading without diagnosis of hypertension, unless patient has an established diagnosis of hypertension. Assign code 642.3x for transient hypertension of pregnancy.

9. Hypertension, Controlled

   Assign appropriate code from categories 401-405. This diagnostic statement usually refers to an existing state of hypertension under control by therapy.

10. Hypertension, Uncontrolled

    Uncontrolled hypertension may refer to untreated hypertension or hypertension not responding to current therapeutic regimen. In either case, assign the appropriate code from categories 401-405 to designate the stage and type of hypertension. Code to the type of hypertension.

11. Elevated Blood Pressure

    For a statement of elevated blood pressure without further specificity, assign code 796.2, Elevated blood pressure reading without diagnosis of hypertension, rather than a code from category 401.

Late Effects of Cerebrovascular Disease Category 438 is used to indicate conditions classifiable to categories 430-437 as the causes of late effects (neurologic deficits), themselves classified elsewhere. These "late effects" include neurologic deficits that persist after initial onset of conditions classifiable to 430-437. The neurologic deficits caused by cerebrovascular disease may be present from the onset or may arise at any time after the onset of the condition classifiable to 430-437. Codes from category 438 may be assigned on a health care record with codes from 430-437, if the patient has a current cerebrovascular accident (CVA) and deficits from an old CVA. Assign code V12.59 (and not a code from category 438) as an additional code for history of cerebrovascular disease when no neurologic deficits are present.

C8. Diseases of Respiratory System

Reserved for future guideline expansion

C9. Diseases of Digestive System

Reserved for future guideline expansion

C10. Diseases of Genitourinary System

Reserved for future guideline expansion

C11. Complications of Pregnancy, Childbirth, and the Puerperium

A. General Rules for Obstetric Cases

1. Obstetric cases require codes from chapter 11, codes in the range 630-677, Complications of Pregnancy, Childbirth, and the Puerperium. Should the physician document that the pregnancy is incidental to the encounter, then code V22.2 should be used in place of any chapter 11 codes. It is the physician's responsibility to state that the condition being treated is not affecting the pregnancy.

2. Chapter 11 codes have sequencing priority over codes from other chapters. Additional codes from other chapters may be used in conjunction with chapter 11 codes to further specify conditions. For example, sepsis and septic shock associated with abortion, ectopic pregnancy, and molar pregnancy are classified to category codes in Chapter 11 (630-639).

3. Chapter 11 codes are to be used only on the maternal record, never on the record of the newborn.

4. Categories 640-648, 651-676 have required fifth-digits, which indicate whether the encounter is antepartum, postpartum and whether a delivery has also occurred.

5. The fifth-digits, which are appropriate for each code number, are listed in brackets under each code. The fifth-digits on each code should all be consistent with each other. That is, should a delivery occur all of the fifth-digits should indicate the delivery.

6. For prenatal outpatient visits for patients with high-risk pregnancies, a code from category V23, Supervision of high-risk pregnancy, should be used as the principal or first-listed diagnosis. Secondary chapter 11 codes may be used in conjunction with these codes if appropriate. A thorough review of any pertinent excludes note is necessary to be certain that these V codes are being used properly.

7. An outcome of delivery code, V27.0-V27.9, should be included on every maternal record when a delivery has occurred. These codes are not to be used on subsequent records or on the newborn record.

8. For routine outpatient prenatal visits when no complications are present codes V22.0, Supervision of normal first pregnancy, and V22.1, Supervision of other normal pregnancy, should be used as the first-listed diagnoses. These codes should not be used in conjunction with chapter 11 codes.

B. Selection of OB Principal or First-listed Diagnosis

1. In episodes when no delivery occurs, the principal diagnosis should correspond to the principal complication of the pregnancy, which necessitated the encounter. Should more than one complication exist, all of which are treated or monitored, any of the complications codes may be sequenced first.
2. When a delivery occurs, the principal diagnosis should correspond to the main circumstances or complication of the delivery.

   In cases of cesarean delivery, the selection of the principal diagnosis should correspond to the reason the cesarean delivery was performed unless the reason for admission/encounter was unrelated to the condition resulting in the cesarean delivery.

C. Fetal Conditions Affecting the Management of the Mother

Codes from category 655, Known or suspected fetal abnormality affecting management of the mother, and category 656, Other fetal and placental problems affecting the management of the mother, are assigned only when the fetal condition is actually responsible for modifying the management of the mother, i.e., by requiring diagnostic studies, additional observation, special care, or termination of pregnancy. The fact that the fetal condition exists does not justify assigning a code from this series to the mother's record.

D. HIV Infection in Pregnancy, Childbirth and the Puerperium

During pregnancy, childbirth or the puerperium, a patient admitted because of an HIV-related illness should receive a principal diagnosis of 647.6X, Other specified infectious and parasitic diseases in the mother classifiable elsewhere, but complicating the pregnancy, childbirth or the puerperium, followed by 042 and the code(s) for the HIV-related illness(es). This is an exception to the sequencing rule found in above.

Patients with asymptomatic HIV infection status admitted during pregnancy, childbirth, or the puerperium should receive codes of 647.6X and V08.

E. Normal Delivery, 650

1. Code 650 is for use in cases when a woman is admitted for a full-term normal delivery and delivers a single, healthy infant without any complications antepartum, during the delivery, or postpartum during the delivery episode.
2. Code 650 may be used if the patient had a complication at some point during her pregnancy but the complication is not present at the time of the admission for delivery.
3. Code 650 is always a principal diagnosis. It is not to be used if any other code from chapter 11 is needed to describe a current complication of the antenatal, delivery, or perinatal period. Additional codes from other chapters may be used with code 650 if they are not related to or are in any way complicating the pregnancy.
4. V27.0, Single liveborn, is the only outcome of delivery code appropriate for use with 650.

F. The Postpartum Period

1. The postpartum period begins immediately after delivery and continues for six weeks following delivery.
2. A postpartum complication is any complication occurring within the six-week period.
3. Chapter 11 codes may also be used to describe pregnancy-related complications after the six-week period should the physician document that a condition is pregnancy related.
4. Postpartum complications that occur during the same admission as the delivery are identified with a fifth digit of "2." Subsequent admissions/encounters for postpartum complications should identified with a fifth digit of "4."
5. When the mother delivers outside the hospital prior to admission and is admitted for routine postpartum care and no complications are noted, code V24.0, Postpartum care and examination immediately after delivery, should be assigned as the principal diagnosis.
6. A delivery diagnosis code should not be used for a woman who has delivered prior to admission to the hospital. Any postpartum procedures should be coded.

G. Code 677, Late effect of complication of pregnancy, childbirth, and the puerperium

1. Code 677, Late effect of complication of pregnancy, childbirth, and the puerperium is for use in those cases when an initial complication of a pregnancy develops a sequelae requiring care or treatment at a future date.
2. This code may be used at any time after the initial postpartum period.
3. This code, like all late effect codes, is to be sequenced following the code describing the sequelae of the complication.

H. Abortions

1. Fifth-digits are required for abortion categories 634-637. Fifth-digit 1, incomplete, indicates that all of the products of conception have not been expelled from the uterus. Fifth-digit 2, complete, indicates that all products of conception have been expelled from the uterus prior to the episode of care.
2. A code from categories 640-648 and 651-657 may be used as additional codes with an abortion code to indicate the complication leading to the abortion.

   Fifth digit 3 is assigned with codes from these categories when used with an abortion code because the other fifth digits will not apply. Codes from the 660-669 series are not to be used for complications of abortion.
3. Code 639 is to be used for all complications following abortion. Code 639 cannot be assigned with codes from categories 634-638.
4. Abortion with Liveborn Fetus.

   When an attempted termination of pregnancy results in a liveborn fetus assign code 644.21, Early onset of delivery, with an appropriate code from category V27, Outcome of Delivery. The procedure code for the attempted termination of pregnancy should also be assigned.
5. Retained Products of Conception following an abortion.

   Subsequent admissions for retained products of conception following a spontaneous or legally induced abortion are assigned the appropriate code from category 634, Spontaneous abortion, or legally induced abortion, with a fifth digit of "1" (incomplete). This advice is appropriate even when the patient was discharged previously with a discharge diagnosis of complete abortion.

C12. Diseases Skin and Subcutaneous Tissue

Reserved for future guideline expansion

C13. Diseases of Musculoskeletal and Connective Tissue

Reserved for future guideline expansion

C14. Congenital Anomalies

Reserved for future guideline expansion

C15. Newborn (Perinatal) Guidelines

For coding and reporting purposes the perinatal period is defined as birth through the 28th day following birth. The following guidelines are provided for reporting purposes. Hospitals may record other diagnoses as needed for internal data use.

A. General Perinatal Rule

All clinically significant conditions noted on routine newborn examination should be coded. A condition is clinically significant if it requires:

clinical evaluation; or

therapeutic treatment; or

diagnostic procedures; or

extended length of hospital stay; or

increased nursing care and/or monitoring; or

has implications for future health care needs.

Note: The perinatal guidelines listed above are the same as the general coding guidelines for "additional diagnoses," except for the final point regarding implications for future health care needs. Whether or not a condition is clinically significant can only be determined by the physician.

B. Use of Codes V30-V39

When coding the birth of an infant, assign a code from categories V30-V39, according to the type of birth. A code from this series is assigned as a principal diagnosis, and assigned only once to a newborn at the time of birth.

C. Newborn Transfers

If the newborn is transferred to another institution, the V30 series is not used at the receiving hospital.

D. Use of Category V29

1. Assign a code from category V29, Observation and evaluation of newborns and infants for suspected conditions not found, to identify those instances when a healthy newborn is evaluated for a suspected condition that is determined after study not to be present. Do not use a code from category V29 when the patient has identified signs or

symptoms of a suspected problem; in such cases, code the sign or symptom.

2. A V29 code is to be used as a secondary code after the V30, Outcome of delivery, code. It may also be assigned as a principal code for readmissions or encounters when the V30 code no longer applies. It is for use only for healthy newborns and infants for which no condition after study is found to be present.

E. Maternal Causes of Perinatal Morbidity

Codes from categories 760-763, Maternal causes of perinatal morbidity and mortality, are assigned only when the maternal condition has actually affected the fetus or newborn. The fact that the mother has an associated medical condition or experiences some complication of pregnancy, labor or delivery does not justify the routine assignment of codes from these categories to the newborn record.

F. Congenital Anomalies

Assign an appropriate code from categories 740-759, Congenital Anomalies, as an additional diagnosis when a specific abnormality is diagnosed for an infant. Congenital anomalies may also be the principal or first listed diagnosis for admissions/encounters subsequent to the newborn admission. Such abnormalities may occur as a set of symptoms or multiple malformations. A code should be assigned for each presenting manifestation of the syndrome if the syndrome is not specifically indexed in ICD-9-CM.

G. Coding of Additional Perinatal Diagnoses

1. Assign codes for conditions that require treatment or further investigation, prolong the length of stay, or require resource utilization.
2. Assign codes for conditions that have been specified by the physician as having implications for future health care needs.

Note: This guideline should not be used for adult patients.

3. Assign a code for Newborn conditions originating in the perinatal period (categories 760-779), as well as complications arising during the current episode of care classified in other chapters, only if the diagnoses have been documented by the responsible physician at the time of transfer or discharge as having affected the fetus or newborn.

H. Prematurity and Fetal Growth Retardation

Codes from category 764 and subcategories 765.0 and 765.1 should not be assigned based solely on recorded birthweight or estimated gestational age, but on the attending physician's clinical assessment of maturity of the infant. NOTE: Since physicians may utilize different criteria in determining prematurity, do not code the diagnosis of prematurity unless the physician documents this condition.

A code from subcategory 765.2, Weeks of gestation, should be assigned as an additional code with category 764 and codes from 765.0 and 765.1 to specify weeks of gestation as documented by the physician.

C16. Signs, Symptoms and Ill-Defined Conditions

Reserved for future guideline expansion

C17. Injury and Poisoning

A. Coding of Injuries

When coding injuries, assign separate codes for each injury unless a combination code is provided, in which case the combination code is assigned. Multiple injury codes are provided in ICD-9-CM, but should not be assigned unless information for a more specific code is not available. These codes are not to be used for normal, healing surgical wounds or to identify complications of surgical wounds.

The code for the most serious injury, as determined by the physician, is sequenced first.

1. Superficial injuries such as abrasions or contusions are not coded when associated with more severe injuries of the same site.
2. When a primary injury results in minor damage to peripheral nerves or blood vessels, the primary injury is sequenced first with additional code(s) from categories 950-957, Injury to nerves and spinal cord, and/or 900-904, Injury to blood vessels. When the primary injury is to the blood vessels or nerves, that injury should be sequenced first.

B. Coding of Fractures

The principles of multiple coding of injuries should be followed in coding fractures. Fractures of specified sites are coded individually by site in accordance with both the provisions within categories 800-829 and the level of detail furnished by medical record content. Combination categories for multiple fractures are provided for use when there is insufficient detail in the medical record (such as trauma cases transferred to another hospital), when the reporting form limits the number of codes that can be used in reporting pertinent clinical data, or when there is insufficient specificity at the fourth-digit or fifth-digit level. More specific guidelines are as follows:

1. Multiple fractures of same limb classifiable to the same three-digit or four-digit category are coded to that category.
2. Multiple unilateral or bilateral fractures of same bone(s) but classified to different fourth-digit subdivisions (bone part) within the same three-digit category are coded individually by site.
3. Multiple fracture categories 819 and 828 classify bilateral fractures of both upper limbs (819) and both lower limbs (828), but without any detail at the fourth-digit level other than open and closed type of fractures.
4. Multiple fractures are sequenced in accordance with the severity of the fracture and the physician should be asked to list the fracture diagnoses in the order of severity.

C. Coding of Burns

Current burns (940-948) are classified by depth, extent and by agent (E code). Burns are classified by depth as first degree (erythema), second degree (blistering), and third degree (full-thickness involvement).

1. Sequence first the code that reflects the highest degree of burn when more than one burn is present.
2. Classify burns of the same local site (three-digit category level, (940-947) but of different degrees to the subcategory identifying the highest degree recorded in the diagnosis.
3. Non-healing burns are coded as acute burns.

   Necrosis of burned skin should be coded as a non-healed burn.
4. Assign code 958.3, Posttraumatic wound infection, not elsewhere classified, as an additional code for any documented infected burn site.
5. When coding burns, assign separate codes for each burn site. Category 946 Burns of Multiple specified sites, should only be used if the location of the burns are not documented.

   Category 949, Burn, unspecified, is extremely vague and should rarely be used.
6. Assign codes from category 948, Burns classified according to extent of body surface involved, when the site of the burn is not specified or when there is a need for additional data. It is advisable to use category 948 as additional coding when needed to provide data for evaluating burn mortality, such as that needed by burn units. It is also advisable to use category 948 as an additional code for reporting purposes when there is mention of a third-degree burn involving 20 percent or more of the body surface.

   In assigning a code from category 948:

   Fourth-digit codes are used to identify the percentage of total body surface involved in a burn (all degree).

   Fifth-digits are assigned to identify the percentage of body surface involved in third-degree burn.

   Fifth-digit zero (0) is assigned when less than 10 percent or when no body surface is involved in a third-degree burn.

   Category 948 is based on the classic "rule of nines" in estimating body surface involved: head and neck are assigned nine percent, each arm nine percent, each leg 18 percent, the anterior trunk 18 percent, posterior trunk 18 percent, and genitalia one percent. Physicians may change these percentage assignments where necessary to accommodate infants and children who have proportionately larger heads than adults and patients who have large buttocks, thighs, or abdomen that involve burns.
7. Encounters for the treatment of the late effects of burns (i.e., scars or joint contractures) should be coded to the residual condition (sequelae) followed by the appropriate late effect code (906.5-906.9). A late effect E code may also be used, if desired.
8. When appropriate, both a sequelae with a late effect code, and a current burn code may be assigned on the same record.

D. Coding of Debridement of Wound, Infection, or Burn

Excisional debridement may be performed by a physician and/or other health care provider and involves an excisional, as opposed to a mechanical (brushing, scrubbing, washing) debridement.

For coding purposes, excisional debridement, 86.22.

Nonexcisional debridement is assigned to 86.28.

Modified based on Coding Clinic, 2nd Quarter 2000, p. 9.

E. Adverse Effects, Poisoning and Toxic Effects

The properties of certain drugs, medicinal and biological substances or combinations of such substances, may cause toxic reactions. The occurrence of drug toxicity is classified in ICD-9-CM as follows:

1. Adverse Effect

When the drug was correctly prescribed and properly administered, code the reaction plus the appropriate code from the E930-E949 series. Codes from the E930-E949 series must be used to identify the causative substance for an adverse effect of drug, medicinal and biological substances, correctly prescribed and properly administered. The effect, such as tachycardia, delirium, gastrointestinal hemorrhaging, vomiting, hypokalemia, hepatitis, renal failure, or respiratory failure, is coded and followed by the appropriate code from the E930-E949 series.

Adverse effects of therapeutic substances correctly prescribed and properly administered (toxicity, synergistic reaction, side effect, and idiosyncratic reaction) may be due to (1) differences among patients, such as age, sex, disease, and genetic factors, and (2) drug-related factors, such as type of drug, route of administration, duration of therapy, dosage, and bioavailability.

2. Poisoning
   a. When an error was made in drug prescription or in the administration of the drug by physician, nurse, patient, or other person, use the appropriate poisoning code from the 960-979 series.
   b. If an overdose of a drug was intentionally taken or administered and resulted in drug toxicity, it would be coded as a poisoning (960-979 series).
   c. If a nonprescribed drug or medicinal agent was taken in combination with a correctly prescribed and properly administered drug, any drug toxicity or other reaction resulting from the interaction of the two drugs would be classified as a poisoning.
   d. When coding a poisoning or reaction to the improper use of a medication (e.g., wrong dose, wrong substance, wrong route of administration) the poisoning code is sequenced first, followed by a code for the manifestation. If there is also a diagnosis of drug abuse or dependence to the substance, the abuse or dependence is coded as an additional code.

C18. Classification of Factors Influencing Health Status and Contact with Health Service

A. ICD-9-CM provides codes to deal with encounters for circumstances other than a disease or injury. The Supplementary Classification of Factors Influencing Health Status and Contact with Health Services (V01.0-V83.89) is provided to deal with occasions when circumstances other than a disease or injury (codes 001-999) are recorded as a diagnosis or problem.

There are four primary circumstances for the use of V codes:

1. When a person who is not currently sick encounters the health services for some specific reason, such as to act as an organ donor, to receive prophylactic care, such as inoculations or health screenings, or to receive counseling on health related issue.
2. When a person with a resolving disease or injury, or a chronic, long-term condition requiring continuous care, encounters the health care system for specific aftercare of that disease or injury (e.g., dialysis for renal disease; chemotherapy for malignancy; cast change). A diagnosis/symptom code should be used whenever a current, acute, diagnosis is being treated or a sign or symptom is being studied.
3. When circumstances or problems influence a person's health status but are not in themselves a current illness or injury.
4. For newborns, to indicate birth status.

B. V codes are for use in both the inpatient and outpatient setting but are generally more applicable to the outpatient setting. V codes may be used as either a first listed (principal diagnosis code in the inpatient setting) or secondary code depending on the circumstances of the encounter. Certain V codes may only be used as first listed, others only as secondary codes.

C. V Codes indicate a reason for an encounter. They are not procedure codes. A corresponding procedure code must accompany a V code to describe the procedure performed.

D. Categories of V Codes

1. Contact/Exposure

Category V01 indicates contact with or

exposure to communicable diseases. These codes are for patients who do not show any sign or symptom of a disease but have been exposed to it by close personal contact with an infected individual or are in an area where a disease is epidemic. These codes may be used as a first listed code to explain an encounter for testing, or, more commonly, as a secondary code to identify a potential risk.

2. Inoculations and vaccinations

   Categories V03-V06 are for encounters for inoculations and vaccinations. They indicate that a patient is being seen to receive a prophylactic inoculation against a disease. The injection itself must be represented by the appropriate procedure code. A code from V03-V06 may be used as a secondary code if the inoculation is given as a routine part of preventive health care, such as a well-baby visit.

3. Status

   Status codes indicate that a patient is either a carrier of a disease or has the sequelae or residual of a past disease or condition. This includes such things as the presence of prosthetic or mechanical devices resulting from past treatment. A status code is informative because the status may affect the course of treatment and its outcome. A status code is distinct from a history code. The history code indicates that the patient no longer has the condition.

   The status V codes/categories are:

   V02 Carrier or suspected carrier of infectious diseases

   Carrier status, indicates that a person harbors the specific organisms of a disease without manifest symptoms and is capable of transmitting the infection.

   V08 Asymptomatic HIV infection status

   This code indicates that a patient has tested positive for HIV but has manifested no signs or symptoms of the disease.

   V09 Infection with drug-resistant microorganisms

   This category indicates that a patient has an infection which is resistant to drug treatment. Sequence the infection code first.

   V21 Constitutional states in development

   V22.2 Pregnant state, incidental

   This code is a secondary code only for use when the pregnancy is in no way complicating the reason for visit. Otherwise, a code from the obstetric chapter is required.

   V26.5x Sterilization status

   V42 Organ or tissue replaced by transplant

   V43 Organ or tissue replaced by other means

   V44 Artificial opening status

   V45 Other postsurgical states

   V46 Other dependence on machines

   V49.6 Upper limb amputation status

   V49.7 Lower limb amputation status

   V48.81 Postmenopausal status

   V49.82 Dental sealant status

   V58.6 Long-term (current) drug use

   This subcategory indicates a patient's continuous use of a prescribed drug (including such things as aspirin therapy) for the long-term treatment of a condition or for prophylactic use. It is not for use for patients who have addictions to drugs.

   V83 Genetic carrier status

   Categories V42-V46, and subcategories V49.6, V49.7 are for use only if there are no complications or malfunctions of the organ or tissue replaced, the amputation site or the equipment on which the patient is dependent. These are always secondary codes.

4. History (of)

   There are two types of history V codes, personal and family. Personal history codes explain a patient's past medical condition that no longer exists and is not receiving any treatment but that has the potential for recurrence, and, therefore, may require continued monitoring. The exceptions to this general rule are category V14, Personal history of allergy to medicinal agents and subcategory V15.0, Allergy, other than to medicinal agents. A person who has had an allergic episode to a substance or food in the past should always be considered allergic to the substance.

Family history codes are for use when a patient has a family member(s) who has had a particular disease that causes the patient to be at higher risk of also contracting the disease.

Personal history codes may be used in conjunction with follow-up codes and family history codes may be use in conjunction with screening codes to explain the need for a test or procedure. History codes are also acceptable on any medical record regardless of the reason for visit. A history of an illness, even if no longer present, is important information that may alter the type of treatment ordered.

The history V code categories are:

V10 Personal history of malignant neoplasm

V12 Personal history of certain other diseases

V13 Personal history of other diseases

Except: V13.4, Personal history of arthritis, and V13.6, Personal history of congenital malformations. These conditions are lifelong so are not true history codes.

V14 Personal history of allergy to medicinal agents

V15 Other personal history presenting hazards to health

Except: V15.7, Personal history of contraception.

V16 Family history of malignant neoplasm

V17 Family history of certain chronic disabling diseases

V18 Family history of certain other specific diseases

V19 Family history of other conditions

5. Screening

Screening is the testing for disease or disease precursors in seemingly well individuals so that early detection and treatment can be provided for those who test positive for the disease. Screenings that are recommended for many subgroups in a population include: routine mammograms for women over 40, a fecal occult blood test for everyone over 50, an amniocentesis to rule out a fetal anomaly for pregnant women over 35, because the incidence of breast cancer and colon cancer in these subgroups is higher than in the general population, as is the incidence of Down's syndrome in older mothers.

The testing of a person to rule out or confirm a suspected diagnosis because the patient has some sign or symptom is a diagnostic examination, not a screening. In these cases, the sign or symptom is used to explain the reason for the test.

A screening code may be a first listed code if the reason for the visit is specifically the screening exam. It may also be used as an additional code if the screening is done during an office visit for other health problems. A screening code is not necessary if the screening is inherent to a routine examination, such as a pap smear done during a routine pelvic examination.

Should a condition be discovered during the screening then the code for the condition may be assigned as an additional diagnosis.

The V code indicates that a screening exam is planned. A procedure code is required to confirm that the screening was performed.

The screening V code categories:

V28 Antenatal screening

V73-V82 Special screening examinations

6. Observation

There are two observation V code categories. They are for use in very limited circumstances when a person is being observed for a suspected condition that is ruled out. The observation codes are not for use if an injury or illness or any signs or symptoms related to the suspected condition are present. In such cases the diagnosis/symptom code is used with the corresponding E code to identify any external cause.

The observation codes are to be used as principal diagnosis only. The only exception to this is when the principal diagnosis is required to be a code from the V30, Live born infant, category. Then the V29 observation code is sequenced after the V30 code. Additional codes may be used in addition to the observation code but only if they are unrelated to the suspected condition being observed.

The observation V code categories:

V29 Observation and evaluation of newborns for suspected condition not found

A code from category V30 should be sequenced before the V29 code.

V71 Observation and evaluation for suspected condition not found

7. Aftercare

Aftercare visit codes cover situations when the initial treatment of a disease or injury has been performed and the patient requires continued care during the healing or recovery phase, or for the long-term consequences of the disease. The aftercare V code should not be used if treatment is directed at a current, acute disease or injury, the diagnosis code is to be used in these cases. Exceptions to this rule are codes V58.0, Radiotherapy, and V58.1, Chemotherapy. These codes are to be first listed, followed by the diagnosis code when a patient's encounter is solely to receive radiation therapy or chemotherapy for the treatment of a neoplasm. Should a patient receive both chemotherapy and radiation therapy during the same encounter code V58.0 and V58.1 may be used together on a record with either one being sequenced first.

The aftercare codes are generally first listed to explain the specific reason for the encounter. An aftercare code may be used as an additional code when some type of aftercare is provided in addition to the reason for admission and no diagnosis code is applicable. An example of this would be the closure of a colostomy during an encounter for treatment of another condition.

Certain aftercare V code categories need a secondary diagnosis code to describe the resolving condition or sequelae, for others, the condition is inherent in the code title.

Additional V code aftercare category terms include, fitting and adjustment, and attention to artificial openings.

The aftercare V category/codes:

V52 Fitting and adjustment of prosthetic device and implant

V53 Fitting and adjustment of other device

V54 Other orthopedic aftercare

V55 Attention to artificial openings

V56 Encounter for dialysis and dialysis catheter care

V57 Care involving the use of rehabilitation procedures

V58.0 Radiotherapy

V58.1 Chemotherapy

V58.3 Attention to surgical dressings and sutures

V58.41 Encounter for planned post-operative wound closure

V53.42 Aftercare, surgery, neoplasm

V53.43 Aftercare, surgery, trauma

V58.49 Other specified aftercare following surgery

V53.71-V53.78 Aftercare following surgery

V58.81 Fitting and adjustment of vascular catheter

V58.82 Fitting and adjustment of nonvascular catheter

V53.83 Monitoring therapeutic drug

V58.89 Other specified aftercare

8. Follow-up

The follow-up codes are for use to explain continuing surveillance following completed treatment of a disease, condition, or injury. They infer that the condition has been fully treated and no longer exists. They should not be confused with aftercare codes which explain current treatment for a healing condition or its sequelae. Follow-up codes may be used in conjunction with history codes to provide the full picture of the healed condition and its treatment. The follow-up code is sequenced first, followed by the history code.

A follow-up code may be used to explain repeated visits. Should a condition be found to have recurred on the follow-up visit, then the diagnosis code should be used in place of the follow-up code.

The follow-up V code categories:

V24 Postpartum care and evaluation

V67 Follow-up examination

9. Donor

Category V59 is the donor codes. They are for use for living individuals who are donating blood or other body tissue. These codes are only for individuals donating for others, not for self donations. They are not for use to identify cadaveric donations.

10. Counseling

Counseling V codes are for use for when a patient or family member receives assistance in the aftermath of an illness or injury, or when support is required in coping with family or social problems. They are not necessary for use in conjunction with a diagnosis code when the counseling component of care is considered integral to standard treatment.

The counseling V categories/codes:

V25.0 General counseling and advice for contraceptive management

V26.3 Genetic counseling

V26.4 General counseling and advice for procreative management

V61 Other family circumstances

V65.1 Person consulted on behalf of another person

V65.3 Dietary surveillance and counseling

V65.4 Other counseling, not elsewhere classified

11. Obstetrics and related conditions

See the Obstetrics guidelines for further instruction on the use of these codes.

V codes for pregnancy are for use in those circumstances when none of the problems or complications included in the codes from the Obstetrics chapter exist (a routine prenatal visit or postpartum care) V22.0, Supervision of normal first pregnancy, and V22.1, Supervision of other normal pregnancy, are always first listed and are not to be used with any other code from the OB chapter.

The outcome of delivery, category V27, should be included on all maternal delivery records. It is always a secondary code.

V codes for family planning (contraceptive) or procreative management and counseling should be included on an obstetric record either during the pregnancy or the postpartum stage, if applicable.

Obstetrics and related conditions V code categories:

V22 Normal pregnancy

V23 Supervision of high-risk pregnancy

Except: V23.2, Pregnancy with history of abortion. Code 646.3, Habitual aborter, from the OB chapter is required to indicate a history of abortion during a pregnancy.

V24 Postpartum care and evaluation

V25 Encounter for contraceptive management

Except V25.0x (See counseling above)

V26 Procreative management

Except V26.5x, Sterilization status, V26.3 and V26.4 (Counseling)

V27 Outcome of delivery

V28 Antenatal screening

See Screening—see section 5 of this article

12. Newborn, infant and child

See the newborn guidelines for further instruction on the use of these codes.

Newborn V code categories:

V20 Health supervision of infant or child

V29 Observation and evaluation of newborns for suspected condition not found—see Observation, section 6 of this article.

V30-V39 Liveborn infant according to type of birth

13. Routine and administrative examinations

The V codes allow for the description of encounters for routine examinations, such as, a general check-up, or, examinations for administrative purposes, such as, a pre-employment physical. The codes are for use as first listed codes only and are not to be used if the examination is for diagnosis of a suspected condition or for treatment purposes. In such cases the diagnosis code is used. During a routine exam, should a diagnosis or condition be discovered, it should be coded as an additional code. Pre-existing and chronic conditions, and history codes may also be included as additional codes as long as the examination is for administrative purposes and not focused on any particular condition.

Pre-operative examination V codes are for use only in those situations when a patient is being cleared for surgery and no treatment is given.

The V codes categories/code for routine and administrative examinations:

V20.2 Routine infant or child health check

Any injections given should have a corresponding procedure code.

V70 General medical examination

V72 Special investigations and examinations

Except V72.5 and V72.6

14. Miscellaneous V codes

The miscellaneous V codes capture a number of other health care encounters that do not fall into one of the other categories. Certain of these codes identify the reason for the encounter, others are for use as additional codes which provide useful information on circumstances which may affect a patient's care and treatment.

Miscellaneous V code categories/codes:

V07 Need for isolation and other prophylactic measures
V50 Elective surgery for purposes other than remedying health states
V58.5 Orthodontics
V60 Housing, household, and economic circumstances
V62 Other psychosocial circumstances
V63 Unavailability of other medical facilities for care
V64 Persons encountering health services for specific procedures, not carried out
V66 Convalescence and Palliative Care
V68 Encounters for administrative purposes
V69 Problems related to lifestyle

15. Nonspecific V codes

Certain V codes are so non-specific, or potentially redundant with other codes in the classification that there can be little justification for their use in the inpatient setting. Their use in the outpatient setting should be limited to those instances when there is no further documentation to permit more precise coding. Otherwise, any sign or symptom or any other reason for visit which is captured in another code should be used.

Nonspecific V code categories/codes:

V29 Personal history of mental disorder

A code from the mental disorders chapter, with an in remission fifth-digit, should be used.

V13.4 Personal history of arthritis
V13.6 Personal history of congenital malformations
V15.7 Personal history of contraception
V23.2 Pregnancy with history of abortion
V40 Mental and behavioral problems
V41 Problems with special senses and other special functions
V47 Other problems with internal organs
V48 Problems with head, neck, and trunk
V49 Problems with limbs and other problems

Exceptions:

V49.6 Upper limb amputation status
V49.7 Lower limb amputation status
V49.81 Postmenopausal status
V49.82 Dental sealant status

V51 Aftercare involving the use of plastic surgery
V58.2 Blood transfusion, without reported diagnosis
V58.9 Unspecified aftercare
V72.5 Radiological examination, NEC
V72.6 Laboratory examination

Codes V72.5 and V72.6 are not to be used if any sign or symptoms, or reason for a test is documented. See section K and L of the outpatient guidelines.

C19. Supplemental Classification of External Causes of Injury and Poisoning (E codes)

Introduction: These guidelines are provided for those who are currently collecting E codes in order that there will be standardization in the process. If your institution plans to begin collecting E codes, these guidelines are to be applied. The use of E codes is supplemental to the application of ICD-9-CM diagnosis codes. E codes are never to be recorded as principal diagnosis (first-listed in noninpatient setting) and are not required for reporting to CMS.

External causes of injury and poisoning codes (E codes) are intended to provide data for injury research and evaluation of injury prevention strategies. E codes capture how the injury or poisoning happened (cause), the intent (unintentional or accidental; or intentional, such as suicide or assault), and the place where the event occurred. Some major categories of E codes include:

transport accidents

poisoning and adverse effects of drugs, medicinal substances and biologicals

accidental falls

accidents caused by fire and flames

accidents due to natural and environmental factors

late effects of accidents, assaults or self injury

assaults or purposely inflicted injury

suicide or self inflicted injury

These guidelines apply for the coding and collection of E codes from records in hospitals, outpatient clinics, emergency departments, other ambulatory care settings and physician offices, and nonacute care settings, except when other specific guidelines apply. (See Section III, Reporting Diagnostic Guidelines for Hospital-based Outpatient Services/ Reporting Requirements for Physician Billing.)

A. General E Code Coding Guidelines

1. An E code may be used with any code in the range of 001-V83.02, which indicates an injury, poisoning, or adverse effect due to an external cause.
2. Assign the appropriate E code for all initial treatments of an injury, poisoning, or adverse effect of drugs.
3. Use a late effect E code for subsequent visits when a late effect of the initial injury or poisoning is being treated. There is no late effect E code for adverse effects of drugs.
4. Use the full range of E codes to completely describe the cause, the intent and the place of occurrence, if applicable, for all injuries, poisonings, and adverse effects of drugs.
5. Assign as many E codes as necessary to fully explain each cause. If only one E code can be recorded, assign the E code most related to the principal diagnosis.
6. The selection of the appropriate E code is guided by the Index to External Causes, which is located after the alphabetical index to diseases and by Inclusion and Exclusion notes in the Tabular List.
7. An E code can never be a principal (first listed) diagnosis.

B. Place of Occurrence Guideline

Use an additional code from category E849 to indicate the Place of Occurrence for injuries and poisonings. The Place of Occurrence describes the place where the event occurred and not the patient's activity at the time of the event.

Do not use E849.9 if the place of occurrence is not stated.

C. Adverse Effects of Drugs, Medicinal and Biological Substances Guidelines

1. Do not code directly from the Table of Drugs and Chemicals. Always refer back to the Tabular List.
2. Use as many codes as necessary to describe completely all drugs, medicinal or biological substances.
3. If the same E code would describe the causative agent for more than one adverse reaction, assign the code only once.
4. If two or more drugs, medicinal or biological substances are reported, code each individually unless the combination code is listed in the Table of Drugs and Chemicals. In that case, assign the E code for the combination.
5. When a reaction results from the interaction of a drug(s) and alcohol, use poisoning codes and E codes for both.
6. If the reporting format limits the number of E codes that can be used in reporting clinical data, code the one most related to the principal diagnosis. Include at least one from each category (cause, intent, place) if possible.

   If there are different fourth digit codes in the same three digit category, use the code for "Other specified" of that category. If there is no "Other specified" code in that category, use the appropriate "Unspecified" code in that category.

   If the codes are in different three digit categories, assign the appropriate E code for other multiple drugs and medicinal substances.
7. Codes from the E930-E949 series must be used to identify the causative substance for an adverse effect of drug, medicinal and biological substances, correctly prescribed and properly administered. The effect, such as tachycardia, delirium, gastrointestinal hemorrhaging, vomiting, hypokalemia, hepatitis, renal failure, or respiratory failure, is coded and followed by the appropriate code from the E930-E949 series.

D. Multiple Cause E Code Coding Guidelines

If two or more events cause separate injuries, an E code should be assigned for each cause. The first listed E code will be selected in the following order:

E codes for child and adult abuse take priority over all other E codes—see Child and Adult abuse guidelines

E codes for terrorism events take priority over all other E codes except child and adult abuse

E codes for cataclysmic events take priority over all other E codes except child and adult abuse and terrorism

E codes for transport accidents take priority over all other E codes except cataclysmic events and child and adult abuse and terrorism

The first-listed E code should correspond to the cause of the most serious diagnosis due to an assault, accident, or self-harm, following the order of hierarchy listed above.

E. Child and Adult Abuse Guideline

1. When the cause of an injury or neglect is intentional child or adult abuse, the first listed E code should be assigned from categories E960-E968, Homicide and injury purposely inflicted by other persons, (except category E967). An E code from category E967, Child and adult battering and other maltreatment, should be added as an additional code to identify the perpetrator, if known.
2. In cases of neglect when the intent is determined to be accidental E code E904.0, Abandonment or neglect of infant and helpless person, should be the first listed E code.

F. Unknown or Suspected Intent Guideline

1. If the intent (accident, self-harm, assault) of the cause of an injury or poisoning is unknown or unspecified, code the intent as undetermined E980-E989.
2. If the intent (accident, self-harm, assault) of the cause of an injury or poisoning is questionable, probable or suspected, code the intent as undetermined E980-E989.

G. Undetermined Cause

When the intent of an injury or poisoning is known, but the cause is unknown, use codes: E928.9, Unspecified accident, E958.9, Suicide and self-inflicted injury by unspecified means, and E968.9, Assault by unspecified means.

These E codes should rarely be used, as the documentation in the medical record, in both the inpatient outpatient and other settings, should normally provide sufficient detail to determine the cause of the injury.

H. Late Effects of External Cause Guidelines

1. Late effect E codes exist for injuries and poisonings but not for adverse effects of drugs, misadventures and surgical complications.
2. A late effect E code (E929, E959, E969, E977, E989, or E999.1) should be used with any report of a late effect or sequela resulting from a previous injury or poisoning (905-909).
3. A late effect E code should never be used with a related current nature of injury code.

I. Misadventures and Complications of Care Guidelines

1. Assign a code in the range of E870-E876 if misadventures are stated by the physician.
2. Assign a code in the range of E878-E879 if the physician attributes an abnormal reaction or later complication to a surgical or medical procedure, but does not mention misadventure at the time of the procedure as the cause of the reaction.

J. Terrorism Guidelines

1. When the cause of an injury is identified by the Federal Government (FBI) as terrorism, the first-listed E-code should be a code from category E979, Terrorism. The definition of terrorism employed by the FBI is found at the inclusion note at E979. The terrorism E-code is the only E-code that should be assigned. Additional E codes from the assault categories should not be assigned.
2. When the cause of an injury is suspected to be the result of terrorism a code from category E979 should not be assigned. Assign a code in the range of E codes based circumstances on the documentation of intent and mechanism.
3. Assign code E979.9, Terrorism, secondary effects, for conditions occurring subsequent to the terrorist event. This code should not be assigned for conditions that are due to the initial terrorist act.
4. For statistical purposes these codes will be tabulated within the category for assault, expanding the current category from E960-E969 to include E979 and E999.1.

Section II Selection of Principal Diagnoses for Acute Care (Inpatient) Facilities

The circumstances of inpatient admission always govern the selection of principal diagnosis. The principal diagnosis is defined in the Uniform Hospital Discharge Data Set (UHDDS) as "that condition established after study to be chiefly responsible for occasioning the admission of the patient to the hospital for care."

The UHDDS definitions are used by acute care short-term hospitals to report inpatient data elements in a standardized manner. These data elements and their definitions can be found in the July 31, 1985, Federal Register (Vol. 50, No, 147), pp. 31038-40.

In determining principal diagnosis the coding conventions in the ICD-9-CM, Volumes I and II take precedence over these official coding guidelines. (See Section IA).

The importance of consistent, complete documentation in the medical record cannot be overemphasized. Without such documentation the application of all coding guidelines is a difficult, if not impossible, task.

A. Codes for symptoms, signs, and ill-defined conditions

Codes for symptoms, signs, and ill-defined conditions from Chapter 16 are not to be used as principal diagnosis when a related definitive diagnosis has been established.

B. Two or more interrelated conditions, each potentially meeting the definition for principal diagnosis.

When there are two or more interrelated conditions (such as diseases in the same ICD-9-CM chapter or manifestations characteristically associated with a certain disease) potentially meeting the definition of principal diagnosis, either condition may be sequenced first, unless the circumstances of the admission, the therapy provided, the Tabular List, or the Alphabetic Index indicate otherwise.

C. Two or more diagnoses that equally meet the definition for principal diagnosis.

In the unusual instance when two or more diagnoses equally meet the criteria for principal diagnosis as determined by the circumstances of admission, diagnostic workup and/or therapy provided, and the Alphabetic Index, Tabular List, or another coding guidelines does not provide sequencing direction, any one of the diagnoses may be sequenced first.

D. Two or more comparative or contrasting conditions.

In those rare instances when two or more contrasting or comparative diagnoses are documented as "either/or" (or similar terminology), they are coded as if the diagnoses were confirmed and the diagnoses are sequenced according to the circumstances of the admission. If no further determination can be made as to which diagnosis should be principal, either diagnosis may be sequenced first.

E. A symptom(s) followed by contrasting/comparative diagnoses.

When a symptom(s) is followed by contrasting/comparative diagnoses, the symptom code is sequenced first. All the contrasting/comparative diagnoses should be coded as additional diagnoses.

F. Original treatment plan not carried out.

Sequence as the principal diagnosis the condition, which after study occasioned the admission to the hospital, even though treatment may not have been carried out due to unforeseen circumstances.

G. Complications of surgery and other medical care.

When the admission is for treatment of a complication resulting from surgery or other medical care, the complication code is sequenced as the principal diagnosis. If the complication is classified to the 996-999 series, an additional code for the specific complication may be assigned.

H. Uncertain Diagnosis.

If the diagnosis documented at the time of discharge is qualified as "probable", "suspected", "likely", "questionable", "possible", or "still to be ruled out", code the condition as if it existed or was established. The bases for these guidelines are the diagnostic workup, arrangements for further workup or observation, and initial therapeutic approach that correspond most closely with the established diagnosis.

Section III Reporting Additional Diagnoses for Inpatient, Short-Term, Acute Care Hospital Records

GENERAL RULES FOR OTHER (ADDITIONAL) DIAGNOSES

For reporting purposes the definition for—other diagnoses" is interpreted as additional conditions that affect patient care in terms of requiring:

clinical evaluation; or

therapeutic treatment; or

diagnostic procedures; or

extended length of hospital stay; or

increased nursing care and/or monitoring.

The UHDDS item #11-b defines Other Diagnoses as "all conditions that coexist at the time of admission, that develop subsequently, or that affect the treatment received and/or the length of stay. Diagnoses that relate to an earlier episode which have no bearing on the current hospital stay are to be excluded."

UHDDS definitions apply to inpatients in acute care, short-term, hospital setting. THe UHDDS definitions are used by acute care short-term hospitals to report inpatient data elements in a standardized manner. These data elements and their definitions can be found in the July 31, 1985, Federal Register (Vol. 50, No, 147), pp. 31038–40.

The following guidelines are to be applied in designating "other diagnoses" when neither the Alphabetic Index nor the Tabular List in ICD-9-CM provide direction. The listing of the diagnoses in the patient record is the responsibility of the attending physician.

A. Previous conditions

If the physician has included a diagnosis in the final diagnostic statement, such as the discharge summary or the face sheet, it should ordinarily be coded. Some physicians include in the diagnostic statement resolved conditions or diagnoses and status-post procedures from previous admission that have no bearing on the current stay. Such conditions are not to be reported and are coded only if required by hospital policy.

However, history codes (V10-V19) may be used as secondary codes if the historical condition or family history has an impact on current care or influences treatment.

B. Abnormal findings

Abnormal findings (laboratory, x-ray, pathologic, and other diagnostic results) are not coded and reported unless the physician indicates their clinical significance. If the findings are outside the normal range and the attending physician has ordered other tests to evaluate the condition or prescribed treatment, it is appropriate to ask the physician whether the abnormal finding should be added.

Please note: This differs from the coding practices in the outpatient setting for coding encounters for diagnostic tests that have been interpreted by a physician.

C. Uncertain Diagnosis

If the diagnosis documented at the time of discharge is qualified as "probable", "suspected", "likely", "questionable", "possible", or "still to be ruled out", code the condition as if it existed or was established. The bases for these guidelines are the diagnostic workup, arrangements for further workup or observation, and initial therapeutic approach that correspond most closely with the established diagnosis.

Section IV Diagnostic Coding and Reporting Guidelines for Outpatient Services

These coding guidelines for outpatient diagnoses have been approved for use by hospitals/physicians in coding and reporting hospital-based outpatient services and physician office visits.

Information about the use of certain abbreviations, punctuation, symbols, and other conventions used in the ICD-9-CM Tabular List (code numbers and titles), can be found in Section IA of these guidelines, under "Conventions Used in the Tabular List." Information about the correct sequence to use in finding a code is also described in Section I.

The terms encounter and visit are often used interchangeably in describing outpatient service contacts and, therefore, appear together in these guidelines without distinguishing one from the other.

Though the conventions and general guidelines apply to all settings, coding guidelines for outpatient and physician reporting of diagnoses will vary in a number of instances from those for inpatient diagnoses, recognizing that:

The Uniform Hospital Discharge Data Set (UHDDS) definition of principal diagnosis applies only to inpatients in acute, short-term, general hospitals.

Coding guidelines for inconclusive diagnoses (probable, suspected, rule out, etc.) were developed for inpatient reporting and do not apply to outpatients.

A. Selection of first-listed condition

In the outpatient setting, the term first-listed diagnosis is used in lieu of principal diagnosis.

In determining the first-listed diagnosis the coding conventions of ICD-9-CM, as well as the general and disease specific guidelines take precedence over the outpatient guidelines.

Diagnoses often are not established at the time of the initial encounter/visit. It may take two or more visits before the diagnosis is confirmed.

The most critical rule involves beginning the search for the correct code assignment through the Alphabetic Index. Never begin searching initially in the Tabular List as this will lead to coding errors.

B. The appropriate code or codes from 001.0 through V83.89 must be used to identify diagnoses, symptoms, conditions, problems, complaints, or other reason(s) for the encounter/visit.

C. For accurate reporting of ICD-9-CM diagnosis codes, the documentation should describe the patient's condition, using terminology which includes specific diagnoses as well as symptoms, problems, or reasons for the encounter. There are ICD-9-CM codes to describe all of these.

D. The selection of codes 001.0 through 999.9 will frequently be used to describe the reason for the encounter. These codes are from the section of ICD-9-CM for the classification of diseases and injuries (e.g. infectious and parasitic diseases; neoplasms; symptoms, signs, and ill-defined conditions, etc.).

E. Codes that describe symptoms and signs, as opposed to diagnoses, are acceptable for reporting purposes when a diagnosis has not been established (confirmed) by the physician. Chapter 16 of ICD-9-CM, Symptoms, Signs, and Ill-defined conditions (codes 780.0 - 799.9) contain many, but not all codes for symptoms.

F. ICD-9-CM provides codes to deal with encounters for circumstances other than a disease or injury. The Supplementary Classification of factors Influencing Health Status and Contact with Health Services (V01.0- V83.89) is provided to deal with occasions when circumstances other than a disease or injury are recorded as diagnosis or problems.

G. Level of Detail in Coding

1. ICD-9-CM is composed of codes with either 3, 4, or 5 digits. Codes with three digits are included in ICD-9-CM as the heading of a category of codes that may be further subdivided by the use of fourth and/or fifth digits, which provide greater specificity.
2. A three-digit code is to be used only if it is not further subdivided. Where fourth-digit subcategories and/or fifth-digit subclassifications are provided, they must be assigned. A code is invalid if it has not been coded to the full number of digits required for that code. See also discussion under Section I, General Coding Guidelines, Level of Detail.

H. List first the ICD-9-CM code for the diagnosis, condition, problem, or other reason for encounter/visit shown in the medical record to be chiefly responsible for the services provided. List additional codes that describe any coexisting conditions.

I. Do not code diagnoses documented as "probable", "suspected," "questionable," "rule out," or "working diagnosis". Rather, code the condition(s) to the highest degree of certainty for that encounter/visit, such as symptoms, signs, abnormal test results, or other reason for the visit.

Please note: This differs from the coding practices used by hospital medical record departments for coding the diagnosis of acute care, short-term hospital inpatients.

J. Chronic diseases treated on an ongoing basis may be coded and reported as many times as the patient receives treatment and care for the condition(s).

K. Code all documented conditions that coexist at the time of the encounter/visit, and require or affect patient care treatment or management. Do not code conditions that were previously treated and no longer exist. However, history codes (V10-V19) may be used as secondary codes if the historical condition or family history has an impact on current care or influences treatment.

L. For patients receiving diagnostic services only during an encounter/visit, sequence first the diagnosis, condition, problem, or other reason for encounter/visit shown in the medical record to be chiefly responsible for the outpatient services provided during the encounter/visit. Codes for other diagnoses (e.g., chronic conditions) may be sequenced as additional diagnoses.

For outpatient encounters for diagnostic tests that have been interpreted by a physician, and the final report is available at the time of coding, code any confirmed or definitive diagnosis(es) documented in the interpretation. Do not code related signs and symptoms as additional diagnoses.

Please note: This differs from the coding practice in the hospital inpatient setting regarding abnormal findings on test results.

M. For patients receiving therapeutic services only during an encounter/visit, sequence first the diagnosis, condition, problem, or other reason for encounter/visit shown in the medical record to be chiefly responsible for the outpatient services provided during the encounter/visit. Codes for other diagnoses (e.g., chronic conditions) may be sequenced as additional diagnoses.

The only exception to this rule is that when the primary reason for the admission/encounter is chemotherapy, radiation therapy, or rehabilitation, the appropriate V code for the service is listed first, and the diagnosis or problem for which the service is being performed listed second.

N. For patients receiving preoperative evaluations only, sequence a code from category V72.8, Other specified examinations, to describe the pre-op consultations. Assign a code for the condition to describe the reason for the surgery as an additional diagnosis. Code also any findings related to the pre-op evaluation.

O. For ambulatory surgery, code the diagnosis for which the surgery was performed. If the postoperative diagnosis is known to be different from the preoperative diagnosis at the time the diagnosis is confirmed, select the postoperative diagnosis for coding, since it is the most definitive.

P. For routine outpatient prenatal visits when no complications are present codes V22.0, Supervision of normal first pregnancy, and V22.1, Supervision of other normal pregnancy, should be used as principal diagnoses. These codes should not be used in conjunction with chapter 11 codes.

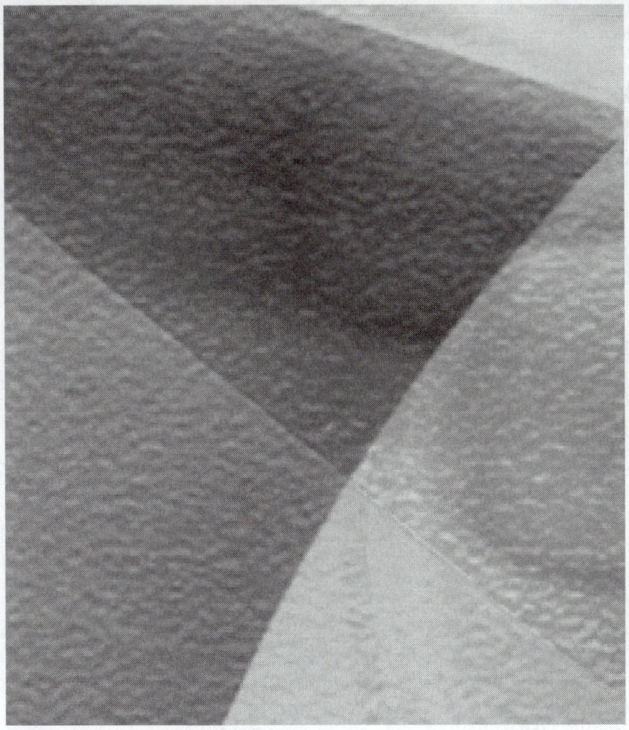

PART II

Alphabetic Index, Volume 2

SECTION I INDEX TO DISEASES

A

- **AAV** (disease) (illness) (infection) - *see* Human immunodeficiency virus (disease) (illness) (infection)
- **Abactio** - *see* Abortion, induced
- **Abactus venter** - *see* Abortion, induced
- **Abarognosis** 781.99
- **Abasia** (-astasia) 307.9
  - atactica 781.3
  - choreic 781.3
  - hysterical 300.11
  - paroxysmal trepidant 781.3
  - spastic 781.3
  - trembling 781.3
  - trepidans 781.3
- **Abderhalden-Kaufmann-Lignac syndrome** (cystinosis) 270.0
- **Abdomen, abdominal** - *see also* condition
  - accordion 306.4
  - acute 789.0
  - angina 557.1
  - burst 868.00
  - convulsive equivalent (*see also* Epilepsy) 345.5
  - heart 746.87
  - muscle deficiency syndrome 756.79
  - obstipum 756.79
- **Abdominalgia** 789.0
  - periodic 277.3
- **Abduction contracture, hip or other joint** - *see* Contraction, joint
- **Abercrombie's syndrome** (amyloid degeneration) 277.3
- **Aberrant** (congenital) - *see also* Malposition, congenital
  - adrenal gland 759.1
  - blood vessel NEC 747.60
    - arteriovenous NEC 747.60
    - cerebrovascular 747.81
    - gastrointestinal 747.61
    - lower limb 747.64
    - renal 747.62
    - spinal 747.82
    - upper limb 747.63
  - breast 757.6
  - endocrine gland NEC 759.2
  - gastrointestinal vessel (peripheral) 747.61
  - hepatic duct 751.69
  - lower limb vessel (peripheral) 747.64
  - pancreas 751.7
  - parathyroid gland 759.2
  - peripheral vascular vessel NEC 747.60
  - pituitary gland (pharyngeal) 759.2
  - renal blood vessel 747.62
  - sebaceous glands, mucous membrane, mouth 750.26
  - spinal vessel 747.82
  - spleen 759.0
  - testis (descent) 752.51
  - thymus gland 759.2
  - thyroid gland 759.2
  - upper limb vessel (peripheral) 747.63
- **Aberratio**
  - lactis 757.6
  - testis 752.51
- **Aberration** - *see also* Anomaly
  - chromosome - *see* Anomaly, chromosome(s)
  - distantial 368.9
  - mental (*see also* Disorder, mental, nonpsychotic) 300.9
- **Abetalipoproteinemia** 272.5
- **Abionarce** 780.79
- **Abiotrophy** 799.89 ⇐
- **Ablatio**
  - placentae - *see* Placenta, ablatio
  - retinae (*see also* Detachment, retina) 361.9
- **Ablation**
  - pituitary (gland) (with hypofunction) 253.7
  - placenta - *see* Placenta, ablatio
  - uterus 621.8
- **Ablepharia, ablepharon, ablephary** 743.62
- **Ablepsia** - *see* Blindness
- **Ablepsy** - *see* Blindness
- **Ablutomania** 300.3
- **Abnormal, abnormality, abnormalities** - *see also* Anomaly
  - acid-base balance 276.4
    - fetus or newborn - *see* Distress, fetal
  - adaptation curve, dark 368.63
  - alveolar ridge 525.9
  - amnion 658.9
    - affecting fetus or newborn 762.9
  - anatomical relationship NEC 759.9
  - apertures, congenital, diaphragm 756.6
  - auditory perception NEC 388.40
  - autosomes NEC 758.5
    - 13 758.1
    - 18 758.2
    - 21 or 22 758.0
    - D_1 758.1
    - E_3 758.2
    - G 758.0
  - ballistocardiogram 794.39
  - basal metabolic rate (BMR) 794.7
  - biosynthesis, testicular androgen 257.2
  - blood level (of)
    - cobalt 790.6
    - copper 790.6
    - iron 790.6
    - lithium 790.6
    - magnesium 790.6
    - mineral 790.6
    - zinc 790.6
  - blood pressure
    - elevated (without diagnosis of hypertension) 796.2
    - low (*see also* Hypotension) 458.9
      - reading (incidental) (isolated) (nonspecific) 796.3
  - bowel sounds 787.5
  - breathing behavior - *see* Respiration
  - caloric test 794.19
  - cervix (acquired) NEC 622.9
    - congenital 752.40
    - in pregnancy or childbirth 654.6
      - causing obstructed labor 660.2
        - affecting fetus or newborn 763.1
  - chemistry, blood NEC 790.6
  - chest sounds 786.7
  - chorion 658.9
    - affecting fetus or newborn 762.9
  - chromosomal NEC 758.89
    - analysis, nonspecific result 795.2
    - autosomes (*see also* Abnormal, autosomes NEC) 758.5
    - fetal (suspected), affecting management of pregnancy 655.1
    - sex 758.81
  - clinical findings NEC 796.4
  - communication - *see* Fistula
  - configuration of pupils 379.49

Abnormal, abnormality, abnormalities *(Continued)*

  - coronary
    - artery 746.85
    - vein 746.9
  - cortisol-binding globulin 255.8
  - course, Eustachian tube 744.24
  - dentofacial NEC 524.9
    - functional 524.5
    - specified type NEC 524.8
  - development, developmental NEC 759.9
    - bone 756.9
    - central nervous system 742.9
  - direction, teeth 524.3
  - dynia (*see also* Defect, coagulation) 286.9
  - Ebstein 746.2
  - echocardiogram 793.2
  - echoencephalogram 794.01
  - echogram NEC - *see* Findings, abnormal, structure
  - electrocardiogram (ECG) (EKG) 794.31
  - electroencephalogram (EEG) 794.02
  - electromyogram (EMG) 794.17
    - ocular 794.14
  - electro-oculogram (EOG) 794.12
  - electroretinogram (ERG) 794.11
  - erythrocytes 289.9
    - congenital, with perinatal jaundice 282.9 *[774.0]*
  - eustachian valve 746.9
  - excitability under minor stress 301.9
  - fat distribution 782.9
  - feces 787.7
  - fetal heart rate - *see* Distress, fetal
  - fetus NEC
    - affecting management of pregnancy - *see* Pregnancy, management affected by, fetal
    - causing disproportion 653.7
      - affecting fetus or newborn 763.1
      - causing obstructed labor 660.1
        - affecting fetus or newborn 763.1
  - findings without manifest disease - *see* Findings, abnormal
  - fluid
    - amniotic 792.3
    - cerebrospinal 792.0
    - peritoneal 792.9
    - pleural 792.9
    - synovial 792.9
    - vaginal 792.9
  - forces of labor NEC 661.9
    - affecting fetus or newborn 763.7
  - form, teeth 520.2
  - function studies
    - auditory 794.15
    - bladder 794.9
    - brain 794.00
    - cardiovascular 794.30
    - endocrine NEC 794.6
    - kidney 794.4
    - liver 794.8
    - nervous system
      - central 794.00
      - peripheral 794.19
    - oculomotor 794.14
    - pancreas 794.9
    - placenta 794.9
    - pulmonary 794.2
    - retina 794.11
    - special senses 794.19

◄ **New** ◄ **Revised Code**

Absence *(Continued)*
- ureter (congenital) 753.4
  - acquired V45.74
- urethra, congenital 753.8
  - acquired V45.74
- urinary system, part NEC, congenital 753.8
  - acquired V45.74
- uterus (acquired) V45.77
  - congenital 752.3
- uvula (congenital) 750.26
- vagina, congenital 752.49
  - acquired V45.77
- vas deferens (congenital) 752.89
  - acquired V45.77
- vein (congenital) (peripheral) NEC (*see also* Anomaly, peripheral vascular system) 747.60
  - brain 747.81
  - great 747.49
  - portal 747.49
  - pulmonary 747.49
- vena cava (congenital) (inferior) (superior) 747.49
- ventral horn cell 742.59
- ventricular septum 745.3
- vermis of cerebellum 742.2
- vertebra, congenital 756.13
- vulva, congenital 752.49

Absentia epileptica (*see also* Epilepsy) 345.0
Absinthemia (*see also* Dependence) 304.6
Absinthism (*see also* Dependence) 304.6
Absorbent system disease 459.89
Absorption
- alcohol, through placenta or breast milk 760.71
- antibiotics, through placenta or breast milk 760.74
- anti-infective, through placenta or breast milk 760.74
- chemical NEC 989.9
  - specified chemical or substance - *see* Table of Drugs and Chemicals
  - through placenta or breast milk (fetus or newborn) 760.70
    - alcohol 760.71
    - anti-infective agents 760.74
    - cocaine 760.75
    - "crack" 760.75
    - diethylstilbestrol [DES] 760.76
    - hallucinogenic agents 760.73
    - medicinal agents NEC 760.79
    - narcotics 760.72
    - obstetric anesthetic or analgesic drug 763.5
    - specified agent NEC 760.79
    - suspected, affecting management of pregnancy 655.5
- cocaine, through placenta or breast milk 760.75
- drug NEC (*see also* Reaction, drug)
  - through placenta or breast milk (fetus or newborn) 760.70
    - alcohol 760.71
    - anti-infective agents 760.74
    - cocaine 760.75
    - "crack" 760.75
    - diethylstilbestrol (DES) 760.76
    - hallucinogenic agents 760.73
    - medicinal agents NEC 760.79
    - narcotics 760.72
    - obstetric anesthetic or analgesic drug 763.5

Absorption *(Continued)*
- drug NEC *(Continued)*
  - through placenta or breast milk *(Continued)*
    - specified agent NEC 760.79
    - suspected, affecting management of pregnancy 655.5
- fat, disturbance 579.8
- hallucinogenic agents, through placenta or breast milk 760.73
- immune sera, through placenta or breast milk 760.79
- lactose defect 271.3
- medicinal agents NEC, through placenta or breast milk 760.79
- narcotics, through placenta or breast milk 760.72
- noxious substance - *see* Absorption, chemical
- protein, disturbance 579.8
- pus or septic, general - *see* Septicemia
- quinine, through placenta or breast milk 760.74
- toxic substance - *see* Absorption, chemical
- uremic - *see* Uremia

Abstinence symptoms or syndrome
- alcohol 291.81
- drug 292.0

Abt-Letterer-Siwe syndrome (acute histiocytosis X) (M9722/3) 202.5
Abulia 799.89
Abulomania 301.6
Abuse
- adult 995.80
  - emotional 995.82
  - multiple forms 995.85
  - neglect (nutritional) 995.84
  - physical 995.81
  - psychological 995.82
  - sexual 995.83
- alcohol (*see also* Alcoholism) 305.0
  - dependent 303.9
  - nondependent 305.0
- child 995.50
  - counseling
    - perpetrator
      - non-parent V62.83
      - parent V61.22
    - victim V61.21
  - emotional 995.51
  - multiple forms 995.59
  - neglect (nutritional) 995.52
  - physical 995.54
    - shaken infant syndrome 995.55
  - psychological 995.51
  - sexual 995.53
- drugs, nondependent 305.9

> Note Use the following fifth-digit subclassification with the following codes: 305.0, 305.2-305.9:
>
> 0 unspecified
> 1 continuous
> 2 episodic
> 3 in remission

  - amphetamine type 305.7
  - antidepressants 305.8
  - barbiturates 305.4
  - caffeine 305.9
  - cannabis 305.2
  - cocaine type 305.6
  - hallucinogens 305.3

Abuse *(Continued)*
- drugs, nondependent *(Continued)*
  - hashish 305.2
  - LSD 305.3
  - marijuana 305.2
  - mixed 305.9
  - morphine type 305.5
  - opioid type 305.5
  - phencyclidine (PCP) 305.9
  - specified NEC 305.9
  - tranquilizers 305.4
- spouse 995.80
- tobacco 305.1

Acalcerosis 275.40
Acalcicosis 275.40
Acalculia 784.69
- developmental 315.1

Acanthocheilonemiasis 125.4
Acanthocytosis 272.5
Acanthokeratodermia 701.1
Acantholysis 701.8
- bullosa 757.39

Acanthoma (benign) (M8070/0) - *see also* Neoplasm, by site, benign
- malignant (M8070/3) - *see* Neoplasm, by site, malignant

Acanthosis (acquired) (nigricans) 701.2
- adult 701.2
- benign (congenital) 757.39
- congenital 757.39
- glycogenic
  - esophagus 530.89
- juvenile 701.2
- tongue 529.8

Acanthrocytosis 272.5
Acapnia 276.3
Acarbia 276.2
Acardia 759.89
Acardiacus amorphus 759.89
Acardiotrophia 429.1
Acardius 759.89
Acariasis 133.9
- sarcoptic 133.0

Acaridiasis 133.9
Acarinosis 133.9
Acariosis 133.9
Acarodermatitis 133.9
- urticarioides 133.9

Acarophobia 300.29
Acatalasemia 277.89
Acatalasia 277.89
Acatamathesia 784.69
Acataphasia 784.5
Acathisia 781.0
- due to drugs 333.99

Acceleration, accelerated
- atrioventricular conduction 426.7
- idioventricular rhythm 427.89

Accessory (congenital)
- adrenal gland 759.1
- anus 751.5
- appendix 751.5
- atrioventricular conduction 426.7
- auditory ossicles 744.04
- auricle (ear) 744.1
- autosome(s) NEC 758.5
  - 21 or 22 758.0
- biliary duct or passage 751.69
- bladder 753.8
- blood vessels (peripheral) (congenital) NEC (*see also* Anomaly, peripheral vascular system) 747.60
  - cerebral 747.81
  - coronary 746.85

◄ New ⬅ Revised Code

Acidemia *(Continued)*
  fetal *(Continued)*
    during labor, in liveborn infant 768.3
    intrauterine—*see* Distress fetal 656.3
    unspecified as to time of onset, in liveborn infant 768.4
  pipecolic 270.7
Acidity, gastric (high) (low) 536.8
  psychogenic 306.4
Acidocytopenia 288.0
Acidocytosis 288.3
Acidopenia 288.0
Acidosis 276.2
  diabetic 250.1
  fetal
    affecting management of pregnancy 656.8
    affecting newborn 768.9
  kidney tubular 588.8
  lactic 276.2
  metabolic NEC 276.2
    with respiratory acidosis 276.4
    late, of newborn 775.7
  renal
    hyperchloremic 588.8
    tubular (distal) (proximal) 588.8
  respiratory 276.2
    complicated by
      metabolic acidosis 276.4
      metabolic alkalosis 276.4
Aciduria 791.9
  arginosuccinic 270.6
  beta-aminoisobutyric (BAIB) 277.2
  glycolic 271.8
  methylmalonic 270.3
    with glycinemia 270.7
  organic 270.9
  orotic (congenital) (hereditary) (pyrimidine deficiency) 281.4
Acladiosis 111.8
  skin 111.8
Aclasis
  diaphyseal 756.4
  tarsoepiphyseal 756.59
Acleistocardia 745.5
Aclusion 524.4
Acmesthesia 782.0
Acne (pustular) (vulgaris) 706.1
  agminata (*see also* Tuberculosis) 017.0
  artificialis 706.1
  atrophica 706.0
  cachecticorum (Hebra) 706.1
  conglobata 706.1
  conjunctiva 706.1
  cystic 706.1
  decalvans 704.09
  erythematosa 695.3
  eyelid 706.1
  frontalis 706.0
  indurata 706.1
  keloid 706.1
  lupoid 706.0
  necrotic, necrotica 706.0
    miliaris 704.8
  nodular 706.1
  occupational 706.1
  papulosa 706.1
  rodens 706.0
  rosacea 695.3
  scorbutica 267
  scrofulosorum (Bazin) (*see also* Tuberculosis) 017.0
  summer 692.72
  tropical 706.1
  varioliformis 706.0
Acneiform drug eruptions 692.3
Acnitis (primary) (*see also* Tuberculosis) 017.0
Acomia 704.00
Acontractile bladder 344.61
Aconuresis (*see also* Incontinence) 788.30
Acosta's disease 993.2
Acousma 780.1
Acoustic - *see* Condition
Acousticophobia 300.29
Acquired - *see* Condition
Acquired immune deficiency syndrome - *see* Human immunodeficiency virus (disease) (illness) (infection)
Acquired immunodeficiency syndrome - *see* Human immunodeficiency virus (disease) (illness) (infection)
Acragnosis 781.99
Acrania 740.0
Acroagnosis 781.99
Acroasphyxia, chronic 443.89
Acrobrachycephaly 756.0
Acrobystiolith 608.89
Acrobystitis 607.2
Acrocephalopolysyndactyly 755.55
Acrocephalosyndactyly 755.55
Acrocephaly 756.0
Acrochondrohyperplasia 759.82
Acrocyanosis 443.89
  newborn 770.83
Acrodermatitis 686.8
  atrophicans (chronica) 701.8
  continua (Hallopeau) 696.1
  enteropathica 686.8
  Hallopeau's 696.1
  perstans 696.1
  pustulosa continua 696.1
  recalcitrant pustular 696.1
Acrodynia 985.0
Acrodysplasia 755.55
Acrohyperhidrosis 780.8
Acrokeratosis verruciformis 757.39
Acromastitis 611.0
Acromegaly, acromegalia (skin) 253.0
Acromelalgia 443.89
Acromicria, acromikria 756.59
Acronyx 703.0
Acropachy, thyroid (*see also* Thyrotoxicosis) 242.9
Acropachyderma 757.39
Acroparesthesia 443.89
  simple (Schultz's type) 443.89
  vasomotor (Nothnagel's type) 443.89
Acropathy thyroid (*see also* Thyrotoxicosis) 242.9
Acrophobia 300.29
Acroposthitis 607.2
Acroscleriasis (*see also* Scleroderma) 710.1
Acroscleroderma (*see also* Scleroderma) 710.1
Acrosclerosis (*see also* Scleroderma) 710.1
Acrosphacelus 785.4
Acrosphenosyndactylia 755.55
Acrospiroma, eccrine (M8402/0) - *see* Neoplasm, skin, benign
Acrostealgia 732.9
Acrosyndactyly (*see also* Syndactylism) 755.10
Acrotrophodynia 991.4
Actinic - *see also* Condition
  cheilitis (due to sun) 692.72
    chronic NEC 692.74
    due to radiation, except from sun 692.82
Actinic *(Continued)*
  conjunctivitis 370.24
  dermatitis (due to sun) (*see also* Dermatitis, actinic) 692.70
    due to
      roentgen rays or radioactive substance 692.82
      ultraviolet radiation, except from sun 692.82
    sun NEC 692.70
  elastosis solare 692.74
  granuloma 692.73
  keratitis 370.24
  ophthalmia 370.24
  reticuloid 692.73
Actinobacillosis, general 027.8
Actinobacillus
  lignieresii 027.8
  mallei 024
  muris 026.1
Actinocutitis NEC (*see also* Dermatitis, actinic) 692.70
Actinodermatitis NEC (*see also* Dermatitis, actinic) 692.70
Actinomyces
  israelii (infection) - *see* Actinomycosis
  muris-ratti (infection) 026.1
Actinomycosis, actinomycotic 039.9
  with
    pneumonia 039.1
  abdominal 039.2
  cervicofacial 039.3
  cutaneous 039.0
  pulmonary 039.1
  specified site NEC 039.8
  thoracic 039.1
Actinoneuritis 357.89
Action, heart
  disorder 427.9
    postoperative 997.1
  irregular 427.9
    postoperative 997.1
    psychogenic 306.2
Active - *see* Condition
Activity decrease, functional 780.99
Acute - *see also* Condition
  abdomen NEC 789.0
  gallbladder (*see also* Cholecystitis, acute) 575.0
Acyanoblepsia 368.53
Acyanopsia 368.53
Acystia 753.8
Acystinervia - *see* Neurogenic, bladder
Acystineuria - *see* Neurogenic, bladder
Adactylia, adactyly (congenital) 755.4
  lower limb (complete) (intercalary) (partial) (terminal) (*see also* Deformity, reduction, lower limb) 755.39
    meaning all digits (complete) (partial) 755.31
    transverse (complete) (partial) 755.31
  upper limb (complete) (intercalary) (partial) (terminal) (*see also* Deformity, reduction, upper limb) 755.29
    meaning all digits (complete) (partial) 755.21
    transverse (complete) (partial) 755.21
Adair-Dighton syndrome (brittle bones and blue sclera, deafness) 756.51
Adamantinoblastoma (M9310/0) - *see* Ameloblastoma
Adamantinoma (M9310/0) - *see* Ameloblastoma

Note The list of adjectival modifiers below is not exhaustive. A description of adenocarcinoma that does not appear in this list should be coded in the same manner as carcinoma with that description. Thus, "mixed acidophil-basophil adenocarcinoma" should be coded in the same manner as "mixed acidophil-basophil carcinoma," which appears in the list under "Carcinoma."

Except where otherwise indicated, the morphological varieties of adenocarcinoma in the list below should be coded by site as for "Neoplasm, malignant."

- **Adenocarcinoma** *(Continued)*
  - in *(Continued)*
    - polypoid adenoma (M8210/3)
    - tubular adenoma (M8210/3)
    - villous adenoma (M8261/3)
  - infiltrating duct (M8500/3)
    - with Paget's disease (M8541/3) - *see* Neoplasm, breast, malignant
    - specified site - *see* Neoplasm, by site, malignant
    - unspecified site 174.9
  - inflammatory (M8530/3)
    - specified site - *see* Neoplasm, by site, malignant
    - unspecified site 174.9
  - in situ (M8140/2) - *see* Neoplasm, by site, in situ
  - intestinal type (M8144/3)
    - specified site - *see* Neoplasm, by site, malignant
    - unspecified site 151.9
  - intraductal (noninfiltrating) (M8500/2)
    - papillary (M8503/2)
      - specified site - *see* Neoplasm, by site, in situ
      - unspecified site 233.0
    - specified site - *see* Neoplasm, by site, in situ
    - unspecified site 233.0
  - islet cell (M8150/3)
    - and exocrine, mixed (M8154/3)
      - specified site - *see* Neoplasm, by site, malignant
      - unspecified site 157.9
    - pancreas 157.4
    - specified site NEC - *see* Neoplasm, by site, malignant
    - unspecified site 157.4
  - lobular (M8520/3)
    - specified site - *see* Neoplasm, by site, malignant
    - unspecified site 174.9
  - medullary (M8510/3)
  - mesonephric (M9110/3)
  - mixed cell (M8323/3)
  - mucinous (M8480/3)
  - mucin-producing (M8481/3)
  - mucoid (M8480/3) - *see also* Neoplasm, by site, malignant
    - cell (M8300/3)
      - specified site - *see* Neoplasm, by site, malignant
      - unspecified site 194.3
  - nonencapsulated sclerosing (M8350/3) 193
  - oncocytic (M8290/3)
  - oxyphilic (M8290/3)
  - papillary (M8260/3)
    - and follicular (M8340/3) 193
    - intraductal (noninfiltrating) (M8503/2)
      - specified site - *see* Neoplasm, by site, in situ
      - unspecified site 233.0
    - serous (M8460/3)
      - specified site - *see* Neoplasm, by site, malignant
      - unspecified site 183.0
  - papillocystic (M8450/3)
    - specified site - *see* Neoplasm, by site, malignant
    - unspecified site 183.0
  - pseudomucinous (M8470/3)
    - specified site - *see* Neoplasm, by site, malignant

- **Adenocarcinoma** *(Continued)*
  - pseudomucinous *(Continued)*
    - unspecified site 183.0
  - renal cell (M8312/3) 189.0
  - sebaceous (M8410/3)
  - serous (M8441/3) - *see also* Neoplasm, by site, malignant
    - papillary
      - specified site - *see* Neoplasm, by site, malignant
      - unspecified site 183.0
  - signet ring cell (M8490/3)
  - superficial spreading (M8143/3)
  - sweat gland (M8400/3) - *see* Neoplasm, skin, malignant
  - trabecular (M8190/3)
  - tubular (M8211/3)
  - villous (M8262/3)
  - water-clear cell (M8322/3) 194.1
- **Adenofibroma** (M9013/0)
  - clear cell (M8313/0) - *see* Neoplasm, by site, benign
  - endometrioid (M8381/0) 220
    - borderline malignancy (M8381/1) 236.2
    - malignant (M8381/3) 183.0
  - mucinous (M9015/0)
    - specified site - *see* Neoplasm, by site, benign
    - unspecified site 220
  - prostate 600.20
    - with urinary retention 600.21
  - serous (M9014/0)
    - specified site - *see* Neoplasm, by site, benign
    - unspecified site 220
  - specified site - *see* Neoplasm, by site, benign
  - unspecified site 220
- **Adenofibrosis**
  - breast 610.2
  - endometrioid 617.0
- **Adenoiditis** 474.01
  - acute 463
  - chronic 474.01
    - with chronic tonsillitis 474.02
- **Adenoids** (congenital) (of nasal fossa) 474.9
  - hypertrophy 474.12
  - vegetations 474.2
- **Adenolipomatosis** (symmetrical) 272.8
- **Adenolymphoma** (M8561/0)
  - specified site - *see* Neoplasm, by site, benign
  - unspecified 210.2
- **Adenoma** (sessile) (M8140/0) - *see also* Neoplasm, by site, benign

> Note Except where otherwise indicated, the morphological varieties of adenoma in the list below should be coded by site as for "Neoplasm, benign."

  - acidophil (M8280/0)
    - specified site - *see* Neoplasm, by site, benign
    - unspecified site 227.3
  - acinar (cell) (M8550/0)
  - acinic cell (M8550/0)
  - adrenal (cortex) (cortical) (functioning) (M8370/0) 227.0
    - clear cell type (M8373/0) 227.0
    - compact cell type (M8371/0) 227.0
    - glomerulosa cell type (M8374/0) 227.0

- **Adenoma** *(Continued)*
  - adrenal (cortex) (cortical) (functioning) *(Continued)*
    - heavily pigmented variant (M8372/0) 227.0
    - mixed cell type (M8375/0) 227.0
  - alpha cell (M8152/0)
    - pancreas 211.7
    - specified site NEC - *see* Neoplasm, by site, benign
    - unspecified site 211.7
  - alveolar (M8251/0)
  - apocrine (M8401/0)
    - breast 217
    - specified site NEC - *see* Neoplasm, skin, benign
    - unspecified site 216.9
  - basal cell (M8147/0)
  - basophil (M8300/0)
    - specified site - *see* Neoplasm, by site, benign
    - unspecified site 227.3
  - beta cell (M8151/0)
    - pancreas 211.7
    - specified site NEC - *see* Neoplasm, by site, benign
    - unspecified site 211.7
  - bile duct (M8160/0) 211.5
  - black (M8372/0) 227.0
  - bronchial (M8140/1) 235.7
    - carcinoid type (M8240/3) - *see* Neoplasm, lung, malignant
    - cylindroid type (M8200/3) - *see* Neoplasm, lung, malignant
  - ceruminous (M8420/0) 216.2
  - chief cell (M8321/0) 227.1
  - chromophobe (M8270/0)
    - specified site - *see* Neoplasm, by site, benign
    - unspecified site 227.3
  - clear cell (M8310/0)
  - colloid (M8334/0)
    - specified site - *see* Neoplasm, by site, benign
    - unspecified site 226
  - cylindroid type, bronchus (M8200/3) - *see* Neoplasm, lung, malignant
  - duct (M8503/0)
  - embryonal (M8191/0)
  - endocrine, multiple (M8360/1)
    - single specified site - *see* Neoplasm, by site, uncertain behavior
    - two or more specified sites 237.4
    - unspecified site 237.4
  - endometrioid (M8380/0) - *see also* Neoplasm, by site, benign
    - borderline malignancy (M8380/1) - *see* Neoplasm, by site, uncertain behavior
  - eosinophil (M8280/0)
    - specified site - *see* Neoplasm, by site, benign
    - unspecified site 227.3
  - fetal (M8333/0)
    - specified site - *see* Neoplasm, by site, benign
    - unspecified site 226
  - follicular (M8330/0)
    - specified site - *see* Neoplasm, by site, benign
    - unspecified site 226
  - hepatocellular (M8170/0) 211.5
  - Hürthle cell (M8290/0) 226
  - intracystic papillary (M8504/0)

◀ New ⬅ Revised Code

Adhesion(s) *(Continued)*
- intestine (postoperative) (*see also* Adhesions, peritoneum) 568.0
  - with obstruction 560.81
    - with hernia - *see also* Hernia, by site, with obstruction
      - gangrenous - *see* Hernia, by site, with gangrene
- intra-abdominal (*see also* Adhesions, peritoneum) 568.0
- iris 364.70
  - to corneal graft 996.79
- joint (*see also* Ankylosis) 718.5
- kidney 593.89
- labium (majus) (minus), congenital 752.49
- liver 572.8
- lung 511.0
- mediastinum 519.3
- meninges 349.2
  - cerebral (any) 349.2
    - congenital 742.4
  - congenital 742.8
  - spinal (any) 349.2
    - congenital 742.59
  - tuberculous (cerebral) (spinal) (*see also* Tuberculosis, meninges) 013.0
- mesenteric (*see also* Adhesions, peritoneum) 568.0
- middle ear (fibrous) 385.10
  - drum head 385.19
    - to
      - incus 385.11
      - promontorium 385.13
      - stapes 385.12
    - specified NEC 385.19
- nasal (septum) (to turbinates) 478.1
- nerve NEC 355.9
  - spinal 355.9
    - root 724.9
      - cervical NEC 723.4
      - lumbar NEC 724.4
      - lumbosacral 724.4
      - thoracic 724.4
- ocular muscle 378.60
- omentum (*see also* Adhesions, peritoneum) 568.0
- organ or site, congenital NEC - *see* Anomaly, specified type NEC
- ovary 614.6
  - congenital (to cecum, kidney, or omentum) 752.0
- parauterine 614.6
- parovarian 614.6
- pelvic (peritoneal)
  - female (postoperative) (postinfection) 614.6
  - male (postoperative) (postinfection) (*see also* Adhesions, peritoneum) 568.0
  - postpartal (old) 614.6
  - tuberculous (*see also* Tuberculosis) 016.9
- penis to scrotum (congenital) 752.69
- periappendiceal (*see also* Adhesions, peritoneum) 568.0
- pericardium (nonrheumatic) 423.1
  - rheumatic 393
  - tuberculous (*see also* Tuberculosis) 017.9 *[420.0]*
- pericholecystic 575.8
- perigastric (*see also* Adhesions, peritoneum) 568.0
- periovarian 614.6

Adhesion(s) *(Continued)*
- periprostatic 602.8
- perirectal (*see also* Adhesions, peritoneum) 568.0
- perirenal 593.89
- peritoneum, peritoneal (fibrous) (postoperative) 568.0
  - with obstruction (intestinal) 560.81
    - with hernia - *see also* Hernia, by site, with obstruction
      - gangrenous - *see* Hernia, by site, with gangrene
  - duodenum 537.3
  - congenital 751.4
  - female (postoperative) (postinfective) 614.6
  - pelvic, female 614.6
  - pelvic, male 568.0
  - postpartal, pelvic 614.6
  - to uterus 614.6
- peritubal 614.6
- periureteral 593.89
- periuterine 621.5
- perivesical 596.8
- perivesicular (seminal vesicle) 608.89
- pleura, pleuritic 511.0
  - tuberculous (*see also* Tuberculosis, pleura) 012.0
- pleuropericardial 511.0
- postoperative (gastrointestinal tract) (*see also* Adhesions, peritoneum)
  - eyelid 997.99
    - surgically created V45.69
  - pelvic female 614.9
  - pelvic, male 568.0
  - urethra 598.2
- postpartal, old 624.4
- preputial, prepuce 605
- pulmonary 511.0
- pylorus (*see also* Adhesions, peritoneum) 568.0
- Rosenmüller's fossa 478.29
- sciatic nerve 355.0
- seminal vesicle 608.89
- shoulder (joint) 726.0
- sigmoid flexure (*see also* Adhesions, peritoneum) 568.0
- spermatic cord (acquired) 608.89
  - congenital 752.89
- spinal canal 349.2
  - nerve 355.9
    - root 724.9
      - cervical NEC 723.4
      - lumbar NEC 724.4
      - lumbosacral 724.4
      - thoracic 724.4
- stomach (*see also* Adhesions, peritoneum) 568.0
- subscapular 726.2
- tendonitis 726.90
  - shoulder 726.0
- testicle 608.89
- tongue (congenital) (to gum or roof of mouth) 750.12
  - acquired 529.8
- trachea 519.1
- tubo-ovarian 614.6
- tunica vaginalis 608.89
- ureter 593.89
- uterus 621.5
  - to abdominal wall 614.6
    - in pregnancy or childbirth 654.4
      - affecting fetus or newborn 763.89

Adhesion(s) *(Continued)*
- vagina (chronic) (postoperative) (postradiation) 623.2
- vaginitis (congenital) 752.49
- vesical 596.8
- vitreous 379.29

Adie (-Holmes) syndrome (tonic pupillary reaction) 379.46
Adiponecrosis neonatorum 778.1
Adiposa dolorosa 272.8
Adiposalgia 272.8
Adiposis
- cerebralis 253.8
- dolorosa 272.8
- tuberosa simplex 272.8

Adiposity 278.00
- heart (*see also* Degeneration, myocardial) 429.1
- localized 278.1

Adiposogenital dystrophy 253.8
Adjustment
- prosthesis or other device - *see* Fitting of
- reaction - *see* Reaction, adjustment

Administration, prophylactic
- antibiotics V07.39
- antitoxin, any V07.2
- antivenin V07.2
- chemotherapeutic agent NEC V07.39
- chemotherapy NEC V07.39
- diphtheria antitoxin V07.2
- fluoride V07.31
- gamma globulin V07.2
- immune sera (gamma globulin) V07.2
- passive immunization agent V07.2
- RhoGAM V07.2

Admission (encounter)
- as organ donor - *see* Donor
- by mistake V68.9
- for
  - adequacy testing (for)
    - hemodialysis V56.31
    - peritoneal dialysis V56.32
  - adjustment (of)
    - artificial
      - arm (complete) (partial) V52.0
      - eye V52.2
      - leg (complete) (partial) V52.1
    - brain neuropacemaker V53.02
    - breast
      - implant V52.4
      - prosthesis V52.4
    - cardiac device V53.39
      - defibrillator, automatic implantable V53.32
      - pacemaker V53.31
        - carotid sinus V53.39
    - catheter
      - non-vascular V58.82
      - vascular V58.81
    - cerebral ventricle (communicating) shunt V53.01
    - colostomy belt V55.3
    - contact lenses V53.1
    - cystostomy device V53.6
    - dental prosthesis V52.3
    - device, unspecified type V53.90
      - abdominal V53.5
      - cardiac V53.39
        - defibrillator, automatic implantable V53.32
        - pacemaker V53.31
      - carotid sinus V53.39
      - cerebral ventricle (communicating) shunt V53.01

- **Admission** *(Continued)*
  - for *(Continued)*
    - adjustment (of) *(Continued)*
      - device NEC *(Continued)*
        - insulin pump V53.91 ◀
        - intrauterine contraceptive V25.1
        - nervous system V53.09
        - orthodontic V53.4
        - other device V53.99 ◀
        - prosthetic V52.9
          - breast V52.4
          - dental V52.3
          - eye V52.2
          - specified type NEC V52.8
        - special senses V53.09
        - substitution
          - auditory V53.09
          - nervous system V53.09
          - visual V53.09
        - urinary V53.6
      - dialysis catheter
        - extracorporeal V56.1
        - peritoneal V56.2
      - diaphragm (contraceptive) V25.02
      - growth rod V54.02 ◀
      - hearing aid V53.2
      - ileostomy device V55.2
      - intestinal appliance or device NEC V53.5
      - intrauterine contraceptive device V25.1
      - neuropacemaker (brain) (peripheral nerve) (spinal cord) V53.02
      - orthodontic device V53.4
      - orthopedic (device) V53.7
        - brace V53.7
        - cast V53.7
        - shoes V53.7
      - pacemaker
        - brain V53.02
        - cardiac V53.31
        - carotid sinus V53.39
        - peripheral nerve V53.02
        - spinal cord V53.02
      - prosthesis V52.9
        - arm (complete) (partial) V52.0
        - breast V52.4
        - dental V52.3
        - eye V52.2
        - leg (complete) (partial) V52.1
        - specified type NEC V52.8
      - spectacles V53.1
      - wheelchair V53.8
    - adoption referral or proceedings V68.89
    - aftercare (*see also* Aftercare) V58.9
      - cardiac pacemaker V53.31
      - chemotherapy V58.1
      - dialysis
        - extracorporeal (renal) V56.0
        - peritoneal V56.8
        - renal V56.0
      - fracture (*see also* Aftercare, fracture) V54.9
      - medical NEC V58.89
      - orthopedic V54.9
        - specified type NEC V54.89
      - pacemaker device
        - brain V53.02
        - cardiac V53.31
        - carotid sinus V53.39
        - nervous system V53.02
        - spinal cord V53.02
      - postoperative NEC V58.49
        - wound closure, planned V58.41
      - postpartum

- **Admission** *(Continued)*
  - for *(Continued)*
    - aftercare (*see also* Aftercare) *(Continued)*
      - postpartum *(Continued)*
        - immediately after delivery V24.0
        - routine follow-up V24.2
      - postradiation V58.0
      - radiation therapy V58.0
      - removal of
        - non-vascular catheter V58.82
        - vascular catheter V58.81
      - specified NEC V58.89
      - surgical NEC V58.49
        - wound closure, planned V58.41
    - artificial insemination V26.1
    - attention to artificial opening (of) V55.9
      - artificial vagina V55.7
      - colostomy V55.3
      - cystostomy V55.5
      - enterostomy V55.4
      - gastrostomy V55.1
      - ileostomy V55.2
      - jejunostomy V55.4
      - nephrostomy V55.6
      - specified site NEC V55.8
        - intestinal tract V55.4
        - urinary tract V55.6
      - tracheostomy V55.0
      - ureterostomy V55.6
      - urethrostomy V55.6
    - battery replacement
      - cardiac pacemaker V53.31
    - boarding V65.0
    - breast
      - augmentation or reduction V50.1
      - removal, prophylactic V50.41
    - change of
      - cardiac pacemaker (battery) V53.31
      - carotid sinus pacemaker V53.39
      - catheter in artificial opening - *see* Attention to, artificial, opening
      - dressing V58.3
      - fixation device
        - external V54.89
        - internal V54.01 ⬅
      - Kirschner wire V54.89
      - neuropacemaker device (brain) (peripheral nerve) (spinal cord) V53.02
      - pacemaker device
        - brain V53.02
        - cardiac V53.31
        - carotid sinus V53.39
        - nervous system V53.02
      - plaster cast V54.89
      - splint, external V54.89
      - Steinmann pin V54.89
      - surgical dressing V58.3
      - traction device V54.89
    - checkup only V70.0
    - chemotherapy V58.1
    - circumcision, ritual or routine (in absence of medical indication) V50.2
    - clinical research investigation (control) (normal comparison) (participant) V70.7
    - closure of artificial opening - *see* Attention to, artificial, opening
    - contraceptive
      - counseling V25.09
        - emergency V25.03 ◀
        - postcoital V25.03 ◀
      - management V25.9
        - specified type NEC V25.8

- **Admission** *(Continued)*
  - for *(Continued)*
    - convalescence following V66.9
      - chemotherapy V66.2
      - psychotherapy V66.3
      - radiotherapy V66.1
      - surgery V66.0
      - treatment (for) V66.5
        - combined V66.6
        - fracture V66.4
        - mental disorder NEC V66.3
        - specified condition NEC V66.5
    - cosmetic surgery NEC V50.1
      - following healed injury or operation V51
    - counseling (*see also* Counseling) V65.40
      - without complaint or sickness V65.49
      - contraceptive management V25.09
        - emergency V25.03 ◀
        - postcoital V25.03 ◀
      - dietary V65.3
      - exercise V65.41
      - for nonattending third party V65.19 ⬅
      - for pediatric pre-birth visit for expectant mother V65.11 ◀
      - genetic V26.3
      - gonorrhea V65.45
      - HIV V65.44
      - human immunodeficiency virus V65.44
      - injury prevention V65.43
      - insulin pump training V65.46 ◀
      - procreative management V26.4
      - sexually transmitted disease NEC V65.45
        - HIV V65.44
      - specified reason NEC V65.49
      - substance use and abuse V65.42
      - syphilis V65.45
      - victim of abuse
        - child V61.21
        - partner or spouse V61.11
    - desensitization to allergens V07.1
    - dialysis V56.0
      - catheter
        - fitting and adjustment
          - extracorporeal V56.1
          - peritoneal V56.2
        - removal or replacement
          - extracorporeal V56.1
          - peritoneal V56.2
      - extracorporeal (renal) V56.0
      - peritoneal V56.8
      - renal V56.0
    - dietary surveillance and counseling V65.3
    - drug monitoring, therapeutic V58.83
    - ear piercing V50.3
    - elective surgery
      - breast
        - augmentation or reduction V50.1
        - removal, prophylactic V50.41
      - circumcision, ritual or routine (in absence of medical indication) V50.2
      - cosmetic NEC V50.1
        - following healed injury or operation V51
      - ear piercing V50.3
      - face-lift V50.1
      - hair transplant V50.0
      - plastic
        - cosmetic NEC V50.1

- **Aftercare** *(Continued)*
  - neuropacemaker (brain) (peripheral nerve) (spinal cord) V53.02
  - occupational therapy V57.21
  - orthodontic V58.5
  - orthopedic V54.9
    - change of external fixation or traction device V54.89
    - following joint replacement V54.81
    - internal fixation device V54.09
    - removal of fixation device
      - external V54.89
      - internal V54.01
    - specified care NEC V54.89
  - orthoptic training V57.4
  - orthotic training V57.81
  - pacemaker
    - brain V53.02
    - cardiac V53.31
    - carotid sinus V53.39
    - peripheral nerve V53.02
    - spinal cord V53.02
  - peritoneal dialysis (intermittent) (treatment) V56.8
  - physical therapy NEC V57.1
    - breathing exercises V57.0
  - radiotherapy session V58.0
  - rehabilitation procedure V57.9
    - breathing exercises V57.0
    - multiple types V57.89
    - occupational V57.21
    - orthoptic V57.4
    - orthotic V57.81
    - physical therapy NEC V57.1
    - remedial exercises V57.1
    - specified type NEC V57.89
    - speech V57.3
    - therapeutic exercises V57.1
    - vocational V57.22
  - renal dialysis (intermittent) (treatment) V56.0
  - specified type NEC V58.89
    - removal of non-vascular cathether V58.82
    - removal of vascular catheter V58.81
  - speech therapy V57.3
  - vocational rehabilitation V57.22
- **After-cataract** 366.50
  - obscuring vision 366.53
  - specified type, not obscuring vision 366.52
- **Agalactia** 676.4
- **Agammaglobulinemia** 279.00
  - with lymphopenia 279.2
  - acquired (primary) (secondary) 279.06
  - Bruton's X-linked 279.04
  - infantile sex-linked (Bruton's) (congenital) 279.04
  - Swiss-type 279.2
- **Aganglionosis** (bowel) (colon) 751.3
- **AGCUS** (atypical glandular cell changes of undetermined significance
  - favor benign 795.01
  - favor dysplasia 795.02
- **Age** (old) (*see also* Senile) 797
- **Agenesis** - *see also* Absence, by site, congenital
  - acoustic nerve 742.8
  - adrenal (gland) 759.1
  - alimentary tract (complete) (partial) NEC 751.8
    - lower 751.2
    - upper 750.8
  - anus, anal (canal) 751.2

- **Agenesis** *(Continued)*
  - aorta 747.22
  - appendix 751.2
  - arm (complete) (partial) (*see also* Deformity, reduction, upper limb) 755.20
  - artery (peripheral) NEC (*see also* Anomaly, peripheral vascular system) 747.60
    - brain 747.81
    - coronary 746.85
    - pulmonary 747.3
    - umbilical 747.5
  - auditory (canal) (external) 744.01
  - auricle (ear) 744.01
  - bile, biliary duct or passage 751.61
  - bone NEC 756.9
  - brain 740.0
    - specified part 742.2
  - breast 757.6
  - bronchus 748.3
  - canaliculus lacrimalis 743.65
  - carpus NEC (*see also* Deformity, reduction, upper limb) 755.28
  - cartilage 756.9
  - cecum 751.2
  - cerebellum 742.2
  - cervix 752.49
  - chin 744.89
  - cilia 743.63
  - circulatory system, part NEC 747.89
  - clavicle 755.51
  - clitoris 752.49
  - coccyx 756.13
  - colon 751.2
  - corpus callosum 742.2
  - cricoid cartilage 748.3
  - diaphragm (with hernia) 756.6
  - digestive organ(s) or tract (complete) (partial) NEC 751.8
    - lower 751.2
    - upper 750.8
  - ductus arteriosus 747.89
  - duodenum 751.1
  - ear NEC 744.09
    - auricle 744.01
    - lobe 744.21
  - ejaculatory duct 752.89
  - endocrine (gland) NEC 759.2
  - epiglottis 748.3
  - esophagus 750.3
  - Eustachian tube 744.24
  - extrinsic muscle, eye 743.69
  - eye 743.00
    - adnexa 743.69
  - eyelid (fold) 743.62
  - face
    - bones NEC 756.0
    - specified part NEC 744.89
  - fallopian tube 752.19
  - femur NEC (*see also* Absence, femur, congenital) 755.34
  - fibula NEC (*see also* Absence, fibula, congenital) 755.37
  - finger NEC (*see also* Absence, finger, congenital) 755.29
  - foot (complete) (*see also* Deformity, reduction, lower limb) 755.31
  - gallbladder 751.69
  - gastric 750.8
  - genitalia, genital (organ)
    - female 752.89
      - external 752.49
      - internal NEC 752.89
    - male 752.89
      - penis 752.69

- **Agenesis** *(Continued)*
  - glottis 748.3
  - gonadal 758.6
  - hair 757.4
  - hand (complete) (*see also* Deformity, reduction, upper limb) 755.21
  - heart 746.89
    - valve NEC 746.89
      - aortic 746.89
      - mitral 746.89
      - pulmonary 746.01
  - hepatic 751.69
  - humerus NEC (*see also* Absence, humerus, congenital) 755.24
  - hymen 752.49
  - ileum 751.1
  - incus 744.04
  - intestine (small) 751.1
    - large 751.2
  - iris (dilator fibers) 743.45
  - jaw 524.09
  - jejunum 751.1
  - kidney(s) (partial) (unilateral) 753.0
  - labium (majus) (minus) 752.49
  - labyrinth, membranous 744.05
  - lacrimal apparatus (congenital) 743.65
  - larynx 748.3
  - leg NEC (*see also* Deformity, reduction, lower limb) 755.30
  - lens 743.35
  - limb (complete) (partial) (*see also* Deformity, reduction) 755.4
    - lower NEC 755.30
    - upper 755.20
  - lip 750.26
  - liver 751.69
  - lung (bilateral) (fissures) (lobe) (unilateral) 748.5
  - mandible 524.09
  - maxilla 524.09
  - metacarpus NEC 755.28
  - metatarsus NEC 755.38
  - muscle (any) 756.81
  - musculoskeletal system NEC 756.9
  - nail(s) 757.5
  - neck, part 744.89
  - nerve 742.8
  - nervous system, part NEC 742.8
  - nipple 757.6
  - nose 748.1
  - nuclear 742.8
  - organ
    - of Corti 744.05
    - or site not listed - *see* Anomaly, specified type NEC
  - osseous meatus (ear) 744.03
  - ovary 752.0
  - oviduct 752.19
  - pancreas 751.7
  - parathyroid (gland) 759.2
  - patella 755.64
  - pelvic girdle (complete) (partial) 755.69
  - penis 752.69
  - pericardium 746.89
  - perineal body 756.81
  - pituitary (gland) 759.2
  - prostate 752.89
  - pulmonary
    - artery 747.3
    - trunk 747.3
    - vein 747.49
  - punctum lacrimale 743.65
  - radioulnar NEC (*see also* Absence, forearm, congenital) 755.25

▶ **New** ⬅ **Revised Code**

Agenesis *(Continued)*
radius NEC (*see also* Absence, radius, congenital) 755.26
rectum 751.2
renal 753.0
respiratory organ NEC 748.9
rib 756.3
roof of orbit 742.0
round ligament 752.89
sacrum 756.13
salivary gland 750.21
scapula 755.59
scrotum 752.89
seminal duct or tract 752.89
septum
atrial 745.69
between aorta and pulmonary artery 745.0
ventricular 745.3
shoulder girdle (complete) (partial) 755.59
skull (bone) 756.0
with
anencephalus 740.0
encephalocele 742.0
hydrocephalus 742.3
with spina bifida (*see also* Spina bifida) 741.0
microcephalus 742.1
spermatic cord 752.89
spinal cord 742.59
spine 756.13
lumbar 756.13
isthmus 756.11
pars articularis 756.11
spleen 759.0
sternum 756.3
stomach 750.7
tarsus NEC 755.38
tendon 756.81
testicular 752.89
testis 752.89
thymus (gland) 759.2
thyroid (gland) 243
cartilage 748.3
tibia NEC (*see also* Absence, tibia, congenital) 755.36
tibiofibular NEC 755.35
toe (complete) (partial) (*see also* Absence, toe, congenital) 755.39
tongue 750.11
trachea (cartilage) 748.3
ulna NEC (*see also* Absence, ulna, congenital) 755.27
ureter 753.4
urethra 753.8
urinary tract NEC 753.8
uterus 752.3
uvula 750.26
vagina 752.49
vas deferens 752.89
vein(s) (peripheral) NEC (*see also* Anomaly, peripheral vascular system) 747.60
brain 747.81
great 747.49
portal 747.49
pulmonary 747.49
vena cava (inferior) (superior) 747.49
vermis of cerebellum 742.2
vertebra 756.13
lumbar 756.13
isthmus 756.11
pars articularis 756.11
vulva 752.49

Ageusia (*see also* Disturbance, sensation) 781.1
Aggressiveness 301.3
Aggressive outburst (*see also* Disturbance, conduct) 312.0
in children and adolescents 313.9
Aging skin 701.8
Agitated - *see* condition
Agitation 307.9
catatonic (*see also* Schizophrenia) 295.2
Aglossia (congenital) 750.11
Aglycogenosis 271.0
Agnail (finger) (with lymphangitis) 681.02
Agnosia (body image) (tactile) 784.69
verbal 784.69
auditory 784.69
secondary to organic lesion 784.69
developmental 315.8
secondary to organic lesion 784.69
visual 784.69
developmental 315.8
secondary to organic lesion 784.69
visual 368.16
developmental 315.31
Agoraphobia 300.22
with panic attacks 300.21
Agrammatism 784.69
Agranulocytopenia 288.0
Agranulocytosis (angina) (chronic) (cyclical) (genetic) (infantile) (periodic) (pernicious) 288.0
Agraphia (absolute) 784.69
with alexia 784.61
developmental 315.39
Agrypnia (*see also* Insomnia) 780.52
Ague (*see also* Malaria) 084.6
brass-founders' 985.8
dumb 084.6
tertian 084.1
Agyria 742.2
Ahumada-del Castillo syndrome (nonpuerperal galactorrhea and amenorrhea) 253.1
AIDS 042
AIDS-associated retrovirus (disease) (illness) 042
infection - *see* Human immunodeficiency virus, infection
AIDS-associated virus (disease) (illness) 042
infection - *see* Human immunodeficiency virus, infection
AIDS-like disease (illness) (syndrome) 042
AIDS-related complex 042
AIDS-related conditions 042
AIDS-related virus (disease) (illness) 042
infection - *see* Human immunodeficiency virus, infection
AIDS virus (disease) (illness) 042
infection - *see* Human immunodeficiency virus, infection
Ailment, heart - *see* Disease, heart
Ailurophobia 300.29
Ainhum (disease) 136.0
Air
anterior mediastinum 518.1
compressed, disease 993.3
embolism (any site) (artery) (cerebral) 958.0
with
abortion - *see* Abortion, by type, with embolism

Air *(Continued)*
embolism *(Continued)*
with *(Continued)*
ectopic pregnancy (*see also* categories 633.0-633.9) 639.6
molar pregnancy (*see also* categories 630-632) 639.6
due to implanted device - *see* Complications, due to (presence of) any device, implant, or graft classified to 996.0-996.5 NEC
following
abortion 639.6
ectopic or molar pregnancy 639.6
infusion, perfusion, or transfusion 999.1
in pregnancy, childbirth, or puerperium 673.0
traumatic 958.0
hunger 786.09
psychogenic 306.1
leak (lung) (pulmonary) (thorax) 512.8
iatrogenic 512.1
postoperative 512.1
rarefied, effects of - *see* Effect, adverse, high altitude
sickness 994.6
Airplane sickness 994.6
Akathisia, acathisia 781.0
due to drugs 333.99
Akinesia algeria 352.6
Akiyami 100.89
Akureyri disease (epidemic neuromyasthenia) 049.8
Alacrima (congenital) 743.65
Alactasia (hereditary) 271.3
Alalia 784.3
developmental 315.31
receptive-expressive 315.32
secondary to organic lesion 784.3
Alaninemia 270.8
Alastrim 050.1
Albarrán's disease (colibacilluria) 791.9
Albers-Schönberg's disease (marble bones) 756.52
Albert's disease 726.71
Albinism, albino (choroid) (cutaneous) (eye) (generalized) (isolated) (ocular) (oculocutaneous) (partial) 270.2
Albinismus 270.2
Albright (-Martin) (-Bantam) disease (pseudohypoparathyroidism) 275.49
Albright (-McCune) (-Sternberg) syndrome (osteitis fibrosa disseminata) 756.59
Albuminous - *see* condition
Albuminuria, albuminuric (acute) (chronic) (subacute) 791.0
Bence-Jones 791.0
cardiac 785.9
complicating pregnancy, childbirth, or puerperium 646.2
with hypertension - *see* Toxemia, of pregnancy
affecting fetus or newborn 760.1
cyclic 593.6
gestational 646.2
gravidarum 646.2
with hypertension - *see* Toxemia, of pregnancy
affecting fetus or newborn 760.1

Albuminuria, albuminuric *(Continued)*
- heart 785.9
- idiopathic 593.6
- orthostatic 593.6
- postural 593.6
- pre-eclamptic (mild) 642.4
  - affecting fetus or newborn 760.0
  - severe 642.5
    - affecting fetus or newborn 760.0
- recurrent physiologic 593.6
- scarlatinal 034.1

Albumosuria 791.0
- Bence-Jones 791.0
- myelopathic (M9730/3) 203.0

Alcaptonuria 270.2

Alcohol, alcoholic
- abstinence 291.81
- acute intoxication 305.0
  - with dependence 303.0
- addiction (*see also* Alcoholism) 303.9
  - maternal
    - with suspected fetal damage affecting management of pregnancy 655.4
    - affecting fetus or newborn 760.71
- amnestic disorder, persisting 291.1
- anxiety 291.89
- brain syndrome, chronic 291.2
- cardiopathy 425.5
- chronic (*see also* Alcoholism) 303.9
- cirrhosis (liver) 571.2
- delirium 291.0
  - acute 291.0
  - chronic 291.1
  - tremens 291.0
  - withdrawal 291.0
- dementia NEC 291.2
- deterioration 291.2
- drunkenness (simple) 305.0
- hallucinosis (acute) 291.3
- insanity 291.9
- intoxication (acute) 305.0
  - with dependence 303.0
  - pathological 291.4
- jealousy 291.5
- Korsakoff's, Korsakov's, Korsakow's 291.1
- liver NEC 571.3
  - acute 571.1
  - chronic 571.2
- mania (acute) (chronic) 291.9
- mood 291.89
- paranoia 291.5
- paranoid (type) psychosis 291.5
- pellagra 265.2
- poisoning, accidental (acute) NEC 980.9
  - specified type of alcohol - *see* Table of Drugs and Chemicals
- psychosis (*see also* Psychosis, alcoholic) 291.9
  - Korsakoff's, Korsakov's, Korsakow's 291.1
  - polyneuritic 291.1
    - with
      - delusions 291.5
      - hallucinations 291.3
- withdrawal symptoms, syndrome NEC 291.81
  - delirium 291.0
  - hallucinosis 291.3

Alcoholism 303.9

> Note Use the following fifth-digit subclassification with category 303:
> 0 unspecified
> 1 continuous
> 2 episodic
> 3 in remission

- with psychosis (*see also* Psychosis, alcoholic) 291.9
- acute 303.0
- chronic 303.9
  - with psychosis 291.9
- complicating pregnancy, childbirth, or puerperium 648.4
  - affecting fetus or newborn 760.71
- history V11.3
- Korsakoff's, Korsakov's, Korsakow's 291.1
- suspected damage to fetus affecting management of pregnancy 655.4

Alder's anomaly or syndrome (leukocyte granulation anomaly) 288.2

Alder-Reilly anomaly (leukocyte granulation) 288.2

Aldosteronism (primary) 255.11 ⬅
- congenital 255.10 ⬅
- familial type I 255.11 ◀
- glucocorticoid-remediable 255.11 ◀
- secondary 255.14 ◀

Aldosteronoma (M8370/1) 237.2

Aldrich (-Wiskott) syndrome (eczema-thrombocytopenia) 279.12

Aleppo boil 085.1

Aleukemic - *see* condition

Aleukia
- congenital 288.0
- hemorrhagica 284.9
  - acquired (secondary) 284.8
  - congenital 284.0
  - idiopathic 284.9
- splenica 289.4

Alexia (congenital) (developmental) 315.01
- secondary to organic lesion 784.61

Algoneurodystrophy 733.7

Algophobia 300.29

Alibert's disease (mycosis fungoides) (M9700/3) 202.1

Alibert-Bazin disease (M9700/3) 202.1

Alice in Wonderland syndrome 293.89

Alienation, mental (*see also* Psychosis) 298.9

Alkalemia 276.3

Alkalosis 276.3
- metabolic 276.3
  - with respiratory acidosis 276.4
- respiratory 276.3

Alkaptonuria 270.2

Allen-Masters syndrome 620.6

Allergic bronchopulmonary aspergillosis 518.6

Allergy, allergic (reaction) 995.3
- air-borne substance (*see also* Fever, hay) 477.9
  - specified allergen NEC 477.8
- alveolitis (extrinsic) 495.9
  - due to
    - Aspergillus clavatus 495.4
    - cryptostroma corticale 495.6
    - organisms (fungal, thermophilic actinomycete, other) growing in ventilation (air conditioning systems) 495.7
  - specified type NEC 495.8

Allergy, allergic *(Continued)*
- anaphylactic shock 999.4
  - due to food - *see* Anaphylactic shock, due to, food
- angioneurotic edema 995.1
- animal (dander) (epidermal) (hair) 477.8
- arthritis (*see also* Arthritis, allergic) 716.2
- asthma - *see* Asthma
- bee sting (anaphylactic shock) 989.5
- biological - *see* Allergy, drug
- bronchial asthma - *see* Asthma
- conjunctivitis (eczematous) 372.14
- dander (animal) 477.8
- dandruff 477.8
- dermatitis (venenata) - *see* Dermatitis
- diathesis V15.09
- drug, medicinal substance, and biological (any) (correct medicinal substance properly administered) (external) (internal) 995.2
  - wrong substance given or taken NEC 977.9
    - specified drug or substance - *see* Table of Drugs and Chemicals
- dust (house) (stock) 477.8
- eczema - *see* Eczema
- endophthalmitis 360.19
- epidermal (animal) 477.8
- feathers 477.8
- food (any) (ingested) 693.1
  - atopic 691.8
  - in contact with skin 692.5
- gastritis 535.4
- gastroenteritis 558.3
- gastrointestinal 558.3
- grain 477.0
- grass (pollen) 477.0
  - asthma (*see also* Asthma) 493.0
  - hay fever 477.0
- hair (animal) 477.8
- hay fever (grass) (pollen) (ragweed) (tree) (*see also* Fever, hay) 477.9
- history (of) V15.09
  - to
    - eggs V15.03
    - food additives V15.05
    - insect bite V15.06
    - latex V15.07
    - milk products V15.02
    - nuts V15.05
      - peanuts V15.01
    - radiographic dye V15.08
    - seafood V15.04
    - specified food NEC V15.05
    - spider bite V15.06
- horse serum - *see* Allergy, serum
- inhalant 477.9
  - dust 477.8
  - pollen 477.0
  - specified allergen other than pollen 477.8
- kapok 477.8
- medicine - *see* Allergy, drug
- migraine 346.2
- milk protein 558.3 ◀
- pannus 370.62
- pneumonia 518.3
- pollen (any) (hay fever) 477.0
  - asthma (*see also* Asthma) 493.0
- primrose 477.0
- primula 477.0
- purpura 287.0

◀ **New** ⬅ **Revised Code**

Allergy, allergic *(Continued)*
- ragweed (pollen) (Senecio jacobae) 477.0
  - asthma (*see also* Asthma) 493.0
  - hay fever 477.0
- respiratory (*see also* Allergy, inhalant) 477.9
  - due to
    - drug - *see* Allergy, drug
    - food - *see* Allergy, food
- rhinitis (*see also* Fever, hay) 477.9
  - due to food 477.1
- rose 477.0
- Senecio jacobae 477.0
- serum (prophylactic) (therapeutic) 999.5
  - anaphylactic shock 999.4
- shock (anaphylactic) (due to adverse effect of correct medicinal substance properly administered) 995.0
  - food - *see* Anaphylactic shock, due to, food
  - from serum or immunization 999.5
    - anaphylactic 999.4
- sinusitis (*see also* Fever, hay) 477.9
- skin reaction 692.9
  - specified substance - *see* Dermatitis, due to
- tree (any) (hay fever) (pollen) 477.0
  - asthma (*see also* Asthma) 493.0
- upper respiratory (*see also* Fever, hay) 477.9
- urethritis 597.89
- urticaria 708.0
- vaccine - *see* Allergy, serum

Allescheriosis 117.6

Alligator skin disease (ichthyosis congenita) 757.1
- acquired 701.1

Allocheiria, allochiria (*see also* Disturbance, sensation) 782.0

Almeida's disease (Brazilian blastomycosis) 116.1

Alopecia (atrophicans) (pregnancy) (premature) (senile) 704.00
- adnata 757.4
- areata 704.01
- celsi 704.01
- cicatrisata 704.09
- circumscripta 704.01
- congenital, congenitalis 757.4
- disseminata 704.01
- effluvium (telogen) 704.02
- febrile 704.09
- generalisata 704.09
- hereditaria 704.09
- marginalis 704.01
- mucinosa 704.09
- postinfectional 704.09
- seborrheica 704.09
- specific 091.82
- syphilitic (secondary) 091.82
- telogen effluvium 704.02
- totalis 704.09
- toxica 704.09
- universalis 704.09
- x-ray 704.09

Alpers' disease 330.8

Alpha-lipoproteinemia 272.4

Alpha thalassemia 282.49

Alphos 696.1

Alpine sickness 993.2

Alport's syndrome (hereditary hematuria-nephropathy-deafness) 759.89

Alteration (of), altered
- awareness 780.09
  - transient 780.02
- consciousness 780.09
  - persistent vegetative state 780.03
  - transient 780.02
- mental status 780.99
  - amnesia (retrograde) 780.93
  - memory loss 780.93

Alternaria (infection) 118

Alternating - *see* condition

Altitude, high (effects) - *see* Effect, adverse, high altitude

Aluminosis (of lung) 503

Alvarez syndrome (transient cerebral ischemia) 435.9

Alveolar capillary block syndrome 516.3

Alveolitis
- allergic (extrinsic) 495.9
  - due to organisms (fungal, thermophilic actinomycete, other) growing in ventilation (air conditioning systems) 495.7
  - specified type NEC 495.8
- due to
  - Aspergillus clavatus 495.4
  - Cryptostroma corticale 495.6
- fibrosing (chronic) (cryptogenic) (lung) 516.3
  - idiopathic 516.3
  - rheumatoid 714.81
- jaw 526.5
- sicca dolorosa 526.5

Alveolus, alveolar - *see* condition

Alymphocytosis (pure) 279.2

Alymphoplasia, thymic 279.2

Alzheimer's
- dementia (senile)
  - with behavioral disturbance 331.0 *[294.11]*
  - without behavioral disturbance 331.0 *[294.10]*
- disease or sclerosis 331.0
  - with dementia - *see* Alzheimer's, dementia

Amastia (*see also* Absence, breast) 611.8

Amaurosis (acquired) (congenital) (*see also* Blindness) 369.00
- fugax 362.34
- hysterical 300.11
- Leber's (congenital) 362.76
- tobacco 377.34
- uremic - *see* Uremia

Amaurotic familial idiocy (infantile) (juvenile) (late) 330.1

Ambisexual 752.7

Amblyopia (acquired) (congenital) (partial) 368.00
- color 368.59
  - acquired 368.55
- deprivation 368.02
- ex anopsia 368.00
- hysterical 300.11
- nocturnal 368.60
  - vitamin A deficiency 264.5
- refractive 368.03
- strabismic 368.01
- suppression 368.01
- tobacco 377.34
- toxic NEC 377.34
- uremic - *see* Uremia

Ameba, amebic (histolytica) - *see also* Amebiasis
- abscess 006.3
  - bladder 006.8

Ameba, amebic *(Continued)*
- abscess *(Continued)*
  - brain (with liver and lung abscess) 006.5
  - liver 006.3
    - with
      - brain abscess (and lung abscess) 006.5
      - lung abscess 006.4
  - lung (with liver abscess) 006.4
    - with brain abscess 006.5
  - seminal vesicle 006.8
  - spleen 006.8
- carrier (suspected of) V02.2
- meningoencephalitis
  - due to Naegleria (gruberi) 136.2
  - primary 136.2

Amebiasis NEC 006.9
- with
  - brain abscess (with liver or lung abscess) 006.5
  - liver abscess (without mention of brain or lung abscess) 006.3
  - lung abscess (with liver abscess) 006.4
    - with brain abscess 006.5
- acute 006.0
- bladder 006.8
- chronic 006.1
- cutaneous 006.6
- cutis 006.6
- due to organism other than Entamoeba histolytica 007.8
- hepatic (*see also* Abscess, liver, amebic) 006.3
- nondysenteric 006.2
- seminal vesicle 006.8
- specified
  - organism NEC 007.8
  - site NEC 006.8

Ameboma 006.8

Amelia 755.4
- lower limb 755.31
- upper limb 755.21

Ameloblastoma (M9310/0) 213.1
- jaw (bone) (lower) 213.1
  - upper 213.0
- long bones (M9261/3) - *see* Neoplasm, bone, malignant
- malignant (M9310/3) 170.1
  - jaw (bone) (lower) 170.1
    - upper 170.0
- mandible 213.1
- tibial (M9261/3) 170.7

Amelogenesis imperfecta 520.5
- nonhereditaria (segmentalis) 520.4

Amenorrhea (primary) (secondary) 626.0
- due to ovarian dysfunction 256.8
- hyperhormonal 256.8

Amentia (*see also* Retardation, mental) 319
- Meynert's (nonalcoholic) 294.0
  - alcoholic 291.1
- nevoid 759.6

American
- leishmaniasis 085.5
- mountain tick fever 066.1
- trypanosomiasis - *see* Trypanosomiasis, American

Ametropia (*see also* Disorder, accommodation) 367.9

Amianthosis 501

Amimia 784.69

ICD-9-CM
A
Vol. 2

- **Amino acid**
  - deficiency 270.9
    - anemia 281.4
  - metabolic disorder (*see also* Disorder, amino acid) 270.9
- **Aminoaciduria** 270.9
  - imidazole 270.5
- **Amnesia** (retrograde) 780.93 ⬅
  - auditory 784.69
    - developmental 315.31
    - secondary to organic lesion 784.69
  - hysterical or dissociative type 300.12
  - psychogenic 300.12
  - transient global 437.7
- **Amnestic** (confabulatory) syndrome 294.0
  - alcohol-induced 291.1
  - drug-induced 292.83
  - posttraumatic 294.0
- **Amniocentesis screening** (for) V28.2
  - alpharetoprotein level, raised V28.1
  - chromosomal anomalies V28.0
- **Amnion, amniotic** - *see also* condition
  - nodosum 658.8
- **Amnionitis** (complicating pregnancy) 658.4
  - affecting fetus or newborn 762.7
- **Amoral trends** 301.7
- **Amotio retinae** (*see also* Detachment, retina) 361.9
- **Ampulla**
  - lower esophagus 530.89
  - phrenic 530.89
- **Amputation**
  - any part of fetus, to facilitate delivery 763.89
  - cervix (supravaginal) (uteri) 622.8
    - in pregnancy or childbirth 654.6
      - affecting fetus or newborn 763.89
  - clitoris - *see* Wound, open, clitoris
  - congenital
    - lower limb 755.31
    - upper limb 755.21
  - neuroma (traumatic) - *see also* Injury, nerve, by site
    - surgical complication (late) 997.61
  - penis - *see* Amputation, traumatic, penis
  - status (without complication) - *see* Absence, by site, acquired
  - stump (surgical) (posttraumatic)
    - abnormal, painful, or with complication (late) 997.60
    - healed or old NEC - *see also* Absence, by site, acquired
      - lower V49.70
      - upper V49.60
  - traumatic (complete) (partial)

> Note "Complicated" includes traumatic amputation with delayed healing, delayed treatment, foreign body, or infection.

- **Amputation** (continued)
  - traumatic (continued)
    - arm 887.4
      - at or above elbow 887.2
        - complicated 887.3
      - below elbow 887.0
        - complicated 887.1
      - both (bilateral) (any level(s)) 887.6
        - complicated 887.7
      - complicated 887.5

Amputation *(Continued)*

- finger(s) (one or both hands) 886.0
  - with thumb(s) 885.0
    - complicated 885.1
  - complicated 886.1
- foot (except toe(s) only) 896.0
  - and other leg 897.6
    - complicated 897.7
  - both (bilateral) 896.2
    - complicated 896.3
  - complicated 896.1
- toe(s) only (one or both feet) 895.0
  - complicated 895.1
- genital organ(s) (external) NEC 878.8
  - complicated 878.9
- hand (except finger(s) only) 887.0
  - and other arm 887.6
    - complicated 887.7
  - both (bilateral) 887.6
    - complicated 887.7
  - complicated 887.1
  - finger(s) (one or both hands) 886.0
    - with thumb(s) 885.0
      - complicated 885.1
    - complicated 886.1
  - thumb(s) (with fingers of either hand) 885.0
    - complicated 885.1
- head 874.9
- late effect - *see* Late, effects (of), amputation
- leg 897.4
  - and other foot 897.6
    - complicated 897.7
  - at or above knee 897.2
    - complicated 897.3
  - below knee 897.0
    - complicated 897.1
  - both (bilateral) 897.6
    - complicated 897.7
  - complicated 897.5
- lower limb(s) except toe(s) - *see* Amputation, traumatic, leg
- nose - *see* Wound, open, nose
- penis 878.0
  - complicated 878.1
- sites other than limbs - *see* Wound, open, by site
- thumb(s) (with finger(s) of either hand) 885.0
  - complicated 885.1
- toe(s) (one or both feet) 895.0
  - complicated 895.1
- upper limb(s) - *see* Amputation, traumatic, arm

- **Amputee** (bilateral) (old) - *see* Absence, by site, acquired V49.70
- **Amusia** 784.69
  - developmental 315.39
  - secondary to organic lesion 784.69
- **Amyelencephalus** 740.0
- **Amyelia** 742.59
- **Amygdalitis** - *see* Tonsillitis
- **Amygdalolith** 474.8
- **Amyloid disease or degeneration** 277.3
  - heart 277.3 *[425.7]*
- **Amyloidosis** (familial) (general) (generalized) (genetic) (primary) (secondary) 277.3
  - with lung involvement 277.3 *[517.8]*
  - heart 277.3 *[425.7]*
  - nephropathic 277.3 *[583.81]*
  - neuropathic (Portuguese) (Swiss) 277.3 *[357.4]*

Amyloidosis *(Continued)*

- pulmonary 277.3 *[517.8]*
- systemic, inherited 277.3

- **Amylopectinosis** (brancher enzyme deficiency) 271.0
- **Amylophagia** 307.52
- **Amyoplasia congenita** 756.89
- **Amyotonia** 728.2
  - congenita 358.8
- **Amyotrophia, amyotrophy, amyotrophic** 728.2
  - congenita 756.89
  - diabetic 250.6 *[358.1]*
  - lateral sclerosis (syndrome) 335.20
  - neuralgic 353.5
  - sclerosis (lateral) 335.20
  - spinal progressive 335.21
- **Anacidity, gastric** 536.0
  - psychogenic 306.4
- **Anaerosis of newborn** 768.9
- **Analbuminemia** 273.8
- **Analgesia** (*see also* Anesthesia) 782.0
- **Analphalipoproteinemia** 272.5
- **Anaphylactic shock or reaction** (correct substance properly administered) 995.0
  - due to
    - food 995.60
      - additives 995.66
      - crustaceans 995.62
      - eggs 995.68
      - fish 995.65
      - fruits 995.63
      - milk products 995.67
      - nuts (tree) 995.64
      - peanuts 995.61
      - seeds 995.64,
      - specified NEC 995.69
      - tree nuts 995.64
      - vegetables 995.63
    - immunization 999.4
    - overdose or wrong substance given or taken 977.9
      - specified drug - *see* Table of Drugs and Chemicals
    - serum 999.4
  - following sting(s) 989.5
  - purpura 287.0
  - serum 999.4
- **Anaphylactoid shock or reaction** - *see* Anaphylactic shock
- **Anaphylaxis** - *see* Anaphylactic shock
- **Anaplasia, cervix** 622.1
- **Anarthria** 784.5
- **Anarthritic rheumatoid disease** 446.5
- **Anasarca** 782.3
  - cardiac (*see also* Failure, heart 428.0
  - fetus or newborn 778.0
  - lung 514
  - nutritional 262
  - pulmonary 514
  - renal (*see also* Nephrosis) 581.9
- **Anaspadias** 752.62
- **Anastomosis**
  - aneurysmal - *see* Aneurysm
  - arteriovenous, congenital NEC (*see also* Anomaly, arteriovenous) 747.60
    - ruptured, of brain (*see also* Hemorrhage, subarachnoid) 430
  - intestinal 569.89
    - complicated NEC 997.4
      - involving urinary tract 997.5
  - retinal and choroidal vessels 743.58
    - acquired 362.17

New Revised Code

Note Use the following fifth-digit subclassification with categories 711-712, 716:

0 site unspecified
1 shoulder region
2 upper arm
3 forearm
4 hand
5 pelvic region and thigh
6 lower leg
7 ankle and foot
8 other specified sites
9 multiple sites

ICD-9-CM
A
Vol. 2

Note Use the following fifth digit subclassification with category 493:

0 unspecified ⟵
1 with status asthmaticus
2 with (acute) exacerbation ⟵

◄ New ⟵ Revised Code

B

ICD-9-CM B Vol. 2

◀ New ⬅ Revised Code

ICD-9-CM B Vol. 2

New   Revised Code

ICD-9-CM B Vol. 2

◄ New ⇐ Revised Code

Note Use the following fifth-digit subclassification with category 948 to indicate the percent of body surface with third degree burn:

0 less than 10 percent or unspecified
1 10-19 percent
2 20-29 percent
3 30-39 percent
4 40-49 percent
5 50-59 percent
6 60-69 percent
7 70-79 percent
8 80-89 percent
9 90 percent or more of body surface

ICD-9-CM B Vol. 2

Burn *(Continued)*
with
blisters - *see* Burn, by site, second degree
erythema - *see* Burn, by site, first degree
skin loss (epidermal) - *see also* Burn, by site, second degree
full thickness - *see also* Burn, by site, third degree
with necrosis of underlying tissues - *see* Burn, by site, third degree, deep
first degree - *see* Burn, by site, first degree
second degree - *see* Burn, by site, second degree
third degree - *see also* Burn, by site, third degree
deep - *see* Burn, by site, third degree, deep
abdomen, abdominal (muscle) (wall) 942.03
with
trunk - *see* Burn, trunk, multiple sites
first degree 942.13
second degree 942.23
third degree 942.33
deep 942.43
with loss of body part 942.53
ankle 945.03
with
lower limb(s) - *see* Burn, leg, multiple sites
first degree 945.13
second degree 945.23
third degree 945.33
deep 945.43
with loss of body part 945.53
anus - *see* Burn, trunk, specified site NEC
arm(s) 943.00
first degree 943.10
second degree 943.20
third degree 943.30
deep 943.40
with loss of body part 943.50
lower - *see* Burn, forearm(s)
multiple sites, except hand(s) or wrist(s) 943.09
first degree 943.19
second degree 943.29
third degree 943.39
deep 943.49
with loss of body part 943.59
upper 943.03
first degree 943.13
second degree 943.23
third degree 943.33
deep 943.43
with loss of body part 943.53
auditory canal (external) - *see* Burn, ear
auricle (ear) - *see* Burn, ear
axilla 943.04
with
upper limb(s), except hand(s) or wrist(s) - *see* Burn, arm(s), multiple sites

Burn *(Continued)*
axilla *(Continued)*
first degree 943.14
second degree 943.24
third degree 943.34
deep 943.44
with loss of body part 943.54
back 942.04
with
trunk - *see* Burn, trunk, multiple sites
first degree 942.14
second degree 942.24
third degree 942.34
deep 942.44
with loss of body part 942.54
biceps
brachii - *see* Burn, arm(s), upper
femoris - *see* Burn, thigh
breast(s) 942.01
with
trunk - *see* Burn, trunk, multiple sites
first degree 942.11
second degree 942.21
third degree 942.31
deep 942.41
with loss of body part 942.51
brow - *see* Burn, forehead
buttock(s) - *see* Burn, back
canthus (eye) 940.1
chemical 940.0
cervix (uteri) 947.4
cheek (cutaneous) 941.07
with
face or head - *see* Burn, head, multiple sites
first degree 941.17
second degree 941.27
third degree 941.37
deep 941.47
with loss of body part 941.57
chest wall (anterior) 942.02
with
trunk - *see* Burn, trunk, multiple sites
first degree 942.12
second degree 942.22
third degree 942.32
deep 942.42
with loss of body part 942.52
chin 941.04
with
face or head - *see* Burn, head, multiple sites
first degree 941.14
second degree 941.24
third degree 941.34
deep 941.44
with loss of body part 941.54
clitoris - *see* Burn, genitourinary organs, external
colon 947.3
conjunctiva (and cornea) 940.4
chemical
acid 940.3
alkaline 940.2
cornea (and conjunctiva) 940.4
chemical
acid 940.3
alkaline 940.2
costal region - *see* Burn, chest wall

Burn *(Continued)*
due to ingested chemical agent - *see* Burn, internal organs
ear (auricle) (canal) (drum) (external) 941.01
with
face or head - *see* Burn, head, multiple sites
first degree 941.11
second degree 941.21
third degree 941.31
deep 941.41
with loss of a body part 941.51
elbow 943.02
with
hand(s) and wrist(s) - *see* Burn, multiple specified sites
upper limb(s), except hand(s) or wrist(s) - *see also* Burn, arm(s), multiple sites
first degree 943.12
second degree 943.22
third degree 943.32
deep 943.42
with loss of body part 943.52
electricity, electric current - *see* Burn, by site
entire body - *see* Burn, multiple, specified sites
epididymis - *see* Burn, genitourinary organs, external
epigastric region - *see* Burn, abdomen
epiglottis 947.1
esophagus 947.2
extent (percent of body surface)
less than 10 percent 948.0
10-19 percent 948.1
20-29 percent 948.2
30-39 percent 948.3
40-49 percent 948.4
50-59 percent 948.5
60-69 percent 948.6
70-79 percent 948.7
80-89 percent 948.8
90 percent or more 948.9
extremity
lower - *see* Burn, leg
upper - *see* Burn, arm(s)
eye(s) (and adnexa) (only) 940.9
with
face, head, or neck 941.02
first degree 941.12
second degree 941.22
third degree 941.32
deep 941.42
with loss of body part 941.52
other sites (classifiable to more than one category in 940-945) - *see* Burn, multiple, specified sites
resulting rupture and destruction of eyeball 940.5
specified part - *see* Burn, by site
eyeball - *see also* Burn, eye
with resulting rupture and destruction of eyeball 940.5
eyelid(s) 940.1
chemical 940.0
face - *see* Burn, head
finger (nail) (subungual) 944.01

ICD-9-CM B Vol. 2

C

ICD-9-CM C Vol. 2

- **Carcinoid** *(Continued)*
  - syndrome (intestinal) (metastatic) 259.2
  - type bronchial adenoma (M8240/3) - *see* Neoplasm, lung, malignant
- **Carcinoidosis** 259.2
- **Carcinoma** (M8010/3) - *see also* Neoplasm, by site, malignant

> Note Except where otherwise indicated, the morphological varieties of carcinoma in the list below should be coded by site as for "Neoplasm, malignant."

  - with
    - apocrine metaplasia (M8573/3)
    - cartilaginous (and osseous) metaplasia (M8571/3)
    - osseous (and cartilaginous) metaplasia (M8571/3)
    - productive fibrosis (M8141/3)
    - spindle cell metaplasia (M8572/3)
    - squamous metaplasia (M8570/3)
  - acidophil (M8280/3)
    - specified site - *see* Neoplasm, by site, malignant
    - unspecified site 194.3
  - acidophil-basophil, mixed (M8281/3)
    - specified site - *see* Neoplasm, by site, malignant
    - unspecified site 194.3
  - acinar (cell) (M8550/3)
  - acinic cell (M8550/3)
  - adenocystic (M8200/3)
  - adenoid
    - cystic (M8200/3)
    - squamous cell (M8075/3)
  - adenosquamous (M8560/3)
  - adnexal (skin) (M8390/3) - *see* Neoplasm, skin, malignant
  - adrenal cortical (M8370/3) 194.0
  - alveolar (M8251/3)
    - cell (M8250/3) - *see* Neoplasm, lung, malignant
  - anaplastic type (M8021/3)
  - apocrine (M8401/3)
    - breast - *see* Neoplasm, breast, malignant
    - specified site NEC - *see* Neoplasm, skin, malignant
    - unspecified site 173.9
  - basal cell (pigmented) (M8090/3) - *see also* Neoplasm, skin, malignant
    - fibro-epithelial type (M8093/3) - *see* Neoplasm, skin, malignant
    - morphea type (M8092/3) - *see* Neoplasm, skin, malignant
    - multicentric (M8091/3) - *see* Neoplasm, skin, malignant
  - basaloid (M8123/3)
  - basal-squamous cell, mixed (M8094/3) - *see* Neoplasm, skin, malignant
  - basophil (M8300/3)
    - specified site - *see* Neoplasm, by site, malignant
    - unspecified site 194.3
  - basophil-acidophil, mixed (M8281/3)
    - specified site - *see* Neoplasm, by site, malignant
    - unspecified site 194.3
  - basosquamous (M8094/3) - *see* Neoplasm, skin, malignant

- **Carcinoma** *(Continued)*
  - bile duct type (M8160/3)
    - and hepatocellular, mixed (M8180/3) 155.0
    - liver 155.1
    - specified site NEC - *see* Neoplasm, by site, malignant
    - unspecified site 155.1
  - branchial or branchiogenic 146.8
  - bronchial or bronchogenic - *see* Neoplasm, lung, malignant
  - bronchiolar (terminal) (M8250/3) - *see* Neoplasm, lung, malignant
  - bronchiolo-alveolar (M8250/3) - *see* Neoplasm, lung, malignant
  - bronchogenic (epidermoid) 162.9
  - C cell (M8510/3)
    - specified site - *see* Neoplasm, by site, malignant
    - unspecified site 193
  - ceruminous (M8420/3) 173.2
  - chorionic (M9100/3)
    - specified site - *see* Neoplasm, by site, malignant
    - unspecified site
      - female 181
      - male 186.9
  - chromophobe (M8270/3)
    - specified site - *see* Neoplasm, by site, malignant
    - unspecified site 194.3
  - clear cell (mesonephroid type) (M8310/3)
  - cloacogenic (M8124/3)
    - specified site - *see* Neoplasm, by site, malignant
    - unspecified site 154.8
  - colloid (M8480/3)
  - cribriform (M8201/3)
  - cylindroid type (M8200/3)
  - diffuse type (M8145/3)
    - specified site - *see* Neoplasm, by site, malignant
    - unspecified site 151.9
  - duct (cell) (M8500/3)
    - with Paget's disease (M8541/3) - *see* Neoplasm, breast, malignant
    - infiltrating (M8500/3)
      - specified site - *see* Neoplasm, by site, malignant
      - unspecified site 174.9
  - ductal (M8500/3)
  - ductular, infiltrating (M8521/3)
  - embryonal (M9070/3)
    - and teratoma, mixed (M9081/3)
    - combined with choriocarcinoma (M9101/3) - *see* Neoplasm, by site, malignant
    - infantile type (M9071/3)
    - liver 155.0
    - polyembryonal type (M9072/3)
  - endometrioid (M8380/3)
  - eosinophil (M8280/3)
    - specified site - *see* Neoplasm, by site, malignant
    - unspecified site 194.3
  - epidermoid (M8070/3) - *see also* Carcinoma, squamous cell
    - and adenocarcinoma, mixed (M8560/3)
    - in situ, Bowen's type (M8081/2) - *see* Neoplasm, skin, in situ
    - intradermal - *see* Neoplasm, skin, in situ

- **Carcinoma** *(Continued)*
  - fibroepithelial type basal cell (M8093/3) - *see* Neoplasm, skin, malignant
  - follicular (M8330/3)
    - and papillary (mixed) (M8340/3) 193
    - moderately differentiated type (M8332/3) 193
    - pure follicle type (M8331/3) 193
    - specified site - *see* Neoplasm, by site, malignant
    - trabecular type (M8332/3) 193
    - unspecified site 193
    - well differentiated type (M8331/3) 193
  - gelatinous (M8480/3)
  - giant cell (M8031/3)
    - and spindle cell (M8030/3)
  - granular cell (M8320/3)
  - granulosa cell (M8620/3) 183.0
  - hepatic cell (M8170/3) 155.0
  - hepatocellular (M8170/3) 155.0
    - and bile duct, mixed (M8180/3) 155.0
  - hepatocholangiolitic (M8180/3) 155.0
  - Hürthle cell (thyroid) 193
  - hypernephroid (M8311/3)
  - in
    - adenomatous
      - polyp (M8210/3)
      - polyposis coli (M8220/3) 153.9
    - pleomorphic adenoma (M8940/3)
    - polypoid adenoma (M8210/3)
    - situ (M8010/3) - *see* Carcinoma, in situ
    - tubular adenoma (M8210/3)
    - villous adenoma (M8261/3)
  - infiltrating duct (M8500/3)
    - with Paget's disease (M8541/3) - *see* Neoplasm, breast, malignant
    - specified site - *see* Neoplasm, by site, malignant
    - unspecified site 174.9
  - inflammatory (M8530/3)
    - specified site - *see* Neoplasm, by site, malignant
    - unspecified site 174.9
  - in situ (M8010/2) - *see also* Neoplasm, by site, in situ
    - epidermoid (M8070/2) - *see also* Neoplasm, by site, in situ
      - with questionable stromal invasion (M8076/2)
        - specified site - *see* Neoplasm, by site, in situ
        - unspecified site 233.1
      - Bowen's type (M8081/2) - *see* Neoplasm, skin, in situ
    - intraductal (M8500/2)
      - specified site - *see* Neoplasm, by site, in situ
      - unspecified site 233.0
    - lobular (M8520/2)
      - specified site - *see* Neoplasm, by site, in situ
      - unspecified site 233.0
    - papillary (M8050/2) - *see* Neoplasm, by site, in situ
    - squamous cell (M8070/2) - *see also* Neoplasm, by site, in situ
      - with questionable stromal invasion (M8076/2)
        - specified site - *see* Neoplasm, by site, in situ
        - unspecified site 233.1

Carcinoma *(Continued)*
- in situ *(Continued)*
  - transitional cell (M8120/2) - *see* Neoplasm, by site, in situ
- intestinal type (M8144/3)
  - specified site - *see* Neoplasm, by site, malignant
  - unspecified site 151.9
- intraductal (noninfiltrating) (M8500/2)
  - papillary (M8503/2)
    - specified site - *see* Neoplasm, by site, in situ
    - unspecified site 233.0
  - specified site - *see* Neoplasm, by site, in situ
  - unspecified site 233.0
- intraepidermal (M8070/2) - *see also* Neoplasm, skin, in situ
  - squamous cell, Bowen's type (M8081/2) - *see* Neoplasm, skin, in situ
- intraepithelial (M8010/2) - *see also* Neoplasm, by site, in situ
  - squamous cell (M8072/2) - *see* Neoplasm, by site, in situ
- intraosseous (M9270/3) 170.1
  - upper jaw (bone) 170.0
- islet cell (M8150/3)
  - and exocrine, mixed (M8154/3)
    - specified site - *see* Neoplasm, by site, malignant
    - unspecified site 157.9
  - pancreas 157.4
  - specified site NEC - *see* Neoplasm, by site, malignant
  - unspecified site 157.4
- juvenile, breast (M8502/3) - *see* Neoplasm, breast, malignant
- Kulchitsky's cell (carcinoid tumor of intestine) 259.2
- large cell (M8012/3)
  - squamous cell, non-keratinizing type (M8072/3)
- Leydig cell (testis) (M8650/3)
  - specified site - *see* Neoplasm, by site, malignant
  - unspecified site 186.9
    - female 183.0
    - male 186.9
- liver cell (M8170/3) 155.0
- lobular (infiltrating) (M8520/3)
  - noninfiltrating (M8520/3)
    - specified site - *see* Neoplasm, by site, in situ
    - unspecified site 233.0
  - specified site - *see* Neoplasm, by site, malignant
  - unspecified site 174.9
- lymphoepithelial (M8082/3)
- medullary (M8510/3)
  - with
    - amyloid stroma (M8511/3)
      - specified site - *see* Neoplasm, by site, malignant
      - unspecified site 193
    - lymphoid stroma (M8512/3)
      - specified site - *see* Neoplasm, by site, malignant
      - unspecified site 174.9
- mesometanephric (M9110/3)
- mesonephric (M9110/3)
- metastatic (M8010/6) - *see* Metastasis, cancer

Carcinoma *(Continued)*
- metatypical (M8095/3) - *see* Neoplasm, skin, malignant
- morphea type basal cell (M8092/3) - *see* Neoplasm, skin, malignant
- mucinous (M8480/3)
- mucin-producing (M8481/3)
- mucin-secreting (M8481/3)
- mucoepidermoid (M8430/3)
- mucoid (M8480/3)
  - cell (M8300/3)
    - specified site - *see* Neoplasm, by site, malignant
    - unspecified site 194.3
- mucous (M8480/3)
- nonencapsulated sclerosing (M8350/3) 193
- noninfiltrating
  - intracystic (M8504/2) - *see* Neoplasm, by site, in situ
  - intraductal (M8500/2)
    - papillary (M8503/2)
      - specified site - *see* Neoplasm, by site, in situ
      - unspecified site 233.0
    - specified site - *see* Neoplasm, by site, in situ
    - unspecified site 233.0
  - lobular (M8520/2)
    - specified site - *see* Neoplasm, by site, in situ
    - unspecified site 233.0
- oat cell (M8042/3)
  - specified site - *see* Neoplasm, by site, malignant
  - unspecified site 162.9
- odontogenic (M9270/3) 170.1
  - upper jaw (bone) 170.0
- oncocytic (M8290/3)
- oxyphilic (M8290/3)
- papillary (M8050/3)
  - and follicular (mixed) (M8340/3) 193
  - epidermoid (M8052/3)
  - intraductal (noninfiltrating) (M8503/2)
    - specified site - *see* Neoplasm, by site, in situ
    - unspecified site 233.0
  - serous (M8460/3)
    - specified site - *see* Neoplasm, by site, malignant
    - surface (M8461/3)
      - specified site - *see* Neoplasm, by site, malignant
      - unspecified site 183.0
    - unspecified site 183.0
  - squamous cell (M8052/3)
  - transitional cell (M8130/3)
- papillocystic (M8450/3)
  - specified site - *see* Neoplasm, by site, malignant
  - unspecified site 183.0
- parafollicular cell (M8510/3)
  - specified site - *see* Neoplasm, by site, malignant
  - unspecified site 193
- pleomorphic (M8022/3)
- polygonal cell (M8034/3)
- prickle cell (M8070/3)
- pseudoglandular, squamous cell (M8075/3)
- pseudomucinous (M8470/3)
  - specified site - *see* Neoplasm, by site, malignant
  - unspecified site 183.0

Carcinoma *(Continued)*
- pseudosarcomatous (M8033/3)
- regaud type (M8082/3) - *see* Neoplasm, nasopharynx, malignant
- renal cell (M8312/3) 189.0
- reserve cell (M8041/3)
- round cell (M8041/3)
- Schmincke (M8082/3) - *see* Neoplasm, nasopharynx, malignant
- Schneiderian (M8121/3)
  - specified site - *see* Neoplasm, by site, malignant
  - unspecified site 160.0
- scirrhous (M8141/3)
- sebaceous (M8410/3) - *see* Neoplasm, skin, malignant
- secondary (M8010/6) - *see* Neoplasm, by site, malignant, secondary
- secretory, breast (M8502/3) - *see* Neoplasm, breast, malignant
- serous (M8441/3)
  - papillary (M8460/3)
    - specified site - *see* Neoplasm, by site, malignant
    - unspecified site 183.0
  - surface, papillary (M8461/3)
    - specified site - *see* Neoplasm, by site, malignant
    - unspecified site 183.0
- Sertoli cell (M8640/3)
  - specified site - *see* Neoplasm, by site, malignant
  - unspecified site 186.9
- signet ring cell (M8490/3)
  - metastatic (M8490/6) - *see* Neoplasm, by site, secondary
- simplex (M8231/3)
- skin appendage (M8390/3) - *see* Neoplasm, skin, malignant
- small cell (M8041/3)
  - fusiform cell type (M8043/3)
  - squamous cell, nonkeratinizing type (M8073/3)
- solid (M8230/3)
  - with amyloid stroma (M8511/3)
    - specified site - *see* Neoplasm, by site, malignant
    - unspecified site 193
- spheroidal cell (M8035/3)
- spindle cell (M8032/3)
  - and giant cell (M8030/3)
- spinous cell (M8070/3)
- squamous (cell) (M8070/3)
  - adenoid type (M8075/3)
  - and adenocarcinoma, mixed (M8560/3)
  - intraepidermal, Bowen's type - *see* Neoplasm, skin, in situ
  - keratinizing type (large cell) (M8071/3)
  - large cell, nonkeratinizing type (M8072/3)
  - microinvasive (M8076/3)
    - specified site - *see* Neoplasm, by site, malignant
    - unspecified site 180.9
  - nonkeratinizing type (M8072/3)
  - papillary (M8052/3)
  - pseudoglandular (M8075/3)
  - small cell, nonkeratinizing type (M8073/3)
  - spindle cell type (M8074/3)
  - verrucous (M8051/3)
- superficial spreading (M8143/3)

Carcinoma *(Continued)*
sweat gland (M8400/3) - *see* Neoplasm, skin, malignant
theca cell (M8600/3) 183.0
thymic (M8580/3) 164.0
trabecular (M8190/3)
transitional (cell) (M8120/3)
papillary (M8130/3)
spindle cell type (M8122/3)
tubular (M8211/3)
undifferentiated type (M8020/3)
urothelial (M8120/3)
ventriculi 151.9
verrucous (epidermoid) (squamous cell) (M8051/3)
villous (M8262/3)
water-clear cell (M8322/3) 194.1
wolffian duct (M9110/3)
Carcinomaphobia 300.29
Carcinomatosis
peritonei (M8010/6) 197.6
specified site NEC (M8010/3) - *see* Neoplasm, by site, malignant
unspecified site (M8010/6) 199.0
Carcinosarcoma (M8980/3) - *see also* Neoplasm, by site, malignant
embryonal type (M8981/3) - *see* Neoplasm, by site, malignant
Cardia, cardial - *see* condition
Cardiac - *see also* condition
death - *see* Disease, heart
device
defibrillator, automatic implantable V45.02
in situ NEC V45.00
pacemaker
cardiac
fitting or adjustment V53.31
in situ V45.01
carotid sinus
fitting or adjustment V53.39
in situ V45.09
pacemaker - *see* Cardiac, device, pacemaker
tamponade 423.9
Cardialgia (*see also* Pain, precordial) 786.51
Cardiectasis - *see* Hypertrophy, cardiac
Cardiochalasia 530.81
Cardiomalacia (*see also* Degeneration, myocardial) 429.1
Cardiomegalia glycogenica diffusa 271.0
Cardiomegaly (*see also* Hypertrophy, cardiac) 429.3
congenital 746.89
glycogen 271.0
hypertensive (*see also* Hypertension, heart) 402.90
idiopathic 425.4
Cardiomyoliposis (*see also* Degeneration, myocardial) 429.1
Cardiomyopathy (congestive) (constrictive) (familial) (infiltrative) (obstructive) (restrictive) (sporadic) 425.4
alcoholic 425.5
amyloid 277.3 *[425.7]*
beriberi 265.0 *[425.7]*
cobalt-beer 425.5
congenital 425.3
due to
amyloidosis 277.3 *[425.7]*
beriberi 265.0 *[425.7]*
cardiac glycogenosis 271.0 *[425.7]*
Chagas' disease 086.0

Cardiomyopathy *(Continued)*
due to *(Continued)*
Friedreich's ataxia 334.0 *[425.8]*
hypertension - *see* Hypertension, with, heart involvement
mucopolysaccharidosis 277.5 *[425.7]*
myotonia atrophica 359.2 *[425.8]*
progressive muscular dystrophy 359.1 *[425.8]*
sarcoidosis 135 *[425.8]*
glycogen storage 271.0 *[425.7]*
hypertensive - *see* Hypertension, with, heart involvement
hypertrophic
nonobstructive 425.4
obstructive 425.1
congenital 746.84
idiopathic (concentric) 425.4
in
Chagas' disease 086.0
sarcoidosis 135 *[425.8]*
ischemic 414.8
metabolic NEC 277.9 *[425.7]*
amyloid 277.3 *[425.7]*
thyrotoxic (*see also* Thyrotoxicosis) 242.9 *[425.7]*
thyrotoxicosis (*see also* Thyrotoxicosis) 242.9 *[425.7]*
nutritional 269.9 *[425.7]*
beriberi 265.0 *[425.7]*
obscure of Africa 425.2
peripartum 674.5 ◀
postpartum 674.5 ⟸
primary 425.4
secondary 425.9
thyrotoxic (*see also* Thyrotoxicosis) 242.9 *[425.7]*
toxic NEC 425.9
tuberculous (*see also* Tuberculosis) 017.9 *[425.8]*
Cardionephritis - *see* Hypertension, cardiorenal
Cardionephropathy - *see* Hypertension, cardiorenal
Cardionephrosis - *see* Hypertension, cardiorenal
Cardioneurosis 306.2
Cardiopathia nigra 416.0
Cardiopathy (*see also* Disease, heart) 429.9
hypertensive (*see also* Hypertension, heart) 402.90
idiopathic 425.4
mucopolysaccharidosis 277.5 *[425.7]*
Cardiopericarditis (*see also* Pericarditis) 423.9
Cardiophobia 300.29
Cardioptosis 746.87
Cardiorenal - *see* condition
Cardiorrhexis (*see also* Infarct, myocardium) 410.9
Cardiosclerosis - *see* Arteriosclerosis, coronary
Cardiosis - *see* Disease, heart
Cardiospasm (esophagus) (reflex) (stomach) 530.0
congenital 750.7
Cardiostenosis - *see* Disease, heart
Cardiosymphysis 423.1
Cardiothyrotoxicosis - *see* Hyperthyroidism
Cardiovascular - *see* condition
Carditis (acute) (bacterial) (chronic) (subacute) 429.89

Carditis *(Continued)*
Coxsackie 074.20
hypertensive (*see also* Hypertension, heart) 402.90
meningococcal 036.40
rheumatic - *see* Disease, heart, rheumatic
rheumatoid 714.2
Care (of)
child (routine) V20.1
convalescent following V66.9
chemotherapy V66.2
medical NEC V66.5
psychotherapy V66.3
radiotherapy V66.1
surgery V66.0
surgical NEC V66.0
treatment (for) V66.5
combined V66.6
fracture V66.4
mental disorder NEC V66.3
specified type NEC V66.5
end-of-life V66.7
family member (handicapped) (sick)
creating problem for family V61.49
provided away from home for holiday relief V60.5
unavailable, due to
absence (person rendering care) (sufferer) V60.4
inability (any reason) of person rendering care V60.4
holiday relief V60.5
hospice V66.7
lack of (at or after birth) (infant) (child) 995.52
adult 995.84
lactation of mother V24.1
palliative V66.7
postpartum
immediately after delivery V24.0
routine follow-up V24.2
prenatal V22.1
first pregnancy V22.0
high-risk pregnancy V23.9
specified problem NEC V23.8
terminal V66.7
unavailable, due to
absence of person rendering care V60.4
inability (any reason) of person rendering care V60.4
well baby V20.1
Caries (bone) (*see also* Tuberculosis, bone) 015.9 *[730.8]*
arrested 521.04
cementum 521.03
cerebrospinal (tuberculous) 015.0 *[730.88]*
dental (acute) (chronic) (incipient) (infected) 521.09
with pulp exposure 521.03
extending to
dentine 521.02
pulp 521.03
other specified NEC 521.09
dentin (acute) (chronic) 521.02
enamel (acute) (chronic) (incipient) 521.01
external meatus 380.89
hip (*see also* Tuberculosis) 015.1 *[730.85]*
knee 015.2 *[730.86]*
labyrinth 386.8

ICD-9-CM
C
Vol. 2

ICD-9-CM
C
Vol. 2

ICD-9-CM
C
Vol. 2

◀ New ⇐ Revised Code

Chylocele *(Continued)*
- tunica vaginalis (nonfilarial) 608.84
  - filarial (*see also* Infestation, filarial) 125.9

Chylomicronemia (fasting) (with hyperprebetalipoproteinemia) 272.3
Chylopericardium (acute) 420.90
Chylothorax (nonfilarial) 457.8
- filarial (*see also* Infestation, filarial) 125.9

Chylous
- ascites 457.8
- cyst of peritoneum 457.8
- hydrocele 603.9
- hydrothorax (nonfilarial) 457.8
  - filarial (*see also* Infestation, filarial) 125.9

Chyluria 791.1
- bilharziasis 120.0
- due to
  - Brugia (malayi) 125.1
  - Wuchereria (bancrofti) 125.0
    - malayi 125.1
- filarial (*see also* Infestation, filarial) 125.9
- filariasis (*see also* Infestation, filarial) 125.9
- nonfilarial 791.1

Cicatricial (deformity) - *see* Cicatrix
Cicatrix (adherent) (contracted) (painful) (vicious) 709.2
- adenoid 474.8
- alveolar process 525.8
- anus 569.49
- auricle 380.89
- bile duct (*see also* Disease, biliary) 576.8
- bladder 596.8
- bone 733.99
- brain 348.8
- cervix (postoperative) (postpartal) 622.3
  - in pregnancy or childbirth 654.6
    - causing obstructed labor 660.2
- chorioretinal 363.30
  - disseminated 363.35
  - macular 363.32
  - peripheral 363.34
  - posterior pole NEC 363.33
- choroid - *see* Cicatrix, chorioretinal
- common duct (*see also* Disease, biliary) 576.8
- congenital 757.39
- conjunctiva 372.64
- cornea 371.00
  - tuberculous (*see also* Tuberculosis) 017.3 *[371.05]*
- duodenum (bulb) 537.3
- esophagus 530.3
- eyelid 374.46
  - with
    - ectropion - *see* Ectropion
    - entropion - *see* Entropion
- hypopharynx 478.29
- knee, semilunar cartilage 717.5
- lacrimal
  - canaliculi 375.53
  - duct
    - acquired 375.56
    - neonatal 375.55
  - punctum 375.52
  - sac 375.54
- larynx 478.79
- limbus (cystoid) 372.64

Cicatrix *(Continued)*
- lung 518.89
- macular 363.32
  - disseminated 363.35
  - peripheral 363.34
- middle ear 385.89
- mouth 528.9
- muscle 728.89
- nasolacrimal duct
  - acquired 375.56
  - neonatal 375.55
- nasopharynx 478.29
- palate (soft) 528.9
- penis 607.89
- prostate 602.8
- rectum 569.49
- retina 363.30
  - disseminated 363.35
  - macular 363.32
  - peripheral 363.34
  - posterior pole NEC 363.33
- semilunar cartilage - *see* Derangement, meniscus
- seminal vesicle 608.89
- skin 709.2
  - infected 686.8
  - postinfectional 709.2
  - tuberculous (*see also* Tuberculosis) 017.0
- specified site NEC 709.2
- throat 478.29
- tongue 529.8
- tonsil (and adenoid) 474.8
- trachea 478.9
- tuberculous NEC (*see also* Tuberculosis) 011.9
- ureter 593.89
- urethra 599.84
- uterus 621.8
- vagina 623.4
  - in pregnancy or childbirth 654.7
    - causing obstructed labor 660.2
- vocal cord 478.5
- wrist, constricting (annular) 709.2

CIN I [cervical intraepithelial neoplasia I] 622.1
CIN II [cervical intraepithelial neoplasia II] 622.1
CIN III [cervical intraepithelial neoplasia III] 233.1
Cinchonism
- correct substance properly administered 386.9
- overdose or wrong substance given or taken 961.4

Circine herpes 110.5
Circle of Willis - *see* condition
Circular - *see also* condition
- hymen 752.49

Circulating anticoagulants 286.5
- following childbirth 666.3
- postpartum 666.3

Circulation
- collateral (venous), any site 459.89
- defective 459.9
  - congenital 747.9
  - lower extremity 459.89
- embryonic 747.9
- failure 799.89
  - fetus or newborn 779.89
  - peripheral 785.59
- fetal, persistent 747.83
- heart, incomplete 747.9

Circulatory system - *see* condition
Circulus senilis 371.41
Circumcision
- in absence of medical indication V50.2
- ritual V50.2
- routine V50.2

Circumscribed - *see* condition
Circumvallata placenta - *see* Placenta, abnormal
Cirrhosis, cirrhotic 571.5
- with alcoholism 571.2
- alcoholic (liver) 571.2
- atrophic (of liver) - *see* Cirrhosis, portal
- Baumgarten-Cruveilhier 571.5
- biliary (cholangiolitic) (cholangitic) (cholestatic) (extrahepatic) (hypertrophic) (intrahepatic) (nonobstructive) (obstructive) (pericholangiolitic) (posthepatic) (primary) (secondary) (xanthomatous) 571.6
  - due to
    - clonorchiasis 121.1
    - flukes 121.3
- brain 331.9
- capsular - *see* Cirrhosis, portal
- cardiac 571.5
  - alcoholic 571.2
- central (liver) - *see* Cirrhosis, liver
- Charcôt's 571.6
- cholangiolitic - *see* Cirrhosis, biliary
- cholangitic - *see* Cirrhosis, biliary
- cholestatic - *see* Cirrhosis, biliary
- clitoris (hypertrophic) 624.2
- coarsely nodular 571.5
- congestive (liver) - *see* Cirrhosis, cardiac
- Cruveilhier-Baumgarten 571.5
- cryptogenic (of liver) 571.5
  - alcoholic 571.2
- dietary (*see also* Cirrhosis, portal) 571.5
- due to
  - bronzed diabetes 275.0
  - congestive hepatomegaly - *see* Cirrhosis, cardiac
  - cystic fibrosis 277.00
  - hemochromatosis 275.0
  - hepatolenticular degeneration 275.1
  - passive congestion (chronic) - *see* Cirrhosis, cardiac
  - Wilson's disease 275.1
  - xanthomatosis 272.2
- extrahepatic (obstructive) - *see* Cirrhosis, biliary
- fatty 571.8
  - alcoholic 571.0
- florid 571.2
- Glisson's - *see* Cirrhosis, portal
- Hanot's (hypertrophic) - *see* Cirrhosis, biliary
- hepatic - *see* Cirrhosis, liver
- hepatolienal - *see* Cirrhosis, liver
- hobnail - *see* Cirrhosis, portal
- hypertrophic - *see also* Cirrhosis, liver
  - biliary - *see* Cirrhosis, biliary
  - Hanot's - *see* Cirrhosis, biliary
- infectious NEC - *see* Cirrhosis, portal
- insular - *see* Cirrhosis, portal
- intrahepatic (obstructive) (primary) (secondary) - *see* Cirrhosis, biliary
- juvenile (*see also* Cirrhosis, portal) 571.5
- kidney (*see also* Sclerosis, renal) 587

ICD-9-CM
C
Vol. 2

◀ New ⟵ Revised Code

Congestion, congestive *(Continued)*
- spleen 289.51
  - chronic 289.51
- stomach 537.89
- trachea 464.11
- urethra 599.84
- uterus 625.5
  - with subinvolution 621.1
- viscera 799.89

Congestive - *see* Congestion

Conical
- cervix 622.6
- cornea 371.60
- teeth 520.2

Conjoined twins 759.4
- causing disproportion (fetopelvic) 653.7

Conjugal maladjustment V61.10
- involving divorce or estrangement V61.0

Conjunctiva - *see* condition

Conjunctivitis (exposure) (infectious) (nondiphtheritic) (pneumococcal) (pustular) (staphylococcal) (streptococcal) NEC 372.30
- actinic 370.24
- acute 372.00
  - atopic 372.05
  - contagious 372.03
  - follicular 372.02
  - hemorrhagic (viral) 077.4
- adenoviral (acute) 077.3
- allergic (chronic) 372.14
  - with hay fever 372.05
- anaphylactic 372.05
- angular 372.03
- Apollo (viral) 077.4
- atopic 372.05
- blennorrhagic (neonatorum) 098.40
- catarrhal 372.03
- chemical 372.05
- chlamydial 077.98
  - due to
    - Chlamydia trachomatis - *see* Trachoma
    - paratrachoma 077.0
- chronic 372.10
  - allergic 372.14
  - follicular 372.12
  - simple 372.11
  - specified type NEC 372.14
  - vernal 372.13
- diphtheritic 032.81
- due to
  - dust 372.05
  - enterovirus type 70 077.4
  - erythema multiforme 695.1 *[372.33]*
  - filariasis (*see also* Filariasis) 125.9 *[372.15]*
  - mucocutaneous
    - disease NEC 372.33
    - leishmaniasis 085.5 *[372.15]*
  - Reiter's disease 099.3 *[372.33]*
  - syphilis 095.8 *[372.10]*
  - toxoplasmosis (acquired) 130.1
    - congenital (active) 771.2
  - trachoma - *see* Trachoma
- dust 372.05
- eczematous 370.31
- epidemic 077.1
  - hemorrhagic 077.4
- follicular (acute) 372.02
  - adenoviral (acute) 077.3
  - chronic 372.12
- glare 370.24
- gonococcal (neonatorum) 098.40

Conjunctivitis *(Continued)*
- granular (trachomatous) 076.1
  - late effect 139.1
- hemorrhagic (acute) (epidemic) 077.4
- herpetic (simplex) 054.43
  - zoster 053.21
- inclusion 077.0
- infantile 771.6
- influenzal 372.03
- Koch-Weeks 372.03
- light 372.05
- medicamentosa 372.05
- membranous 372.04
- meningococcic 036.89
- Morax-Axenfeld 372.02
- mucopurulent NEC 372.03
- neonatal 771.6
  - gonococcal 098.40
- Newcastle's 077.8
- nodosa 360.14
- of Beal 077.3
- parasitic 372.15
  - filariasis (*see also* Filariasis) 125.9 *[372.15]*
  - mucocutaneous leishmaniasis 085.5 *[372.15]*
- Parinaud's 372.02
- petrificans 372.39
- phlyctenular 370.31
- pseudomembranous 372.04
  - diphtheritic 032.81
- purulent 372.03
- Reiter's 099.3 *[372.33]*
- rosacea 695.3 *[372.31]*
- serous 372.01
  - viral 077.99
- simple chronic 372.11
- specified NEC 372.39
- sunlamp 372.04
- swimming pool 077.0
- trachomatous (follicular) 076.1
  - acute 076.0
  - late effect 139.1
- traumatic NEC 372.39
- tuberculous (*see also* Tuberculosis) 017.3 *[370.31]*
- tularemic 021.3
- tularensis 021.3
- vernal 372.13
  - limbar 372.13 *[370.32]*
- viral 077.99
  - acute hemorrhagic 077.4
  - specified NEC 077.8

Conjunctivochalasis 372.81

Conjunctoblepharitis - *see* Conjunctivitis

Conn (-Louis) syndrome (primary aldosteronism) 255.12

Connective tissue - *see* condition

Conradi (-Hünermann) syndrome or disease (chondrodysplasia calcificans congenita) 756.59

Consanguinity V19.7

Consecutive - *see* condition

Consolidated lung (base) - *see* Pneumonia, lobar

Constipation 564.00
- atonic 564.09
- drug induced
  - correct substance properly administered 564.09
  - overdose or wrong substance given or taken 977.9
    - specified drug - *see* Table of Drugs and Chemicals

Constipation *(Continued)*
- neurogenic 564.09
- other specified NEC 564.09
- outlet dysfunction 564.02
- psychogenic 306.4
- simple 564.00
- slow transit 564.01
- spastic 564.09

Constitutional - *see also* condition
- arterial hypotension (*see also* Hypotension) 458.9
- obesity 278.00
  - morbid 278.01
- psychopathic state 301.9
- short stature in childhood 783.43
- state, developmental V21.9
  - specified development NEC V21.8
- substandard 301.6

Constitutionally substandard 301.6

Constriction
- anomalous, meningeal bands or folds 742.8
- aortic arch (congenital) 747.10
- asphyxiation or suffocation by 994.7
- bronchus 519.1
- canal, ear (*see also* Stricture, ear canal, acquired) 380.50
- duodenum 537.3
- gallbladder (*see also* Obstruction, gallbladder) 575.2
  - congenital 751.69
- intestine (*see also* Obstruction, intestine) 560.9
- larynx 478.74
  - congenital 748.3
- meningeal bands or folds, anomalous 742.8
- organ or site, congenital NEC - *see* Atresia
- prepuce (congenital) 605
- pylorus 537.0
  - adult hypertrophic 537.0
  - congenital or infantile 750.5
  - newborn 750.5
- ring (uterus) 661.4
  - affecting fetus or newborn 763.7
- spastic - *see also* Spasm
  - ureter 593.3
  - urethra - *see* Stricture, urethra
- stomach 537.89
- ureter 593.3
- urethra - *see* Stricture, urethra
- visual field (functional) (peripheral) 368.45

Constrictive - *see* condition

Consultation V65.9
- medical - *see also* Counseling, medical
- specified reason NEC V65.8
- without complaint or sickness V65.9
  - feared complaint unfounded V65.5
  - specified reason NEC V65.8

Consumption - *see* Tuberculosis

Contact
- with
  - AIDS virus V01.7
  - anthrax V01.81
  - cholera V01.0
  - communicable disease V01.9
    - specified type NEC V01.89
    - viral NEC V01.7
  - German measles V01.4
  - gonorrhea V01.6
  - HIV V01.7
  - human immunodeficiency virus V01.7
  - parasitic disease NEC V01.89

ICD-9-CM C Vol. 2

Note Use the following fifth-digit subclassification with categories 851-854:

0 unspecified state of consciousness
1 with no loss of consciousness
2 with brief [less than one hour] loss of consciousness
3 with moderate [1-24 hours] loss of consciousness
4 with prolonged [more than 24 hours] loss of consciousness and return to pre-existing conscious level
5 with prolonged [more than 24 hours] loss of consciousness, without return to pre-existing conscious level

Use fifth-digit 5 to designate when a patient is unconscious and dies before regaining consciousness, regardless of the duration of the loss of consciousness

6 with loss of consciousness of unspecified duration
9 with concussion, unspecified

Contusion *(Continued)*
- mandibular joint (and other part(s) of neck, scalp, or face, except eye) 920
- mastoid region (and other part(s) of neck, scalp, or face, except eye) 920
- membrane, brain - *see* Contusion, brain
- midthoracic region 922.1
- mouth (and other part(s) of neck, scalp, or face, except eye) 920
- multiple sites (not classifiable to same three-digit category) 924.8
  - lower limb 924.4
  - trunk 922.8
  - upper limb 923.8
- muscle NEC 924.9
- myocardium - *see* Contusion, cardiac
- nasal (septum) (and other part(s) of neck, scalp, or face, except eye) 920
- neck (and scalp, or face, any part, except eye) 920
- nerve - *see* Injury, nerve, by site
- nose (and other part(s) of neck, scalp, or face, except eye) 920
- occipital region (scalp) (and neck or face, except eye) 920
  - lobe - *see* Contusion, brain, occipital lobe
- orbit (region) (tissues) 921.2
- palate (soft) (and other part(s) of neck, scalp, or face, except eye) 920
- parietal region (scalp) (and neck, or face, except eye) 920
  - lobe - *see* Contusion, brain
- penis 922.4
- pericardium - *see* Contusion, cardiac
- perineum 922.4
- periocular area 921.1
- pharynx (and other part(s) of neck, scalp, or face, except eye) 920
- popliteal space (*see also* Contusion, knee) 924.11
- prepuce 922.4
- pubic region 922.4
- pudenda 922.4
- pulmonary - *see* Contusion, lung
- quadriceps femoralis 924.00
- rib cage 922.1
- sacral region 922.32
- salivary ducts or glands (and other part(s) of neck, scalp, or face, except eye) 920
- scalp (and neck, or face, any part, except eye) 920
- scapular region 923.01
  - with shoulder or upper arm 923.09
- sclera (eye) 921.3
- scrotum 922.4
- shoulder 923.00
  - with upper arm or axillary regions 923.09
- skin NEC 924.9
- skull 920
- spermatic cord 922.4
- spinal cord - *see also* Injury, spinal, by site
  - cauda equina 952.4
  - conus medullaris 952.4
- spleen 865.01
  - with open wound into cavity 865.11
- sternal region 922.1
- stomach - *see* Injury, internal, stomach
- subconjunctival 921.1
- subcutaneous NEC 924.9
- submaxillary region (and other part(s) of neck, scalp, or face, except eye) 920
- submental region (and other part(s) of neck, scalp, or face, except eye) 920
- subperiosteal NEC 924.9
- supraclavicular fossa (and other part(s) of neck, scalp, or face, except eye) 920
- supraorbital (and other part(s) of neck, scalp, or face, except eye) 920
- temple (region) (and other part(s) of neck, scalp, or face, except eye) 920
- testis 922.4
- thigh (and hip) 924.00
- thorax 922.1
  - organ - *see* Injury, internal, intrathoracic
- throat (and other part(s) of neck, scalp, or face, except eye) 920
- thumb(s) (nail) (subungual) 923.3
- toe(s) (nail) (subungual) 924.3
- tongue (and other part(s) of neck, scalp, or face, except eye) 920
- trunk 922.9
  - multiple sites 922.8
  - specified site - *see* Contusion, by site
- tunica vaginalis 922.4
- tympanum (membrane) (and other part(s) of neck, scalp, or face, except eye) 920
- upper extremity 923.9
  - multiple sites 923.8
- uvula (and other part(s) of neck, scalp, or face, except eye) 920
- vagina 922.4
- vocal cord(s) (and other part(s) of neck, scalp, or face, except eye) 920
- vulva 922.4
- wrist 923.21
  - with hand(s), except finger(s) alone 923.20

Conus (any type) (congenital) 743.57
- acquired 371.60
- medullaris syndrome 336.8

Convalescence (following) V66.9
- chemotherapy V66.2
- medical NEC V66.5
- psychotherapy V66.3
- radiotherapy V66.1
- surgery NEC V66.0
- treatment (for) NEC V66.5
  - combined V66.6
  - fracture V66.4
  - mental disorder NEC V66.3
  - specified disorder NEC V66.5

Conversion
- closed surgical procedure to open procedure ⬅
  - arthroscopic V64.43 ◄
  - laparoscopic V64.41 ◄
  - thoracoscopic V64.42 ◄
- hysteria, hysterical, any type 300.11
- neurosis, any 300.11
- reaction, any 300.11

Converter, tuberculosis (test reaction) 795.5

Convulsions (idiopathic) 780.39
- apoplectiform (*see also* Disease, cerebrovascular, acute) 436
- brain 780.39
- cerebral 780.39
- cerebrospinal 780.39
- due to trauma NEC - *see* Injury, intracranial
- eclamptic (*see also* Eclampsia) 780.39
- epileptic (*see also* Epilepsy) 345.9
- epileptiform (*see also* Seizure, epileptiform) 780.39
- epileptoid (*see also* Seizure, epileptiform) 780.39
- ether
  - anesthetic
    - correct substance properly administered 780.39
    - overdose or wrong substance given 968.2
  - other specified type - *see* Table of Drugs and Chemicals
- febrile 780.31
- generalized 780.39
- hysterical 300.11
- infantile 780.39
  - epilepsy - *see* Epilepsy
- internal 780.39
- jacksonian (*see also* Epilepsy) 345.5
- myoclonic 333.2
- newborn 779.0
- paretic 094.1
- pregnancy (nephritic) (uremic) - *see* Eclampsia, pregnancy
- psychomotor (*see also* Epilepsy) 345.4
- puerperal, postpartum - *see* Eclampsia, pregnancy
- recurrent 780.39
  - epileptic - *see* Epilepsy
- reflex 781.0
- repetitive 780.39
  - epileptic - *see* Epilepsy
- salaam (*see also* Epilepsy) 345.6
- scarlatinal 034.1
- spasmodic 780.39
- tetanus, tetanic (*see also* Tetanus) 037
- thymic 254.8
- uncinate 780.39
- uremic 586

Convulsive - *see also* Convulsions
- disorder or state 780.39
  - epileptic - *see* Epilepsy
- equivalent, abdominal (*see also* Epilepsy) 345.5

Cooke-Apert-Gallais syndrome (adrenogenital) 255.2

Cooley's anemia (erythroblastic) 282.49 ⬅

Coolie itch 126.9

Cooper's
- disease 610.1
- hernia - *see* Hernia, Cooper's

Coordination disturbance 781.3

Copper wire arteries, retina 362.13

Copra itch 133.8

Coprolith 560.39

Coprophilia 302.89

Coproporphyria, hereditary 277.1

Coprostasis 560.39
- with hernia - *see also* Hernia, by site, with obstruction
  - gangrenous - *see* Hernia, by site, with gangrene

Cor
- biloculare 745.7
- bovinum - *see* Hypertrophy, cardiac
- bovis - *see* Hypertrophy, cardiac
- pulmonale (chronic) 416.9
  - acute 415.0

ICD-9-CM
C
Vol. 2

ICD-9-CM
C
Vol. 2

D

- **Death** *(Continued)*
  - brain 348.8
  - cardiac - *see* Disease, heart
  - cause unknown 798.2
  - cot (infant) 798.0
  - crib (infant) 798.0
  - fetus, fetal (cause not stated) (intrauterine) 779.9
    - early, with retention (before 22 completed weeks' gestation) 632
    - from asphyxia or anoxia (before labor) 768.0
      - during labor 768.1
    - late, affecting management of pregnancy (after 22 completed weeks' gestation) 656.4
  - from pregnancy NEC 646.9
  - instantaneous 798.1
  - intrauterine (*see also* Death, fetus) 779.9
    - complicating pregnancy 656.4
  - maternal, affecting fetus or newborn 761.6
  - neonatal NEC 779.9
  - sudden (cause unknown) 798.1
    - during delivery 669.9
      - under anesthesia NEC 668.9
    - infant, syndrome (SIDS) 798.0
    - puerperal, during puerperium 674.9
  - unattended (cause unknown) 798.9
  - under anesthesia NEC
    - due to
      - correct substance properly administered 995.4
      - overdose or wrong substance given 968.4
        - specified anesthetic - *see* Table of Drugs and Chemicals
    - during delivery 668.9
  - violent 798.1
- **de Beurmann-Gougerot disease** (sporotrichosis) 117.1
- **Debility** (general) (infantile) (postinfectional) 799.3
  - with nutritional difficulty 269.9
  - congenital or neonatal NEC 779.9
  - nervous 300.5
  - old age 797
  - senile 797
- **Débove's disease** (splenomegaly) 789.2
- **Decalcification**
  - bone (*see also* Osteoporosis) 733.00
  - teeth 521.8
- **Decapitation** 874.9
  - fetal (to facilitate delivery) 763.89
- **Decapsulation, kidney** 593.89
- **Decay**
  - dental 521.00
  - senile 797
  - tooth, teeth 521.00
- **Decensus, uterus** - *see* Prolapse, uterus
- **Deciduitis** (acute)
  - with
    - abortion - *see* Abortion, by type, with sepsis
    - ectopic pregnancy (*see also* categories 633.0-633.9) 639.0
    - molar pregnancy (*see also* categories 630-632) 639.0
  - affecting fetus or newborn 760.8
  - following
    - abortion 639.0
    - ectopic or molar pregnancy 639.0
  - in pregnancy 646.6
  - puerperal, postpartum 670
- **Deciduoma malignum** (M9100/3) 181
- **Deciduous tooth** (retained) 520.6
- **Decline** (general) (*see also* Debility) 799.3
- **Decompensation**
  - cardiac (acute) (chronic) (*see also* Disease, heart) 429.9
    - failure - *see* Failure, heart
  - cardiorenal (*see also* Hypertension, cardiorenal) 404.90
  - cardiovascular (*see also* Disease, cardiovascular) 429.2
  - heart (*see also* Disease, heart) 429.9
    - failure - *see* Failure, heart
  - hepatic 572.2
  - myocardial (acute) (chronic) (*see also* Disease, heart) 429.9
    - failure - *see* Failure, heart
  - respiratory 519.9
- **Decompression sickness** 993.3
- **Decrease, decreased**
  - blood
    - platelets (*see also* Thrombocytopenia) 287.5
    - pressure 796.3
      - due to shock following
        - injury 958.4
        - operation 998.0
  - cardiac reserve - *see* Disease, heart
  - estrogen 256.39
    - postablative 256.2
  - fetal movements 655.7
  - fragility of erythrocytes 289.89 ⬅
  - function
    - adrenal (cortex) 255.4
      - medulla 255.5
    - ovary in hypopituitarism 253.4
    - parenchyma of pancreas 577.8
    - pituitary (gland) (lobe) (anterior) 253.2
      - posterior (lobe) 253.8
  - functional activity 780.99
  - glucose 790.29 ⬅
  - haptoglobin (serum) NEC 273.8
  - libido 799.81 ◀
  - platelets (*see also* Thrombocytopenia) 287.5
  - pulse pressure 785.9
  - respiration due to shock following injury 958.4
  - sexual desire 799.81 ◀
  - tear secretion NEC 375.15
  - tolerance
    - fat 579.8
    - salt and water 276.9
  - vision NEC 369.9
- **Decubial gangrene** 707.0 *[785.4]*
- **Decubiti** (*see also* Decubitus) 707.0
- **Decubitus** (ulcer) 707.0
  - with gangrene 707.0 *[785.4]*
- **Deepening acetabulum** 718.85
- **Defect, defective** 759.9
  - 3-beta-hydroxysteroid dehydrogenase 255.2
  - 11-hydroxylase 255.2
  - 21-hydroxylase 255.2
  - abdominal wall, congenital 756.70
  - aorticopulmonary septum 745.0
  - aortic septal 745.0
  - atrial septal (ostium secundum type) 745.5
    - acquired 429.71
    - ostium primum type 745.61
    - sinus venosus 745.8
  - atrioventricular
    - canal 745.69
- **Defect, defective** *(Continued)*
  - atrioventricular *(Continued)*
    - septum 745.4
      - acquired 429.71
  - atrium secundum 745.5
    - acquired 429.71
  - auricular septal 745.5
    - acquired 429.71
  - bilirubin excretion 277.4
  - biosynthesis, testicular androgen 257.2
  - bulbar septum 745.0
  - butanol-insoluble iodide 246.1
  - chromosome - *see* Anomaly, chromosome
  - circulation (acquired) 459.9
    - congenital 747.9
    - newborn 747.9
  - clotting NEC (*see also* Defect, coagulation) 286.9
  - coagulation (factor) (*see also* Deficiency, coagulation factor) 286.9
    - with
      - abortion - *see* Abortion, by type, with hemorrhage
      - ectopic pregnancy (*see also* categories 634-638) 639.1
      - molar pregnancy (*see also* categories 630-632) 639.1
    - acquired (any) 286.7
    - antepartum or intrapartum 641.3
      - affecting fetus or newborn 762.1
    - causing hemorrhage of pregnancy or delivery 641.3
    - due to
      - liver disease 286.7
      - vitamin K deficiency 286.7
    - newborn, transient 776.3
    - postpartum 666.3
    - specified type NEC 286.3
  - conduction (heart) 426.9
    - bone (*see also* Deafness, conductive) 389.00
  - congenital, organ or site NEC - *see also* Anomaly
    - circulation 747.9
    - Descemet's membrane 743.9
      - specified type NEC 743.49
    - diaphragm 756.6
    - ectodermal 757.9
    - esophagus 750.9
    - pulmonic cusps - *see* Anomaly, heart valve
    - respiratory system 748.9
      - specified type NEC 748.8
  - cushion endocardial 745.60
  - dentin (hereditary) 520.5
  - Descemet's membrane (congenital) 743.9
    - acquired 371.30
    - specific type NEC 743.49
  - deutan 368.52
  - developmental - *see also* Anomaly, by site
    - cauda equina 742.59
    - left ventricle 746.9
      - with atresia or hypoplasia of aortic orifice or valve, with hypoplasia of ascending aorta 746.7
      - in hypoplastic left heart syndrome 746.7
    - testis 752.9
    - vessel 747.9

Deficiency, deficient *(Continued)*
- coagulation factor NEC *(Continued)*
  - due to
    - liver disease 286.7
    - vitamin K deficiency 286.7
  - newborn, transient 776.3
  - postpartum 666.3
  - specified type NEC 286.3
- color vision (congenital) 368.59
  - acquired 368.55
- combined, two or more coagulation factors (*see also* Defect, coagulation) 286.9
- complement factor NEC 279.8
- contact factor (*see also* Defect, coagulation) 286.3
- copper NEC 275.1
- corticoadrenal 255.4
- craniofacial axis 756.0
- cyanocobalamin (vitamin B_{12}) 266.2
- debrancher enzyme (limit dextrinosis) 271.0
- desmolase 255.2
- diet 269.9
- dihydrofolate reductase 281.2
- dihydropteridine reductase 270.1
- disaccharidase (intestinal) 271.3
- disease NEC 269.9
- ear(s) V48.8
- edema 262
- endocrine 259.9
- enzymes, circulating NEC (*see also* Deficiency, by specific enzyme) 277.6
- ergosterol 268.9
  - with
    - osteomalacia 268.2
    - rickets (*see also* Rickets) 268.0
- erythrocytic glutathione (anemia) 282.2
- eyelid(s) V48.8
- factor (*see also* Defect, coagulation) 286.9
  - I (congenital) (fibrinogen) 286.3
    - antepartum or intrapartum 641.3
      - affecting fetus or newborn 762.1
    - newborn, transient 776.3
    - postpartum 666.3
  - II (congenital) (prothrombin) 286.3
  - V (congenital) (labile) 286.3
  - VII (congenital) (stable) 286.3
  - VIII (congenital) (functional) 286.0
    - with
      - functional defect 286.0
      - vascular defect 286.4
  - IX (Christmas) (congenital) (functional) 286.1
  - X (congenital) (Stuart-Prower) 286.3
  - XI (congenital) (plasma thromboplastin antecedent) 286.2
  - XII (congenital) (Hageman) 286.3
  - XIII (congenital) (fibrin stabilizing) 286.3
  - Hageman 286.3
  - multiple (congenital) 286.9
    - acquired 286.7
- fibrinase (*see also* Defect, coagulation) 286.3
- fibrinogen (congenital) (*see also* Defect, coagulation) 286.3
  - acquired 286.6
- fibrin-stabilizing factor (congenital) (*see also* Defect, coagulation) 286.3
  - acquired 286.7
- finger - *see* Absence, finger

Deficiency, deficient *(Continued)*
- fletcher factor (*see also* Defect, coagulation) 286.9
- fluorine 269.3
- folate, anemia 281.2
- folic acid (vitamin B_C) 266.2
  - anemia 281.2
- follicle-stimulating hormone (FSH) 253.4
- fructokinase 271.2
- fructose-1, 6-diphosphate 271.2
- fructose-1-phosphate aldolase 271.2
- FSH (follicle-stimulating hormone) 253.4
- fucosidase 271.8
- galactokinase 271.1
- galactose-1-phosphate uridyl transferase 271.1
- gamma globulin in blood 279.00
- glass factor (*see also* Defect, coagulation) 286.3
- glucocorticoid 255.4
- glucose-6-phosphatase 271.0
- glucose-6-phosphate dehydrogenase anemia 282.2
- glucuronyl transferase 277.4
- glutathione-reductase (anemia) 282.2
- glycogen synthetase 271.0
- growth hormone 253.3
- Hageman factor (congenital) (*see also* Defect, coagulation) 286.3
- head V48.0
- hemoglobin (*see also* Anemia) 285.9
- hepatophosphorylase 271.0
- hexose monophosphate (HMP) shunt 282.2
- hGH (human growth hormone) 253.3
- HG-PRT 277.2
- homogentisic acid oxidase 270.2
- hormone - *see also* Deficiency, by specific hormone
  - anterior pituitary (isolated) (partial) NEC 253.4
    - growth (human) 253.3
  - follicle-stimulating 253.4
  - growth (human) (isolated) 253.3
  - human growth 253.3
  - interstitial cell-stimulating 253.4
  - luteinizing 253.4
  - melanocyte-stimulating 253.4
  - testicular 257.2
- human growth hormone 253.3
- humoral 279.00
  - with
    - hyper-IgM 279.05
      - autosomal recessive 279.05
      - X-linked 279.05
    - increased IgM 279.05
  - congenital hypogammaglobulinemia 279.04
    - non-sex-linked 279.06
  - selective immunoglobulin NEC 279.03
    - IgA 279.01
    - IgG 279.03
    - IgM 279.02
      - increased 279.05
  - specified NEC 279.09
- hydroxylase 255.2
- hypoxanthine-guanine phosphoribosyltransferase (HG-PRT) 277.2
- ICSH (interstitial cell-stimulating hormone) 253.4

Deficiency, deficient *(Continued)*
- immunity NEC 279.3
  - cell-mediated 279.10
    - with
      - hyperimmunoglobulinemia 279.2
      - thrombocytopenia and eczema 279.12
    - specified NEC 279.19
  - combined (severe) 279.2
    - syndrome 279.2
  - common variable 279.06
  - humoral NEC 279.00
  - IgA (secretory) 279.01
  - IgG 279.03
  - IgM 279.02
- immunoglobulin, selective NEC 279.03
  - IgA 279.01
  - IgG 279.03
  - IgM 279.02
- inositol (B complex) 266.2
- interferon 279.4
- internal organ V47.0
- interstitial cell-stimulating hormone (ICSH) 253.4
- intrinsic factor (Castle's) (congenital) 281.0
- intrinsic (urethral) sphincter (ISD) 599.82
- invertase 271.3
- iodine 269.3
- iron, anemia 280.9
- labile factor (congenital) (*see also* Defect, coagulation) 286.3
  - acquired 286.7
- lacrimal fluid (acquired) 375.15
  - congenital 743.64
- lactase 271.3
- Laki-Lorand factor (*see also* Defect, coagulation) 286.3
- lecithin-cholesterol acyltranferase 272.5
- LH (luteinizing hormone) 253.4
- limb V49.0
  - lower V49.0
    - congenital (*see also* Deficiency, lower limb, congenital) 755.30
  - upper V49.0
    - congenital (*see also* Deficiency, upper limb, congenital) 755.20
- lipocaic 577.8
- lipoid (high-density) 272.5
- lipoprotein (familial) (high-density) 272.5
- liver phosphorylase 271.0
- lower limb V49.0
  - congenital 755.30
    - with complete absence of distal elements 755.31
    - longitudinal (complete) (partial) (with distal deficiencies, incomplete) 755.32
      - with complete absence of distal elements 755.31
      - combined femoral, tibial, fibular (incomplete) 755.33
      - femoral 755.34
      - fibular 755.37
      - metatarsal(s) 755.38
      - phalange(s) 755.39
        - meaning all digits 755.31
      - tarsal(s) 755.38
      - tibia 755.36
      - tibiofibular 755.35
    - transverse 755.31

ICD-9-CM
D
Vol. 2

◀ New ◀ Revised Code

- **Deformity** *(Continued)*
  - eyebrow (congenital) 744.89
  - eyelid (congenital) 743.9
    - acquired 374.89
    - specified type NEC 743.62
  - face (acquired) 738.19
    - congenital (any part) 744.9
      - due to intrauterine malposition and pressure 754.0
  - fallopian tube (congenital) 752.10
    - acquired 620.8
  - femur (acquired) 736.89
    - congenital 755.60
  - fetal
    - with fetopelvic disproportion 653.7
      - affecting fetus or newborn 763.1
    - causing obstructed labor 660.1
      - affecting fetus or newborn 763.1
    - known or suspected, affecting management of pregnancy 655.9
  - finger (acquired) 736.20
    - boutonniere type 736.21
    - congenital 755.50
    - flexion contracture 718.44
    - swan neck 736.22
  - flexion (joint) (acquired) 736.9
    - congenital NEC 755.9
    - hip or thigh (acquired) 736.39
      - congenital (*see also* Subluxation, congenital, hip) 754.32
  - foot (acquired) 736.70
    - cavovarus 736.75
      - congenital 754.59
    - congenital NEC 754.70
      - specified type NEC 754.79
    - valgus (acquired) 736.79
      - congenital 754.60
        - specified type NEC 754.69
    - varus (acquired) 736.79
      - congenital 754.50
        - specified type NEC 754.59
  - forearm (acquired) 736.00
    - congenital 755.50
  - forehead (acquired) 738.19
    - congenital (*see also* Deformity, skull, congenital) 756.0
  - frontal bone (acquired) 738.19
    - congenital (*see also* Deformity, skull, congenital) 756.0
  - gallbladder (congenital) 751.60
    - acquired 575.8
  - gastrointestinal tract (congenital) NEC 751.9
    - acquired 569.89
    - specified type NEC 751.8
  - genitalia, genital organ(s) or system NEC
    - congenital 752.9
    - female (congenital) 752.9
      - acquired 629.8
      - external 752.40
      - internal 752.9
    - male (congenital) 752.9
      - acquired 608.89
  - globe (eye) (congenital) 743.9
    - acquired 360.89
  - gum (congenital) 750.9
    - acquired 523.9
  - gunstock 736.02
  - hand (acquired) 736.00
    - claw 736.06
    - congenital 755.50
    - minus (and plus) (intrinsic) 736.09
    - pill roller (intrinsic) 736.09

- **Deformity** *(Continued)*
  - hand (acquired) *(Continued)*
    - plus (and minus) (intrinsic) 736.09
    - swan neck (intrinsic) 736.09
  - head (acquired) 738.10
    - congenital (*see also* Deformity, skull, congenital) 756.0
    - specified NEC 738.19
  - heart (congenital) 746.9
    - auricle (congenital) 746.9
    - septum 745.9
      - auricular 745.5
      - specified type NEC 745.8
      - ventricular 745.4
    - valve (congenital) NEC 746.9
      - acquired - *see* Endocarditis
      - pulmonary (congenital) 746.00
      - specified type NEC 746.89
    - ventricle (congenital) 746.9
  - heel (acquired) 736.76
    - congenital 755.67
  - hepatic duct (congenital) 751.60
    - acquired 576.8
      - with calculus, choledocholithiasis, or stones - *see* Choledocholithiasis
  - hip (joint) (acquired) 736.30
    - congenital NEC 755.63
    - flexion 718.45
      - congenital (*see also* Subluxation, congenital, hip) 754.32
  - hourglass - *see* Contraction, hourglass
  - humerus (acquired) 736.89
    - congenital 755.50
  - hymen (congenital) 752.40
  - hypophyseal (congenital) 759.2
  - ileocecal (coil) (valve) (congenital) 751.5
    - acquired 569.89
  - ileum (intestine) (congenital) 751.5
    - acquired 569.89
  - ilium (acquired) 738.6
    - congenital 755.60
  - integument (congenital) 757.9
  - intervertebral cartilage or disc (acquired) - *see also* Displacement, intervertebral disc
    - congenital 756.10
  - intestine (large) (small) (congenital) 751.5
    - acquired 569.89
  - iris (acquired) 364.75
    - congenital 743.9
    - prolapse 364.8
  - ischium (acquired) 738.6
    - congenital 755.60
  - jaw (acquired) (congenital) NEC 524.9
    - due to intrauterine malposition and pressure 754.0
  - joint (acquired) NEC 738.8
    - congenital 755.9
    - contraction (abduction) (adduction) (extension) (flexion) - *see* Contraction, joint
  - kidney(s) (calyx) (pelvis) (congenital) 753.9
    - acquired 593.89
    - vessel 747.62
      - acquired 459.9
  - Klippel-Feil (brevicollis) 756.16
  - knee (acquired) NEC 736.6
    - congenital 755.64
  - labium (majus) (minus) (congenital) 752.40
    - acquired 624.8

- **Deformity** *(Continued)*
  - lacrimal apparatus or duct (congenital) 743.9
    - acquired 375.69
  - larynx (muscle) (congenital) 748.3
    - acquired 478.79
    - web (glottic) (subglottic) 748.2
  - leg (lower) (upper) (acquired) NEC 736.89
    - congenital 755.60
      - reduction - *see* Deformity, reduction, lower limb
  - lens (congenital) 743.9
    - acquired 379.39
  - lid (fold) (congenital) 743.9
    - acquired 374.89
  - ligament (acquired) 728.9
    - congenital 756.9
  - limb (acquired) 736.9
    - congenital, except reduction deformity 755.9
      - lower 755.60
        - reduction (*see also* Deformity, reduction, lower limb) 755.30
      - upper 755.50
        - reduction (*see also* Deformity, reduction, lower limb) 755.20
    - specified NEC 736.89
  - lip (congenital) NEC 750.9
    - acquired 528.5
    - specified type NEC 750.26
  - liver (congenital) 751.60
    - acquired 573.8
    - duct (congenital) 751.60
      - acquired 576.8
        - with calculus, choledocholithiasis, or stones - *see* Choledocholithiasis
  - lower extremity - *see* Deformity, leg
  - lumbosacral (joint) (region) (congenital) 756.10
    - acquired 738.5
  - lung (congenital) 748.60
    - acquired 518.89
    - specified type NEC 748.69
  - lymphatic system, congenital 759.9
  - Madelung's (radius) 755.54
  - maxilla (acquired) (congenital) 524.9
  - meninges or membrane (congenital) 742.9
    - brain 742.4
      - acquired 349.2
    - spinal (cord) 742.59
      - acquired 349.2
  - mesentery (congenital) 751.9
    - acquired 568.89
  - metacarpus (acquired) 736.00
    - congenital 755.50
  - metatarsus (acquired) 736.70
    - congenital 754.70
  - middle ear, except ossicles (congenital) 744.03
    - ossicles 744.04
  - mitral (leaflets) (valve) (congenital) 746.9
    - acquired - *see* Endocarditis, mitral
    - Ebstein's 746.89
    - parachute 746.5
    - specified type NEC 746.89
    - stenosis, congenital 746.5
  - mouth (acquired) 528.9
    - congenital NEC 750.9
      - specified type NEC 750.26
  - multiple, congenital NEC 759.7

ICD-9-CM

D

Vol. 2

Degeneration, degenerative *(Continued)*
- changes, spine or vertebra (*see also* Spondylosis) 721.90
- chitinous 277.3
- chorioretinal 363.40
  - congenital 743.53
  - hereditary 363.50
- choroid (colloid) (drusen) 363.40
  - hereditary 363.50
  - senile 363.41
    - diffuse secondary 363.42
- cochlear 386.8
- collateral ligament (knee) (medial) 717.82
  - lateral 717.81
- combined (spinal cord) (subacute) 266.2 *[336.2]*
  - with anemia (pernicious) 281.0 *[336.2]*
    - due to dietary deficiency 281.1 *[336.2]*
  - due to vitamin B_{12} deficiency anemia (dietary) 281.1 [336.2]
- conjunctiva 372.50
  - amyloid 277.3 *[372.50]*
- cornea 371.40
  - calcerous 371.44
  - familial (hereditary) (*see also* Dystrophy, cornea) 371.50
    - macular 371.55
    - reticular 371.54
  - hyaline (of old scars) 371.41
  - marginal (Terrien's) 371.48
  - mosaic (shagreen) 371.41
  - nodular 371.46
  - peripheral 371.48
  - senile 371.41
- cortical (cerebellar) (parenchymatous) 334.2
  - alcoholic 303.9 *[334.4]*
  - diffuse, due to arteriopathy 437.0
- corticostriatal-spinal 334.8
- cretinoid 243
- cruciate ligament (knee) (posterior) 717.84
  - anterior 717.83
- cutis 709.3
  - amyloid 277.3
- dental pulp 522.2
- disc disease - *see* Degeneration, intervertebral disc
- dorsolateral (spinal cord) - *see* Degeneration, combined
- endocardial 424.90
- extrapyramidal NEC 333.90
- eye NEC 360.40
  - macular (*see also* Degeneration, macula) 362.50
    - congenital 362.75
    - hereditary 362.76
- fatty (diffuse) (general) 272.8
  - liver 571.8
    - alcoholic 571.0
  - localized site - *see* Degeneration, by site, fatty
  - placenta - *see* Placenta, abnormal
- globe (eye) NEC 360.40
  - macular - *see* Degeneration, macula
- grey matter 330.8
- heart (brown) (calcareous) (fatty) (fibrous) (hyaline) (mural) (muscular) (pigmentary) (senile) (with arteriosclerosis) (*see also* Degeneration, myocardial) 429.1

Degeneration, degenerative *(Continued)*
- heart *(Continued)*
  - amyloid 277.3 *[425.7]*
  - atheromatous - *see* Arteriosclerosis, coronary
  - gouty 274.82
  - hypertensive (*see also* Hypertension, heart) 402.90
  - ischemic 414.9
  - valve, valvular - *see* Endocarditis
- hepatolenticular (Wilson's) 275.1
- hepatorenal 572.4
- heredofamilial
  - brain NEC 331.89
  - spinal cord NEC 336.8
- hyaline (diffuse) (generalized) 728.9
  - localized - *see also* Degeneration, by site
    - cornea 371.41
    - keratitis 371.41
- hypertensive vascular - *see* Hypertension
- infrapatellar fat pad 729.31
- internal semilunar cartilage 717.3
- intervertebral disc 722.6
  - with myelopathy 722.70
  - cervical, cervicothoracic 722.4
    - with myelopathy 722.71
  - lumbar, lumbosacral 722.52
    - with myelopathy 722.73
  - thoracic, thoracolumbar 722.51
    - with myelopathy 722.72
- intestine 569.89
  - amyloid 277.3
  - lardaceous 277.3
- iris (generalized) (*see also* Atrophy, iris) 364.59
  - pigmentary 364.53
  - pupillary margin 364.54
- ischemic - *see* Ischemia
- joint disease (*see also* Osteoarthrosis) 715.9
  - multiple sites 715.09
  - spine (*see also* Spondylosis) 721.90
- kidney (*see also* Sclerosis, renal) 587
  - amyloid 277.3 *[583.81]*
  - cyst, cystic (multiple) (solitary) 593.2
    - congenital (*see also* Cystic, disease, kidney) 753.10
  - fatty 593.89
  - fibrocystic (congenital) 753.19
  - lardaceous 277.3 *[583.81]*
  - polycystic (congenital) 753.12
    - adult type (APKD) 753.13
    - autosomal dominant 753.13
    - autosomal recessive 753.14
    - childhood type (CPKD) 753.14
    - infantile type 753.14
  - waxy 277.3 *[583.81]*
- Kuhnt-Junius (retina) 362.52
- labyrinth, osseous 386.8
- lacrimal passages, cystic 375.12
- lardaceous (any site) 277.3
- lateral column (posterior), spinal cord (*see also* Degeneration, combined) 266.2 [336.2]
- lattice 362.63
- lens 366.9
  - infantile, juvenile, or presenile 366.00
  - senile 366.10
- lenticular (familial) (progressive) (Wilson's) (with cirrhosis of liver) 275.1
  - striate artery 437.0

Degeneration, degenerative *(Continued)*
- lethal ball, prosthetic heart valve 996.02
- ligament
  - collateral (knee) (medial) 717.82
    - lateral 717.81
  - cruciate (knee) (posterior) 717.84
    - anterior 717.83
- liver (diffuse) 572.8
  - amyloid 277.3
  - congenital (cystic) 751.62
  - cystic 572.8
    - congenital 751.62
  - fatty 571.8
    - alcoholic 571.0
  - hypertrophic 572.8
  - lardaceous 277.3
  - parenchymatous, acute or subacute (*see also* Necrosis, liver) 570
  - pigmentary 572.8
  - toxic (acute) 573.8
  - waxy 277.3
- lung 518.89
- lymph gland 289.3
  - hyaline 289.3
  - lardaceous 277.3
- macula (acquired) (senile) 362.50
  - atrophic 362.51
  - Best's 362.76
  - congenital 362.75
  - cystic 362.54
  - cystoid 362.53
  - disciform 362.52
  - dry 362.51
  - exudative 362.52
  - familial pseudoinflammatory 362.77
  - hereditary 362.76
  - hole 362.54
  - juvenile (Stargardt's) 362.75
  - nonexudative 362.51
  - pseudohole 362.54
  - wet 362.52
- medullary - *see* Degeneration, brain
- membranous labyrinth, congenital (causing impairment of hearing) 744.05
- meniscus - *see* Derangement, joint
- microcystoid 362.62
- mitral - *see* Insufficiency, mitral
- Mönckeberg's (*see also* Arteriosclerosis, extremities) 440.20
- moral 301.7
- motor centers, senile 331.2
- mural (*see also* Degeneration, myocardial) 429.1
  - heart, cardiac (*see also* Degeneration, myocardial) 429.1
  - myocardium, myocardial (*see also* Degeneration, myocardial) 429.1
- muscle 728.9
  - fatty 728.9
  - fibrous 728.9
  - heart (*see also* Degeneration, myocardial) 429.1
  - hyaline 728.9
- muscular progressive 728.2
- myelin, central nervous system NEC 341.9
- myocardium, myocardial (brown) (calcareous) (fatty) (fibrous) (hyaline) (mural) (muscular) (pigmentary) (senile) (with arteriosclerosis) 429.1

ICD-9-CM
D
Vol. 2

Note Use the following fifth-digit subclassification with categories 640-648, 651-676:

0 unspecified as to episode of care
1 delivered, with or without mention of antepartum condition
2 delivered, with mention of postpartum complication
3 antepartum condition or complication
4 postpartum condition or complication

ICD-9-CM
D
Vol. 2

Dementia *(Continued)*
  presenile *(Continued)*
    depressed type 290.13
    paranoid type 290.12
    simple type 290.10
    uncomplicated 290.10
  primary (acute) (*see also* Schizophrenia) 295.0
  progressive, syphilitic 094.1
  puerperal - *see* Psychosis, puerperal
  schizophrenic (*see also* Schizophrenia) 295.9
  senile 290.0
    with
      acute confusional state 290.3
      delirium 290.3
      delusional features 290.20
      depressive features 290.21
    depressed type 290.21
    exhaustion 290.0
    paranoid type 290.20
  simple type (acute) (*see also* Schizophrenia) 295.0
  simplex (acute) (*see also* Schizophrenia) 295.0
  syphilitic 094.1
  uremic - *see* Uremia
  vascular 290.40
Demerol dependence (*see also* Dependence) 304.0
Demineralization, ankle (*see also* Osteoporosis) 733.00
Demodex folliculorum (infestation) 133.8
de Morgan's spots (senile angiomas) 448.1
Demyelinating
  polyneuritis, chronic inflammatory 357.81
Demyelination, demyelinization
  central nervous system 341.9
    specified NEC 341.8
  corpus callosum (central) 341.8
  global 340
Dengue (fever) 061
  sandfly 061
  vaccination, prophylactic (against) V05.1
  virus hemorrhagic fever 065.4
Dens
  evaginatus 520.2
  in dente 520.2
  invaginatus 520.2
Density
  increased, bone (disseminated) (generalized) (spotted) 733.99
  lung (nodular) 518.89
Dental - *see also* condition
  examination only V72.2
Dentia praecox 520.6
Denticles (in pulp) 522.2
Dentigerous cyst 526.0
Dentin
  irregular (in pulp) 522.3
  opalescent 520.5
  secondary (in pulp) 522.3
  sensitive 521.8
Dentinogenesis imperfecta 520.5
Dentinoma (M9271/0) 213.1
  upper jaw (bone) 213.0
Dentition 520.7
  abnormal 520.6
  anomaly 520.6
  delayed 520.6
  difficult 520.7
  disorder of 520.6
  precocious 520.6
  retarded 520.6
Denture sore (mouth) 528.9
Dependence

> Note Use the following fifth-digit subclassification with category 304:
>
> 0 unspecified
> 1 continuous
> 2 episodic
> 3 in remission

  with
    withdrawal symptoms
      alcohol 291.81
      drug 292.0
  14-hydroxy-dihydromorphinone 304.0
  absinthe 304.6
  acemorphan 304.0
  acetanilid(e) 304.6
  acetophenetidin 304.6
  acetorphine 304.0
  acetyldihydrocodeine 304.0
  acetyldihydrocodeinone 304.0
  Adalin 304.1
  Afghanistan black 304.3
  agrypnal 304.1
  alcohol, alcoholic (ethyl) (methyl) (wood) 303.9
    maternal, with suspected fetal damage affecting management of pregnancy 655.4
  allobarbitone 304.1
  allonal 304.1
  allylisopropylacetylurea 304.1
  alphaprodine (hydrochloride) 304.0
  Alurate 304.1
  Alvodine 304.0
  amethocaine 304.6
  amidone 304.0
  amidopyrine 304.6
  aminopyrine 304.6
  amobarbital 304.1
  amphetamine(s) (type) (drugs classifiable to 969.7) 304.4
  amylene hydrate 304.6
  amylobarbitone 304.1
  amylocaine 304.6
  Amytal (sodium) 304.1
  analgesic (drug) NEC 304.6
    synthetic with morphine-like effect 304.0
  anesthetic (agent) (drug) (gas) (general) (local) NEC 304.6
  Angel dust 304.6
  anileridine 304.0
  antipyrine 304.6
  aprobarbital 304.1
  aprobarbitone 304.1
  atropine 304.6
  Avertin (bromide) 304.6
  barbenyl 304.1
  barbital(s) 304.1
  barbitone 304.1
  barbiturate(s) (compounds) (drugs classifiable to 967.0) 304.1
  barbituric acid (and compounds) 304.1
  benzedrine 304.4
  benzylmorphine 304.0
  Beta-chlor 304.1
  bhang 304.3
  blue velvet 304.0
  Brevital 304.1
  bromal (hydrate) 304.1
  bromide(s) NEC 304.1
  bromine compounds NEC 304.1
  bromisovalum 304.1
Dependence *(Continued)*
  bromoform 304.1
  Bromo-seltzer 304.1
  bromural 304.1
  butabarbital (sodium) 304.1
  butabarpal 304.1
  butallylonal 304.1
  butethal 304.1
  buthalitone (sodium) 304.1
  Butisol 304.1
  butobarbitone 304.1
  butyl chloral (hydrate) 304.1
  caffeine 304.4
  cannabis (indica) (sativa) (resin) (derivatives) (type) 304.3
  carbamazepine 304.6
  Carbrital 304.1
  carbromal 304.1
  carisoprodol 304.6
  Catha (edulis) 304.4
  chloral (betaine) (hydrate) 304.1
  chloralamide 304.1
  chloralformamide 304.1
  chloralose 304.1
  chlordiazepoxide 304.1
  Chloretone 304.1
  chlorobutanol 304.1
  chlorodyne 304.1
  chloroform 304.6
  Cliradon 304.0
  coca (leaf) and derivatives 304.2
  cocaine 304.2
    hydrochloride 304.2
    salt (any) 304.2
  codeine 304.0
  combination of drugs (excluding morphine or opioid type drug) NEC 304.8
    morphine or opioid type drug with any other drug 304.7
  croton-chloral 304.1
  cyclobarbital 304.1
  cyclobarbitone 304.1
  dagga 304.3
  Delvinal 304.1
  Demerol 304.0
  desocodeine 304.0
  desomorphine 304.0
  desoxyephedrine 304.4
  DET 304.5
  dexamphetamine 304.4
  dexedrine 304.4
  dextromethorphan 304.0
  dextromoramide 304.0
  dextronorpseudoephedrine 304.4
  dextrorphan 304.0
  diacetylmorphine 304.0
  Dial 304.1
  diallylbarbituric acid 304.1
  diamorphine 304.0
  diazepam 304.1
  dibucaine 304.6
  dichloroethane 304.6
  diethyl barbituric acid 304.1
  diethylsulfone-diethylmethane 304.1
  difencloxazine 304.0
  dihydrocodeine 304.0
  dihydrocodeinone 304.0
  dihydrohydroxycodeinone 304.0
  dihydroisocodeine 304.0
  dihydromorphine 304.0
  dihydromorphinone 304.0
  dihydroxcodeinone 304.0
  Dilaudid 304.0

◀ New ⟵ Revised Code

ICD-9-CM

D

Vol. 2

- **Dermatitis** *(Continued)*
  - eyelid *(Continued)*
    - infective *(Continued)*
      - due to *(Continued)*
        - leprosy (*see also* Leprosy) 030.0 *[373.4]*
        - lupus vulgaris (tuberculous) (*see also* Tuberculosis) 017.0 *[373.4]*
        - mycotic dermatitis (*see also* Dermatomycosis) 111.9 *[373.5]*
        - vaccinia 051.0 *[373.5]*
          - postvaccination 999.0 *[373.5]*
      - yaws (*see also* Yaws) 102.9 *[373.4]*
  - facta, factitia 698.4
    - psychogenic 316 *[698.4]*
  - ficta 698.4
    - psychogenic 316 *[698.4]*
  - flexural 691.8
  - follicularis 704.8
  - friction 709.8
  - fungus 111.9
    - specified type NEC 111.8
  - gangrenosa, gangrenous (infantum) (*see also* Gangrene) 785.4
  - gestationis 646.8
  - gonococcal 098.89
  - gouty 274.89
  - harvest mite 133.8
  - heat 692.89
  - herpetiformis (bullous) (erythematous) (pustular) (vesicular) 694.0
    - juvenile 694.2
    - senile 694.5
  - hiemalis 692.89
  - hypostatic, hypostatica 454.1
    - with ulcer 454.2
  - impetiginous 684
  - infantile (acute) (chronic) (intertriginous) (intrinsic) (seborrheic) 690.12
  - infectiosa eczematoides 690.8
  - infectious (staphylococcal) (streptococcal) 686.9
    - eczematoid 690.8
  - infective eczematoid 690.8
  - Jacquet's (diaper dermatitis) 691.0
  - leptus 133.8
  - lichenified NEC 692.9
  - lichenoid, chronic 701.0
  - lichenoides purpurica pigmentosa 709.1
  - meadow 692.6
  - medicamentosa (correct substance properly administered) (internal use) (*see also* Dermatitis, due to, drugs or medicinals) 693.0
    - due to contact with skin 692.3
  - mite 133.8
  - multiformis 694.0
    - juvenile 694.2
    - senile 694.5
  - napkin 691.0
  - neuro 698.3
  - neurotica 694.0
  - nummular NEC 692.9
  - osteatosis, osteatotic 706.8
  - papillaris capillitii 706.1
  - pellagrous 265.2
  - perioral 695.3
  - perstans 696.1
  - photosensitivity (sun) 692.72
    - other light 692.82
  - pigmented purpuric lichenoid 709.1
  - polymorpha dolorosa 694.0
  - primary irritant 692.9
  - pruriginosa 694.0
- **Dermatitis** *(Continued)*
  - pruritic NEC 692.9
  - psoriasiform nodularis 696.2
  - psychogenic 316
  - purulent 686.00
  - pustular contagious 051.2
  - pyococcal 686.00
  - pyocyaneus 686.09
  - pyogenica 686.00
  - radiation 692.82
  - repens 696.1
  - Ritter's (exfoliativa) 695.81
  - Schamberg's (progressive pigmentary dermatosis) 709.09
  - schistosome 120.3
  - seasonal bullous 694.8
  - seborrheic 690.10
    - infantile 690.12
  - sensitization NEC 692.9
  - septic (*see also* Septicemia) 686.00
    - gonococcal 098.89
  - solar, solare NEC (*see also* Dermatitis, due to, sun) 692.70
  - stasis 459.81
    - due to
      - postphlebitic syndrome 459.12
        - with ulcer 459.13
      - varicose veins - *see* Varicose
    - ulcerated or with ulcer (varicose) 454.2
  - sunburn (*see also* Sunburn) 692.71
  - suppurative 686.00
  - traumatic NEC 709.8
  - trophoneurotica 694.0
  - ultraviolet, except from sun 692.82
    - due to sun NEC (*see also* Dermatitis, due to, sun) 692.70
  - varicose 454.1
    - with ulcer 454.2
  - vegetans 686.8
  - verrucosa 117.2
  - xerotic 706.8
- **Dermatoarthritis, lipoid** 272.8 *[713.0]*
- **Dermatochalasia, dermatochalasis** 374.87
- **Dermatofibroma** (lenticulare) (M8832/0) - *see also* Neoplasm, skin, benign
  - protuberans (M8832/1) - *see* Neoplasm, skin, uncertain behavior
- **Dermatofibrosarcoma** (protuberans) (M8832/3) - *see* Neoplasm, skin, malignant
- **Dermatographia** 708.3
- **Dermatolysis** (congenital) (exfoliativa) 757.39
  - acquired 701.8
  - eyelids 374.34
  - palpebrarum 374.34
  - senile 701.8
- **Dermatomegaly NEC** 701.8
- **Dermatomucomyositis** 710.3
- **Dermatomycosis** 111.9
  - furfuracea 111.0
  - specified type NEC 111.8
- **Dermatomyositis** (acute) (chronic) 710.3
- **Dermatoneuritis of children** 985.0
- **Dermatophiliasis** 134.1
- **Dermatophytide** - *see* Dermatophytosis
- **Dermatophytosis** (Epidermophyton) (infection) (microsporum) (tinea) (Trichophyton) 110.9
  - beard 110.0
  - body 110.5
  - deep seated 110.6
  - fingernails 110.1
  - foot 110.4
  - groin 110.3
- **Dermatophytosis** *(Continued)*
  - hand 110.2
  - nail 110.1
  - perianal (area) 110.3
  - scalp 110.0
  - scrotal 110.8
  - specified site NEC 110.8
  - toenails 110.1
  - vulva 110.8
- **Dermatopolyneuritis** 985.0
- **Dermatorrhexis** 756.83
  - acquired 701.8
- **Dermatosclerosis** (*see also* Scleroderma) 710.1
  - localized 701.0
- **Dermatosis** 709.9
  - Andrews' 686.8
  - atopic 691.8
  - Bowen's (M8081/2) - *see* Neoplasm, skin, in situ
  - bullous 694.9
    - specified type NEC 694.8
  - erythematosquamous 690.8
  - exfoliativa 695.89
  - factitial 698.4
  - gonococcal 098.89
  - herpetiformis 694.0
    - juvenile 694.2
    - senile 694.5
  - hysterical 300.11
  - Linear IgA 694.8
  - menstrual NEC 709.8
  - neutrophilic, acute febrile 695.89
  - occupational (*see also* Dermatitis) 692.9
  - papulosa nigra 709.8
  - pigmentary NEC 709.00
    - progressive 709.09
    - Schamberg's 709.09
    - Siemens-Bloch 757.33
  - progressive pigmentary 709.09
  - psychogenic 316
  - pustular subcorneal 694.1
  - Schamberg's (progressive pigmentary) 709.09
  - senile NEC 709.3
  - specified NEC 702.8
  - Unna's (seborrheic dermatitis) 690.10
- **Dermographia** 708.3
- **Dermographism** 708.3
- **Dermoid** (cyst) (M9084/0) - *see also* Neoplasm, by site, benign
  - with malignant transformation (M9084/3) 183.0
- **Dermopathy**
  - infiltrative, with thyrotoxicosis 242.0
  - senile NEC 709.3
- **Dermophytosis** - *see* Dermatophytosis
- **Descemet's membrane** - *see* condition
- **Descemetocele** 371.72
- **Descending** - *see* condition
- **Descensus uteri** (complete) (incomplete) (partial) (without vaginal wall prolapse) 618.1
  - with mention of vaginal wall prolapse - *see* Prolapse, uterovaginal
- **Desensitization to allergens** V07.1
- **Desert**
  - rheumatism 114.0
  - sore (*see also* Ulcer, skin) 707.9
- **Desertion** (child) (newborn) 995.52
  - adult 995.84
- **Desmoid** (extra-abdominal) (tumor) (M8821/1) - *see also* Neoplasm, connective tissue, uncertain behavior
  - abdominal (M8822/1) - *see* Neoplasm, connective tissue, uncertain behavior

Diabetes, diabetic *(Continued)*

> Note Use the following fifth-digit subclassification with category 250:
>
> 0 type II [non-insulin dependent type] [NIDDM type] [adult-onset type] or unspecified type, not stated as uncontrolled
>
> Fifth-digit 0 is for use for type II, adult-onset diabetic patients, even if the patient requires insulin
>
> 1 type I [insulin dependent type] [IDDM type] [juvenile type], not stated as uncontrolled
>
> 2 type II [non-insulin dependent type] [NIDDM type] [adult-onset type] or unspecified type, uncontrolled
>
> Fifth-digit 2 is for use for type II, adult-onset diabetic patients, even if the patient requires insulin
>
> 3 type I [insulin dependent type] [IDDM type] [juvenile type], uncontrolled

- with
  - coma (with ketoacidosis) 250.3
    - hyperosmolar (nonketotic) 250.2
  - complication NEC 250.9
    - specified NEC 250.8
  - gangrene 250.7 *[785.4]*
  - hyperosmolarity 250.2
  - ketosis, ketoacidosis 250.1
  - osteomyelitis 250.8 *[731.8]*
  - specified manifestations NEC 250.8
- acetonemia 250.1
- acidosis 250.1
- amyotrophy 250.6 *[358.1]*
- angiopathy, peripheral 250.7 *[443.81]*
- asymptomatic 790.29
- autonomic neuropathy (peripheral) 250.6 *[337.1]*
- bone change 250.8 *[731.8]*
- bronze, bronzed 275.0
- cataract 250.5 *[366.41]*
- chemical 790.29
  - complicating pregnancy, childbirth, or puerperium 648.8
- coma (with ketoacidosis) 250.3
  - hyperglycemic 250.3
  - hyperosmolar (nonketotic) 250.2
  - hypoglycemic 250.3
  - insulin 250.3
- complicating pregnancy, childbirth, or puerperium (maternal) 648.0
  - affecting fetus or newborn 775.0
- complication NEC 250.9
  - specified NEC 250.8
- dorsal sclerosis 250.6 *[340]*
- dwarfism-obesity syndrome 258.1
- gangrene 250.7 *[785.4]*
- gastroparesis 250.6 *[536.3]*
- gestational 648.8
  - complicating pregnancy, childbirth, or puerperium 648.8
- glaucoma 250.5 *[365.44]*
- glomerulosclerosis (intercapillary) 250.4 *[581.81]*
- glycogenosis, secondary 250.8 *[259.8]*
- hemochromatosis 275.0

Diabetes, diabetic *(Continued)*

- hyperosmolar coma 250.2
- hyperosmolarity 250.2
- hypertension-nephrosis syndrome 250.4 *[581.81]*
- hypoglycemia 250.8
- hypoglycemic shock 250.8
- insipidus 253.5
  - nephrogenic 588.1
  - pituitary 253.5
  - vasopressin-resistant 588.1
- intercapillary glomerulosclerosis 250.4 *[581.81]*
- iritis 250.5 *[364.42]*
- ketosis, ketoacidosis 250.1
- Kimmelstiel (-Wilson) disease or syndrome (intercapillary glomerulosclerosis) 250.4 *[581.81]*
- Lancereaux's (diabetes mellitus with marked emaciation) 250.8 *[261]*
- latent (chemical) 790.29
  - complicating pregnancy, childbirth, or puerperium 648.8
- lipoidosis 250.8 *[272.7]*
- macular edema 250.5 *[362.01]*
- maternal
  - with manifest disease in the infant 775.1
  - affecting fetus or newborn 775.0
- microaneurysms, retinal 250.5 *[362.01]*
- mononeuropathy 250.6 *[355.9]*
- neonatal, transient 775.1
- nephropathy 250.4 *[583.81]*
- nephrosis (syndrome) 250.4 *[581.81]*
- neuralgia 250.6 *[357.2]*
- neuritis 250.6 *[357.2]*
- neurogenic arthropathy 250.6 *[713.5]*
- neuropathy 250.6 *[357.2]*
- nonclinical 790.29
- osteomyelitis 250.8 *[731.8]*
- peripheral autonomic neuropathy 250.6 *[337.1]*
- phosphate 275.3
- polyneuropathy 250.6 *[357.2]*
- renal (true) 271.4
- retinal
  - edema 250.5 *[362.01]*
  - hemorrhage 250.5 *[362.01]*
  - microaneurysms 250.5 *[362.01]*
- retinitis 250.5 *[362.01]*
- retinopathy 250.5 *[362.01]*
  - background 250.5 *[362.01]*
  - proliferative 250.5 *[362.02]*
- steroid induced
  - correct substance properly administered 251.8
  - overdose or wrong substance given or taken 962.0
- stress 790.29
- subclinical 790.29
- subliminal 790.29
- sugar 250.0
- ulcer (skin) 250.8 *[707.9]*
  - lower extremity 250.8 *[707.10]*
    - ankle 250.8 *[707.13]*
    - calf 250.8 *[707.12]*
    - foot 250.8 *[707.15]*
    - heel 250.8 *[707.14]*
    - knee 250.8 *[707.19]*
    - specified site NEC 250.8 *[707.19]*
    - thigh 250.8 *[707.11]*
    - toes 250.8 *[707.15]*
  - specified site NEC 250.8 *[707.8]*
- xanthoma 250.8 *[272.2]*

Diacyclothrombopathia 287.1

Diagnosis deferred 799.9

Dialysis (intermittent) (treatment)
- anterior retinal (juvenile) (with detachment) 361.04
- extracorporeal V56.0
- peritoneal V56.8
- renal V56.0
  - status only V45.1
- specified type NEC V56.8

Diamond-Blackfan anemia or syndrome (congenital hypoplastic anemia) 284.0

Diamond-Gardener syndrome (autoerythrocyte sensitization) 287.2

Diaper rash 691.0

Diaphoresis (excessive) NEC 780.8

Diaphragm - *see* condition

Diaphragmalgia 786.52

Diaphragmitis 519.4

Diaphyseal aclasis 756.4

Diaphysitis 733.99

Diarrhea, diarrheal (acute) (autumn) (bilious) (bloody) (catarrhal) (choleraic) (chronic) (gravis) (green) (infantile) (lienteric) (noninfectious) (presumed noninfectious) (putrefactive) (secondary) (sporadic) (summer) (symptomatic) (thermic) 787.91
- achlorhydric 536.0
- allergic 558.3
- amebic (*see also* Amebiasis) 006.9
  - with abscess - *see* Abscess, amebic
  - acute 006.0
  - chronic 006.1
  - nondysenteric 006.2
- bacillary - *see* Dysentery, bacillary
- bacterial NEC 008.5
- balantidial 007.0
- bile salt-induced 579.8
- cachectic NEC 787.91
- chilomastix 007.8
- choleriformis 001.1
- coccidial 007.2
- Cochin-China 579.1
  - anguilluliasis 127.2
  - psilosis 579.1
- Dientamoeba 007.8
- dietetic 787.91
- due to
  - achylia gastrica 536.8
  - Aerobacter aerogenes 008.2
  - Bacillus coli - *see* Enteritis, E. coli
  - bacteria NEC 008.5
  - bile salts 579.8
  - Capillaria
    - hepatica 128.8
    - philippinensis 127.5
  - Clostridium perfringens (C) (F) 008.46
  - Enterobacter aerogenes 008.2
  - enterococci 008.49
  - Escherichia coli - *see* Enteritis, E. coli
  - Giardia lamblia 007.1
  - Heterophyes heterophyes 121.6
  - irritating foods 787.91
  - Metagonimus yokogawai 121.5
  - Necator americanus 126.1
  - Paracolobactrum arizonae 008.1
  - Paracolon bacillus NEC 008.47
    - Arizona 008.1
  - Proteus (bacillus) (mirabilis) (Morganii) 008.3
  - Pseudomonas aeruginosa 008.42
  - S. japonicum 120.2

ICD-9-CM
D
Vol. 2

◄ **New** **Revised Code**

ICD-9-CM D Vol. 2

Disease, diseased *(Continued)*
- heart (organic) 429.9
  - with
    - acute pulmonary edema (*see also* Failure, ventricular, left) 428.1
      - hypertensive 402.91
        - with renal failure 404.92
        - benign 402.11
          - with renal failure 404.12
        - malignant 402.01
          - with renal failure 404.02
    - kidney disease - *see* Hypertension, cardiorenal
    - rheumatic fever (conditions classifiable to 390)
      - active 391.9
        - with chorea 392.0
      - inactive or quiescent (with chorea) 398.90
  - amyloid 277.3 *[425.7]*
  - aortic (valve) (*see also* Endocarditis, aortic) 424.1
  - arteriosclerotic or sclerotic (minimal) (senile) - *see* Arteriosclerosis, coronary
  - artery, arterial - *see* Arteriosclerosis, coronary
  - atherosclerotic - *see* Arteriosclerosis, coronary
  - beer drinkers' 425.5
  - beriberi 265.0 *[425.7]*
  - black 416.0
  - congenital NEC 746.9
    - cyanotic 746.9
    - maternal, affecting fetus or newborn 760.3
    - specified type NEC 746.89
  - congestive (*see also* Failure, heart 428.0
  - coronary 414.9
  - cryptogenic 429.9
  - due to
    - amyloidosis 277.3 *[425.7]*
    - beriberi 265.0 *[425.7]*
    - cardiac glycogenosis 271.0 *[425.7]*
    - Friedreich's ataxia 334.0 *[425.8]*
    - gout 274.82
    - mucopolysaccharidosis 277.5 *[425.7]*
    - myotonia atrophica 359.2 *[425.8]*
    - progressive muscular dystrophy 359.1 *[425.8]*
    - sarcoidosis 135 *[425.8]*
  - fetal 746.9
    - inflammatory 746.89
  - fibroid (*see also* Myocarditis) 429.0
  - functional 427.9
    - postoperative 997.1
    - psychogenic 306.2
  - glycogen storage 271.0 *[425.7]*
  - gonococcal NEC 098.85
  - gouty 274.82
  - hypertensive (*see also* Hypertension, heart) 402.90
    - benign 402.10
    - malignant 402.00
  - hyperthyroid (*see also* Hyperthyroidism) 242.9 *[425.7]*
  - incompletely diagnosed - *see* Disease, heart
  - ischemic (chronic) (*see also* Ischemia, heart) 414.9
    - acute (*see also* Infarct, myocardium) 410.9
      - without myocardial infarction 411.89
        - with coronary (artery) occlusion 411.81

Disease, diseased *(Continued)*
- heart *(Continued)*
  - ischemic *(Continued)*
    - asymptomatic 412
    - diagnosed on ECG or other special investigation but currently presenting no symptoms 412
  - kyphoscoliotic 416.1
  - mitral (*see also* Endocarditis, mitral) 394.9
  - muscular (*see also* Degeneration, myocardial) 429.1
  - postpartum 674.8
  - psychogenic (functional) 306.2
  - pulmonary (chronic) 416.9
    - acute 415.0
    - specified NEC 416.8
  - rheumatic (chronic) (inactive) (old) (quiescent) (with chorea) 398.90
    - active or acute 391.9
      - with chorea (active) (rheumatic) (Sydenham's) 392.0
    - specified type NEC 391.8
  - maternal, affecting fetus or newborn 760.3
  - rheumatoid - *see* Arthritis, rheumatoid
  - sclerotic - *see* Arteriosclerosis, coronary
  - senile (*see also* Myocarditis) 429.0
  - specified type NEC 429.89
  - syphilitic 093.89
    - aortic 093.1
      - aneurysm 093.0
    - asymptomatic 093.89
    - congenital 090.5
  - thyroid (gland) (*see also* Hyperthyroidism) 242.9 *[425.7]*
  - thyrotoxic (*see also* Thyrotoxicosis) 242.9 *[425.7]*
  - tuberculous (*see also* Tuberculosis) 017.9 *[425.8]*
  - valve, valvular (obstructive) (regurgitant) - *see also* Endocarditis
    - congenital NEC (*see also* Anomaly, heart, valve) 746.9
      - pulmonary 746.00
      - specified type NEC 746.89
  - vascular - *see* Disease, cardiovascular
- heavy-chain (gamma G) 273.2
- Heberden's 715.04
- Hebra's
  - dermatitis exfoliativa 695.89
  - erythema multiforme exudativum 695.1
  - pityriasis
    - maculata et circinata 696.3
    - rubra 695.89
      - pilaris 696.4
  - prurigo 698.2
- Heerfordt's (uveoparotitis) 135
- Heidenhain's 290.10
  - with dementia 290.10
- Heilmeyer-Schöner (M9842/3) 207.1
- Heine-Medin (*see also* Poliomyelitis) 045.9
- Heller's (*see also* Psychosis, childhood) 299.1
- Heller-Döhle (syphilitic aortitis) 093.1
- hematopoietic organs 289.9
- hemoglobin (Hb) 282.7
  - with thalassemia 282.49
  - abnormal (mixed) NEC 282.7
    - with thalassemia 282.49
  - AS genotype 282.5
  - Bart's 282.7

Disease, diseased *(Continued)*
- hemoglobin *(Continued)*
  - C (Hb-C) 282.7
    - with other abnormal hemoglobin NEC 282.7
    - elliptocytosis 282.7
    - Hb-S (without crisis) 282.63
      - with
        - crisis 282.64
        - vaso-occlusive pain 282.64
    - sickle-cell (without crisis) 282.63
      - with
        - crisis 282.64
        - vaso-occlusive pain 282.64
    - thalassemia 282.49
  - constant spring 282.7
  - D (Hb-D) 282.7
    - with other abnormal hemoglobin NEC 282.7
    - Hb-S (without crisis) 282.68
      - with crisis 282.69
    - sickle-cell (without crisis) 282.69
      - with crisis 282.69
    - thalassemia 282.49
  - E (Hb-E) 282.7
    - with other abnormal hemoglobin NEC 282.7
    - Hb-S (without crisis) 282.69
      - with crisis 282.69
    - sickle-cell (without crisis) 282.69
      - with crisis 282.69
    - thalassemia 282.49
  - elliptocytosis 282.7
  - F (Hb-F) 282.7
  - G (Hb-G) 282.7
  - H (Hb-H) 282.49
  - hereditary persistence, fetal (HPFH) ("Swiss variety") 282.7
  - high fetal gene 282.7
  - I thalassemia 282.49
  - M 289.7
  - S - *see also* Disease, sickle-cell, Hb-S
    - thalassemia (without crisis) 282.41
      - with
        - crisis 282.42
        - vaso-occlusive pain 282.42
  - spherocytosis 282.7
  - unstable, hemolytic 282.7
  - Zurich (Hb-Zurich) 282.7
- hemolytic (fetus) (newborn) 773.2
  - autoimmune (cold type) (warm type) 283.0
  - due to or with
    - incompatibility
      - ABO (blood group) 773.1
      - blood (group) (Duffy) (Kell) (Kidd) (Lewis) (M) (S) NEC 773.2
      - Rh (blood group) (factor) 773.0
    - Rh negative mother 773.0
  - unstable hemoglobin 282.7
- hemorrhagic 287.9
  - newborn 776.0
- Henoch (-Schönlein) (purpura nervosa) 287.0
- hepatic - *see* Disease, liver
- hepatolenticular 275.1
- heredodegenerative NEC
  - brain 331.89
  - spinal cord 336.8
- Hers' (glycogenosis VI) 271.0
- Herter (-Gee) (-Heubner) (nontropical sprue) 579.0
- Herxheimer's (diffuse idiopathic cutaneous atrophy) 701.8
- Heubner's 094.89

ICD-9-CM

D

Vol. 2

ICD-9-CM D Vol. 2

New   Revised Code

> Note
>
> "Closed" includes simple, complete, partial, uncomplicated, and unspecified dislocation.
>
> "Open" includes dislocation specified as infected or compound and dislocation with foreign body.
>
> "Chronic," "habitual," "old," or "recurrent" dislocations should be coded as indicated under the entry "Dislocation, recurrent"; and "pathological" as indicated under the entry "Dislocation, pathological."
>
> For late effect of dislocation see Late, effect, dislocation.

ICD-9-CM D Vol. 2

Dislocation *(Continued)*
humerus (closed) *(Continued)*
proximal end (closed) *(Continued)*
anterior *(Continued)*
open 831.11
inferior (closed) 831.03
open 831.13
open 831.10
posterior (closed) 831.02
open 831.12
implant - *see* Complications, mechanical
incus 385.23
infracoracoid (closed) 831.01
open 831.11
innominate (pubic junction) (sacral junction) (closed) 839.69
acetabulum (*see also* Dislocation, hip) 835.00
open 839.79
interphalangeal (joint)
finger or hand (closed) 834.02
open 834.12
foot or toe (closed) 838.06
open 838.16
jaw (cartilage) (meniscus) (closed) 830.0
open 830.1
recurrent 524.69
joint NEC (closed) 839.8
developmental 718.7
open 839.9
pathological - *see* Dislocation, pathological
recurrent - *see* Dislocation, recurrent
knee (closed) 836.50
anterior 836.51
open 836.61
congenital (with genu recurvatum) 754.41
habitual 718.36
lateral 836.54
open 836.64
medial 836.53
open 836.63
old 718.36
open 836.60
posterior 836.52
open 836.62
recurrent 718.36
rotatory 836.59
open 836.69
lacrimal gland 375.16
leg (closed) 839.8
open 839.9
lens (crystalline) (complete) (partial) 379.32
anterior 379.33
congenital 743.37
ocular implant 996.53
posterior 379.34
traumatic 921.3
ligament - *see* Dislocation, by site
lumbar (vertebrae) (closed) 839.20
open 839.30
lumbosacral (vertebrae) (closed) 839.20
congenital 756.19
open 839.30
mandible (closed) 830.0
open 830.1
maxilla (inferior) (closed) 830.0
open 830.1
meniscus (knee) - *see also* Tear, meniscus
other sites - *see* Dislocation, by site

Dislocation *(Continued)*
metacarpal (bone)
distal end (closed) 834.01
open 834.11
proximal end (closed) 833.05
open 833.15
metacarpophalangeal (joint) (closed) 834.01
open 834.11
metatarsal (bone) (closed) 838.04
open 838.14
metatarsophalangeal (joint) (closed) 838.05
open 838.15
midcarpal (joint) (closed) 833.03
open 833.13
midtarsal (joint) (closed) 838.02
open 838.12
Monteggia's - *see* Dislocation, hip
multiple locations (except fingers only or toes only) (closed) 839.8
open 839.9
navicular (bone) foot (closed) 837.0
open 837.1
neck (*see also* Dislocation, vertebra, cervical) 839.00
Nélaton's - *see* Dislocation, ankle
nontraumatic (joint) - *see* Dislocation, pathological
nose (closed) 839.69
open 839.79
not recurrent, not current injury - *see* Dislocation, pathological
occiput from atlas (closed) 839.01
open 839.11
old - *see* Dislocation, recurrent
open (compound) NEC 839.9
ossicle, ear 385.23
paralytic (flaccid) (spastic) - *see* Dislocation, pathological
patella (closed) 836.3
congenital 755.64
open 836.4
pathological NEC 718.20
ankle 718.27
elbow 718.22
foot 718.27
hand 718.24
hip 718.25
knee 718.26
lumbosacral joint 724.6
multiple sites 718.29
pelvic region 718.25
sacroiliac 724.6
shoulder (region) 718.21
specified site NEC 718.28
spine 724.8
sacroiliac 724.6
wrist 718.23
pelvis (closed) 839.69
acetabulum (*see also* Dislocation, hip) 835.00
open 839.79
phalanx
foot or toe (closed) 838.09
open 838.19
hand or finger (*see also* Dislocation, finger) 834.00
postpoliomyelitic - *see* Dislocation, pathological
prosthesis, internal - *see* Complications, mechanical
radiocarpal (joint) (closed) 833.02
open 833.12

Dislocation *(Continued)*
radioulnar (joint)
distal end (closed) 833.01
open 833.11
proximal end (*see also* Dislocation, elbow) 832.00
radius
distal end (closed) 833.00
open 833.10
proximal end (closed) 832.01
open 832.11
recurrent (*see also* Derangement, joint, recurrent) 718.3
elbow 718.32
hip 718.35
joint NEC 718.38
knee 718.36
lumbosacral (joint) 724.6
patella 718.36
sacroiliac 724.6
shoulder 718.31
temporomandibular 524.69
rib (cartilage) (closed) 839.69
congenital 756.3
open 839.79
sacrococcygeal (closed) 839.42
open 839.52
sacroiliac (joint) (ligament) (closed) 839.42
congenital 755.69
open 839.52
recurrent 724.6
sacrum (closed) 839.42
open 839.52
scaphoid (bone)
ankle or foot (closed) 837.0
open 837.1
wrist (closed) (*see also* Dislocation, wrist) 833.00
open 833.10
scapula (closed) 831.09
open 831.19
semilunar cartilage, knee - *see* Tear, meniscus
septal cartilage (nose) (closed) 839.69
open 839.79
septum (nasal) (old) 470
sesamoid bone - *see* Dislocation, by site
shoulder (blade) (ligament) (closed) 831.00
anterior (subclavicular) (subcoracoid) (subglenoid) (closed) 831.01
open 831.11
chronic 718.31
inferior 831.03
open 831.13
open 831.10
posterior (closed) 831.02
open 831.12
recurrent 718.31
skull - *see* Injury, intracranial
Smith's - *see* Dislocation, foot
spine (articular process) (*see also* Dislocation, vertebra) (closed) 839.40
atlanto-axial (closed) 839.01
open 839.11
recurrent 723.8
cervical, cervicodorsal, cervicothoracic (closed) (*see also* Dislocation, vertebrae, cervical) 839.00
open 839.10
recurrent 723.8

ICD-9-CM
D
Vol. 2

◀ New ⟸ Revised Code

ICD-9-CM
D
Vol. 2

> Note Use the following fifth-digit subclassification with categories 312.0-312.2:
>
> 0 unspecified
> 1 mild
> 2 moderate
> 3 severe

ICD-9-CM D Vol. 2

ICD-9-CM
D
Vol. 2

E

ICD-9-CM E Vol. 2

Encephalitis *(Continued)*
- postimmunization 323.5
- postinfectious NEC 136.9 *[323.6]*
- postmeasles 055.0
- posttraumatic 323.8
- postvaccinal (smallpox) 323.5
- postvaricella 052.0
- postviral NEC 079.99 *[323.6]*
  - postexanthematous 057.9 *[323.6]*
    - specified NEC 057.8 *[323.6]*
- Powassan 063.8
- progressive subcortical (Binswanger's) 290.12
- Rio Bravo 049.8
- rubella 056.01
- Russian
  - autumnal 062.0
  - spring-summer type (taiga) 063.0
- saturnine 984.9 *[323.7]*
- Semliki Forest 062.8
- serous 048
- slow-acting virus NEC 046.8
- specified cause NEC 323.8
- St. Louis type 062.3
- subacute sclerosing 046.2
- subcorticalis chronica 290.12
- summer 062.0
- suppurative 324.0
- syphilitic 094.81
  - congenital 090.41
- tick-borne 063.9
- torula, torular 117.5 *[323.4]*
- toxic NEC 989.9 *[323.7]*
- toxoplasmic (acquired) 130.0
  - congenital (active) 771.2 *[323.4]*
- trichinosis 124 *[323.4]*
- Trypanosomiasis (*see also* Trypanosomiasis) 086.9 *[323.2]*
- tuberculous (*see also* Tuberculosis) 013.6
- type B (Japanese) 062.0
- type C 062.3
- van Bogaert's 046.2
- Venezuelan 066.2
- Vienna type 049.8
- viral, virus 049.9
  - arthropod-borne NEC 064
    - mosquito-borne 062.9
      - Australian X disease 062.4
      - California virus 062.5
      - Eastern equine 062.2
      - Ilheus virus 062.8
      - Japanese (B type) 062.0
      - Murray Valley 062.4
      - specified type NEC 062.8
      - St. Louis 062.3
      - type B 062.0
      - type C 062.3
      - Western equine 062.1
    - tick-borne 063.9
      - biundulant 063.2
      - Central European 063.2
      - Czechoslovakian 063.2
      - diphasic meningoencephalitis 063.2
      - Far Eastern 063.0
      - Langat 063.8
      - louping ill 063.1
      - Powassan 063.8
      - Russian spring-summer (taiga) 063.0
      - specified type NEC 063.8
    - vector unknown 064
  - slow acting NEC 046.8
  - specified type NEC 049.8

Encephalitis *(Continued)*
- viral, virus *(Continued)*
  - vaccination, prophylactic (against) V05.0
- von Economo's 049.8
- Western equine 062.1
- West Nile type 066.4

Encephalocele 742.0
- orbit 376.81

Encephalocystocele 742.0

Encephalomalacia (brain) (cerebellar) (cerebral) (cerebrospinal) (*see also* Softening, brain) 434.9
- due to
  - hemorrhage (*see also* Hemorrhage, brain) 431
  - recurrent spasm of artery 435.9
- embolic (cerebral) (*see also* Embolism, brain) 434.1
- subcorticalis chronicus arteriosclerotica 290.12
- thrombotic (*see also* Thrombosis, brain) 434.0

Encephalomeningitis - *see* Meningoencephalitis

Encephalomeningocele 742.0

Encephalomeningomyelitis - *see* Meningoencephalitis

Encephalomeningopathy (*see also* Meningoencephalitis) 349.9

Encephalomyelitis (chronic) (granulomatous) (hemorrhagic necrotizing, acute) (myalgic, benign) (*see also* Encephalitis) 323.9
- abortive disseminated 049.8
- acute disseminated (postinfectious) 136.9 *[323.6]*
  - postimmunization 323.5
- due to or resulting from vaccination (any) 323.5
- equine (acute) (infectious) 062.9
  - eastern 062.2
  - Venezuelan 066.2
  - western 062.1
- funicularis infectiosa 049.8
- late effect - *see* Late, effect, encephalitis
- Munch-Peterson's 049.8
- postchickenpox 052.0
- postimmunization 323.5
- postmeasles 055.0
- postvaccinal (smallpox) 323.5
- rubella 056.01
- specified cause NEC 323.8
- syphilitic 094.81

Encephalomyelocele 742.0

Encephalomyelomeningitis - *see* Meningoencephalitis

Encephalomyeloneuropathy 349.9

Encephalomyelopathy 349.9
- subacute necrotizing (infantile) 330.8

Encephalomyeloradiculitis (acute) 357.0

Encephalomyeloradiculoneuritis (acute) 357.0

Encephalomyeloradiculopathy 349.9

Encephalomyocarditis 074.23

Encephalopathia hyperbilirubinemica, newborn 774.7
- due to isoimmunization (conditions classifiable to 773.0-773.2) 773.4

Encephalopathy (acute) 348.30
- alcoholic 291.2
- anoxic - *see* Damage, brain, anoxic

Encephalopathy *(Continued)*
- arteriosclerotic 437.0
  - late effect - *see* Late effect(s) (of) cerebrovascular disease
- bilirubin, newborn 774.7
  - due to isoimmunization 773.4
- congenital 742.9
- demyelinating (callosal) 341.8
- due to
  - birth injury (intracranial) 767.8
  - dialysis 294.8
    - transient 293.9
  - hyperinsulinism - *see* Hyperinsulinism
  - influenza (virus) 487.8
  - lack of vitamin (*see also* Deficiency, vitamin) 269.2
  - nicotinic acid deficiency 291.2
  - serum (nontherapeutic) (therapeutic) 999.5
  - syphilis 094.81
  - trauma (postconcussional) 310.2
    - current (*see also* Concussion, brain) 850.9
      - with skull fracture - *see* Fracture, skull, by site, with intracranial injury
  - vaccination 323.5
- hepatic 572.2
- hyperbilirubinemic, newborn 774.7
  - due to isoimmunization (conditions classifiable to 773.0-773.2) 773.4
- hypertensive 437.2
- hypoglycemic 251.2
- hypoxic - *see* Damage, brain, anoxic
- infantile cystic necrotizing (congenital) 341.8
- lead 984.9 *[323.7]*
- leukopolio 330.0
- metabolic - *see also* Delirium 348.31
  - toxic 349.82
- necrotizing, subacute 330.8
- other specified type NEC 348.39
- pellagrous 265.2
- portal-systemic 572.2
- postcontusional 310.2
- posttraumatic 310.2
- saturnine 984.9 *[323.7]*
- septic 348.31
- spongioform, subacute (viral) 046.1
- subacute
  - necrotizing 330.8
  - spongioform 046.1
  - viral, spongioform 046.1
- subcortical progressive (Schilder) 341.1
  - chronic (Binswanger's) 290.12
- toxic 349.82
  - metabolic - *see* Delirium
- traumatic (postconcussional) 310.2
  - current (*see also* Concussion, brain) 850.9
    - with skull fracture - *see* Fracture, skull, by site, with intracranial injury
- vitamin B deficiency NEC 266.9
- Wernicke's (superior hemorrhagic polioencephalitis) 265.1

Encephalorrhagia (*see also* Hemorrhage, brain) 432.9
- healed or old V12.59
- late effect - *see* Late effect(s) (of) cerebrovascular disease

Encephalosis, posttraumatic 310.2

Enchondroma (M9220/0) - *see also* Neoplasm, bone, benign
- multiple, congenital 756.4

Note use the following fifth-digit subclassifications with categories 345.0, 345.1, 345.4-345.9

0 without mention of intractable epilepsy
1 with intractable epilepsy

- **Eructation** 787.3
  - nervous 306.4
  - psychogenic 306.4
- **Eruption**
  - creeping 126.9
  - drug - *see* Dermatitis, due to, drug
  - Hutchinson, summer 692.72
  - Kaposi's varicelliform 054.0
  - napkin (psoriasiform) 691.0
  - polymorphous
    - light (sun) 692.72
      - other source 692.82
  - psoriasiform, napkin 691.0
  - recalcitrant pustular 694.8
  - ringed 695.89
  - skin (*see also* Dermatitis) 782.1
    - creeping (meaning hookworm) 126.9
    - due to
      - chemical(s) NEC 692.4
        - internal use 693.8
      - drug - *see* Dermatitis, due to, drug
      - prophylactic inoculation or vaccination against disease - *see* Dermatitis, due to, vaccine
      - smallpox vaccination NEC - *see* Dermatitis, due to, vaccine
    - erysipeloid 027.1
    - feigned 698.4
    - Hutchinson, summer 692.72
    - Kaposi's, varicelliform 054.0
      - vaccinia 999.0
    - lichenoid, axilla 698.3
    - polymorphous, due to light 692.72
    - toxic NEC 695.0
    - vesicular 709.8
  - teeth, tooth
    - accelerated 520.6
    - delayed 520.6
    - difficult 520.6
    - disturbance of 520.6
    - in abnormal sequence 520.6
    - incomplete 520.6
    - late 520.6
    - natal 520.6
    - neonatal 520.6
    - obstructed 520.6
    - partial 520.6
    - persistent primary 520.6
    - premature 520.6
  - vesicular 709.8
- **Erysipelas** (gangrenous) (infantile) (newborn) (phlegmonous) (suppurative) 035
  - external ear 035 *[380.13]*
  - puerperal, postpartum, childbirth 670
- **Erysipelatoid** (Rosenbach's) 027.1
- **Erysipeloid** (Rosenbach's) 027.1
- **Erythema, erythematous** (generalized) 695.9
  - ab igne - *see* Burn, by site, first degree
  - annulare (centrifugum) (rheumaticum) 695.0
  - arthriticum epidemicum 026.1
  - brucellum (*see also* Brucellosis) 023.9
  - bullosum 695.1
  - caloricum - *see* Burn, by site, first degree
  - chronicum migrans 088.81
  - circinatum 695.1
  - diaper 691.0
  - due to
    - chemical (contact) NEC 692.4
      - internal 693.8
    - drug (internal use) 693.0
      - contact 692.3

- **Erythema, erythematous** *(Continued)*
  - elevatum diutinum 695.89
  - endemic 265.2
  - epidemic, arthritic 026.1
  - figuratum perstans 695.0
  - gluteal 691.0
  - gyratum (perstans) (repens) 695.1
  - heat - *see* Burn, by site, first degree
  - ichthyosiforme congenitum 757.1
  - induratum (primary) (scrofulosorum) (*see also* Tuberculosis) 017.1
    - nontuberculous 695.2
  - infantum febrile 057.8
  - infectional NEC 695.9
  - infectiosum 057.0
  - inflammation NEC 695.9
  - intertrigo 695.89
  - iris 695.1
  - lupus (discoid) (localized) (*see also* Lupus, erythematosus) 695.4
  - marginatum 695.0
    - rheumaticum - *see* Fever, rheumatic
  - medicamentosum - *see* Dermatitis, due to, drug
  - migrans 529.1
    - chronicum 088.81
  - multiforme 695.1
    - bullosum 695.1
    - conjunctiva 695.1
    - exudativum (Hebra) 695.1
    - pemphigoides 694.5
  - napkin 691.0
  - neonatorum 778.8
  - nodosum 695.2
    - tuberculous (*see also* Tuberculosis) 017.1
  - nummular, nummulare 695.1
  - palmar 695.0
  - palmaris hereditarium 695.0
  - pernio 991.5
  - perstans solare 692.72
  - rash, newborn 778.8
  - scarlatiniform (exfoliative) (recurrent) 695.0
  - simplex marginatum 057.8
  - solare (*see also* Sunburn) 692.71
  - streptogenes 696.5
  - toxic, toxicum NEC 695.0
    - newborn 778.8
  - tuberculous (primary) (*see also* Tuberculosis) 017.0
  - venenatum 695.0
- **Erythematosus** - *see* condition
- **Erythematous** - *see* condition
- **Erythermalgia** (primary) 443.89
- **Erythralgia** 443.89
- **Erythrasma** 039.0
- **Erythredema** 985.0
  - polyneuritica 985.0
  - polyneuropathy 985.0
- **Erythremia** (acute) (M9841/3) 207.0
  - chronic (M9842/3) 207.1
  - secondary 289.0
- **Erythroblastopenia** (acquired) 284.8
  - congenital 284.0
- **Erythroblastophthisis** 284.0
- **Erythroblastosis** (fetalis) (newborn) 773.2
  - due to
    - ABO
      - antibodies 773.1
      - incompatibility, maternal/fetal 773.1
      - isoimmunization 773.1

- **Erythroblastosis** *(Continued)*
  - due to *(Continued)*
    - Rh
      - antibodies 773.0
      - incompatibility, maternal/fetal 773.0
      - isoimmunization 773.0
- **Erythrocyanosis** (crurum) 443.89
- **Erythrocythemia** - *see* Erythremia
- **Erythrocytopenia** 285.9
- **Erythrocytosis** (megalosplenic)
  - familial 289.6
  - oval, hereditary (*see also* Elliptocytosis) 282.1
  - secondary 289.0
  - stress 289.0
- **Erythroderma** (*see also* Erythema) 695.9
  - desquamativa (in infants) 695.89
  - exfoliative 695.89
  - ichthyosiform, congenital 757.1
  - infantum 695.89
  - maculopapular 696.2
  - neonatorum 778.8
  - psoriaticum 696.1
  - secondary 695.9
- **Erythrogenesis imperfecta** 284.0
- **Erythroleukemia** (M9840/3) 207.0
- **Erythromelalgia** 443.89
- **Erythromelia** 701.8
- **Erythropenia** 285.9
- **Erythrophagocytosis** 289.9
- **Erythrophobia** 300.23
- **Erythroplakia**
  - oral mucosa 528.7
  - tongue 528.7
- **Erythroplasia** (Queyrat) (M8080/2)
  - specified site - *see* Neoplasm, skin, in situ
  - unspecified site 233.5
- **Erythropoiesis, idiopathic ineffective** 285.0
- **Escaped beats, heart** 427.60
  - postoperative 997.1
- **Esoenteritis** - *see* Enteritis
- **Esophagalgia** 530.89
- **Esophagectasis** 530.89
  - due to cardiospasm 530.0
- **Esophagismus** 530.5
- **Esophagitis** (alkaline) (chemical) (chronic) (infectional) (necrotic) (peptic) (postoperative) (regurgitant) 530.10
  - acute 530.12
  - candidal 112.84
  - reflux 530.11
  - specified NEC 530.19
  - tuberculous (*see also* Tuberculosis) 017.8
  - ulcerative 530.19
- **Esophagocele** 530.6
- **Esophagodynia** 530.89
- **Esophagomalacia** 530.89
- **Esophagoptosis** 530.89
- **Esophagospasm** 530.5
- **Esophagostenosis** 530.3
- **Esophagostomiasis** 127.7
- **Esophagotracheal** - *see* condition
- **Esophagus** - *see* condition
- **Esophoria** 378.41
  - convergence, excess 378.84
  - divergence, insufficiency 378.85
- **Esotropia** (nonaccommodative) 378.00
  - accommodative 378.35
  - alternating 378.05
    - with
      - A pattern 378.06
      - specified noncomitancy NEC 378.08
      - V pattern 378.07

Esotropia *(Continued)*
- alternating *(Continued)*
  - with *(Continued)*
    - X pattern 378.08
    - Y pattern 378.08
  - intermittent 378.22
- intermittent 378.20
  - alternating 378.22
  - monocular 378.21
- monocular 378.01
  - with
    - A pattern 378.02
    - specified noncomitancy NEC 378.04
    - V pattern 378.03
    - X pattern 378.04
    - Y pattern 378.04
  - intermittent 378.21

Espundia 085.5
Essential - *see* condition
Esterapenia 289.89 ◄
Esthesioneuroblastoma (M9522/3) 160.0
Esthesioneurocytoma (M9521/3) 160.0
Esthesioneuroepithelioma (M9523/3) 160.0
Esthiomene 099.1
Estivo-autumnal
- fever 084.0
- malaria 084.0

Estrangement V61.0
Estriasis 134.0
Ethanolaminuria 270.8
Ethanolism (*see also* Alcoholism) 303.9
Ether dependence, dependency (*see also* Dependence) 304.6
Etherism (*see also* Dependence) 304.6
Ethmoid, ethmoidal - *see* condition
Ethmoiditis (chronic) (nonpurulent) (purulent) (*see also* Sinusitis, ethmoidal) 473.2
- influenzal 487.1
- Woakes' 471.1

Ethylism (*see also* Alcoholism) 303.9
Eulenburg's disease (congenital paramyotonia) 359.2
Eunuchism 257.2
Eunuchoidism 257.2
- hypogonadotropic 257.2

European blastomycosis 117.5
Eustachian - *see* condition
Euthyroid sick syndrome 790.94
Euthyroidism 244.9
Evaluation
- fetal lung maturity 659.8
- for suspected condition (*see also* Observation) V71.9
  - abuse V71.81
  - exposure
    - anthrax 471.82
    - biological agent NEC 471.83
  - neglect V71.81
  - newborn - *see* Observation, suspected, condition, newborn
  - specified condition NEC V71.89
- mental health V70.2
  - requested by authority V70.1
- nursing care V63.8
- social service V63.8

Evan's syndrome (thrombocytopenic purpura) 287.3
Eventration
- colon into chest - *see* Hernia, diaphragm
- diaphragm (congenital) 756.6

Eversion
- bladder 596.8

Eversion *(Continued)*
- cervix (uteri) 622.0
  - with mention of cervicitis 616.0
- foot NEC 736.79
  - congenital 755.67
- lacrimal punctum 375.51
- punctum lacrimale (postinfectional) (senile) 375.51
- ureter (meatus) 593.89
- urethra (meatus) 599.84
- uterus 618.1
  - complicating delivery 665.2
    - affecting fetus or newborn 763.89
  - puerperal, postpartum 674.8

Evisceration
- birth injury 767.8
- bowel (congenital) - *see* Hernia, ventral
- congenital (*see also* Hernia, ventral) 553.29
- operative wound 998.32
- traumatic NEC 869.1
  - eye 871.3

Evulsion - *see* Avulsion
Ewing's
- angioendothelioma (M9260/3) - *see* Neoplasm, bone, malignant
- sarcoma (M9260/3) - *see* Neoplasm, bone, malignant
- tumor (M9260/3) - *see* Neoplasm, bone, malignant

Exaggerated lumbosacral angle (with impinging spine) 756.12
Examination (general) (routine) (of) (for) V70.9
- allergy V72.7
- annual V70.0
- cardiovascular preoperative V72.81
- cervical Papanicolaou smear V76.2
  - as a part of routine gynecological examination V72.3
- child care (routine) V20.2
- clinical research investigation (normal control patient) (participant) V70.7
- dental V72.2
- developmental testing (child) (infant) V20.2
- donor (potential) V70.8
- ear V72.1
- eye V72.0
- following
  - accident (motor vehicle) V71.4
  - alleged rape or seduction (victim or culprit) V71.5
  - inflicted injury (victim or culprit) NEC V71.6
  - rape or seduction, alleged (victim or culprit) V71.5
  - treatment (for) V67.9
    - combined V67.6
    - fracture V67.4
    - involving high-risk medication NEC V67.51
    - mental disorder V67.3
    - specified condition NEC V67.59
- follow-up (routine) (following) V67.9
  - cancer chemotherapy V67.2
  - chemotherapy V67.2
  - disease NEC V67.59
  - high-risk medication NEC V67.51
  - injury NEC V67.59
  - population survey V70.6
  - postpartum V24.2
  - psychiatric V67.3
  - psychotherapy V67.3
  - radiotherapy V67.1

Examination *(Continued)*
- follow-up *(Continued)*
  - specified surgery NEC V67.09
  - surgery V67.00
    - vaginal pap smear V67.01
- gynecological V72.3
  - for contraceptive maintenance V25.40
    - intrauterine device V25.42
    - pill V25.41
    - specified method NEC V25.49
- health (of)
  - armed forces personnel V70.5
  - checkup V70.0
  - child, routine V20.2
  - defined subpopulation NEC V70.5
  - inhabitants of institutions V70.5
  - occupational V70.5
  - pre-employment screening V70.5
  - preschool children V70.5
    - for admission to school V70.3
  - prisoners V70.5
    - for entrance into prison V70.3
  - prostitutes V70.5
  - refugees V70.5
  - school children V70.5
  - students V70.5
- hearing V72.1
- infant V20.2
- laboratory V72.6
- lactating mother V24.1
- medical (for) (of) V70.9
  - administrative purpose NEC V70.3
  - admission to
    - old age home V70.3
    - prison V70.3
    - school V70.3
  - adoption V70.3
  - armed forces personnel V70.5
  - at health care facility V70.0
  - camp V70.3
  - child, routine V20.2
  - clinical research investigation, (control) (normal comparison) (participant) V70.7
  - defined subpopulation NEC V70.5
  - donor (potential) V70.8
  - driving license V70.3
  - general V70.9
    - routine V70.0
    - specified reason NEC V70.8
  - immigration V70.3
  - inhabitants of institutions V70.5
  - insurance certification V70.3
  - marriage V70.3
  - medicolegal reasons V70.4
  - naturalization V70.3
  - occupational V70.5
  - population survey V70.6
  - pre-employment V70.5
  - preschool children V70.5
    - for admission to school V70.3
  - prison V70.3
  - prisoners V70.5
    - for entrance into prison V70.3
  - prostitutes V70.5
  - refugees V70.5
  - school children V70.5
  - specified reason NEC V70.8
  - sport competition V70.3
  - students V70.5
- medicolegal reason V70.4
- pelvic (annual) (periodic) V72.3
- periodic (annual) (routine) V70.0

ICD-9-CM
E
Vol. 2

F

ICD-9-CM

F

Vol. 2

ICD-9-CM
F
Vol. 2

◄ New ⬅ Revised Code

ICD-9-CM F Vol. 2

ICD-9-CM F Vol. 2

ICD-9-CM
F
Vol. 2

Note Multiple fractures of sites classifiable to the same three- or four-digit category are coded to that category, except for sites classifiable to 810-818 or 820-827 in different limbs.

Multiple fractures of sites classifiable to different fourth-digit subdivisions within the same three-digit category should be dealt with according to coding rules.

Multiple fractures of sites classifiable to different three-digit categories (identifiable from the listing under "Fracture"), and of sites classifiable to 810-818 or 820-827 in different limbs should be coded according to the following list, which should be referred to in the following priority order: skull or face bones, pelvis or vertebral column, legs, arms.

Note Use the following fifth-digit subclassification with categories 800, 801, 803, and 804:

- 0 unspecified state of consciousness
- 1 with no loss of consciousness
- 2 with brief [less than one hour] loss of consciousness
- 3 with moderate [1-24 hours] loss of consciousness
- 4 with prolonged [more than 24 hours] loss of consciousness and return to pre-existing conscious level
- 5 with prolonged [more than 24 hours] loss of consciousness, without return to pre-existing conscious level

Use fifth-digit 5 to designate when a patient is unconscious and dies before regaining consciousness, regardless of the duration of the loss of consciousness

- 6 with loss of consciousness of unspecified duration
- 9 with concussion, unspecified

G

Note Use the following fifth-digit subclassification for category 535:

0 without mention of hemorrhage
1 with hemorrhage

ICD-9-CM G Vol. 2

Note Use the following fifth-digit subclassification with category 242:

0 without mention of thyrotoxic crisis or storm
1 with mention of thyrotoxic crisis or storm

Granuloma NEC *(Continued)*
- annulare 695.89
- anus 569.49
- apical 522.6
- appendix 543.9
- aural 380.23
- beryllium (skin) 709.4
  - lung 503
- bone (*see also* Osteomyelitis) 730.1
  - eosinophilic 277.89
  - from residual foreign body 733.99
- canaliculus lacrimalis 375.81
- cerebral 348.8
- cholesterin, middle ear 385.82
- coccidioidal (progressive) 114.3
  - lung 114.4
  - meninges 114.2
  - primary (lung) 114.0
- colon 569.89
- conjunctiva 372.61
- dental 522.6
- ear, middle (cholesterin) 385.82
  - with otitis media - *see* Otitis media
- eosinophilic 277.89
  - bone 277.89
  - lung 277.89
  - oral mucosa 528.9
- exuberant 701.5
- eyelid 374.89
- facial
  - lethal midline 446.3
  - malignant 446.3
- faciale 701.8
- fissuratum (gum) 523.8
- foot NEC 686.1
- foreign body (in soft tissue) NEC 728.82
  - bone 733.99
  - in operative wound 998.4
  - muscle 728.82
  - skin 709.4
  - subcutaneous tissue 709.4
- fungoides 202.1
- gangraenescens 446.3
- giant cell (central) (jaw) (reparative) 526.3
  - gingiva 523.8
  - peripheral (gingiva) 523.8
- gland (lymph) 289.3
- Hodgkin's (M9661/3) 201.1
- ileum 569.89
- infectious NEC 136.9
- inguinale (Donovan) 099.2
  - venereal 099.2
- intestine 569.89
- iridocyclitis 364.10
- jaw (bone) 526.3
  - reparative giant cell 526.3
- kidney (*see also* Infection, kidney) 590.9
- lacrimal sac 375.81
- larynx 478.79
- lethal midline 446.3
- lipid 277.89
- lipoid 277.89
- liver 572.8
- lung (infectious) (*see also* Fibrosis, lung) 515
  - coccidioidal 114.4
  - eosinophilic 277.89
- lymph gland 289.3
- Majocchi's 110.6
- malignant, face 446.3
- mandible 526.3
- mediastinum 519.3

Granuloma NEC *(Continued)*
- midline 446.3
- monilial 112.3
- muscle 728.82
  - from residual foreign body 728.82
- nasal sinus (*see also* Sinusitis) 473.9
- operation wound 998.59
  - foreign body 998.4
  - stitch (external) 998.89
    - internal wound 998.89
  - talc 998.7
- oral mucosa, eosinophilic or pyogenic 528.9
- orbit, orbital 376.11
- paracoccidioidal 116.1
- penis, venereal 099.2
- periapical 522.6
- peritoneum 568.89
  - due to ova of helminths NEC (*see also* Helminthiasis) 128.9
- postmastoidectomy cavity 383.33
- postoperative - *see* Granuloma, operation wound
- prostate 601.8
- pudendi (ulcerating) 099.2
- pudendorum (ulcerative) 099.2
- pulp, internal (tooth) 521.4
- pyogenic, pyogenicum (skin) 686.1
  - maxillary alveolar ridge 522.6
  - oral mucosa 528.9
- rectum 569.49
- reticulohistiocytic 277.89
- rubrum nasi 705.89
- sarcoid 135
- Schistosoma 120.9
- septic (skin) 686.1
- silica (skin) 709.4
- sinus (accessory) (infectional) (nasal) (*see also* Sinusitis) 473.9
- skin (pyogenicum) 686.1
  - from foreign body or material 709.4
- sperm 608.89
- spine
  - syphilitic (epidural) 094.89
  - tuberculous (*see also* Tuberculosis) 015.0 *[730.88]*
- stitch (postoperative) 998.89
  - internal wound 998.89
- suppurative (skin) 686.1
- suture (postoperative) 998.89
  - internal wound 998.89
- swimming pool 031.1
- talc 728.82
  - in operation wound 998.7
- telangiectaticum (skin) 686.1
- trichophyticum 110.6
- tropicum 102.4
- umbilicus 686.1
  - newborn 771.4
- urethra 599.84
- uveitis 364.10
- vagina 099.2
- venereum 099.2
- vocal cords 478.5
- Wegener's (necrotizing respiratory granulomatosis) 446.4

Granulomatosis NEC 686.1
- disciformis chronica et progressiva 709.3
- infantiseptica 771.2
- lipoid 277.89
- lipophagic, intestinal 040.2
- miliary 027.0

Granulomatosis NEC *(Continued)*
- necrotizing, respiratory 446.4
- progressive, septic 288.1
- Wegener's (necrotizing respiratory) 446.4

Granulomatous tissue - *see* Granuloma
Granulosis rubra nasi 705.89
Graphite fibrosis (of lung) 503
Graphospasm 300.89
- organic 333.84

Grating scapula 733.99
Gravel (urinary) (*see also* Calculus) 592.9
Graves' disease (exophthalmic goiter) (*see also* Goiter, toxic) 242.0
Gravis - *see* condition
Grawitz's tumor (hypernephroma) (M8312/3) 189.0
Grayness, hair (premature) 704.3
- congenital 757.4

Gray or grey syndrome (chloramphenicol) (newborn) 779.4
Greenfield's disease 330.0
Green sickness 280.9
Greenstick fracture - *see* Fracture, by site
Greig's syndrome (hypertelorism) 756.0
Griesinger's disease (*see also* Ancylostomiasis) 126.9
Grinders'
- asthma 502
- lung 502
- phthisis (*see also* Tuberculosis) 011.4

Grinding, teeth 306.8
Grip
- Dabney's 074.1
- devil's 074.1

Grippe, grippal - *see also* Influenza
- Balkan 083.0
- intestinal 487.8
- summer 074.8

Grippy cold 487.1
Grisel's disease 723.5
Groin - *see* condition
Grooved
- nails (transverse) 703.8
- tongue 529.5
  - congenital 750.13

Ground itch 126.9
Growing pains, children 781.99
Growth (fungoid) (neoplastic) (new) (M8000/1) - *see also* Neoplasm, by site, unspecified nature
- adenoid (vegetative) 474.12
- benign (M8000/0) - *see* Neoplasm, by site, benign
- fetal, poor 764.9
  - affecting management of pregnancy 656.5
- malignant (M8000/3) - *see* Neoplasm, by site, malignant
- rapid, childhood V21.0
- secondary (M8000/6) - *see* Neoplasm, by site, malignant, secondary

Gruber's hernia - *see* Hernia, Gruber's
Gruby's disease (tinea tonsurans) 110.0
G-trisomy 758.0
Guama fever 066.3
Gubler (-Millard) paralysis or syndrome 344.89
Guérin-Stern syndrome (arthrogryposis multiplex congenita) 754.89
Guertin's disease (electric chorea) 049.8

ICD-9-CM
G
Vol. 2

H

ICD-9-CM
H
Vol. 2

- **Hemiplegia** *(Continued)*
  - late effect
    - birth injury, intracranial or spinal 343.4
    - cerebrovascular lesion - *see* Late effect(s) (of) cerebrovascular disease
    - viral encephalitis 139.0
  - middle alternating NEC 344.89
  - newborn NEC 767.0
  - seizure (current episode) (*see also* Disease, cerebrovascular, acute) 436
  - spastic 342.1
    - congenital or infantile 343.1
  - specified NEC 342.8
  - thrombotic (current) (*see also* Thrombosis, brain) 434.0
    - late effect - *see* Late effect(s) (of) cerebrovascular disease
- **Hemisection, spinal cord** - *see* Fracture, vertebra, by site, with spinal cord injury
- **Hemispasm** 781.0
  - facial 781.0
- **Hemispatial neglect** 781.8
- **Hemisporosis** 117.9
- **Hemitremor** 781.0
- **Hemivertebra** 756.14
- **Hemobilia** 576.8
- **Hemocholecyst** 575.8
- **Hemochromatosis** (acquired) (diabetic) (hereditary) (liver) (myocardium) (primary idiopathic) (secondary) 275.0
  - with refractory anemia 285.0
- **Hemodialysis** V56.0
- **Hemoglobin** - *see also* condition
  - abnormal (disease) - *see* Disease, hemoglobin
  - AS genotype 282.5
  - fetal, hereditary persistence 282.7
  - high-oxygen-affinity 289.0
  - low NEC 285.9
  - S (Hb-S), heterozygous 282.5
- **Hemoglobinemia** 283.2
  - due to blood transfusion NEC 999.8
    - bone marrow 996.85
  - paroxysmal 283.2
- **Hemoglobinopathy** (mixed) (*see also* Disease, hemoglobin) 282.7
  - with thalassemia 282.49
  - sickle-cell 282.60
    - with thalassemia (without crisis) 282.41
      - with
        - crisis 282.42
        - vaso-occlusive pain 282.42
- **Hemoglobinuria, hemoglobinuric** 791.2
  - with anemia, hemolytic, acquired (chronic) NEC 283.2
  - cold (agglutinin) (paroxysmal) (with Raynaud's syndrome) 283.2
  - due to
    - exertion 283.2
    - hemolysis (from external causes) NEC 283.2
  - exercise 283.2
  - fever (malaria) 084.8
  - infantile 791.2
  - intermittent 283.2
  - malarial 084.8
  - march 283.2
  - nocturnal (paroxysmal) 283.2
  - paroxysmal (cold) (nocturnal) 283.2
- **Hemolymphangioma** (M9175/0) 228.1
- **Hemolysis**
  - fetal - *see* Jaundice, fetus or newborn
  - intravascular (disseminated) NEC 286.6
    - with
      - abortion - *see* Abortion, by type, with hemorrhage, delayed or excessive
      - ectopic pregnancy (*see also* categories 633.0-633.9) 639.1
      - hemorrhage of pregnancy 641.3
        - affecting fetus or newborn 762.1
      - molar pregnancy (*see also* categories 630-632) 639.1
    - acute 283.2
    - following
      - abortion 639.1
      - ectopic or molar pregnancy 639.1
  - neonatal - *see* Jaundice, fetus or newborn
  - transfusion NEC 999.8
    - bone marrow 996.85
- **Hemolytic** - *see also* condition
  - anemia - *see* Anemia, hemolytic
  - uremic syndrome 283.11
- **Hemometra** 621.4
- **Hemopericardium** (with effusion) 423.0
  - newborn 772.8
  - traumatic (*see also* Hemothorax, traumatic) 860.2
    - with open wound into thorax 860.3
- **Hemoperitoneum** 568.81
  - infectional (*see also* Peritonitis) 567.2
  - traumatic - *see* Injury, internal, peritoneum
- **Hemophilia** (familial) (hereditary) 286.0
  - A 286.0
    - carrier (asymptomatic) V83.01
      - symptomatic V83.02
  - acquired 286.5
  - B (Leyden) 286.1
  - C 286.2
  - calcipriva (*see also* Fibrinolysis) 286.7
  - classical 286.0
  - nonfamilial 286.7
  - vascular 286.4
- **Hemophilus influenzae NEC** 041.5
  - arachnoiditis (basic) (brain) (spinal) 320.0
    - late effect - *see* category 326
  - bronchopneumonia 482.2
  - cerebral ventriculitis 320.0
    - late effect - *see* category 326
  - cerebrospinal inflammation 320.0
    - late effect - *see* category 326
  - infection NEC 041.5
  - leptomeningitis 320.0
    - late effect - *see* category 326
  - meningitis (cerebral) (cerebrospinal) (spinal) 320.0
    - late effect - *see* category 326
  - meningomyelitis 320.0
    - late effect - *see* category 326
  - pachymeningitis (adhesive) (fibrous) (hemorrhagic) (hypertrophic) (spinal) 320.0
    - late effect - *see* category 326
  - pneumonia (broncho-) 482.2
- **Hemophthalmos** 360.43
- **Hemopneumothorax** (*see also* Hemothorax) 511.8
  - traumatic 860.4
    - with open wound into thorax 860.5
- **Hemoptysis** 786.3
  - due to Paragonimus (westermani) 121.2
  - newborn 770.3
  - tuberculous (*see also* Tuberculosis, pulmonary) 011.9
- **Hemorrhage, hemorrhagic** (nontraumatic) 459.0
  - abdomen 459.0
  - accidental (antepartum) 641.2
    - affecting fetus or newborn 762.1
  - adenoid 474.8
  - adrenal (capsule) (gland) (medulla) 255.4
    - newborn 772.5
  - after labor - *see* Hemorrhage, postpartum
  - alveolar
    - lung, newborn 770.3
    - process 525.8
  - alveolus 525.8
  - amputation stump (surgical) 998.11
    - secondary, delayed 997.69
  - anemia (chronic) 280.0
    - acute 285.1
  - antepartum - *see* Hemorrhage, pregnancy
  - anus (sphincter) 569.3
  - apoplexy (stroke) 432.9
  - arachnoid - *see* Hemorrhage, subarachnoid
  - artery NEC 459.0
    - brain (*see also* Hemorrhage, brain) 431
    - middle meningeal - *see* Hemorrhage, subarachnoid
  - basilar (ganglion) (*see also* Hemorrhage, brain) 431
  - bladder 596.8
  - blood dyscrasia 289.9
  - bowel 578.9
    - newborn 772.4
  - brain (miliary) (nontraumatic) 431
    - with
      - birth injury 767.0
    - arachnoid - *see* Hemorrhage, subarachnoid
    - due to
      - birth injury 767.0
      - rupture of aneurysm (congenital) (*see also* Hemorrhage, subarachnoid) 430
      - mycotic 431
    - syphilis 094.89
    - epidural or extradural - *see* Hemorrhage, extradural
    - fetus or newborn (anoxic) (hypoxic) (due to birth trauma) (nontraumatic) 767.0
      - intraventricular 772.10
        - grade I 772.11
        - grade II 772.12
        - grade III 772.13
        - grade IV 772.14
    - iatrogenic 997.02
    - postoperative 997.02
    - puerperal, postpartum, childbirth 674.0
    - stem 431
    - subarachnoid, arachnoid, or meningeal - *see* Hemorrhage, subarachnoid
    - subdural - *see* Hemorrhage, subdural
    - traumatic NEC 853.0

> Note Use the following fifth-digit subclassification with categories 851-854:
>
> 0 unspecified state of consciousness
>
> 1 with no loss of consciousness

ICD-9-CM **H** Vol. 2

New   Revised Code

- **High** *(Continued)*
  - output failure (cardiac) (*see also* Failure, heart) 428.9
  - oxygen-affinity hemoglobin 289.0
  - palate 750.26
  - risk
    - behavior - *see* problem
    - family situation V61.9
      - specified circumstance NEC V61.8
    - individual NEC V62.89
    - infant NEC V20.1
    - patient taking drugs (prescribed) V67.51
      - nonprescribed (*see also* Abuse, drugs, nondependent) 305.9
    - pregnancy V23.9
      - inadequate prenatal care V23.7
      - specified problem NEC V23.8
  - temperature (of unknown origin) (*see also* Pyrexia) 780.6
  - thoracic rib 756.3
- **Hildenbrand's disease** (typhus) 081.9
- **Hilger's syndrome** 337.0
- **Hill diarrhea** 579.1
- **Hilliard's lupus** (*see also* Tuberculosis) 017.0
- **Hilum** - *see* condition
- **Hip** - *see* condition
- **Hippel's disease** (retinocerebral angiomatosis) 759.6
- **Hippus** 379.49
- **Hirschfeld's disease** (acute diabetes mellitus) (*see also* Diabetes) 250.0
- **Hirschsprung's disease or megacolon** (congenital) 751.3
- **Hirsuties** (*see also* Hypertrichosis) 704.1
- **Hirsutism** (*see also* Hypertrichosis) 704.1
- **Hirudiniasis** (external) (internal) 134.2
- **His-Werner disease** (trench fever) 083.1
- **Hiss-Russell dysentery** 004.1
- **Histamine cephalgia** 346.2
- **Histidinemia** 270.5
- **Histidinuria** 270.5
- **Histiocytoma** (M8832/0) - (*see also* Neoplasm, skin, benign)
  - fibrous (M8830/0) - (*see also* Neoplasm, skin, benign)
    - atypical (M8830/1) - *see* Neoplasm, connective tissue, uncertain behavior
    - malignant (M8830/3) - *see* Neoplasm, connective tissue, malignant
- **Histiocytosis** (acute) (chronic) (subacute) 277.89
  - acute differentiated progressive (M9722/3) 202.5
  - cholesterol 277.89
  - essential 277.89
  - lipid, lipoid (essential) 272.7
  - lipochrome (familial) 288.1
  - malignant (M9720/3) 202.3
  - X (chronic) 277.89
    - acute (progressive) (M9722/3) 202.5
- **Histoplasmosis** 115.90
  - with
    - endocarditis 115.94
    - meningitis 115.91
    - pericarditis 115.93
    - pneumonia 115.95
    - retinitis 115.92
    - specified manifestation NEC 115.99
  - African (due to Histoplasma duboisii) 115.10

- **Histoplasmosis** *(Continued)*
  - African *(Continued)*
    - with
      - endocarditis 115.14
      - meningitis 115.11
      - pericarditis 115.13
      - pneumonia 115.15
      - retinitis 115.12
      - specified manifestation NEC 115.19
  - American (due to Histoplasma capsulatum) 115.00
    - with
      - endocarditis 115.04
      - meningitis 115.01
      - pericarditis 115.03
      - pneumonia 115.05
      - retinitis 115.02
      - specified manifestation NEC 115.09
  - Darling's - *see* Histoplasmosis, American
  - large form (*see also* Histoplasmosis, African) 115.10
  - lung 115.05
  - small form (*see also* Histoplasmosis, American) 115.00
- **History** (personal) of
  - abuse
    - emotional V15.42
    - neglect V15.42
    - physical V15.41
    - sexual V15.41
  - affective psychosis V11.1
  - alcoholism V11.3
    - specified as drinking problem (*see also* Abuse, drugs, nondependent) 305.0
  - allergy to
    - analgesic agent NEC V14.6
    - anesthetic NEC V14.4
    - antibiotic agent NEC V14.1
      - penicillin V14.0
    - anti-infective agent NEC V14.3
    - diathesis V15.09
    - drug V14.9
      - specified type NEC V14.8
    - eggs V15.03
    - food additives V15.05
    - insect bite V15.06
    - latex V15.07
    - medicinal agents V14.9
      - specified type NEC V14.8
    - milk products V15.02
    - narcotic agent NEC V14.5
    - nuts V15.05
      - peanuts V15.01
    - penicillin V14.0
    - radiographic dye V15.08
    - seafood V15.04
    - serum V14.7
    - specified food NEC V15.05
    - specified nonmedicinal agents NEC V15.09
    - spider bite V15.06
    - sulfa V14.2
    - sulfonamides V14.2
    - therapeutic agent NEC V15.09
    - vaccine V14.7
  - anemia V12.3
  - arthritis V13.4
  - benign neoplasm of brain V12.41
  - blood disease V12.3
  - calculi, urinary V13.01
  - cardiovascular disease V12.50
    - myocardial infarction 412
  - child abuse V15.41
  - cigarette smoking V15.82

- **History (personal) of** *(Continued)*
  - circulatory system disease V12.50
    - myocardial infarction 412
  - congenital malformation V13.69
  - contraception V15.7
  - diathesis, allergic V15.09
  - digestive system disease V12.70
    - peptic ulcer V12.71
    - polyps, colonic V12.72
    - specified NEC V12.79
  - disease (of) V13.9
    - blood V12.3
    - blood-forming organs V12.3
    - cardiovascular system V12.50
    - circulatory system V12.50
    - digestive system V12.70
      - peptic ulcer V12.71
      - polyps, colonic V12.72
      - specified NEC V12.79
    - infectious V12.00
    - malaria V12.03
      - poliomyelitis V12.02
      - specified NEC V12.09
      - tuberculosis V12.01
    - parasitic V12.00
      - specified NEC V12.09
    - respiratory system V12.6
    - skin V13.3
    - specified site NEC V13.8
    - subcutaneous tissue V13.3
    - trophoblastic V13.1
      - affecting management of pregnancy V23.1
  - disorder (of) V13.9
    - endocrine V12.2
    - genital system V13.29
    - hematological V12.3
    - immunity V12.2
    - mental V11.9
      - affective type V11.1
      - manic-depressive V11.1
      - neurosis V11.2
      - schizophrenia V11.0
      - specified type NEC V11.8
    - metabolic V12.2
    - musculoskeletal NEC V13.5
    - nervous system V12.40
      - specified type NEC V12.49
    - obstetric V13.29
      - affecting management of current pregnancy V23.49
        - pre-term labor V23.41
      - pre-term labor V13.21
    - sense organs V12.40
      - specified type NEC V12.49
    - specified site NEC V13.8
    - urinary system V13.00
      - calculi V13.01
      - specified NEC V13.09
  - drug use
    - nonprescribed (*see also* Abuse, drugs, nondependent) 305.9
    - patent (*see also* Abuse, drugs, nondependent) 305.9
  - effect NEC of external cause V15.89
  - embolism (pulmonary) V12.51
  - emotional abuse V15.42
  - endocrine disorder V12.2
  - extracorporeal membrane oxygenation (ECMO) V15.87
  - family
    - allergy V19.6
    - anemia V18.2
    - arteriosclerosis V17.4
    - arthritis V17.7
    - asthma V17.5
    - blindness V19.0

ICD-9-CM
H
Vol. 2

ICD-9-CM

H

Vol. 2

- **Hydropneumopericardium** (*see also* Pericarditis) 423.9
- **Hydropneumothorax** 511.8
  - nontuberculous 511.8
    - bacterial 511.1
  - pneumococcal 511.1
  - staphylococcal 511.1
  - streptococcal 511.1
  - traumatic 860.0
    - with open wound into thorax 860.1
  - tuberculous (*see also* Tuberculosis, pleura) 012.0
- **Hydrops** 782.3
  - abdominis 789.5
  - amnii (complicating pregnancy) (*see also* Hydramnios) 657
  - articulorum intermittens (*see also* Rheumatism, palindromic) 719.3
  - cardiac (*see also* Failure, heart) 428.0
  - congenital - *see* Hydrops, fetalis
  - endolymphatic (*see also* Disease, Meniere's) 386.00
  - fetal(is) or newborn 778.0
    - due to isoimmunization 773.3
    - not due to isoimmunization 778.0
  - gallbladder 575.3
  - idiopathic (fetus or newborn) 778.0
  - joint (*see also* Effusion, joint) 719.0
  - labyrinth (*see also* Disease, Meniere's) 386.00
  - meningeal NEC 331.4
  - nutritional 262
  - pericardium - *see* Pericarditis
  - pleura (*see also* Hydrothorax) 511.8
  - renal (*see also* Nephrosis) 581.9
  - spermatic cord (*see also* Hydrocele) 603.9
- **Hydropyonephrosis** (*see also* Pyelitis) 590.80
  - chronic 590.00
- **Hydrorachis** 742.53
- **Hydrorrhea** (nasal) 478.1
  - gravidarum 658.1
  - pregnancy 658.1
- **Hydrosadenitis** 705.83
- **Hydrosalpinx** (fallopian tube) (follicularis) 614.1
- **Hydrothorax** (double) (pleural) 511.8
  - chylous (nonfilarial) 457.8
    - filaria (*see also* Infestation, filarial) 125.9
  - nontuberculous 511.8
    - bacterial 511.1
  - pneumococcal 511.1
  - staphylococcal 511.1
  - streptococcal 511.1
  - traumatic 862.29
    - with open wound into thorax 862.39
  - tuberculous (*see also* Tuberculosis, pleura) 012.0
- **Hydroureter** 593.5
  - congenital 753.22
- **Hydroureteronephrosis** (*see also* Hydronephrosis) 591
- **Hydrourethra** 599.84
- **Hydroxykynureninuria** 270.2
- **Hydroxyprolinemia** 270.8
- **Hydroxyprolinuria** 270.8
- **Hygroma** (congenital) (cystic) (M9173/0) 228.1
  - prepatellar 727.3
  - subdural - *see* Hematoma, subdural
- **Hymen** - *see* condition
- **Hymenolepiasis** (diminuta) (infection) (infestation) (nana) 123.6
- **Hymenolepsis** (diminuta) (infection) (infestation) (nana) 123.6
- **Hypalgesia** (*see also* Disturbance, sensation) 782.0
- **Hyperabduction syndrome** 447.8
- **Hyperacidity, gastric** 536.8
  - psychogenic 306.4
- **Hyperactive, hyperactivity**
  - basal cell, uterine cervix 622.1
  - bladder 596.51
  - bowel (syndrome) 564.9
    - sounds 787.5
  - cervix epithelial (basal) 622.1
  - child 314.01
  - colon 564.9
  - gastrointestinal 536.8
    - psychogenic 306.4
  - intestine 564.9
  - labyrinth (unilateral) 386.51
    - with loss of labyrinthine reactivity 386.58
    - bilateral 386.52
  - nasal mucous membrane 478.1
  - stomach 536.8
  - thyroid (gland) (*see also* Thyrotoxicosis) 242.9
- **Hyperacusis** 388.42
- **Hyperadrenalism** (cortical) 255.3
  - medullary 255.6
- **Hyperadrenocorticism** 255.3
  - congenital 255.2
  - iatrogenic
    - correct substance properly administered 255.3
    - overdose or wrong substance given or taken 962.0
- **Hyperaffectivity** 301.11
- **Hyperaldosteronism** (atypical) (hyperplastic) (normoaldosteronal) (normotensive) (primary) 255.10 ⬅
  - seconday 255.14 ◄
- **Hyperalgesia** (*see also* Disturbance, sensation) 782.0
- **Hyperalimentation** 783.6
  - carotene 278.3
  - specified NEC 278.8
  - vitamin A 278.2
  - vitamin D 278.4
- **Hyperaminoaciduria** 270.9
  - arginine 270.6
  - citrulline 270.6
  - cystine 270.0
  - glycine 270.0
  - lysine 270.7
  - ornithine 270.6
  - renal (types I, II, III) 270.0
- **Hyperammonemia** (congenital) 270.6
- **Hyperamnesia** 780.9
- **Hyperamylasemia** 790.5
- **Hyperamnesia** 780.99
- **Hyperaphia** 782.0
- **Hyperazotemia** 791.9
- **Hyperbetalipoproteinemia** (acquired) (essential) (familial) (hereditary) (primary) (secondary) 272.0
  - with prebetalipoproteinemia 272.2
- **Hyperbilirubinemia** 782.4
  - congenital 277.4
  - constitutional 277.4
  - neonatal (transient) (*see also* Jaundice, fetus or newborn) 774.6
    - of prematurity 774.2
- **Hyperbilirubinemica encephalopathia, newborn** 774.7
  - due to isoimmunization 773.4
- **Hypercalcemia, hypercalcemic** (idiopathic) 275.42
  - nephropathy 588.8
- **Hypercalcinuria** 275.40
- **Hypercapnia** 786.09
  - with mixed acid-base disorder 276.4
  - fetal, affecting newborn 770.89
- **Hypercarotinemia** 278.3
- **Hypercementosis** 521.5
- **Hyperchloremia** 276.9
- **Hyperchlorhydria** 536.8
  - neurotic 306.4
  - psychogenic 306.4
- **Hypercholesterinemia** - *see* Hypercholesterolemia
- **Hypercholesterolemia** 272.0
  - with hyperglyceridemia, endogenous 272.2
  - essential 272.0
  - familial 272.0
  - hereditary 272.0
  - primary 272.0
  - pure 272.0
- **Hypercholesterolosis** 272.0
- **Hyperchylia gastrica** 536.8
  - psychogenic 306.4
- **Hyperchylomicronemia** (familial) (with hyperbetalipoproteinemia) 272.3
- **Hypercoagulation (primary) syndrome** 289.81 ◄
  - secondary 289.82 ◄
- **Hypercorticosteronism**
  - correct substance properly administered 255.3
  - overdose or wrong substance given or taken 962.0
- **Hypercortisonism**
  - correct substance properly administered 255.3
  - overdose or wrong substance given or taken 962.0
- **Hyperdynamic beta-adrenergic state or syndrome** (circulatory) 429.82
- **Hyperelectrolytemia** 276.9
- **Hyperemesis** 536.2
  - arising during pregnancy - *see* Hyperemesis, gravidarum
  - gravidarum (mild) (before 22 completed weeks' gestation) 643.0
    - with
      - carbohydrate depletion 643.1
      - dehydration 643.1
      - electrolyte imbalance 643.1
      - metabolic disturbance 643.1
    - affecting fetus or newborn 761.8
    - severe (with metabolic disturbance) 643.1
  - psychogenic 306.4
- **Hyperemia** (acute) 780.99
  - anal mucosa 569.49
  - bladder 596.7
  - cerebral 437.8
  - conjunctiva 372.71
  - ear, internal, acute 386.30
  - enteric 564.89
  - eye 372.71
  - eyelid (active) (passive) 374.82
  - intestine 564.89
  - iris 364.41
  - kidney 593.81
  - labyrinth 386.30
  - liver (active) (passive) 573.8

◀ New ⇐ Revised Code

ICD-9-CM

H

Vol. 2

◄ New ⇐ Revised Code

	Malignant	Benign	Unspecified
Hypertension, hypertensive (arterial) (arteriolar) (crisis) (degeneration) (disease) (essential) (fluctuating) (idiopathic) (intermittent) (labile) (low renin) (orthostatic) (paroxysmal) (primary) (systemic) (uncontrolled) (vascular)	401.0	401.1	401.9
with			
heart involvement (conditions classifiable to 428, 429.0-429.3, 429.8, 429.9 due to hypertension) (*see also* Hypertension, heart)	402.00	402.10	402.90
with kidney involvement-*see* Hypertension, cardiorenal			
renal involvement (only conditions classifiable to 585, 586, 587) (excludes conditions classifiable to 584) (*see also* Hypertension, kidney)	403.00	403.10	403.90
with heart involvement-*see* Hypertension, cardiorenal			
failure (and sclerosis) (*see also* Hypertension, kidney)	403.01	403.11	403.91
sclerosis without failure (*see also* Hypertension, kidney)	403.00	403.10	403.90
accelerated (*see also* Hypertension, by type, malignant)	401.0	-	-
antepartum-see Hypertension, complicating pregnancy, childbirth, or the puerperium			
cardiorenal (disease)	404.00	404.10	404.90
with			
heart failure	404.01	404.11	404.91
and renal failure	404.03	404.13	404.93
renal failure	404.02	404.12	404.92
and heart failure	404.03	404.13	404.93
cardiovascular disease (arteriosclerotic) (sclerotic)	402.00	402.10	402.90
with			
heart failure	402.01	402.11	402.91
renal involvement (conditions classifiable to 403) (*see also* Hypertension, cardiorenal)	404.00	404.10	404.90
cardiovascular renal (disease) (sclerosis) (*see also* Hypertension, cardiorenal)	404.00	404.10	404.90
cerebrovascular disease NEC	437.2	437.2	437.2
complicating pregnancy, childbirth, or the puerperium	642.2	642.0	642.9
with			
albuminuria (and edema) (mild)	-	-	642.4
severe	-	-	642.5
edema (mild)	-	-	642.4
severe	-	-	642.5
heart disease	642.2	642.2	642.2
and renal disease	642.2	642.2	642.2
renal disease	642.2	642.2	642.2
and heart disease	642.2	642.2	642.2
chronic	642.2	642.0	642.0
with pre-eclampsia or eclampsia	642.7	642.7	642.7
fetus or newborn	760.0	760.0	760.0
essential	-	642.0	642.0
with pre-eclampsia or eclampsia	-	642.7	642.7
fetus or newborn	760.0	760.0	760.0
fetus or newborn	760.0	760.0	760.0
gestational	-	-	642.3
pre-existing	642.2	642.0	642.0
with pre-eclampsia or eclampsia	642.7	642.7	642.7
fetus or newborn	760.0	760.0	760.0
secondary to renal disease	642.1	642.1	642.1
with pre-eclampsia or eclampsia	642.7	642.7	642.7
fetus or newborn	760.0	760.0	760.0
transient	-	-	642.3
due to			
aldosteronism, primary	405.09	405.19	405.99
brain tumor	405.09	405.19	405.99
bulbar poliomyelitis	405.09	405.19	405.99
calculus			
kidney	405.09	405.19	405.99
ureter	405.09	405.19	405.99
coarctation, aorta	405.09	405.19	405.99
Cushing's disease	405.09	405.19	405.99
glomerulosclerosis (*see also* Hypertension, kidney)	403.00	403.10	403.90
periarteritis nodosa	405.09	405.19	405.99
pheochromocytoma	405.09	405.19	405.99
polycystic kidney(s)	405.09	405.19	405.99
polycythemia	405.09	405.19	405.99
porphyria	405.09	405.19	405.99
pyelonephritis	405.09	405.19	405.99
renal (artery)			
aneurysm	405.01	405.11	405.91
anomaly	405.01	405.11	405.91
embolism	405.01	405.11	405.91
fibromuscular hyperplasia	405.01	405.11	405.91
occlusion	405.01	405.11	405.91

	Malignant	Benign	Unspecified
Hypertension *(Continued)*			
due to *(Continued)*			
renal *(Continued)*			
stenosis	405.01	405.11	405.91
thrombosis	405.01	405.11	405.91
encephalopathy	437.2	437.2	437.2
gestational (transient) NEC	-	-	642.3
Goldblatt's	440.1	440.1	440.1
heart (disease) (conditions classifiable to 428, 429.0-429.3, 429.8, 429.9 due to hypertension)	402.00	402.10	402.90
with			
heart failure	402.01	402.11	402.91
hypertensive kidney disease (conditions classifiable to 403) (*see also* Hypertension, cardiorenal)	404.00	404.10	404.90
renal sclerosis (*see also* Hypertension, cardiorenal)	404.00	404.10	404.90
intracranial, benign	-	348.2	-
intraocular	-	-	365.04
kidney	403.00	403.10	403.90
with			
heart involvement (conditions classifiable to 428, 429.0-429.3, 429.8, 429.9 due to hypertension) (*see also* Hypertension, cardiorenal)	404.00	404.10	404.90
hypertensive heart (disease) (conditions classifiable to 402) (*see also* Hypertension, cardiorenal)	404.00	404.10	404.90
renal failure (conditions classifiable to 585, 586)	403.01	403.11	403.91
lesser circulation	-	-	416.0
necrotizing	401.0	-	-
ocular	-	-	365.04
portal (due to chronic liver disease)	-	-	572.3
postoperative			997.91
psychogenic	-	-	306.2
puerperal, postpartum- *see* Hypertension, complicating pregnancy, childbirth, or the puerperium			
pulmonary (artery)	-	-	416.8
with cor pulmonale (chronic)	-	-	416.8
acute	-	-	415.0
idiopathic	-	-	416.0
primary	-	-	416.0
of newborn	-	-	747.83
secondary	-	-	416.8
renal (disease) (*see also* Hypertension, kidney)	403.00	403.10	403.90
renovascular NEC	405.01	405.11	405.91
secondary NEC	405.09	405.19	405.99
due to			
aldosteronism, primary	405.09	405.19	405.99
brain tumor	405.09	405.19	405.99
bulbar poliomyelitis	405.09	405.19	405.99
calculus			
kidney	405.09	405.19	405.99
ureter	405.09	405.19	405.99
coarctation, aorta	405.09	405.19	405.99
Cushing's disease	405.09	405.19	405.99
glomerulosclerosis (*see also* Hypertension, kidney)	403.00	403.10	403.90
periarteritis nodosa	405.09	405.19	405.99
pheochromocytoma	405.09	405.19	405.99
polycystic kidney(s)	405.09	405.19	405.99
polycythemia	405.09	405.19	405.99
porphyria	405.09	405.19	405.99
pyelonephritis	405.09	405.19	405.99
renal (artery)			
aneurysm	405.01	405.11	405.91
anomaly	405.01	405.11	405.91
embolism	405.01	405.11	405.91
fibromuscular hyperplasia	405.01	405.11	405.91
occlusion	405.01	405.11	405.91
stenosis	405.01	405.11	405.91
thrombosis	405.01	405.11	405.91
transient	-	-	796.2
of pregnancy	-	-	642.3
venous, chronic (asymptomatic) (idiopathic)	-	-	459.30
due to			
deep vein thrombosis (*see also* Syndrome, postphlebitic)	-	-	459.10
with			
complication, NEC	-	-	459.39
inflammation	-	-	459.32
with ulcer	-	-	459.33
ulcer	-	-	459.31
with inflammation	-	-	459.33

I

ICD-9-CM
I
Vol. 2

Note Use the following fifth-digit subclassification with category 410:

0 episode unspecified
1 initial episode
2 subsequent episode without recurrence

ICD-9-CM
I
Vol. 2

◄ New ⟵ Revised Code

Inflammation, inflamed, inflammatory *(Continued)*
- tympanic membrane - *see* Myringitis
- umbilicus, umbilical 686.9
  - newborn NEC 771.4
- uterine ligament (*see also* Disease, pelvis, inflammatory) 614.4
  - acute 614.3
- uterus (catarrhal) (*see also* Endometritis) 615.9
- uveal tract (anterior) (*see also* Iridocyclitis) 364.3
  - posterior - *see* Chorioretinitis
  - sympathetic 360.11
- vagina (*see also* Vaginitis) 616.10
- vas deferens 608.4
- vein (*see also* Phlebitis) 451.9
  - thrombotic 451.9
    - cerebral (*see also* Thrombosis, brain) 434.0
    - leg 451.2
      - deep (vessels) NEC 451.19
      - superficial (vessels) 451.0
    - lower extremity 451.2
      - deep (vessels) NEC 451.19
      - superficial (vessels) 451.0
- vocal cord 478.5
- vulva (*see also* Vulvitis) 616.10

Inflation, lung imperfect (newborn) 770.5

Influenza, influenzal 487.1
- with
  - bronchitis 487.1
  - bronchopneumonia 487.0
  - cold (any type) 487.1
  - digestive manifestations 487.8
  - hemoptysis 487.1
  - involvement of
    - gastrointestinal tract 487.8
    - nervous system 487.8
  - laryngitis 487.1
  - manifestations NEC 487.8
    - respiratory 487.1
      - pneumonia 487.0
  - pharyngitis 487.1
  - pneumonia (any form classifiable to 480-483, 485-486) 487.0
  - respiratory manifestations NEC 487.1
  - sinusitis 487.1
  - sore throat 487.1
  - tonsillitis 487.1
  - tracheitis 487.1
  - upper respiratory infection (acute) 487.1
- abdominal 487.8
- Asian 487.1
- bronchial 487.1
- bronchopneumonia 487.0
- catarrhal 487.1
- epidemic 487.1
- gastric 487.8
- intestinal 487.8
- laryngitis 487.1
- maternal affecting fetus or newborn 760.2
  - manifest influenza in infant 771.2
- pharyngitis 487.1
- pneumonia (any form) 487.0
- respiratory (upper) 487.1
- stomach 487.8
- vaccination, prophylactic (against) V04.81

Influenza-like disease 487.1

Infraction, Freiberg's (metatarsal head) 732.5

Infusion complication, misadventure, or reaction - *see* Complication, infusion

Ingestion
- chemical - *see* Table of Drugs and Chemicals
- drug or medicinal substance
  - overdose or wrong substance given or taken 977.9
    - specified drug - *see* Table of Drugs and Chemicals
- foreign body NEC (*see also* Foreign body) 938

Ingrowing
- hair 704.8
- nail (finger) (toe) (infected) 703.0

Inguinal - *see also* condition
- testis 752.51

Inhalation
- carbon monoxide 986
- flame
  - mouth 947.0
  - lung 947.1
- food or foreign body (*see also* Asphyxia, food or foreign body) 933.1
- gas, fumes, or vapor (noxious) 987.9
  - specified agent - *see* Table of Drugs and Chemicals
- liquid or vomitus (*see also* Asphyxia, food or foreign body) 933.1
  - lower respiratory tract NEC 934.9
- meconium (fetus or newborn) 770.1
- mucus (*see also* Asphyxia, mucus) 933.1
- oil (causing suffocation) (*see also* Asphyxia, food or foreign body) 933.1
- pneumonia - *see* Pneumonia, aspiration
- smoke 987.9
- steam 987.9
- stomach contents or secretions (*see also* Asphyxia, food or foreign body) 933.1
  - in labor and delivery 668.0

Inhibition, inhibited
- academic as adjustment reaction 309.23
- orgasm
  - female 302.73
  - male 302.74
- sexual
  - desire 302.71
  - excitement 302.72
- work as adjustment reaction 309.23

Inhibitor, systemic lupus erythematosus (presence of) 286.5

Iniencephalus, iniencephaly 740.2

Injected eye 372.74

Injury 959.9

> Note For abrasion, insect bite (nonvenomous), blister, or scratch, *see* Injury, superficial.
>
> For laceration, traumatic rupture, tear, or penetrating wound of internal organs, such as heart, lung, liver, kidney, pelvic organs, whether or not accompanied by open wound in the same region, *see* Injury, internal.
>
> For nerve injury, *see* Injury, nerve.
>
> For late effect of injuries classifiable to 850-854, 860-869, 900-919, 950-959, *see* Late, effect, injury, by type.

Injury *(Continued)*
- abdomen, abdominal (viscera) - *see also* Injury, internal, abdomen
  - muscle or wall 959.12
- acoustic, resulting in deafness 951.5
- adenoid 959.09
- adrenal (gland) - *see* Injury, internal, adrenal
- alveolar (process) 959.09
- ankle (and foot) (and knee) (and leg, except thigh) 959.7
- anterior chamber, eye 921.3
- anus 959.19
- aorta (thoracic) 901.0
  - abdominal 902.0
- appendix - *see* Injury, internal, appendix
- arm, upper (and shoulder) 959.2
- artery (complicating trauma) (*see also* Injury, blood vessel, by site) 904.9
  - cerebral or meningeal (*see also* Hemorrhage, brain, traumatic, subarachnoid) 852.0
- auditory canal (external) (meatus) 959.09
- auricle, auris, ear 959.09
- axilla 959.2
- back 959.19
- bile duct - *see* Injury, internal, bile duct
- birth - *see also* Birth, injury
  - canal NEC, complicating delivery 665.9
- bladder (sphincter) - *see* Injury, internal, bladder
- blast (air) (hydraulic) (immersion) (underwater) NEC 869.0
  - with open wound into cavity NEC 869.1
  - abdomen or thorax - *see* Injury, internal, by site
  - brain - *see* Concussion, brain
  - ear (acoustic nerve trauma) 951.5
    - with perforation of tympanic membrane - *see* Wound, open, ear, drum
- blood vessel NEC 904.9
  - abdomen 902.9
    - multiple 902.87
    - specified NEC 902.89
  - aorta (thoracic) 901.0
    - abdominal 902.0
  - arm NEC 903.9
  - axillary 903.00
    - artery 903.1
    - vein 903.02
  - azygos vein 901.89
  - basilic vein 903.1
  - brachial (artery) (vein) 903.1
  - bronchial 901.89
  - carotid artery 900.00
    - common 900.01
    - external 900.02
    - internal 900.03
  - celiac artery 902.20
    - specified branch NEC 902.24
  - cephalic vein (arm) 903.1
  - colica dextra 902.26
  - cystic
    - artery 902.24
    - vein 902.39
  - deep plantar 904.6
  - digital (artery) (vein) 903.5
  - due to accidental puncture or laceration during procedure 998.2

ICD-9-CM

Vol. 2

- **Injury** *(Continued)*
  - blood vessel NEC *(Continued)*
    - extremity
      - lower 904.8
        - multiple 904.7
        - specified NEC 904.7
      - upper 903.9
        - multiple 903.8
        - specified NEC 903.8
    - femoral
      - artery (superficial) 904.1
        - above profunda origin 904.0
        - common 904.0
      - vein 904.2
    - gastric
      - artery 902.21
      - vein 902.39
    - head 900.9
      - intracranial - *see* Injury, intracranial
      - multiple 900.82
      - specified NEC 900.89
    - hemiazygos vein 901.89
    - hepatic
      - artery 902.22
      - vein 902.11
    - hypogastric 902.59
      - artery 902.51
      - vein 902.52
    - ileocolic
      - artery 902.26
      - vein 902.31
    - iliac 902.50
      - artery 902.53
      - specified branch NEC 902.59
      - vein 902.54
    - innominate
      - artery 901.1
      - vein 901.3
    - intercostal (artery) (vein) 901.81
    - jugular vein (external) 900.81
      - internal 900.1
    - leg NEC 904.8
    - mammary (artery) (vein) 901.82
    - mesenteric
      - artery 902.20
        - inferior 902.27
        - specified branch NEC 902.29
        - superior (trunk) 902.25
          - branches, primary 902.26
      - vein 902.39
        - inferior 902.32
        - superior (and primary subdivisions) 902.31
    - neck 900.9
      - multiple 900.82
      - specified NEC 900.89
    - ovarian 902.89
      - artery 902.81
      - vein 902.82
    - palmar artery 903.4
    - pelvis 902.9
      - multiple 902.87
      - specified NEC 902.89
    - plantar (deep) (artery) (vein) 904.6
    - popliteal 904.40
      - artery 904.41
      - vein 904.42
    - portal 902.33
    - pulmonary 901.40
      - artery 901.41
      - vein 901.42
    - radial (artery) (vein) 903.2
    - renal 902.40

- **Injury** *(Continued)*
  - blood vessel NEC *(Continued)*
    - renal *(Continued)*
      - artery 902.41
      - specified NEC 902.49
      - vein 902.42
    - saphenous
      - artery 904.7
      - vein (greater) (lesser) 904.3
    - splenic
      - artery 902.23
      - vein 902.34
    - subclavian
      - artery 901.1
      - vein 901.3
    - suprarenal 902.49
    - thoracic 901.9
      - multiple 901.83
      - specified NEC 901.89
    - tibial 904.50
      - artery 904.50
        - anterior 904.51
        - posterior 904.53
      - vein 904.50
        - anterior 904.52
        - posterior 904.54
    - ulnar (artery) (vein) 903.3
    - uterine 902.59
      - artery 902.55
      - vein 902.56
    - vena cava
      - inferior 902.10
        - specified branches NEC 902.19
      - superior 901.2
  - brachial plexus 953.4
    - newborn 767.6
  - brain NEC (*see also* Injury, intracranial) 854.0
  - breast 959.19
  - broad ligament - *see* Injury, internal, broad ligament
  - bronchus, bronchi - *see* Injury, internal, bronchus
  - brow 959.09
  - buttock 959.19
  - canthus, eye 921.1
  - cathode ray 990
  - cauda equina 952.4
    - with fracture, vertebra - *see* Fracture, vertebra, sacrum
  - cavernous sinus (*see also* Injury, intracranial) 854.0
  - cecum - *see* Injury, internal, cecum
  - celiac ganglion or plexus 954.1
  - cerebellum (*see also* Injury, intracranial) 854.0
  - cervix (uteri) - *see* Injury, internal, cervix
  - cheek 959.09
  - chest - *see* Injury, internal, chest
    - wall 959.11
  - childbirth - *see also* Birth, injury
    - maternal NEC 665.9
  - chin 959.09
  - choroid (eye) 921.3
  - clitoris 959.14
  - coccyx 959.19
    - complicating delivery 665.6
  - colon - *see* Injury, internal, colon
  - common duct - *see* Injury, internal, common duct
  - conjunctiva 921.1
    - superficial 918.2

- **Injury** *(Continued)*
  - cord
    - spermatic - *see* Injury, internal, spermatic cord
    - spinal - *see* Injury, spinal, by site
  - cornea 921.3
    - abrasion 918.1
    - due to contact lens 371.82
    - penetrating - *see* Injury, eyeball, penetrating
    - superficial 918.1
      - due to contact lens 371.82
  - cortex (cerebral) (*see also* Injury, intracranial) 854.0
    - visual 950.3
  - costal region 959.11
  - costochondral 959.11
  - cranial
    - bones - *see* Fracture, skull, by site
    - cavity (*see also* Injury, intracranial) 854.0
    - nerve - *see* Injury, nerve, cranial
  - crushing - *see* Crush
  - cutaneous sensory nerve
    - lower limb 956.4
    - upper limb 955.5
  - delivery - *see also* Birth, injury
    - maternal NEC 665.9
  - Descemet's membrane - *see* Injury, eyeball, penetrating
  - diaphragm - *see* Injury, internal, diaphragm
  - duodenum - *see* Injury, internal, duodenum
  - ear (auricle) (canal) (drum) (external) 959.09
  - elbow (and forearm) (and wrist) 959.3
  - epididymis 959.14
  - epigastric region 959.12
  - epiglottis 959.09
  - epiphyseal, current - *see* Fracture, by site
  - esophagus - *see* Injury, internal, esophagus
  - eustachian tube 959.09
  - extremity (lower) (upper) NEC 959.8
  - eye 921.9
    - penetrating eyeball - *see* Injury, eyeball, penetrating
    - superficial 918.9
  - eyeball 921.3
    - penetrating 871.7
      - with
        - partial loss (of intraocular tissue) 871.2
        - prolapse or exposure (of intraocular tissue) 871.1
      - without prolapse 871.0
      - foreign body (nonmagnetic) 871.6
        - magnetic 871.5
    - superficial 918.9
  - eyebrow 959.09
  - eyelid(s) 921.1
    - laceration - *see* Laceration, eyelid
    - superficial 918.0
  - face (and neck) 959.09
  - fallopian tube - *see* Injury, internal, fallopian tube
  - fingers(s) (nail) 959.5
  - flank 959.19
  - foot (and ankle) (and knee) (and leg, except thigh) 959.7
  - forceps NEC 767.9
    - scalp 767.19
  - forearm (and elbow) (and wrist) 959.3

- **Injury** *(Continued)*
  - forehead 959.09
  - gallbladder - *see* Injury, internal, gallbladder
  - gasserian ganglion 951.2
  - gastrointestinal tract - *see* Injury, internal, gastrointestinal tract
  - genital organ(s)
    - with
      - abortion - *see* Abortion, by type, with, damage to pelvic organs
      - ectopic pregnancy (*see also* categories 633.0-633.9) 639.2
      - molar pregnancy (*see also* categories 630-632) 639.2
    - external 959.14 ⇐
    - fracture of corpus cavernosum penis 959.13 ◄
    - following
      - abortion 639.2
      - ectopic or molar pregnancy 639.2
    - internal - *see* Injury, internal, genital organs
    - obstetrical trauma NEC 665.9
      - affecting fetus or newborn 763.89
  - gland
    - lacrimal 921.1
      - laceration 870.8
    - parathyroid 959.09
    - salivary 959.09
    - thyroid 959.09
  - globe (eye) (*see also* Injury, eyeball) 921.3
  - grease gun - *see* Wound, open, by site, complicated
  - groin 959.19 ⇐
  - gum 959.09
  - hand(s) (except fingers) 959.4
  - head NEC 959.01
    - with
      - loss of consciousness 850.5
      - skull fracture - *see* Fracture, skull, by site
  - heart - *see* Injury, internal, heart
  - heel 959.7
  - hip (and thigh) 959.6
  - hymen 959.14 ⇐
  - hyperextension (cervical) (vertebra) 847.0
  - ileum - *see* Injury, internal, ileum
  - iliac region 959.19 ⇐
  - infrared rays NEC 990
  - instrumental (during surgery) 998.2
    - birth injury - *see* Birth, injury
    - nonsurgical (*see also* Injury, by site) 959.9
    - obstetrical 665.9
      - affecting fetus or newborn 763.89
      - bladder 665.5
      - cervix 665.3
      - high vaginal 665.4
      - perineal NEC 664.9
      - urethra 665.5
      - uterus 665.5
  - internal 869.0

> Note For injury of internal organ(s) by foreign body entering through a natural orifice (e.g., inhaled, ingested, or swallowed)-*see* Foreign body, entering through orifice.
>
> For internal injury of any of the following sites with internal injury of any other of the sites-*see* Injury, internal, multiple.

- **Injury** *(Continued)*
  - internal *(Continued)*
    - with
      - fracture
        - pelvis - *see* Fracture, pelvis
        - specified site, except pelvis - *see* Injury, internal, by site
      - open wound into cavity 869.1
    - abdomen, abdominal (viscera) NEC 868.00
      - with
        - fracture, pelvis - *see* Fracture, pelvis
        - open wound into cavity 868.10
      - specified site NEC 868.09
        - with open wound into cavity 868.19
    - adrenal (gland) 868.01
      - with open wound into cavity 868.11
    - aorta (thoracic) 901.0
      - abdominal 902.0
    - appendix 863.85
      - with open wound into cavity 863.95
    - bile duct 868.02
      - with open wound into cavity 868.12
    - bladder (sphincter) 867.0
      - with
        - abortion - *see* Abortion, by type, with, damage to pelvic organs
        - ectopic pregnancy (*see also* categories 633.0-633.9) 639.2
        - molar pregnancy (*see also* categories 630-632) 639.2
        - open wound into cavity 867.1
      - following
        - abortion 639.2
        - ectopic or molar pregnancy 639.2
      - obstetrical trauma 665.5
        - affecting fetus or newborn 763.89
    - blood vessel - *see* Injury, blood vessel, by site
    - broad ligament 867.6
      - with open wound into cavity 867.7
    - bronchus, bronchi 862.21
      - with open wound into cavity 862.31
    - cecum 863.89
      - with open wound into cavity 863.99
    - cervix (uteri) 867.4
      - with
        - abortion - *see* Abortion, by type, with damage to pelvic organs
        - ectopic pregnancy (*see also* categories 633.0-633.9) 639.2
        - molar pregnancy (*see also* categories 630-632) 639.2
        - open wound into cavity 867.5
      - following
        - abortion 639.2
        - ectopic or molar pregnancy 639.2
      - obstetrical trauma 665.3
        - affecting fetus or newborn 763.89
    - chest (*see also* Injury, internal, intrathoracic organs) 862.8

- **Injury** *(Continued)*
  - internal *(Continued)*
    - chest *(Continued)*
      - with open wound into cavity 862.9
    - colon 863.40
      - with
        - open wound into cavity 863.50
        - rectum 863.46
          - with open wound into cavity 863.56
      - ascending (right) 863.41
        - with open wound into cavity 863.51
      - descending (left) 863.43
        - with open wound into cavity 863.53
      - multiple sites 863.46
        - with open wound into cavity 863.56
      - sigmoid 863.44
        - with open wound into cavity 863.54
      - specified site NEC 863.49
        - with open wound into cavity 863.59
      - transverse 863.42
        - with open wound into cavity 863.52
    - common duct 868.02
      - with open wound into cavity 868.12
    - complicating delivery 665.9
      - affecting fetus or newborn 763.89
    - diaphragm 862.0
      - with open wound into cavity 862.1
    - duodenum 863.21
      - with open wound into cavity 863.31
    - esophagus (intrathoracic) 862.22
      - with open wound into cavity 862.32
      - cervical region 874.4
        - complicated 874.5
    - fallopian tube 867.6
      - with open wound into cavity 867.7
    - gallbladder 868.02
      - with open wound into cavity 868.12
    - gastrointestinal tract NEC 863.80
      - with open wound into cavity 863.90
    - genital organ NEC 867.6
      - with open wound into cavity 867.7
    - heart 861.00
      - with open wound into thorax 861.10
    - ileum 863.29
      - with open wound into cavity 863.39
    - intestine NEC 863.89
      - with open wound into cavity 863.99
      - large NEC 863.40
        - with open wound into cavity 863.50
      - small NEC 863.20
        - with open wound into cavity 863.30
    - intra-abdominal (organ) 868.00

Note Multiple internal injuries of sites classifiable to the same three- or four-digit category should be classified to that category.

Multiple injuries classifiable to different fourth-digit subdivisions of 861.- (heart and lung injuries) should be dealt with according to coding rules.

- **Injury** *(Continued)*
  - internal *(Continued)*
    - thymus (gland) 862.29
      - with open wound into cavity 862.39
    - trachea (intrathoracic) 862.29
      - with open wound into cavity 862.39
      - cervical region (*see also* Wound, open, trachea) 874.02
    - ureter 867.2
      - with open wound into cavity 867.3
    - urethra (sphincter) 867.0
      - with
        - abortion - *see* Abortion, by type, with, damage to pelvic organs
        - ectopic pregnancy (*see also* categories 633.0-633.9) 639.2
        - molar pregnancy (*see also* categories 630-632) 639.2
        - open wound into cavity 867.1
      - following
        - abortion 639.2
        - ectopic or molar pregnancy 639.2
      - obstetrical trauma 665.5
        - affecting fetus or newborn 763.89
    - uterus 867.4
      - with
        - abortion - *see* Abortion, by type, with, damage to pelvic organs
        - ectopic pregnancy (*see also* categories 633.0-633.9) 639.2
        - molar pregnancy (*see also* categories 630-632) 639.2
        - open wound into cavity 867.5
      - following
        - abortion 639.2
        - ectopic or molar pregnancy 639.2
      - obstetrical trauma NEC 665.5
        - affecting fetus or newborn - 763.89
    - vas deferens 867.6
      - with open wound into cavity 867.7
    - vesical (sphincter) 867.0
      - with open wound into cavity 867.1
    - viscera (abdominal) (*see also* Injury, internal, multiple) 868.00
      - with
        - fracture, pelvis - *see* Fracture, pelvis
        - open wound into cavity 868.10
      - thoracic NEC (*see also* Injury, internal, intrathoracic organs) 862.8
        - with open wound into cavity 862.9
  - interscapular region 959.19
  - intervertebral disc 959.19
  - intestine - *see* Injury, internal, intestine
  - intra-abdominal (organs) NEC - *see* Injury, internal, intra-abdominal
  - intracranial 854.0

> Note Use the following fifth-digit subclassification with categories 851-854:
>
> 0 unspecified state of consciousness
> 1 with no loss of consciousness
> 2 with brief [less than one hour] loss of consciousness
> 3 with moderate [1-24 hours] loss of consciousness
> 4 with prolonged [more than 24 hours] loss of consciousness and return to pre-existing conscious level
> 5 with prolonged [more than 24 hours] loss of consciousness, without return to pre-existing conscious level
>
> Use fifth-digit 5 to designate when a patient is unconscious and dies before regaining consciousness, regardless of the duration of the loss of consciousness
>
> 6 with loss of consciousness of unspecified duration
> 9 with concussion, unspecified

- **Injury** *(Continued)*
  - intracranial *(Continued)*
    - with
      - open intracranial wound 854.1
      - skull fracture - *see* Fracture, skull, by site
    - contusion 851.8
      - with open intracranial wound 851.9
      - brain stem 851.4
        - with open intracranial wound 851.5
      - cerebellum 851.4
        - with open intracranial wound 851.5
      - cortex (cerebral) 851.0
        - with open intracranial wound 851.2
    - hematoma - *see* Injury, intracranial, hemorrhage
    - hemorrhage 853.0
      - with
        - laceration - *see* Injury, intracranial, laceration
        - open intracranial wound 853.1
      - extradural 852.4
        - with open intracranial wound 852.5
      - subarachnoid 852.0
        - with open intracranial wound 852.1
      - subdural 852.2
        - with open intracranial wound 852.3
    - laceration 851.8
      - with open intracranial wound 851.9
      - brain stem 851.6
        - with open intracranial wound 851.7
      - cerebellum 851.6
        - with open intracranial wound 851.7
      - cortex (cerebral) 851.2
        - with open intracranial wound 851.3
  - intraocular - *see* Injury, eyeball, penetrating
  - intrathoracic organs (multiple) - *see* Injury, internal, intrathoracic organs
  - intrauterine - *see* Injury, internal, intrauterine
  - iris 921.3
    - penetrating - *see* Injury, eyeball, penetrating

- **Injury** *(Continued)*
  - jaw 959.09
  - jejunum - *see* Injury, internal, jejunum
  - joint NEC 959.9
    - old or residual 718.80
      - ankle 718.87
      - elbow 718.82
      - foot 718.87
      - hand 718.84
      - hip 718.85
      - knee 718.86
      - multiple sites 718.89
      - pelvic region 718.85
      - shoulder (region) 718.81
      - specified site NEC 718.88
      - wrist 718.83
  - kidney - *see* Injury, internal, kidney
  - knee (and ankle) (and foot) (and leg, except thigh) 959.7
  - labium (majus) (minus) 959.14
  - labyrinth, ear 959.09
  - lacrimal apparatus, gland, or sac 921.1
    - laceration 870.8
  - larynx 959.09
  - late effect - *see* Late, effects (of), injury
  - leg, except thigh (and ankle) (and foot) (and knee) 959.7
    - upper or thigh 959.6
  - lens, eye 921.3
    - penetrating - *see* Injury, eyeball, penetrating
  - lid, eye - *see* Injury, eyelid
  - lip 959.09
  - liver - *see* Injury, internal, liver
  - lobe, parietal - *see* Injury, intracranial
  - lumbar (region) 959.19
    - plexus 953.5
  - lumbosacral (region) 959.19
    - plexus 953.5
  - lung - *see* Injury, internal, lung
  - malar region 959.09
  - mastoid region 959.09
  - maternal, during pregnancy, affecting fetus or newborn 760.5
  - maxilla 959.09
  - mediastinum - *see* Injury, internal, mediastinum
  - membrane
    - brain (*see also* Injury, intracranial) 854.0
    - tympanic 959.09
  - meningeal artery - *see* Hemorrhage, brain, traumatic, subarachnoid
  - meninges (cerebral) - *see* Injury, intracranial
  - mesenteric
    - artery - *see* Injury, blood vessel, mesenteric, artery
    - plexus, inferior 954.1
    - vein - *see* Injury, blood vessel, mesenteric, vein
  - mesentery - *see* Injury, internal, mesentery
  - mesosalpinx - *see* Injury, internal, mesosalpinx
  - middle ear 959.09
  - midthoracic region 959.11
  - mouth 959.09
  - multiple (sites not classifiable to the same four-digit category in 959.0-959.7) 959.8
    - internal 869.0
      - with open wound into cavity 869.1
  - musculocutaneous nerve 955.4

ICD-9-CM I Vol. 2

◀ New ⟸ Revised Code

Injury *(Continued)*
- retroperitoneal - *see* Injury, internal, retroperitoneum
- roentgen rays NEC 990
- round ligament - *see* Injury, internal, round ligament
- sacral (region) 959.19
  - plexus 953.5
- sacroiliac ligament NEC 959.19
- sacrum 959.19
- salivary ducts or glands 959.09
- scalp 959.09
  - due to birth trauma 767.19
  - fetus or newborn 767.19
- scapular region 959.2
- sclera 921.3
  - penetrating - *see* Injury, eyeball, penetrating
  - superficial 918.2
- scrotum 959.14
- seminal vesicle - *see* Injury, internal, seminal vesicle
- shoulder (and upper arm) 959.2
- sinus
  - cavernous (*see also* Injury, intracranial) 854.0
  - nasal 959.09
- skeleton NEC, birth injury 767.3
- skin NEC 959.9
- skull - *see* Fracture, skull, by site
- soft tissue (of external sites) (severe) - *see* Wound, open, by site
- specified site NEC 959.8
- spermatic cord - *see* Injury, internal, spermatic cord
- spinal (cord) 952.9
  - with fracture, vertebra - *see* Fracture, vertebra, by site, with spinal cord injury
  - cervical (C_1-C_4) 952.00
    - with
      - anterior cord syndrome 952.02
      - central cord syndrome 952.03
      - complete lesion of cord 952.01
      - incomplete lesion NEC 952.04
      - posterior cord syndrome 952.04
    - C_5-C_7 level 952.05
      - with
        - anterior cord syndrome 952.07
        - central cord syndrome 952.08
        - complete lesion of cord 952.06
        - incomplete lesion NEC 952.09
        - posterior cord syndrome 952.09
      - specified type NEC 952.09
    - specified type NEC 952.04
  - dorsal (D_1-D_6) (T_1-T_6) (thoracic) 952.10
    - with
      - anterior cord syndrome 952.12
      - central cord syndrome 952.13
      - complete lesion of cord 952.11
      - incomplete lesion NEC 952.14
      - posterior cord syndrome 952.14
    - D_7-D_{12} level (T_7-T_{12}) 952.15
      - with
        - anterior cord syndrome 952.17
        - central cord syndrome 952.18
        - complete lesion of cord 952.16
        - incomplete lesion NEC 952.19
        - posterior cord syndrome 952.19
      - specified type NEC 952.19
    - specified type NEC 952.14

Injury *(Continued)*
- spinal *(Continued)*
  - lumbar 952.2
  - multiple sites 952.8
  - nerve (root) NEC - *see* Injury, nerve, spinal, root
  - plexus 953.9
    - brachial 953.4
    - lumbosacral 953.5
    - multiple sites 953.8
  - sacral 952.3
  - thoracic (*see also* Injury, spinal, dorsal) 952.10
- spleen - *see* Injury, internal, spleen
- stellate ganglion 954.1
- sternal region 959.11
- stomach - *see* Injury, internal, stomach
- subconjunctival 921.1
- subcutaneous 959.9
- subdural - *see* Injury, intracranial
- submaxillary region 959.09
- submental region 959.09
- subungual
  - fingers 959.5
  - toes 959.7
- superficial 919

> Note Use the following fourth-digit subdivisions with categories 910-919:
>
> .0 abrasion or friction burn without mention of infection
> .1 abrasion or friction burn, infected
> .2 blister without mention of infection
> .3 blister, infected
> .4 insect bite, nonvenomous, without mention of infection
> .5 insect bite, nonvenomous, infected
> .6 superficial foreign body (splinter) without major open wound and without mention of infection
> .7 superficial foreign body (splinter) without major open wound, infected
> .8 other and unspecified superficial injury without mention of infection
> .9 other and unspecified superficial injury, infected
>
> For late effects of superficial injury, *see* category 906.2.

  - abdomen, abdominal (muscle) (wall) (and other part(s) of trunk) 911
  - ankle (and hip, knee, leg, or thigh) 916
  - anus (and other part(s) of trunk) 911
  - arm 913
    - upper (and shoulder) 912
  - auditory canal (external) (meatus) (and other part(s) of face, neck, or scalp, except eye) 910
  - axilla (and upper arm) 912
  - back (and other part(s) of trunk) 911
  - breast (and other part(s) of trunk) 911
  - brow (and other part(s) of face, neck, or scalp, except eye) 910
  - buttock (and other part(s) of trunk) 911

Injury *(Continued)*
- superficial *(Continued)*
  - canthus, eye 918.0
  - cheek(s) (and other part(s) of face, neck, or scalp, except eye) 910
  - chest wall (and other part(s) of trunk) 911
  - chin (and other part(s) of face, neck, or scalp, except eye) 910
  - clitoris (and other part(s) of trunk) 911
  - conjunctiva 918.2
  - cornea 918.1
    - due to contact lens 371.82
  - costal region (and other part(s) of trunk) 911
  - ear(s) (auricle) (canal) (drum) (external) (and other part(s) of face, neck, or scalp, except eye) 910
  - elbow (and forearm) (and wrist) 913
  - epididymis (and other part(s) of trunk) 911
  - epigastric region (and other part(s) of trunk) 911
  - epiglottis (and other part(s) of face, neck, or scalp, except eye) 910
  - eye(s) (and adnexa) NEC 918.9
  - eyelid(s) (and periocular area) 918.0
  - face (any part(s), except eye) (and neck or scalp) 910
  - finger(s) (nail) (any) 915
  - flank (and other part(s) of trunk) 911
  - foot (phalanges) (and toe(s)) 917
  - forearm (and elbow) (and wrist) 913
  - forehead (and other part(s) of face, neck, or scalp, except eye) 910
  - globe (eye) 918.9
  - groin (and other part(s) of trunk) 911
  - gum(s) (and other part(s) of face, neck, or scalp, except eye) 910
  - hand(s) (except fingers alone) 914
  - head (and other part(s) of face, neck, or scalp, except eye) 910
  - heel (and foot or toe) 917
  - hip (and ankle, knee, leg, or thigh) 916
  - iliac region (and other part(s) of trunk) 911
  - interscapular region (and other part(s) of trunk) 911
  - iris 918.9
  - knee (and ankle, hip, leg, or thigh) 916
  - labium (majus) (minus) (and other part(s) of trunk) 911
  - lacrimal (apparatus) (gland) (sac) 918.0
  - leg (lower) (upper) (and ankle, hip, knee, or thigh) 916
  - lip(s) (and other part(s) of face, neck, or scalp, except eye) 910
  - lower extremity (except foot) 916
  - lumbar region (and other part(s) of trunk) 911
  - malar region (and other part(s) of face, neck, or scalp, except eye) 910
  - mastoid region (and other part(s) of face, neck, or scalp, except eye) 910
  - midthoracic region (and other part(s) of trunk) 911

ICD-9-CM

I

Vol. 2

Injury *(Continued)*
- superficial *(Continued)*
  - mouth (and other part(s) of face, neck, or scalp, except eye) 910
  - multiple sites (not classifiable to the same three-digit category) 919
  - nasal (septum) (and other part(s) of face, neck, or scalp, except eye) 910
  - neck (and face or scalp, any part(s), except eye) 910
  - nose (septum) (and other part(s) of face, neck, or scalp, except eye) 910
  - occipital region (and other part(s) of face, neck, or scalp, except eye) 910
  - orbital region 918.0
  - palate (soft) (and other part(s) of face, neck, or scalp, except eye) 910
  - parietal region (and other part(s) of face, neck, or scalp, except eye) 910
  - penis (and other part(s) of trunk) 911
  - perineum (and other part(s) of trunk) 911
  - periocular area 918.0
  - pharynx (and other part(s) of face, neck, or scalp, except eye) 910
  - popliteal space (and ankle, hip, leg, or thigh) 916
  - prepuce (and other part(s) of trunk) 911
  - pubic region (and other part(s) of trunk) 911
  - pudenda (and other part(s) of trunk) 911
  - sacral region (and other part(s) of trunk) 911
  - salivary (ducts) (glands) (and other part(s) of face, neck, or scalp, except eye) 910
  - scalp (and other part(s) of face or neck, except eye) 910
  - scapular region (and upper arm) 912
  - sclera 918.2
  - scrotum (and other part(s) of trunk) 911
  - shoulder (and upper arm) 912
  - skin NEC 919
  - specified site(s) NEC 919
  - sternal region (and other part(s) of trunk) 911
  - subconjunctival 918.2
  - subcutaneous NEC 919
  - submaxillary region (and other part(s) of face, neck, or scalp, except eye) 910
  - submental region (and other part(s) of face, neck, or scalp, except eye) 910
  - supraclavicular fossa (and other part(s) of face, neck, or scalp, except eye) 910
  - supraorbital 918.0
  - temple (and other part(s) of face, neck, or scalp, except eye) 910
  - temporal region (and other part(s) of face, neck, or scalp, except eye) 910

Injury *(Continued)*
- superficial *(Continued)*
  - testis (and other part(s) of trunk) 911
  - thigh (and ankle, hip, knee, or leg) 916
  - thorax, thoracic (external) (and other part(s) of trunk) 911
  - throat (and other part(s) of face, neck, or scalp, except eye) 910
  - thumb(s) (nail) 915
  - toe(s) (nail) (subungual) (and foot) 917
  - tongue (and other part(s) of face, neck, or scalp, except eye) 910
  - tooth, teeth 521.2
  - trunk (any part(s)) 911
  - tunica vaginalis (and other part(s) of trunk) 911
  - tympanum, tympanic membrane (and other part(s) of face, neck, or scalp, except eye) 910
  - upper extremity NEC 913
  - uvula (and other part(s) of face, neck, or scalp, except eye) 910
  - vagina (and other part(s) of trunk) 911
  - vulva (and other part(s) of trunk) 911
  - wrist (and elbow) (and forearm) 913
- supraclavicular fossa 959.19
- supraorbital 959.09
- surgical complication (external or internal site) 998.2
- symphysis pubis 959.19
  - complicating delivery 665.6
    - affecting fetus or newborn 763.89
- temple 959.09
- temporal region 959.09
- testis 959.14
- thigh (and hip) 959.6
- thorax, thoracic (external) 959.11
  - cavity - *see* Injury, internal, thorax
  - internal - *see* Injury, internal, intrathoracic organs
- throat 959.09
- thumb(s) (nail) 959.5
- thymus - *see* Injury, internal, thymus
- thyroid (gland) 959.09
- toe (nail) (any) 959.7
- tongue 959.09
- tonsil 959.09
- tooth NEC 873.63
  - complicated 873.73
- trachea - *see* Injury, internal, trachea
- trunk 959.19
- tunica vaginalis 959.19
- tympanum, tympanic membrane 959.09
- ultraviolet rays NEC 990
- ureter - *see* Injury, internal, ureter
- urethra (sphincter) - *see* Injury, internal, urethra
- uterus - *see* Injury, internal, uterus
- uvula 959.09
- vagina 959.14
- vascular - *see* Injury, blood vessel
- vas deferens - *see* Injury, internal, vas deferens
- vein (*see also* Injury, blood vessel, by site) 904.9
- vena cava
  - inferior 902.10
  - superior 901.2

Injury *(Continued)*
- vesical (sphincter) - *see* Injury, internal, vesical
- viscera (abdominal) - *see* Injury, internal, viscera
  - with fracture, pelvis - *see* Fracture, pelvis
- visual 950.9
  - cortex 950.3
- vitreous (humor) 871.2
- vulva 959.14
- whiplash (cervical spine) 847.0
- wringer - *see* Crush, by site
- wrist (and elbow) (and forearm) 959.3
- x-ray NEC 990

Inoculation - *see also* Vaccination
- complication or reaction - *see* Complication, vaccination

Insanity, insane (*see also* Psychosis) 298.9
- adolescent (*see also* Schizophrenia) 295.9
- alternating (*see also* Psychosis, affective, circular) 296.7
- confusional 298.9
  - acute 293.0
  - subacute 293.1
- delusional 298.9
- paralysis, general 094.1
  - progressive 094.1
- paresis, general 094.1
- senile 290.20

Insect
- bite - *see* Injury, superficial, by site
- venomous, poisoning by 989.5

Insemination, artificial V26.1

Insertion
- cord (umbilical) lateral or velamentous 663.8
  - affecting fetus or newborn 762.6
- intrauterine contraceptive device V25.1
- placenta, vicious - *see* Placenta, previa
- subdermal implantable contraceptive V25.5
- velamentous, umbilical cord 663.8
  - affecting fetus or newborn 762.6

Insolation 992.0
- meaning sunstroke 992.0

Insomnia 780.52
- with sleep apnea 780.51
- nonorganic origin 307.41
  - persistent (primary) 307.42
  - transient 307.41
- subjective complaint 307.49

Inspiration
- food or foreign body (*see also* Asphyxia, food or foreign body) 933.1
- mucus (*see also* Asphyxia, mucus) 933.1

Inspissated bile syndrome, newborn 774.4

Instability
- detrusor 596.59
- emotional (excessive) 301.3
- joint (posttraumatic) 718.80
  - ankle 718.87
  - elbow 718.82
  - foot 718.87
  - hand 718.84
  - hip 718.85
  - knee 718.86
  - lumbosacral 724.6
  - multiple sites 718.89
  - pelvic region 718.85
  - sacroiliac 724.6

ICD-9-CM
I
Vol. 2

- **Insufficiency, insufficient** *(Continued)*
  - vascular *(Continued)*
    - peripheral 443.9
    - renal (*see also* Hypertension, kidney) 403.90
  - velopharyngeal
    - acquired 528.9
    - congenital 750.29
  - venous (peripheral) 459.81
  - ventricular - *see* Insufficiency, myocardial
  - vertebral artery 435.1
  - vertebrobasilar artery 435.3
  - weight gain during pregnancy 646.8
  - zinc 269.3
- **Insufflation**
  - fallopian
    - fertility testing V26.21
    - following sterilization reversal V26.22
  - meconium 770.1
- **Insular** - *see* condition
- **Insulinoma** (M8151/0)
  - malignant (M8151/3)
    - pancreas 157.4
    - specified site - *see* Neoplasm, by site, malignant
    - unspecified site 157.4
  - pancreas 211.7
  - specified site - *see* Neoplasm, by site, benign
  - unspecified site 211.7
- **Insuloma** - *see* Insulinoma
- **Insult**
  - brain 437.9
    - acute 436
  - cerebral 437.9
    - acute 436
  - cerebrovascular 437.9
    - acute 436
  - vascular NEC 437.9
    - acute 436
- **Insurance examination** (certification) V70.3
- **Intemperance** (*see also* Alcoholism) 303.9
- **Interception of pregnancy** (menstrual extraction) V25.3
- **Intermenstrual**
  - bleeding 626.6
    - irregular 626.6
    - regular 626.5
  - hemorrhage 626.6
    - irregular 626.6
    - regular 626.5
  - pain(s) 625.2
- **Intermittent** - *see* condition
- **Internal** - *see* condition
- **Interproximal wear** 521.1
- **Interruption**
  - aortic arch 747.11
  - bundle of His 426.50
  - fallopian tube (for sterilization) V25.2
  - phase-shift, sleep cycle 307.45
  - repeated REM-sleep 307.48
  - sleep
    - due to perceived environmental disturbances 307.48
    - phase-shift, of 24-hour sleep-wake cycle 307.45
    - repeated REM-sleep type 307.48
  - vas deferens (for sterilization) V25.2
- **Intersexuality** 752.7
- **Interstitial** - *see* condition
- **Intertrigo** 695.89
  - labialis 528.5
- **Intervertebral disc** - *see* condition
- **Intestine, intestinal** - *see also* condition
  - flu 487.8
- **Intolerance**
  - carbohydrate NEC 579.8
  - cardiovascular exercise, with pain (at rest) (with less than ordinary activity) (with ordinary activity) V47.2
  - cold 780.99
  - dissacharide (hereditary) 271.3
  - drug
    - correct substance properly administered 995.2
    - wrong substance given or taken in error 977.9
      - specified drug - *see* Table of Drugs and Chemicals
  - effort 306.2
  - fat NEC 579.8
  - foods NEC 579.8
  - fructose (hereditary) 271.2
  - glucose (-galactose) (congenital) 271.3
  - gluten 579.0
  - lactose (hereditary) (infantile) 271.3
  - lysine (congenital) 270.7
  - milk NEC 579.8
  - protein (familial) 270.7
  - starch NEC 579.8
  - sucrose (-isomaltose) (congenital) 271.3
- **Intoxicated NEC** (*see also* Alcoholism) 305.0
- **Intoxication**
  - acid 276.2
  - acute
    - alcoholic 305.0
      - with alcoholism 303.0
      - hangover effects 305.0
    - caffeine 305.9
    - hallucinogenic (*see also* Abuse, drugs, nondependent) 305.3
  - alcohol (acute) 305.0
    - with alcoholism 303.0
    - hangover effects 305.0
    - idiosyncratic 291.4
    - pathological 291.4
  - alimentary canal 558.2
  - ammonia (hepatic) 572.2
  - chemical - *see also* Table of Drugs and Chemicals
    - via placenta or breast milk 760.70
      - alcohol 760.71
      - anti-infective agents 760.74
      - cocaine 760.75
      - "crack" 760.75
      - hallucinogenic agents NEC 760.73
      - medicinal agents NEC 760.79
      - narcotics 760.72
      - obstetric anesthetic or analgesic drug 763.5
      - specified agent NEC 760.79
      - suspected, affecting management of pregnancy 655.5
  - cocaine, through placenta or breast milk 760.75
  - delirium
    - alcohol 291.0
    - drug 292.81
  - drug
    - with delirium 292.81
    - correct substance properly administered (*see also* Allergy, drug) 995.2
- **Intoxication** *(Continued)*
  - drug *(Continued)*
    - newborn 779.4
    - obstetric anesthetic or sedation 668.9
      - affecting fetus or newborn 763.5
    - overdose or wrong substance given or taken - *see* Table of Drugs and Chemicals
    - pathologic 292.2
    - specific to newborn 779.4
    - via placenta or breast milk 760.70
      - alcohol 760.71
      - anti-infective agents 760.74
      - cocaine 760.75
      - "crack" 760.75
      - hallucinogenic agents 760.73
      - medicinal agents NEC 760.79
      - narcotics 760.72
      - obstetric anesthetic or analgesic drug 763.5
      - specified agent NEC 760.79
      - suspected, affecting management of pregnancy 655.5
  - enteric - *see* Intoxication, intestinal
  - fetus or newborn, via placenta or breast milk 760.70
    - alcohol 760.71
    - anti-infective agents 760.74
    - cocaine 760.75
    - "crack" 760.75
    - hallucinogenic agents 760.73
    - medicinal agents NEC 760.79
    - narcotics 760.72
    - obstetric anesthetic or analgesic drug 763.5
    - specified agent NEC 760.79
    - suspected, affecting management of pregnancy 655.5
  - food - *see* Poisoning, food
  - gastrointestinal 558.2
  - hallucinogenic (acute) 305.3
  - hepatocerebral 572.2
  - idiosyncratic alcohol 291.4
  - intestinal 569.89
    - due to putrefaction of food 005.9
  - methyl alcohol (*see also* Alcoholism) 305.0
    - with alcoholism 303.0
  - pathologic 291.4
    - drug 292.2
  - potassium (K) 276.7
  - septic
    - with
      - abortion - *see* Abortion, by type, with sepsis
      - ectopic pregnancy (*see also* categories 633.0-633.9) 639.0
      - molar pregnancy (*see also* categories 630-632) 639.0
    - during labor 659.3
    - following
      - abortion 639.0
      - ectopic or molar pregnancy 639.0
    - generalized - *see* Septicemia
    - puerperal, postpartum, childbirth 670
  - serum (prophylactic) (therapeutic) 999.5
  - uremic - *see* Uremia
  - water 276.6
- **Intracranial** - *see* condition
- **Intrahepatic gallbladder** 751.69
- **Intraligamentous** - *see also* condition
  - pregnancy - *see* Pregnancy, cornual
- **Intraocular** - *see also* condition
  - sepsis 360.00

J

K

◄ New ⟸ Revised Code

L

- **Labia, labium** - *see* condition
- **Labiated hymen** 752.49
- **Labile**
  - blood pressure 796.2
  - emotions, emotionality 301.3
  - vasomotor system 443.9
- **Labioglossal paralysis** 335.22
- **Labium leporinum** (*see also* Cleft, lip) 749.10
- **Labor** (*see also* Delivery)
  - with complications - *see* Delivery, complicated
  - abnormal NEC 661.9
    - affecting fetus or newborn 763.7
  - arrested active phase 661.1
    - affecting fetus or newborn 763.7
  - desultory 661.2
    - affecting fetus or newborn 763.7
  - dyscoordinate 661.4
    - affecting fetus or newborn 763.7
  - early onset (22-36 weeks gestation) 644.2
  - failed
    - induction 659.1
      - mechanical 659.0
      - medical 659.1
      - surgical 659.0
    - trial (vaginal delivery) 660.6
  - false 644.1
  - forced or induced, affecting fetus or newborn 763.89
  - hypertonic 661.4
    - affecting fetus or newborn 763.7
  - hypotonic 661.2
    - affecting fetus or newborn 763.7
    - primary 661.0
      - affecting fetus or newborn 763.7
    - secondary 661.1
      - affecting fetus or newborn 763.7
  - incoordinate 661.4
    - affecting fetus or newborn 763.7
  - irregular 661.2
    - affecting fetus or newborn 763.7
  - long - *see* Labor, prolonged
  - missed (at or near term) 656.4
  - obstructed NEC 660.9
    - affecting fetus or newborn 763.1
    - specified cause NEC 660.8
      - affecting fetus or newborn 763.1
  - pains, spurious 644.1
  - precipitate 661.3
    - affecting fetus or newborn 763.6
  - premature 644.2
    - threatened 644.0
  - prolonged or protracted 662.1
    - affecting fetus or newborn 763.89
    - first stage 662.0
      - affecting fetus or newborn 763.89
    - second stage 662.2
      - affecting fetus or newborn 763.89
  - threatened NEC 644.1
  - undelivered 644.1
- **Labored breathing** (*see also* Hyperventilation) 786.09
- **Labyrinthitis** (inner ear) (destructive) (latent) 386.30
  - circumscribed 386.32
  - diffuse 386.31
  - focal 386.32
  - purulent 386.33
  - serous 386.31
  - suppurative 386.33
  - syphilitic 095.8
  - toxic 386.34
  - viral 386.35
- **Laceration** - *see also* Wound, open, by site
  - accidental, complicating surgery 998.2
  - Achilles tendon 845.09
    - with open wound 892.2
  - anus (sphincter) 879.6
    - with
      - abortion - *see* Abortion, by type, with damage to pelvic organs
      - ectopic pregnancy (*see also* categories 633.0-633.9) 639.2
      - molar pregnancy (*see also* categories 630-632) 639.2
    - complicated 879.7
    - complicating delivery 664.2
      - with laceration of anal or rectal mucosa 664.3
    - following
      - abortion 639.2
      - ectopic or molar pregnancy 639.2
    - nontraumatic, nonpuerperal 565.0
  - bladder (urinary)
    - with
      - abortion - *see* Abortion, by type, with damage to pelvic organs
      - ectopic pregnancy (*see also* categories 633.0-633.9) 639.2
      - molar pregnancy (*see also* categories 630-632) 639.2
    - following
      - abortion 639.2
      - ectopic or molar pregnancy 639.2
    - obstetrical trauma 665.5
  - blood vessel - *see* Injury, blood vessel, by site
  - bowel
    - with
      - abortion - *see* Abortion, by type, with damage to pelvic organs
      - ectopic pregnancy (*see also* categories 633.0-633.9) 639.2
      - molar pregnancy (*see also* categories 630-632) 639.2
    - following
      - abortion 639.2
      - ectopic or molar pregnancy 639.2
    - obstetrical trauma 665.5
  - brain (cerebral) (membrane) (with hemorrhage) 851.8

> Note Use the following fifth-digit subclassification with categories 851-854:
>
> 0 unspecified state of consciousness
> 1 with no loss of consciousness
> 2 with brief [less than one hour] loss of consciousness
> 3 with moderate [1-24 hours] loss of consciousness
> 4 with prolonged [more than 24 hours] loss of consciousness and return to pre-existing conscious level
> 5 with prolonged [more than 24 hours] loss of consciousness, without return to pre-existing conscious level

Laceration (*Continued*)
brain (*Continued*)

> Use fifth-digit 5 to designate when a patient is unconscious and dies before regaining consciousness, regardless of the duration of the loss of consciousness
>
> 6 with loss of consciousness of unspecified duration
> 9 with concussion, unspecified

- with
  - open intracranial wound 851.9
  - skull fracture - *see* Fracture, skull, by site
- cerebellum 851.6
  - with open intracranial wound 851.7
- cortex 851.2
  - with open intracranial wound 851.3
- during birth 767.0
- stem 851.6
  - with open intracranial wound 851.7

- broad ligament
  - with
    - abortion - *see* Abortion, by type, with damage to pelvic organs
    - ectopic pregnancy (*see also* categories 633.0-633.9) 639.2
    - molar pregnancy (*see also* categories 630-632) 639.2
  - following
    - abortion 639.2
    - ectopic or molar pregnancy 639.2
  - nontraumatic 620.6
  - obstetrical trauma 665.6
  - syndrome (nontraumatic) 620.6
- capsule, joint - *see* Sprain, by site
- cardiac - *see* Laceration, heart
- causing eversion of cervix uteri (old) 622.0
- central, complicating delivery 664.4
- cerebellum - *see* Laceration, brain, cerebellum
- cerebral - *see also* Laceration, brain
  - during birth 767.0
- cervix (uteri)
  - with
    - abortion - *see* Abortion, by type, with damage to pelvic organs
    - ectopic pregnancy (*see also* categories 633.0-633.9) 639.2
    - molar pregnancy (*see also* categories 630-632) 639.2
  - following
    - abortion 639.2
    - ectopic or molar pregnancy 639.2
  - nonpuerperal, nontraumatic 622.3
  - obstetrical trauma (current) 665.3
  - old (postpartal) 622.3
  - traumatic - *see* Injury, internal, cervix
- chordae heart 429.5
- complicated 879.9
- cornea - *see* Laceration, eyeball
  - superficial 918.1
- cortex (cerebral) - *see* Laceration, brain, cortex
- esophagus 530.89
- eye(s) - *see* Laceration, ocular
- eyeball NEC 871.4
  - with prolapse or exposure of intraocular tissue 871.1
  - penetrating - *see* Penetrating wound, eyeball

L

Labia, labium - *see* condition
Labiated hymen 752.49
Labile
  blood pressure 796.2
  emotions, emotionality 301.3
  vasomotor system 443.9
Labioglossal paralysis 335.22
Labium leporinum (*see also* Cleft, lip) 749.10
Labor (*see also* Delivery)
  with complications - *see* Delivery, complicated
  abnormal NEC 661.9
    affecting fetus or newborn 763.7
  arrested active phase 661.1
    affecting fetus or newborn 763.7
  desultory 661.2
    affecting fetus or newborn 763.7
  dyscoordinate 661.4
    affecting fetus or newborn 763.7
  early onset (22-36 weeks gestation) 644.2
  failed
    induction 659.1
      mechanical 659.0
      medical 659.1
      surgical 659.0
    trial (vaginal delivery) 660.6
  false 644.1
  forced or induced, affecting fetus or newborn 763.89
  hypertonic 661.4
    affecting fetus or newborn 763.7
  hypotonic 661.2
    affecting fetus or newborn 763.7
    primary 661.0
      affecting fetus or newborn 763.7
    secondary 661.1
      affecting fetus or newborn 763.7
  incoordinate 661.4
    affecting fetus or newborn 763.7
  irregular 661.2
    affecting fetus or newborn 763.7
  long - *see* Labor, prolonged
  missed (at or near term) 656.4
  obstructed NEC 660.9
    affecting fetus or newborn 763.1
    specified cause NEC 660.8
      affecting fetus or newborn 763.1
  pains, spurious 644.1
  precipitate 661.3
    affecting fetus or newborn 763.6
  premature 644.2
    threatened 644.0
  prolonged or protracted 662.1
    affecting fetus or newborn 763.89
    first stage 662.0
      affecting fetus or newborn 763.89
    second stage 662.2
      affecting fetus or newborn 763.89
  threatened NEC 644.1
  undelivered 644.1
Labored breathing (*see also* Hyperventilation) 786.09
Labyrinthitis (inner ear) (destructive) (latent) 386.30
  circumscribed 386.32
  diffuse 386.31
  focal 386.32
  purulent 386.33
Labyrinthitis (*Continued*)
  serous 386.31
  suppurative 386.33
  syphilitic 095.8
  toxic 386.34
  viral 386.35
Laceration - *see also* Wound, open, by site
  accidental, complicating surgery 998.2
  Achilles tendon 845.09
    with open wound 892.2
  anus (sphincter) 879.6 ◄ (Revised Code)
    with
      abortion - *see* Abortion, by type, with damage to pelvic organs
      ectopic pregnancy (*see also* categories 633.0-633.9) 639.2
      molar pregnancy (*see also* categories 630-632) 639.2
    complicated 879.7 ◄ (New)
    complicating delivery 664.2
      with laceration of anal or rectal mucosa 664.3
    following
      abortion 639.2
      ectopic or molar pregnancy 639.2
    nontraumatic, nonpuerperal 565.0
  bladder (urinary)
    with
      abortion - *see* Abortion, by type, with damage to pelvic organs
      ectopic pregnancy (*see also* categories 633.0-633.9) 639.2
      molar pregnancy (*see also* categories 630-632) 639.2
    following
      abortion 639.2
      ectopic or molar pregnancy 639.2
    obstetrical trauma 665.5
  blood vessel - *see* Injury, blood vessel, by site
  bowel
    with
      abortion - *see* Abortion, by type, with damage to pelvic organs
      ectopic pregnancy (*see also* categories 633.0-633.9) 639.2
      molar pregnancy (*see also* categories 630-632) 639.2
    following
      abortion 639.2
      ectopic or molar pregnancy 639.2
    obstetrical trauma 665.5
  brain (cerebral) (membrane) (with hemorrhage) 851.8

> Note Use the following fifth-digit subclassification with categories 851-854:
>
> 0 unspecified state of consciousness
> 1 with no loss of consciousness
> 2 with brief [less than one hour] loss of consciousness
> 3 with moderate [1-24 hours] loss of consciousness
> 4 with prolonged [more than 24 hours] loss of consciousness and return to pre-existing conscious level
> 5 with prolonged [more than 24 hours] loss of consciousness, without return to pre-existing conscious level
> Use fifth-digit 5 to designate when a patient is unconscious and dies before regaining consciousness, regardless of the duration of the loss of consciousness
> 6 with loss of consciousness of unspecified duration
> 9 with concussion, unspecified

Laceration (*Continued*)
  brain (*Continued*)
    with
      open intracranial wound 851.9
      skull fracture - *see* Fracture, skull, by site
    cerebellum 851.6
      with open intracranial wound 851.7
    cortex 851.2
      with open intracranial wound 851.3
    during birth 767.0
    stem 851.6
      with open intracranial wound 851.7
  broad ligament
    with
      abortion - *see* Abortion, by type, with damage to pelvic organs
      ectopic pregnancy (*see also* categories 633.0-633.9) 639.2
      molar pregnancy (*see also* categories 630-632) 639.2
    following
      abortion 639.2
      ectopic or molar pregnancy 639.2
    nontraumatic 620.6
    obstetrical trauma 665.6
    syndrome (nontraumatic) 620.6
  capsule, joint - *see* Sprain, by site
  cardiac - *see* Laceration, heart
  causing eversion of cervix uteri (old) 622.0
  central, complicating delivery 664.4
  cerebellum - *see* Laceration, brain, cerebellum
  cerebral - *see also* Laceration, brain
    during birth 767.0
  cervix (uteri)
    with
      abortion - *see* Abortion, by type, with damage to pelvic organs
      ectopic pregnancy (*see also* categories 633.0-633.9) 639.2
      molar pregnancy (*see also* categories 630-632) 639.2
    following
      abortion 639.2
      ectopic or molar pregnancy 639.2
    nonpuerperal, nontraumatic 622.3
    obstetrical trauma (current) 665.3
    old (postpartal) 622.3
    traumatic - *see* Injury, internal, cervix
  chordae heart 429.5
  complicated 879.9
  cornea - *see* Laceration, eyeball
    superficial 918.1
  cortex (cerebral) - *see* Laceration, brain, cortex
  esophagus 530.89
  eye(s) - *see* Laceration, ocular
  eyeball NEC 871.4
    with prolapse or exposure of intraocular tissue 871.1
    penetrating - *see* Penetrating wound, eyeball

- **Leukemia, leukemic** *(Continued)*
  - basophilic (M9870/3) 205.1
  - blast (cell) (M9801/3) 208.0
  - blastic (M9801/3) 208.0
    - granulocytic (M9861/3) 205.0
  - chronic NEC (M9803/3) 208.1
  - compound (M9810/3) 207.8
  - eosinophilic (M9880/3) 205.1
  - giant cell (M9910/3) 207.2
  - granulocytic (M9860/3) 205.9
    - acute (M9861/3) 205.0
    - aleukemic (M9864/3) 205.8
    - blastic (M9861/3) 205.0
    - chronic (M9863/3) 205.1
    - subacute (M9862/3) 205.2
    - subleukemic (M9864/3) 205.8
  - hairy cell (M9940/3) 202.4
  - hemoblastic (M9801/3) 208.0
  - histiocytic (M9890/3) 206.9
  - lymphatic (M9820/3) 204.9
    - acute (M9821/3) 204.0
    - aleukemic (M9824/3) 204.8
    - chronic (M9823/3) 204.1
    - subacute (M9822/3) 204.2
    - subleukemic (M9824/3) 204.8
  - lymphoblastic (M9821/3) 204.0
  - lymphocytic (M9820/3) 204.9
    - acute (M9821/3) 204.0
    - aleukemic (M9824/3) 204.8
    - chronic (M9823/3) 204.1
    - subacute (M9822/3) 204.2
    - subleukemic (M9824/3) 204.8
  - lymphogenous (M9820/3) - *see* Leukemia, lymphoid
  - lymphoid (M9820/3) 204.9
    - acute (M9821/3) 204.0
    - aleukemic (M9824/3) 204.8
    - blastic (M9821/3) 204.0
    - chronic (M9823/3) 204.1
    - subacute (M9822/3) 204.2
    - subleukemic (M9824/3) 204.8
  - lymphosarcoma cell (M9850/3) 207.8
  - mast cell (M9900/3) 207.8
  - megakaryocytic (M9910/3) 207.2
  - megakaryocytoid (M9910/3) 207.2
  - mixed (cell) (M9810/3) 207.8
  - monoblastic (M9891/3) 206.0
  - monocytic (Schilling-type) (M9890/3) 206.9
    - acute (M9891/3) 206.0
    - aleukemic (M9894/3) 206.8
    - chronic (M9893/3) 206.1
    - Naegeli-type (M9863/3) 205.1
    - subacute (M9892/3) 206.2
    - subleukemic (M9894/3) 206.8
  - monocytoid (M9890/3) 206.9
    - acute (M9891/3) 206.0
    - aleukemic (M9894/3) 206.8
    - chronic (M9893/3) 206.1
    - myelogenous (M9863/3) 205.1
    - subacute (M9892/3) 206.2
    - subleukemic (M9894/3) 206.8
  - monomyelocytic (M9860/3) - *see* Leukemia, myelomonocytic
  - myeloblastic (M9861/3) 205.0
  - myelocytic (M9863/3) 205.1
    - acute (M9861/3) 205.0
  - myelogenous (M9860/3) 205.9
    - acute (M9861/3) 205.0
    - aleukemic (M9864/3) 205.8
    - chronic (M9863/3) 205.1
    - monocytoid (M9863/3) 205.1
    - subacute (M9862/3) 205.2
    - subleukemic (M9864) 205.8
  - myeloid (M9860/3) 205.9

- **Leukemia, leukemic** *(Continued)*
  - myeloid (M9860/3) *(Continued)*
    - acute (M9861/3) 205.0
    - aleukemic (M9864/3) 205.8
    - chronic (M9863/3) 205.1
    - subacute (M9862/3) 205.2
    - subleukemic (M9864/3) 205.8
  - myelomonocytic (M9860/3) 205.9
    - acute (M9861/3) 205.0
    - chronic (M9863/3) 205.1
  - Naegeli-type monocytic (M9863/3) 205.1
  - neutrophilic (M9865/3) 205.1
  - plasma cell (M9830/3) 203.1
  - plasmacytic (M9830/3) 203.1
  - prolymphocytic (M9825/3) - *see* Leukemia, lymphoid
  - promyelocytic, acute (M9866/3) 205.0
  - Schilling-type monocytic (M9890/3) - *see* Leukemia, monocytic
  - stem cell (M9801/3) 208.0
  - subacute NEC (M9802/3) 208.2
  - subleukemic NEC (M9804/3) 208.8
  - thrombocytic (M9910/3) 207.2
  - undifferentiated (M9801/3) 208.0
- **Leukemoid reaction** (lymphocytic) (monocytic) (myelocytic) 288.8
- **Leukoclastic vasculitis** 446.29
- **Leukocoria** 360.44
- **Leukocythemia** - *see* Leukemia
- **Leukocytosis** 288.8
  - basophilic 288.8
  - eosinophilic 288.3
  - lymphocytic 288.8
  - monocytic 288.8
  - neutrophilic 288.8
- **Leukoderma** 709.09
  - syphilitic 091.3
    - late 095.8
- **Leukodermia** (*see also* Leukoderma) 709.09
- **Leukodystrophy** (cerebral) (globoid cell) (metachromatic) (progressive) (sudanophilic) 330.0
- **Leukoedema, mouth or tongue** 528.7
- **Leukoencephalitis**
  - acute hemorrhagic (postinfectious) NEC 136.9 *[323.6]*
    - postimmunization or postvaccinal 323.5
  - subacute sclerosing 046.2
    - van Bogaert's 046.2
  - van Bogaert's (sclerosing) 046.2
- **Leukoencephalopathy** (*see also* Encephalitis) 323.9
  - acute necrotizing hemorrhagic (postinfectious) 136.9 *[323.6]*
    - postimmunization or postvaccinal 323.5
  - metachromatic 330.0
  - multifocal (progressive) 046.3
  - progressive multifocal 046.3
- **Leukoerythroblastosis** 289.0
- **Leukoerythrosis** 289.0
- **Leukokeratosis** (*see also* Leukoplakia) 702.8
  - mouth 528.6
  - nicotina palati 528.7
  - tongue 528.6
- **Leukokoria** 360.44
- **Leukokraurosis vulva, vulvae** 624.0
- **Leukolymphosarcoma** (M9850/3) 207.8
- **Leukoma** (cornea) (interfering with central vision) 371.03
  - adherent 371.04
- **Leukomalacia, periventricular** 779.7
- **Leukomelanopathy, hereditary** 288.2

- **Leukonychia** (punctata) (striata) 703.8
  - congenital 757.5
- **Leukopathia**
  - unguium 703.8
    - congenital 757.5
- **Leukopenia** 288.0
  - cyclic 288.0
  - familial 288.0
  - malignant 288.0
  - periodic 288.0
  - transitory neonatal 776.7
- **Leukopenic** - *see* condition
- **Leukoplakia** 702.8
  - anus 569.49
  - bladder (postinfectional) 596.8
  - buccal 528.6
  - cervix (uteri) 622.2
  - esophagus 530.83
  - gingiva 528.6
  - kidney (pelvis) 593.89
  - larynx 478.79
  - lip 528.6
  - mouth 528.6
  - oral soft tissue (including tongue) (mucosa) 528.6
  - palate 528.6
  - pelvis (kidney) 593.89
  - penis (infectional) 607.0
  - rectum 569.49
  - syphilitic 095.8
  - tongue 528.6
  - tonsil 478.29
  - ureter (postinfectional) 593.89
  - urethra (postinfectional) 599.84
  - uterus 621.8
  - vagina 623.1
  - vesical 596.8
  - vocal cords 478.5
  - vulva 624.0
- **Leukopolioencephalopathy** 330.0
- **Leukorrhea** (vagina) 623.5
  - due to Trichomonas (vaginalis) 131.00
  - trichomonal (Trichomonas vaginalis) 131.00
- **Leukosarcoma** (M9850/3) 207.8
- **Leukosis** (M9800/3) - *see* Leukemia
- **Lev's disease or syndrome** (acquired complete heart block) 426.0
- **Levi's syndrome** (pituitary dwarfism) 253.3
- **Levocardia** (isolated) 746.87
  - with situs inversus 759.3
- **Levulosuria** 271.2
- **Lewandowski's disease** (primary) (*see also* Tuberculosis) 017.0
- **Lewandowski-Lutz disease** (epidermodysplasia verruciformis) 078.19
- **Lewy body dementia** 331.82 ◀
- **Lewy body disease** 331.82 ◀
- **Leyden's disease** (periodic vomiting) 536.2
- **Leyden-Möbius dystrophy** 359.1
- **Leydig cell**
  - carcinoma (M8650/3)
    - specified site - *see* Neoplasm, by site, malignant
    - unspecified site
      - female 183.0
      - male 186.9
  - tumor (M8650/1)
    - benign (M8650/0)
      - specified site - *see* Neoplasm, by site, benign
      - unspecified site
        - female 220
        - male 222.0

◀ New ⇐ Revised Code

Note Use the following fifth-digit subclassification with categories 200-202:

0	unspecified site
1	lymph nodes of head, face, and neck
2	intrathoracic lymph nodes
3	intra-abdominal lymph nodes
4	lymph nodes of axilla and upper limb
5	lymph nodes of inguinal region and lower limb
6	intrapelvic lymph nodes
7	spleen
8	lymph nodes of multiple sites

M

- **Macacus ear** 744.29
- **Maceration**
  - fetus (cause not stated) 779.9
  - wet feet, tropical (syndrome) 991.4
- **Machado-Joseph disease** 334.8
- **Machupo virus hemorrhagic fever** 078.7
- **Macleod's syndrome** (abnormal transradiancy, one lung) 492.8
- **Macrocephalia, macrocephaly** 756.0
- **Macrocheilia** (congenital) 744.81
- **Macrochilia** (congenital) 744.81
- **Macrocolon** (congenital) 751.3
- **Macrocornea** 743.41
  - associated with buphthalmos 743.22
- **Macrocytic** - *see* condition
- **Macrocytosis** 289.89
- **Macrodactylia, macrodactylism** (fingers) (thumbs) 755.57
  - toes 755.65
- **Macrodontia** 520.2
- **Macroencephaly** 742.4
- **Macrogenia** 524.05
- **Macrogenitosomia** (female) (male) (praecox) 255.2
- **Macrogingivae** 523.8
- **Macroglobulinemia** (essential) (idiopathic) (monoclonal) (primary) (syndrome) (Waldenström's) 273.3
- **Macroglossia** (congenital) 750.15
  - acquired 529.8
- **Macrognathia, macrognathism** (congenital) 524.00
  - mandibular 524.02
    - alveolar 524.72
  - maxillary 524.01
    - alveolar 524.71
- **Macrogyria** (congenital) 742.4
- **Macrohydrocephalus** (*see also* Hydrocephalus) 331.4
- **Macromastia** (*see also* Hypertrophy, breast) 611.1
- **Macropsia** 368.14
- **Macrosigmoid** 564.7
  - congenital 751.3
- **Macrospondylitis, acromegalic** 253.0
- **Macrostomia** (congenital) 744.83
- **Macrotia** (external ear) (congenital) 744.22
- **Macula**
  - cornea, corneal
    - congenital 743.43
      - interfering with vision 743.42
    - interfering with central vision 371.03
    - not interfering with central vision 371.02
  - degeneration (*see also* Degeneration, macula) 362.50
    - hereditary (*see also* Dystrophy, retina) 362.70
  - edema, cystoid 362.53
- **Maculae ceruleae** 132.1
- **Macules and papules** 709.8
- **Maculopathy, toxic** 362.55
- **Madarosis** 374.55
- **Madelung's**
  - deformity (radius) 755.54
  - disease (lipomatosis) 272.8
  - lipomatosis 272.8
- **Madness** (*see also* Psychosis) 298.9
  - myxedema (acute) 293.0
    - subacute 293.1
- **Madura**
  - disease (actinomycotic) 039.9
    - mycotic 117.4
  - foot (actinomycotic) 039.4
    - mycotic 117.4
- **Maduromycosis** (actinomycotic) 039.9
  - mycotic 117.4
- **Maffucci's syndrome** (dyschondroplasia with hemangiomas) 756.4
- **Magenblase syndrome** 306.4
- **Main en griffe** (acquired) 736.06
  - congenital 755.59
- **Maintenance**
  - chemotherapy regimen or treatment V58.1
  - dialysis regimen or treatment
    - extracorporeal (renal) V56.0
    - peritoneal V56.8
    - renal V56.0
  - drug therapy or regimen V58.1
  - external fixation NEC V54.89
  - radiotherapy V58.0
  - traction NEC V54.89
- **Majocchi's**
  - disease (purpura annularis telangiectodes) 709.1
  - granuloma 110.6
- **Major** - *see* condition
- **Mal**
  - cerebral (idiopathic) (*see also* Epilepsy) 345.9
  - comital (*see also* Epilepsy) 345.9
  - de los pintos (*see also* Pinta) 103.9
  - de Meleda 757.39
  - de mer 994.6
  - lie - *see* Presentation, fetal
  - perforant (*see also* Ulcer, lower extremity) 707.15
- **Malabar itch** 110.9
  - beard 110.0
  - foot 110.4
  - scalp 110.0
- **Malabsorption** 579.9
  - calcium 579.8
  - carbohydrate 579.8
  - disaccharide 271.3
  - drug-induced 579.8
  - due to bacterial overgrowth 579.8
  - fat 579.8
  - folate, congenital 281.2
  - galactose 271.1
  - glucose-galactose (congenital) 271.3
  - intestinal 579.9
  - isomaltose 271.3
  - lactose (hereditary) 271.3
  - methionine 270.4
  - monosaccharide 271.8
  - postgastrectomy 579.3
  - postsurgical 579.3
  - protein 579.8
  - sucrose (-isomaltose) (congenital) 271.3
  - syndrome 579.9
    - postgastrectomy 579.3
    - postsurgical 579.3
- **Malacia, bone** 268.2
  - juvenile (*see also* Rickets) 268.0
  - Kienböck's (juvenile) (lunate) (wrist) 732.3
    - adult 732.8
- **Malacoplakia**
  - bladder 596.8
  - colon 569.89
  - pelvis (kidney) 593.89
  - ureter 593.89
- **Malacoplakia** *(Continued)*
  - urethra 599.84
- **Malacosteon** 268.2
  - juvenile (*see also* Rickets) 268.0
- **Maladaptation** - *see* Maladjustment
- **Maladie de Roger** 745.4
- **Maladjustment**
  - conjugal V61.10
    - involving divorce or estrangement V61.0
  - educational V62.3
  - family V61.9
    - specified circumstance NEC V61.8
  - marital V61.10
    - involving divorce or estrangement V61.0
  - occupational V62.2
  - simple, adult (*see also* Reaction, adjustment) 309.9
  - situational acute (*see also* Reaction, adjustment) 309.9
  - social V62.4
- **Malaise** 780.79
- **Malakoplakia** - *see* Malacoplakia
- **Malaria, malarial** (fever) 084.6
  - algid 084.9
  - any type, with
    - algid malaria 084.9
    - blackwater fever 084.8
    - fever
      - blackwater 084.8
      - hemoglobinuric (bilious) 084.8
    - hemoglobinuria, malarial 084.8
    - hepatitis 084.9 *[573.2]*
    - nephrosis 084.9 *[581.81]*
    - pernicious complication NEC 084.9
      - cardiac 084.9
      - cerebral 084.9
  - cardiac 084.9
  - carrier (suspected) of V02.9
  - cerebral 084.9
  - complicating pregnancy, childbirth, or puerperium 647.4
  - congenital 771.2
  - congestion, congestive 084.6
    - brain 084.9
  - continued 084.0
  - estivo-autumnal 084.0
  - falciparum (malignant tertian) 084.0
  - hematinuria 084.8
  - hematuria 084.8
  - hemoglobinuria 084.8
  - hemorrhagic 084.6
  - induced (therapeutically) 084.7
    - accidental - *see* Malaria, by type
  - liver 084.9 *[573.2]*
  - malariae (quartan) 084.2
  - malignant (tertian) 084.0
  - mixed infections 084.5
  - monkey 084.4
  - ovale 084.3
  - pernicious, acute 084.0
  - Plasmodium, P.
    - falciparum 084.0
    - malariae 084.2
    - ovale 084.3
    - vivax 084.1
  - quartan 084.2
  - quotidian 084.0
  - recurrent 084.6
    - induced (therapeutically) 084.7
      - accidental - *see* Malaria, by type
  - remittent 084.6
  - specified types NEC 084.4

◄ New ⟸ Revised Code

- **Lesion** *(Continued)*
  - cranial nerve *(Continued)*
    - eleventh 352.4
    - twelfth 352.5
  - cystic - *see* Cyst
  - degenerative - *see* Degeneration
  - dermal (skin) 709.9
  - Dieulafoy (hemorrhagic)
    - of
      - duodenum 537.84
      - intestine 569.86
      - stomach 537.84
  - duodenum 537.89
    - with obstruction 537.3
  - eyelid 373.9
  - gasserian ganglion 350.8
  - gastric 537.89
  - gastroduodenal 537.89
  - gastrointestinal 569.89
  - glossopharyngeal nerve 352.2
  - heart (organic) - *see also* Disease, heart
    - vascular - *see* Disease, cardiovascular
  - helix (ear) 709.9
  - hyperchromic, due to pinta (carate) 103.1
  - hyperkeratotic (*see also* Hyperkeratosis) 701.1
  - hypoglossal nerve 352.5
  - hypopharynx 478.29
  - hypothalamic 253.9
  - ileocecal coil 569.89
  - ileum 569.89
  - iliohypogastric nerve 355.79
  - ilioinguinal nerve 355.79
  - in continuity - *see* Injury, nerve, by site
  - inflammatory - *see* Inflammation
  - intestine 569.89
  - intracerebral - *see* Lesion, brain
  - intrachiasmal (optic) (*see also* Lesion, chiasmal) 377.54
  - intracranial, space-occupying NEC 784.2
  - joint 719.90
    - ankle 719.97
    - elbow 719.92
    - foot 719.97
    - hand 719.94
    - hip 719.95
    - knee 719.96
    - multiple sites 719.99
    - pelvic region 719.95
    - sacroiliac (old) 724.6
    - shoulder (region) 719.91
    - specified site NEC 719.98
    - wrist 719.93
  - keratotic (*see also* Keratosis) 701.1
  - kidney (*see also* Disease, renal) 593.9
  - laryngeal nerve (recurrent) 352.3
  - leonine 030.0
  - LGSIL (low grade squamous intraepithelial dysplasia 622.1
  - lip 528.5
  - liver 573.8
  - lumbosacral
    - plexus 353.1
    - root (nerve) NEC 353.4
  - lung 518.89
    - coin 793.1
  - maxillary sinus 473.0
  - mitral - *see* Endocarditis, mitral
  - motor cortex 348.8
  - nerve (*see also* Disorder, nerve) 355.9
  - nervous system 349.9
    - congenital 742.9

- **Lesion** *(Continued)*
  - nonallopathic NEC 739.9
    - in region (of)
      - abdomen 739.9
      - acromioclavicular 739.7
      - cervical, cervicothoracic 739.1
      - costochondral 739.8
      - costovertebral 739.8
      - extremity
        - lower 739.6
        - upper 739.7
      - head 739.0
      - hip 739.5
      - lower extremity 739.6
      - lumbar, lumbosacral 739.3
      - occipitocervical 739.0
      - pelvic 739.5
      - pubic 739.5
      - rib cage 739.8
      - sacral, sacrococcygeal, sacroiliac 739.4
      - sternochondral 739.8
      - sternoclavicular 739.7
      - thoracic, thoracolumbar 739.2
      - upper extremity 739.7
  - nose (internal) 478.1
  - obstructive - *see* Obstruction
  - obturator nerve 355.79
  - occlusive
    - artery - *see* Embolism, artery
  - organ or site NEC - *see* Disease, by site
  - osteolytic 733.90
  - paramacular, of retina 363.32
  - peptic 537.89
  - periodontal, due to traumatic occlusion 523.8
  - perirectal 569.49
  - peritoneum (granulomatous) 568.89
  - pigmented (skin) 709.00
  - pinta - *see* Pinta, lesions
  - polypoid - *see* Polyp
  - prechiasmal (optic) (*see also* Lesion, chiasmal) 377.54
  - primary - *see also* Syphilis, primary
    - carate 103.0
    - pinta 103.0
    - yaws 102.0
  - pulmonary 518.89
    - valve (*see also* Endocarditis, pulmonary) 424.3
  - pylorus 537.89
  - radiation NEC 990
  - radium NEC 990
  - rectosigmoid 569.89
  - retina, retinal - *see also* Retinopathy
    - vascular 362.17
  - retroperitoneal 568.89
  - romanus 720.1
  - sacroiliac (joint) 724.6
  - salivary gland 527.8
    - benign lymphoepithelial 527.8
  - saphenous nerve 355.79
  - secondary - *see* Syphilis, secondary
  - sigmoid 569.89
  - sinus (accessory) (nasal) (*see also* Sinusitis) 473.9
  - skin 709.9
    - suppurative 686.00
  - SLAP (superior glenoid labrum) 840.7
  - space-occupying, intracranial NEC 784.2
  - spinal cord 336.9
    - congenital 742.9

- **Lesion** *(Continued)*
  - spinal cord *(Continued)*
    - traumatic (complete) (incomplete) (transverse) - *see also* Injury, spinal, by site
      - with
        - broken
          - back - *see* Fracture, vertebra, by site, with spinal cord injury
          - neck - *see* Fracture, vertebra, cervical, with spinal cord injury
        - fracture, vertebra - *see* Fracture, vertebra, by site, with spinal cord injury
  - spleen 289.50
  - stomach 537.89
  - superior glenoid labrum (SLAP) 840.7
  - syphilitic - *see* Syphilis
  - tertiary - *see* Syphilis, tertiary
  - thoracic root (nerve) 353.3
  - tonsillar fossa 474.9
  - tooth, teeth 525.8
    - white spot 521.01
  - traumatic NEC (*see also* nature and site of injury) 959.9
  - tricuspid (valve) - *see* Endocarditis, tricuspid
  - trigeminal nerve 350.9
  - ulcerated or ulcerative - *see* Ulcer
  - uterus NEC 621.9
  - vagina 623.8
  - vagus nerve 352.3
  - valvular - *see* Endocarditis
  - vascular 459.9
    - affecting central nervous system (*see also* Lesion, cerebrovascular) 437.9
    - following trauma (*see also* Injury, blood vessel, by site) 904.9
    - retina 362.17
    - traumatic - *see* Injury, blood vessel, by site
    - umbilical cord 663.6
      - affecting fetus or newborn 762.6
  - visual
    - cortex NEC (*see also* Disorder, visual, cortex) 377.73
    - pathway NEC (*see also* Disorder, visual, pathway) 377.63
  - warty - *see* Verruca
  - white spot, on teeth 521.01
  - x-ray NEC 990
- **Lethargic** - *see* condition
- **Lethargy** 780.79
- **Letterer-Siwe disease** (acute histiocytosis X) (M9722/3) 202.5
- **Leucinosis** 270.3
- **Leucocoria** 360.44
- **Leucosarcoma** (M9850/3) 207.8
- **Leukasmus** 270.2
- **Leukemia, leukemic** (congenital) (M9800/3) 208.9

> Note Use the following fifth-digit subclassification for categories 203-208:
>
> 0 without mention of remission
> 1 with remission

  - acute NEC (M9801/3) 208.0
  - aleukemic NEC (M9804/3) 208.8
    - granulocytic (M9864/3) 205.8

N

	Malignant					
	Primary	Secondary	Ca in stiu	Benign	Uncertain Behavior	Unspecified
Neoplasm, neoplastic	199.1	199.1	234.9	229.9	238.9	239.9

Notes — 1. The list below gives the code numbers for neoplasms by anatomical site. For each site there are six possible code numbers according to whether the neoplasm in question is malignant, benign, in situ, of uncertain behavior, or of unspecified nature. The description of the neoplasm will often indicate which of the six columns is appropriate; e.g., malignant melanoma of skin, benign fibroadenoma of breast, carcinoma in situ of cervix uteri.

Where such descriptors are not present, the remainder of the Index should be consulted where guidance is given to the appropriate column for each morphological (histological) variety listed; e.g., Mesonephroma—*see* Neoplasm, malignant; Embryoma—*see also* Neoplasm, uncertain behavior; Disease, Bowen's—*see* Neoplasm, skin, in situ. However, the guidance in the Index can be overridden if one of the descriptors mentioned above is present; e.g., malignant adenoma of colon is coded to 153.9 and not to 211.3 as the adjective "malignant" overrides the Index entry "Adenoma—*see also* Neoplasm, benign."

2. Sites marked with the sign * (e.g., face NEC*) should be classified to malignant neoplasm of skin of these sites if the variety of neoplasm is a squamous cell carcinoma or an epidermoid carcinoma and to benign neoplasm of skin of these sites if the variety of neoplasm is a papilloma (any type).

Site	Primary	Secondary	Ca in stiu	Benign	Uncertain Behavior	Unspecified
abdomen, abdominal	195.2	198.89	234.8	229.8	238.8	239.8
cavity	195.2	198.89	234.8	229.8	238.8	239.8
organ	195.2	198.89	234.8	229.8	238.8	239.8
viscera	195.2	198.89	234.8	229.8	238.8	239.8
wall	173.5	198.2	232.5	216.5	238.2	239.2
connective tissue	171.5	198.89	—	215.5	238.1	239.2
abdominopelvic	195.8	198.89	234.8	229.8	238.8	239.8
accessory sinus-*see* Neoplasm, sinus						
acoustic nerve	192.0	198.4	—	225.1	237.9	239.7
acromion (process)	170.4	198.5	—	213.4	238.0	239.2
adenoid (pharynx) (tissue)	147.1	198.89	230.0	210.7	235.1	239.0
adipose tissue (*see also* Neoplasm, connective tissue)	171.9	198.89	—	215.9	238.1	239.2
adnexa (uterine)	183.9	198.82	233.3	221.8	236.3	239.5
adrenal (cortex) (gland) (medulla)	194.0	198.7	234.8	227.0	237.2	239.7
ala nasi (external)	173.3	198.2	232.3	216.3	238.2	239.2
alimentary canal or tract NEC	159.9	197.8	230.9	211.9	235.5	239.0
alveolar	143.9	198.89	230.0	210.4	235.1	239.0
mucosa	143.9	198.89	230.0	210.4	235.1	239.0
lower	143.1	198.89	230.0	210.4	235.1	239.0
upper	143.0	198.89	230.0	210.4	235.1	239.0
ridge or process	170.1	198.5	—	213.1	238.0	239.2
carcinoma	143.9	—	—	—	—	—
lower	143.1	—	—	—	—	—
upper	143.0	—	—	—	—	—
lower	170.1	198.5	—	213.1	238.0	239.2
mucosa	143.9	198.89	230.0	210.4	235.1	239.0
lower	143.1	198.89	230.0	210.4	235.1	239.0
upper	143.0	198.89	230.0	210.4	235.1	239.0
upper	170.0	198.5	—	213.0	238.0	239.2
sulcus	145.1	198.89	230.0	210.4	235.1	239.0
alveolus	143.9	198.89	230.0	210.4	235.1	239.0
lower	143.1	198.89	230.0	210.4	235.1	239.0
upper	143.0	198.89	230.0	210.4	235.1	239.0
ampulla of Vater	156.2	197.8	230.8	211.5	235.3	239.0
ankle NEC*	195.5	198.89	232.7	229.8	238.8	239.8
anorectum, anorectal (junction)	154.8	197.5	230.7	211.4	235.2	239.0
antecubital fossa or space*	195.4	198.89	232.6	229.8	238.8	239.8
antrum (Highmore) (maxillary)	160.2	197.3	231.8	212.0	235.9	239.1
pyloric	151.2	197.8	230.2	211.1	235.2	239.0
tympanicum	160.1	197.3	231.8	212.0	235.9	239.1
anus, anal	154.3	197.5	230.6	211.4	235.5	239.0
canal	154.2	197.5	230.5	211.4	235.5	239.0
contiguous sites with rectosigmoid junction or rectum	154.8	—	—	—	—	—
margin	173.5	198.2	232.5	216.5	238.2	239.2
skin	173.5	198.2	232.5	216.5	238.2	239.2
sphincter	154.2	197.5	230.5	211.4	235.5	239.0
aorta (thoracic)	171.4	198.89	—	215.4	238.1	239.2
abdominal	171.5	198.89	—	215.5	238.1	239.2
aortic body	194.6	198.89	—	227.6	237.3	239.7
aponeurosis	171.9	198.89	—	215.9	238.1	239.2
palmar	171.2	198.89	—	215.2	238.1	239.2
plantar	171.3	198.89	—	215.3	238.1	239.2

	Malignant					
	Primary	Secondary	Ca in stiu	Benign	Uncertain Behavior	Unspecified
Neoplasm *(Continued)*						
appendix	153.5	197.5	230.3	211.3	235.2	239.0
arachnoid (cerebral)	192.1	198.4	—	225.2	237.6	239.7
spinal	192.3	198.4	—	225.4	237.6	239.7
areola (female)	174.0	198.81	233.0	217	238.3	239.3
male	175.0	198.81	233.0	217	238.3	239.3
arm NEC*	195.4	198.89	232.6	229.8	238.8	239.8
artery-*see* Neoplasm, connective tissue						
aryepiglottic fold	148.2	198.89	230.0	210.8	235.1	239.0
hypopharyngeal aspect	148.2	198.89	230.0	210.8	235.1	239.0
laryngeal aspect	161.1	197.3	231.0	212.1	235.6	239.1
marginal zone	148.2	198.89	230.0	210.8	235.1	239.0
arytenoid (cartilage)	161.3	197.3	231.0	212.1	235.6	239.1
fold-*see* Neoplasm, aryepiglottic						
atlas	170.2	198.5	—	213.2	238.0	239.2
atrium, cardiac	164.1	198.89	—	212.7	238.8	239.8
auditory						
canal (external) (skin)	173.2	198.2	232.2	216.2	238.2	239.2
internal	160.1	197.3	231.8	212.0	235.9	239.1
nerve	192.0	198.4	—	225.1	237.9	239.7
tube	160.1	197.3	231.8	212.0	235.9	239.1
opening	147.2	198.89	230.0	210.7	235.1	239.0
auricle, ear	173.2	198.2	232.2	216.2	238.2	239.2
cartilage	171.0	198.89	—	215.0	238.1	239.2
auricular canal (external)	173.2	198.2	232.2	216.2	238.2	239.2
internal	160.1	197.3	231.8	212.0	235.9	239.1
autonomic nerve or nervous system NEC	171.9	198.89	—	215.9	238.1	239.2
axilla, axillary	195.1	198.89	234.8	229.8	238.8	239.8
fold	173.5	198.2	232.5	216.5	238.2	239.2
back NEC*	195.8	198.89	232.5	229.8	238.8	239.8
Bartholin's gland	184.1	198.82	233.3	221.2	236.3	239.5
basal ganglia	191.0	198.3	—	225.0	237.5	239.6
basis pedunculi	191.7	198.3	—	225.0	237.5	239.6
bile or biliary (tract)	156.9	197.8	230.8	211.5	235.3	239.0
canaliculi (biliferi) (intrahepatic)	155.1	197.8	230.8	211.5	235.3	239.0
canals, interlobular	155.1	197.8	230.8	211.5	235.3	239.0
contiguous sites	156.8	—	—	—	—	—
duct or passage (common) (cystic) (extrahepatic)	156.1	197.8	230.8	211.5	235.3	239.0
contiguous sites						
with gallbladder	156.8	—	—	—	—	—
interlobular	155.1	197.8	230.8	211.5	235.3	239.0
intrahepatic	155.1	197.8	230.8	211.5	235.3	239.0
and extrahepatic	156.9	197.8	230.8	211.5	235.3	239.0
bladder (urinary)	188.9	198.1	233.7	223.3	236.7	239.4
contiguous sites	188.8	—	—	—	—	—
dome	188.1	198.1	233.7	223.3	236.7	239.4
neck	188.5	198.1	233.7	223.3	236.7	239.4
orifice	188.9	198.1	233.7	223.3	236.7	239.4
ureteric	188.6	198.1	233.7	223.3	236.7	239.4
urethral	188.5	198.1	233.7	223.3	236.7	239.4
sphincter	188.8	198.1	233.7	223.3	236.7	239.4
trigone	188.0	198.1	233.7	223.3	236.7	239.4
urachus	188.7	—	233.7	223.3	236.7	239.4
wall	188.9	198.1	233.7	223.3	236.7	239.4
anterior	188.3	198.1	233.7	223.3	236.7	239.4
lateral	188.2	198.1	233.7	223.3	236.7	239.4
posterior	188.4	198.1	233.7	223.3	236.7	239.4
blood vessel-*see* Neoplasm, connective tissue						
bone (periosteum)	170.9	198.5	—	213.9	238.0	239.2

Note-Carcinomas and adenocarcinomas, of any type other than intraosseous or odontogenic, of the sites listed under "Neoplasm, bone" should be considered as constituting metastatic spread from an unspecified primary site and coded to 198.5 for morbidity coding and to 199.1 for underlying cause of death coding.

	Primary	Secondary	Ca in stiu	Benign	Uncertain Behavior	Unspecified
acetabulum	170.6	198.5	—	213.6	238.0	239.2

	Malignant					
	Primary	Secondary	Ca in stiu	Benign	Uncertain Behavior	Unspecified
Neoplasm *(Continued)*						
bone *(Continued)*						
acromion (process)	170.4	198.5	—	213.4	238.0	239.2
ankle	170.8	198.5	—	213.8	238.0	239.2
arm NEC	170.4	198.5	—	213.4	238.0	239.2
astragalus	170.8	198.5	—	213.8	238.0	239.2
atlas	170.2	198.5	—	213.2	238.0	239.2
axis	170.2	198.5	—	213.2	238.0	239.2
back NEC	170.2	198.5	—	213.2	238.0	239.2
calcaneus	170.8	198.5	—	213.8	238.0	239.2
calvarium	170.0	198.5	—	213.0	238.0	239.2
carpus (any)	170.5	198.5	—	213.5	238.0	239.2
cartilage NEC	170.9	198.5	—	213.9	238.0	239.2
clavicle	170.3	198.5	—	213.3	238.0	239.2
clivus	170.0	198.5	—	213.0	238.0	239.2
coccygeal vertebra	170.6	198.5	—	213.6	238.0	239.2
coccyx	170.6	198.5	—	213.6	238.0	239.2
costal cartilage	170.3	198.5	—	213.3	238.0	239.2
costovertebral joint	170.3	198.5	—	213.3	238.0	239.2
cranial	170.0	198.5	—	213.0	238.0	239.2
cuboid	170.8	198.5	—	213.8	238.0	239.2
cuneiform	170.9	198.5	—	213.9	238.0	239.2
ankle	170.8	198.5	—	213.8	238.0	239.2
wrist	170.5	198.5	—	213.5	238.0	239.2
digital	170.9	198.5	—	213.9	238.0	239.2
finger	170.5	198.5	—	213.5	238.0	239.2
toe	170.8	198.5	—	213.8	238.0	239.2
elbow	170.4	198.5	—	213.4	238.0	239.2
ethmoid (labyrinth)	170.0	198.5	—	213.0	238.0	239.2
face	170.0	198.5	—	213.0	238.0	239.2
lower jaw	170.1	198.5	—	213.1	238.0	239.2
femur (any part)	170.7	198.5	—	213.7	238.0	239.2
fibula (any part)	170.7	198.5	—	213.7	238.0	239.2
finger (any)	170.5	198.5	—	213.5	238.0	239.2
foot	170.8	198.5	—	213.8	238.0	239.2
forearm	170.4	198.5	—	213.4	238.0	239.2
frontal	170.0	198.5	—	213.0	238.0	239.2
hand	170.5	198.5	—	213.5	238.0	239.2
heel	170.8	198.5	—	213.8	238.0	239.2
hip	170.6	198.5	—	213.6	238.0	239.2
humerus (any part)	170.4	198.5	—	213.4	238.0	239.2
hyoid	170.0	198.5	—	213.0	238.0	239.2
ilium	170.6	198.5	—	213.6	238.0	239.2
innominate	170.6	198.5	—	213.6	238.0	239.2
intervertebral cartilage or disc	170.2	198.5	—	213.2	238.0	239.2
ischium	170.6	198.5	—	213.6	238.0	239.2
jaw (lower)	170.1	198.5	—	213.1	238.0	239.2
upper	170.0	198.5	—	213.0	238.0	239.2
knee	170.7	198.5	—	213.7	238.0	239.2
leg NEC	170.7	198.5	—	213.7	238.0	239.2
limb NEC	170.9	198.5	—	213.9	238.0	239.2
lower (long bones)	170.7	198.5	—	213.7	238.0	239.2
short bones	170.8	198.5	—	213.8	238.0	239.2
upper (long bones)	170.4	198.5	—	213.4	238.0	239.2
short bones	170.5	198.5	—	213.5	238.0	239.2
long	170.9	198.5	—	213.9	238.0	239.2
lower limbs NEC	170.7	198.5	—	213.7	238.0	239.2
upper limbs NEC	170.4	198.5	—	213.4	238.0	239.2
malar	170.0	198.5	—	213.0	238.0	239.2
mandible	170.1	198.5	—	213.1	238.0	239.2
marrow NEC	202.9	198.5	—	—	—	238.7
mastoid	170.0	198.5	—	213.0	238.0	239.2
maxilla, maxillary (superior)	170.0	198.5	—	213.0	238.0	239.2
inferior	170.1	198.5	—	213.1	238.0	239.2

◀ New ⟸ Revised Code

	Malignant					
	Primary	**Secondary**	**Ca in stiu**	**Benign**	**Uncertain Behavior**	**Unspecified**
Neoplasm *(Continued)*						
bone *(Continued)*						
metacarpus (any)	170.5	198.5	—	213.5	238.0	239.2
metatarsus (any)	170.8	198.5	—	213.8	238.0	239.2
navicular (ankle)	170.8	198.5	—	213.8	238.0	239.2
hand	170.5	198.5	—	213.5	238.0	239.2
nose, nasal	170.0	198.5	—	213.0	238.0	239.2
occipital	170.0	198.5	—	213.0	238.0	239.2
orbit	170.0	198.5	—	213.0	238.0	239.2
parietal	170.0	198.5	—	213.0	238.0	239.2
patella	170.8	198.5	—	213.8	238.0	239.2
pelvic	170.6	198.5	—	213.6	238.0	239.2
phalanges	170.9	198.5	—	213.9	238.0	239.2
foot	170.8	198.5	—	213.8	238.0	239.2
hand	170.5	198.5	—	213.5	238.0	239.2
pubic	170.6	198.5	—	213.6	238.0	239.2
radius (any part)	170.4	198.5	—	213.4	238.0	239.2
rib	170.3	198.5	—	213.3	238.0	239.2
sacral vertebra	170.6	198.5	—	213.6	238.0	239.2
sacrum	170.6	198.5	—	213.6	238.0	239.2
scaphoid (of hand)	170.5	198.5	—	213.5	238.0	239.2
of ankle	170.8	198.5	—	213.8	238.0	239.2
scapula (any part)	170.4	198.5	—	213.4	238.0	239.2
sella turcica	170.0	198.5	—	213.0	238.0	239.2
short	170.9	198.5	—	213.9	238.0	239.2
lower limb	170.8	198.5	—	213.8	238.0	239.2
upper limb	170.5	198.5	—	213.5	238.0	239.2
shoulder	170.4	198.5	—	213.4	238.0	239.2
skeleton, skeletal NEC	170.9	198.5	—	213.9	238.0	239.2
skull	170.0	198.5	—	213.0	238.0	239.2
sphenoid	170.0	198.5	—	213.0	238.0	239.2
spine, spinal (column)	170.2	198.5	—	213.2	238.0	239.2
coccyx	170.6	198.5	—	213.6	238.0	239.2
sacrum	170.6	198.5	—	213.6	238.0	239.2
sternum	170.3	198.5	—	213.3	238.0	239.2
tarsus (any)	170.8	198.5	—	213.8	238.0	239.2
temporal	170.0	198.5	—	213.0	238.0	239.2
thumb	170.5	198.5	—	213.5	238.0	239.2
tibia (any part)	170.7	198.5	—	213.7	238.0	239.2
toe (any)	170.8	198.5	—	213.8	238.0	239.2
trapezium	170.5	198.5	—	213.5	238.0	239.2
trapezoid	170.5	198.5	—	213.5	238.0	239.2
turbinate	170.0	198.5	—	213.0	238.0	239.2
ulna (any part)	170.4	198.5	—	213.4	238.0	239.2
unciform	170.5	198.5	—	213.5	238.0	239.2
vertebra (column)	170.2	198.5	—	213.2	238.0	239.2
coccyx	170.6	198.5	—	213.6	238.0	239.2
sacrum	170.6	198.5	—	213.6	238.0	239.2
vomer	170.0	198.5	—	213.0	238.0	239.2
wrist	170.5	198.5	—	213.5	238.0	239.2
xiphoid process	170.3	198.5	—	213.3	238.0	239.2
zygomatic	170.0	198.5	—	213.0	238.0	239.2
book-leaf (mouth)	145.8	198.89	230.0	210.4	235.1	239.0
bowel - *see* Neoplasm, intestine						
brachial plexus	171.2	198.89	—	215.2	238.1	239.2
brain NEC	191.9	198.3	—	225.0	237.5	239.6
basal ganglia	191.0	198.3	—	225.0	237.5	239.6
cerebellopontine angle	191.6	198.3	—	225.0	237.5	239.6
cerebellum NOS	191.6	198.3	—	225.0	237.5	239.6
cerebrum	191.0	198.3	—	225.0	237.5	239.6
choroid plexus	191.5	198.3	—	225.0	237.5	239.6
contiguous sites	191.8	—	—	—	—	—
corpus callosum	191.8	198.3	—	225.0	237.5	239.6
corpus striatum	191.0	198.3	—	225.0	237.5	239.6

	Malignant					
	Primary	Secondary	Ca in stiu	Benign	Uncertain Behavior	Unspecified
Neoplasm *(Continued)*						
brain *(Continued)*						
cortex (cerebral)	191.0	198.3	—	225.0	237.5	239.6
frontal lobe	191.1	198.3	—	225.0	237.5	239.6
globus pallidus	191.0	198.3	—	225.0	237.5	239.6
hippocampus	191.2	198.3	—	225.0	237.5	239.6
hypothalamus	191.0	198.3	—	225.0	237.5	239.6
internal capsule	191.0	198.3	—	225.0	237.5	239.6
medulla oblongata	191.7	198.3	—	225.0	237.5	239.6
meninges	192.1	198.4	—	225.2	237.6	239.7
midbrain	191.7	198.3	—	225.0	237.5	239.6
occipital lobe	191.4	198.3	—	225.0	237.5	239.6
parietal lobe	191.3	198.3	—	225.0	237.5	239.6
peduncle	191.7	198.3	—	225.0	237.5	239.6
pons	191.7	198.3	—	225.0	237.5	239.6
stem	191.7	198.3	—	225.0	237.5	239.6
tapetum	191.8	198.3	—	225.0	237.5	239.6
temporal lobe	191.2	198.3	—	225.0	237.5	239.6
thalamus	191.0	198.3	—	225.0	237.5	239.6
uncus	191.2	198.3	—	225.0	237.5	239.6
ventricle (floor)	191.5	198.3	—	225.0	237.5	239.6
branchial (cleft) (vestiges)	146.8	198.89	230.0	210.6	235.1	239.0
breast (connective tissue) (female) (glandular tissue) (soft parts)	174.9	198.81	233.0	217	238.3	239.3
areola	174.0	198.81	233.0	217	238.3	239.3
male	175.0	198.81	233.0	217	238.3	239.3
axillary tail	174.6	198.81	233.0	217	238.3	239.3
central portion	174.1	198.81	233.0	217	238.3	239.3
contiguous sites	174.8	—	—	—	—	—
ectopic sites	174.8	198.81	233.0	217	238.3	239.3
inner	174.8	198.81	233.0	217	238.3	239.3
lower	174.8	198.81	233.0	217	238.3	239.3
lower-inner quadrant	174.3	198.81	233.0	217	238.3	239.3
lower-outer quadrant	174.5	198.81	233.0	217	238.3	239.3
male	175.9	198.81	233.0	217	238.3	239.3
areola	175.0	198.81	233.0	217	238.3	239.3
ectopic tissue	175.9	198.81	233.0	217	238.3	239.3
nipple	175.0	198.81	233.0	217	238.3	239.3
mastectomy site (skin)	173.5	198.2	—	—	—	—
specified as breast tissue	174.8	198.81	—	—	—	—
midline	174.8	198.81	233.0	217	238.3	239.3
nipple	174.0	198.81	233.0	217	238.3	239.3
male	175.0	198.81	233.0	217	238.3	239.3
outer	174.8	198.81	233.0	217	238.3	239.3
skin	173.5	198.2	232.5	216.5	238.2	239.2
tail (axillary)	174.6	198.81	233.0	217	238.3	239.3
upper	174.8	198.81	233.0	217	238.3	239.3
upper-inner quadrant	174.2	198.81	233.0	217	238.3	239.3
upper-outer quadrant	174.4	198.81	233.0	217	238.3	239.3
broad ligament	183.3	198.82	233.3	221.0	236.3	239.5
bronchiogenic, bronchogenic (lung)	162.9	197.0	231.2	212.3	235.7	239.1
bronchiole	162.9	197.0	231.2	212.3	235.7	239.1
bronchus	162.9	197.0	231.2	212.3	235.7	239.1
carina	162.2	197.0	231.2	212.3	235.7	239.1
contiguous sites with lung or trachea	162.8	—	—	—	—	—
lower lobe of lung	162.5	197.0	231.2	212.3	235.7	239.1
main	162.2	197.0	231.2	212.3	235.7	239.1
middle lobe of lung	162.4	197.0	231.2	212.3	235.7	239.1
upper lobe of lung	162.3	197.0	231.2	212.3	235.7	239.1
brow	173.3	198.2	232.3	216.3	238.2	239.2
buccal (cavity)	145.9	198.89	230.0	210.4	235.1	239.0
commissure	145.0	198.89	230.0	210.4	235.1	239.0
groove (lower) (upper)	145.1	198.89	230.0	210.4	235.1	239.0
mucosa	145.0	198.89	230.0	210.4	235.1	239.0
sulcus (lower) (upper)	145.1	198.89	230.0	210.4	235.1	239.0

	Malignant					
	Primary	Secondary	Ca in stiu	Benign	Uncertain Behavior	Unspecified
Neoplasm *(Continued)*						
bulbourethral gland	189.3	198.1	233.9	223.81	236.99	239.5
bursa-*see* Neoplasm, connective tissue						
buttock NEC*	195.3	198.89	232.5	229.8	238.8	239.8
calf*	195.5	198.89	232.7	229.8	238.8	239.8
calvarium	170.0	198.5	—	213.0	238.0	239.2
calyx, renal	189.1	198.0	233.9	223.1	236.91	239.5
canal						
anal	154.2	197.5	230.5	211.4	235.5	239.0
auditory (external)	173.2	198.2	232.2	216.2	238.2	239.2
auricular (external)	173.2	198.2	232.2	216.2	238.2	239.2
canaliculi, biliary (biliferi) (intrahepatic)	155.1	197.8	230.8	211.5	235.3	239.0
canthus (eye) (inner) (outer)	173.1	198.2	232.1	216.1	238.2	239.2
capillary-*see* Neoplasm, connective tissue						
caput coli	153.4	197.5	230.3	211.3	235.2	239.0
cardia (gastric)	151.0	197.8	230.2	211.1	235.2	239.0
cardiac orifice (stomach)	151.0	197.8	230.2	211.1	235.2	239.0
cardio-esophageal junction	151.0	197.8	230.2	211.1	235.2	239.0
cardio-esophagus	151.0	197.8	230.2	211.1	235.2	239.0
carina (bronchus) (trachea)	162.2	197.0	231.2	212.3	235.7	239.1
carotid (artery)	171.0	198.89	—	215.0	238.1	239.2
body	194.5	198.89	—	227.5	237.3	239.7
carpus (any bone)	170.5	198.5	—	213.5	238.0	239.2
cartilage (articular) (joint) NEC-*see also* Neoplasm, bone	170.9	198.5	—	213.9	238.0	239.2
arytenoid	161.3	197.3	231.0	212.1	235.6	239.1
auricular	171.0	198.89	—	215.0	238.1	239.2
bronchi	162.2	197.3	—	212.3	235.7	239.1
connective tissue-*see* Neoplasm, connective tissue						
costal	170.3	198.5	—	213.3	238.0	239.2
cricoid	161.3	197.3	231.0	212.1	235.6	239.1
cuneiform	161.3	197.3	231.0	212.1	235.6	239.1
ear (external)	171.0	198.89	—	215.0	238.1	239.2
ensiform	170.3	198.5	—	213.3	238.0	239.2
epiglottis	161.1	197.3	231.0	212.1	235.6	239.1
anterior surface	146.4	198.89	230.0	210.6	235.1	239.0
eyelid	171.0	198.89	—	215.0	238.1	239.2
intervertebral	170.2	198.5	—	213.2	238.0	239.2
larynx, laryngeal	161.3	197.3	231.0	212.1	235.6	239.1
nose, nasal	160.0	197.3	231.8	212.0	235.9	239.1
pinna	171.0	198.89	—	215.0	238.1	239.2
rib	170.3	198.5	—	213.3	238.0	239.2
semilunar (knee)	170.7	198.5	—	213.7	238.0	239.2
thyroid	161.3	197.3	231.0	212.1	235.6	239.1
trachea	162.0	197.3	231.1	212.2	235.7	239.1
cauda equina	192.2	198.3	—	225.3	237.5	239.7
cavity						
buccal	145.9	198.89	230.0	210.4	235.1	239.0
nasal	160.0	197.3	231.8	212.0	235.9	239.1
oral	145.9	198.89	230.0	210.4	235.1	239.0
peritoneal	158.9	197.6	—	211.8	235.4	239.0
tympanic	160.1	197.3	231.8	212.0	235.9	239.1
cecum	153.4	197.5	230.3	211.3	235.2	239.0
central nervous system-*see* Neoplasm, white matter	191.0	198.3	—	225.0	237.5	239.6
cerebellopontine (angle)	191.6	198.3	—	225.0	237.5	239.6
cerebellum, cerebellar	191.6	198.3	—	225.0	237.5	239.6
cerebrum, cerebral (cortex) (hemisphere) (white matter)	191.0	198.3	—	225.0	237.5	239.6
meninges	192.1	198.4	—	225.2	237.6	239.7
peduncle	191.7	198.3	—	225.0	237.5	239.6
ventricle (any)	191.5	198.3	—	225.0	237.5	239.6
cervical region	195.0	198.89	234.8	229.8	238.8	239.8
cervix (cervical) (uteri) (uterus)	180.9	198.82	233.1	219.0	236.0	239.5

	Malignant					
	Primary	Secondary	Ca in stiu	Benign	Uncertain Behavior	Unspecified
Neoplasm *(Continued)*						
cervix *(Continued)*						
canal	180.0	198.82	233.1	219.0	236.0	239.5
contiguous sites	180.8	—	—	—	—	—
endocervix (canal) (gland)	180.0	198.82	233.1	219.0	236.0	239.5
exocervix	180.1	198.82	233.1	219.0	236.0	239.5
external os	180.1	198.82	233.1	219.0	236.0	239.5
internal os	180.0	198.82	233.1	219.0	236.0	239.5
nabothian gland	180.0	198.82	233.1	219.0	236.0	239.5
squamocolumnar junction	180.8	198.82	233.1	219.0	236.0	239.5
stump	180.8	198.82	233.1	219.0	236.0	239.5
cheek	195.0	198.89	234.8	229.8	238.8	239.8
external	173.3	198.2	232.3	216.3	238.2	239.2
inner aspect	145.0	198.89	230.0	210.4	235.1	239.0
internal	145.0	198.89	230.0	210.4	235.1	239.0
mucosa	145.0	198.89	230.0	210.4	235.1	239.0
chest (wall) NEC	195.1	198.89	234.8	229.8	238.8	239.8
chiasma opticum	192.0	198.4	—	225.1	237.9	239.7
chin	173.3	198.2	232.3	216.3	238.2	239.2
choana	147.3	198.89	230.0	210.7	235.1	239.0
cholangiole	155.1	197.8	230.8	211.5	235.3	239.0
choledochal duct	156.1	197.8	230.8	211.5	235.3	239.0
choroid	190.6	198.4	234.0	224.6	238.8	239.8
plexus	191.5	198.3	—	225.0	237.5	239.6
ciliary body	190.0	198.4	234.0	224.0	238.8	239.8
clavicle	170.3	198.5	—	213.3	238.0	239.2
clitoris	184.3	198.82	233.3	221.2	236.3	239.5
clivus	170.0	198.5	—	213.0	238.0	239.2
cloacogenic zone	154.8	197.5	230.7	211.4	235.5	239.0
coccygeal						
body or glomus	194.6	198.89	—	227.6	237.3	239.7
vertebra	170.6	198.5	—	213.6	238.0	239.2
coccyx	170.6	198.5	—	213.6	238.0	239.2
colon-*see also* Neoplasm, intestine, large and rectum	154.0	197.5	230.4	211.4	235.2	239.0
column, spinal-*see* Neoplasm, spine						
columnella	173.3	198.2	232.3	216.3	238.2	239.2
commissure						
labial, lip	140.6	198.89	230.0	210.4	235.1	239.0
laryngeal	161.0	197.3	231.0	212.1	235.6	239.1
common (bile) duct	156.1	197.8	230.8	211.5	235.3	239.0
concha	173.2	198.2	232.2	216.2	238.2	239.2
nose	160.0	197.3	231.8	212.0	235.9	239.1
conjunctiva	190.3	198.4	234.0	224.3	238.8	239.8
connective tissue NEC	171.9	198.89	—	215.9	238.1	239.2

Note-For neoplasms of connective tissue (blood vessel, bursa, fascia, ligament, muscle, peripheral nerves, sympathetic and parasympathetic nerves and ganglia, synovia, tendon, etc.) or of morphological types that indicate connective tissue, code according to the list under "Neoplasm, connective tissue;" for sites that do not appear in this list, code to neoplasm of that site; e.g.,

	Primary	Secondary	Ca in stiu	Benign	Uncertain Behavior	Unspecified
liposarcoma, shoulder	171.2					
leiomyosarcoma, stomach	151.9					
neurofibroma, chest wall	215.4					

Morphological types that indicate connective tissue appear in their proper place in the alphabetic index with the instruction "*see* Neoplasm, connective tissue ...."

	Primary	Secondary	Ca in stiu	Benign	Uncertain Behavior	Unspecified
abdomen	171.5	198.89	—	215.5	238.1	239.2
abdominal wall	171.5	198.89	—	215.5	238.1	239.2
ankle	171.3	198.89	—	215.3	238.1	239.2
antecubital fossa or space	171.2	198.89	—	215.2	238.1	239.2
arm	171.2	198.89	—	215.2	238.1	239.2
auricle (ear)	171.0	198.89	—	215.0	238.1	239.2
axilla	171.4	198.89	—	215.4	238.1	239.2
back	171.7	198.89	—	215.7	238.1	239.2
breast (female) (*see also* Neoplasm, breast)	174.9	198.81	233.0	217	238.3	239.3
male	175.9	198.81	233.0	217	238.3	239.3

	Malignant					
	Primary	Secondary	Ca in stiu	Benign	Uncertain Behavior	Unspecified
Neoplasm *(Continued)*						
connective tissue NEC *(Continued)*						
buttock	171.6	198.89	—	215.6	238.1	239.2
calf	171.3	198.89	—	215.3	238.1	239.2
cervical region	171.0	198.89	—	215.0	238.1	239.2
cheek	171.0	198.89	—	215.0	238.1	239.2
chest (wall)	171.4	198.89	—	215.4	238.1	239.2
chin	171.0	198.89	—	215.0	238.1	239.2
contiguous sites	171.8	—	—	—	—	—
diaphragm	171.4	198.89	—	215.4	238.1	239.2
ear (external)	171.0	198.89	—	215.0	238.1	239.2
elbow	171.2	198.89	—	215.2	238.1	239.2
extrarectal	171.6	198.89	—	215.6	238.1	239.2
extremity	171.8	198.89	—	215.8	238.1	239.2
lower	171.3	198.89	—	215.3	238.1	239.2
upper	171.2	198.89	—	215.2	238.1	239.2
eyelid	171.0	198.89	—	215.0	238.1	239.2
face	171.0	198.89	—	215.0	238.1	239.2
finger	171.2	198.89	—	215.2	238.1	239.2
flank	171.7	198.89	—	215.7	238.1	239.2
foot	171.3	198.89	—	215.3	238.1	239.2
forearm	171.2	198.89	—	215.2	238.1	239.2
forehead	171.0	198.89	—	215.0	238.1	239.2
gluteal region	171.6	198.89	—	215.6	238.1	239.2
great vessels NEC	171.4	198.89	—	215.4	238.1	239.2
groin	171.6	198.89	—	215.6	238.1	239.2
hand	171.2	198.89	—	215.2	238.1	239.2
head	171.0	198.89	—	215.0	238.1	239.2
heel	171.3	198.89	—	215.3	238.1	239.2
hip	171.3	198.89	—	215.3	238.1	239.2
hypochondrium	171.5	198.89	—	215.5	238.1	239.2
iliopsoas muscle	171.6	198.89	—	215.5	238.1	239.2
infraclavicular region	171.4	198.89	—	215.4	238.1	239.2
inguinal (canal) (region)	171.6	198.89	—	215.6	238.1	239.2
intrathoracic	171.4	198.89	—	215.4	238.1	239.2
ischorectal fossa	171.6	198.89	—	215.6	238.1	239.2
jaw	143.9	198.89	230.0	210.4	235.1	239.0
knee	171.3	198.89	—	215.3	238.1	239.2
leg	171.3	198.89	—	215.3	238.1	239.2
limb NEC	171.9	198.89	—	215.8	238.1	239.2
lower	171.3	198.89	—	215.3	238.1	239.2
upper	171.2	198.89	—	215.2	238.1	239.2
nates	171.6	198.89	—	215.6	238.1	239.2
neck	171.0	198.89	—	215.0	238.1	239.2
orbit	190.1	198.4	234.0	224.1	238.8	239.8
pararectal	171.6	198.89	—	215.6	238.1	239.2
para-urethral	171.6	198.89	—	215.6	238.1	239.2
paravaginal	171.6	198.89	—	215.6	238.1	239.2
pelvis (floor)	171.6	198.89	—	215.6	238.1	239.2
pelvo-abdominal	171.8	198.89	—	215.8	238.1	239.2
perineum	171.6	198.89	—	215.6	238.1	239.2
perirectal (tissue)	171.6	198.89	—	215.6	238.1	239.2
periurethral (tissue)	171.6	198.89	—	215.6	238.1	239.2
popliteal fossa or space	171.3	198.89	—	215.3	238.1	239.2
presacral	171.6	198.89	—	215.6	238.1	239.2
psoas muscle	171.5	198.89	—	215.5	238.1	239.2
pterygoid fossa	171.0	198.89	—	215.0	238.1	239.2
rectovaginal septum or wall	171.6	198.89	—	215.6	238.1	239.2
rectovesical	171.6	198.89	—	215.6	238.1	239.2
retroperitoneum	158.0	197.6	—	211.8	235.4	239.0
sacrococcygeal region	171.6	198.89	—	215.6	238.1	239.2
scalp	171.0	198.89	—	215.0	238.1	239.2
scapular region	171.4	198.89	—	215.4	238.1	239.2
shoulder	171.2	198.89	—	215.2	238.1	239.2

	Malignant					
	Primary	Secondary	Ca in stiu	Benign	Uncertain Behavior	Unspecified
Neoplasm *(Continued)*						
connective tissue NEC *(Continued)*						
skin (dermis) NEC	173.9	198.2	232.9	216.9	238.2	239.2
submental	171.0	198.89	—	215.0	238.1	239.2
supraclavicular region	171.0	198.89	—	215.0	238.1	239.2
temple	171.0	198.89	—	215.0	238.1	239.2
temporal region	171.0	198.89	—	215.0	238.1	239.2
thigh	171.3	198.89	—	215.3	238.1	239.2
thoracic (duct) (wall)	171.4	198.89	—	215.4	238.1	239.2
thorax	171.4	198.89	—	215.4	238.1	239.2
thumb	171.2	198.89	—	215.2	238.1	239.2
toe	171.3	198.89	—	215.3	238.1	239.2
trunk	171.7	198.89	—	215.7	238.1	239.2
umbilicus	171.5	198.89	—	215.5	238.1	239.2
vesicorectal	171.6	198.89	—	215.6	238.1	239.2
wrist	171.2	198.89	—	215.2	238.1	239.2
conus medullaris	192.2	198.3	—	225.3	237.5	239.7
cord (true) (vocal)	161.0	197.3	231.0	212.1	235.6	239.1
false	161.1	197.3	231.0	212.1	235.6	239.1
spermatic	187.6	198.82	233.6	222.8	236.6	239.5
spinal (cervical) (lumbar) (thoracic)	192.2	198.3	—	225.3	237.5	239.7
cornea (limbus)	190.4	198.4	234.0	224.4	238.8	239.8
corpus						
albicans	183.0	198.6	233.3	220	236.2	239.5
callosum, brain	191.8	198.3	—	225.0	237.5	239.6
cavernosum	187.3	198.82	233.5	222.1	236.6	239.5
gastric	151.4	197.8	230.2	211.1	235.2	239.0
penis	187.3	198.82	233.5	222.1	236.6	239.5
striatum, cerebrum	191.0	198.3	—	225.0	237.5	239.6
uteri	182.0	198.82	233.2	219.1	236.0	239.5
isthmus	182.1	198.82	233.2	219.1	236.0	239.5
cortex						
adrenal	194.0	198.7	234.8	227.0	237.2	239.7
cerebral	191.0	198.3	—	225.0	237.5	239.6
costal cartilage	170.3	198.5	—	213.3	238.0	239.2
costovertebral joint	170.3	198.5	—	213.3	238.0	239.2
Cowper's gland	189.3	198.1	233.9	223.81	236.99	239.5
cranial (fossa, any)	191.9	198.3	—	225.0	237.5	239.6
meninges	192.1	198.4	—	225.2	237.6	239.7
nerve (any)	192.0	198.4	—	225.1	237.9	239.7
craniobuccal pouch	194.3	198.89	234.8	227.3	237.0	239.7
craniopharyngeal (duct) (pouch)	194.3	198.89	234.8	227.3	237.0	239.7
cricoid	148.0	198.89	230.0	210.8	235.1	239.0
cartilage	161.3	197.3	231.0	212.1	235.6	239.1
cricopharynx	148.0	198.89	230.0	210.8	235.1	239.0
crypt of Morgagni	154.8	197.5	230.7	211.4	235.2	239.0
crystalline lens	190.0	198.4	234.0	224.0	238.8	239.8
cul-de-sac (Douglas')	158.8	197.6	—	211.8	235.4	239.0
cuneiform cartilage	161.3	197.3	231.0	212.1	235.6	239.1
cutaneous-*see* Neoplasm, skin						
cutis-*see* Neoplasm, skin						
cystic (bile) duct (common)	156.1	197.8	230.8	211.5	235.3	239.0
dermis-*see* Neoplasm, skin						
diaphragm	171.4	198.89	—	215.4	238.1	239.2
digestive organs, system, tube, or tract NEC	159.9	197.8	230.9	211.9	235.5	239.0
contiguous sites with peritoneum	159.8	—	—	—	—	—
disc, intervertebral	170.2	198.5	—	213.2	238.0	239.2
disease, generalized	199.0	199.0	234.9	229.9	238.9	199.0
disseminated	199.0	199.0	234.9	229.9	238.9	199.0
Douglas' cul-de-sac or pouch	158.8	197.6	—	211.8	235.4	239.0
duodenojejunal junction	152.8	197.4	230.7	211.2	235.2	239.0
duodenum	152.0	197.4	230.7	211.2	235.2	239.0
dura (cranial) (mater)	192.1	198.4	—	225.2	237.6	239.7

◀ New ⟸ Revised Code

	Malignant					
	Primary	Secondary	Ca in stiu	Benign	Uncertain Behavior	Unspecified
Neoplasm *(Continued)*						
dura *(Continued)*						
cerebral	192.1	198.4	—	225.2	237.6	239.7
spinal	192.3	198.4	—	225.4	237.6	239.7
ear (external)	173.2	198.2	232.2	216.2	238.2	239.2
auricle or auris	173.2	198.2	232.2	216.2	238.2	239.2
canal, external	173.2	198.2	232.2	216.2	238.2	239.2
cartilage	171.0	198.89	—	215.0	238.1	239.2
external meatus	173.2	198.2	232.2	216.2	238.2	239.2
inner	160.1	197.3	231.8	212.0	235.9	239.8
lobule	173.2	198.2	232.2	216.2	238.2	239.2
middle	160.1	197.3	231.8	212.0	235.9	239.8
contiguous sites with accessory sinuses or nasal cavities	160.8	—	—	—	—	—
skin	173.2	198.2	232.2	216.2	238.2	239.2
earlobe	173.2	198.2	232.2	216.2	238.2	239.2
ejaculatory duct	187.8	198.82	233.6	222.8	236.6	239.5
elbow NEC*	195.4	198.89	232.6	229.8	238.8	239.8
endocardium	164.1	198.89	—	212.7	238.8	239.8
endocervix (canal) (gland)	180.0	198.82	233.1	219.0	236.0	239.5
endocrine gland NEC	194.9	198.89	—	227.9	237.4	239.7
pluriglandular NEC	194.8	198.89	234.8	227.8	237.4	239.7
endometrium (gland) (stroma)	182.0	198.82	233.2	219.1	236.0	239.5
ensiform cartilage	170.3	198.5	—	213.3	238.0	239.2
enteric-*see* Neoplasm, intestine						
ependyma (brain)	191.5	198.3	—	225.0	237.5	239.6
epicardium	164.1	198.89	—	212.7	238.8	239.8
epididymis	187.5	198.82	233.6	222.3	236.6	239.5
epidural	192.9	198.4	—	225.9	237.9	239.7
epiglottis	161.1	197.3	231.0	212.1	235.6	239.1
anterior aspect or surface	146.4	198.89	230.0	210.6	235.1	239.0
cartilage	161.3	197.3	231.0	212.1	235.6	239.1
free border (margin)	146.4	198.89	230.0	210.6	235.1	239.0
junctional region	146.5	198.89	230.0	210.6	235.1	239.0
posterior (laryngeal) surface	161.1	197.3	231.0	212.1	235.6	239.1
suprahyoid portion	161.1	197.3	231.0	212.1	235.6	239.1
esophagogastric junction	151.0	197.8	230.2	211.1	235.2	239.0
esophagus	150.9	197.8	230.1	211.0	235.5	239.0
abdominal	150.2	197.8	230.1	211.0	235.5	239.0
cervical	150.0	197.8	230.1	211.0	235.5	239.0
contiguous sites	150.8	—	—	—	—	—
distal (third)	150.5	197.8	230.1	211.0	235.5	239.0
lower (third)	150.5	197.8	230.1	211.0	235.5	239.0
middle (third)	150.4	197.8	230.1	211.0	235.5	239.0
proximal (third)	150.3	197.8	230.1	211.0	235.5	239.0
specified part NEC	150.8	197.8	230.1	211.0	235.5	239.0
thoracic	150.1	197.8	230.1	211.0	235.5	239.0
upper (third)	150.3	197.8	230.1	211.0	235.5	239.0
ethmoid (sinus)	160.3	197.3	231.8	212.0	235.9	239.1
bone or labyrinth	170.0	198.5	—	213.0	238.0	239.2
Eustachian tube	160.1	197.3	231.8	212.0	235.9	239.1
exocervix	180.1	198.82	233.1	219.0	236.0	239.5
external						
meatus (ear)	173.2	198.2	232.2	216.2	238.2	239.2
os, cervix uteri	180.1	198.82	233.1	219.0	236.0	239.5
extradural	192.9	198.4	—	225.9	237.9	239.7
extrahepatic (bile) duct	156.1	197.8	230.8	211.5	235.3	239.0
contiguous sites with gallbladder	156.8	—	—	—	—	—
extraocular muscle	190.1	198.4	234.0	224.1	238.8	239.8
extrarectal	195.3	198.89	234.8	229.8	238.8	239.8
extremity*	195.8	198.89	232.8	229.8	238.8	239.8
lower*	195.5	198.89	232.7	229.8	238.8	239.8
upper*	195.4	198.89	232.6	229.8	238.8	239.8
eye NEC	190.9	198.4	234.0	224.9	238.8	239.8

	Malignant					
	Primary	Secondary	Ca in stiu	Benign	Uncertain Behavior	Unspecified
Neoplasm *(Continued)*						
eye NEC *(Continued)*						
contiguous sites	190.8	—	—	—	—	—
specified sites NEC	190.8	198.4	234.0	224.8	238.8	239.8
eyeball	190.0	198.4	234.0	224.0	238.8	239.8
eyebrow	173.3	198.2	232.3	216.3	238.2	239.2
eyelid (lower) (skin) (upper)	173.1	198.2	232.1	216.1	238.2	239.2
cartilage	171.0	198.89	—	215.0	238.1	239.2
face NEC*	195.0	198.89	232.3	229.8	238.8	239.8
Fallopian tube (accessory)	183.2	198.82	233.3	221.0	236.3	239.5
falx (cerebella) (cerebri)	192.1	198.4	—	225.2	237.6	239.7
fascia-*see also* Neoplasm, connective tissue						
palmar	171.2	198.89	—	215.2	238.1	239.2
plantar	171.3	198.89	—	215.3	238.1	239.2
fatty tissue-*see* Neoplasm, connective tissue						
fauces, faucial NEC	146.9	198.89	230.0	210.6	235.1	239.0
pillars	146.2	198.89	230.0	210.6	235.1	239.0
tonsil	146.0	198.89	230.0	210.5	235.1	239.0
femur (any part)	170.7	198.5	—	213.7	238.0	239.2
fetal membrane	181	198.82	233.2	219.8	236.1	239.5
fibrous tissue-*see* Neoplasm, connective tissue						
fibula (any part)	170.7	198.5	—	213.7	238.0	239.2
filum terminale	192.2	198.3	—	225.3	237.5	239.7
finger NEC*	195.4	198.89	232.6	229.8	238.8	239.8
flank NEC*	195.8	198.89	232.5	229.8	238.8	239.8
follicle, nabothian	180.0	198.82	233.1	219.0	236.0	239.5
foot NEC*	195.5	198.89	232.7	229.8	238.8	239.8
forearm NEC*	195.4	198.89	232.6	229.8	238.8	239.8
forehead (skin)	173.3	198.2	232.3	216.3	238.2	239.2
foreskin	187.1	198.82	233.5	222.1	236.6	239.5
fornix						
pharyngeal	147.3	198.89	230.0	210.7	235.1	239.0
vagina	184.0	198.82	233.3	221.1	236.3	239.5
fossa (of)						
anterior (cranial)	191.9	198.3	—	225.0	237.5	239.6
cranial	191.9	198.3	—	225.0	237.5	239.6
ischiorectal	195.3	198.89	234.8	229.8	238.8	239.8
middle (cranial)	191.9	198.3	—	225.0	237.5	239.6
pituitary	194.3	198.89	234.8	227.3	237.0	239.7
posterior (cranial)	191.9	198.3	—	225.0	237.5	239.6
pterygoid	171.0	198.89	—	215.0	238.1	239.2
pyriform	148.1	198.89	230.0	210.8	235.1	239.0
Rosenmüller	147.2	198.89	230.0	210.7	235.1	239.0
tonsillar	146.1	198.89	230.0	210.6	235.1	239.0
fourchette	184.4	198.82	233.3	221.2	236.3	239.5
frenulum						
labii-*see* Neoplasm, lip, internal						
linguae	141.3	198.89	230.0	210.1	235.1	239.0
frontal						
bone	170.0	198.5	—	213.0	238.0	239.2
lobe, brain	191.1	198.3	—	225.0	237.5	239.6
meninges	192.1	198.4	—	225.2	237.6	239.7
pole	191.1	198.3	—	225.0	237.5	239.6
sinus	160.4	197.3	231.8	212.0	235.9	239.1
fundus						
stomach	151.3	197.8	230.2	211.1	235.2	239.0
uterus	182.0	198.82	233.2	219.1	236.0	239.5
gall duct (extrahepatic)	156.1	197.8	230.8	211.5	235.3	239.0
intrahepatic	155.1	197.8	230.8	211.5	235.3	239.0
gallbladder	156.0	197.8	230.8	211.5	235.3	239.0
contiguous sites with extrahepatic bile ducts	156.8	—	—	—	—	—
ganglia (*see also* Neoplasm, connective tissue)	171.9	198.89	—	215.9	238.1	239.2
basal	191.0	198.3	—	225.0	237.5	239.6

◀ New ⬅ Revised Code

	Malignant					
	Primary	Secondary	Ca in stiu	Benign	Uncertain Behavior	Unspecified
Neoplasm *(Continued)*						
ganglion (*see also* Neoplasm, connective tissue)	171.9	198.89	—	215.9	238.1	239.2
cranial nerve	192.0	198.4	—	225.1	237.9	239.7
Gartner's duct	184.0	198.82	233.3	221.1	236.3	239.5
gastric-*see* Neoplasm, stomach						
gastrocolic	159.8	197.8	230.9	211.9	235.5	239.0
gastroesophageal junction	151.0	197.8	230.2	211.1	235.2	239.0
gastrointestinal (tract) NEC	159.9	197.8	230.9	211.9	235.5	239.0
generalized	199.0	199.0	234.9	229.9	238.9	199.0
genital organ or tract						
female NEC	184.9	198.82	233.3	221.9	236.3	239.5
contiguous sites	184.8					
specified site NEC	184.8	198.82	233.3	221.8	236.3	239.5
male NEC	187.9	198.82	233.6	222.9	236.6	239.5
contiguous sites	187.8	—	—	—	—	—
specified site NEC	187.8	198.82	233.6	222.8	236.6	239.5
genitourinary tract						
female	184.9	198.82	233.3	221.9	236.3	239.5
male	187.9	198.82	233.6	222.9	236.6	239.5
gingiva (alveolar) (marginal)	143.9	198.89	230.0	210.4	235.1	239.0
lower	143.1	198.89	230.0	210.4	235.1	239.0
mandibular	143.1	198.89	230.0	210.4	235.1	239.0
maxillary	143.0	198.89	230.0	210.4	235.1	239.0
upper	143.0	198.89	230.0	210.4	235.1	239.0
gland, glandular (lymphatic) (system)-*see also* Neoplasm, lymph gland						
endocrine NEC	194.9	198.89	—	227.9	237.4	239.7
salivary-*see* Neoplasm, salivary, gland						
glans penis	187.2	198.82	233.5	222.1	236.6	239.5
globus pallidus	191.0	198.3	—	225.0	237.5	239.6
glomus						
coccygeal	194.6	198.89	—	227.6	237.3	239.7
jugularis	194.6	198.89	—	227.6	237.3	239.7
glosso-epiglottic fold(s)	146.4	198.89	230.0	210.6	235.1	239.0
glossopalatine fold	146.2	198.89	230.0	210.6	235.1	239.0
glossopharyngeal sulcus	146.1	198.89	230.0	210.6	235.1	239.0
glottis	161.0	197.3	231.0	212.1	235.6	239.1
gluteal region*	195.3	198.89	232.5	229.8	238.8	239.8
great vessels NEC	171.4	198.89	—	215.4	238.1	239.2
groin NEC	195.3	198.89	232.5	229.8	238.8	239.8
gum	143.9	198.89	230.0	210.4	235.1	239.0
contiguous sites	143.8	—	—	—	—	—
lower	143.1	198.89	230.0	210.4	235.1	239.0
upper	143.0	198.89	230.0	210.4	235.1	239.0
hand NEC*	195.4	198.89	232.6	229.8	238.8	239.8
head NEC*	195.0	198.89	232.4	229.8	238.8	239.8
heart	164.1	198.89	—	212.7	238.8	239.8
contiguous sites with mediastinum or thymus	164.8	—	—	—	—	—
heel NEC*	195.5	198.89	232.7	229.8	238.8	239.8
helix	173.2	198.2	232.2	216.2	238.2	239.2
hematopoietic, hemopoietic tissue NEC	202.8	198.89	—	—	—	238.7
hemisphere, cerebral	191.0	198.3	—	225.0	237.5	239.6
hemorrhoidal zone	154.2	197.5	230.5	211.4	235.5	239.0
hepatic	155.2	197.7	230.8	211.5	235.3	239.0
duct (bile)	156.1	197.8	230.8	211.5	235.3	239.0
flexure (colon)	153.0	197.5	230.3	211.3	235.2	239.0
primary	155.0	—	—	—	—	—
hilus of lung	162.2	197.0	231.2	212.3	235.7	239.1
hip NEC*	195.5	198.89	232.7	229.8	238.8	239.8
hippocampus, brain	191.2	198.3	—	225.0	237.5	239.6
humerus (any part)	170.4	198.5	—	213.4	238.0	239.2
hymen	184.0	198.82	233.3	221.1	236.3	239.5
hypopharynx, hypopharyngeal NEC	148.9	198.89	230.0	210.8	235.1	239.0
contiguous sites	148.8	—	—	—	—	—

	Malignant					
	Primary	Secondary	Ca in stiu	Benign	Uncertain Behavior	Unspecified
Neoplasm *(Continued)*						
hypopharynx, hypopharyngeal NEC *(Continued)*						
postcricoid region	148.0	198.89	230.0	210.8	235.1	239.0
posterior wall	148.3	198.89	230.0	210.8	235.1	239.0
pyriform fossa (sinus)	148.1	198.89	230.0	210.8	235.1	239.0
specified site NEC	148.8	198.89	230.0	210.8	235.1	239.0
wall	148.9	198.89	230.0	210.8	235.1	239.0
posterior	148.3	198.89	230.0	210.8	235.1	239.0
hypophysis	194.3	198.89	234.8	227.3	237.0	239.7
hypothalamus	191.0	198.3	—	225.0	237.5	239.6
ileocecum, ileocecal (coil) (junction) (valve)	153.4	197.5	230.3	211.3	235.2	239.0
ileum	152.2	197.4	230.7	211.2	235.2	239.0
ilium	170.6	198.5	—	213.6	238.0	239.2
immunoproliferative NEC	203.8	—	—	—	—	—
infraclavicular (region)*	195.1	198.89	232.5	229.8	238.8	239.8
inguinal (region)*	195.3	198.89	232.5	229.8	238.8	239.8
insula	191.0	198.3	—	225.0	237.5	239.6
insular tissue (pancreas)	157.4	197.8	230.9	211.7	235.5	239.0
brain	191.0	198.3	—	225.0	237.5	239.6
interarytenoid fold	148.2	198.89	230.0	210.8	235.1	239.0
hypopharyngeal aspect	148.2	198.89	230.0	210.8	235.1	239.0
laryngeal aspect	161.1	197.3	231.0	212.1	235.6	239.1
marginal zone	148.2	198.89	230.0	210.8	235.1	239.0
interdental papillae	143.9	198.89	230.0	210.4	235.1	239.0
lower	143.1	198.89	230.0	210.4	235.1	239.0
upper	143.0	198.89	230.0	210.4	235.1	239.0
internal						
capsule	191.0	198.3	—	225.0	237.5	239.6
os (cervix)	180.0	198.82	233.1	219.0	236.0	239.5
intervertebral cartilage or disc	170.2	198.5	—	213.2	238.0	239.2
intestine, intestinal	159.0	197.8	230.7	211.9	235.2	239.0
large	153.9	197.5	230.3	211.3	235.2	239.0
appendix	153.5	197.5	230.3	211.3	235.2	239.0
caput coli	153.4	197.5	230.3	211.3	235.2	239.0
cecum	153.4	197.5	230.3	211.3	235.2	239.0
colon	153.9	197.5	230.3	211.3	235.2	239.0
and rectum	154.0	197.5	230.4	211.4	235.2	239.0
ascending	153.6	197.5	230.3	211.3	235.2	239.0
caput	153.4	197.5	230.3	211.3	235.2	239.0
contiguous sites	153.8	—	—	—	—	—
descending	153.2	197.5	230.3	211.3	235.2	239.0
distal	153.2	197.5	230.3	211.3	235.2	239.0
left	153.2	197.5	230.3	211.3	235.2	239.0
pelvic	153.3	197.5	230.3	211.3	235.2	239.0
right	153.6	197.5	230.3	211.3	235.2	239.0
sigmoid (flexure)	153.3	197.5	230.3	211.3	235.2	239.0
transverse	153.1	197.5	230.3	211.3	235.2	239.0
contiguous sites	153.8	—	—	—	—	—
hepatic flexure	153.0	197.5	230.3	211.3	235.2	239.0
ileocecum, ileocecal (coil) (valve)	153.4	197.5	230.3	211.3	235.2	239.0
sigmoid flexure (lower) (upper)	153.3	197.5	230.3	211.3	235.2	239.0
splenic flexure	153.7	197.5	230.3	211.3	235.2	239.0
small	152.9	197.4	230.7	211.2	235.2	239.0
contiguous sites	152.8	—	—	—	—	—
duodenum	152.0	197.4	230.7	211.2	235.2	239.0
ileum	152.2	197.4	230.7	211.2	235.2	239.0
jejunum	152.1	197.4	230.7	211.2	235.2	239.0
tract NEC	159.0	197.8	230.7	211.9	235.2	239.0
intra-abdominal	195.2	198.89	234.8	229.8	238.8	239.8
intracranial NEC	191.9	198.3	—	225.0	237.5	239.6
intrahepatic (bile) duct	155.1	197.8	230.8	211.5	235.3	239.0
intraocular	190.0	198.4	234.0	224.0	238.8	239.8
intraorbital	190.1	198.4	234.0	224.1	238.8	239.8

	Malignant					
	Primary	Secondary	Ca in stiu	Benign	Uncertain Behavior	Unspecified
Neoplasm *(Continued)*						
intrasellar	194.3	198.89	234.8	227.3	237.0	239.7
intrathoracic (cavity) (organs NEC)	195.1	198.89	234.8	229.8	238.8	239.8
contiguous sites with respiratory organs	165.8	—	—	—	—	—
iris	190.0	198.4	234.0	224.0	238.8	239.8
ischiorectal (fossa)	195.3	198.89	234.8	229.8	238.8	239.8
ischium	170.6	198.5	—	213.6	238.0	239.2
island of Reil	191.0	198.3	—	225.0	237.5	239.6
islands or islets of Langerhans	157.4	197.8	230.9	211.7	235.5	239.0
isthmus uteri	182.1	198.82	233.2	219.1	236.0	239.5
jaw	195.0	198.89	234.8	229.8	238.8	239.8
bone	170.1	198.5	—	213.1	238.0	239.2
carcinoma	143.9	—	—	—	—	—
lower	143.1	—	—	—	—	—
upper	143.0	—	—	—	—	—
lower	170.1	198.5	—	213.1	238.0	239.2
upper	170.0	198.5	—	213.0	238.0	239.2
carcinoma (any type) (lower) (upper)	195.0	—	—	—	—	—
skin	173.3	198.2	232.3	216.3	238.2	239.2
soft tissues	143.9	198.89	230.0	210.4	235.1	239.0
lower	143.1	198.89	230.0	210.4	235.1	239.0
upper	143.0	198.89	230.0	210.4	235.1	239.0
jejunum	152.1	197.4	230.7	211.2	235.2	239.0
joint NEC (*see also* Neoplasm, bone)	170.9	198.5	—	213.9	238.0	239.2
acromioclavicular	170.4	198.5	—	213.4	238.0	239.2
bursa or synovial membrane-*see* Neoplasm, connective tissue						
costovertebral	170.3	198.5	—	213.3	238.0	239.2
sternocostal	170.3	198.5	—	213.3	238.0	239.2
temporomandibular	170.1	198.5	—	213.1	238.0	239.2
junction						
anorectal	154.8	197.5	230.7	211.4	235.5	239.0
cardioesophageal	151.0	197.8	230.2	211.1	235.2	239.0
esophagogastric	151.0	197.8	230.2	211.1	235.2	239.0
gastroesophageal	151.0	197.8	230.2	211.1	235.2	239.0
hard and soft palate	145.5	198.89	230.0	210.4	235.1	239.0
ileocecal	153.4	197.5	230.3	211.3	235.2	239.0
pelvirectal	154.0	197.5	230.4	211.4	235.2	239.0
pelviureteric	189.1	198.0	233.9	223.1	236.91	239.5
rectosigmoid	154.0	197.5	230.4	211.4	235.2	239.0
squamocolumnar, of cervix	180.8	198.82	233.1	219.0	236.0	239.5
kidney (parenchymal)	189.0	198.0	233.9	223.0	236.91	239.5
calyx	189.1	198.0	233.9	223.1	236.91	239.5
hilus	189.1	198.0	233.9	223.1	236.91	239.5
pelvis	189.1	198.0	233.9	223.1	236.91	239.5
knee NEC*	195.5	198.89	232.7	229.8	238.8	239.8
labia (skin)	184.4	198.82	233.3	221.2	236.3	239.5
majora	184.1	198.82	233.3	221.2	236.3	239.5
minora	184.2	198.82	233.3	221.2	236.3	239.5
labial-*see also* Neoplasm, lip sulcus (lower) (upper)	145.1	198.89	230.0	210.4	235.1	239.0
labium (skin)	184.4	198.82	233.3	221.2	236.3	239.5
majus	184.1	198.82	233.3	221.2	236.3	239.5
minus	184.2	198.82	233.3	221.2	236.3	239.5
lacrimal						
canaliculi	190.7	198.4	234.0	224.7	238.8	239.8
duct (nasal)	190.7	198.4	234.0	224.7	238.8	239.8
gland	190.2	198.4	234.0	224.2	238.8	239.8
punctum	190.7	198.4	234.0	224.7	238.8	239.8
sac	190.7	198.4	234.0	224.7	238.8	239.8
Langerhans, islands or islets	157.4	197.8	230.9	211.7	235.5	239.0
laryngopharynx	148.9	198.89	230.0	210.8	235.1	239.0
larynx, laryngeal NEC	161.9	197.3	231.0	212.1	235.6	239.1
aryepiglottic fold	161.1	197.3	231.0	212.1	235.6	239.1
cartilage (arytenoid) (cricoid) (cuneiform) (thyroid)	161.3	197.3	231.0	212.1	235.6	239.1

	Malignant					
	Primary	Secondary	Ca in stiu	Benign	Uncertain Behavior	Unspecified
Neoplasm *(Continued)*						
larynx, laryngeal NEC *(Continued)*						
commissure (anterior) (posterior)	161.0	197.3	231.0	212.1	235.6	239.1
contiguous sites	161.8	—	—	—	—	—
extrinsic NEC	161.1	197.3	231.0	212.1	235.6	239.1
meaning hypopharynx	148.9	198.89	230.0	210.8	235.1	239.0
interarytenoid fold	161.1	197.3	231.0	212.1	235.6	239.1
intrinsic	161.0	197.3	231.0	212.1	235.6	239.1
ventricular band	161.1	197.3	231.0	212.1	235.6	239.1
leg NEC*	195.5	198.89	232.7	229.8	238.8	239.8
lens, crystalline	190.0	198.4	234.0	224.0	238.8	239.8
lid (lower) (upper)	173.1	198.2	232.1	216.1	238.2	239.2
ligament-*see also* Neoplasm, connective tissue						
broad	183.3	198.82	233.3	221.0	236.3	239.5
Mackenrodt's	183.8	198.82	233.3	221.8	236.3	239.5
non-uterine-*see* Neoplasm, connective tissue						
round	183.5	198.82	—	221.0	236.3	239.5
sacro-uterine	183.4	198.82	—	221.0	236.3	239.5
uterine	183.4	198.82	—	221.0	236.3	239.5
utero-ovarian	183.8	198.82	233.3	221.8	236.3	239.5
uterosacral	183.4	198.82	—	221.0	236.3	239.5
limb*	195.8	198.89	232.8	229.8	238.8	239.8
lower*	195.5	198.89	232.7	229.8	238.8	239.8
upper*	195.4	198.89	232.6	229.8	238.8	239.8
limbus of cornea	190.4	198.4	234.0	224.4	238.8	239.8
lingual NEC (*see also* Neoplasm, tongue)	141.9	198.89	230.0	210.1	235.1	239.0
lingula, lung	162.3	197.0	231.2	212.3	235.7	239.1
lip (external) (lipstick area) (vermillion border)	140.9	198.89	230.0	210.0	235.1	239.0
buccal aspect-*see* Neoplasm, lip, internal						
commissure	140.6	198.89	230.0	210.4	235.1	239.0
contiguous sites	140.8	—	—	—	—	—
with oral cavity or pharynx	149.8	—	—	—	—	—
frenulum-*see* Neoplasm, lip, internal						
inner aspect-*see* Neoplasm, lip, internal						
internal (buccal) (frenulum) (mucosa) (oral)	140.5	198.89	230.0	210.0	235.1	239.0
lower	140.4	198.89	230.0	210.0	235.1	239.0
upper	140.3	198.89	230.0	210.0	235.1	239.0
lower	140.1	198.89	230.0	210.0	235.1	239.0
internal (buccal) (frenulum) (mucosa) (oral)	140.4	198.89	230.0	210.0	235.1	239.0
mucosa-*see* Neoplasm, lip, internal						
oral aspect-*see* Neoplasm, lip, internal						
skin (commissure) (lower) (upper)	173.0	198.2	232.0	216.0	238.2	239.2
upper	140.0	198.89	230.0	210.0	235.1	239.0
internal (buccal) (frenulum) (mucosa) (oral)	140.3	198.89	230.0	210.0	235.1	239.0
liver	155.2	197.7	230.8	211.5	235.3	239.0
primary	155.0	—	—	—	—	—
lobe						
azygos	162.3	197.0	231.2	212.3	235.7	239.1
frontal	191.1	198.3	—	225.0	237.5	239.6
lower	162.5	197.0	231.2	212.3	235.7	239.1
middle	162.4	197.0	231.2	212.3	235.7	239.1
occipital	191.4	198.3	—	225.0	237.5	239.6
parietal	191.3	198.3	—	225.0	237.5	239.6
temporal	191.2	198.3	—	225.0	237.5	239.6
upper	162.3	197.0	231.2	212.3	235.7	239.1
lumbosacral plexus	171.6	198.4	—	215.6	238.1	239.2
lung	162.9	197.0	231.2	212.3	235.7	239.1
azygos lobe	162.3	197.0	231.2	212.3	235.7	239.1
carina	162.2	197.0	231.2	212.3	235.7	239.1
contiguous sites with bronchus or trachea	162.8	—	—	—	—	—
hilus	162.2	197.0	231.2	212.3	235.7	239.1
lingula	162.3	197.0	231.2	212.3	235.7	239.1
lobe NEC	162.9	197.0	231.2	212.3	235.7	239.1

	Malignant					
	Primary	**Secondary**	**Ca in stiu**	**Benign**	**Uncertain Behavior**	**Unspecified**
Neoplasm *(Continued)*						
lung *(Continued)*						
lower lobe	162.5	197.0	231.2	212.3	235.7	239.1
main bronchus	162.2	197.0	231.2	212.3	235.7	239.1
middle lobe	162.4	197.0	231.2	212.3	235.7	239.1
upper lobe	162.3	197.0	231.2	212.3	235.7	239.1
lymph, lymphatic channel NEC (*see also* Neoplasm, connective tissue)	171.9	198.89	—	215.9	238.1	239.2
gland (secondary)	—	196.9	—	229.0	238.8	239.8
abdominal	—	196.2	—	229.0	238.8	239.8
aortic	—	196.2	—	229.0	238.8	239.8
arm	—	196.3	—	229.0	238.8	239.8
auricular (anterior) (posterior)	—	196.0	—	229.0	238.8	239.8
axilla, axillary	—	196.3	—	229.0	238.8	239.8
brachial	—	196.3	—	229.0	238.8	239.8
bronchial	—	196.1	—	229.0	238.8	239.8
bronchopulmonary	—	196.1	—	229.0	238.8	239.8
celiac	—	196.2	—	229.0	238.8	239.8
cervical	—	196.0	—	229.0	238.8	239.8
cervicofacial	—	196.0	—	229.0	238.8	239.8
Cloquet	—	196.5	—	229.0	238.8	239.8
colic	—	196.2	—	229.0	238.8	239.8
common duct	—	196.2	—	229.0	238.8	239.8
cubital	—	196.3	—	229.0	238.8	239.8
diaphragmatic	—	196.1	—	229.0	238.8	239.8
epigastric, inferior	—	196.6	—	229.0	238.8	239.8
epitrochlear	—	196.3	—	229.0	238.8	239.8
esophageal	—	196.1	—	229.0	238.8	239.8
face	—	196.0	—	229.0	238.8	239.8
femoral	—	196.5	—	229.0	238.8	239.8
gastric	—	196.2	—	229.0	238.8	239.8
groin	—	196.5	—	229.0	238.8	239.8
head	—	196.0	—	229.0	238.8	239.8
hepatic	—	196.2	—	229.0	238.8	239.8
hilar (pulmonary)	—	196.1	—	229.0	238.8	239.8
splenic	—	196.2	—	229.0	238.8	239.8
hypogastric	—	196.6	—	229.0	238.8	239.8
ileocolic	—	196.2	—	229.0	238.8	239.8
iliac	—	196.6	—	229.0	238.8	239.8
infraclavicular	—	196.3	—	229.0	238.8	239.8
inguina, inguinal	—	196.5	—	229.0	238.8	239.8
innominate	—	196.1	—	229.0	238.8	239.8
intercostal	—	196.1	—	229.0	238.8	239.8
intestinal	—	196.2	—	229.0	238.8	239.8
intrabdominal	—	196.2	—	229.0	238.8	239.8
intrapelvic	—	196.6	—	229.0	238.8	239.8
intrathoracic	—	196.1	—	229.0	238.8	239.9
jugular	—	196.0	—	229.0	238.8	239.8
leg	—	196.5	—	229.0	238.8	239.8
limb						
lower	—	196.5	—	229.0	238.8	239.8
upper	—	196.3	—	229.0	238.8	239.8
lower limb	—	196.5	—	229.0	238.8	238.9
lumbar	—	196.2	—	229.0	238.8	239.8
mandibular	—	196.0	—	229.0	238.8	239.8
mediastinal	—	196.1	—	229.0	238.8	239.8
mesenteric (inferior) (superior)	—	196.2	—	229.0	238.8	239.8
midcolic	—	196.2	—	229.0	238.8	239.8
multiple sites in categories 196.0-196.6	—	196.8	—	229.0	238.8	239.8
neck	—	196.0	—	229.0	238.8	239.8
obturator	—	196.6	—	229.0	238.8	239.8
occipital	—	196.0	—	229.0	238.8	239.8
pancreatic	—	196.2	—	229.0	238.8	239.8
para-aortic	—	196.2	—	229.0	238.8	239.8

	Malignant					
	Primary	Secondary	Ca in stiu	Benign	Uncertain Behavior	Unspecified
Neoplasm *(Continued)*						
lymph, lymphatic channel NEC *(Continued)*						
gland *(Continued)*						
paracervical	—	196.6	—	229.0	238.8	239.8
parametrial	—	196.6	—	229.0	238.8	239.8
parasternal	—	196.1	—	229.0	238.8	239.8
parotid	—	196.0	—	229.0	238.8	239.8
pectoral	—	196.3	—	229.0	238.8	239.8
pelvic	—	196.6	—	229.0	238.8	239.8
peri-aortic	—	196.2	—	229.0	238.8	239.8
peripancreatic	—	196.2	—	229.0	238.8	239.8
popliteal	—	196.5	—	229.0	238.8	239.8
porta hepatis	—	196.2	—	229.0	238.8	239.8
portal	—	196.2	—	229.0	238.8	239.8
preauricular	—	196.0	—	229.0	238.8	239.8
prelaryngeal	—	196.0	—	229.0	238.8	239.8
presymphysial	—	196.6	—	229.0	238.8	239.8
pretracheal	—	196.0	—	229.0	238.8	239.8
primary (any site) NEC	202.9	—	—	—	—	—
pulmonary (hiler)	—	196.1	—	229.0	238.8	239.8
pyloric	—	196.2	—	229.0	238.8	239.8
retroperitoneal	—	196.2	—	229.0	238.8	239.8
retropharyngeal	—	196.0	—	229.0	238.8	239.8
Rosenmüller's	—	196.5	—	229.0	238.8	239.8
sacral	—	196.6	—	229.0	238.8	239.8
scalene	—	196.0	—	229.0	238.8	239.8
site NEC	—	196.9	—	229.0	238.8	239.8
splenic (hilar)	—	196.2	—	229.0	238.8	239.8
subclavicular	—	196.3	—	229.0	238.8	239.8
subinguinal	—	196.5	—	229.0	238.8	239.8
sublingual	—	196.0	—	229.0	238.8	239.8
submandibular	—	196.0	—	229.0	238.8	239.8
submaxillary	—	196.0	—	229.0	238.8	239.8
submental	—	196.0	—	229.0	238.8	239.8
subscapular	—	196.3	—	229.0	238.8	239.8
supraclavicular	—	196.0	—	229.0	238.8	239.8
thoracic	—	196.1	—	229.0	238.8	239.8
tibial	—	196.5	—	229.0	238.8	239.8
tracheal		196.1	—	229.0	238.8	239.8
tracheobronchial	—	196.1	—	229.0	238.8	239.8
upper limb	—	196.3	—	229.0	238.8	239.8
Virchow's	—	196.0	—	229.0	238.8	239.8
node-*see also* Neoplasm, lymph gland primary NEC	202.9	—	—	—	—	—
vessel (*see also* Neoplasm, connective tissue)	171.9	198.89	—	215.9	238.1	239.2
Mackenrodt's ligament	183.8	198.82	233.3	221.8	236.3	239.5
malar region-*see* Neoplasm, cheek	170.0	198.5	—	213.0	238.0	239.2
mammary gland-*see* Neoplasm, breast						
mandible	170.1	198.5	—	213.1	238.0	239.2
alveolar						
mucosa	143.1	198.89	230.0	210.4	235.1	239.0
ridge or process	170.1	198.5	—	213.1	238.0	239.2
carcinoma	143.1	—	—	—	—	—
carcinoma	143.1	—	—	—	—	—
marrow (bone) NEC	202.9	198.5	—	—	—	238.7
mastectomy site (skin)	173.5	198.2	—	—	—	—
specified as breast tissue	174.8	198.81	—	—	—	—
mastoid (air cells) (antrum) (cavity)	160.1	197.3	231.8	212.0	235.9	239.1
bone or process	170.0	198.5	—	213.0	238.0	239.2
maxilla, maxillary (superior)	170.0	198.5	—	213.0	238.0	239.2
alveolar						
mucosa	143.0	198.89	230.0	210.4	235.1	239.0
ridge or process	170.0	198.5	—	213.0	238.0	239.2
carcinoma	143.0	—	—	—	—	—

	Malignant					
	Primary	Secondary	Ca in stiu	Benign	Uncertain Behavior	Unspecified
Neoplasm *(Continued)*						
maxilla, maxillary *(Continued)*						
antrum	160.2	197.3	231.8	212.0	235.9	239.1
carcinoma	143.0	—	—	—	—	—
inferior-*see* Neoplasm, mandible						
sinus	160.2	197.3	231.8	212.0	235.9	239.1
meatus						
external (ear)	173.2	198.2	232.2	216.2	238.2	239.2
Meckel's diverticulum	152.3	197.4	230.7	211.2	235.2	239.0
mediastinum, mediastinal	164.9	197.1	—	212.5	235.8	239.8
anterior	164.2	197.1	—	212.5	235.8	239.8
contiguous sites with heart and thymus	164.8	—	—	—	—	—
posterior	164.3	197.1	—	212.5	235.8	239.8
medulla						
adrenal	194.0	198.7	234.8	227.0	237.2	239.7
oblongata	191.7	198.3	—	225.0	237.5	239.6
meibomian gland	173.1	198.2	232.1	216.1	238.2	239.2
melanoma-*see* Melanoma						
meninges (brain) (cerebral) (cranial) (intracranial)	192.1	198.4	—	225.2	237.6	239.7
spinal (cord)	192.3	198.4	—	225.4	237.6	239.7
meniscus, knee joint (lateral) (medial)	170.7	198.5	—	213.7	238.0	239.2
mesentery, mesenteric	158.8	197.6	—	211.8	235.4	239.0
mesoappendix	158.8	197.6	—	211.8	235.4	239.0
mesocolon	158.8	197.6	—	211.8	235.4	239.0
mesopharynx-*see* Neoplasm, oropharynx						
mesosalpinx	183.3	198.82	233.3	221.0	236.3	239.5
mesovarium	183.3	198.82	233.3	221.0	236.3	239.5
metacarpus (any bone)	170.5	198.5	—	213.5	238.0	239.2
metastatic NEC-*see also* Neoplasm, by site, secondary	—	199.1	—	—	—	—
metatarsus (any bone)	170.8	198.5	—	213.8	238.0	239.2
midbrain	191.7	198.3	—	225.0	237.5	239.6
milk duct-*see* Neoplasm, breast						
mons						
pubis	184.4	198.82	233.3	221.2	236.3	239.5
veneris	184.4	198.82	233.3	221.2	236.3	239.5
motor tract	192.9	198.4	—	225.9	237.9	239.7
brain	191.9	198.3	—	225.0	237.5	239.6
spinal	192.2	198.3	—	225.3	237.5	239.7
mouth	145.9	198.89	230.0	210.4	235.1	239.0
contiguous sites	145.8	—	—	—	—	—
floor	144.9	198.89	230.0	210.3	235.1	239.0
anterior portion	144.0	198.89	230.0	210.3	235.1	239.0
contiguous sites	144.8	—	—	—	—	—
lateral portion	144.1	198.89	230.0	210.3	235.1	239.0
roof	145.5	198.89	230.0	210.4	235.1	239.0
specified part NEC	145.8	198.89	230.0	210.4	235.1	239.0
vestibule	145.1	198.89	230.0	210.4	235.1	239.0
mucosa						
alveolar (ridge or process)	143.9	198.89	230.0	210.4	235.1	239.0
lower	143.1	198.89	230.0	210.4	235.1	239.0
upper	143.0	198.89	230.0	210.4	235.1	239.0
buccal	145.0	198.89	230.0	210.4	235.1	239.0
cheek	145.0	198.89	230.0	210.4	235.1	239.0
lip-*see* Neoplasm, lip, internal						
nasal	160.0	197.3	231.8	212.0	235.9	239.1
oral	145.0	198.89	230.0	210.4	235.1	239.0
Müllerian duct						
female	184.8	198.82	233.3	221.8	236.3	239.5
male	187.8	198.82	233.6	222.8	236.6	239.5
multiple sites NEC	199.0	199.0	234.9	229.9	238.9	199.0
muscle-*see also* Neoplasm, connective tissue extraocular	190.1	198.4	234.0	224.1	238.8	239.8
myocardium	164.1	198.89	—	212.7	238.8	239.8
myometrium	182.0	198.82	233.2	219.1	236.0	239.5

	Malignant					
	Primary	Secondary	Ca in stiu	Benign	Uncertain Behavior	Unspecified
Neoplasm *(Continued)*						
myopericardium	164.1	198.89	—	212.7	238.8	239.8
nabothian gland (follicle)	180.0	198.82	233.1	219.0	236.0	239.5
nail	173.9	198.2	232.9	216.9	238.2	239.2
finger	173.6	198.2	232.6	216.6	238.2	239.2
toe	173.7	198.2	232.7	216.7	238.2	239.2
nares, naris (anterior) (posterior)	160.0	197.3	231.8	212.0	235.9	239.1
nasal-*see* Neoplasm, nose						
nasolabial groove	173.3	198.2	232.3	216.3	238.2	239.2
nasolacrimal duct	190.7	198.4	234.0	224.7	238.8	239.8
nasopharynx, nasopharyngeal	147.9	198.89	230.0	210.7	235.1	239.0
contiguous sites	147.8	—	—	—	—	—
floor	147.3	198.89	230.0	210.7	235.1	239.0
roof	147.0	198.89	230.0	210.7	235.1	239.0
specified site NEC	147.8	198.89	230.0	210.7	235.1	239.0
wall	147.9	198.89	230.0	210.7	235.1	239.0
anterior	147.3	198.89	230.0	210.7	235.1	239.0
lateral	147.2	198.89	230.0	210.7	235.1	239.0
posterior	147.1	198.89	230.0	210.7	235.1	239.0
superior	147.0	198.89	230.0	210.7	235.1	239.0
nates	173.5	198.2	232.5	216.5	238.2	239.2
neck NEC*	195.0	198.89	234.8	229.8	238.8	239.8
nerve (autonomic) (parasympathetic) (peripheral) (sympathetic) - *see also* Neoplasm, connective tissue						
abducens	192.0	198.4	—	225.1	237.9	239.7
accessory (spinal)	192.0	198.4	—	225.1	237.9	239.7
acoustic	192.0	198.4	—	225.1	237.9	239.7
auditory	192.0	198.4	—	225.1	237.9	239.7
brachial	171.2	198.89	—	215.2	238.1	239.2
cranial (any)	192.0	198.4	—	225.1	237.9	239.7
facial	192.0	198.4	—	225.1	237.9	239.7
femoral	171.3	198.89	—	215.3	238.1	239.2
glossopharyngeal	192.0	198.4	—	225.1	237.9	239.7
hypoglossal	192.0	198.4	—	225.1	237.9	239.7
intercostal	171.4	198.89	—	215.4	238.1	239.2
lumbar	171.7	198.89	—	215.7	238.1	239.2
median	171.2	198.89	—	215.2	238.1	239.2
obturator	171.3	198.89	—	215.3	238.1	239.2
oculomotor	192.0	198.4	—	225.1	237.9	239.7
olfactory	192.0	198.4	—	225.1	237.9	239.7
optic	192.0	198.4	—	225.1	237.9	239.7
peripheral NEC	171.9	198.89	—	215.9	238.1	239.2
radial	171.2	198.89	—	215.2	238.1	239.2
sacral	171.6	198.89	—	215.6	238.1	239.2
sciatic	171.3	198.89	—	215.3	238.1	239.2
spinal NEC	171.9	198.89	—	215.9	238.1	239.2
trigeminal	192.0	198.4	—	225.1	237.9	239.7
trochlear	192.0	198.4	—	225.1	237.9	239.7
ulnar	171.2	198.89	—	215.2	238.1	239.2
vagus	192.0	198.4	—	225.1	237.9	239.7
nervous system (central) NEC	192.9	198.4	—	225.9	237.9	239.7
autonomic NEC	171.9	198.89	—	215.9	238.1	239.2
brain-*see also* Neoplasm, brain membrane or meninges	192.1	198.4	—	225.2	237.6	239.7
contiguous sites	192.8	—	—	—	—	—
parasympathetic NEC	171.9	198.89	—	215.9	238.1	239.2
sympathetic NEC	171.9	198.89	—	215.9	238.1	239.2
nipple (female)	174.0	198.81	233.0	217	238.3	239.3
male	175.0	198.81	233.0	217	238.3	239.3
nose, nasal	195.0	198.89	234.8	229.8	238.8	239.8
ala (external)	173.3	198.2	232.3	216.3	238.2	239.2
bone	170.0	198.5	—	213.0	238.0	239.2
cartilage	160.0	197.3	231.8	212.0	235.9	239.1
cavity	160.0	197.3	231.8	212.0	235.9	239.1
contiguous sites with accessory sinuses or middle ear	160.8	—	—	—	—	—

◀ New ⟸ Revised Code

	Malignant					
	Primary	Secondary	Ca in stiu	Benign	Uncertain Behavior	Unspecified
Neoplasm *(Continued)*						
nose, nasal *(Continued)*						
choana	147.3	198.89	230.0	210.7	235.1	239.0
external (skin)	173.3	198.2	232.3	216.3	238.2	239.2
fossa	160.0	197.3	231.8	212.0	235.9	239.1
internal	160.0	197.3	231.8	212.0	235.9	239.1
mucosa	160.0	197.3	231.8	212.0	235.9	239.1
septum	160.0	197.3	231.8	212.0	235.9	239.1
posterior margin	147.3	198.89	230.0	210.7	235.1	239.0
sinus-*see* Neoplasm, sinus						
skin	173.3	198.2	232.3	216.3	238.2	239.2
turbinate (mucosa)	160.0	197.3	231.8	212.0	235.9	239.1
bone	170.0	198.5	—	2130	238.0	239.2
vestibule	160.0	197.3	231.8	212.0	235.9	239.1
nostril	160.0	197.3	231.8	212.0	235.9	239.1
nucleus pulposus	170.2	198.5	—	213.2	238.0	230.2
occipital						
bone	170.0	198.5	—	213.0	238.0	239.2
lobe or pole, brain	191.4	198.3	—	225.0	237.5	239.6
odontogenic-*see* Neoplasm, jaw bone						
oesophagus-*see* Neoplasm, esophagus						
olfactory nerve or bulb	192.0	198.4	—	225.1	237.9	239.7
olive (brain)	191.7	198.3	—	225.0	237.5	239.6
omentum	158.8	197.6	—	211.8	235.4	239.0
operculum (brain)	191.0	198.3	—	225.0	237.5	239.6
optic nerve, chiasm, or tract	192.0	198.4	—	225.1	237.9	239.7
oral (cavity)	145.9	198.89	230.0	210.4	235.1	239.0
contiguous sites with lip or pharynx	149.8	—	—	—	—	—
ill-defined	149.9	198.89	230.0	210.4	235.1	239.0
mucosa	145.9	198.89	230.0	210.4	235.1	239.0
orbit	190.1	198.4	234.0	224.1	238.8	239.8
bone	170.0	198.5	—	213.0	238.0	239.2
eye	190.1	198.4	234.0	224.1	238.8	239.8
soft parts	190.1	198.4	234.0	224.1	238.8	239.8
organ of Zuckerkandl	194.6	198.89	—	227.6	237.3	239.7
oropharynx	146.9	198.89	230.0	210.6	235.1	239.0
branchial cleft (vestige)	146.8	198.89	230.0	210.6	235.1	239.0
contiguous sites	146.8	—	—	—	—	—
junctional region	146.5	198.89	230.0	210.6	235.1	239.0
lateral wall	146.6	198.89	230.0	210.6	235.1	239.0
pillars of fauces	146.2	198.89	230.0	210.6	235.1	239.0
posterior wall	146.7	198.89	230.0	210.6	235.1	239.0
specified part NEC	146.8	198.89	230.0	210.6	235.1	239.0
vallecula	146.3	198.89	230.0	210.6	235.1	239.0
os						
external	180.1	198.82	233.1	219.0	236.0	239.5
internal	180.0	198.82	233.1	219.0	236.0	239.5
ovary	183.0	198.6	233.3	220	236.2	239.5
oviduct	183.2	198.82	233.3	221.0	236.3	239.5
palate	145.5	198.89	230.0	210.4	235.1	239.0
hard	145.2	198.89	230.0	210.4	235.1	239.0
junction of hard and soft palate	145.5	198.89	230.0	210.4	235.1	239.0
soft	145.3	198.89	230.0	210.4	235.1	239.0
nasopharyngeal surface	147.3	198.89	230.0	210.7	235.1	239.0
posterior surface	147.3	198.89	230.0	210.7	235.1	239.0
superior surface	147.3	198.89	230.0	210.7	235.1	239.0
palatoglossal arch	146.2	198.89	230.0	210.6	235.1	239.0
palatopharyngeal arch	146.2	198.89	230.0	210.6	235.1	239.0
pallium	191.0	198.3	—	225.0	237.5	239.6
palpebra	173.1	198.2	232.1	216.1	238.2	239.2
pancreas	157.9	197.8	230.9	211.6	235.5	239.0
body	157.1	197.8	230.9	211.6	235.5	239.0
contiguous sites	157.8	—	—	—	—	—

	Malignant					
	Primary	Secondary	Ca in stiu	Benign	Uncertain Behavior	Unspecified
Neoplasm *(Continued)*						
pancreas *(Continued)*						
duct (of Santorini) (of Wirsung)	157.3	197.8	230.9	211.6	235.5	239.0
ectopic tissue	157.8	197.8				
head	157.0	197.8	230.9	211.6	235.5	239.0
islet cells	157.4	197.8	230.9	211.7	235.5	239.0
neck	157.8	197.8	230.9	211.6	235.5	239.0
tail	157.2	197.8	230.9	211.6	235.5	239.0
para-aortic body	194.6	198.89	—	227.6	237.3	239.7
paraganglion NEC	194.6	198.89	—	227.6	237.3	239.7
parametrium	183.4	198.82	—	221.0	236.3	239.5
paranephric	158.0	197.6	—	211.8	235.4	239.0
pararectal	195.3	198.89	—	229.8	238.8	239.8
parasagittal (region)	195.0	198.89	234.8	229.8	238.8	239.8
parasellar	192.9	198.4	—	225.9	237.9	239.7
parathyroid (gland)	194.1	198.89	234.8	227.1	237.4	239.7
paraurethral	195.3	198.89	—	229.8	238.8	239.8
gland	189.4	198.1	233.9	223.89	236.99	239.5
paravaginal	195.3	198.89	—	229.8	238.8	239.8
parenchyma, kidney	189.0	198.0	233.9	223.0	236.91	239.5
parietal						
bone	170.0	198.5	—	213.0	238.0	239.2
lobe, brain	191.3	198.3	—	225.0	237.5	239.6
paroophoron	183.3	198.82	233.3	221.0	236.3	239.5
parotid (duct) (gland)	142.0	198.89	230.0	210.2	235.0	239.0
parovarium	183.3	198.82	233.3	221.0	236.3	239.5
patella	170.8	198.5	—	213.8	238.0	239.2
peduncle, cerebral	191.7	198.3	—	225.0	237.5	239.6
pelvirectal junction	154.0	197.5	230.4	211.4	235.2	239.0
pelvis, pelvic	195.3	198.89	234.8	229.8	238.8	239.8
bone	170.6	198.5	—	213.6	238.0	239.2
floor	195.3	198.89	234.8	229.8	238.8	239.8
renal	189.1	198.0	233.9	223.1	236.91	239.5
viscera	195.3	198.89	234.8	229.8	238.8	239.8
wall	195.3	198.89	234.8	229.8	238.8	239.8
pelvo-abdominal	195.8	198.89	234.8	229.8	238.8	239.8
penis	187.4	198.82	233.5	222.1	236.6	239.5
body	187.3	198.82	233.5	222.1	236.6	239.5
corpus (cavernosum)	187.3	198.82	233.5	222.1	236.6	239.5
glans	187.2	198.82	233.5	222.1	236.6	239.5
skin NEC	187.4	198.82	233.5	222.1	236.6	239.5
periadrenal (tissue)	158.0	197.6	—	211.8	235.4	239.0
perianal (skin)	173.5	198.2	232.5	216.5	238.2	239.2
pericardium	164.1	198.89	—	212.7	238.8	239.8
perinephric	158.0	197.6	—	211.8	235.4	239.0
perineum	195.3	198.89	234.8	229.8	238.8	239.8
periodontal tissue NEC	143.9	198.89	230.0	210.4	235.1	239.0
periosteum-*see* Neoplasm, bone						
peripancreatic	158.0	197.6	—	211.8	235.4	239.0
peripheral nerve NEC	171.9	198.89	—	215.9	238.1	239.2
perirectal (tissue)	195.3	198.89	—	229.8	238.8	239.8
perirenal (tissue)	158.0	197.6	—	211.8	235.4	239.0
peritoneum, peritoneal (cavity)	158.9	197.6	—	211.8	235.4	239.0
contiguous sites	158.8	—	—	—	—	—
with digestive organs	159.8	—	—	—	—	—
parietal	158.8	197.6	—	211.8	235.4	239.0
pelvic	158.8	197.6	—	211.8	235.4	239.0
specified part NEC	158.8	197.6	—	211.8	235.4	239.0
peritonsillar (tissue)	195.0	198.89	234.8	229.8	238.8	239.8
periurethral tissue	195.3	198.89	—	229.8	238.8	239.8
phalanges	170.9	198.5	—	213.9	238.0	239.2
foot	170.8	198.5	—	213.8	238.0	239.2
hand	170.5	198.5	—	213.5	238.0	239.2

	Malignant					
	Primary	Secondary	Ca in stiu	Benign	Uncertain Behavior	Unspecified
Neoplasm *(Continued)*						
pharynx, pharyngeal	149.0	198.89	230.0	210.9	235.1	239.0
bursa	147.1	198.89	230.0	210.7	235.1	239.0
fornix	147.3	198.89	230.0	210.7	235.1	239.0
recess	147.2	198.89	230.0	210.7	235.1	239.0
region	149.0	198.89	230.0	210.9	235.1	239.0
tonsil	147.1	198.89	230.0	210.7	235.1	239.0
wall (lateral) (posterior)	149.0	198.89	230.0	210.9	235.1	239.0
pia mater (cerebral) (cranial)	192.1	198.4	—	225.2	237.6	239.7
spinal	192.3	198.4	—	225.4	237.6	239.7
pillars of fauces	146.2	198.89	230.0	210.6	235.1	239.0
pineal (body) (gland)	194.4	198.89	234.8	227.4	237.1	239.7
pinna (ear) NEC	173.2	198.2	232.2	216.2	238.2	239.2
cartilage	171.0	198.89	—	215.0	238.1	239.2
piriform fossa or sinus	148.1	198.89	230.0	210.8	235.1	239.0
pituitary (body) (fossa) (gland) (lobe)	194.3	198.89	234.8	227.3	237.0	239.7
placenta	181	198.82	233.2	219.8	236.1	239.5
pleura, pleural (cavity)	163.9	197.2	—	212.4	235.8	239.1
contiguous sites	163.8	—	—	—	—	—
parietal	163.0	197.2	—	212.4	235.8	239.1
visceral	163.1	197.2	—	212.4	235.8	239.1
plexus						
brachial	171.2	198.89	—	215.2	238.1	239.2
cervical	171.0	198.89	—	215.0	238.1	239.2
choroid	191.5	198.3	—	225.0	237.5	239.6
lumbosacral	171.6	198.89	—	215.6	238.1	239.2
sacral	171.6	198.89	—	215.6	238.1	239.2
pluri-endocrine	194.8	198.89	234.8	227.8	237.4	239.7
pole						
frontal	191.1	198.3	—	225.0	237.5	239.6
occipital	191.4	198.3	—	225.0	237.5	239.6
pons (varolii)	191.7	198.3	—	225.0	237.5	239.6
popliteal fossa or space*	195.5	198.89	234.8	229.8	238.8	239.8
postcricoid (region)	148.0	198.89	230.0	210.8	235.1	239.0
posterior fossa (cranial)	191.6	198.3	—	225.0	237.5	239.6
postnasal space	147.9	198.89	230.0	210.7	235.1	239.0
prepuce	187.1	198.82	233.5	222.1	236.6	239.5
prepylorus	151.1	197.8	230.2	211.1	235.2	239.0
presacral (region)	195.3	198.89	—	229.8	238.8	239.8
prostate (gland)	185	198.82	233.4	222.2	236.5	239.5
utricle	189.3	198.1	233.9	223.81	236.99	239.5
pterygoid fossa	171.0	198.89	—	215.0	238.1	239.2
pubic bone	170.6	198.5	—	213.6	238.0	239.2
pudenda, pudendum (female)	184.4	198.82	233.3	221.2	236.3	239.5
pulmonary	162.9	197.0	231.2	212.3	235.7	239.1
putamen	191.0	198.3	—	225.0	237.5	239.6
pyloric						
antrum	151.2	197.8	230.2	211.1	235.2	239.0
canal	151.1	197.8	230.2	211.1	235.2	239.0
pylorus	151.1	197.8	230.2	211.1	235.2	239.0
pyramid (brain)	191.7	198.3	—	225.0	237.5	239.6
pyriform fossa or sinus	148.1	198.89	230.0	210.8	235.1	239.0
radius (any part)	170.4	198.5	—	213.4	238.0	239.2
Rathke's pouch	194.3	198.89	234.8	227.3	237.0	239.7
rectosigmoid (colon) (junction)	154.0	197.5	230.4	211.4	235.2	239.0
contiguous sites with anus or rectum	154.8	—	—	—	—	—
rectouterine pouch	158.8	197.6	—	211.8	235.4	239.0
rectovaginal septum or wall	195.3	198.89	234.8	229.8	238.8	239.8
rectovesical septum	195.3	198.89	234.8	229.8	238.8	239.8
rectum (ampulla)	154.1	197.5	230.4	211.4	235.2	239.0
and colon	154.0	197.5	230.4	211.4	235.2	239.0
contiguous sites with anus or rectosigmoid junction	154.8	—	—	—	—	—
renal	189.0	198.0	233.9	223.0	236.91	239.5

	Malignant					
	Primary	Secondary	Ca in stiu	Benign	Uncertain Behavior	Unspecified
Neoplasm *(Continued)*						
renal *(Continued)*						
calyx	189.1	198.0	233.9	223.1	236.91	239.5
hilus	189.1	198.0	233.9	223.1	236.91	239.5
parenchyma	189.0	198.0	233.9	223.0	236.91	239.5
pelvis	189.1	198.0	233.9	223.1	236.91	239.5
respiratory						
organs or system NEC	165.9	197.3	231.9	212.9	235.9	239.1
contiguous sites with intrathoracic organs	165.8	—	—	—	—	—
specified sites NEC	165.8	197.3	231.8	212.8	235.9	239.1
tract NEC	165.9	197.3	231.9	212.9	235.9	239.1
upper	165.0	197.3	231.9	212.9	235.9	239.1
retina	190.5	198.4	234.0	224.5	238.8	239.8
retrobulbar	190.1	198.4	—	224.1	238.8	239.8
retrocecal	158.0	197.6	—	211.8	235.4	239.0
retromolar (area) (triangle) (trigone)	145.6	198.89	230.0	210.4	235.1	239.0
retro-orbital	195.0	198.89	234.8	229.8	238.8	239.8
retroperitoneal (space) (tissue)	158.0	197.6	—	211.8	235.4	239.0
contiguous sites	158.8	—	—	—	—	—
retroperitoneum	158.0	197.6	—	211.8	235.4	239.0
contiguous sites	158.8	—	—	—	—	—
retropharyngeal	149.0	198.89	230.0	210.9	235.1	239.0
retrovesical (septum)	195.3	198.89	234.8	229.8	238.8	239.8
rhinencephalon	191.0	198.3	—	225.0	237.5	239.6
rib	170.3	198.5	—	213.3	238.0	239.2
Rosenmüller's fossa	147.2	198.89	230.0	210.7	235.1	239.0
round ligament	183.5	198.82	—	221.0	236.3	239.5
sacrococcyx, sacrococcygeal	170.6	198.5	—	213.6	238.0	239.2
region	195.3	198.89	234.8	229.8	238.8	239.8
sacrouterine ligament	183.4	198.82	—	221.0	236.3	239.5
sacrum, sacral (vertebra)	170.6	198.5	—	213.6	238.0	239.2
salivary gland or duct (major)	142.9	198.89	230.0	210.2	235.0	239.0
contiguous sites	142.8	—	—	—	—	—
minor NEC	145.9	198.89	230.0	210.4	235.1	239.0
parotid	142.0	198.89	230.0	210.2	235.0	239.0
pluriglandular	142.8	198.89	230.0	210.2	235.0	239.0
sublingual	142.2	198.89	230.0	210.2	235.0	239.0
submandibular	142.1	198.89	230.0	210.2	235.0	239.0
submaxillary	142.1	198.89	230.0	210.2	235.0	239.0
salpinx (uterine)	183.2	198.82	233.3	221.0	236.3	239.5
Santorini's duct	157.3	197.8	230.9	211.6	235.5	239.0
scalp	173.4	198.2	232.4	216.4	238.2	239.2
scapula (any part)	170.4	198.5	—	213.4	238.0	239.2
scapular region	195.1	198.89	234.8	229.8	238.8	239.8
scar NEC (*see also* Neoplasm, skin)	173.9	198.2	232.9	216.9	238.2	239.2
sciatic nerve	171.3	198.89	—	215.3	238.1	239.2
sclera	190.0	198.4	234.0	224.0	238.8	239.8
scrotum (skin)	187.7	198.82	233.6	222.4	236.6	239.5
sebaceous gland-*see* Neoplasm, skin						
sella turcica	194.3	198.89	234.8	227.3	237.0	239.7
bone	170.0	198.5	—	213.0	238.0	239.2
semilunar cartilage (knee)	170.7	198.5	—	213.7	238.0	239.2
seminal vesicle	187.8	198.82	233.6	222.8	236.6	239.5
septum						
nasal	160.0	197.3	231.8	212.0	235.9	239.1
posterior margin	147.3	198.89	230.0	210.7	235.1	239.0
rectovaginal	195.3	198.89	234.8	229.8	238.8	239.8
rectovesical	195.3	198.89	234.8	229.8	238.8	239.8
urethrovaginal	184.9	198.82	233.3	221.9	236.3	239.5
vesicovaginal	184.9	198.82	233.3	221.9	236.3	239.5
shoulder NEC*	195.4	198.89	232.6	229.8	238.8	239.8
sigmoid flexure (lower) (upper)	153.3	197.5	230.3	211.3	235.2	239.0
sinus (accessory)	160.9	197.3	231.8	212.0	235.9	239.1
bone (any)	170.0	198.5	—	213.0	238.0	239.2

	Malignant					
	Primary	Secondary	Ca in stiu	Benign	Uncertain Behavior	Unspecified
Neoplasm *(Continued)*						
sinus *(Continued)*						
contiguous sites with middle ear or nasal cavities	160.8	—	—	—	—	—
ethmoidal	160.3	197.3	231.8	212.0	235.9	239.1
frontal	160.4	197.3	231.8	212.0	235.9	239.1
maxillary	160.2	197.3	231.8	212.0	235.9	239.1
nasal, paranasal NEC	160.9	197.3	231.8	212.0	235.9	239.1
pyriform	148.1	198.89	230.0	210.8	235.1	239.0
sphenoidal	160.5	197.3	231.8	212.0	235.9	239.1
skeleton, skeletal NEC	170.9	198.5	—	213.9	238.0	239.2
Skene's gland	189.4	198.1	233.9	223.89	236.99	239.5
skin NEC	173.9	198.2	232.9	216.9	238.2	239.2
abdominal wall	173.5	198.2	232.5	216.5	238.2	239.2
ala nasi	173.3	198.2	232.3	216.3	238.2	239.2
ankle	173.7	198.2	232.7	216.7	238.2	239.2
antecubital space	173.6	198.2	232.6	216.6	238.2	239.2
anus	173.5	198.2	232.5	216.5	238.2	239.2
arm	173.6	198.2	232.6	216.6	238.2	239.2
auditory canal (external)	173.2	198.2	232.2	216.2	238.2	239.2
auricle (ear)	173.2	198.2	232.2	216.2	238.2	239.2
auricular canal (external)	173.2	198.2	232.2	216.2	238.2	239.2
axilla, axillary fold	173.5	198.2	232.5	216.5	238.2	239.2
back	173.5	198.2	232.5	216.5	238.2	239.2
breast	173.5	198.2	232.5	216.5	238.2	239.2
brow	173.3	198.2	232.3	216.3	238.2	239.2
buttock	173.5	198.2	232.5	216.5	238.2	239.2
calf	173.7	198.2	232.7	216.7	238.2	239.2
canthus (eye) (inner) (outer)	173.1	198.2	232.1	216.1	238.2	239.2
cervical region	173.4	198.2	232.4	216.4	238.2	239.2
cheek (external)	173.3	198.2	232.3	216.3	238.2	239.2
chest (wall)	173.5	198.2	232.5	216.5	238.2	239.2
chin	173.3	198.2	232.3	216.3	238.2	239.2
clavicular area	173.5	198.2	232.5	216.5	238.2	239.2
clitoris	184.3	198.82	233.3	221.2	236.3	239.5
columnella	173.3	198.2	232.3	216.3	238.2	239.2
concha	173.2	198.2	232.2	216.2	238.2	239.2
contiguous sites	173.8	—	—	—	—	—
ear (external)	173.2	198.2	232.2	216.2	238.2	239.2
elbow	173.6	198.2	232.6	216.6	238.2	239.2
eyebrow	173.3	198.2	232.3	216.3	238.2	239.2
eyelid	173.1	198.2	232.1	216.1	238.2	239.2
face NEC	173.3	198.2	232.3	216.3	238.2	239.2
female genital organs (external)	184.4	198.82	233.3	221.2	236.3	239.5
clitoris	184.3	198.82	233.3	221.2	236.3	239.5
labium NEC	184.4	198.82	233.3	221.2	236.3	239.5
majus	184.1	198.82	233.3	221.2	236.3	239.5
minus	184.2	198.82	233.3	221.2	236.3	239.5
pudendum	184.4	198.82	233.3	221.2	236.3	239.5
vulva	184.4	198.82	233.3	221.2	236.3	239.5
finger	173.6	198.2	232.6	216.6	238.2	239.2
flank	173.5	198.2	232.5	216.5	238.2	239.2
foot	173.7	198.2	232.7	216.7	238.2	239.2
forearm	173.6	198.2	232.6	216.6	238.2	239.2
forehead	173.3	198.2	232.3	216.3	238.2	239.2
glabella	173.3	198.2	232.3	216.3	238.2	239.2
gluteal region	173.5	198.2	232.5	216.5	238.2	239.2
groin	173.5	198.2	232.5	216.5	238.2	239.2
hand	173.6	198.2	232.6	216.6	238.2	239.2
head NEC	173.4	198.2	232.4	216.4	238.2	239.2
heel	173.7	198.2	232.7	216.7	238.2	239.2
helix	173.2	198.2	232.2	216.2	238.2	239.2
hip	173.7	198.2	232.7	216.7	238.2	239.2
infraclavicular region	173.5	198.2	232.5	216.5	238.2	239.2

	Malignant					
	Primary	Secondary	Ca in stiu	Benign	Uncertain Behavior	Unspecified
Neoplasm *(Continued)*						
skin NEC *(Continued)*						
inguinal region	173.5	198.2	232.5	216.5	238.2	239.2
jaw	173.3	198.2	232.3	216.3	238.2	239.2
knee	173.7	198.2	232.7	216.7	238.2	239.2
labia						
majora	184.1	198.82	233.3	221.2	236.3	239.5
minora	184.2	198.82	233.3	221.2	236.3	239.5
leg	173.7	198.2	232.7	216.7	238.2	239.2
lid (lower) (upper)	173.1	198.2	232.1	216.1	238.2	239.2
limb NEC	173.9	198.2	232.9	216.9	238.2	239.5
lower	173.7	198.2	232.7	216.7	238.2	239.2
upper	173.6	198.2	232.6	216.6	238.2	239.2
lip (lower) (upper)	173.0	198.2	232.0	216.0	238.2	239.2
male genital organs	187.9	198.82	233.6	222.9	236.6	239.5
penis	187.4	198.82	233.5	222.1	236.6	239.5
prepuce	187.1	198.82	233.5	222.1	236.6	239.5
scrotum	187.7	198.82	233.6	222.4	236.6	239.5
mastectomy site	173.5	198.2	—	—	—	—
specified as breast tissue	174.8	198.81	—	—	—	—
meatus, acoustic (external)	173.2	198.2	232.2	216.2	238.2	239.2
nates	173.5	198.2	232.5	216.5	238.2	239.2
neck	173.4	198.2	232.4	216.4	238.2	239.2
nose (external)	173.3	198.2	232.3	216.3	238.2	239.2
palm	173.6	198.2	232.6	216.6	238.2	239.2
palpebra	173.1	198.2	232.1	216.1	238.2	239.2
penis NEC	187.4	198.82	233.5	222.1	236.6	239.5
perianal	173.5	198.2	232.5	216.5	238.2	239.2
perineum	173.5	198.2	232.5	216.5	238.2	239.2
pinna	173.2	198.2	232.2	216.2	238.2	239.2
plantar	173.7	198.2	232.7	216.7	238.2	239.2
popliteal fossa or space	173.7	198.2	232.7	216.7	238.2	239.2
prepuce	187.1	198.82	233.5	222.1	236.6	239.5
pubes	173.5	198.2	232.5	216.5	238.2	239.2
sacrococcygeal region	173.5	198.2	232.5	216.5	238.2	239.2
scalp	173.4	198.2	232.4	216.4	238.2	239.2
scapular region	173.5	198.2	232.5	216.5	238.2	239.2
scrotum	187.7	198.82	233.6	222.4	236.6	239.5
shoulder	173.6	198.2	232.6	216.6	238.2	239.2
sole (foot)	173.7	198.2	232.7	216.7	238.2	239.2
specified sites NEC	173.8	198.2	232.8	216.8	232.8	239.2
submammary fold	173.5	198.2	232.5	216.5	238.2	239.2
supraclavicular region	173.4	198.2	232.4	216.4	238.2	239.2
temple	173.3	198.2	232.3	216.3	238.2	239.2
thigh	173.7	198.2	232.7	216.7	238.2	239.2
thoracic wall	173.5	198.2	232.5	216.5	238.2	239.2
thumb	173.6	198.2	232.6	216.6	238.2	239.2
toe	173.7	198.2	232.7	216.7	238.2	239.2
tragus	173.2	198.2	232.2	216.2	238.2	239.2
trunk	173.5	198.2	232.5	216.5	238.2	239.2
umbilicus	173.5	198.2	232.5	216.5	238.2	239.2
vulva	184.4	198.82	233.3	221.2	236.3	239.5
wrist	173.6	198.2	232.6	216.6	238.2	239.2
skull	170.0	198.5	—	213.0	238.0	239.2
soft parts or tissues-*see* Neoplasm, connective tissue						
specified site NEC	195.8	198.89	234.8	229.8	238.8	239.8
spermatic cord	187.6	198.82	233.6	222.8	236.6	239.5
sphenoid	160.5	197.3	231.8	212.0	235.9	239.1
bone	170.0	198.5	—	213.0	238.0	239.2
sinus	160.5	197.3	231.8	212.0	235.9	239.1
sphincter						
anal	154.2	197.5	230.5	211.4	235.5	239.0
of Oddi	156.1	197.8	230.8	211.5	235.3	239.0

	Malignant					
	Primary	Secondary	Ca in stiu	Benign	Uncertain Behavior	Unspecified
Neoplasm *(Continued)*						
spine, spinal (column)	170.2	198.5	—	213.2	238.0	239.2
bulb	191.7	198.3	—	225.0	237.5	239.6
coccyx	170.6	198.5	—	213.6	238.0	239.2
cord (cervical) (lumbar) (sacral) (thoracic)	192.2	198.3	—	225.3	237.5	239.7
dura mater	192.3	198.4	—	225.4	237.6	239.7
lumbosacral	170.2	198.5	—	213.2	238.0	239.2
membrane	192.3	198.4	—	225.4	237.6	239.7
meninges	192.3	198.4	—	225.4	237.6	239.7
nerve (root)	171.9	198.89	—	215.9	238.1	239.2
pia mater	192.3	198.4	—	225.4	237.6	239.7
root	171.9	198.89	—	215.9	238.1	239.2
sacrum	170.6	198.5	—	213.6	238.0	239.2
spleen, splenic NEC	159.1	197.8	230.9	211.9	235.5	239.0
flexure (colon)	153.7	197.5	230.3	211.3	235.2	239.0
stem, brain	191.7	198.3	—	225.0	237.5	239.6
Stensen's duct	142.0	198.89	230.0	210.2	235.0	239.0
sternum	170.3	198.5	—	213.3	238.0	239.2
stomach	151.9	197.8	230.2	211.1	235.2	239.0
antrum (pyloric)	151.2	197.8	230.2	211.1	235.2	239.0
body	151.4	197.8	230.2	211.1	235.2	239.0
cardia	151.0	197.8	230.2	211.1	235.2	239.0
cardiac orifice	151.0	197.8	230.2	211.1	235.2	239.0
contiguous sites	151.8	—	—	—	—	—
corpus	151.4	197.8	230.2	211.1	235.2	239.0
fundus	151.3	197.8	230.2	211.1	235.2	239.0
greater curvature NEC	151.6	197.8	230.2	211.1	235.2	239.0
lesser curvature NEC	151.5	197.8	230.2	211.1	235.2	239.0
prepylorus	151.1	197.8	230.2	211.1	235.2	239.0
pylorus	151.1	197.8	230.2	211.1	235.2	239.0
wall NEC	151.9	197.8	230.2	211.1	235.2	239.0
anterior NEC	151.8	197.8	230.2	211.1	235.2	239.0
posterior NEC	151.8	197.8	230.2	211.1	235.2	239.0
stroma, endometrial	182.0	198.82	233.2	219.1	236.0	239.5
stump, cervical	180.8	198.82	233.1	219.0	236.0	239.5
subcutaneous (nodule) (tissue) NEC-*see* Neoplasm, connective tissue						
subdural	192.1	198.4	—	225.2	237.6	239.7
subglottis, subglottic	161.2	197.3	231.0	212.1	235.6	239.1
sublingual	144.9	198.89	230.0	210.3	235.1	239.0
gland or duct	142.2	198.89	230.0	210.2	235.0	239.0
submandibular gland	142.1	198.89	230.0	210.2	235.0	239.0
submaxillary gland or duct	142.1	198.89	230.0	210.2	235.0	239.0
submental	195.0	198.89	234.8	229.8	238.8	239.8
subpleural	162.9	197.0	—	212.3	235.7	239.1
substernal	164.2	197.1	—	212.5	235.8	239.8
sudoriferous, sudoriparous gland, site unspecified	173.9	198.2	232.9	216.9	238.2	239.2
specified site-*see* Neoplasm, skin						
supraclavicular region	195.0	198.89	234.8	229.8	238.8	239.8
supraglottis	161.1	197.3	231.0	212.1	235.6	239.1
suprarenal (capsule) (cortex) (gland) (medulla)	194.0	198.7	234.8	227.0	237.2	239.7
suprasellar (region)	191.9	198.3	—	225.0	237.5	239.6
sweat gland (apocrine) (eccrine), site unspecified	173.9	198.2	232.9	216.9	238.2	239.2
specified site-*see* Neoplasm, skin						
sympathetic nerve or nervous system NEC	171.9	198.89	—	215.9	238.1	239.2
symphysis pubis	170.6	198.5	—	213.6	238.0	239.2
synovial membrane-*see* Neoplasm, connective tissue						
tapetum, brain	191.8	198.3	—	225.0	237.5	239.6
tarsus (any bone)	170.8	198.5	—	213.8	238.0	239.2
temple (skin)	173.3	198.2	232.3	216.3	238.2	239.2
temporal						
bone	170.0	198.5	—	213.0	238.0	239.2
lobe or pole	191.2	198.3	—	225.0	237.5	239.6
region	195.0	198.89	234.8	229.8	238.8	239.8
skin	173.3	198.2	232.3	216.3	238.2	239.2

	Malignant					
	Primary	Secondary	Ca in stiu	Benign	Uncertain Behavior	Unspecified
Neoplasm *(Continued)*						
tendon (sheath)-*see* Neoplasm, connective tissue						
tentorium (cerebelli)	192.1	198.4	—	225.2	237.6	239.7
testis, testes (descended) (scrotal)	186.9	198.82	233.6	222.0	236.4	239.5
ectopic	186.0	198.82	233.6	222.0	236.4	239.5
retained	186.0	198.82	233.6	222.0	236.4	239.5
undescended	186.0	198.82	233.6	222.0	236.4	239.5
thalamus	191.0	198.3	—	225.0	237.5	239.6
thigh NEC*	195.5	198.89	234.8	229.8	238.8	239.8
thorax, thoracic (cavity) (organs NEC)	195.1	198.89	234.8	229.8	238.8	239.8
duct	171.4	198.89	—	215.4	238.1	239.2
wall NEC	195.1	198.89	234.8	229.8	238.8	239.8
throat	149.0	198.89	230.0	210.9	235.1	239.0
thumb NEC*	195.4	198.89	232.6	229.8	238.8	239.8
thymus (gland)	164.0	198.89	—	212.6	235.8	239.8
contiguous sites with heart and mediastinum	164.8	—	—	—	—	—
thyroglossal duct	193	198.89	234.8	226	237.4	239.7
thyroid (gland)	193	198.89	234.8	226	237.4	239.7
cartilage	161.3	197.3	231.0	212.1	235.6	239.1
tibia (any part)	170.7	198.5	—	213.7	238.0	239.2
toe NEC*	195.5	198.89	232.7	229.8	238.8	239.8
tongue	141.9	198.89	230.0	210.1	235.1	239.0
anterior (two-thirds) NEC	141.4	198.89	230.0	210.1	235.1	239.0
dorsal surface	141.1	198.89	230.0	210.1	235.1	239.0
ventral surface	141.3	198.89	230.0	210.1	235.1	239.0
base (dorsal surface)	141.0	198.89	230.0	210.1	235.1	239.0
border (lateral)	141.2	198.89	230.0	210.1	235.1	239.0
contiguous sites	141.8	—	—	—	—	—
dorsal surface NEC	141.1	198.89	230.0	210.1	235.1	239.0
fixed part NEC	141.0	198.89	230.0	210.1	235.1	239.0
foramen cecum	141.1	198.89	230.0	210.1	235.1	239.0
frenulum linguae	141.3	198.89	230.0	210.1	235.1	239.0
junctional zone	141.5	198.89	230.0	210.1	235.1	239.0
margin (lateral)	141.2	198.89	230.0	210.1	235.1	239.0
midline NEC	141.1	198.89	230.0	210.1	235.1	239.0
mobile part NEC	141.4	198.89	230.0	210.1	235.1	239.0
posterior (third)	141.0	198.89	230.0	210.1	235.1	239.0
root	141.0	198.89	230.0	210.1	235.1	239.0
surface (dorsal)	141.1	198.89	230.0	210.1	235.1	239.0
base	141.0	198.89	230.0	210.1	235.1	239.0
ventral	141.3	198.89	230.0	210.1	235.1	239.0
tip	141.2	198.89	230.0	210.1	235.1	239.0
tonsil	141.6	198.89	230.0	210.1	235.1	239.0
tonsil	146.0	198.89	230.0	210.5	235.1	239.0
fauces, faucial	146.0	198.89	230.0	210.5	235.1	239.0
lingual	141.6	198.89	230.0	210.1	235.1	239.0
palatine	146.0	198.89	230.0	210.5	235.1	239.0
pharyngeal	147.1	198.89	230.0	210.7	235.1	239.0
pillar (anterior) (posterior)	146.2	198.89	230.0	210.6	235.1	239.0
tonsillar fossa	146.1	198.89	230.0	210.6	235.1	239.0
tooth socket NEC	143.9	198.89	230.0	210.4	235.1	239.0
trachea (cartilage) (mucosa)	162.0	197.3	231.1	212.2	235.7	239.1
contiguous sites with bronchus or lung	162.8	—	—	—	—	—
tracheobronchial	162.8	197.3	231.1	212.2	235.7	239.1
contiguous sites with lung	162.8	—	—	—	—	—
tragus	173.2	198.2	232.2	216.2	238.2	239.2
trunk NEC*	195.8	198.89	232.5	229.8	238.8	239.8
tubo-ovarian	183.8	198.82	233.3	221.8	236.3	239.5
tunica vaginalis	187.8	198.82	233.6	222.8	236.6	239.5
turbinate (bone)	170.0	198.5	—	213.0	238.0	239.2
nasal	160.0	197.3	231.8	212.0	235.9	239.1
tympanic cavity	160.1	197.3	231.8	212.0	235.9	239.1
ulna (any part)	170.4	198.5	—	213.4	238.0	239.2

	Malignant					
	Primary	Secondary	Ca in stiu	Benign	Uncertain Behavior	Unspecified
Neoplasm *(Continued)*						
umbilicus, umbilical	173.5	198.2	232.5	216.5	238.2	239.2
uncus, brain	191.2	198.3	—	225.0	237.5	239.6
unknown site or unspecified	199.1	199.1	234.9	229.9	238.9	239.9
urachus	188.7	198.1	233.7	223.3	236.7	239.4
ureter, ureteral	189.2	198.1	233.9	223.2	236.91	239.5
orifice (bladder)	188.6	198.1	233.7	223.3	236.7	239.4
ureter-bladder (junction)	188.6	198.1	233.7	223.3	236.7	239.4
urethra, urethral (gland)	189.3	198.1	233.9	223.81	236.99	239.5
orifice, internal	188.5	198.1	233.7	223.3	236.7	239.4
urethrovaginal (septum)	184.9	198.82	233.3	221.9	236.3	239.5
urinary organ or system NEC	189.9	198.1	233.9	223.9	236.99	239.5
bladder-*see* Neoplasm, bladder						
contiguous sites	189.8	—	—	—	—	—
specified sites NEC	189.8	198.1	233.9	223.89	236.99	239.5
utero-ovarian	183.8	198.82	233.3	221.8	236.3	239.5
ligament	183.3	198.82	—	221.0	236.3	239.5
uterosacral ligament	183.4	198.82	—	221.0	236.3	239.5
uterus, uteri, uterine	179	198.82	233.2	219.9	236.0	239.5
adnexa NEC	183.9	198.82	233.3	221.8	236.3	239.5
contiguous sites	183.8	—	—	—	—	—
body	182.0	198.82	233.2	219.1	236.0	239.5
contiguous sites	182.8	—	—	—	—	—
cervix	180.9	198.82	233.1	219.0	236.0	239.5
cornu	182.0	198.82	233.2	219.1	236.0	239.5
corpus	182.0	198.82	233.2	219.1	236.0	239.5
endocervix (canal) (gland)	180.0	198.82	233.1	219.0	236.0	239.5
endometrium	182.0	198.82	233.2	219.1	236.0	239.5
exocervix	180.1	198.82	233.1	219.0	236.0	239.5
external os	180.1	198.82	233.1	219.0	236.0	239.5
fundus	182.0	198.82	233.2	219.1	236.0	239.5
internal os	180.0	198.82	233.1	219.0	236.0	239.5
isthmus	182.1	198.82	233.2	219.1	236.0	239.5
ligament	183.4	198.82	—	221.0	236.3	239.5
broad	183.3	198.82	233.3	221.0	236.3	239.5
round	183.5	198.82	—	221.0	236.3	239.5
lower segment	182.1	198.82	233.2	219.1	236.0	239.5
myometrium	182.0	198.82	233.2	219.1	236.0	239.5
squamocolumnar junction	180.8	198.82	233.1	219.0	236.0	239.5
tube	183.2	198.82	233.3	221.0	236.3	239.5
utricle, prostatic	189.3	198.1	233.9	223.81	236.99	239.5
uveal tract	190.0	198.4	234.0	224.0	238.8	239.8
uvula	145.4	198.89	230.0	210.4	235.1	239.0
vagina, vaginal (fornix) (vault) (wall)	184.0	198.82	233.3	221.1	236.3	239.5
vaginovesical	184.9	198.82	233.3	221.9	236.3	239.5
septum	194.9	198.82	233.3	221.9	236.3	239.5
vallecula (epiglottis)	146.3	198.89	230.0	210.6	235.1	239.0
vascular-*see* Neoplasm, connective tissue						
vas deferens	187.6	198.82	233.6	222.8	236.6	239.5
Vater's ampulla	156.2	197.8	230.8	211.5	235.3	239.0
vein, venous-*see* Neoplasm, connective tissue						
vena cava (abdominal) (inferior)	171.5	198.89	—	215.5	238.1	239.2
superior	171.4	198.89	—	215.4	238.1	239.2
ventricle (cerebral) (floor) (fourth) (lateral) (third)	191.5	198.3	—	225.0	237.5	239.6
cardiac (left) (right)	164.1	198.89	—	212.7	238.8	239.8
ventricular band of larynx	161.1	197.3	231.0	212.1	235.6	239.1
ventriculus-*see* Neoplasm, stomach						
vermillion border-*see* Neoplasm, lip						
vermis, cerebellum	191.6	198.3	—	225.0	237.5	239.6
vertebra (column)	170.2	198.5	—	213.2	238.0	239.2
coccyx	170.6	198.5	—	213.6	238.0	239.2
sacrum	170.6	198.5	—	213.6	238.0	239.2
vesical-*see* Neoplasm, bladder						

	Malignant					
	Primary	Secondary	Ca in stiu	Benign	Uncertain Behavior	Unspecified
Neoplasm *(Continued)*						
vesicle, seminal	187.8	198.82	233.6	222.8	236.6	239.5
vesicocervical tissue	184.9	198.82	233.3	221.9	236.3	239.5
vesicorectal	195.3	198.89	234.8	229.8	238.8	239.8
vesicovaginal	184.9	198.82	233.3	221.9	236.3	239.5
septum	184.9	198.82	233.3	221.9	236.3	239.5
vessel (blood)-*see* Neoplasm, connective tissue						
vestibular gland, greater	184.1	198.82	233.3	221.2	236.3	239.5
vestibule						
mouth	145.1	198.89	230.0	210.4	235.1	239.0
nose	160.0	197.3	231.8	212.0	235.9	239.1
Virchow's gland	—	196.0	—	229.0	238.8	239.8
viscera NEC	195.8	198.89	234.8	229.8	238.8	239.8
vocal cords (true)	161.0	197.3	231.0	212.1	235.6	239.1
false	161.1	197.3	231.0	212.1	235.6	239.1
vomer	170.0	198.5	—	213.0	238.0	239.2
vulva	184.4	198.82	233.3	221.2	236.3	239.5
vulvovaginal gland	184.4	198.82	233.3	221.2	236.3	239.5
Waldeyer's ring	149.1	198.89	230.0	210.9	235.1	239.0
Wharton's duct	142.1	198.89	230.0	210.2	235.0	239.0
white matter (central) (cerebral)	191.0	198.3	—	225.0	237.5	239.6
windpipe	162.0	197.3	231.1	212.2	235.7	239.1
Wirsung's duct	157.3	197.8	230.9	211.6	235.5	239.0
wolffian (body) (duct)						
female	184.8	198.82	233.3	221.8	236.3	239.5
male	187.8	198.82	233.6	222.8	236.6	239.5
womb-*see* Neoplasm, uterus						
wrist NEC*	195.4	198.89	232.6	229.8	238.8	239.8
xiphoid process	170.3	198.5	—	213.3	238.0	239.2
Zuckerkandl's organ	194.6	198.89	—	227.6	237.3	239.7

Note Except where otherwise indicated, varieties of nevus in the list below that are followed by a morphology code number (M-/0) should be coded by site as for "Neoplasm, skin, benign."

ICD-9-CM
N
Vol. 2

O

ICD-9-CM O Vol. 2

ICD-9-CM O Vol. 2

◀ New ⬅ Revised Code

ICD-9-CM
O
Vol. 2

P

◄ **New** ⟸ **Revised Code**

ICD-9-CM

P

Vol. 2

ICD-9-CM
P
Vol. 2

◄ New ⇐ Revised Code

ICD-9-CM
P
Vol. 2

Perforation, perforative *(Continued)*
- gastric (ulcer) - *see* Ulcer, stomach, with perforation
- heart valve - *see* Endocarditis
- ileum (*see also* Perforation, intestine) 569.83
- instrumental
  - external - *see* Wound, open, by site
  - pregnant uterus, complicating delivery 665.9
  - surgical (accidental) (blood vessel) (nerve) (organ) 998.2
- intestine 569.83
  - with
    - abortion - *see* Abortion, by type, with damage to pelvic organs
    - ectopic pregnancy (*see also* categories 633.0-633.9) 639.2
    - molar pregnancy (*see also* categories 630-632) 639.2
  - fetus or newborn 777.6
  - obstetrical trauma 665.5
  - ulcerative NEC 569.83
- jejunum, jejunal 569.83
  - ulcer - *see* Ulcer, gastrojejunal, with perforation
- mastoid (antrum) (cell) 383.89
- maxillary sinus (*see also* Sinusitis, maxillary) 473.0
- membrana tympani - *see* Perforation, tympanum
- nasal
  - septum 478.1
    - congenital 748.1
    - syphilitic 095.8
  - sinus (*see also* Sinusitis) 473.9
    - congenital 748.1
- palate (hard) 526.89
  - soft 528.9
    - syphilitic 095.8
  - syphilitic 095.8
- palatine vault 526.89
  - syphilitic 095.8
    - congenital 090.5
- pelvic
  - floor
    - with
      - abortion - *see* Abortion, by type, with damage to pelvic organs
      - ectopic pregnancy (*see also* categories 633.0-633.9) 639.2
      - molar pregnancy (*see also* categories 630-632) 639.2
    - obstetrical trauma 664.1
  - organ
    - with
      - abortion - *see* Abortion, by type, with damage to pelvic organs
      - ectopic pregnancy (*see also* categories 633.0-633.9) 639.2
      - molar pregnancy (*see also* categories 630-632) 639.2
    - following
      - abortion 639.2
      - ectopic or molar pregnancy 639.2
    - obstetrical trauma 665.5
- perineum - *see* Laceration, perineum
- periurethral tissue
  - with
    - abortion - *see* Abortion, by type, with damage to pelvic organs

Perforation, perforative *(Continued)*
- periurethral tissue *(Continued)*
  - with *(Continued)*
    - ectopic pregnancy (*see also* categories 630-632) 639.2
    - molar pregnancy (*see also* categories 630-632) 639.2
- pharynx 478.29
- pylorus, pyloric (ulcer) - *see* Ulcer, stomach, with perforation
- rectum 569.49
- sigmoid 569.83
- sinus (accessory) (chronic) (nasal) (*see also* Sinusitis) 473.9
- sphenoidal sinus (*see also* Sinusitis, sphenoidal) 473.3
- stomach (due to ulcer) - *see* Ulcer, stomach, with perforation
- surgical (accidental) (by instrument) (blood vessel) (nerve) (organ) 998.2
- traumatic
  - external - *see* Wound, open, by site
  - eye (*see also* Penetrating wound, ocular) 871.7
  - internal organ - *see* Injury, internal, by site
- tympanum (membrane) (persistent posttraumatic) (postinflammatory) 384.20
  - with
    - otitis media - *see* Otitis media
  - attic 384.22
  - central 384.21
  - healed 384.81
  - marginal NEC 384.23
  - multiple 384.24
  - pars flaccida 384.22
  - total 384.25
  - traumatic - *see* Wound, open, ear, drum
- typhoid, gastrointestinal 002.0
- ulcer - *see* Ulcer, by site, with perforation
- ureter 593.89
- urethra
  - with
    - abortion - *see* Abortion, by type, with damage to pelvic organs
    - ectopic pregnancy (*see also* categories 633.0-633.9) 639.2
    - molar pregnancy (*see also* categories 630-632) 639.2
  - following
    - abortion 639.2
    - ectopic or molar pregnancy 639.2
  - obstetrical trauma 665.5
- uterus - *see also* Injury, internal, uterus
  - with
    - abortion - *see* Abortion, by type, with damage to pelvic organs
    - ectopic pregnancy (*see also* categories 633.0-633.9) 639.2
    - molar pregnancy (*see also* categories 630-632) 639.2
  - by intrauterine contraceptive device 996.32
  - following
    - abortion 639.2
    - ectopic or molar pregnancy 639.2
  - obstetrical trauma - *see* Injury, internal, uterus, obstetrical trauma
- uvula 528.9
  - syphilitic 095.8

Perforation, perforative *(Continued)*
- vagina - *see* Laceration, vagina
- viscus NEC 799.89 ⬅
  - traumatic 868.00
    - with open wound into cavity 868.10

Periadenitis mucosa necrotica recurrens 528.2

Periangiitis 446.0

Periantritis 535.4

Periappendicitis (acute) (*see also* Appendicitis) 541

Periarteritis (disseminated) (infectious) (necrotizing) (nodosa) 446.0

Periarthritis (joint) 726.90
- Duplay's 726.2
- gonococcal 098.50
- humeroscapularis 726.2
- scapulohumeral 726.2
- shoulder 726.2
- wrist 726.4

Periarthrosis (angioneural) - *see* Periarthritis

Peribronchitis 491.9
- tuberculous (*see also* Tuberculosis) 011.3

Pericapsulitis, adhesive (shoulder) 726.0

Pericarditis (granular) (with decompensation) (with effusion) 423.9
- with
  - rheumatic fever (conditions classifiable to 390)
    - active (*see also* Pericarditis, rheumatic) 391.0
    - inactive or quiescent 393
- actinomycotic 039.8 *[420.0]*
- acute (nonrheumatic) 420.90
  - with chorea (acute) (rheumatic) (Sydenham's) 392.0
  - bacterial 420.99
  - benign 420.91
  - hemorrhagic 420.90
  - idiopathic 420.91
  - infective 420.90
  - nonspecific 420.91
  - rheumatic 391.0
    - with chorea (acute) (rheumatic) (Sydenham's) 392.0
  - sicca 420.90
  - viral 420.91
- adhesive or adherent (external) (internal) 423.1
  - acute - *see* Pericarditis, acute
  - rheumatic (external) (internal) 393
- amebic 006.8 *[420.0]*
- bacterial (acute) (subacute) (with serous or seropurulent effusion) 420.99
- calcareous 423.2
- cholesterol (chronic) 423.8
  - acute 420.90
- chronic (nonrheumatic) 423.8
  - rheumatic 393
- constrictive 423.2
- Coxsackie 074.21
- due to
  - actinomycosis 039.8 *[420.0]*
  - amebiasis 006.8 *[420.0]*
  - Coxsackie (virus) 074.21
  - histoplasmosis (*see also* Histoplasmosis) 115.93
  - nocardiosis 039.8 *[420.0]*
  - tuberculosis (*see also* Tuberculosis) 017.9 *[420.0]*
- fibrinocaseous (*see also* Tuberculosis) 017.9 *[420.0]*
- fibrinopurulent 420.99

- **Phlebectasia** (*see also* Varicose, vein) 454.9
  - congenital NEC 747.60
  - esophagus (*see also* Varix, esophagus) 456.1
    - with hemorrhage (*see also* Varix, esophagus, bleeding) 456.0
- **Phlebitis** (infective) (pyemic) (septic) (suppurative) 451.9
  - antecubital vein 451.82
  - arm NEC 451.84
    - axillary vein 451.89
    - basilic vein 451.82
    - deep 451.83
    - superficial 451.82
  - basilic vein 451.82
  - blue 451.9
  - brachial vein 451.83
  - breast, superficial 451.89
  - cavernous (venous) sinus - *see* Phlebitis, intracranial sinus
  - cephalic vein 451.82
  - cerebral (venous) sinus - *see* Phlebitis, intracranial sinus
  - chest wall, superficial 451.89
  - complicating pregnancy or puerperium 671.9
    - affecting fetus or newborn 760.3
  - cranial (venous) sinus - *see* Phlebitis, intracranial sinus
  - deep (vessels) 451.19
    - femoral vein 451.11
    - specified vessel NEC 451.19
  - due to implanted device - *see* Complications, due to (presence of) any device, implant, or graft classified to 996.0-996.5 NEC
  - during or resulting from a procedure 997.2
  - femoral vein (deep) (superficial) 451.11
  - femoropopliteal 451.19
  - following infusion, perfusion, or transfusion 999.2
  - gouty 274.89 *[451.9]*
  - hepatic veins 451.89
  - iliac vein 451.81
  - iliofemoral 451.11
  - intracranial sinus (any) (venous) 325
    - late effect - *see* category 326
    - nonpyogenic 437.6
      - in pregnancy or puerperium 671.5
  - jugular vein 451.89
  - lateral (venous) sinus - *see* Phlebitis, intracranial sinus
  - leg 451.2
    - deep (vessels) 451.19
      - specified vessel NEC 451.19
    - superficial (vessels) 451.0
      - femoral vein 451.11
  - longitudinal sinus - *see* Phlebitis, intracranial sinus
  - lower extremity 451.2
    - deep (vessels) 451.19
      - femoral vein 451.11
      - specified vessel NEC 451.19
    - superficial (vessels) 451.0
      - femoral vein 451.11
  - migrans, migrating (superficial) 453.1
  - pelvic
    - with
      - abortion - *see* Abortion, by type, with sepsis
      - ectopic pregnancy (*see also* categories 633.0-633.9) 639.0
      - molar pregnancy (*see also* categories 630-632) 639.0

Phlebitis *(Continued)*

- pelvic *(Continued)*
  - following
    - abortion 639.0
    - ectopic or molar pregnancy 639.0
  - puerperal, postpartum 671.4
- popliteal vein 451.19
- portal (vein) 572.1
- postoperative 997.2
- pregnancy 671.9
  - deep 671.3
  - specified type NEC 671.5
- superficial 671.2
- puerperal, postpartum, childbirth 671.9
  - deep 671.4
  - lower extremities 671.2
  - pelvis 671.4
  - specified site NEC 671.5
  - superficial 671.2
- radial vein 451.83
- retina 362.18
- saphenous (great) (long) 451.0
  - accessory or small 451.0
- sinus (meninges) - *see* Phlebitis, intracranial sinus
- specified site NEC 451.89
- subclavian vein 451.89
- syphilitic 093.89
- tibial vein 451.19
- ulcer, ulcerative 451.9
  - leg 451.2
    - deep (vessels) 451.19
      - femoral vein 451.11
      - specified vessel NEC 451.19
    - superficial (vessels) 451.0
      - femoral vein 451.11
  - lower extremity 451.2
    - deep (vessels) 451.19
      - femoral vein 451.11
      - specified vessel NEC 451.19
    - superficial (vessels) 451.0
- ulnar vein 451.83
- umbilicus 451.89
- upper extremity - *see* Phlebitis, arm
  - deep (veins) 451.83
    - brachial vein 451.83
    - radial vein 451.83
    - ulnar vein 451.83
  - superficial (veins) 451.82
    - antecubital vein 451.82
    - basilic vein 451.82
    - cephalic vein 451.82
- uterus (septic) (*see also* Endometritis) 615.9
- varicose (leg) (lower extremity) (*see also* Varicose, vein) 454.1

- **Phlebofibrosis** 459.89
- **Phleboliths** 459.89
- **Phlebosclerosis** 459.89
- **Phlebothrombosis** - *see* Thrombosis
- **Phlebotomus fever** 066.0
- **Phlegm, choked on** 933.1
- **Phlegmasia**
  - alba dolens (deep vessels) 451.19
    - complicating pregnancy 671.3
    - nonpuerperal 451.19
    - puerperal, postpartum, childbirth 671.4
  - cerulea dolens 451.19
- **Phlegmon** (*see also* Abscess) 682.9
  - erysipelatous (*see also* Erysipelas) 035
  - iliac 682.2
    - fossa 540.1
  - throat 478.29
- **Phlegmonous** - *see* condition
- **Phlyctenulosis** (allergic) (keratoconjunctivitis) (nontuberculous) 370.31
  - cornea 370.31
    - with ulcer (*see also* Ulcer, cornea) 370.00
  - tuberculous (*see also* Tuberculosis) 017.3 *[370.31]*
- **Phobia, phobic** (reaction) 300.20
  - animal 300.29
  - isolated NEC 300.29
  - obsessional 300.3
  - simple NEC 300.29
  - social 300.23
  - specified NEC 300.29
  - state 300.20
- **Phocas' disease** 610.1
- **Phocomelia** 755.4
  - lower limb 755.32
    - complete 755.33
    - distal 755.35
    - proximal 755.34
  - upper limb 755.22
    - complete 755.23
    - distal 755.25
    - proximal 755.24
- **Phoria** (*see also* Heterophoria) 378.40
- **Phosphate-losing tubular disorder** 588.0
- **Phosphatemia** 275.3
- **Phosphaturia** 275.3
- **Photoallergic response** 692.72
- **Photocoproporphyria** 277.1
- **Photodermatitis** (sun) 692.72
  - light other than sun 692.82
- **Photokeratitis** 370.24
- **Photo-ophthalmia** 370.24
- **Photophobia** 368.13
- **Photopsia** 368.15
- **Photoretinitis** 363.31
- **Photoretinopathy** 363.31
- **Photosensitiveness** (sun) 692.72
  - light other than sun 692.82
- **Photosensitization skin** (sun) 692.72
  - light other than sun 692.82
- **Phototoxic response** 692.72
- **Phrenitis** 323.9
- **Phrynoderma** 264.8
- **Phthiriasis** (pubis) (any site) 132.2
  - with any infestation classifiable to 132.0 and 132.1 132.3
- **Phthirus infestation** - *see* Phthiriasis
- **Phthisis** (*see also* Tuberculosis) 011.9
  - bulbi (infectional) 360.41
  - colliers' 011.4
  - cornea 371.05
  - eyeball (due to infection) 360.41
  - millstone makers' 011.4
  - miners' 011.4
  - potters' 011.4
  - sandblasters' 011.4
  - stonemasons' 011.4
- **Phycomycosis** 117.7
- **Physalopteriasis** 127.7
- **Physical therapy NEC** V57.1
  - breathing exercises V57.0
- **Physiological cup, optic papilla**
  - borderline, glaucoma suspect 365.00
  - enlarged 377.14
  - glaucomatous 377.14
- **Phytobezoar** 938
  - intestine 936
  - stomach 935.2
- **Pian** (*see also* Yaws) 102.9
- **Pianoma** 102.1

ICD-9-CM
P
Vol. 2

◀ **New** ⟸ **Revised Code**

- **Pneumonitis** *(Continued)*
  - interstitial (chronic) (*see also* Fibrosis, lung) 515
    - lymphoid 516.8
  - lymphoid, interstitial 516.8
  - meconium 770.1
  - postanesthetic
    - correct substance properly administered 507.0
    - obstetric 668.0
    - overdose or wrong substance given 968.4
      - specified anesthetic - *see* Table of Drugs and Chemicals
  - postoperative 997.3
    - obstetric 668.0
  - radiation 508.0
  - rubella, congenital 771.0
  - "ventilation" 495.7
  - wood-dust 495.8
- **Pneumonoconiosis** - *see* Pneumoconiosis
- **Pneumoparotid** 527.8
- **Pneumopathy NEC** 518.89
  - alveolar 516.9
    - specified NEC 516.8
  - due to dust NEC 504
  - parietoalveolar 516.9
    - specified condition NEC 516.8
- **Pneumopericarditis** (*see also* Pericarditis) 423.9
  - acute 420.90
- **Pneumopericardium** - *see also* Pericarditis
  - congenital 770.2
  - fetus or newborn 770.2
  - traumatic (post) (*see also* Pneumothorax, traumatic) 860.0
    - with open wound into thorax 860.1
- **Pneumoperitoneum** 568.89
  - fetus or newborn 770.2
- **Pneumophagia** (psychogenic) 306.4
- **Pneumopleurisy, pneumopleuritis** (*see also* Pneumonia) 486
- **Pneumopyopericardium** 420.99
- **Pneumopyothorax** (*see also* Pyopneumothorax) 510.9
  - with fistula 510.0
- **Pneumorrhagia** 786.3
  - newborn 770.3
  - tuberculous (*see also* Tuberculosis, pulmonary) 011.9
- **Pneumosiderosis** (occupational) 503
- **Pneumothorax** (acute) (chronic) 512.8
  - congenital 770.2
  - due to operative injury of chest wall or lung 512.1
    - accidental puncture or laceration 512.1
  - fetus or newborn 770.2
  - iatrogenic 512.1
  - postoperative 512.1
  - spontaneous 512.8
    - fetus or newborn 770.2
    - tension 512.0
  - sucking 512.8
    - iatrogenic 512.1
    - postoperative 512.1
  - tense valvular, infectional 512.0
  - tension 512.0
    - iatrogenic 512.1
    - postoperative 512.1
    - spontaneous 512.0
  - traumatic 860.0
    - with
      - hemothorax 860.4
        - with open wound into thorax 860.5

- **Pneumothorax** *(Continued)*
  - traumatic *(Continued)*
    - with *(Continued)*
      - open wound into thorax 860.1
  - tuberculous (*see also* Tuberculosis) 011.7
- **Pocket**(s)
  - endocardial (*see also* Endocarditis) 424.90
  - periodontal 523.8
- **Podagra** 274.9
- **Podencephalus** 759.89
- **Poikilocytosis** 790.09
- **Poikiloderma** 709.09
  - Civatte's 709.09
  - congenital 757.33
  - vasculare atrophicans 696.2
- **Poikilodermatomyositis** 710.3
- **Pointed ear** 744.29
- **Poise imperfect** 729.9
- **Poisoned** - *see* Poisoning
- **Poisoning** (acute) - *see also* Table of Drugs and Chemicals
  - Bacillus, B.
    - aertrycke (*see also* Infection, Salmonella) 003.9
    - botulinus 005.1
    - cholerae (suis) (*see also* Infection, Salmonella) 003.9
    - paratyphosus (*see also* Infection, Salmonella) 003.9
    - suipestifer (*see also* Infection, Salmonella) 003.9
  - bacterial toxins NEC 005.9
  - berries, noxious 988.2
  - blood (general) - *see* Septicemia
  - botulism 005.1
  - bread, moldy, mouldy - *see* Poisoning, food
  - damaged meat - *see* Poisoning, food
  - death-cap (Amanita phalloides) (Amanita verna) 988.1
  - decomposed food - *see* Poisoning, food
  - diseased food - *see* Poisoning, food
  - drug - *see* Table of Drugs and Chemicals
  - epidemic, fish, meat, or other food - *see* Poisoning, food
  - fava bean 282.2
  - fish (bacterial) - *see also* Poisoning, food
    - noxious 988.0
  - food (acute) (bacterial) (diseased) (infected) NEC 005.9
    - due to
      - bacillus
        - aertrycke (*see also* Poisoning, food, due to Salmonella) 003.9
        - botulinus 005.1
        - cereus 005.89
        - choleraesuis (*see also* Poisoning, food, due to Salmonella) 003.9
        - paratyphosus (*see also* Poisoning, food, due to Salmonella) 003.9
        - suipestifer (*see also* Poisoning, food, due to Salmonella) 003.9
      - Clostridium 005.3
        - botulinum 005.1
        - perfringens 005.2
        - welchii 005.2
      - Salmonella (aertrycke) (callinarum) (choleraesuis) (enteritidis) (paratyphi) (suipestifer) 003.9

- **Poisoning** *(Continued)*
  - food *(Continued)*
    - due to *(Continued)*
      - Salmonella *(Continued)*
        - with
          - gastroenteritis 003.0
          - localized infection(s) (*see also* Infection, Salmonella) 003.20
          - septicemia 003.1
          - specified manifestation NEC 003.8
      - specified bacterium NEC 005.89
      - Staphylococcus 005.0
      - Streptococcus 005.0
      - Vibrio parahaemolyticus 005.4
      - Vibrio vulnificus 005.81
    - noxious or naturally toxic 988.0
      - berries 988.2
      - fish 988.0
      - mushroom 988.1
      - plants NEC 988.2
  - ice cream - *see* Poisoning, food
  - ichthyotoxism (bacterial) 005.9
  - kreotoxism, food 005.9
  - malarial - *see* Malaria
  - meat - *see* Poisoning, food
  - mushroom (noxious) 988.1
  - mussel - *see also* Poisoning, food
    - noxious 988.0
  - noxious foodstuffs (*see also* Poisoning, food, noxious) 988.9
    - specified type NEC 988.8
  - plants, noxious 988.2
  - pork - *see also* Poisoning, food
    - specified NEC 988.8
    - Trichinosis 124
  - ptomaine - *see* Poisoning, food
  - putrefaction, food - *see* Poisoning, food
  - radiation 508.0
  - Salmonella (*see also* Infection, Salmonella) 003.9
  - sausage - *see also* Poisoning, food
    - Trichinosis 124
  - saxitoxin 988.0
  - shellfish - *see also* Poisoning, food
    - noxious 988.0
  - Staphylococcus, food 005.0
  - toxic, from disease NEC 799.89 ⬅
  - truffles - *see* Poisoning, food
  - uremic - *see* Uremia
  - uric acid 274.9
- **Poison ivy, oak, sumac or other plant dermatitis** 692.6
- **Poker spine** 720.0
- **Policeman's disease** 729.2
- **Polioencephalitis** (acute) (bulbar) (*see also* Poliomyelitis, bulbar) 045.0
  - inferior 335.22
  - influenzal 487.8
  - superior hemorrhagic (acute) (Wernicke's) 265.1
  - Wernicke's (superior hemorrhagic) 265.1
- **Polioencephalomyelitis** (acute) (anterior) (bulbar) (*see also* Polioencephalitis) 045.0
- **Polioencephalopathy, superior hemorrhagic** 265.1
  - with
    - beriberi 265.0
    - pellagra 265.2
- **Poliomeningoencephalitis** - *see* Meningoencephalitis

Note Use the following fifth-digit subclassification with categories 640-648, 651-676:

0 unspecified as to episode of care
1 delivered, with or without mention of antepartum condition
2 delivered, with mention of postpartum complication
3 antepartum condition or complication
4 postpartum condition or complication

ICD-9-CM
P
Vol. 2

◀ New ⬅ Revised Code

- **Pregnancy** *(Continued)*
  - intraperitoneal - *see* Pregnancy, abdominal
  - isthmian - *see* Pregnancy, tubal
  - management affected by
    - abnormal, abnormality
      - fetus (suspected) 655.9
        - specified NEC 655.8
      - placenta 656.7
    - advanced maternal age NEC 659.6
      - multigravida 659.6
      - primigravida 659.5
    - antibodies (maternal)
      - anti-c 656.1
      - anti-d 656.1
      - anti-e 656.1
      - blood group (ABO) 656.2
        - rh(esus) 656.1
    - elderly multigravida 659.6
    - elderly primigravida 659.5
    - fetal (suspected)
      - abnormality 655.9
        - acid-base balance 656.8
        - heart rate or rhythm 659.7
        - specified NEC 655.8
      - acidemia 656.3
      - anencephaly 655.0
      - bradycardia 659.7
      - central nervous system malformation 655.0
      - chromosomal abnormalities (conditions classifiable to 758.0-758.9) 655.1
      - damage from
        - drugs 655.5
          - obstetric, anesthetic, or sedative 655.5
        - environmental toxins 655.8
        - intrauterine contraceptive device 655.8
        - maternal
          - alcohol addiction 655.4
          - disease NEC 655.4
          - drug use 655.5
          - listeriosis 655.4
          - rubella 655.3
          - toxoplasmosis 655.4
          - viral infection 655.3
        - radiation 655.6
      - death (near term) 656.4
        - early (before 22 completed weeks' gestation) 632
      - distress 656.8
      - excessive growth 656.6
      - growth retardation 656.5
      - hereditary disease 655.2
      - hydrocephalus 655.0
      - intrauterine death 656.4
      - poor growth 656.5
      - spina bifida (with myelomeningocele) 655.0
    - fetal-maternal hemorrhage 656.0
    - hereditary disease in family (possibly) affecting fetus 655.2
    - incompatibility, blood groups (ABO) 656.2
      - Rh(esus) 656.1
    - insufficient prenatal care V23.7
    - intrauterine death 656.4
    - isoimmunization (ABO) 656.2
      - Rh(esus) 656.1
    - large-for-dates fetus 656.6
    - light-for-dates fetus 656.5
    - meconium in liquor 656.8

- **Pregnancy** *(Continued)*
  - management affected by *(Continued)*
    - mental disorder (conditions classifiable to 290-303, 305-316, 317-319) 648.4
    - multiparity (grand) 659.4
    - poor obstetric history V23.49
      - pre-term labor V25.41
    - postmaturity
      - post term 645.1
      - prolonged 645.2
    - post term pregnancy 645.1
    - previous
      - abortion V23.2
        - habitual 646.3
      - cesarean delivery 654.2
      - difficult delivery V23.49
      - forceps delivery V23.49
      - habitual abortions 646.3
      - hemorrhage, antepartum or postpartum V23.49
      - hydatidiform mole V23.1
      - infertility V23.0
      - malignancy NEC V23.8
      - nonobstetrical conditions V23.8
      - premature delivery V23.41
      - trophoblastic disease (conditions in 630) V23.1
      - vesicular mole V23.1
    - prolonged pregnancy 645.2
    - small-for-dates fetus 656.5
    - young maternal age 659.8
  - maternal death NEC 646.9
  - mesometric (mural) - *see* Pregnancy, cornual
  - molar 631
    - hydatidiform (*see also* Hydatidiform mole) 630
      - previous, affecting management of pregnancy V23.1
    - previous, affecting management of pregnancy V23.49
  - multiple NEC 651.9
    - with fetal loss and retention of one or more fetus(es) 651.6
    - affecting fetus or newborn 761.5
    - specified type NEC 651.8
      - with fetal loss and retention of one or more fetus(es) 651.6
  - mural - *see* Pregnancy, cornual
  - observation NEC V22.1
    - first pregnancy V22.0
    - high-risk V23.9
      - specified problem NEC V23.8
  - ovarian 633.20
    - with intrauterine pregnancy 633.21
    - affecting fetus or newborn 761.4
  - postmature
    - post-term 645.1
    - prolonged 645.2
  - post term 645.1
  - prenatal care only V22.1
    - first pregnancy V22.0
    - high-risk V23.9
      - specified problem NEC V23.8
  - prolonged 645.2
  - quadruplet NEC 651.2
    - with fetal loss and retention of one or more fetus(es) 651.5
    - affecting fetus or newborn 761.5
  - quintuplet NEC 651.8
    - with fetal loss and retention of one or more fetus(es) 651.6
    - affecting fetus or newborn 761.5

- **Pregnancy** *(Continued)*
  - sextuplet NEC 651.8
    - with fetal loss and retention of one or more fetus(es) 651.6
    - affecting fetus or newborn 761.5
  - spurious 300.11
  - superfecundation NEC 651.9
    - with fetal loss and retention of one or more fetus(es) 651.6
  - superfetation NEC 651.9
    - with fetal loss and retention of one or more fetus(es) 651.6
  - supervision (of) (for) - *see also* Pregnancy, management affected by elderly
    - multigravida V23.82
    - primigravida V23.81
    - high-risk V23.9
      - insufficient prenatal care V23.7
      - specified problem NEC V23.8
    - multiparity V23.3
    - normal NEC V22.1
      - first V22.0
    - poor
      - obstetric history V23.49
        - pre-term labor V23.41
      - reproductive history V23.5
    - previous
      - abortion V23.2
      - hydatidiform mole V23.1
      - infertility V23.0
      - neonatal death V23.5
      - stillbirth V23.5
      - trophoblastic disease V23.1
      - vesicular mole V23.1
    - specified problem NEC V23.8
    - young
      - multigravida V23.84
      - primigravida V23.83
  - triplet NEC 651.1
    - with fetal loss and retention of one or more fetus(es) 651.4
    - affecting fetus or newborn 761.5
  - tubal (with rupture) 633.10
    - with intrauterine pregnancy 633.11
    - affecting fetus or newborn 761.4
  - twin NEC 651.0
    - with fetal loss and retention of one fetus 651.3
    - affecting fetus or newborn 761.5
  - unconfirmed V72.4
  - undelivered (no other diagnosis) V22.2
    - with false labor 644.1
    - high-risk V23.9
      - specified problem NEC V23.8
  - unwanted NEC V61.7
- **Pregnant uterus** - *see* condition
- **Preiser's disease** (osteoporosis) 733.09
- **Prekwashiorkor** 260
- **Preleukemia** 238.7
- **Preluxation of hip, congenital** (*see also* Subluxation, congenital, hip) 754.32
- **Premature** - *see also* condition
  - beats (nodal) 427.60
    - atrial 427.61
    - auricular 427.61
    - postoperative 997.1
    - specified type NEC 427.69
    - supraventricular 427.61
    - ventricular 427.69
  - birth NEC 765.1
  - closure
    - cranial suture 756.0
    - fontanel 756.0
    - foramen ovale 745.8

ICD-9-CM

P

Vol. 2

Note Use the following fifth-digit subclassification with categories 296.0-296.6:

0 unspecified
1 mild
2 moderate
3 severe, without mention of psychotic behavior

◀ New ⬅ Revised Code

ICD-9-CM
P
Vol. 2

- **Punch drunk** 310.2
- **Puncta lacrimalia occlusion** 375.52
- **Punctiform hymen** 752.49
- **Puncture** (traumatic) - *see also* Wound, open, by site
  - accidental, complicating surgery 998.2
  - bladder, nontraumatic 596.6
  - by
    - device, implant, or graft - *see* Complications, mechanical
    - foreign body
      - internal organs - *see also* Injury, internal, by site
      - by ingested object - *see* Foreign body
      - left accidentally in operation wound 998.4
    - instrument (any) during a procedure, accidental 998.2
  - internal organs, abdomen, chest, or pelvis - *see* Injury, internal, by site
  - kidney, nontraumatic 593.89
- **Pupil** - *see* condition
- **Pupillary membrane** 364.74
  - persistent 743.46
- **Pupillotonia** 379.46
  - pseudotabetic 379.46
- **Purpura** 287.2
  - abdominal 287.0
  - allergic 287.0
  - anaphylactoid 287.0
  - annularis telangiectodes 709.1
  - arthritic 287.0
  - autoerythrocyte sensitization 287.2
  - autoimmune 287.0
  - bacterial 287.0
  - Bateman's (senile) 287.2
  - capillary fragility (hereditary) (idiopathic) 287.8
  - cryoglobulinemic 273.2
  - devil's pinches 287.2
  - fibrinolytic (*see also* Fibrinolysis) 286.6
  - fulminans, fulminous 286.6
  - gangrenous 287.0
  - hemorrhagic (*see also* Purpura, thrombocytopenic) 287.3
    - nodular 272.7
    - nonthrombocytopenic 287.0
    - thrombocytopenic 287.3
  - Henoch's (purpura nervosa) 287.0
  - Henoch-Schönlein (allergic) 287.0
  - hypergammaglobulinemic (benign primary) (Waldenström's) 273.0
  - idiopathic 287.3
    - nonthrombocytopenic 287.0
    - thrombocytopenic 287.3
  - infectious 287.0
  - malignant 287.0
  - neonatorum 772.6
  - nervosa 287.0
  - newborn NEC 772.6
  - nonthrombocytopenic 287.2
    - hemorrhagic 287.0
    - idiopathic 287.0
  - nonthrombopenic 287.2
  - peliosis rheumatica 287.0
  - pigmentaria, progressiva 709.09
  - posttransfusion 287.4
  - primary 287.0
  - primitive 287.0
  - red cell membrane sensitivity 287.2
  - rheumatica 287.0
  - Schönlein (-Henoch) (allergic) 287.0
  - scorbutic 267

Purpura *(Continued)*
  - senile 287.2
  - simplex 287.2
  - symptomatica 287.0
  - telangiectasia annularis 709.1
  - thrombocytopenic (congenital) (essential) (hereditary) (idiopathic) (primary) (*see also* Thrombocytopenia) 287.3
    - neonatal, transitory (*see also* Thrombocytopenia, neonatal transitory) 776.1
    - puerperal, postpartum 666.3
    - thrombotic 446.6
  - thrombohemolytic (*see also* Fibrinolysis) 286.6
  - thrombopenic (congenital) (essential) (*see also* Thrombocytopenia) 287.3
  - thrombotic 446.6
    - thrombocytic 446.6
    - thrombocytopenic 446.6
  - toxic 287.0
  - variolosa 050.0
  - vascular 287.0
  - visceral symptoms 287.0
  - Werlhof's (*see also* Purpura, thrombocytopenic) 287.3
- **Purpuric spots** 782.7
- **Purulent** - *see* condition
- **Pus**
  - absorption, general - *see* Septicemia
  - in
    - stool 792.1
    - urine 791.9
  - tube (rupture) (*see also* Salpingo-oophoritis) 614.2
- **Pustular rash** 782.1
- **Pustule** 686.9
  - malignant 022.0
  - nonmalignant 686.9
- **Putnam's disease** (subacute combined sclerosis with pernicious anemia) 281.0 *[336.2]*
- **Putnam-Dana syndrome** (subacute combined sclerosis with pernicious anemia) 281.0 *[336.2]*
- **Putrefaction, intestinal** 569.89
- **Putrescent pulp** (dental) 522.1
- **Pyarthritis** - *see* Pyarthrosis
- **Pyarthrosis** (*see also* Arthritis, pyogenic) 711.0
  - tuberculous - *see* Tuberculosis, joint
- **Pycnoepilepsy, pycnolepsy** (idiopathic) (*see also* Epilepsy) 345.0
- **Pyelectasia** 593.89
- **Pyelectasis** 593.89
- **Pyelitis** (congenital) (uremic) 590.80
  - with
    - abortion - *see* Abortion, by type, with specified complication NEC
    - contracted kidney 590.00
    - ectopic pregnancy (*see also* categories 633.0-633.9) 639.8
    - molar pregnancy (*see also* categories 630-632) 639.8
  - acute 590.10
    - with renal medullary necrosis 590.11
  - chronic 590.00
    - with
      - renal medullary necrosis 590.01
  - complicating pregnancy, childbirth, or puerperium 646.6
    - affecting fetus or newborn 760.1
  - cystica 590.3

Pyelitis *(Continued)*
  - following
    - abortion 639.8
    - ectopic or molar pregnancy 639.8
  - gonococcal 098.19
    - chronic or duration of 2 months or over 098.39
  - tuberculous (*see also* Tuberculosis) 016.0 *[590.81]*
- **Pyelocaliectasis** 593.89
- **Pyelocystitis** (*see also* Pyelitis) 590.80
- **Pyelohydronephrosis** 591
- **Pyelonephritis** (*see also* Pyelitis) 590.80
  - acute 590.10
    - with renal medullary necrosis 590.11
  - chronic 590.00
  - syphilitic (late) 095.4
  - tuberculous (*see also* Tuberculosis) 016.0 *[590.81]*
- **Pyelonephrosis** (*see also* Pyelitis) 590.80
  - chronic 590.00
- **Pyelophlebitis** 451.89
- **Pyelo-ureteritis cystica** 590.3
- **Pyemia, pyemic** (purulent) (*see also* Septicemia) 038.9
  - abscess - *see* Abscess
  - arthritis (*see also* Arthritis, pyogenic) 711.0
  - Bacillus coli 038.42
  - embolism - *see* Embolism, pyemic
  - fever 038.9
  - infection 038.9
  - joint (*see also* Arthritis, pyogenic) 711.0
  - liver 572.1
  - meningococcal 036.2
  - newborn 771.81
  - phlebitis - *see* Phlebitis
  - pneumococcal 038.2
  - portal 572.1
  - postvaccinal 999.3
  - specified organism NEC 038.8
  - staphylococcal 038.10
    - aureus 038.11
    - specified organism NEC 038.19
  - streptococcal 038.0
  - tuberculous - *see* Tuberculosis, miliary
- **Pygopagus** 759.4
- **Pykno-epilepsy, pyknolepsy** (idiopathic) (*see also* Epilepsy) 345.0
- **Pyle** (-Cohn) disease (craniometaphyseal dysplasia) 756.89
- **Pylephlebitis** (suppurative) 572.1
- **Pylethrombophlebitis** 572.1
- **Pylethrombosis** 572.1
- **Pyloritis** (*see also* Gastritis) 535.5
- **Pylorospasm** (reflex) 537.81
  - congenital or infantile 750.5
  - neurotic 306.4
  - newborn 750.5
  - psychogenic 306.4
- **Pylorus, pyloric** - *see* condition
- **Pyoarthrosis** - *see* Pyarthrosis
- **Pyocele**
  - mastoid 383.00
  - sinus (accessory) (nasal) (*see also* Sinusitis) 473.9
  - turbinate (bone) 473.9
  - urethra (*see also* Urethritis) 597.0
- **Pyococcal dermatitis** 686.00
- **Pyococcide, skin** 686.00
- **Pyocolpos** (*see also* Vaginitis) 616.10
- **Pyocyaneus dermatitis** 686.09
- **Pyocystitis** (*see also* Cystitis) 595.9

Q

Q

R

Note Use the following subclassification for categories V09.5, V09.7, V09.8, V09.9:

0 without mention of resistance to multiple drugs
1 with resistance to multiple drugs
V09.5 quinolones and fluoroquinolones
V09.7 antimycobacterial agents
V09.8 specified drugs NEC
V09.9 unspecified drugs
9 multiple sites

◀ New ⬅ Revised Code

ICD-9-CM
R
Vol. 2

S

Schistosomiasis 120.9
Asiatic 120.2
bladder 120.0
chestermani 120.8
colon 120.1
cutaneous 120.3
due to
S. hematobium 120.0
S. japonicum 120.2
S. mansoni 120.1
S. mattheii 120.8
eastern 120.2
genitourinary tract 120.0
intestinal 120.1
lung 120.2
Manson's (intestinal) 120.1
Oriental 120.2
pulmonary 120.2
specified type NEC 120.8
vesical 120.0
Schizencephaly 742.4
Schizo-affective psychosis (*see also* Schizophrenia) 295.7
Schizodontia 520.2
Schizoid personality 301.20
introverted 301.21
schizotypal 301.22
Schizophrenia, schizophrenic (reaction) 295.9

Note Use the following fifth-digit subclassification with category 295:

0 unspecified
1 subchronic
2 chronic
3 subchronic with acute exacerbation
4 chronic with acute exacerbation
5 in remission

acute (attack) NEC 295.8
episode 295.4
atypical form 295.8
borderline 295.5
catalepsy 295.2
catatonic (type) (acute) (excited) (withdrawn) 295.2
childhood (type) (*see also* Psychosis, childhood) 299.9
chronic NEC 295.6
coenesthesiopathic 295.8
cyclic (type) 295.7
disorganized (type) 295.1
flexibilitas cerea 295.2
hebephrenic (type) (acute) 295.1
incipient 295.5
latent 295.5
paranoid (type) (acute) 295.3
paraphrenic (acute) 295.3
prepsychotic 295.5
primary (acute) 295.0
prodromal 295.5
pseudoneurotic 295.5
pseudopsychopathic 295.5
reaction 295.9
residual (state) (type) 295.6
restzustand 295.6
schizo-affective (type) (depressed) (excited) 295.7
schizophreniform type 295.4
simple (type) (acute) 295.0
simplex (acute) 295.0
specified type NEC 295.8

Schizophrenia, schizophrenic (*Continued*)
syndrome of childhood NEC (*see also* Psychosis, childhood) 299.9
undifferentiated 295.9
acute 295.8
chronic 295.6
Schizothymia 301.20
introverted 301.21
schizotypal 301.22
Schlafkrankheit 086.5
Schlatter's tibia (osteochondrosis) 732.4
Schlatter-Osgood disease (osteochondrosis, tibial tubercle) 732.4
Schloffer's tumor (*see also* Peritonitis) 567.2
Schmidt's syndrome
sphallo-pharyngo-laryngeal hemiplegia 352.6
thyroid-adrenocortical insufficiency 258.1
vagoaccessory 352.6
Schmincke
carcinoma (M8082/3) - *see* Neoplasm, nasopharynx, malignant
tumor (M8082/3) - *see* Neoplasm, nasopharynx, malignant
Schmitz (-Stutzer) dysentery 004.0
Schmorl's disease or nodes 722.30
lumbar, lumbosacral 722.32
specified region NEC 722.39
thoracic, thoracolumbar 722.31
Schneider's syndrome 047.9
Schneiderian
carcinoma (M8121/3)
specified site - *see* Neoplasm, by site, malignant
unspecified site 160.0
papilloma (M8121/0)
specified site - *see* Neoplasm, by site, benign
unspecified site 212.0
Schoffer's tumor (*see also* Peritonitis) 567.2
Scholte's syndrome (malignant carcinoid) 259.2
Scholz's disease 330.0
Scholz (-Bielschowsky-Henneberg) syndrome 330.0
Schönlein (-Henoch) disease (primary) (purpura) (rheumatic) 287.0
School examination V70.3
Schottmüller's disease (*see also* Fever, paratyphoid) 002.9
Schroeder's syndrome (endocrine-hypertensive) 255.3
Schüller-Christian disease or syndrome (chronic histiocytosis X) 277.89 ⬅
Schultz's disease or syndrome (agranulocytosis) 288.0
Schultze's acroparesthesia, simple 443.89
Schwalbe-Ziehen-Oppenheimer disease 333.6
Schwannoma (M9560/0) - *see also* Neoplasm, connective tissue, benign
malignant (M9560/3) - *see* Neoplasm, connective tissue, malignant
Schwartz (-Jampel) syndrome 756.89
Schwartz-Bartter syndrome (inappropriate secretion of antidiuretic hormone) 253.6
Schweninger-Buzzi disease (macular atrophy) 701.3
Sciatic - *see* condition

Sciatica (infectional) 724.3
due to
displacement of intervertebral disc 722.10
herniation, nucleus pulposus 722.10
Scimitar syndrome (anomalous venous drainage, right lung to inferior vena cava) 747.49
Sclera - *see* condition
Sclerectasia 379.11
Scleredema
adultorum 710.1
Buschke's 710.1
newborn 778.1
Sclerema
adiposum (newborn) 778.1
adultorum 710.1
edematosum (newborn) 778.1
neonatorum 778.1
newborn 778.1
Scleriasis - *see* Scleroderma
Scleritis 379.00
with corneal involvement 379.05
anterior (annular) (localized) 379.03
brawny 379.06
granulomatous 379.09
posterior 379.07
specified NEC 379.09
suppurative 379.09
syphilitic 095.0
tuberculous (nodular) (*see also* Tuberculosis) 017.3 *[379.09]*
Sclerochoroiditis (*see also* Scleritis) 379.00
Scleroconjunctivitis (*see also* Scleritis) 379.00
Sclerocystic ovary (syndrome) 256.4
Sclerodactylia 701.0
Scleroderma, sclerodermia (acrosclerotic) (diffuse) (generalized) (progressive) (pulmonary) 710.1
circumscribed 701.0
linear 701.0
localized (linear) 701.0
newborn 778.1
Sclerokeratitis 379.05
meaning sclerosing keratitis 370.54
tuberculous (*see also* Tuberculosis) 017.3 *[379.09]*
Scleroma, trachea 040.1
Scleromalacia
multiple 731.0
perforans 379.04
Scleromyxedema 701.8
Scleroperikeratitis 379.05
Sclerose en plaques 340
Sclerosis, sclerotic
adrenal (gland) 255.8
Alzheimer's 331.0
with dementia - *see* Alzheimer's, dementia
amyotrophic (lateral) 335.20
annularis fibrosi
aortic 424.1
mitral 424.0
aorta, aortic 440.0
valve (*see also* Endocarditis, aortic) 424.1
artery, arterial, arteriolar, arteriovascular - *see* Arteriosclerosis
ascending multiple 340
Baló's (concentric) 341.1
basilar - *see* Sclerosis, brain

◀ New ⬅ Revised Code

ICD-9-CM S Vol. 2

Shock *(Continued)*
  hemorrhagic *(Continued)*
    due to *(Continued)*
      surgery (intraoperative) (postoperative) 998.0
      trauma 958.4
  hypovolemic NEC 785.59
    surgical 998.0
    traumatic 958.4
  insulin 251.0
    therapeutic misadventure 962.3
  kidney 584.5
    traumatic (following crushing) 958.5
  lightning 994.0
  lung 518.5
  nervous (*see also* Reaction, stress, acute) 308.9
  obstetric 669.1
    with
      abortion - *see* Abortion, by type, with shock
      ectopic pregnancy (*see also* categories 633.0-633.9) 639.5
      molar pregnancy (*see also* categories 630-632) 639.5
    following
      abortion 639.5
      ectopic or molar pregnancy 639.5
  paralysis, paralytic (*see also* Disease, cerebrovascular, acute) 436
    late effect - *see* Late effect(s) (of) cerebrovascular disease
  pleural (surgical) 998.0
    due to trauma 958.4
  postoperative 998.0
    with
      abortion - *see* Abortion, by type, with shock
      ectopic pregnancy (*see also* categories 633.0-633.9) 639.5
      molar pregnancy (*see also* categories 630-632) 639.5
    following
      abortion 639.5
      ectopic or molar pregnancy 639.5
  psychic (*see also* Reaction, stress, acute) 308.9
    past history (of) V15.49
  psychogenic (*see also* Reaction, stress, acute) 308.9
  septic 785.52
    with
      abortion - *see* Abortion, by type, with shock
      ectopic pregnancy (*see also* categories 633.0-633.9) 639.5
      molar pregnancy (*see also* categories 630-632) 639.5
    due to
      surgical procedure 998.0
      transfusion NEC 999.8
        bone marrow 996.85
    following
      abortion 639.5
      ectopic or molar pregnancy 639.5
      surgical procedure 998.0
      transfusion NEC 999.8
        bone marrow 996.85
  spinal - *see also* Injury, spinal, by site
    with spinal bone injury - *see* Fracture, vertebra, by site, with spinal cord injury
  surgical 998.0
  therapeutic misadventure NEC (*see also* Complications) 998.89
  thyroxin 962.7

Shock *(Continued)*
  toxic 040.82
  transfusion - *see* Complications, transfusion
  traumatic (immediate) (delayed) 958.4
Shoemakers' chest 738.3
Short, shortening, shortness
  Achilles tendon (acquired) 727.81
  arm 736.89
    congenital 755.20
  back 737.9
  bowel syndrome 579.3
  breath 786.05
  common bile duct, congenital 751.69
  cord (umbilical) 663.4
    affecting fetus or newborn 762.6
  cystic duct, congenital 751.69
  esophagus (congenital) 750.4
  femur (acquired) 736.81
    congenital 755.34
  frenulum linguae 750.0
  frenum, lingual 750.0
  hamstrings 727.81
  hip (acquired) 736.39
    congenital 755.63
  leg (acquired) 736.81
    congenital 755.30
  metatarsus (congenital) 754.79
    acquired 736.79
  organ or site, congenital NEC - *see* Distortion
  palate (congenital) 750.26
  P-R interval syndrome 426.81
  radius (acquired) 736.09
    congenital 755.26
  round ligament 629.8
  sleeper 307.49
  stature, constitutional (hereditary) 783.43
  tendon 727.81
    Achilles (acquired) 727.81
      congenital 754.79
    congenital 756.89
  thigh (acquired) 736.81
    congenital 755.34
  tibialis anticus 727.81
  umbilical cord 663.4
    affecting fetus or newborn 762.6
  urethra 599.84
  uvula (congenital) 750.26
  vagina 623.8
Shortsightedness 367.1
Shoshin (acute fulminating beriberi) 265.0
Shoulder - *see* condition
Shovel-shaped incisors 520.2
Shower, thromboembolic - *see* Embolism
Shunt (status)
  aortocoronary bypass V45.81
  arterial-venous (dialysis) V45.1
  arteriovenous, pulmonary (acquired) 417.0
    congenital 747.3
    traumatic (complication) 901.40
  cerebral ventricle (communicating) in situ V45.2
  coronary artery bypass V45.81
  surgical, prosthetic, with complications - *see* Complications, shunt
  vascular NEC V45.89
Shutdown
  renal 586
    with
      abortion - *see* Abortion, by type, with renal failure
      ectopic pregnancy (*see also* categories 633.0-633.9) 639.3

Shutdown *(Continued)*
  renal *(Continued)*
    with *(Continued)*
      molar pregnancy (*see also* categories 630-632) 639.3
    complicating
      abortion 639.3
      ectopic or molar pregnancy 639.3
    following labor and delivery 669.3
Shwachman's syndrome 288.0
Shy-Drager syndrome (orthostatic hypotension with multisystem degeneration) 333.0
Sialadenitis (any gland) (chronic) (suppurative) 527.2
  epidemic - *see* Mumps
Sialadenosis, periodic 527.2
Sialaporia 527.7
Sialectasia 527.8
Sialitis 527.2
Sialoadenitis (*see also* Sialadenitis) 527.2
Sialoangitis 527.2
Sialodochitis (fibrinosa) 527.2
Sialodocholithiasis 527.5
Sialolithiasis 527.5
Sialorrhea (*see also* Ptyalism) 527.7
  periodic 527.2
Sialosis 527.8
  rheumatic 710.2
Siamese twin 759.4
Sicard's syndrome 352.6
Sicca syndrome (keratoconjunctivitis) 710.2
Sick 799.9
  cilia syndrome 759.89
  or handicapped person in family V61.49
Sickle-cell
  anemia (*see also* Disease, sickle-cell) 282.60
  disease (*see also* Disease, sickle-cell) 282.60
  hemoglobin
    C disease (without crisis) 282.63
      with
        crisis 282.64
        vaso-occlusive pain 282.64
    D disease (without crisis) 282.68
      with crisis 282.69
    E disease (without crisis) 282.68
      with crisis 282.69
    thalassemia (without crisis) 282.41
      with
        crisis 282.42
        vaso-occlusive pain 282.42
  trait 282.5
Sicklemia (*see also* Disease, sickle-cell) 282.60
  trait 282.5
Sickness
  air (travel) 994.6
  airplane 994.6
  alpine 993.2
  altitude 993.2
  Andes 993.2
  aviators' 993.2
  balloon 993.2
  car 994.6
  compressed air 993.3
  decompression 993.3
  green 280.9
  harvest 100.89
  milk 988.8
  morning 643.0
  motion 994.6
  mountain 993.2
    acute 289.0
  protein (*see also* Complications, vaccination) 999.5

New   Revised Code

ICD-9-CM
S
Vol. 2

- **Sprue** *(Continued)*
  - tropical 579.1
- **Spur** - *see also* Exostosis
  - bone 726.91
    - calcaneal 726.73
  - calcaneal 726.73
  - iliac crest 726.5
  - nose (septum) 478.1
    - bone 726.91
  - septal 478.1
- **Spuria placenta** - *see* Placenta, abnormal
- **Spurway's syndrome** (brittle bones and blue sclera) 756.51
- **Sputum, abnormal** (amount) (color) (excessive) (odor) (purulent) 786.4
  - bloody 786.3
- **Squamous** - *see also* condition
  - cell metaplasia
    - bladder 596.8
    - cervix - *see* condition
  - epithelium in
    - cervical canal (congenital) 752.49
    - uterine mucosa (congenital) 752.3
  - metaplasia
    - bladder 596.8
    - cervix - *see* condition
- **Squashed nose** 738.0
  - congenital 754.0
- **Squeeze, divers'** 993.3
- **Squint** (*see also* Strabismus) 378.9
  - accommodative (*see also* Esotropia) 378.00
  - concomitant (*see also* Heterotropia) 378.30
- **Stab** - *see also* Wound, open, by site
  - internal organs - *see* Injury, internal, by site, with open wound
- **Staggering gait** 781.2
  - hysterical 300.11
- **Staghorn calculus** 592.0
- **Stähl's**
  - ear 744.29
  - pigment line (cornea) 371.11
- **Stähli's pigment lines** (cornea) 371.11
- **Stain**
  - port wine 757.32
  - tooth, teeth (hard tissues) 521.7
    - due to
      - accretions 523.6
      - deposits (betel) (black) (green) (materia alba) (orange) (tobacco) 523.6
      - metals (copper) (silver) 521.7
      - nicotine 523.6
      - pulpal bleeding 521.7
      - tobacco 523.6
- **Stammering** 307.0
- **Standstill**
  - atrial 426.6
  - auricular 426.6
  - cardiac (*see also* Arrest, cardiac) 427.5
  - sinoatrial 426.6
  - sinus 426.6
  - ventricular (*see also* Arrest, cardiac) 427.5
- **Stannosis** 503
- **Stanton's disease** (melioidosis) 025
- **Staphylitis** (acute) (catarrhal) (chronic) (gangrenous) (membranous) (suppurative) (ulcerative) 528.3
- **Staphylococcemia** 038.10
  - aureus 038.11
  - specified organism NEC 038.19
- **Staphylococcus, staphylococcal** - *see* condition
- **Staphyloderma** (skin) 686.00
- **Staphyloma** 379.11
  - anterior, localized 379.14
  - ciliary 379.11
  - cornea 371.73
  - equatorial 379.13
  - posterior 379.12
  - posticum 379.12
  - ring 379.15
  - sclera NEC 379.11
- **Starch eating** 307.52
- **Stargardt's disease** 362.75
- **Starvation** (inanition) (due to lack of food) 994.2
  - edema 262
  - voluntary NEC 307.1
- **Stasis**
  - bile (duct) (*see also* Disease, biliary) 576.8
  - bronchus (*see also* Bronchitis) 490
  - cardiac (*see also* Failure, heart) 428.0
  - cecum 564.89
  - colon 564.89
  - dermatitis (*see also* Varix, with stasis dermatitis) 454.1
  - duodenal 536.8
  - eczema (*see also* Varix, with stasis dermatitis) 454.1
  - edema (*see also* Hypertension, venous) 459.30
  - foot 991.4
  - gastric 536.3
  - ileocecal coil 564.89
  - ileum 564.89
  - intestinal 564.89
  - jejunum 564.89
  - kidney 586
  - liver 571.9
    - cirrhotic - *see* Cirrhosis, liver
  - lymphatic 457.8
  - pneumonia 514
  - portal 571.9
  - pulmonary 514
  - rectal 564.89
  - renal 586
    - tubular 584.5
  - stomach 536.3
  - ulcer
    - with varicose veins 454.0
    - without varicose veins 459.81
  - urine NEC (*see also* Retention, urine) 788.20
  - venous 459.81
- **State**
  - affective and paranoid, mixed, organic psychotic 294.8
  - agitated 307.9
    - acute reaction to stress 308.2
  - anxiety (neurotic) (*see also* Anxiety) 300.00
    - specified type NEC 300.09
  - apprehension (*see also* Anxiety) 300.00
    - specified type NEC 300.09
  - climacteric, female 627.2
    - following induced menopause 627.4
  - clouded
    - epileptic (*see also* Epilepsy) 345.9
    - paroxysmal (idiopathic) (*see also* Epilepsy) 345.9
  - compulsive (mixed) (with obsession) 300.3
  - confusional 298.9
    - acute 293.0
      - with
        - arteriosclerotic dementia 290.41
        - presenile brain disease 290.11
        - senility 290.3
- **State** *(Continued)*
  - confusional *(Continued)*
    - acute *(Continued)*
      - alcoholic 291.0
      - drug-induced 292.81
    - epileptic 293.0
    - postoperative 293.9
    - reactive (emotional stress) (psychological trauma) 298.2
    - subacute 293.1
  - constitutional psychopathic 301.9
  - convulsive (*see also* Convulsions) 780.39
  - depressive NEC 311
    - induced by drug 292.84
    - neurotic 300.4
  - dissociative 300.15
  - hallucinatory 780.1
    - induced by drug 292.12
  - hypercoagulable (primary) 289.81 ◀
    - secondary 289.82 ◀
  - hyperdynamic beta-adrenergic circulatory 429.82
  - locked-in 344.81
  - menopausal 627.2
    - artificial 627.4
    - following induced menopause 627.4
  - neurotic NEC 300.9
    - with depersonalization episode 300.6
  - obsessional 300.3
  - oneiroid (*see also* Schizophrenia) 295.4
  - panic 300.01
  - paranoid 297.9
    - alcohol-induced 291.5
    - arteriosclerotic 290.42
    - climacteric 297.2
    - drug-induced 292.11
    - in
      - presenile brain disease 290.12
      - senile brain disease 290.20
    - involutional 297.2
    - menopausal 297.2
    - senile 290.20
    - simple 297.0
  - postleukotomy 310.0
  - pregnant (*see also* Pregnancy) V22.2
  - psychogenic, twilight 298.2
  - psychotic, organic (*see also* Psychosis, organic) 294.9
    - mixed paranoid and affective 294.8
    - senile or presenile NEC 290.9
    - transient NEC 293.9
      - with
        - anxiety 293.84
        - delusions 293.81
        - depression 293.83
        - hallucinations 293.82
  - residual schizophrenic (*see also* Schizophrenia) 295.6
  - tension (*see also* Anxiety) 300.9
  - transient organic psychotic 293.9
    - anxiety type 293.84
    - depressive type 293.83
    - hallucinatory type 293.83
    - paranoid type 293.81
    - specified type NEC 293.89
  - twilight
    - epileptic 293.0
    - psychogenic 298.2
  - vegetative (persistent) 780.03
- **Status** (post)
  - absence
    - epileptic (*see also* Epilepsy) 345.2
    - of organ, acquired (postsurgical) - *see* Absence, by site, acquired
  - anastomosis of intestine (for bypass) V45.3

◀ New ⟵ Revised Code

◄ **New** ⇐ **Revised Code**

ICD-9-CM S Vol. 2

T

◀ New ⟸ Revised Code

Tenderness *(Continued)*
- rebound 789.6
- skin 782.0

Tendinitis, tendonitis (*see also* Tenosynovitis) 726.90
- Achilles 726.71
- adhesive 726.90
  - shoulder 726.0
- calcific 727.82
  - shoulder 726.11
- gluteal 726.5
- patellar 726.64
- peroneal 726.79
- pes anserinus 726.61
- psoas 726.5
- tibialis (anterior) (posterior) 726.72
- trochanteric 726.5

Tendon - *see* condition

Tendosynovitis - *see* Tenosynovitis

Tendovaginitis - *see* Tenosynovitis

Tenesmus 787.99
- rectal 787.99
- vesical 788.9

Tenia - *see* Taenia

Teniasis - *see* Taeniasis

Tennis elbow 726.32

Tenonitis - *see also* Tenosynovitis
- eye (capsule) 376.04

Tenontosynovitis - *see* Tenosynovitis

Tenontothecitis - *see* Tenosynovitis

Tenophyte 727.9

Tenosynovitis 727.00
- adhesive 726.90
  - shoulder 726.0
- ankle 727.06
- bicipital (calcifying) 726.12
- buttock 727.09
- due to crystals - *see* Arthritis, due to crystals
- elbow 727.09
- finger 727.05
- foot 727.06
- gonococcal 098.51
- hand 727.05
- hip 727.09
- knee 727.09
- radial styloid 727.04
- shoulder 726.10
  - adhesive 726.0
- spine 720.1
- supraspinatus 726.10
- toe 727.06
- tuberculous - *see* Tuberculosis, tenosynovitis
- wrist 727.05

Tenovaginitis - *see* Tenosynovitis

Tension
- arterial, high (*see also* Hypertension) 401.9
  - without diagnosis of hypertension 796.2
- headache 307.81
- intraocular (elevated) 365.00
- nervous 799.2
- ocular (elevated) 365.00
- pneumothorax 512.0
  - iatrogenic 512.1
  - postoperative 512.1
  - spontaneous 512.0
- premenstrual 625.4
- state 300.9

Tentorium - *see* condition

Teratencephalus 759.89

Teratism 759.7

Teratoblastoma (malignant) (M9080/3) - *see* Neoplasm, by site, malignant

Teratocarcinoma (M9081/3) - *see also* Neoplasm, by site, malignant
- liver 155.0

Teratoma (solid) (M9080/1) - *see also* Neoplasm, by site, uncertain behavior
- adult (cystic) (M9080/0) - *see* Neoplasm, by site, benign
- and embryonal carcinoma, mixed (M9081/3) - *see* Neoplasm, by site, malignant
- benign (M9080/0) - *see* Neoplasm, by site, benign
- combined with choriocarcinoma (M9101/3) - *see* Neoplasm, by site, malignant
- cystic (adult) (M9080/0) - *see* Neoplasm, by site, benign
- differentiated type (M9080/0) - *see* Neoplasm, by site, benign
- embryonal (M9080/3) - *see also* Neoplasm, by site, malignant
  - liver 155.0
- fetal
  - sacral, causing fetopelvic disproportion 653.7
- immature (M9080/3) - *see* Neoplasm, by site, malignant
- liver (M9080/3) 155.0
  - adult, benign, cystic, differentiated type, or mature (M9080/0) 211.5
- malignant (M9080/3) - *see also* Neoplasm, by site, malignant
  - anaplastic type (M9082/3) - *see* Neoplasm, by site, malignant
  - intermediate type (M9083/3) - *see* Neoplasm, by site, malignant
  - liver (M9080/3) 155.0
  - trophoblastic (M9102/3)
    - specified site - *see* Neoplasm, by site, malignant
    - unspecified site 186.9
  - undifferentiated type (M9082/3) - *see* Neoplasm, by site, malignant
- mature (M9080/0) - *see* Neoplasm, by site, benign
- ovary (M9080/0) 220
  - embryonal, immature, or malignant (M9080/3) 183.0
- suprasellar (M9080/3) - *see* Neoplasm, by site, malignant
- testis (M9080/3) 186.9
  - adult, benign, cystic, differentiated type or mature (M9080/0) 222.0
  - undescended 186.0

Terminal care V66.7

Termination
- anomalous - *see also* Malposition, congenital
  - portal vein 747.49
  - right pulmonary vein 747.42
- pregnancy (legal) (therapeutic) (*see* Abortion, legal) 635.9
  - fetus NEC 779.6
  - illegal (*see also* Abortion, illegal) 636.9

Ternidens diminutus infestation 127.7

Terrors, night (child) 307.46

Terry's syndrome 362.21

Tertiary - *see* condition

Tessellated fundus, retina (tigroid) 362.89

Test(s)
- adequacy
  - hemodialysis V56.31
  - peritoneal dialysis V56.32
- AIDS virus V72.6
- allergen V72.7
- bacterial disease NEC (*see also* Screening, by name of disease) V74.9
- basal metabolic rate V72.6
- blood-alcohol V70.4
- blood-drug V70.4
  - for therapeutic drug monitoring V58.83
- developmental, infant or child V20.2
- Dick V74.8
- fertility V26.21
- genetic V26.3
- hearing V72.1
- HIV V72.6
- human immunodeficiency virus V72.6
- Kveim V82.89
- laboratory V72.6
  - for medicolegal reason V70.4
- Mantoux (for tuberculosis) V74.1
- mycotic organism V75.4
- parasitic agent NEC V75.8
- paternity V70.4
- peritoneal equilibration V56.32
- pregnancy
  - positive V22.1
    - first pregnancy V22.0
  - unconfirmed V72.4
- preoperative V72.84
  - cardiovascular V72.81
  - respiratory V72.82
  - specified NEC V72.83
- procreative management NEC V26.29
- sarcoidosis V82.89
- Schick V74.3
- Schultz-Charlton V74.8
- skin, diagnostic
  - allergy V72.7
  - bacterial agent NEC (*see also* Screening, by name of disease) V74.9
  - Dick V74.8
  - hypersensitivity V72.7
  - Kveim V82.89
  - Mantoux V74.1
  - mycotic organism V75.4
  - parasitic agent NEC V75.8
  - sarcoidosis V82.89
  - Schick V74.3
  - Schultz-Charlton V74.8
  - tuberculin V74.1
- specified type NEC V72.85
- tuberculin V74.1
- vision V72.0
- Wassermann
  - positive (*see also* Serology for syphilis, positive) 097.1
    - false 795.6

Testicle, testicular, testis - *see also* condition
- feminization (syndrome) 257.8

Tetanus, tetanic (cephalic) (convulsions) 037
- with
  - abortion - *see* Abortion, by type, with sepsis
  - ectopic pregnancy (*see also* categories 633.0-633.9) 639.0
  - molar pregnancy (*see* categories 630-632) 639.0
- following
  - abortion 639.0
  - ectopic or molar pregnancy 639.0

ICD-9-CM

T

Vol. 2

Tetanus, tetanic *(Continued)*
- inoculation V03.7
  - reaction (due to serum) - *see* Complications, vaccination
- neonatorum 771.3
- puerperal, postpartum, childbirth 670

Tetany, tetanic 781.7
- alkalosis 276.3
- associated with rickets 268.0
- convulsions 781.7
  - hysterical 300.11
- functional (hysterical) 300.11
- hyperkinetic 781.7
  - hysterical 300.11
- hyperpnea 786.01
  - hysterical 300.11
  - psychogenic 306.1
- hyperventilation 786.01
  - hysterical 300.11
  - psychogenic 306.1
- hypocalcemic, neonatal 775.4
- hysterical 300.11
- neonatal 775.4
- parathyroid (gland) 252.1
- parathyroprival 252.1
- postoperative 252.1
- postthyroidectomy 252.1
- pseudotetany 781.7
  - hysterical 300.11
- psychogenic 306.1
  - specified as conversion reaction 300.11

Tetralogy of Fallot 745.2

Tetraplegia - *see* Quadriplegia

Thailand hemorrhagic fever 065.4

Thalassanemia 282.49

Thalassemia (alpha) (beta) (disease) (Hb-C) (Hb-D) (Hb-E) (Hb-H) (Hb-I) (Hb-S) (high fetal gene) (high fetal hemoglobin) (intermedia) (major) (minima) (minor) (mixed) (sickle-cell) (trait) (with other hemoglobinopathy) 282.49
- Hb-S (without crisis) 282.41
  - with
    - crisis 282.42
    - vaso-occlusive pain 282.42
- sickle-cell (without crisis) 282.41
  - with
    - crisis 282.42
    - vaso-occlusive pain 282.42

Thalassemic variants 282.49

Thaysen-Gee disease (nontropical sprue) 579.0

Thecoma (M8600/0) 220
- malignant (M8600/3) 183.0

Thelarche, precocious 259.1

Thelitis 611.0
- puerperal, postpartum 675.0

Therapeutic - *see* condition

Therapy V57.9
- blood transfusion, without reported diagnosis V58.2
- breathing V57.0
- chemotherapy V58.1
  - fluoride V07.31
  - prophylactic NEC V07.39
- dialysis (intermittent) (treatment)
  - extracorporeal V56.0
  - peritoneal V56.8
  - renal V56.0
  - specified type NEC V56.8
- exercise NEC V57.1
  - breathing V57.0
- extracorporeal dialysis (renal) V56.0
- fluoride prophylaxis V07.31
- hemodialysis V56.0
- long term oxygen therapy V46.2

Therapy *(Continued)*
- occupational V57.21
- orthoptic V57.4
- orthotic V57.81
- peritoneal dialysis V56.8
- physical NEC V57.1
- postmenopausal hormone replacement V07.4
- radiation V58.0
- speech V57.3
- vocational V57.22

Thermalgesia 782.0

Thermalgia 782.0

Thermanalgesia 782.0

Thermanesthesia 782.0

Thermic - *see* condition

Thermography (abnormal) 793.9
- breast 793.89

Thermoplegia 992.0

Thesaurismosis
- amyloid 277.3
- bilirubin 277.4
- calcium 275.40
- cystine 270.0
- glycogen (*see also* Disease, glycogen storage) 271.0
- kerasin 272.7
- lipoid 272.7
- melanin 255.4
- phosphatide 272.7
- urate 274.9

Thiaminic deficiency 265.1
- with beriberi 265.0

Thibierge-Weissenbach syndrome (cutaneous systemic sclerosis) 710.1

Thickened endometrium 793.5

Thickening
- bone 733.99
  - extremity 733.99
- breast 611.79
- hymen 623.3
- larynx 478.79
- nail 703.8
  - congenital 757.5
- periosteal 733.99
- pleura (*see also* Pleurisy) 511.0
- skin 782.8
- subepiglottic 478.79
- tongue 529.8
- valve, heart - *see* Endocarditis

Thiele syndrome 724.6

Thigh - *see* condition

Thinning vertebra (*see also* Osteoporosis) 733.00

Thirst, excessive 783.5
- due to deprivation of water 994.3

Thomsen's disease 359.2

Thomson's disease (congenital poikiloderma) 757.33

Thoracic - *see also* condition
- kidney 753.3
- outlet syndrome 353.0
- stomach - *see* Hernia, diaphragm

Thoracogastroschisis (congenital) 759.89

Thoracopagus 759.4

Thoracoschisis 756.3

Thoracoscopic surgical procedure converted to open procedure V64.42

Thorax - *see* condition

Thorn's syndrome (*see also* Disease, renal) 593.9

Thornwaldt's, Tornwaldt's
- bursitis (pharyngeal) 478.29
- cyst 478.26
- disease (pharyngeal bursitis) 478.29

Thorson-Biörck syndrome (malignant carcinoid) 259.2

Threadworm (infection) (infestation) 127.4

Threatened
- abortion or miscarriage 640.0
  - with subsequent abortion (*see also* Abortion, spontaneous) 634.9
  - affecting fetus 762.1
- labor 644.1
  - affecting fetus or newborn 761.8
  - premature 644.0
- miscarriage 640.0
  - affecting fetus 762.1
- premature
  - delivery 644.2
    - affecting fetus or newborn 761.8
  - labor 644.0
    - before 22 completed weeks of gestation 640.0

Three-day fever 066.0

Threshers' lung 495.0

Thrix annulata (congenital) 757.4

Throat - *see* condition

Thrombasthenia (Glanzmann's) (hemorrhagic) (hereditary) 287.1

Thromboangiitis 443.1
- obliterans (general) 443.1
  - cerebral 437.1
  - vessels
    - brain 437.1
    - spinal cord 437.1

Thromboarteritis - *see* Arteritis

Thromboasthenia (Glanzmann's) (hemorrhagic) (hereditary) 287.1

Thrombocytasthenia (Glanzmann's) 287.1

Thrombocythemia (essential) (hemorrhagic) (primary) (M9962/1) 238.7
- idiopathic (M9962/1) 238.7

Thrombocytopathy (dystrophic) (granulopenic) 287.1

Thrombocytopenia, thrombocytopenic 287.5
- with giant hemangioma 287.3
- amegakaryocytic, congenital 287.3
- congenital 287.3
- cyclic 287.3
- dilutional 287.4
- due to
  - drugs 287.4
  - extracorporeal circulation of blood 287.4
  - massive blood transfusion 287.4
  - platelet alloimmunization 287.4
- essential 287.3
- hereditary 287.3
- Kasabach-Merritt 287.3
- neonatal, transitory 776.1
  - due to
    - exchange transfusion 776.1
    - idiopathic maternal thrombocytopenia 776.1
    - isoimmunization 776.1
- primary 287.3
- puerperal, postpartum 666.3
- purpura (*see also* Purpura, thrombocytopenic) 287.3
  - thrombotic 446.6
- secondary 287.4
- sex-linked 287.3

Thrombocytosis, essential 289.9

Thromboembolism - *see* Embolism

Thrombopathy (Bernard-Soulier) 287.1
- constitutional 286.4
- Willebrand-Jürgens (angiohemophilia) 286.4

Thrombopenia (*see also* Thrombocytopenia) 287.5

◀ New ⬅ Revised Code

ICD-9-CM
T
Vol. 2

Note Use the following fifth-digit subclassification with category 242:

0 without mention of thyrotoxic crisis or storm
1 with mention of thyrotoxic crisis or storm

ICD-9-CM
T
Vol. 2

◀ New ⟸ Revised Code

Note Use the following fifth-digit subclassification with categories 010-018:

0 unspecified
1 bacteriological or histological examination not done
2 bacteriological or histological examination unknown (at present)
3 tubercle bacilli found (in sputum) by microscopy
4 tubercle bacilli not found (in sputum) by microscopy, but found by bacterial culture
5 tubercle bacilli not found by bacteriological examination, but tuberculosis confirmed histologically
6 tubercle bacilli not found by bacteriological or histological examination, but tuberculosis confirmed by other methods [inoculation of animals]

For tuberculous conditions specified as late effects or sequelae, *see* category 137.

◀ New ⟸ Revised Code

ICD-9-CM
T
Vol. 2

ICD-9-CM
T
Vol. 2

ICD-9-CM
T
Vol. 2

U

Note Use the following fifth-digit subclassification with categories 531-534:

0 without mention of obstruction
1 with obstruction

V

ICD-9-CM V Vol. 2

W

X

Y

Z

SECTION II TABLE OF DRUGS AND CHEMICALS

ALPHABETIC INDEX TO POISONING AND EXTERNAL CAUSES OF ADVERSE EFFECTS OF DRUGS AND OTHER CHEMICAL SUBSTANCES

This table contains a classification of drugs and other chemical substances to identify poisoning states and external causes of adverse effects.

Each of the listed substances in the table is assigned a code according to the poisoning classification (960-989). These codes are used when there is a statement of poisoning, overdose, wrong substance given or taken, or intoxication.

The table also contains a listing of external causes of adverse effects. An adverse effect is a pathologic manifestation due to ingestion or exposure to drugs or other chemical substances (e.g., dermatitis, hypersensitivity reaction, aspirin gastritis). The adverse effect is to be identified by the appropriate code found in Section I, Index to Diseases and Injuries. An external cause code can then be used to identify the circumstances involved. The table headings pertaining to external causes are defined below:

Accidental poisoning (E850-E869)-accidental overdose of drug, wrong substance given or taken, drug taken inadvertently, accidents in the usage of drugs and biologicals in medical and surgical procedures, and to show external causes of poisonings classifiable to 980-989.

Therapeutic use (E930-E949)-a correct substance properly administered in therapeutic or prophylactic dosage as the external cause of adverse effects.

Suicide attempt (E950-E952)-instances in which self-inflicted injuries or poisonings are involved.

Assault (E961-E962)-injury or poisoning inflicted by another person with the intent to injure or kill.

Undetermined (E980-E982)-to be used when the intent of the poisoning or injury cannot be determined whether it was intentional or accidental.

The American Hospital Formulary Service (AHFS) list numbers are included in the table to help classify new drugs not identified in the table by name. The AHFS list numbers are keyed to the continually revised AHFS (American Hospital Formulary Service, 2 vol. Washington, D.C.: American Society of Hospital Pharmacists, 1959-). These listings are found in the table under the main term **Drug.**

Excluded from the table are radium and other radioactive substances. The classification of adverse effects and complications pertaining to these substances will be found in Index to Diseases and Injuries, and Index to External Causes of Injuries.

Although certain substances are indexed with one or more subentries, the majority are listed according to one use or state. It is recognized that many substances may be used in various ways, in medicine and in industry, and may cause adverse effects whatever the state of the agent (solid, liquid, or fumes arising from a liquid). In cases in which the reported data indicate a use or state not in the table, or which is clearly different from the one listed, an attempt should be made to classify the substance in the form which most nearly expresses the reported facts.

Substance	Poisoning	External Cause (E-Code)				
		Accident	Therapeutic Use	Suicide Attempt	Assault	Undetermined
1-propanol	980.3	E860.4	—	E950.9	E962.1	E980.9
2-propanol	980.2	E860.3	—	E950.9	E962.1	E980.9
2,4-D (dichlorophenoxyacetic acid)	989.4	E863.5	—	E950.6	E962.1	E980.7
2,4-toluene diisocyanate	983.0	E864.0	—	E950.7	E962.1	E980.6
2,4,5-T (trichlorophenoxyacetic acid)	989.2	E863.5	—	E950.6	E962.1	E980.7
14-hydroxydihydromorphinone	965.09	E850.2	E935.2	E950.0	E962.0	E980.0
ABOB	961.7	E857	E931.7	E950.4	E962.0	E980.4
Abrus (seed)	988.2	E865.3	—	E950.9	E962.1	E980.9
Absinthe	980.0	E860.1	—	E950.9	E962.1	E980.9
beverage	980.0	E860.0	—	E950.9	E962.1	E980.9
Acenocoumarin, acenocoumarol	964.2	E858.2	E934.2	E950.4	E962.0	E980.4
Acepromazine	969.1	E853.0	E939.1	E950.3	E962.0	E980.3
Acetal	982.8	E862.4	—	E950.9	E962.1	E980.9
Acetaldehyde (vapor)	987.8	E869.8	—	E952.8	E962.2	E982.8
liquid	989.89	E866.8	—	E950.9	E962.1	E980.9
Acetaminophen	965.4	E850.4	E935.4	E950.0	E962.0	E980.0
Acetaminosalol	965.1	E850.3	E935.3	E950.0	E962.0	E980.0
Acetanilid(e)	965.4	E850.4	E935.4	E950.0	E962.0	E980.0
Acetarsol, acetarsone	961.1	E857	E931.1	E950.4	E962.0	E980.4
Acetazolamide	974.2	E858.5	E944.2	E950.4	E962.0	E980.4
Acetic	—	—	—	—	—	—
acid	983.1	E864.1	—	E950.7	E962.1	E980.6
with sodium acetate (ointment)	976.3	E858.7	E946.3	E950.4	E962.0	E980.4
irrigating solution	974.5	E858.5	E944.5	E950.4	E962.0	E980.4
lotion	976.2	E858.7	E946.2	E950.4	E962.0	E980.4
anhydride	983.1	E864.1	—	E950.7	E962.1	E980.6
ether (vapor)	982.8	E862.4	—	E950.9	E962.1	E980.9
Acetohexamide	962.3	E858.0	E932.3	E950.4	E962.0	E980.4
Acetomenaphthone	964.3	E858.2	E934.3	E950.4	E962.0	E980.4
Acetomorphine	965.01	E850.0	E935.0	E950.0	E962.0	E980.0
Acetone (oils) (vapor)	982.8	E862.4	—	E950.9	E962.1	E980.9
Acetophenazine (maleate)	969.1	E853.0	E939.1	E950.3	E962.0	E980.3
Acetophenetidin	965.4	E850.4	E935.4	E950.0	E962.0	E980.0
Acetophenone	982.0	E862.4	—	E950.9	E962.1	E980.9
Acetorphine	965.09	E850.2	E935.2	E950.0	E962.0	E980.0
Acetosulfone (sodium)	961.8	E857	E931.8	E950.4	E962.0	E980.4
Acetrizoate (sodium)	977.8	E858.8	E947.8	E950.4	E962.0	E980.4
Acetylcarbromal	967.3	E852.2	E937.3	E950.2	E962.0	E980.2
Acetylcholine (chloride)	971.0	E855.3	E941.0	E950.4	E962.0	E980.4
Acetylcysteine	975.5	E858.6	E945.5	E950.4	E962.0	E980.4
Acetyldigitoxin	972.1	E858.3	E942.1	E950.4	E962.0	E980.4
Acetyldihydrocodeine	965.09	E850.2	E935.2	E950.0	E962.0	E980.0
Acetyldihydrocodeinone	965.09	E850.2	E935.2	E950.0	E962.0	E980.0
Acetylene (gas) (industrial)	987.1	E868.1	—	E951.8	E962.2	E981.8
incomplete combustion of - *see* Carbon monoxide, fuel, utility	—	—	—	—	—	—
tetrachloride (vapor)	982.3	E862.4	—	E950.9	E962.1	E980.9
Acetyliodosalicylic acid	965.1	E850.3	E935.3	E950.0	E962.0	E980.0
Acetylphenylhydrazine	965.8	E850.8	E935.8	E950.0	E962.0	E980.0
Acetylsalicylic acid	965.1	E850.3	E935.3	E950.0	E962.0	E980.0
Achromycin	960.4	E856	E930.4	E950.4	E962.0	E980.4
ophthalmic preparation	976.5	E858.7	E946.5	E950.4	E962.0	E980.4
topical NEC	976.0	E858.7	E946.0	E950.4	E962.0	E980.4
Acidifying agents	963.2	E858.1	E933.2	E950.4	E962.0	E980.4
Acids (corrosive) NEC	983.1	E864.1	—	E950.7	E962.1	E980.6
Aconite (wild)	988.2	E865.4	—	E950.9	E962.1	E980.9
Aconitine (liniment)	976.8	E858.7	E946.8	E950.4	E962.0	E980.4
Aconitum ferox	988.2	E865.4	—	E950.9	E962.1	E980.9
Acridine	983.0	E864.0	—	E950.7	E962.1	E980.6
vapor	987.8	E869.8	—	E952.8	E962.2	E982.8
Acriflavine	961.9	E857	E931.9	E950.4	E962.0	E980.4
Acrisorcin	976.0	E858.7	E946.0	E950.4	E962.0	E980.4

Substance	Poisoning	External Cause (E-Code) Accident	Therapeutic Use	Suicide Attempt	Assault	Undetermined
Acrolein (gas)	987.8	E869.8	—	E952.8	E962.2	E982.8
liquid	989.89	E866.8	—	E950.9	E962.1	E980.9
Actaea spicata	988.2	E865.4	—	E950.9	E962.1	E980.9
Acterol	961.5	E857	E931.5	E950.4	E962.0	E980.4
ACTH	962.4	E858.0	E932.4	E950.4	E962.0	E980.4
Acthar	962.4	E858.0	E932.4	E950.4	E962.0	E980.4
Actinomycin (C) (D)	960.7	E856	E930.7	E950.4	E962.0	E980.4
Adalin (acetyl)	967.3	E852.2	E937.3	E950.2	E962.0	E980.2
Adenosine (phosphate)	977.8	E858.8	E947.8	E950.4	E962.0	E980.4
Adhesives	989.89	E866.6	—	E950.9	E962.1	E980.9
ADH	962.5	E858.0	E932.5	E950.4	E962.0	E980.4
Adicillin	960.0	E856	E930.0	E950.4	E962.0	E980.4
Adiphenine	975.1	E855.6	E945.1	E950.4	E962.0	E980.4
Adjunct, pharmaceutical	977.4	E858.8	E947.4	E950.4	E962.0	E980.4
Adrenal (extract, cortex or medulla) (glucocorticoids) (hormones) (mineralocorticoids)	962.0	E858.0	E932.0	E950.4	E962.0	E980.4
ENT agent	976.6	E858.7	E946.6	E950.4	E962.0	E980.4
ophthalmic preparation	976.5	E858.7	E946.5	E950.4	E962.0	E980.4
topical NEC	976.0	E858.7	E946.0	E950.4	E962.0	E980.4
Adrenalin	971.2	E855.5	E941.2	E950.4	E962.0	E980.4
Adrenergic blocking agents	971.3	E855.6	E941.3	E950.4	E962.0	E980.4
Adrenergics	971.2	E855.5	E941.2	E950.4	E962.0	E980.4
Adrenochrome (derivatives)	972.8	E858.3	E942.8	E950.4	E962.0	E980.4
Adrenocorticotropic hormone	962.4	E858.0	E932.4	E950.4	E962.0	E980.4
Adrenocorticotropin	962.4	E858.0	E932.4	E950.4	E962.0	E980.4
Adriamycin	960.7	E856	E930.7	E950.4	E962.0	E980.4
Aerosol spray - *see* Sprays	—	—	—	—	—	—
Aerosporin	960.8	E856	E930.8	E950.4	E962.0	E980.4
ENT agent	976.6	E858.7	E946.6	E950.4	E962.0	E980.4
ophthalmic preparation	976.5	E858.7	E946.5	E950.4	E962.0	E980.4
topical NEC	976.0	E858.7	E946.0	E950.4	E962.0	E980.4
Aethusa cynapium	988.2	E865.4	—	E950.9	E962.1	E980.9
Afghanistan black	969.6	E854.1	E939.6	E950.3	E962.0	E980.3
Aflatoxin	989.7	E865.9	—	E950.9	E962.1	E980.9
African boxwood	988.2	E865.4	—	E950.9	E962.1	E980.9
Agar (-agar)	973.3	E858.4	E943.3	E950.4	E962.0	E980.4
Agricultural agent NEC	989.89	E863.9	—	E950.6	E962.1	E980.7
Agrypnal	967.0	E851	E937.0	E950.1	E962.0	E980.1
Air contaminant(s), source or type not specified	—	—	—	—	—	—
specified type - *see* specific substance	987.9	E869.9	—	E952.9	E962.2	E982.9
Akee	988.2	E865.4	—	E950.9	E962.1	E980.9
Akrinol	976.0	E858.7	E946.0	E950.4	E962.0	E980.4
Alantolactone	961.6	E857	E931.6	E950.4	E962.0	E980.4
Albamycin	960.8	E856	E930.8	E950.4	E962.0	E980.4
Albumin (normal human serum)	964.7	E858.2	E934.7	E950.4	E962.0	E980.4
Albuterol	975.7	E858.6	E945.7	E950.4	E962.0	E980.4
Alcohol	980.9	E860.9	—	E950.9	E962.1	E980.9
absolute	980.0	E860.1	—	E950.9	E962.1	E980.9
beverage	980.0	E860.0	E947.8	E950.9	E962.1	E980.9
amyl	980.3	E860.4	—	E950.9	E962.1	E980.9
antifreeze	980.1	E860.2	—	E950.9	E962.1	E980.9
butyl	980.3	E860.4	—	E950.9	E962.1	E980.9
dehydrated	980.0	E860.1	—	E950.9	E862.1	E980.9
beverage	980.0	E860.0	E947.8	E950.9	E962.1	E980.9
denatured	980.0	E860.1	—	E950.9	E962.1	E980.9
deterrents	977.3	E858.8	E947.3	E950.4	E962.0	E980.4
diagnostic (gastric function)	977.8	E858.8	E947.8	E950.4	E962.0	E980.4
ethyl	980.0	E860.1	—	E950.9	E962.1	E980.9
beverage	980.0	E860.0	E947.8	E950.9	E962.1	E980.9
grain	980.0	E860.1	—	E950.9	E962.1	E980.9
beverage	980.0	E860.0	E947.8	E950.9	E962.1	E980.9
industrial	980.9	E860.9	—	E950.9	E962.1	E980.9

◀ New ⟸ Revised Code

Substance	Poisoning	External Cause (E-Code)				
		Accident	Therapeutic Use	Suicide Attempt	Assault	Undetermined
Alcohol *(Continued)*						
isopropyl	980.2	E860.3	—	E950.9	E962.1	E980.9
methyl	980.1	E860.2	—	E950.9	E962.1	E980.9
preparation for consumption	980.0	E860.0	E947.8	E950.9	E962.1	E980.9
propyl	980.3	E860.4	—	E950.9	E962.1	E980.9
secondary	980.2	E860.3	—	E950.9	E962.1	E980.9
radiator	980.1	E860.2	—	E950.9	E962.1	E980.9
rubbing	980.2	E860.3	—	E950.9	E962.1	E980.9
specified type NEC	980.8	E860.8	—	E950.9	E962.1	E980.9
surgical	980.9	E860.9	—	E950.9	E962.1	E980.9
vapor (from any type of alcohol)	987.8	E869.8	—	E952.8	E962.2	E982.8
wood	980.1	E860.2	—	E950.9	E962.1	E980.9
Alcuronium chloride	975.2	E858.6	E945.2	E950.4	E962.0	E980.4
Aldactone	974.4	E858.5	E944.4	E950.4	E962.0	E980.4
Aldicarb	989.3	E863.2	—	E950.6	E962.1	E980.7
Aldomet	972.6	E858.3	E942.6	E950.4	E962.0	E980.4
Aldosterone	962.0	E858.0	E932.0	E950.4	E962.0	E980.4
Aldrin (dust)	989.2	E863.0	—	E950.6	E962.1	E980.7
Aleve - *see* Naproxen	—	—	—	—	—	—
Algeldrate	973.0	E858.4	E943.0	E950.4	E962.0	E980.4
Alidase	963.4	E858.1	E933.4	E950.4	E962.0	E980.4
Aliphatic thiocyanates	989.0	E866.8	—	E950.9	E962.1	E980.9
Alkaline antiseptic solution (aromatic)	976.6	E858.7	E946.6	E950.4	E962.0	E980.4
Alkalinizing agents (medicinal)	963.3	E858.1	E933.3	E950.4	E962.0	E980.4
Alkalis, caustic	983.2	E864.2	—	E950.7	E962.1	E980.6
Alkalizing agents (medicinal)	963.3	E858.1	E933.3	E950.4	E962.0	E980.4
Alka-seltzer	965.1	E850.3	E935.3	E950.0	E962.0	E980.0
Alkavervir	972.6	E858.3	E942.6	E950.4	E962.0	E980.4
Allegron	969.0	E854.0	E939.0	E950.3	E962.0	E980.3
Allobarbital, allobarbitone	967.0	E851	E937.0	E950.1	E962.0	E980.1
Allopurinol	974.7	E858.5	E944.7	E950.4	E962.0	E980.4
Allylestrenol	962.2	E858.0	E932.2	E950.4	E962.0	E980.4
Allylisopropylacetylurea	967.8	E852.8	E937.8	E950.2	E962.0	E980.2
Allylisopropylmalonylurea	967.0	E851	E937.0	E950.1	E962.0	E980.1
Allyltribromide	967.3	E852.2	E937.3	E950.2	E962.0	E980.2
Aloe, aloes, aloin	973.1	E858.4	E943.1	E950.4	E962.0	E980.4
Alosetron	973.8	E858.4	E943.8	E950.4	E962.0	E980.4
Aloxidone	966.0	E855.0	E936.0	E950.4	E962.0	E980.4
Aloxiprin	965.1	E850.3	E935.3	E950.0	E962.0	E980.0
Alpha amylase	963.4	E858.1	E933.4	E950.4	E962.0	E980.4
Alphaprodine (hydrochloride)	965.09	E850.2	E935.2	E950.0	E962.0	E980.0
Alpha tocopherol	963.5	E858.1	E933.5	E950.4	E962.0	E980.4
Alseroxylon	972.6	E858.3	E942.6	E950.4	E962.0	E980.4
Alum (ammonium) (potassium)	983.2	E864.2	—	E950.7	E962.1	E980.6
medicinal (astringent) NEC	976.2	E858.7	E946.2	E950.4	E962.0	E980.4
Aluminium, aluminum (gel) (hydroxide)	973.0	E858.4	E943.0	E950.4	E962.0	E980.4
acetate solution	976.2	E858.7	E946.2	E950.4	E962.0	E980.4
aspirin	965.1	E850.3	E935.3	E950.0	E962.0	E980.0
carbonate	973.0	E858.4	E943.0	E950.4	E962.0	E980.4
glycinate	973.0	E858.4	E943.0	E950.4	E962.0	E980.4
nicotinate	972.2	E858.3	E942.2	E950.4	E962.0	E980.4
ointment (surgical) (topical)	976.3	E858.7	E946.3	E950.4	E962.0	E980.4
phosphate	973.0	E858.4	E943.0	E950.4	E962.0	E980.4
subacetate	976.2	E858.7	E946.2	E950.4	E962.0	E980.4
topical NEC	976.3	E858.7	E946.3	E950.4	E962.0	E980.4
Alurate	967.0	E851	E937.0	E950.1	E962.0	E980.1
Alverine (citrate)	975.1	E858.6	E945.1	E950.4	E962.0	E980.4
Alvodine	965.09	E850.2	E935.2	E950.0	E962.0	E980.0
Amanita phalloides	988.1	E865.5	—	E950.9	E962.1	E980.9
Amantadine (hydrochloride)	966.4	E855.0	E936.4	E950.4	E962.0	E980.4
Ambazone	961.9	E857	E931.9	E950.4	E962.0	E980.4
Ambenonium	971.0	E855.3	E941.0	E950.4	E962.0	E980.4

Substance	Poisoning	External Cause (E-Code) Accident	Therapeutic Use	Suicide Attempt	Assault	Undetermined
Ambutonium bromide	971.1	E855.4	E941.1	E950.4	E962.0	E990.4
Ametazole	977.8	E858.8	E947.8	E950.4	E962.0	E980.4
Amethocaine (infiltration) (topical)	968.5	E855.2	E938.5	E950.4	E962.0	E980.4
nerve block (peripheral) (plexus)	968.6	E855.2	E938.6	E950.4	E962.0	E980.4
spinal	968.7	E855.2	E938.7	E950.4	E962.0	E980.4
Amethopterin	963.1	E858.1	E933.1	E950.4	E962.0	E980.4
Amfepramone	977.0	E858.8	E947.0	E950.4	E962.0	E980.4
Amidone	965.02	E850.1	E935.1	E950.0	E962.0	E980.0
Amidopyrine	965.5	E850.5	E935.5	E950.0	E962.0	E980.0
Aminacrine	976.0	E858.7	E946.0	E950.4	E962.0	E980.4
Aminitrozole	961.5	E857	E931.5	E950.4	E962.0	E980.4
Aminoacetic acid	974.5	E858.5	E944.5	E950.4	E962.0	E980.4
Amino acids	974.5	E858.5	E944.5	E950.4	E962.0	E980.4
Aminocaproic acid	964.4	E858.2	E934.4	E950.4	E962.0	E980.4
Aminoethylisothiourium	963.8	E858.1	E933.8	E950.4	E962.0	E980.4
Aminoglutethimide	966.3	E855.0	E936.3	E950.4	E962.0	E980.4
Aminometradine	974.3	E858.5	E944.3	E950.4	E962.0	E980.4
Aminopentamide	971.1	E855.4	E941.1	E950.4	E962.0	E980.4
Aminophenazone	965.5	E850.5	E935.5	E950.0	E962.0	E980.0
Aminophenol	983.0	E864.0	—	E950.7	E962.1	E980.6
Aminophenylpyridone	969.5	E853.8	E939.5	E950.3	E962.0	E980.3
Aminophylline	975.7	E858.6	E945.7	E950.4	E962.0	E980.4
Aminopterin	963.1	E858.1	E933.1	E950.4	E962.0	E980.4
Aminopyrine	965.5	E850.5	E935.5	E950.0	E962.0	E980.0
Aminosalicylic acid	961.8	E857	E931.8	E950.4	E962.0	E980.4
Amiphenazole	970.1	E854.3	E940.1	E950.4	E962.0	E980.4
Amiquinsin	972.6	E858.3	E942.6	E950.4	E962.0	E980.4
Amisometradine	974.3	E858.5	E944.3	E950.4	E962.0	E980.4
Amitriptyline	969.0	E854.0	E939.0	E950.3	E962.0	E980.3
Ammonia (fumes) (gas) (vapor)	987.8	E869.8	—	E952.8	E962.2	E982.8
liquid (household) NEC	983.2	E861.4	—	E950.7	E962.1	E980.6
spirit, aromatic	970.8	E854.3	E940.8	E950.4	E962.0	E980.4
Ammoniated mercury	976.0	E858.7	E946.0	E950.4	E962.0	E980.4
Ammonium	—	—	—	—	—	—
carbonate	983.2	E864.2	—	E950.7	E962.1	E980.6
chloride (acidifying agent)	963.2	E858.1	E933.2	E950.4	E962.0	E980.4
expectorant	975.5	E858.6	E945.5	E950.4	E962.0	E980.4
compounds (household) NEC	983.2	E861.4	—	E950.7	E962.1	E980.6
fumes (any usage)	987.8	E869.8	—	E952.8	E962.2	E982.8
industrial	983.2	E864.2	—	E950.7	E962.1	E980.6
ichthosulfonate	976.4	E858.7	E946.4	E950.4	E962.0	E980.4
mandelate	961.9	E857	E931.9	E950.4	E962.0	E980.4
Amobarbital	967.0	E851	E937.0	E950.1	E962.0	E980.1
Amodiaquin(e)	961.4	E857	E931.4	E950.4	E962.0	E980.4
Amopyroquin(e)	961.4	E857	E931.4	E950.4	E962.0	E980.4
Amphenidone	969.5	E853.8	E939.5	E950.3	E962.0	E980.3
Amphetamine	969.7	E854.2	E939.7	E950.3	E962.0	E980.3
Amphomycin	960.8	E856	E930.8	E950.4	E962.0	E980.4
Amphotericin B	960.1	E856	E930.1	E950.4	E962.0	E980.4
topical	976.0	E858.7	E946.0	E950.4	E962.0	E980.4
Ampicillin	960.0	E856	E930.0	E950.4	E962.0	E980.4
Amprotropine	971.1	E855.4	E941.1	E950.4	E962.0	E980.4
Amygdalin	977.8	E858.8	E947.8	E950.4	E962.0	E980.4
Amyl	—	—	—	—	—	—
acetate (vapor)	982.8	E862.4	—	E950.9	E962.1	E980.9
alcohol	980.3	E860.4	—	E950.9	E962.1	E980.9
nitrite (medicinal)	972.4	E858.3	E942.4	E950.4	E962.0	E980.4
Amylase (alpha)	963.4	E858.1	E933.4	E950.4	E962.0	E980.4
Amylene hydrate	980.8	E860.8	—	E950.9	E962.1	E980.9
Amylobarbitone	967.0	E851	E937.0	E950.1	E962.0	E980.1
Amylocaine	968.9	E855.2	E938.9	E950.4	E962.0	E980.4

◀ New ⟸ Revised Code

Substance	Poisoning	External Cause (E-Code) Accident	Therapeutic Use	Suicide Attempt	Assault	Undetermined
Amylocaine *(Continued)*						
infiltration (subcutaneous)	968.5	E855.2	E938.5	E950.4	E962.0	E980.4
nerve block (peripheral) (plexus)	968.6	E855.2	E938.6	E950.4	E962.0	E980.4
spinal	968.7	E855.2	E938.7	E950.4	E962.0	E980.4
topical (surface)	968.5	E855.2	E938.5	E950.4	E962.0	E980.4
Amytal (sodium)	967.0	E851	E937.0	E950.1	E962.0	E980.1
Analeptics	970.0	E854.3	E940.0	E950.4	E962.0	E980.4
Analgesics	965.9	E850.9	E935.9	E950.0	E962.0	E980.0
aromatic NEC	965.4	E850.4	E935.4	E950.0	E962.0	E980.0
non-narcotic NEC	965.7	E850.7	E935.7	E950.0	E962.0	E980.0
specified NEC	965.8	E850.8	E935.8	E950.0	E962.0	E980.0
Anamirta cocculus	988.2	E865.3	—	E950.9	E962.1	E980.9
Ancillin	960.0	E856	E930.0	E950.4	E962.0	E980.4
Androgens (anabolic congeners)	962.1	E858.0	E932.1	E950.4	E962.0	E980.4
Androstalone	962.1	E858.0	E932.1	E950.4	E962.0	E980.4
Androsterone	962.1	E858.0	E932.1	E950.4	E962.0	E980.4
Anemone pulsatilla	988.2	E865.4	—	E950.9	E962.1	E980.9
Anesthesia, anesthetic (general) NEC	968.4	E855.1	E938.4	E950.4	E962.0	E980.4
block (nerve) (plexus)	968.6	E855.2	E938.6	E950.4	E962.0	E980.4
gaseous NEC	968.2	E855.1	E938.2	E950.4	E962.0	E980.4
halogenated hydrocarbon derivatives NEC	968.2	E855.1	E938.2	E950.4	E962.0	E980.4
infiltration (intradermal) (subcutaneous) (submucosal)	968.5	E855.2	E938.5	E950.4	E962.0	E980.4
intravenous	968.3	E855.1	E938.3	E950.4	E962.0	E980.4
local NEC	968.9	E855.2	E938.9	E950.4	E962.0	E980.4
nerve blocking (peripheral) (plexus)	968.6	E855.2	E938.6	E950.4	E962.0	E980.4
rectal NEC	968.3	E855.1	E938.3	E950.4	E962.0	E980.4
spinal	968.7	E855.2	E938.7	E950.4	E962.0	E980.4
surface	968.5	E855.2	E938.5	E950.4	E962.0	E980.4
topical	968.5	E855.2	E938.5	E950.4	E962.0	E980.4
Aneurine	963.5	E858.1	E933.5	E950.4	E962.0	E980.4
Angio-Conray	977.8	E858.8	E947.8	E950.4	E962.0	E980.4
Angiotensin	971.2	E855.5	E941.2	E950.4	E962.0	E980.4
Anhydrohydroxyprogesterone	962.2	E858.0	E932.2	E950.4	E962.0	E980.4
Anhydron	974.3	E858.5	E944.3	E950.4	E962.0	E980.4
Anileridine	965.09	E850.2	E935.2	E950.0	E962.0	E980.0
Aniline (dye) (liquid)	983.0	E864.0	—	E950.7	E962.1	E980.6
analgesic	965.4	E850.4	E935.4	E950.0	E962.0	E980.0
derivatives, therapeutic NEC	965.4	E850.4	E935.4	E950.0	E962.0	E980.0
vapor	987.8	E869.8	—	E952.8	E962.2	E982.8
Aniscoropine	971.1	E855.4	E941.1	E950.4	E962.0	E980.4
Anisindione	964.2	E858.2	E934.2	E950.4	E962.0	E980.4
Anorexic agents	977.0	E858.8	E947.0	E950.4	E962.0	E980.4
Ant (bite) (sting)	989.5	E905.5	—	E950.9	E962.1	E980.9
Antabuse	977.3	E858.8	E947.3	E950.4	E962.0	E980.4
Antacids	973.0	E858.4	E943.0	E950.4	E962.0	E980.4
Antazoline	963.0	E858.1	E933.0	E950.4	E962.0	E980.4
Anthelmintics	961.6	E857	E931.6	E950.4	E962.0	E980.4
Anthralin	976.4	E858.7	E946.4	E950.4	E962.0	E980.4
Anthramycin	960.7	E856	E930.7	E950.4	E962.0	E980.4
Antiadrenergics	971.3	E855.6	E941.3	E950.4	E962.0	E980.4
Antiallergic agents	963.0	E858.1	E933.0	E950.4	E962.0	E980.4
Antianemic agents NEC	964.1	E858.2	E934.1	E950.4	E962.0	E980.4
Antiaris toxicaria	988.2	E865.4	—	E950.9	E962.1	E980.9
Antiarteriosclerotic agents	972.2	E858.3	E942.2	E950.4	E962.0	E980.4
Antiasthmatics	975.7	E858.6	E945.7	E950.4	E962.0	E980.4
Antibiotics	960.9	E856	E930.9	E950.4	E962.0	E980.4
antifungal	960.1	E856	E930.1	E950.4	E962.0	E980.4
antimycobacterial	960.6	E856	E930.6	E950.4	E962.0	E980.4
antineoplastic	960.7	E856	E930.7	E950.4	E962.0	E980.4
cephalosporin (group)	960.5	E856	E930.5	E950.4	E962.0	E980.4
chloramphenicol (group)	960.2	E856	E930.2	E950.4	E962.0	E980.4
macrolides	960.3	E856	E930.3	E950.4	E962.0	E980.4

Substance	Poisoning	External Cause (E-Code) Accident	Therapeutic Use	Suicide Attempt	Assault	Undetermined
Antibiotics *(Continued)*						
specified NEC	960.8	E856	E930.8	E950.4	E962.0	E980.4
tetracycline (group)	960.4	E856	E930.4	E950.4	E962.0	E980.4
Anticancer agents NEC	963.1	E858.1	E933.1	E950.4	E962.0	E980.4
antibiotics	960.7	E856	E930.7	E950.4	E962.0	E980.4
Anticholinergics	971.1	E855.4	E941.1	E950.4	E962.0	E980.4
Anticholinesterase (organophosphorus) (reversible)	971.0	E855.3	E941.0	E950.4	E962.0	E980.4
Anticoagulants	964.2	E858.2	E934.2	E950.4	E962.0	E980.4
antagonists	964.5	E858.2	E934.5	E950.4	E962.0	E980.4
Anti-common cold agents NEC	975.6	E858.6	E945.6	E950.4	E962.0	E980.4
Anticonvulsants NEC	966.3	E855.0	E936.3	E950.4	E962.0	E980.4
Antidepressants	969.0	E854.0	E939.0	E950.3	E962.0	E980.3
Antidiabetic agents	962.3	E858.0	E932.3	E950.4	E962.0	E980.4
Antidiarrheal agents	973.5	E858.4	E943.5	E950.4	E962.0	E980.4
Antidiuretic hormone	962.5	E858.0	E932.5	E950.4	E962.0	E980.4
Antidotes NEC	977.2	E858.8	E947.2	E950.4	E962.0	E980.4
Antiemetic agents	963.0	E858.1	E933.0	E950.4	E962.0	E980.4
Antiepilepsy agent NEC	966.3	E855.0	E936.3	E950.4	E962.0	E980.4
Antifertility pills	962.2	E858.0	E932.2	E950.4	E962.0	E980.4
Antiflatulents	973.8	E858.4	E943.8	E950.4	E962.0	E980.4
Antifreeze	989.89	E866.8	—	E950.9	E962.1	E980.9
alcohol	980.1	E860.2	—	E950.9	E962.1	E980.9
ethylene glycol	982.8	E862.4	—	E950.9	E962.1	E980.9
Antifungals (nonmedicinal) (sprays)	989.4	E863.6	—	E950.6	E962.1	E980.7
medicinal NEC	961.9	E857	E931.9	E950.4	E962.0	E980.4
antibiotic	960.1	E856	E930.1	E950.4	E962.0	E980.4
topical	976.0	E858.7	E946.0	E950.4	E962.0	E980.4
Antigastric secretion agents	973.0	E858.4	E943.0	E950.4	E962.0	E980.4
Antihelmintics	961.6	E857	E931.6	E950.4	E962.0	E980.4
Antihemophilic factor (human)	964.7	E858.2	E934.7	E950.4	E962.0	E980.4
Antihistamine	963.0	E858.1	E933.0	E950.4	E962.0	E980.4
Antihypertensive agents NEC	972.6	E858.3	E942.6	E950.4	E962.0	E980.4
Anti-infectives NEC	961.9	E857	E931.9	E950.4	E962.0	E980.4
antibiotics	960.9	E856	E930.9	E950.4	E962.0	E980.4
specified NEC	960.8	E856	E930.8	E950.4	E962.0	E980.4
anthelmintic	961.6	E857	E931.6	E950.4	E962.0	E980.4
antimalarial	961.4	E857	E931.4	E950.4	E962.0	E980.4
antimycobacterial NEC	961.8	E857	E931.8	E950.4	E962.0	E980.4
antibiotics	960.6	E856	E930.6	E950.4	E962.0	E980.4
antiprotozoal NEC	961.5	E857	E931.5	E950.4	E962.0	E980.4
blood	961.4	E857	E931.4	E950.4	E962.0	E980.4
antiviral	961.7	E857	E931.7	E950.4	E962.0	E980.4
arsenical	961.1	E857	E931.1	E950.4	E962.0	E980.4
ENT agents	976.6	E858.7	E946.6	E950.4	E962.0	E980.4
heavy metals NEC	961.2	E857	E931.2	E950.4	E962.0	E980.4
local	976.0	E858.7	E946.0	E950.4	E962.0	E980.4
ophthalmic preparation	976.5	E858.7	E946.5	E950.4	E962.0	E980.4
topical NEC	976.0	E858.7	E946.0	E950.4	E962.0	E980.4
Anti-inflammatory agents (topical)	976.0	E858.7	E946.0	E950.4	E962.0	E980.4
Antiknock (tetraethyl lead)	984.1	E862.1	—	E950.9	E962.1	E980.9
Antilipemics	972.2	E858.3	E942.2	E950.4	E962.0	E980.4
Antimalarials	961.4	E857	E931.4	E950.4	E962.0	E980.4
Antimony (compounds) (vapor) NEC	985.4	E866.2	—	E950.9	E962.1	E980.9
anti-infectives	961.2	E857	E931.2	E950.4	E962.0	E980.4
pesticides (vapor)	985.4	E863.4	—	E950.6	E962.2	E980.7
potassium tartrate	961.2	E857	E931.2	E950.4	E962.0	E980.4
tartrated	961.2	E857	E931.2	E950.4	E962.0	E980.4
Antimuscarinic agents	971.1	E855.4	E941.1	E950.4	E962.0	E980.4
Antimycobacterials NEC	961.8	E857	E931.8	E950.4	E962.0	E980.4
antibiotics	960.6	E856	E930.6	E950.4	E962.0	E980.4
Antineoplastic agents	963.1	E858.1	E933.1	E950.4	E962.0	E980.4
antibiotics	960.7	E856	E930.7	E950.4	E962.0	E980.4
Anti-Parkinsonism agents	966.4	E855.0	E936.4	E950.4	E962.0	E980.4

Substance	Poisoning	External Cause (E-Code) Accident	Therapeutic Use	Suicide Attempt	Assault	Undetermined
Antiphlogistics	965.69	E850.6	E935.6	E950.0	E962.0	E980.0
Antiprotozoals NEC	961.5	E857	E931.5	E950.4	E962.0	E980.4
blood	961.4	E857	E931.4	E950.4	E962.0	E980.4
Antipruritics (local)	976.1	E858.7	E946.1	E950.4	E962.0	E980.4
Antipsychotic agents NEC	969.3	E853.8	E939.3	E950.3	E962.0	E980.3
Antipyretics	965.9	E850.9	E935.9	E950.0	E962.0	E980.0
specified NEC	965.8	E850.8	E935.8	E950.0	E962.0	E980.0
Antipyrine	965.5	E850.5	E935.5	E950.0	E962.0	E980.0
Antirabies serum (equine)	979.9	E858.8	E949.9	E950.4	E962.0	E980.4
Antirheumatics	965.69	E850.6	E935.6	E950.0	E962.0	E980.0
Antiseborrheics	976.4	E858.7	E946.4	E950.4	E962.0	E980.4
Antiseptics (external) (medicinal)	976.0	E858.7	E946.0	E950.4	E962.0	E980.4
Antistine	963.0	E858.1	E933.0	E950.4	E962.0	E980.4
Antithyroid agents	962.8	E858.0	E932.8	E950.4	E962.0	E980.4
Antitoxin, any	979.9	E858.8	E949.9	E950.4	E962.0	E980.4
Antituberculars	961.8	E857	E931.8	E950.4	E962.0	E980.4
antibiotics	960.6	E856	E930.6	E950.4	E962.0	E980.4
Antitussives	975.4	E858.6	E945.4	E950.4	E962.0	E980.4
Antivaricose agents (sclerosing)	972.7	E858.3	E942.7	E950.4	E962.0	E980.4
Antivenin (crotaline) (spider-bite)	979.9	E858.8	E949.9	E950.4	E962.0	E980.4
Antivert	963.0	E858.1	E933.0	E950.4	E962.0	E980.4
Antivirals NEC	961.7	E857	E931.7	E950.4	E962.0	E980.4
Ant poisons - *see* Pesticides	—	—	—	—	—	—
Antrol	989.4	E863.4	—	E950.6	E962.1	E980.7
fungicide	989.4	E863.6	—	E950.6	E962.1	E980.7
Apomorphine hydrochloride (emetic)	973.6	E858.4	E943.6	E950.4	E962.0	E980.4
Appetite depressants, central	977.0	E858.8	E947.0	E950.4	E962.0	E980.4
Apresoline	972.6	E858.3	E942.6	E950.4	E962.0	E980.4
Aprobarbital, aprobarbitone	967.0	E851	E937.0	E950.1	E962.0	E980.1
Apronalide	967.8	E852.8	E937.8	E950.2	E962.0	E980.2
Aqua fortis	983.1	E864.1	—	E950.7	E962.1	E980.6
Arachis oil (topical)	976.3	E858.7	E946.3	E950.4	E962.0	E980.4
cathartic	973.2	E858.4	E943.2	E950.4	E962.0	E980.4
Aralen	961.4	E857	E931.4	E950.4	E962.0	E980.4
Arginine salts	974.5	E858.5	E944.5	E950.4	E962.0	E980.4
Argyrol	976.0	E858.7	E946.0	E950.4	E962.0	E980.4
ENT agent	976.6	E858.7	E946.6	E950.4	E962.0	E980.4
ophthalmic preparation	976.5	E858.7	E946.5	E950.4	E962.0	E980.4
Aristocort	962.0	E858.0	E932.0	E950.4	E962.0	E980.4
ENT agent	976.6	E858.7	E946.6	E950.4	E962.0	E980.4
ophthalmic preparation	976.5	E858.7	E946.5	E950.4	E962.0	E980.4
topical NEC	976.0	E858.7	E946.0	E950.4	E962.0	E980.4
Aromatics, corrosive	983.0	E864.0	—	E950.7	E962.1	E980.6
disinfectants	983.0	E861.4	—	E950.7	E962.1	E980.6
Arsenate of lead (insecticide)	985.1	E863.4	—	E950.8	E962.1	E980.8
herbicide	985.1	E863.5	—	E950.8	E962.1	E980.8
Arsenic, arsenicals (compounds) (dust) (fumes) (vapor) NEC	985.1	E866.3	—	E950.8	E962.1	E980.8
anti-infectives	961.1	E857	E931.1	E950.4	E962.0	E980.4
pesticide (dust) (fumes)	985.1	E863.4	—	E950.8	E962.1	E980.8
Arsine (gas)	985.1	E866.3	—	E950.8	E962.1	E980.8
Arsphenamine (silver)	961.1	E857	E931.1	E950.4	E962.0	E980.4
Arsthinol	961.1	E857	E931.1	E950.4	E962.0	E980.4
Artane	971.1	E855.4	E941.1	E950.4	E962.0	E980.4
Arthropod (venomous) NEC	989.5	E905.5	—	E950.9	E962.1	E980.9
Asbestos	989.81	E866.8	—	E950.9	E962.1	E980.9
Ascaridole	961.6	E857	E931.6	E950.4	E962.0	E980.4
Ascorbic acid	963.5	E858.1	E933.5	E950.4	E962.0	E980.4
Asiaticoside	976.0	E858.7	E946.0	E950.4	E962.0	E980.4
Aspidium (oleoresin)	961.6	E857	E931.6	E950.4	E962.0	E980.4
Aspirin	965.1	E850.3	E935.3	E950.0	E962.0	E980.0

Substance	Poisoning	External Cause (E-Code) Accident	Therapeutic Use	Suicide Attempt	Assault	Undetermined
Astringents (local)	976.2	E858.7	E946.2	E950.4	E962.0	E980.4
Atabrine	961.3	E857	E931.3	E950.4	E962.0	E980.4
Ataractics	969.5	E853.8	E939.5	E950.3	E962.0	E980.3
Atonia drug, intestinal	973.3	E858.4	E943.3	E950.4	E962.0	E980.4
Atophan	974.7	E858.5	E944.7	E950.4	E962.0	E980.4
Atropine	971.1	E855.4	E941.1	E950.4	E962.0	E980.4
Attapulgite	973.5	E858.4	E943.5	E950.4	E962.0	E980.4
Attenuvax	979.4	E858.8	E949.4	E950.4	E962.0	E980.4
Aureomycin	960.4	E856	E930.4	E950.4	E962.0	E980.4
ophthalmic preparation	976.5	E858.7	E946.5	E950.4	E962.0	E980.4
topical NEC	976.0	E858.7	E946.0	E950.4	E962.0	E980.4
Aurothioglucose	965.69	E850.6	E935.6	E950.0	E962.0	E980.0
Aurothioglycanide	965.69	E850.6	E935.6	E950.0	E962.0	E980.0
Aurothiomalate	965.69	E850.6	E935.6	E950.0	E962.0	E980.0
Automobile fuel	981	E862.1	—	E950.9	E962.1	E980.9
Autonomic nervous system agents NEC	971.9	E855.9	E941.9	E950.4	E962.0	E980.4
Avlosulfon	961.8	E857	E931.8	E950.4	E962.0	E980.4
Avomine	967.8	E852.8	E937.8	E950.2	E962.0	E980.2
Azacyclonol	969.5	E853.8	E939.5	E950.3	E962.0	E980.3
Azapetine	971.3	E855.6	E941.3	E950.4	E962.0	E980.4
Azaribine	963.1	E858.1	E933.1	E950.4	E962.0	E980.4
Azaserine	960.7	E856	E930.7	E950.4	E962.0	E980.4
Azathioprine	963.1	E858.1	E933.1	E950.4	E962.0	E980.4
Azosulfamide	961.0	E857	E931.0	E950.4	E962.0	E980.4
Azulfidine	961.0	E857	E931.0	E950.4	E962.0	E980.4
Azuresin	977.8	E858.8	E947.8	E950.4	E962.0	E980.4
Bacimycin	976.0	E858.7	E946.0	E950.4	E962.0	E980.4
ophthalmic preparation	976.5	E858.7	E946.5	E950.4	E962.0	E980.4
Bacitracin	960.8	E856	E930.8	E950.4	E962.0	E980.4
ENT agent	976.6	E858.7	E946.6	E950.4	E962.0	E980.4
ophthalmic preparation	976.5	E858.7	E946.5	E950.4	E962.0	E980.4
topical NEC	976.0	E858.7	E946.0	E950.4	E962.0	E980.4
Baking soda	963.3	E858.1	E933.3	E950.4	E962.0	E980.4
BAL	963.8	E858.1	E933.8	E950.4	E962.0	E980.4
Bamethan (sulfate)	972.5	E858.3	E942.5	E950.4	E962.0	E980.4
Bamipine	963.0	E858.1	E933.0	E950.4	E962.0	E980.4
Baneberry	988.2	E865.4	—	E950.9	E962.1	E980.9
Banewort	988.2	E865.4	—	E950.9	E962.1	E980.9
Barbenyl	967.0	E851	E937.0	E950.1	E962.0	E980.1
Barbital, barbitone	967.0	E851	E937.0	E950.1	E962.0	E980.1
Barbiturates, barbituric acid	967.0	E851	E937.0	E950.1	E962.0	E980.1
anesthetic (intravenous)	968.3	E855.1	E938.3	E950.4	E962.0	E980.4
Barium (carbonate) (chloride) (sulfate)	985.8	E866.4	—	E950.9	E962.1	E980.9
diagnostic agent	977.8	E858.8	E947.8	E950.4	E962.0	E980.4
pesticide	985.8	E863.4	—	E950.6	E962.1	E980.7
rodenticide	985.8	E863.7	—	E950.6	E962.1	E980.7
Barrier cream	976.3	E858.7	E946.3	E950.4	E962.0	E980.4
Battery acid or fluid	983.1	E864.1	—	E950.7	E962.1	E980.6
Bay rum	980.8	E860.8	—	E950.9	E962.1	E980.9
BCG vaccine	978.0	E858.8	E948.0	E950.4	E962.0	E980.4
Bearsfoot	988.2	E865.4	—	E950.9	E962.1	E980.9
Beclamide	966.3	E855.0	E936.3	E950.4	E962.0	E980.4
Bee (sting) (venom)	989.5	E905.3	—	E950.9	E962.1	E980.9
Belladonna (alkaloids)	971.1	E855.4	E941.1	E950.4	E962.0	E980.4
Bemegride	970.0	E854.3	E940.0	E950.4	E962.0	E980.4
Benactyzine	969.8	E855.8	E939.8	E950.3	E962.0	E980.3
Benadryl	963.0	E858.1	E933.0	E950.4	E962.0	E980.4

Substance	Poisoning	External Cause (E-Code) Accident	Therapeutic Use	Suicide Attempt	Assault	Undetermined
Bendrofluazide	974.3	E858.5	E944.3	E950.4	E962.0	E980.4
Bendroflumethiazide	974.3	E858.5	E944.3	E950.4	E962.0	E980.4
Benemid	974.7	E858.5	E944.7	E950.4	E962.0	E980.4
Benethamine penicillin G	960.0	E856	E930.0	E950.4	E962.0	E980.4
Benisone	976.0	E858.7	E946.0	E950.4	E962.0	E980.4
Benoquin	976.8	E858.7	E946.8	E950.4	E962.0	E980.4
Benoxinate	968.5	E855.2	E938.5	E950.4	E962.0	E980.4
Bentonite	976.3	E858.7	E946.3	E950.4	E962.0	E980.4
Benzalkonium (chloride)	976.0	E858.7	E946.0	E950.4	E962.0	E980.4
ophthalmic preparation	976.5	E858.7	E946.5	E950.4	E962.0	E980.4
Benzamidosalicylate (calcium)	961.8	E857	E931.8	E950.4	E962.0	E980.4
Benzathine penicillin	960.0	E856	E930.0	E950.4	E962.0	E980.4
Benzcarbimine	963.1	E858.1	E933.1	E950.4	E962.0	E980.4
Benzedrex	971.2	E855.5	E941.2	E950.4	E962.0	E980.4
Benzedrine (amphetamine)	969.7	E854.2	E939.7	E950.3	E962.0	E980.3
Benzene (acetyl) (dimethyl) (methyl) (solvent) (vapor)	982.0	E862.4	—	E950.9	E962.1	E980.9
hexachloride (gamma) (insecticide) (vapor)	989.2	E863.0	—	E950.6	E962.1	E980.7
Benzethonium	976.0	E858.7	E946.0	E950.4	E962.0	E980.4
Benzhexol (chloride)	966.4	E855.0	E936.4	E950.4	E962.0	E980.4
Benzilonium	971.1	E855.4	E941.1	E950.4	E962.0	E980.4
Benzin(e) - *see* Ligroin	—	—	—	—	—	—
Benziodarone	972.4	E858.3	E942.4	E950.4	E962.0	E980.4
Benzocaine	968.5	E855.2	E938.5	E950.4	E962.0	E980.4
Benzodiapin	969.4	E853.2	E939.4	E950.3	E962.0	E980.3
Benzodiazepines (tranquilizers) NEC	969.4	E853.2	E939.4	E950.3	E962.0	E980.3
Benzoic acid (with salicylic acid) (anti-infective)	976.0	E858.7	E946.0	E950.4	E962.0	E980.4
Benzoin	976.3	E858.7	E946.3	E950.4	E962.0	E980.4
Benzol (vapor)	982.0	E862.4	—	E950.9	E962.1	E980.9
Benzomorphan	965.09	E850.2	E935.2	E950.0	E962.0	E980.0
Benzonatate	975.4	E858.6	E945.4	E950.4	E962.0	E980.4
Benzothiadiazides	974.3	E858.5	E944.3	E950.4	E962.0	E980.4
Benzoylpas	961.8	E857	E931.8	E950.4	E962.0	E980.4
Benzperidol	969.5	E853.8	E939.5	E950.3	E962.0	E980.3
Benzphetamine	977.0	E858.8	E947.0	E950.4	E962.0	E980.4
Benzpyrinium	971.0	E855.3	E941.0	E950.4	E962.0	E980.4
Benzquinamide	963.0	E858.1	E933.0	E950.4	E962.0	E980.4
Benzthiazide	974.3	E858.5	E944.3	E950.4	E962.0	E980.4
Benztropine	971.1	E855.4	E941.1	E950.4	E962.0	E980.4
Benzyl	—	—	—	—	—	—
acetate	982.8	E862.4	—	E950.9	E962.1	E980.9
benzoate (anti-infective)	976.0	E858.7	E946.0	E950.4	E962.0	E980.4
morphine	965.09	E850.2	E935.2	E950.0	E962.0	E980.0
penicillin	960.0	E856	E930.0	E950.4	E962.0	E980.4
Bephenium	—	—	—	—	—	—
hydroxynapthoate	961.6	E857	E931.6	E950.4	E962.0	E980.4
Bergamot oil	989.89	E866.8	—	E950.9	E962.1	E980.9
Berries, poisonous	988.2	E865.3	—	E950.9	E962.1	E980.9
Beryllium (compounds) (fumes)	985.3	E866.4	—	E950.9	E962.1	E980.9
Beta-carotene	976.3	E858.7	E946.3	E950.4	E962.0	E980.4
Beta-Chlor	967.1	E852.0	E937.1	E950.2	E962.0	E980.2
Betamethasone	962.0	E858.0	E932.0	E950.4	E962.0	E980.4
topical	976.0	E858.7	E946.0	E950.4	E962.0	E980.4
Betazole	977.8	E858.8	E947.8	E950.4	E962.0	E980.4
Bethanechol	971.0	E855.3	E941.0	E950.4	E962.0	E980.4
Bethanidine	972.6	E858.3	E942.6	E950.4	E962.0	E980.4
Betula oil	976.3	E858.7	E946.3	E950.4	E962.0	E980.4
Bhang	969.6	E854.1	E939.6	E950.3	E962.0	E980.3
Bialamicol	961.5	E857	E931.5	E950.4	E962.0	E980.4
Bichloride of mercury - *see* Mercury, chloride	—	—	—	—	—	—
Bichromates (calcium) (crystals) (potassium) (sodium)	983.9	E864.3	—	E950.7	E962.1	E980.6
fumes	987.8	E869.8	—	E952.8	E962.2	E982.8
Biguanide derivatives, oral	962.3	E858.0	E932.3	E950.4	E962.0	E980.4
Biligrafin	977.8	E858.8	E947.8	E950.4	E962.0	E980.4

Substance	Poisoning	External Cause (E-Code)				
		Accident	Therapeutic Use	Suicide Attempt	Assault	Undetermined
Bilopaque	977.8	E858.8	E947.8	E950.4	E962.0	E980.4
Bioflavonoids	972.8	E858.3	E942.8	E950.4	E962.0	E980.4
Biological substance NEC	979.9	E858.8	E949.9	E950.4	E962.0	E980.4
Biperiden	966.4	E855.0	E936.4	E950.4	E962.0	E980.4
Bisacodyl	973.1	E858.4	E943.1	E950.4	E962.0	E980.4
Bishydroxycoumarin	964.2	E858.2	E934.2	E950.4	E962.0	E980.4
Bismarsen	961.1	E857	E931.1	E950.4	E962.0	E980.4
Bismuth (compounds) NEC	985.8	E866.4	—	E950.9	E962.1	E980.9
anti-infectives	961.2	E857	E931.2	E950.4	E962.0	E980.4
subcarbonate	973.5	E858.4	E943.5	E950.4	E962.0	E980.4
sulfarsphenamine	961.1	E857	E931.1	E950.4	E962.0	E980.4
Bithionol	961.6	E857	E931.6	E950.4	E962.0	E980.4
Bitter almond oil	989.0	E866.8	—	E950.9	E962.1	E980.9
Bittersweet	988.2	E865.4	—	E950.9	E962.1	E930.9
Black	—	—	—	—	—	—
flag	989.4	E863.4	—	E950.6	E962.1	E980.7
henbane	988.2	E865.4	—	E950.9	E962.1	E980.9
leaf (40)	989.4	E863.4	—	E950.6	E962.1	E980.7
widow spider (bite)	989.5	E905.1	—	E950.9	E962.1	E980.9
antivenin	979.9	E858.8	E949.9	E950.4	E962.0	E980.4
Blast furnace gas (carbon monoxide from)	986	E868.8	—	E952.1	E962.2	E982.1
Bleach NEC	983.9	E864.3	—	E950.7	E962.1	E980.6
Bleaching solutions	983.9	E864.3	—	E950.7	E962.1	E980.6
Bleomycin (sulfate)	960.7	E856	E930.7	E950.4	E962.0	E980.4
Blockain	968.9	E855.2	E938.9	E950.4	E962.0	E980.4
infiltration (subcutaneous)	968.5	E855.2	E938.5	E950.4	E962.0	E980.4
nerve block (peripheral) (plexus)	968.6	E855.2	E938.6	E950.4	E962.0	E980.4
topical (surface)	968.5	E855.2	E938.5	E950.4	E962.0	E980.4
Blood (derivatives) (natural) (plasma) (whole)	964.7	E858.2	E934.7	E950.4	E962.0	E980.4
affecting agent	964.9	E858.2	E934.9	E950.4	E962.0	E980.4
specified NEC	964.8	E858.2	E934.8	E950.4	E962.0	E980.4
substitute (macromolecular)	964.8	E858.2	E934.8	E950.4	E962.0	E980.4
Blue velvet	965.09	E850.2	E935.2	E950.0	E962.0	E980.0
Bone meal	989.89	E866.5	—	E950.9	E962.1	E980.9
Bonine	963.0	E858.1	E933.0	E950.4	E962.0	E980.4
Boracic acid	976.0	E858.7	E946.0	E950.4	E962.0	E980.4
ENT agent	976.6	E858.7	E946.6	E950.4	E962.0	E980.4
ophthalmic preparation	976.5	E858.7	E946.5	E950.4	E962.0	E980.4
Borate (cleanser) (sodium)	989.6	E861.3	—	E950.9	E962.1	E980.9
Borax (cleanser)	989.6	E861.3	—	E950.9	E962.1	E980.9
Boric acid	976.0	E858.7	E946.0	E950.4	E962.0	E980.4
ENT agent	976.6	E858.7	E946.6	E950.4	E962.0	E980.4
ophthalmic preparation	976.5	E858.7	E946.5	E950.4	E962.0	E980.4
Boron hydride NEC	989.89	E866.8	—	E950.9	E962.1	E980.9
fumes or gas	987.8	E869.8	—	E952.8	E962.2	E982.8
Botox	975.3	E858.6	E945.3	E950.4	E962.0	E980.4 ◄
Brake fluid vapor	987.8	E869.8	—	E952.8	E962.2	E982.8
Brass (compounds) (fumes)	985.8	E866.4	—	E950.9	E962.1	E980.9
Brasso	981	E861.3	—	E950.9	E962.1	E980.9
Bretylium (tosylate)	972.6	E858.3	E942.6	E950.4	E962.0	E980.4
Brevital (sodium)	968.3	E855.1	E938.3	E950.4	E962.0	E980.4
British antilewisite	963.8	E858.1	E933.8	E950.4	E962.0	E980.4
Bromal (hydrate)	967.3	E852.2	E937.3	E950.2	E962.0	E980.2
Bromelains	963.4	E858.1	E933.4	E950.4	E962.0	E980.4
Bromides NEC	967.3	E852.2	E937.3	E950.2	E962.0	E980.2
Bromine (vapor)	987.8	E869.8	—	E952.8	E962.2	E982.8
compounds (medicinal)	967.3	E852.2	E937.3	E950.2	E962.0	E980.2
Bromisovalum	967.3	E852.2	E937.3	E950.2	E962.0	E980.2
Bromobenzyl cyanide	987.5	E869.3	—	E952.8	E962.2	E982.8
Bromodiphenhydramine	963.0	E858.1	E933.0	E950.4	E962.0	E980.4
Bromoform	967.3	E852.2	E937.3	E950.2	E962.0	E980.2
Bromophenol blue reagent	977.8	E858.8	E947.8	E950.4	E962.0	E980.4
Bromosalicylhydroxamic acid	961.8	E857	E931.8	E950.4	E962.0	E980.4

Substance	Poisoning	External Cause (E-Code) Accident	Therapeutic Use	Suicide Attempt	Assault	Undetermined
Bromo-seltzer	965.4	E850.4	E935.4	E950.0	E962.0	E980.0
Brompheniramine	963.0	E858.1	E933.0	E950.4	E962.0	E980.4
Bromural	967.3	E852.2	E937.3	E950.2	E962.0	E980.2
Brown spider (bite) (venom)	989.5	E905.1	—	E950.9	E962.1	E980.9
Brucia	988.2	E865.3	—	E950.9	E962.1	E980.9
Brucine	989.1	E863.7	—	E950.6	E962.1	E980.7
Brunswick green - *see* Copper	—	—	—	—	—	—
Bruten - *see* Ibuprofen	—	—	—	—	—	—
Bryonia (alba) (dioica)	988.2	E865.4	—	E950.9	E962.1	E980.9
Buclizine	969.5	E853.8	E939.5	E950.3	E962.0	E980.3
Bufferin	965.1	E850.3	E935.3	E950.0	E962.0	E980.0
Bufotenine	969.6	E854.1	E939.6	E950.3	E962.0	E980.3
Buphenine	971.2	E855.5	E941.2	E950.4	E962.0	E980.4
Bupivacaine	968.9	E855.2	E938.9	E950.4	E962.0	E980.4
infiltration (subcutaneous)	968.5	E855.2	E938.5	E950.4	E962.0	E980.4
nerve block (peripheral) (plexus)	968.6	E855.2	E938.6	E950.4	E962.0	E980.4
Busulfan	963.1	E858.1	E933.1	E950.4	E962.0	E980.4
Butabarbital (sodium)	967.0	E851	E937.0	E950.1	E962.0	E980.1
Butabarbitone	967.0	E851	E937.0	E950.1	E962.0	E980.1
Butabarpal	967.0	E851	E937.0	E950.1	E962.0	E980.1
Butacaine	968.5	E855.2	E938.5	E950.4	E962.0	E980.4
Butallylonal	967.0	E851	E937.0	E950.1	E962.0	E980.1
Butane (distributed in mobile container)	987.0	E868.0	—	E951.1	E962.2	E981.1
distributed through pipes	987.0	E867	—	E951.0	E962.2	E981.0
incomplete combustion of - *see* Carbon monoxide, butane	—	—	—	—	—	—
Butanol	980.3	E860.4	—	E950.9	E962.1	E980.9
Butanone	982.8	E862.4	—	E950.9	E962.1	E980.9
Butaperazine	969.1	E853.0	E939.1	E950.3	E962.0	E980.3
Butazolidin	965.5	E850.5	E935.5	E950.0	E962.0	E980.0
Butethal	967.0	E851	E937.0	E950.1	E962.0	E980.1
Butethamate	971.1	E855.4	E941.1	E950.4	E962.0	E980.4
Buthalitone (sodium)	968.3	E855.1	E938.3	E950.4	E962.0	E980.4
Butisol (sodium)	967.0	E851	E937.0	E950.1	E962.0	E980.1
Butobarbital, butobarbitone	967.0	E851	E937.0	E950.1	E962.0	E980.1
Butriptyline	969.0	E854.0	E939.0	E950.3	E962.0	E980.3
Buttercups	988.2	E865.4	—	E950.9	E962.1	E980.9
Butter of antimony - *see* Antimony	—	—	—	—	—	—
Butyl	—	—	—	—	—	—
acetate (secondary)	982.8	E862.4	—	E950.9	E962.1	E980.9
alcohol	980.3	E860.4	—	E950.9	E962.1	E980.9
carbinol	980.8	E860.8	—	E950.9	E962.1	E980.9
carbitol	982.8	E862.4	—	E950.9	E962.1	E980.9
cellosolve	982.8	E862.4	—	E950.9	E962.1	E980.9
chloral (hydrate)	967.1	E852.0	E937.1	E950.2	E962.0	E980.2
formate	982.8	E862.4	—	E950.9	E962.1	E980.9
scopolammonium bromide	971.1	E855.4	E941.1	E950.4	E962.0	E980.4
Butyn	968.5	E855.2	E938.5	E950.4	E962.0	E980.4
Butyrophenone (-based tranquilizers)	969.2	E853.1	E939.2	E950.3	E962.0	E980.3
Cacodyl, cacodylic acid - *see* Arsenic	—	—	—	—	—	—
Cactinomycin	960.7	E856	E930.7	E950.4	E962.0	E980.4
Cade oil	976.4	E858.7	E946.4	E950.4	E962.0	E980.4
Cadmium (chloride) (compounds) (dust) (fumes) (oxide)	985.5	E866.4	—	E950.9	E962.1	E980.9
sulfide (medicinal) NEC	976.4	E858.7	E946.4	E950.4	E962.0	E980.4
Caffeine	969.7	E854.2	E939.7	E950.3	E962.0	E980.3
Calabar bean	988.2	E865.4	—	E950.9	E962.1	E980.9
Caladium seguinium	988.2	E865.4	—	E950.9	E962.1	E980.9
Calamine (liniment) (lotion)	976.3	E858.7	E946.3	E950.4	E962.0	E980.4
Calciferol	963.5	E858.1	E933.5	E950.4	E962.0	E980.4
Calcium (salts) NEC	974.5	E858.5	E944.5	E950.4	E962.0	E980.4
acetylsalicylate	965.1	E850.3	E935.3	E950.0	E962.0	E980.0
benzamidosalicylate	961.8	E857	E931.8	E950.4	E962.0	E980.4
carbaspirin	965.1	E850.3	E935.3	E950.0	E962.0	E980.0
carbimide (citrated)	977.3	E858.8	E947.3	E950.4	E962.0	E980.4

Substance	Poisoning	External Cause (E-Code) Accident	Therapeutic Use	Suicide Attempt	Assault	Undetermined
Calcium *(Continued)*						
carbonate (antacid)	973.0	E858.4	E943.0	E950.4	E962.0	E980.4
cyanide (citrated)	977.3	E858.8	E947.3	E950.4	E962.0	E980.4
dioctyl sulfosuccinate	973.2	E858.4	E943.2	E950.4	E962.0	E980.4
disodium edathamil	963.8	E858.1	E933.8	E950.4	E962.0	E980.4
disodium edetate	963.8	E858.1	E933.8	E950.4	E962.0	E980.4
EDTA	963.8	E858.1	E933.8	E950.4	E962.0	E980.4
hydrate, hydroxide	983.2	E864.2	—	E950.7	E962.1	E980.6
mandelate	961.9	E857	E931.9	E950.4	E962.0	E980.4
oxide	983.2	E864.2	—	E950.7	E962.1	E980.6
Calomel - *see* Mercury, chloride	—	—	—	—	—	—
Caloric agents NEC	974.5	E858.5	E944.5	E950.4	E962.0	E980.4
Calusterone	963.1	E858.1	E933.1	E950.4	E962.0	E980.4
Camoquin	961.4	E857	E931.4	E950.4	E962.0	E980.4
Camphor (oil)	976.1	E858.7	E946.1	E950.4	E962.0	E980.4
Candeptin	976.0	E858.7	E946.0	E950.4	E962.0	E980.4
Candicidin	976.0	E858.7	E946.0	E950.4	E962.0	E980.4
Cannabinols	969.6	E854.1	E939.6	E950.3	E962.0	E980.3
Cannabis (derivatives) (indica) (sativa)	969.6	E854.1	E939.6	E950.3	E962.0	E980.3
Canned heat	980.1	E860.2	—	E950.9	E962.1	E980.9
Cantharides, cantharidin, cantharis	976.8	E858.7	E946.8	E950.4	E962.0	E980.4
Capillary agents	972.8	E858.3	E942.8	E950.4	E962.0	E980.4
Capreomycin	960.6	E856	E930.6	E950.4	E962.0	E980.4
Captodiame, captodiamine	969.5	E853.8	E939.5	E950.3	E962.0	E980.3
Caramiphen (hydrochloride)	971.1	E855.4	E941.1	E950.4	E962.0	E980.4
Carbachol	971.0	E855.3	E941.0	E950.4	E962.0	E980.4
Carbacrylamine resins	974.5	E858.5	E944.5	E950.4	E962.0	E980.4
Carbamate (sedative)	967.8	E852.8	E937.8	E950.2	E962.0	E980.2
herbicide	989.3	E863.5	—	E950.6	E962.1	E980.7
insecticide	989.3	E863.2	—	E950.6	E962.1	E980.7
Carbamazepine	966.3	E855.0	E936.3	E950.4	E962.0	E980.4
Carbamic esters	967.8	E852.8	E937.8	E950.2	E962.0	E980.2
Carbamide	974.4	E858.5	E944.4	E950.4	E962.0	E980.4
topical	976.8	E858.7	E946.8	E950.4	E962.0	E980.4
Carbamylcholine chloride	971.0	E855.3	E941.0	E950.4	E962.0	E980.4
Carbarsone	961.1	E857	E931.1	E950.4	E962.0	E980.4
Carbaryl	989.3	E863.2	—	E950.6	E962.1	E980.7
Carbaspirin	965.1	E850.3	E935.3	E950.0	E962.0	E980.0
Carbazochrome	972.8	E858.3	E942.8	E950.4	E962.0	E980.4
Carbenicillin	960.0	E856	E930.0	E950.4	E962.0	E980.4
Carbenoxolone	973.8	E858.4	E943.8	E950.4	E962.0	E980.4
Carbetapentane	975.4	E858.6	E945.4	E950.4	E962.0	E980.4
Carbimazole	962.8	E858.0	E932.8	E950.4	E962.0	E980.4
Carbinol	980.1	E860.2	—	E950.9	E962.1	E980.9
Carbinoxamine	963.0	E858.1	E933.0	E950.4	E962.0	E980.4
Carbitol	982.8	E862.4	—	E950.9	E962.1	E980.9
Carbocaine	968.9	E855.2	E938.9	E950.4	E962.0	E980.4
infiltration (subcutaneous)	968.5	E855.2	E938.5	E950.4	E962.0	E980.4
nerve block (peripheral) (plexus)	968.6	E855.2	E938.6	E950.4	E962.0	E980.4
topical (surface)	968.5	E855.2	E938.5	E950.4	E962.0	E980.4
Carbol-fuchsin solution	976.0	E858.7	E946.0	E950.4	E962.0	E980.4
Carbolic acid (*see also* Phenol)	983.0	E864.0	—	E950.7	E962.1	E980.6
Carbomycin	960.8	E856	E930.8	E950.4	E962.0	E980.4
Carbon	—	—	—	—	—	—
bisulfide (liquid) (vapor)	982.2	E862.4	—	E950.9	E962.1	E980.9
dioxide (gas)	987.8	E869.8	—	E952.8	E962.2	E982.8
disulfide (liquid) (vapor)	982.2	E862.4	—	E950.9	E962.1	E980.9
monoxide (from incomplete combustion of) (in) NEC	986	E868.9	—	E952.1	E962.2	E982.1
blast furnace gas	986	E868.8	—	E952.1	E962.2	E982.1
butane (distributed in mobile container)	986	E868.0	—	E951.1	E962.2	E981.1
distributed through pipes	986	E867	—	E951.0	E962.2	E981.0
charcoal fumes	986	E868.3	—	E952.1	E962.2	E982.1

Substance	Poisoning	External Cause (E-Code)				
		Accident	Therapeutic Use	Suicide Attempt	Assault	Undetermined
Carbon *(Continued)*						
coal						
gas (piped)	986	E867	—	E951.0	E962.2	E981.0
solid (in domestic stoves, fireplaces)	986	E868.3	—	E952.1	E962.2	E982.1
coke (in domestic stoves, fireplaces)	986	E868.3	—	E952.1	E962.2	E982.1
exhaust gas (motor) not in transit	986	E868.2	—	E952.0	E962.2	E982.0
combustion engine, any not in watercraft	986	E868.2	—	E952.0	E962.2	E982.0
farm tractor, not in transit	986	E868.2	—	E952.0	E962.2	E982.0
gas engine	986	E868.2	—	E952.0	E962.2	E982.0
motor pump	986	E868.2	—	E952.0	E962.2	E982.0
motor vehicle, not in transit	986	E868.2	—	E952.0	E962.2	E982.0
fuel (in domestic use)	986	E868.3	—	E952.1	E962.2	E982.1
gas (piped)	986	E867	—	E951.0	E962.2	E981.0
in mobile container	986	E868.0	—	E951.1	E962.2	E981.1
utility	986	E868.1	—	E951.8	E962.2	E981.1
in mobile container	986	E868.0	—	E951.1	E962.2	E981.1
piped (natural)	986	E867	—	E951.0	E962.2	E981.0
illuminating gas	986	E868.1	—	E951.8	E962.2	E981.8
industrial fuels or gases, any	986	E868.8	—	E952.1	E962.2	E982.1
kerosene (in domestic stoves, fireplaces)	986	E868.3	—	E952.1	E962.2	E982.1
kiln gas or vapor	986	E868.8	—	E952.1	E962.2	E982.1
motor exhaust gas, not in transit	986	E868.2	—	E952.0	E962.2	E982.0
piped gas (manufactured) (natural)	986	E867	—	E951.0	E962.2	E981.0
producer gas	986	E868.8	—	E952.1	E962.2	E982.1
propane (distributed in mobile container)	986	E868.0	—	E951.1	E962.2	E981.1
distributed through pipes	986	E867	—	E951.0	E962.2	E981.0
specified source NEC	986	E868.8	—	E952.1	E962.2	E982.1
stove gas	986	E868.1	—	E951.8	E962.2	E981.8
piped	986	E867	—	E951.0	E962.2	E981.0
utility gas	986	E868.1	—	E951.8	E962.2	E981.8
piped	986	E867	—	E951.0	E962.2	E981.0
water gas	986	E868.1	—	E951.8	E962.2	E981.8
wood (in domestic stoves, fireplaces)	986	E868.3	—	E952.1	E962.2	E982.1
tetrachloride (vapor) NEC	987.8	E869.8	—	E952.8	E962.2	E982.8
liquid (cleansing agent) NEC	982.1	E861.3	—	E950.9	E962.1	E980.9
solvent	982.1	E862.4	—	E950.9	E962.1	E980.9
Carbonic acid (gas)	987.8	E869.8	—	E952.8	E962.2	E982.8
anhydrase inhibitors	974.2	E858.5	E944.2	E950.4	E962.0	E980.4
Carbowax	976.3	E858.7	E946.3	E950.4	E962.0	E980.4
Carbrital	967.0	E851	E937.0	E950.1	E962.0	E980.1
Carbromal (derivatives)	967.3	E852.2	E937.3	E950.2	E962.0	E980.2
Cardiac	—	—	—	—	—	—
depressants	972.0	E858.3	E942.0	E950.4	E962.0	E980.4
rhythm regulators	972.0	E858.3	E942.0	E950.4	E962.0	E980.4
Cardiografin	977.8	E858.8	E947.8	E950.4	E962.0	E980.4
Cardio-green	977.8	E858.8	E947.8	E950.4	E962.0	E980.4
Cardiotonic glycosides	972.1	E858.3	E942.1	E950.4	E962.0	E980.4
Cardiovascular agents NEC	972.9	E858.3	E942.9	E950.4	E962.0	E980.4
Cardrase	974.2	E858.5	E944.2	E950.4	E962.0	E980.4
Carfusin	976.0	E858.7	E946.0	E950.4	E962.0	E980.4
Carisoprodol	968.0	E855.1	E938.0	E950.4	E962.0	E980.4
Carmustine	963.1	E858.1	E933.1	E950.4	E962.0	E980.4
Carotene	963.5	E858.1	E933.5	E950.4	E962.0	E980.4
Carphenazine (maleate)	969.1	E853.0	E939.1	E950.3	E962.0	E980.3
Carter's Little Pills	973.1	E858.4	E943.1	E950.4	E962.0	E980.4
Cascara (sagrada)	973.1	E858.4	E943.1	E950.4	E962.0	E980.4
Cassava	988.2	E865.4	—	E950.9	E962.1	E980.9
Castellani's paint	976.0	E858.7	E946.0	E950.4	E962.0	E980.4
Castor	—	—	—	—	—	—
bean	988.2	E865.3	—	E950.9	E962.1	E980.9
oil	973.1	E858.4	E943.1	E950.4	E962.0	E980.4
Caterpillar (sting)	989.5	E905.5	—	E950.9	E962.1	E980.9
Catha (edulis)	970.8	E854.3	E940.8	E950.4	E962.0	E980.4

Substance	Poisoning	External Cause (E-Code)				
		Accident	Therapeutic Use	Suicide Attempt	Assault	Undetermined
Cathartics NEC	973.3	E858.4	E943.3	E950.4	E962.0	E980.4
contact	973.1	E858.4	E943.1	E950.4	E962.0	E980.4
emollient	973.2	E858.4	E943.2	E950.4	E962.0	E980.4
intestinal irritants	973.1	E858.4	E943.1	E950.4	E962.0	E980.4
saline	973.3	E858.4	E943.3	E950.4	E962.0	E980.4
Cathomycin	960.8	E856	E930.8	E950.4	E962.0	E980.4
Caustic(s)	983.9	E864.4	—	E950.7	E962.1	E980.6
alkali	983.2	E864.2	—	E950.7	E962.1	E980.6
hydroxide	983.2	E864.2	—	E950.7	E962.1	E980.6
potash	983.2	E864.2	—	E950.7	E962.1	E980.6
soda	983.2	E864.2	—	E950.7	E962.1	E980.6
specified NEC	983.9	E864.3	—	E950.7	E962.1	E980.6
Ceepryn	976.0	E858.7	E946.0	E950.4	E962.0	E980.4
ENT agent	976.6	E858.7	E946.6	E950.4	E962.0	E980.4
lozenges	976.6	E858.7	E946.6	E950.4	E962.0	E980.4
Celestone	962.0	E858.0	E932.0	E950.4	E962.0	E980.4
topical	976.0	E858.7	E946.0	E950.4	E962.0	E980.4
Cellosolve	982.8	E862.4	—	E950.9	E962.1	E980.9
Cell stimulants and proliferants	976.8	E858.7	E946.8	E950.4	E962.0	E980.4
Cellulose derivatives, cathartic	973.3	E858.4	E943.3	E950.4	E962.0	E980.4
nitrates (topical)	976.3	E858.7	E946.3	E950.4	E962.0	E980.4
Centipede (bite)	989.5	E905.4	—	E950.9	E962.1	E980.9
Central nervous system	—	—	—	—	—	—
depressants	968.4	E855.1	E938.4	E950.4	E962.0	E980.4
anesthetic (general) NEC	968.4	E855.1	E938.4	E950.4	E962.0	E980.4
gases NEC	968.2	E855.1	E938.2	E950.4	E962.0	E980.4
intravenous	968.3	E855.1	E938.3	E950.4	E962.0	E980.4
barbiturates	967.0	E851	E937.0	E950.1	E962.0	E980.1
bromides	967.3	E852.2	E937.3	E950.2	E962.0	E980.2
cannabis sativa	969.6	E854.1	E939.6	E950.3	E962.0	E980.3
chloral hydrate	967.1	E852.0	E937.1	E950.2	E962.0	E980.2
hallucinogenics	969.6	E854.1	E939.6	E950.3	E962.0	E980.3
hypnotics	967.9	E852.9	E937.9	E950.2	E962.0	E980.2
specified NEC	967.8	E852.8	E937.8	E950.2	E962.0	E980.2
muscle relaxants	968.0	E855.1	E938.0	E950.4	E962.0	E980.4
paraldehyde	967.2	E852.1	E937.2	E950.2	E962.0	E980.2
sedatives	967.9	E852.9	E937.9	E950.2	E962.0	E980.2
mixed NEC	967.6	E852.5	E937.6	E950.2	E962.0	E980.2
specified NEC	967.8	E852.8	E937.8	E950.2	E962.0	E980.2
muscle-tone depressants	968.0	E855.1	E938.0	E950.4	E962.0	E980.4
stimulants	970.9	E854.3	E940.9	E950.4	E962.0	E980.4
amphetamines	969.7	E854.2	E939.7	E950.3	E962.0	E980.3
analeptics	970.0	E854.3	E940.0	E950.4	E962.0	E980.4
antidepressants	969.0	E854.0	E939.0	E950.3	E962.0	E980.3
opiate antagonists	970.1	E854.3	E940.0	E950.4	E962.0	E980.4
specified NEC	970.8	E854.3	E940.8	E950.4	E962.0	E980.4
Cephalexin	960.5	E856	E930.5	E950.4	E962.0	E980.4
Cephaloglycin	960.5	E856	E930.5	E950.4	E962.0	E980.4
Cephaloridine	960.5	E856	E930.5	E950.4	E962.0	E980.4
Cephalosporins NEC	960.5	E856	E930.5	E950.4	E962.0	E980.4
N (adicillin)	960.0	E856	E930.0	E950.4	E962.0	E980.4
Cephalothin (sodium)	960.5	E856	E930.5	E950.4	E962.0	E980.4
Cerbera (odallam)	988.2	E865.4	—	E950.9	E962.1	E980.9
Cerberin	972.1	E858.3	E942.1	E950.4	E962.0	E980.4
Cerebral stimulants	970.9	E854.3	E940.9	E950.4	E962.0	E980.4
psychotherapeutic	969.7	E854.2	E939.7	E950.3	E962.0	E980.3
specified NEC	970.8	E854.3	E940.8	E950.4	E962.0	E980.4
Cetalkonium (chloride)	976.0	E858.7	E946.0	E950.4	E962.0	E980.4
Cetoxime	963.0	E858.1	E933.0	E950.4	E962.0	E980.4
Cetrimide	976.2	E858.7	E946.2	E950.4	E962.0	E980.4

Substance	Poisoning	External Cause (E-Code)				
		Accident	Therapeutic Use	Suicide Attempt	Assault	Undetermined
Cetylpyridinium	976.0	E858.7	E946.0	E950.4	E962.0	E980.4
ENT agent	976.6	E858.7	E946.6	E950.4	E962.0	E980.4
lozenges	976.6	E858.7	E946.6	E950.4	E962.0	E980.4
Cevadilla - *see* Sabadilla	—	—	—	—	—	—
Cevitamic acid	963.5	E858.1	E933.5	E950.4	E962.0	E980.4
Chalk, precipitated	973.0	E858.4	E943.0	E950.4	E962.0	E980.4
Charcoal	—	—	—	—	—	—
fumes (carbon monoxide)	986	E868.3	—	E952.1	E962.2	E982.1
industrial	986	E868.8	—	E952.1	E962.2	E982.1
medicinal (activated)	973.0	E858.4	E943.0	E950.4	E962.0	E980.4
Chelating agents NEC	977.2	E858.8	E947.2	E950.4	E962.0	E980.4
Chelidonium majus	988.2	E865.4	—	E950.9	E962.1	E980.9
Chemical substance	989.9	E866.9	—	E950.9	E962.1	E980.9
specified NEC	989.89	E866.8	—	E950.9	E962.1	E980.9
Chemotherapy, antineoplastic	963.1	E858.1	E933.1	E950.4	E962.0	E980.4
Chenopodium (oil)	961.6	E857	E931.6	E950.4	E962.0	E980.4
Cherry laurel	988.2	E865.4	—	E950.9	E962.1	E980.9
Chiniofon	961.3	E857	E931.3	E950.4	E962.0	E980.4
Chlophedianol	975.4	E858.6	E945.4	E950.4	E962.0	E980.4
Chloral (betaine) (formamide) (hydrate)	967.1	E852.0	E937.1	E950.2	E962.0	E980.2
Chloralamide	967.1	E852.0	E937.1	E950.2	E962.0	E980.2
Chlorambucil	963.1	E858.1	E933.1	E950.4	E962.0	E980.4
Chloramphenicol	960.2	E856	E930.2	E950.4	E962.0	E980.4
ENT agent	976.6	E858.7	E946.6	E950.4	E962.0	E980.4
ophthalmic preparation	976.5	E858.7	E946.5	E950.4	E962.0	E980.4
topical NEC	976.0	E858.7	E946.0	E950.4	E962.0	E980.4
Chlorate(s) (potassium) (sodium) NEC	983.9	E864.3	—	E950.7	E962.1	E980.6
herbicides	989.4	E863.5	—	E950.6	E962.1	E980.7
Chlorcyclizine	963.0	E858.1	E933.0	E950.4	E962.0	E980.4
Chlordan(e) (dust)	989.2	E863.0	—	E950.6	E962.1	E980.7
Chlordantoin	976.0	E858.7	E946.0	E950.4	E962.0	E980.4
Chlordiazepoxide	969.4	E853.2	E939.4	E950.3	E962.0	E980.3
Chloresium	976.8	E858.7	E946.8	E950.4	E962.0	E980.4
Chlorethiazol	967.1	E852.0	E937.1	E950.2	E962.0	E980.2
Chlorethyl - *see* Ethyl, chloride	—	—	—	—	—	—
Chloretone	967.1	E852.0	E937.1	E950.2	E962.0	E980.2
Chlorex	982.3	E862.4	—	E950.9	E962.1	E980.9
Chlorhexadol	967.1	E852.0	E937.1	E950.2	E962.0	E980.2
Chlorhexidine (hydrochloride)	976.0	E858.7	E946.0	E950.4	E962.0	E980.4
Chlorhydroxyquinolin	976.0	E858.7	E946.0	E950.4	E962.0	E980.4
Chloride of lime (bleach)	983.9	E864.3	—	E950.7	E962.1	E980.6
Chlorinated	—	—	—	—	—	—
camphene	989.2	E863.0	—	E950.6	E962.1	E980.7
diphenyl	989.89	E866.8	—	E950.9	E962.1	E980.9
hydrocarbons NEC	989.2	E863.0	—	E950.6	E962.1	E980.7
solvent	982.3	E862.4	—	E950.9	E962.1	E980.9
lime (bleach)	983.9	E864.3	—	E950.7	E962.1	E980.6
naphthalene - *see* Naphthalene	—	—	—	—	—	—
pesticides NEC	989.2	E863.0	—	E950.6	E962.1	E980.7
soda - *see* Sodium, hypochlorite	—	—	—	—	—	—
Chlorine (fumes) (gas)	987.6	E869.8	—	E952.8	E962.2	E982.8
bleach	983.9	E864.3	—	E950.7	E962.1	E980.6
compounds NEC	983.9	E864.3	—	E950.7	E962.1	E980.6
disinfectant	983.9	E861.4	—	E950.7	E962.1	E980.6
releasing agents NEC	983.9	E864.3	—	E950.7	E962.1	E980.6
Chlorisondamine	972.3	E858.3	E942.3	E950.4	E962.0	E980.4
Chlormadinone	962.2	E858.0	E932.2	E950.4	E962.0	E980.4
Chlormerodrin	974.0	E858.5	E944.0	E950.4	E962.0	E980.4
Chlormethiazole	967.1	E852.0	E937.1	E950.2	E962.0	E980.2
Chlormethylenecycline	960.4	E856	E930.4	E950.4	E962.0	E980.4
Chlormezanone	969.5	E853.8	E939.5	E950.3	E962.0	E980.3
Chloroacetophenone	987.5	E869.3	—	E952.8	E962.2	E982.8

Substance	Poisoning	External Cause (E-Code)				
		Accident	Therapeutic Use	Suicide Attempt	Assault	Undetermined
Chloroaniline	983.0	E864.0	—	E950.7	E962.1	E980.6
Chlorobenzene, chlorobenzol	982.0	E862.4	—	E950.9	E962.1	E980.9
Chlorobutanol	967.1	E852.0	E937.1	E950.2	E962.0	E980.2
Chlorodinitrobenzene	983.0	E864.0	—	E950.7	E962.1	E980.6
dust or vapor	987.8	E869.8	—	E952.8	E962.2	E982.8
Chloroethane - *see* Ethyl, chloride	—	—	—	—	—	—
Chloroform (fumes) (vapor)	987.8	E869.8	—	E952.8	E962.2	E982.8
anesthetic (gas)	968.2	E855.1	E938.2	E950.4	E962.0	E980.4
liquid NEC	968.4	E855.1	E938.4	E950.4	E962.0	E980.4
solvent	982.3	E862.4	—	E950.9	E962.1	E980.9
Chloroguanide	961.4	E857	E931.4	E950.4	E962.0	E980.4
Chloromycetin	960.2	E856	E930.2	E950.4	E962.0	E980.4
ENT agent	976.6	E858.7	E946.6	E950.4	E962.0	E980.4
ophthalmic preparation	976.5	E858.7	E946.5	E950.4	E962.0	E980.4
otic solution	976.6	E858.7	E946.6	E950.4	E962.0	E980.4
topical NEC	976.0	E858.7	E946.0	E950.4	E962.0	E980.4
Chloronitrobenzene	983.0	E864.0	—	E950.7	E962.1	E980.6
dust or vapor	987.8	E869.8	—	E952.8	E962.2	E982.8
Chlorophenol	983.0	E864.0	—	E950.7	E962.1	E980.6
Chlorophenothane	989.2	E863.0	—	E950.6	E962.1	E980.7
Chlorophyll (derivatives)	976.8	E858.7	E946.8	E950.4	E962.0	E980.4
Chloropicrin (fumes)	987.8	E869.8	—	E952.8	E962.2	E982.8
fumigant	989.4	E863.8	—	E950.6	E962.1	E980.7
fungicide	989.4	E863.6	—	E950.6	E962.1	E980.7
pesticide (fumes)	989.4	E863.4	—	E950.6	E962.1	E980.7
Chloroprocaine	968.9	E855.2	E938.9	E950.4	E962.0	E980.4
infiltration (subcutaneous)	968.5	E855.2	E938.5	E950.4	E962.0	E980.4
nerve block (peripheral) (plexus)	968.6	E855.2	E938.6	E950.4	E962.0	E980.4
Chloroptic	976.5	E858.7	E946.5	E950.4	E962.0	E980.4
Chloropurine	963.1	E858.1	E933.1	E950.4	E962.0	E980.4
Chloroquine (hydrochloride) (phosphate)	961.4	E857	E931.4	E950.4	E962.0	E980.4
Chlorothen	963.0	E858.1	E933.0	E950.4	E962.0	E980.4
Chlorothiazide	974.3	E858.5	E944.3	E950.4	E962.0	E980.4
Chlorotrianisene	962.2	E858.0	E932.2	E950.4	E962.0	E980.4
Chlorovinyldichloroarsine	985.1	E866.3	—	E950.8	E962.1	E980.8
Chloroxylenol	976.0	E858.7	E946.0	E950.4	E962.0	E980.4
Chlorphenesin (carbamate)	968.0	E855.1	E938.0	E950.4	E962.0	E980.4
topical (antifungal)	976.0	E858.7	E946.0	E950.4	E962.0	E980.4
Chlorpheniramine	963.0	E858.1	E933.0	E950.4	E962.0	E980.4
Chlorphenoxamine	966.4	E855.0	E936.4	E950.4	E962.0	E980.4
Chlorphentermine	977.0	E858.8	E947.0	E950.4	E962.0	E980.4
Chlorproguanil	961.4	E857	E931.4	E950.4	E962.0	E980.4
Chlorpromazine	969.1	E853.0	E939.1	E950.3	E962.0	E980.3
Chlorpropamide	962.3	E858.0	E932.3	E950.4	E962.0	E980.4
Chlorprothixene	969.3	E853.8	E939.3	E950.3	E962.0	E980.3
Chlorquinaldol	976.0	E858.7	E946.0	E950.4	E962.0	E980.4
Chlortetracycline	960.4	E856	E930.4	E950.4	E962.0	E980.4
Chlorthalidone	974.4	E858.5	E944.4	E950.4	E962.0	E980.4
Chlortrianisene	962.2	E858.0	E932.2	E950.4	E962.0	E980.4
Chlor-Trimeton	963.0	E858.1	E933.0	E950.4	E962.0	E980.4
Chlorzoxazone	968.0	E855.1	E938.0	E950.4	E962.0	E980.4
Choke damp	987.8	E869.8	—	E952.8	E962.2	E982.8
Cholebrine	977.8	E858.8	E947.8	E950.4	E962.0	E980.4
Cholera vaccine	978.2	E858.8	E948.2	E950.4	E962.0	E980.4
Cholesterol-lowering agents	972.2	E858.3	E942.2	E950.4	E962.0	E980.4
Cholestyramine (resin)	972.2	E858.3	E942.2	E950.4	E962.0	E980.4
Cholic acid	973.4	E858.4	E943.4	E950.4	E962.0	E980.4
Choline	—	—	—	—	—	—
dihydrogen citrate	977.1	E858.8	E947.1	E950.4	E962.0	E980.4
salicylate	965.1	E850.3	E935.3	E950.0	E962.0	E980.0
theophyllinate	974.1	E858.5	E944.1	E950.4	E962.0	E980.4

Substance	Poisoning	External Cause (E-Code) Accident	Therapeutic Use	Suicide Attempt	Assault	Undetermined
Cholinergics	971.0	E855.3	E941.0	E950.4	E962.0	E980.4
Chografin	977.8	E858.8	E947.8	E950.4	E962.0	E980.4
Chorionic gonadotropin	962.4	E858.0	E932.4	E950.4	E962.0	E980.4
Chromates	983.9	E864.3	—	E950.7	E962.1	E980.6
dust or mist	987.8	E869.8	—	E952.8	E962.2	E982.8
lead	984.0	E866.0	—	E950.9	E962.1	E980.9
paint	984.0	E861.5	—	E950.9	E962.1	E980.9
Chromic acid	983.9	E864.3	—	E950.7	E962.1	E980.6
dust or mist	987.8	E869.8	—	E952.8	E962.2	E982.8
Chromium	985.6	E866.4	—	E950.9	E962.1	E980.9
compounds - *see* Chromates	—	—	—	—	—	—
Chromonar	972.4	E858.3	E942.4	E950.4	E962.0	E980.4
Chromyl chloride	983.9	E864.3	—	E950.7	E962.1	E980.6
Chrysarobin (ointment)	976.4	E858.7	E946.4	E950.4	E962.0	E980.4
Chrysazin	973.1	E858.4	E943.1	E950.4	E962.0	E980.4
Chymar	963.4	E858.1	E933.4	E950.4	E962.0	E980.4
ophthalmic preparation	976.5	E858.7	E946.5	E950.4	E962.0	E980.4
Chymotrypsin	963.4	E858.1	E933.4	E950.4	E962.0	E980.4
ophthalmic preparation	976.5	E858.7	E946.5	E950.4	E962.0	E980.4
Cicuta maculata or virosa	988.2	E865.4	—	E950.9	E962.1	E980.9
Cigarette lighter fluid	981	E862.1	—	E950.9	E962.1	E980.9
Cinchocaine (spinal)	968.7	E855.2	E938.7	E950.4	E962.0	E980.4
topical (surface)	968.5	E855.2	E938.5	E950.4	E962.0	E980.4
Cinchona	961.4	E857	E931.4	E950.4	E962.0	E980.4
Cinchonine alkaloids	961.4	E857	E931.4	E950.4	E962.0	E980.4
Cinchophen	974.7	E858.5	E944.7	E950.4	E962.0	E980.4
Cinnarizine	963.0	E858.1	E933.0	E950.4	E962.0	E980.4
Citanest	968.9	E855.2	E938.9	E950.4	E962.0	E980.4
infiltration (subcutaneous)	968.5	E855.2	E938.5	E950.4	E962.0	E980.4
nerve block (peripheral) (plexus)	968.6	E855.2	E938.6	E950.4	E962.0	E980.4
Citric acid	989.89	E866.8	—	E950.9	E962.1	E980.9
Citrovorum factor	964.1	E858.2	E934.1	E950.4	E962.0	E980.4
Claviceps purpurea	988.2	E865.4	—	E950.9	E962.1	E980.9
Cleaner, cleansing agent NEC	989.89	E861.3	—	E950.9	E962.1	E980.9
of paint or varnish	982.8	E862.9	—	E950.9	E962.1	E980.9
Clematis vitalba	988.2	E865.4	—	E950.9	E962.1	E980.9
Clemizole	963.0	E858.1	E933.0	E950.4	E962.0	E980.4
penicillin	960.0	E856	E930.0	E950.4	E962.0	E980.4
Clidinium	971.1	E855.4	E941.1	E950.4	E962.0	E980.4
Clindamycin	960.8	E856	E930.8	E950.4	E962.0	E980.4
Cliradon	965.09	E850.2	E935.2	E950.0	E962.0	E980.0
Clocortolone	962.0	E858.0	E932.0	E950.4	E962.0	E980.4
Clofedanol	975.4	E858.6	E945.4	E950.4	E962.0	E980.4
Clofibrate	972.2	E858.3	E942.2	E950.4	E962.0	E980.4
Clomethiazole	967.1	E852.0	E937.1	E950.2	E962.0	E980.2
Clomiphene	977.8	E858.8	E947.8	E950.4	E962.0	E980.4
Clonazepam	969.4	E853.2	E939.4	E950.3	E962.0	E980.3
Clonidine	972.6	E858.3	E942.6	E950.4	E962.0	E980.4
Clopamide	974.3	E858.5	E944.3	E950.4	E962.0	E980.4
Clorazepate	969.4	E853.2	E939.4	E950.3	E962.0	E980.3
Clorexolone	974.4	E858.5	E944.4	E950.4	E962.0	E980.4
Clorox (bleach)	983.9	E864.3	—	E950.7	E962.1	E980.6
Clortermine	977.0	E858.8	E947.0	E950.4	E962.0	E980.4
Clotrimazole	976.0	E858.7	E946.0	E950.4	E962.0	E980.4
Cloxacillin	960.0	E856	E930.0	E950.4	E962.0	E980.4
Coagulants NEC	964.5	E858.2	E934.5	E950.4	E962.0	E980.4
Coal (carbon monoxide from) - *see also* Carbon, monoxide, coal	—	—	—	—	—	—
oil - *see* Kerosene	—	—	—	—	—	—
tar NEC	983.0	E864.0	—	E950.7	E962.1	E980.6
fumes	987.8	E869.8	—	E952.8	E962.2	E982.8
medicinal (ointment)	976.4	E858.7	E946.4	E950.4	E962.0	E980.4

Substance	Poisoning	External Cause (E-Code) Accident	Therapeutic Use	Suicide Attempt	Assault	Undetermined
Coal *(Continued)*						
analgesics NEC	965.5	E850.5	E935.5	E950.0	E962.0	E980.0
naphtha (solvent)	981	E862.0	—	E950.9	E962.1	E980.9
Cobalt (fumes) (industrial)	985.8	E866.4	—	E950.9	E962.1	E980.9
Cobra (venom)	989.5	E905.0	—	E950.9	E962.1	E980.9
Coca (leaf)	970.8	E854.3	E940.8	E950.4	E962.0	E980.4
Cocaine (hydrochloride) (salt)	970.8	E854.3	E940.8	E950.4	E962.0	E980.4
topical anesthetic	968.5	E855.2	E938.5	E950.4	E962.0	E980.4
Coccidioidin	977.8	E858.8	E947.8	E950.4	E962.0	E980.4
Cocculus indicus	988.2	E865.3	—	E950.9	E962.1	E980.9
Cochineal	989.89	E866.8	—	E950.9	E962.1	E980.9
medicinal products	977.4	E858.8	E947.4	E950.4	E962.0	E980.4
Codeine	965.09	E850.2	E935.2	E950.0	E962.0	E980.0
Coffee	989.89	E866.8	—	E950.9	E962.1	E980.9
Cogentin	971.1	E855.4	E941.1	E950.4	E962.0	E980.4
Coke fumes or gas (carbon monoxide)	986	E868.3	—	E952.1	E962.2	E982.1
industrial use	986	E868.8	—	E952.1	E962.2	E982.1
Colace	973.2	E858.4	E943.2	E950.4	E962.0	E980.4
Colchicine	974.7	E858.5	E944.7	E950.4	E962.0	E980.4
Colchicum	988.2	E865.3	—	E950.9	E962.1	E980.9
Cold cream	976.3	E858.7	E946.3	E950.4	E962.0	E980.4
Colestipol	972.2	E858.3	E942.2	E950.4	E962.0	E980.4
Colistimethate	960.8	E856	E930.8	E950.4	E962.0	E980.4
Colistin	960.8	E856	E930.8	E950.4	E962.0	E980.4
Collagen	977.8	E866.8	E947.8	E950.9	E962.1	E980.9
Collagenase	976.8	E858.7	E946.8	E950.4	E962.0	E980.4
Collodion (flexible)	976.3	E858.7	E946.3	E950.4	E962.0	E980.4
Colocynth	973.1	E858.4	E943.1	E950.4	E962.0	E980.4
Coloring matter - *see* Dye(s)	—	—	—	—	—	—
Combustion gas - *see* Carbon, monoxide	—	—	—	—	—	—
Compazine	969.1	E853.0	E939.1	E950.3	E962.0	E980.3
Compound	—	—	—	—	—	—
42 (warfarin)	989.4	E863.7	—	E950.6	E962.1	E980.7
269 (endrin)	989.2	E863.0	—	E950.6	E962.1	E980.7
497 (dieldrin)	989.2	E863.0	—	E950.6	E962.1	E980.7
1080 (sodium fluoroacetate)	989.4	E863.7	—	E950.6	E962.1	E980.7
3422 (parathion)	989.3	E863.1	—	E950.6	E962.1	E980.7
3911 (phorate)	989.3	E863.1	—	E950.6	E962.1	E980.7
3956 (toxaphene)	989.2	E863.0	—	E950.6	E962.1	E980.7
4049 (malathion)	989.3	E863.1	—	E950.6	E962.1	E980.7
4124 (dicapthon)	989.4	E863.4	—	E950.6	E962.1	E980.7
E (cortisone)	962.0	E858.0	E932.0	E950.4	E962.0	E980.4
F (hydrocortisone)	962.0	E858.0	E932.0	E950.4	E962.0	E980.4
Congo red	977.8	E858.8	E947.8	E950.4	E962.0	E980.4
Coniine, conine	965.7	E850.7	E935.7	E950.0	E962.0	E980.0
Conium (maculatum)	988.2	E865.4	—	E950.9	E962.1	E980.9
Conjugated estrogens (equine)	962.2	E858.0	E932.2	E950.4	E962.0	E980.4
Contac	975.6	E858.6	E945.6	E950.4	E962.0	E980.4
Contact lens solution	976.5	E858.7	E946.5	E950.4	E962.0	E980.4
Contraceptives (oral)	962.2	E858.0	E932.2	E950.4	E962.0	E980.4
vaginal	976.8	E858.7	E946.8	E950.4	E962.0	E980.4
Contrast media (roentgenographic)	977.8	E858.8	E947.8	E950.4	E962.0	E980.4
Convallaria majalis	988.2	E865.4	—	E950.9	E962.1	E980.9
Copper (dust) (fumes) (salts) NEC	985.8	E866.4	—	E950.9	E962.1	E980.9
arsenate, arsenite	985.1	E866.3	—	E950.8	E962.1	E980.8
insecticide	985.1	E863.4	—	E950.8	E962.1	E980.8
emetic	973.6	E858.4	E943.6	E950.4	E962.0	E980.4
fungicide	985.8	E863.6	—	E950.6	E962.1	E980.7
insecticide	985.8	E863.4	—	E950.6	E962.1	E980.7
oleate	976.0	E858.7	E946.0	E950.4	E962.0	E980.4
sulfate	983.9	E864.3	—	E950.7	E962.1	E980.6
fungicide	983.9	E863.6	—	E950.7	E962.1	E980.6

Substance	Poisoning	External Cause (E-Code) Accident	Therapeutic Use	Suicide Attempt	Assault	Undetermined
Copper *(Continued)*						
cupric	973.6	E858.4	E943.6	E950.4	E962.0	E980.4
cuprous	983.9	E864.3	—	E950.7	E962.1	E980.6
Copperhead snake (bite) (venom)	989.5	E905.0	—	E950.9	E962.1	E980.9
Coral (sting)	989.5	E905.6	—	E950.9	E962.1	E980.9
snake (bite) (venom)	989.5	E905.0	—	E950.9	E962.1	E980.9
Cordran	976.0	E858.7	E946.0	E950.4	E962.0	E980.4
Corn cures	976.4	E858.7	E946.4	E950.4	E962.0	E980.4
Cornhusker's lotion	976.3	E858.7	E946.3	E950.4	E962.0	E980.4
Corn starch	976.3	E858.7	E946.3	E950.4	E962.0	E980.4
Corrosive	983.9	E864.4	—	E950.7	E962.1	E980.6
acids NEC	983.1	E864.1	—	E950.7	E962.1	E980.6
aromatics	983.0	E864.0	—	E950.7	E962.1	E980.6
disinfectant	983.0	E861.4	—	E950.7	E962.1	E980.6
fumes NEC	987.9	E869.9	—	E952.9	E962.2	E982.9
specified NEC	983.9	E864.3	—	E950.7	E962.1	E980.6
sublimate - *see* Mercury, chloride	—	—	—	—	—	—
Cortate	962.0	E858.0	E932.0	E950.4	E962.0	E980.4
Cort-Dome	962.0	E858.0	E932.0	E950.4	E962.0	E980.4
ENT agent	976.6	E858.7	E946.6	E950.4	E962.0	E980.4
ophthalmic preparation	976.5	E858.7	E946.5	E950.4	E962.0	E980.4
topical NEC	976.0	E858.7	E946.0	E950.4	E962.0	E980.4
Cortef	962.0	E858.0	E932.0	E950.4	E962.0	E980.4
ENT agent	976.6	E858.7	E946.6	E950.4	E962.0	E980.4
ophthalmic preparation	976.5	E858.7	E946.5	E950.4	E962.0	E980.4
topical NEC	976.0	E858.7	E946.0	E950.4	E962.0	E980.4
Corticosteroids (fluorinated)	962.0	E858.0	E932.0	E950.4	E962.0	E980.4
ENT agent	976.6	E858.7	E946.6	E950.4	E962.0	E980.4
ophthalmic preparation	976.5	E858.7	E946.5	E950.4	E962.0	E980.4
topical NEC	976.0	E858.7	E946.0	E950.4	E962.0	E980.4
Corticotropin	962.4	E858.0	E932.4	E950.4	E962.0	E980.4
Cortisol	962.0	E858.0	E932.0	E950.4	E962.0	E980.4
ENT agent	976.6	E858.7	E946.6	E950.4	E962.0	E980.4
ophthalmic preparation	976.5	E858.7	E946.5	E950.4	E962.0	E980.4
topical NEC	976.0	E858.7	E946.0	E950.4	E962.0	E980.4
Cortisone derivatives (acetate)	962.0	E858.0	E932.0	E950.4	E962.0	E980.4
ENT agent	976.6	E858.7	E946.6	E950.4	E962.0	E980.4
ophthalmic preparation	976.5	E858.7	E946.5	E950.4	E962.0	E980.4
topical NEC	976.0	E858.7	E946.0	E950.4	E962.0	E980.4
Cortogen	962.0	E858.0	E932.0	E950.4	E962.0	E980.4
ENT agent	976.6	E858.7	E946.6	E950.4	E962.0	E980.4
ophthalmic preparation	976.5	E858.7	E946.5	E950.4	E962.0	E980.4
Cortone	962.0	E858.0	E932.0	E950.4	E962.0	E980.4
ENT agent	976.6	E858.7	E946.6	E950.4	E962.0	E980.4
ophthalmic preparation	976.5	E858.7	E946.5	E950.4	E962.0	E980.4
Cortril	962.0	E858.0	E932.0	E950.4	E962.0	E980.4
ENT agent	976.6	E858.7	E946.6	E950.4	E962.0	E980.4
ophthalmic preparation	976.5	E858.7	E946.5	E950.4	E962.0	E980.4
topical NEC	976.0	E858.7	E946.0	E950.4	E962.0	E980.4
Cosmetics	989.89	E866.7	—	E950.9	E962.1	E980.9
Cosyntropin	977.8	E858.8	E947.8	E950.4	E962.0	E980.4
Cotarnine	964.5	E858.2	E934.5	E950.4	E962.0	E980.4
Cottonseed oil	976.3	E858.7	E946.3	E950.4	E962.0	E980.4
Cough mixtures (antitussives)	975.4	E858.6	E945.4	E950.4	E962.0	E980.4
containing opiates	965.09	E850.2	E935.2	E950.0	E962.0	E980.0
expectorants	975.5	E858.6	E945.5	E950.4	E962.0	E980.4
Coumadin	964.2	E858.2	E934.2	E950.4	E962.0	E980.4
rodenticide	989.4	E863.7	—	E950.6	E962.1	E980.7
Coumarin	964.2	E858.2	E934.2	E950.4	E962.0	E980.4
Coumetarol	964.2	E858.2	E934.2	E950.4	E962.0	E980.4
Cowbane	988.2	E865.4	—	E950.9	E962.1	E980.9
Cozyme	963.5	E858.1	E933.5	E950.4	E962.0	E980.4
Crack	970.8	E854.3	E940.8	E950.4	E962.0	E980.4

Substance	Poisoning	External Cause (E-Code) Accident	Therapeutic Use	Suicide Attempt	Assault	Undetermined
Creolin	983.0	E864.0	—	E950.7	E962.1	E980.6
disinfectant	983.0	E861.4	—	E950.7	E962.1	E980.6
Creosol (compound)	983.0	E864.0	—	E950.7	E962.1	E980.6
Creosote (beechwood) (coal tar)	983.0	E864.0	—	E950.7	E962.1	E980.6
medicinal (expectorant)	975.5	E858.6	E945.5	E950.4	E962.0	E980.4
syrup	975.5	E858.6	E945.5	E950.4	E962.0	E980.4
Cresol	983.0	E864.0	—	E950.7	E962.1	E980.6
disinfectant	983.0	E861.4	—	E950.7	E962.1	E980.6
Cresylic acid	983.0	E864.0	—	E950.7	E962.1	E980.6
Cropropamide	965.7	E850.7	E935.7	E950.0	E962.0	E980.0
with crotethamide	970.0	E854.3	E940.0	E950.4	E962.0	E980.4
Crotamiton	976.0	E858.7	E946.0	E950.4	E962.0	E980.4
Crotethamide	965.7	E850.7	E935.7	E950.0	E962.0	E980.0
with cropropamide	970.0	E854.3	E940.0	E950.4	E962.0	E980.4
Croton (oil)	973.1	E858.4	E943.1	E950.4	E962.0	E980.4
chloral	967.1	E852.0	E937.1	E950.2	E962.0	E980.2
Crude oil	981	E862.1	—	E950.9	E962.1	E980.9
Cryogenine	965.8	E850.8	E935.8	E950.0	E962.0	E980.0
Cryolite (pesticide)	989.4	E863.4	—	E950.6	E962.1	E980.7
Cryptenamine	972.6	E858.3	E942.6	E950.4	E962.0	E980.4
Crystal violet	976.0	E858.7	E946.0	E950.4	E962.0	E980.4
Cuckoopint	988.2	E865.4	—	E950.9	E962.1	E980.9
Cumetharol	964.2	E858.2	E934.2	E950.4	E962.0	E980.4
Cupric sulfate	973.6	E858.4	E943.6	E950.4	E962.0	E980.4
Cuprous sulfate	983.9	E864.3	—	E950.7	E962.1	E980.6
Curare, curarine	975.2	E858.6	E945.2	E950.4	E962.0	E980.4
Cyanic acid - *see* Cyanide(s)	—	—	—	—	—	—
Cyanide(s) (compounds) (hydrogen) (potassium) (sodium) NEC	989.0	E866.8	—	E950.9	E962.1	E980.9
dust or gas (inhalation) NEC	987.7	E869.8	—	E952.8	E962.2	E982.8
fumigant	989.0	E863.8	—	E950.6	E962.1	E980.7
mercuric - *see* Mercury	—	—	—	—	—	—
pesticide (dust) (fumes)	989.0	E863.4	—	E950.6	E962.1	E980.7
Cyanocobalamin	964.1	E858.2	E934.1	E950.4	E962.0	E980.4
Cyanogen (chloride) (gas)	—	—	—	—	—	—
NEC	987.8	E869.8	—	E952.8	E962.2	E982.8
Cyclaine	968.5	E855.2	E938.5	E950.4	E962.0	E980.4
Cyclamen europaeum	988.2	E865.4	—	E950.9	E962.1	E980.9
Cyclandelate	972.5	E858.3	E942.5	E950.4	E962.0	E980.4
Cyclazocine	965.09	E850.2	E935.2	E950.0	E962.0	E980.0
Cyclizine	963.0	E858.1	E933.0	E950.4	E962.0	E980.4
Cyclobarbital, cyclobarbitone	967.0	E851	E937.0	E950.1	E962.0	E980.1
Cycloguanil	961.4	E857	E931.4	E950.4	E962.0	E980.4
Cyclohexane	982.0	E862.4	—	E950.9	E962.1	E980.9
Cyclohexanol	980.8	E860.8	—	E950.9	E962.1	E980.9
Cyclohexanone	982.8	E862.4	—	E950.9	E962.1	E980.9
Cyclomethycaine	968.5	E855.2	E938.5	E950.4	E962.0	E980.4
Cyclopentamine	971.2	E855.5	E941.2	E950.4	E962.0	E980.4
Cyclopenthiazide	974.3	E858.5	E944.3	E950.4	E962.0	E980.4
Cyclopentolate	971.1	E855.4	E941.1	E950.4	E962.0	E980.4
Cyclophosphamide	963.1	E858.1	E933.1	E950.4	E962.0	E980.4
Cyclopropane	968.2	E855.1	E938.2	E950.4	E962.0	E980.4
Cycloserine	960.6	E856	E930.6	E950.4	E962.0	E980.4
Cyclothiazide	974.3	E858.5	E944.3	E950.4	E962.0	E980.4
Cycrimine	966.4	E855.0	E936.4	E950.4	E962.0	E980.4
Cymarin	972.1	E858.3	E942.1	E950.4	E962.0	E980.4
Cyproheptadine	963.0	E858.1	E933.0	E950.4	E962.0	E980.4
Cyprolidol	969.0	E854.0	E939.0	E950.3	E962.0	E980.3
Cytarabine	963.1	E858.1	E933.1	E950.4	E962.0	E980.4
Cytisus	—	—	—	—	—	—
laburnum	988.2	E865.4	—	E950.9	E962.1	E980.9
scoparius	988.2	E865.4	—	E950.9	E962.1	E980.9

Substance	Poisoning	External Cause (E-Code) Accident	Therapeutic Use	Suicide Attempt	Assault	Undetermined
Cytomel	962.7	E858.0	E932.7	E950.4	E962.0	E980.4
Cytosine (antineoplastic)	963.1	E858.1	E933.1	E950.4	E962.0	E980.4
Cytoxan	963.1	E858.1	E933.1	E950.4	E962.0	E980.4
Dacarbazine	963.1	E858.1	E933.1	E950.4	E962.0	E980.4
Dactinomycin	960.7	E856	E930.7	E950.4	E962.0	E980.4
DADPS	961.8	E857	E931.8	E950.4	E962.0	E980.4
Dakin's solution (external)	976.0	E858.7	E946.0	E950.4	E962.0	E980.4
Dalmane	969.4	E853.2	E939.4	E950.3	E962.0	E980.3
DAM	977.2	E858.8	E947.2	E950.4	E962.0	E980.4
Danilone	964.2	E858.2	E934.2	E950.4	E962.0	E980.4
Danthron	973.1	E858.4	E943.1	E950.4	E962.0	E980.4
Dantrolene	975.2	E858.6	E945.2	E950.4	E962.0	E980.4
Daphne (gnidium) (mezereum)	988.2	E865.4	—	E950.9	E962.1	E980.9
berry	988.2	E865.3	—	E950.9	E962.1	E980.9
Dapsone	961.8	E857	E931.8	E950.4	E962.0	E980.4
Daraprim	961.4	E857	E931.4	E950.4	E962.0	E980.4
Darnel	988.2	E865.3	—	E950.9	E962.1	E980.9
Darvon	965.8	E850.8	E935.8	E950.0	E962.0	E980.0
Daunorubicin	960.7	E856	E930.7	E950.4	E962.0	E980.4
DBI	962.3	E858.0	E932.3	E950.4	E962.0	E980.4
D-Con (rodenticide)	989.4	E863.7	—	E950.6	E962.1	E980.7
DDS	961.8	E857	E931.8	E950.4	E962.0	E980.4
DDT	989.2	E863.0	—	E950.6	E962.1	E980.7
Deadly nightshade	988.2	E865.4	—	E950.9	E962.1	E980.9
berry	988.2	E865.3	—	E950.9	E962.1	E980.9
Deanol	969.7	E854.2	E939.7	E950.3	E962.0	E980.3
Debrisoquine	972.6	E858.3	E942.6	E950.4	E962.0	E980.4
Decaborane	989.89	E866.8	—	E950.9	E962.1	E980.9
fumes	987.8	E869.8	—	E952.8	E962.2	E982.8
Decadron	962.0	E858.0	E932.0	E950.4	E962.0	E980.4
ENT agent	976.6	E858.7	E946.6	E950.4	E962.0	E980.4
ophthalmic preparation	976.5	E858.7	E946.5	E950.4	E962.0	E980.4
topical NEC	976.0	E858.7	E946.0	E950.4	E962.0	E980.4
Decahydronaphthalene	982.0	E862.4	—	E950.9	E962.1	E980.9
Decalin	982.0	E862.4	—	E950.9	E962.1	E980.9
Decamethonium	975.2	E858.6	E945.2	E950.4	E962.0	E980.4
Decholin	973.4	E858.4	E943.4	E950.4	E962.0	E980.4
sodium (diagnostic)	977.8	E858.8	E947.8	E950.4	E962.0	E980.4
Declomycin	960.4	E856	E930.4	E950.4	E962.0	E980.4
Deferoxamine	963.8	E858.1	E933.8	E950.4	E962.0	E980.4
Dehydrocholic acid	973.4	E858.4	E943.4	E950.4	E962.0	E980.4
DeKalin	982.0	E862.4	—	E950.9	E962.1	E980.9
Delalutin	962.2	E858.0	E932.2	E950.4	E962.0	E980.4
Delphinium	988.2	E865.3	—	E950.9	E962.1	E980.9
Deltasone	962.0	E858.0	E932.0	E950.4	E962.0	E980.4
Deltra	962.0	E858.0	E932.0	E950.4	E962.0	E980.4
Delvinal	967.0	E851	E937.0	E950.1	E962.0	E980.1
Demecarium (bromide)	971.0	E855.3	E941.0	E950.4	E962.0	E980.4
Demeclocycline	960.4	E856	E930.4	E950.4	E962.0	E980.4
Demecolcine	963.1	E858.1	E933.1	E950.4	E962.0	E980.4
Demelanizing agents	976.8	E858.7	E946.8	E950.4	E962.0	E980.4
Demerol	965.09	E850.2	E935.2	E950.0	E962.0	E980.0
Demethylchlortetracycline	960.4	E856	E930.4	E950.4	E962.0	E980.4
Demethyltetracycline	960.4	E856	E930.4	E950.4	E962.0	E980.4
Demeton	989.3	E863.1	—	E950.6	E962.1	E980.7
Demulcents	976.3	E858.7	E946.3	E950.4	E962.0	E980.4
Demulen	962.2	E858.0	E932.2	E950.4	E962.0	E980.4
Denatured alcohol	980.0	E860.1	—	E950.9	E962.1	E980.9
Dendrid	976.5	E858.7	E946.5	E950.4	E962.0	E980.4
Dental agents, topical	976.7	E858.7	E946.7	E950.4	E962.0	E980.4
Deodorant spray (feminine hygiene)	976.8	E858.7	E946.8	E950.4	E962.0	E980.4

		External Cause (E-Code)				
Substance	**Poisoning**	**Accident**	**Therapeutic Use**	**Suicide Attempt**	**Assault**	**Undetermined**
Deoxyribonuclease	963.4	E858.1	E933.4	E950.4	E962.0	E980.4
Depressants	—	—	—	—	—	—
appetite, central	977.0	E858.8	E947.0	E950.4	E962.0	E980.4
cardiac	972.0	E858.3	E942.0	E950.4	E962.0	E980.4
central nervous system (anesthetic)	968.4	E855.1	E938.4	E950.4	E962.0	E980.4
psychotherapeutic	969.5	E853.9	E939.5	E950.3	E962.0	E980.3
Dequalinium	976.0	E858.7	E946.0	E950.4	E962.0	E980.4
Dermolate	976.2	E858.7	E946.2	E950.4	E962.0	E980.4
DES	962.2	E858.0	E932.2	E950.4	E962.0	E980.4
Desenex	976.0	E858.7	E946.0	E950.4	E962.0	E980.4
Deserpidine	972.6	E858.3	E942.6	E950.4	E962.0	E980.4
Desipramine	969.0	E854.0	E939.0	E950.3	E962.0	E980.3
Deslanoside	972.1	E858.3	E942.1	E950.4	E962.0	E980.4
Desocodeine	965.09	E850.2	E935.2	E950.0	E962.0	E980.0
Desomorphine	965.09	E850.2	E935.2	E950.0	E962.0	E980.0
Desonide	976.0	E858.7	E946.0	E950.4	E962.0	E980.4
Desoxycorticosterone derivatives	962.0	E858.0	E932.0	E950.4	E962.0	E980.4
Desoxyephedrine	969.7	E854.2	E939.7	E950.3	E962.0	E980.3
DET	969.6	E854.1	E939.6	E950.3	E962.0	E980.3
Detergents (ingested) (synthetic)	989.6	E861.0	—	E950.9	E962.1	E980.9
external medication	976.2	E858.7	E946.2	E950.4	E962.0	E980.4
Deterrent, alcohol	977.3	E858.8	E947.3	E950.4	E962.0	E980.4
Detrothyronine	962.7	E858.0	E932.7	E950.4	E962.0	E980.4
Dettol (external medication)	976.0	E858.7	E946.0	E950.4	E962.0	E980.4
Dexamethasone	962.0	E858.0	E932.0	E950.4	E962.0	E980.4
ENT agent	976.6	E858.7	E946.6	E950.4	E962.0	E980.4
ophthalmic preparation	976.5	E858.7	E946.5	E950.4	E962.0	E980.4
topical NEC	976.0	E858.7	E946.0	E950.4	E962.0	E980.4
Dexamphetamine	969.7	E854.2	E939.7	E950.3	E962.0	E980.3
Dexedrine	969.7	E854.2	E939.7	E950.3	E962.0	E980.3
Dexpanthenol	963.5	E858.1	E933.5	E950.4	E962.0	E980.4
Dextran	964.8	E858.2	E934.8	E950.4	E962.0	E980.4
Dextriferron	964.0	E858.2	E934.0	E950.4	E962.0	E980.4
Dextroamphetamine	969.7	E854.2	E939.7	E950.3	E962.0	E980.3
Dextro calcium pantothenate	963.5	E858.1	E933.5	E950.4	E962.0	E980.4
Dextromethorphan	975.4	E858.6	E945.4	E950.4	E962.0	E980.4
Dextromoramide	965.09	E850.2	E935.2	E950.0	E962.0	E980.0
Dextro pantothenyl alcohol	963.5	E858.1	E933.5	E950.4	E962.0	E980.4
topical	976.8	E858.7	E946.8	E950.4	E962.0	E980.4
Dextropropoxyphene (hydrochloride)	965.8	E850.8	E935.8	E950.0	E962.0	E980.0
Dextrorphan	965.09	E850.2	E935.2	E950.0	E962.0	E980.0
Dextrose NEC	974.5	E858.5	E944.5	E950.4	E962.0	E980.4
Dextrothyroxine	962.7	E858.0	E932.7	E950.4	E962.0	E980.4
DFP	971.0	E855.3	E941.0	E950.4	E962.0	E980.4
DHE-45	972.9	E858.3	E942.9	E950.4	E962.0	E980.4
Diabinese	962.3	E858.0	E932.3	E950.4	E962.0	E980.4
Diacetyl monoxime	977.2	E858.8	E947.2	E950.4	E962.0	E980.4
Diacetylmorphine	965.01	E850.0	E935.0	E950.0	E962.0	E980.0
Diagnostic agents	977.8	E858.8	E947.8	E950.4	E962.0	E980.4
Dial (soap)	976.2	E858.7	E946.2	E950.4	E962.0	E980.4
sedative	967.0	E851	E937.0	E950.1	E962.0	E980.1
Diallylbarbituric acid	967.0	E851	E937.0	E950.1	E962.0	E980.1
Diaminodiphenyisulfone	961.8	E857	E931.8	E950.4	E962.0	E980.4
Diamorphine	965.01	E850.0	E935.0	E950.0	E962.0	E980.0
Diamox	974.2	E858.5	E944.2	E950.4	E962.0	E980.4
Diamthazole	976.0	E858.7	E946.0	E950.4	E962.0	E980.4
Diaphenyisulfone	961.8	E857	E931.8	E950.4	E962.0	E980.4
Diasone (sodium)	961.8	E857	E931.8	E950.4	E962.0	E980.4
Diazepam	969.4	E853.2	E939.4	E950.3	E962.0	E980.3
Diazinon	989.3	E863.1	—	E950.6	E962.1	E980.7
Diazomethane (gas)	987.8	E869.8	—	E952.8	E962.2	E982.8

Substance	Poisoning	Accident	Therapeutic Use	Suicide Attempt	Assault	Undetermined
		External Cause (E-Code)				
Diazoxide	972.5	E858.3	E942.5	E950.4	E962.0	E980.4
Dibenamine	971.3	E855.6	E941.3	E950.4	E962.0	E980.4
Dibenzheptropine	963.0	E858.1	E933.0	E950.4	E962.0	E980.4
Dibenzyline	971.3	E855.6	E941.3	E950.4	E962.0	E980.4
Diborane (gas)	987.8	E869.8	—	E952.8	E962.2	E982.8
Dibromomannitol	963.1	E858.1	E933.1	E950.4	E962.0	E980.4
Dibucaine (spinal)	968.7	E855.2	E938.7	E950.4	E962.0	E980.4
topical (surface)	968.5	E855.2	E938.5	E950.4	E962.0	E980.4
Dibunate sodium	975.4	E858.6	E945.4	E950.4	E962.0	E980.4
Dibutoline	971.1	E855.4	E941.1	E950.4	E962.0	E980.4
Dicapthon	989.4	E863.4	—	E950.6	E962.1	E980.7
Dichloralphenazone	967.1	E852.0	E937.1	E950.2	E962.0	E980.2
Dichlorodifluoromethane	987.4	E869.2	—	E952.8	E962.2	E982.8
Dichloroethane	982.3	E862.4	—	E950.9	E962.1	E980.9
Dichloroethylene	982.3	E862.4	—	E950.9	E962.1	E980.9
Dichloroethyl sulfide	987.8	E869.8	—	E952.8	E962.2	E982.8
Dichlorohydrin	982.3	E862.4	—	E950.9	E962.1	E980.9
Dichloromethane (solvent) (vapor)	982.3	E862.4	—	E950.9	E962.1	E980.9
Dichlorophen(e)	961.6	E857	E931.6	E950.4	E962.0	E980.4
Dichlorphenamide	974.2	E858.5	E944.2	E950.4	E962.0	E980.4
Dichlorvos	989.3	E863.1	—	E950.6	E962.1	E980.7
Diclofenac sodium	965.69	E850.6	E935.6	E950.0	E962.0	E980.0
Dicoumarin, dicumarol	964.2	E858.2	E934.2	E950.4	E962.0	E980.4
Dicyanogen (gas)	987.8	E869.8	—	E952.8	E962.2	E982.8
Dicyclomine	971.1	E855.4	E941.1	E950.4	E962.0	E980.4
Dieldrin (vapor)	989.2	E863.0	—	E950.6	E962.1	E980.7
Dienestrol	962.2	E858.0	E932.2	E950.4	E962.0	E980.4
Dietetics	977.0	E858.8	E947.0	E950.4	E962.0	E980.4
Diethazine	966.4	E855.0	E936.4	E950.4	E962.0	E980.4
Diethyl	—	—	—	—	—	—
barbituric acid	967.0	E851	E937.0	E950.1	E962.0	E980.1
carbamazine	961.6	E857	E931.6	E950.4	E962.0	E980.4
carbinol	980.8	E860.8	—	E950.9	E962.1	E980.9
carbonate	982.8	E862.4	—	E950.9	E962.1	E980.9
ether (vapor) - *see* Ether(s)	—	—	—	—	—	—
propion	977.0	E858.8	E947.0	E950.4	E962.0	E980.4
stilbestrol	962.2	E858.0	E932.2	E950.4	E962.0	E980.4
Diethylene	—	—	—	—	—	—
dioxide	982.8	E862.4	—	E950.9	E962.1	E980.9
glycol (monoacetate) (monoethyl ether)	982.8	E862.4	—	E950.9	E962.1	E980.9
Diethylsulfone-diethylmethane	967.8	E852.8	E937.8	E950.2	E962.0	E980.2
Difencloxazine	965.09	E850.2	E935.2	E950.0	E962.0	E980.0
Diffusin	963.4	E858.1	E933.4	E950.4	E962.0	E980.4
Diflos	971.0	E855.3	E941.0	E950.4	E962.0	E980.4
Digestants	973.4	E858.4	E943.4	E950.4	E962.0	E980.4
Digitalin(e)	972.1	E858.3	E942.1	E950.4	E962.0	E980.4
Digitalis glycosides	972.1	E858.3	E942.1	E950.4	E962.0	E980.4
Digitoxin	972.1	E858.3	E942.1	E950.4	E962.0	E980.4
Digoxin	972.1	E858.3	E942.1	E950.4	E962.0	E980.4
Dihydrocodeine	965.09	E850.2	E935.2	E950.0	E962.0	E980.0
Dihydrocodeinone	965.09	E850.2	E935.2	E950.0	E962.0	E980.0
Dihydroergocristine	972.9	E858.3	E942.9	E950.4	E962.0	E980.4
Dihydroergotamine	972.9	E858.3	E942.9	E950.4	E962.0	E980.4
Dihydroergotoxine	972.9	E858.3	E942.9	E950.4	E962.0	E980.4
Dihydrohydroxycodeinone	965.09	E850.2	E935.2	E950.0	E962.0	E980.0
Dihydrohydroxymorphinone	965.09	E850.2	E935.2	E950.0	E962.0	E980.0
Dihydroisocodeine	965.09	E850.2	E935.2	E950.0	E962.0	E980.0
Dihydromorphine	965.09	E850.2	E935.2	E950.0	E962.0	E980.0
Dihydromorphinone	965.09	E850.2	E935.2	E950.0	E962.0	E980.0
Dihydrostreptomycin	960.6	E856	E930.6	E950.4	E962.0	E980.4
Dihydrotachysterol	962.6	E858.0	E932.6	E950.4	E962.0	E980.4

Substance	Poisoning	External Cause (E-Code) Accident	Therapeutic Use	Suicide Attempt	Assault	Undetermined
Dihydroxyanthraquinone	973.1	E858.4	E943.1	E950.4	E962.0	E980.4
Dihydroxycodeinone	965.09	E850.2	E935.2	E950.0	E962.0	E980.0
Diiodohydroxyquin	961.3	E857	E931.3	E950.4	E962.0	E980.4
topical	976.0	E858.7	E946.0	E950.4	E962.0	E980.4
Diiodohydroxyquinoline	961.3	E857	E931.3	E950.4	E962.0	E980.4
Dilantin	966.1	E855.0	E936.1	E950.4	E962.0	E980.4
Dilaudid	965.09	E850.2	E935.2	E950.0	E962.0	E980.0
Diloxanide	961.5	E857	E931.5	E950.4	E962.0	E980.4
Dimefline	970.0	E854.3	E940.0	E950.4	E962.0	E980.4
Dimenhydrinate	963.0	E858.1	E933.0	E950.4	E962.0	E980.4
Dimercaprol	963.8	E858.1	E933.8	E950.4	E962.0	E980.4
Dimercaptopropanol	963.8	E858.1	E933.8	E950.4	E962.0	E980.4
Dimetane	963.0	E858.1	E933.0	E950.4	E962.0	E980.4
Dimethicone	976.3	E858.7	E946.3	E950.4	E962.0	E980.4
Dimethindene	963.0	E858.1	E933.0	E950.4	E962.0	E980.4
Dimethisoquin	968.5	E855.2	E938.5	E950.4	E962.0	E980.4
Dimethisterone	962.2	E858.0	E932.2	E950.4	E962.0	E980.4
Dimethoxanate	975.4	E858.6	E945.4	E950.4	E962.0	E980.4
Dimethyl	—	—	—	—	—	—
arsine, arsinic acid - *see* Arsenic	—	—	—	—	—	—
carbinol	980.2	E860.3	—	E950.9	E962.1	E980.9
diguanide	962.3	E858.0	E932.3	E950.4	E962.0	E980.4
ketone	982.8	E862.4	—	E950.9	E962.1	E980.9
vapor	987.8	E869.8	—	E952.8	E962.2	E982.8
meperidine	965.09	E850.2	E935.2	E950.0	E962.0	E980.0
parathion	989.3	E863.1	—	E950.6	E962.1	E980.7
polysiloxane	973.8	E858.4	E943.8	E950.4	E962.0	E980.4
sulfate (fumes)	987.8	E869.8	—	E952.8	E962.2	E982.8
liquid	983.9	E864.3	—	E950.7	E962.1	E980.6
sulfoxide NEC	982.8	E862.4	—	E950.9	E962.1	E980.9
medicinal	976.4	E858.7	E946.4	E950.4	E962.0	E980.4
triptamine	969.6	E854.1	E939.6	E950.3	E962.0	E980.3
tubocurarine	975.2	E858.6	E945.2	E950.4	E962.0	E980.4
Dindevan	964.2	E858.2	E934.2	E950.4	E962.0	E980.4
Dinitro (-ortho-) cresol (herbicide) (spray)	989.4	E863.5	—	E950.6	E962.1	E980.7
insecticide	989.4	E863.4	—	E950.6	E962.1	E980.7
Dinitrobenzene	983.0	E864.0	—	E950.7	E962.1	E980.6
vapor	987.8	E869.8	—	E952.8	E962.2	E982.8
Dinitro-orthocresol (herbicide)	989.4	E863.5	—	E950.6	E962.1	E980.7
insecticide	989.4	E863.4	—	E950.6	E962.1	E980.7
Dinitrophenol (herbicide) (spray)	989.4	E863.5	—	E950.6	E962.1	E980.7
insecticide	989.4	E863.4	—	E950.6	E962.1	E980.7
Dinoprost	975.0	E858.6	E945.0	E950.4	E962.0	E980.4
Dioctyl sulfosuccinate (calcium) (sodium)	973.2	E858.4	E943.2	E950.4	E962.0	E980.4
Diodoquin	961.3	E857	E931.3	E950.4	E962.0	E980.4
Dione derivatives NEC	966.3	E855.0	E936.3	E950.4	E962.0	E980.4
Dionin	965.09	E850.2	E935.2	E950.0	E962.0	E980.0
Dioxane	982.8	E862.4	—	E950.9	E962.1	E980.9
Dioxin - *see* herbicide	—	—	—	—	—	—
Dioxyline	972.5	E858.3	E942.5	E950.4	E962.0	E980.4
Dipentene	982.8	E862.4	—	E950.9	E962.1	E980.9
Diphemanil	971.1	E855.4	E941.1	E950.4	E962.0	E980.4
Diphenadione	964.2	E858.2	E934.2	E950.4	E962.0	E980.4
Diphenhydramine	963.0	E858.1	E933.0	E950.4	E962.0	E980.4
Diphenidol	963.0	E858.1	E933.0	E950.4	E962.0	E980.4
Diphenoxylate	973.5	E858.4	E943.5	E950.4	E962.0	E980.4
Diphenylchlorarsine	985.1	E866.3	—	E950.8	E962.1	E980.8
Diphenylhydantoin (sodium)	966.1	E855.0	E936.1	E950.4	E962.0	E980.4
Diphenylpyraline	963.0	E858.1	E933.0	E950.4	E962.0	E980.4
Diphtheria	—	—	—	—	—	—
antitoxin	979.9	E858.8	E949.9	E950.4	E962.0	E980.4

Substance	Poisoning	External Cause (E-Code) Accident	Therapeutic Use	Suicide Attempt	Assault	Undetermined
Diphtheria *(Continued)*						
toxoid	978.5	E858.8	E948.5	E950.4	E962.0	E980.4
with tetanus toxoid	978.9	E858.8	E948.9	E950.4	E962.0	E980.4
with pertussis component	978.6	E858.8	E948.6	E950.4	E962.0	E980.4
vaccine	978.5	E858.8	E948.5	E950.4	E962.0	E980.4
Dipipanone	965.09	E850.2	E935.2	E950.0	E962.0	E980.0
Diplovax	979.5	E858.8	E949.5	E950.4	E962.0	E980.4
Diprophylline	975.1	E858.6	E945.1	E950.4	E962.0	E980.4
Dipyridamole	972.4	E858.3	E942.4	E950.4	E962.0	E980.4
Dipyrone	965.5	E850.5	E935.5	E950.0	E962.0	E980.0
Diquat	989.4	E863.5	—	E950.6	E962.1	E980.7
Disinfectant NEC	983.9	E861.4	—	E950.7	E962.1	E980.6
alkaline	983.2	E861.4	—	E950.7	E962.1	E980.6
aromatic	983.0	E861.4	—	E950.7	E962.1	E980.6
Disipal	966.4	E855.0	E936.4	E950.4	E962.0	E980.4
Disodium edetate	963.8	E858.1	E933.8	E950.4	E962.0	E980.4
Disulfamide	974.4	E858.5	E944.4	E950.4	E962.0	E980.4
Disulfanilamide	961.0	E857	E931.0	E950.4	E962.0	E980.4
Disulfiram	977.3	E858.8	E947.3	E950.4	E962.0	E980.4
Dithiazanine	961.6	E857	E931.6	E950.4	E962.0	E980.4
Dithioglycerol	963.8	E858.1	E933.8	E950.4	E962.0	E980.4
Dithranol	976.4	E858.7	E946.4	E950.4	E962.0	E980.4
Diucardin	974.3	E858.5	E944.3	E950.4	E962.0	E980.4
Diupres	974.3	E858.5	E944.3	E950.4	E962.0	E980.4
Diuretics NEC	974.4	E858.5	E944.4	E950.4	E962.0	E980.4
carbonic acid anhydrase inhibitors	974.2	E858.5	E944.2	E950.4	E962.0	E980.4
mercurial	974.0	E858.5	E944.0	E950.4	E962.0	E980.4
osmotic	974.4	E858.5	E944.4	E950.4	E962.0	E980.4
purine derivatives	974.1	E858.5	E944.1	E950.4	E962.0	E980.4
saluretic	974.3	E858.5	E944.3	E950.4	E962.0	E980.4
Diuril	974.3	E858.5	E944.3	E950.4	E962.0	E980.4
Divinyl ether	968.2	E855.1	E938.2	E950.4	E962.0	E980.4
D-lysergic acid diethylamide	969.6	E854.1	E939.6	E950.3	E962.0	E980.3
DMCT	960.4	E856	E930.4	E950.4	E962.0	E980.4
DMSO	982.8	E862.4	—	E950.9	E962.1	E980.9
DMT	969.6	E854.1	E939.6	E950.3	E962.0	E980.3
DNOC	989.4	E863.5	—	E950.6	E962.1	E980.7
DOCA	962.0	E858.0	E932.0	E950.4	E962.0	E980.4
Dolophine	965.02	E850.1	E935.1	E950.0	E962.0	E980.0
Doloxene	965.8	E850.8	E935.8	E950.0	E962.0	E980.0
DOM	969.6	E854.1	E939.6	E950.3	E962.0	E980.3
Domestic gas - *see* Gas, utility	—	—	—	—	—	—
Domiphen (bromide) (lozenges)	976.6	E858.7	E946.6	E950.4	E962.0	E980.4
Dopa (levo)	966.4	E855.0	E936.4	E950.4	E962.0	E980.4
Dopamine	971.2	E855.5	E941.2	E950.4	E962.0	E980.4
Doriden	967.5	E852.4	E937.5	E950.2	E962.0	E980.2
Dormiral	967.0	E851	E937.0	E950.1	E962.0	E980.1
Dormison	967.8	E852.8	E937.8	E950.2	E962.0	E980.2
Dornase	963.4	E858.1	E933.4	E950.4	E962.0	E980.4
Dorsacaine	968.5	E855.2	E938.5	E950.4	E962.0	E980.4
Dothiepin hydrochloride	969.0	E854.0	E939.0	E950.3	E962.0	E980.3
Doxapram	970.0	E854.3	E940.0	E950.4	E962.0	E980.4
Doxepin	969.0	E854.0	E939.0	E950.3	E962.0	E980.3
Doxorubicin	960.7	E856	E930.7	E950.4	E962.0	E980.4
Doxycycline	960.4	E856	E930.4	E950.4	E962.0	E980.4
Doxylamine	963.0	E858.1	E933.0	E950.4	E962.0	E980.4
Dramamine	963.0	E858.1	E933.0	E950.4	E962.0	E980.4
Drano (drain cleaner)	983.2	E864.2	—	E950.7	E962.1	E980.6
Dromoran	965.09	E850.2	E935.2	E950.0	E962.0	E980.0
Dromostanolone	962.1	E858.0	E932.1	E950.4	E962.0	E980.4
Droperidol	969.2	E853.1	E939.2	E950.3	E962.0	E980.3
Drotrecogin alfa	964.2	E858.2	E934.2	E950.4	E962.0	E980.4 ◀

◀ New ⟸ Revised Code

Substance	Poisoning	External Cause (E-Code) Accident	Therapeutic Use	Suicide Attempt	Assault	Undetermined
Drug	977.9	E858.9	E947.9	E950.5	E962.0	E980.5
specified NEC	977.8	E858.8	E947.8	E950.4	E962.0	E980.4
AHFS List	—	—	—	—	—	—
4:00 antihistamine drugs	963.0	E858.1	E933.0	E950.4	E962.0	E980.4
8:04 amebacides	961.5	E857	E931.5	E950.4	E962.0	E980.4
arsenical anti-infectives	961.1	E857	E931.1	E950.4	E962.0	E980.4
quinoline derivatives	961.3	E857	E931.3	E950.4	E962.0	E980.4
8:08 anthelmintics	961.6	E857	E931.6	E950.4	E962.0	E980.4
quinoline derivatives	961.3	E857	E931.3	E950.4	E962.0	E980.4
8:12.04 antifungal antibiotics	960.1	E856	E930.1	E950.4	E962.0	E980.4
8:12.06 cephalosporins	960.5	E856	E930.5	E950.4	E962.0	E980.4
8:12.08 chloramphenicol	960.2	E856	E930.2	E950.4	E962.0	E980.4
8:12.12 erythromycins	960.3	E856	E930.3	E950.4	E962.0	E980.4
8:12.16 penicillins	960.0	E856	E930.0	E950.4	E962.0	E980.4
8:12.20 streptomycins	960.6	E856	E930.6	E950.4	E962.0	E980.4
8:12.24 tetracyclines	960.4	E856	E930.4	E950.4	E962.0	E980.4
8:12.28 other antibiotics	960.8	E856	E930.8	E950.4	E962.0	E980.4
antimycobacterial	960.6	E856	E930.6	E950.4	E962.0	E980.4
macrolides	960.3	E856	E930.3	E950.4	E962.0	E980.4
8:16 antituberculars	961.8	E857	E931.8	E950.4	E962.0	E980.4
antibiotics	960.6	E856	E930.6	E950.4	E962.0	E980.4
8:18 antivirals	961.7	E857	E931.7	E950.4	E962.0	E980.4
8:20 plasmodicides (antimalarials)	961.4	E857	E931.4	E950.4	E962.0	E980.4
8:24 sulfonamides	961.0	E857	E931.0	E950.4	E962.0	E980.4
8:26 sulfones	961.8	E857	E931.8	E950.4	E962.0	E980.4
8:28 treponemicides	961.2	E857	E931.2	E950.4	E962.0	E980.4
8:32 trichomonacides	961.5	E857	E931.5	E950.4	E962.0	E980.4
quinoline derivatives	961.3	E857	E931.3	E950.4	E962.0	E980.4
nitrofuran derivatives	961.9	E857	E931.9	E950.4	E962.0	E980.4
8:36 urinary germicides	961.9	E857	E931.9	E950.4	E962.0	E980.4
quinoline derivatives	961.3	E857	E931.3	E950.4	E962.0	E980.4
8:40 other anti-infectives	961.9	E857	E931.9	E950.4	E962.0	E980.4
10:00 antineoplastic agents	963.1	E858.1	E933.1	E950.4	E962.0	E980.4
antibiotics	960.7	E856	E930.7	E950.4	E962.0	E980.4
progestogens	962.2	E858.0	E932.2	E950.4	E962.0	E980.4
12:04 parasympathomimetic (cholinergic) agents	971.0	E855.3	E941.0	E950.4	E962.0	E980.4
12:08 parasympatholytic (cholinergic-blocking) agents	971.1	E855.4	E941.1	E950.4	E962.0	E980.4
12:12 sympathomimetic (adrenergic) agents	971.2	E855.5	E941.2	E950.4	E962.0	E980.4
12:16 sympatholytic (adrenergic-blocking) agents	971.3	E855.6	E941.3	E950.4	E962.0	E980.4
12:20 skeletal muscle relaxants	—	—	—	—	—	—
central nervous system muscle-tone depressants	968.0	E855.1	E938.0	E950.4	E962.0	E980.4
myoneural blocking agents	975.2	E858.6	E945.2	E950.4	E962.0	E980.4
16:00 blood derivatives	964.7	E858.2	E934.7	E950.4	E962.0	E980.4
20:04 antianemia drugs	964.1	E858.2	E934.1	E950.4	E962.0	E980.4
20:04.04 iron preparations	964.0	E858.2	E934.0	E950.4	E962.0	E980.4
20:04.08 liver and stomach preparations	964.1	E858.2	E934.1	E950.4	E962.0	E980.4
20:12.04 anticoagulants	964.2	E858.2	E934.2	E950.4	E962.0	E980.4
20:12.08 antiheparin agents	964.5	E858.2	E934.5	E950.4	E962.0	E980.4
20:12.12 coagulants	964.5	E858.2	E934.5	E950.4	E962.0	E980.4
20:12.16 hemostatics NEC	964.5	E858.2	E934.5	E950.4	E962.0	E980.4
capillary active drugs	972.8	E858.3	E942.8	E950.4	E962.0	E980.4
24:04 cardiac drugs	972.9	E858.3	E942.9	E950.4	E962.0	E980.4
cardiotonic agents	972.1	E858.3	E942.1	E950.4	E962.0	E980.4
rhythm regulators	972.0	E858.3	E942.0	E950.4	E962.0	E980.4
24:06 antilipemic agents	972.2	E858.3	E942.2	E950.4	E962.0	E980.4
thyroid derivatives	962.7	E858.0	E932.7	E950.4	E962.0	E980.4
24:08 hypotensive agents	972.6	E858.3	E942.6	E950.4	E962.0	E980.4
adrenergic blocking agents	971.3	E855.6	E941.3	E950.4	E962.0	E980.4
ganglion blocking agents	972.3	E858.3	E942.3	E950.4	E962.0	E980.4
vasodilators	972.5	E858.3	E942.5	E950.4	E962.0	E980.4

Substance	Poisoning	Accident	Therapeutic Use	Suicide Attempt	Assault	Undetermined
		External Cause (E-Code)				
Drug *(Continued)*						
24:12 vasodilating agents NEC	972.5	E858.3	E942.5	E950.4	E962.0	E980.4
coronary	972.4	E858.3	E942.4	E950.4	E962.0	E980.4
nicotinic acid derivatives	972.2	E858.3	E942.2	E950.4	E962.0	E980.4
24:16 sclerosing agents	972.7	E858.3	E942.7	E950.4	E962.0	E980.4
28:04 general anesthetics	968.4	E855.1	E938.4	E950.4	E962.0	E980.4
gaseous anesthetics	968.2	E855.1	E938.2	E950.4	E962.0	E980.4
halothane	968.1	E855.1	E938.1	E950.4	E962.0	E980.4
intravenous anesthetics	968.3	E855.1	E938.3	E950.4	E962.0	E980.4
28:08 analgesics and antipyretics	965.9	E850.9	E935.9	E950.0	E962.0	E980.0
antirheumatics	965.69	E850.6	E935.6	E950.0	E962.0	E980.0
aromatic analgesics	965.4	E850.4	E935.4	E950.0	E962.0	E980.0
non-narcotic NEC	965.7	E850.7	E935.7	E950.0	E962.0	E980.0
opium alkaloids	965.00	E850.2	E935.2	E950.0	E962.0	E980.0
heroin	965.01	E850.0	E935.0	E950.0	E962.0	E980.0
methadone	965.02	E850.1	E935.1	E950.0	E962.0	E980.0
specified type NEC	965.09	E850.2	E935.2	E950.0	E962.0	E980.0
pyrazole derivatives	965.5	E850.5	E935.5	E950.0	E962.0	E980.0
salicylates	965.1	E850.3	E935.3	E950.0	E962.0	E980.0
specified NEC	965.8	E850.8	E935.8	E950.0	E962.0	E980.0
28:10 narcotic antagonists	970.1	E854.3	E940.1	E950.4	E962.0	E980.4
28:12 anticonvulsants	966.3	E855.0	E936.3	E950.4	E962.0	E980.4
barbiturates	967.0	E851	E937.0	E950.1	E962.0	E980.1
benzodiazepine-based tranquilizers	969.4	E853.4	E939.4	E950.3	E962.0	E980.3
bromides	967.3	E852.2	E937.3	E950.2	E962.0	E980.2
hydantoin derivatives	966.1	E855.0	E936.1	E950.4	E962.0	E980.4
oxazolidine (derivatives)	966.0	E855.0	E936.0	E950.4	E962.0	E980.4
succinimides	966.2	E855.0	E936.2	E950.4	E962.0	E980.4
28:16.04 antidepressants	969.0	E854.0	E939.0	E950.3	E962.0	E980.3
28:16.08 tranquilizers	969.5	E853.9	E939.5	E950.3	E962.0	E980.3
benzodiazepine-based	969.4	E853.2	E939.4	E950.3	E962.0	E980.3
butyrophenone-based	969.2	E853.1	E939.2	E950.3	E962.0	E980.3
major NEC	969.3	E853.8	E939.3	E950.3	E962.0	E980.3
phenothiazine-based	969.1	E853.0	E939.1	E950.3	E962.0	E980.3
28:16.12 other psychotherapeutic agents	969.8	E855.8	E939.8	E950.3	E962.0	E980.3
28:20 respiratory and cerebral stimulants	970.9	E854.3	E940.9	E950.4	E962.0	E980.4
analeptics	970.0	E854.3	E940.0	E950.4	E962.0	E980.4
anorexigenic agents	977.0	E858.8	E947.0	E950.4	E962.0	E980.4
psychostimulants	969.7	E854.2	E939.7	E950.3	E962.0	E980.3
specified NEC	970.8	E854.3	E940.8	E950.4	E962.0	E980.4
28:24 sedatives and hypnotics	967.9	E852.9	E937.9	E950.2	E962.0	E980.2
barbiturates	967.0	E851	E937.0	E950.1	E962.0	E980.1
benzodiazepine-based tranquilizers	969.4	E853.2	E939.4	E950.3	E962.0	E980.3
chloral hydrate (group)	967.1	E852.0	E937.1	E950.2	E962.0	E980.2
glutethimide group	967.5	E852.4	E937.5	E950.2	E962.0	E980.2
intravenous anesthetics	968.3	E855.1	E938.3	E950.4	E962.0	E980.4
methaqualone (compounds)	967.4	E852.3	E937.4	E950.2	E962.0	E980.2
paraldehyde	967.2	E852.1	E937.2	E950.2	E962.0	E980.2
phenothiazine-based tranquilizers	969.1	E853.0	E939.1	E950.3	E962.0	E980.3
specified NEC	967.8	E852.8	E937.8	E950.2	E962.0	E980.2
thiobarbiturates	968.3	E855.1	E938.3	E950.4	E962.0	E980.4
tranquilizer NEC	969.5	E853.9	E939.5	E950.3	E962.0	E980.3
36:04 to 36:88 diagnostic agents	977.8	E858.8	E947.8	E950.4	E962.0	E980.4
40:00 electrolyte, caloric, and water balance agents NEC	974.5	E858.5	E944.5	E950.4	E962.0	E980.4
40:04 acidifying agents	963.2	E858.1	E933.2	E950.4	E962.0	E980.4
40:08 alkalinizing agents	963.3	E858.1	E933.3	E950.4	E962.0	E980.4
40:10 ammonia detoxicants	974.5	E858.5	E944.5	E950.4	E962.0	E980.4
40:12 replacement solutions	974.5	E858.5	E944.5	E950.4	E962.0	E980.4
plasma expanders	964.8	E858.2	E934.8	E950.4	E962.0	E980.4
40:16 sodium-removing resins	974.5	E858.5	E944.5	E950.4	E962.0	E980.4
40:18 potassium-removing resins	974.5	E858.5	E944.5	E950.4	E962.0	E980.4
40:20 caloric agents	974.5	E858.5	E944.5	E950.4	E962.0	E980.4

Substance	Poisoning	Accident	Therapeutic Use	Suicide Attempt	Assault	Undetermined
		External Cause (E-Code)				
Drug *(Continued)*						
40:24 salt and sugar substitutes	974.5	E858.5	E944.5	E950.4	E962.0	E980.4
40:28 diuretics NEC	974.4	E858.5	E944.4	E950.4	E962.0	E980.4
carbonic acid anhydrase inhibitors	974.2	E858.5	E944.2	E950.4	E962.0	E980.4
mercurials	974.0	E858.5	E944.0	E950.4	E962.0	E980.4
purine derivatives	974.1	E858.5	E944.1	E950.4	E962.0	E980.4
saluretics	974.3	E858.5	E944.3	E950.4	E962.0	E980.4
thiazides	974.3	E858.5	E944.3	E950.4	E962.0	E980.4
40:36 irrigating solutions	974.5	E858.5	E944.5	E950.4	E962.0	E980.4
40:40 uricosuric agents	974.7	E858.5	E944.7	E950.4	E962.0	E980.4
44:00 enzymes	963.4	E858.1	E933.4	E950.4	E962.0	E980.4
fibrinolysis-affecting agents	964.4	E858.2	E934.4	E950.4	E962.0	E980.4
gastric agents	973.4	E858.4	E943.4	E950.4	E962.0	E980.4
48:00 expectorants and cough preparations	—	—	—	—	—	—
antihistamine agents	963.0	E858.1	E933.0	E950.4	E962.0	E980.4
antitussives	975.4	E858.6	E945.4	E950.4	E962.0	E980.4
codeine derivatives	965.09	E850.2	E935.2	E950.0	E962.0	E980.0
expectorants	975.5	E858.6	E945.5	E950.4	E962.0	E980.4
narcotic agents NEC	965.09	E850.2	E935.2	E950.0	E962.0	E980.0
52:04 anti-infectives (EENT)	—	—	—	—	—	—
ENT agent	976.6	E858.7	E946.6	E950.4	E962.0	E980.4
ophthalmic preparation	976.5	E858.7	E946.5	E950.4	E962.0	E980.4
52:04.04 antibiotics (EENT)	—	—	—	—	—	—
ENT agent	976.6	E858.7	E946.6	E950.4	E962.0	E980.4
ophthalmic preparation	976.5	E858.7	E946.5	E950.4	E962.0	E980.4
52:04.06 antivirals (EENT)	—	—	—	—	—	—
ENT agent	976.6	E858.7	E946.6	E950.4	E962.0	E980.4
ophthalmic preparation	976.5	E858.7	E946.5	E950.4	E962.0	E980.4
2:04.08 sulfonamides (EENT)	—	—	—	—	—	—
ENT agent	976.6	E858.7	E946.6	E950.4	E962.0	E980.4
ophthalmic preparation	976.5	E858.7	E946.5	E950.4	E962.0	E980.4
52:04.12 miscellaneous anti-infectives (EENT)	—	—	—	—	—	—
ENT agent	976.6	E858.7	E946.6	E950.4	E962.0	E980.4
ophthalmic preparation	976.5	E858.7	E946.5	E950.4	E962.0	E980.4
52:08 anti-inflammatory agents (EENT)	—	—	—	—	—	—
ENT agent	976.6	E858.7	E946.6	E950.4	E962.0	E980.4
ophthalmic preparation	976.5	E858.7	E946.5	E950.4	E962.0	E980.4
52:10 carbonic anhydrase inhibitors	974.2	E858.5	E944.2	E950.4	E962.0	E980.4
52:12 contact lens solutions	976.5	E858.7	E946.5	E950.4	E962.0	E980.4
52:16 local anesthetics (EENT)	968.5	E855.2	E938.5	E950.4	E962.0	E980.4
52:20 miotics	971.0	E855.3	E941.0	E950.4	E962.0	E980.4
52:24 mydriatics	—	—	—	—	—	—
adrenergics	971.2	E855.5	E941.2	E950.4	E962.0	E980.4
anticholinergics	971.1	E855.4	E941.1	E950.4	E962.0	E980.4
antimuscarinics	971.1	E855.4	E941.1	E950.4	E962.0	E980.4
parasympatholytics	971.1	E855.4	E941.1	E950.4	E962.0	E980.4
spasmolytics	971.1	E855.4	E941.1	E950.4	E962.0	E980.4
sympathomimetics	971.2	E855.5	E941.2	E950.4	E962.0	E980.4
52:28 mouth washes and gargles	976.6	E858.7	E946.6	E950.4	E962.0	E980.4
52:32 vasoconstrictors (EENT)	971.2	E855.5	E941.2	E950.4	E962.0	E980.4
52:36 unclassified agents (EENT)	—	—	—	—	—	—
ENT agent	976.6	E858.7	E946.6	E950.4	E962.0	E980.4
ophthalmic preparation	976.5	E858.7	E946.5	E950.4	E962.0	E980.4
56:04 antacids and adsorbents	973.0	E858.4	E943.0	E950.4	E962.0	E980.4
56:08 antidiarrhea agents	973.5	E858.4	E943.5	E950.4	E962.0	E980.4
56:10 antiflatulents	973.8	E858.4	E943.8	E950.4	E962.0	E980.4
56:12 cathartics NEC	973.3	E858.4	E943.3	E950.4	E962.0	E980.4
emollients	973.2	E858.4	E943.2	E950.4	E962.0	E980.4
irritants	973.1	E858.4	E943.1	E950.4	E962.0	E980.4
56:16 digestants	973.4	E858.4	E943.4	E950.4	E962.0	E980.4
56:20 emetics and antiemetics	—	—	—	—	—	—
antiemetics	963.0	E858.1	E933.0	E950.4	E962.0	E980.4
emetics	973.6	E858.4	E943.6	E950.4	E962.0	E980.4

Substance	Poisoning	External Cause (E-Code) Accident	Therapeutic Use	Suicide Attempt	Assault	Undetermined
Drug *(Continued)*						
56:24 lipotropic agents	977.1	E858.8	E947.1	E950.4	E962.0	E980.4
56:40 miscellaneous G.I. drugs	973.8	E858.4	E943.8	E950.4	E962.0	E980.4
60:00 gold compounds	965.69	E850.6	E935.6	E950.0	E962.0	E980.0
64:00 heavy metal antagonists	963.8	E858.1	E933.8	E950.4	E962.0	E980.4
68:04 adrenals	962.0	E858.0	E932.0	E950.4	E962.0	E980.4
68:08 androgens	962.1	E858.0	E932.1	E950.4	E962.0	E980.4
68:12 contraceptives, oral	962.2	E858.0	E932.2	E950.4	E962.0	E980.4
68:16 estrogens	962.2	E858.0	E932.2	E950.4	E962.0	E980.4
68:18 gonadotropins	962.4	E858.0	E932.4	E950.4	E962.0	E980.4
68:20 insulins and antidiabetic agents	962.3	E858.0	E932.3	E950.4	E962.0	E980.4
68:20.08 insulins	962.3	E858.0	E932.3	E950.4	E962.0	E980.4
68:24 parathyroid	962.6	E858.0	E932.6	E950.4	E962.0	E980.4
68:28 pituitary (posterior)	962.5	E858.0	E932.5	E950.4	E962.0	E980.4
anterior	962.4	E858.0	E932.4	E950.4	E962.0	E980.4
68:32 progestogens	962.2	E858.0	E932.2	E950.4	E962.0	E980.4
68:34 other corpus luteum hormones NEC	962.2	E858.0	E932.2	E950.4	E962.0	E980.4
68:36 thyroid and antithyroid	—	—	—	—	—	—
antithyroid	962.8	E858.0	E932.8	E950.4	E962.0	E980.4
thyroid (derivatives)	962.7	E858.0	E932.7	E950.4	E962.0	E980.4
72:00 local anesthetics NEC	968.9	E855.2	E938.9	E950.4	E962.0	E980.4
topical (surface)	968.5	E855.2	E938.5	E950.4	E962.0	E980.4
infiltration (intradermal) (subcutaneous) (submucosal)	968.5	E855.2	E938.5	E950.4	E962.0	E980.4
nerve blocking (peripheral) (plexus) (regional)	968.6	E855.2	E938.6	E950.4	E962.0	E980.4
spinal	968.7	E855.2	E938.7	E950.4	E962.0	E980.4
76:00 oxytocics	975.0	E858.6	E945.0	E950.4	E962.0	E980.4
78:00 radioactive agents	990	—	—	—	—	—
80:04 serums NEC	979.9	E858.8	E949.9	E950.4	E962.0	E980.4
immune gamma globulin (human)	964.6	E858.2	E934.6	E950.4	E962.0	E980.4
80:08 toxoids NEC	978.8	E858.8	E948.8	E950.4	E962.0	E980.4
diphtheria	978.5	E858.8	E948.5	E950.4	E962.0	E980.4
and tetanus	978.9	E858.8	E948.9	E950.4	E962.0	E980.4
with pertussis component	978.6	E858.8	E948.6	E950.4	E962.0	E980.4
tetanus	978.4	E858.8	E948.4	E950.4	E962.0	E980.4
and diphtheria	978.9	E858.8	E948.9	E950.4	E962.0	E980.4
with pertussis component	978.6	E858.8	E948.6	E950.4	E962.0	E980.4
80:12 vaccines	979.9	E858.8	E949.9	E950.4	E962.0	E980.4
bacterial NEC	978.8	E858.8	E948.8	E950.4	E962.0	E980.4
with	—	—	—	—	—	—
other bacterial components	978.9	E858.8	E948.9	E950.4	E962.0	E980.4
pertussis component	978.6	E858.8	E948.6	E950.4	E962.0	E980.4
viral and rickettsial components	979.7	E858.8	E949.7	E950.4	E962.0	E980.4
rickettsial NEC	979.6	E858.8	E949.6	E950.4	E962.0	E980.4
with	—	—	—	—	—	—
bacterial component	979.7	E858.8	E949.7	E950.4	E962.0	E980.4
pertussis component	978.6	E858.8	E948.6	E950.4	E962.0	E980.4
viral component	979.7	E858.8	E949.7	E950.4	E962.0	E980.4
viral NEC	979.6	E858.8	E949.6	E950.4	E962.0	E980.4
with	—	—	—	—	—	—
bacterial component	979.7	E858.8	E949.7	E950.4	E962.0	E980.4
pertussis component	978.6	E858.8	E948.6	E950.4	E962.0	E980.4
rickettsial component	979.7	E858.8	E949.7	E950.4	E962.0	E980.4
84:04.04 antibiotics (skin and mucous membrane)	976.0	E858.7	E946.0	E950.4	E962.0	E980.4
84:04.08 fungicides (skin and mucous membrane)	976.0	E858.7	E946.0	E950.4	E962.0	E980.4
84:04.12 scabicides and pediculicides (skin and mucous membrane)	976.0	E858.7	E946.0	E950.4	E962.0	E980.4
84:04.16 miscellaneous local anti-infectives (skin and mucous membrane)	976.0	E858.7	E946.0	E950.4	E962.0	E980.4
84:06 anti-inflammatory agents (skin and mucous membrane)	976.0	E858.7	E946.0	E950.4	E962.0	E980.4
84:08 antipruritics and local anesthetics	—	—	—	—	—	—
antipruritics	976.1	E858.7	E946.1	E950.4	E962.0	E980.4
local anesthetics	968.5	E855.2	E938.5	E950.4	E962.0	E980.4
84:12 astringents	976.2	E858.7	E946.2	E950.4	E962.0	E980.4
84:16 cell stimulants and proliferants	976.8	E858.7	E946.8	E950.4	E962.0	E980.4
84:20 detergents	976.2	E858.7	E946.2	E950.4	E962.0	E980.4

Substance	Poisoning	External Cause (E-Code) Accident	Therapeutic Use	Suicide Attempt	Assault	Undetermined
Drug *(Continued)*						
84:24 emollients, demulcents, and protectants	976.3	E858.7	E946.3	E950.4	E962.0	E980.4
84:28 keratolytic agents	976.4	E858.7	E946.4	E950.4	E962.0	E980.4
84:32 keratoplastic agents	976.4	E858.7	E946.4	E950.4	E962.0	E980.4
84:36 miscellaneous agents (skin and mucous membrane)	976.8	E858.7	E946.8	E950.4	E962.0	E980.4
86:00 spasmolytic agents	975.1	E858.6	E945.1	E950.4	E962.0	E980.4
antiasthmatics	975.7	E858.6	E945.7	E950.4	E962.0	E980.4
papaverine	972.5	E858.3	E942.5	E950.4	E962.0	E980.4
theophylline	974.1	E858.5	E944.1	E950.4	E962.0	E980.4
88:04 vitamin A	963.5	E858.1	E933.5	E950.4	E962.0	E980.4
88:08 vitamin B complex	963.5	E858.1	E933.5	E950.4	E962.0	E980.4
hematopoietic vitamin	964.1	E858.2	E934.1	E950.4	E962.0	E980.4
nicotinic acid derivatives	972.2	E858.3	E942.2	E950.4	E962.0	E980.4
88:12 vitamin C	963.5	E858.1	E933.5	E950.4	E962.0	E980.4
88:16 vitamin D	963.5	E858.1	E933.5	E950.4	E962.0	E980.4
88:20 vitamin E	963.5	E858.1	E933.5	E950.4	E962.0	E980.4
88:24 vitamin K activity	964.3	E858.2	E934.3	E950.4	E962.0	E980.4
88:28 multivitamin preparations	963.5	E858.1	E933.5	E950.4	E962.0	E980.4
92:00 unclassified therapeutic agents	977.8	E858.8	E947.8	E950.4	E962.0	E980.4
Duboisine	971.1	E855.4	E941.1	E950.4	E962.0	E980.4
Dulcolax	973.1	E858.4	E943.1	E950.4	E962.0	E980.4
Duponol (C) (EP)	976.2	E858.7	E946.2	E950.4	E962.0	E980.4
Durabolin	962.1	E858.0	E932.1	E950.4	E962.0	E980.4
Dyclone	968.5	E855.2	E938.5	E950.4	E962.0	E980.4
Dyclonine	968.5	E855.2	E938.5	E950.4	E962.0	E980.4
Dydrogesterone	962.2	E858.0	E932.2	E950.4	E962.0	E980.4
Dyes NEC	989.89	E866.8	—	E950.9	E962.1	E980.9
diagnostic agents	977.8	E858.8	E947.8	E950.4	E962.0	E980.4
pharmaceutical NEC	977.4	E858.8	E947.4	E950.4	E962.0	E980.4
Dyflos	971.0	E855.3	E941.0	E950.4	E962.0	E980.4
Dymelor	962.3	E858.0	E932.3	E950.4	E962.0	E980.4
Dynamite	989.89	E866.8	—	E950.9	E962.1	E980.9
fumes	987.8	E869.8	—	E952.8	E962.2	E982.8
Dyphylline	975.1	E858.6	E945.1	E950.4	E962.0	E980.4
Ear preparations	976.6	E858.7	E946.6	E950.4	E962.0	E980.4
Echothiopate, ecothiopate	971.0	E855.3	E941.0	E950.4	E962.0	E980.4
Ecstasy	969.7	E854.2	E939.7	E950.3	E962.0	E980.3
Ectylurea	967.8	E852.8	E937.8	E950.2	E962.0	E980.2
Edathamil disodium	963.8	E858.1	E933.8	E950.4	E962.0	E980.4
Edecrin	974.4	E858.5	E944.4	E950.4	E962.0	E980.4
Edetate, disodium (calcium)	963.8	E858.1	E933.8	E950.4	E962.0	E980.4
Edrophonium	971.0	E855.3	E941.0	E950.4	E962.0	E980.4
Elase	976.8	E858.7	E946.8	E950.4	E962.0	E980.4
Elaterium	973.1	E858.4	E943.1	E950.4	E962.0	E980.4
Elder	988.2	E865.4	—	E950.9	E962.1	E980.9
berry (unripe)	988.2	E865.3	—	E950.9	E962.1	E980.9
Electrolytes NEC	974.5	E858.5	E944.5	E950.4	E962.0	E980.4
Electrolytic agent NEC	974.5	E858.5	E944.5	E950.4	E962.0	E980.4
Embramine	963.0	E858.1	E933.0	E950.4	E962.0	E980.4
Emetics	973.6	E858.4	E943.6	E950.4	E962.0	E980.4
Emetine (hydrochloride)	961.5	E857	E931.5	E950.4	E962.0	E980.4
Emollients	976.3	E858.7	E946.3	E950.4	E962.0	E980.4
Emylcamate	969.5	E853.8	E939.5	E950.3	E962.0	E980.3
Encyprate	969.0	E854.0	E939.0	E950.3	E962.0	E980.3
Endocaine	968.5	E855.2	E938.5	E950.4	E962.0	E980.4
Endrin	989.2	E863.0	—	E950.6	E962.1	E980.7
Enflurane	968.2	E855.1	E938.2	E950.4	E962.0	E980.4
Enovid	962.2	E858.0	E932.2	E950.4	E962.0	E980.4
ENT preparations (anti-infectives)	976.6	E858.7	E946.6	E950.4	E962.0	E980.4
Enzodase	963.4	E858.1	E933.4	E950.4	E962.0	E980.4
Enzymes NEC	963.4	E858.1	E933.4	E950.4	E962.0	E980.4
Epanutin	966.1	E855.0	E936.1	E950.4	E962.0	E980.4
Ephedra (tincture)	971.2	E855.5	E941.2	E950.4	E962.0	E980.4

Substance	Poisoning	External Cause (E-Code)				
		Accident	Therapeutic Use	Suicide Attempt	Assault	Undetermined
Ephedrine	971.2	E855.5	E941.2	E950.4	E962.0	E980.4
Epiestriol	962.2	E858.0	E932.2	E950.4	E962.0	E980.4
Epilim - *see* Sodium valproate	—	—	—	—	—	—
Epinephrine	971.2	E855.5	E941.2	E950.4	E962.0	E980.4
Epsom salt	973.3	E858.4	E943.3	E950.4	E962.0	E980.4
Equanil	969.5	E853.8	E939.5	E950.3	E962.0	E980.3
Equisetum (diuretic)	974.4	E858.5	E944.4	E950.4	E962.0	E980.4
Ergometrine	975.0	E858.6	E945.0	E950.4	E962.0	E980.4
Ergonovine	975.0	E858.6	E945.0	E950.4	E962.0	E980.4
Ergot NEC	988.2	E865.4	—	E950.9	E962.1	E980.9
medicinal (alkaloids)	975.0	E858.6	E945.0	E950.4	E962.0	E980.4
Ergotamine (tartrate) (for migraine) NEC	972.9	E858.3	E942.9	E950.4	E962.0	E980.4
Ergotrate	975.0	E858.6	E945.0	E950.4	E962.0	E980.4
Erythrityl tetranitrate	972.4	E858.3	E942.4	E950.4	E962.0	E980.4
Erythrol tetranitrate	972.4	E858.3	E942.4	E950.4	E962.0	E980.4
Erythromycin	960.3	E856	E930.3	E950.4	E962.0	E980.4
ophthalmic preparation	976.5	E858.7	E946.5	E950.4	E962.0	E980.4
topical NEC	976.0	E858.7	E946.0	E950.4	E962.0	E980.4
Eserine	971.0	E855.3	E941.0	E950.4	E962.0	E980.4
Eskabarb	967.0	E851	E937.0	E950.1	E962.0	E980.1
Eskalith	969.8	E855.8	E939.8	E950.3	E962.0	E980.3
Estradiol (cypionate) (dipropionate) (valerate)	962.2	E858.0	E932.2	E950.4	E962.0	E980.4
Estriol	962.2	E858.0	E932.2	E950.4	E962.0	E980.4
Estrogens (with progestogens)	962.2	E858.0	E932.2	E950.4	E962.0	E980.4
Estrone	962.2	E858.0	E932.2	E950.4	E962.0	E980.4
Etafedrine	971.2	E855.5	E941.2	E950.4	E962.0	E980.4
Ethacrynate sodium	974.4	E858.5	E944.4	E950.4	E962.0	E980.4
Ethacrynic acid	974.4	E858.5	E944.4	E950.4	E962.0	E980.4
Ethambutol	961.8	E857	E931.8	E950.4	E962.0	E980.4
Ethamide	974.2	E858.5	E944.2	E950.4	E962.0	E980.4
Ethamivan	970.0	E854.3	E940.0	E950.4	E962.0	E980.4
Ethamsylate	964.5	E858.2	E934.5	E950.4	E962.0	E980.4
Ethanol	980.0	E860.1	—	E950.9	E962.1	E980.9
beverage	980.0	E860.0	—	E950.9	E962.1	E980.9
Ethchlorvynol	967.8	E852.8	E937.8	E950.2	E962.0	E980.2
Ethebenecid	974.7	E858.5	E944.7	E950.4	E962.0	E980.4
Ether(s) (diethyl) (ethyl) (vapor)	987.8	E869.8	—	E952.8	E962.2	E982.8
anesthetic	968.2	E855.1	E938.2	E950.4	E962.0	E980.4
petroleum - *see* Ligroin solvent	982.8	E862.4	—	E950.9	E962.1	E980.9
Ethidine chloride (vapor)	987.8	E869.8	—	E952.8	E962.2	E982.8
liquid (solvent)	982.3	E862.4	—	E950.9	E962.1	E980.9
Ethinamate	967.8	E852.8	E937.8	E950.2	E962.0	E980.2
Ethinylestradiol	962.2	E858.0	E932.2	E950.4	E962.0	E980.4
Ethionamide	961.8	E857	E931.8	E950.4	E962.0	E980.4
Ethisterone	962.2	E858.0	E932.2	E950.4	E962.0	E980.4
Ethobral	967.0	E851	E937.0	E950.1	E962.0	E980.1
Ethocaine (infiltration) (topical)	968.5	E855.2	E938.5	E950.4	E962.0	E980.4
nerve block (peripheral) (plexus)	968.6	E855.2	E938.6	E950.4	E962.0	E980.4
spinal	968.7	E855.2	E938.7	E950.4	E962.0	E980.4
Ethoheptazine (citrate)	965.7	E850.7	E935.7	E950.0	E962.0	E980.0
Ethopropazine	966.4	E855.0	E936.4	E950.4	E962.0	E980.4
Ethosuximide	966.2	E855.0	E936.2	E950.4	E962.0	E980.4
Ethotoin	966.1	E855.0	E936.1	E950.4	E962.0	E980.4
Ethoxazene	961.9	E857	E931.9	E950.4	E962.0	E980.4
Ethoxzolamide	974.2	E858.5	E944.2	E950.4	E962.0	E980.4
Ethyl	—	—	—	—	—	—
acetate (vapor)	982.8	E862.4	—	E950.9	E962.1	E980.9
alcohol	980.0	E860.1	—	E950.9	E962.1	E980.9
beverage	980.0	E860.0	—	E950.9	E962.1	E980.9
aldehyde (vapor)	987.8	E869.8	—	E952.8	E962.2	E982.8
liquid	989.89	E866.8	—	E950.9	E962.1	E980.9
aminobenzoate	968.5	E855.2	E938.5	E950.4	E962.0	E980.4

Substance	Poisoning	Accident	Therapeutic Use	Suicide Attempt	Assault	Undetermined
		External Cause (E-Code)				
Ethyl *(Continued)*						
biscoumacetate	964.2	E858.2	E934.2	E950.4	E962.0	E980.4
bromide (anesthetic)	968.2	E855.1	E938.2	E950.4	E962.0	E980.4
carbamate (antineoplastic)	963.1	E858.1	E933.1	E950.4	E962.0	E980.4
carbinol	980.3	E860.4	—	E950.9	E962.1	E980.9
chaulmoograte	961.8	E857	E931.8	E950.4	E962.0	E980.4
chloride (vapor)	987.8	E869.8	—	E952.8	E962.2	E982.8
anesthetic (local)	968.5	E855.2	E938.5	E950.4	E962.0	E980.4
inhaled	968.2	E855.1	E938.2	E950.4	E962.0	E980.4
solvent	982.3	E862.4	—	E950.9	E962.1	E980.9
estranol	962.1	E858.0	E932.1	E950.4	E962.0	E980.4
ether - *see* Ether(s)	—	—	—	—	—	—
formate (solvent) NEC	982.8	E862.4	—	E950.9	E962.1	E980.9
iodoacetate	987.5	E869.3	—	E952.8	E962.2	E982.8
lactate (solvent) NEC	982.8	E862.4	—	E950.9	E962.1	E980.9
methylcarbinol	980.8	E860.8	—	E950.9	E962.1	E980.9
morphine	965.09	E850.2	E935.2	E950.0	E962.0	E980.0
Ethylene (gas)	987.1	E869.8	—	E952.8	E962.2	E982.8
anesthetic (general)	968.2	E855.1	E938.2	E950.4	E962.0	E980.4
chlorohydrin (vapor)	982.3	E862.4	—	E950.9	E962.1	E980.9
dichloride (vapor)	982.3	E862.4	—	E950.9	E962.1	E980.9
glycol(s) (any) (vapor)	982.8	E862.4	—	E950.9	E962.1	E980.9
Ethylidene	—	—	—	—	—	—
chloride NEC	982.3	E862.4	—	E950.9	E962.1	E980.9
diethyl ether	982.8	E862.4	—	E950.9	E962.1	E980.9
Ethynodiol	962.2	E858.0	E932.2	E950.4	E962.0	E980.4
Etidocaine	968.9	E855.2	E938.9	E950.4	E962.0	E980.4
infiltration (subcutaneous)	968.5	E855.2	E938.5	E950.4	E962.0	E980.4
nerve (peripheral) (plexus)	968.6	E855.2	E938.6	E950.4	E962.0	E980.4
Etilfen	967.0	E851	E937.0	E950.1	E962.0	E980.1
Etomide	965.7	E850.7	E935.7	E950.0	E962.0	E980.0
Etorphine	965.09	E850.2	E935.2	E950.0	E962.0	E980.0
Etoval	967.0	E851	E937.0	E950.1	E962.0	E980.1
Etryptamine	969.0	E854.0	E939.0	E950.3	E962.0	E980.3
Eucaine	968.5	E855.2	E938.5	E950.4	E962.0	E980.4
Eucalyptus (oil) NEC	975.5	E858.6	E945.5	E950.4	E962.0	E980.4
Eucatropine	971.1	E855.4	E941.1	E950.4	E962.0	E980.4
Eucodal	965.09	E850.2	E935.2	E950.0	E962.0	E980.0
Euneryl	967.0	E851	E937.0	E950.1	E962.0	E980.1
Euphthalmine	971.1	E855.4	E941.1	E950.4	E962.0	E980.4
Eurax	976.0	E858.7	E946.0	E950.4	E962.0	E980.4
Euresol	976.4	E858.7	E946.4	E950.4	E962.0	E980.4
Euthroid	962.7	E858.0	E932.7	E950.4	E962.0	E980.4
Evans blue	977.8	E858.8	E947.8	E950.4	E962.0	E980.4
Evipal	967.0	E851	E937.0	E950.1	E962.0	E980.1
sodium	968.3	E855.1	E938.3	E950.4	E962.0	E980.4
Evipan	967.0	E851	E937.0	E950.1	E962.0	E980.1
sodium	968.3	E855.1	E938.3	E950.4	E962.0	E980.4
Exalgin	965.4	E850.4	E935.4	E950.0	E962.0	E980.0
Excipients, pharmaceutical	977.4	E858.8	E947.4	E950.4	E962.0	E980.4
Exhaust gas - *see* Carbon, monoxide	—	—	—	—	—	—
Ex-Lax (phenolphthalein)	973.1	E858.4	E943.1	E950.4	E962.0	E980.4
Expectorants	975.5	E858.6	E945.5	E950.4	E962.0	E980.4
External medications (skin) (mucous membrane)	976.9	E858.7	E946.9	E950.4	E962.0	E980.4
dental agent	976.7	E858.7	E946.7	E950.4	E962.0	E980.4
ENT agent	976.6	E858.7	E946.6	E950.4	E962.0	E980.4
ophthalmic preparation	976.5	E858.7	E946.5	E950.4	E962.0	E980.4
specified NEC	976.8	E858.7	E946.8	E950.4	E962.0	E980.4
Eye agents (anti-infective)	976.5	E858.7	E946.5	E950.4	E962.0	E980.4
Factor IX complex (human)	964.5	E858.2	E934.5	E950.4	E962.0	E980.4
Fecal softeners	973.2	E858.4	E943.2	E950.4	E962.0	E980.4
Fenbutrazate	977.0	E858.8	E947.0	E950.4	E962.0	E980.4

Substance	Poisoning	External Cause (E-Code)				
		Accident	Therapeutic Use	Suicide Attempt	Assault	Undetermined
Fencamfamin	970.8	E854.3	E940.8	E950.4	E962.0	E980.4
Fenfluramine	977.0	E858.8	E947.0	E950.4	E962.0	E980.4
Fenoprofen	965.61	E850.6	E935.6	E950.0	E962.0	E980.0
Fentanyl	965.09	E850.2	E935.2	E950.0	E962.0	E980.0
Fentazin	969.1	E853.0	E939.1	E930.3	E962.0	E980.3
Fenticlor, fentichlor	976.0	E858.7	E946.0	E950.4	E962.0	E980.4
Fer de lance (bite) (venom)	989.5	E905.0	—	E950.9	E962.1	E980.9
Ferric - *see* Iron	—	—	—	—	—	—
Ferrocholinate	964.0	E858.2	E934.0	E950.4	E962.0	E980.4
Ferrous fumerate, gluconate, lactate, salt NEC, sulfate (medicinal)	964.0	E858.2	E934.0	E950.4	E962.0	E980.4
Ferrum - *see* Iron	—	—	—	—	—	—
Fertilizers NEC	989.89	E866.5	—	E950.9	E962.1	E980.4
with herbicide mixture	989.4	E863.5	—	E950.6	E962.1	E980.7
Fibrinogen (human)	964.7	E858.2	E934.7	E950.4	E962.0	E980.4
Fibrinolysin	964.4	E858.2	E934.4	E950.4	E962.0	E980.4
Fibrinolysis-affecting agents	964.4	E858.2	E934.4	E950.4	E962.0	E980.4
Filix mas	961.6	E857	E931.6	E950.4	E962.0	E980.4
Fiorinal	965.1	E850.3	E935.3	E950.0	E962.0	E980.0
Fire damp	987.1	E869.8	—	E952.8	E962.2	E982.8
Fish, nonbacterial or noxious	988.0	E865.2	—	E950.9	E962.1	E980.9
shell	988.0	E865.1	—	E950.9	E962.1	E980.9
Flagyl	961.5	E857	E931.5	E950.4	E962.0	E980.4
Flavoxate	975.1	E858.6	E945.1	E950.4	E962.0	E980.4
Flaxedil	975.2	E858.6	E945.2	E950.4	E962.0	E980.4
Flaxseed (medicinal)	976.3	E858.7	E946.3	E950.4	E962.0	E980.4
Florantyrone	973.4	E858.4	E943.4	E950.4	E962.0	E980.4
Floraquin	961.3	E857	E931.3	E950.4	E962.0	E980.4
Florinef	962.0	E858.0	E932.0	E950.4	E962.0	E980.4
ENT agent	976.6	E858.7	E946.6	E950.4	E962.0	E980.4
ophthalmic preparation	976.5	E858.7	E946.5	E950.4	E962.0	E980.4
topical NEC	976.0	E858.7	E946.0	E950.4	E962.0	E980.4
Flowers of sulfur	976.4	E858.7	E946.4	E950.4	E962.0	E980.4
Floxuridine	963.1	E858.1	E933.1	E950.4	E962.0	E980.4
Flucytosine	961.9	E857	E931.9	E950.4	E962.0	E980.4
Fludrocortisone	962.0	E858.0	E932.0	E950.4	E962.0	E980.4
ENT agent	976.6	E858.7	E946.6	E950.4	E962.0	E980.4
ophthalmic preparation	976.5	E858.7	E946.5	E950.4	E962.0	E980.4
topical NEC	976.0	E858.7	E946.0	E950.4	E962.0	E980.4
Flumethasone	976.0	E858.7	E946.0	E950.4	E962.0	E980.4
Flumethiazide	974.3	E858.5	E944.3	E950.4	E962.0	E980.4
Flumidin	961.7	E857	E931.7	E950.4	E962.0	E980.4
Flunitrazepam	969.4	E853.2	E939.4	E950.3	E962.0	E980.3
Fluocinolone	976.0	E858.7	E946.0	E950.4	E962.0	E980.4
Fluocortolone	962.0	E858.0	E932.0	E950.4	E962.0	E980.4
Fluohydrocortisone	962.0	E858.0	E932.0	E950.4	E962.0	E980.4
ENT agent	976.6	E858.7	E946.6	E950.4	E962.0	E980.4
ophthalmic preparation	976.5	E858.7	E946.5	E950.4	E962.0	E980.4
topical NEC	976.0	E858.7	E946.0	E950.4	E962.0	E980.4
Fluonid	976.0	E858.7	E946.0	E950.4	E962.0	E980.4
Fluopromazine	969.1	E853.0	E939.1	E950.3	E962.0	E980.3
Fluoracetate	989.4	E863.7	—	E950.6	E962.1	E980.7
Fluorescein (sodium)	977.8	E858.8	E947.8	E950.4	E962.0	E980.4
Fluoride(s) (pesticides) (sodium) NEC	989.4	E863.4	—	E950.6	E962.1	E980.7
hydrogen - *see* Hydrofluoric acid	—	—	—	—	—	—
medicinal	976.7	E858.7	E946.7	E950.4	E962.0	E980.4
not pesticide NEC	983.9	E864.4	—	E950.7	E962.1	E980.6
stannous	976.7	E858.7	E946.7	E950.4	E962.0	E980.4
Fluorinated corticosteroids	962.0	E858.0	E932.0	E950.4	E962.0	E980.4
Fluorine (compounds) (gas)	987.8	E869.8	—	E952.8	E962.2	E982.8
salt - *see* Fluoride(s)	—	—	—	—	—	—
Fluoristan	976.7	E858.7	E946.7	E950.4	E962.0	E980.4
Fluoroacetate	989.4	E863.7	—	E950.6	E962.1	E980.7
Fluorodeoxyuridine	963.1	E858.1	E933.1	E950.4	E962.0	E980.4

Substance	Poisoning	External Cause (E-Code) Accident	Therapeutic Use	Suicide Attempt	Assault	Undetermined
Fluorometholone (topical) NEC	976.0	E858.7	E946.0	E950.4	E962.0	E980.4
ophthalmic preparation	976.5	E858.7	E946.5	E950.4	E962.0	E980.4
Fluorouracil	963.1	E858.1	E933.1	E950.4	E962.0	E980.4
Fluothane	968.1	E855.1	E938.1	E950.4	E962.0	E980.4
Fluoxetine hydrochloride	969.0	E854.0	E939.0	E950.3	E962.0	E980.3
Fluoxymesterone	962.1	E858.0	E932.1	E950.4	E962.0	E980.4
Fluphenazine	969.1	E853.0	E939.1	E950.3	E962.0	E980.3
Fluprednisolone	962.0	E858.0	E932.0	E950.4	E962.0	E980.4
Flurandrenolide	976.0	E858.7	E946.0	E950.4	E962.0	E980.4
Flurazepam (hydrochloride)	969.4	E853.2	E939.4	E950.3	E962.0	E980.3
Flurbiprofen	965.61	E850.6	E935.6	E950.0	E962.0	E980.0
Flurobate	976.0	E858.7	E946.0	E950.4	E962.0	E980.4
Flurothyl	969.8	E855.8	E939.8	E950.3	E962.0	E980.3
Fluroxene	968.2	E855.1	E938.2	E950.4	E962.0	E980.4
Folacin	964.1	E858.2	E934.1	E950.4	E962.0	E980.4
Folic acid	964.1	E858.2	E934.1	E950.4	E962.0	E980.4
Follicle stimulating hormone	962.4	E858.0	E932.4	E950.4	E962.0	E980.4
Food, foodstuffs, nonbacterial or noxious	988.9	E865.9	—	E950.9	E962.1	E980.9
berries, seeds	988.2	E865.3	—	E950.9	E962.1	E980.9
fish	988.0	E865.2	—	E950.9	E962.1	E980.9
mushrooms	988.1	E865.5	—	E950.9	E962.1	E980.9
plants	988.2	E865.9	—	E950.9	E962.1	E980.9
specified type NEC	988.2	E865.4	—	E950.9	E962.1	E980.9
shellfish	988.0	E865.1	—	E950.9	E962.1	E980.9
specified NEC	988.8	E865.8	—	E950.9	E962.1	E980.9
Fool's parsley	988.2	E865.4	—	E950.9	E962.1	E980.9
Formaldehyde (solution)	989.89	E861.4	—	E950.9	E962.1	E980.9
fungicide	989.4	E863.6	—	E950.6	E962.1	E980.7
gas or vapor	987.8	E869.8	—	E952.8	E962.2	E982.8
Formalin	989.89	E861.4	—	E950.9	E962.1	E980.9
fungicide	989.4	E863.6	—	E950.6	E962.1	E980.7
vapor	987.8	E869.8	—	E952.8	E962.2	E982.8
Formic acid	983.1	E864.1	—	E950.7	E962.1	E980.6
vapor	987.8	E869.8	—	E952.8	E962.2	E982.8
Fowler's solution	985.1	E866.3	—	E950.8	E962.1	E980.8
Foxglove	988.2	E865.4	—	E950.9	E962.1	E980.9
Fox green	977.8	E858.8	E947.8	E950.4	E962.0	E980.4
Framycetin	960.8	E856	E930.8	E950.4	E962.0	E980.4
Frangula (extract)	973.1	E858.4	E943.1	E950.4	E962.0	E980.4
Frei antigen	977.8	E858.8	E947.8	E950.4	E962.0	E980.4
Freons	987.4	E869.2	—	E952.8	E962.2	E982.8
Fructose	974.5	E858.5	E944.5	E950.4	E962.0	E980.4
Frusemide	974.4	E858.5	E944.4	E950.4	E962.0	E980.4
FSH	962.4	E858.0	E932.4	E950.4	E962.0	E980.4
Fuel	—	—	—	—	—	—
automobile	981	E862.1	—	E950.9	E962.1	E980.9
exhaust gas, not in transit	986	E868.2	—	E952.0	E962.2	E982.0
vapor NEC	987.1	E869.8	—	E952.8	E962.2	E982.8
gas (domestic use) - *see also* Carbon, monoxide, fuel	—	—	—	—	—	—
utility	987.1	E868.1	—	E951.8	E962.2	E981.8
incomplete combustion of - *see* Carbon, monoxide, fuel, utility	—	—	—	—	—	—
in mobile container	987.0	E868.0	—	E951.1	E962.2	E981.1
piped (natural)	987.1	E867	—	E951.0	E962.2	E981.0
industrial, incomplete combustion	986	E868.3	—	E952.1	E962.2	E982.1
Fugillin	960.8	E856	E930.8	E950.4	E962.0	E980.4
Fulminate of mercury	985.0	E866.1	—	E950.9	E962.1	E980.9
Fulvicin	960.1	E856	E930.1	E950.4	E962.0	E980.4
Fumadil	960.8	E856	E930.8	E950.4	E962.0	E980.4
Fumagillin	960.8	E856	E930.8	E950.4	E962.0	E980.4
Fumes (from)	987.9	E869.9	—	E952.9	E962.2	E982.9
carbon monoxide - *see* Carbon, monoxide	—	—	—	—	—	—
charcoal (domestic use)	986	E868.3	—	E952.1	E962.2	E982.1

Substance	Poisoning	Accident	Therapeutic Use	Suicide Attempt	Assault	Undetermined
		External Cause (E-Code)				
Fumes *(Continued)*						
chloroform - *see* Chloroform						
coke (in domestic stoves, fireplaces)	986	E868.3	—	E952.1	E962.2	E982.1
corrosive NEC	987.8	E869.8	—	E952.8	E962.2	E982.8
ether - *see* Ether(s)						
freons	987.4	E869.2	—	E952.8	E962.2	E982.8
hydrocarbons	987.1	E869.8	—	E952.8	E962.2	E982.8
petroleum (liquefied)	987.0	E868.0	—	E951.1	E962.2	E981.1
distributed through pipes (pure or mixed with air)	987.0	E867	—	E951.0	E962.2	E981.0
lead - *see* Lead	—	—	—	—	—	—
metals - *see* specified metal	—	—	—	—	—	—
nitrogen dioxide	987.2	E869.0	—	E952.8	E962.2	E982.8
pesticides - *see* Pesticides	—	—	—	—	—	—
petroleum (liquefied)	987.0	E868.0	—	E951.1	E962.2	E981.1
distributed through pipes (pure or mixed with air)	987.0	E867	—	E951.0	E962.2	E981.0
polyester	987.8	E869.8	—	E952.8	E962.2	E982.8
specified source, other (*see also* substance specified)	987.8	E869.8	—	E952.8	E962.2	E982.8
sulfur dioxide	987.3	E869.1	—	E952.8	E962.2	E982.8
Fumigants	989.4	E863.8	—	E950.6	E962.1	E980.7
Fungi, noxious, used as food	988.1	E865.5	—	E950.9	E962.1	E980.9
Fungicides (*see also* Antifungals)	989.4	E863.6	—	E950.6	E962.1	E980.7
Fungizone	960.1	E856	E930.1	E950.4	E962.0	E980.4
topical	976.0	E858.7	E946.0	E950.4	E962.0	E980.4
Furacin	976.0	E858.7	E946.0	E950.4	E962.0	E980.4
Furadantin	961.9	E857	E931.9	E950.4	E962.0	E980.4
Furazolidone	961.9	E857	E931.9	E950.4	E962.0	E980.4
Furnace (coal burning) (domestic), gas from	986	E868.3	—	E952.1	E962.2	E982.1
industrial	986	E868.8	—	E952.1	E962.2	E982.1
Furniture polish	989.89	E861.2	—	E950.9	E962.1	E980.9
Furosemide	974.4	E858.5	E944.4	E950.4	E962.0	E980.4
Furoxone	961.9	E857	E931.9	E950.4	E962.0	E980.4
Fusel oil (amyl) (butyl) (propyl)	980.3	E860.4	—	E950.9	E962.1	E980.9
Fusidic acid	960.8	E856	E930.8	E950.4	E962.0	E980.4
Gallamine	975.2	E858.6	E945.2	E950.4	E962.0	E980.4
Gallotannic acid	976.2	E858.7	E946.2	E950.4	E962.0	E980.4
Gamboge	973.1	E858.4	E943.1	E950.4	E962.0	E980.4
Gamimune	964.6	E858.2	E934.6	E950.4	E962.0	E980.4
Gamma-benzene hexachloride (vapor)	989.2	E863.0	—	E950.6	E962.1	E980.7
Gamma globulin	964.6	E858.2	E934.6	E950.4	E962.0	E980.4
Gamma hydroxy butyrate (GHB)	968.4	E855.1	E938.4	E950.4	E962.0	E980.4
Gamulin	964.6	E858.2	E934.6	E950.4	E962.0	E980.4
Ganglionic blocking agents	972.3	E858.3	E942.3	E950.4	E962.0	E980.4
Ganja	969.6	E854.1	E939.6	E950.3	E962.0	E980.3
Garamycin	960.8	E856	E930.8	E950.4	E962.0	E980.4
ophthalmic preparation	976.5	E858.7	E946.5	E950.4	E962.0	E980.4
topical NEC	976.0	E858.7	E946.0	E950.4	E962.0	E980.4
Gardenal	967.0	E851	E937.0	E950.1	E962.0	E980.1
Gardepanyl	967.0	E851	E937.0	E950.1	E962.0	E980.1
Gas	987.9	E869.9	—	E952.9	E962.2	E982.9
acetylene	987.1	E868.1	—	E951.8	E962.2	E981.8
incomplete combustion of - *see* Carbon, monoxide, fuel, utility	—	—	—	—	—	—
air contaminants, source or type not specified	987.9	E869.9	—	E952.9	E962.2	E982.9
anesthetic (general) NEC	968.2	E855.1	E938.2	E950.4	E962.0	E980.4
blast furnace	986	E868.8	—	E952.1	E962.2	E982.1
butane - *see* Butane	—	—	—	—	—	—
carbon monoxide - *see* Carbon, monoxide, chlorine	987.6	E869.8	—	E952.8	E962.2	E982.8
coal - *see* Carbon, monoxide, coal	—	—	—	—	—	—
cyanide	987.7	E869.8	—	E952.8	E962.2	E982.8
dicyanogen	987.8	E869.8	—	E952.8	E962.2	E982.8
domestic - *see* Gas, utility	—	—	—	—	—	—
exhaust - *see* Carbon, monoxide, exhaust gas	—	—	—	—	—	—
from wood- or coal-burning stove or fireplace	986	E868.3	—	E952.1	E962.2	E982.1

Substance	Poisoning	External Cause (E-Code)				
		Accident	**Therapeutic Use**	**Suicide Attempt**	**Assault**	**Undetermined**
Gas *(Continued)*	—	—	—	—	—	—
fuel (domestic use) - *see also* Carbon, monoxide, fuel						
industrial use	986	E868.8	—	E952.1	E962.2	E982.1
utility	987.1	E868.1	—	E951.8	E962.2	E981.8
incomplete combustion of - *see* Carbon, monoxide, fuel, utility	—	—	—	—	—	—
in mobile container	987.0	E868.0	—	E951.1	E962.2	E981.1
piped (natural)	987.1	E867	—	E951.0	E962.2	E981.0
garage	986	E868.2	—	E952.0	E962.2	E982.0
hydrocarbon NEC	987.1	E869.8	—	E952.8	E962.2	E982.8
incomplete combustion of - *see* Carbon, monoxide, fuel, utility	—	—	—	—	—	—
liquefied (mobile container)	987.0	E868.0	—	E951.1	E962.2	E981.1
piped	987.0	E867	—	E951.0	E962.2	E981.0
hydrocyanic acid	987.7	E869.8	—	E952.8	E962.2	E982.8
illuminating - *see* Gas, utility	—	—	—	—	—	—
incomplete combustion, any - *see* Carbon, monoxide	—	—	—	—	—	—
kiln	986	E868.8	—	E952.1	E962.2	E982.1
lacrimogenic	987.5	E869.3	—	E952.8	E962.2	E982.8
marsh	987.1	E869.8	—	E952.8	E962.2	E982.8
motor exhaust, not in transit	986	E868.8	—	E952.1	E962.2	E982.1
mustard - *see* Mustard, gas	—	—	—	—	—	—
natural	987.1	E867	—	E951.0	E962.2	E981.0
nerve (war)	987.9	E869.9	—	E952.9	E962.2	E982.9
oils	981	E862.1	—	E950.9	E962.1	E980.9
petroleum (liquefied) (distributed in mobile containers)	987.0	E868.0	—	E951.1	E962.2	E981.1
piped (pure or mixed with air)	987.0	E867	—	E951.1	E962.2	E981.1
piped (manufactured) (natural) NEC	987.1	E867	—	E951.0	E962.2	E981.0
producer	986	E868.8	—	E952.1	E962.2	E982.1
propane - *see* Propane	—	—	—	—	—	—
refrigerant (freon)	987.4	E869.2	—	E952.8	E962.2	E982.8
not freon	987.9	E869.9	—	E952.9	E962.2	E982.9
sewer	987.8	E869.8	—	E952.8	E962.2	E982.8
specified source NEC (*see also* substance specified)	987.8	E869.8	—	E952.8	E962.2	E982.8
stove - *see* Gas, utility	—	—	—	—	—	—
tear	987.5	E869.3	—	E952.8	E962.2	E982.8
utility (for cooking, heating, or lighting) (piped) NEC	987.1	E868.1	—	E951.8	E962.2	E981.8
incomplete combustion of - *see* Carbon, monoxide, fuel, utilty	—	—	—	—	—	—
in mobile container	987.0	E868.0	—	E951.1	E962.2	E981.1
piped (natural)	987.1	E867	—	E951.0	E962.2	E981.0
water	987.1	E868.1	—	E951.8	E962.2	E981.8
incomplete combustion of - *see* Carbon, monoxide, fuel, utility	—	—	—	—	—	—
Gaseous substance - *see* Gas	—	—	—	—	—	—
Gasoline, gasolene	981	E862.1	—	E950.9	E962.1	E980.9
vapor	987.1	E869.8	—	E952.8	E962.2	E982.8
Gastric enzymes	973.4	E858.4	E943.4	E950.4	E962.0	E980.4
Gastrografin	977.8	E858.8	E947.8	E950.4	E962.0	E980.4
Gastrointestinal agents	973.9	E858.4	E943.9	E950.4	E962.0	E980.4
specified NEC	973.8	E858.4	E943.8	E950.4	E962.0	E980.4
Gaultheria procumbens	988.2	E865.4	—	E950.9	E962.1	E980.9
Gelatin (intravenous)	964.8	E858.2	E934.8	E950.4	E962.0	E980.4
absorbable (sponge)	964.5	E858.2	E934.5	E950.4	E962.0	E980.4
Gelfilm	976.8	E858.7	E946.8	E950.4	E962.0	E980.4
Gelfoam	964.5	E858.2	E934.5	E950.4	E962.0	E980.4
Gelsemine	970.8	E854.3	E940.8	E950.4	E962.0	E980.4
Gelsemium (sempervirens)	988.2	E865.4	—	E950.9	E962.1	E980.9
Gemonil	967.0	E851	E937.0	E950.1	E962.0	E980.1
Gentamicin	960.8	E856	E930.8	E950.4	E962.0	E980.4
ophthalmic preparation	976.5	E858.7	E946.5	E950.4	E962.0	E980.4
topical NEC	976.0	E858.7	E946.0	E950.4	E962.0	E980.4
Gentian violet	976.0	E858.7	E946.0	E950.4	E962.0	E980.4
Gexane	976.0	E858.7	E946.0	E950.4	E962.0	E980.4
Gila monster (venom)	989.5	E905.0	—	E950.9	E962.1	E980.9
Ginger, Jamaica	989.89	E866.8	—	E950.9	E962.1	E980.9
Gitalin	972.1	E858.3	E942.1	E950.4	E962.0	E980.4

Substance	Poisoning	External Cause (E-Code) Accident	Therapeutic Use	Suicide Attempt	Assault	Undetermined
Gitoxin	972.1	E858.3	E942.1	E950.4	E962.0	E980.4
Glandular extract (medicinal) NEC	977.9	E858.9	E947.9	E950.5	E962.0	E980.5
Glaucarubin	961.5	E857	E931.5	E950.4	E962.0	E980.4
Globin zinc insulin	962.3	E858.0	E932.3	E950.4	E962.0	E980.4
Glucagon	962.3	E858.0	E932.3	E950.4	E962.0	E980.4
Glucochloral	967.1	E852.0	E937.1	E950.2	E962.0	E980.2
Glucocorticoids	962.0	E858.0	E932.0	E950.4	E962.0	E980.4
Glucose	974.5	E858.5	E944.5	E950.4	E962.0	E980.4
oxidase reagent	977.8	E858.8	E947.8	E950.4	E962.0	E980.4
Glucosulfone sodium	961.8	E857	E931.8	E950.4	E962.0	E980.4
Glue(s)	989.89	E866.6	—	E950.9	E962.1	E980.9
Glutamic acid (hydrochloride)	973.4	E858.4	E943.4	E950.4	E962.0	E980.4
Glutaraldehyde	989.89	E861.4	—	E950.9	E962.1	E980.9 ◀
Glutathione	963.8	E858.1	E933.8	E950.4	E962.0	E980.4
Glutethimide (group)	967.5	E852.4	E937.5	E950.2	E962.0	E980.2
Glycerin (lotion)	976.3	E858.7	E946.3	E950.4	E962.0	E980.4
Glycerol (topical)	976.3	E858.7	E946.3	E950.4	E962.0	E980.4
Glyceryl	—	—	—	—	—	—
guaiacolate	975.5	E858.6	E945.5	E950.4	E962.0	E980.4
triacetate (topical)	976.0	E858.7	E946.0	E950.4	E962.0	E980.4
trinitrate	972.4	E858.3	E942.4	E950.4	E962.0	E980.4
Glycine	974.5	E858.5	E944.5	E950.4	E962.0	E980.4
Glycobiarsol	961.1	E857	E931.1	E950.4	E962.0	E980.4
Glycols (ether)	982.8	E862.4	—	E950.9	E962.1	E980.9
Glycopyrrolate	971.1	E855.4	E941.1	E950.4	E962.0	E980.4
Glymidine	962.3	E858.0	E932.3	E950.4	E962.0	E980.4
Gold (compounds) (salts)	965.69	E850.6	E935.6	E950.0	E962.0	E980.0
Golden sulfide of antimony	985.4	E866.2	—	E950.9	E962.1	E980.9
Goldylocks	988.2	E865.4	—	E950.9	E962.1	E980.9
Gonadal tissue extract	962.9	E858.0	E932.9	E950.4	E962.0	E980.4
female	962.2	E858.0	E932.2	E950.4	E962.0	E980.4
male	962.1	E858.0	E932.1	E950.4	E962.0	E980.4
Gonadotropin	962.4	E858.0	E932.4	E950.4	E962.0	E980.4
Grain alcohol	980.0	E860.1	—	E950.9	E962.1	E980.9
beverage	980.0	E860.0	—	E950.9	E962.1	E980.9
Gramicidin	960.8	E856	E930.8	E950.4	E962.0	E980.4
Gratiola officinalis	988.2	E865.4	—	E950.9	E962.1	E980.9
Grease	989.89	E866.8	—	E950.9	E962.1	E980.9
Green hellebore	988.2	E865.4	—	E950.9	E962.1	E980.9
Green soap	976.2	E858.7	E946.2	E950.4	E962.0	E980.4
Grifulvin	960.1	E856	E930.1	E950.4	E962.0	E980.4
Griseofulvin	960.1	E856	E930.1	E950.4	E962.0	E980.4
Growth hormone	962.4	E858.0	E932.4	E950.4	E962.0	E980.4
Guaiacol	975.5	E858.6	E945.5	E950.4	E962.0	E980.4
Giuaiac reagent	977.8	E858.8	E947.8	E950.4	E962.0	E980.4
Guaifenesin	975.5	E858.6	E945.5	E950.4	E962.0	E980.4
Guaiphenesin	975.5	E858.6	E945.5	E950.4	E962.0	E980.4
Guanatol	961.4	E857	E931.4	E950.4	E962.0	E980.4
Guanethidine	972.6	E858.3	E942.6	E950.4	E962.0	E980.4
Guano	989.89	E866.5	—	E950.9	E962.1	E980.9
Guanochlor	972.6	E858.3	E942.6	E950.4	E962.0	E980.4
Guanoctine	972.6	E858.3	E942.6	E950.4	E962.0	E980.4
Guanoxan	972.6	E858.3	E942.6	E950.4	E962.0	E980.4
Hair treatment agent NEC	976.4	E858.7	E946.4	E950.4	E962.0	E980.4
Halcinonide	976.0	E858.7	E946.0	E950.4	E962.0	E980.4
Halethazole	976.0	E858.7	E946.0	E950.4	E962.0	E980.4
Hallucinogens	969.6	E854.1	E939.6	E950.3	E962.0	E980.3
Haloperidol	969.2	E853.1	E939.2	E950.3	E962.0	E980.3
Haloprogin	976.0	E858.7	E946.0	E950.4	E962.0	E980.4
Halotex	976.0	E858.7	E946.0	E950.4	E962.0	E980.4
Halothane	968.1	E855.1	E938.1	E950.4	E962.0	E980.4
Halquinols	976.0	E858.7	E946.0	E950.4	E962.0	E980.4
Harmonyl	972.6	E858.3	E942.6	E950.4	E962.0	E980.4

Substance	Poisoning	External Cause (E-Code) Accident	Therapeutic Use	Suicide Attempt	Assault	Undetermined
Hartmann's solution	974.5	E858.5	E944.5	E950.4	E962.0	E980.4
Hashish	969.6	E854.1	E939.6	E950.3	E962.0	E980.3
Hawaiian wood rose seeds	969.6	E854.1	E939.6	E950.3	E962.0	E980.3
Headache cures, drugs, powders NEC	977.9	E858.9	E947.9	E950.5	E962.0	E980.9
Heavenly Blue (morning glory)	969.6	E854.1	E939.6	E950.3	E962.0	E980.3
Heavy metal antagonists	963.8	E858.1	E933.8	E950.4	E962.0	E980.4
anti-infectives	961.2	E857	E931.2	E950.4	E962.0	E980.4
Hedaquinium	976.0	E858.7	E946.0	E950.4	E962.0	E980.4
Hedge hyssop	988.2	E865.4	—	E950.9	E962.1	E980.9
Heet	976.8	E858.7	E946.8	E950.4	E962.0	E980.4
Helenin	961.6	E857	E931.6	E950.4	E962.0	E980.4
Hellebore (black) (green) (white)	988.2	E865.4	—	E950.9	E962.1	E980.9
Hemlock	988.2	E865.4	—	E950.9	E962.1	E980.9
Hemostatics	964.5	E858.2	E934.5	E950.4	E962.0	E980.4
capillary active drugs	972.8	E858.3	E942.8	E950.4	E962.0	E980.4
Henbane	988.2	E865.4	—	E950.9	E962.1	E980.9
Heparin (sodium)	964.2	E858.2	E934.2	E950.4	E962.0	E980.4
Heptabarbital, heptabarbitone	967.0	E851	E937.0	E950.1	E962.0	E980.1
Heptachlor	989.2	E863.0	—	E950.6	E962.1	E980.7
Heptalgin	965.09	E850.2	E935.2	E950.0	E962.0	E980.0
Herbicides	989.4	E863.5	—	E950.6	E962.1	E980.7
Heroin	965.01	E850.0	E935.0	E950.0	E962.0	E980.0
Herplex	976.5	E858.7	E946.5	E950.4	E962.0	E980.4
HES	964.8	E858.2	E934.8	E950.4	E962.0	E980.4
Hetastarch	964.8	E858.2	E934.8	E950.4	E962.0	E980.7
Hexachlorocyclohexane	989.2	E863.0	—	E950.6	E962.1	E980.7
Hexachlorophene	976.2	E858.7	E946.2	E950.4	E962.0	E980.4
Hexadimethrine (bromide)	964.5	E858.2	E934.5	E950.4	E962.0	E980.4
Hexafluorenium	975.2	E858.6	E945.2	E950.4	E962.0	E980.4
Hexa-germ	976.2	E858.7	E946.2	E950.4	E962.0	E980.4
Hexahydrophenol	980.8	E860.8	—	E950.9	E962.1	E980.9
Hexalen	980.8	E860.8	—	E950.9	E962.1	E980.9
Hexamethonium	972.3	E858.3	E942.3	E950.4	E962.0	E980.4
Hexamethylenamine	961.9	E857	E931.9	E950.4	E962.0	E980.4
Hexamine	961.9	E857	E931.9	E950.4	E962.0	E980.4
Hexanone	982.8	E862.4	—	E950.9	E962.1	E980.9
Hexapropymate	967.8	E852.8	E937.8	E950.2	E962.0	E980.2
Hexestrol	962.2	E858.0	E932.2	E950.4	E962.0	E980.4
Hexethal (sodium)	967.0	E851	E937.0	E950.1	E962.0	E980.1
Hexetidine	976.0	E858.7	E946.0	E950.4	E962.0	E980.4
Hexobarbital, hexobarbitone	967.0	E851	E937.0	E950.1	E962.0	E980.1
sodium (anesthetic)	968.3	E855.1	E938.3	E950.4	E962.0	E980.4
soluble	968.3	E855.1	E938.3	E950.4	E962.0	E980.4
Hexocyclium	971.1	E855.4	E941.1	E950.4	E962.0	E980.4
Hexoestrol	962.2	E858.0	E932.2	E950.4	E962.0	E980.4
Hexone	982.8	E862.4	—	E950.9	E962.1	E980.9
Hexylcaine	968.5	E855.2	E938.5	E950.4	E962.0	E980.4
Hexylresorcinol	961.6	E857	E931.6	E950.4	E962.0	E980.4
Hinkle's pills	973.1	E858.4	E943.1	E950.4	E962.0	E980.4
Histalog	977.8	E858.8	E947.8	E950.4	E962.0	E980.4
Histamine (phosphate)	972.5	E858.3	E942.5	E950.4	E962.0	E980.4
Histoplasmin	977.8	E858.8	E947.8	E950.4	E962.0	E980.4
Holly berries	988.2	E865.3	—	E950.9	E962.1	E980.9
Homatropine	971.1	E855.4	E941.1	E950.4	E962.0	E980.4
Homo-tet	964.6	E858.2	E934.6	E950.4	E962.0	E980.4
Hormones (synthetic substitute) NEC	962.9	E858.0	E932.9	E950.4	E962.0	E980.4
adrenal cortical steroids	962.0	E858.0	E932.0	E950.4	E962.0	E980.4
antidiabetic agents	962.3	E858.0	E932.3	E950.4	E962.0	E980.4
follicle stimulating	962.4	E858.0	E932.4	E950.4	E962.0	E980.4
gonadotropic	962.4	E858.0	E932.4	E950.4	E962.0	E980.4
growth	962.4	E858.0	E932.4	E950.4	E962.0	E980.4

◀ New ⟸ Revised Code

Substance	Poisoning	Accident	Therapeutic Use	Suicide Attempt	Assault	Undetermined
		External Cause (E-Code)				
Hormones *(Continued)*						
ovarian (substitutes)	962.2	E858.0	E932.2	E950.4	E962.0	E980.4
parathyroid (derivatives)	962.6	E858.0	E932.6	E950.4	E962.0	E980.4
pituitary (posterior)	962.5	E858.0	E932.5	E950.4	E962.0	E980.4
anterior	962.4	E858.0	E932.4	E950.4	E962.0	E980.4
thyroid (derivative)	962.7	E858.0	E932.7	E950.4	E962.0	E980.4
Hornet (sting)	989.5	E905.3	—	E950.9	E962.1	E980.9
Horticulture agent NEC	989.4	E863.9	—	E950.6	E962.1	E980.7
Hyaluronidase	963.4	E858.1	E933.4	E950.4	E962.0	E980.4
Hyazyme	963.4	E858.1	E933.4	E950.4	E962.0	E980.4
Hycodan	965.09	E850.2	E935.2	E950.0	E962.0	E980.0
Hydantoin derivatives	966.1	E855.0	E936.1	E950.4	E962.0	E980.4
Hydeltra	962.0	E858.0	E932.0	E950.4	E962.0	E980.4
Hydergine	971.3	E855.6	E941.3	E950.4	E962.0	E980.4
Hydrabamine penicillin	960.0	E856	E930.0	E950.4	E962.0	E980.4
Hydralazine, hydrallazine	972.6	E858.3	E942.6	E950.4	E962.0	E980.4
Hydrargaphen	976.0	E858.7	E946.0	E950.4	E962.0	E980.4
Hydrazine	983.9	E864.3	—	E950.7	E962.1	E980.6
Hydriodic acid	975.5	E858.6	E945.5	E950.4	E962.0	E980.4
Hydrocarbon gas	987.1	E869.8	—	E952.8	E962.2	E982.8
incomplete combustion of - *see* Carbon, monoxide, fuel, utility	—	—	—	—	—	—
liquefied (mobile container)	987.0	E868.0	—	E951.1	E962.2	E981.1
piped (natural)	987.0	E867	—	E951.0	E962.2	E981.0
Hydrochloric acid (liquid)	983.1	E864.1	—	E950.7	E962.1	E980.6
medicinal	973.4	E858.4	E943.4	E950.4	E962.0	E980.4
vapor	987.8	E869.8	—	E952.8	E962.2	E982.8
Hydrochlorothiazide	974.3	E858.5	E944.3	E950.4	E962.0	E980.4
Hydrocodone	965.09	E850.2	E935.2	E950.0	E962.0	E980.0
Hydrocortisone	962.0	E858.0	E932.0	E950.4	E962.0	E980.4
ENT agent	976.6	E858.7	E946.6	E950.4	E962.0	E980.4
ophthalmic preparation	976.5	E858.7	E946.5	E950.4	E962.0	E980.4
topical NEC	976.0	E858.7	E946.0	E950.4	E962.0	E980.4
Hydrocortone	962.0	E858.0	E932.0	E950.4	E962.0	E980.4
ENT agent	976.6	E858.7	E946.6	E950.4	E962.0	E980.4
ophthalmic preparation	976.5	E858.7	E946.5	E950.4	E962.0	E980.4
topical NEC	976.0	E858.7	E946.0	E950.4	E962.0	E980.4
Hydrocyanic acid - *see* Cyanide(s)	—	—	—	—	—	—
Hydroflumethiazide	974.3	E858.5	E944.3	E950.4	E962.0	E980.4
Hydrofluoric acid (liquid)	983.1	E864.1	—	E950.7	E962.1	E980.6
vapor	987.8	E869.8	—	E952.8	E962.2	E982.8
Hydrogen	987.8	E869.8	—	E952.8	E962.2	E982.8
arsenide	985.1	E866.3	—	E950.8	E962.1	E980.8
arseniurated	985.1	E866.3	—	E950.8	E962.1	E980.8
cyanide (salts)	989.0	E866.8	—	E950.9	E962.1	E980.9
gas	987.7	E869.8	—	E952.8	E962.2	E982.8
fluoride (liquid)	983.1	E864.1	—	E950.7	E962.1	E980.6
vapor	987.8	E869.8	—	E952.8	E962.2	E982.8
peroxide (solution)	976.6	E858.7	E946.6	E950.4	E962.0	E980.4
phosphorated	987.8	E869.8	—	E952.8	E962.2	E982.8
sulfide (gas)	987.8	E869.8	—	E952.8	E962.2	E982.8
arseniurated	985.1	E866.3	—	E950.8	E962.1	E980.8
sulfureted	987.8	E869.8	—	E952.8	E962.2	E982.8
Hydromorphinol	965.09	E850.2	E935.2	E950.0	E962.0	E980.0
Hydromorphinone	965.09	E850.2	E935.2	E950.0	E962.0	E980.0
Hydromorphone	965.09	E850.2	E935.2	E950.0	E962.0	E980.0
Hydromox	974.3	E858.5	E944.3	E950.4	E962.0	E980.4
Hydrophilic lotion	976.3	E858.7	E946.3	E950.4	E962.0	E980.4
Hydroquinone	983.0	E864.0	—	E950.7	E962.1	E980.6
vapor	987.8	E869.8	—	E952.8	E962.2	E982.8
Hydrosulfuric acid (gas)	987.8	E869.8	—	E952.8	E962.2	E982.8
Hydrous wool fat (lotion)	976.3	E858.7	E946.3	E950.4	E962.0	E980.4
Hydroxide, caustic	983.2	E864.2	—	E950.7	E962.1	E980.6

Substance	Poisoning	External Cause (E-Code)				
		Accident	Therapeutic Use	Suicide Attempt	Assault	Undetermined
Hydroxocobalamin	964.1	E858.2	E934.1	E950.4	E962.0	E980.4
Hydroxyamphetamine	971.2	E855.5	E941.2	E950.4	E962.0	E980.4
Hydroxychloroquine	961.4	E857	E931.4	E950.4	E962.0	E980.4
Hydroxydihydrocodeinone	965.09	E850.2	E935.2	E950.0	E962.0	E980.0
Hydroxyethyl starch	964.8	E858.2	E934.8	E950.4	E962.0	E980.4
Hydroxyphenamate	969.5	E853.8	E939.5	E950.3	E962.0	E980.3
Hydroxyphenylbutazone	965.5	E850.5	E935.5	E950.0	E962.0	E980.0
Hydroxyprogesterone	962.2	E858.0	E932.2	E950.4	E962.0	E980.4
Hydroxyquinoline derivatives	961.3	E857	E931.3	E950.4	E962.0	E980.4
Hydroxystilbamidine	961.5	E857	E931.5	E950.4	E962.0	E980.4
Hydroxyurea	963.1	E858.1	E933.1	E950.4	E962.0	E980.4
Hydroxyzine	969.5	E853.8	E939.5	E950.3	E962.0	E980.3
Hyoscine (hydrobromide)	971.1	E855.4	E941.1	E950.4	E962.0	E980.4
Hyoscyamine	971.1	E855.4	E941.1	E950.4	E962.0	E980.4
Hyoscyamus (albus) (niger)	988.2	E865.4	—	E950.9	E962.1	E980.9
Hypaque	977.8	E858.8	E947.8	E950.4	E962.0	E980.4
Hypertussis	964.6	E858.2	E934.6	E950.4	E962.0	E980.4
Hypnotics NEC	967.9	E852.9	E937.9	E950.2	E962.0	E980.2
Hypochlorites - *see* Sodium, hypochlorite	—	—	—	—	—	—
Hypotensive agents NEC	972.6	E858.3	E942.6	E950.4	E962.0	E980.4
Ibufenac	965.69	E850.6	E935.6	E950.0	E962.0	E980.0
Ibuprofen	965.61	E850.6	E935.6	E950.0	E962.0	E980.0
ICG	977.8	E858.8	E947.8	E950.4	E962.0	E980.4
Ichthammol	976.4	E858.7	E946.4	E950.4	E962.0	E980.4
Ichthyol	976.4	E858.7	E946.4	E950.4	E962.0	E980.4
Idoxuridine	976.5	E858.7	E946.5	E950.4	E962.0	E980.4
IDU	976.5	E858.7	E946.5	E950.4	E962.0	E980.4
Iletin	962.3	E858.0	E932.3	E950.4	E962.0	E980.4
Ilex	988.2	E865.4	—	E950.9	E962.1	E980.9
Illuminating gas - *see* Gas, utility	—	—	—	—	—	—
Ilopan	963.5	E858.1	E933.5	E950.4	E962.0	E980.4
Ilotycin	960.3	E856	E930.3	E950.4	E962.0	E980.4
ophthalmic preparation	976.5	E858.7	E946.5	E950.4	E962.0	E980.4
topical NEC	976.0	E858.7	E946.0	E950.4	E962.0	E980.4
Imipramine	969.0	E854.0	E939.0	E950.3	E962.0	E980.3
Immu-G	964.6	E858.2	E934.6	E950.4	E962.0	E980.4
Immuglobin	964.6	E858.2	E934.6	E950.4	E962.0	E980.4
Immune serum globulin	964.6	E858.2	E934.6	E950.4	E962.0	E980.4
Immunosuppressive agents	963.1	E858.1	E933.1	E950.4	E962.0	E980.4
Immu-tetanus	964.6	E858.2	E934.6	E950.4	E962.0	E980.4
Indandione (derivatives)	964.2	E858.2	E934.2	E950.4	E962.0	E980.4
Inderal	972.0	E858.3	E942.0	E950.4	E962.0	E980.4
Indian	—	—	—	—	—	—
hemp	969.6	E854.1	E939.6	E950.3	E962.0	E980.3
tobacco	988.2	E865.4	—	E950.9	E962.1	E980.9
Indigo carmine	977.8	E858.8	E947.8	E950.4	E962.0	E980.4
Indocin	965.69	E850.6	E935.6	E950.0	E962.0	E980.0
Indocyanine green	977.8	E858.8	E947.8	E950.4	E962.0	E980.4
Indomethacin	965.69	E850.6	E935.6	E950.0	E962.0	E980.0
Industrial	—	—	—	—	—	—
alcohol	980.9	E860.9	—	E950.9	E962.1	E980.9
fumes	987.8	E869.8	—	E952.8	E962.2	E982.8
solvents (fumes) (vapors)	982.8	E862.9	—	E950.9	E962.1	E980.9
Influenza vaccine	979.6	E858.8	E949.6	E950.4	E962.0	E982.8
Ingested substances NEC	989.9	E866.9	—	E950.9	E962.1	E980.9
INH (isoniazid)	961.8	E857	E931.8	E950.4	E962.0	E980.4
Inhalation, gas (noxious) - *see* Gas	—	—	—	—	—	—
Ink	989.89	E866.8	—	E950.9	E962.1	E980.9
Innovar	967.6	E852.5	E937.6	E950.2	E962.0	E980.2
Inositol niacinate	972.2	E858.3	E942.2	E950.4	E962.0	E980.4
Inproquone	963.1	E858.1	E933.1	E950.4	E962.0	E980.4

Substance	Poisoning	External Cause (E-Code) Accident	Therapeutic Use	Suicide Attempt	Assault	Undetermined
Insect (sting), venomous	989.5	E905.5	—	E950.9	E962.1	E980.9
Insecticides (*see also* Pesticides)	989.4	E863.4	—	E950.6	E962.1	E980.7
chlorinated	989.2	E863.0	—	E950.6	E962.1	E980.7
mixtures	989.4	E863.3	—	E950.6	E962.1	E980.7
organochlorine (compounds)	989.2	E863.0	—	E950.6	E962.1	E980.7
organophosphorus (compounds)	989.3	E863.1	—	E950.6	E962.1	E980.7
Insular tissue extract	962.3	E858.0	E932.3	E950.4	E962.0	E980.4
Insulin (amorphous) (globin) (isophane) (Lente) (NPH) (Protamine) (Semilente) (Ultralente) (zinc)	962.3	E858.0	E932.3	E950.4	E962.0	E980.4
Intranarcon	968.3	E855.1	E938.3	E950.4	E962.0	E980.4
Inulin	977.8	E858.8	E947.8	E950.4	E962.0	E980.4
Invert sugar	974.5	E858.5	E944.5	E950.4	E962.0	E980.4
Inza - see Naproxen	—	—	—	—	—	—
Iodide NEC (*see also* Iodine)	976.0	E858.7	E946.0	E950.4	E962.0	E980.4
mercury (ointment)	976.0	E858.7	E946.0	E950.4	E962.0	E980.4
methylate	976.0	E858.7	E946.0	E950.4	E962.0	E980.4
potassium (expectorant) NEC	975.5	E858.6	E945.5	E950.4	E962.0	E980.4
Iodinated glycerol	975.5	E858.6	E945.5	E950.4	E962.0	E980.4
Iodine (antiseptic, external) (tincture) NEC	976.0	E858.7	E946.0	E950.4	E962.0	E980.4
diagnostic	977.8	E858.8	E947.8	E950.4	E962.0	E980.4
for thyroid conditions (antithyroid)	962.8	E858.0	E932.8	E950.4	E962.0	E980.4
vapor	987.8	E869.8	—	E952.8	E962.2	E982.8
Iodized oil	977.8	E858.8	E947.8	E950.4	E962.0	E980.4
Iodobismitol	961.2	E857	E931.2	E950.4	E962.0	E980.4
Iodochlorhydroxyquin	961.3	E857	E931.3	E950.4	E962.0	E980.4
topical	976.0	E858.7	E946.0	E950.4	E962.0	E980.4
Iodoform	976.0	E858.7	E946.0	E950.4	E962.0	E980.4
Iodopanoic acid	977.8	E858.8	E947.8	E950.4	E962.0	E980.4
Iodophthalein	977.8	E858.8	E947.8	E950.4	E962.0	E980.4
Ion exchange resins	974.5	E858.5	E944.5	E950.4	E962.0	E980.4
Iopanoic acid	977.8	E858.8	E947.8	E950.4	E962.0	E980.4
Iophendylate	977.8	E858.8	E947.8	E950.4	E962.0	E980.4
Iothiouracil	962.8	E858.0	E932.8	E950.4	E962.0	E980.4
Ipecac	973.6	E858.4	E943.6	E950.4	E962.0	E980.4
Ipecacuanha	973.6	E858.4	E943.6	E950.4	E962.0	E980.4
Ipodate	977.8	E858.8	E947.8	E950.4	E962.0	E980.4
Ipral	967.0	E851	E937.0	E950.1	E962.0	E980.1
Ipratropium	975.1	E858.6	E945.1	E950.4	E962.0	E980.4
Iproniazid	969.0	E854.0	E939.0	E950.3	E962.0	E980.3
Iron (compounds) (medicinal) (preparations)	964.0	E858.2	E934.0	E950.4	E962.0	E980.4
dextran	964.0	E858.2	E934.0	E950.4	E962.0	E980.4
nonmedicinal (dust) (fumes) NEC	985.8	E866.4	—	E950.9	E962.1	E980.9
Irritant drug	977.9	E858.9	E947.9	E950.5	E962.0	E980.5
Ismelin	972.6	E858.3	E942.6	E950.4	E962.0	E980.4
Isoamyl nitrite	972.4	E858.3	E942.4	E950.4	E962.0	E980.4
Isobutyl acetate	982.8	E862.4	—	E950.9	E962.1	E980.9
Isocarboxazid	969.0	E854.0	E939.0	E950.3	E962.0	E980.3
Isoephedrine	971.2	E855.5	E941.2	E950.4	E962.0	E980.4
Isoetharine	971.2	E855.5	E941.2	E950.4	E962.0	E980.4
Isofluorophate	971.0	E855.3	E941.0	E950.4	E962.0	E980.4
Isoniazid (INH)	961.8	E857	E931.8	E950.4	E962.0	E980.4
Isopentaquine	961.4	E857	E931.4	E950.4	E962.0	E980.4
Isophane insulin	962.3	E858.0	E932.3	E950.4	E962.0	E980.4
Isopregnenone	962.2	E858.0	E932.2	E950.4	E962.0	E980.4
Isoprenaline	971.2	E855.5	E941.2	E950.4	E962.0	E980.4
Isopropamide	971.1	E855.4	E941.1	E950.4	E962.0	E980.4
Isopropanol	980.2	E860.3	—	E950.9	E962.1	E980.9
topical (germicide)	976.0	E858.7	E946.0	E950.4	E962.0	E980.4
Isopropyl	—	—	—	—	—	—
acetate	982.8	E862.4	—	E950.9	E962.1	E980.9
alcohol	980.2	E860.3	—	E950.9	E962.1	E980.9
topical (germicide)	976.0	E858.7	E946.0	E950.4	E962.0	E980.4
ether	982.8	E862.4	—	E950.9	E962.1	E980.9

Substance	Poisoning	External Cause (E-Code) Accident	Therapeutic Use	Suicide Attempt	Assault	Undetermined
Isoproterenol	971.2	E855.5	E941.2	E950.4	E962.0	E980.4
Isosorbide dinitrate	972.4	E858.3	E942.4	E950.4	E962.0	E980.4
Isothipendyl	963.0	E858.1	E933.0	E950.4	E962.0	E980.4
Isoxazolyl penicillin	960.0	E856	E930.0	E950.4	E962.0	E980.4
Isoxsuprine hydrochloride	972.5	E858.3	E942.5	E950.4	E962.0	E980.4
I-thyroxine sodium	962.7	E858.0	E932.7	E950.4	E962.0	E980.4
Jaborandi (pilocarpus) (extract)	971.0	E855.3	E941.0	E950.4	E962.0	E980.4
Jalap	973.1	E858.4	E943.1	E950.4	E962.0	E980.4
Jamaica	—	—	—	—	—	—
dogwood (bark)	965.7	E850.7	E935.7	E950.0	E962.0	E980.0
ginger	989.89	E866.8	—	E950.9	E962.1	E980.9
Jatropha	988.2	E865.4	—	E950.9	E962.1	E980.9
curcas	988.2	E865.3	—	E950.9	E962.1	E980.9
Jectofer	964.0	E858.2	E934.0	E950.4	E962.0	E980.4
Jellyfish (sting)	989.5	E905.6	—	E950.9	E962.1	E980.9
Jequirity (bean)	988.2	E865.3	—	E950.9	E962.1	E980.9
Jimson weed	988.2	E865.4	—	E950.9	E962.1	E980.9
seeds	988.2	E865.3	—	E950.9	E962.1	E980.9
Juniper tar (oil) (ointment)	976.4	E858.7	E946.4	E950.4	E962.0	E980.4
Kallikrein	972.5	E858.3	E942.5	E950.4	E962.0	E980.4
Kanamycin	960.6	E856	E930.6	E950.4	E962.0	E980.4
Kantrex	960.6	E856	E930.6	E950.4	E962.0	E980.4
Kaolin	973.5	E858.4	E943.5	E950.4	E962.0	E980.4
Karaya (gum)	973.3	E858.4	E943.3	E950.4	E962.0	E980.4
Kemithal	968.3	E855.1	E938.3	E950.4	E962.0	E980.4
Kenacort	962.0	E858.0	E932.0	E950.4	E962.0	E980.4
Keratolytics	976.4	E858.7	E946.4	E950.4	E962.0	E980.4
Keratoplastics	976.4	E858.7	E946.4	E950.4	E962.0	E980.4
Kerosene, kerosine (fuel) (solvent) NEC	981	E862.1	—	E950.9	E962.1	E980.9
insecticide	981	E863.4	—	E950.6	E962.1	E980.7
vapor	987.1	E869.8	—	E952.8	E962.2	E982.8
Ketamine	968.3	E855.1	E938.3	E950.4	E962.0	E980.4
Ketobemidone	965.09	E850.2	E935.2	E950.0	E962.0	E980.0
Ketols	982.8	E862.4	—	E950.9	E962.1	E980.9
Ketone oils	982.8	E862.4	—	E950.9	E962.1	E980.9
Ketoprofen	965.61	E850.6	E935.6	E950.0	E962.0	E980.0
Kiln gas or vapor (carbon monoxide)	986	E868.8	—	E952.1	E962.2	E982.1
Konsyl	973.3	E858.4	E943.3	E950.4	E962.0	E980.4
Kosam seed	988.2	E865.3	—	E950.9	E962.1	E980.9
Krait (venom)	989.5	E905.0	—	E950.9	E962.1	E980.9
Kwell (insecticide)	989.2	E863.0	—	E950.6	E962.1	E980.7
anti-infective (topical)	976.0	E858.7	E946.0	E950.4	E962.0	E980.4
Laburnum (flowers) (seeds)	988.2	E865.3	—	E950.9	E962.1	E980.9
leaves	988.2	E865.4	—	E950.9	E962.1	E980.9
Lacquers	989.89	E861.6	—	E950.9	E962.1	E980.9
Lacrimogenic gas	987.5	E869.3	—	E952.8	E962.2	E982.8
Lactic acid	983.1	E864.1	—	E950.7	E962.1	E980.6
Lactobacillus acidophilus	973.5	E858.4	E943.5	E950.4	E962.0	E980.4
Lactoflavin	963.5	E858.1	E933.5	E950.4	E962.0	E980.4
Lactuca (virosa) (extract)	967.8	E852.8	E937.8	E950.2	E962.0	E980.2
Lactucarium	967.8	E852.8	E937.8	E950.2	E962.0	E980.2
Laevulose	974.5	E858.5	E944.5	E950.4	E962.0	E980.4
Lanatoside (C)	972.1	E858.3	E942.1	E950.4	E962.0	E980.4
Lanolin (lotion)	976.3	E858.7	E946.3	E950.4	E962.0	E980.4
Largactil	969.1	E853.0	E939.1	E950.3	E962.0	E980.3
Larkspur	988.2	E865.3	—	E950.9	E962.1	E980.9
Laroxyl	969.0	E854.0	E939.0	E950.3	E962.0	E980.3
Lasix	974.4	E858.5	E944.4	E950.4	E962.0	E980.4
Latex	989.82	E866.8	—	E950.9	E962.1	E980.9
Lathyrus (seed)	988.2	E865.3	—	E950.9	E962.1	E980.9
Laudanum	965.09	E850.2	E935.2	E950.0	E962.0	E980.0
Laudexium	975.2	E858.6	E945.2	E950.4	E962.0	E980.4

Substance	Poisoning	Accident	Therapeutic Use	Suicide Attempt	Assault	Undetermined
		External Cause (E-Code)				
Laurel, black or cherry	988.2	E865.4	—	E950.9	E962.1	E980.9
Laurolinium	976.0	E858.7	E946.0	E950.4	E962.0	E980.4
Lauryl sulfoacetate	976.2	E858.7	E946.2	E950.4	E962.0	E980.4
Laxatives NEC	973.3	E858.4	E943.3	E950.4	E962.0	E980.4
emollient	973.2	E858.4	E943.2	E950.4	E962.0	E980.4
L-dopa	966.4	E855.0	E936.4	E950.4	E962.0	E980.4
L-Tryptophan - *see* amino acid	—	—	—	—	—	—
Lead (dust) (fumes) (vapor) NEC	984.9	E866.0	—	E950.9	E962.1	E980.9
acetate (dust)	984.1	E866.0	—	E950.9	E962.1	E980.9
anti-infectives	961.2	E857	E931.2	E950.4	E962.0	E980.4
antiknock compound (tetra-ethyl)	984.1	E862.1	—	E950.9	E962.1	E980.9
arsenate, arsenite (dust) (insecticide) (vapor)	985.1	E863.4	—	E950.8	E962.1	E980.8
herbicide	985.1	E863.5	—	E950.8	E962.1	E980.8
carbonate	984.0	E866.0	—	E950.9	E962.1	E980.9
paint	984.0	E861.5	—	E950.9	E962.1	E980.9
chromate	984.0	E866.0	—	E950.9	E962.1	E980.9
paint	984.0	E861.5	—	E950.9	E962.1	E980.9
dioxide	984.0	E866.0	—	E950.9	E962.1	E980.9
inorganic (compound)	984.0	E866.0	—	E950.9	E962.1	E980.9
paint	984.0	E861.5	—	E950.9	E962.1	E980.9
iodide	984.0	E866.0	—	E950.9	E962.1	E980.9
pigment (paint)	984.0	E861.5	—	E950.9	E962.1	E980.9
monoxide (dust)	984.0	E866.0	—	E950.9	E962.1	E980.9
paint	984.0	E861.5	—	E950.9	E962.1	E980.9
organic	984.1	E866.0	—	E950.9	E962.1	E980.9
oxide	984.0	E866.0	—	E950.9	E962.1	E980.9
paint	984.0	E861.5	—	E950.9	E962.1	E980.9
paint	984.0	E861.5	—	E950.9	E962.1	E980.9
salts	984.0	E866.0	—	E950.9	E962.1	E980.9
specified compound NEC	984.8	E866.0	—	E950.9	E962.1	E980.9
tetra-ethyl	984.1	E862.1	—	E950.9	E962.1	E980.9
Lebanese red	969.6	E854.1	E939.6	E950.3	E962.0	E980.3
Lente Iletin (insulin)	962.3	E858.0	E932.3	E950.4	E962.0	E980.4
Leptazol	970.0	E854.3	E940.0	E950.4	E962.0	E980.4
Leritine	965.09	E850.2	E935.2	E950.0	E962.0	E980.0
Letter	962.7	E858.0	E932.7	E950.4	E962.0	E980.4
Lettuce opium	967.8	E852.8	E937.8	E950.2	E962.0	E980.2
Leucovorin (factor)	964.1	E858.2	E934.1	E950.4	E962.0	E980.4
Leukeran	963.1	E858.1	E933.1	E950.4	E962.0	E980.4
Levalbuterol	975.7	E858.6	E945.7	E950.4	E962.0	E980.4
Levallorphan	970.1	E854.3	E940.1	E950.4	E962.0	E980.4
Levanil	967.8	E852.8	E937.8	E950.2	E962.0	E980.2
Levarterenol	971.2	E855.5	E941.2	E950.4	E962.0	E980.4
Levodopa	966.4	E855.0	E936.4	E950.4	E962.0	E980.4
Levo-dromoran	965.09	E850.2	E935.2	E950.0	E962.0	E980.0
Levoid	962.7	E858.0	E932.7	E950.4	E962.0	E980.4
Levo-iso-methadone	965.02	E850.1	E935.1	E950.0	E962.0	E980.0
Levomepromazine	967.8	E852.8	E937.8	E950.2	E962.0	E980.2
Levoprome	967.8	E852.8	E937.8	E950.2	E962.0	E980.2
Levopropoxyphene	975.4	E858.6	E945.4	E950.4	E962.0	E980.4
Levorphan, levophanol	965.09	E850.2	E935.2	E950.0	E962.0	E980.0
Levothyroxine (sodium)	962.7	E858.0	E932.7	E950.4	E962.0	E980.4
Levsin	971.1	E855.4	E941.1	E950.4	E962.0	E980.4
Levulose	974.5	E858.5	E944.5	E950.4	E962.0	E980.4
Lewisite (gas)	985.1	E866.3	—	E950.8	E962.1	E980.8
Librium	969.4	E853.2	E939.4	E950.3	E962.0	E980.3
Lidex	976.0	E858.7	E946.0	E950.4	E962.0	E980.4
Lidocaine (infiltration) (topical)	968.5	E855.2	E938.5	E950.4	E962.0	E980.4
nerve block (peripheral) (plexus)	968.6	E855.2	E938.6	E950.4	E962.0	E980.4
spinal	968.7	E855.2	E938.7	E950.4	E962.0	E980.4
Lighter fluid	981	E862.1	—	E950.9	E962.1	E980.9

Substance	Poisoning	External Cause (E-Code)				
		Accident	Therapeutic Use	Suicide Attempt	Assault	Undetermined
Lignocaine (infiltration) (topical)	968.5	E855.2	E938.5	E950.4	E962.0	E980.4
nerve block (peripheral) (plexus)	968.6	E855.2	E938.6	E950.4	E962.0	E980.4
spinal	968.7	E855.2	E938.7	E950.4	E962.0	E980.4
Ligroin(e) (solvent)	981	E862.0	—	E950.9	E962.1	E980.9
vapor	987.1	E869.8	—	E952.8	E962.2	E982.8
Ligustrum vulgare	988.2	E865.3	—	E950.9	E962.1	E980.9
Lily of the valley	988.2	E865.4	—	E950.9	E962.1	E980.9
Lime (chloride)	983.2	E864.2	—	E950.7	E962.1	E980.6
solution, sulferated	976.4	E858.7	E946.4	E950.4	E962.0	E980.4
Limonene	982.8	E862.4	—	E950.9	E962.1	E980.9
Lincomycin	960.8	E856	E930.8	E950.4	E962.0	E980.4
Lindane (insecticide) (vapor)	989.2	E863.0	—	E950.6	E962.1	E980.7
anti-infective (topical)	976.0	E858.7	E946.0	E950.4	E962.0	E980.4
Liniments NEC	976.9	E858.7	E946.9	E950.4	E962.0	E980.4
Linoleic acid	972.2	E858.3	E942.2	E950.4	E962.0	E980.4
Liothyronine	962.7	E858.0	E932.7	E950.4	E962.0	E980.4
Liotrix	962.7	E858.0	E932.7	E950.4	E962.0	E980.4
Lipancreatin	973.4	E858.4	E943.4	E950.4	E962.0	E980.4
Lipo-Lutin	962.2	E858.0	E932.2	E950.4	E962.0	E980.4
Lipotropic agents	977.1	E858.8	E947.1	E950.4	E962.0	E980.4
Liquefied petroleum gases	987.0	E868.0	—	E951.1	E962.2	E981.1
piped (pure or mixed with air)	987.0	E867	—	E951.0	E962.2	E981.0
Liquid petrolatum	973.2	E858.4	E943.2	E950.4	E962.0	E980.4
substance	989.9	E866.9	—	E950.9	E962.1	E980.9
specified NEC	989.89	E866.8	—	E950.9	E962.1	E980.9
Lirugen	979.4	E858.8	E949.4	E950.4	E962.0	E980.4
Lithane	969.8	E855.8	E939.8	E950.3	E962.0	E980.3
Lithium	985.8	E866.4	—	E950.9	E962.1	E980.9
carbonate	969.8	E855.8	E939.8	E950.3	E962.0	E980.3
Lithonate	969.8	E855.8	E939.8	E950.3	E962.0	E980.3
Liver (extract) (injection) (preparations)	964.1	E858.2	E934.1	E950.4	E962.0	E980.4
Lizard (bite) (venom)	989.5	E905.0	—	E950.9	E962.1	E980.9
LMD	964.8	E858.2	E934.8	E950.4	E962.0	E980.4
Lobelia	988.2	E865.4	—	E950.9	E962.1	E980.9
Lobeline	970.0	E854.3	E940.0	E950.4	E962.0	E980.4
Locorten	976.0	E858.7	E946.0	E950.4	E962.0	E980.4
Lolium temulentum	988.2	E865.3	—	E950.9	E962.1	E980.9
Lomotil	973.5	E858.4	E943.5	E950.4	E962.0	E980.4
Lomustine	963.1	E858.1	E933.1	E950.4	E962.0	E980.4
Lophophora williamsii	969.6	E854.1	E939.6	E950.3	E962.0	E980.3
Lorazepam	969.4	E853.2	E939.4	E950.3	E962.0	E980.3
Lotions NEC	976.9	E858.7	E946.9	E950.4	E962.0	E980.4
Lotronex	973.8	E858.4	E943.8	E950.4	E962.0	E980.4
Lotusate	967.0	E851	E937.0	E950.1	E962.0	E980.1
Lowila	976.2	E858.7	E946.2	E950.4	E962.0	E980.4
Loxapine	969.3	E853.8	E939.3	E950.3	E962.0	E980.3
Lozenges (throat)	976.6	E858.7	E946.6	E950.4	E962.0	E980.4
LSD (25)	969.6	E854.1	E939.6	E950.3	E962.0	E980.3
Lubricating oil NEC	981	E862.2	—	E950.9	E962.1	E980.9
Lucanthone	961.6	E857	E931.6	E950.4	E962.0	E980.4
Luminal	967.0	E851	E937.0	E950.1	E962.0	E980.1
Lung irritant (gas) NEC	987.9	E869.9	—	E952.9	E962.2	E982.9
Lutocylol	962.2	E858.0	E932.2	E950.4	E962.0	E980.4
Lutromone	962.2	E858.0	E932.2	E950.4	E962.0	E980.4
Lututrin	975.0	E858.6	E945.0	E950.4	E962.0	E980.4
Lye (concentrated)	983.2	E864.2	—	E950.7	E962.1	E980.6
Lygranum (skin test)	977.8	E858.8	E947.8	E950.4	E962.0	E980.4
Lymecycline	960.4	E856	E930.4	E950.4	E962.0	E980.4
Lymphogranuloma venereum antigen	977.8	E858.8	E947.8	E950.4	E962.0	E980.4
Lynestrenol	962.2	E858.0	E932.2	E950.4	E962.0	E980.4
Lyovac Sodium Edecrin	974.4	E858.5	E944.4	E950.4	E962.0	E980.4
Lypressin	962.5	E858.0	E932.5	E950.4	E962.0	E980.4

◀ New ⟸ Revised Code

Substance	Poisoning	External Cause (E-Code) Accident	Therapeutic Use	Suicide Attempt	Assault	Undetermined
Lysergic acid (amide) (diethylamide)	969.6	E854.1	E939.6	E950.3	E962.0	E980.3
Lysergide	969.6	E854.1	E939.6	E950.3	E962.0	E980.3
Lysine vasopressin	962.5	E858.0	E932.5	E950.4	E962.0	E980.4
Lysol	983.0	E864.0	—	E950.7	E962.1	E980.6
Lytta (vitatta)	976.8	E858.7	E946.8	E950.4	E962.0	E980.4
Mace	987.5	E869.3	—	E952.8	E962.2	E982.8
Macrolides (antibiotics)	960.3	E856	E930.3	E950.4	E962.0	E980.4
Mafenide	976.0	E858.7	E946.0	E950.4	E962.0	E980.4
Magaldrate	973.0	E858.4	E943.0	E950.4	E962.0	E980.4
Magic mushroom	969.6	E854.1	E939.6	E950.3	E962.0	E980.3
Magnamycin	960.8	E856	E930.8	E950.4	E962.0	E980.4
Magnesia magma	973.0	E858.4	E943.0	E950.4	E962.0	E980.4
Magnesium (compounds) (fumes) NEC	985.8	E866.4	—	E950.9	E962.1	E980.9
antacid	973.0	E858.4	E943.0	E950.4	E962.0	E980.4
carbonate	973.0	E858.4	E943.0	E950.4	E962.0	E980.4
cathartic	973.3	E858.4	E943.3	E950.4	E962.0	E980.4
citrate	973.3	E858.4	E943.3	E950.4	E962.0	E980.4
hydroxide	973.0	E858.4	E943.0	E950.4	E962.0	E980.4
oxide	973.0	E858.4	E943.0	E950.4	E962.0	E980.4
sulfate (oral)	973.3	E858.4	E943.3	E950.4	E962.0	E980.4
intravenous	966.3	E855.0	E936.3	E950.4	E962.0	E980.4
trisilicate	973.0	E858.4	E943.0	E950.4	E962.0	E980.4
Malathion (insecticide)	989.3	E863.1	—	E950.6	E962.1	E980.7
Male fern (oleoresin)	961.6	E857	E931.6	E950.4	E962.0	E980.4
Mandelic acid	961.9	E857	E931.9	E950.4	E962.0	E980.4
Manganese compounds (fumes) NEC	985.2	E866.4	—	E950.9	E962.1	E980.9
Mannitol (diuretic) (medicinal) NEC	974.4	E858.5	E944.4	E950.4	E962.0	E980.4
hexanitrate	972.4	E858.3	E942.4	E950.4	E962.0	E980.4
mustard	963.1	E858.1	E933.1	E950.4	E962.0	E980.4
Mannomustine	963.1	E858.1	E933.1	E950.4	E962.0	E980.4
MAO inhibitors	969.0	E854.0	E939.0	E950.3	E962.0	E980.3
Mapharsen	961.1	E857	E931.1	E950.4	E962.0	E980.4
Marcaine	968.9	E855.2	E938.9	E950.4	E962.0	E980.4
infiltration (subcutaneous)	968.5	E855.2	E938.5	E950.4	E962.0	E980.4
nerve block (peripheral) (plexus)	968.6	E855.2	E938.6	E950.4	E962.0	E980.4
Marezine	963.0	E858.1	E933.0	E950.4	E962.0	E980.4
Marihuana, marijuana (derivatives)	969.6	E854.1	E939.6	E950.3	E962.0	E980.3
Marine animals or plants (sting)	989.5	E905.6	—	E950.9	E962.1	E980.9
Marplan	969.0	E854.0	E939.0	E950.3	E962.0	E980.3
Marsh gas	987.1	E869.8	—	E952.8	E962.2	E982.8
Marsilid	969.0	E854.0	E939.0	E950.3	E962.0	E980.3
Matulane	963.1	E858.1	E933.1	E950.4	E962.0	E980.4
Mazindol	977.0	E858.8	E947.0	E950.4	E962.0	E980.4
MDMA	969.7	E854.2	E939.7	E950.3	E962.0	E980.3 ◀
Meadow saffron	988.2	E865.3	—	E950.9	E962.1	E980.9
Measles vaccine	979.4	E858.8	E949.4	E950.4	E962.0	E980.4
Meat, noxious or nonbacterial	988.8	E865.0	—	E950.9	E962.1	E980.9
Mebanazine	969.0	E854.0	E939.0	E950.3	E962.0	E980.3
Mebaral	967.0	E851	E937.0	E950.1	E962.0	E980.1
Mebendazole	961.6	E857	E931.6	E950.4	E962.0	E980.4
Mebeverine	975.1	E858.6	E945.1	E950.4	E962.0	E980.4
Mebhydroline	963.0	E858.1	E933.0	E950.4	E962.0	E980.4
Mebrophenhydramine	963.0	E858.1	E933.0	E950.4	E962.0	E980.4
Mebutamate	969.5	E853.8	E939.5	E950.3	E962.0	E980.3
Mecamylamine (chloride)	972.3	E858.3	E942.3	E950.4	E962.0	E980.4
Mechlorethamine hydrochloride	963.1	E858.1	E933.1	E950.4	E962.0	E980.4
Meclizene (hydrochloride)	963.0	E858.1	E933.0	E950.4	E962.0	E980.4
Meclofenoxate	970.0	E854.3	E940.0	E950.4	E962.0	E980.4
Meclozine (hydrochloride)	963.0	E858.1	E933.0	E950.4	E962.0	E980.4
Medazepam	969.4	E853.2	E939.4	E950.3	E962.0	E980.3
Medicine, medicinal substance	977.9	E858.9	E947.9	E950.5	E962.0	E980.5
specified NEC	977.8	E858.8	E947.8	E950.4	E962.0	E980.4

Substance	Poisoning	External Cause (E-Code) Accident	Therapeutic Use	Suicide Attempt	Assault	Undetermined
Medinal	967.0	E851	E937.0	E950.1	E962.0	E980.1
Medomin	967.0	E851	E937.0	E950.1	E962.0	E980.1
Medroxyprogesterone	962.2	E858.0	E932.2	E950.4	E962.0	E980.4
Medrysone	976.5	E858.7	E946.5	E950.4	E962.0	E980.4
Mefenamic acid	965.7	E850.7	E935.7	E950.0	E962.0	E980.0
Megahallucinogen	969.6	E854.1	E939.6	E950.3	E962.0	E980.3
Megestrol	962.2	E858.0	E932.2	E950.4	E962.0	E980.4
Meglumine	977.8	E858.8	E947.8	E950.4	E962.0	E980.4
Meladinin	976.3	E858.7	E946.3	E950.4	E962.0	E980.4
Melanizing agents	976.3	E858.7	E946.3	E950.4	E962.0	E980.4
Melarsoprol	961.1	E857	E931.1	E950.4	E962.0	E980.4
Melia azedarach	988.2	E865.3	—	E950.9	E962.1	E980.9
Mellaril	969.1	E853.0	E939.1	E950.3	E962.0	E980.3
Meloxine	976.3	E858.7	E946.3	E950.4	E962.0	E980.4
Melphalan	963.1	E858.1	E933.1	E950.4	E962.0	E980.4
Menadiol sodium diphosphate	964.3	E858.2	E934.3	E950.4	E962.0	E980.4
Menadione (sodium bisulfite)	964.3	E858.2	E934.3	E950.4	E962.0	E980.4
Menaphthone	964.3	E858.2	E934.3	E950.4	E962.0	E980.4
Meningococcal vaccine	978.8	E858.8	E948.8	E950.4	E962.0	E980.4
Menningovax-C	978.8	E858.8	E948.8	E950.4	E962.0	E980.4
Menotropins	962.4	E858.0	E932.4	E950.4	E962.0	E980.4
Menthol NEC	976.1	E858.7	E946.1	E950.4	E962.0	E980.4
Mepacrine	961.3	E857	E931.3	E950.4	E962.0	E980.4
Meparfynol	967.8	E852.8	E937.8	E950.2	E962.0	E980.2
Mepazine	969.1	E853.0	E939.1	E950.3	E962.0	E980.3
Mepenzolate	971.1	E855.4	E941.1	E950.4	E962.0	E980.4
Meperidine	965.09	E850.2	E935.2	E950.0	E962.0	E980.0
Mephenamin(e)	966.4	E855.0	E936.4	E950.4	E962.0	E980.4
Mephenesin (carbamate)	968.0	E855.1	E938.0	E950.4	E962.0	E980.4
Mephenoxalone	969.5	E853.8	E939.5	E950.3	E962.0	E980.3
Mephentermine	971.2	E855.5	E941.2	E950.4	E962.0	E980.4
Mephenytoin	966.1	E855.0	E936.1	E950.4	E962.0	E980.4
Mephobarbital	967.0	E851	E937.0	E950.1	E962.0	E980.1
Mepiperphenidol	971.1	E855.4	E941.1	E950.4	E962.0	E980.4
Mepivacaine	968.9	E855.2	E938.9	E950.4	E962.0	E980.4
infiltration (subcutaneous)	968.5	E855.2	E938.5	E950.4	E962.0	E980.4
nerve block (peripheral) (plexus)	968.6	E855.2	E938.6	E950.4	E962.0	E980.4
topical (surface)	968.5	E855.2	E938.5	E950.4	E962.0	E980.4
Meprednisone	962.0	E858.0	E932.0	E950.4	E962.0	E980.4
Meprobam	969.5	E853.8	E939.5	E950.3	E962.0	E980.3
Meprobamate	969.5	E853.8	E939.5	E950.3	E962.0	E980.3
Mepyramine (maleate)	963.0	E858.1	E933.0	E950.4	E962.0	E980.4
Meralluride	974.0	E858.5	E944.0	E950.4	E962.0	E980.4
Merbaphen	974.0	E858.5	E944.0	E950.4	E962.0	E980.4
Merbromin	976.0	E858.7	E946.0	E950.4	E962.0	E980.4
Mercaptomerin	974.0	E858.5	E944.0	E950.4	E962.0	E980.4
Mercaptopurine	963.1	E858.1	E933.1	E950.4	E962.0	E980.4
Mercumatilin	974.0	E858.5	E944.0	E950.4	E962.0	E980.4
Mercuramide	974.0	E858.5	E944.0	E950.4	E962.0	E980.4
Mercuranin	976.0	E858.7	E946.0	E950.4	E962.0	E980.4
Mercurochrome	976.0	E858.7	E946.0	E950.4	E962.0	E980.4
Mercury, mercuric, mercurous (compounds) (cyanide) (fumes) (nonmedicinal) (vapor) NEC	985.0	E866.1	—	E950.9	E962.1	E980.9
ammoniated	976.0	E858.7	E946.0	E950.4	E962.0	E980.4
anti-infective	961.2	E857	E931.2	E950.4	E962.0	E980.4
topical	976.0	E858.7	E946.0	E950.4	E962.0	E980.4
chloride (antiseptic) NEC	976.0	E858.7	E946.0	E950.4	E962.0	E980.4
fungicide	985.0	E863.6	—	E950.6	E962.1	E980.7
diuretic compounds	974.0	E858.5	E944.0	E950.4	E962.0	E980.4
fungicide	985.0	E863.6	—	E950.6	E962.1	E980.7
organic (fungicide)	985.0	E863.6	—	E950.6	E962.1	E980.7
Merethoxylline	974.0	E858.5	E944.0	E950.4	E962.0	E980.4

Substance	Poisoning	External Cause (E-Code)				
		Accident	Therapeutic Use	Suicide Attempt	Assault	Undetermined
Mersalyl	974.0	E858.5	E944.0	E950.4	E962.0	E980.4
Merthiolate (topical)	976.0	E858.7	E946.0	E950.4	E962.0	E980.4
ophthalmic preparation	976.5	E858.7	E946.5	E950.4	E962.0	E980.4
Meruvax	979.4	E858.8	E949.4	E950.4	E962.0	E980.4
Mescal buttons	969.6	E854.1	E939.6	E950.3	E962.0	E980.3
Mescaline (salts)	969.6	E854.1	E939.6	E950.3	E962.0	E980.3
Mesoridazine besylate	969.1	E853.0	E939.1	E950.3	E962.0	E980.3
Mestanolone	962.1	E858.0	E932.1	E950.4	E962.0	E980.4
Mestranol	962.2	E858.0	E932.2	E950.4	E962.0	E980.4
Metactesylacetate	976.0	E858.7	E946.0	E950.4	E962.0	E980.4
Metaldehyde (snail killer) NEC	989.4	E863.4	—	E950.6	E962.1	E980.7
Metals (heavy) (nonmedicinal) NEC	985.9	E866.4	—	E950.9	E962.1	E980.9
dust, fumes, or vapor NEC	985.9	E866.4	—	E950.9	E962.1	E980.9
light NEC	985.9	E866.4	—	E950.9	E962.1	E980.9
dust, fumes, or vapor NEC	985.9	E866.4	—	E950.9	E962.1	E980.9
pesticides (dust) (vapor)	985.9	E863.4	—	E950.6	E962.1	E980.7
Metamucil	973.3	E858.4	E943.3	E950.4	E962.0	E980.4
Metaphen	976.0	E858.7	E946.0	E950.4	E962.0	E980.4
Metaproterenol	975.1	E858.6	E945.1	E950.4	E962.0	E980.4
Metaraminol	972.8	E858.3	E942.8	E950.4	E962.0	E980.4
Metaxalone	968.0	E855.1	E938.0	E950.4	E962.0	E980.4
Metformin	962.3	E858.0	E932.3	E950.4	E962.0	E980.4
Methacycline	960.4	E856	E930.4	E950.4	E962.0	E980.4
Methadone	965.02	E850.1	E935.1	E950.0	E962.0	E980.0
Methallenestril	962.2	E858.0	E932.2	E950.4	E962.0	E980.4
Methamphetamine	969.7	E854.2	E939.7	E950.3	E962.0	E980.3
Methandienone	962.1	E858.0	E932.1	E950.4	E962.0	E980.4
Methandriol	962.1	E858.0	E932.1	E950.4	E962.0	E980.4
Methandrostenolone	962.1	E858.0	E932.1	E950.4	E962.0	E980.4
Methane gas	987.1	E869.8	—	E952.8	E962.2	E982.8
Methanol	980.1	E860.2	—	E950.9	E962.1	E980.9
vapor	987.8	E869.8	—	E952.8	E962.2	E982.8
Methantheline	971.1	E855.4	E941.1	E950.4	E962.0	E980.4
Methaphenilene	963.0	E858.1	E933.0	E950.4	E962.0	E980.4
Methapyrilene	963.0	E858.1	E933.0	E950.4	E962.0	E980.4
Methaqualone (compounds)	967.4	E852.3	E937.4	E950.2	E962.0	E980.2
Metharbital, metharbitone	967.0	E851	E937.0	E950.1	E962.0	E980.1
Methazolamide	974.2	E858.5	E944.2	E950.4	E962.0	E980.4
Methdilazine	963.0	E858.1	E933.0	E950.4	E962.0	E980.4
Methedrine	969.7	E854.2	E939.7	E950.3	E962.0	E980.3
Methenamine (mandelate)	961.9	E857	E931.9	E950.4	E962.0	E980.4
Methenolone	962.1	E858.0	E932.1	E950.4	E962.0	E980.4
Methergine	975.0	E858.6	E945.0	E950.4	E962.0	E980.4
Methiacil	962.8	E858.0	E932.8	E950.4	E962.0	E980.4
Methicillin (sodium)	960.0	E856	E930.0	E950.4	E962.0	E980.4
Methimazole	962.8	E858.0	E932.8	E950.4	E962.0	E980.4
Methionine	977.1	E858.8	E947.1	E950.4	E962.0	E980.4
Methisazone	961.7	E857	E931.7	E950.4	E962.0	E980.4
Methitural	967.0	E851	E937.0	E950.1	E962.0	E980.1
Methixene	971.1	E855.4	E941.1	E950.4	E962.0	E980.4
Methobarbital, methobarbitone	967.0	E851	E937.0	E950.1	E962.0	E980.1
Methocarbamol	968.0	E855.1	E938.0	E950.4	E962.0	E980.4
Methohexital, methohexitone (sodium)	968.3	E855.1	E938.3	E950.4	E962.0	E980.4
Methoin	966.1	E855.0	E936.1	E950.4	E962.0	E980.4
Methopholine	965.7	E850.7	E935.7	E950.0	E962.0	E980.0
Methorate	975.4	E858.6	E945.4	E950.4	E962.0	E980.4
Methoserpidine	972.6	E858.3	E942.6	E950.4	E962.0	E980.4
Methotrexate	963.1	E858.1	E933.1	E950.4	E962.0	E980.4
Methotrimeprazine	967.8	E852.8	E937.8	E950.2	E962.0	E980.2
Methoxa-Dome	976.3	E858.7	E946.3	E950.4	E962.0	E980.4
Methoxamine	971.2	E855.5	E941.2	E950.4	E962.0	E980.4

Substance	Poisoning	External Cause (E-Code) Accident	Therapeutic Use	Suicide Attempt	Assault	Undetermined
Methoxsalen	976.3	E858.7	E946.3	E950.4	E962.0	E980.4
Methoxybenzyl penicillin	960.0	E856	E930.0	E950.4	E962.0	E980.4
Methoxychlor	989.2	E863.0	—	E950.6	E962.1	E980.7
Methoxyflurane	968.2	E855.1	E938.2	E950.4	E962.0	E980.4
Methoxyphenamine	971.2	E855.5	E941.2	E950.4	E962.0	E980.4
Methoxypromazine	969.1	E853.0	E939.1	E950.3	E962.0	E980.3
Methoxypsoralen	976.3	E858.7	E946.3	E950.4	E962.0	E980.4
Methscopolamine (bromide)	971.1	E855.4	E941.1	E950.4	E962.0	E980.4
Methsuximide	966.2	E855.0	E936.2	E950.4	E962.0	E980.4
Methyclothiazide	974.3	E858.5	E944.3	E950.4	E962.0	E980.4
Methyl	—	—	—	—	—	—
acetate	982.8	E862.4	—	E950.9	E962.1	E980.9
acetone II	982.8	E862.4	—	E950.9	E962.1	E980.9
alcohol	980.1	E860.2	—	E950.9	E962.1	E980.9
amphetamine	969.7	E854.2	E939.7	E950.3	E962.0	E980.3
androstanolone	962.1	E858.0	E932.1	E950.4	E962.0	E980.4
atropine	971.1	E855.4	E941.1	E950.4	E962.0	E980.4
benzene	982.0	E862.4	—	E950.9	E962.1	E980.9
bromide (gas)	987.8	E869.8	—	E952.8	E962.2	E982.8
fumigant	987.8	E863.8	—	E950.6	E962.2	E980.7
butanol	980.8	E860.8	—	E950.9	E962.1	E980.9
carbinol	980.1	E860.2	—	E950.9	E962.1	E980.9
cellosolve	982.8	E862.4	—	E950.9	E962.1	E980.9
cellulose	973.3	E858.4	E943.3	E950.4	E961.0	E980.4
chloride (gas)	987.8	E869.8	—	E952.8	E962.2	E982.8
cyclohexane	982.8	E862.4	—	E950.9	E962.1	E980.9
cyclohexanone	982.8	E862.4	—	E950.9	E962.1	E980.9
dihydromorphinone	965.09	E850.2	E935.2	E950.0	E962.0	E980.0
ergometrine	975.0	E858.6	E945.0	E950.4	E962.0	E980.4
ergonovine	975.0	E858.6	E945.0	E950.4	E962.0	E980.4
ethyl ketone	982.8	E862.4	—	E950.9	E962.1	E980.9
hydrazine	983.9	E864.3	—	E950.7	E962.1	E980.6
isobutyl ketone	982.8	E862.4	—	E950.9	E962.1	E980.9
morphine NEC	965.09	E850.2	E935.2	E950.0	E962.0	E980.0
parafynol	967.8	E852.8	E937.8	E950.2	E962.0	E980.2
parathion	989.3	E863.1	—	E950.6	E962.1	E980.7
pentynol NEC	967.8	E852.8	E937.8	E950.2	E962.0	E980.2
peridol	969.2	E853.1	E939.2	E950.3	E962.0	E980.3
phenidate	969.7	E854.2	E939.7	E950.3	E962.0	E980.3
prednisolone	962.0	E858.0	E932.0	E950.4	E962.0	E980.4
ENT agent	976.6	E858.7	E946.6	E950.4	E962.0	E980.4
ophthalmic preparation	976.5	E858.7	E946.5	E950.4	E962.0	E980.4
topical NEC	976.0	E858.7	E946.0	E950.4	E962.0	E980.4
propylcarbinol	980.8	E860.8	—	E950.9	E962.1	E980.9
rosaniline NEC	976.0	E858.7	E946.0	E950.4	E962.0	E980.4
salicylate NEC	976.3	E858.7	E946.3	E950.4	E962.0	E980.4
sulfate (fumes)	987.8	E869.8	—	E952.8	E962.2	E982.8
liquid	983.9	E864.3	—	E950.7	E962.1	E980.6
sulfonal	967.8	E852.8	E937.8	E950.2	E962.0	E980.2
testosterone	962.1	E858.0	E932.1	E950.4	E962.0	E980.4
thiouracil	962.8	E858.0	E932.8	E950.4	E962.0	E980.4
Methylated spirit	980.0	E860.1	—	E950.9	E962.1	E980.9
Methyldopa	972.6	E858.3	E942.6	E950.4	E962.0	E980.4
Methylene blue	961.9	E857	E931.9	E950.4	E962.0	E980.4
chloride or dichloride (solvent) NEC	982.3	E862.4	—	E950.9	E962.1	E980.9
Methylhexabital	967.0	E851	E937.0	E950.1	E962.0	E980.1
Methylparaben (ophthalmic)	976.5	E858.7	E946.5	E950.4	E962.0	E980.4
Methyprylon	967.5	E852.4	E937.5	E950.2	E962.0	E980.2
Methysergide	971.3	E855.6	E941.3	E950.4	E962.0	E980.4
Metoclopramide	963.0	E858.1	E933.0	E950.4	E962.0	E980.4
Metofoline	965.7	E850.7	E935.7	E950.0	E962.0	E980.0

◀ New ⟸ Revised Code

Substance	Poisoning	External Cause (E-Code)				
		Accident	Therapeutic Use	Suicide Attempt	Assault	Undetermined
Metopon	965.09	E850.2	E935.2	E950.0	E962.0	E980.0
Metronidazole	961.5	E857	E931.5	E950.4	E962.0	E980.4
Metycaine	968.9	E855.2	E938.9	E950.4	E962.0	E980.4
infiltration (subcutaneous)	968.5	E855.2	E938.5	E950.4	E962.0	E980.4
nerve block (peripheral) (plexus)	968.6	E855.2	E938.6	E950.4	E962.0	E980.4
topical (surface)	968.5	E855.2	E938.5	E950.4	E962.0	E980.4
Metyrapone	977.8	E858.8	E947.8	E950.4	E962.0	E980.4
Mevinphos	989.3	E863.1	—	E950.6	E962.1	E980.7
Mezereon (berries)	988.2	E865.3	—	E950.9	E962.1	E980.9
Micatin	976.0	E858.7	E946.0	E950.4	E962.0	E980.4
Miconazole	976.0	E858.7	E946.0	E950.4	E962.0	E980.4
Midol	965.1	E850.3	E935.3	E950.0	E962.0	E980.0
Mifepristone	962.9	E858.0	E932.9	E950.4	E962.0	E980.4
Milk of magnesia	973.0	E858.4	E943.0	E950.4	E962.0	E980.4
Millipede (tropical) (venomous)	989.5	E905.4	—	E950.9	E962.1	E980.9
Miltown	969.5	E853.8	E939.5	E950.3	E962.0	E980.3
Mineral	—	—	—	—	—	—
oil (medicinal)	973.2	E858.4	E943.2	E950.4	E962.0	E980.4
nonmedicinal	981	E862.1	—	E950.9	E962.1	E980.9
topical	976.3	E858.7	E946.3	E950.4	E962.0	E980.4
salts NEC	974.6	E858.5	E944.6	E950.4	E962.0	E980.4
spirits	981	E862.0	—	E950.9	E962.1	E980.9
Minocycline	960.4	E856	E930.4	E950.4	E962.0	E980.4
Mithramycin (antineoplastic)	960.7	E856	E930.7	E950.4	E962.0	E980.4
Mitobronitol	963.1	E858.1	E933.1	E950.4	E962.0	E980.4
Mitomycin (antineoplastic)	960.7	E856	E930.7	E950.4	E962.0	E980.4
Mitotane	963.1	E858.1	E933.1	E950.4	E962.0	E980.4
Moderil	972.6	E858.3	E942.6	E950.4	E962.0	E980.4
Mogadon - *see* Nitrazepam	—	—	—	—	—	—
Molindone	969.3	E853.8	E939.3	E950.3	E962.0	E980.3
Monistat	976.0	E858.7	E946.0	E950.4	E962.0	E980.4
Monkshood	988.2	E865.4	—	E950.9	E962.1	E980.9
Monoamine oxidase inhibitors	969.0	E854.0	E939.0	E950.3	E962.0	E980.3
Monochlorobenzene	982.0	E862.4	—	E950.9	E962.1	E980.9
Monosodium glutamate	989.89	E866.8	—	E950.9	E962.1	E980.9
Monoxide, carbon - *see* Carbon, monoxide	—	—	—	—	—	—
Moperone	969.2	E853.1	E939.2	E950.3	E962.0	E980.3
Morning glory seeds	969.6	E854.1	E939.6	E950.3	E962.0	E980.3
Moroxydine (hydrochloride)	961.7	E857	E931.7	E950.4	E962.0	E980.4
Morphazinamide	961.8	E857	E931.8	E950.4	E962.0	E980.4
Morphinans	965.09	E850.2	E935.2	E950.0	E962.0	E980.0
Morphine NEC	965.09	E850.2	E935.2	E950.0	E962.0	E980.0
antagonists	970.1	E854.3	E940.1	E950.4	E962.0	E980.4
Morpholinylethyl morphine	965.09	E850.2	E935.2	E950.0	E962.0	E980.0
Morrhuate sodium	972.7	E858.3	E942.7	E950.4	E962.0	E980.4
Moth balls (*see also* Pesticides)	989.4	E863.4	—	E950.6	E962.1	E980.7
naphthalene	983.0	E863.4	—	E950.7	E962.1	E980.6
Motor exhaust gas - *see* Carbon, monoxide, exhaust gas	—	—	—	—	—	—
Mouth wash	976.6	E858.7	E946.6	E950.4	E962.0	E980.4
Mucolytic agent	975.5	E858.6	E945.5	E950.4	E962.0	E980.4
Mucomyst	975.5	E858.6	E945.5	E950.4	E962.0	E980.4
Mucous membrane agents (external)	976.9	E858.7	E946.9	E950.4	E962.0	E980.4
specified NEC	976.8	E858.7	E946.8	E950.4	E962.0	E980.4
Mumps	—	—	—	—	—	—
immune globulin (human)	964.6	E858.2	E934.6	E950.4	E962.0	E980.4
skin test antigen	977.8	E858.8	E947.8	E950.4	E962.0	E980.4
vaccine	979.6	E858.8	E949.6	E950.4	E962.0	E980.4
Mumpsvax	979.6	E858.8	E949.6	E950.4	E962.0	E980.4
Muriatic acid - *see* Hydrochloric acid	—	—	—	—	—	—
Muscarine	971.0	E855.3	E941.0	E950.4	E962.0	E980.4
Muscle affecting agents NEC	975.3	E858.6	E945.3	E950.4	E962.0	E980.4
oxytocic	975.0	E858.6	E945.0	E950.4	E962.0	E980.4

Substance	Poisoning	External Cause (E-Code) Accident	Therapeutic Use	Suicide Attempt	Assault	Undetermined
Muscle affecting agents NEC *(Continued)*						
relaxants	975.3	E858.6	E945.3	E950.4	E962.0	E980.4
central nervous system	968.0	E855.1	E938.0	E950.4	E962.0	E980.4
skeletal	975.2	E858.6	E945.2	E950.4	E962.0	E980.4
smooth	975.1	E858.6	E945.1	E950.4	E962.0	E980.4
Mushrooms, noxious	988.1	E865.5	—	E950.9	E962.1	E980.9
Mussel, noxious	988.0	E865.1	—	E950.9	E962.1	E980.9
Mustard (emetic)	973.6	E858.4	E943.6	E950.4	E962.0	E980.4
gas	987.8	E869.8	—	E952.8	E962.2	E982.8
nitrogen	963.1	E858.1	E933.1	E950.4	E962.0	E980.4
Mustine	963.1	E858.1	E933.1	E950.4	E962.0	E980.4
M-vac	979.4	E858.8	E949.4	E950.4	E962.0	E980.4
Mycifradin	960.8	E856	E930.8	E950.4	E962.0	E980.4
topical	976.0	E858.7	E946.0	E950.4	E962.0	E980.4
Mycitracin	960.8	E856	E930.8	E950.4	E962.0	E980.4
ophthalmic preparation	976.5	E858.7	E946.5	E950.4	E962.0	E980.4
Mycostatin	960.1	E856	E930.1	E950.4	E962.0	E980.4
topical	976.0	E858.7	E946.0	E950.4	E962.0	E980.4
Mydriacyl	971.1	E855.4	E941.1	E950.4	E962.0	E980.4
Myelobromal	963.1	E858.1	E933.1	E950.4	E962.0	E980.4
Myleran	963.1	E858.1	E933.1	E950.4	E962.0	E980.4
Myochrysin(e)	965.69	E850.6	E935.6	E950.0	E962.0	E980.0
Myoneural blocking agents	975.2	E858.6	E945.2	E950.4	E962.0	E980.4
Myristica fragrans	988.2	E865.3	—	E950.9	E962.1	E980.9
Myristicin	988.2	E865.3	—	E950.9	E962.1	E980.9
Mysoline	966.3	E855.0	E936.3	E950.4	E962.0	E980.4
Nafcillin (sodium)	960.0	E856	E930.0	E950.4	E962.0	E980.4
Nail polish remover	982.8	E862.4	—	E950.9	E962.1	E980.9
Nalidixic acid	961.9	E857	E931.9	E950.4	E962.0	E980.4
Nalorphine	970.1	E854.3	E940.1	E950.4	E962.0	E980.4
Naloxone	970.1	E854.3	E940.1	E950.4	E962.0	E980.4
Nandrolone (decanoate) (phenpropionate)	962.1	E858.0	E932.1	E950.4	E962.0	E980.4
Naphazoline	971.2	E855.5	E941.2	E950.4	E962.0	E980.4
Naphtha (painter's) (petroleum)	981	E862.0	—	E950.9	E962.1	E980.9
solvent	981	E862.0	—	E950.9	E962.1	E980.9
vapor	987.1	E869.8	—	E952.8	E962.2	E982.8
Naphthalene (chlorinated)	983.0	E864.0	—	E950.7	E962.1	E980.6
insecticide or moth repellent	983.0	E863.4	—	E950.7	E962.1	E980.6
vapor	987.8	E869.8	—	E952.8	E962.2	E982.8
Naphthol	983.0	E864.0	—	E950.7	E962.1	E980.6
Naphthylamine	983.0	E864.0	—	E950.7	E962.1	E980.6
Naprosyn - *see* Naproxen	—	—	—	—	—	—
Naproxen	965.61	E850.6	E935.6	E950.0	E962.0	E980.0
Narcotic (drug)	967.9	E852.9	E937.9	E950.2	E962.0	E980.2
analgesic NEC	965.8	E850.8	E935.8	E950.0	E962.0	E980.0
antagonist	970.1	E854.3	E940.1	E950.4	E962.0	E980.4
specified NEC	967.8	E852.8	E937.8	E950.2	E962.0	E980.2
Narcotine	975.4	E858.6	E945.4	E950.4	E962.0	E980.4
Nardil	969.0	E854.0	E939.0	E950.3	E962.0	E980.3
Natrium cyanide - *see* Cyanide(s)	—	—	—	—	—	—
Natural	—	—	—	—	—	—
blood (product)	964.7	E858.2	E934.7	E950.4	E962.0	E980.4
gas (piped)	987.1	E867	—	E951.0	E962.2	E981.0
incomplete combustion	986	E867	—	E951.0	E962.2	E981.0
Nealbarbital, nealbarbitone	967.0	E851	E937.0	E950.1	E962.0	E980.1
Nectadon	975.4	E858.6	E945.4	E950.4	E962.0	E980.4
Nematocyst (sting)	989.5	E905.6	—	E950.9	E962.1	E980.9
Nembutal	967.0	E851	E937.0	E950.1	E962.0	E980.1
Neoarsphenamine	961.1	E857	E931.1	E950.4	E962.0	E980.4
Neocinchophen	974.7	E858.5	E944.7	E950.4	E962.0	E980.4
Neomycin	960.8	E856	E930.8	E950.4	E962.0	E980.4
ENT agent	976.6	E858.7	E946.6	E950.4	E962.0	E980.4
ophthalmic preparation	976.5	E858.7	E946.5	E950.4	E962.0	E980.4

◄ New ⟵ Revised Code

Substance	Poisoning	External Cause (E-Code) Accident	Therapeutic Use	Suicide Attempt	Assault	Undetermined
Neomycin *(Continued)*						
topical NEC	976.0	E858.7	E946.0	E950.4	E962.0	E980.4
Neonal	967.0	E851	E937.0	E950.1	E962.0	E980.1
Neoprontosil	961.0	E857	E931.0	E950.4	E962.0	E980.4
Neosalvarsan	961.1	E857	E931.1	E950.4	E962.0	E980.4
Neosilversalvarsan	961.1	E857	E931.1	E950.4	E962.0	E980.4
Neosporin	960.8	E856	E930.8	E950.4	E962.0	E980.4
ENT agent	976.6	E858.7	E946.6	E950.4	E962.0	E980.4
ophthalmic preparation	976.5	E858.7	E946.5	E950.4	E962.0	E980.4
topical NEC	976.0	E858.7	E946.0	E950.4	E962.0	E980.4
Neostigmine	971.0	E855.3	E941.0	E950.4	E962.0	E980.4
Neraval	967.0	E851	E937.0	E950.1	E962.0	E980.1
Neravan	967.0	E851	E937.0	E950.1	E962.0	E980.1
Nerium oleander	988.2	E865.4	—	E950.9	E962.1	E980.9
Nerve gases (war)	987.9	E869.9	—	E952.9	E962.2	E982.9
Nesacaine	968.9	E855.2	E938.9	E950.4	E962.0	E980.4
infiltration (subcutaneous)	968.5	E855.2	E938.5	E950.4	E962.0	E980.4
nerve block (peripheral) (plexus)	968.6	E855.2	E938.6	E950.4	E962.0	E980.4
Neurobarb	967.0	E851	E937.0	E950.1	E962.0	E980.1
Neuroleptics NEC	969.3	E853.8	E939.3	E950.3	E962.0	E980.3
Neuroprotective agent	977.8	E858.8	E947.8	E950.4	E962.0	E980.4
Neutral spirits	980.0	E860.1	—	E950.9	E962.1	E980.9
beverage	980.0	E860.0	—	E950.9	E962.1	E980.9
Niacin, niacinamide	972.2	E858.3	E942.2	E950.4	E962.0	E980.4
Nialamide	969.0	E854.0	E939.0	E950.3	E962.0	E980.3
Nickle (carbonyl) (compounds) (fumes) (tetracarbonyl) (vapor)	985.8	E866.4	—	E950.9	E962.1	E980.9
Niclosamide	961.6	E857	E931.6	E950.4	E962.0	E980.4
Nicomorphine	965.09	E850.2	E935.2	E950.0	E962.0	E980.0
Nicotinamide	972.2	E858.3	E942.2	E950.4	E962.0	E980.4
Nicotine (insecticide) (spray) (sulfate) NEC	989.4	E863.4	—	E950.6	E962.1	E980.7
not insecticide	989.89	E866.8	—	E950.9	E962.1	E980.9
Nicotinic acid (derivatives)	972.2	E858.3	E942.2	E950.4	E962.0	E980.4
Nicotinyl alcohol	972.2	E858.3	E942.2	E950.4	E962.0	E980.4
Nicoumalone	964.2	E858.2	E934.2	E950.4	E962.0	E980.4
Nifenazone	965.5	E850.5	E935.5	E950.0	E962.0	E980.0
Nifuraldezone	961.9	E857	E931.9	E950.4	E962.0	E980.4
Nightshade (deadly)	988.2	E865.4	—	E950.9	E962.1	E980.9
Nikethamide	970.0	E854.3	E940.0	E950.4	E962.0	E980.4
Nilstat	960.1	E856	E930.1	E950.4	E962.0	E980.4
topical	976.0	E858.7	E946.0	E950.4	E962.0	E980.4
Nimodipine	977.8	E858.8	E947.8	E950.4	E962.0	E980.4
Niridazole	961.6	E857	E931.6	E950.4	E962.0	E980.4
Nisentil	965.09	E850.2	E935.2	E950.0	E962.0	E980.0
Nitrates	972.4	E858.3	E942.4	E950.4	E962.0	E980.4
Nitrazepam	969.4	E853.2	E939.4	E950.3	E962.0	E980.3
Nitric	—	—	—	—	—	—
acid (liquid)	983.1	E864.1	—	E950.7	E962.1	E980.6
vapor	987.8	E869.8	—	E952.8	E962.2	E982.8
oxide (gas)	987.2	E869.0	—	E952.8	E962.2	E982.8
Nitrite, amyl (medicinal) (vapor)	972.4	E858.3	E942.4	E950.4	E962.0	E980.4
Nitroaniline	983.0	E864.0	—	E950.7	E962.1	E980.6
vapor	987.8	E869.8	—	E952.8	E962.2	E982.8
Nitrobenzene, nitrobenzol	983.0	E864.0	—	E950.7	E962.1	E980.6
vapor	987.8	E869.8	—	E952.8	E962.2	E982.8
Nitrocellulose	976.3	E858.7	E946.3	E950.4	E962.0	E980.4
Nitrofuran derivatives	961.9	E857	E931.9	E950.4	E962.0	E980.4
Nitrofurantoin	961.9	E857	E931.9	E950.4	E962.0	E980.4
Nitrofurazone	976.0	E858.7	E946.0	E950.4	E962.0	E980.4
Nitrogen (dioxide) (gas) (oxide)	987.2	E869.0	—	E952.8	E962.2	E982.8
mustard (antineoplastic)	963.1	E858.1	E933.1	E950.4	E962.0	E980.4
Nitroglycerin, nitroglycerol (medicinal)	972.4	E858.3	E942.4	E950.4	E962.0	E980.4
nonmedicinal	989.89	E866.8	—	E950.9	E962.1	E980.9
fumes	987.8	E869.8	—	E952.8	E962.2	E982.8

Substance	Poisoning	External Cause (E-Code) Accident	Therapeutic Use	Suicide Attempt	Assault	Undetermined
Nitrohydrochloric acid	983.1	E864.1	—	E950.7	E962.1	E980.6
Nitromersol	976.0	E858.7	E946.0	E950.4	E962.0	E980.4
Nitronaphthalene	983.0	E864.0	—	E950.7	E962.2	E980.6
Nitrophenol	983.0	E864.0	—	E950.7	E962.2	E980.6
Nitrothiazol	961.6	E857	E931.6	E950.4	E962.0	E980.4
Nitrotoluene, nitrotoluol	983.0	E864.0	—	E950.7	E962.1	E980.6
vapor	987.8	E869.8	—	E952.8	E962.2	E982.8
Nitrous	968.2	E855.1	E938.2	E950.4	E962.0	E980.4
acid (liquid)	983.1	E864.1	—	E950.7	E962.1	E980.6
fumes	987.2	E869.0	—	E952.8	E962.2	E982.8
oxide (anesthetic) NEC	968.2	E855.1	E938.2	E950.4	E962.0	E980.4
Nitrozone	976.0	E858.7	E946.0	E950.4	E962.0	E980.4
Noctec	967.1	E852.0	E937.1	E950.2	E962.0	E980.2
Noludar	967.5	E852.4	E937.5	E950.2	E962.0	E980.2
Noptil	967.0	E851	E937.0	E950.1	E962.0	E980.1
Noradrenalin	971.2	E855.5	E941.2	E950.4	E962.0	E980.4
Noramidopyrine	965.5	E850.5	E935.5	E950.0	E962.0	E980.0
Norepinephrine	971.2	E855.5	E941.2	E950.4	E962.0	E980.4
Norethandrolone	962.1	E858.0	E932.1	E950.4	E962.0	E980.4
Norethindrone	962.2	E858.0	E932.2	E950.4	E962.0	E980.4
Norethisterone	962.2	E858.0	E932.2	E950.4	E962.0	E980.4
Norethynodrel	962.2	E858.0	E932.2	E950.4	E962.0	E980.4
Norlestrin	962.2	E858.0	E932.2	E950.4	E962.0	E980.4
Norlutin	962.2	E858.0	E932.2	E950.4	E962.0	E980.4
Normison - *see* Benzodiazepines	—	—	—	—	—	—
Normorphine	965.09	E850.2	E935.2	E950.0	E962.0	E980.0
Nortriptyline	969.0	E854.0	E939.0	E950.3	E962.0	E980.3
Noscapine	975.4	E858.6	E945.4	E950.4	E962.0	E980.4
Nose preparations	976.6	E858.7	E946.6	E950.4	E962.0	E980.4
Novobiocin	960.8	E856	E930.8	E950.4	E962.0	E980.4
Novocain (infiltration) (topical)	968.5	E855.2	E938.5	E950.4	E962.0	E980.4
nerve block (peripheral) (plexus)	968.6	E855.2	E938.6	E950.4	E962.0	E980.4
spinal	968.7	E855.2	E938.7	E950.4	E962.0	E980.4
Noxythiolin	961.9	E857	E931.9	E950.4	E962.0	E980.4
NPH Iletin (insulin)	962.3	E858.0	E932.3	E950.4	E962.0	E980.4
Numorphan	965.09	E850.2	E935.2	E950.0	E962.0	E980.0
Nunol	967.0	E851	E937.0	E950.1	E962.0	E980.1
Nupercaine (spinal anesthetic)	968.7	E855.2	E938.7	E950.4	E962.0	E980.4
topical (surface)	968.5	E855.2	E938.5	E950.4	E962.0	E980.4
Nutmeg oil (liniment)	976.3	E858.7	E946.3	E950.4	E962.0	E980.4
Nux vomica	989.1	E863.7	—	E950.6	E962.1	E980.7
Nydrazid	961.8	E857	E931.8	E950.4	E962.0	E980.4
Nylidrin	971.2	E855.5	E941.2	E950.4	E962.0	E980.4
Nystatin	960.1	E856	E930.1	E950.4	E962.0	E980.4
topical	976.0	E858.7	E946.0	E950.4	E962.0	E980.4
Nytol	963.0	E858.1	E933.0	E950.4	E962.0	E980.4
Oblivion	967.8	E852.8	E937.8	E950.2	E962.0	E980.2
Octyl nitrite	972.4	E858.3	E942.4	E950.4	E962.0	E980.4
Oestradiol (cypionate) (dipropionate) (valerate)	962.2	E858.0	E932.2	E950.4	E962.0	E980.4
Oestriol	962.2	E858.0	E932.2	E950.4	E962.0	E980.4
Oestrone	962.2	E858.0	E932.2	E950.4	E962.0	E980.4
Oil (of) NEC	989.89	E866.8	—	E950.9	E962.1	E980.9
bitter almond	989.0	E866.8	—	E950.9	E962.1	E980.9
camphor	976.1	E858.7	E946.1	E950.4	E962.0	E980.4
colors	989.89	E861.6	—	E950.9	E962.1	E980.9
fumes	987.8	E869.8	—	E952.8	E962.2	E982.8
lubricating	981	E862.2	—	E950.9	E962.1	E980.9
specified source, other - *see* substance specified	—	—	—	—	—	—
vitriol (liquid)	983.1	E864.1	—	E950.7	E962.1	E980.6
fumes	987.8	E869.8	—	E952.8	E962.2	E982.8
wintergreen (bitter) NEC	976.3	E858.7	E946.3	E950.4	E962.0	E980.4

◀ New ◀ Revised Code

Substance	Poisoning	External Cause (E-Code)				
		Accident	Therapeutic Use	Suicide Attempt	Assault	Undetermined
Ointments NEC	976.9	E858.7	E946.9	E950.4	E962.0	E980.4
Oleander	988.2	E865.4	—	E950.9	E962.1	E980.9
Oleandomycin	960.3	E856	E930.3	E950.4	E962.0	E980.4
Oleovitamin A	963.5	E858.1	E933.5	E950.4	E962.0	E980.4
Oleum ricini	973.1	E858.4	E943.1	E950.4	E962.0	E980.4
Olive oil (medicinal) NEC	973.2	E858.4	E943.2	E950.4	E962.0	E980.4
OMPA	989.3	E863.1	—	E950.6	E962.1	E980.7
Oncovin	963.1	E858.1	E933.1	E950.4	E962.0	E980.4
Ophthaine	968.5	E855.2	E938.5	E950.4	E962.0	E980.4
Ophthetic	968.5	E855.2	E938.5	E950.4	E962.0	E980.4
Opiates, opioids, opium NEC	965.00	E850.2	E935.2	E950.0	E962.0	E980.0
antagonists	970.1	E854.3	E940.1	E950.4	E962.0	E980.4
Oracon	962.2	E858.0	E932.2	E950.4	E962.0	E980.4
Oragrafin	977.8	E858.8	E947.8	E950.4	E962.0	E980.4
Oral contraceptives	962.2	E858.0	E932.2	E950.4	E962.0	E980.4
Orciprenaline	975.1	E858.6	E945.1	E950.4	E962.0	E980.4
Organidin	975.5	E858.6	E945.5	E950.4	E962.0	E980.4
Organophosphates	989.3	E863.1	—	E950.6	E962.1	E980.7
Orimune	979.5	E858.8	E949.5	E950.4	E962.0	E980.4
Orinase	962.3	E858.0	E932.3	E950.4	E962.0	E980.4
Orphenadrine	966.4	E855.0	E936.4	E950.4	E962.0	E980.4
Ortal (sodium)	967.0	E851	E937.0	E950.1	E962.0	E980.1
Orthoboric acid	976.0	E858.7	E946.0	E950.4	E962.0	E980.4
ENT agent	976.6	E858.7	E946.6	E950.4	E962.0	E980.4
ophthalmic preparation	976.5	E858.7	E946.5	E950.4	E962.0	E980.4
Orthocaine	968.5	E855.2	E938.5	E950.4	E962.0	E980.4
Ortho-Novum	962.2	E858.0	E932.2	E950.4	E962.0	E980.4
Orthotolidine (reagent)	977.8	E858.8	E947.8	E950.4	E962.0	E980.4
Osmic acid (liquid)	983.1	E864.1	—	E950.7	E962.1	E980.6
fumes	987.8	E869.8	—	E952.8	E962.2	E982.8
Osmotic diuretics	974.4	E858.5	E944.4	E950.4	E962.0	E980.4
Ouabain	972.1	E858.3	E942.1	E950.4	E962.0	E980.4
Ovarian hormones (synthetic substitutes)	962.2	E858.0	E932.2	E950.4	E962.0	E980.4
Ovral	962.2	E858.0	E932.2	E950.4	E962.0	E980.4
Ovulation suppressants	962.2	E858.0	E932.2	E950.4	E962.0	E980.4
Ovulen	962.2	E858.0	E932.2	E950.4	E962.0	E980.4
Oxacillin (sodium)	960.0	E856	E930.0	E950.4	E962.0	E980.4
Oxalic acid	983.1	E864.1	—	E950.7	E962.1	E980.6
Oxanamide	969.5	E853.8	E939.5	E950.3	E962.0	E980.3
Oxandrolone	962.1	E858.0	E932.1	E950.4	E962.0	E980.4
Oxaprozin	965.61	E850.6	E935.6	E950.0	E962.0	E980.0
Oxazepam	969.4	E853.2	E939.4	E950.3	E962.0	E980.3
Oxazolidine derivatives	966.0	E855.0	E936.0	E950.4	E962.0	E980.4
Ox bile extract	973.4	E858.4	E943.4	E950.4	E962.0	E980.4
Oxedrine	971.2	E855.5	E941.2	E950.4	E962.0	E980.4
Oxeladin	975.4	E858.6	E945.4	E950.4	E962.0	E980.4
Oxethazaine NEC	968.5	E855.2	E938.5	E950.4	E962.0	E980.4
Oxidizing agents NEC	983.9	E864.3	—	E950.7	E962.1	E980.6
Oxolinic acid	961.3	E857	E931.3	E950.4	E962.0	E980.4
Oxophenarsine	961.1	E857	E931.1	E950.4	E962.0	E980.4
Oxsoralen	976.3	E858.7	E946.3	E950.4	E962.0	E980.4
Oxtriphylline	976.7	E858.6	E945.7	E950.4	E962.0	E980.4
Oxybuprocaine	968.5	E855.2	E938.5	E950.4	E962.0	E980.4
Oxybutynin	975.1	E858.6	E945.1	E950.4	E962.0	E980.4
Oxycodone	965.09	E850.2	E935.2	E950.0	E962.0	E980.0
Oxygen	987.8	E869.8	—	E952.8	E962.2	E982.8
Oxylone	976.0	E858.7	E946.0	E950.4	E962.0	E980.4
ophthalmic preparation	976.5	E858.7	E946.5	E950.4	E962.0	E980.4
Oxymesterone	962.1	E858.0	E932.1	E950.4	E962.0	E980.4
Oxymetazoline	971.2	E855.5	E941.2	E950.4	E962.0	E980.4
Oxymetholone	962.1	E858.0	E932.1	E950.4	E962.0	E980.4
Oxymorphone	965.09	E850.2	E935.2	E950.0	E962.0	E980.0

Substance	Poisoning	External Cause (E-Code)				
		Accident	Therapeutic Use	Suicide Attempt	Assault	Undetermined
Oxypertine	969.0	E854.0	E939.0	E950.3	E962.0	E980.3
Oxyphenbutazone	965.5	E850.5	E935.5	E950.0	E962.0	E980.0
Oxyphencyclimine	971.1	E855.4	E941.1	E950.4	E962.0	E980.4
Oxyphenisatin	973.1	E858.4	E943.1	E950.4	E962.0	E980.4
Oxyphenonium	971.1	E855.4	E941.1	E950.4	E962.0	E980.4
Oxyquinoline	961.3	E857	E931.3	E950.4	E962.0	E980.4
Oxytetracycline	960.4	E856	E930.4	E950.4	E962.0	E980.4
Oxytocics	975.0	E858.6	E945.0	E950.4	E962.0	E980.4
Oxytocin	975.0	E858.6	E945.0	E950.4	E962.0	E980.4
Ozone	987.8	E869.8	—	E952.8	E962.2	E982.8
PABA	976.3	E858.7	E946.3	E950.4	E962.0	E980.4
Packed red cells	964.7	E858.2	E934.7	E950.4	E962.0	E980.4
Paint NEC	989.89	E861.6	—	E950.9	E962.1	E980.9
cleaner	982.8	E862.9	—	E950.9	E962.1	E980.9
fumes NEC	987.8	E869.8	—	E952.8	E962.1	E982.8
lead (fumes)	984.0	E861.5	—	E950.9	E962.1	E980.9
solvent NEC	982.8	E862.9	—	E950.9	E962.1	E980.9
stripper	982.8	E862.9	—	E950.9	E962.1	E980.9
Palfium	965.09	E850.2	E935.2	E950.0	E962.0	E980.0
Palivizumab	979.9	E858.8	E949.6	E950.4	E962.0	E980.4
Paludrine	961.4	E857	E931.4	E950.4	E962.0	E980.4
PAM	977.2	E855.8	E947.2	E950.4	E962.0	E980.4
Pamaquine (napthoate)	961.4	E857	E931.4	E950.4	E962.0	E980.4
Pamprin	965.1	E850.3	E935.3	E950.0	E962.0	E980.0
Panadol	965.4	E850.4	E935.4	E950.0	E962.0	E980.0
Pancreatic dornase (mucolytic)	963.4	E858.1	E933.4	E950.4	E962.0	E980.4
Pancreatin	973.4	E858.4	E943.4	E950.4	E962.0	E980.4
Pancrelipase	973.4	E858.4	E943.4	E950.4	E962.0	E980.4
Pangamic acid	963.5	E858.1	E933.5	E950.4	E962.0	E980.4
Panthenol	963.5	E858.1	E933.5	E950.4	E962.0	E980.4
topical	976.8	E858.7	E946.8	E950.4	E962.0	E980.4
Pantopaque	977.8	E858.8	E947.8	E950.4	E962.0	E980.4
Pantopon	965.00	E850.2	E935.2	E950.0	E962.0	E980.0
Pantothenic acid	963.5	E858.1	E933.5	E950.4	E962.0	E980.4
Panwarfin	964.2	E858.2	E934.2	E950.4	E962.0	E980.4
Papain	973.4	E858.4	E943.4	E950.4	E962.0	E980.4
Papaverine	972.5	E858.3	E942.5	E950.4	E962.0	E980.4
Para-aminobenzoic acid	976.3	E858.7	E946.3	E950.4	E962.0	E980.4
Para-aminophenol derivatives	965.4	E850.4	E935.4	E950.0	E962.0	E980.0
Para-aminosalicylic acid (derivatives)	961.8	E857	E931.8	E950.4	E962.0	E980.4
Paracetaldehyde (medicinal)	967.2	E852.1	E937.2	E950.2	E962.0	E980.2
Paracetamol	965.4	E850.4	E935.4	E950.0	E962.0	E980.0
Paracodin	965.09	E850.2	E935.2	E950.0	E962.0	E980.0
Paradione	966.0	E855.0	E936.0	E950.4	E962.0	E980.4
Paraffin(s) (wax)	981	E862.3	—	E950.9	E962.1	E980.9
liquid (medicinal)	973.2	E858.4	E943.2	E950.4	E962.0	E980.4
nonmedicinal (oil)	981	E962.1	—	E950.9	E962.1	E980.9
Paraldehyde (medicinal)	967.2	E852.1	E937.2	E950.2	E962.0	E980.2
Paramethadione	966.0	E855.0	E936.0	E950.4	E962.0	E980.4
Paramethasone	962.0	E858.0	E932.0	E950.4	E962.0	E980.4
Paraquat	989.4	E863.5	—	E950.6	E962.1	E980.7
Parasympatholytics	971.1	E855.4	E941.1	E950.4	E962.0	E980.4
Parasympathomimetics	971.0	E855.3	E941.0	E950.4	E962.0	E980.4
Parathion	989.3	E863.1	—	E950.6	E962.1	E980.7
Parathormone	962.6	E858.0	E932.6	E950.4	E962.0	E980.4
Parathyroid (derivatives)	962.6	E858.0	E932.6	E950.4	E962.0	E980.4
Paratyphoid vaccine	978.1	E858.8	E948.1	E950.4	E962.0	E980.4
Paredrine	971.2	E855.5	E941.2	E950.4	E962.0	E980.4
Paregoric	965.00	E850.2	E935.2	E950.0	E962.0	E980.0
Pargyline	972.3	E858.3	E942.3	E950.4	E962.0	E980.4
Paris green	985.1	E866.3	—	E950.8	E962.1	E980.8
insecticide	985.1	E863.4	—	E950.8	E962.1	E980.8

Substance	Poisoning	External Cause (E-Code)				
		Accident	Therapeutic Use	Suicide Attempt	Assault	Undetermined
Parnate	969.0	E854.0	E939.0	E950.3	E962.0	E980.3
Paromomycin	960.8	E856	E930.8	E950.4	E962.0	E980.4
Paroxypropione	963.1	E858.1	E933.1	E950.4	E962.0	E980.4
Parzone	965.09	E850.2	E935.2	E950.0	E962.0	E980.0
PAS	961.8	E857	E931.8	E950.4	E962.0	E980.4
PCBs	981	E862.3	—	E950.9	E962.1	E980.9
PCP (pentachlorophenol)	989.4	E863.6	—	E950.6	E962.1	E980.7
herbicide	989.4	E863.5	—	E950.6	E962.1	E980.7
insecticide	989.4	E863.4	—	E950.6	E962.1	E980.7
phencyclidine	968.3	E855.1	E938.3	E950.4	E962.0	E980.4
Peach kernel oil (emulsion)	973.2	E858.4	E943.2	E950.4	E962.0	E980.4
Peanut oil (emulsion) NEC	973.2	E858.4	E943.2	E950.4	E962.0	E980.4
topical	976.3	E858.7	E946.3	E950.4	E962.0	E980.4
Pearly Gates (morning glory seeds)	969.6	E854.1	E939.6	E950.3	E962.0	E980.3
Pecazine	969.1	E853.0	E939.1	E950.3	E962.0	E980.3
Pecilocin	960.1	E856	E930.1	E950.4	E962.0	E980.4
Pectin (with kaolin) NEC	973.5	E858.4	E943.5	E950.4	E962.0	E980.4
Pelletierine tannate	961.6	E857	E931.6	E950.4	E962.0	E980.4
Pemoline	969.7	E854.2	E939.7	E950.3	E962.0	E980.3
Pempidine	972.3	E858.3	E942.3	E950.4	E962.0	E980.4
Penamecillin	960.0	E856	E930.0	E950.4	E962.0	E980.4
Penethamate hydriodide	960.0	E856	E930.0	E950.4	E962.0	E980.4
Penicillamine	963.8	E858.1	E933.8	E950.4	E962.0	E980.4
Penicillin (any type)	960.0	E856	E930.0	E950.4	E962.0	E980.4
Penicillinase	963.4	E858.1	E933.4	E950.4	E962.0	E980.4
Pentachlorophenol (fungicide)	989.4	E863.6	—	E950.6	E962.1	E980.7
herbicide	989.4	E863.5	—	E950.6	E962.1	E980.7
insecticide	989.4	E863.4	—	E950.6	E962.1	E980.7
Pentaerythritol	972.4	E858.3	E942.4	E950.4	E962.0	E980.4
chloral	967.1	E852.0	E937.1	E950.2	E962.0	E980.2
tetranitrate NEC	972.4	E858.3	E942.4	E950.4	E962.0	E980.4
Pentagastrin	977.8	E858.8	E947.8	E950.4	E962.0	E980.4
Pentalin	982.3	E862.4	—	E950.9	E962.1	E980.9
Pentamethonium (bromide)	972.3	E858.3	E942.3	E950.4	E962.0	E980.4
Pentamidine	961.5	E857	E931.5	E950.4	E962.0	E980.4
Pentanol	980.8	E860.8	—	E950.9	E962.1	E980.9
Pentaquine	961.4	E857	E931.4	E950.4	E962.0	E980.4
Pentazocine	965.8	E850.8	E935.8	E950.0	E962.0	E980.0
Penthienate	971.1	E855.4	E941.1	E950.4	E962.0	E980.4
Pentobarbital, pentobarbitone (sodium)	967.0	E851	E937.0	E950.1	E962.0	E980.1
Pentolinium (tartrate)	972.3	E858.3	E942.3	E950.4	E962.0	E980.4
Pentothal	968.3	E855.1	E938.3	E950.4	E962.0	E980.4
Pentylenetetrazol	970.0	E854.3	E940.0	E950.4	E962.0	E980.4
Pentylsalicylamide	961.8	E857	E931.8	E950.4	E962.0	E980.4
Pepsin	973.4	E858.4	E943.4	E950.4	E962.0	E980.4
Peptavlon	977.8	E858.8	E947.8	E950.4	E962.0	E980.4
Percaine (spinal)	968.7	E855.2	E938.7	E950.4	E962.0	E980.4
topical (surface)	968.5	E855.2	E938.5	E950.4	E962.0	E980.4
Perchloroethylene (vapor)	982.3	E862.4	—	E950.9	E962.1	E980.9
medicinal	961.6	E857	E931.6	E950.4	E962.0	E980.4
Percodan	965.09	E850.2	E935.2	E950.0	E962.0	E980.0
Percogesic	965.09	E850.2	E935.2	E950.0	E962.0	E980.0
Percorten	962.0	E858.0	E932.0	E950.4	E962.0	E980.4
Pergonal	962.4	E858.0	E932.4	E950.4	E962.0	E980.4
Perhexiline	972.4	E858.3	E942.4	E950.4	E962.0	E980.4
Periactin	963.0	E858.1	E933.0	E950.4	E962.0	E980.4
Periclor	967.1	E852.0	E937.1	E950.2	E962.0	E980.2
Pericyazine	969.1	E853.0	E939.1	E950.3	E962.0	E980.3
Peritrate	972.4	E858.3	E942.4	E950.4	E962.0	E980.4
Permanganates NEC	983.9	E864.3	—	E950.7	E962.1	E980.6
potassium (topical)	976.0	E858.7	E946.0	E950.4	E962.0	E980.4

Substance	Poisoning	External Cause (E-Code)				
		Accident	Therapeutic Use	Suicide Attempt	Assault	Undetermined
Pernocton	967.0	E851	E937.0	E950.1	E962.0	E980.1
Pernoston	967.0	E851	E937.0	E950.1	E962.0	E980.1
Peronin(e)	965.09	E850.2	E935.2	E950.0	E962.0	E980.0
Perphenazine	969.1	E853.0	E939.1	E950.3	E962.0	E980.3
Pertofrane	969.0	E854	E939.0	E950.3	E962.0	E980.3
Pertussis	—	—	—	—	—	—
immune serum (human)	964.6	E858.2	E934.6	E950.4	E962.0	E980.4
vaccine (with diphtheria toxoid) (with tetanus toxoid)	978.6	E858.8	E948.6	E950.4	E962.0	E980.4
Peruvian balsam	976.8	E858.7	E946.8	E950.4	E962.0	E980.4
Pesticides (dust) (fumes) (vapor)	989.4	E863.4	—	E950.6	E962.1	E980.7
arsenic	985.1	E863.4	—	E950.8	E962.1	E980.8
chlorinated	989.2	E863.0	—	E950.6	E962.1	E980.7
cyanide	989.0	E863.4	—	E950.6	E962.1	E980.7
kerosene	981	E863.4	—	E950.6	E962.1	E980.7
mixture (of compounds)	989.4	E863.3	—	E950.6	E962.1	E980.7
naphthalene	983.0	E863.4	—	E950.7	E962.1	E980.6
organochlorine (compounds)	989.2	E863.0	—	E950.6	E962.1	E980.7
petroleum (distillate) (products) NEC	981	E863.4	—	E950.6	E962.1	E980.7
specified ingredient NEC	989.4	E863.4	—	E950.6	E962.1	E980.7
strychnine	989.1	E863.4	—	E950.6	E962.1	E980.7
thallium	985.8	E863.7	—	E950.6	E962.1	E980.7
Pethidine (hydrochloride)	965.09	E850.2	E935.2	E950.0	E962.0	E980.0
Petrichloral	967.1	E852.0	E937.1	E950.2	E962.0	E980.2
Petrol	981	E862.1	—	E950.9	E962.1	E980.9
vapor	987.1	E869.8	—	E952.8	E962.2	E982.8
Petrolatum (jelly) (ointment)	976.3	E858.7	E946.3	E950.4	E962.0	E980.4
hydrophilic	976.3	E858.7	E946.3	E950.4	E962.0	E980.4
liquid	973.2	E858.4	E943.2	E950.4	E962.0	E980.4
topical	976.3	E858.7	E946.3	E950.4	E962.0	E980.4
nonmedicinal	981	E862.1	—	E950.9	E962.1	E980.9
Petroleum (cleaners) (fuels) (products) NEC	981	E862.1	—	E950.9	E962.1	E980.9
benzin(e) - *see* Ligroin	—	—	—	—	—	—
ether - *see* Ligroin	—	—	—	—	—	—
jelly - *see* Petrolatum	—	—	—	—	—	—
aphtha - *see* Ligroin	—	—	—	—	—	—
pesticide	981	E863.4	—	E950.6	E962.1	E980.7
solids	981	E862.3	—	E950.9	E962.1	E980.9
solvents	981	E862.0	—	E950.9	E962.1	E980.9
vapor	987.1	E869.8	—	E952.8	E962.2	E982.8
Peyote	969.6	E854.1	E939.6	E950.3	E962.0	E980.3
Phanodorm, phanodorn	967.0	E851	E937.0	E950.1	E962.0	E980.1
Phanquinone, phanquone	961.5	E857	E931.5	E950.4	E962.0	E980.4
Pharmaceutical excipient or adjunct	977.4	E858.8	E947.4	E950.4	E962.0	E980.4
Phenacemide	966.3	E855.0	E936.3	E950.4	E962.0	E980.4
Phenacetin	965.4	E850.4	E935.4	E950.0	E962.0	E980.0
Phenadoxone	965.09	E850.2	E935.2	E950.0	E962.0	E980.0
Phenaglycodol	969.5	E853.8	E939.5	E950.3	E962.0	E980.3
Phenantoin	966.1	E855.0	E936.1	E950.4	E962.0	E980.4
Phenaphthazine reagent	977.8	E858.8	E947.8	E950.4	E962.0	E980.4
Phenazocine	965.09	E850.2	E935.2	E950.0	E962.0	E980.0
Phenazone	965.5	E850.5	E935.5	E950.0	E962.0	E980.0
Phenazopyridine	976.1	E858.7	E946.1	E950.4	E962.0	E980.4
Phenbenicillin	960.0	E856	E930.0	E950.4	E962.0	E980.4
Phenbutrazate	977.0	E858.8	E947.0	E950.4	E962.0	E980.4
Phencyclidine	968.3	E855.1	E938.3	E950.4	E962.0	E980.4
Phendimetrazine	977.0	E858.8	E947.0	E950.4	E962.0	E980.4
Phenelzine	969.0	E854.0	E939.0	E950.3	E962.0	E980.3
Phenergan	967.8	E852.8	E937.8	E950.2	E962.0	E980.2
Phenethicillin (potassium)	960.0	E856	E930.0	E950.4	E962.0	E980.4
Phenetsal	965.1	E850.3	E935.3	E950.0	E962.0	E980.0
Pheneturide	966.3	E855.0	E936.3	E950.4	E962.0	E980.4

Substance	Poisoning	External Cause (E-Code) Accident	Therapeutic Use	Suicide Attempt	Assault	Undetermined
Phenformin	962.3	E858.0	E932.3	E950.4	E962.0	E980.4
Phenglutarimide	971.1	E855.4	E941.1	E950.4	E962.0	E980.4
Phenicarbazide	965.8	E850.8	E935.8	E950.0	E962.0	E980.0
Phenindamine (tartrate)	963.0	E858.1	E933.0	E950.4	E962.0	E980.4
Phenindione	964.2	E858.2	E934.2	E950.4	E962.0	E980.4
Pheniprazine	969.0	E854.0	E939.0	E950.3	E962.0	E980.3
Pheniramine (maleate)	963.0	E858.1	E933.0	E950.4	E962.0	E980.4
Phenmetrazine	977.0	E858.8	E947.0	E950.4	E962.0	E980.4
Phenobal	967.0	E851	E937.0	E950.1	E962.0	E980.1
Phenobarbital	967.0	E851	E937.0	E950.1	E962.0	E980.1
Phenobarbitone	967.0	E851	E937.0	E950.1	E962.0	E980.1
Phenoctide	976.0	E858.7	E946.0	E950.4	E962.0	E980.4
Phenol (derivatives) NEC	983.0	E864.0	—	E950.7	E962.1	E980.6
disinfectant	983.0	E864.0	—	E950.7	E962.1	E980.6
pesticide	989.4	E863.4	—	E950.6	E962.1	E980.7
red	977.8	E858.8	E947.8	E950.4	E962.0	E980.4
Phenolphthalein	973.1	E858.4	E943.1	E950.4	E962.0	E980.4
Phenolsulfonphthalein	977.8	E858.8	E947.8	E950.4	E962.0	E980.4
Phenomorphan	965.09	E850.2	E935.2	E950.0	E962.0	E980.0
Phenonyl	967.0	E851	E937.0	E950.1	E962.0	E980.1
Phenoperidine	965.09	E850.2	E935.2	E950.0	E962.0	E980.0
Phenoquin	974.7	E858.5	E944.7	E950.4	E962.0	E980.4
Phenothiazines (tranquilizers) NEC	969.1	E853.0	E939.1	E950.3	E962.0	E980.3
insecticide	989.3	E863.4	—	E950.6	E962.1	E980.7
Phenoxybenzamine	971.3	E855.6	E941.3	E950.4	E962.0	E980.4
Phenoxymethyl penicillin	960.0	E856	E930.0	E950.4	E962.0	E980.4
Phenprocoumon	964.2	E858.2	E934.2	E950.4	E962.0	E980.4
Phensuximide	966.2	E855.0	E936.2	E950.4	E962.0	E980.4
Phentermine	977.0	E858.8	E947.0	E950.4	E962.0	E980.4
Phentolamine	971.3	E855.6	E941.3	E950.4	E962.0	E980.4
Phenyl	—	—	—	—	—	—
butazone	965.5	E850.5	E935.5	E950.0	E962.0	E980.0
enediamine	983.0	E864.0	—	E950.7	E962.1	E980.6
hydrazine	983.0	E864.0	—	E950.7	E962.1	E980.6
antineoplastic	963.1	E858.1	E933.1	E950.4	E962.0	E980.4
mercuric compounds - *see* Mercury	—	—	—	—	—	—
salicylate	976.3	E858.7	E946.3	E950.4	E962.0	E980.4
Phenylephrine	971.2	E855.5	E941.2	E950.4	E962.0	E980.4
Phenylethylbiguanide	962.3	E858.0	E932.3	E950.4	E962.0	E980.4
Phenylpropanolamine	971.2	E855.5	E941.2	E950.4	E962.0	E980.4
Phenylsulfthion	989.3	E863.1	—	E950.6	E962.1	E980.7
Phenyramidol, phenyramidon	965.7	E850.7	E935.7	E950.0	E962.0	E980.0
Phenytoin	966.1	E855.0	E936.1	E950.4	E962.0	E980.4
pHisoHex	976.2	E858.7	E946.2	E950.4	E962.0	E980.4
Pholcodine	965.09	E850.2	E935.2	E950.0	E962.0	E980.0
Phorate	989.3	E863.1	—	E950.6	E962.1	E980.7
Phosdrin	989.3	E863.1	—	E950.6	E962.1	E980.7
Phosgene (gas)	987.8	E869.8	—	E952.8	E962.2	E982.8
Phosphate (tricresyl)	989.89	E866.8	—	E950.9	E962.1	E980.9
organic	989.3	E863.1	—	E950.6	E962.1	E980.7
solvent	982.8	E862.4	—	E950.9	E962.1	E980.9
Phosphine	987.8	E869.8	—	E952.8	E962.2	E982.8
fumigant	987.8	E863.8	—	E950.6	E962.2	E980.7
Phospholine	971.0	E855.3	E941.0	E950.4	E962.0	E980.4
Phosphoric acid	983.1	E864.1	—	E950.7	E962.1	E980.6
Phosphorus (compounds) NEC	983.9	E864.3	—	E950.7	E962.1	E980.6
rodenticide	983.9	E863.7	—	E950.7	E962.1	E980.6
Phthalimidoglutarimide	967.8	E852.8	E937.8	E950.2	E962.0	E980.2
Phthalylsulfathiazole	961.0	E857	E931.0	E950.4	E962.0	E980.4
Phylloquinone	964.3	E858.2	E934.3	E950.4	E962.0	E980.4
Physeptone	965.02	E850.1	E935.1	E950.0	E962.0	E980.0

Substance	Poisoning	External Cause (E-Code)				
		Accident	Therapeutic Use	Suicide Attempt	Assault	Undetermined
Physostigma venenosum	988.2	E865.4	—	E950.9	E962.1	E980.9
Physostigmine	971.0	E855.3	E941.0	E950.4	E962.0	E980.4
Phytolacca decandra	988.2	E865.4	—	E950.9	E962.1	E980.9
Phytomenadione	964.3	E858.2	E934.3	E950.4	E962.0	E980.4
Phytonadione	964.3	E858.2	E934.3	E950.4	E962.0	E980.4
Picric (acid)	983.0	E864.0	—	E950.7	E962.1	E980.6
Picrotoxin	970.0	E854.3	E940.0	E950.4	E962.0	E980.4
Pilocarpine	971.0	E855.3	E941.0	E950.4	E962.0	E980.4
Pilocarpus (jaborandi) extract	971.0	E855.3	E941.0	E950.4	E962.0	E980.4
Pimaricin	960.1	E856	E930.1	E950.4	E962.0	E980.4
Piminodine	965.09	E850.2	E935.2	E950.0	E962.0	E980.0
Pine oil, pinesol (disinfectant)	983.9	E861.4	—	E950.7	E962.1	E980.6
Pinkroot	961.6	E857	E931.6	E950.4	E962.0	E980.4
Pipadone	965.09	E850.2	E935.2	E950.0	E962.0	E980.0
Pipamazine	963.0	E858.1	E933.0	E950.4	E962.0	E980.4
Pipazethate	975.4	E858.6	E945.4	E950.4	E962.0	E980.4
Pipenzolate	971.1	E855.4	E941.1	E950.4	E962.0	E980.4
Piperacetazine	969.1	E853.0	E939.1	E950.3	E962.0	E980.3
Piperazine NEC	961.6	E857	E931.6	E950.4	E962.0	E980.4
estrone sulfate	962.2	E858.0	E932.2	E950.4	E962.0	E980.4
Piper cubeba	988.2	E865.4	—	E950.9	E962.1	E980.9
Piperidione	975.4	E858.6	E945.4	E950.4	E962.0	E980.4
Piperidolate	971.1	E855.4	E941.1	E950.4	E962.0	E980.4
Piperocaine	968.9	E855.2	E938.9	E950.4	E962.0	E980.4
infiltration (subcutaneous)	968.5	E855.2	E938.5	E950.4	E962.0	E980.4
nerve block (peripheral) (plexus)	968.6	E855.2	E938.6	E950.4	E962.0	E980.4
topical (surface)	968.5	E855.2	E938.5	E950.4	E962.0	E980.4
Pipobroman	963.1	E858.1	E933.1	E950.4	E962.0	E980.4
Pipradrol	970.8	E854.3	E940.8	E950.4	E962.0	E980.4
Piscidia (bark) (erythrina)	965.7	E850.7	E935.7	E950.0	E962.0	E980.0
Pitch	983.0	E864.0	—	E950.7	E962.1	E980.6
Pitkin's solution	968.7	E855.2	E938.7	E950.4	E962.0	E980.4
Pitocin	975.0	E858.6	E945.0	E950.4	E962.0	E980.4
Pitressin (tannate)	962.5	E858.0	E932.5	E950.4	E962.0	E980.4
Pituitary extracts (posterior)	962.5	E858.0	E932.5	E950.4	E962.0	E980.4
anterior	962.4	E858.0	E932.4	E950.4	E962.0	E980.4
Pituitrin	962.5	E858.0	E932.5	E950.4	E962.0	E980.4
Placental extract	962.9	E858.0	E932.9	E950.4	E962.0	E980.4
Placidyl	967.8	E852.8	E937.8	E950.2	E962.0	E980.2
Plague vaccine	978.3	E858.8	E948.3	E950.4	E962.0	E980.4
Plant foods or fertilizers NEC	989.89	E866.5	—	E950.9	E962.1	E980.9
mixed with herbicides	989.4	E863.5	—	E950.6	E962.1	E930.7
Plants, noxious, used as food	988.2	E865.9	—	E950.9	E962.1	E980.9
berries and seeds	988.2	E865.3	—	E950.9	E962.1	E980.9
specified type NEC	988.2	E865.4	—	E950.9	E962.1	E980.9
Plasma (blood)	964.7	E858.2	E934.7	E950.4	E962.0	E980.4
expanders	964.8	E858.2	E934.8	E950.4	E962.0	E980.4
Plasmanate	964.7	E858.2	E934.7	E950.4	E962.0	E980.4
Plegicil	969.1	E853.0	E939.1	E950.3	E962.0	E980.3
Podophyllin	976.4	E858.7	E946.4	E950.4	E962.0	E980.4
Podophyllum resin	976.4	E858.7	E946.4	E950.4	E962.0	E980.4
Poison NEC	989.9	E866.9	—	E950.9	E962.1	E980.9
Poisonous berries	988.2	E865.3	—	E950.9	E962.1	E980.9
Pokeweed (any part)	988.2	E865.4	—	E950.9	E962.1	E980.9
Poldine	971.1	E855.4	E941.1	E950.4	E962.0	E980.4
Poliomyelitis vaccine	979.5	E858.8	E949.5	E950.4	E962.0	E980.4
Poliovirus vaccine	979.5	E858.8	E949.5	E950.4	E962.0	E980.4
Polish (car) (floor) (furniture) (metal) (silver)	989.89	E861.2	—	E950.9	E962.1	E980.9
abrasive	989.89	E861.3	—	E950.9	E962.1	E980.9
porcelain	989.89	E861.3	—	E950.9	E962.1	E980.9
Poloxalkol	973.2	E858.4	E943.2	E950.4	E962.0	E980.4

Substance	Poisoning	External Cause (E-Code) Accident	Therapeutic Use	Suicide Attempt	Assault	Undetermined
Polyaminostyrene resins	974.5	E858.5	E944.5	E950.4	E962.0	E980.4
Polychlorinated biphenyl - *see* PCBs	—	—	—	—	—	—
Polycycline	960.4	E856	E930.4	E950.4	E962.0	E980.4
Polyester resin hardener	982.8	E862.4	—	E950.9	E962.1	E980.9
fumes	987.8	E869.8	—	E952.8	E962.2	E982.8
Polyestradiol (phosphate)	962.2	E858.0	E932.2	E950.4	E962.0	E980.4
Polyethanolamine alkyl sulfate	976.2	E858.7	E946.2	E950.4	E962.0	E980.4
Polyethylene glycol	976.3	E858.7	E946.3	E950.4	E962.0	E980.4
Polyferose	964.0	E858.2	E934.0	E950.4	E962.0	E980.4
Polymyxin B	960.8	E856	E930.8	E950.4	E962.0	E980.4
ENT agent	976.6	E858.7	E946.6	E950.4	E962.0	E980.4
ophthalmic preparation	976.5	E858.7	E946.5	E950.4	E962.0	E980.4
topical NEC	976.0	E858.7	E946.0	E950.4	E962.0	E980.4
Polynoxylin(e)	976.0	E858.7	E946.0	E950.4	E962.0	E980.4
Polyoxymethyleneurea	976.0	E858.7	E946.0	E950.4	E962.0	E980.4
Polytetrafluoroethylene (inhaled)	987.8	E869.8	—	E952.8	E962.2	E982.8
Polythiazide	974.3	E858.5	E944.3	E950.4	E962.0	E980.4
Polyvinylpyrrolidone	964.8	E858.2	E934.8	E950.4	E962.0	E980.4
Pontocaine (hydrochloride) (infiltration) (topical)	968.5	E855.2	E938.5	E950.4	E962.0	E980.4
nerve block (peripheral) (plexus)	968.6	E855.2	E938.6	E950.4	E962.0	E980.4
spinal	968.7	E855.2	E938.7	E950.4	E962.0	E980.4
Pot	969.6	E854.1	E939.6	E950.3	E962.0	E980.3
Potash (caustic)	983.2	E864.2	—	E950.7	E962.1	E980.6
Potassic saline injection (lactated)	974.5	E858.5	E944.5	E950.4	E962.0	E980.4
Potassium (salts) NEC	974.5	E858.5	E944.5	E950.4	E962.0	E980.4
aminosalicylate	961.8	E857	E931.8	E950.4	E962.0	E980.4
arsenite (solution)	985.1	E866.3	—	E950.8	E962.1	E980.8
bichromate	983.9	E864.3	—	E950.7	E962.1	E980.6
bisulfate	983.9	E864.3	—	E950.7	E962.1	E980.6
bromide (medicinal) NEC	967.3	E852.2	E937.3	E950.2	E962.0	E980.2
carbonate	983.2	E864.2	—	E950.7	E962.1	E980.6
chlorate NEC	983.9	E864.3	—	E950.7	E962.1	E980.6
cyanide - *see* Cyanide	—	—	—	—	—	—
hydroxide	983.2	E864.2	—	E950.7	E962.1	E980.6
iodide (expectorant) NEC	975.5	E858.6	E945.5	E950.4	E962.0	E980.4
nitrate	989.89	E866.8	—	E950.9	E962.1	E980.9
oxalate	983.9	E864.3	—	E950.7	E962.1	E980.6
perchlorate NEC	977.8	E858.8	E947.8	E950.4	E962.0	E980.4
antithyroid	962.8	E858.0	E932.8	E950.4	E962.0	E980.4
permanganate	976.0	E858.7	E946.0	E950.4	E962.0	E980.4
nonmedicinal	983.9	E864.3	—	E950.7	E962.1	E980.6
Povidone-iodine (anti-infective) NEC	976.0	E858.7	E946.0	E950.4	E962.0	E980.4
Practolol	972.0	E858.3	E942.0	E950.4	E962.0	E980.4
Pralidoxime (chloride)	977.2	E858.8	E947.2	E950.4	E962.0	E980.4
Pramoxine	968.5	E855.2	E938.5	E950.4	E962.0	E980.4
Prazosin	972.6	E858.3	E942.6	E950.4	E962.0	E980.4
Prednisolone	962.0	E858.0	E932.0	E950.4	E962.0	E980.4
ENT agent	976.6	E858.7	E946.6	E950.4	E962.0	E980.4
ophthalmic preparation	976.5	E858.7	E946.5	E950.4	E962.0	E980.4
topical NEC	976.0	E858.7	E946.0	E950.4	E962.0	E980.4
Prednisone	962.0	E858.0	E932.0	E950.4	E962.0	E980.4
Pregnanediol	962.2	E858.0	E932.2	E950.4	E962.0	E990.4
Pregneninolone	962.2	E858.0	E932.2	E950.4	E962.0	E980.4
Preludin	977.0	E858.8	E947.0	E950.4	E962.0	E980.4
Premarin	962.2	E858.0	E932.2	E950.4	E962.0	E980.4
Prenylamine	972.4	E858.3	E942.4	E950.4	E962.0	E980.4
Preparation H	976.8	E858.7	E946.8	E950.4	E962.0	E980.4
Preservatives	989.89	E866.8	—	E950.9	E962.1	E980.9
Pride of China	988.2	E865.3	—	E950.9	E962.1	E980.9
Prilocaine	968.9	E855.2	E938.9	E950.4	E962.0	E980.4
infiltration (subcutaneous)	968.5	E855.2	E938.5	E950.4	E962.0	E980.4
nerve block (peripheral) (plexus)	968.6	E855.2	E938.6	E950.4	E962.0	E980.4

Substance	Poisoning	External Cause (E-Code) Accident	Therapeutic Use	Suicide Attempt	Assault	Undetermined
Primaquine	961.4	E857	E931.4	E950.4	E962.0	E980.4
Primidone	966.3	E855.0	E936.3	E950.4	E962.0	E980.4
Primula (veris)	988.2	E865.4	—	E950.9	E962.1	E980.9
Prinodol	965.09	E850.2	E935.2	E950.0	E962.0	E980.0
Priscol, Priscoline	971.3	E855.6	E941.3	E950.4	E962.0	E980.4
Privet	988.2	E865.4	—	E950.9	E962.1	E980.9
Privine	971.2	E855.5	E941.2	E950.4	E962.0	E980.4
Pro-Banthine	971.1	E855.4	E941.1	E950.4	E962.0	E980.4
Probarbital	967.0	E851	E937.0	E950.1	E962.0	E980.1
Probenecid	974.7	E858.5	E944.7	E950.4	E962.0	E990.4
Procainamide (hydrochloride)	972.0	E858.3	E942.0	E950.4	E962.0	E980.4
Procaine (hydrochloride) (infiltration) (topical)	968.5	E855.2	E938.5	E950.4	E962.0	E980.4
nerve block (periphreal) (plexus)	968.6	E855.2	E938.6	E950.4	E962.0	E980.4
penicillin G	960.0	E856	E930.0	E950.4	E962.0	E980.4
spinal	968.7	E855.2	E938.7	E950.4	E962.0	E980.4
Procalmidol	969.5	E853.8	E939.5	E950.3	E962.0	E980.3
Procarbazine	963.1	E858.1	E933.1	E950.4	E962.0	E980.4
Prochlorperazine	969.1	E853.0	E939.1	E950.3	E962.0	E980.3
Procyclidine	966.4	E855.0	E936.4	E950.4	E962.0	E980.4
Producer gas	986	E868.8	—	E952.1	E962.2	E982.1
Profenamine	966.4	E855.0	E936.4	E950.4	E962.0	E980.4
Profenil	975.1	E858.6	E945.1	E950.4	E962.0	E980.4
Progesterones	962.2	E858.0	E932.2	E950.4	E962.0	E980.4
Progestin	962.2	E858.0	E932.2	E950.4	E962.0	E980.4
Progestogens (with estrogens)	962.2	E858.0	E932.2	E950.4	E962.0	E980.4
Progestone	962.2	E858.0	E932.2	E950.4	E962.0	E980.4
Proguanil	961.4	E857	E931.4	E950.4	E962.0	E980.4
Prolactin	962.4	E858.0	E932.4	E950.4	E962.0	E980.4
Proloid	962.7	E858.0	E932.7	E950.4	E962.0	E980.4
Proluton	962.2	E858.0	E932.2	E950.4	E962.0	E980.4
Promacetin	961.8	E857	E931.8	E950.4	E962.0	E980.4
Promazine	969.1	E853.0	E939.1	E950.3	E962.0	E980.3
Promedrol	965.09	E850.2	E935.2	E950.0	E962.0	E980.0
Promethazine	967.8	E852.8	E937.8	E950.2	E962.0	E980.2
Promine	961.8	E857	E931.8	E950.4	E962.0	E980.4
Pronestyl (hydrochloride)	972.0	E858.3	E942.0	E950.4	E962.0	E980.4
Pronetalol, pronethalol	972.0	E858.3	E942.0	E950.4	E962.0	E980.4
Prontosil	961.0	E857	E931.0	E950.4	E962.0	E980.4
Propamidine isethionate	961.5	E857	E931.5	E950.4	E962.0	E980.4
Propanal (medicinal)	967.8	E852.8	E937.8	E950.2	E962.0	E980.2
Propane (gas) (distributed in mobile container)	987.0	E868.0	—	E951.1	E962.2	E981.1
distributed through pipes	987.0	E867	—	E951.0	E962.2	E981.0
incomplete combustion of - *see* Carbon monoxide, Propane	—	—	—	—	—	—
Propanidid	968.3	E855.1	E938.3	E950.4	E962.0	E980.4
Propanol	980.3	E860.4	—	E950.9	E962.1	E980.9
Propantheline	971.1	E855.4	E941.1	E950.4	E962.0	E980.4
Proparacaine	968.5	E855.2	E938.5	E950.4	E962.0	E980.4
Propatyl nitrate	972.4	E858.3	E942.4	E950.4	E962.0	E980.4
Propicillin	960.0	E856	E930.0	E950.4	E962.0	E980.4
Propiolactone (vapor)	987.8	E869.8	—	E952.8	E962.2	E982.8
Propiomazine	967.8	E852.8	E937.8	E950.2	E962.0	E980.2
Propionaldehyde (medicinal)	967.8	E852.8	E937.8	E950.2	E962.0	E980.2
Propionate compound	976.0	E858.7	E946.0	E950.4	E962.0	E980.4
Propion gel	976.0	E858.7	E946.0	E950.4	E962.0	E980.4
Propitocaine	968.9	E855.2	E938.9	E950.4	E962.0	E980.4
infiltration (subcutaneous)	968.5	E855.2	E938.5	E950.4	E962.0	E980.4
nerve block (peripheral) (plexus)	968.6	E855.2	E938.6	E950.4	E962.0	E980.4
Propoxur	989.3	E863.2	—	E950.6	E962.1	E980.7
Propoxycaine	968.9	E855.2	E938.9	E950.4	E962.0	E980.4
infiltration (subcutaneous)	968.5	E855.2	E938.5	E950.4	E962.0	E980.4
nerve block (peripheral) (plexus)	968.6	E855.2	E938.6	E950.4	E962.0	E980.4
topical (surface)	968.5	E855.2	E938.5	E950.4	E962.0	E980.4

Substance	Poisoning	External Cause (E-Code) Accident	Therapeutic Use	Suicide Attempt	Assault	Undetermined
Propoxyphene (hydrochloride)	965.8	E850.8	E935.8	E950.0	E962.0	E980.0
Propranolol	972.0	E858.3	E942.0	E950.4	E962.0	E980.4
Propyl	—	—	—	—	—	—
alcohol	980.3	E860.4	—	E950.9	E962.1	E980.9
carbinol	980.3	E860.4	—	E950.9	E962.1	E980.9
hexadrine	971.2	E855.5	E941.2	E950.4	E962.0	E980.4
iodone	977.8	E858.8	E947.8	E950.4	E962.0	E980.4
thiouracil	962.8	E858.0	E932.8	E950.4	E962.0	E980.4
Propylene	987.1	E869.8	—	E952.8	E962.2	E982.8
Propylparaben (ophthalmic)	976.5	E858.7	E946.5	E950.4	E962.0	E980.4
Proscillaridin	972.1	E858.3	E942.1	E950.4	E962.0	E980.4
Prostaglandins	975.0	E858.6	E945.0	E950.4	E962.0	E980.4
Prostigmin	971.0	E855.3	E941.0	E950.4	E962.0	E980.4
Protamine (sulfate)	964.5	E858.2	E934.5	E950.4	E962.0	E980.4
zinc insulin	962.3	E858.0	E932.3	E950.4	E962.0	E980.4
Protectants (topical)	976.3	E858.7	E946.3	E950.4	E962.0	E980.4
Protein hydrolysate	974.5	E858.5	E944.5	E950.4	E962.0	E980.4
Prothiaden - *see* Dothiepin hydrochloride	—	—	—	—	—	—
Prothionamide	961.8	E857	E931.8	E950.4	E962.0	E980.4
Prothipendyl	969.5	E853.8	E939.5	E950.3	E962.0	E980.3
Protokylol	971.2	E855.5	E941.2	E950.4	E962.0	E980.4
Protopam	977.2	E858.8	E947.2	E950.4	E962.0	E980.4
Protoveratrine(s) (A) (B)	972.6	E858.3	E942.6	E950.4	E962.0	E980.4
Protriptyline	969.0	E854.0	E939.0	E950.3	E962.0	E980.3
Provera	962.2	E858.0	E932.2	E950.4	E962.0	E980.4
Provitamin A	963.5	E858.1	E933.5	E950.4	E962.0	E980.4
Proxymetacaine	968.5	E855.2	E938.5	E950.4	E962.0	E980.4
Proxyphylline	975.1	E858.6	E945.1	E950.4	E962.0	E980.4
Prozac - *see* Fluoxetine hydrochloride	—	—	—	—	—	—
Prunus	—	—	—	—	—	—
laurocerasus	988.2	E865.4	—	E950.9	E962.1	E980.9
virginiana	988.2	E865.4	—	E950.9	E962.1	E980.9
Prussic acid	989.0	E866.8	—	E950.9	E962.1	E980.9
vapor	987.7	E869.8	—	E952.8	E962.2	E982.8
Pseudoephedrine	971.2	E855.5	E941.2	E950.4	E962.0	E980.4
Psilocin	969.6	E854.1	E939.6	E950.3	E962.0	E980.3
Psilocybin	969.6	E854.1	E939.6	E950.3	E962.0	E980.3
PSP	977.8	E858.8	E947.8	E950.4	E962.0	E980.4
Psychedelic agents	969.6	E854.1	E939.6	E950.3	E962.0	E980.3
Psychodysleptics	969.6	E854.1	E939.6	E950.3	E962.0	E980.3
Psychostimulants	969.7	E854.2	E939.7	E950.3	E962.0	E980.3
Psychotherapeutic agents	969.9	E855.9	E939.9	E950.3	E962.0	E980.3
antidepressants	969.0	E854.0	E939.0	E950.3	E962.0	E980.3
specified NEC	969.8	E855.8	E939.8	E950.3	E962.0	E980.3
tranquilizers NEC	969.5	E853.9	E939.5	E950.3	E962.0	E980.3
Psychotomimetic agents	969.6	E854.1	E939.6	E950.3	E962.0	E980.3
Psychotropic agents	969.9	E854.8	E939.9	E950.3	E962.0	E980.3
specified NEC	969.8	E854.8	E939.8	E950.3	E962.0	E980.3
Psyllium	973.3	E858.4	E943.3	E950.4	E962.0	E980.4
Pteroylglutamic acid	964.1	E858.2	E934.1	E950.4	E962.0	E980.4
Pteroyltriglutamate	963.1	E858.1	E933.1	E950.4	E962.0	E980.4
PTFE	987.8	E869.8	—	E952.8	E962.2	E982.8
Pulsatilla	988.2	E865.4	—	E950.9	E962.1	E980.9
Purex (bleach)	983.9	E864.3	—	E950.7	E962.1	E980.6
Purine diuretics	974.1	E858.5	E944.1	E950.4	E962.0	E980.4
Purinethol	963.1	E858.1	E933.1	E950.4	E962.0	E980.4
PVP	964.8	E858.2	E934.8	E950.4	E962.0	E980.4
Pyrabital	965.7	E850.7	E935.7	E950.0	E962.0	E980.0
Pyramidon	965.5	E850.5	E935.5	E950.0	E962.0	E980.0
Pyrantel (pamoate)	961.6	E857	E931.6	E950.4	E962.0	E980.4
Pyrathiazine	963.0	E858.1	E933.0	E950.4	E962.0	E980.4

Substance	Poisoning	External Cause (E-Code) Accident	Therapeutic Use	Suicide Attempt	Assault	Undetermined
Pyrazinamide	961.8	E857	E931.8	E950.4	E962.0	E980.4
Pyrazinoic acid (amide)	961.8	E857	E931.8	E950.4	E962.0	E980.4
Pyrazole (derivatives)	965.5	E850.5	E935.5	E950.0	E962.0	E980.0
Pyrazolone (analgesics)	965.5	E850.5	E935.5	E950.0	E962.0	E980.0
Pyrethrins, pyrethrum	989.4	E863.4	—	E950.6	E962.1	E980.7
Pyribenzamine	963.0	E858.1	E933.0	E950.4	E962.0	E980.4
Pyridine (liquid) (vapor)	982.0	E862.4	—	E950.9	E962.1	E980.9
aldoxime chloride	977.2	E858.8	E947.2	E950.4	E962.0	E980.4
Pyridium	976.1	E858.7	E946.1	E950.4	E962.0	E980.4
Pyridostigmine	971.0	E855.3	E941.0	E950.4	E962.0	E980.4
Pyridoxine	963.5	E858.1	E933.5	E950.4	E962.0	E980.4
Pyrilamine	963.0	E858.1	E933.0	E950.4	E962.0	E980.4
Pyrimethamine	961.4	E857	E931.4	E950.4	E962.0	E980.4
Pyrogallic acid	983.0	E864.0	—	E950.7	E962.1	E980.6
Pyroxylin	976.3	E858.7	E946.3	E950.4	E962.0	E980.4
Pyrrobutamine	963.0	E858.1	E933.0	E950.4	E962.0	E980.4
Pyrrocitine	968.5	E855.2	E938.5	E950.4	E962.0	E980.4
Pyrvinium (pamoate)	961.6	E857	E931.6	E950.4	E962.0	E980.4
PZI	962.3	E858.0	E932.3	E950.4	E962.0	E980.4
Quaalude	967.4	E852.3	E937.4	E950.2	E962.0	E980.2
Quaternary ammonium derivatives	971.1	E855.4	E941.1	E950.4	E962.0	E980.4
Quicklime	983.2	E864.2	—	E950.7	E962.1	E980.6
Quinacrine	961.3	E857	E931.3	E950.4	E962.0	E980.4
Quinaglute	972.0	E858.3	E942.0	E950.4	E962.0	E980.4
Quinalbarbitone	967.0	E851	E937.0	E950.1	E962.0	E980.1
Quinestradiol	962.2	E858.0	E932.2	E950.4	E962.0	E980.4
Quinethazone	974.3	E858.5	E944.3	E950.4	E962.0	E980.4
Quinidine (gluconate) (polygalacturonate) (salts) (sulfate)	972.0	E858.3	E942.0	E950.4	E962.0	E980.4
Quinine	961.4	E857	E931.4	E950.4	E962.0	E980.4
Quiniobine	961.3	E857	E931.3	E950.4	E962.0	E980.4
Quinolines	961.3	E857	E931.3	E950.4	E962.0	E980.4
Quotane	968.5	E855.2	E938.5	E950.4	E962.0	E980.4
Rabies	—	—	—	—	—	—
immune globulin (human)	964.6	E858.2	E934.6	E950.4	E962.0	E980.4
vaccine	979.1	E858.8	E949.1	E950.4	E962.0	E980.4
Racemoramide	965.09	E850.2	E935.2	E950.0	E962.0	E980.0
Racemorphan	965.09	E850.2	E935.2	E950.0	E962.0	E980.0
Radiator alcohol	980.1	E860.2	—	E950.9	E962.1	E980.9
Radio-opaque (drugs) (materials)	977.8	E858.8	E947.8	E950.4	E962.0	E980.4
Ranunculus	988.2	E865.4	—	E950.9	E962.1	E980.9
Rat poison	989.4	E863.7	—	E950.6	E962.1	E980.7
Rattlesnake (venom)	989.5	E905.0	—	E950.9	E962.1	E980.9
Raudixin	972.6	E858.3	E942.6	E950.4	E962.0	E980.4
Rautensin	972.6	E858.3	E942.6	E950.4	E962.0	E980.4
Rautina	972.6	E858.3	E942.6	E950.4	E962.0	E980.4
Rautotal	972.6	E858.3	E942.6	E950.4	E962.0	E980.4
Rauwiloid	972.6	E858.3	E942.6	E950.4	E962.0	E980.4
Rauwoldin	972.6	E858.3	E942.6	E950.4	E962.0	E980.4
Rauwolfia (alkaloids)	972.6	E858.3	E942.6	E950.4	E962.0	E980.4
Realgar	985.1	E866.3	—	E950.8	E962.1	E980.8
Red cells, packed	964.7	E858.2	E934.7	E950.4	E962.0	E980.4
Reducing agents, industrial NEC	983.9	E864.3	—	E950.7	E962.1	E980.6
Refrigerant gas (freon)	987.4	E869.2	—	E952.8	E962.2	E982.8
not freon	987.9	E869.9	—	E952.9	E962.2	E982.9
Regroton	974.4	E858.5	E944.4	E950.4	E962.0	E980.4
Rela	968.0	E855.1	E938.0	E950.4	E962.0	E980.4
Relaxants, skeletal muscle (autonomic)	975.2	E858.6	E945.2	E950.4	E962.0	E980.4
central nervous system	968.0	E855.1	E938.0	E950.4	E962.0	E980.4
Renese	974.3	E858.5	E944.3	E950.4	E962.0	E980.4
Renografin	977.8	E858.8	E947.8	E950.4	E962.0	E980.4
Replacement solutions	974.5	E858.5	E944.5	E950.4	E962.0	E980.4

Substance	Poisoning	External Cause (E-Code) Accident	Therapeutic Use	Suicide Attempt	Assault	Undetermined
Rescinnamine	972.6	E858.3	E942.6	E950.4	E962.0	E980.4
Reserpine	972.6	E858.3	E942.6	E950.4	E962.0	E980.4
Resorcin, resorcinol	976.4	E858.7	E946.4	E950.4	E962.0	E980.4
Respaire	975.5	E858.6	E945.5	E950.4	E962.0	E980.4
Respiratory agents NEC	975.8	E858.6	E945.8	E950.4	E962.0	E980.4
Retinoic acid	976.8	E858.7	E946.8	E950.4	E962.0	E980.4
Retinol	963.5	E858.1	E933.5	E950.4	E962.0	E980.4
Rh (D) immune globulin (human)	964.6	E858.2	E934.6	E950.4	E962.0	E980.4
Rhodine	965.1	E850.3	E935.3	E950.0	E962.0	E980.0
RhoGAM	964.6	E858.2	E934.6	E950.4	E962.0	E980.4
Riboflavin	963.5	E858.1	E933.5	E950.4	E962.0	E980.4
Ricin	989.89	E866.8	—	E950.9	E962.1	E980.9
Ricinus communis	988.2	E865.3	—	E950.9	E962.1	E980.9
Rickettsial vaccine NEC	979.6	E858.8	E949.6	E950.4	E962.0	E980.4
with viral and bacterial vaccine	979.7	E858.8	E949.7	E950.4	E962.0	E980.4
Rifampin	960.6	E856	E930.6	E950.4	E962.0	E980.4
Rimifon	961.8	E857	E931.8	E950.4	E962.0	E980.4
Ringer's injection (lactated)	974.5	E858.5	E944.5	E950.4	E962.0	E980.4
Ristocetin	960.8	E856	E930.8	E950.4	E962.0	E980.4
Ritalin	969.7	E854.2	E939.7	E950.3	E962.0	E980.3
Roach killers - *see* Pesticides	—	—	—	—	—	—
Rocky Mountain spotted fever vaccine	979.6	E858.8	E949.6	E950.4	E962.0	E980.4
Rodenticides	989.4	E863.7	—	E950.6	E962.1	E980.7
Rohypnol	969.4	E853.2	E939.4	E950.3	E962.0	E980.3
Rolaids	973.0	E858.4	E943.0	E950.4	E962.0	E980.4
Rolitetracycline	960.4	E856	E930.4	E950.4	E962.0	E980.4
Romilar	975.4	E858.6	E945.4	E950.4	E962.0	E980.4
Rose water ointment	976.3	E858.7	E946.3	E950.4	E962.0	E980.4
Rotenone	989.4	E863.7	—	E950.6	E962.1	E980.7
Rotoxamine	963.0	E858.1	E933.0	E950.4	E962.0	E980.4
Rough-on-rats	989.4	E863.7	—	E950.6	E962.1	E980.7
RU486	962.9	E858.0	E932.9	E950.4	E962.0	E980.4
Rubbing alcohol	980.2	E860.3	—	E950.9	E962.1	E980.9
Rubella virus vaccine	979.4	E858.8	E949.4	E950.4	E962.0	E980.4
Rubelogen	979.4	E858.8	E949.4	E950.4	E962.0	E980.4
Rubeovax	979.4	E858.8	E949.4	E950.4	E962.0	E980.4
Rubidomycin	960.7	E856	E930.7	E950.4	E962.0	E980.4
Rue	988.2	E865.4	—	E950.9	E962.1	E980.9
Ruta	988.2	E865.4	—	E950.9	E962.1	E980.9
Sabadilla (medicinal)	976.0	E858.7	E946.0	E950.4	E962.0	E980.4
pesticide	989.4	E863.4	—	E950.6	E962.1	E980.7
Sabin oral vaccine	979.5	E858.8	E949.5	E950.4	E962.0	E980.4
Saccharated iron oxide	964.0	E858.2	E934.0	E950.4	E962.0	E980.4
Saccharin	974.5	E858.5	E944.5	E950.4	E962.0	E980.4
Safflower oil	972.2	E858.3	E942.2	E950.4	E962.0	E980.4
Salbutamol sulfate	975.7	E858.6	E945.7	E950.4	E962.0	E980.4
Salicylamide	965.1	E850.3	E935.3	E950.0	E962.0	E980.0
Salicylate(s)	965.1	E850.3	E935.3	E950.0	E962.0	E980.0
methyl	976.3	E858.7	E946.3	E950.4	E962.0	E980.4
theobromine calcium	974.1	E858.5	E944.1	E950.4	E962.0	E980.4
Salicylazosulfapyridine	961.0	E857	E931.0	E950.4	E962.0	E980.4
Salicylhydroxamic acid	976.0	E858.7	E946.0	E950.4	E962.0	E980.4
Salicylic acid (keratolytic) NEC	976.4	E858.7	E946.4	E950.4	E962.0	E980.4
congeners	965.1	E850.3	E935.3	E950.0	E962.0	E980.0
salts	965.1	E850.3	E935.3	E950.0	E962.0	E980.0
Saliniazid	961.8	E857	E931.8	E950.4	E962.0	E980.4
Salol	976.3	E858.7	E946.3	E950.4	E962.0	E980.4
Salt (substitute) NEC	974.5	E858.5	E944.5	E950.4	E962.0	E980.4
Saluretics	974.3	E858.5	E944.3	E950.4	E962.0	E980.4
Saluron	974.3	E858.5	E944.3	E950.4	E962.0	E980.4
Salvarsan 606 (neosilver) (silver)	961.1	E857	E931.1	E950.4	E962.0	E980.4
Sambucus canadensis	988.2	E865.4	—	E950.9	E962.1	E980.9
berry	988.2	E865.3	—	E950.9	E962.1	E980.9

Substance	Poisoning	External Cause (E-Code) Accident	Therapeutic Use	Suicide Attempt	Assault	Undetermined
Sandril	972.6	E858.3	E942.6	E950.4	E962.0	E980.4
Sanguinaria canadensis	988.2	E865.4	—	E950.9	E962.1	E980.9
Saniflush (cleaner)	983.9	E861.3	—	E950.7	E962.1	E980.6
Santonin	961.6	E857	E931.6	E950.4	E962.0	E980.4
Santyl	976.8	E858.7	E946.8	E950.4	E962.0	E980.4
Sarkomycin	960.7	E856	E930.7	E950.4	E962.0	E980.4
Saroten	969.0	E854.0	E939.0	E950.3	E962.0	E980.3
Saturnine - *see* Lead	—	—	—	—	—	—
Savin (oil)	976.4	E858.7	E946.4	E950.4	E962.0	E980.4
Scammony	973.1	E858.4	E943.1	E950.4	E962.0	E980.4
Scarlet red	976.8	E858.7	E946.8	E950.4	E962.0	E980.4
Scheele's green	985.1	E866.3	—	E950.8	E962.1	E980.8
insecticide	985.1	E863.4	—	E950.8	E962.1	E980.8
Schradan	989.3	E863.1	—	E950.6	E962.1	E980.7
Schweinfurt(h) green	985.1	E866.3	—	E950.8	E962.1	E980.8
insecticide	985.1	E863.4	—	E950.8	E962.1	E980.8
Scilla - *see* Squill	—	—	—	—	—	—
Sclerosing agents	972.7	E858.3	E942.7	E950.4	E962.0	E980.4
Scopolamine	971.1	E855.4	E941.1	E950.4	E962.0	E980.4
Scouring powder	989.89	E861.3	—	E950.9	E962.1	E980.9
Sea	—	—	—	—	—	—
anemone (sting)	989.5	E905.6	—	E950.9	E962.1	E980.9
cucumber (sting)	989.5	E905.6	—	E950.9	E962.1	E980.9
snake (bite) (venom)	989.5	E905.0	—	E950.9	E962.1	E980.9
urchin spine (puncture)	989.5	E905.6	—	E950.9	E962.1	E980.9
Secbutabarbital	967.0	E851	E937.0	E950.1	E962.0	E980.1
Secbutabarbitone	967.0	E851	E937.0	E950.1	E962.0	E980.1
Secobarbital	967.0	E851	E937.0	E950.1	E962.0	E980.1
Seconal	967.0	E851	E937.0	E950.1	E962.0	E980.1
Secretin	977.8	E858.8	E947.8	E950.4	E962.0	E980.4
Sedatives, nonbarbiturate	967.9	E852.9	E937.9	E950.2	E962.0	E980.2
specified NEC	967.8	E852.8	E937.8	E950.2	E962.0	E980.2
Sedormid	967.8	E852.8	E937.8	E950.2	E962.0	E980.2
Seed (plant)	988.2	E865.3	—	E950.9	E962.1	E980.9
disinfectant or dressing	989.89	E866.5	—	E950.9	E962.1	E980.9
Selenium (fumes) NEC	985.8	E866.4	—	E950.9	E962.1	E980.9
disulfide or sulfide	976.4	E858.7	E946.4	E950.4	E962.0	E980.4
Selsun	976.4	E858.7	E946.4	E950.4	E962.0	E980.4
Senna	973.1	E858.4	E943.1	E950.4	E962.0	E980.4
Septisol	976.2	E858.7	E946.2	E950.4	E962.0	E980.4
Serax	969.4	E853.2	E939.4	E950.3	E962.0	E980.3
Serenesil	967.8	E852.8	E937.8	E950.2	E962.0	E980.2
Serenium (hydrochloride)	961.9	E857	E931.9	E950.4	E962.0	E980.4
Serepax - *see* Oxazepam	—	—	—	—	—	—
Sernyl	968.3	E855.1	E938.3	E950.4	E962.0	E980.4
Serotonin	977.8	E858.8	E947.8	E950.4	E962.0	E980.4
Serpasil	972.6	E858.3	E942.6	E950.4	E962.0	E980.4
Sewer gas	987.8	E869.8	—	E952.8	E962.2	E982.8
Shampoo	989.6	E861.0	—	E950.9	E962.1	E980.9
Shellfish, nonbacterial or noxious	988.0	E865.1	—	E950.9	E962.1	E980.9
Silicones NEC	989.83	E866.8	E947.8	E950.9	E962.1	E980.9
Silvadene	976.0	E858.7	E946.0	E950.4	E962.0	E980.4
Silver (compound) (medicinal) NEC	976.0	E858.7	E946.0	E950.4	E962.0	E980.4
anti-infectives	976.0	E858.7	E946.0	E950.4	E962.0	E980.4
arsphenamine	961.1	E857	E931.1	E950.4	E962.0	E980.4
nitrate	976.0	E858.7	E946.0	E950.4	E962.0	E980.4
ophthalmic preparation	976.5	E858.7	E946.5	E950.4	E962.0	E980.4
toughened (keratolytic)	976.4	E858.7	E946.4	E950.4	E962.0	E980.4
nonmedicinal (dust)	985.8	E866.4	—	E950.9	E962.1	E980.9
protein (mild) (strong)	976.0	E858.7	E946.0	E950.4	E962.0	E980.4
salvarsan	961.1	E857	E931.1	E950.4	E962.0	E980.4

Substance	Poisoning	External Cause (E-Code) Accident	Therapeutic Use	Suicide Attempt	Assault	Undetermined
Simethicone	973.8	E858.4	E943.8	E950.4	E962.0	E980.4
Sinequan	969.0	E854.0	E939.0	E950.3	E962.0	E980.3
Singoserp	972.6	E858.3	E942.6	E950.4	E962.0	E980.4
Sintrom	964.2	E858.2	E934.2	E950.4	E962.0	E980.4
Sitosterols	972.2	E858.3	E942.2	E950.4	E962.0	E980.4
Skeletal muscle relaxants	975.2	E858.6	E945.2	E950.4	E962.0	E980.4
Skin	—	—	—	—	—	—
agents (external)	976.9	E858.7	E946.9	E950.4	E962.0	E980.4
specified NEC	976.8	E858.7	E946.8	E950.4	E962.0	E980.4
test antigen	977.8	E858.8	E947.8	E950.4	E962.0	E980.4
Sleep-eze	963.0	E858.1	E933.0	E950.4	E962.0	E980.4
Sleeping draught (drug) (pill) (tablet)	967.9	E852.9	E937.9	E950.2	E962.0	E980.2
Smallpox vaccine	979.0	E858.8	E949.0	E950.4	E962.0	E980.4
Smelter fumes NEC	985.9	E866.4	—	E950.9	E962.1	E980.9
Smog	987.3	E869.1	—	E952.8	E962.2	E982.8
Smoke NEC	987.9	E869.9	—	E952.9	E962.2	E982.9
Smooth muscle relaxant	975.1	E858.6	E945.1	E950.4	E962.0	E980.4
Snail killer	989.4	E863.4	—	E950.6	E962.1	E980.7
Snake (bite) (venom)	989.5	E905.0	—	E950.9	E962.1	E980.9
Snuff	989.89	E866.8	—	E950.9	E962.1	E980.9
Soap (powder) (product)	989.6	E861.1	—	E950.9	E962.1	E980.9
medicinal, soft	976.2	E858.7	E946.2	E950.4	E962.0	E980.4
Soda (caustic)	983.2	E864.2	—	E950.7	E962.1	E980.6
bicarb	963.3	E858.1	E933.3	E950.4	E962.0	E980.4
chlorinated - *see* Sodium, hypochlorite	—	—	—	—	—	—
Sodium	—	—	—	—	—	—
acetosulfone	961.8	E857	E931.8	E950.4	E962.0	E980.4
acetrizoate	977.8	E858.8	E947.8	E950.4	E962.0	E980.4
amytal	967.0	E851	E937.0	E950.1	E962.0	E980.1
arsenate - *see* Arsenic	—	—	—	—	—	—
bicarbonate	963.3	E858.1	E933.3	E950.4	E962.0	E980.4
bichromate	983.9	E864.3	—	E950.7	E962.1	E980.6
biphosphate	963.2	E858.1	E933.2	E950.4	E962.0	E980.4
bisulfate	983.9	E864.3	—	E950.7	E962.1	E980.6
borate (cleanser)	989.6	E861.3	—	E950.9	E962.1	E980.9
bromide NEC	967.3	E852.2	E937.3	E950.2	E962.0	E980.2
cacodylate (nonmedicinal) NEC	978.8	E858.8	E948.8	E950.4	E962.0	E980.4
anti-infective	961.1	E857	E931.1	E950.4	E962.0	E980.4
herbicide	989.4	E863.5	—	E950.6	E962.1	E980.7
calcium edetate	963.8	E858.1	E933.8	E950.4	E962.0	E980.4
carbonate NEC	983.2	E864.2	—	E950.7	E962.1	E980.6
chlorate NEC	983.9	E864.3	—	E950.7	E962.1	E980.6
herbicide	983.9	E863.5	—	E950.7	E962.1	E980.6
chloride NEC	974.5	E858.5	E944.5	E950.4	E962.0	E980.4
chromate	983.9	E864.3	—	E950.7	E962.1	E980.6
citrate	963.3	E858.1	E933.3	E950.4	E962.0	E980.4
cyanide - *see* Cyanide(s)	—	—	—	—	—	—
cyclamate	974.5	E858.5	E944.5	E950.4	E962.0	E980.4
diatrizoate	977.8	E858.8	E947.8	E950.4	E962.0	E980.4
dibunate	975.4	E858.6	E945.4	E950.4	E962.0	E980.4
dioctyl sulfosuccinate	973.2	E858.4	E943.2	E950.4	E962.0	E980.4
edetate	963.8	E858.1	E933.8	E950.4	E962.0	E980.4
ethacrynate	974.4	E858.5	E944.4	E950.4	E962.0	E980.4
fluoracetate (dust) (rodenticide)	989.4	E863.7	—	E950.6	E962.1	E980.7
fluoride - *see* Fluoride(s)	—	—	—	—	—	—
free salt	974.5	E858.5	E944.5	E950.4	E962.0	E980.4
glucosulfone	961.8	E857	E931.8	E950.4	E962.0	E980.4
hydroxide	983.2	E864.2	—	E950.7	E962.1	E980.6
hypochlorite (bleach) NEC	983.9	E864.3	—	E950.7	E962.1	E980.6
disinfectant	983.9	E861.4	—	E950.7	E962.1	E980.6
medicinal (anti-infective) (external)	976.0	E858.7	E946.0	E950.4	E962.0	E980.4
vapor	987.8	E869.8	—	E952.8	E962.2	E982.8

Substance	Poisoning	External Cause (E-Code) Accident	Therapeutic Use	Suicide Attempt	Assault	Undetermined
Sodium *(Continued)*						
hyposulfite	976.0	E858.7	E946.0	E950.4	E962.0	E980.4
indigotindisulfonate	977.8	E858.8	E947.8	E950.4	E962.0	E980.4
iodide	977.8	E858.8	E947.8	E950.4	E962.0	E980.4
iothalamate	977.8	E858.8	E947.8	E950.4	E962.0	E980.4
iron edetate	964.0	E858.2	E934.0	E950.4	E962.0	E980.4
lactate	963.3	E858.1	E933.3	E950.4	E962.0	E980.4
lauryl sulfate	976.2	E858.7	E946.2	E950.4	E962.0	E980.4
L-triiodothyronine	962.7	E858.0	E932.7	E950.4	E962.0	E980.4
metrizoate	977.8	E858.8	E947.8	E950.4	E962.0	E980.4
monofluoracetate (dust) (rodenticide)	989.4	E863.7	—	E950.6	E962.1	E980.7
morrhuate	972.7	E858.3	E942.7	E950.4	E962.0	E980.4
nafcillin	960.0	E856	E930.0	E950.4	E962.0	E980.4
nitrate (oxidizing agent)	983.9	E864.3	—	E950.7	E962.1	E980.6
nitrite (medicinal)	972.4	E858.3	E942.4	E950.4	E962.0	E980.4
nitroferricyanide	972.6	E858.3	E942.6	E950.4	E962.0	E980.4
nitroprusside	972.6	E858.3	E942.6	E950.4	E962.0	E980.4
para-aminohippurate	977.8	E858.8	E947.8	E950.4	E962.0	E980.4
perborate (nonmedicinal) NEC	989.89	E866.8	—	E950.9	E962.1	E980.9
medicinal	976.6	E858.7	E946.6	E950.4	E962.0	E980.4
soap	989.6	E861.1	—	E950.9	E962.1	E980.9
percarbonate - *see* Sodium, perborate	—	—	—	—	—	—
phosphate	973.3	E858.4	E943.3	E950.4	E962.0	E980.4
polystyrene sulfonate	974.5	E858.5	E944.5	E950.4	E962.0	E980.4
propionate	976.0	E858.7	E946.0	E950.4	E962.0	E980.4
psylliate	972.7	E858.3	E942.7	E950.4	E962.0	E980.4
removing resins	974.5	E858.5	E944.5	E950.4	E962.0	E980.4
salicylate	965.1	E850.3	E935.3	E950.0	E962.0	E980.0
sulfate	973.3	E858.4	E943.3	E950.4	E962.0	E980.4
sulfoxone	961.8	E857	E931.8	E950.4	E962.0	E980.4
tetradecyl sulfate	972.7	E858.3	E942.7	E950.4	E962.0	E980.4
thiopental	968.3	E855.1	E938.3	E950.4	E962.0	E980.4
thiosalicylate	965.1	E850.3	E935.3	E950.0	E962.0	E980.0
thiosulfate	976.0	E858.7	E946.0	E950.4	E962.0	E980.4
tolbutamide	977.8	E858.8	E947.8	E950.4	E962.0	E980.4
tyropanoate	977.8	E858.8	E947.8	E950.4	E962.0	E980.4
valproate	966.3	E855.0	E936.3	E950.4	E962.0	E980.4
Solanine	977.8	E858.8	E947.8	E950.4	E962.0	E980.4
Solanum dulcamara	988.2	E865.4	—	E950.9	E962.1	E980.9
Solapsone	961.8	E857	E931.8	E950.4	E962.0	E980.4
Solasulfone	961.8	E857	E931.8	E950.4	E962.0	E980.4
Soldering fluid	983.1	E864.1	—	E950.7	E962.1	E980.6
Solid substance	989.9	E866.9	—	E950.9	E962.1	E980.9
specified NEC	989.9	E866.8	—	E950.9	E962.1	E980.9
Solvents, industrial	982.8	E862.9	—	E950.9	E962.1	E980.9
naphtha	981	E862.0	—	E950.9	E962.1	E980.9
petroleum	981	E862.0	—	E950.9	E962.1	E980.9
specified NEC	982.8	E862.4	—	E950.9	E962.1	E980.9
Soma	968.0	E855.1	E938.0	E950.4	E962.0	E980.4
Somatotropin	962.4	E858.0	E932.4	E950.4	E962.0	E980.4
Sominex	963.0	E858.1	E933.0	E950.4	E962.0	E980.4
Somnos	967.1	E852.0	E937.1	E950.2	E962.0	E980.2
Somonal	967.0	E851	E937.0	E950.1	E962.0	E980.1
Soneryl	967.0	E851	E937.0	E950.1	E962.0	E980.1
Soothing syrup	977.9	E858.9	E947.9	E950.5	E962.0	E980.5
Sopor	967.4	E852.3	E937.4	E950.2	E962.0	E980.2
Soporific drug	967.9	E852.9	E937.9	E950.2	E962.0	E980.2
specified type NEC	967.8	E852.8	E937.8	E950.2	E962.0	E980.2
Sorbitol NEC	977.4	E858.8	E947.4	E950.4	E962.0	E980.4
Sotradecol	972.7	E858.3	E942.7	E950.4	E962.0	E980.4
Spacoline	975.1	E858.6	E945.1	E950.4	E962.0	E980.4
Spanish fly	976.8	E858.7	E946.8	E950.4	E962.0	E980.4

◀ New ⬅ Revised Code

Substance	Poisoning	External Cause (E-Code) Accident	Therapeutic Use	Suicide Attempt	Assault	Undetermined
Sparine	969.1	E853.0	E939.1	E950.3	E962.0	E980.3
Sparteine	975.0	E858.6	E945.0	E950.4	E962.0	E980.4
Spasmolytics	975.1	E858.6	E945.1	E950.4	E962.0	E980.4
anticholinergics	971.1	E855.4	E941.1	E950.4	E962.0	E980.4
Spectinomycin	960.8	E856	E930.8	E950.4	E962.0	E980.4
Speed	969.7	E854.2	E939.7	E950.3	E962.0	E980.3
Spermicides	976.8	E858.7	E946.8	E950.4	E962.0	E980.4
Spider (bite) (venom)	989.5	E905.1	—	E950.9	E962.1	E980.9
antivenin	979.9	E858.8	E949.9	E950.4	E962.0	E980.4
Spigelia (root)	961.6	E857	E931.6	E950.4	E962.0	E980.4
Spiperone	969.2	E853.1	E939.2	E950.3	E962.0	E980.3
Spiramycin	960.3	E856	E930.3	E950.4	E962.0	E980.4
Spirilene	969.5	E853.8	E939.5	E950.3	E962.0	E980.3
Spirit(s) (neutral) NEC	980.0	E860.1	—	E950.9	E962.1	E980.9
beverage	980.0	E860.0	—	E950.9	E962.1	E980.9
industrial	980.9	E860.9	—	E950.9	E962.1	E980.9
mineral	981	E862.0	—	E950.9	E962.1	E980.9
of salt - *see* Hydrochloric acid	—	—	—	—	—	—
surgical	980.9	E860.9	—	E950.9	E962.1	E980.9
Spironolactone	974.4	E858.5	E944.4	E950.4	E962.0	E980.4
Sponge, absorbable (gelatin)	964.5	E858.2	E934.5	E950.4	E962.0	E980.4
Sporostacin	976.0	E858.7	E946.0	E950.4	E962.0	E980.4
Sprays (aerosol)	989.89	E866.8	—	E950.9	E962.1	E980.9
cosmetic	989.89	E866.7	—	E950.9	E962.1	E980.9
medicinal NEC	977.9	E858.9	E947.9	E950.5	E962.0	E980.5
pesticides - *see* Pesticides	—	—	—	—	—	—
specified content - *see* substance specified	—	—	—	—	—	—
Spurge flax	988.2	E865.4	—	E950.9	E962.1	E980.9
Spurges	988.2	E865.4	—	E950.9	E962.1	E980.9
Squill (expectorant) NEC	975.5	E858.6	E945.5	E950.4	E962.0	E980.4
rat poison	989.4	E863.7	—	E950.6	E962.1	E980.7
Squirting cucumber (cathartic)	973.1	E858.4	E943.1	E950.4	E962.0	E980.4
Stains	989.89	E866.8	—	E950.9	E962.1	E980.9
Stannous - *see also* Tin fluoride	976.7	E858.7	E946.7	E950.4	E962.0	E980.4
Stanolone	962.1	E858.0	E932.1	E950.4	E962.0	E980.4
Stanozolol	962.1	E858.0	E932.1	E950.4	E962.0	E980.4
Staphisagria or stavesacre (pediculicide)	976.0	E858.7	E946.0	E950.4	E962.0	E980.4
Stelazine	969.1	E853.0	E939.1	E950.3	E962.0	E980.3
Stemetil	969.1	E853.0	E939.1	E950.3	E962.0	E980.3
Sterculia (cathartic) (gum)	973.3	E858.4	E943.3	E950.4	E962.0	E980.4
Sternutator gas	987.8	E869.8	—	E952.8	E962.2	E982.8
Steroids NEC	962.0	E858.0	E932.0	E950.4	E962.0	E980.4
ENT agent	976.6	E858.7	E946.6	E950.4	E962.0	E980.4
ophthalmic preparation	976.5	E858.7	E946.5	E950.4	E962.0	E980.4
topical NEC	976.0	E858.7	E946.0	E950.4	E962.0	E980.4
Stibine	985.8	E866.4	—	E950.9	E962.1	E980.9
Stibophen	961.2	E857	E931.2	E950.4	E962.0	E980.4
Stilbamide, stilbamidine	961.5	E857	E931.5	E950.4	E962.0	E980.4
Stilbestrol	962.2	E858.0	E932.2	E950.4	E962.0	E980.4
Stimulants (central nervous system)	970.9	E854.3	E940.9	E950.4	E962.0	E980.4
analeptics	970.0	E854.3	E940.0	E950.4	E962.0	E980.4
opiate antagonist	970.1	E854.3	E940.1	E950.4	E962.0	E980.4
psychotherapeutic NEC	969.0	E854.0	E939.0	E950.3	E962.0	E980.3
specified NEC	970.8	E854.3	E940.8	E950.4	E962.0	E980.4
Storage batteries (acid) (cells)	983.1	E864.1	—	E950.7	E962.1	E980.6
Stovaine	968.9	E855.2	E938.9	E950.4	E962.0	E980.4
infiltration (subcutaneous)	968.5	E855.2	E938.5	E950.4	E962.0	E980.4
nerve block (peripheral) (plexus)	968.6	E855.2	E938.6	E950.4	E962.0	E980.4
spinal	968.7	E855.2	E938.7	E950.4	E962.0	E980.4
topical (surface)	968.5	E855.2	E938.5	E950.4	E962.0	E980.4
Stovarsal	961.1	E857	E931.1	E950.4	E962.0	E980.4

Substance	Poisoning	External Cause (E-Code) Accident	Therapeutic Use	Suicide Attempt	Assault	Undetermined
Stove gas - *see* Gas, utility	—	—	—	—	—	—
Stoxil	976.5	E858.7	E946.5	E950.4	E962.0	E980.4
STP	969.6	E854.1	E939.6	E950.3	E962.0	E980.3
Stramonium (medicinal) NEC	971.1	E855.4	E941.1	E950.4	E962.0	E980.4
natural state	988.2	E865.4	—	E950.9	E962.1	E980.9
Streptodornase	964.4	E858.2	E934.4	E950.4	E962.0	E980.4
Streptoduocin	960.6	E856	E930.6	E950.4	E962.0	E980.4
Streptokinase	964.4	E858.2	E934.4	E950.4	E962.0	E980.4
Streptomycin	960.6	E856	E930.6	E950.4	E962.0	E980.4
Streptozocin	960.7	E856	E930.7	E950.4	E962.0	E980.4
Stripper (paint) (solvent)	982.8	E862.9	—	E950.9	E962.1	E980.9
Strobane	989.2	E863.0	—	E950.6	E962.1	E980.7
Strophanthin	972.1	E858.3	E942.1	E950.4	E962.0	E980.4
Strophanthus hispidus or kombe	988.2	E865.4	—	E950.9	E962.1	E980.9
Strychnine (rodenticide) (salts)	989.1	E863.7	—	E950.6	E962.1	E980.7
medicinal NEC	970.8	E854.3	E940.8	E950.4	E962.0	E980.4
Strychnos (ignatii) - *see* Strychnine	—	—	—	—	—	—
Styramate	968.0	E855.1	E938.0	E950.4	E962.0	E980.4
Styrene	983.0	E864.0	—	E950.7	E962.1	E980.6
Succinimide (anticonvulsant)	966.2	E855.0	E936.2	E950.4	E962.0	E980.4
mercuric - *see* Mercury	—	—	—	—	—	—
Succinylcholine	975.2	E858.6	E945.2	E950.4	E962.0	E980.4
Succinylsulfathiazole	961.0	E857	E931.0	E950.4	E962.0	E980.4
Sucrose	974.5	E858.5	E944.5	E950.4	E962.0	E980.4
Sulfacetamide	961.0	E857	E931.0	E950.4	E962.0	E980.4
ophthalmic preparation	976.5	E858.7	E946.5	E950.4	E962.0	E980.4
Sulfachlorpyridazine	961.0	E857	E931.0	E950.4	E962.0	E980.4
Sulfacytine	961.0	E857	E931.0	E950.4	E962.0	E980.4
Sulfadiazine	961.0	E857	E931.0	E950.4	E962.0	E980.4
silver (topical)	976.0	E858.7	E946.0	E950.4	E962.0	E980.4
Sulfadimethoxine	961.0	E857	E931.0	E950.4	E962.0	E980.4
Sulfadimidine	961.0	E857	E931.0	E950.4	E962.0	E980.4
Sulfaethidole	961.0	E857	E931.0	E950.4	E962.0	E980.4
Sulfafurazole	961.0	E857	E931.0	E950.4	E962.0	E980.4
Sulfaguanidine	961.0	E857	E931.0	E950.4	E962.0	E980.4
Sulfamerazine	961.0	E857	E931.0	E950.4	E962.0	E980.4
Sulfameter	961.0	E857	E931.0	E950.4	E962.0	E980.4
Sulfamethizole	961.0	E857	E931.0	E950.4	E962.0	E980.4
Sulfamethoxazole	961.0	E857	E931.0	E950.4	E962.0	E980.4
Sulfamethoxydiazine	961.0	E857	E931.0	E950.4	E962.0	E980.4
Sulfamethoxypyridazine	961.0	E857	E931.0	E950.4	E962.0	E980.4
Sulfamethylthiazole	961.0	E857	E931.0	E950.4	E962.0	E980.4
Sulfamylon	976.0	E858.7	E946.0	E950.4	E962.0	E980.4
Sulfan blue (diagnostic dye)	977.8	E858.8	E947.8	E950.4	E962.0	E980.4
Sulfanilamide	961.0	E857	E931.0	E950.4	E962.0	E980.4
Sulfanilylguanidine	961.0	E857	E931.0	E950.4	E962.0	E980.4
Sulfaphenazole	961.0	E857	E931.0	E950.4	E962.0	E980.4
Sulfaphenylthiazole	961.0	E857	E931.0	E950.4	E962.0	E980.4
Sulfaproxyline	961.0	E857	E931.0	E950.4	E962.0	E980.4
Sulfapyridine	961.0	E857	E931.0	E950.4	E962.0	E980.4
Sulfapyrimidine	961.0	E857	E931.0	E950.4	E962.0	E980.4
Sulfarsphenamine	961.1	E857	E931.1	E950.4	E962.0	E980.4
Sulfasalazine	961.0	E857	E931.0	E950.4	E962.0	E980.4
Sulfasomizole	961.0	E857	E931.0	E950.4	E962.0	E980.4
Sulfasuxidine	961.0	E857	E931.0	E950.4	E962.0	E980.4
Sulfinpyrazone	974.7	E858.5	E944.7	E950.4	E962.0	E980.4
Sulfisoxazole	961.0	E857	E931.0	E950.4	E962.0	E980.4
ophthalmic preparation	976.5	E858.7	E946.5	E950.4	E962.0	E980.4
Sulfomyxin	960.8	E856	E930.8	E950.4	E962.0	E980.4
Sulfonal	967.8	E852.8	E937.8	E950.2	E962.0	E980.2
Sulfonamides (mixtures)	961.0	E857	E931.0	E950.4	E962.0	E980.4

Substance	Poisoning	External Cause (E-Code)				
		Accident	Therapeutic Use	Suicide Attempt	Assault	Undetermined
Sulfones	961.8	E857	E931.8	E950.4	E962.0	E980.4
Sulfonethylmethane	967.8	E852.8	E937.8	E950.2	E962.0	E980.2
Sulfonmethane	967.8	E852.8	E937.8	E950.2	E962.0	E980.2
Sulfonphthal, sulfonphthol	977.8	E858.8	E947.8	E950.4	E962.0	E980.4
Sulfonylurea derivatives, oral	962.3	E858.0	E932.3	E950.4	E962.0	E980.4
Sulfoxone	961.8	E857	E931.8	E950.4	E962.0	E980.4
Sulfur, sulfureted, sulfuric, sulfurous, sulfuryl (compounds) NEC	989.89	E866.8	—	E950.9	E962.1	E980.9
acid	983.1	E864.1	—	E950.7	E962.1	E980.6
dioxide	987.3	E869.1	—	E952.8	E962.2	E982.8
ether - *see* Ether(s)	—	—	—	—	—	—
hydrogen	987.8	E869.8	—	E952.8	E962.2	E982.8
medicinal (keratolytic) (ointment) NEC	976.4	E858.7	E946.4	E950.4	E962.0	E980.4
pesticide (vapor)	989.4	E863.4	—	E950.6	E962.1	E980.7
vapor NEC	987.8	E869.8	—	E952.8	E962.2	E982.8
Sulkowitch's reagent	977.8	E858.8	E947.8	E950.4	E962.0	E980.4
Sulph - *see also* Sulf-	—	—	—	—	—	—
Sulphadione	961.8	E857	E931.8	E950.4	E962.0	E980.4
Sulthiame, sultiame	966.3	E855.0	E936.3	E950.4	E962.0	E980.4
Superinone	975.5	E858.6	E945.5	E950.4	E962.0	E980.4
Suramin	961.5	E857	E931.5	E950.4	E962.0	E980.4
Surfacaine	968.5	E855.2	E938.5	E950.4	E962.0	E980.4
Surital	968.3	E855.1	E938.3	E950.4	E962.0	E980.4
Sutilains	976.8	E858.7	E946.8	E950.4	E962.0	E980.4
Suxamethonium (bromide) (chloride) (iodide)	975.2	E858.6	E945.2	E950.4	E962.0	E980.4
Suxethonium (bromide)	975.2	E858.6	E945.2	E950.4	E962.0	E980.4
Sweet oil (birch)	976.3	E858.7	E946.3	E950.4	E962.0	E980.4
Sym-dichloroethyl ether	982.3	E862.4	—	E950.9	E962.1	E980.9
Sympatholytics	971.3	E855.6	E941.3	E950.4	E962.0	E980.4
Sympathomimetics	971.2	E855.5	E941.2	E950.4	E962.0	E980.4
Synagis	979.6	E858.8	E949.6	E950.4	E962.0	E980.4
Synalar	976.0	E858.7	E946.0	E950.4	E962.0	E980.4
Synthroid	962.7	E858.0	E932.7	E950.4	E962.0	E980.4
Syntocinon	975.0	E858.6	E945.0	E950.4	E962.0	E950.4
Syrosingopine	972.6	E858.3	E942.6	E950.4	E962.0	E980.4
Systemic agents (primarily)	963.9	E858.1	E933.9	E950.4	E962.0	E980.4
specified NEC	963.8	E858.1	E933.8	E950.4	E962.0	E980.4
Tablets (*see also* specified substance)	977.9	E858.9	E947.9	E950.5	E962.0	E980.5
Tace	962.2	E858.0	E932.2	E950.4	E962.0	E980.4
Tacrine	971.0	E855.3	E941.0	E950.4	E962.0	E980.4
Talbutal	967.0	E851	E937.0	E950.1	E962.0	E980.1
Talc	976.3	E858.7	E946.3	E950.4	E962.0	E980.4
Talcum	976.3	E858.7	E946.3	E950.4	E962.0	E980.4
Tandearil, tanderil	965.5	E850.5	E935.5	E950.0	E962.0	E980.0
Tannic acid	983.1	E864.1	—	E950.7	E962.1	E980.6
medicinal (astringent)	976.2	E858.7	E946.2	E950.4	E962.0	E980.4
Tannin - *see* Tannic acid	—	—	—	—	—	—
Tansy	988.2	E865.4	—	E950.9	E962.1	E980.9
TAO	960.3	E856	E930.3	E950.4	E962.0	E980.4
Tapazole	962.8	E858.0	E932.8	E950.4	E962.0	E980.4
Tar NEC	983.0	E864.0	—	E950.7	E962.1	E980.6
camphor - *see* Naphthalene	—	—	—	—	—	—
fumes	987.8	E869.8	—	E952.8	E962.2	E982.8
Taractan	969.3	E853.8	E939.3	E950.3	E962.0	E980.3
Tarantula (venomous)	989.5	E905.1	—	E950.9	E962.1	E980.9
Tartar emetic (anti-infective)	961.2	E857	E931.2	E950.4	E962.0	E980.4
Tartaric acid	983.1	E864.1	—	E950.7	E962.1	E980.6
Tartrated antimony (anti-infective)	961.2	E857	E931.2	E950.4	E962.0	E980.4
TCA - *see* Trichloroacetic acid	—	—	—	—	—	—
TDI	983.0	E864.0	—	E950.7	E962.1	E980.6
vapor	987.8	E869.8	—	E952.8	E962.2	E982.8
Tear gas	987.5	E869.3	—	E952.8	E962.2	E982.8
Teclothiazide	974.3	E858.5	E944.3	E950.4	E962.0	E980.4

Substance	Poisoning	External Cause (E-Code) Accident	Therapeutic Use	Suicide Attempt	Assault	Undetermined
Tegretol	966.3	E855.0	E936.3	E950.4	E962.0	E980.4
Telepaque	977.8	E858.8	E947.8	E950.4	E962.0	E980.4
Tellurium	985.8	E866.4	—	E950.9	E962.1	E980.9
fumes	985.8	E866.4	—	E950.9	E962.1	E980.9
TEM	963.1	E858.1	E933.1	E950.4	E962.0	E980.4
Temazepam - *see* Benzodiazepines	—	—	—	—	—	—
TEPA	963.1	E858.1	E933.1	E950.4	E962.0	E980.4
TEPP	989.3	E863.1	—	E950.6	E962.1	E980.7
Terbutaline	971.2	E855.5	E941.2	E950.4	E962.0	E980.4
Teroxalene	961.6	E857	E931.6	E950.4	E962.0	E980.4
Terpin hydrate	975.5	E858.6	E945.5	E950.4	E962.0	E980.4
Terramycin	960.4	E856	E930.4	E950.4	E962.0	E980.4
Tessalon	975.4	E858.6	E945.4	E950.4	E962.0	E980.4
Testosterone	962.1	E858.0	E932.1	E950.4	E962.0	E980.4
Tetanus (vaccine)	978.4	E858.8	E948.4	E950.4	E962.0	E980.4
antitoxin	979.9	E858.8	E949.9	E950.4	E962.0	E980.4
immune globulin (human)	964.6	E858.2	E934.6	E950.4	E962.0	E980.4
toxoid	978.4	E858.8	E948.4	E950.4	E962.0	E980.4
with diphtheria toxoid	978.9	E858.8	E948.9	E950.4	E962.0	E980.4
with pertussis	978.6	E858.8	E948.6	E950.4	E962.0	E980.4
Tetrabenazine	969.5	E853.8	E939.5	E950.3	E962.0	E980.3
Tetracaine (infiltration) (topical)	968.5	E855.2	E938.5	E950.4	E962.0	E980.4
nerve block (peripheral) (plexus)	968.6	E855.2	E938.6	E950.4	E962.0	E980.4
spinal	968.7	E855.2	E938.7	E950.4	E962.0	E980.4
Tetrachlorethylene - *see* Tetrachloroethylene	—	—	—	—	—	—
Tetrachlormethiazide	974.3	E858.5	E944.3	E950.4	E962.0	E980.4
Tetrachloroethane (liquid) (vapor)	982.3	E862.4	—	E950.9	E962.1	E980.9
paint or varnish	982.3	E861.6	—	E950.9	E962.1	E980.9
Tetrachloroethylene (liquid) (vapor)	982.3	E862.4	—	E950.9	E962.1	E980.9
medicinal	961.6	E857	E931.6	E950.4	E962.0	E980.4
Tetrachloromethane - *see* Carbon, tetrachloride	—	—	—	—	—	—
Tetracycline	960.4	E856	E930.4	E950.4	E962.0	E980.4
ophthalmic preparation	976.5	E858.7	E946.5	E950.4	E962.0	E980.4
topical NEC	976.0	E858.7	E946.0	E950.4	E962.0	E980.4
Tetraethylammonium chloride	972.3	E858.3	E942.3	E950.4	E962.0	E980.4
Tetraethyl lead (antiknock compound)	984.1	E862.1	—	E950.9	E962.1	E980.9
Tetraethyl pyrophosphate	989.3	E863.1	—	E950.6	E962.1	E980.7
Tetraethylthiuram disulfide	977.3	E858.8	E947.3	E950.4	E962.0	E980.4
Tetrahydroaminoacridine	971.0	E855.3	E941.0	E950.4	E962.0	E980.4
Tetrahydrocannabinol	969.6	E854.1	E939.6	E950.3	E962.0	E980.3
Tetrahydronaphthalene	982.0	E862.4	—	E950.9	E962.1	E980.9
Tetrahydrozoline	971.2	E855.5	E941.2	E950.4	E962.0	E980.4
Tetralin	982.0	E862.4	—	E950.9	E962.1	E980.9
Tetramethylthiuram (disulfide) NEC	989.4	E863.6	—	E950.6	E962.1	E980.7
medicinal	976.2	E858.7	E946.2	E950.4	E962.0	E980.4
Tetronal	967.8	E852.8	E937.8	E950.2	E962.0	E980.2
Tetryl	983.0	E864.0	—	E950.7	E962.1	E980.6
Thalidomide	967.8	E852.8	E937.8	E950.2	E962.0	E980.2
Thallium (compounds) (dust) NEC	985.8	E866.4	—	E950.9	E962.1	E980.9
pesticide (rodenticide)	985.8	E863.7	—	E950.6	E962.1	E980.7
THC	969.6	E854.1	E939.6	E950.3	E962.0	E980.3
Thebacon	965.09	E850.2	E935.2	E950.0	E962.0	E980.0
Thebaine	965.09	E850.2	E935.2	E950.0	E962.0	E980.0
Theobromine (calcium salicylate)	974.1	E858.5	E944.1	E950.4	E962.0	E980.4
Theophylline (diuretic)	974.1	E858.5	E944.1	E950.4	E962.0	E980.4
ethylenediamine	975.7	E858.6	E945.7	E950.4	E962.0	E980.4
Thiabendazole	961.6	E857	E931.6	E950.4	E962.0	E980.4
Thialbarbital, thialbarbitone	968.3	E855.1	E938.3	E950.4	E962.0	E980.4
Thiamine	963.5	E858.1	E933.5	E950.4	E962.0	E980.4
Thiamylal (sodium)	968.3	E855.1	E938.3	E950.4	E962.0	E980.4
Thiazesim	969.0	E854.0	E939.0	E950.3	E962.0	E980.3

Substance	Poisoning	External Cause (E-Code) Accident	Therapeutic Use	Suicide Attempt	Assault	Undetermined
Thiazides (diuretics)	974.3	E858.5	E944.3	E950.4	E962.0	E980.4
Thiethylperazine	963.0	E858.1	E933.0	E950.4	E962.0	E980.4
Thimerosal (topical)	976.0	E858.7	E946.0	E950.4	E962.0	E980.4
ophthalmic preparation	976.5	E858.7	E946.5	E950.4	E962.0	E980.4
Thioacetazone	961.8	E857	E931.8	E950.4	E962.0	E980.4
Thiobarbiturates	968.3	E855.1	E938.3	E950.4	E962.0	E980.4
Thiobismol	961.2	E857	E931.2	E950.4	E962.0	E980.4
Thiocarbamide	962.8	E858.0	E932.8	E950.4	E962.0	E980.4
Thiocarbarsone	961.1	E857	E931.1	E950.4	E962.0	E980.4
Thiocarlide	961.8	E857	E931.8	E950.4	E962.0	E980.4
Thioguanine	963.1	E858.1	E933.1	E950.4	E962.0	E980.4
Thiomercaptomerin	974.0	E858.5	E944.0	E950.4	E962.0	E980.4
Thiomerin	974.0	E858.5	E944.0	E950.4	E962.0	E980.4
Thiopental, thiopentone (sodium)	968.3	E855.1	E938.3	E950.4	E962.0	E980.4
Thiopropazate	969.1	E853.0	E939.1	E950.3	E962.0	E980.3
Thioproperazine	969.1	E853.0	E939.1	E950.3	E962.0	E980.3
Thioridazine	969.1	E853.0	E939.1	E950.3	E962.0	E980.3
Thio-TEPA, thiotepa	963.1	E858.1	E933.1	E950.4	E962.0	E980.4
Thiothixene	969.3	E853.8	E939.3	E950.3	E962.0	E980.3
Thiouracil	962.8	E858.0	E932.8	E950.4	E962.0	E980.4
Thiourea	962.8	E858.0	E932.8	E950.4	E962.0	E980.4
Thiphenamil	971.1	E855.4	E941.1	E950.4	E962.0	E980.4
Thiram NEC	989.4	E863.	—	E950.6	E962.1	E980.7
medicinal	976.2	E858.7	E946.2	E950.4	E962.0	E980.4
Thonzylamine	963.0	E858.1	E933.0	E950.4	E962.0	E980.4
Thorazine	969.1	E853.0	E939.1	E950.3	E962.0	E980.3
Thornapple	988.2	E865.4	—	E950.9	E962.1	E980.9
Throat preparation (lozenges) NEC	976.6	E858.7	E946.6	E950.4	E962.0	E980.4
Thrombin	964.5	E858.2	E934.5	E950.4	E962.0	E980.4
Thrombolysin	964.4	E858.2	E934.4	E950.4	E962.0	E980.4
Thymol	983.0	E864.0	—	E950.7	E962.1	E980.6
Thymus extract	962.9	E858.0	E932.9	E950.4	E962.0	E980.4
Thyroglobulin	962.7	E858.0	E932.7	E950.4	E962.0	E980.4
Thyroid (derivatives) (extract)	962.7	E858.0	E932.7	E950.4	E962.0	E980.4
Thyrolar	962.7	E858.0	E932.7	E950.4	E962.0	E980.4
Thyrotrophin, thyrotropin	977.8	E858.8	E947.8	E950.4	E962.0	E980.4
Thyroxin(e)	962.7	E858.0	E932.7	E950.4	E962.0	E980.4
Tigan	963.0	E858.1	E933.0	E950.4	E962.0	E980.4
Tigloidine	968.0	E855.1	E938.0	E950.4	E962.0	E980.4
Tin (chloride) (dust) (oxide) NEC	985.8	E866.4	—	E950.9	E962.1	E980.9
anti-infectives	961.2	E857	E931.2	E950.4	E962.0	E980.4
Tinactin	976.0	E858.7	E946.0	E950.4	E962.0	E980.4
Tincture, iodine - *see* Iodine	—	—	—	—	—	—
Tindal	969.1	E853.0	E939.1	E950.3	E962.0	E980.3
Titanium (compounds) (vapor)	985.8	E866.4	—	E950.9	E962.1	E980.9
ointment	976.3	E858.7	E946.3	E950.4	E962.0	E980.4
Titroid	962.7	E858.0	E932.7	E950.4	E962.0	E980.4
TMTD - *see* Tetramethylthiuram disulfide	—	—	—	—	—	—
TNT	989.89	E866.8	—	E950.9	E962.1	E980.9
fumes	987.8	E869.8	—	E952.8	E962.2	E982.8
Toadstool	988.1	E865.5	—	E950.9	E962.1	E980.9
Tobacco NEC	989.84	E866.8	—	E950.9	E962.1	E980.9
Indian	988.2	E865.4	—	E950.9	E962.1	E980.9
smoke, second-hand	987.8	E869.4	—	—	—	—
Tocopherol	963.5	E858.1	E933.5	E950.4	E962.0	E980.4
Tocosamine	975.0	E858.6	E945.0	E950.4	E962.0	E980.4
Tofranil	969.0	E854.0	E939.0	E950.3	E962.0	E980.3
Toilet deodorizer	989.89	E866.8	—	E950.9	E962.1	E980.9
Tolazamide	962.3	E858.0	E932.3	E950.4	E962.0	E980.4
Tolazoline	971.3	E855.6	E941.3	E950.4	E962.0	E980.4
Tolbutamide	962.3	E858.0	E932.3	E950.4	E962.0	E980.4
sodium	977.8	E858.8	E947.8	E950.4	E962.0	E980.4

Substance	Poisoning	External Cause (E-Code) Accident	Therapeutic Use	Suicide Attempt	Assault	Undetermined
Tolmetin	965.69	E856.0	E935.6	E950.0	E962.0	E980.0
Tolnaftate	976.0	E858.7	E946.0	E950.4	E962.0	E980.4
Tolpropamine	976.1	E858.7	E946.1	E950.4	E962.0	E980.4
Tolserol	968.0	E855.1	E938.0	E950.4	E962.0	E980.4
Toluene (liquid) (vapor)	982.0	E862.4	—	E950.9	E962.1	E980.9
diisocyanate	983.0	E864.0	—	E950.7	E962.1	E980.6
Toluidine	983.0	E864.0	—	E950.7	E962.1	E980.6
vapor	987.8	E869.8	—	E952.8	E962.2	E982.8
Toluol (liquid) (vapor)	982.0	E862.4	—	E950.9	E962.1	E980.9
Tolylene-2,4-diisocyanate	983.0	E864.0	—	E950.7	E962.1	E980.6
Tonics, cardiac	972.1	E858.3	E942.1	E950.4	E962.0	E980.4
Toxaphene (dust) (spray)	989.2	E863.0	—	E950.6	E962.1	E980.7
Toxoids NEC	978.8	E858.8	E948.8	E950.4	E962.0	E980.4
Tractor fuel NEC	981	E862.1	—	E950.9	E962.1	E980.9
Tragacanth	973.3	E858.4	E943.3	E950.4	E962.0	E980.4
Tramazoline	971.2	E855.5	E941.2	E950.4	E962.0	E980.4
Tranquilizers	969.5	E853.9	E939.5	E950.3	E962.0	E980.3
benzodiazepine-based	969.4	E853.2	E939.4	E950.3	E962.0	E980.3
butyrophenone-based	969.2	E853.1	E939.2	E950.3	E962.0	E980.3
major NEC	969.3	E853.8	E939.3	E950.3	E962.0	E980.3
phenothiazine-based	969.1	E853.0	E939.1	E950.3	E962.0	E980.3
specified NEC	969.5	E853.8	E939.5	E950.3	E962.0	E980.3
Trantoin	961.9	E857	E931.9	E950.4	E962.0	E980.4
Tranxene	969.4	E853.2	E939.4	E950.3	E962.0	E980.3
Tranylcypromine (sulfate)	969.0	E854.0	E939.0	E950.3	E962.0	E980.3
Trasentine	975.1	E858.6	E945.1	E950.4	E962.0	E980.4
Travert	974.5	E858.5	E944.5	E950.4	E962.0	E980.4
Trecator	961.8	E857	E931.8	E950.4	E962.0	E980.4
Tretinoin	976.8	E858.7	E946.8	E950.4	E962.0	E980.4
Triacetin	976.0	E858.7	E946.0	E950.4	E962.0	E980.4
Triacetyloleandomycin	960.3	E856	E930.3	E950.4	E962.0	E980.4
Triamcinolone	962.0	E858.0	E932.0	E950.4	E962.0	E980.4
ENT agent	976.6	E858.7	E946.6	E950.4	E962.0	E980.4
ophthalmic preparation	976.5	E858.7	E946.5	E950.4	E962.0	E980.4
topical NEC	976.0	E858.7	E946.0	E950.4	E962.0	E980.4
Triamterene	974.4	E858.5	E944.4	E950.4	E962.0	E980.4
Triaziquone	963.1	E858.1	E933.1	E950.4	E962.0	E980.4
Tribromacetaldehyde	967.3	E852.2	E937.3	E950.2	E962.0	E980.2
Tribromoethanol	968.2	E855.1	E938.2	E950.4	E962.0	E980.4
Tribromomethane	967.3	E852.2	E937.3	E950.2	E962.0	E980.2
Trichlorethane	982.3	E862.4	—	E950.9	E962.1	E980.9
Trichlormethiazide	974.3	E858.5	E944.3	E950.4	E962.0	E980.4
Trichloroacetic acid	983.1	E864.1	—	E950.7	E962.1	E980.6
medicinal (keratolytic)	976.4	E858.7	E946.4	E950.4	E962.0	E980.4
Trichloroethanol	967.1	E852.0	E937.1	E950.2	E962.0	E980.2
Trichloroethylene (liquid) (vapor)	982.3	E862.4	—	E950.9	E962.1	E980.9
anesthetic (gas)	968.2	E855.1	E938.2	E950.4	E962.0	E980.4
Trichloroethyl phosphate	967.1	E852.0	E937.1	E950.2	E962.0	E980.2
Trichlorofluoromethane NEC	987.4	E869.2	—	E952.8	E962.2	E982.8
Trichlorotriethylamine	963.1	E858.1	E933.1	E950.4	E962.0	E980.4
Trichomonacides NEC	961.5	E857	E931.5	E950.4	E962.0	E980.4
Trichomycin	960.1	E856	E930.1	E950.4	E962.0	E980.4
Triclofos	967.1	E852.0	E937.1	E950.2	E962.0	E980.2
Tricresyl phosphate	989.89	E866.8	—	E950.9	E962.1	E980.9
solvent	982.8	E862.4	—	E950.9	E962.1	E980.9
Tricyclamol	966.4	E855.0	E936.4	E950.4	E962.0	E980.4
Tridesilon	976.0	E858.7	E946.0	E950.4	E962.0	E980.4
Tridihexethyl	971.1	E855.4	E941.1	E950.4	E962.0	E980.4
Tridione	966.0	E855.0	E936.0	E950.4	E962.0	E980.4

Substance	Poisoning	External Cause (E-Code) Accident	Therapeutic Use	Suicide Attempt	Assault	Undetermined
Triethanolamine NEC	983.2	E864.2	—	E950.7	E962.1	E980.6
detergent	983.2	E861.0	—	E950.7	E962.1	E980.6
trinitrate	972.4	E858.3	E942.4	E950.4	E962.0	E980.4
Triethanomelamine	963.1	E858.1	E933.1	E950.4	E962.0	E980.4
Triethylene melamine	963.1	E858.1	E933.1	E950.4	E962.0	E980.4
Triethylenephosphoramide	963.1	E858.1	E933.1	E950.4	E962.0	E980.4
Triethylenethiophosphoramide	963.1	E858.1	E933.1	E950.4	E962.0	E980.4
Trifluoperazine	969.1	E853.0	E939.1	E950.3	E962.0	E980.3
Trifluperidol	969.2	E853.1	E939.2	E950.3	E962.0	E980.3
Triflupromazine	969.1	E853.0	E939.1	E950.3	E962.0	E980.3
Trihexyphenidyl	971.1	E855.4	E941.1	E950.4	E962.0	E980.4
Triiodothyronine	962.7	E858.0	E932.7	E950.4	E962.0	E980.4
Trilene	968.2	E855.1	E938.2	E950.4	E962.0	E980.4
Trimeprazine	963.0	E858.1	E933.0	E950.4	E962.0	E980.4
Trimetazidine	972.4	E858.3	E942.4	E950.4	E962.0	E980.4
Trimethadione	966.0	E855.0	E936.0	E950.4	E962.0	E980.4
Trimethaphan	972.3	E858.3	E942.3	E950.4	E962.0	E980.4
Trimethidinium	972.3	E858.3	E942.3	E950.4	E962.0	E980.4
Trimethobenzamide	963.0	E858.1	E933.0	E950.4	E962.0	E980.4
Trimethylcarbinol	980.8	E860.8	—	E950.9	E962.1	E980.9
Trimethylpsoralen	976.3	E858.7	E946.3	E950.4	E962.0	E980.4
Trimeton	963.0	E858.1	E933.0	E950.4	E962.0	E980.4
Trimipramine	969.0	E854.0	E939.0	E950.3	E962.0	E980.3
Trimustine	963.1	E858.1	E933.1	E950.4	E962.0	E980.4
Trinitrin	972.4	E858.3	E942.4	E950.4	E962.0	E980.4
Trinitrophenol	983.0	E864.0	—	E950.7	E962.1	E980.6
Trinitrotoluene	989.89	E866.8	—	E950.9	E962.1	E980.9
fumes	987.8	E869.8	—	E952.8	E962.2	E982.8
Trional	967.8	E852.8	E937.8	E950.2	E962.0	E980.2
Trioxide of arsenic - *see* Arsenic	—	—	—	—	—	—
Trioxsalen	976.3	E858.7	E946.3	E950.4	E962.0	E980.4
Tripelennamine	963.0	E858.1	E933.0	E950.4	E962.0	E980.4
Triperidol	969.2	E853.1	E939.2	E950.3	E962.0	E980.3
Triprolidine	963.0	E858.1	E933.0	E950.4	E962.0	E980.4
Trisoralen	976.3	E858.7	E946.3	E950.4	E962.0	E980.4
Troleandomycin	960.3	E856	E930.3	E950.4	E962.0	E980.4
Trolnitrate (phosphate)	972.4	E858.3	E942.4	E950.4	E962.0	E980.4
Trometamol	963.3	E858.1	E933.3	E950.4	E962.0	E980.4
Tromethamine	963.3	E858.1	E933.3	E950.4	E962.0	E980.4
Tronothane	968.5	E855.2	E938.5	E950.4	E962.0	E980.4
Tropicamide	971.1	E855.4	E941.1	E950.4	E962.0	E980.4
Troxidone	966.0	E855.0	E936.0	E950.4	E962.0	E980.4
Tryparsamide	961.1	E857	E931.1	E950.4	E962.0	E980.4
Trypsin	963.4	E858.1	E933.4	E950.4	E962.0	E980.4
Tryptizol	969.0	E854.0	E939.0	E950.3	E962.0	E980.3
Tuaminoheptane	971.2	E855.5	E941.2	E950.4	E962.0	E980.4
Tuberculin (old)	977.8	E858.8	E947.8	E950.4	E962.0	E980.4
Tubocurare	975.2	E858.6	E945.2	E950.4	E962.0	E980.4
Tubocurarine	975.2	E858.6	E945.2	E950.4	E962.0	E980.4
Turkish green	969.6	E854.1	E939.6	E950.3	E962.0	E980.3
Turpentine (spirits of) (liquid) (vapor)	982.8	E862.4	—	E950.9	E962.1	E980.9
Tybamate	969.5	E853.8	E939.5	E950.3	E962.0	E980.3
Tyloxapol	975.5	E858.6	E945.5	E950.4	E962.0	E980.4
Tymazoline	971.2	E855.5	E941.2	E950.4	E962.0	E980.4
Typhoid vaccine	978.1	E858.8	E948.1	E950.4	E962.0	E980.4
Typhus vaccine	979.2	E858.8	E949.2	E950.4	E962.0	E980.4
Tyrothricin	976.0	E858.7	E946.0	E950.4	E962.0	E980.4
ENT agent	976.6	E858.7	E946.6	E950.4	E962.0	E980.4
ophthalmic preparation	976.5	E858.7	E946.5	E950.4	E962.0	E980.4
Undecenoic acid	976.0	E858.7	E946.0	E950.4	E962.0	E980.4
Undecylenic acid	976.0	E858.7	E946.0	E950.4	E962.0	E980.4

Substance	Poisoning	External Cause (E-Code) Accident	Therapeutic Use	Suicide Attempt	Assault	Undetermined
Unna's boot	976.3	E858.7	E946.3	E950.4	E962.0	E980.4
Uracil mustard	963.1	E858.1	E933.1	E950.4	E962.0	E980.4
Uramustine	963.1	E858.1	E933.1	E950.4	E962.0	E980.4
Urari	975.2	E858.6	E945.2	E950.4	E962.0	E980.4
Urea	974.4	E858.5	E944.4	E950.4	E962.0	E980.4
topical	976.8	E858.7	E946.8	E950.4	E962.0	E980.4
Urethan(e) (antineoplastic)	963.1	E858.1	E933.1	E950.4	E962.0	E980.4
Urginea (maritima) (scilla) - *see* Squill	—	—	—	—	—	—
Uric acid metabolism agents NEC	974.7	E858.5	E944.7	E950.4	E962.0	E980.4
Urokinase	964.4	E858.2	E934.4	E950.4	E962.0	E980.4
Urokon	977.8	E858.8	E947.8	E950.4	E962.0	E980.4
Urotropin	961.9	E857	E931.9	E950.4	E962.0	E980.4
Urtica	988.2	E865.4	—	E950.9	E962.1	E980.9
Utility gas - *see* Gas, utility	—	—	—	—	—	—
Vaccine NEC	979.9	E858.8	E949.9	E950.4	E962.0	E980.4
bacterial NEC	978.8	E858.8	E948.8	E950.4	E962.0	E980.4
with	—	—	—	—	—	—
other bacterial component	978.9	E858.8	E948.9	E950.4	E962.0	E980.4
pertussis component	978.6	E858.8	E948.6	E950.4	E962.0	E980.4
viral-rickettsial component	979.7	E858.8	E949.7	E950.4	E962.0	E980.4
mixed NEC	978.9	E858.8	E948.9	E950.4	E962.0	E980.4
BCG	978.0	E858.8	E948.0	E950.4	E962.0	E980.4
cholera	978.2	E858.8	E948.2	E950.4	E962.0	E980.4
diphtheria	978.5	E858.8	E948.5	E950.4	E962.0	E980.4
influenza	979.6	E858.8	E949.6	E950.4	E962.0	E980.4
measles	979.4	E858.8	E949.4	E950.4	E962.0	E980.4
meningococcal	978.8	E858.8	E948.8	E950.4	E962.0	E980.4
mumps	979.6	E858.8	E949.6	E950.4	E962.0	E980.4
paratyphoid	978.1	E858.8	E948.1	E950.4	E962.0	E980.4
pertussis (with diphtheria toxoid) (with tetanus toxoid)	978.6	E858.8	E948.6	E950.4	E962.0	E980.4
plague	978.3	E858.8	E948.3	E950.4	E962.0	E980.4
poliomyelitis	979.5	E858.8	E949.5	E950.4	E962.0	E980.4
poliovirus	979.5	E858.8	E949.5	E950.4	E962.0	E980.4
rabies	979.1	E858.8	E949.1	E950.4	E962.0	E980.4
respiratory syncytial virus	979.6	E858.8	E949.6	E950.4	E962.0	E980.4
rickettsial NEC	979.6	E858.8	E949.6	E950.4	E962.0	E980.4
with	—	—	—	—	—	—
bacterial component	979.7	E858.8	E949.7	E950.4	E962.0	E980.4
pertussis component	978.6	E858.8	E948.6	E950.4	E962.0	E980.4
viral component	979.7	E858.8	E949.7	E950.4	E962.0	E980.4
Rocky Mountain spotted fever	979.6	E858.8	E949.6	E950.4	E962.0	E980.4
rotavirus	979.6	E858.8	E949.6	E950.4	E962.0	E980.4
rubella virus	979.4	E858.8	E949.4	E950.4	E962.0	E980.4
sabin oral	979.5	E858.8	E949.5	E950.4	E962.0	E980.4
smallpox	979.0	E858.8	E949.0	E950.4	E962.0	E980.4
tetanus	978.4	E858.8	E948.4	E950.4	E962.0	E980.4
typhoid	978.1	E858.8	E948.1	E950.4	E962.0	E980.4
typhus	979.2	E858.8	E949.2	E950.4	E962.0	E980.4
viral NEC	979.6	E858.8	E949.6	E950.4	E962.0	E980.4
with	—	—	—	—	—	—
bacterial component	979.7	E858.8	E949.7	E950.4	E962.0	E980.4
pertussis component	978.6	E858.8	E948.6	E950.4	E962.0	E980.4
rickettsial component	979.7	E858.8	E949.7	E950.4	E962.0	E980.4
yellow fever	979.3	E858.8	E949.3	E950.4	E962.0	E980.4
Vaccinia immune globulin (human)	964.6	E858.2	E934.6	E950.4	E962.0	E980.4
Vaginal contraceptives	976.8	E858.7	E946.8	E950.4	E962.0	E980.4
Valethamate	971.1	E855.4	E941.1	E950.4	E962.0	E980.4
Valisone	976.0	E858.7	E946.0	E950.4	E962.0	E980.4
Valium	969.4	E853.2	E939.4	E950.3	E962.0	E980.3
Valmid	967.8	E852.8	E937.8	E950.2	E962.0	E980.2
Vanadium	985.8	E866.4	—	E950.9	E962.1	E980.9
Vancomycin	960.8	E856	E930.8	E950.4	E962.0	E980.4

◀ New ⟸ Revised Code

Substance	Poisoning	External Cause (E-Code): Accident	Therapeutic Use	Suicide Attempt	Assault	Undetermined
Vapor (*see also* Gas)	987.9	E869.9	—	E952.9	E962.2	E982.9
kiln (carbon monoxide)	986	E868.8	—	E952.1	E962.2	E982.1
lead - *see* Lead	—	—	—	—	—	—
specified source NEC - (*see also* specific substance)	987.8	E869.8	—	E952.8	E962.2	E982.8
Varidase	964.4	E858.2	E934.4	E950.4	E962.0	E980.4
Varnish	989.89	E861.6	—	E950.9	E962.1	E980.9
cleaner	982.8	E862.9	—	E950.9	E962.1	E980.9
Vaseline	976.3	E858.7	E946.3	E950.4	E962.0	E980.4
Vasodilan	972.5	E858.3	E942.5	E950.4	E962.0	E980.4
Vasodilators NEC	972.5	E858.3	E942.5	E950.4	E962.0	E980.4
coronary	972.4	E858.3	E942.4	E950.4	E962.0	E980.4
Vasopressin	962.5	E858.0	E932.5	E950.4	E962.0	E980.4
Vasopressor drugs	962.5	E858.0	E932.5	E950.4	E962.0	E980.4
Venom, venomous (bite) (sting)	989.5	E905.9	—	E950.9	E962.1	E980.9
arthropod NEC	989.5	E905.5	—	E950.9	E962.1	E980.9
bee	989.5	E905.3	—	E950.9	E962.1	E980.9
centipede	989.5	E905.4	—	E950.9	E962.1	E980.9
hornet	989.5	E905.3	—	E950.9	E962.1	E980.9
lizard	989.5	E905.0	—	E950.9	E962.1	E980.9
marine animals or plants	989.5	E905.6	—	E950.9	E962.1	E980.9
millipede (tropical)	989.5	E905.4	—	E950.9	E962.1	E980.9
plant NEC	989.5	E905.7	—	E950.9	E962.1	E980.9
marine	989.5	E905.6	—	E950.9	E962.1	E980.9
scorpion	989.5	E905.2	—	E950.9	E962.1	E980.9
snake	989.5	E905.0	—	E950.9	E962.1	E980.9
specified NEC	989.5	E905.8	—	E950.9	E962.1	E980.9
spider	989.5	E905.1	—	E950.9	E962.1	E980.9
wasp	989.5	E905.3	—	E950.9	E962.1	E980.9
Ventolin - *see* Salbutamol sulfate	—	—	—	—	—	—
Veramon	967.0	E851	E937.0	E950.1	E962.0	E980.1
Veratrum	—	—	—	—	—	—
album	988.2	E865.4	—	E950.9	E962.1	E980.9
alkaloids	972.6	E858.3	E942.6	E950.4	E962.0	E980.4
viride	988.2	E865.4	—	E950.9	E962.1	E980.9
Verdigris (*see also* Copper)	985.8	E866.4	—	E950.9	E962.1	E980.9
Veronal	967.0	E851	E937.0	E950.1	E962.0	E980.1
Veroxil	961.6	E857	E931.6	E950.4	E962.0	E980.4
Versidyne	965.7	E850.7	E935.7	E950.0	E962.0	E980.0
Viagra	972.5	E858.3	E942.5	E950.4	E962.0	E980.4
Vienna	—	—	—	—	—	—
green	985.1	E866.3	—	E950.8	E962.1	E980.8
insecticide	985.1	E863.4	—	E950.6	E962.1	E980.7
red	989.89	E866.8	—	E950.9	E962.1	E980.9
pharmaceutical dye	977.4	E858.8	E947.4	E950.4	E962.0	E980.4
Vinbarbital, vinbarbitone	967.0	E851	E937.0	E950.1	E962.0	E980.1
Vinblastine	963.1	E858.1	E933.1	E950.4	E962.0	E980.4
Vincristine	963.1	E858.1	E933.1	E950.4	E962.0	E980.4
Vinesthene, vinethene	968.2	E855.1	E938.2	E950.4	E962.0	E980.4
Vinyl	—	—	—	—	—	—
bital	967.0	E851	E937.0	E950.1	E962.0	E980.1
ether	968.2	E855.1	E938.2	E950.4	E962.0	E980.4
Vioform	961.3	E857	E931.3	E950.4	E962.0	E980.4
topical	976.0	E858.7	E946.0	E950.4	E962.0	E980.4
Viomycin	960.6	E856	E930.6	E950.4	E962.0	E980.4
Viosterol	963.5	E858.1	E933.5	E950.4	E962.0	E980.4
Viper (venom)	989.5	E905.0	—	E950.9	E962.1	E980.9
Viprynium (embonate)	961.6	E857	E931.6	E950.4	E962.0	E980.4
Virugon	961.7	E857	E931.7	E950.4	E962.0	E980.4
Visine	976.5	E858.7	E946.5	E950.4	E962.0	E980.4
Vitamins NEC	963.5	E858.1	E933.5	E950.4	E962.0	E980.4
B_{12}	964.1	E858.2	E934.1	E950.4	E962.0	E980.4

Substance	Poisoning	External Cause (E-Code) Accident	Therapeutic Use	Suicide Attempt	Assault	Undetermined
Vitamins NEC *(Continued)*						
hematopoietic	964.1	E858.2	E934.1	E950.4	E962.0	E980.4
K	964.3	E858.2	E934.3	E950.4	E962.0	E980.4
Vleminckx's solution	976.4	E858.7	E946.4	E950.4	E962.0	E980.4
Voltaren - *see* Diclofenac sodium	—	—	—	—	—	—
Warfarin (potassium) (sodium)	964.2	E858.2	E934.2	E950.4	E962.0	E980.4
rodenticide	989.4	E863.7	—	E950.6	E962.1	E980.7
Wasp (sting)	989.5	E905.3	—	E950.9	E962.1	E980.9
Water	—	—	—	—	—	—
balance agents NEC	974.5	E858.5	E944.5	E950.4	E962.0	E980.4
gas	987.1	E868.1	—	E951.8	E962.2	E981.8
incomplete combustion of - *see* Carbon, monoxide, fuel, utility	—	—	—	—	—	—
hemlock	988.2	E865.4	—	E950.9	E962.1	E980.9
moccasin (venom)	989.5	E905.0	—	E950.9	E962.1	E980.9
Wax (paraffin) (petroleum)	981	E862.3	—	E950.9	E962.1	E980.9
automobile	989.89	E861.2	—	E950.9	E962.1	E980.9
floor	981	E862.0	—	E950.9	E962.1	E980.9
Weed killers NEC	989.4	E863.5	—	E950.6	E962.1	E980.7
Welldorm	967.1	E852.0	E937.1	E950.2	E962.0	E980.2
White	—	—	—	—	—	—
arsenic - *see* Arsenic	—	—	—	—	—	—
hellebore	988.2	E865.4	—	E950.9	E962.1	E980.9
lotion (keratolytic)	976.4	E858.7	E946.4	E950.4	E962.0	E980.4
spirit	981	E862.0	—	E950.9	E962.1	E980.9
Whitewashes	989.89	E861.6	—	E950.9	E962.1	E980.9
Whole blood	964.7	E858.2	E934.7	E950.4	E962.0	E980.4
Wild	—	—	—	—	—	—
black cherry	988.2	E865.4	—	E950.9	E962.1	E980.9
poisonous plants NEC	988.2	E865.4	—	E950.9	E962.1	E980.9
Window cleaning fluid	989.89	E861.3	—	E950.9	E962.1	E980.9
Wintergreen (oil)	976.3	E858.7	E946.3	E950.4	E962.0	E980.4
Witch hazel	976.2	E858.7	E946.2	E950.4	E962.0	E980.4
Wood	—	—	—	—	—	—
alcohol	980.1	E860.2	—	E950.9	E962.1	E980.9
spirit	980.1	E860.2	—	E950.9	E962.1	E980.9
Woorali	975.2	E858.6	E945.2	E950.4	E962.0	E980.4
Wormseed, American	961.6	E857	E931.6	E950.4	E962.0	E980.4
Xanthine diuretics	974.1	E858.5	E944.1	E950.4	E962.0	E980.4
Xanthocillin	960.0	E856	E930.0	E950.4	E962.0	E980.4
Xanthotoxin	976.3	E858.7	E946.3	E950.4	E962.0	E980.4
Xigris ◀	964.2	E858.2	E934.2	E950.4	E962.0	E980.4
Xylene (liquid) (vapor)	982.0	E862.4	—	E950.9	E962.1	E980.9
Xylocaine (infiltration) (topical)	968.5	E855.2	E938.5	E950.4	E962.0	E980.4
nerve block (peripheral) (plexus)	968.6	E855.2	E938.6	E950.4	E962.0	E980.4
spinal	968.7	E855.2	E938.7	E950.4	E962.0	E980.4
Xylol (liquid) (vapor)	982.0	E862.4	—	E950.9	E962.1	E980.9
Xylometazoline	971.2	E855.5	E941.2	E950.4	E962.0	E980.4
Yellow	—	—	—	—	—	—
fever vaccine	979.3	E858.8	E949.3	E950.4	E962.0	E980.4
jasmine	988.2	E865.4	—	E950.9	E962.1	E980.9
Yew	988.2	E865.4	—	E950.9	E962.1	E980.9
Zactane	965.7	E850.7	E935.7	E950.0	E962.0	E980.0
Zaroxolyn	974.3	E858.5	E944.3	E950.4	E962.0	E980.4
Zephiran (topical)	976.0	E858.7	E946.0	E950.4	E962.0	E980.4
ophthalmic preparation	976.5	E858.7	E946.5	E950.4	E962.0	E980.4
Zerone	980.1	E860.2	—	E950.9	E962.1	E980.9
Zinc (compounds) (fumes) (salts) (vapor) NEC	985.8	E866.4	—	E950.9	E962.1	E980.9
anti-infectives	976.0	E858.7	E946.0	E950.4	E962.0	E980.4
antivaricose	972.7	E858.3	E942.7	E950.4	E962.0	E980.4
bacitracin	976.0	E858.7	E946.0	E950.4	E962.0	E980.4
chloride	976.2	E858.7	E946.2	E950.4	E962.0	E980.4
gelatin	976.3	E858.7	E946.3	E950.4	E962.0	E980.4
oxide	976.3	E858.7	E946.3	E950.4	E962.0	E980.4

Substance	Poisoning	External Cause (E-Code)				
		Accident	Therapeutic Use	Suicide Attempt	Assault	Undetermined
Zinc *(Continued)*						
peroxide	976.0	E858.7	E946.0	E950.4	E962.0	E980.4
pesticides	985.8	E863.4	—	E950.6	E962.1	E980.7
phosphide (rodenticide)	985.8	E863.7	—	E950.6	E962.1	E980.7
stearate	976.3	E858.7	E946.3	E950.4	E962.0	E980.4
sulfate (antivaricose)	972.7	E858.3	E942.7	E950.4	E962.0	E980.4
ENT agent	976.6	E858.7	E946.6	E950.4	E962.0	E980.4
ophthalmic solution	976.5	E858.7	E946.5	E950.4	E962.0	E980.4
topical NEC	976.0	E858.7	E946.0	E950.4	E962.0	E980.4
undecylenate	976.0	E858.7	E946.0	E950.4	E962.0	E980.4
Zovant ◀	964.2	E858.2	E934.2	E950.4	E962.0	E980.4
Zoxazolamine	968.0	E855.1	E938.0	E950.4	E962.0	E980.4
Zygadenus (venenosus)	988.2	E865.4	—	E950.9	E962.1	E980.9

SECTION III

INDEX TO EXTERNAL CAUSES OF INJURY (E CODE)

This section contains the index to the codes which classify environmental events, circumstances, and other conditions as the cause of injury and other adverse effects. Where a code from the section Supplementary Classification of External Causes of Injury and Poisoning (E800-E998) is applicable, it is intended that the E code shall be used in addition to a code from the main body of the classification, Chapters 1 to 17.

The alphabetic index to the E codes is organized by main terms which describe the accident, circumstance, event, or specific agent which caused the injury or other adverse effect.

Note Transport accidents (E800-E848) include accidents involving:

- aircraft and spacecraft (E840-E845)
- watercraft (E830-E838)
- motor vehicle (E810-E825)
- railway (E800-E807)
- other road vehicles (E826-E829)

For definitions and examples related to transport accidents - see Supplementary Classification of External Causes of Injury and Poisoning (E800-E999).

The fourth-digit subdivisions for use with categories E800-E848 to identify the injured person are found at the end of this section.

For identifying the place in which an accident or poisoning occurred (circumstances classifiable to categories E850-E869 and E880-E928) - see the listing in this section under "Accident, occurring."

See the Table of Drugs and Chemicals (Section 2 of this volume) for identifying the specific agent involved in drug overdose or a wrong substance given or taken in error, and for intoxication or poisoning by a drug or other chemical substance.

The specific adverse effect, reaction, or localized toxic effect of a correct drug or substance properly administered in therapeutic or prophylactic dosage should be classified according to the nature of the adverse effect (e.g., allergy, dermatitis, tachycardia) listed in Section I of this volume.

◀ New ⬅ Revised Code

A

◀ New ⟸ Revised Code

- **Burning, burns** *(Continued)*
  - inflicted by other person *(Continued)*
    - stated as *(Continued)*
      - undetermined whether accidental or intentional (*see also* Burn, stated as undetermined whether accidental or intentional) E988.1
  - internal, from swallowed caustic, corrosive liquid, substance - *see* Table of Drugs and Chemicals
  - in
    - terrorism E979.3
      - from nuclear explosion E979.5
      - petrol bomb E979.3
    - war operations (from fire-producing device or conventional weapon) E990.9
      - from nuclear explosion E996
      - petrol bomb E990.0
    - from nuclear explosion E996
    - petrol bomb E990.0
  - lamp (*see also* Fire, specified NEC) E898.1
  - late effect of NEC E929.4
  - lighter (cigar) (cigarette) (*see also* Fire, specified NEC) E898.1
  - lightning E907
  - liquid (boiling) (hot) (molten) E924.0
    - caustic, corrosive (external) E924.1
      - swallowed - *see* Table of Drugs and Chemicals
  - local application of externally applied substance in medical or surgical care E873.5
  - machinery - *see* Accident, machine
  - matches (*see also* Fire, specified NEC) E898.1
  - medicament, externally applied E873.5
  - metal, molten E924.0
  - object (hot) E924.8
    - producing fire or flames - *see* Fire
  - oven (electric) (gas) E924.8
  - pipe (smoking) (*see also* Fire, specified NEC) E898.1
  - radiation - *see* Radiation
  - railway engine, locomotive, train (*see also* Explosion, railway engine) E803
  - self-inflicted (unspecified whether accidental or intentional) E988.1
    - caustic or corrosive substance NEC E988.7
    - stated as intentional, purposeful E958.1
      - caustic or corrosive substance NEC E958.7
  - stated as undetermined whether accidental or intentional E988.1
    - caustic or corrosive substance NEC E988.7
  - steam E924.0
    - pipe E924.8
  - substance (hot) E924.9
    - boiling or molten E924.0
    - caustic, corrosive (external) E924.1
      - swallowed - *see* Table of Drugs and Chemicals
  - suicidal (attempt) NEC E958.1
    - caustic substance E958.7
    - late effect of E959
  - tanning bed E926.2
  - therapeutic misadventure
    - overdose of radiation E873.2
  - torch, welding (*see also* Fire, specified NEC) E898.1
  - trash fire (*see also* Burning, bonfire) E897
  - vapor E924.0
  - vitriol E924.1
  - x-rays E926.3
    - in medical, surgical procedure - *see* Misadventure, failure, in dosage, radiation operations
- **Butted by animal** E906.8

C

- **Cachexia, lead or saturnine** E866.0
  - from pesticide NEC (*see also* Table of Drugs and Chemicals) E863.4
- **Caisson disease** E902.2
- **Capital punishment** (any means) E978
- **Car sickness** E903
- **Casualty** (not due to war) NEC E928.9
  - terrorism E979.8
  - war (*see also* War operations) E995
- **Cat**
  - bite E906.3
  - scratch E906.8
- **Cataclysmic** (any injury)
  - earth surface movement or eruption E909.9
    - specified type NEC E909.8
  - storm or flood resulting from storm E908.9
    - specified type NEC E909.8
- **Catching fire** - *see* Ignition
- **Caught**
  - between
    - objects (moving) (stationary and moving) E918
      - and machinery - *see* Accident, machine
  - by cable car, not on rails E847
  - in
    - machinery (moving parts of) - *see* Accident, machine
    - object E918
- **Cave-in** (causing asphyxia, suffocation (by pressure)) (*see also* Suffocation, due to, cave-in) E913.3
  - with injury other than asphyxia or suffocation E916
    - with asphyxia or suffocation (*see also* Suffocation, due to, cave-in) E913.3
  - struck or crushed by E916
    - with asphyxia or suffocation (*see also* Suffocation, due to, cave-in) E913.3
- **Change(s) in air pressure** - *see also* Effects of, air pressure
  - sudden, in aircraft (ascent) (descent) (causing aeroneurosis or aviators' disease) E902.1
- **Chilblains** E901.0
  - due to manmade conditions E901.1
- **Choking** (on) (any object except food or vomitus) E912
  - apple E911
  - bone E911
  - food, any type (regurgitated) E911
  - mucus or phlegm E912
  - seed E911
- **Civil insurrection** - *see* War operations
- **Cloudburst** E908.8
- **Cold, exposure to** (accidental) (excessive) (extreme) (place) E901.9
  - causing chilblains or immersion foot E901.0
  - due to
    - manmade conditions E901.1
    - specified cause NEC E901.8
    - weather (conditions) E901.0
  - late effect of NEC E929.5
  - self-inflicted (undetermined whether accidental or intentional) E988.3
    - suicidal E958.3
  - suicide E958.3
- **Colic, lead, painters', or saturnine** - *see* category E866
- **Collapse**
  - burning (uncontrolled fire) E891.8
    - in terrorism E979.3
    - private E890.8 higher
  - dam E909.3
  - due to heat - *see* Heat
  - machinery - *see* Accident, machine or vehicle
  - man-made structure E909.3
  - postoperative NEC E878.9
  - structure, burning NEC E891.8
    - burning (uncontrolled fire)
      - in terrorism E979.3
- **Collision** (accidental)

> Note In the case of collisions between different types of vehicles, persons and objects, priority in classification is in the following order:
>
> Aircraft
> Watercraft
> Motor vehicle
> Railway vehicle
> Pedal cycle
> Animal-drawn vehicle
> Animal being ridden
> Streetcar or other nonmotor road vehicle
> Other vehicle
> Pedestrian or person using pedestrian conveyance
> Object (except where falling from or set in motion by vehicle, etc. listed above)
>
> In the listing below, the combinations are listed only under the vehicle, etc., having priority. For definitions, *see* Supplementary Classification of External Causes of Injury and Poisoning (E800-E999).

  - aircraft (with object or vehicle) (fixed)-entrance (on (movable) (moving)) E841
    - with
      - person (while landing, taking off) vehicle off the (without accident to aircraft) E844
    - powered (in transit) (with unpowered aircraft) E841
      - while landing, taking off E840
    - unpowered E842
      - while landing, taking off E840
  - animal being ridden (in sport or transport) E828
    - and
      - animal (being ridden) (herded) (unattended) E828

◄ **New** ⟸ **Revised Code**

◀ New ⟸ Revised Code

G

H

I

J

ICD-9-CM E Codes Vol. 2

M

N

O

P

ICD-9-CM E Codes Vol. 2

S

ICD-9-CM
E Codes
Vol. 2

ICD-9-CM
E Codes
Vol. 2

T

◄ New ⟸ Revised Code

V

W

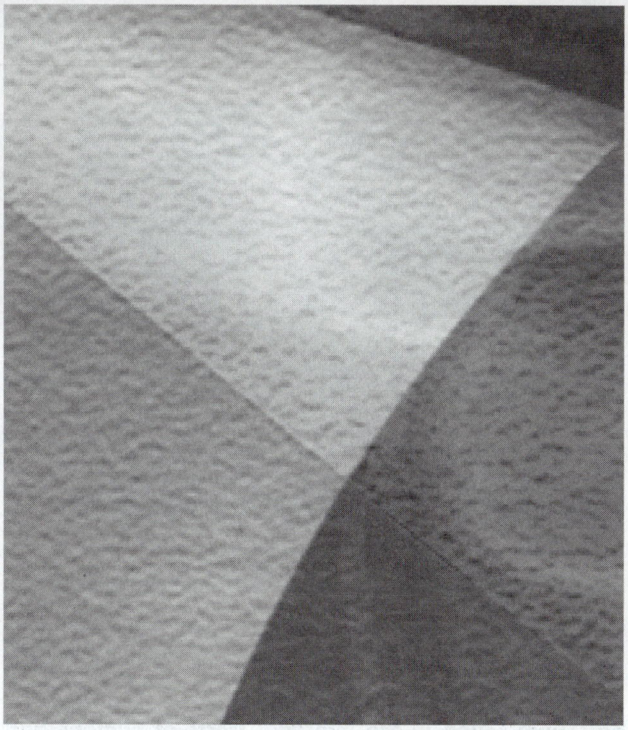

PART III

Diseases: Tabular List Volume 1

1. INFECTIOUS AND PARASITIC DISEASES (001–139)

Note: Categories for "late effects" of infectious and parasitic diseases are to be found at 137–139.

Includes: diseases generally recognized as communicable or transmissible as well as a few diseases of unknown but possibly infectious origin

Excludes *acute respiratory infections (460–466)*
carrier or suspected carrier of infectious organism (V02.0–V02.9)
certain localized infections
influenza (487.0–487.8)

INTESTINAL INFECTIOUS DISEASES (001–009)

Excludes *helminthiases (120.0–129)*

● **001 Cholera**

001.0 Due to Vibrio cholerae

001.1 Due to Vibrio cholerae el tor

❑ **001.9 Cholera, unspecified**

● **002 Typhoid and paratyphoid fevers**

002.0 Typhoid fever
Typhoid (fever) (infection) [any site]

002.1 Paratyphoid fever A

002.2 Paratyphoid fever B

002.3 Paratyphoid fever C

❑ **002.9 Paratyphoid fever, unspecified**

● **003 Other salmonella infections**

Includes: infection or food poisoning by Salmonella [any serotype]

003.0 Salmonella gastroenteritis
Salmonellosis

003.1 Salmonella septicemia

● **003.2 Localized salmonella infections**

❑ **003.20 Localized salmonella infection, unspecified**

003.21 Salmonella meningitis

003.22 Salmonella pneumonia

003.23 Salmonella arthritis

003.24 Salmonella osteomyelitis

❑ **003.29 Other**

❑ **003.8 Other specified salmonella infections**

❑ **003.9 Salmonella infection, unspecified**

● **004 Shigellosis**

Includes: bacillary dysentery

004.0 Shigella dysenteriae
Infection by group A Shigella (Schmitz) (Shiga)

004.1 Shigella flexneri
Infection by group B Shigella

004.2 Shigella boydii
Infection by group C Shigella

004.3 Shigella sonnei
Infection by group D Shigella

❑ **004.8 Other specified shigella infections**

❑ **004.9 Shigellosis, unspecified**

● **005 Other food poisoning (bacterial)**

Excludes *salmonella infections (003.0–003.9)*
toxic effect of:
food contaminants (989.7)
noxious foodstuffs (988.0–988.9)

005.0 Staphylococcal food poisoning
Staphylococcal toxemia specified as due to food

005.1 Botulism
Food poisoning due to Clostridium botulinum

005.2 Food poisoning due to Clostridium perfringens [C. welchii]
Enteritis necroticans

005.3 **Food poisoning due to other Clostridia**

005.4 **Food poisoning due to Vibrio parahaemolyticus**

● 005.8 **Other bacterial food poisoning**

Excludes *salmonella food poisoning (003.0–003.9)*

005.81 **Food poisoning due to Vibrio vulnificus**

❑ 005.89 **Other bacterial food poisoning**
Food poisoning due to Bacillus cereus

❑ 005.9 **Food poisoning, unspecified**

● 006 **Amebiasis**

Includes: infection due to Entamoeba histolytica

Excludes *amebiasis due to organisms other than Entamoeba histolytica (007.8)*

006.0 **Acute amebic dysentery without mention of abscess**
Acute amebiasis

006.1 **Chronic intestinal amebiasis without mention of abscess**
Chronic:
amebiasis
amebic dysentery

006.2 **Amebic nondysenteric colitis**

006.3 **Amebic liver abscess**
Hepatic amebiasis

006.4 **Amebic lung abscess**
Amebic abscess of lung (and liver)

006.5 **Amebic brain abscess**
Amebic abscess of brain (and liver) (and lung)

006.6 **Amebic skin ulceration**
Cutaneous amebiasis

❑ 006.8 **Amebic infection of other sites**
Amebic:
appendicitis
balanitis
Ameboma

Excludes *specific infections by free-living amebae (136.2)*

❑ 006.9 **Amebiasis, unspecified**
Amebiasis NOS

● 007 **Other protozoal intestinal diseases**

Includes: protozoal:
colitis
diarrhea
dysentery

007.0 **Balantidiasis**
Infection by Balantidium coli

007.1 **Giardiasis**
Infection by Giardia lamblia
Lambliasis

007.2 **Coccidiosis**
Infection by Isospora belli and Isospora hominis
Isosporiasis

007.3 **Intestinal trichomoniasis**

007.4 **Cryptosporidiosis**

007.5 **Cyclosporiasis**

❑ 007.8 **Other specified protozoal intestinal diseases**
Amebiasis due to organisms other than Entamoeba histolytica

❑ 007.9 **Unspecified protozoal intestinal disease**
Flagellate diarrhea
Protozoal dysentery NOS

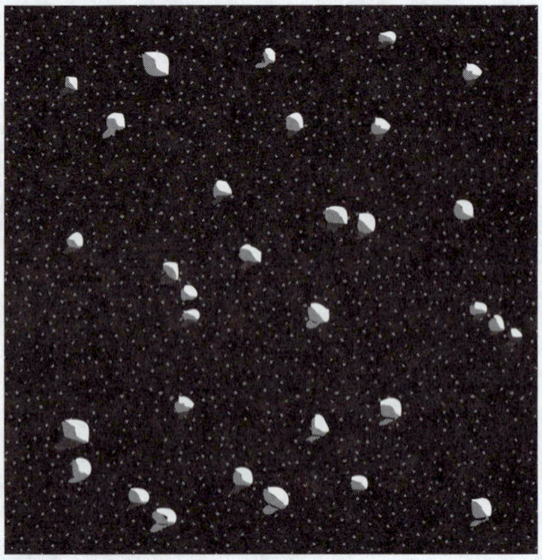

Figure 1-1 *E. coli* particles.

Item 1-1 *Escherichia coli [E. coli]* is a gram-negative bacterium found in the intestinal tracts of humans and animals and is usually nonpathogenic. Pathogenic strains can cause diarrhea or pyogenic (pus-producing) infections.

● 008 **Intestinal infections due to other organisms**

Includes: any condition classifiable to 009.0–009.3 with mention of the responsible organisms

Excludes *food poisoning by these organisms (005.0–005.9)*

● 008.0 **Escherichia coli [E. coli]**

❑ 008.00 **E. coli, unspecified**
E. coli enteritis NOS

008.01 **Enteropathogenic E. coli**

008.02 **Enterotoxigenic E. coli**

008.03 **Enteroinvasive E. coli**

008.04 **Enterohemorrhagic E. coli**

❑ 008.09 **Other intestinal E. coli infections**

008.1 **Arizona group of paracolon bacilli**

008.2 **Aerobacter aerogenes**
Enterobacter aerogenes

008.3 **Proteus (mirabilis) (morganii)**

● 008.4 **Other specified bacteria**

008.41 **Staphylococcus**
Staphylococcal enterocolitis

008.42 **Pseudomonas**

008.43 **Campylobacter**

008.44 **Yersinia enterocolitica**

008.45 **Clostridium difficile**
Pseudomembranous colitis

❑ 008.46 **Other anaerobes**
Anaerobic enteritis NOS
Bacteroides (fragilis)
Gram-negative anaerobes

❑ 008.47 **Other gram-negative bacteria**
Gram-negative enteritis NOS

Excludes *gram-negative anaerobes (008.46)*

❑ 008.49 **Other**

❑ 008.5 **Bacterial enteritis, unspecified**

● **008.6 Enteritis due to specified virus**

008.61 Rotavirus

008.62 Adenovirus

008.63 Norwalk virus
Norwalk-like agent

❑ **008.64 Other small round viruses [SRVs]**
Small round virus NOS

008.65 Calcivirus

008.66 Astrovirus

008.67 Enterovirus NEC
Coxsackie virus
Echovirus

Excludes *poliovirus (045.0–045.9)*

❑ **008.69 Other viral enteritis**
Torovirus

❑ **008.8 Other organism, not elsewhere classified**
Viral:
enteritis NOS
gastroenteritis

Excludes *influenza with involvement of gastrointestinal tract (487.8)*

● **009 Ill-defined intestinal infections**

Excludes *diarrheal disease or intestinal infection due to specified organism (001.0–008.8)*
diarrhea following gastrointestinal surgery (564.4)
intestinal malabsorption (579.0–579.9)
ischemic enteritis (557.0–557.9)
other noninfectious gastroenteritis and colitis (558.1–558.9)
regional enteritis (555.0–555.9)
ulcerative colitis (556)

009.0 Infectious colitis, enteritis, and gastroenteritis
Colitis (septic)
Dysentery:
NOS
catarrhal
hemorrhagic
Enteritis (septic)
Gastroenteritis (septic)

009.1 Colitis, enteritis, and gastroenteritis of presumed infectious origin

Excludes *colitis NOS (558.9)*
enteritis NOS (558.9)
gastroenteritis NOS (558.9)

009.2 Infectious diarrhea
Diarrhea:
dysenteric
epidemic
Infectious diarrheal disease NOS

009.3 Diarrhea of presumed infectious origin

Excludes *diarrhea NOS (787.91)*

Item 1-2 Tuberculosis is caused by the *Mycobacterium tuberculosis* organism. The first tuberculosis infection is called the primary infection. A Ghon lesion is the initial lesion. A secondary lesion occurs when the tubercle bacilli are carried to other areas.

TUBERCULOSIS (010–018)

Includes: infection by Mycobacterium tuberculosis (human) (bovine)

Excludes *congenital tuberculosis (771.2)*
late effects of tuberculosis (137.0–137.4)

The following fifth-digit subclassification is for use with categories 010–018:

❑ **0 unspecified**
1 bacteriological or histological examination not done
2 bacteriological or histological examination unknown (at present)
3 tubercle bacilli found (in sputum) by microscopy
4 tubercle bacilli not found (in sputum) by microscopy, but found by bacterial culture
5 tubercle bacilli not found by bacteriological examination, but tuberculosis confirmed histologically
6 tubercle bacilli not found by bacteriological or histological examination, but tuberculosis confirmed by other methods [inoculation of animals]

● **010 Primary tuberculous infection**

Requires fifth digit. See beginning of section 010–018 for codes and definitions.

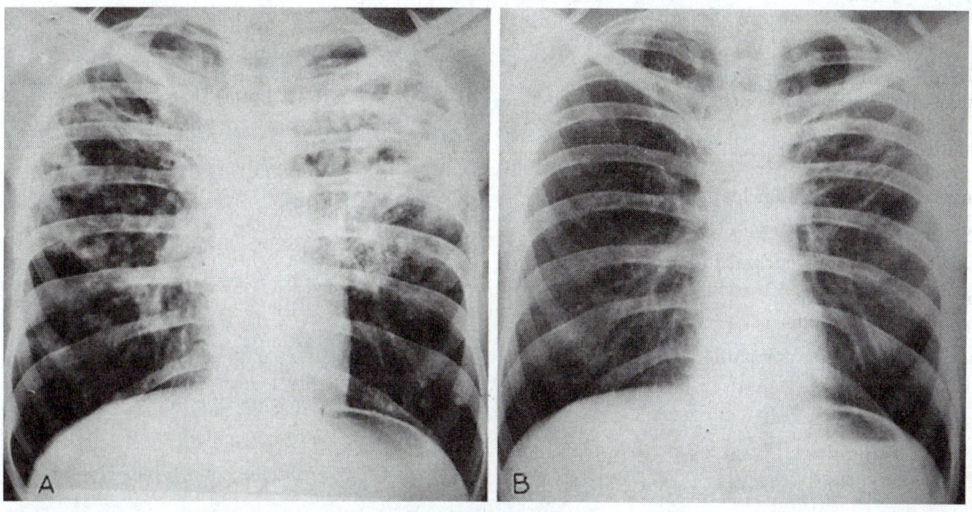

Figure 1-2 Far advanced bilateral pulmonary tuberculosis before and after 8 months of treatment with streptomycin, PAS, and isoniazid. (From Hinshaw HC, Garland LH: Diseases of the Chest, 2nd ed. Philadelphia, WB Saunders, 1963, p. 538.)

● 010.0 Primary tuberculous infection

Excludes *nonspecific reaction to tuberculin skin test without active tuberculosis (795.5)*
positive PPD (795.5)
positive tuberculin skin test without active tuberculosis (795.5)

● 010.1 Tuberculous pleurisy in primary progressive tuberculosis

● ❑ 010.8 Other primary progressive tuberculosis

Excludes *tuberculous erythema nodosum (017.1)*

● ❑ 010.9 Primary tuberculous infection, unspecified

● 011 Pulmonary tuberculosis

Requires fifth digit. See beginning of section 010–018 for codes and definitions.

Use additional code to identify any associated silicosis (502)

● 011.0 Tuberculosis of lung, infiltrative

● 011.1 Tuberculosis of lung, nodular

● 011.2 Tuberculosis of lung with cavitation

● 011.3 Tuberculosis of bronchus

Excludes *isolated bronchial tuberculosis (012.2)*

● 011.4 Tuberculous fibrosis of lung

● 011.5 Tuberculous bronchiectasis

● 011.6 Tuberculous pneumonia [any form]

● 011.7 Tuberculous pneumothorax

● ❑ 011.8 Other specified pulmonary tuberculosis

● ❑ 011.9 Pulmonary tuberculosis, unspecified
Respiratory tuberculosis NOS
Tuberculosis of lung NOS

● 012 Other respiratory tuberculosis

Requires fifth digit. See beginning of section 010–018 for codes and definitions.

Excludes *respiratory tuberculosis, unspecified (011.9)*

● 012.0 Tuberculous pleurisy
Tuberculosis of pleura
Tuberculous empyema
Tuberculous hydrothorax

Excludes *pleurisy with effusion without mention of cause (511.9)*
tuberculous pleurisy in primary progressive tuberculosis (010.1)

● 012.1 Tuberculosis of intrathoracic lymph nodes
Tuberculosis of lymph nodes:
hilar
mediastinal
tracheobronchial
Tuberculous tracheobronchial adenopathy

Excludes *that specified as primary (010.0–010.9)*

● 012.2 Isolated tracheal or bronchial tuberculosis

● 012.3 Tuberculous laryngitis
Tuberculosis of glottis

● ❑ 012.8 Other specified respiratory tuberculosis
Tuberculosis of:
mediastinum
nasopharynx
nose (septum)
sinus [any nasal]

● 013 Tuberculosis of meninges and central nervous system

Requires fifth digit. See beginning of section 010–018 for codes and definitions.

● 013.0 Tuberculous meningitis
Tuberculosis of meninges (cerebral) (spinal)
Tuberculous:
leptomeningitis
meningoencephalitis

Excludes *tuberculoma of meninges (013.1)*

● 013.1 Tuberculoma of meninges

● 013.2 Tuberculoma of brain
Tuberculosis of brain (current disease)

● 013.3 Tuberculous abscess of brain

● 013.4 Tuberculoma of spinal cord

● 013.5 Tuberculous abscess of spinal cord

● 013.6 Tuberculous encephalitis or myelitis

● ❑ 013.8 Other specified tuberculosis of central nervous system

● ❑ 013.9 Unspecified tuberculosis of central nervous system
Tuberculosis of central nervous system NOS

● 014 Tuberculosis of intestines, peritoneum, and mesenteric glands

Requires fifth digit. See beginning of section 010–018 for codes and definitions.

● 014.0 Tuberculous peritonitis
Tuberculous ascites

● ❑ 014.8 Other
Tuberculosis (of):
anus
intestine (large) (small)
mesenteric glands
rectum
retroperitoneal (lymph nodes)
Tuberculous enteritis

● 015 Tuberculosis of bones and joints

Requires fifth digit. See beginning of section 010–018 for codes and definitions.

Use additional code to identify manifestation, as:
tuberculous:
arthropathy (711.4)
necrosis of bone (730.8)
osteitis (730.8)
osteomyelitis (730.8)
synovitis (727.01)
tenosynovitis (727.01)

● 015.0 Vertebral column
Pott's disease
Use additional code to identify manifestation, as:
curvature of spine [Pott's] (737.4)
kyphosis (737.4)
spondylitis (720.81)

● 015.1 Hip

● 015.2 Knee

● 015.5 Limb bones
Tuberculous dactylitis

● 015.6 Mastoid
Tuberculous mastoiditis

● ❑ 015.7 Other specified bone

● ❑ 015.8 Other specified joint

● ❑ 015.9 Tuberculosis of unspecified bones and joints

● 016 Tuberculosis of genitourinary system

Requires fifth digit. See beginning of section 010–018 for codes and definitions.

016.0 Kidney
Renal tuberculosis

Use additional code to identify manifestation, as:
tuberculous:
nephropathy (583.81)
pyelitis (590.81)
pyelonephritis (590.81)

016.1 Bladder

016.2 Ureter

016.3 Other urinary organs

016.4 Epididymis

016.5 Other male genital organs
Use additional code to identify manifestation, as:
tuberculosis of:
prostate (601.4)
seminal vesicle (608.81)
testis (608.81)

016.6 Tuberculous oophoritis and salpingitis

016.7 Other female genital organs
Tuberculous:
cervicitis
endometritis

016.9 Genitourinary tuberculosis, unspecified

017 Tuberculosis of other organs

Requires fifth digit. See beginning of section 010–018 for codes and definitions.

017.0 Skin and subcutaneous cellular tissue

Lupus:	Tuberculosis:
exedens	colliquativa
vulgaris	cutis
Scrofuloderma	lichenoides
	papulonecrotica
	verrucosa cutis

Excludes *lupus erythematosus (695.4)*
disseminated (710.0)
lupus NOS (710.0)
nonspecific reaction to tuberculin skin test without active tuberculosis (795.5)
positive PPD (795.5)
positive tuberculin skin test without active tuberculosis (795.5)

017.1 Erythema nodosum with hypersensitivity reaction in tuberculosis
Bazin's disease
Erythema:
induratum
nodosum, tuberculous
Tuberculosis indurativa

Excludes *erythema nodosum NOS (695.2)*

017.2 Peripheral lymph nodes
Scrofula
Scrofulous abscess
Tuberculous adenitis

Excludes *tuberculosis of lymph nodes:*
bronchial and mediastinal (012.1)
mesenteric and retroperitoneal (014.8)
tuberculous tracheobronchial adenopathy (012.1)

017.3 Eye
Use additional code to identify manifestation, as:
tuberculous:
chorioretinitis, disseminated (363.13)
episcleritis (379.09)
interstitial keratitis (370.59)
iridocyclitis, chronic (364.11)
keratoconjunctivitis (phlyctenular) (370.31)

017.4 Ear
Tuberculosis of ear
Tuberculous otitis media

Excludes *tuberculous mastoiditis (015.6)*

017.5 Thyroid gland

017.6 Adrenal glands
Addison's disease, tuberculous

017.7 Spleen

017.8 Esophagus

017.9 Other specified organs
Use additional code to identify manifestation, as:
tuberculosis of:
endocardium [any valve] (424.91)
myocardium (422.0)
pericardium (420.0)

ICD-9-CM 001-099 Vol. 1

018 Miliary tuberculosis

Requires fifth digit. See beginning of section 010–018 for codes and definitions.

Includes: tuberculosis:
disseminated
generalized
miliary, whether of a single specified site, multiple sites, or unspecified site
polyserositis

018.0 Acute miliary tuberculosis

018.8 Other specified miliary tuberculosis

018.9 Miliary tuberculosis, unspecified

ZOONOTIC BACTERIAL DISEASES (020–027)

020 Plague

Includes: infection by Yersinia [Pasteurella] pestis

020.0 Bubonic

020.1 Cellulocutaneous

020.2 Septicemic

020.3 Primary pneumonic

020.4 Secondary pneumonic

020.5 Pneumonic, unspecified

020.8 Other specified types of plague
Abortive plague
Ambulatory plague
Pestis minor

020.9 Plague, unspecified

021 Tularemia

Includes: deerfly fever
infection by Francisella [Pasteurella] tularensis
rabbit fever

021.0 Ulceroglandular tularemia

021.1 Enteric tularemia
Tularemia:
cryptogenic
intestinal
typhoidal

021.2 Pulmonary tularemia
Bronchopneumonic tularemia

021.3 Oculoglandular tularemia

021.8 Other specified tularemia
Tularemia:
generalized or disseminated
glandular

021.9 Unspecified tularemia

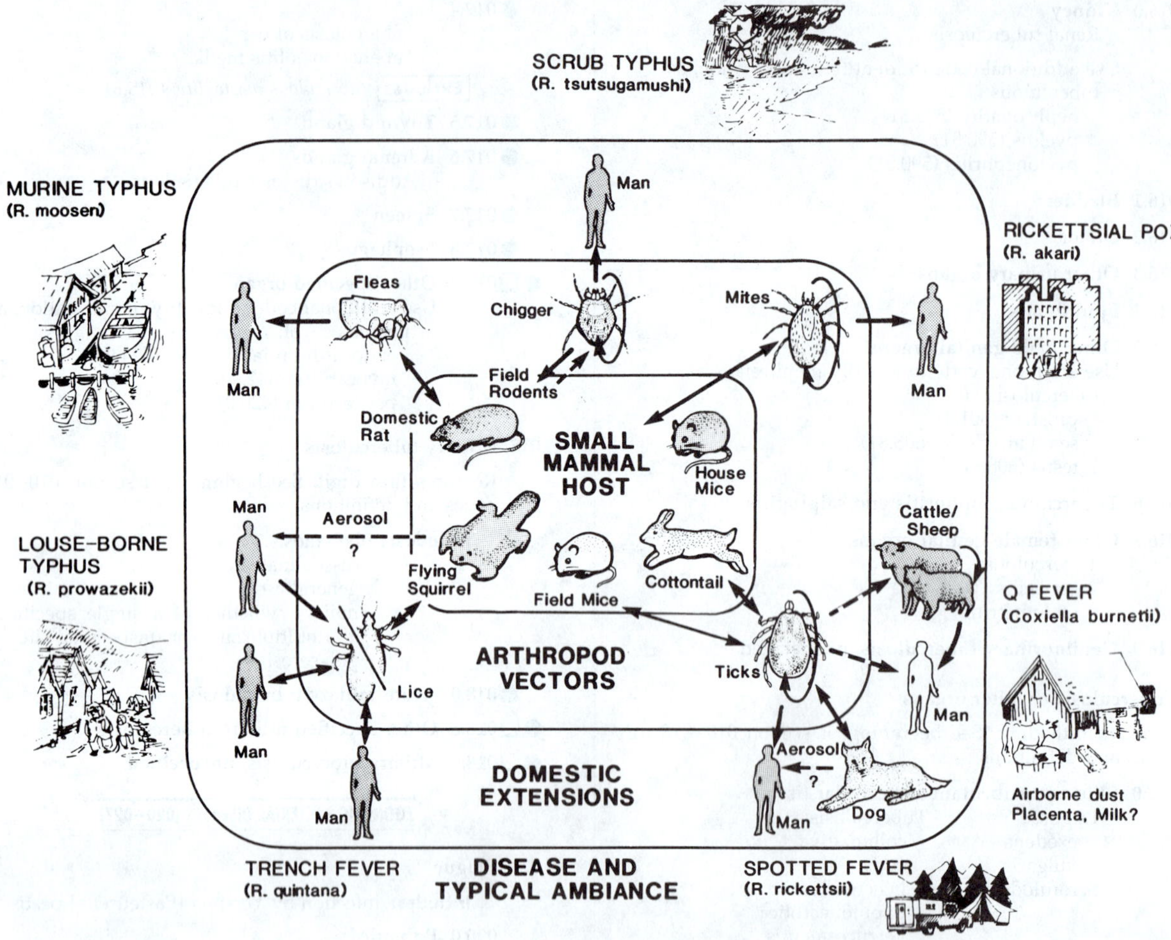

Figure 1–3 Schematic summary of some major interactions between rickettsial organisms and their small animal hosts and arthropod vectors, the participation of domestic animals, and examples of the typical ambiance under which each rickettsial infection is contacted by humans. (From Strickland GT: Hunter's Tropical Medicine, 7th ed. Philadelphia, WB Saunders, 1991, p. 261. Courtesy of Dr. J. K. Frenkel, University of Kansas Medical Center, Kansas City, KS.)

● **022 Anthrax**

022.0 Cutaneous anthrax
Malignant pustule

022.1 Pulmonary anthrax
Respiratory anthrax
Wool-sorters' disease

022.2 Gastrointestinal anthrax

022.3 Anthrax septicemia

❑ **022.8 Other specified manifestations of anthrax**

❑ **022.9 Anthrax, unspecified**

● **023 Brucellosis**

Includes: fever:
Malta
Mediterranean
undulant

023.0 Brucella melitensis

023.1 Brucella abortus

023.2 Brucella suis

023.3 Brucella canis

❑ **023.8 Other brucellosis**
Infection by more than one organism

❑ **023.9 Brucellosis, unspecified**

024 Glanders
Infection by:
Actinobacillus mallei
Malleomyces mallei
Pseudomonas mallei
Farcy
Malleus

025 Melioidosis
Infection by:
Malleomyces pseudomallei
Pseudomonas pseudomallei
Whitmore's bacillus
Pseudoglanders

● **026 Rat-bite fever**

026.0 Spirillary fever
Rat-bite fever due to Spirillum minor [S. minus]
Sodoku

026.1 Streptobacillary fever
Epidemic arthritic erythema
Haverhill fever
Rat-bite fever due to Streptobacillus moniliformis

❑ **026.9 Unspecified rat-bite fever**

● **027 Other zoonotic bacterial diseases**

027.0 Listeriosis
Infection by Listeria monocytogenes
Septicemia by Listeria monocytogenes

Use additional code to identify manifestations, as meningitis (320.7)

Excludes *congenital listeriosis (771.2)*

027.1 Erysipelothrix infection
Erysipeloid (of Rosenbach)
Infection by Erysipelothrix insidiosa [E. rhusiopathiae]
Septicemia by Erysipelothrix insidiosa [E. rhusiopathiae]

027.2 Pasteurellosis
Pasteurella pseudotuberculosis infection by Pasteurella multocida [P. septica]
Mesenteric adenitis by Pasteurella multocida [P. septica]
Septic infection (cat bite) (dog bite) by Pasteurella multocida [P. septica]

Excludes *infection by:*
Francisella [Pasteurella] tularensis (021.0–021.9)
Yersinia [Pasteurella] pestis (020.0–020.9)

❑ **027.8 Other specified zoonotic bacterial diseases**

❑ **027.9 Unspecified zoonotic bacterial disease**

OTHER BACTERIAL DISEASES (030–041)

Excludes *bacterial venereal diseases (098.0–099.9)*
bartonellosis (088.0)

● **030 Leprosy**

Includes: Hansen's disease
infection by Mycobacterium leprae

030.0 Lepromatous [type L]
Lepromatous leprosy (macular) (diffuse) (infiltrated) (nodular) (neuritic)

030.1 Tuberculoid [type T]
Tuberculoid leprosy (macular) (maculoanesthetic) (major) (minor) (neuritic)

030.2 Indeterminate [group I]
Indeterminate [uncharacteristic] leprosy (macular) (neuritic)

030.3 Borderline [group B]
Borderline or dimorphous leprosy (infiltrated) (neuritic)

❑ **030.8 Other specified leprosy**

❑ **030.9 Leprosy, unspecified**

● **031 Diseases due to other mycobacteria**

031.0 Pulmonary
Battey disease
Infection by Mycobacterium:
avium
intracellulare [Battey bacillus]
kansasii

031.1 Cutaneous
Buruli ulcer
Infection by Mycobacterium:
marinum [M. balnei]
ulcerans

031.2 Disseminated
Disseminated mycobacterium avium-intracellulare complex (DMAC)
Mycobacterium avium-intracellulare complex (MAC) bacteremia

❑ **031.8 Other specified mycobacterial diseases**

❑ **031.9 Unspecified diseases due to mycobacteria**
Atypical mycobacterium infection NOS

● **032 Diphtheria**

Includes: infection by Corynebacterium diphtheriae

032.0 Faucial diphtheria
Membranous angina, diphtheritic

032.1 Nasopharyngeal diphtheria

032.2 Anterior nasal diphtheria

032.3 Laryngeal diphtheria
Laryngotracheitis, diphtheritic

● **032.8 Other specified diphtheria**

032.81 Conjunctival diphtheria
Pseudomembranous diphtheritic conjunctivitis

032.82 Diphtheritic myocarditis

032.83 Diphtheritic peritonitis

032.84 Diphtheritic cystitis

032.85 Cutaneous diphtheria

❑ **032.89 Other**

❑ **032.9 Diphtheria, unspecified**

● **033 Whooping cough**

Includes: pertussis

Use additional code to identify any associated pneumonia (484.3)

033.0 Bordetella pertussis [B. pertussis]

033.1 Bordetella parapertussis [B. parapertussis]

❑ **033.8 Whooping cough due to other specified organism**
Bordetella bronchiseptica [B. bronchiseptica]

❑ **033.9 Whooping cough, unspecified organism**

● **034 Streptococcal sore throat and scarlet fever**

034.0 Streptococcal sore throat
Septic:
angina
sore throat
Streptococcal:
angina
laryngitis
pharyngitis
tonsillitis

034.1 Scarlet fever
Scarlatina

Excludes *parascarlatina (057.8)*

035 Erysipelas

Excludes *postpartum or puerperal erysipelas (670)*

● **036 Meningococcal infection**

036.0 Meningococcal meningitis
Cerebrospinal fever (meningococcal)
Meningitis:
cerebrospinal
epidemic

036.1 Meningococcal encephalitis

036.2 Meningococcemia
Meningococcal septicemia

036.3 Waterhouse-Friderichsen syndrome, meningococcal
Meningococcal hemorrhagic adrenalitis
Meningococcic adrenal syndrome
Waterhouse-Friderichsen syndrome NOS

● 036.4 **Meningococcal carditis**

❑ 036.40 **Meningococcal carditis, unspecified**

036.41 **Meningococcal pericarditis**

036.42 **Meningococcal endocarditis**

036.43 **Meningococcal myocarditis**

● 036.8 **Other specified meningococcal infections**

036.81 **Meningococcal optic neuritis**

036.82 **Meningococcal arthropathy**

❑ 036.89 **Other**

❑ 036.9 **Meningococcal infection, unspecified**
Meningococcal infection NOS

037 **Tetanus**

Excludes *tetanus:*
complicating:
abortion (634–638 with .0, 639.0)
ectopic or molar pregnancy (639.0)
neonatorum (771.3)
puerperal (670)

● 038 **Septicemia**

Note: Use additional code for systemic inflammatory response syndrome (SIRS), 995.91-995.92 ◄

Excludes *bacteremia (790.7)*
septicemia (sepsis) of newborn (771.81)

038.0 **Streptococcal septicemia**

● 038.1 **Staphylococcal septicemia**

❑ 038.10 **Staphylococcal septicemia, unspecified**

038.11 **Staphylococcus aureus septicemia**

❑ 038.19 **Other staphylococcal septicemia**

038.2 **Pneumococcal septicemia [Streptococcus pneumoniae septicemia]**

038.3 **Septicemia due to anaerobes**
Septicemia due to Bacteroides

Excludes *gas gangrene (040.0)*
that due to anaerobic streptococci (038.0)

● 038.4 **Septicemia due to other gram-negative organisms**

❑ 038.40 **Gram-negative organism, unspecified**
Gram-negative septicemia NOS

038.41 **Hemophilus influenzae [H. influenzae]**

038.42 **Escherichia coli [E. coli]**

038.43 **Pseudomonas**

038.44 **Serratia**

❑ 038.49 **Other**

❑ 038.8 **Other specified septicemias**

Excludes *septicemia (due to):*
anthrax (022.3)
gonococcal (098.89)
herpetic (054.5)
meningococcal (036.2)
septicemic plague (020.2)

❑ 038.9 **Unspecified septicemia**
Septicemia NOS

Excludes *bacteremia NOS (790.7)*

● 039 **Actinomycotic infections**

Includes: actinomycotic mycetoma
infection by Actinomycetales, such as species of Actinomyces, Actinomadura, Nocardia, Streptomyces
maduromycosis (actinomycotic)
schizomycetoma (actinomycotic)

039.0 **Cutaneous**
Erythrasma
Trichomycosis axillaris

039.1 **Pulmonary**
Thoracic actinomycosis

039.2 **Abdominal**

039.3 **Cervicofacial**

039.4 **Madura foot**

Excludes *madura foot due to mycotic infection (117.4)*

❑ 039.8 **Of other specified sites**

❑ 039.9 **Of unspecified site**
Actinomycosis NOS
Maduromycosis NOS
Nocardiosis NOS

● 040 **Other bacterial diseases**

Excludes *bacteremia NOS (790.7)*
bacterial infection NOS (041.9)

040.0 **Gas gangrene**
Gas bacillus infection or gangrene
Infection by Clostridium:
histolyticum
oedematiens
perfringens [welchii]
septicum
sordellii
Malignant edema
Myonecrosis, clostridial
Myositis, clostridial

040.1 **Rhinoscleroma**

040.2 **Whipple's disease**
Intestinal lipodystrophy

040.3 **Necrobacillosis**

● 040.8 **Other specified bacterial diseases**

040.81 **Tropical pyomyositis**

040.82 **Toxic shock syndrome**

Use additional code to identify the organism

❑ 040.89 **Other**

● 041 **Bacterial infection in conditions classified elsewhere and of unspecified site**

Note: This category is provided to be used as an additional code to identify the bacterial agent in diseases classified elsewhere. This category will also be used to classify bacterial infections of unspecified nature or site.

Excludes *bacteremia NOS (790.7)*
septicemia (038.0–038.9)

● 041.0 **Streptococcus**

❑ 041.00 **Streptococcus, unspecified**

041.01 **Group A**

041.02 **Group B**

041.03 **Group C**

041.04 **Group D [Enterococcus]**

041.05 **Group G**

❑ 041.09 **Other Streptococcus**

● 041.1 **Staphylococcus**

❑ 041.10 **Staphylococcus, unspecified**

041.11 **Staphylococcus aureus**

❑ 041.19 **Other Staphylococcus**

041.2 **Pneumococcus**

041.3 **Friedländer's bacillus**
Infection by Klebsiella pneumoniae

041.4 **Escherichia coli [E. coli]**

041.5 **Hemophilus influenzae [H. influenzae]**

041.6 **Proteus (mirabilis) (morganii)**

041.7 **Pseudomonas**

● 041.8 **Other specified bacterial infections**

041.81 **Mycoplasma**
Eaton's agent
Pleuropneumonia-like organisms [PPLO]

041.82 **Bacillus fragilis**

041.83 **Clostridium perfringens**

❑ 041.84 **Other anaerobes**
Bacteroides (fragilis)
Gram-negative anaerobes

Excludes *Helicobacter pylori (041.86)*

041.85 **Other gram-negative organisms**
Aerobacter aerogenes
Gram-negative bacteria NOS
Mima polymorpha
Serratia

Excludes *gram-negative anaerobes (041.84)*

041.86 **Helicobacter pylori (H. pylori)**

❑ 041.89 **Other specified bacteria**

❑ 041.9 **Bacterial infection, unspecified**

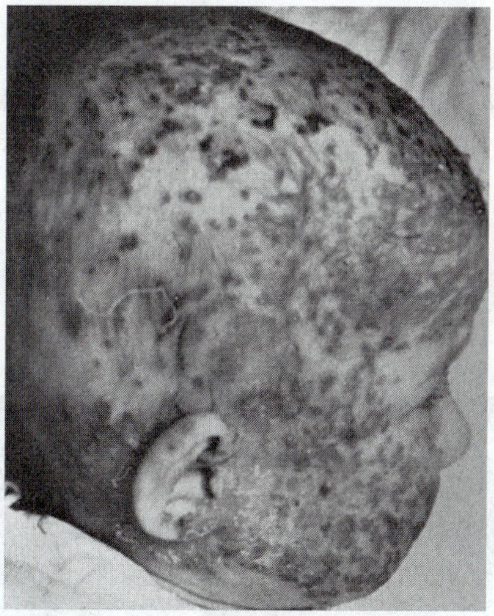

Figure 1–4 Vesicular, pustular, scabby, and necrotic lesions in Kaposi's sarcoma. (From Debre R, Celers J: Clinical Virology—The Evaluation and Management of Human Viral Infections. Philadelphia, WB Saunders, 1970, p. 460.)

Item 1–3 AIDS (acquired immune deficiency syndrome) is caused by HIV (human immunodeficiency virus). HIV affects certain white blood cells (T-4 lymphocytes) and destroys the ability of the cells to fight infections, making patients susceptible to a host of infectious diseases, e.g., *Pneumocystis carinii* pneumonia (PCP), Kaposi's sarcoma, and lymphoma. AIDS-related complex (ARC) is an early stage of AIDS in which tests for HIV are positive but the symptoms are mild.

HUMAN IMMUNODEFICIENCY VIRUS (HIV) INFECTION (042)

042 **Human immunodeficiency virus [HIV] disease**
Acquired immune deficiency syndrome
Acquired immunodeficiency syndrome
AIDS
AIDS-like syndrome
AIDS-related complex
ARC
HIV infection, symptomatic

Use additional code(s) to identify all manifestations of HIV

Use additional code to identify HIV-2 infection (079.53)

Excludes *asymptomatic HIV infection status (V08)*
exposure to HIV virus (V01.7)
nonspecific serologic evidence of HIV (795.71)

POLIOMYELITIS AND OTHER NON-ARTHROPOD-BORNE VIRAL DISEASES OF CENTRAL NERVOUS SYSTEM (045–049)

● 045 **Acute poliomyelitis**

Excludes *late effects of acute poliomyelitis (138)*

The following fifth-digit subclassification is for use with category 045:
❑ 0 **poliovirus, unspecified type**
1 **poliovirus type I**
2 **poliovirus type II**
3 **poliovirus type III**

● 045.0 **Acute paralytic poliomyelitis specified as bulbar**
Infantile paralysis (acute) specified as bulbar
Poliomyelitis (acute) (anterior) specified as bulbar
Polioencephalitis (acute) (bulbar)
Polioencephalomyelitis (acute) (anterior) (bulbar)

● ❑ 045.1 **Acute poliomyelitis with other paralysis**
Paralysis:
acute atrophic, spinal
infantile, paralytic
Poliomyelitis (acute) with paralysis except bulbar
anterior with paralysis except bulbar
epidemic with paralysis except bulbar

● 045.2 **Acute nonparalytic poliomyelitis**
Poliomyelitis (acute) specified as nonparalytic
anterior specified as nonparalytic
epidemic specified as nonparalytic

● ❑ 045.9 **Acute poliomyelitis, unspecified**
Infantile paralysis unspecified whether paralytic or nonparalytic
Poliomyelitis (acute) unspecified whether paralytic or nonparalytic
anterior unspecified whether paralytic or nonparalytic
epidemic unspecified whether paralytic or nonparalytic

● 046 **Slow virus infection of central nervous system**

046.0 **Kuru**

046.1 **Jakob-Creutzfeldt disease**
Subacute spongiform encephalopathy

046.2 **Subacute sclerosing panencephalitis**
Dawson's inclusion body encephalitis
Van Bogaert's sclerosing leukoencephalitis

046.3 **Progressive multifocal leukoencephalopathy**
Multifocal leukoencephalopathy NOS

❑ 046.8 **Other specified slow virus infection of central nervous system**

❑ 046.9 **Unspecified slow virus infection of central nervous system**

● 047 **Meningitis due to enterovirus**

Includes: meningitis:
abacterial
aseptic
viral

Excludes *meningitis due to:*
adenovirus (049.1)
arthropod-borne virus (060.0–066.9)
leptospira (100.81)
virus of:
herpes simplex (054.72)
herpes zoster (053.0)
lymphocytic choriomeningitis (049.0)
mumps (072.1)
poliomyelitis (045.0–045.9)
any other infection specifically classified elsewhere

047.0 **Coxsackie virus**

047.1 **ECHO virus**
Meningo-eruptive syndrome

❑ 047.8 **Other specified viral meningitis**

❑ 047.9 **Unspecified viral meningitis**
Viral meningitis NOS

❑ 048 **Other enterovirus diseases of central nervous system**
Boston exanthem

● 049 **Other non-arthropod-borne viral diseases of central nervous system**

Excludes *late effects of viral encephalitis (139.0)*

049.0 **Lymphocytic choriomeningitis**
Lymphocytic:
meningitis (serous) (benign)
meningoencephalitis (serous) (benign)

049.1 **Meningitis due to adenovirus**

❑ 049.8 **Other specified non-arthropod-borne viral diseases of central nervous system**
Encephalitis:
acute:
inclusion body
necrotizing
epidemic
lethargica
Rio Bravo
von Economo's disease

❑ 049.9 **Unspecified non-arthropod-borne viral diseases of central nervous system**
Viral encephalitis NOS

VIRAL DISEASES ACCOMPANIED BY EXANTHEM (050–057)

Excludes *arthropod-borne viral diseases (060.0–066.9)*
Boston exanthem (048)

● 050 **Smallpox**

050.0 **Variola major**
Hemorrhagic (pustular) smallpox
Malignant smallpox
Purpura variolosa

050.1 **Alastrim**
Variola minor

050.2 **Modified smallpox**
Varioloid

❑ 050.9 **Smallpox, unspecified**

● 051 **Cowpox and paravaccinia**

051.0 **Cowpox**
Vaccinia not from vaccination

Excludes *vaccinia (generalized) (from vaccination) (999.0)*

051.1 **Pseudocowpox**
Milkers' node

051.2 **Contagious pustular dermatitis**
Ecthyma contagiosum
Orf

❑ 051.9 **Paravaccinia, unspecified**

● 052 **Chickenpox**

052.0 **Postvaricella encephalitis**
Postchickenpox encephalitis

052.1 **Varicella (hemorrhagic) pneumonitis**

❑ 052.7 **With other specified complications**

❑ 052.8 **With unspecified complication**

052.9 **Varicella without mention of complication**
Chickenpox NOS
Varicella NOS

● 053 **Herpes zoster**

Includes: shingles
zona

053.0 **With meningitis**

● 053.1 **With other nervous system complications**

❑ 053.10 **With unspecified nervous system complication**

053.11 **Geniculate herpes zoster**
Herpetic geniculate ganglionitis

053.12 **Postherpetic trigeminal neuralgia**

053.13 **Postherpetic polyneuropathy**

❑ 053.19 **Other**

● 053.2 **With ophthalmic complications**

053.20 **Herpes zoster dermatitis of eyelid**
Herpes zoster ophthalmicus

053.21 **Herpes zoster keratoconjunctivitis**

053.22 **Herpes zoster iridocyclitis**

❑ 053.29 **Other**

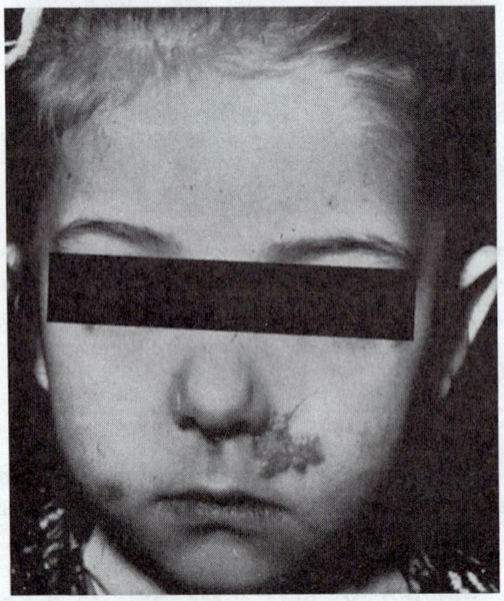

Figure 1–5 Grouped outbursts of herpes vesicles on the face. (From Debre R, Celers J: Clinical Virology—The Evaluation and Management of Human Viral Infections. Philadelphia, WB Saunders, 1970, p. 460.)

Item 1-4 Herpes is a viral disease for which there is no cure. There are two types of the herpes simplex virus: Type I causes cold sores or fever blisters and Type II causes genital herpes. The virus can be spread from a sore on the lips to the genitals or from the genitals to the lips.

● **053.7 With other specified complications**
053.71 Otitis externa due to herpes zoster
❑ **053.79 Other**
❑ **053.8 With unspecified complication**
053.9 Herpes zoster without mention of complication
Herpes zoster NOS

● **054 Herpes simplex**
Excludes *congenital herpes simplex (771.2)*
054.0 Eczema herpeticum
Kaposi's varicelliform eruption
● **054.1 Genital herpes**
❑ **054.10 Genital herpes, unspecified**
Herpes progenitalis
054.11 Herpetic vulvovaginitis
054.12 Herpetic ulceration of vulva
054.13 Herpetic infection of penis
❑ **054.19 Other**
054.2 Herpetic gingivostomatitis
054.3 Herpetic meningoencephalitis
Herpes encephalitis
Simian B disease
● **054.4 With ophthalmic complications**
❑ **054.40 With unspecified ophthalmic complication**
054.41 Herpes simplex dermatitis of eyelid
054.42 Dendritic keratitis
054.43 Herpes simplex disciform keratitis
054.44 Herpes simplex iridocyclitis
❑ **054.49 Other**
054.5 Herpetic septicemia
054.6 Herpetic whitlow
Herpetic felon
● **054.7 With other specified complications**
054.71 Visceral herpes simplex
054.72 Herpes simplex meningitis
054.73 Herpes simplex otitis externa
❑ **054.79 Other**
❑ **054.8 With unspecified complication**
054.9 Herpes simplex without mention of complication

● **055 Measles**
Includes: morbilli
rubeola
055.0 Postmeasles encephalitis
055.1 Postmeasles pneumonia
055.2 Postmeasles otitis media
● **055.7 With other specified complications**
055.71 Measles keratoconjunctivitis
Measles keratitis
❑ **055.79 Other**
❑ **055.8 With unspecified complication**
055.9 Measles without mention of complication

● **056 Rubella**
Includes: German measles
Excludes *congenital rubella (771.0)*
● **056.0 With neurological complications**
❑ **056.00 With unspecified neurological complication**
056.01 Encephalomyelitis due to rubella
Encephalitis due to rubella
Meningoencephalitis due to rubella
❑ **056.09 Other**
● **056.7 With other specified complications**
056.71 Arthritis due to rubella
❑ **056.79 Other**
❑ **056.8 With unspecified complications**
056.9 Rubella without mention of complication

● **057 Other viral exanthemata**
057.0 Erythema infectiosum [fifth disease]
❑ **057.8 Other specified viral exanthemata**
Dukes (-Filatow) disease
Exanthema subitum [sixth disease]
Fourth disease
Parascarlatina
Pseudoscarlatina
Roseola infantum
❑ **057.9 Viral exanthem, unspecified**

ARTHROPOD-BORNE VIRAL DISEASES (060–066)

Use additional code to identify any associated meningitis (321.2)

Excludes *late effects of viral encephalitis (139.0)*

● **060 Yellow fever**
060.0 Sylvatic
Yellow fever:
jungle
sylvan
060.1 Urban
❑ **060.9 Yellow fever, unspecified**

061 Dengue
Breakbone fever
Excludes *hemorrhagic fever caused by dengue virus (065.4)*

● **062 Mosquito-borne viral encephalitis**
062.0 Japanese encephalitis
Japanese B encephalitis
062.1 Western equine encephalitis
062.2 Eastern equine encephalitis
Excludes *Venezuelan equine encephalitis (066.2)*
062.3 St. Louis encephalitis
062.4 Australian encephalitis
Australian arboencephalitis
Australian X disease
Murray Valley encephalitis
062.5 California virus encephalitis
Encephalitis:
California
La Crosse
Tahyna fever

ICD-9-CM 001-099 Vol. 1

❑ **062.8 Other specified mosquito-borne viral encephalitis**
Encephalitis by Ilheus virus
Excludes *West Nile virus (066.4)*

❑ **062.9 Mosquito-borne viral encephalitis, unspecified**

● **063 Tick-borne viral encephalitis**

Includes: diphasic meningoencephalitis

063.0 Russian spring-summer [taiga] encephalitis

063.1 Louping ill

063.2 Central European encephalitis

❑ **063.8 Other specified tick-borne viral encephalitis**
Langat encephalitis
Powassan encephalitis

❑ **063.9 Tick-borne viral encephalitis, unspecified**

064 Viral encephalitis transmitted by other and unspecified arthropods
Arthropod-borne viral encephalitis, vector unknown
Negishi virus encephalitis
Excludes *viral encephalitis NOS (049.9)*

● **065 Arthropod-borne hemorrhagic fever**

065.0 Crimean hemorrhagic fever [CHF Congo virus]
Central Asian hemorrhagic fever

065.1 Omsk hemorrhagic fever

065.2 Kyasanur Forest disease

❑ **065.3 Other tick-borne hemorrhagic fever**

065.4 Mosquito-borne hemorrhagic fever
Chikungunya hemorrhagic fever
Dengue hemorrhagic fever
Excludes *Chikungunya fever (066.3)*
dengue (061)
yellow fever (060.0–060.9)

❑ **065.8 Other specified arthropod-borne hemorrhagic fever**
Mite-borne hemorrhagic fever

❑ **065.9 Arthropod-borne hemorrhagic fever, unspecified**
Arbovirus hemorrhagic fever NOS

● **066 Other arthropod-borne viral diseases**

066.0 Phlebotomus fever
Changuinola fever
Sandfly fever

066.1 Tick-borne fever
Nairobi sheep disease
Tick fever:
American mountain
Colorado
Kemerovo
Quaranfil

066.2 Venezuelan equine fever
Venezuelan equine encephalitis

❑ **066.3 Other mosquito-borne fever**
Fever (viral):
Bunyamwera
Bwamba
Chikungunya
Guama
Mayaro
Mucambo
O' Nyong-Nyong
Fever (viral):
Oropouche
Pixuna
Rift valley
Ross river
Wesselsbron
Zika
Excludes *dengue (061)*
yellow fever (060.0–060.9)

❑ **066.4 West Nile fever**
West Nile encephalitis
West Nile encephalomyelitis
West Nile virus

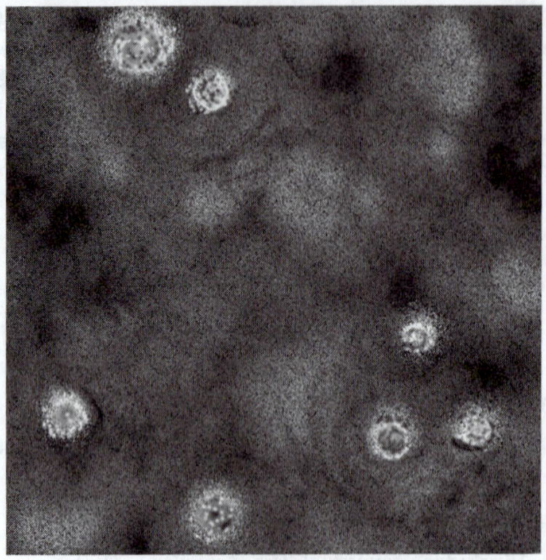

Figure 1–6 Hepatitis B virions (Dane particles).

Item 1–5 Hepatitis A (HAV) was formerly called epidemic, infectious, short-incubation, or acute catarrhal jaundice hepatitis. The primary transmission mode is the oral–fecal route.

Item 1–6 Hepatitis B (HBV) was formerly called long-incubation period, serum, or homologous serum hepatitis. Transmission modes are through body fluids and from mother to neonate.

Item 1–7 Hepatitis C, caused by the hepatitis C virus, is primarily transfusion associated.

Item 1–8 Hepatitis D, also called delta hepatitis, is caused by the hepatitis D virus in patients formerly or currently infected with hepatitis B.

Item 1–9 Hepatitis E is also called enterically transmitted non-A, non-B hepatitis. The primary transmission mode is the oral–fecal route, usually through contaminated water.

❑ **066.8 Other specified arthropod-borne viral diseases**
Chandipura fever
Piry fever

❑ **066.9 Arthropod-borne viral disease, unspecified**
Arbovirus infection NOS

OTHER DISEASES DUE TO VIRUSES AND CHLAMYDIAE (070–079)

● **070 Viral hepatitis**

Includes: viral hepatitis (acute) (chronic)
Excludes *cytomegalic inclusion virus hepatitis (078.5)*

The following fifth-digit subclassification is for use with categories 070.2 and 070.3:

❑ **0 acute or unspecified, without mention of hepatitis delta**
❑ **1 acute or unspecified, with hepatitis delta**
2 chronic, without mention of hepatitis delta
3 chronic, with hepatitis delta

070.0 Viral hepatitis A with hepatic coma

070.1 Viral hepatitis A without mention of hepatic coma
Infectious hepatitis

● **070.2 Viral hepatitis B with hepatic coma**

● **070.3 Viral hepatitis B without mention of hepatic coma**
Serum hepatitis

● **070.4 Other specified viral hepatitis with hepatic coma**

❑ **070.41 Acute or unspecified hepatitis C with hepatic coma**

070.42 Hepatitis delta without mention of active hepatitis B disease with hepatic coma
Hepatitis delta with hepatitis B carrier state

070.43 Hepatitis E with hepatic coma

070.44 Chronic hepatitis C with hepatic coma

❑ **070.49 Other specified viral hepatitis with hepatic coma**

● **070.5 Other specified viral hepatitis without mention of hepatic coma**

❑ **070.51 Acute or unspecified hepatitis C without mention of hepatic coma**

070.52 Hepatitis delta without mention of active hepatitis B disease or hepatic coma

070.53 Hepatitis E without mention of hepatic coma

070.54 Chronic hepatitis C without mention of hepatic coma

❑ **070.59 Other specified viral hepatitis without mention of hepatic coma**

❑ **070.6 Unspecified viral hepatitis with hepatic coma**

❑ **070.9 Unspecified viral hepatitis without mention of hepatic coma**
Viral hepatitis NOS

071 Rabies
Hydrophobia
Lyssa

● **072 Mumps**

072.0 Mumps orchitis

072.1 Mumps meningitis

072.2 Mumps encephalitis
Mumps meningoencephalitis

072.3 Mumps pancreatitis

● **072.7 Mumps with other specified complications**

072.71 Mumps hepatitis

072.72 Mumps polyneuropathy

❑ **072.79 Other**

❑ **072.8 Mumps with unspecified complication**

❑ **072.9 Mumps without mention of complication**
Epidemic parotitis
Infectious parotitis

● **073 Ornithosis**

Includes: parrot fever
psittacosis

073.0 With pneumonia
Lobular pneumonitis due to ornithosis

❑ **073.7 With other specified complications**

❑ **073.8 With unspecified complication**

❑ **073.9 Ornithosis, unspecified**

● **074 Specific diseases due to Coxsackie virus**

Excludes *Coxsackie virus:*
infection NOS (079.2)
meningitis (047.0)

074.0 Herpangina
Vesicular pharyngitis

074.1 Epidemic pleurodynia
Bornholm disease
Devil's grip
Epidemic:
myalgia
myositis

● **074.2 Coxsackie carditis**

❑ **074.20 Coxsackie carditis, unspecified**

074.21 Coxsackie pericarditis

074.22 Coxsackie endocarditis

074.23 Coxsackie myocarditis
Aseptic myocarditis of newborn

074.3 Hand, foot, and mouth disease
Vesicular stomatitis and exanthem

❑ **074.8 Other specified diseases due to Coxsackie virus**
Acute lymphonodular pharyngitis

075 Infectious mononucleosis
Glandular fever
Monocytic angina
Pfeiffer's disease

● **076 Trachoma**

Excludes *late effect of trachoma (139.1)*

076.0 Initial stage
Trachoma dubium

076.1 Active stage
Granular conjunctivitis (trachomatous)
Trachomatous:
follicular conjunctivitis
pannus

❑ **076.9 Trachoma, unspecified**
Trachoma NOS

● **077 Other diseases of conjunctiva due to viruses and Chlamydiae**

Excludes *ophthalmic complications of viral diseases classified elsewhere*

077.0 Inclusion conjunctivitis
Paratrachoma
Swimming pool conjunctivitis

Excludes *inclusion blennorrhea (neonatal) (771.6)*

077.1 Epidemic keratoconjunctivitis
Shipyard eye

077.2 Pharyngoconjunctival fever
Viral pharyngoconjunctivitis

❑ **077.3 Other adenoviral conjunctivitis**
Acute adenoviral follicular conjunctivitis

077.4 Epidemic hemorrhagic conjunctivitis
Apollo:
conjunctivitis
disease
Conjunctivitis due to enterovirus type 70
Hemorrhagic conjunctivitis (acute) (epidemic)

❑077.8 **Other viral conjunctivitis**
Newcastle conjunctivitis

● 077.9 **Unspecified diseases of conjunctiva due to viruses and Chlamydiae**

❑077.98 **Due to Chlamydiae**

❑077.99 **Due to viruses**
Viral conjunctivitis NOS

● 078 **Other diseases due to viruses and Chlamydiae**

Excludes *viral infection NOS (079.0–079.9)*
viremia NOS (790.8)

078.0 **Molluscum contagiosum**

● 078.1 **Viral warts**
Viral warts due to human papillomavirus

❑078.10 **Viral warts, unspecified**
Condyloma NOS
Verruca NOS:
NOS
Vulgaris
Warts (infectious)

078.11 **Condyloma acuminatum**

❑078.19 **Other specified viral warts**
Genital warts NOS
Verruca
plana
plantaris

078.2 **Sweating fever**
Miliary fever
Sweating disease

078.3 **Cat-scratch disease**
Benign lymphoreticulosis (of inoculation)
Cat-scratch fever

078.4 **Foot and mouth disease**
Aphthous fever
Epizootic:
aphthae
stomatitis

078.5 **Cytomegaloviral disease**
Cytomegalic inclusion disease
Salivary gland virus disease

Use additional code to identify manifestation, as:
cytomegalic inclusion virus:
hepatitis (573.1)
pneumonia (484.1)

Excludes *congenital cytomegalovirus infection (771.1)*

078.6 **Hemorrhagic nephrosonephritis**
Hemorrhagic fever:
epidemic
Korean
Russian with renal syndrome

078.7 **Arenaviral hemorrhagic fever**
Hemorrhagic fever:
Argentine
Bolivian
Junin virus
Machupo virus

● 078.8 **Other specified diseases due to viruses and Chlamydiae**

Excludes *epidemic diarrhea (009.2)*
lymphogranuloma venereum (099.1)

078.81 **Epidemic vertigo**

078.82 **Epidemic vomiting syndrome**
Winter vomiting disease

❑078.88 **Other specified diseases due to Chlamydiae**

❑078.89 **Other specified diseases due to viruses**
Epidemic cervical myalgia
Marburg disease
Tanapox

Item 1-10 Retrovirus develops by copying its RNA, genetic materials, into the DNA, which then produces new virus particles. It is from the Retroviridae virus family.
Human T-cell lymphotropic virus, Type I (HTLV-I) is also called human T-cell leukemia virus, Type I, and is a retrovirus thought to cause T-cell leukemia/lymphoma.
Human T-cell lymphotropic virus, Type II (HTLV-II), is also called human T-cell leukemia virus, Type II, and is a retrovirus associated with hematologic disorders.
HIV-2 is one of the serotypes of HIV and is usually confined to West Africa, whereas HIV-1 is found worldwide.

● 079 **Viral and chlamydial infection in conditions classified elsewhere and of unspecified site**

Note: This category is provided to be used as an additional code to identify the viral agent in diseases classifiable elsewhere. This category will also be used to classify virus infection of unspecified nature or site.

079.0 **Adenovirus**

079.1 **ECHO virus**

079.2 **Coxsackie virus**

079.3 **Rhinovirus**

079.4 **Human papillomavirus**

● 079.5 **Retrovirus**

Excludes *human immunodeficiency virus, type 1 [HIV-1] (042)*
human T-cell lymphotropic virus, type III [HTLV-III] (042)
lymphadenopathy-associated virus [LAV] (042)

❑079.50 **Retrovirus, unspecified**

079.51 **Human T-cell lymphotropic virus, type I [HTLV-I]**

079.52 **Human T-cell lymphotropic virus, type II [HTLV-II]**

079.53 **Human immunodeficiency virus, type 2 [HIV-2]**

❑079.59 **Other specified retrovirus**

079.6 **Respiratory syncytial virus (RSV)**

● 079.8 **Other specified viral and chlamydial infections**

079.81 **Hantavirus**

❑079.88 **Other specified chlamydial infection**

❑079.89 **Other specified viral infection**

● 079.9 **Unspecified viral and chlamydial infections**

Excludes *viremia NOS (790.8)*

❑079.98 **Unspecified chlamydial infection**
Chlamydial infection NOS

❑079.99 **Unspecified viral infection**
Viral infection NOS

Item 1-11 Rickettsioses are diseases spread from ticks, lice, fleas, or mites to humans. See Figure 1-3. Typhus is spread to humans chiefly by the fleas of rats. Endemic identifies a disease as being present in low numbers of humans at all times, whereas, epidemic identifies a disease as being present in high numbers of humans at a specific time. Morbidity (death) is higher in epidemic diseases. Brill's disease, also known as Brill-Zinsser disease, is spread from human to human by body lice and also from the lice of flying squirrels. Scrub typhus is spread in the same ways as Brill's disease. Malaria is spread to humans by mosquitos.

RICKETTSIOSES AND OTHER ARTHROPOD-BORNE DISEASES (080–088)

Excludes *arthropod-borne viral diseases (060.0–066.9)*

080 **Louse-borne [epidemic] typhus**
Typhus (fever):
classical
epidemic
exanthematic NOS
louse-borne

● 081 **Other typhus**

081.0 **Murine [endemic] typhus**
Typhus (fever):
endemic
flea-borne

081.1 **Brill's disease**
Brill-Zinsser disease
Recrudescent typhus (fever)

081.2 **Scrub typhus**
Japanese river fever
Kedani fever
Mite-borne typhus
Tsutsugamushi

❑ 081.9 **Typhus, unspecified**
Typhus (fever) NOS

● 082 **Tick-borne rickettsioses**

082.0 **Spotted fevers**
Rocky mountain spotted fever
São Paulo fever

082.1 **Boutonneuse fever**
African tick typhus
India tick typhus
Kenya tick typhus
Marseilles fever
Mediterranean tick fever

082.2 **North Asian tick fever**
Siberian tick typhus

082.3 **Queensland tick typhus**

● 082.4 **Ehrlichiosis**

❑ 082.40 **Ehrlichiosis, unspecified**

082.41 **Ehrlichiosis chafeensis (E. chafeensis)**

❑ 082.49 **Other ehrlichiosis**

❑ 082.8 **Other specified tick-borne rickettsioses**
Lone star fever

❑ 082.9 **Tick-borne rickettsiosis, unspecified**
Tick-borne typhus NOS

● 083 **Other rickettsioses**

083.0 **Q fever**

083.1 **Trench fever**
Quintan fever
Wolhynian fever

083.2 **Rickettsialpox**
Vesicular rickettsiosis

❑ 083.8 **Other specified rickettsioses**

❑ 083.9 **Rickettsiosis, unspecified**

● 084 **Malaria**

Note: Subcategories 084.0–084.6 exclude the listed conditions with mention of pernicious complications (084.8–084.9).

Excludes *congenital malaria (771.2)*

084.0 **Falciparum malaria [malignant tertian]**
Malaria (fever):
by Plasmodium falciparum
subtertian

084.1 **Vivax malaria [benign tertian]**
Malaria (fever) by Plasmodium vivax

084.2 **Quartan malaria**
Malaria (fever) by Plasmodium malariae
Malariae malaria

084.3 **Ovale malaria**
Malaria (fever) by Plasmodium ovale

❑ 084.4 **Other malaria**
Monkey malaria

084.5 **Mixed malaria**
Malaria (fever) by more than one parasite

❑ 084.6 **Malaria, unspecified**
Malaria (fever) NOS

084.7 **Induced malaria**
Therapeutically induced malaria

Excludes *accidental infection from syringe, blood transfusion, etc. (084.0–084.6, above, according to parasite species)*
transmission from mother to child during delivery (771.2)

084.8 **Blackwater fever**
Hemoglobinuric:
fever (bilious)
malaria
Malarial hemoglobinuria

❑ 084.9 **Other pernicious complications of malaria**
Algid malaria
Cerebral malaria

Use additional code to identify complication, as:
malarial:
hepatitis (573.2)
nephrosis (581.81)

● 085 **Leishmaniasis**

085.0 **Visceral [kala-azar]**
Dumdum fever
Infection by Leishmania:
donovani
infantum
Leishmaniasis:
dermal, post-kala-azar
Mediterranean
visceral (Indian)

085.1 **Cutaneous, urban**
Aleppo boil
Baghdad boil
Delhi boil
Infection by Leishmania tropica (minor)
Leishmaniasis, cutaneous:
dry form
late
recurrent
ulcerating
Oriental sore

085.2 **Cutaneous, Asian desert**
Infection by Leishmania tropica major
Leishmaniasis, cutaneous:
acute necrotizing
rural
wet form
zoonotic form

085.3 **Cutaneous, Ethiopian**
Infection by Leishmania ethiopica
Leishmaniasis, cutaneous:
diffuse
lepromatous

085.4 **Cutaneous, American**
Chiclero ulcer
Infection by Leishmania mexicana
Leishmaniasis tegumentaria diffusa

085.5 **Mucocutaneous (American)**
Espundia
Infection by Leishmania braziliensis
Uta

❑ 085.9 **Leishmaniasis, unspecified**

● 086 **Trypanosomiasis**

Use additional code to identify manifestations, as:
trypanosomiasis:
encephalitis (323.2)
meningitis (321.3)

086.0 **Chagas' disease with heart involvement**
American trypanosomiasis with heart involvement
Infection by Trypanosoma cruzi with heart involvement
Any condition classifiable to 086.2 with heart involvement

086.1 **Chagas' disease with other organ involvement**
American trypanosomiasis with involvement of organ other than heart
Infection by Trypanosoma cruzi with involvement of organ other than heart
Any condition classifiable to 086.2 with involvement of organ other than heart

086.2 **Chagas' disease without mention of organ involvement**
American trypanosomiasis
Infection by Trypanosoma cruzi

086.3 **Gambian trypanosomiasis**
Gambian sleeping sickness
Infection by Trypanosoma gambiense

086.4 **Rhodesian trypanosomiasis**
Infection by Trypanosoma rhodesiense
Rhodesian sleeping sickness

❑ 086.5 **African trypanosomiasis, unspecified**
Sleeping sickness NOS

❑ 086.9 **Trypanosomiasis, unspecified**

● 087 **Relapsing fever**

Includes: recurrent fever

087.0 **Louse-borne**

087.1 **Tick-borne**

❑ 087.9 **Relapsing fever, unspecified**

● 088 **Other arthropod-borne diseases**

088.0 **Bartonellosis**
Carrión's disease
Oroya fever
Verruga peruana

● ❑ 088.8 **Other specified arthropod-borne diseases**

088.81 **Lyme disease**
Erythema chronicum migrans

088.82 **Babesiosis**
Babesiasis

❑ 088.89 **Other**

❑ 088.9 **Arthropod-borne disease, unspecified**

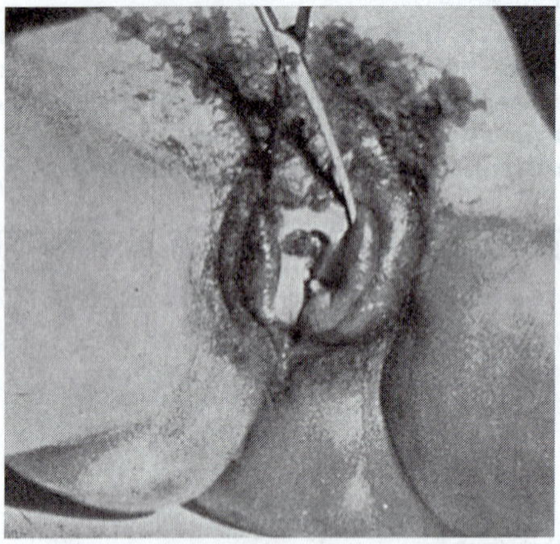

Figure 1–7 Chancre. (From Delp MH, Manning RT: Major Physical Diagnosis, 8th ed. Philadelphia, WB Saunders, 1975, p. 613.)

Item 1–12 Syphilis, also known as lues, is the most serious of the venereal diseases caused by ***Treponema pallidum***. The **primary** stage is characterized by an ulceration known as **chancre,** which usually appears on the genitals but can also develop on the anus, lips, tonsils, breasts, or fingers.
The **secondary** stage is characterized by a rash that can affect any area of the body. **Latent** syphilis is divided into **early,** which is diagnosed within two years of infection, and **late,** which is diagnosed two years or more after infection. **Congenital** syphilis is also labeled **early** or **late** based on the time of diagnosis.

SYPHILIS AND OTHER VENEREAL DISEASES (090–099)

Excludes *nonvenereal endemic syphilis (104.0)*
urogenital trichomoniasis (131.0)

● 090 **Congenital syphilis**

090.0 **Early congenital syphilis, symptomatic**
Congenital syphilitic:
choroiditis
coryza (chronic)
hepatomegaly
mucous patches
periostitis
splenomegaly
Syphilitic (congenital):
epiphysitis
osteochondritis
pemphigus
Any congenital syphilitic condition specified as early or manifesting less than two years after birth

090.1 **Early congenital syphilis, latent**
Congenital syphilis without clinical manifestations, with positive serological reaction and negative spinal fluid test, less than two years after birth

❑ **090.2 Early congenital syphilis, unspecified**
Congenital syphilis NOS, less than two years after birth

090.3 Syphilitic interstitial keratitis
Syphilitic keratitis:
parenchymatous
punctata profunda

Excludes *interstitial keratitis NOS (370.50)*

● **090.4 Juvenile neurosyphilis**
Use additional code to identify any associated mental disorder

❑ **090.40 Juvenile neurosyphilis, unspecified**
Congenital neurosyphilis
Dementia paralytica juvenilis
Juvenile:
general paresis
tabes
taboparesis

090.41 Congenital syphilitic encephalitis

090.42 Congenital syphilitic meningitis

❑ **090.49 Other**

❑ **090.5 Other late congenital syphilis, symptomatic**
Gumma due to congenital syphilis
Hutchinson's teeth
Syphilitic saddle nose
Any congenital syphilitic condition specified as late or manifesting two years or more after birth

090.6 Late congenital syphilis, latent
Congenital syphilis without clinical manifestations, with positive serological reaction and negative spinal fluid test, two years or more after birth

❑ **090.7 Late congenital syphilis, unspecified**
Congenital syphilis NOS, two years or more after birth

❑ **090.9 Congenital syphilis, unspecified**

● **091 Early syphilis, symptomatic**

Excludes *early cardiovascular syphilis (093.0–093.9)*
early neurosyphilis (094.0–094.9)

091.0 Genital syphilis (primary)
Genital chancre

091.1 Primary anal syphilis

❑ **091.2 Other primary syphilis**
Primary syphilis of:
breast
fingers
lip
tonsils

091.3 Secondary syphilis of skin or mucous membranes
Condyloma latum
Secondary syphilis of:
anus
mouth
pharynx
skin
tonsils
vulva

091.4 Adenopathy due to secondary syphilis
Syphilitic adenopathy (secondary)
Syphilitic lymphadenitis (secondary)

● **091.5 Uveitis due to secondary syphilis**

❑ **091.50 Syphilitic uveitis, unspecified**

091.51 Syphilitic chorioretinitis (secondary)

091.52 Syphilitic iridocyclitis (secondary)

● **091.6 Secondary syphilis of viscera and bone**

091.61 Secondary syphilitic periostitis

091.62 Secondary syphilitic hepatitis
Secondary syphilis of liver

❑ **091.69 Other viscera**

091.7 Secondary syphilis, relapse
Secondary syphilis, relapse (treated) (untreated)

● **091.8 Other forms of secondary syphilis**

091.81 Acute syphilitic meningitis (secondary)

091.82 Syphilitic alopecia

❑ **091.89 Other**

❑ **091.9 Unspecified secondary syphilis**

● **092 Early syphilis, latent**

Includes: syphilis (acquired) without clinical manifestations, with positive serological reaction and negative spinal fluid test, less than two years after infection

092.0 Early syphilis, latent, serological relapse after treatment

❑ **092.9 Early syphilis, latent, unspecified**

● **093 Cardiovascular syphilis**

093.0 Aneurysm of aorta, specified as syphilitic
Dilatation of aorta, specified as syphilitic

093.1 Syphilitic aortitis

● **093.2 Syphilitic endocarditis**

❑ **093.20 Valve, unspecified**
Syphilitic ostial coronary disease

093.21 Mitral valve

093.22 Aortic valve
Syphilitic aortic incompetence or stenosis

093.23 Tricuspid valve

093.24 Pulmonary valve

● **093.8 Other specified cardiovascular syphilis**

093.81 Syphilitic pericarditis

093.82 Syphilitic myocarditis

❑ **093.89 Other**

❑ **093.9 Cardiovascular syphilis, unspecified**

● **094 Neurosyphilis**

Use additional code to identify any associated mental disorder

094.0 Tabes dorsalis
Locomotor ataxia (progressive)
Posterior spinal sclerosis (syphilitic)
Tabetic neurosyphilis

Use additional code to identify manifestation, as:
neurogenic arthropathy [Charcot's joint disease] (713.5)

094.1 General paresis
Dementia paralytica
General paralysis (of the insane) (progressive)
Paretic neurosyphilis
Taboparesis

094.2 Syphilitic meningitis
Meningovascular syphilis

Excludes *acute syphilitic meningitis (secondary) (091.81)*

094.3 Asymptomatic neurosyphilis

● **094.8 Other specified neurosyphilis**

094.81 Syphilitic encephalitis

ICD-9-CM 001-099 Vol. 1

094.82 **Syphilitic Parkinsonism**

094.83 **Syphilitic disseminated retinochoroiditis**

094.84 **Syphilitic optic atrophy**

094.85 **Syphilitic retrobulbar neuritis**

094.86 **Syphilitic acoustic neuritis**

094.87 **Syphilitic ruptured cerebral aneurysm**

❑ 094.89 **Other**

❑ 094.9 **Neurosyphilis, unspecified**
Gumma (syphilitic) of central nervous system NOS
Syphilis (early) (late) of central nervous system NOS
Syphiloma of central nervous system NOS

● 095 **Other forms of late syphilis, with symptoms**

Includes: gumma (syphilitic)
tertiary, or unspecified stage

095.0 **Syphilitic episcleritis**

095.1 **Syphilis of lung**

095.2 **Syphilitic peritonitis**

095.3 **Syphilis of liver**

095.4 **Syphilis of kidney**

095.5 **Syphilis of bone**

095.6 **Syphilis of muscle**
Syphilitic myositis

095.7 **Syphilis of synovium, tendon, and bursa**
Syphilitic:
bursitis
synovitis

❑ 095.8 **Other specified forms of late symptomatic syphilis**

Excludes *cardiovascular syphilis (093.0–093.9)*
neurosyphilis (094.0–094.9)

❑ 095.9 **Late symptomatic syphilis, unspecified**

096 **Late syphilis, latent**
Syphilis (acquired) without clinical manifestations, with positive serological reaction and negative spinal fluid test, two years or more after infection

● 097 **Other and unspecified syphilis**

❑ 097.0 **Late syphilis, unspecified**

❑ 097.1 **Latent syphilis, unspecified**
Positive serological reaction for syphilis

❑ 097.9 **Syphilis, unspecified**
Syphilis (acquired) NOS

Excludes *syphilis NOS causing death under two years of age (090.9)*

● 098 **Gonococcal infections**

098.0 **Acute, of lower genitourinary tract**
Gonococcal:
Bartholinitis (acute)
urethritis (acute)
vulvovaginitis (acute)
Gonorrhea (acute):
NOS
genitourinary (tract) NOS

● 098.1 **Acute, of upper genitourinary tract**

❑ 098.10 **Gonococcal infection (acute) of upper genitourinary tract, site unspecified**

098.11 **Gonococcal cystitis (acute)**
Gonorrhea (acute) of bladder

098.12 **Gonococcal prostatitis (acute)**

098.13 **Gonococcal epididymo-orchitis (acute)**
Gonococcal orchitis (acute)

098.14 **Gonococcal seminal vesiculitis (acute)**
Gonorrhea (acute) of seminal vesicle

098.15 **Gonococcal cervicitis (acute)**
Gonorrhea (acute) of cervix

098.16 **Gonococcal endometritis (acute)**
Gonorrhea (acute) of uterus

098.17 **Gonococcal salpingitis, specified as acute**

❑ 098.19 **Other**

098.2 **Chronic, of lower genitourinary tract**
Gonococcal specified as chronic or with duration of two months or more:
Bartholinitis specified as chronic or with duration of two months or more
urethritis specified as chronic or with duration of two months or more
vulvovaginitis specified as chronic or with duration of two months or more
Gonorrhea specified as chronic or with duration of two months or more:
NOS specified as chronic or with duration of two months or more
genitourinary (tract) specified as chronic or with duration of two months or more
Any condition classifiable to 098.0 specified as chronic or with duration of two months or more

● 098.3 **Chronic, of upper genitourinary tract**
Includes: any condition classifiable to 098.1 stated as chronic or with a duration of two months or more

❑ 098.30 **Chronic gonococcal infection of upper genitourinary tract, site unspecified**

098.31 **Gonococcal cystitis, chronic**
Any condition classifiable to 098.11, specified as chronic
Gonorrhea of bladder, chronic

098.32 **Gonococcal prostatitis, chronic**
Any condition classifiable to 098.12, specified as chronic

098.33 **Gonococcal epididymo-orchitis, chronic**
Any condition classifiable to 098.13, specified as chronic
Chronic gonococcal orchitis

098.34 **Gonococcal seminal vesiculitis, chronic**
Any condition classifiable to 098.14, specified as chronic
Gonorrhea of seminal vesicle, chronic

098.35 **Gonococcal cervicitis, chronic**
Any condition classifiable to 098.15, specified as chronic
Gonorrhea of cervix, chronic

098.36 **Gonococcal endometritis, chronic**
Any condition classifiable to 098.16, specified as chronic

098.37 **Gonococcal salpingitis (chronic)**

❑ 098.39 **Other**

● 098.4 **Gonococcal infection of eye**

098.40 **Gonococcal conjunctivitis (neonatorum)**
Gonococcal ophthalmia (neonatorum)

098.41 **Gonococcal iridocyclitis**

098.42 **Gonococcal endophthalmia**

098.43 **Gonococcal keratitis**

❑ 098.49 **Other**

● 098.5 **Gonococcal infection of joint**
- 098.50 **Gonococcal arthritis**
  - Gonococcal infection of joint NOS
- 098.51 **Gonococcal synovitis and tenosynovitis**
- 098.52 **Gonococcal bursitis**
- 098.53 **Gonococcal spondylitis**
- ❑ 098.59 **Other**
  - Gonococcal rheumatism

098.6 **Gonococcal infection of pharynx**

098.7 **Gonococcal infection of anus and rectum**
- Gonococcal proctitis

● 098.8 **Gonococcal infection of other specified sites**
- 098.81 **Gonococcal keratosis (blennorrhagica)**
- 098.82 **Gonococcal meningitis**
- 098.83 **Gonococcal pericarditis**
- 098.84 **Gonococcal endocarditis**
- ❑ 098.85 **Other gonococcal heart disease**
- 098.86 **Gonococcal peritonitis**
- ❑ 098.89 **Other**
  - Gonococcemia

● 099 **Other venereal diseases**

099.0 **Chancroid**
- Bubo (inguinal):
  - chancroidal
  - due to Hemophilus ducreyi
- Chancre:
  - Ducrey's simple soft
- Ulcus molle (cutis) (skin)

099.1 **Lymphogranuloma venereum**
- Climatic or tropical bubo
- (Durand-) Nicolas-Favre disease
- Esthiomene
- Lymphogranuloma inguinale

099.2 **Granuloma inguinale**
- Donovanosis
- Granuloma pudendi (ulcerating)
- Granuloma venereum
- Pudendal ulcer

099.3 **Reiter's disease**
- Reiter's syndrome

Use additional code for associated:
- arthropathy (711.1)
- conjunctivitis (372.33)

● 099.4 **Other nongonococcal urethritis [NGU]**
- ❑ 099.40 **Unspecified**
  - Nonspecific urethritis
- 099.41 **Chlamydia trachomatis**
- ❑ 099.49 **Other specified organism**

● 099.5 **Other venereal diseases due to Chlamydia trachomatis**

Excludes *Chlamydia trachomatis infection of conjunctiva (076.0–076.9, 077.0, 077.9)*
Lymphogranuloma venereum (099.1)

- ❑ 099.50 **Unspecified site**
- 099.51 **Pharynx**
- 099.52 **Anus and rectum**
- 099.53 **Lower genitourinary sites**

Excludes *urethra (099.41)*

Use additional code to specify site of infection, such as:
- bladder (595.4)
- cervix (616.0)
- vagina and vulva (616.11)

- ❑ 099.54 **Other genitourinary sites**

Use additional code to specify site of infection, such as:
- pelvic inflammatory disease NOS (614.9)
- testis and epididymis (604.91)

- ❑ 099.55 **Unspecified genitourinary site**
- 099.56 **Peritoneum**
  - Perihepatitis
- ❑ 099.59 **Other specified site**

❑ 099.8 **Other specified venereal diseases**

❑ 099.9 **Venereal disease, unspecified**

OTHER SPIROCHETAL DISEASES (100–104)

● 100 **Leptospirosis**

100.0 **Leptospirosis icterohemorrhagica**
- Leptospiral or spirochetal jaundice (hemorrhagic)
- Weil's disease

● 100.8 **Other specified leptospiral infections**
- 100.81 **Leptospiral meningitis (aseptic)**
- ❑ 100.89 **Other**
  - Fever:
    - Fort Bragg
    - pretibial
    - swamp
  - Infection by Leptospira:
    - australis
    - bataviae
    - pyrogenes

❑ 100.9 **Leptospirosis, unspecified**

101 **Vincent's angina**
- Acute necrotizing ulcerative:
  - gingivitis
  - stomatitis
- Fusospirochetal pharyngitis
- Spirochetal stomatitis
- Trench mouth
- Vincent's:
  - gingivitis
  - infection [any site]

● 102 **Yaws**

Includes: frambesia
pian

102.0 **Initial lesions**
- Chancre of yaws
- Frambesia, initial or primary
- Initial frambesial ulcer
- Mother yaw

102.1 **Multiple papillomata and wet crab yaws**
- Butter yaws
- Frambesioma
- Pianoma
- Plantar or palmar papilloma of yaws

❑ 102.2 **Other early skin lesions**
- Cutaneous yaws, less than five years after infection
- Early yaws (cutaneous) (macular) (papular) (maculopapular) (micropapular)
- Frambeside of early yaws

102.3 **Hyperkeratosis**
- Ghoul hand
- Hyperkeratosis, palmar or plantar (early) (late) due to yaws
- Worm-eaten soles

102.4 Gummata and ulcers
Nodular late yaws (ulcerated)
Gummatous frambeside

102.5 Gangosa
Rhinopharyngitis mutilans

102.6 Bone and joint lesions
Goundou of yaws (late)
Gumma, bone of yaws (late)
Gummatous osteitis or periostitis of yaws (late)
Hydrarthrosis of yaws (early) (late)
Osteitis of yaws (early) (late)
Periostitis (hypertrophic) of yaws (early) (late)

❑ **102.7 Other manifestations**
Juxta-articular nodules of yaws
Mucosal yaws

102.8 Latent yaws
Yaws without clinical manifestations, with positive serology

❑ **102.9 Yaws, unspecified**

● **103 Pinta**

103.0 Primary lesions
Chancre (primary) of pinta [carate]
Papule (primary) of pinta [carate]
Pintid of pinta [carate]

103.1 Intermediate lesions
Erythematous plaques of pinta [carate]
Hyperchromic lesions of pinta [carate]
Hyperkeratosis of pinta [carate]

103.2 Late lesions
Cardiovascular lesions of pinta [carate]
Skin lesions of pinta [carate]:
achromic of pinta [carate]
cicatricial of pinta [carate]
dyschromic of pinta [carate]
Vitiligo of pinta [carate]

103.3 Mixed lesions
Achromic and hyperchromic skin lesions of pinta [carate]

❑ **103.9 Pinta, unspecified**

● **104 Other spirochetal infection**

104.0 Nonvenereal endemic syphilis
Bejel
Njovera

❑ **104.8 Other specified spirochetal infections**
Excludes *relapsing fever (087.0–087.9)*
syphilis (090.0–097.9)

❑ **104.9 Spirochetal infection, unspecified**

MYCOSES (110–118)

Use additional code to identify manifestation, as:
arthropathy (711.6)
meningitis (321.0–321.1)
otitis externa (380.15)

Excludes *infection by Actinomycetales, such as species of Actinomyces, Actinomadura, Nocardia, Streptomyces (039.0–039.9)*

● **110 Dermatophytosis**

Includes: infection by species of Epidermophyton, Microsporum, and Trichophyton
tinea, any type except those in 111

110.0 Of scalp and beard
Kerion
Sycosis, mycotic
Trichophytic tinea [black dot tinea], scalp

110.1 Of nail
Dermatophytic onychia
Onychomycosis
Tinea unguium

110.2 Of hand
Tinea manuum

110.3 Of groin and perianal area
Dhobie itch
Eczema marginatum
Tinea cruris

110.4 Of foot
Athlete's foot
Tinea pedis

110.5 Of the body
Herpes circinatus
Tinea imbricata [Tokelau]

110.6 Deep seated dermatophytosis
Granuloma trichophyticum
Majocchi's granuloma

❑ **110.8 Of other specified sites**

❑ **110.9 Of unspecified site**
Favus NOS
Microsporic tinea NOS
Ringworm NOS

● **111 Dermatomycosis, other and unspecified**

111.0 Pityriasis versicolor
Infection by Malassezia [Pityrosporum] furfur
Tinea flava
Tinea versicolor

111.1 Tinea nigra
Infection by Cladosporium species
Keratomycosis nigricans
Microsporosis nigra
Pityriasis nigra
Tinea palmaris nigra

111.2 Tinea blanca
Infection by Trichosporon (beigelii) cutaneum
White piedra

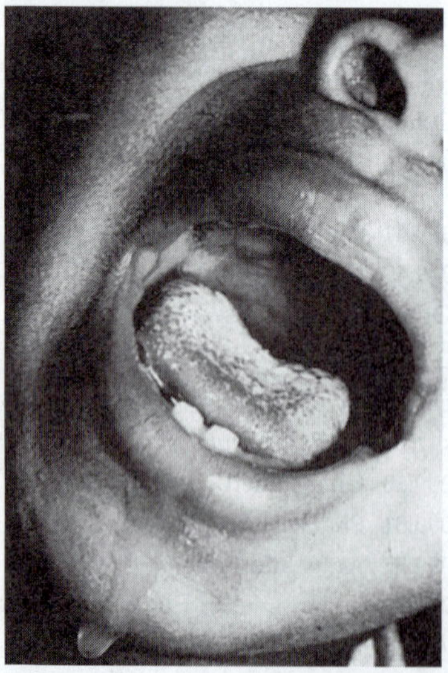

Figure 1-8 Oral candidiasis, also called thrush. (From Rippon JW: Medical Mycology, 3rd ed. Philadelphia, WB Saunders, 1988, p. 542.)

Item 1-13 Candidiasis, also called oidiomycosis or moniliasis, is a fungal infection. It most often appears on moist cutaneous areas of the body, but can also be responsible for a variety of systemic infections such as endocarditis, meningitis, arthritis, and myositis.

111.3 Black piedra
Infection by Piedraia hortai

❑**111.8 Other specified dermatomycoses**

❑**111.9 Dermatomycosis, unspecified**

● **112 Candidiasis**

Includes: infection by Candida species
moniliasis

Excludes *neonatal monilial infection (771.7)*

112.0 Of mouth
Thrush (oral)

112.1 Of vulva and vagina
Candidal vulvovaginitis
Monilial vulvovaginitis

❑**112.2 Of other urogenital sites**
Candidal balanitis

112.3 Of skin and nails
Candidal intertrigo
Candidal onychia
Candidal perionyxis [paronychia]

112.4 Of lung
Candidal pneumonia

112.5 Disseminated
Systemic candidiasis

● **112.8 Of other specified sites**

112.81 Candidal endocarditis

112.82 Candidal otitis externa
Otomycosis in moniliasis

112.83 Candidal meningitis

112.84 Candidal esophagitis

112.85 Candidal enteritis

❑**112.89 Other**

❑**112.9 Of unspecified site**

● **114 Coccidioidomycosis**

Includes: infection by Coccidioides (immitis)
Posada-Wernicke disease

114.0 Primary coccidioidomycosis (pulmonary)
Acute pulmonary coccidioidomycosis
Coccidioidomycotic pneumonitis
Desert rheumatism
Pulmonary coccidioidomycosis
San Joaquin Valley fever

114.1 Primary extrapulmonary coccidioidomycosis
Chancriform syndrome
Primary cutaneous coccidioidomycosis

114.2 Coccidioidal meningitis

❑**114.3 Other forms of progressive coccidioidomycosis**
Coccidioidal granuloma
Disseminated coccidioidomycosis

114.4 Chronic pulmonary coccidioidomycosis

❑**114.5 Pulmonary coccidioidomycosis, unspecified**

❑**114.9 Coccidioidomycosis, unspecified**

● **115 Histoplasmosis**

The following fifth-digit subclassification is for use with category 115:
0 **without mention of manifestation**
1 **meningitis**
2 **retinitis**
3 **pericarditis**
4 **endocarditis**
5 **pneumonia**
❑ 9 **other**

● **115.0 Infection by Histoplasma capsulatum**
American histoplasmosis
Darling's disease
Reticuloendothelial cytomycosis
Small form histoplasmosis

● **115.1 Infection by Histoplasma duboisii**
African histoplasmosis
Large form histoplasmosis

● ❑**115.9 Histoplasmosis, unspecified**
Histoplasmosis NOS

● **116 Blastomycotic infection**

116.0 Blastomycosis
Blastomycotic dermatitis
Chicago disease
Cutaneous blastomycosis
Disseminated blastomycosis
Gilchrist's disease
Infection by Blastomyces [Ajellomyces] dermatitidis
North American blastomycosis
Primary pulmonary blastomycosis

116.1 Paracoccidioidomycosis
Brazilian blastomycosis
Infection by Paracoccidioides [Blastomyces] brasiliensis
Lutz-Splendore-Almeida disease
Mucocutaneous-lymphangitic paracoccidioidomycosis
Pulmonary paracoccidioidomycosis
South American blastomycosis
Visceral paracoccidioidomycosis

116.2 Lobomycosis
Infections by Loboa [Blastomyces] loboi
Keloidal blastomycosis
Lobo's disease

● **117 Other mycoses**

117.0 Rhinosporidiosis
Infection by Rhinosporidium seeberi

117.1 Sporotrichosis
Cutaneous sporotrichosis
Disseminated sporotrichosis
Infection by Sporothrix [Sporotrichum] schenckii
Lymphocutaneous sporotrichosis
Pulmonary sporotrichosis
Sporotrichosis of the bones

117.2 Chromoblastomycosis
Chromomycosis
Infection by Cladosporidium carrionii, Fonsecaea compactum, Fonsecaea pedrosoi, Phialophora verrucosa

117.3 Aspergillosis
Infection by Aspergillus species, mainly A. fumigatus, A. flavus group, A. terreus group

117.4 **Mycotic mycetomas**
Infection by various genera and species of Ascomycetes and Deuteromycetes, such as Acremonium [Cephalosporium] falciforme, Neotestudina rosatii, Madurella grisea, Madurella mycetomii, Pyrenochaeta romeroi, Zopfia [Leptosphaeria] senegalensis
Madura foot, mycotic
Maduromycosis, mycotic

Excludes *actinomycotic mycetomas (039.0–039.9)*

117.5 **Cryptococcosis**
Busse-Buschke's disease
European cryptococcosis
Infection by Cryptococcus neoformans
Pulmonary cryptococcosis
Systemic cryptococcosis
Torula

117.6 **Allescheriosis [Petriellidosis]**
Infections by Allescheria [Petriellidium] boydii [Monosporium apiospermum]

Excludes *mycotic mycetoma (117.4)*

117.7 **Zygomycosis [Phycomycosis or Mucormycosis]**
Infection by species of Absidia, Basidiobolus, Conidiobolus, Cunninghamella, Entomophthora, Mucor, Rhizopus, Saksenaea

117.8 **Infection by dematiacious fungi [Phaehyphomycosis]**
Infection by dematiacious fungi, such as Cladosporium trichoides [bantianum], Dreschlera hawaiiensis, Phialophora gougerotii, Phialophora jeanselmi

❑117.9 **Other and unspecified mycoses**

118 **Opportunistic mycoses**
Infection of skin, subcutaneous tissues, and/or organs by a wide variety of fungi generally considered to be pathogenic to compromised hosts only (e.g., infection by species of Alternaria, Dreschlera, Fusarium)

HELMINTHIASES (120–129)

● 120 **Schistosomiasis [bilharziasis]**

120.0 **Schistosoma haematobium**
Vesical schistosomiasis NOS

120.1 **Schistosoma mansoni**
Intestinal schistosomiasis NOS

120.2 **Schistosoma japonicum**
Asiatic schistosomiasis NOS
Katayama disease or fever

120.3 **Cutaneous**
Cercarial dermatitis
Infection by cercariae of Schistosoma
Schistosome dermatitis
Swimmers' itch

❑120.8 **Other specified schistosomiasis**
Infection by Schistosoma:
bovis
intercalatum
mattheii
spindale
Schistosomiasis chestermani

❑120.9 **Schistosomiasis, unspecified**
Blood flukes NOS
Hemic distomiasis

● 121 **Other trematode infections**

121.0 **Opisthorchiasis**
Infection by:
cat liver fluke
Opisthorchis (felineus) (tenuicollis) (viverrini)

121.1 **Clonorchiasis**
Biliary cirrhosis due to clonorchiasis
Chinese liver fluke disease
Hepatic distomiasis due to Clonorchis sinensis
Oriental liver fluke disease

121.2 **Paragonimiasis**
Infection by Paragonimus
Lung fluke disease (oriental)
Pulmonary distomiasis

121.3 **Fascioliasis**
Infection by Fasciola:
gigantica
hepatica
Liver flukes NOS
Sheep liver fluke infection

121.4 **Fasciolopsiasis**
Infection by Fasciolopsis (buski)
Intestinal distomiasis

121.5 **Metagonimiasis**
Infection by Metagonimus yokogawai

121.6 **Heterophyiasis**
Infection by:
Heterophyes heterophyes
Stellantchasmus falcatus

❑121.8 **Other specified trematode infections**
Infection by:
Dicrocoelium dendriticum
Echinostoma ilocanum
Gastrodiscoides hominis

❑121.9 **Trematode infection, unspecified**
Distomiasis NOS
Fluke disease NOS

● 122 **Echinococcosis**

Includes: echinococciasis
hydatid disease
hydatidosis

122.0 **Echinococcus granulosus infection of liver**

122.1 **Echinococcus granulosus infection of lung**

122.2 **Echinococcus granulosus infection of thyroid**

❑122.3 **Echinococcus granulosus infection, other**

❑122.4 **Echinococcus granulosus infection, unspecified**

122.5 **Echinococcus multilocularis infection of liver**

❑122.6 **Echinococcus multilocularis infection, other**

❑122.7 **Echinococcus multilocularis infection, unspecified**

❑122.8 **Echinococcosis, unspecified, of liver**

❑122.9 **Echinococcosis, other and unspecified**

● 123 **Other cestode infection**

123.0 **Taenia solium infection, intestinal form**
Pork tapeworm (adult) (infection)

123.1 **Cysticercosis**
Cysticerciasis
Infection by Cysticercus cellulosae [larval form of Taenia solium]

123.2 **Taenia saginata infection**
Beef tapeworm (infection)
Infection by Taeniarhynchus saginatus

❑123.3 **Taeniasis, unspecified**

123.4 **Diphyllobothriasis, intestinal**
Diphyllobothrium (adult) (latum) (pacificum) infection
Fish tapeworm (infection)

123.5 Sparganosis [larval diphyllobothriasis]
Infection by:
Diphyllobothrium larvae
Sparganum (mansoni) (proliferum)
Spirometra larvae

123.6 Hymenolepiasis
Dwarf tapeworm (infection)
Hymenolepis (diminuta) (nana) infection
Rat tapeworm (infection)

❑ **123.8 Other specified cestode infection**
Diplogonoporus (grandis) infection
Dipylidium (caninum) infection
Dog tapeworm (infection)

❑ **123.9 Cestode infection, unspecified**
Tapeworm (infection) NOS

124 Trichinosis
Trichinella spiralis infection
Trichinellosis
Trichiniasis

● **125 Filarial infection and dracontiasis**

125.0 Bancroftian filariasis
Chyluria due to Wuchereria bancrofti
Elephantiasis due to Wuchereria bancrofti
Infection due to Wuchereria bancrofti
Lymphadenitis due to Wuchereria bancrofti
Lymphangitis due to Wuchereria bancrofti
Wuchereriasis

125.1 Malayan filariasis
Brugia filariasis due to Brugia [Wuchereria] malayi
Chyluria due to Brugia [Wuchereria] malayi
Elephantiasis due to Brugia [Wuchereria] malayi
Infection due to Brugia [Wuchereria] malayi
Lymphadenitis due to Brugia [Wuchereria] malayi
Lymphangitis due to Brugia [Wuchereria] malayi

125.2 Loiasis
Eyeworm disease of Africa
Loa loa infection

125.3 Onchocerciasis
Onchocerca volvulus infection
Onchocercosis

125.4 Dipetalonemiasis
Infection by:
Acanthocheilonema perstans
Dipetalonema perstans

125.5 Mansonella ozzardi infection
Filariasis ozzardi

❑ **125.6 Other specified filariasis**
Dirofilaria infection
Infection by:
Acanthocheilonema streptocerca
Dipetalonema streptocerca

125.7 Dracontiasis
Guinea-worm infection
Infection by Dracunculus medinensis

❑ **125.9 Unspecified filariasis**

● **126 Ancylostomiasis and necatoriasis**

Includes: cutaneous larva migrans due to Ancylostoma
hookworm (disease) (infection)
uncinariasis

126.0 Ancylostoma duodenale

126.1 Necator americanus

126.2 Ancylostoma braziliense

126.3 Ancylostoma ceylanicum

❑ **126.8 Other specified Ancylostoma**

❑ **126.9 Ancylostomiasis and necatoriasis, unspecified**
Creeping eruption NOS
Cutaneous larva migrans NOS

● **127 Other intestinal helminthiases**

127.0 Ascariasis
Ascaridiasis
Infection by Ascaris lumbricoides
Roundworm infection

127.1 Anisakiasis
Infection by Anisakis larva

127.2 Strongyloidiasis
Infection by Strongyloides stercoralis

Excludes *trichostrongyliasis (127.6)*

127.3 Trichuriasis
Infection by Trichuris trichiuria
Trichocephaliasis
Whipworm (disease) (infection)

127.4 Enterobiasis
Infection by Enterobius vermicularis
Oxyuriasis
Oxyuris vermicularis infection
Pinworm (disease) (infection)
Threadworm infection

127.5 Capillariasis
Infection by Capillaria philippinensis

Excludes *infection by Capillaria hepatica (128.8)*

127.6 Trichostrongyliasis
Infection by Trichostrongylus species

❑ **127.7 Other specified intestinal helminthiasis**
Infection by:
Oesophagostomum apiostomum and related species
Ternidens diminutus
Other specified intestinal helminth
Physalopteriasis

127.8 Mixed intestinal helminthiasis
Infection by intestinal helminths classified to more than one of the categories 120.0–127.7
Mixed helminthiasis NOS

❑ **127.9 Intestinal helminthiasis, unspecified**

● **128 Other and unspecified helminthiases**

128.0 Toxocariasis
Larva migrans visceralis
Toxocara (canis) (cati) infection
Visceral larva migrans syndrome

128.1 Gnathostomiasis
Infection by Gnathostoma spinigerum and related species

❑ **128.8 Other specified helminthiasis**
Infection by:
Angiostrongylus cantonensis
Capillaria hepatica
Other specified helminth

❑ **128.9 Helminth infection, unspecified**
Helminthiasis NOS
Worms NOS

❑ **129 Intestinal parasitism, unspecified**

Item 1-14 Toxoplasmosis is caused by the protozoa Toxoplasma gondii, of which the house cat can be a host. Human infection occurs when contact is made with materials containing the pathogen, such as feces or contaminated soil.
Infection can also occur with ingestion of lamb, goat, and pork meat, especially when the meat contains infected cysts.

OTHER INFECTIOUS AND PARASITIC DISEASES (130–136)

● **130 Toxoplasmosis**

Includes: infection by toxoplasma gondii
toxoplasmosis (acquired)

Excludes *congenital toxoplasmosis (771.2)*

130.0 Meningoencephalitis due to toxoplasmosis
Encephalitis due to acquired toxoplasmosis

130.1 Conjunctivitis due to toxoplasmosis

130.2 Chorioretinitis due to toxoplasmosis
Focal retinochoroiditis due to acquired toxoplasmosis

130.3 Myocarditis due to toxoplasmosis

130.4 Pneumonitis due to toxoplasmosis

130.5 Hepatitis due to toxoplasmosis

❑ **130.7 Toxoplasmosis of other specified sites**

130.8 Multisystemic disseminated toxoplasmosis
Toxoplasmosis of multiple sites

❑ **130.9 Toxoplasmosis, unspecified**

● **131 Trichomoniasis**

Includes: infection due to Trichomonas (vaginalis)

● **131.0 Urogenital trichomoniasis**

❑ **131.00 Urogenital trichomoniasis, unspecified**
Fluor (vaginalis) trichomonal or due to Trichomonas (vaginalis)
Leukorrhea (vaginalis) trichomonal or due to Trichomonas (vaginalis)

131.01 Trichomonal vulvovaginitis
Vaginitis, trichomonal or due to Trichomonas (vaginalis)

131.02 Trichomonal urethritis

131.03 Trichomonal prostatitis

❑ **131.09 Other**

❑ **131.8 Other specified sites**

Excludes *intestinal (007.3)*

❑ **131.9 Trichomoniasis, unspecified**

● **132 Pediculosis and Phthirus infestation**

132.0 Pediculus capitis [head louse]

132.1 Pediculus corporis [body louse]

132.2 Phthirus pubis [pubic louse]
Pediculus pubis

132.3 Mixed infestation
Infestation classifiable to more than one of the categories 132.0–132.2

❑ **132.9 Pediculosis, unspecified**

● **133 Acariasis**

133.0 Scabies
Infestation by Sarcoptes scabiei
Norwegian scabies
Sarcoptic itch

❑ **133.8 Other acariasis**
Chiggers
Infestation by:
Demodex folliculorum
Trombicula

❑ **133.9 Acariasis, unspecified**
Infestation by mites NOS

● **134 Other infestation**

134.0 Myiasis
Infestation by:
Dermatobia (hominis)
fly larvae
Gasterophilus (intestinalis)
maggots
Oestrus ovis

❑ **134.1 Other arthropod infestation**
Infestation by:
chigoe
sand flea
Tunga penetrans
Jigger disease
Scarabiasis
Tungiasis

134.2 Hirudiniasis
Hirudiniasis (external) (internal)
Leeches (aquatic) (land)

❑ **134.8 Other specified infestations**

❑ **134.9 Infestation, unspecified**
Infestation (skin) NOS
Skin parasites NOS

135 Sarcoidosis
Besnier-Boeck-Schaumann disease
Lupoid (miliary) of Boeck
Lupus pernio (Besnier)
Lymphogranulomatosis, benign (Schaumann's)
Sarcoid (any site):
NOS
Boeck
Darier-Roussy
Uveoparotid fever

● **136 Other and unspecified infectious and parasitic diseases**

136.0 Ainhum
Dactylolysis spontanea

136.1 Behçet's syndrome

136.2 Specific infections by free-living amebae
Meningoencephalitis due to Naegleria

136.3 Pneumocystosis
Pneumonia due to Pneumocystis carinii

136.4 Psorospermiasis

136.5 Sarcosporidiosis
Infection by Sarcocystis lindemanni

❑ **136.8 Other specified infectious and parasitic diseases**
Candiru infestation

❑ **136.9 Unspecified infectious and parasitic diseases**
Infectious disease NOS
Parasitic disease NOS

LATE EFFECTS OF INFECTIOUS AND PARASITIC DISEASES (137–139)

● **137 Late effects of tuberculosis**

Note: This category is to be used to indicate conditions classifiable to 010–018 as the cause of late effects, which are themselves classified elsewhere. The "late effects" include those specified as such, as sequelae, or as due to old or inactive tuberculosis, without evidence of active disease.

❑137.0 **Late effects of respiratory or unspecified tuberculosis**

❑137.1 **Late effects of central nervous system tuberculosis**

❑137.2 **Late effects of genitourinary tuberculosis**

❑137.3 **Late effects of tuberculosis of bones and joints**

❑137.4 **Late effects of tuberculosis of other specified organs**

138 Late effects of acute poliomyelitis

Note: This category is to be used to indicate conditions classifiable to 045 as the cause of late effects, which are themselves classified elsewhere. The "late effects" include conditions specified as such, or as sequelae, or as due to old or inactive poliomyelitis, without evidence of active disease.

● ❑139 **Late effects of other infectious and parasitic diseases**

Note: This category is to be used to indicate conditions classifiable to categories 001–009, 020–041, 046–136 as the cause of late effects, which are themselves classified elsewhere. The "late effects" include conditions specified as such; they also include sequelae of diseases classifiable to the above categories if there is evidence that the disease itself is no longer present.

139.0 Late effects of viral encephalitis

Late effects of conditions classifiable to 049.8–049.9, 062–064

❑139.1 **Late effects of trachoma**

Late effects of conditions classifiable to 076

❑139.8 **Late effects of other and unspecified infectious and parasitic diseases**

2. NEOPLASMS (140–239)

1. Content:
   This chapter contains the following broad groups:
   140–195 Malignant neoplasms, stated or presumed to be primary, of specified sites, except of lymphatic and hematopoietic tissue
   196–198 Malignant neoplasms, stated or presumed to be secondary, of specified sites
   199 Malignant neoplasms, without specification of site
   200–208 Malignant neoplasms, stated or presumed to be primary, of lymphatic and hematopoietic tissue
   210–229 Benign neoplasms
   230–234 Carcinoma in situ
   235–238 Neoplasms of uncertain behavior [see Note, at beginning of section 235–238]
   239 Neoplasms of unspecified nature
2. Functional activity
   All neoplasms are classified in this chapter, whether or not functionally active. An additional code from Chapter 3 may be used to identify such functional activity associated with any neoplasm, e.g.:
   catecholamine-producing malignant pheochromocytoma of adrenal:
   code 194.0, additional code 255.6
   basophil adenoma of pituitary with Cushing's syndrome:
   code 227.3, additional code 255.0
3. Morphology [Histology]
   For those wishing to identify the histological type of neoplasms, a comprehensive coded nomenclature, which comprises the morphology rubrics of the ICD-Oncology, is given after the E-code chapter.
4. Malignant neoplasms overlapping site boundaries
   Categories 140–195 are for the classification of primary malignant neoplasms according to their point of origin. A malignant neoplasm that overlaps two or more subcategories within a three-digit rubric and whose point of origin cannot be determined should be classified to the subcategory .8 "Other." For example, "carcinoma involving tip and ventral surface of tongue" should be assigned to 141.8. On the other hand, "carcinoma of tip of tongue, extending to involve the ventral surface" should be coded to 141.2, as the point of origin, the tip, is known. Three subcategories (149.8, 159.8, 165.8) have been provided for malignant neoplasms that overlap the boundaries of three-digit rubrics within certain systems. Overlapping malignant neoplasms that cannot be classified as indicated above should be assigned to the appropriate subdivision of category 195 (Malignant neoplasm of other and ill-defined sites).

MALIGNANT NEOPLASM OF LIP, ORAL CAVITY, AND PHARYNX (140–149)

Excludes *carcinoma in situ (230.0)*

● **140 Malignant neoplasm of lip**

Excludes *skin of lip (173.0)*

140.0 Upper lip, vermilion border
Upper lip:
NOS
external
Upper lip:
lipstick area

140.1 Lower lip, vermilion border
Lower lip:
NOS
external
Lower lip:
lipstick area

140.3 Upper lip, inner aspect
Upper lip:
buccal aspect
frenulum
Upper lip:
mucosa
oral aspect

140.4 Lower lip, inner aspect
Lower lip:
buccal aspect
frenulum
Lower lip:
mucosa
oral aspect

❑ **140.5 Lip, unspecified, inner aspect**
Lip, not specified whether upper or lower:
buccal aspect
frenulum
mucosa
oral aspect

140.6 Commissure of lip
Labial commissure

❑ **140.8 Other sites of lip**
Malignant neoplasm of contiguous or overlapping sites of lip whose point of origin cannot be determined

❑ **140.9 Lip, unspecified, vermilion border**
Lip, not specified as upper or lower:
NOS
external
lipstick area

● **141 Malignant neoplasm of tongue**

141.0 Base of tongue
Dorsal surface of base of tongue
Fixed part of tongue NOS

141.1 Dorsal surface of tongue
Anterior two-thirds of tongue, dorsal surface
Dorsal tongue NOS
Midline of tongue

Excludes *dorsal surface of base of tongue (141.0)*

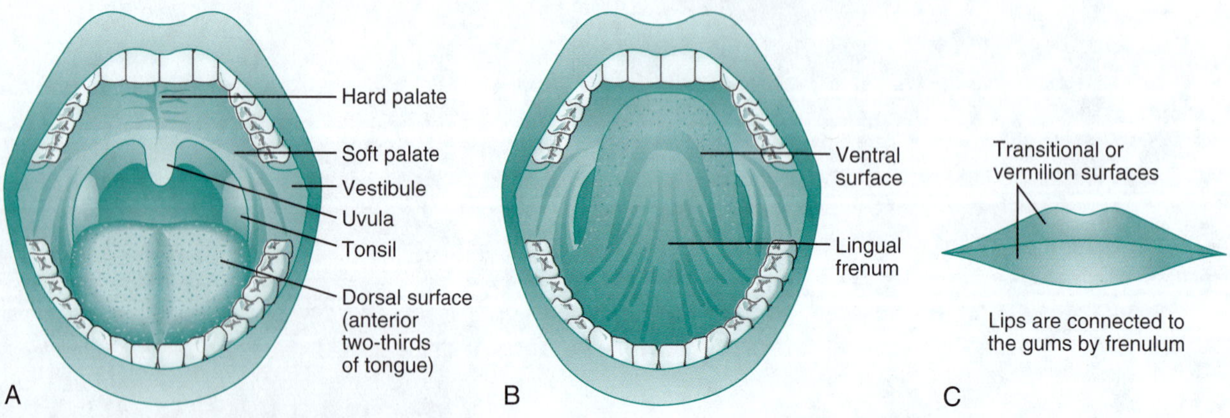

Figure 2–1 Anatomical structures of the mouth and lips. **A.** Dorsal surface. **B.** Ventral surface. **C.** Transitional or vermilion borders. Lips are connected to the gums by frenulum.

141.2 **Tip and lateral border of tongue**

141.3 **Ventral surface of tongue**
Anterior two-thirds of tongue, ventral surface
Frenulum linguae

❑141.4 **Anterior two-thirds of tongue, part unspecified**
Mobile part of tongue NOS

141.5 **Junctional zone**
Border of tongue at junction of fixed and mobile parts at insertion of anterior tonsillar pillar

141.6 **Lingual tonsil**

❑141.8 **Other sites of tongue**
Malignant neoplasm of contiguous or overlapping sites of tongue whose point of origin cannot be determined

❑141.9 **Tongue, unspecified**
Tongue NOS

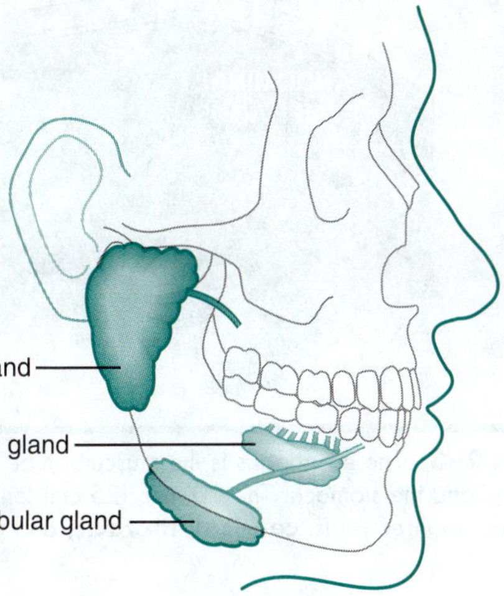

Figure 2–2 Major salivary glands.

● 142 **Malignant neoplasm of major salivary glands**

Includes: salivary ducts

Excludes *malignant neoplasm of minor salivary glands:*
NOS (145.9)
buccal mucosa (145.0)
soft palate (145.3)
tongue (141.0–141.9)
tonsil, palatine (146.0)

142.0 **Parotid gland**

142.1 **Submandibular gland**
Submaxillary gland

142.2 **Sublingual gland**

❑142.8 **Other major salivary glands**
Malignant neoplasm of contiguous or overlapping sites of salivary glands and ducts whose point of origin cannot be determined

❑142.9 **Salivary gland, unspecified**
Salivary gland (major) NOS

● 143 **Malignant neoplasm of gum**

Includes: alveolar (ridge) mucosa
gingiva (alveolar) (marginal)
interdental papillae

Excludes *malignant odontogenic neoplasms (170.0–170.1)*

143.0 **Upper gum**

143.1 **Lower gum**

❑143.8 **Other sites of gum**
Malignant neoplasm of contiguous or overlapping sites of gum whose point of origin cannot be determined

❑143.9 **Gum, unspecified**

● 144 **Malignant neoplasm of floor of mouth**

144.0 **Anterior portion**
Anterior to the premolar-canine junction

144.1 **Lateral portion**

❑144.8 **Other sites of floor of mouth**
Malignant neoplasm of contiguous or overlapping sites of floor of mouth whose point of origin cannot be determined

❑144.9 **Floor of mouth, part unspecified**

● 145 **Malignant neoplasm of other and unspecified parts of mouth**

Excludes *mucosa of lips (140.0–140.9)*

145.0 **Cheek mucosa**
Buccal mucosa
Cheek, inner aspect

145.1 **Vestibule of mouth**
Buccal sulcus (upper) (lower)
Labial sulcus (upper) (lower)

145.2 **Hard palate**

145.3 **Soft palate**

Excludes *nasopharyngeal [posterior] [superior] surface of soft palate (147.3)*

145.4 **Uvula**

❑145.5 **Palate, unspecified**
Junction of hard and soft palate
Roof of mouth

145.6 **Retromolar area**

❑145.8 **Other specified parts of mouth**
Malignant neoplasm of contiguous or overlapping sites of mouth whose point of origin cannot be determined

❑145.9 **Mouth, unspecified**
Buccal cavity NOS
Minor salivary gland, unspecified site
Oral cavity NOS

● 146 **Malignant neoplasm of oropharynx**

146.0 **Tonsil**

Tonsil:	Tonsil:
NOS	palatine
faucial	

Excludes *lingual tonsil (141.6)*
pharyngeal tonsil (147.1)

146.1 **Tonsillar fossa**

146.2 **Tonsillar pillars (anterior) (posterior)**
Faucial pillar
Glossopalatine fold
Palatoglossal arch
Palatopharyngeal arch

146.3 **Vallecula**
Anterior and medial surface of the pharyngoepiglottic fold

146.4 **Anterior aspect of epiglottis**
Epiglottis, free border [margin]
Glossoepiglottic fold(s)

Excludes *epiglottis:*
NOS (161.1)
suprahyoid portion (161.1)

146.5 **Junctional region**
Junction of the free margin of the epiglottis, the aryepiglottic fold, and the pharyngoepiglottic fold

146.6 **Lateral wall of oropharynx**

146.7 **Posterior wall of oropharynx**

❑146.8 **Other specified sites of oropharynx**
Branchial cleft
Malignant neoplasm of contiguous or overlapping sites of oropharynx whose point of origin cannot be determined

❑146.9 **Oropharynx, unspecified**

● 147 **Malignant neoplasm of nasopharynx**

147.0 **Superior wall**
Roof of nasopharynx

147.1 **Posterior wall**
Adenoid
Pharyngeal tonsil

147.2 **Lateral wall**
Fossa of Rosenmüller
Opening of auditory tube
Pharyngeal recess

147.3 **Anterior wall**
Floor of nasopharynx
Nasopharyngeal [posterior] [superior] surface of soft palate
Posterior margin of nasal septum and choanae

❑147.8 **Other specified sites of nasopharynx**
Malignant neoplasm of contiguous or overlapping sites of nasopharynx whose point of origin cannot be determined

❑147.9 **Nasopharynx, unspecified**
Nasopharyngeal wall NOS

● 148 **Malignant neoplasm of hypopharynx**

148.0 **Postcricoid region**

148.1 **Pyriform sinus**
Pyriform fossa

148.2 **Aryepiglottic fold, hypopharyngeal aspect**
Aryepiglottic fold or interarytenoid fold:
NOS
marginal zone

Excludes *aryepiglottic fold or interarytenoid fold, laryngeal aspect (161.1)*

148.3 **Posterior hypopharyngeal wall**

❑148.8 **Other specified sites of hypopharynx**
Malignant neoplasm of contiguous or overlapping sites of hypopharynx whose point of origin cannot be determined

❑148.9 **Hypopharynx, unspecified**
Hypopharyngeal wall NOS
Hypopharynx NOS

● 149 **Malignant neoplasm of other and ill-defined sites within the lip, oral cavity, and pharynx**

❑149.0 **Pharynx, unspecified**

149.1 **Waldeyer's ring**

❑149.8 **Other**
Malignant neoplasms of lip, oral cavity, and pharynx whose point of origin cannot be assigned to any one of the categories 140–148

Excludes *"book leaf" neoplasm [ventral surface of tongue and floor of mouth] (145.8)*

❑149.9 **Ill-defined**

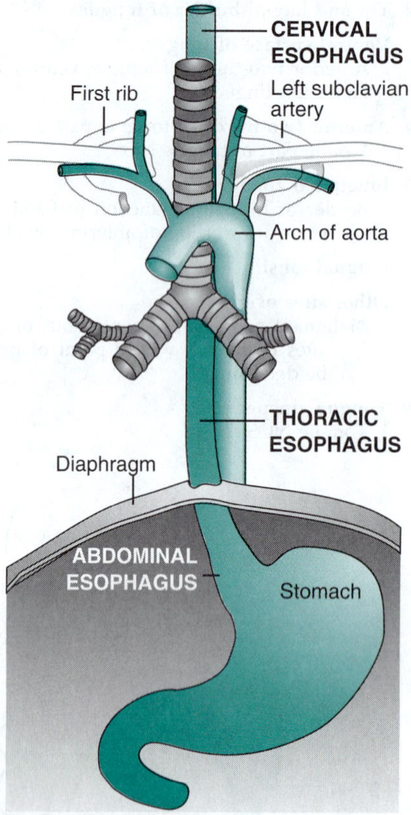

Figure 2–3 The esophagus is the muscular tube that connects the pharynx and the stomach. The 10 inch (25 cm) long esophagus is divided into three parts: **cervical, thoracic,** and **abdominal.**

MALIGNANT NEOPLASM OF DIGESTIVE ORGANS AND PERITONEUM (150–159)

Excludes *carcinoma in situ (230.1–230.9)*

● 150 **Malignant neoplasm of esophagus**

150.0 **Cervical esophagus**

150.1 **Thoracic esophagus**

150.2 **Abdominal esophagus**

Excludes *adenocarcinoma (151.0)*
cardioesophageal junction (151.0)

150.3 **Upper third of esophagus**
Proximal third of esophagus

150.4 **Middle third of esophagus**

150.5 **Lower third of esophagus**
Distal third of esophagus

Excludes *adenocarcinoma (151.0)*
cardioesophageal junction (151.0)

❑150.8 **Other specified part**
Malignant neoplasm of contiguous or overlapping sites of esophagus whose point of origin cannot be determined

❑150.9 **Esophagus, unspecified**

161.1 Supraglottis
Aryepiglottic fold or interarytenoid fold, laryngeal aspect
Epiglottis (suprahyoid portion) NOS
Extrinsic larynx
False vocal cords
Posterior (laryngeal) surface of epiglottis
Ventricular bands

Excludes *anterior aspect of epiglottis (146.4)*
aryepiglottic fold or interarytenoid fold:
NOS (148.2)
hypopharyngeal aspect (148.2)
marginal zone (148.2)

161.2 Subglottis

161.3 Laryngeal cartilages

Cartilage:	Cartilage:
arytenoid	cuneiform
cricoid	thyroid

❑ **161.8 Other specified sites of larynx**
Malignant neoplasm of contiguous or overlapping sites of larynx whose point of origin cannot be determined

❑ **161.9 Larynx, unspecified**

● **162 Malignant neoplasm of trachea, bronchus, and lung**

162.0 Trachea
Cartilage of trachea
Mucosa of trachea

162.2 Main bronchus
Carina
Hilus of lung

162.3 Upper lobe, bronchus or lung

162.4 Middle lobe, bronchus or lung

162.5 Lower lobe, bronchus or lung

❑ **162.8 Other parts of bronchus or lung**
Malignant neoplasm of contiguous or overlapping sites of bronchus or lung whose point of origin cannot be determined

❑ **162.9 Bronchus and lung, unspecified**

● **163 Malignant neoplasm of pleura**

163.0 Parietal pleura

163.1 Visceral pleura

❑ **163.8 Other specified sites of pleura**
Malignant neoplasm of contiguous or overlapping sites of pleura whose point of origin cannot be determined

❑ **163.9 Pleura, unspecified**

● **164 Malignant neoplasm of thymus, heart, and mediastinum**

164.0 Thymus

164.1 Heart
Endocardium
Epicardium
Myocardium
Pericardium

Excludes *great vessels (171.4)*

164.2 Anterior mediastinum

164.3 Posterior mediastinum

❑ **164.8 Other**
Malignant neoplasm of contiguous or overlapping sites of thymus, heart, and mediastinum whose point of origin cannot be determined

❑ **164.9 Mediastinum, part unspecified**

● **165 Malignant neoplasm of other and ill-defined sites within the respiratory system and intrathoracic organs**

❑ **165.0 Upper respiratory tract, part unspecified**

❑ **165.8 Other**
Malignant neoplasm of respiratory and intrathoracic organs whose point of origin cannot be assigned to any one of the categories 160–164

❑ **165.9 Ill-defined sites within the respiratory system**
Respiratory tract NOS

Excludes *intrathoracic NOS (195.1)*
thoracic NOS (195.1)

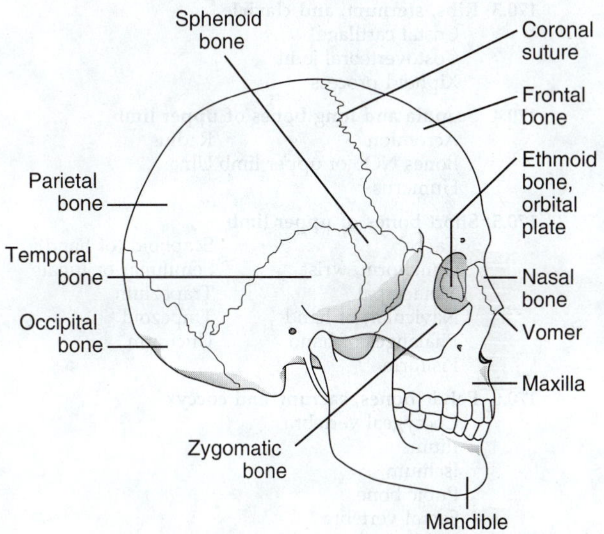

Figure 2–6 Bones of the skull and face.

MALIGNANT NEOPLASM OF BONE, CONNECTIVE TISSUE, SKIN, AND BREAST (170–176)

Excludes *carcinoma in situ:*
breast (233.0)
skin (232.0–232.9)

● **170 Malignant neoplasm of bone and articular cartilage**

Includes: cartilage (articular) (joint)
periosteum

Excludes *bone marrow NOS (202.9)*
cartilage:
ear (171.0)
eyelid (171.0)
larynx (161.3)
nose (160.0)
synovia (171.0–171.9)

170.0 Bones of skull and face, except mandible

Bone:	Bone:
ethmoid	sphenoid
frontal	temporal
malar	zygomatic
nasal	Maxilla (superior)
occipital	Turbinate
orbital	Upper jaw bone
parietal	Vomer

Excludes *carcinoma, any type except intraosseous or odontogenic:*
maxilla, maxillary (sinus) (160.2)
upper jaw bone (143.0)
jaw bone (lower) (170.1)

ICD-9-CM 100-199 Vol. 1

170.1 Mandible
Inferior maxilla
Jaw bone NOS
Lower jaw bone

Excludes *carcinoma, any type except intraosseous or odontogenic:*
jaw bone NOS (143.9)
lower (143.1)
upper jaw bone (170.0)

170.2 Vertebral column, excluding sacrum and coccyx
Spinal column
Spine
Vertebra

Excludes *sacrum and coccyx (170.6)*

170.3 Ribs, sternum, and clavicle
Costal cartilage
Costovertebral joint
Xiphoid process

170.4 Scapula and long bones of upper limb
Acromion
Bones NOS of upper limb
Humerus
Radius
Ulna

170.5 Short bones of upper limb
Carpal
Cuneiform, wrist
Metacarpal
Navicular, of hand
Phalanges of hand
Pisiform
Scaphoid (of hand)
Semilunar or lunate
Trapezium
Trapezoid
Unciform

170.6 Pelvic bones, sacrum, and coccyx
Coccygeal vertebra
Ilium
Ischium
Pubic bone
Sacral vertebra

170.7 Long bones of lower limb
Bones NOS of lower limb
Femur
Fibula
Tibia

170.8 Short bones of lower limb
Astragalus [talus]
Calcaneus
Cuboid
Cuneiform, ankle
Metatarsal
Navicular (of ankle)
Patella
Phalanges of foot
Tarsal

❑ **170.9 Bone and articular cartilage, site unspecified**

● **171 Malignant neoplasm of connective and other soft tissue**

Includes: blood vessel
bursa
fascia
fat
ligament, except uterine
muscle
peripheral, sympathetic, and parasympathetic nerves and ganglia
synovia
tendon (sheath)

Excludes *cartilage (of):*
articular (170.0–170.9)
larynx (161.3)
nose (160.0)
connective tissue:
breast (174.0–175.9)
internal organs - code to malignant neoplasm of the site [e.g., leiomyosarcoma of stomach, 151.9]
heart (164.1)
uterine ligament (183.4)

171.0 Head, face, and neck
Cartilage of:
ear
eyelid

171.2 Upper limb, including shoulder
Arm
Finger
Forearm
Hand

171.3 Lower limb, including hip
Foot
Leg
Popliteal space
Thigh
Toe

171.4 Thorax
Axilla
Diaphragm
Great vessels

Excludes *heart (164.1)*
mediastinum (164.2–164.9)
thymus (164.0)

171.5 Abdomen
Abdominal wall
Hypochondrium

Excludes *peritoneum (158.8)*
retroperitoneum (158.0)

171.6 Pelvis
Buttock
Groin
Inguinal region
Perineum

Excludes *pelvic peritoneum (158.8)*
retroperitoneum (158.0)
uterine ligament, any (183.3–183.5)

❑ **171.7 Trunk, unspecified**
Back NOS
Flank NOS

❑ **171.8 Other specified sites of connective and other soft tissue**
Malignant neoplasm of contiguous or overlapping sites of connective tissue whose point of origin cannot be determined

❑ **171.9 Connective and other soft tissue, site unspecified**

● **172 Malignant melanoma of skin**

Includes: melanocarcinoma
melanoma (skin) NOS

Excludes *skin of genital organs (184.0–184.9, 187.1–187.9)*
sites other than skin - code to malignant neoplasm of the site

172.0 Lip

Excludes *vermilion border of lip (140.0–140.1, 140.9)*

172.1 Eyelid, including canthus

172.2 Ear and external auditory canal
Auricle (ear)
Auricular canal, external
External [acoustic] meatus
Pinna

❑ **172.3 Other and unspecified parts of face**
Cheek (external)
Chin
Eyebrow
Forehead
Nose, external
Temple

172.4 **Scalp and neck**

172.5 **Trunk, except scrotum**

Axilla
Breast
Buttock
Groin
Perianal skin
Perineum
Umbilicus

Excludes *anal canal (154.2)*
anus NOS (154.3)
scrotum (187.7)

172.6 **Upper limb, including shoulder**

Arm
Finger
Forearm
Hand

172.7 **Lower limb, including hip**

Ankle
Foot
Heel
Knee
Leg
Popliteal area
Thigh
Toe

❑172.8 **Other specified sites of skin**

Malignant melanoma of contiguous or overlapping sites of skin whose point of origin cannot be determined

❑172.9 **Melanoma of skin, site unspecified**

● 173 **Other malignant neoplasm of skin**

Includes: malignant neoplasm of:
sebaceous glands
sudoriferous, sudoriparous glands
sweat glands

Excludes *Kaposi's sarcoma (176.0–176.9)*
malignant melanoma of skin (172.0–172.9)
skin of genital organs (184.0–184.9, 187.1–187.9)

173.0 **Skin of lip**

Excludes *vermilion border of lip (140.0–140.1, 140.9)*

173.1 **Eyelid, including canthus**

Excludes *cartilage of eyelid (171.0)*

173.2 **Skin of ear and external auditory canal**

Auricle (ear)
Auricular canal, external
External meatus
Pinna

Excludes *cartilage of ear (171.0)*

❑173.3 **Skin of other and unspecified parts of face**

Cheek, external
Chin
Eyebrow
Forehead
Nose, external
Temple

173.4 **Scalp and skin of neck**

173.5 **Skin of trunk, except scrotum**

Axillary fold
Perianal skin
Skin of:
abdominal wall
anus
back
breast
buttock
chest wall
groin
perineum
umbilicus

Excludes *anal canal (154.2)*
anus NOS (154.3)
skin of scrotum (187.7)

173.6 **Skin of upper limb, including shoulder**

Arm
Finger
Forearm
Hand

173.7 **Skin of lower limb, including hip**

Ankle
Foot
Heel
Knee
Leg
Popliteal area
Thigh
Toe

❑173.8 **Other specified sites of skin**

Malignant neoplasm of contiguous or overlapping sites of skin whose point of origin cannot be determined

❑173.9 **Skin, site unspecified**

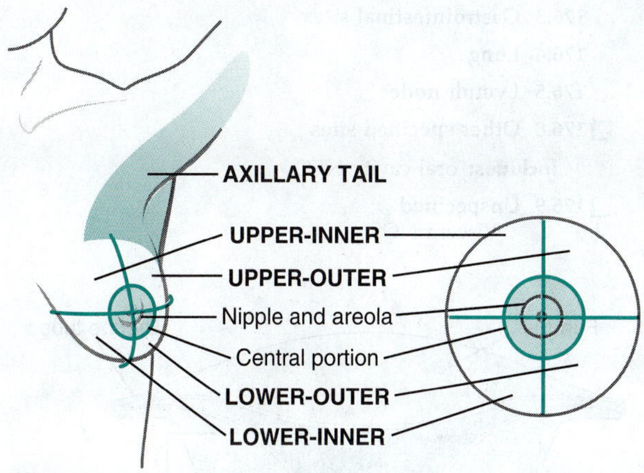

Figure 2–7 Female breast quadrants and axillary tail.

● 174 **Malignant neoplasm of female breast**

Includes: breast (female)
connective tissue
soft parts
Paget's disease of:
breast
nipple

Excludes *skin of breast (172.5, 173.5)*

174.0 **Nipple and areola**

174.1 **Central portion**

174.2 **Upper-inner quadrant**

174.3 **Lower-inner quadrant**

174.4 **Upper-outer quadrant**

174.5 **Lower-outer quadrant**

174.6 **Axillary tail**

❑174.8 **Other specified sites of female breast**

Ectopic sites
Inner breast
Lower breast
Malignant neoplasm of contiguous or overlapping sites of breast whose point of origin cannot be determined
Midline of breast
Outer breast
Upper breast

❑ **174.9 Breast (female), unspecified**

● **175 Malignant neoplasm of male breast**

Excludes *skin of breast (172.5, 173.5)*

175.0 Nipple and areola

❑ **175.9 Other and unspecified sites of male breast**
Ectopic breast tissue, male

● **176 Kaposi's sarcoma**

176.0 Skin

176.1 Soft tissue

Includes: blood vessel
connective tissue
fascia
ligament
lymphatic(s) NEC
muscle

Excludes *lymph glands and nodes (176.5)*

176.2 Palate

176.3 Gastrointestinal sites

176.4 Lung

176.5 Lymph nodes

❑ **176.8 Other specified sites**

Includes: oral cavity NEC

❑ **176.9 Unspecified**
Viscera NOS

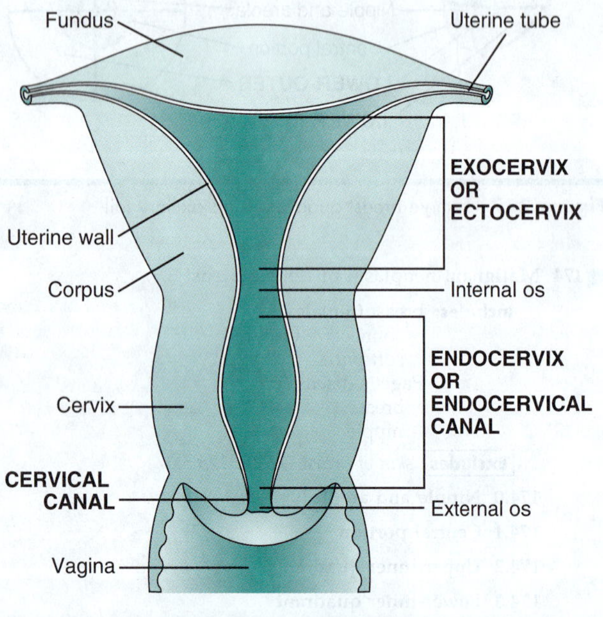

Figure 2-8 Cervix uteri.

MALIGNANT NEOPLASM OF GENITOURINARY ORGANS (179–189)

Excludes *carcinoma in situ (233.1–233.9)*

❑ **179 Malignant neoplasm of uterus, part unspecified**

● **180 Malignant neoplasm of cervix uteri**

Includes: invasive malignancy [carcinoma]

Excludes *carcinoma in situ (233.1)*

180.0 Endocervix
Cervical canal NOS
Endocervical canal
Endocervical gland

180.1 Exocervix

❑ **180.8 Other specified sites of cervix**
Cervical stump
Squamocolumnar junction of cervix
Malignant neoplasm of contiguous or overlapping sites of cervix uteri whose point of origin cannot be determined

❑ **180.9 Cervix uteri, unspecified**

181 Malignant neoplasm of placenta
Choriocarcinoma NOS
Chorioepithelioma NOS

Excludes *chorioadenoma (destruens) (236.1)*
hydatidiform mole (630)
malignant (236.1)
invasive mole (236.1)
male choriocarcinoma NOS (186.0–186.9)

● **182 Malignant neoplasm of body of uterus**

Excludes *carcinoma in situ (233.2)*

182.0 Corpus uteri, except isthmus
Cornu
Endometrium
Fundus
Myometrium

182.1 Isthmus
Lower uterine segment

❑ **182.8 Other specified sites of body of uterus**
Malignant neoplasm of contiguous or overlapping sites of body of uterus whose point of origin cannot be determined

Excludes *uterus NOS (179)*

● **183 Malignant neoplasm of ovary and other uterine adnexa**

Excludes *Douglas' cul-de-sac (158.8)*

183.0 Ovary

Use additional code to identify any functional activity

183.2 Fallopian tube
Oviduct
Uterine tube

183.3 Broad ligament
Mesovarium
Parovarian region

183.4 Parametrium
Uterine ligament NOS
Uterosacral ligament

183.5 Round ligament

❑ **183.8 Other specified sites of uterine adnexa**
Tubo-ovarian
Utero-ovarian
Malignant neoplasm of contiguous or overlapping sites of ovary and other uterine adnexa whose point of origin cannot be determined

❑ **183.9 Uterine adnexa, unspecified**

● **184 Malignant neoplasm of other and unspecified female genital organs**

Excludes *carcinoma in situ (233.3)*

184.0 Vagina
Gartner's duct
Vaginal vault

184.1 **Labia majora**
Greater vestibular [Bartholin's] gland

184.2 **Labia minora**

184.3 **Clitoris**

❑184.4 **Vulva, unspecified**
External female genitalia NOS
Pudendum

❑184.8 **Other specified sites of female genital organs**
Malignant neoplasm of contiguous or overlapping sites of female genital organs whose point of origin cannot be determined

❑184.9 **Female genital organ, site unspecified**
Female genitourinary tract NOS

185 **Malignant neoplasm of prostate**
Excludes *seminal vesicles (187.8)*

● 186 **Malignant neoplasm of testis**
Use additional code to identify any functional activity

186.0 **Undescended testis**
Ectopic testis
Retained testis

❑186.9 **Other and unspecified testis**
Testis:
NOS
descended
scrotal

● 187 **Malignant neoplasm of penis and other male genital organs**

187.1 **Prepuce**
Foreskin

187.2 **Glans penis**

187.3 **Body of penis**
Corpus cavernosum

❑187.4 **Penis, part unspecified**
Skin of penis NOS

187.5 **Epididymis**

187.6 **Spermatic cord**
Vas deferens

187.7 **Scrotum**
Skin of scrotum

❑187.8 **Other specified sites of male genital organs**
Seminal vesicle
Tunica vaginalis
Malignant neoplasm of contiguous or overlapping sites of penis and other male genital organs whose point of origin cannot be determined

❑187.9 **Male genital organ, site unspecified**
Male genital organ or tract NOS

● 188 **Malignant neoplasm of bladder**
Excludes *carcinoma in situ (233.7)*

188.0 **Trigone of urinary bladder**

188.1 **Dome of urinary bladder**

188.2 **Lateral wall of urinary bladder**

188.3 **Anterior wall of urinary bladder**

188.4 **Posterior wall of urinary bladder**

188.5 **Bladder neck**
Internal urethral orifice

188.6 **Ureteric orifice**

188.7 **Urachus**

❑188.8 **Other specified sites of bladder**
Malignant neoplasm of contiguous or overlapping sites of bladder whose point of origin cannot be determined

❑188.9 **Bladder, part unspecified**
Bladder wall NOS

● 189 **Malignant neoplasm of kidney and other and unspecified urinary organs**

189.0 **Kidney, except pelvis**
Kidney NOS
Kidney parenchyma

189.1 **Renal pelvis**
Renal calyces
Ureteropelvic junction

189.2 **Ureter**
Excludes *ureteric orifice of bladder (188.6)*

189.3 **Urethra**
Excludes *urethral orifice of bladder (188.5)*

189.4 **Paraurethral glands**

❑189.8 **Other specified sites of urinary organs**
Malignant neoplasm of contiguous or overlapping sites of kidney and other urinary organs whose point of origin cannot be determined

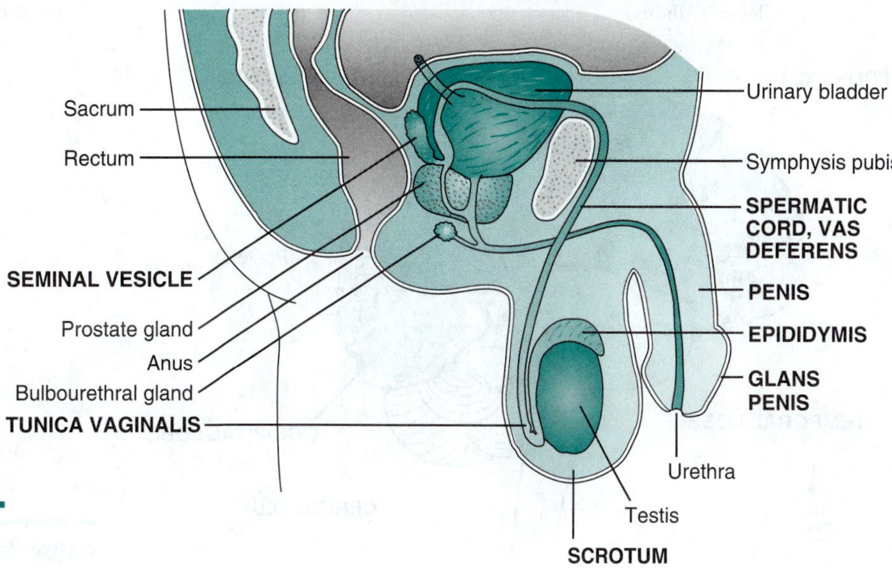

Figure 2–9 Penis and other male genital organs.

❑ **189.9 Urinary organ, site unspecified**
Urinary system NOS

MALIGNANT NEOPLASM OF OTHER AND UNSPECIFIED SITES (190–199)

Excludes *carcinoma in situ (234.0–234.9)*

● **190 Malignant neoplasm of eye**

Excludes *carcinoma in situ (234.0)*
eyelid (skin) (172.1, 173.1)
cartilage (171.0)
optic nerve (192.0)
orbital bone (170.0)

190.0 Eyeball, except conjunctiva, cornea, retina, and choroid
Ciliary body
Crystalline lens
Iris
Sclera
Uveal tract

190.1 Orbit
Connective tissue of orbit
Extraocular muscle
Retrobulbar

Excludes *bone of orbit (170.0)*

190.2 Lacrimal gland

190.3 Conjunctiva

190.4 Cornea

190.5 Retina

190.6 Choroid

190.7 Lacrimal duct
Lacrimal sac
Nasolacrimal duct

❑ **190.8 Other specified sites of eye**
Malignant neoplasm of contiguous or overlapping sites of eye whose point of origin cannot be determined

❑ **190.9 Eye, part unspecified**

● **191 Malignant neoplasm of brain**

Excludes *cranial nerves (192.0)*
retrobulbar area (190.1)

191.0 Cerebrum, except lobes and ventricles
Basal ganglia
Cerebral cortex
Corpus striatum
Globus pallidus
Hypothalamus
Thalamus

191.1 Frontal lobe

191.2 Temporal lobe
Hippocampus
Uncus

191.3 Parietal lobe

191.4 Occipital lobe

191.5 Ventricles
Choroid plexus
Floor of ventricle

191.6 Cerebellum NOS
Cerebellopontine angle

191.7 Brain stem
Cerebral peduncle
Medulla oblongata
Midbrain
Pons

❑ **191.8 Other parts of brain**
Corpus callosum
Tapetum
Malignant neoplasm of contiguous or overlapping sites of brain whose point of origin cannot be determined

❑ **191.9 Brain, unspecified**
Cranial fossa NOS

● **192 Malignant neoplasm of other and unspecified parts of nervous system**

Excludes *peripheral, sympathetic, and parasympathetic nerves and ganglia (171.0–171.9)*

192.0 Cranial nerves
Olfactory bulb

192.1 Cerebral meninges
Dura (mater)
Falx (cerebelli) (cerebri)
Meninges NOS
Tentorium

192.2 Spinal cord
Cauda equina

192.3 Spinal meninges

❑ **192.8 Other specified sites of nervous system**
Malignant neoplasm of contiguous or overlapping sites of other parts of nervous system whose point of origin cannot be determined

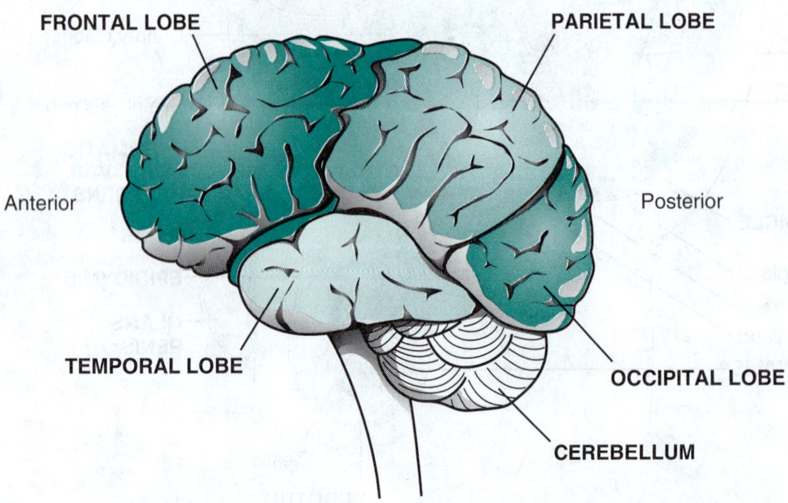

Figure 2–10 The brain.

❑ **192.9 Nervous system, part unspecified**
Nervous system (central) NOS
Excludes *meninges NOS (192.1)*

193 Malignant neoplasm of thyroid gland
Sipple's syndrome
Thyroglossal duct
Use additional code to identify any functional activity

● **194 Malignant neoplasm of other endocrine glands and related structures**
Use additional code to identify any functional activity
Excludes *islets of Langerhans (157.4)*
ovary (183.0)
testis (186.0–186.9)
thymus (164.0)

194.0 Adrenal gland
Adrenal cortex
Adrenal medulla
Suprarenal gland

194.1 Parathyroid gland

194.3 Pituitary gland and craniopharyngeal duct
Craniobuccal pouch
Hypophysis
Rathke's pouch
Sella turcica

194.4 Pineal gland

194.5 Carotid body

194.6 Aortic body and other paraganglia
Coccygeal body
Glomus jugulare
Para-aortic body

❑ **194.8 Other**
Pluriglandular involvement NOS
Note: If the sites of multiple involvements are known, they should be coded separately.

❑ **194.9 Endocrine gland, site unspecified**

● **195 Malignant neoplasm of other and ill-defined sites**
Includes: malignant neoplasms of contiguous sites, not elsewhere classified, whose point of origin cannot be determined
Excludes *malignant neoplasm:*
lymphatic and hematopoietic tissue (200.0–208.9)
secondary sites (196.0–198.8)
unspecified site (199.0–199.1)

195.0 Head, face, and neck
Cheek NOS
Jaw NOS
Nose NOS
Supraclavicular region NOS

195.1 Thorax
Axilla
Chest (wall) NOS
Intrathoracic NOS

195.2 Abdomen
Intra-abdominal NOS

195.3 Pelvis
Groin
Inguinal region NOS
Presacral region
Sacrococcygeal region
Sites overlapping systems within pelvis, as:
rectovaginal (septum)
rectovesical (septum)

195.4 Upper limb

195.5 Lower limb

❑ **195.8 Other specified sites**
Back NOS
Flank NOS
Trunk NOS

● **196 Secondary and unspecified malignant neoplasm of lymph nodes**
Excludes *any malignant neoplasm of lymph nodes, specified as primary (200.0–202.9)*
Hodgkin's disease (201.0–201.9)
lymphosarcoma (200.1)
reticulosarcoma (200.0)
other forms of lymphoma (202.0–202.9)

196.0 Lymph nodes of head, face, and neck
Cervical
Cervicofacial
Scalene
Supraclavicular

196.1 Intrathoracic lymph nodes
Bronchopulmonary
Intercostal
Mediastinal
Tracheobronchial

196.2 Intra-abdominal lymph nodes
Intestinal
Mesenteric
Retroperitoneal

196.3 Lymph nodes of axilla and upper limb
Brachial
Epitrochlear
Infraclavicular
Pectoral

196.5 Lymph nodes of inguinal region and lower limb
Femoral
Groin
Popliteal
Tibial

196.6 Intrapelvic lymph nodes
Hypogastric
Iliac
Obturator
Parametrial

❑ **196.8 Lymph nodes of multiple sites**

❑ **196.9 Site unspecified**
Lymph nodes NOS

● **197 Secondary malignant neoplasm of respiratory and digestive systems**
Excludes *lymph node metastasis (196.0–196.9)*

197.0 Lung
Bronchus

197.1 Mediastinum

197.2 Pleura

❑ **197.3 Other respiratory organs**
Trachea

197.4 Small intestine, including duodenum

197.5 Large intestine and rectum

197.6 Retroperitoneum and peritoneum

197.7 Liver, specified as secondary

❑ **197.8 Other digestive organs and spleen**

● **198 Secondary malignant neoplasm of other specified sites**
Excludes *lymph node metastasis (196.0–196.9)*

198.0 Kidney

❑ **198.1 Other urinary organs**

198.2 Skin
Skin of breast

198.3 Brain and spinal cord

❑ **198.4 Other parts of nervous system**
Meninges (cerebral) (spinal)

198.5 Bone and bone marrow

198.6 Ovary

198.7 Adrenal gland
Suprarenal gland

● **198.8 Other specified sites**

198.81 Breast

Excludes *skin of breast (198.2)*

198.82 Genital organs

❑ **198.89 Other**

Excludes *retroperitoneal lymph nodes (196.2)*

● **199 Malignant neoplasm without specification of site**

199.0 Disseminated
Carcinomatosis unspecified site (primary) (secondary)
Generalized:
cancer unspecified site (primary) (secondary)
malignancy unspecified site (primary) (secondary)
Multiple cancer unspecified site (primary) (secondary)

❑ **199.1 Other**
Cancer unspecified site (primary) (secondary)
Carcinoma unspecified site (primary) (secondary)
Malignancy unspecified site (primary) (secondary)

MALIGNANT NEOPLASM OF LYMPHATIC AND HEMATOPOIETIC TISSUE (200–208)

Excludes *secondary neoplasm of:*
bone marrow (198.5)
spleen (197.8)
secondary and unspecified neoplasm of lymph nodes (196.0–196.9)

The following fifth-digit subclassification is for use with categories 200–202:

❑ **0 unspecified site, extranodal and solid organ sites**
1 lymph nodes of head, face, and neck
2 intrathoracic lymph nodes
3 intra-abdominal lymph nodes
4 lymph nodes of axilla and upper limb
5 lymph nodes of inguinal region and lower limb
6 intrapelvic lymph nodes
7 spleen
8 lymph nodes of multiple sites

● **200 Lymphosarcoma and reticulosarcoma**

Requires fifth digit. See note before section 200 for codes and definitions.

● **200.0 Reticulosarcoma**
Lymphoma (malignant):
histiocytic (diffuse):
nodular
pleomorphic cell type
reticulum cell type
Reticulum cell sarcoma:
NOS
pleomorphic cell type

● **200.1 Lymphosarcoma**
Lymphoblastoma (diffuse)
Lymphoma (malignant):
lymphoblastic (diffuse)
lymphocytic (cell type) (diffuse)
lymphosarcoma type
Lymphosarcoma:
NOS
diffuse NOS
lymphoblastic (diffuse)
lymphocytic (diffuse)
prolymphocytic

Excludes *lymphosarcoma:*
follicular or nodular (202.0)
mixed cell type (200.8)
lymphosarcoma cell leukemia (207.8)

● **200.2 Burkitt's tumor or lymphoma**
Malignant lymphoma, Burkitt's type

● ❑ **200.8 Other named variants**
Lymphoma (malignant):
lymphoplasmacytoid type
mixed lymphocytic-histiocytic (diffuse)
Lymphosarcoma, mixed cell type (diffuse)
Reticulolymphosarcoma (diffuse)

● **201 Hodgkin's disease**

Requires fifth digit. See note before section 200 for codes and definitions.

● **201.0 Hodgkin's paragranuloma**

● **201.1 Hodgkin's granuloma**

● **201.2 Hodgkin's sarcoma**

● **201.4 Lymphocytic-histiocytic predominance**

● **201.5 Nodular sclerosis**
Hodgkin's disease, nodular sclerosis:
NOS
cellular phase

● **201.6 Mixed cellularity**

● **201.7 Lymphocytic depletion**
Hodgkin's disease, lymphocytic depletion:
NOS
diffuse fibrosis
reticular type

● ❑ **201.9 Hodgkin's disease, unspecified**
Hodgkin's:
disease NOS
lymphoma NOS
Malignant:
lymphogranuloma
lymphogranulomatosis

● **202 Other malignant neoplasms of lymphoid and histiocytic tissue**

Requires fifth digit. See note before section 200 for codes and definitions.

● **202.0 Nodular lymphoma**
Brill-Symmers disease
Lymphoma:
follicular (giant)
lymphocytic, nodular
Lymphosarcoma:
follicular (giant)
nodular
Reticulosarcoma, follicular or nodular

● **202.1 Mycosis fungoides**

● **202.2 Sézary's disease**

● **202.3 Malignant histiocytosis**
Histiocytic medullary reticulosis
Malignant:
reticuloendotheliosis
reticulosis

● **202.4 Leukemic reticuloendotheliosis**
Hairy-cell leukemia

● **202.5 Letterer-Siwe disease**
Acute:
differentiated progressive histiocytosis
histiocytosis X (progressive)
infantile reticuloendotheliosis
reticulosis of infancy

Excludes *Hand-Schüller-Christian disease (277.89)* ⇐
histiocytosis (acute) (chronic) (277.89) ⇐
histiocytosis X (chronic) (277.89) ⇐

202.6 Malignant mast cell tumors
Malignant:
mastocytoma
mastocytosis
Mast cell sarcoma
Systemic tissue mast cell disease
Excludes *mast cell leukemia (207.8)*

202.8 Other lymphomas
Lymphoma (malignant):
NOS
diffuse
Excludes *benign lymphoma (229.0)*

202.9 Other and unspecified malignant neoplasms of lymphoid and histiocytic tissue
Follicular dendritic cell sarcoma ◀
Interdigitating dendritic cell sarcoma ◀
Langerhans cell sarcoma ◀
Malignant neoplasm of bone marrow NOS

203 Multiple myeloma and immunoproliferative neoplasms

The following fifth-digit subclassification is for use with category 203:
0 without mention of remission
1 in remission

203.0 Multiple myeloma
Kahler's disease
Myelomatosis
Excludes *solitary myeloma (238.6)*

203.1 Plasma cell leukemia
Plasmacytic leukemia

203.8 Other immunoproliferative neoplasms

204 Lymphoid leukemia

Includes: leukemia:
lymphatic
lymphoblastic
leukemia:
lymphocytic
lymphogenous

The following fifth-digit subclassification is for use with category 204:
0 without mention of remission
1 in remission

204.0 Acute
Excludes *acute exacerbation of chronic lymphoid leukemia (204.1)*

204.1 Chronic

204.2 Subacute

204.8 Other lymphoid leukemia
Aleukemic leukemia:
lymphatic
lymphocytic
lymphoid

204.9 Unspecified lymphoid leukemia

205 Myeloid leukemia

Includes: leukemia:
granulocytic
myeloblastic
myelocytic
myelogenous
myelomonocytic
myelosclerotic
myelosis

The following fifth-digit subclassification is for use with category 205:
0 without mention of remission
1 in remission

205.0 Acute
Acute promyelocytic leukemia
Excludes *acute exacerbation of chronic myeloid leukemia (205.1)*

205.1 Chronic
Eosinophilic leukemia
Neutrophilic leukemia

205.2 Subacute

205.3 Myeloid sarcoma
Chloroma
Granulocytic sarcoma

205.8 Other myeloid leukemia
Aleukemic leukemia:
granulocytic
myelogenous
myeloid
Aleukemic myelosis

205.9 Unspecified myeloid leukemia

206 Monocytic leukemia

Includes: leukemia:
histiocytic
monoblastic
monocytoid

The following fifth-digit subclassification is for use with category 206:
0 without mention of remission
1 in remission

206.0 Acute
Excludes *acute exacerbation of chronic monocytic leukemia (206.1)*

206.1 Chronic

206.2 Subacute

206.8 Other monocytic leukemia
Aleukemic:
monocytic leukemia
monocytoid leukemia

206.9 Unspecified monocytic leukemia

207 Other specified leukemia

Excludes *leukemic reticuloendotheliosis (202.4)*
plasma cell leukemia (203.1)

The following fifth-digit subclassification is for use with category 207:
0 without mention of remission
1 in remission

207.0 Acute erythremia and erythroleukemia
Acute erythremic myelosis
Di Guglielmo's disease
Erythremic myelosis

207.1 Chronic erythremia
Heilmeyer-Schöner disease

207.2 Megakaryocytic leukemia
Megakaryocytic myelosis
Thrombocytic leukemia

207.8 Other specified leukemia
Lymphosarcoma cell leukemia

208 Leukemia of unspecified cell type

The following fifth-digit subclassification is for use with category 208:
0 without mention of remission
1 in remission

208.0 Acute
Acute leukemia NOS
Blast cell leukemia
Stem cell leukemia
Excludes *acute exacerbation of chronic unspecified leukemia (208.1)*

●❑ 208.1 **Chronic**
Chronic leukemia NOS

●❑ 208.2 **Subacute**
Subacute leukemia NOS

●❑ 208.8 **Other leukemia of unspecified cell type**

●❑ 208.9 **Unspecified leukemia**
Leukemia NOS

BENIGN NEOPLASMS (210–229)

● 210 **Benign neoplasm of lip, oral cavity, and pharynx**

Excludes *cyst (of):*
jaw (526.0–526.2, 526.89)
oral soft tissue (528.4)
radicular (522.8)

210.0 **Lip**
Frenulum labii
Lip (inner aspect) (mucosa) (vermilion border)

Excludes *labial commissure (210.4)*
skin of lip (216.0)

210.1 **Tongue**
Lingual tonsil

210.2 **Major salivary glands**
Gland:
parotid
sublingual
submandibular

Excludes *benign neoplasms of minor salivary glands:*
NOS (210.4)
buccal mucosa (210.4)
lips (210.0)
palate (hard) (soft) (210.4)
tongue (210.1)
tonsil, palatine (210.5)

210.3 **Floor of mouth**

❑ 210.4 **Other and unspecified parts of mouth**
Gingiva
Gum (upper) (lower)
Labial commissure
Oral cavity NOS
Oral mucosa
Palate (hard) (soft)
Uvula

Excludes *benign odontogenic neoplasms of bone (213.0–213.1)*
developmental odontogenic cysts (526.0)
mucosa of lips (210.0)
nasopharyngeal [posterior] [superior] surface of soft palate (210.7)

210.5 **Tonsil**
Tonsil (faucial) (palatine)

Excludes *lingual tonsil (210.1)*
pharyngeal tonsil (210.7)
tonsillar:
fossa (210.6)
pillars (210.6)

❑ 210.6 **Other parts of oropharynx**
Branchial cleft or vestiges
Epiglottis, anterior aspect
Fauces NOS
Mesopharynx NOS
Tonsillar:
fossa
pillars
Vallecula

Excludes *epiglottis:*
NOS (212.1)
suprahyoid portion (212.1)

210.7 **Nasopharynx**
Adenoid tissue
Lymphadenoid tissue
Pharyngeal tonsil
Posterior nasal septum

210.8 **Hypopharynx**
Arytenoid fold
Laryngopharynx
Postcricoid region
Pyriform fossa

❑ 210.9 **Pharynx, unspecified**
Throat NOS

● 211 **Benign neoplasm of other parts of digestive system**

211.0 **Esophagus**

211.1 **Stomach**
Body of stomach
Cardia of stomach
Fundus of stomach
Cardiac orifice
Pylorus

211.2 **Duodenum, jejunum, and ileum**
Small intestine NOS

Excludes *ampulla of Vater (211.5)*
ileocecal valve (211.3)

211.3 **Colon**
Appendix
Cecum
Ileocecal valve
Large intestine NOS

Excludes *rectosigmoid junction (211.4)*

211.4 **Rectum and anal canal**
Anal canal or sphincter
Anus NOS
Rectosigmoid junction

Excludes *anus:*
margin (216.5)
skin (216.5)
perianal skin (216.5)

211.5 **Liver and biliary passages**
Ampulla of Vater
Common bile duct
Cystic duct
Gallbladder
Hepatic duct
Sphincter of Oddi

211.6 **Pancreas, except islets of Langerhans**

211.7 **Islets of Langerhans**
Islet cell tumor

Use additional code to identify any functional activity

211.8 **Retroperitoneum and peritoneum**
Mesentery
Mesocolon
Omentum
Retroperitoneal tissue

❑ 211.9 **Other and unspecified site**
Alimentary tract NOS
Digestive system NOS
Gastrointestinal tract NOS
Intestinal tract NOS
Intestine NOS
Spleen, not elsewhere classified

● 212 **Benign neoplasm of respiratory and intrathoracic organs**

212.0 **Nasal cavities, middle ear, and accessory sinuses**
Cartilage of nose
Eustachian tube
Nares
Septum of nose
Sinus:
ethmoidal
frontal
maxillary
sphenoidal

Excludes *auditory canal (external) (216.2)*
bone of:
ear (213.0)
nose [turbinates] (213.0)
cartilage of ear (215.0)
ear (external) (skin) (216.2)
nose NOS (229.8)
skin (216.3)
olfactory bulb (225.1)
polyp of:
accessory sinus (471.8)
ear (385.30–385.35)
nasal cavity (471.0)
posterior margin of septum and choanae (210.7)

212.1 Larynx
Cartilage:
arytenoid
cricoid
cuneiform
thyroid
Epiglottis (suprahyoid portion) NOS
Glottis
Vocal cords (false) (true)

Excludes *epiglottis, anterior aspect (210.6)*
polyp of vocal cord or larynx (478.4)

212.2 Trachea

212.3 Bronchus and lung
Carina
Hilus of lung

212.4 Pleura

212.5 Mediastinum

212.6 Thymus

212.7 Heart

Excludes *great vessels (215.4)*

❑ **212.8 Other specified sites**

❑ **212.9 Site unspecified**
Respiratory organ NOS
Upper respiratory tract NOS

Excludes *intrathoracic NOS (229.8)*
thoracic NOS (229.8)

● **213 Benign neoplasm of bone and articular cartilage**

Includes: cartilage (articular) (joint)
periosteum

Excludes *cartilage of:*
ear (215.0)
eyelid (215.0)
larynx (212.1)
cartilage of:
nose (212.0)
exostosis NOS (726.91)
synovia (215.0–215.9)

213.0 Bones of skull and face

Excludes *lower jaw bone (213.1)*

213.1 Lower jaw bone

213.2 Vertebral column, excluding sacrum and coccyx

213.3 Ribs, sternum, and clavicle

213.4 Scapula and long bones of upper limb

213.5 Short bones of upper limb

213.6 Pelvic bones, sacrum, and coccyx

213.7 Long bones of lower limb

213.8 Short bones of lower limb

❑ **213.9 Bone and articular cartilage, site unspecified**

● **214 Lipoma**

Includes: angiolipoma
fibrolipoma
hibernoma
lipoma (fetal) (infiltrating) (intramuscular)
myelolipoma
myxolipoma

214.0 Skin and subcutaneous tissue of face

❑ **214.1 Other skin and subcutaneous tissue**

214.2 Intrathoracic organs

214.3 Intra-abdominal organs

214.4 Spermatic cord

❑ **214.8 Other specified sites**

❑ **214.9 Lipoma, unspecified site**

● **215 Other benign neoplasm of connective and other soft tissue**

Includes: blood vessel
bursa
fascia
ligament
muscle
peripheral, sympathetic, and parasympathetic nerves and ganglia
synovia
tendon (sheath)

Excludes *cartilage:*
articular (213.0–213.9)
larynx (212.1)
nose (212.0)
connective tissue of:
breast (217)
internal organ, except lipoma and hemangioma - code to benign neoplasm of the site
lipoma (214.0–214.9)

215.0 Head, face, and neck

215.2 Upper limb, including shoulder

215.3 Lower limb, including hip

215.4 Thorax

Excludes *heart (212.7)*
mediastinum (212.5)
thymus (212.6)

215.5 Abdomen
Abdominal wall
Hypochondrium

215.6 Pelvis
Buttock
Groin
Inguinal region
Perineum

Excludes *uterine:*
leiomyoma (218.0–218.9)
ligament, any (221.0)

❑ **215.7 Trunk, unspecified**
Back NOS
Flank NOS

❑ **215.8 Other specified sites**

❑ **215.9 Site unspecified**

● **216 Benign neoplasm of skin**

Includes: blue nevus
dermatofibroma
hydrocystoma
pigmented nevus
syringoadenoma
syringoma

Excludes *skin of genital organs (221.0–222.9)*

ICD-9-CM 200-299 Vol. 1

216.0 Skin of lip

Excludes *vermilion border of lip (210.0)*

216.1 Eyelid, including canthus

Excludes *cartilage of eyelid (215.0)*

216.2 Ear and external auditory canal
Auricle (ear)
Auricular canal, external
External meatus
Pinna

Excludes *cartilage of ear (215.0)*

❑216.3 Skin of other and unspecified parts of face
Cheek, external
Eyebrow
Nose, external
Temple

216.4 Scalp and skin of neck

216.5 Skin of trunk, except scrotum
Axillary fold
Perianal skin
Skin of:
abdominal wall
anus
back
breast
buttock
chest wall
groin
perineum
Umbilicus

Excludes *anal canal (211.4)*
anus NOS (211.4)
skin of scrotum (222.4)

216.6 Skin of upper limb, including shoulder

216.7 Skin of lower limb, including hip

❑216.8 Other specified sites of skin

❑216.9 Skin, site unspecified

217 Benign neoplasm of breast
Breast (male) (female)
connective tissue
glandular tissue
soft parts

Excludes *adenofibrosis (610.2)*
benign cyst of breast (610.0)
fibrocystic disease (610.1)
skin of breast (216.5)

● 218 Uterine leiomyoma

Includes: fibroid (bleeding) (uterine)
uterine:
fibromyoma
myoma

218.0 Submucous leiomyoma of uterus

218.1 Intramural leiomyoma of uterus
Interstitial leiomyoma of uterus

218.2 Subserous leiomyoma of uterus
Subperitoneal leiomyoma of uterus

❑218.9 Leiomyoma of uterus, unspecified

● 219 Other benign neoplasm of uterus

219.0 Cervix uteri

219.1 Corpus uteri
Endometrium
Fundus
Myometrium

❑219.8 Other specified parts of uterus

❑219.9 Uterus, part unspecified

220 Benign neoplasm of ovary

Use additional code to identify any functional activity (256.0–256.1)

Excludes *cyst:*
corpus albicans (620.2)
corpus luteum (620.1)
endometrial (617.1)
follicular (atretic) (620.0)
graafian follicle (620.0)
ovarian NOS (620.2)
retention (620.2)

● 221 Benign neoplasm of other female genital organs

Includes: adenomatous polyp
benign teratoma

Excludes *cyst:*
epoophoron (752.11)
fimbrial (752.11)
Gartner's duct (752.11)
parovarian (752.11)

221.0 Fallopian tube and uterine ligaments
Oviduct
Parametrium
Uterine ligament (broad) (round) (uterosacral)
Uterine tube

221.1 Vagina

221.2 Vulva
Clitoris
External female genitalia NOS
Greater vestibular [Bartholin's] gland
Labia (majora) (minora)
Pudendum

Excludes *Bartholin's (duct) (gland) cyst (616.2)*

❑221.8 Other specified sites of female genital organs

❑221.9 Female genital organ, site unspecified
Female genitourinary tract NOS

● 222 Benign neoplasm of male genital organs

222.0 Testis

Use additional code to identify any functional activity

222.1 Penis
Corpus cavernosum
Glans penis
Prepuce

222.2 Prostate

Excludes *adenomatous hyperplasia of prostate (600.20–600.21)* ⬅
prostatic:
adenoma (600.20–600.21) ⬅
enlargement (600.00–600.21) ⬅
hypertrophy (600.00–600.21) ⬅

222.3 Epididymis

222.4 Scrotum
Skin of scrotum

❑222.8 Other specified sites of male genital organs
Seminal vesicle
Spermatic cord

❑222.9 Male genital organ, site unspecified
Male genitourinary tract NOS

● 223 **Benign neoplasm of kidney and other urinary organs**

223.0 **Kidney, except pelvis**
Kidney NOS

Excludes *renal:*
calyces (223.1)
pelvis (223.1)

223.1 **Renal pelvis**

223.2 **Ureter**

Excludes *ureteric orifice of bladder (223.3)*

223.3 **Bladder**

● 223.8 **Other specified sites of urinary organs**

223.81 **Urethra**

Excludes *urethral orifice of bladder (223.3)*

❑ 223.89 **Other**
Paraurethral glands

❑ 223.9 **Urinary organ, site unspecified**
Urinary system NOS

● 224 **Benign neoplasm of eye**

Excludes *cartilage of eyelid (215.0)*
eyelid (skin) (216.1)
optic nerve (225.1)
orbital bone (213.0)

224.0 **Eyeball, except conjunctiva, cornea, retina, and choroid**
Ciliary body
Iris
Sclera
Uveal tract

224.1 **Orbit**

Excludes *bone of orbit (213.0)*

224.2 **Lacrimal gland**

224.3 **Conjunctiva**

224.4 **Cornea**

224.5 **Retina**

Excludes *hemangioma of retina (228.03)*

224.6 **Choroid**

224.7 **Lacrimal duct**
Lacrimal sac
Nasolacrimal duct

❑ 224.8 **Other specified parts of eye**

❑ 224.9 **Eye, part unspecified**

● 225 **Benign neoplasm of brain and other parts of nervous system**

Excludes *hemangioma (228.02)*
neurofibromatosis (237.7)
peripheral, sympathetic, and parasympathetic nerves and ganglia (215.0–215.9)
retrobulbar (224.1)

225.0 **Brain**

225.1 **Cranial nerves**

225.2 **Cerebral meninges**
Meninges NOS
Meningioma (cerebral)

225.3 **Spinal cord**
Cauda equina

225.4 **Spinal meninges**
Spinal meningioma

❑ 225.8 **Other specified sites of nervous system**

❑ 225.9 **Nervous system, part unspecified**
Nervous system (central) NOS

Excludes *meninges NOS (225.2)*

226 **Benign neoplasm of thyroid glands**

Use additional code to identify any functional activity

● 227 **Benign neoplasm of other endocrine glands and related structures**

Use additional code to identify any functional activity

Excludes *ovary (220)*
pancreas (211.6)
testis (222.0)

227.0 **Adrenal gland**
Suprarenal gland

227.1 **Parathyroid gland**

227.3 **Pituitary gland and craniopharyngeal duct (pouch)**
Craniobuccal pouch
Hypophysis
Rathke's pouch
Sella turcica

227.4 **Pineal gland**
Pineal body

227.5 **Carotid body**

227.6 **Aortic body and other paraganglia**
Coccygeal body
Glomus jugulare
Para-aortic body

❑ 227.8 **Other**

❑ 227.9 **Endocrine gland, site unspecified**

● 228 **Hemangioma and lymphangioma, any site**

Includes: angioma (benign) (cavernous) (congenital) NOS
cavernous nevus
glomus tumor
hemangioma (benign) (congenital)

Excludes *benign neoplasm of spleen, except hemangioma and lymphangioma (211.9)*
glomus jugulare (227.6)
nevus:
NOS (216.0–216.9)
blue or pigmented (216.0–216.9)
vascular (757.32)

● 228.0 **Hemangioma, any site**

❑ 228.00 **Of unspecified site**

228.01 **Of skin and subcutaneous tissue**

228.02 **Of intracranial structures**

228.03 **Of retina**

228.04 **Of intra-abdominal structures**
Peritoneum
Retroperitoneal tissue

❑ 228.09 **Of other sites**
Systemic angiomatosis

228.1 **Lymphangioma, any site**
Congenital lymphangioma
Lymphatic nevus

● 229 **Benign neoplasm of other and unspecified sites**

229.0 **Lymph nodes**

Excludes *lymphangioma (228.1)*

❑ 229.8 **Other specified sites**
Intrathoracic NOS
Thoracic NOS

ICD-9-CM 200-299 Vol. 1

❑ 229.9 Site unspecified

CARCINOMA IN SITU (230–234)

Includes: Bowen's disease
erythroplasia
Queyrat's erythroplasia

Excludes *leukoplakia - see Alphabetic Index*

● 230 Carcinoma in situ of digestive organs

230.0 Lip, oral cavity, and pharynx
Gingiva
Hypopharynx
Mouth [any part]
Nasopharynx
Oropharynx
Salivary gland or duct
Tongue

Excludes *aryepiglottic fold or interarytenoid fold, laryngeal aspect (231.0)*
epiglottis:
NOS (231.0)
suprahyoid portion (231.0)
skin of lip (232.0)

230.1 Esophagus

230.2 Stomach
Body of stomach
Cardia of stomach
Fundus of stomach
Cardiac orifice
Pylorus

230.3 Colon
Appendix
Cecum
Ileocecal valve
Large intestine NOS

Excludes *rectosigmoid junction (230.4)*

230.4 Rectum
Rectosigmoid junction

230.5 Anal canal
Anal sphincter

❑ 230.6 Anus, unspecified

Excludes *anus:*
margin (232.5)
skin (232.5)
perianal skin (232.5)

❑ 230.7 Other and unspecified parts of intestine
Duodenum
Ileum
Jejunum
Small intestine NOS

Excludes *ampulla of Vater (230.8)*

230.8 Liver and biliary system
Ampulla of Vater
Common bile duct
Cystic duct
Gallbladder
Hepatic duct
Sphincter of Oddi

❑ 230.9 Other and unspecified digestive organs
Digestive organ NOS
Gastrointestinal tract NOS
Pancreas
Spleen

● 231 Carcinoma in situ of respiratory system

231.0 Larynx
Cartilage:
arytenoid
cricoid
cuneiform
thyroid
Epiglottis:
NOS
posterior surface
suprahyoid portion
Vocal cords (false) (true)

Excludes *aryepiglottic fold or interarytenoid fold:*
NOS (230.0)
hypopharyngeal aspect (230.0)
marginal zone (230.0)

231.1 Trachea

231.2 Bronchus and lung
Carina
Hilus of lung

❑ 231.8 Other specified parts of respiratory system
Accessory sinuses
Middle ear
Nasal cavities
Pleura

Excludes *ear (external) (skin) (232.2)*
nose NOS (234.8)
skin (232.3)

❑ 231.9 Respiratory system, part unspecified
Respiratory organ NOS

● 232 Carcinoma in situ of skin

Includes: pigment cells

232.0 Skin of lip

Excludes *vermilion border of lip (230.0)*

232.1 Eyelid, including canthus

232.2 Ear and external auditory canal

❑ 232.3 Skin of other and unspecified parts of face

232.4 Scalp and skin of neck

232.5 Skin of trunk, except scrotum
Anus, margin
Axillary fold
Perianal skin
Skin of:
abdominal wall
anus
back
breast
buttock
chest wall
groin
perineum
Umbilicus

Excludes *anal canal (230.5)*
anus NOS (230.6)
skin of genital organs (233.3, 233.5–233.6)

232.6 Skin of upper limb, including shoulder

232.7 Skin of lower limb, including hip

❑ 232.8 Other specified sites of skin

❑ 232.9 Skin, site unspecified

● 233 Carcinoma in situ of breast and genitourinary system

233.0 Breast

Excludes *Paget's disease (174.0–174.9)*
skin of breast (232.5)

233.1 Cervix uteri

❑ 233.2 Other and unspecified parts of uterus

❑ 233.3 Other and unspecified female genital organs

233.4 Prostate

233.5 Penis

❑ 233.6 **Other and unspecified male genital organs**

233.7 **Bladder**

❑ 233.9 **Other and unspecified urinary organs**

● 234 **Carcinoma in situ of other and unspecified sites**

234.0 **Eye**

Excludes *cartilage of eyelid (234.8)*
eyelid (skin) (232.1)
optic nerve (234.8)
orbital bone (234.8)

❑ 234.8 **Other specified sites**
Endocrine gland [any]

❑ 234.9 **Site unspecified**
Carcinoma in situ NOS

NEOPLASMS OF UNCERTAIN BEHAVIOR (235–238)

Note: Categories 235–238 classify by site certain histomorphologically well-defined neoplasms, the subsequent behavior of which cannot be predicted from the present appearance.

● 235 **Neoplasm of uncertain behavior of digestive and respiratory systems**

235.0 **Major salivary glands**
Gland:
parotid
sublingual
submandibular

Excludes *minor salivary glands (235.1)*

235.1 **Lip, oral cavity, and pharynx**
Gingiva
Hypopharynx
Minor salivary glands
Mouth
Nasopharynx
Oropharynx
Tongue

Excludes *aryepiglottic fold or interarytenoid fold, laryngeal aspect (235.6)*
epiglottis:
NOS (235.6)
suprahyoid portion (235.6)
skin of lip (238.2)

235.2 **Stomach, intestines, and rectum**

235.3 **Liver and biliary passages**
Ampulla of Vater
Bile ducts [any]
Gallbladder
Liver

235.4 **Retroperitoneum and peritoneum**

❑ 235.5 **Other and unspecified digestive organs**
Anal:
canal
sphincter
Anus NOS
Esophagus
Pancreas
Spleen

Excludes *anus:*
margin (238.2)
skin (238.2)
perianal skin (238.2)

235.6 **Larynx**

Excludes *aryepiglottic fold or interarytenoid fold:*
NOS (235.1)
hypopharyngeal aspect (235.1)
marginal zone (235.1)

235.7 **Trachea, bronchus, and lung**

235.8 **Pleura, thymus, and mediastinum**

❑ 235.9 **Other and unspecified respiratory organs**
Accessory sinuses
Middle ear
Nasal cavities
Respiratory organ NOS

Excludes *ear (external) (skin) (238.2)*
nose (238.8)
skin (238.2)

● 236 **Neoplasm of uncertain behavior of genitourinary organs**

236.0 **Uterus**

236.1 **Placenta**
Chorioadenoma (destruens)
Invasive mole
Malignant hydatid(iform) mole

236.2 **Ovary**

Use additional code to identify any functional activity

❑ 236.3 **Other and unspecified female genital organs**

236.4 **Testis**

Use additional code to identify any functional activity

236.5 **Prostate**

❑ 236.6 **Other and unspecified male genital organs**

236.7 **Bladder**

● 236.9 **Other and unspecified urinary organs**

❑ 236.90 **Urinary organ, unspecified**

236.91 **Kidney and ureter**

❑ 236.99 **Other**

● 237 **Neoplasm of uncertain behavior of endocrine glands and nervous system**

237.0 **Pituitary gland and craniopharyngeal duct**

Use additional code to identify any functional activity

237.1 **Pineal gland**

237.2 **Adrenal gland**
Suprarenal gland

Use additional code to identify any functional activity

237.3 **Paraganglia**
Aortic body
Carotid body
Coccygeal body
Glomus jugulare

❑ 237.4 **Other and unspecified endocrine glands**
Parathyroid gland
Thyroid gland

237.5 **Brain and spinal cord**

237.6 **Meninges**
Meninges:
NOS
cerebral
spinal

● 237.7 **Neurofibromatosis**
von Recklinghausen's disease

❑ 237.70 **Neurofibromatosis, unspecified**

237.71 **Neurofibromatosis, type 1 [von Recklinghausen's disease]**

237.72 **Neurofibromatosis, type 2 [acoustic neurofibromatosis]**

ICD-9-CM 200-299 Vol. 1

❑ 237.9 Other and unspecified parts of nervous system
Cranial nerves
Excludes *peripheral, sympathetic, and parasympathetic nerves and ganglia (238.1)*

● 238 Neoplasm of uncertain behavior of other and unspecified sites and tissues

238.0 Bone and articular cartilage
Excludes *cartilage:*
ear (238.1)
eyelid (238.1)
larynx (235.6)
nose (235.9)
synovia (238.1)

❑ 238.1 Connective and other soft tissue
Peripheral, sympathetic, and parasympathetic nerves and ganglia
Excludes *cartilage (of):*
articular (238.0)
larynx (235.6)
nose (235.9)
connective tissue of breast (238.3)

238.2 Skin
Excludes *anus NOS (235.5)*
skin of genital organs (236.3, 236.6)
vermilion border of lip (235.1)

238.3 Breast
Excludes *skin of breast (238.2)*

238.4 Polycythemia vera

238.5 Histiocytic and mast cells
Mast cell tumor NOS
Mastocytoma NOS

238.6 Plasma cells
Plasmacytoma NOS
Solitary myeloma

❑ 238.7 Other lymphatic and hematopoietic tissues
Disease:
lymphoproliferative (chronic) NOS
myeloproliferative (chronic) NOS
Idiopathic thrombocythemia
Megakaryocytic myelosclerosis
Myelodysplastic syndrome
Myelosclerosis with myeloid metaplasia
Panmyelosis (acute)
Excludes *myelofibrosis (289.89)* ⇐
myelosclerosis NOS (289.89) ⇐
myelosis:
NOS (205.9)
megakaryocytic (207.2)

❑ 238.8 Other specified sites
Eye
Heart
Excludes *eyelid (skin) (238.2)*
cartilage (238.1)

❑ 238.9 Site unspecified

NEOPLASMS OF UNSPECIFIED NATURE (239)

● 239 Neoplasms of unspecified nature

Note: Category 239 classifies by site neoplasms of unspecified morphology and behavior. The term "mass," unless otherwise stated, is not to be regarded as a neoplastic growth.

Includes: "growth" NOS
neoplasm NOS
new growth NOS
tumor NOS

❑ 239.0 Digestive system
Excludes *anus:*
margin (239.2)
skin (239.2)
perianal skin (239.2)

❑ 239.1 Respiratory system

❑ 239.2 Bone, soft tissue, and skin
Excludes *anal canal (239.0)*
anus NOS (239.0)
bone marrow (202.9)
cartilage:
larynx (239.1)
nose (239.1)
connective tissue of breast (239.3)
skin of genital organs (239.5)
vermilion border of lip (239.0)

❑ 239.3 Breast
Excludes *skin of breast (239.2)*

❑ 239.4 Bladder

❑ 239.5 Other genitourinary organs

❑ 239.6 Brain
Excludes *cerebral meninges (239.7)*
cranial nerves (239.7)

❑ 239.7 Endocrine glands and other parts of nervous system
Excludes *peripheral, sympathetic, and parasympathetic nerves and ganglia (239.2)*

❑ 239.8 Other specified sites
Excludes *eyelid (skin) (239.2)*
cartilage (239.2)
great vessels (239.2)
optic nerve (239.7)

❑ 239.9 Site unspecified

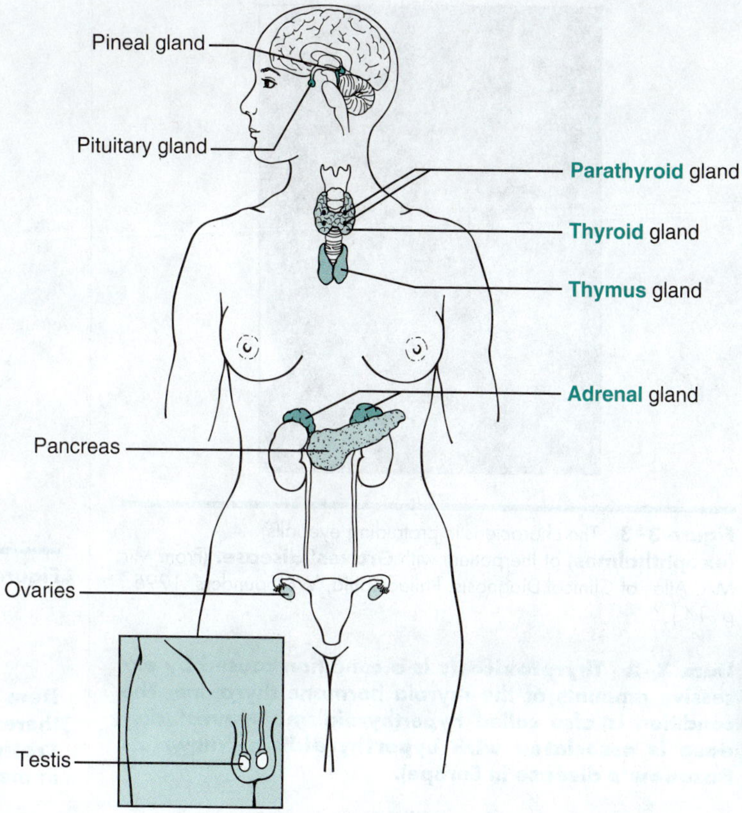

Figure 3-1 The endocrine system. (From Buck CJ: Step-by-Step Medical Coding, 3rd ed. Philadelphia, WB Saunders, 2000, p. 198.)

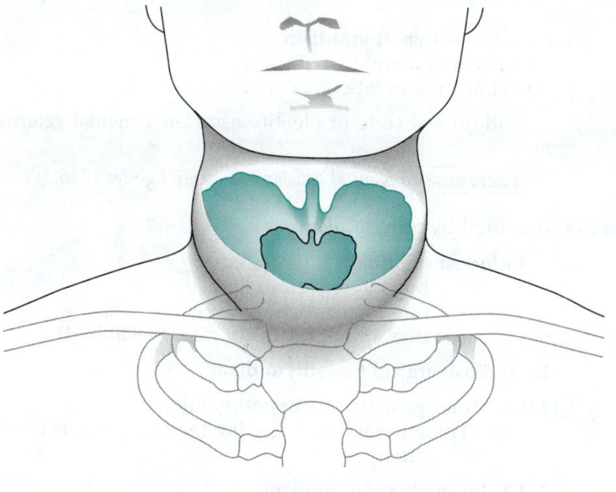

Figure 3-2 **Goiter** is an enlargement of the thyroid gland.

Item 3-1 Simple indicates no nodules are present. The most common type of goiter is a diffuse colloidal, also called a nontoxic or endemic goiter. Goiters classifiable to 240.0 or 240.9 are those goiters without mention of nodules.

3. ENDOCRINE, NUTRITIONAL AND METABOLIC DISEASES, AND IMMUNITY DISORDERS (240–279)

Excludes *endocrine and metabolic disturbances specific to the fetus and newborn (775.0–775.9)*

Note: All neoplasms, whether functionally active or not, are classified in Chapter 2. Codes in Chapter 3 (i.e., 242.8, 246.0, 251–253, 255–259) may be used to identify such functional activity associated with any neoplasm, or by ectopic endocrine tissue.

DISORDERS OF THYROID GLAND (240–246)

● **240 Simple and unspecified goiter**

240.0 Goiter, specified as simple
Any condition classifiable to 240.9, specified as simple

❑ **240.9 Goiter, unspecified**
Enlargement of thyroid
Goiter or struma:
NOS
diffuse colloid
endemic
Goiter or struma:
hyperplastic
nontoxic (diffuse)
parenchymatous
sporadic

Excludes *congenital (dyshormonogenic) goiter (246.1)*

● **241 Nontoxic nodular goiter**

Excludes *adenoma of thyroid (226)*
cystadenoma of thyroid (226)

241.0 Nontoxic uninodular goiter
Thyroid nodule
Uninodular goiter (nontoxic)

241.1 Nontoxic multinodular goiter
Multinodular goiter (nontoxic)

❑ **241.9 Unspecified nontoxic nodular goiter**
Adenomatous goiter
Nodular goiter (nontoxic) NOS
Struma nodosa (simplex)

ICD-9-CM 200-299 Vol. 1

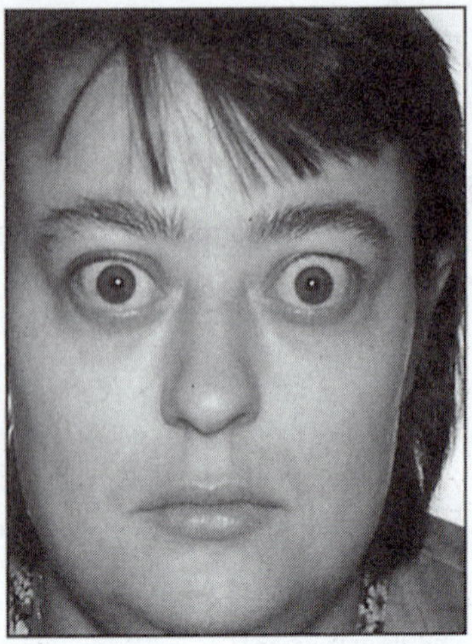

Figure 3–3 The characteristic protruding eyeballs **(exophthalmos)** of the patient with **Graves' disease.** (From Mir MA: Atlas of Clinical Diagnosis. Philadelphia, WB Saunders, 1995, p. 14.)

Item 3–2 Thyrotoxicosis is a condition caused by excessive amounts of the thyroid hormone thyroxine. The condition is also called hyperthyroidism. Graves' disease is associated with hyperthyroidism (known as Basedow's disease in Europe).

● 242 **Thyrotoxicosis with or without goiter**

Excludes *neonatal thyrotoxicosis (775.3)*

The following fifth-digit subclassification is for use with category 242:

0 **without mention of thyrotoxic crisis or storm**

1 **with mention of thyrotoxic crisis or storm**

● 242.0 **Toxic diffuse goiter**
Basedow's disease
Exophthalmic or toxic goiter NOS
Graves'disease
Primary thyroid hyperplasia

● 242.1 **Toxic uninodular goiter**
Thyroid nodule, toxic or with hyperthyroidism
Uninodular goiter, toxic or with hyperthyroidism

● 242.2 **Toxic multinodular goiter**
Secondary thyroid hyperplasia

● ❑ 242.3 **Toxic nodular goiter, unspecified**
Adenomatous goiter, toxic or with hyperthyroidism
Nodular goiter, toxic or with hyperthyroidism
Struma nodosa, toxic or with hyperthyroidism
Any condition classifiable to 241.9 specified as toxic or with hyperthyroidism

● 242.4 **Thyrotoxicosis from ectopic thyroid nodule**

● ❑ 242.8 **Thyrotoxicosis of other specified origin**
Overproduction of thyroid-stimulating hormone [TSH]
Thyrotoxicosis:
factitia from ingestion of excessive thyroid material

Use additional E code to identify cause, if drug-induced

● ❑ 242.9 **Thyrotoxicosis without mention of goiter or other cause**
Hyperthyroidism NOS
Thyrotoxicosis NOS

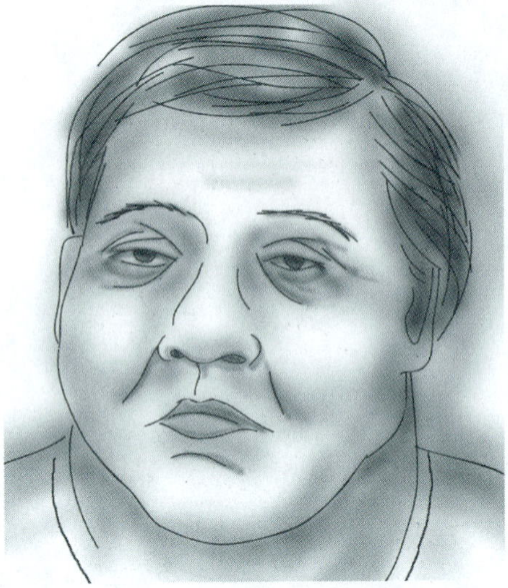

Figure 3–4 Myxedema is severe hypothyroidism.

Item 3–3 Hypothyroidism is a condition in which there are insufficient levels of thyroxine. Cretinism is congenital hypothyroidism, which can result in mental and physical retardation.

243 **Congenital hypothyroidism**
Congenital thyroid insufficiency
Cretinism (athyrotic) (endemic)

Use additional code to identify associated mental retardation

Excludes *congenital (dyshormonogenic) goiter (246.1)*

● 244 **Acquired hypothyroidism**

Includes: athyroidism (acquired)
hypothyroidism (acquired)
myxedema (adult) (juvenile)
thyroid (gland) insufficiency (acquired)

244.0 **Postsurgical hypothyroidism**

❑ 244.1 **Other postablative hypothyroidism**
Hypothyroidism following therapy, such as irradiation

244.2 **Iodine hypothyroidism**
Hypothyroidism resulting from administration or ingestion of iodide

Use additional E to identify drug

❑ 244.3 **Other iatrogenic hypothyroidism**
Hypothyroidism resulting from:
P-aminosalicylic acid [PAS]
Phenylbutazone
Resorcinol
Iatrogenic hypothyroidism NOS

Use additional E to identify drug

❑ 244.8 **Other specified acquired hypothyroidism**
Secondary hypothyroidism NEC

❑ 244.9 **Unspecified hypothyroidism**
Hypothyroidism, primary or NOS
Myxedema, primary or NOS

● 245 Thyroiditis

245.0 Acute thyroiditis
Abscess of thyroid
Thyroiditis:
nonsuppurative, acute
pyogenic
suppurative
Use additional code to identify organism

245.1 Subacute thyroiditis
Thyroiditis:
de Quervain's
giant cell
granulomatous
viral

245.2 Chronic lymphocytic thyroiditis
Hashimoto's disease
Struma lymphomatosa
Thyroiditis:
autoimmune
lymphocytic (chronic)

245.3 Chronic fibrous thyroiditis
Struma fibrosa
Thyroiditis:
invasive (fibrous)
ligneous
Riedel's

245.4 Iatrogenic thyroiditis
Use additional E to identify cause

❑ 245.8 Other and unspecified chronic thyroiditis
Chronic thyroiditis:
NOS
nonspecific

❑ 245.9 Thyroiditis, unspecified
Thyroiditis NOS

● 246 Other disorders of thyroid

246.0 Disorders of thyrocalcitonin secretion
Hypersecretion of calcitonin or thyrocalcitonin

246.1 Dyshormonogenic goiter
Congenital (dyshormonogenic) goiter
Goiter due to enzyme defect in synthesis of thyroid hormone
Goitrous cretinism (sporadic)

246.2 Cyst of thyroid
Excludes *cystadenoma of thyroid (226)*

246.3 Hemorrhage and infarction of thyroid

❑ 246.8 Other specified disorders of thyroid
Abnormality of thyroid-binding globulin
Atrophy of thyroid
Hyper-TBG-nemia
Hypo-TBG-nemia

❑ 246.9 Unspecified disorder of thyroid

DISEASES OF OTHER ENDOCRINE GLANDS (250–259)

● 250 Diabetes mellitus

Excludes *gestational diabetes (648.8)*
hyperglycemia NOS (790.6)
neonatal diabetes mellitus (775.1)
nonclinical diabetes (790.29) ⇐

The following fifth-digit subclassification is for use with category 250:

0 type II [non-insulin dependent type] [NIDDM type] [adult-onset type] or unspecified type, not stated as uncontrolled
Fifth-digit 0 is for use for type II, adult-onset, diabetic patients, even if the patient requires insulin

1 type I [insulin dependent type] [IDDM] [juvenile type], not stated as uncontrolled

2 type II [non-insulin dependent type] [NIDDM type] [adult-onset type] or unspecified type, uncontrolled
Fifth-digit 2 is for use for type II, adult-onset, diabetic patients, even if the patient requires insulin

3 type I [insulin dependent type] [IDDM] [juvenile type], uncontrolled

● 250.0 Diabetes mellitus without mention of complication
Diabetes mellitus without mention of complication or manifestation classifiable to 250.1–250.9
Diabetes (mellitus) NOS

● 250.1 Diabetes with ketoacidosis
Diabetic:
acidosis without mention of coma
ketosis without mention of coma

● 250.2 Diabetes with hyperosmolarity
Hyperosmolar (nonketotic) coma

● 250.3 Diabetes with other coma
Diabetic coma (with ketoacidosis)
Diabetic hypoglycemic coma
Insulin coma NOS
Excludes *diabetes with hyperosmolar coma (250.2)*

● 250.4 Diabetes with renal manifestations
Use additional code to identify manifestation, as:
diabetic:
nephropathy NOS (583.81)
nephrosis (581.81)
intercapillary glomerulosclerosis (581.81)
Kimmelstiel-Wilson syndrome (581.81)

● 250.5 Diabetes with ophthalmic manifestations
Use additional code to identify manifestation, as:
diabetic:
blindness (369.00–369.9)
cataract (366.41)
glaucoma (365.44)
retinal edema (362.01) ⇐
retinopathy (362.01–362.02)

● 250.6 Diabetes with neurological manifestations
Use additional code to identify manifestation, as:
diabetic:
amyotrophy (358.1)
mononeuropathy (354.0–355.9)
neurogenic arthropathy (713.5)
peripheral autonomic neuropathy (337.1)
polyneuropathy (357.2)

● 250.7 Diabetes with peripheral circulatory disorders
Use additional code to identify manifestation, as:
diabetic:
gangrene (785.4)
peripheral angiopathy (443.81)

● ❑ 250.8 Diabetes with other specified manifestations
Diabetic hypoglycemia
Hypoglycemic shock
Use additional code to identify manifestation, as:
any associated ulceration (707.10–707.9)
diabetic bone changes (731.8)
Use additional E code to identify cause, if drug-induced

● ❑ 250.9 Diabetes with unspecified complication

● 251 Other disorders of pancreatic internal secretion

ICD-9-CM 200-299 Vol. 1

251.0 Hypoglycemic coma
Iatrogenic hyperinsulinism
Non-diabetic insulin coma

Use additional E code to identify cause, if drug-induced

Excludes *hypoglycemic coma in diabetes mellitus (250.3)*

❑**251.1 Other specified hypoglycemia**
Hyperinsulinism:
NOS
ectopic
functional
Hyperplasia of pancreatic islet beta cells NOS

Excludes *hypoglycemia in diabetes mellitus (250.8)*
hypoglycemia in infant of diabetic mother (775.0)
hypoglycemic coma (251.0)
neonatal hypoglycemia (775.6)

Use additional E code to identify cause, if drug-induced

❑**251.2 Hypoglycemia, unspecified**
Hypoglycemia:
NOS
reactive
spontaneous

Excludes *hypoglycemia:*
with coma (251.0)
in diabetes mellitus (250.8)
leucine-induced (270.3)

251.3 Postsurgical hypoinsulinemia
Hypoinsulinemia following complete or partial pancreatectomy
Postpancreatectomy hyperglycemia

251.4 Abnormality of secretion of glucagon
Hyperplasia of pancreatic islet alpha cells with glucagon excess

251.5 Abnormality of secretion of gastrin
Hyperplasia of pancreatic alpha cells with gastrin excess
Zollinger-Ellison syndrome

❑**251.8 Other specified disorders of pancreatic internal secretion**

❑**251.9 Unspecified disorder of pancreatic internal secretion**
Islet cell hyperplasia NOS

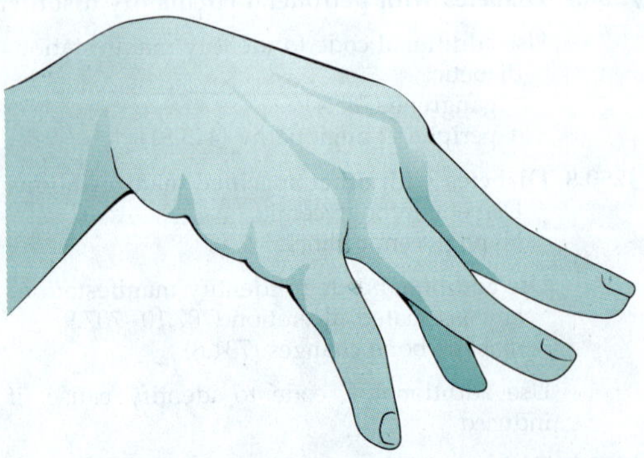

Figure 3-5 Tetany caused by hypoparathyroidism.

Item 3-4 Hyperparathyroidism is an overactive parathyroid gland that secretes excessive parathormone, causing increased levels of circulating calcium. This results in a loss of calcium in the bone.
Hypoparathyroidism is an underactive parathyroid gland that results in decreased levels of circulating calcium. The primary manifestation is tetany, a continuous muscle spasm.

●**252 Disorders of parathyroid gland**

252.0 Hyperparathyroidism
Hyperplasia of parathyroid
Osteitis fibrosa cystica generalisata
von Recklinghausen's disease of bone

Excludes *ectopic hyperparathyroidism (259.3)*
secondary hyperparathyroidism (of renal origin) (588.8)

252.1 Hypoparathyroidism
Parathyroiditis (autoimmune)
Tetany:
parathyroid
parathyroprival

Excludes *pseudohypoparathyroidism (275.4)*
pseudopseudohypoparathyroidism (275.4)
tetany NOS (781.7)
transitory neonatal hypoparathyroidism (775.4)

❑**252.8 Other specified disorders of parathyroid gland**
Cyst of parathyroid gland
Hemorrhage of parathyroid gland

❑**252.9 Unspecified disorder of parathyroid gland**

●**253 Disorders of the pituitary gland and its hypothalamic control**

Includes: the listed conditions whether the disorder is in the pituitary or the hypothalamus

Excludes *Cushing's syndrome (255.0)*

253.0 Acromegaly and gigantism
Overproduction of growth hormone

❑**253.1 Other and unspecified anterior pituitary hyperfunction**
Forbes-Albright syndrome

Excludes *overproduction of:*
ACTH (255.3)
thyroid-stimulating hormone [TSH] (242.8)

253.2 Panhypopituitarism
Cachexia, pituitary
Necrosis of pituitary (postpartum)
Pituitary insufficiency NOS
Sheehan's syndrome
Simmonds' disease

Excludes *iatrogenic hypopituitarism (253.7)*

253.3 Pituitary dwarfism
Isolated deficiency of (human) growth hormone [HGH]
Lorain-Levi dwarfism

❑**253.4 Other anterior pituitary disorders**
Isolated or partial deficiency of an anterior pituitary hormone, other than growth hormone
Prolactin deficiency

253.5 Diabetes insipidus
Vasopressin deficiency

Excludes *nephrogenic diabetes insipidus (588.1)*

❑253.6 **Other disorders of neurohypophysis**
Syndrome of inappropriate secretion of antidiuretic hormone [ADH]
Excludes *ectopic antidiuretic hormone secretion (259.3)*

253.7 **Iatrogenic pituitary disorders**
Hypopituitarism:
hormone-induced
hypophysectomy-induced
postablative
radiotherapy-induced
Use additional E code to identify cause

❑253.8 **Other disorders of the pituitary and other syndromes of diencephalohypophyseal origin**
Abscess of pituitary
Adiposogenital dystrophy
Cyst of Rathke's pouch
Fröhlich's syndrome
Excludes *craniopharyngioma (237.0)*

❑253.9 **Unspecified**
Dyspituitarism

● 254 **Diseases of thymus gland**
Excludes *aplasia or dysplasia with immunodeficiency (279.2)*
hypoplasia with immunodeficiency (279.2)
myasthenia gravis (358.00) ⇐

254.0 **Persistent hyperplasia of thymus**
Hypertrophy of thymus

254.1 **Abscess of thymus**

❑254.8 **Other specified diseases of thymus gland**
Atrophy of thymus
Cyst of thymus
Excludes *thymoma (212.6)*

❑254.9 **Unspecified disease of thymus gland**

Item 3-5 Hyperadrenalism is overactivity of the adrenal cortex, which secretes a variety of hormones. Excessive glucocorticoid hormone results in hyperglycemia (Cushing's syndrome), and excessive aldosterone results in Conn's syndrome. Adrenogenital syndrome is the result of excessive secretion of androgens, male hormones, which stimulates premature sexual development. Hypoadrenalism, Addison's disease, is a condition in which the adrenal glands atrophy.

● 255 **Disorders of adrenal glands**
Includes: the listed conditions whether the basic disorder is in the adrenals or is pituitary-induced

255.0 **Cushing's syndrome**
Adrenal hyperplasia due to excess ACTH
Cushing's syndrome:
NOS
iatrogenic
idiopathic
pituitary-dependent
Ectopic ACTH syndrome
Iatrogenic syndrome of excess cortisol
Overproduction of cortisol
Use additional E code to identify cause, if drug-induced
Excludes *congenital adrenal hyperplasia (255.2)*

● 255.1 **Hyperaldosteronism**

255.10 **Primary aldosteronism** ◄
Aldosteronism NOS ◄
Hyperaldosteronism, unspecified ◄

255.11 **Glucocorticoid-remediable aldosteronism** ◄
Familial aldosteronism type I ◄

255.12 **Conn's syndrome** ◄

255.13 **Bartter's syndrome** ◄

255.14 **Other secondary aldosteronism** ◄

255.2 **Adrenogenital disorders**
Achard-Thiers syndrome
Adrenogenital syndromes, virilizing or feminizing, whether acquired or associated with congenital adrenal hyperplasia consequent on inborn enzyme defects in hormone synthesis
Congenital adrenal hyperplasia
Female adrenal pseudohermaphroditism
Male:
macrogenitosomia praecox
sexual precocity with adrenal hyperplasia
Virilization (female) (suprarenal)
Excludes *adrenal hyperplasia due to excess ACTH (255.0)*
isosexual virilization (256.4)

ICD-9-CM 200-299 Vol. 1

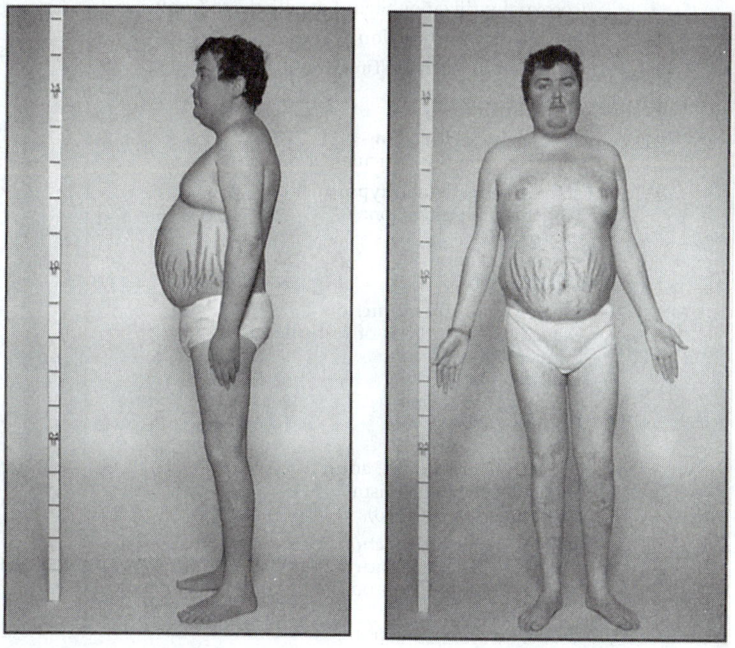

Figure 3-6 Cushing's syndrome, showing characteristic purple striae and abdominal obesity. (From Mir MA: Atlas of Clinical Diagnosis. Philadelphia, WB Saunders, 1995, p. 10.)

❑255.3 **Other corticoadrenal overactivity**
Acquired benign adrenal androgenic overactivity
Overproduction of ACTH

255.4 **Corticoadrenal insufficiency**
Addisonian crisis
Addison's disease NOS
Adrenal:
atrophy (autoimmune)
calcification
Adrenal:
crisis
hemorrhage
infarction
insufficiency NOS
Excludes *tuberculous Addison's disease (017.6)*

❑255.5 **Other adrenal hypofunction**
Adrenal medullary insufficiency
Excludes *Waterhouse-Friderichsen syndrome (meningococcal) (036.3)*

255.6 **Medulloadrenal hyperfunction**
Catecholamine secretion by pheochromocytoma

❑255.8 **Other specified disorders of adrenal glands**
Abnormality of cortisol-binding globulin

❑255.9 **Unspecified disorder of adrenal glands**

● 256 **Ovarian dysfunction**

256.0 **Hyperestrogenism**

❑256.1 **Other ovarian hyperfunction**
Hypersecretion of ovarian androgens

256.2 **Postablative ovarian failure**
Ovarian failure:
iatrogenic
postirradiation
postsurgical

Use additional code for states associated with artificial menopause (627.4)

Excludes *acquired absence of ovary (V45.77)*
asymptomatic age-related (natural) postmenopausal status (V49.81)

● 256.3 **Other ovarian failure**
Excludes *asymptomatic age-related (natural) postmenopausal status (V49.81)*

Use additional code for states associated with natural menopause (627.2)

256.31 **Premature menopause**

❑256.39 **Other ovarian failure**
Delayed menarche
Ovarian hypofunction
Primary ovarian failure NOS

256.4 **Polycystic ovaries**
Isosexual virilization Stein-Leventhal syndrome

❑256.8 **Other ovarian dysfunction**

❑256.9 **Unspecified ovarian dysfunction**

● 257 **Testicular dysfunction**

257.0 **Testicular hyperfunction**
Hypersecretion of testicular hormones

257.1 **Postablative testicular hypofunction**
Testicular hypofunction:
iatrogenic
postirradiation
postsurgical

❑257.2 **Other testicular hypofunction**
Defective biosynthesis of testicular androgen
Eunuchoidism:
NOS
hypogonadotropic
Failure:
Leydig's cell, adult
seminiferous tubule, adult
Testicular hypogonadism
Excludes *azoospermia (606.0)*

❑257.8 **Other testicular dysfunction**
Goldberg-Maxwell syndrome
Male pseudohermaphroditism with testicular feminization
Testicular feminization

❑257.9 **Unspecified testicular dysfunction**

● 258 **Polyglandular dysfunction and related disorders**

258.0 **Polyglandular activity in multiple endocrine adenomatosis**
Wermer's syndrome

❑258.1 **Other combinations of endocrine dysfunction**
Lloyd's syndrome
Schmidt's syndrome

❑258.8 **Other specified polyglandular dysfunction**

❑258.9 **Polyglandular dysfunction, unspecified**

● 259 **Other endocrine disorders**

259.0 **Delay in sexual development and puberty, not elsewhere classified**
Delayed puberty

259.1 **Precocious sexual development and puberty, not elsewhere classified**
Sexual precocity:
NOS
constitutional
cryptogenic
idiopathic

259.2 **Carcinoid syndrome**
Hormone secretion by carcinoid tumors

259.3 **Ectopic hormone secretion, not elsewhere classified**
Ectopic:
antidiuretic hormone secretion [ADH]
hyperparathyroidism
Excludes *ectopic ACTH syndrome (255.0)*

259.4 **Dwarfism, not elsewhere classified**
Dwarfism:
NOS
constitutional
Excludes *dwarfism:*
achondroplastic (756.4)
intrauterine (759.7)
nutritional (263.2)
pituitary (253.3)
renal (588.0)
progeria (259.8)

❑259.8 **Other specified endocrine disorders**
Pineal gland dysfunction
Progeria
Werner's syndrome

❑259.9 **Unspecified endocrine disorder**
Disturbance:
endocrine NOS
hormone NOS
Infantilism NOS

NUTRITIONAL DEFICIENCIES (260–269)

Excludes *deficiency anemias (280.0–281.9)*

260 **Kwashiorkor**
Nutritional edema with dyspigmentation of skin and hair

261 **Nutritional marasmus**
Nutritional atrophy
Severe calorie deficiency
Severe malnutrition NOS

❑262 **Other severe protein-calorie malnutrition**
Nutritional edema without mention of dyspigmentation of skin and hair

● 263 **Other and unspecified protein-calorie malnutrition**

263.0 **Malnutrition of moderate degree**

263.1 **Malnutrition of mild degree**

263.2 **Arrested development following protein-calorie malnutrition**
Nutritional dwarfism
Physical retardation due to malnutrition

❑ 263.8 **Other protein-calorie malnutrition**

❑ 263.9 **Unspecified protein-calorie malnutrition**
Dystrophy due to malnutrition
Malnutrition (calorie) NOS

Excludes *nutritional deficiency NOS (269.9)*

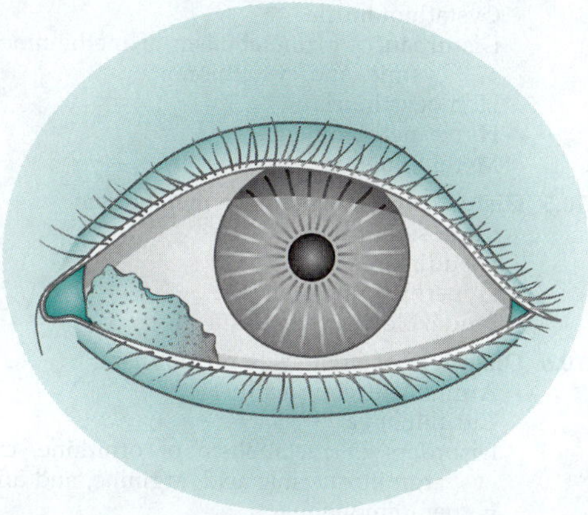

Figure 3–7 Bitot's spot on the conjunctiva.

Item 3–6 Bitot's spot is a gray, foamy erosion on the conjunctiva, usually associated with vitamin A deficiency. The disease may progress to keratomalacia, which can result in eventual prolapse of the iris and loss of the lens.

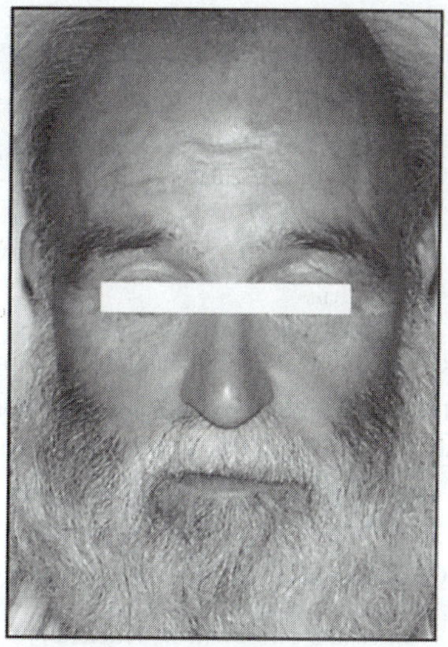

Figure 3–8 In chronic **pellagra,** the skin changes include thickening, scaling, pigmentation, and hyperkeratinization. (From Mir MA: Atlas of Clinical Diagnosis. Philadelphia, WB Saunders, 1995, p. 57.)

Item 3–7 Pellagra is associated with a deficiency of niacin and its precursor, tryptophan. Characteristics of the condition include dermatitis on exposed skin surfaces. Beriberi is associated with thiamin deficiency.

● 264 **Vitamin A deficiency**

264.0 **With conjunctival xerosis**

264.1 **With conjunctival xerosis and Bitot's spot**
Bitot's spot in the young child

264.2 **With corneal xerosis**

264.3 **With corneal ulceration and xerosis**

264.4 **With keratomalacia**

264.5 **With night blindness**

264.6 **With xerophthalmic scars of cornea**

❑ 264.7 **Other ocular manifestations of vitamin A deficiency**
Xerophthalmia due to vitamin A deficiency

❑ 264.8 **Other manifestations of vitamin A deficiency**
Follicular keratosis due to vitamin A deficiency
Xeroderma due to vitamin A deficiency

❑ 264.9 **Unspecified vitamin A deficiency**
Hypovitaminosis A NOS

● 265 **Thiamine and niacin deficiency states**

265.0 **Beriberi**

❑ 265.1 **Other and unspecified manifestations of thiamine deficiency**
Other vitamin B_1 deficiency states

265.2 **Pellagra**
Deficiency:
niacin (-tryptophan)
nicotinamide
nicotinic acid
vitamin PP
Pellagra (alcoholic)

● 266 **Deficiency of B-complex components**

266.0 **Ariboflavinosis**
Riboflavin [vitamin B_2] deficiency

266.1 **Vitamin B_6 deficiency**
Deficiency:
pyridoxal
pyridoxamine
pyridoxine
Vitamin B_6 deficiency syndrome

Excludes *vitamin B_6-responsive sideroblastic anemia (285.0)*

❑ 266.2 **Other B-complex deficiencies**
Deficiency:
cyanocobalamin
folic acid
vitamin B_{12}

Excludes *combined system disease with anemia (281.0–281.1)*
deficiency anemias (281.0–281.9)
subacute degeneration of spinal cord with anemia (281.0–281.1)

❑ 266.9 **Unspecified vitamin B deficiency**

267 **Ascorbic acid deficiency**
Deficiency of vitamin C
Scurvy

Excludes *scorbutic anemia (281.8)*

● 268 **Vitamin D deficiency**

Excludes *vitamin D-resistant:*
osteomalacia (275.3)
rickets (275.3)

268.0 **Rickets, active**

Excludes *celiac rickets (579.0)*
renal rickets (588.0)

❑ 268.1 **Rickets, late effect**
Any condition specified as due to rickets and stated to be a late effect or sequela of rickets

Use additional code to identify the nature of late effect

ICD-9-CM 200-299 Vol. 1

❑268.2 **Osteomalacia, unspecified**

❑268.9 **Unspecified vitamin D deficiency**
Avitaminosis D

● 269 **Other nutritional deficiencies**

269.0 **Deficiency of vitamin K**

Excludes *deficiency of coagulation factor due to vitamin K deficiency (286.7)*
vitamin K deficiency of newborn (776.0)

❑269.1 **Deficiency of other vitamins**
Deficiency:
vitamin E
vitamin P

❑269.2 **Unspecified vitamin deficiency**
Multiple vitamin deficiency NOS

269.3 **Mineral deficiency, not elsewhere classified**
Deficiency:
calcium, dietary
iodine

Excludes *deficiency:*
calcium NOS (275.4)
potassium (276.8)
sodium (276.1)

❑269.8 **Other nutritional deficiency**

Excludes *adult failure to thrive (783.7)*
failure to thrive in childhood (783.41)
feeding problems (783.3)
newborn (779.3)

❑269.9 **Unspecified nutritional deficiency**

OTHER METABOLIC AND IMMUNITY DISORDERS (270–279)

Use additional code to identify any associated mental retardation

● 270 **Disorders of amino-acid transport and metabolism**

Excludes *abnormal findings without manifest disease (790.0–796.9)*
disorders of purine and pyrimidine metabolism (277.1–277.2)
gout (274.0–274.9)

270.0 **Disturbances of amino-acid transport**
Cystinosis
Cystinuria
Fanconi (-de Toni) (-Debré) syndrome
Glycinuria (renal)
Hartnup disease

270.1 **Phenylketonuria [PKU]**
Hyperphenylalaninemia

❑270.2 **Other disturbances of aromatic amino-acid metabolism**
Albinism
Alkaptonuria
Alkaptonuric ochronosis
Disturbances of metabolism of tyrosine and tryptophan
Homogentisic acid defects
Hydroxykynureninuria
Hypertyrosinemia
Indicanuria
Kynureninase defects
Oasthouse urine disease
Ochronosis
Tyrosinosis
Tyrosinuria
Waardenburg syndrome

Excludes *vitamin B_6-deficiency syndrome (266.1)*

270.3 **Disturbances of branched-chain amino-acid metabolism**
Disturbances of metabolism of leucine, isoleucine, and valine
Hypervalinemia
Intermittent branched-chain ketonuria
Leucine-induced hypoglycemia
Leucinosis
Maple syrup urine disease

270.4 **Disturbances of sulphur-bearing amino-acid metabolism**
Cystathioninemia
Cystathioninuria
Disturbances of metabolism of methionine, homocystine, and cystathionine
Homocystinuria
Hypermethioninemia
Methioninemia

270.5 **Disturbances of histidine metabolism**
Carnosinemia
Histidinemia
Hyperhistidinemia
Imidazole aminoaciduria

270.6 **Disorders of urea cycle metabolism**
Argininosuccinic aciduria
Citrullinemia
Disorders of metabolism of ornithine, citrulline, argininosuccinic acid, arginine, and ammonia
Hyperammonemia
Hyperornithinemia

❑270.7 **Other disturbances of straight-chain amino-acid metabolism**
Glucoglycinuria
Glycinemia (with methylmalonic acidemia)
Hyperglycinemia
Hyperlysinemia
Pipecolic acidemia
Saccharopinuria
Other disturbances of metabolism of glycine, threonine, serine, glutamine, and lysine

❑270.8 **Other specified disorders of amino-acid metabolism**
Alaninemia
Ethanolaminuria
Glycoprolinuria
Hydroxyprolinemia
Hyperprolinemia
Iminoacidopathy
Prolinemia
Prolinuria
Sarcosinemia

❑270.9 **Unspecified disorder of amino-acid metabolism**

● 271 **Disorders of carbohydrate transport and metabolism**

Excludes *abnormality of secretion of glucagon (251.4)*
diabetes mellitus (250.0–250.9)
hypoglycemia NOS (251.2)
mucopolysaccharidosis (277.5)

271.0 **Glycogenosis**
Amylopectinosis
Glucose-6-phosphatase deficiency
Glycogen storage disease
McArdle's disease
Pompe's disease
von Gierke's disease

271.1 **Galactosemia**
Galactose-1-phosphate uridyl transferase deficiency
Galactosuria

271.2 **Hereditary fructose intolerance**
Essential benign fructosuria
Fructosemia

271.3 **Intestinal disaccharidase deficiencies and disaccharide malabsorption**
Intolerance or malabsorption (congenital) (of):
glucose-galactose
lactose
sucrose-isomaltose

271.4 **Renal glycosuria**
Renal diabetes

❑ 271.8 **Other specified disorders of carbohydrate transport and metabolism**
Essential benign pentosuria
Fucosidosis
Glycolic aciduria
Hyperoxaluria (primary)
Mannosidosis
Oxalosis
Xylosuria
Xylulosuria

❑ 271.9 **Unspecified disorder of carbohydrate transport and metabolism**

● 272 **Disorders of lipoid metabolism**
Excludes *localized cerebral lipidoses (330.1)*

272.0 **Pure hypercholesterolemia**
Familial hypercholesterolemia
Fredrickson Type IIa hyperlipoproteinemia
Hyperbetalipoproteinemia
Hyperlipidemia, Group A
Low-density-lipoid-type [LDL] hyperlipoproteinemia

272.1 **Pure hyperglyceridemia**
Endogenous hyperglyceridemia
Fredrickson Type IV hyperlipoproteinemia
Hyperlipidemia, Group B
Hyperprebetalipoproteinemia
Hypertriglyceridemia, essential
Very-low-density-lipoid-type [VLDL] hyperlipoproteinemia

272.2 **Mixed hyperlipidemia**
Broad- or floating-betalipoproteinemia
Fredrickson Type IIb or III hyperlipoproteinemia
Hypercholesterolemia with endogenous hyperglyceridemia
Hyperbetalipoproteinemia with prebetalipoproteinemia
Tubo-eruptive xanthoma
Xanthoma tuberosum

272.3 **Hyperchylomicronemia**
Bürger-Grütz syndrome
Fredrickson type I or V hyperlipoproteinemia
Hyperlipidemia, Group D
Mixed hyperglyceridemia

❑ 272.4 **Other and unspecified hyperlipidemia**
Alpha-lipoproteinemia
Combined hyperlipidemia
Hyperlipidemia NOS
Hyperlipoproteinemia NOS

272.5 **Lipoprotein deficiencies**
Abetalipoproteinemia
Bassen-Kornzweig syndrome
High-density lipoid deficiency
Hypoalphalipoproteinemia
Hypobetalipoproteinemia (familial)

272.6 **Lipodystrophy**
Barraquer-Simons disease
Progressive lipodystrophy

Use additional E code to identify cause, if iatrogenic
Excludes *intestinal lipodystrophy (040.2)*

272.7 **Lipidoses**
Chemically induced lipidosis
Disease:
Anderson's
Fabry's
Gaucher's
I cell [mucolipidosis I]
lipoid storage NOS
Niemann-Pick
pseudo-Hurler's or mucolipidosis III
triglyceride storage, Type I or II
Wolman's or triglyceride storage, Type III
Mucolipidosis II
Primary familial xanthomatosis
Excludes *cerebral lipidoses (330.1)*
Tay-Sachs disease (330.1)

❑ 272.8 **Other disorders of lipoid metabolism**
Hoffa's disease or liposynovitis prepatellaris
Launois-Bensaude's lipomatosis
Lipoid dermatoarthritis

❑ 272.9 **Unspecified disorder of lipoid metabolism**

● 273 **Disorders of plasma protein metabolism**
Excludes *agammaglobulinemia and hypogammaglobulinemia (279.0–279.2)*
coagulation defects (286.0–286.9)
hereditary hemolytic anemias (282.0–282.9)

273.0 **Polyclonal hypergammaglobulinemia**
Hypergammaglobulinemic purpura:
benign primary
Waldenström's

273.1 **Monoclonal paraproteinemia**
Benign monoclonal hypergammaglobulinemia [BMH]
Monoclonal gammopathy:
NOS
associated with lymphoplasmacytic dyscrasias
benign
Paraproteinemia:
benign (familial)
secondary to malignant or inflammatory disease

❑ 273.2 **Other paraproteinemias**
Cryoglobulinemic:
purpura
vasculitis
Mixed cryoglobulinemia

273.3 **Macroglobulinemia**
Macroglobulinemia (idiopathic) (primary)
Waldenström's macroglobulinemia

❑ 273.8 **Other disorders of plasma protein metabolism**
Abnormality of transport protein
Bisalbuminemia

❑ 273.9 **Unspecified disorder of plasma protein metabolism**

● 274 **Gout**
Excludes *lead gout (984.0–984.9)*

274.0 **Gouty arthropathy**

● 274.1 **Gouty nephropathy**

❑ 274.10 **Gouty nephropathy, unspecified**

274.11 **Uric acid nephrolithiasis**

❑ 274.19 **Other**

● 274.8 **Gout with other specified manifestations**

274.81 **Gouty tophi of ear**

❑ 274.82 **Gouty tophi of other sites**
Gouty tophi of heart

❑274.89 Other

Use additional code to identify manifestations, as:
gouty:
iritis (364.11)
neuritis (357.4)

❑274.9 Gout, unspecified

● 275 Disorders of mineral metabolism

Excludes *abnormal findings without manifest disease (790.0–796.9)*

275.0 Disorders of iron metabolism
Bronzed diabetes
Hemochromatosis
Pigmentary cirrhosis (of liver)

Excludes *anemia:*
iron deficiency (280.0–280.9)
sideroblastic (285.0)

275.1 Disorders of copper metabolism
Hepatolenticular degeneration
Wilson's disease

275.2 Disorders of magnesium metabolism
Hypermagnesemia
Hypomagnesemia

275.3 Disorders of phosphorus metabolism
Familial hypophosphatemia
Hypophosphatasia
Vitamin D-resistant:
osteomalacia
rickets

● 275.4 Disorders of calcium metabolism

Excludes *parathyroid disorders (252.0–252.9)*
vitamin D deficiency (268.0–268.9)

❑275.40 Unspecified disorder of calcium metabolism

275.41 Hypocalcemia

275.42 Hypercalcemia

❑275.49 Other disorders of calcium metabolism
Nephrocalcinosis
Pseudohypoparathyroidism
Pseudopseudohypoparathyroidism

❑275.8 Other specified disorders of mineral metabolism

❑275.9 Unspecified disorder of mineral metabolism

● 276 Disorders of fluid, electrolyte, and acid-base balance

Excludes *diabetes insipidus (253.5)*
familial periodic paralysis (359.3)

276.0 Hyperosmolality and/or hypernatremia
Sodium [Na] excess
Sodium [Na] overload

276.1 Hyposmolality and/or hyponatremia
Sodium [Na] deficiency

276.2 Acidosis
Acidosis:
NOS
lactic
metabolic
respiratory

Excludes *diabetic acidosis (250.1)*

276.3 Alkalosis
Alkalosis:
NOS
metabolic
respiratory

276.4 Mixed acid-base balance disorder
Hypercapnia with mixed acid-base disorder

276.5 Volume depletion
Dehydration
Depletion of volume of plasma or extracellular fluid
Hypovolemia

Excludes *hypovolemic shock:*
postoperative (998.0)
traumatic (958.4)

276.6 Fluid overload
Fluid retention

Excludes *ascites (789.5)*
localized edema (782.3)

276.7 Hyperpotassemia
Hyperkalemia
Potassium [K]:
excess
intoxication
overload

276.8 Hypopotassemia
Hypokalemia
Potassium [K] deficiency

❑276.9 Electrolyte and fluid disorders not elsewhere classified
Electrolyte imbalance
Hyperchloremia
Hypochloremia

Excludes *electrolyte imbalance:*
associated with hyperemesis gravidarum (643.1)
complicating labor and delivery (669.0)
following abortion and ectopic or molar pregnancy (634–638 with .4, 639.4)

● 277 Other and unspecified disorders of metabolism

● 277.0 Cystic fibrosis
Fibrocystic disease of the pancreas
Mucoviscidosis

277.00 Without mention of meconium ileus
Cystic fibrosis NOS

277.01 With meconium ileus
Meconium:
ileus (of newborn)
obstruction of intestine in mucoviscidosis

277.02 With pulmonary manifestations
Cystic fibrosis with pulmonary exacerbation
Use additional code to identify any infectious organism present, such as:
pseudomonas (041.7)

277.03 With gastrointestinal manifestations

Excludes *with meconium ileus (277.01)*

❑277.09 With other manifestations

277.1 Disorders of porphyrin metabolism
Hematoporphyria
Hematoporphyrinuria
Hereditary coproporphyria
Porphyria
Porphyrinuria
Protocoproporphyria
Protoporphyria
Pyrroloporphyria

❑277.2 Other disorders of purine and pyrimidine metabolism
Hypoxanthine-guanine-phosphoribosyltransferase deficiency [HG-PRT deficiency]
Lesch-Nyhan syndrome
Xanthinuria

Excludes *gout (274.0–274.9)*
orotic aciduric anemia (281.4)

277.3 Amyloidosis
Amyloidosis:
NOS
inherited systemic
nephropathic
neuropathic (Portuguese) (Swiss)
secondary
Benign paroxysmal peritonitis
Familial Mediterranean fever
Hereditary cardiac amyloidosis

277.4 Disorders of bilirubin excretion
Hyperbilirubinemia:
congenital
constitutional
Syndrome:
Crigler-Najjar
Dubin-Johnson
Gilbert's
Rotor's

Excludes *hyperbilirubinemias specific to the perinatal period (774.0–774.7)*

277.5 Mucopolysaccharidosis
Gargoylism
Hunter's syndrome
Hurler's syndrome
Lipochondrodystrophy
Maroteaux-Lamy syndrome
Morquio-Brailsford disease
Osteochondrodystrophy
Sanfilippo's syndrome
Scheie's syndrome

❑**277.6 Other deficiencies of circulating enzymes**
Alpha 1-antitrypsin deficiency
Hereditary angioedema

277.7 Dysmetabolic syndrome X
Use additional code for associated manifestation, such as:
cardiovascular disease (414.00–414.07) ⬅
obesity (278.00–278.01)

● **277.8 Other specified disorders of metabolism**

277.81 Primary carnitine deficiency ◀

277.82 Carnitine deficiency due to inborn errors of metabolism ◀

277.83 Iatrogenic carnitine deficiency ◀
Carnitine deficiency due to: ◀
hemodialysis ◀
valproic acid therapy ◀

277.84 Other secondary carnitine deficiency ◀

❑**277.89 Other specified disorders of metabolism** ◀
Hand-Schüller-Christian disease ◀
Histiocytosis (acute) (chronic) ◀
Histiocytosis X (chronic) ◀

Excludes *histiocytosis:*
acute differentiated progressive (202.5) ◀
X, acute (progressive) (202.5) ◀

❑**277.9 Unspecified disorder of metabolism**
Enzymopathy NOS

● **278 Obesity and other hyperalimentation**

Excludes *hyperalimentation NOS (783.6)*
poisoning by vitamins NOS (963.5)
polyphagia (783.6)

● **278.0 Obesity**

Excludes *adiposogenital dystrophy (253.8)*
obesity of endocrine origin NOS (259.9)

❑**278.00 Obesity, unspecified**
Obesity NOS

278.01 Morbid obesity
Severe obesity ◀

278.1 Localized adiposity
Fat pad

278.2 Hypervitaminosis A

278.3 Hypercarotinemia

278.4 Hypervitaminosis D

❑**278.8 Other hyperalimentation**

● **279 Disorders involving the immune mechanism**

● **279.0 Deficiency of humoral immunity**

❑**279.00 Hypogammaglobulinemia, unspecified**
Agammaglobulinemia NOS

279.01 Selective IgA immunodeficiency

279.02 Selective IgM immunodeficiency

❑**279.03 Other selective immunoglobulin deficiencies**
Selective deficiency of IgG

279.04 Congenital hypogammaglobulinemia
Agammaglobulinemia:
Bruton's type
X-linked

279.05 Immunodeficiency with increased IgM
Immunodeficiency with hyper-IgM:
autosomal recessive
X-linked

279.06 Common variable immunodeficiency
Dysgammaglobulinemia (acquired) (congenital) (primary)
Hypogammaglobulinemia:
acquired primary
congenital non-sex-linked
sporadic

❑**279.09 Other**
Transient hypogammaglobulinemia of infancy

● **279.1 Deficiency of cell-mediated immunity**

❑**279.10 Immunodeficiency with predominant T-cell defect, unspecified**

279.11 DiGeorge's syndrome
Pharyngeal pouch syndrome
Thymic hypoplasia

279.12 Wiskott-Aldrich syndrome

279.13 Nezelof's syndrome
Cellular immunodeficiency with abnormal immunoglobulin deficiency

❑**279.19 Other**

Excludes *ataxia-telangiectasia (334.8)*

279.2 Combined immunity deficiency
Agammaglobulinemia:
autosomal recessive
Swiss-type
X-linked recessive
Severe combined immunodeficiency [SCID]
Thymic:
alymphoplasia
aplasia or dysplasia with immunodeficiency

Excludes *thymic hypoplasia (279.11)*

❑**279.3 Unspecified immunity deficiency**

❑**279.4 Autoimmune disease, not elsewhere classified**
Autoimmune disease NOS

Excludes *transplant failure or rejection (996.80–996.89)*

❑**279.8 Other specified disorders involving the immune mechanism**
Single complement [C_1-C_9] deficiency or dysfunction

❑**279.9 Unspecified disorder of immune mechanism**

4. DISEASES OF THE BLOOD AND BLOOD-FORMING ORGANS (280–289)

Excludes *anemia complicating pregnancy or the puerperium (648.2)*

● **280 Iron deficiency anemias**

Includes: anemia:
asiderotic
hypochromic-microcytic
sideropenic

Excludes *familial microcytic anemia (282.49)* ⬅

280.0 Secondary to blood loss (chronic)
Normocytic anemia due to blood loss

Excludes *acute posthemorrhagic anemia (285.1)*

280.1 Secondary to inadequate dietary iron intake

❑ **280.8 Other specified iron deficiency anemias**
Paterson-Kelly syndrome
Plummer-Vinson syndrome
Sideropenic dysphagia

❑ **280.9 Iron deficiency anemia, unspecified**
Anemia:
achlorhydric
chlorotic
idiopathic hypochromic
iron [Fe] deficiency NOS

● **281 Other deficiency anemias**

281.0 Pernicious anemia
Anemia:
Addison's
Biermer's
congenital pernicious
Congenital intrinsic factor [Castle's] deficiency

Excludes *combined system disease without mention of anemia (266.2)*
subacute degeneration of spinal cord without mention of anemia (266.2)

❑ **281.1 Other vitamin B_{12} deficiency anemia**
Anemia:
vegan's
vitamin B_{12} deficiency (dietary)
due to selective vitamin B_{12} malabsorption with proteinuria
Syndrome:
Imerslund's
Imerslund-Gräsbeck

Excludes *combined system disease without mention of anemia (266.2)*
subacute degeneration of spinal cord without mention of anemia (266.2)

281.2 Folate-deficiency anemia
Congenital folate malabsorption
Folate or folic acid deficiency anemia:
NOS
dietary
drug-induced
Goat's milk anemia
Nutritional megaloblastic anemia (of infancy)
Use additional E code to identify drug

❑ **281.3 Other specified megaloblastic anemias, not elsewhere classified**
Combined B_{12} and folate-deficiency anemia
Refractory megaloblastic anemia

281.4 Protein-deficiency anemia
Amino-acid-deficiency anemia

❑ **281.8 Anemia associated with other specified nutritional deficiency**
Scorbutic anemia

❑ **281.9 Unspecified deficiency anemia**
Anemia:
dimorphic
macrocytic
megaloblastic NOS
nutritional NOS
simple chronic

● **282 Hereditary hemolytic anemias**

282.0 Hereditary spherocytosis
Acholuric (familial) jaundice
Congenital hemolytic anemia (spherocytic)
Congenital spherocytosis
Minkowski-Chauffard syndrome
Spherocytosis (familial)

Excludes *hemolytic anemia of newborn (773.0–773.5)*

282.1 Hereditary elliptocytosis
Elliptocytosis (congenital)
Ovalocytosis (congenital) (hereditary)

282.2 Anemias due to disorders of glutathione metabolism
Anemia:
6-phosphogluconic dehydrogenase deficiency
enzyme deficiency, drug-induced
erythrocytic glutathione deficiency
glucose-6-phosphate dehydrogenase [G-6-PD] deficiency
glutathione-reductase deficiency
hemolytic nonspherocytic (hereditary), type I
Disorder of pentose phosphate pathway
Favism

❑ **282.3 Other hemolytic anemias due to enzyme deficiency**
Anemia:
hemolytic nonspherocytic (hereditary), type II
hexokinase deficiency
pyruvate kinase [PK] deficiency
triosephosphate isomerase deficiency

● **282.4 Thalassemias**

Excludes *sickle-cell:*
disease (282.60–282.69) ⬅
trait (282.5)

282.41 Sickle-cell thalassemia without crisis ◀
Sickle-cell thalassemia NOS ◀
Thalassemia Hb-S disease without crisis ◀

282.42 Sickle-cell thalassemia with crisis ◀
Sickle-cell thalassemia with vasco-occlusive pain ◀
Thalassemia Hb-S disease with crisis ◀
Use additional code for types of crisis, such as: ◀
acute chest syndrome (517.3) ◀
splenic sequestration (289.52) ◀

❑ **282.49 Other thalassemia** ◀
Cooley's anemia ◀
Hereditary leptocytosis ◀
Mediterranean anemia (with other hemoglobinopathy) ◀
Microdrepanocytosis ◀
Thalassemia (alpha) (beta) (intermedia) (major) (minima) (minor) (mixed) (trait) (with other hemoglobinopathy) ◀
Thalassemia NOS ◀

282.5 Sickle-cell trait
Hb-AS genotype
Hemoglobin S [Hb-S] trait
Heterozygous:
hemoglobin S
Hb-S

Excludes *that with other hemoglobinopathy (282.60–282.69)*
that with thalassemia (282.49)

● 282.6 **Sickle-cell disease**
Sickle-cell anemia

Excludes *sickle-cell thalassemia (282.41–282.42)*
sickle-cell trait (282.5)

❑ 282.60 **Sickle-cell disease, unspecified**
Sickle-cell anemia NOS

282.61 **Hb-SS disease without crisis**

282.62 **Hb-SS disease with crisis**
Hb-SS disease with vaso-occlusive pain

Use additional code for types of crisis, such as:
acute chest syndrome (517.3)
splenic sequestration (289.52)

282.63 **Sickle-cell/Hb-C disease without crisis**
Hb-S/Hb-C disease without crisis

282.64 **Sickle-cell/Hb-C disease with crisis**
Hb-S/Hb-C disease with crisis
Sickle-cell/Hb-C disease with vaso-occlusive pain

Use additional code for types of crisis, such as:
acute chest syndrome (517.3)
splenic sequestration (289.52)

282.68 **Other sickle-cell disease without crisis**
Hb-S/Hb-D disease without crisis
Hb-S/Hb-E disease without crisis
Sickle-cell/Hb-D disease without crisis
Sickle-cell/Hb-E disease without crisis

❑ 282.69 **Other sickle-cell disease with crisis**
Hb-S/Hb-D disease with crisis
Hb-S/Hb-E disease with crisis
Other sickle-cell disease with vaso-occlusive pain
Sickle-cell/Hb-D disease with crisis
Sickle-cell/Hb-E disease with crisis

Use additional code for types of crisis, such as:
acute chest syndrome (517.3)
splenic sequestration (289.52)

❑ 282.7 **Other hemoglobinopathies**
Abnormal hemoglobin NOS
Congenital Heinz-body anemia
Disease:
Hb-Bart's
hemoglobin C [Hb-C]
hemoglobin D [Hb-D]
hemoglobin E [Hb-E]
hemoglobin Zurich [Hb-Zurich]
Hemoglobinopathy NOS
Hereditary persistence of fetal hemoglobin [HPFH]
Unstable hemoglobin hemolytic disease

Excludes *familial polycythemia (289.6)*
hemoglobin M [Hb-M] disease (289.7)
high-oxygen-affinity hemoglobin (289.0)

❑ 282.8 **Other specified hereditary hemolytic anemias**
Stomatocytosis

❑ 282.9 **Hereditary hemolytic anemia, unspecified**
Hereditary hemolytic anemia NOS

● 283 **Acquired hemolytic anemias**

283.0 **Autoimmune hemolytic anemias**
Autoimmune hemolytic disease (cold type) (warm type)
Chronic cold hemagglutinin disease
Cold agglutinin disease or hemoglobinuria
Hemolytic anemia:
cold type (secondary) (symptomatic)
drug-induced
warm type (secondary) (symptomatic)

Use additional E code to identify cause, if drug-induced

Excludes *Evans' syndrome (287.3)*
hemolytic disease of newborn (773.0–773.5)

● 283.1 **Non-autoimmune hemolytic anemias**

❑ 283.10 **Non-autoimmune hemolytic anemia, unspecified**

283.11 **Hemolytic-uremic syndrome**

❑ 283.19 **Other non-autoimmune hemolytic anemias**
Hemolytic anemia:
mechanical
microangiopathic
toxic

Use additional E code to identify cause

283.2 **Hemoglobinuria due to hemolysis from external causes**
Acute intravascular hemolysis
Hemoglobinuria:
from exertion
march
paroxysmal (cold) (nocturnal)
due to other hemolysis
Marchiafava-Micheli syndrome

Use additional E code to identify cause

❑ 283.9 **Acquired hemolytic anemia, unspecified**
Acquired hemolytic anemia NOS
Chronic idiopathic hemolytic anemia

● 284 **Aplastic anemia**

284.0 **Constitutional aplastic anemia**
Aplasia, (pure) red cell:
congenital
of infants
primary
Blackfan-Diamond syndrome
Familial hypoplastic anemia
Fanconi's anemia
Pancytopenia with malformations

❑ 284.8 **Other specified aplastic anemias**
Aplastic anemia (due to):
chronic systemic disease
drugs
infection
radiation
toxic (paralytic)
Pancytopenia (acquired)
Red cell aplasia (acquired) (adult) (pure) (with thymoma)

Use additional E code to identify cause

❑ 284.9 **Aplastic anemia, unspecified**
Anemia:
aplastic (idiopathic) NOS
aregenerative
hypoplastic NOS
nonregenerative
refractory
Medullary hypoplasia

● **285 Other and unspecified anemias**

285.0 Sideroblastic anemia
Anemia:
hypochromic with iron loading
sideroachrestic
sideroblastic
acquired
congenital
hereditary
primary
refractory
secondary (drug-induced) (due to disease)
sex-linked hypochromic
vitamin B_6-responsive
Pyridoxine-responsive (hypochromic) anemia

Use additional E code to identify cause, if drug-induced

285.1 Acute posthemorrhagic anemia
Anemia due to acute blood loss

Excludes *anemia due to chronic blood loss (280.0)*
blood loss anemia NOS (280.0)

● **285.2 Anemia in chronic illness**

285.21 Anemia in end-stage renal disease
Erythropoietin-resistant anemia (EPO resistant anemia) ◀

285.22 Anemia in neoplastic disease

285.29 Anemia of other chronic illness

❑ **285.8 Other specified anemias**
Anemia:
dyserythropoietic (congenital)
dyshematopoietic (congenital)
leukoerythroblastic
von Jaksch's
Infantile pseudoleukemia

❑ **285.9 Anemia, unspecified**
Anemia:
NOS
essential
normocytic, not due to blood loss
profound
progressive
secondary
Oligocythemia

Excludes *anemia (due to):*
blood loss:
acute (285.1)
chronic or unspecified (280.0)
iron deficiency (280.0–280.9)

● **286 Coagulation defects**

286.0 Congenital factor VIII disorder
Antihemophilic globulin [AHG] deficiency
Factor VIII (functional) deficiency
Hemophilia:
NOS
A
classical
familial
hereditary
Subhemophilia

Excludes *factor VIII deficiency with vascular defect (286.4)*

286.1 Congenital factor IX disorder
Christmas disease
Deficiency:
factor IX (functional)
plasma thromboplastin component [PTC]
Hemophilia B

286.2 Congenital factor XI deficiency
Hemophilia C
Plasma thromboplastin antecedent [PTA] deficiency
Rosenthal's disease

❑ **286.3 Congenital deficiency of other clotting factors**
Congenital afibrinogenemia
Deficiency:
AC globulin factor:
I [fibrinogen]
II [prothrombin]
V [labile]
VII [stable]
X [Stuart-Prower]
XII [Hageman]
XIII [fibrin stabilizing]
Laki-Lorand factor
proaccelerin
Disease:
Owren's
Stuart-Prower
Dysfibrinogenemia (congenital)
Dysprothrombinemia (constitutional)
Hypoproconvertinemia
Hypoprothrombinemia (hereditary)
Parahemophilia

286.4 von Willebrand's disease
Angiohemophilia (A) (B)
Constitutional thrombopathy
Factor VIII deficiency with vascular defect
Pseudohemophilia type B
Vascular hemophilia
von Willebrand's (-Jürgens') disease

Excludes *factor VIII deficiency:*
NOS (286.0)
with functional defect (286.0)
hereditary capillary fragility (287.8)

286.5 Hemorrhagic disorder due to circulating anticoagulants
Antithrombinemia
Antithromboplastinemia
Antithromboplastinogenemia
Hyperheparinemia
Increase in:
anti-VIIIa
anti-IXa
anti-Xa
anti-XIa
antithrombin
Systemic lupus erythematosus [SLE] inhibitor

Use additional E code to identify cause, if drug-induced

286.6 Defibrination syndrome
Afibrinogenemia, acquired
Consumption coagulopathy
Diffuse or disseminated intravascular coagulation [DIC syndrome]
Fibrinolytic hemorrhage, acquired
Hemorrhagic fibrinogenolysis
Pathologic fibrinolysis
Purpura:
fibrinolytic
fulminans

Excludes *that complicating:*
abortion (634–638 with .1, 639.1)
pregnancy or the puerperium (641.3, 666.3)
disseminated intravascular coagulation in newborn (776.2)

286.7 Acquired coagulation factor deficiency
Deficiency of coagulation factor due to:
liver disease
vitamin K deficiency
Hypoprothrombinemia, acquired
Excludes *vitamin K deficiency of newborn (776.0)*
Use additional E code to identify cause, if drug-induced

❑ **286.9 Other and unspecified coagulation defects**
Defective coagulation NOS
Deficiency, coagulation factor NOS
Delay, coagulation
Disorder:
coagulation
hemostasis
Excludes *abnormal coagulation profile (790.92)*
hemorrhagic disease of newborn (776.0)
that complicating:
abortion (634–638 with .1, 639.1)
pregnancy or the puerperium (641.3, 666.3)

● **287 Purpura and other hemorrhagic conditions**
Excludes *hemorrhagic thrombocythemia (238.7)*
purpura fulminans (286.6)

287.0 Allergic purpura
Peliosis rheumatica
Purpura:
anaphylactoid
autoimmune
Henoch's
nonthrombocytopenic:
hemorrhagic
idiopathic
rheumatica
Schönlein-Henoch
vascular
Vasculitis, allergic
Excludes *hemorrhagic purpura (287.3)*
purpura annularis telangiectodes (709.1)

287.1 Qualitative platelet defects
Thrombasthenia (hemorrhagic) (hereditary)
Thrombocytasthenia
Thrombocytopathy (dystrophic)
Thrombopathy (Bernard-Soulier)
Excludes *von Willebrand's disease (286.4)*

❑ **287.2 Other nonthrombocytopenic purpuras**
Purpura:
NOS
senile
simplex

287.3 Primary thrombocytopenia
Evans'syndrome
Megakaryocytic hypoplasia
Purpura, thrombocytopenic
congenital
hereditary
idiopathic
Thrombocytopenia:
congenital
hereditary
primary
Tidal platelet dysgenesis
Excludes *thrombotic thrombocytopenic purpura (446.6)*
transient thrombocytopenia of newborn (776.1)

287.4 Secondary thrombocytopenia
Posttransfusion purpura
Thrombocytopenia (due to):
dilutional
drugs
extracorporeal circulation of blood
massive blood transfusion
platelet alloimmunization
Use additional E code to identify cause
Excludes *transient thrombocytopenia of newborn (776.1)*

❑ **287.5 Thrombocytopenia, unspecified**

❑ **287.8 Other specified hemorrhagic conditions**
Capillary fragility (hereditary)
Vascular pseudohemophilia

❑ **287.9 Unspecified hemorrhagic conditions**
Hemorrhagic diathesis (familial)

● **288 Diseases of white blood cells**
Excludes *leukemia (204.0–208.9)*

288.0 Agranulocytosis
Infantile genetic agranulocytosis
Kostmann's syndrome
Neutropenia:
NOS
cyclic
drug-induced
Neutropenia:
immune
periodic
toxic
Neutropenic splenomegaly
Use additional E code to identify drug or other cause
Excludes *transitory neonatal neutropenia (776.7)*

288.1 Functional disorders of polymorphonuclear neutrophils
Chronic (childhood) granulomatous disease
Congenital dysphagocytosis
Job's syndrome
Lipochrome histiocytosis (familial)
Progressive septic granulomatosis

288.2 Genetic anomalies of leukocytes
Anomaly (granulation) (granulocyte) or syndrome:
Alder's (-Reilly)
Chédiak-Steinbrinck (-Higashi)
Jordan's
May-Hegglin
Pelger-Huet
Hereditary:
hypersegmentation
hyposegmentation
leukomelanopathy

288.3 Eosinophilia
Eosinophilia
allergic
hereditary
idiopathic
secondary
Eosinophilic leukocytosis
Excludes *Löffler's syndrome (518.3)*
pulmonary eosinophilia (518.3)

❑ **288.8 Other specified disease of white blood cells**
Leukemoid reaction
lymphocytic
monocytic
myelocytic
Leukocytosis
Lymphocytopenia
Lymphocytosis (symptomatic)
Lymphopenia
Monocytosis (symptomatic)
Plasmacytosis
Excludes *immunity disorders (279.0–279.9)*

❑ **288.9 Unspecified disease of white blood cells**

ICD-9-CM 200-299 Vol. 1

● **289 Other diseases of blood and blood-forming organs**

289.0 Polycythemia, secondary
High-oxygen-affinity hemoglobin
Polycythemia:
acquired
benign
due to:
fall in plasma volume
high altitude
emotional
erythropoietin
hypoxemic
nephrogenous
relative
spurious
stress

Excludes *polycythemia:*
neonatal (776.4)
primary (238.4)
vera (238.4)

289.1 Chronic lymphadenitis
Chronic:
adenitis any lymph node, except mesenteric
lymphadenitis any lymph node, except mesenteric

Excludes *acute lymphadenitis (683)*
mesenteric (289.2)
enlarged glands NOS (785.6)

❑ **289.2 Nonspecific mesenteric lymphadenitis**
Mesenteric lymphadenitis (acute) (chronic)

❑ **289.3 Lymphadenitis, unspecified, except mesenteric**

289.4 Hypersplenism
"Big spleen" syndrome
Dyssplenism
Hypersplenia

Excludes *primary splenic neutropenia (288.0)*

● **289.5 Other diseases of spleen**

❑ **289.50 Disease of spleen, unspecified**

289.51 Chronic congestive splenomegaly

289.52 Splenic sequestration ◄
Code first sickle-cell disease in crisis (282.42, 282.62, 282.64, 282.69) ◄

❑ **289.59 Other**
Lien migrans
Perisplenitis
Splenic:
abscess
atrophy
cyst
fibrosis
infarction
rupture, nontraumatic
Splenitis
Wandering spleen

Excludes *bilharzial splenic fibrosis (120.0–120.9)*
hepatolienal fibrosis (571.5)
splenomegaly NOS (789.2)

289.6 Familial polycythemia
Familial:
benign polycythemia
erythrocytosis

289.7 Methemoglobinemia
Congenital NADH [DPNH]-methemoglobin-reductase deficiency
Hemoglobin M [Hb-M] disease
Methemoglobinemia:
NOS
acquired (with sulfhemoglobinemia)
hereditary
toxic
Stokvis' disease
Sulfhemoglobinemia

Use additional E code to identify cause

● **289.8 Other specified diseases of blood and blood-forming organs**

289.81 Primary hypercoagulable state ◄
Activated protein C resistance ◄
Antithrombin III deficiency ◄
Factor V Leiden mutation ◄
Lupus anticoagulant ◄
Protein C deficiency ◄
Protein S deficiency ◄
Prothombin gene mutation ◄

289.82 Secondary hypercoagulable state ◄

❑ **289.89 Other specified disease of blood and blood-forming organs** ◄
Hypergammaglobulinemia ◄
Myelofibrosis ◄
Pseudocholinesterase deficiency ◄

❑ **289.9 Unspecified diseases of blood and blood-forming organs**
Blood dyscrasia NOS
Erythroid hyperplasia

5. MENTAL DISORDERS (290–319)

In the International Classification of Diseases, 9th Revision (ICD-9), the corresponding Chapter V, "Mental Disorders," includes a glossary which defines the contents of each category. The introduction to Chapter V in ICD-9 indicates that the glossary is intended so that psychiatrists can make the diagnosis based on the descriptions provided rather than from the category titles. Lay coders are instructed to code whatever diagnosis the physician records.

Chapter 5, "Mental Disorders," in ICD-9-CM uses the standard classification format with inclusion and exclusion terms, omitting the glossary as part of the main text.

The mental disorders section of ICD-9-CM has been expanded to incorporate additional psychiatric disorders not listed in ICD-9. The glossary from ICD-9 does not contain all these terms. It now appears in Appendix B, which also contains descriptions and definitions for the terms added in ICD-9-CM. Some of these were provided by the American Psychiatric Association's Task Force on Nomenclature and Statistics who are preparing the Diagnostic and Statistical Manual, Third Edition (DSM-III), and others from A Psychiatric Glossary.

The American Psychiatric Association provided invaluable assistance in modifying Chapter 5 of ICD-9-CM to incorporate detail useful to American clinicians and gave permission to use material from the aforementioned sources.

1. Manual of the International Statistical Classification of Diseases, Injuries, and Causes of Death, 9th Revision, World Health Organization, Geneva, Switzerland, 1975.
2. American Psychiatric Association, Task Force on Nomenclature and Statistics, Robert L. Spitzer, M.D., Chairman.
3. A Psychiatric Glossary, Fourth Edition, American Psychiatric Association, Washington, D.C., 1975.

PSYCHOSES (290–299)

Excludes *mental retardation (317–319)*

ORGANIC PSYCHOTIC CONDITIONS (290–294)

Includes: psychotic organic brain syndrome

Excludes *nonpsychotic syndromes of organic etiology (310.0–310.9)*
psychoses classifiable to 295–298 and without impairment of orientation, comprehension, calculation, learning capacity, and judgment, but associated with physical disease, injury, or condition affecting the brain [e.g., following childbirth] (295.0–298.8)

● **290 Senile and presenile organic psychotic conditions**

Code first the associated neurological condition

Excludes *dementia not classified as senile, presenile, or arteriosclerotic (294.10–294.11)*
psychoses classifiable to 295–298 occurring in the senium without dementia or delirium (295.0–298.8)
senility with mental changes of nonpsychotic severity (310.1)
transient organic psychotic conditions (293.0–293.9)

290.0 Senile dementia, uncomplicated

Senile dementia:
NOS
simple type

Excludes *mild memory disturbances, not amounting to dementia, associated with senile brain disease (310.1)*
senile dementia with:
delirium or confusion (290.3)
delusional [paranoid] features (290.20)
depressive features (290.21)

● **290.1 Presenile dementia**

Brain syndrome with presenile brain disease

Excludes *arteriosclerotic dementia (290.40–290.43)*
dementia associated with other cerebral conditions (294.10–294.11)

290.10 Presenile dementia, uncomplicated

Presenile dementia:
NOS
simple type

290.11 Presenile dementia with delirium

Presenile dementia with acute confusional state

290.12 Presenile dementia with delusional features

Presenile dementia, paranoid type

290.13 Presenile dementia with depressive features

Presenile dementia, depressed type

● **290.2 Senile dementia with delusional or depressive features**

Excludes *senile dementia:*
NOS (290.0)
with delirium and/or confusion (290.3)

290.20 Senile dementia with delusional features

Senile dementia, paranoid type
Senile psychosis NOS

290.21 Senile dementia with depressive features

290.3 Senile dementia with delirium

Senile dementia with acute confusional state

Excludes *senile:*
dementia NOS (290.0)
psychosis NOS (290.20)

● **290.4 Arteriosclerotic dementia**

Multi-infarct dementia or psychosis

Use additional code to identify cerebral atherosclerosis (437.0)

Excludes *suspected cases with no clear evidence of arteriosclerosis (290.9)*

290.40 Arteriosclerotic dementia, uncomplicated

Arteriosclerotic dementia:
NOS
simple type

290.41 Arteriosclerotic dementia with delirium

Arteriosclerotic dementia with acute confusional state

290.42 Arteriosclerotic dementia with delusional features

Arteriosclerotic dementia, paranoid type

290.43 Arteriosclerotic dementia with depressive features

Arteriosclerotic dementia, depressed type

❑ **290.8 Other specified senile psychotic conditions**

Presbyophrenic psychosis

❑ **290.9 Unspecified senile psychotic condition**

● **291 Alcoholic psychoses**

Excludes *alcoholism without psychosis (303.0–303.9)*

291.0 Alcohol withdrawal delirium

Alcoholic delirium
Delirium tremens

Excludes *alcohol withdrawal (291.81)*

291.1 Alcoholic amnestic syndrome

Alcoholic polyneuritic psychosis
Korsakoff's psychosis, alcoholic
Wernicke-Korsakoff syndrome (alcoholic)

ICD-9-CM 200-299 Vol. 1

❑ **291.2 Other alcoholic dementia**
Alcoholic dementia NOS
Alcoholism associated with dementia NOS
Chronic alcoholic brain syndrome

291.3 Alcohol withdrawal hallucinosis
Alcoholic:
hallucinosis (acute)
psychosis with hallucinosis

Excludes *alcohol withdrawal with delirium (291.0)*
schizophrenia (295.0–295.9) and paranoid states (297.0–297.9) taking the form of chronic hallucinosis with clear consciousness in an alcoholic

291.4 Idiosyncratic alcohol intoxication
Pathologic:
alcohol intoxication
drunkenness

Excludes *acute alcohol intoxication (305.0)*
in alcoholism (303.0)
simple drunkenness (305.0)

291.5 Alcoholic jealousy
Alcoholic:
paranoia
psychosis, paranoid type

Excludes *nonalcoholic paranoid states (297.0–297.9)*
schizophrenia, paranoid type (295.3)

● **291.8 Other specified alcoholic psychosis**

291.81 Alcohol withdrawal
Alcohol:
abstinence syndrome or symptoms
withdrawal syndrome or symptoms

Excludes *alcohol withdrawal:*
delirium (291.0)
hallucinosis (291.3)
delirium tremens (291.0)

❑ **291.89 Other**

❑ **291.9 Unspecified alcoholic psychosis**
Alcoholic:
mania NOS
psychosis NOS
Alcoholism (chronic) with psychosis

● **292 Drug psychoses**

Includes: drug-induced mental disorders
organic brain syndrome associated with consumption of drugs

Use additional code for any associated drug dependence (304.0–304.9)

Use additional E code to identify drug

292.0 Drug withdrawal syndrome
Drug:
abstinence syndrome or symptoms
withdrawal syndrome or symptoms

● **292.1 Paranoid and/or hallucinatory states induced by drugs**

292.11 Drug-induced organic delusional syndrome
Paranoid state induced by drugs

292.12 Drug-induced hallucinosis
Hallucinatory state induced by drugs

Excludes *states following LSD or other hallucinogens, lasting only a few days or less ["bad trips"] (305.3)*

292.2 Pathological drug intoxication
Drug reaction: resulting in brief psychotic states
NOS
idiosyncratic
pathologic

Excludes *expected brief psychotic reactions to hallucinogens ["bad trips"] (305.3)*
physiological side-effects of drugs (e.g., dystonias)

● **292.8 Other specified drug-induced mental disorders**

292.81 Drug-induced delirium

292.82 Drug-induced dementia

292.83 Drug-induced amnestic syndrome

292.84 Drug-induced organic affective syndrome
Depressive state induced by drugs

❑ **292.89 Other**
Drug-induced organic personality syndrome

❑ **292.9 Unspecified drug-induced mental disorder**
Organic psychosis NOS due to or associated with drugs

● **293 Transient organic psychotic conditions**

Includes: transient organic mental disorders not associated with alcohol or drugs

Code first the associated physical or neurological condition

Excludes *confusional state or delirium superimposed on senile dementia (290.3)*
dementia due to:
alcohol (291.0–291.9)
arteriosclerosis (290.40–290.43)
drugs (292.82)
senility (290.0)

293.0 Acute delirium
Acute:
confusional state
infective psychosis
organic reaction
posttraumatic organic psychosis
psycho-organic syndrome
Acute psychosis associated with endocrine, metabolic, or cerebrovascular disorder
Epileptic:
confusional state
twilight state

293.1 Subacute delirium
Subacute:
confusional state
infective psychosis
organic reaction
posttraumatic organic psychosis
psycho-organic syndrome
psychosis associated with endocrine or metabolic disorder

● **293.8 Other specified transient organic mental disorders**

293.81 Organic delusional syndrome
Transient organic psychotic condition, paranoid type

293.82 Organic hallucinosis syndrome
Transient organic psychotic condition, hallucinatory type

293.83 Organic affective syndrome
Transient organic psychotic condition, depressive type

293.84 Organic anxiety syndrome

❑ **293.89 Other**

❑ **293.9 Unspecified transient organic mental disorder**
Organic psychosis:
infective NOS
posttraumatic NOS
transient NOS
Psycho-organic syndrome

● **294 Other organic psychotic conditions (chronic)**

Includes: organic psychotic brain syndromes (chronic), not elsewhere classified

294.0 Amnestic syndrome

Korsakoff's psychosis or syndrome (nonalcoholic)

Excludes *alcoholic:*
amnestic syndrome (291.1)
Korsakoff's psychosis (291.1)

● **294.1 Dementia in conditions classified elsewhere**

Code first any underlying physical condition as:
dementia in:
Alzheimer's disease (331.0)
cerebral lipidoses (330.1)
dementia with Lewy bodies (331.82) ◀
dementia with Parkinsonism (331.82) ◀
epilepsy (345.0–345.9)
frontal dementia (331.19) ◀
frontotemporal dementia (331.19) ◀
general paresis [syphilis] (094.1)
hepatolenticular degeneration (275.1)
Huntington's chorea (333.4)
Jakob-Creutzfeldt disease (046.1)
multiple sclerosis (340)
Pick's disease of the brain (331.11)
polyarteritis nodosa (446.0)
syphilis (094.1)

Excludes *dementia:*
arteriosclerotic (290.40–290.43)
presenile (290.10–290.13)
senile (290.0)
epileptic psychosis NOS (294.8)

294.10 Dementia in conditions classified elsewhere without behavioral disturbance

Dementia in conditions classified elsewhere NOS

294.11 Dementia in conditions classified elsewhere with behavioral disturbance

Aggressive behavior
Combative behavior
Violent behavior
Wandering off

❑ **294.8 Other specified organic brain syndromes (chronic)**

Epileptic psychosis NOS
Mixed paranoid and affective organic psychotic states

Use additional code for associated epilepsy (345.0–345.9)

Excludes *mild memory disturbances, not amounting to dementia (310.1)*

❑ **294.9 Unspecified organic brain syndrome (chronic)**

Organic psychosis (chronic)

OTHER PSYCHOSES (295–299)

Use additional code to identify any associated physical disease, injury, or condition affecting the brain with psychoses classifiable to 295–298

● **295 Schizophrenic disorders**

Includes: schizophrenia of the types described in 295.0–295.9 occurring in children

Excludes *childhood type schizophrenia (299.9)*
infantile autism (299.0)

The following fifth-digit subclassification is for use with category 295:

❑ **0 unspecified**
1 subchronic
2 chronic
3 subchronic with acute exacerbation
4 chronic with acute exacerbation
5 in remission

● **295.0 Simple type**

Schizophrenia simplex

Excludes *latent schizophrenia (295.5)*

● **295.1 Disorganized type**

Hebephrenia
Hebephrenic type schizophrenia

● **295.2 Catatonic type**

Catatonic (schizophrenia):	Schizophrenic:
agitation	catalepsy
excitation	catatonia
excited type	flexibilitas cerea
stupor	
withdrawn type	

● **295.3 Paranoid type**

Paraphrenic schizophrenia

Excludes *involutional paranoid state (297.2)*
paranoia (297.1)
paraphrenia (297.2)

● **295.4 Acute schizophrenic episode**

Oneirophrenia
Schizophreniform:
attack
disorder
psychosis, confusional type

Excludes *acute forms of schizophrenia of:*
catatonic type (295.2)
hebephrenic type (295.1)
paranoid type (295.3)
simple type (295.0)
undifferentiated type (295.8)

● **295.5 Latent schizophrenia**

Latent schizophrenic reaction
Schizophrenia:
borderline
incipient
prepsychotic
prodromal
pseudoneurotic
pseudopsychopathic

Excludes *schizoid personality (301.20–301.22)*

● **295.6 Residual schizophrenia**

Chronic undifferentiated schizophrenia
Restzustand (schizophrenic)
Schizophrenic residual state

● **295.7 Schizo-affective type**

Cyclic schizophrenia
Mixed schizophrenic and affective psychosis
Schizo-affective psychosis
Schizophreniform psychosis, affective type

● ❑ **295.8 Other specified types of schizophrenia**

Acute (undifferentiated) schizophrenia
Atypical schizophrenia
Cenesthopathic schizophrenia

Excludes *infantile autism (299.0)*

● ❑ **295.9 Unspecified schizophrenia**

Schizophrenia:
NOS
mixed NOS
undifferentiated NOS
Schizophrenic reaction NOS
Schizophreniform psychosis NOS

● **296 Affective psychoses**

Includes: episodic affective disorders

Excludes *neurotic depression (300.4)*
reactive depressive psychosis (298.0)
reactive excitation (298.1)

The following fifth-digit subclassification is for use with categories 296.0–296.6:

❑ 0 unspecified
1 mild
2 moderate
3 severe, without mention of psychotic behavior
4 severe, specified as with psychotic behavior
5 in partial or unspecified remission
6 in full remission

● **296.0 Manic disorder, single episode**
Hypomania (mild) NOS single episode or unspecified
Hypomanic psychosis single episode or unspecified
Mania (monopolar) NOS single episode or unspecified
Manic-depressive psychosis or reaction, single episode or unspecified:
hypomanic, single episode or unspecified
manic, single episode or unspecified

Excludes *circular type, if there was a previous attack of depression (296.4)*

● **296.1 Manic disorder, recurrent episode**
Any condition classifiable to 296.0, stated to be recurrent

Excludes *circular type, if there was a previous attack of depression (296.4)*

● **296.2 Major depressive disorder, single episode**
Depressive psychosis, single episode or unspecified
Endogenous depression, single episode or unspecified
Involutional melancholia, single episode or unspecified
Manic-depressive psychosis or reaction, depressed type, single episode or unspecified
Monopolar depression, single episode or unspecified
Psychotic depression, single episode or unspecified

Excludes *circular type, if previous attack was of manic type (296.5)*
depression NOS (311)
reactive depression (neurotic) (300.4)
psychotic (298.0)

● **296.3 Major depressive disorder, recurrent episode**
Any condition classifiable to 296.2, stated to be recurrent

Excludes *circular type, if previous attack was of manic type (296.5)*
depression NOS (311)
reactive depression (neurotic) (300.4)
psychotic (298.0)

● **296.4 Bipolar affective disorder, manic**
Bipolar disorder, now manic
Manic-depressive psychosis, circular type but currently manic

Excludes *brief compensatory or rebound mood swings (296.99)*

● **296.5 Bipolar affective disorder, depressed**
Bipolar disorder, now depressed
Manic-depressive psychosis, circular type but currently depressed

Excludes *brief compensatory or rebound mood swings (296.99)*

● **296.6 Bipolar affective disorder, mixed**
Manic-depressive psychosis, circular type, mixed

❑ **296.7 Bipolar affective disorder, unspecified**
Atypical bipolar affective disorder NOS
Manic-depressive psychosis, circular type, current condition not specified as either manic or depressive

● **296.8 Manic-depressive psychosis, other and unspecified**

❑ **296.80 Manic-depressive psychosis, unspecified**
Manic-depressive:
reaction NOS
syndrome NOS

296.81 Atypical manic disorder

296.82 Atypical depressive disorder

❑ **296.89 Other**
Manic-depressive psychosis, mixed type

● **296.9 Other and unspecified affective psychoses**

Excludes *psychogenic affective psychoses (298.0–298.8)*

❑ **296.90 Unspecified affective psychosis**
Affective psychosis NOS
Melancholia NOS

❑ **296.99 Other specified affective psychoses**
Mood swings:
brief compensatory
rebound

● **297 Paranoid states (Delusional disorders)**

Includes: paranoid disorders

Excludes *acute paranoid reaction (298.3)*
alcoholic jealousy or paranoid state (291.5)
paranoid schizophrenia (295.3)

297.0 Paranoid state, simple

297.1 Paranoia
Chronic paranoid psychosis
Sander's disease
Systematized delusions

Excludes *paranoid personality disorder (301.0)*

297.2 Paraphrenia
Involutional paranoid state
Late paraphrenia
Paraphrenia (involutional)

297.3 Shared paranoid disorder
Folie à deux
Induced psychosis or paranoid disorder

❑ **297.8 Other specified paranoid states**
Paranoia querulans
Sensitiver Beziehungswahn

Excludes *acute paranoid reaction or state (298.3)*
senile paranoid state (290.20)

❑ **297.9 Unspecified paranoid state**
Paranoid:
disorder NOS
psychosis NOS
Paranoid:
reaction NOS
state NOS

● **298 Other nonorganic psychoses**

Includes: psychotic conditions due to or provoked by:
emotional stress
environmental factors as major part of etiology

298.0 Depressive type psychosis
Psychogenic depressive psychosis
Psychotic reactive depression
Reactive depressive psychosis

Excludes *manic-depressive psychosis, depressed type (296.2–296.3)*
neurotic depression (300.4)
reactive depression NOS (300.4)

298.1 Excitative type psychosis
Acute hysterical psychosis
Psychogenic excitation
Reactive excitation

Excludes *manic-depressive psychosis, manic type (296.0–296.1)*

298.2 Reactive confusion
Psychogenic confusion
Psychogenic twilight state
Excludes *acute confusional state (293.0)*

298.3 Acute paranoid reaction
Acute psychogenic paranoid psychosis
Bouffée délirante
Excludes *paranoid states (297.0–297.9)*

298.4 Psychogenic paranoid psychosis
Protracted reactive paranoid psychosis

❑ **298.8 Other and unspecified reactive psychosis**
Brief reactive psychosis NOS
Hysterical psychosis
Psychogenic psychosis NOS
Psychogenic stupor
Excludes *acute hysterical psychosis (298.1)*

❑ **298.9 Unspecified psychosis**
Atypical psychosis
Psychosis NOS

● **299 Psychoses with origin specific to childhood**
Includes: pervasive developmental disorders
Excludes *adult type psychoses occurring in childhood, as:*
affective disorders (296.0–296.9)
manic-depressive disorders (296.0–296.9)
schizophrenia (295.0–295.9)

The following fifth-digit subclassification is for use with category 299:
0 current or active state
1 residual state

● **299.0 Infantile autism**
Childhood autism
Infantile psychosis
Kanner's syndrome
Excludes *disintegrative psychosis (299.1)*
Heller's syndrome (299.1)
schizophrenic syndrome of childhood (299.9)

● **299.1 Disintegrative psychosis**
Heller's syndrome
Use additional code to identify any associated neurological disorder
Excludes *infantile autism (299.0)*
schizophrenic syndrome of childhood (299.9)

● ❑ **299.8 Other specified early childhood psychoses**
Atypical childhood psychosis
Borderline psychosis of childhood
Excludes *simple stereotypes without psychotic disturbance (307.3)*

● ❑ **299.9 Unspecified**
Child psychosis NOS
Schizophrenia, childhood type NOS
Schizophrenic syndrome of childhood NOS
Excludes *schizophrenia of adult type occurring in childhood (295.0–295.9)*

NEUROTIC DISORDERS, PERSONALITY DISORDERS, AND OTHER NONPSYCHOTIC MENTAL DISORDERS (300–316)

● **300 Neurotic disorders**

● **300.0 Anxiety states**
Excludes *anxiety in:*
acute stress reaction (308.0)
transient adjustment reaction (309.24)
neurasthenia (300.5)
psychophysiological disorders (306.0–306.9)
separation anxiety (309.21)

❑ **300.00 Anxiety state, unspecified**
Anxiety:
neurosis
reaction
state (neurotic)
Atypical anxiety disorder

300.01 Panic disorder
Panic:
attack
state

300.02 Generalized anxiety disorder

❑ **300.09 Other**

● **300.1 Hysteria**
Excludes *adjustment reaction (309.0–309.9)*
anorexia nervosa (307.1)
gross stress reaction (308.0–308.9)
hysterical personality (301.50–301.59)
psychophysiologic disorders (306.0–306.9)

❑ **300.10 Hysteria, unspecified**

300.11 Conversion disorder
Astasia-abasia, hysterical
Conversion hysteria or reaction
Hysterical:
blindness
deafness
paralysis

300.12 Psychogenic amnesia
Hysterical amnesia

300.13 Psychogenic fugue
Hysterical fugue

300.14 Multiple personality
Dissociative identity disorder

❑ **300.15 Dissociative disorder or reaction, unspecified**

300.16 Factitious illness with psychological symptoms
Compensation neurosis
Ganser's syndrome, hysterical

❑ **300.19 Other and unspecified factitious illness**
Factitious illness (with physical symptoms) NOS
Excludes *multiple operations or hospital addiction syndrome (301.51)*

● **300.2 Phobic disorders**
Excludes *anxiety state not associated with a specific situation or object (300.00–300.09)*
obsessional phobias (300.3)

❑ **300.20 Phobia, unspecified**
Anxiety-hysteria NOS
Phobia NOS

300.21 Agoraphobia with panic attacks
Fear of:
open spaces with panic attacks
streets with panic attacks
travel with panic attacks

300.22 Agoraphobia without mention of panic attacks
Any condition classifiable to 300.21 without mention of panic attacks

300.23 Social phobia
Fear of:
eating in public
public speaking
Fear of:
washing in public

❑ **300.29 Other isolated or simple phobias**
Acrophobia
Animal phobias
Claustrophobia
Fear of crowds

300.3 Obsessive-compulsive disorders
Anancastic neurosis
Compulsive neurosis
Obsessional phobia [any]

Excludes *obsessive-compulsive symptoms occurring in:*
endogenous depression (296.2–296.3)
organic states (e.g., encephalitis)
schizophrenia (295.0–295.9)

300.4 Neurotic depression
Anxiety depression
Depression with anxiety
Depressive reaction
Dysthymic disorder
Neurotic depressive state
Reactive depression

Excludes *adjustment reaction with depressive symptoms (309.0–309.1)*
depression NOS (311)
manic-depressive psychosis, depressed type (296.2–296.3)
reactive depressive psychosis (298.0)

300.5 Neurasthenia
Fatigue neurosis
Nervous debility
Psychogenic:
asthenia
general fatigue

Use additional code to identify any associated physical disorder

Excludes *anxiety state (300.00–300.09)*
neurotic depression (300.4)
psychophysiological disorders (306.0–306.9)
specific nonpsychotic mental disorders following organic brain damage (310.0–310.9)

300.6 Depersonalization syndrome
Depersonalization disorder
Derealization (neurotic)
Neurotic state with depersonalization episode

Excludes *depersonalization associated with:*
anxiety (300.00–300.09)
depression (300.4)
manic-depressive disorder or psychosis (296.0–296.9)
schizophrenia (295.0–295.9)

300.7 Hypochondriasis
Body dysmorphic disorder

Excludes *hypochondriasis in:*
hysteria (300.10–300.19)
manic-depressive psychosis, depressed type (296.2–296.3)
neurasthenia (300.5)
obsessional disorder (300.3)
schizophrenia (295.0–295.9)

● **300.8 Other neurotic disorders**

300.81 Somatization disorder
Briquet's disorder
Severe somatoform disorder

300.82 Undifferentiated somatoform disorder
Atypical somatoform disorder
Somatoform disorder NOS

❑ **300.89 Other**
Occupational neurosis, including writers' cramp
Psychasthenia
Psychasthenic neurosis

❑ **300.9 Unspecified neurotic disorder**
Neurosis NOS
Psychoneurosis NOS

● **301 Personality disorders**

Includes: character neurosis

Use additional code to identify any associated neurosis or psychosis, or physical condition

Excludes *nonpsychotic personality disorder associated with organic brain syndromes (310.0–310.9)*

301.0 Paranoid personality disorder
Fanatic personality
Paranoid personality (disorder)
Paranoid traits

Excludes *acute paranoid reaction (298.3)*
alcoholic paranoia (291.5)
paranoid schizophrenia (295.3)
paranoid states (297.0–297.9)

● **301.1 Affective personality disorder**

Excludes *affective psychotic disorders (296.0–296.9)*
neurasthenia (300.5)
neurotic depression (300.4)

301.10 Affective personality disorder, unspecified

301.11 Chronic hypomanic personality disorder
Chronic hypomanic disorder
Hypomanic personality

301.12 Chronic depressive personality disorder
Chronic depressive disorder
Depressive character or personality

301.13 Cyclothymic disorder
Cycloid personality
Cyclothymia
Cyclothymic personality

● **301.2 Schizoid personality disorder**

Excludes *schizophrenia (295.0–295.9)*

❑ **301.20 Schizoid personality disorder, unspecified**

301.21 Introverted personality

301.22 Schizotypal personality

301.3 Explosive personality disorder
Aggressive:
personality
reaction
Aggressiveness
Emotional instability (excessive)
Pathological emotionality
Quarrelsomeness

Excludes *dyssocial personality (301.7)*
hysterical neurosis (300.10–300.19)

301.4 Compulsive personality disorder
Anancastic personality
Obsessional personality

Excludes *obsessive-compulsive disorder (300.3)*
phobic state (300.20–300.29)

● **301.5 Histrionic personality disorder**

Excludes *hysterical neurosis (300.10–300.19)*

❑ **301.50 Histrionic personality disorder, unspecified**
Hysterical personality NOS

301.51 Chronic factitious illness with physical symptoms
Hospital addiction syndrome
Multiple operations syndrome
Munchausen syndrome

❑ **301.59 Other histrionic personality disorder**
Personality:
emotionally unstable
labile
psychoinfantile

301.6 Dependent personality disorder
Asthenic personality
Inadequate personality
Passive personality

Excludes *neurasthenia (300.5)*
passive-aggressive personality (301.84)

301.7 Antisocial personality disorder
Amoral personality
Asocial personality
Dyssocial personality
Personality disorder with predominantly sociopathic or asocial manifestation

Excludes *disturbance of conduct without specifiable personality disorder (312.0–312.9)*
explosive personality (301.3)

● **301.8 Other personality disorders**

301.81 Narcissistic personality

301.82 Avoidant personality

301.83 Borderline personality

301.84 Passive-aggressive personality

❑ **301.89 Other**
Personality:
eccentric
"haltlose" type
immature
masochistic
psychoneurotic

Excludes *psychoinfantile personality (301.59)*

❑ **301.9 Unspecified personality disorder**
Pathological personality NOS
Personality disorder NOS
Psychopathic:
constitutional state
personality (disorder)

● **302 Sexual deviations and disorders**

Excludes *sexual disorder manifest in:*
organic brain syndrome (290.0–294.9, 310.0–310.9)
psychosis (295.0–298.9)

302.0 Ego-dystonic homosexuality
Ego-dystonic lesbianism
Homosexual conflict disorder

Excludes *homosexual pedophilia (302.2)*

302.1 Zoophilia
Bestiality

302.2 Pedophilia

302.3 Transvestism

Excludes *trans-sexualism (302.5)*

302.4 Exhibitionism

● **302.5 Trans-sexualism**

Excludes *transvestism (302.3)*

❑ **302.50 With unspecified sexual history**

302.51 With asexual history

302.52 With homosexual history

302.53 With heterosexual history

302.6 Disorders of psychosexual identity
Feminism in boys
Gender identity disorder of childhood

Excludes *gender identity disorder in adult (302.85)*
homosexuality (302.0)
trans-sexualism (302.50–302.53)
transvestism (302.3)

● **302.7 Psychosexual dysfunction**

Excludes *impotence of organic origin (607.84)*
normal transient symptoms from ruptured hymen
transient or occasional failures of erection due to fatigue, anxiety, alcohol, or drugs

❑ **302.70 Psychosexual dysfunction, unspecified**

302.71 With inhibited sexual desire

Excludes *decreased sexual desire NOS (799.81)* ◄

302.72 With inhibited sexual excitement
Frigidity
Impotence

302.73 With inhibited female orgasm

302.74 With inhibited male orgasm

302.75 With premature ejaculation

302.76 With functional dyspareunia
Dyspareunia, psychogenic

❑ **302.79 With other specified psychosexual dysfunctions**

● **302.8 Other specified psychosexual disorders**

302.81 Fetishism

302.82 Voyeurism

302.83 Sexual masochism

302.84 Sexual sadism

302.85 Gender identity disorder of adolescent or adult life

❑ **302.89 Other**
Nymphomania
Satyriasis

❑ **302.9 Unspecified psychosexual disorder**
Pathologic sexuality NOS
Sexual deviation NOS

● **303 Alcohol dependence syndrome**

Use additional code to identify any associated condition, as:
alcoholic psychoses (291.0–291.9)
drug dependence (304.0–304.9)
physical complications of alcohol, such as:
cerebral degeneration (331.7)
cirrhosis of liver (571.2)
epilepsy (345.0–345.9)
gastritis (535.3)
hepatitis (571.1)
liver damage NOS (571.3)

Excludes *drunkenness NOS (305.0)*

The following fifth-digit subclassification is for use with category 303:
❑ **0 unspecified**
1 continuous
2 episodic
3 in remission

● **303.0 Acute alcoholic intoxication**
Acute drunkenness in alcoholism

● ❑ **303.9 Other and unspecified alcohol dependence**
Chronic alcoholism
Dipsomania

● **304 Drug dependence**

Excludes *nondependent abuse of drugs (305.1–305.9)*

The following fifth-digit subclassification is for use with category 304:
❑ **0 unspecified**
1 continuous
2 episodic
3 in remission

ICD-9-CM 300–399 Vol. 1

● 304.0 **Opioid type dependence**
Heroin
Meperidine
Methadone
Morphine
Opium
Opium alkaloids and their derivatives
Synthetics with morphine-like effects

● 304.1 **Barbiturate and similarly acting sedative or hypnotic dependence**
Barbiturates
Nonbarbiturate sedatives and tranquilizers with a similar effect:
chlordiazepoxide
diazepam
glutethimide
meprobamate
methaqualone

● 304.2 **Cocaine dependence**
Coca leaves and derivatives

● 304.3 **Cannabis dependence**
Hashish
Hemp
Marihuana

● 304.4 **Amphetamine and other psychostimulant dependence**
Methylphenidate
Phenmetrazine

● 304.5 **Hallucinogen dependence**
Dimethyltryptamine [DMT]
Lysergic acid diethylamide [LSD] and derivatives
Mescaline
Psilocybin

● ❑ 304.6 **Other specified drug dependence**
Absinthe addiction
Glue sniffing

Excludes *tobacco dependence (305.1)*

● 304.7 **Combinations of opioid type drug with any other**

● 304.8 **Combinations of drug dependence excluding opioid type drug**

● ❑ 304.9 **Unspecified drug dependence**
Drug addiction NOS
Drug dependence NOS

● 305 **Nondependent abuse of drugs**

Note: Includes cases where a person, for whom no other diagnosis is possible, has come under medical care because of the maladaptive effect of a drug on which he is not dependent and that he has taken on his own initiative to the detriment of his health or social functioning.

Excludes *alcohol dependence syndrome (303.0–303.9)*
drug dependence (304.0–304.9)
drug withdrawal syndrome (292.0)
poisoning by drugs or medicinal substances (960.0–979.9)

The following fifth-digit subclassification is for use with codes 305.0, 305.2–305.9:

❑ 0 **unspecified**
1 **continuous**
2 **episodic**
3 **in remission**

● 305.0 **Alcohol abuse**
Drunkenness NOS
Excessive drinking of alcohol NOS
"Hangover" (alcohol)
Inebriety NOS

Excludes *acute alcohol intoxication in alcoholism (303.0)*
alcoholic psychoses (291.0–291.9)

305.1 **Tobacco use disorder**
Tobacco dependence

Excludes *history of tobacco use (V15.82)*

● 305.2 **Cannabis abuse**

● 305.3 **Hallucinogen abuse**
Acute intoxication from hallucinogens ["bad trips"]
LSD reaction

● 305.4 **Barbiturate and similarly acting sedative or hypnotic abuse**

● 305.5 **Opioid abuse**

● 305.6 **Cocaine abuse**

● 305.7 **Amphetamine or related acting sympathomimetic abuse**

● 305.8 **Antidepressant type abuse**

● ❑ 305.9 **Other, mixed, or unspecified drug abuse**
"Laxative habit"
Misuse of drugs NOS
Nonprescribed use of drugs or patent medicinals

● 306 **Physiological malfunction arising from mental factors**

Includes: psychogenic:
physical symptoms not involving tissue damage
physiological manifestations not involving tissue damage

Excludes *hysteria (300.11–300.19)*
physical symptoms secondary to a psychiatric disorder classified elsewhere
psychic factors associated with physical conditions involving tissue damage classified elsewhere (316)
specific nonpsychotic mental disorders following organic brain damage (310.0–310.9)

306.0 **Musculoskeletal**
Psychogenic paralysis
Psychogenic torticollis

Excludes *Gilles de la Tourette's syndrome (307.23)*
paralysis as hysterical or conversion reaction (300.11)
tics (307.20–307.22)

306.1 **Respiratory**
Psychogenic:
air hunger
cough
hiccough
Psychogenic:
hyperventilation
yawning

Excludes *psychogenic asthma (316 and 493.9)*

306.2 **Cardiovascular**
Cardiac neurosis
Cardiovascular neurosis
Neurocirculatory asthenia
Psychogenic cardiovascular disorder

Excludes *psychogenic paroxysmal tachycardia (316 and 427.2)*

306.3 **Skin**
Psychogenic pruritus

Excludes *psychogenic:*
alopecia (316 and 704.00)
dermatitis (316 and 692.9)
eczema (316 and 691.8 or 692.9)
urticaria (316 and 708.0–708.9)

306.4 Gastrointestinal
Aerophagy
Cyclical vomiting, psychogenic
Diarrhea, psychogenic
Nervous gastritis
Psychogenic dyspepsia
Excludes *cyclical vomiting NOS (536.2)*
globus hystericus (300.11)
mucous colitis (316 and 564.9)
psychogenic:
cardiospasm (316 and 530.0)
duodenal ulcer (316 and 532.0–532.9)
gastric ulcer (316 and 531.0–531.9)
peptic ulcer NOS (316 and 533.0–533.9)
vomiting NOS (307.54)

● **306.5 Genitourinary**
Excludes *enuresis, psychogenic (307.6)*
frigidity (302.72)
impotence (302.72)
psychogenic dyspareunia (302.76)

❑ **306.50 Psychogenic genitourinary malfunction, unspecified**

306.51 Psychogenic vaginismus
Functional vaginismus

306.52 Psychogenic dysmenorrhea

306.53 Psychogenic dysuria

❑ **306.59 Other**

306.6 Endocrine

306.7 Organs of special sense
Excludes *hysterical blindness or deafness (300.11)*
psychophysical visual disturbances (368.16)

❑ **306.8 Other specified psychophysiological malfunction**
Bruxism
Teeth grinding

❑ **306.9 Unspecified psychophysiological malfunction**
Psychophysiologic disorder NOS
Psychosomatic disorder NOS

● **307 Special symptoms or syndromes, not elsewhere classified**

Note: This category is intended for use if the psychopathology is manifested by a single specific symptom or group of symptoms which are not part of an organic illness or other mental disorder classifiable elsewhere.

Excludes *those due to mental disorders classified elsewhere*
those of organic origin

307.0 Stammering and stuttering
Excludes *dysphasia (784.5)*
lisping or lalling (307.9)
retarded development of speech (315.31–315.39)

307.1 Anorexia nervosa
Excludes *eating disturbance NOS (307.50)*
feeding problem (783.3)
of nonorganic origin (307.59)
loss of appetite (783.0)
of nonorganic origin (307.59)

● **307.2 Tics**
Excludes *nail-biting or thumb-sucking (307.9)*
stereotypes occurring in isolation (307.3)
tics of organic origin (333.3)

❑ **307.20 Tic disorder, unspecified**

307.21 Transient tic disorder of childhood

307.22 Chronic motor tic disorder

307.23 Gilles de la Tourette's disorder
Motor-verbal tic disorder

307.3 Stereotyped repetitive movements
Body-rocking
Head banging
Spasmus nutans
Stereotypes NOS
Excludes *tics (307.20–307.23)*
of organic origin (333.3)

● **307.4 Specific disorders of sleep of nonorganic origin**
Excludes *narcolepsy (347)*
those of unspecified cause (780.50–780.59)

❑ **307.40 Nonorganic sleep disorder, unspecified**

307.41 Transient disorder of initiating or maintaining sleep
Hyposomnia associated with acute or intermittent emotional reactions or conflicts
Insomnia associated with acute or intermittent emotional reactions or conflicts
Sleeplessness associated with acute or intermittent emotional reactions or conflicts

307.42 Persistent disorder of initiating or maintaining sleep
Hyposomnia, insomnia, or sleeplessness associated with:
anxiety
conditioned arousal
depression (major) (minor)
psychosis

307.43 Transient disorder of initiating or maintaining wakefulness
Hypersomnia associated with acute or intermittent emotional reactions or conflicts

307.44 Persistent disorder of initiating or maintaining wakefulness
Hypersomnia associated with depression (major) (minor)

307.45 Phase-shift disruption of 24-hour sleep-wake cycle
Irregular sleep-wake rhythm, nonorganic origin
Jet lag syndrome
Rapid time-zone change
Shifting sleep-work schedule

307.46 Somnambulism or night terrors

❑ **307.47 Other dysfunctions of sleep stages or arousal from sleep**
Nightmares:
NOS
REM-sleep type
Sleep drunkenness

307.48 Repetitive intrusions of sleep
Repetitive intrusions of sleep with:
atypical polysomnographic features
environmental disturbances
repeated REM-sleep interruptions

❑ **307.49 Other**
"Short-sleeper"
Subjective insomnia complaint

● **307.5 Other and unspecified disorders of eating**
Excludes *anorexia:*
nervosa (307.1)
of unspecified cause (783.0)
overeating, of unspecified cause (783.6)
vomiting:
NOS (787.0)
cyclical (536.2)
psychogenic (306.4)

ICD-9-CM 300-399 Vol. 1

❑ 307.50 **Eating disorder, unspecified**

307.51 **Bulimia**
Overeating of nonorganic origin

307.52 **Pica**
Perverted appetite of nonorganic origin

307.53 **Psychogenic rumination**
Regurgitation, of nonorganic origin, of food with reswallowing

Excludes *obsessional rumination (300.3)*

307.54 **Psychogenic vomiting**

❑ 307.59 **Other**
Infantile feeding disturbances of nonorganic origin
Loss of appetite of nonorganic origin

307.6 **Enuresis**
Enuresis (primary) (secondary) of nonorganic origin

Excludes *enuresis of unspecified cause (788.3)*

307.7 **Encopresis**
Encopresis (continuous) (discontinuous) of nonorganic origin

Excludes *encopresis of unspecified cause (787.6)*

● 307.8 **Psychalgia**

❑ 307.80 **Psychogenic pain, site unspecified**

307.81 **Tension headache**

Excludes *headache:*
NOS (784.0)
migraine (346.0–346.9)

❑ 307.89 **Other**
Psychogenic backache

Excludes *pains not specifically attributable to a psychological cause (in):*
back (724.5)
joint (719.4)
limb (729.5)
lumbago (724.2)
rheumatic (729.0)

❑ 307.9 **Other and unspecified special symptoms or syndromes, not elsewhere classified**
Hair plucking
Lalling
Lisping
Masturbation
Nail-biting
Thumb-sucking

● 308 **Acute reaction to stress**

Includes: catastrophic stress
combat fatigue
gross stress reaction (acute)
transient disorders in response to exceptional physical or mental stress which usually subside within hours or days

Excludes *adjustment reaction or disorder (309.0–309.9)*
chronic stress reaction (309.1–309.9)

308.0 **Predominant disturbance of emotions**
Anxiety as acute reaction to exceptional [gross] stress
Emotional crisis as acute reaction to exceptional [gross] stress
Panic state as acute reaction to exceptional [gross] stress

308.1 **Predominant disturbance of consciousness**
Fugues as acute reaction to exceptional [gross] stress

308.2 **Predominant psychomotor disturbance**
Agitation states as acute reaction to exceptional [gross] stress
Stupor as acute reaction to exceptional [gross] stress

❑ 308.3 **Other acute reactions to stress**
Acute situational disturbance
Brief or acute posttraumatic stress disorder

Excludes *prolonged posttraumatic emotional disturbance (309.81)*

308.4 **Mixed disorders as reaction to stress**

❑ 308.9 **Unspecified acute reaction to stress**

● 309 **Adjustment reaction**

Includes: adjustment disorders
reaction (adjustment) to chronic stress

Excludes *acute reaction to major stress (308.0–308.9)*
neurotic disorders (300.0–300.9)

309.0 **Brief depressive reaction**
Adjustment disorder with depressed mood
Grief reaction

Excludes *affective psychoses (296.0–296.9)*
neurotic depression (300.4)
prolonged depressive reaction (309.1)
psychogenic depressive psychosis (298.0)

309.1 **Prolonged depressive reaction**

Excludes *affective psychoses (296.0–296.9)*
brief depressive reaction (309.0)
neurotic depression (300.4)
psychogenic depressive psychosis (298.0)

● 309.2 **With predominant disturbance of other emotions**

309.21 **Separation anxiety disorder**

309.22 **Emancipation disorder of adolescence and early adult life**

309.23 **Specific academic or work inhibition**

309.24 **Adjustment reaction with anxious mood**

309.28 **Adjustment reaction with mixed emotional features**
Adjustment reaction with anxiety and depression

❑ 309.29 **Other**
Culture shock

309.3 **With predominant disturbance of conduct**
Conduct disturbance as adjustment reaction
Destructiveness as adjustment reaction

Excludes *destructiveness in child (312.9)*
disturbance of conduct NOS (312.9)
dyssocial behavior without manifest psychiatric disorder (V71.01–V71.02)
personality disorder with predominantly sociopathic or asocial manifestations (301.7)

309.4 **With mixed disturbance of emotions and conduct**

● 309.8 **Other specified adjustment reactions**

309.81 **Prolonged posttraumatic stress disorder**
Chronic posttraumatic stress disorder
Concentration camp syndrome

Excludes *posttraumatic brain syndrome:*
nonpsychotic (310.2)
psychotic (293.0–293.9)

309.82 **Adjustment reaction with physical symptoms**

309.83 **Adjustment reaction with withdrawal**
Elective mutism as adjustment reaction
Hospitalism (in children) NOS

❑ 309.89 **Other**

❑ 309.9 **Unspecified adjustment reaction**
Adaptation reaction NOS
Adjustment reaction NOS

● **310 Specific nonpsychotic mental disorders due to organic brain damage**

Excludes *neuroses, personality disorders, or other nonpsychotic conditions occurring in a form similar to that seen with functional disorders but in association with a physical condition (300.0–300.9, 301.0–301.9)*

310.0 Frontal lobe syndrome
Lobotomy syndrome
Postleucotomy syndrome [state]

Excludes *postcontusion syndrome (310.2)*

310.1 Organic personality syndrome
Cognitive or personality change of other type, of nonpsychotic severity
Mild memory disturbance
Organic psychosyndrome of nonpsychotic severity
Presbyophrenia NOS
Senility with mental changes of nonpsychotic severity

Excludes *memory loss of unknown cause (780.93)* ◀

310.2 Postconcussion syndrome
Postcontusion syndrome or encephalopathy
Posttraumatic brain syndrome, nonpsychotic
Status postcommotio cerebri

Excludes *any organic psychotic conditions following head injury (293.0–294.0)*
frontal lobe syndrome (310.0)
postencephalitic syndrome (310.8)

❑ **310.8 Other specified nonpsychotic mental disorders following organic brain damage**
Postencephalitic syndrome
Other focal (partial) organic psychosyndromes

❑ **310.9 Unspecified nonpsychotic mental disorder following organic brain damage**

311 Depressive disorder, not elsewhere classified
Depressive disorder NOS
Depression NOS
Depressive state NOS

Excludes *acute reaction to major stress with depressive symptoms (308.0)*
affective personality disorder (301.10–301.13)
affective psychoses (296.0–296.9)
brief depressive reaction (309.0)
depressive states associated with stressful events (309.0–309.1)
disturbance of emotions specific to childhood and adolescence, with misery and unhappiness (313.1)
mixed adjustment reaction with depressive symptoms (309.4)
neurotic depression (300.4)
prolonged depressive adjustment reaction (309.1)
psychogenic depressive psychosis (298.0)

● **312 Disturbance of conduct, not elsewhere classified**

Excludes *adjustment reaction with disturbance of conduct (309.3)*
drug dependence (304.0–304.9)
dyssocial behavior without manifest psychiatric disorder (V71.01–V71.02)
personality disorder with predominantly sociopathic or asocial manifestations (301.7)
sexual deviations (302.0–302.9)

The following fifth-digit subclassification is for use with categories 312.0–312.2:

❑ **0 unspecified**
1 mild
2 moderate
3 severe

● **312.0 Undersocialized conduct disorder, aggressive type**
Aggressive outburst
Anger reaction
Unsocialized aggressive disorder

● **312.1 Undersocialized conduct disorder, unaggressive type**
Childhood truancy, unsocialized
Solitary stealing
Tantrums

● **312.2 Socialized conduct disorder**
Childhood truancy, socialized
Group delinquency

Excludes *gang activity without manifest psychiatric disorder (V71.01)*

● **312.3 Disorders of impulse control, not elsewhere classified**

❑ **312.30 Impulse control disorder, unspecified**
312.31 Pathological gambling
312.32 Kleptomania
312.33 Pyromania
312.34 Intermittent explosive disorder
312.35 Isolated explosive disorder
❑ **312.39 Other**

312.4 Mixed disturbance of conduct and emotions
Neurotic delinquency

Excludes *compulsive conduct disorder (312.3)*

● **312.8 Other specified disturbances of conduct, not elsewhere classified**
312.81 Conduct disorder, childhood onset type
312.82 Conduct disorder, adolescent onset type
❑ **312.89 Other conduct disorder**

❑ **312.9 Unspecified disturbance of conduct**
Delinquency (juvenile)

● **313 Disturbance of emotions specific to childhood and adolescence**

Excludes *adjustment reaction (309.0–309.9)*
emotional disorder of neurotic type (300.0–300.9)
masturbation, nail-biting, thumb-sucking, and other isolated symptoms (307.0–307.9)

313.0 Overanxious disorder
Anxiety and fearfulness of childhood and adolescence
Overanxious disorder of childhood and adolescence

Excludes *abnormal separation anxiety (309.21)*
anxiety states (300.00–300.09)
hospitalism in children (309.83)
phobic state (300.20–300.29)

313.1 Misery and unhappiness disorder

Excludes *depressive neurosis (300.4)*

● **313.2 Sensitivity, shyness, and social withdrawal disorder**

Excludes *infantile autism (299.0)*
schizoid personality (301.20–301.22)
schizophrenia (295.0–295.9)

313.21 Shyness disorder of childhood
Sensitivity reaction of childhood or adolescence

313.22 Introverted disorder of childhood
Social withdrawal of childhood or adolescence
Withdrawal reaction of childhood or adolescence

ICD-9-CM 300-399 Vol. 1

313.23 Elective mutism
Excludes *elective mutism as adjustment reaction (309.83)*

313.3 Relationship problems
Sibling jealousy
Excludes *relationship problems associated with aggression, destruction, or other forms of conduct disturbance (312.0–312.9)*

● 313.8 Other or mixed emotional disturbances of childhood or adolescence

313.81 Oppositional disorder

313.82 Identity disorder

313.83 Academic underachievement disorder

❑ 313.89 Other

❑ 313.9 Unspecified emotional disturbance of childhood or adolescense

● 314 Hyperkinetic syndrome of childhood
Excludes *hyperkinesis as symptom of underlying disorder-code the underlying disorder*

● 314.0 Attention deficit disorder
Adult
Child

314.00 Without mention of hyperactivity
Predominantly inattentive type

314.01 With hyperactivity
Combined type
Overactivity NOS
Predominantly hyperactive/impulsive type
Simple disturbance of attention with overactivity

314.1 Hyperkinesis with developmental delay
Developmental disorder of hyperkinesis

Use additional code to identify any associated neurological disorder

314.2 Hyperkinetic conduct disorder
Hyperkinetic conduct disorder without developmental delay
Excludes *hyperkinesis with significant delays in specific skills (314.1)*

❑ 314.8 Other specified manifestations of hyperkinetic syndrome

❑ 314.9 Unspecified hyperkinetic syndrome
Hyperkinetic reaction of childhood or adolescence NOS
Hyperkinetic syndrome NOS

● 315 Specific delays in development
Excludes *that due to a neurological disorder (320.0–389.9)*

● 315.0 Specific reading disorder

❑ 315.00 Reading disorder, unspecified

315.01 Alexia

315.02 Developmental dyslexia

❑ 315.09 Other
Specific spelling difficulty

315.1 Specific arithmetical disorder
Dyscalculia

❑ 315.2 Other specific learning difficulties
Excludes *specific arithmetical disorder (315.1)*
specific reading disorder (315.00–315.09)

● 315.3 Developmental speech or language disorder

315.31 Developmental language disorder
Developmental aphasia
Expressive language disorder
Word deafness
Excludes *acquired aphasia (784.3)*
elective mutism (309.83, 313.0, 313.23)

315.32 Receptive language disorder (mixed)
Receptive expressive language disorder

❑ 315.39 Other
Developmental articulation disorder
Dyslalia
Excludes *lisping and lalling (307.9)*
stammering and stuttering (307.0)

315.4 Coordination disorder
Clumsiness syndrome
Dyspraxia syndrome
Specific motor development disorder

315.5 Mixed development disorder

❑ 315.8 Other specified delays in development

❑ 315.9 Unspecified delay in development
Developmental disorder NOS

316 Psychic factors associated with diseases classified elsewhere
Psychologic factors in physical conditions classified elsewhere

Use additional code to identify the associated physical condition, as:
psychogenic:
asthma (493.9)
dermatitis (692.9)
duodenal ulcer (532.0–532.9)
eczema (691.8, 692.9)
gastric ulcer (531.0–531.9)
mucous colitis (564.9)
paroxysmal tachycardia (427.2)
ulcerative colitis (556)
urticaria (708.0–708.9)
psychosocial dwarfism (259.4)
Excludes *physical symptoms and physiological malfunctions, not involving tissue damage, of mental origin (306.0–306.9)*

MENTAL RETARDATION (317–319)

Use additional code (s) to identify any associated psychiatric or physical condition(s)

317 Mild mental retardation
High-grade defect
IQ 50–70
Mild mental subnormality

● 318 Other specified mental retardation

318.0 Moderate mental retardation
IQ 35–49
Moderate mental subnormality

318.1 Severe mental retardation
IQ 20–34
Severe mental subnormality

318.2 Profound mental retardation
IQ under 20
Profound mental subnormality

❑ 319 Unspecified mental retardation
Mental deficiency NOS
Mental subnormality NOS

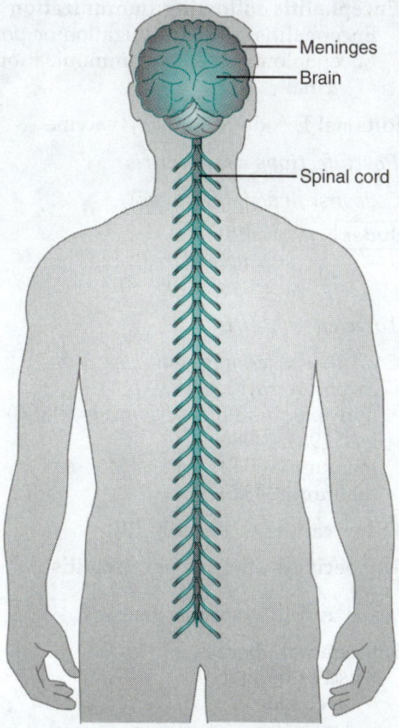

Figure 6–1 The brain and spinal cord make up the central nervous system.

Item 6–1 The two major classifications of the nervous system are the peripheral nervous system and the central nervous system (CNS). The central nervous system contains the brain and the spinal cord. Encephalitis is the swelling of the brain. Meningitis is swelling of the covering of the brain, the meninges. Types and causes of brain infections are:

Type	Cause
purulent	bacterial
aseptic/abacterial	viral
chronic meningitis	mycobacterial and fungal

6. DISEASES OF THE NERVOUS SYSTEM AND SENSE ORGANS (320–389)

INFLAMMATORY DISEASES OF THE CENTRAL NERVOUS SYSTEM (320–326)

● **320 Bacterial meningitis**

Includes: arachnoiditis bacterial
leptomeningitis bacterial
meningitis bacterial
meningoencephalitis bacterial
meningomyelitis bacterial
pachymeningitis bacterial

320.0 Haemophilus meningitis
Meningitis due to Haemophilus influenzae [H. influenzae]

320.1 Pneumococcal meningitis

320.2 Streptococcal meningitis

320.3 Staphylococcal meningitis

● ***320.7 Meningitis in other bacterial diseases classified elsewhere***
Code first underlying disease as:
actinomycosis (039.8)
listeriosis (027.0)
typhoid fever (002.0)
whooping cough (033.0–033.9)

Excludes *meningitis (in):*
epidemic (036.0)
gonococcal (098.82)
meningococcal (036.0)
salmonellosis (003.21)
syphilis:
NOS (094.2)
congenital (090.42)
meningovascular (094.2)
secondary (091.81)
tuberculosis (013.0)

● **320.8 Meningitis due to other specified bacteria**

320.81 Anaerobic meningitis
Bacteroides (fragilis)
Gram-negative anaerobes

320.82 Meningitis due to gram-negative bacteria, not elsewhere classified
Aerobacter aerogenes
Escherichia coli [E. coli]
Friedlander bacillus
Klebsiella pneumoniae
Proteus morganii
Pseudomonas

Excludes *gram-negative anaerobes (320.81)*

❑ **320.89 Meningitis due to other specified bacteria**
Bacillus pyocyaneus

❑ **320.9 Meningitis due to unspecified bacterium**
Meningitis:
bacterial NOS
purulent NOS
pyogenic NOS
suppurative NOS

● **321 Meningitis due to other organisms**

Includes: arachnoiditis due to organisms other than bacteria
leptomeningitis due to organisms other than bacteria
meningitis due to organisms other than bacteria
pachymeningitis due to organisms other than bacteria

● ***321.0 Cryptococcal meningitis***
Code first underlying disease (117.5)

●❑ ***321.1 Meningitis in other fungal diseases***
Code first underlying disease (110.0–118)

Excludes *meningitis in:*
candidiasis (112.83)
coccidioidomycosis (114.2)
histoplasmosis (115.01, 115.11, 115.91)

● ***321.2 Meningitis due to viruses not elsewhere classified***
Code first underlying disease, as:
meningitis due to arbovirus (060.0–066.9)

Excludes *meningitis (due to):*
abacterial (047.0–047.9)
adenovirus (049.1)
aseptic NOS (047.9)
Coxsackie (virus) (047.0)
ECHO virus (047.1)
enterovirus (047.0–047.9)
herpes simplex virus (054.72)
herpes zoster virus (053.0)
lymphocytic choriomeningitis virus (049.0)
mumps (072.1)
viral NOS (047.9)
meningo-eruptive syndrome (047.1)

● ***321.3 Meningitis due to trypanosomiasis***
Code first underlying disease (086.0–086.9)

● *321.4 Meningitis in sarcoidosis*

Code first underlying disease (135)

●❑ *321.8 Meningitis due to other nonbacterial organisms classified elsewhere*

Code first underlying disease

Excludes *leptospiral meningitis (100.81)*

● **322 Meningitis of unspecified cause**

Includes: arachnoiditis with no organism specified as cause
leptomeningitis with no organism specified as cause
meningitis with no organism specified as cause
pachymeningitis with no organism specified as cause

322.0 Nonpyogenic meningitis
Meningitis with clear cerebrospinal fluid

322.1 Eosinophilic meningitis

322.2 Chronic meningitis

❑ **322.9 Meningitis, unspecified**

● **323 Encephalitis, myelitis, and encephalomyelitis**

Includes: acute disseminated encephalomyelitis
meningoencephalitis, except bacterial
meningomyelitis, except bacterial
myelitis (acute):
ascending
transverse

Excludes *bacterial:*
meningoencephalitis (320.0–320.9)
meningomyelitis (320.0–320.9)

● *323.0 Encephalitis in viral diseases classified elsewhere*

Code first underlying disease, as:
cat-scratch disease (078.3)
infectious mononucleosis (075)
ornithosis (073.7)

Excludes *encephalitis (in):*
arthropod-borne viral (062.0–064)
herpes simplex (054.3)
mumps (072.2)
poliomyelitis (045.0–045.9)
rubella (056.01)
slow virus infections of central nervous system (046.0–046.9)
other viral diseases of central nervous system (049.8–049.9)
viral NOS (049.9)

● *323.1 Encephalitis in rickettsial diseases classified elsewhere*

Code first underlying disease (080–083.9)

● *323.2 Encephalitis in protozoal diseases classified elsewhere*

Code first underlying disease, as:
malaria (084.0–084.9)
trypanosomiasis (086.0–086.9)

●❑ *323.4 Other encephalitis due to infection classified elsewhere*

Code first underlying disease

Excludes *encephalitis (in):*
meningococcal (036.1)
syphilis:
NOS (094.81)
congenital (090.41)
toxoplasmosis (130.0)
tuberculosis (013.6)
meningoencephalitis due to free-living ameba [Naegleria] (136.2)

323.5 Encephalitis following immunization procedures
Encephalitis postimmunization or postvaccinal
Encephalomyelitis postimmunization or postvaccinal

Use additional E code to identify vaccine

● *323.6 Postinfectious encephalitis*

Code first underlying disease

Excludes *encephalitis:*
postchickenpox (052.0)
postmeasles (055.0)

● *323.7 Toxic encephalitis*

Code first underlying cause, as:
carbon tetrachloride (982.1)
hydroxyquinoline derivatives (961.3)
lead (984.0–984.9)
mercury (985.0)
thallium (985.8)

❑ **323.8 Other causes of encephalitis**

❑ **323.9 Unspecified cause of encephalitis**

● **324 Intracranial and intraspinal abscess**

324.0 Intracranial abscess
Abscess (embolic):
cerebellar
cerebral
Abscess (embolic) of brain [any part]:
epidural
extradural
otogenic
subdural

Excludes *tuberculous (013.3)*

324.1 Intraspinal abscess
Abscess (embolic) of spinal cord [any part]:
epidural
extradural
subdural

Excludes *tuberculous (013.5)*

❑ **324.9 Of unspecified site**
Extradural or subdural abscess NOS

325 Phlebitis and thrombophlebitis of intracranial venous sinuses

Embolism of cavernous, lateral, or other intracranial or unspecified intracranial venous sinus
Endophlebitis of cavernous, lateral, or other intracranial or unspecified intracranial venous sinus
Phlebitis, septic or suppurative of cavernous, lateral, or other intracranial or unspecified intracranial venous sinus
Thrombophlebitis of cavernous, lateral, or other intracranial or unspecified intracranial venous sinus
Thrombosis of cavernous, lateral, or other intracranial or unspecified intracranial venous sinus

Excludes *that specified as:*
complicating pregnancy, childbirth, or the puerperium (671.5)
of nonpyogenic origin (437.6)

❑ **326 Late effects of intracranial abscess or pyogenic infection**

Note: This category is to be used to indicate conditions whose primary classification is to 320–325 [excluding 320.7, 321.0–321.8, 323.0–323.4, 323.6–323.7] as the cause of late effects, themselves classifiable elsewhere. The "late effects" include conditions specified as such, or as sequelae, which may occur at any time after the resolution of the causal condition.

Use additional code to identify condition, as:
hydrocephalus (331.4)
paralysis (342.0–342.9, 344.0–344.9)

Item 6-2 Leukodystrophy is characterized by degeneration and/or failure of the myelin formation of the central nervous system and sometimes of the peripheral nervous system. The disease is inherited and progressive.

HEREDITARY AND DEGENERATIVE DISEASES OF THE CENTRAL NERVOUS SYSTEM (330–337)

Excludes *hepatolenticular degeneration (275.1)*
multiple sclerosis (340)
other demyelinating diseases of central nervous system (341.0–341.9)

● **330 Cerebral degenerations usually manifest in childhood**
Use additional code to identify associated mental retardation

330.0 Leukodystrophy
Krabbe's disease
Leukodystrophy:
NOS
globoid cell
metachromatic
sudanophilic
Pelizaeus-Merzbacher disease
Sulfatide lipidosis

330.1 Cerebral lipidoses
Amaurotic (familial) idiocy
Disease:
Batten
Jansky-Bielschowsky
Kufs'
Spielmeyer-Vogt
Tay-Sachs
Gangliosidosis

● *330.2 Cerebral degeneration in generalized lipidoses*
Code first underlying disease, as:
Fabry's disease (272.7)
Gaucher's disease (272.7)
Niemann-Pick disease (272.7)
sphingolipidosis (272.7)

●❑ *330.3 Cerebral degeneration of childhood in other diseases classified elsewhere*
Code first underlying disease, as:
Hunter's disease (277.5)
mucopolysaccharidosis (277.5)

❑ **330.8 Other specified cerebral degenerations in childhood**
Alpers' disease or gray-matter degeneration
Infantile necrotizing encephalomyelopathy
Leigh's disease
Subacute necrotizing encephalopathy or encephalomyelopathy

❑ **330.9 Unspecified cerebral degeneration in childhood**

Item 6-3 Pick's disease is the atrophy of the frontal and temporal lobes, causing dementia; Alzheimer's is characterized by a more diffuse cerebral atrophy.

● **331 Other cerebral degenerations**

331.0 Alzheimer's disease

● **331.1 Frontotemporal dementia** ⬅
Use additional code for associated behavioral disturbance (294.10–294.11) ◀

331.11 Pick's disease ◀

331.19 Other frontotemporal dementia ◀
Frontal dementia ◀

331.2 Senile degeneration of brain
Excludes *senility NOS (797)*

331.3 Communicating hydrocephalus
Excludes *congenital hydrocephalus (741.0, 742.3)*

331.4 Obstructive hydrocephalus
Acquired hydrocephalus NOS
Excludes *congenital hydrocephalus (741.0, 742.3)*

● *331.7 Cerebral degeneration in diseases classified elsewhere*
Code first underlying disease, as:
alcoholism (303.0–303.9)
beriberi (265.0)
cerebrovascular disease (430–438)
congenital hydrocephalus (741.0, 742.3)
neoplastic disease (140.0–239.9)
myxedema (244.0–244.9)
vitamin B_{12} deficiency (266.2)
Excludes *cerebral degeneration in:*
Jakob-Creutzfeldt disease (046.1)
progressive multifocal leukoencephalopathy (046.3)
subacute spongiform encephalopathy (046.1)

● **331.8 Other cerebral degeneration**

331.81 Reye's syndrome

331.82 Dementia with Lewy bodies ◀
Dementia with Parkinsonism ◀
Lewy body dementia ◀
Lewy body disease ◀
Use additional code for associated behavioral disturbance (294.10–294.11) ◀

❑ **331.89 Other**
Cerebral ataxia

❑ **331.9 Cerebral degeneration, unspecified**

● **332 Parkinson's disease**
Excludes *dementia with Parkinsonism (331.82)* ◀

332.0 Paralysis agitans
Parkinsonism or Parkinson's disease:
NOS
idiopathic
primary

332.1 Secondary Parkinsonism
Parkinsonism due to drugs
Use additional E code to identify drug, if drug-induced
Excludes *Parkinsonism (in):*
Huntington's disease (333.4)
progressive supranuclear palsy (333.0)
Shy-Drager syndrome (333.0)
syphilitic (094.82)

● **333 Other extrapyramidal disease and abnormal movement disorders**
Includes: other forms of extrapyramidal, basal ganglia, or striatopallidal disease
Excludes *abnormal movements of head NOS (781.0)*

❑ **333.0 Other degenerative diseases of the basal ganglia**
Atrophy or degeneration:
olivopontocerebellar [Déjérine-Thomas syndrome]
pigmentary pallidal [Hallervorden-Spatz disease] striatonigral
Parkinsonian syndrome associated with:
idiopathic orthostatic hypotension
symptomatic orthostatic hypotension
Progressive supranuclear ophthalmoplegia
Shy-Drager syndrome

❑ **333.1 Essential and other specified forms of tremor**
Benign essential tremor
Familial tremor
Use additional E code to identify drug, if drug-induced
Excludes *tremor NOS (781.0)*

ICD-9-CM 300-399 Vol. 1

333.2 Myoclonus
Familial essential myoclonus
Progressive myoclonic epilepsy
Unverricht-Lundborg disease

Use additional E code to identify drug, if drug-induced

333.3 Tics of organic origin

Excludes *Gilles de la Tourette's syndrome (307.23)*
habit spasm (307.22)
tic NOS (307.20)

Use additional E code to identify drug, if drug-induced

Item 6-4 Huntington's disease is characterized by ceaseless, jerky movements and progressive cognitive and behavioral deterioration.

333.4 Huntington's chorea

❑ **333.5 Other choreas**
Hemiballism(us)
Paroxysmal choreo-athetosis

Excludes *Sydenham's or rheumatic chorea (392.0–392.9)*

Use additional E code to identify drug, if drug-induced

333.6 Idiopathic torsion dystonia
Dystonia:
deformans progressiva
musculorum deformans
(Schwalbe-) Ziehen-Oppenheim disease

333.7 Symptomatic torsion dystonia
Athetoid cerebral palsy [Vogt's disease]
Double athetosis (syndrome)

Use additional E code to identify drug, if drug-induced

● **333.8 Fragments of torsion dystonia**

Use additional E code to identify drug, if drug-induced

333.81 Blepharospasm

333.82 Orofacial dyskinesia

333.83 Spasmodic torticollis

Excludes *torticollis:*
NOS (723.5)
hysterical (300.11)
psychogenic (306.0)

333.84 Organic writers' cramp

Excludes *psychogenic (300.89)*

❑ **333.89 Other**

● **333.9 Other and unspecified extrapyramidal diseases and abnormal movement disorders**

❑ **333.90 Unspecified extrapyramidal disease and abnormal movement disorder**

333.91 Stiff-man syndrome

333.92 Neuroleptic malignant syndrome
Use additional E to identify drug

333.93 Benign shuddering attacks

❑ **333.99 Other**
Restless legs

● **334 Spinocerebellar disease**

Excludes *olivopontocerebellar degeneration (333.0)*
peroneal muscular atrophy (356.1)

334.0 Friedreich's ataxia

334.1 Hereditary spastic paraplegia

334.2 Primary cerebellar degeneration
Cerebellar ataxia:
Marie's
Sanger-Brown
Dyssynergia cerebellaris myoclonica
Primary cerebellar degeneration:
NOS
hereditary
sporadic

❑ **334.3 Other cerebellar ataxia**
Cerebellar ataxia NOS

Use additional E code to identify drug, if drug-induced

● 334.4 *Cerebellar ataxia in diseases classified elsewhere*

Code first underlying disease, as:
alcoholism (303.0–303.9)
myxedema (244.0–244.9)
neoplastic disease (140.0–239.9)

❑ **334.8 Other spinocerebellar diseases**
Ataxia-telangiectasia [Louis-Bar syndrome]
Corticostriatal-spinal degeneration

❑ **334.9 Spinocerebellar disease, unspecified**

● **335 Anterior horn cell disease**

335.0 Werdnig-Hoffmann disease
Infantile spinal muscular atrophy
Progressive muscular atrophy of infancy

● **335.1 Spinal muscular atrophy**

❑ **335.10 Spinal muscular atrophy, unspecified**

335.11 Kugelberg-Welander disease
Spinal muscular atrophy:
familial
juvenile

❑ **335.19 Other**
Adult spinal muscular atrophy

● **335.2 Motor neuron disease**

335.20 Amyotrophic lateral sclerosis
Motor neuron disease (bulbar) (mixed type)

335.21 Progressive muscular atrophy
Duchenne-Aran muscular atrophy
Progressive muscular atrophy (pure)

335.22 Progressive bulbar palsy

335.23 Pseudobulbar palsy

335.24 Primary lateral sclerosis

❑ **335.29 Other**

❑ **335.8 Other anterior horn cell diseases**

❑ **335.9 Anterior horn cell disease, unspecified**

● **336 Other diseases of spinal cord**

336.0 Syringomyelia and syringobulbia

336.1 Vascular myelopathies
Acute infarction of spinal cord (embolic) (nonembolic)
Arterial thrombosis of spinal cord
Edema of spinal cord
Hematomyelia
Subacute necrotic myelopathy

● 336.2 *Subacute combined degeneration of spinal cord in diseases classified elsewhere*

Code first underlying disease, as:
pernicious anemia (281.0)
other vitamin B_{12} deficiency anemia (281.1)
vitamin B_{12} deficiency (266.2)

● *336.3 Myelopathy in other diseases classified elsewhere*

Code first underlying disease, as:
myelopathy in neoplastic disease (140.0–239.9)

Excludes *myelopathy in:*
intervertebral disc disorder (722.70–722.73)
spondylosis (721.1, 721.41–721.42, 721.91)

❑ **336.8 Other myelopathy**

Myelopathy:
drug-induced
radiation-induced

Use additional E code to identify cause

❑ **336.9 Unspecified disease of spinal cord**

Cord compression NOS
Myelopathy NOS

Excludes *myelitis (323.0–323.9)*
spinal (canal) stenosis (723.0, 724.00–724.09)

● **337 Disorders of the autonomic nervous system**

Includes: disorders of peripheral autonomic, sympathetic, parasympathetic, or vegetative system

Excludes *familial dysautonomia [Riley-Day syndrome] (742.8)*

337.0 Idiopathic peripheral autonomic neuropathy

Carotid sinus syncope or syndrome
Cervical sympathetic dystrophy or paralysis

● *337.1 Peripheral autonomic neuropathy in disorders classified elsewhere*

Code first underlying disease, as:
amyloidosis (277.3)
diabetes (250.6)

● **337.2 Reflex sympathetic dystrophy**

❑ **337.20 Reflex sympathetic dystrophy, unspecified**

337.21 Reflex sympathetic dystrophy of the upper limb

337.22 Reflex sympathetic dystrophy of the lower limb

❑ **337.29 Reflex sympathetic dystrophy of other specified site**

337.3 Autonomic dysreflexia

Use additional code to identify the cause, such as:
decubitus ulcer (707.0)
fecal impaction (560.39)
urinary tract infection (599.0)

❑ **337.9 Unspecified disorder of autonomic nervous system**

OTHER DISORDERS OF THE CENTRAL NERVOUS SYSTEM (340–349)

340 Multiple sclerosis

Disseminated or multiple sclerosis:
NOS
brain stem
cord
generalized

● **341 Other demyelinating diseases of central nervous system**

341.0 Neuromyelitis optica

341.1 Schilder's disease

Balo's concentric sclerosis
Encephalitis periaxialis:
concentrica [Balo's]
diffusa [Schilder's]

❑ **341.8 Other demyelinating diseases of central nervous system**

Central demyelination of corpus callosum
Central pontine myelinosis
Marchiafava (-Bignami) disease

❑ **341.9 Demyelinating disease of central nervous system, unspecified**

● **342 Hemiplegia and hemiparesis**

Note: This category is to be used when hemiplegia (complete) (incomplete) is reported without further specification, or is stated to be old or long-standing but of unspecified cause. The category is also for use in multiple coding to identify these types of hemiplegia resulting from any cause.

Excludes *congenital (343.1)*
hemiplegia due to late effect of cerebrovascular accident (438.20–438.22)
infantile NOS (343.4)

The following fifth digits are for use with codes 342.0–342.9

❑ **0 affecting unspecified side**
1 affecting dominant side
2 affecting nondominant side

● **342.0 Flaccid hemiplegia**

● **342.1 Spastic hemiplegia**

● ❑ **342.8 Other specified hemiplegia**

● ❑ **342.9 Hemiplegia, unspecified**

● **343 Infantile cerebral palsy**

Includes: cerebral:
palsy NOS
spastic infantile paralysis
congenital spastic paralysis (cerebral)
Little's disease
paralysis (spastic) due to birth injury:
intracranial
spinal

Excludes *hereditary cerebral paralysis, such as:*
hereditary spastic paraplegia (334.1)
Vogt's disease (333.7)
spastic paralysis specified as noncongenital or noninfantile (344.0–344.9)

343.0 Diplegic

Congenital diplegia
Congenital paraplegia

343.1 Hemiplegic

Congenital hemiplegia

Excludes *infantile hemiplegia NOS (343.4)*

343.2 Quadriplegic

Tetraplegic

343.3 Monoplegic

343.4 Infantile hemiplegia

Infantile hemiplegia (postnatal) NOS

❑ **343.8 Other specified infantile cerebral palsy**

❑ **343.9 Infantile cerebral palsy, unspecified**

Cerebral palsy NOS

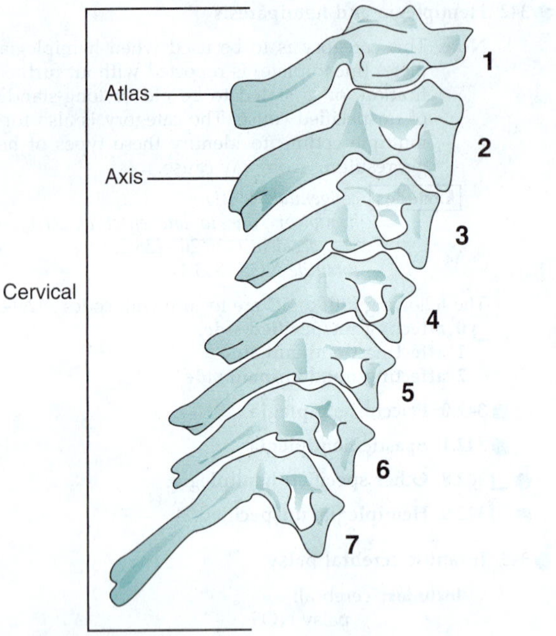

Figure 6–2 Cervical vertebrae.

Item 6–5 Quadriplegia, also called tetraplegia, is the paralysis of all four limbs. Quadriparesis is the incomplete paralysis of all four limbs. Nerve damage in C1–C4 is associated with lower limb paralysis and C5–C7 damage is associated with upper limb paralysis. Diplegia is the paralysis of the upper limbs. Monoplegia is the paralysis of the lower limbs.
Cauda equina syndrome is due to pressure on the roots of the spinal nerves and causes paresthesia (abnormal sensations).

● **344 Other paralytic syndromes**

Note: This category is to be used when the listed conditions are reported without further specification or are stated to be old or long-standing but of unspecified cause. The category is also for use in multiple coding to identify these conditions resulting from any cause.

Includes: paralysis (complete) (incomplete), except as classifiable to 342 and 343

Excludes *congenital or infantile cerebral palsy (343.0–343.9)*
hemiplegia (342.0–342.9)
congenital or infantile (343.1, 343.4)

● **344.0 Quadriplegia and quadriparesis**

❑ **344.00 Quadriplegia, unspecified**

344.01 C_1-C_4, complete

344.02 C_1-C_4, incomplete

344.03 C_5-C_7, complete

344.04 C_5-C_7, incomplete

❑ **344.09 Other**

344.1 Paraplegia
Paralysis of both lower limbs
Paraplegia (lower)

344.2 Diplegia of upper limbs
Diplegia (upper)
Paralysis of both upper limbs

● **344.3 Monoplegia of lower limb**
Paralysis of lower limb

Excludes *Monoplegia of lower limb due to late effect of cerebrovascular accident (438.40–438.42)*

❑ **344.30 Affecting unspecified side**

344.31 Affecting dominant side

344.32 Affecting nondominant side

● **344.4 Monoplegia of upper limb**
Paralysis of upper limb

Excludes *monoplegia of upper limb due to late effect of cerebrovascular accident (438.30–438.32)*

❑ **344.40 Affecting unspecified side**

344.41 Affecting dominant side

344.42 Affecting nondominant side

❑ **344.5 Unspecified monoplegia**

● **344.6 Cauda equina syndrome**

344.60 Without mention of neurogenic bladder

344.61 With neurogenic bladder
Acontractile bladder
Autonomic hyperreflexia of bladder
Cord bladder
Detrusor hyperreflexia

● **344.8 Other specified paralytic syndromes**

344.81 Locked-in state

❑ **344.89 Other specified paralytic syndrome**

❑ **344.9 Paralysis, unspecified**

● **345 Epilepsy**
The following fifth-digit subclassification is for use with categories 345.0, .1, .4-.9:
0 without mention of intractable epilepsy
1 with intractable epilepsy

Excludes *progressive myoclonic epilepsy (333.2)*

● **345.0 Generalized nonconvulsive epilepsy**
Absences:
atonic
typical
Minor epilepsy
Petit mal
Pykno-epilepsy
Seizures:
akinetic
atonic

● **345.1 Generalized convulsive epilepsy**
Epileptic seizures:
clonic
myoclonic
tonic
Epileptic seizures:
tonic-clonic
Grand mal
Major epilepsy

Excludes *convulsions:*
NOS (780.3)
infantile (780.3)
newborn (779.0)
infantile spasms (345.6)

345.2 Petit mal status
Epileptic absence status

345.3 Grand mal status
Status epilepticus NOS

Excludes *epilepsia partialis continua (345.7) status:*
psychomotor (345.7)
temporal lobe (345.7)

● **345.4 Partial epilepsy, with impairment of consciousness**
Epilepsy:
limbic system
partial:
secondarily generalized
with memory and ideational disturbances
psychomotor
psychosensory
temporal lobe
Epileptic automatism

● 345.5 **Partial epilepsy, without mention of impairment of consciousness**
Epilepsy:
Bravais-Jacksonian NOS
focal (motor) NOS
Jacksonian NOS
motor partial
partial NOS
Epilepsy:
sensory-induced
somatomotor
somatosensory
visceral
visual

● 345.6 **Infantile spasms**
Hypsarrhythmia
Lightning spasms
Salaam attacks
Excludes *salaam tic (781.0)*

● 345.7 **Epilepsia partialis continua**
Kojevnikov's epilepsy

● ❑ 345.8 **Other forms of epilepsy**
Epilepsy:
cursive [running]
Epilepsy:
gelastic

● ❑ 345.9 **Epilepsy, unspecified**
Epileptic convulsions, fits, or seizures NOS
Excludes *convulsive seizure or fit NOS (780.3)*

● 346 **Migraine**
The following fifth-digit subclassification is for use with category 346:
0 without mention of intractable migraine
1 with intractable migraine, so stated

● 346.0 **Classical migraine**
Migraine preceded or accompanied by transient focal neurological phenomena
Migraine with aura

● 346.1 **Common migraine**
Atypical migraine
Sick headache

● 346.2 **Variants of migraine**
Cluster headache
Histamine cephalgia
Horton's neuralgia
Migraine:
abdominal
basilar
Migraine:
lower half
retinal
Neuralgia:
ciliary
migrainous

● ❑ 346.8 **Other forms of migraine**
Migraine:
hemiplegic
Migraine:
ophthalmoplegic

● ❑ 346.9 **Migraine, unspecified**

347 **Cataplexy and narcolepsy**

● 348 **Other conditions of brain**

348.0 **Cerebral cysts**
Arachnoid cyst
Porencephalic cyst
Porencephaly, acquired
Pseudoporencephaly
Excludes *porencephaly (congenital) (724.4)*

348.1 **Anoxic brain damage**
Excludes *that occurring in:*
abortion (634–638 with .7, 639.8)
ectopic or molar pregnancy (639.8)
labor or delivery (668.2, 669.4)
that of newborn (767.0, 768.0–768.9, 772.1–772.2)
Use additional E code to identify cause

348.2 **Benign intracranial hypertension**
Pseudotumor cerebri
Excludes *hypertensive encephalopathy (437.2)*

● 348.3 **Encephalopathy, not elsewhere classified** ⬅ (Revised Code)

❑ 348.30 **Encephalopathy, unspecified** ◀

348.31 **Metabolic encephalopathy** ◀
Septic encephalopathy ◀

❑ 348.39 **Other encephalopathy** ◀
Excludes *alcoholic (291.2)* ◀
hepatic encephalopathy (572.2) ◀
hypertensive (437.2) ◀
toxic encephalopathy (349.82) ◀

348.4 **Compression of brain**
Compression brain (stem)
Herniation brain (stem)
Posterior fossa compression syndrome

348.5 **Cerebral edema**

❑ 348.8 **Other conditions of brain**
Cerebral:
calcification
Cerebral:
fungus

❑ 348.9 **Unspecified condition of brain**

● 349 **Other and unspecified disorders of the nervous system**

349.0 **Reaction to spinal or lumbar puncture**
Headache following lumbar puncture

349.1 **Nervous system complications from surgically implanted device**
Excludes *immediate postoperative complications (997.00–997.09)*
mechanical complications of nervous system device (996.2)

❑ 349.2 **Disorders of meninges, not elsewhere classified**
Adhesions, meningeal (cerebral) (spinal)
Cyst, spinal meninges
Meningocele, acquired
Pseudomeningocele, acquired

● 349.8 **Other specified disorders of nervous system**

349.81 **Cerebrospinal fluid rhinorrhea**
Excludes *cerebrospinal fluid otorrhea (388.61)*

349.82 **Toxic encephalopathy**
Use additional E code to identify cause

❑ 349.89 **Other**

❑ 349.9 **Unspecified disorders of nervous system**
Disorder of nervous system (central) NOS

ICD-9-CM 300-399 Vol. 1

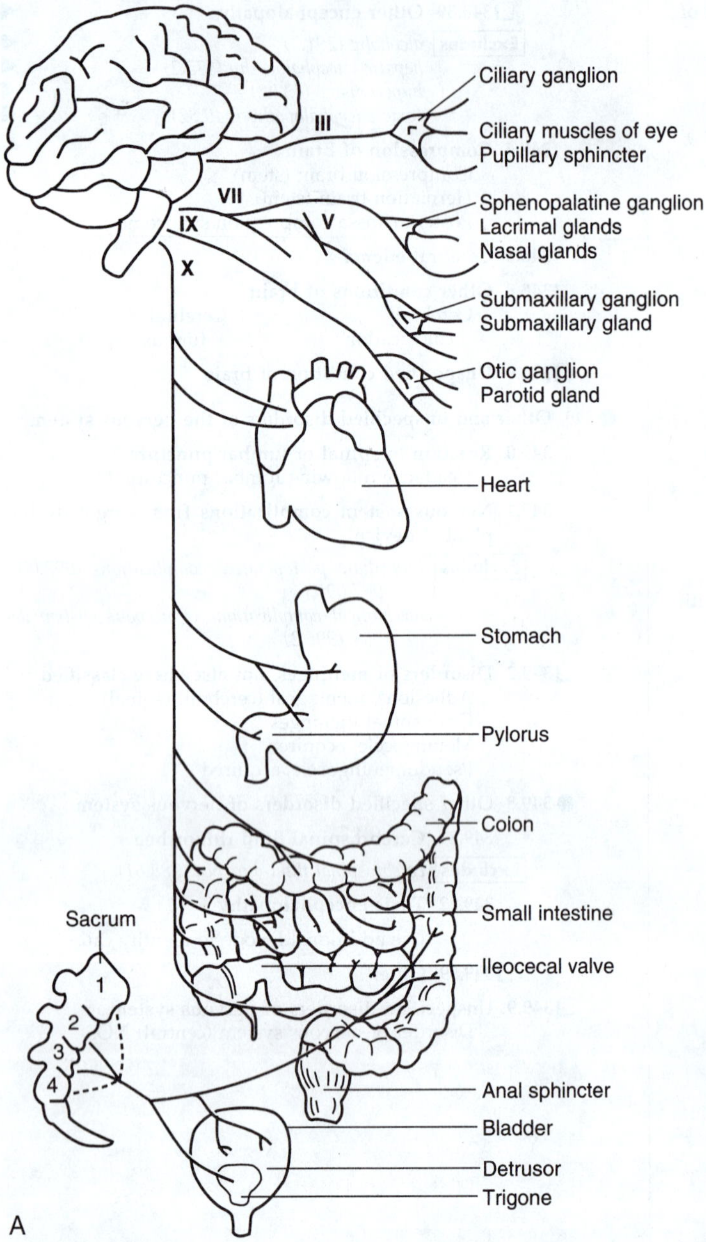

Figure 6–3 **A.** Parasympathetic nervous system.

Item 6–6 The peripheral nervous system consists of 31 pairs of spinal nerves, 12 pairs of cranial nerves, and the autonomic nerves, which are divided into the parasympathetic and sympathetic nerves. The cranial nerves are: olfactory (I), optic (II), oculomotor (III), trochlear (IV), trigeminal (V), abducens (VI), facial (VII), vestibulocochlear (VIII), glossopharyngeal (IX), vagus (X), accessory (XI), and hypoglossal (XII).

DISORDERS OF THE PERIPHERAL NERVOUS SYSTEM (350–359)

Excludes *diseases of:*
acoustic [8th] nerve (388.5)
oculomotor [3rd, 4th, 6th] nerves (378.0–378.9)
optic [2nd] nerve (377.0–377.9)
peripheral autonomic nerves (337.0–337.9)
neuralgia NOS or "rheumatic" (729.2)
neuritis NOS or "rheumatic" (729.2)
radiculitis NOS or "rheumatic" (729.2)
peripheral neuritis in pregnancy (646.4)

● **350 Trigeminal nerve disorders**
Includes: disorders of 5th cranial nerve

350.1 Trigeminal neuralgia
Tic douloureux
Trifacial neuralgia
Trigeminal neuralgia NOS
Excludes *postherpetic (053.12)*

350.2 Atypical face pain

❑ **350.8 Other specified trigeminal nerve disorders**

❑ **350.9 Trigeminal nerve disorder, unspecified**

● **351 Facial nerve disorders**
Includes: disorders of 7th cranial nerve
Excludes *that in newborn (767.5)*

351.0 Bell's palsy
Facial palsy

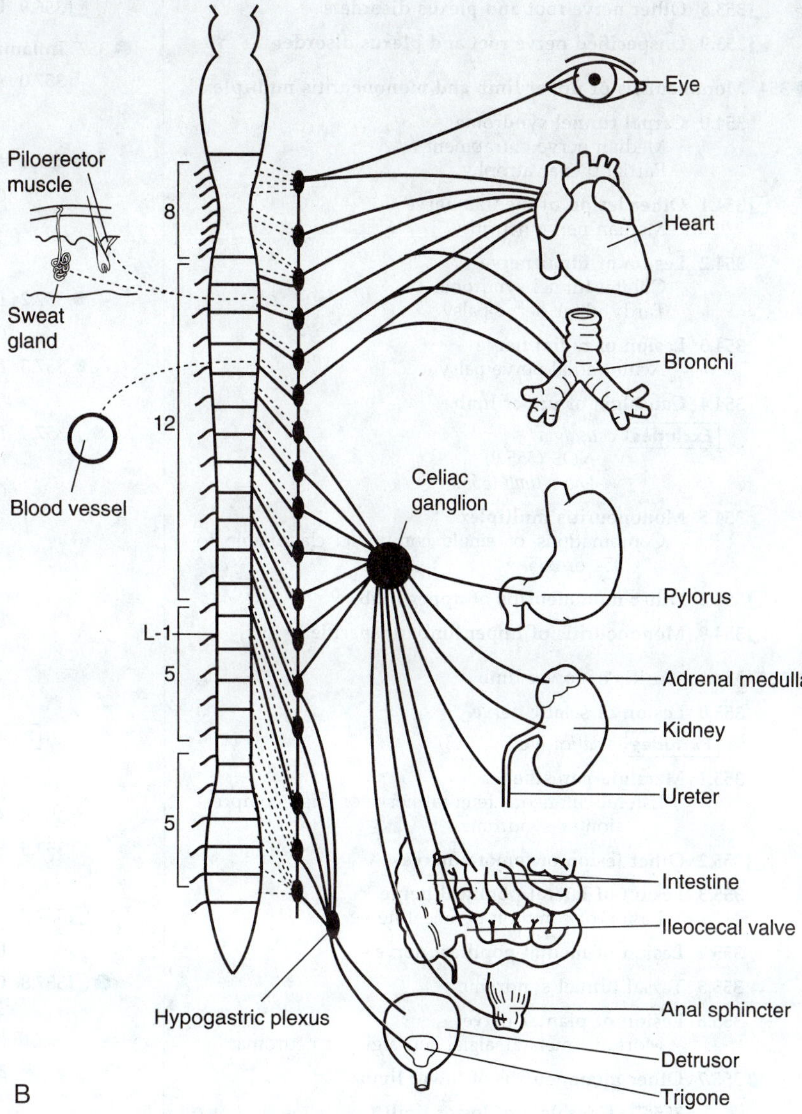

Figure 6–3 B. Sympathetic nervous system. (From Buck CJ: Step-by-Step Medical Coding, 2nd ed. Philadelphia, WB Saunders, 1998, pp 186 and 187.)

351.1 Geniculate ganglionitis
Geniculate ganglionitis NOS
Excludes *herpetic (053.11)*

❑ **351.8 Other facial nerve disorders**
Facial myokymia
Melkersson's syndrome

❑ **351.9 Facial nerve disorder, unspecified**

● **352 Disorders of other cranial nerves**

352.0 Disorders of olfactory [1st] nerve

352.1 Glossopharyngeal neuralgia

❑ **352.2 Other disorders of glossopharyngeal [9th] nerve**

352.3 Disorders of pneumogastric [10th] nerve
Disorders of vagal nerve
Excludes *paralysis of vocal cords or larynx (478.30–478.34)*

352.4 Disorders of accessory [11th] nerve

352.5 Disorders of hypoglossal [12th] nerve

352.6 Multiple cranial nerve palsies
Collet-Sicard syndrome
Polyneuritis cranialis

❑ **352.9 Unspecified disorder of cranial nerves**

● **353 Nerve root and plexus disorders**
Excludes *conditions due to:*
intervertebral disc disorders (722.0–722.9)
spondylosis (720.0–721.9)
vertebrogenic disorders (723.0–724.9)

353.0 Brachial plexus lesions
Cervical rib syndrome
Costoclavicular syndrome
Scalenus anticus syndrome
Thoracic outlet syndrome
Excludes *brachial neuritis or radiculitis NOS (723.4)*
that in newborn (767.6)

353.1 Lumbosacral plexus lesions

353.2 Cervical root lesions, not elsewhere classified

353.3 Thoracic root lesions, not elsewhere classified

353.4 Lumbosacral root lesions, not elsewhere classified

353.5 Neuralgic amyotrophy
Parsonage-Aldren-Turner syndrome

353.6 Phantom limb (syndrome)

ICD-9-CM 300-399 Vol. 1

❑353.8 **Other nerve root and plexus disorders**

❑353.9 **Unspecified nerve root and plexus disorder**

● 354 **Mononeuritis of upper limb and mononeuritis multiplex**

354.0 **Carpal tunnel syndrome**
Median nerve entrapment
Partial thenar atrophy

❑354.1 **Other lesion of median nerve**
Median nerve neuritis

354.2 **Lesion of ulnar nerve**
Cubital tunnel syndrome
Tardy ulnar nerve palsy

354.3 **Lesion of radial nerve**
Acute radial nerve palsy

354.4 **Causalgia of upper limb**

Excludes *causalgia:*
NOS (355.9)
lower limb (355.71)

354.5 **Mononeuritis multiplex**
Combinations of single conditions classifiable to 354 or 355

❑354.8 **Other mononeuritis of upper limb**

❑354.9 **Mononeuritis of upper limb, unspecified**

● 355 **Mononeuritis of lower limb**

355.0 **Lesion of sciatic nerve**

Excludes *sciatica NOS (724.3)*

355.1 **Meralgia paresthetica**
Lateral cutaneous femoral nerve of thigh compression or syndrome

❑355.2 **Other lesion of femoral nerve**

355.3 **Lesion of lateral popliteal nerve**
Lesion of common peroneal nerve

355.4 **Lesion of medial popliteal nerve**

355.5 **Tarsal tunnel syndrome**

355.6 **Lesion of plantar nerve**
Morton's metatarsalgia, neuralgia, or neuroma

● 355.7 **Other mononeuritis of lower limb**

355.71 **Causalgia of lower limb**

Excludes *causalgia:*
NOS (355.9)
upper limb (354.4)

❑355.79 **Other mononeuritis of lower limb**

❑355.8 **Mononeuritis of lower limb, unspecified**

❑355.9 **Mononeuritis of unspecified site**
Causalgia NOS

Excludes *causalgia:*
lower limb (355.71)
upper limb (354.4)

● 356 **Hereditary and idiopathic peripheral neuropathy**

356.0 **Hereditary peripheral neuropathy**
Déjérine-Sottas disease

356.1 **Peroneal muscular atrophy**
Charcot-Marie-Tooth disease
Neuropathic muscular atrophy

356.2 **Hereditary sensory neuropathy**

356.3 **Refsum's disease**
Heredopathia atactica polyneuritiformis

356.4 **Idiopathic progressive polyneuropathy**

❑356.8 **Other specified idiopathic peripheral neuropathy**
Supranuclear paralysis

❑356.9 **Unspecified**

● 357 **Inflammatory and toxic neuropathy**

357.0 **Acute infective polyneuritis**
Guillain-Barre syndrome
Postinfectious polyneuritis

● 357.1 ***Polyneuropathy in collagen vascular disease***

Code first underlying disease, as:
disseminated lupus erythematosus (710.0)
polyarteritis nodosa (446.0)
rheumatoid arthritis (714.0)

● 357.2 ***Polyneuropathy in diabetes***

Code first underlying disease (250.6)

● 357.3 ***Polyneuropathy in malignant disease***

Code first underlying disease (140.0–208.9)

●❑357.4 ***Polyneuropathy in other diseases classified elsewhere***

Code first underlying disease, as:
amyloidosis (277.3)
beriberi (265.0)
deficiency of B vitamins (266.0–266.9)
diphtheria (032.0–032.9)
hypoglycemia (251.2)
pellagra (265.2)
porphyria (277.1)
sarcoidosis (135)
uremia (585)

Excludes *polyneuropathy in:*
herpes zoster (053.13)
mumps (072.72)

357.5 **Alcoholic polyneuropathy**

357.6 **Polyneuropathy due to drugs**

Use additional E code to identify drug

❑357.7 **Polyneuropathy due to other toxic agents**

Use additional E code to identify toxic agent

●❑357.8 **Other**

357.81 **Chronic inflammatory demyelinating polyneuritis**

357.82 **Critical illness polyneuropathy**
Acute motor neuropathy

❑357.89 **Other inflammatory and toxic neuropathy**

❑357.9 **Unspecified**

● 358 **Myoneural disorders**

● 358.0 **Myasthenia gravis** ⬅

358.00 **Myasthenia gravis without (acute) exacerbation** ◀
Myasthenia gravis NOS ◀

358.01 **Myasthenia gravis with acute exacerbation** ◀
Myasthenia gravis in crisis ◀

● 358.1 ***Myasthenic syndromes in diseases classified elsewhere***
Amyotrophy from stated cause classified elsewhere
Eaton-Lambert syndrome from stated cause classified elsewhere

Code first underlying disease, as:
botulism (005.1)
diabetes mellitus (250.6)
hypothyroidism (244.0–244.9)
malignant neoplasm (140.0–208.9)
pernicious anemia (281.0)
thyrotoxicosis (242.0–242.9)

358.2 **Toxic myoneural disorders**

Use additional E code to identify toxic agent

❑ **358.8 Other specified myoneural disorders**

❑ **358.9 Myoneural disorders, unspecified**

● **359 Muscular dystrophies and other myopathies**

Excludes *idiopathic polymyositis (710.4)*

359.0 Congenital hereditary muscular dystrophy
Benign congenital myopathy
Central core disease
Centronuclear myopathy
Myotubular myopathy
Nemaline body disease

Excludes *arthrogryposis multiplex congenita (754.89)*

359.1 Hereditary progressive muscular dystrophy
Muscular dystrophy:
NOS
distal
Duchenne
Erb's
fascioscapulohumeral
Gower's
Landouzy-Déjérine
limb-girdle
ocular
oculopharyngeal

359.2 Myotonic disorders
Dystrophia myotonica
Eulenburg's disease
Myotonia congenita
Paramyotonia congenita
Steinert's disease
Thomsen's disease

359.3 Familial periodic paralysis
Hypokalemic familial periodic paralysis

359.4 Toxic myopathy
Use additional E code to identify toxic agent

● ***359.5 Myopathy in endocrine diseases classified elsewhere***
Code first underlying disease, as:
Addison's disease (255.4)
Cushing's syndrome (255.0)
hypopituitarism (253.2)
myxedema (244.0–244.9)
thyrotoxicosis (242.0–242.9)

● ***359.6 Symptomatic inflammatory myopathy in diseases classified elsewhere***
Code first underlying disease, as:
amyloidosis (277.3)
disseminated lupus erythematosus (710.0)
malignant neoplasm (140.0–208.9)
polyarteritis nodosa (446.0)
rheumatoid arthritis (714.0)
sarcoidosis (135)
scleroderma (710.1)
Sjögren's disease (710.2)

● ❑ **359.8 Other myopathies**

359.81 Critical illness myopathy
Acute necrotizing myopathy
Acute quadriplegic myopathy
Intensive care (ICU) myopathy
Myopathy of critical illness

❑ **359.89 Other myopathies**

❑ **359.9 Myopathy, unspecified**

ICD-9-CM 300-399 Vol. 1

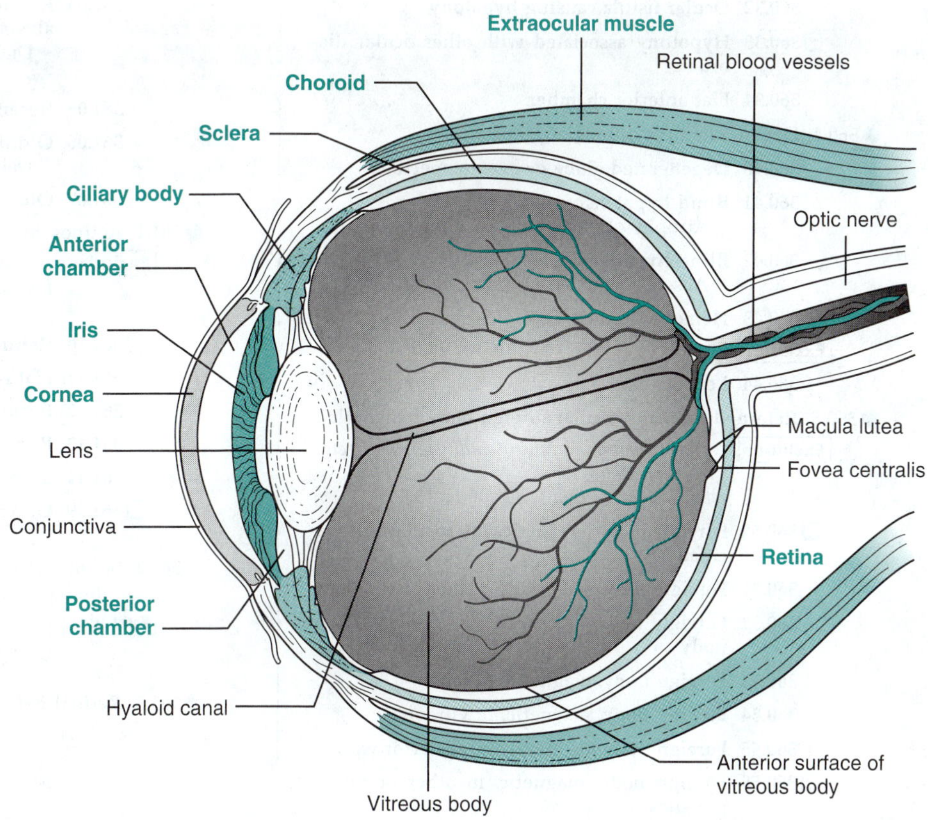

Figure 6–4 Eye and ocular adnexa. (From Buck CJ: Step-by-Step Medical Coding, 3rd ed. Philadelphia, WB Saunders, 2000, p. 205.)

DISORDERS OF THE EYE AND ADNEXA (360–379)

● **360 Disorders of the globe**
Includes: disorders affecting multiple structures of eye

● **360.0 Purulent endophthalmitis**
❑ **360.00 Purulent endophthalmitis, unspecified**
360.01 Acute endophthalmitis
360.02 Panophthalmitis
360.03 Chronic endophthalmitis
360.04 Vitreous abscess

● **360.1 Other endophthalmitis**
360.11 Sympathetic uveitis
360.12 Panuveitis
360.13 Parasitic endophthalmitis NOS
360.14 Ophthalmia nodosa
❑ **360.19 Other**
Phacoanaphylactic endophthalmitis

● **360.2 Degenerative disorders of globe**
❑ **360.20 Degenerative disorder of globe, unspecified**
360.21 Progressive high (degenerative) myopia
Malignant myopia
360.23 Siderosis
❑ **360.24 Other metallosis**
Chalcosis
❑ **360.29 Other**
Excludes *xerophthalmia (264.7)*

● **360.3 Hypotony of eye**
❑ **360.30 Hypotony, unspecified**
360.31 Primary hypotony
360.32 Ocular fistula causing hypotony
❑ **360.33 Hypotony associated with other ocular disorders**
360.34 Flat anterior chamber

● **360.4 Degenerated conditions of globe**
❑ **360.40 Degenerated globe or eye, unspecified**
360.41 Blind hypotensive eye
Atrophy of globe   Phthisis bulbi
360.42 Blind hypertensive eye
Absolute glaucoma
360.43 Hemophthalmos, except current injury
Excludes *traumatic (871.0–871.9, 921.0–921.9)*
360.44 Leucocoria

● **360.5 Retained (old) intraocular foreign body, magnetic**
Excludes *current penetrating injury with magnetic foreign body (871.5)*
retained (old) foreign body of orbit (376.6)
❑ **360.50 Foreign body, magnetic, intraocular, unspecified**
360.51 Foreign body, magnetic, in anterior chamber
360.52 Foreign body, magnetic, in iris or ciliary body
360.53 Foreign body, magnetic, in lens
360.54 Foreign body, magnetic, in vitreous
360.55 Foreign body, magnetic, in posterior wall
❑ **360.59 Foreign body, magnetic, in other or multiple sites**

● **360.6 Retained (old) intraocular foreign body, nonmagnetic**
Retained (old) foreign body:
NOS
nonmagnetic
Excludes *current penetrating injury with (nonmagnetic) foreign body (871.6)*
retained (old) foreign body in orbit (376.6)
❑ **360.60 Foreign body, intraocular, unspecified**
360.61 Foreign body in anterior chamber
360.62 Foreign body in iris or ciliary body
360.63 Foreign body in lens
360.64 Foreign body in vitreous
360.65 Foreign body in posterior wall
❑ **360.69 Foreign body in other or multiple sites**

● **360.8 Other disorders of globe**
360.81 Luxation of globe
❑ **360.89 Other**

❑ **360.9 Unspecified disorder of globe**

● **361 Retinal detachments and defects**

● **361.0 Retinal detachment with retinal defect**
Rhegmatogenous retinal detachment
Excludes *detachment of retinal pigment epithelium (362.42–362.43)*
retinal detachment (serous) (without defect) (361.2)
❑ **361.00 Retinal detachment with retinal defect, unspecified**
361.01 Recent detachment, partial, with single defect
361.02 Recent detachment, partial, with multiple defects
361.03 Recent detachment, partial, with giant tear
361.04 Recent detachment, partial, with retinal dialysis
Dialysis (juvenile) of retina (with detachment)
361.05 Recent detachment, total or subtotal
361.06 Old detachment, partial
Delimited old retinal detachment
361.07 Old detachment, total or subtotal

● **361.1 Retinoschisis and retinal cysts**
Excludes *juvenile retinoschisis (362.73)*
microcystoid degeneration of retina (362.62)
parasitic cyst of retina (360.13)
❑ **361.10 Retinoschisis, unspecified**
361.11 Flat retinoschisis
361.12 Bullous retinoschisis
361.13 Primary retinal cysts
361.14 Secondary retinal cysts
❑ **361.19 Other**
Pseudocyst of retina

361.2 Serous retinal detachment
Retinal detachment without retinal defect
Excludes *central serous retinopathy (362.41)*
retinal pigment epithelium detachment (362.42–362.43)

● **361.3 Retinal defects without detachment**
Excludes *chorioretinal scars after surgery for detachment (363.30–363.35)*
peripheral retinal degeneration without defect (362.60–362.66)

❑ 361.30 **Retinal defect, unspecified**
Retinal break(s) NOS

361.31 **Round hole of retina without detachment**

361.32 **Horseshoe tear of retina without detachment**
Operculum of retina without mention of detachment

❑ 361.33 **Multiple defects of retina without detachment**

● 361.8 **Other forms of retinal detachment**

361.81 **Traction detachment of retina**
Traction detachment with vitreoretinal organization

❑ 361.89 **Other**

❑ 361.9 **Unspecified retinal detachment**

● 362 **Other retinal disorders**

Excludes *chorioretinal scars (363.30–363.35)*
chorioretinitis (363.0–363.2)

● 362.0 ***Diabetic retinopathy***
Code first diabetes (250.5)

● 362.01 ***Background diabetic retinopathy***
Diabetic macular edema
Diabetic retinal edema
Diabetic retinal microaneurysms
Diabetic retinopathy NOS

● 362.02 ***Proliferative diabetic retinopathy***

● 362.1 **Other background retinopathy and retinal vascular changes**

❑ 362.10 **Background retinopathy, unspecified**

362.11 **Hypertensive retinopathy**

362.12 **Exudative retinopathy**
Coats'syndrome

362.13 **Changes in vascular appearance**
Vascular sheathing of retina

Use additional code for any associated atherosclerosis (440.8)

362.14 **Retinal microaneurysms NOS**

362.15 **Retinal telangiectasia**

362.16 **Retinal neovascularization NOS**
Neovascularization:
choroidal
subretinal

❑ 362.17 **Other intraretinal microvascular abnormalities**
Retinal varices

362.18 **Retinal vasculitis**
Eales' disease
Retinal:
arteritis
endarteritis
perivasculitis
phlebitis

● 362.2 **Other proliferative retinopathy**

362.21 **Retrolental fibroplasia**

❑ 362.29 **Other nondiabetic proliferative retinopathy**

● 362.3 **Retinal vascular occlusion**

❑ 362.30 **Retinal vascular occlusion, unspecified**

362.31 **Central retinal artery occlusion**

362.32 **Arterial branch occlusion**

362.33 **Partial arterial occlusion**
Hollenhorst plaque
Retinal microembolism

362.34 **Transient arterial occlusion**
Amaurosis fugax

362.35 **Central retinal vein occlusion**

362.36 **Venous tributary (branch) occlusion**

362.37 **Venous engorgement**
Occlusion:
of retinal vein
incipient of retinal vein
partial of retinal vein

● 362.4 **Separation of retinal layers**

Excludes *retinal detachment (serous) (361.2)*
rhegmatogenous (361.00–361.07)

❑ 362.40 **Retinal layer separation, unspecified**

362.41 **Central serous retinopathy**

362.42 **Serous detachment of retinal pigment epithelium**
Exudative detachment of retinal pigment epithelium

362.43 **Hemorrhagic detachment of retinal pigment epithelium**

● 362.5 **Degeneration of macula and posterior pole**

Excludes *degeneration of optic disc (377.21–377.24)*
hereditary retinal degeneration [dystrophy] (362.70–362.77)

❑ 362.50 **Macular degeneration (senile), unspecified**

362.51 **Nonexudative senile macular degeneration**
Senile macular degeneration:
atrophic
dry

362.52 **Exudative senile macular degeneration**
Kuhnt-Junius degeneration
Senile macular degeneration:
disciform
wet

362.53 **Cystoid macular degeneration**
Cystoid macular edema

362.54 **Macular cyst, hole, or pseudohole**

362.55 **Toxic maculopathy**

Use additional E code to identify drug, if drug induced

362.56 **Macular puckering**
Preretinal fibrosis

362.57 **Drusen (degenerative)**

● 362.6 **Peripheral retinal degenerations**

Excludes *hereditary retinal degeneration [dystrophy] (362.70–362.77)*
retinal degeneration with retinal defect (361.00–361.07)

❑ 362.60 **Peripheral retinal degeneration, unspecified**

362.61 **Paving stone degeneration**

362.62 **Microcystoid degeneration**
Blessig's cysts
Iwanoff's cysts

362.63 **Lattice degeneration**
Palisade degeneration of retina

362.64 **Senile reticular degeneration**

362.65 **Secondary pigmentary degeneration**
Pseudoretinitis pigmentosa

362.66 **Secondary vitreoretinal degenerations**

● 362.7 **Hereditary retinal dystrophies**

❑ 362.70 **Hereditary retinal dystrophy, unspecified**

● 362.71 ***Retinal dystrophy in systemic or cerebroretinal lipidoses***
Code first underlying disease, as:
cerebroretinal lipidoses (330.1)
systemic lipidoses (272.7)

●❑362.72 ***Retinal dystrophy in other systemic disorders and syndromes***
Code first underlying disease, as:
Bassen-Kornzweig syndrome (272.5)
Refsum's disease (356.3)

362.73 **Vitreoretinal dystrophies**
Juvenile retinoschisis

362.74 **Pigmentary retinal dystrophy**
Retinal dystrophy, albipunctate
Retinitis pigmentosa

❑362.75 **Other dystrophies primarily involving the sensory retina**
Progressive cone (-rod) dystrophy
Stargardt's disease

362.76 **Dystrophies primarily involving the retinal pigment epithelium**
Fundus flavimaculatus
Vitelliform dystrophy

362.77 **Dystrophies primarily involving Bruch's membrane**
Dystrophy:
hyaline
pseudoinflammatory foveal
Hereditary drusen

● 362.8 **Other retinal disorders**
Excludes *chorioretinal inflammations (363.0–363.2)*
chorioretinal scars (363.30–363.35)

362.81 **Retinal hemorrhage**
Hemorrhage:
preretinal
retinal (deep) (superficial)
subretinal

362.82 **Retinal exudates and deposits**

362.83 **Retinal edema**
Retinal:
cotton wool spots
edema (localized) (macular) (peripheral)

362.84 **Retinal ischemia**

362.85 **Retinal nerve fiber bundle defects**

❑362.89 **Other retinal disorders**

❑362.9 **Unspecified retinal disorder**

● 363 **Chorioretinal inflammations, scars, and other disorders of choroid**

● 363.0 **Focal chorioretinitis and focal retinochoroiditis**
Excludes *focal chorioretinitis or retinochoroiditis in:*
histoplasmosis (115.02, 115.12, 115.92)
toxoplasmosis (130.2)
congenital infection (771.2)

❑363.00 **Focal chorioretinitis, unspecified**
Focal:
choroiditis or chorioretinitis NOS
retinitis or retinochoroiditis NOS

363.01 **Focal choroiditis and chorioretinitis, juxtapapillary**

❑363.03 **Focal choroiditis and chorioretinitis of other posterior pole**

363.04 **Focal choroiditis and chorioretinitis, peripheral**

363.05 **Focal retinitis and retinochoroiditis, juxtapapillary**
Neuroretinitis

363.06 **Focal retinitis and retinochoroiditis, macular or paramacular**

❑363.07 **Focal retinitis and retinochoroiditis of other posterior pole**

363.08 **Focal retinitis and retinochoroiditis, peripheral**

● 363.1 **Disseminated chorioretinitis and disseminated retinochoroiditis**
Excludes *disseminated choroiditis or chorioretinitis in secondary syphilis (091.51)*
neurosyphilitic disseminated retinitis or retinochoroiditis (094.83)
retinal (peri)vasculitis (362.18)

❑363.10 **Disseminated chorioretinitis, unspecified**
Disseminated:
choroiditis or chorioretinitis NOS
retinitis or retinochoroiditis NOS

363.11 **Disseminated choroiditis and chorioretinitis, posterior pole**

363.12 **Disseminated choroiditis and chorioretinitis, peripheral**

363.13 **Disseminated choroiditis and chorioretinitis, generalized**
Code first any underlying disease, as:
tuberculosis (017.3)

363.14 **Disseminated retinitis and retinochoroiditis, metastatic**

363.15 **Disseminated retinitis and retinochoroiditis, pigment epitheliopathy**
Acute posterior multifocal placoid pigment epitheliopathy

● 363.2 **Other and unspecified forms of chorioretinitis and retinochoroiditis**
Excludes *panophthalmitis (360.02)*
sympathetic uveitis (360.11)
uveitis NOS (364.3)

❑363.20 **Chorioretinitis, unspecified**
Choroiditis NOS
Retinitis NOS
Uveitis, posterior NOS

363.21 **Pars planitis**
Posterior cyclitis

363.22 **Harada's disease**

● 363.3 **Chorioretinal scars**
Scar (postinflammatory) (postsurgical) (posttraumatic):
choroid
retina

❑363.30 **Chorioretinal scar, unspecified**

363.31 **Solar retinopathy**

❑363.32 **Other macular scars**

❑363.33 **Other scars of posterior pole**

363.34 **Peripheral scars**

363.35 **Disseminated scars**

● 363.4 **Choroidal degenerations**

❑363.40 **Choroidal degeneration, unspecified**
Choroidal sclerosis NOS

363.41 **Senile atrophy of choroid**

363.42 **Diffuse secondary atrophy of choroid**

363.43 **Angioid streaks of choroid**

● 363.5 **Hereditary choroidal dystrophies**
Hereditary choroidal atrophy:
partial [choriocapillaris]
total [all vessels]

❑ 363.50 **Hereditary choroidal dystrophy or atrophy, unspecified**

363.51 **Circumpapillary dystrophy of choroid, partial**

363.52 **Circumpapillary dystrophy of choroid, total**
Helicoid dystrophy of choroid

363.53 **Central dystrophy of choroid, partial**
Dystrophy, choroidal:
central areolar
circinate

363.54 **Central choroidal atrophy, total**
Dystrophy, choroidal:
central gyrate
serpiginous

363.55 **Choroideremia**

❑ 363.56 **Other diffuse or generalized dystrophy, partial**
Diffuse choroidal sclerosis

❑ 363.57 **Other diffuse or generalized dystrophy, total**
Generalized gyrate atrophy, choroid

● 363.6 **Choroidal hemorrhage and rupture**

❑ 363.61 **Choroidal hemorrhage, unspecified**

363.62 **Expulsive choroidal hemorrhage**

363.63 **Choroidal rupture**

● 363.7 **Choroidal detachment**

❑ 363.70 **Choroidal detachment, unspecified**

363.71 **Serous choroidal detachment**

363.72 **Hemorrhagic choroidal detachment**

❑ 363.8 **Other disorders of choroid**

❑ 363.9 **Unspecified disorder of choroid**

● 364 **Disorders of iris and ciliary body**

● 364.0 **Acute and subacute iridocyclitis**
Anterior uveitis, acute, subacute
Cyclitis, acute, subacute
Iridocyclitis, acute, subacute
Iritis, acute, subacute

Excludes *gonococcal (098.41)*
herpes simplex (054.44)
herpes zoster (053.22)

❑ 364.00 **Acute and subacute iridocyclitis, unspecified**

364.01 **Primary iridocyclitis**

364.02 **Recurrent iridocyclitis**

364.03 **Secondary iridocyclitis, infectious**

364.04 **Secondary iridocyclitis, noninfectious**
Aqueous:
cells
fibrin
flare

364.05 **Hypopyon**

● 364.1 **Chronic iridocyclitis**

Excludes *posterior cyclitis (363.21)*

❑ 364.10 **Chronic iridocyclitis, unspecified**

● *364.11* ***Chronic iridocyclitis in diseases classified elsewhere***
Code first underlying disease, as:
sarcoidosis (135)
tuberculosis (017.3)

Excludes *syphilitic iridocyclitis (091.52)*

● 364.2 **Certain types of iridocyclitis**

Excludes *posterior cyclitis (363.21)*
sympathetic uveitis (360.11)

364.21 **Fuchs' heterochromic cyclitis**

364.22 **Glaucomatocyclitic crises**

364.23 **Lens-induced iridocyclitis**

364.24 **Vogt-Koyanagi syndrome**

❑ 364.3 **Unspecified iridocyclitis**
Uveitis NOS

● 364.4 **Vascular disorders of iris and ciliary body**

364.41 **Hyphema**
Hemorrhage of iris or ciliary body

364.42 **Rubeosis iridis**
Neovascularization of iris or ciliary body

● 364.5 **Degenerations of iris and ciliary body**

364.51 **Essential or progressive iris atrophy**

364.52 **Iridoschisis**

364.53 **Pigmentary iris degeneration**
Acquired heterochromia of iris
Pigment dispersion syndrome of iris
Translucency of iris

364.54 **Degeneration of pupillary margin**
Atrophy of sphincter of iris
Ectropion of pigment epithelium of iris

364.55 **Miotic cysts of pupillary margin**

364.56 **Degenerative changes of chamber angle**

364.57 **Degenerative changes of ciliary body**

❑ 364.59 **Other iris atrophy**
Iris atrophy (generalized) (sector shaped)

● 364.6 **Cysts of iris, ciliary body, and anterior chamber**

Excludes *miotic pupillary cyst (364.55)*
parasitic cyst (360.13)

364.60 **Idiopathic cysts**

364.61 **Implantation cysts**
Epithelial down-growth, anterior chamber
Implantation cysts (surgical) (traumatic)

364.62 **Exudative cysts of iris or anterior chamber**

364.63 **Primary cyst of pars plana**

364.64 **Exudative cyst of pars plana**

● 364.7 **Adhesions and disruptions of iris and ciliary body**

Excludes *flat anterior chamber (360.34)*

❑ 364.70 **Adhesions of iris, unspecified**
Synechiae (iris) NOS

364.71 **Posterior synechiae**

364.72 **Anterior synechiae**

364.73 **Goniosynechiae**
Peripheral anterior synechiae

364.74 **Pupillary membranes**
Iris bombé
Pupillary:
occlusion
seclusion

364.75 **Pupillary abnormalities**
Deformed pupil
Ectopic pupil
Rupture of sphincter, pupil

364.76 **Iridodialysis**

364.77 **Recession of chamber angle**

ICD-9-CM 300-399 Vol. 1

❑ 364.8 **Other disorders of iris and ciliary body**
Prolapse of iris NOS
Excludes *prolapse of iris in recent wound (871.1)*

❑ 364.9 **Unspecified disorder of iris and ciliary body**

● 365 **Glaucoma**
Excludes *hypertensive eye [absolute glaucoma] (360.42)*
congenital glaucoma (743.20–743.22)

● 365.0 **Borderline glaucoma [glaucoma suspect]**

❑ 365.00 **Preglaucoma, unspecified**

365.01 **Open angle with borderline findings**
Open angle with:
borderline intraocular pressure
cupping of optic discs

365.02 **Anatomical narrow angle**

365.03 **Steroid responders**

❑ 365.04 **Ocular hypertension**

● 365.1 **Open-angle glaucoma**

❑ 365.10 **Open-angle glaucoma, unspecified**
Wide-angle glaucoma NOS

365.11 **Primary open angle glaucoma**
Chronic simple glaucoma

365.12 **Low tension glaucoma**

365.13 **Pigmentary glaucoma**

365.14 **Glaucoma of childhood**
Infantile or juvenile glaucoma

365.15 **Residual stage of open angle glaucoma**

● 365.2 **Primary angle-closure glaucoma**

❑ 365.20 **Primary angle-closure glaucoma, unspecified**

365.21 **Intermittent angle-closure glaucoma**
Angle-closure glaucoma:
interval
subacute

365.22 **Acute angle-closure glaucoma**

365.23 **Chronic angle-closure glaucoma**

365.24 **Residual stage of angle-closure glaucoma**

● 365.3 **Corticosteroid-induced glaucoma**

365.31 **Glaucomatous stage**

365.32 **Residual stage**

● 365.4 **Glaucoma associated with congenital anomalies, dystrophies, and systemic syndromes**

● *365.41* ***Glaucoma associated with chamber angle anomalies***
Code first associated disorder, as:
Axenfeld's anomaly (743.44)
Rieger's anomaly or syndrome (743.44)

● *365.42* ***Glaucoma associated with anomalies of iris***
Code first associated disorder, as:
aniridia (743.45)
essential iris atrophy (364.51)

●❑ *365.43* ***Glaucoma associated with other anterior segment anomalies***
Code first associated disorder, as:
microcornea (743.41)

● *365.44* ***Glaucoma associated with systemic syndromes***
Code first associated disease, as:
neurofibromatosis (237.7)
Sturge-Weber (-Dimitri) syndrome (759.6)

● 365.5 **Glaucoma associated with disorders of the lens**

365.51 **Phacolytic glaucoma**
Use additional code for associated hypermature cataract (366.18)

365.52 **Pseudoexfoliation glaucoma**
Use additional code for associated pseudoexfoliation of capsule (366.11)

❑ 365.59 **Glaucoma associated with other lens disorders**
Use additional code for associated disorder, as:
dislocation of lens (379.33–379.34)
spherophakia (743.36)

● 365.6 **Glaucoma associated with other ocular disorders**

❑ 365.60 **Glaucoma associated with unspecified ocular disorder**

365.61 **Glaucoma associated with pupillary block**
Use additional code for associated disorder, as:
seclusion of pupil [iris bombé] (364.74)

365.62 **Glaucoma associated with ocular inflammations**
Use additional code for associated disorder, as:
glaucomatocyclitic crises (364.22)
iridocyclitis (364.0–364.3)

365.63 **Glaucoma associated with vascular disorders**
Use additional code for associated disorder, as:
central retinal vein occlusion (362.35)
hyphema (364.41)

365.64 **Glaucoma associated with tumors or cysts**
Use additional code for associated disorder, as:
benign neoplasm (224.0–224.9)
epithelial down-growth (364.61)
malignant neoplasm (190.0–190.9)

365.65 **Glaucoma associated with ocular trauma**
Use additional code for associated condition, as:
contusion of globe (921.3)
recession of chamber angle (364.77)

● 365.8 **Other specified forms of glaucoma**

365.81 **Hypersecretion glaucoma**

365.82 **Glaucoma with increased episcleral venous pressure**

365.83 **Aqueous misdirection**
Malignant glaucoma

❑ 365.89 **Other specified glaucoma**

❑ 365.9 **Unspecified glaucoma**

● 366 **Cataract**
Excludes *congenital cataract (743.30–743.34)*

● 366.0 **Infantile, juvenile, and presenile cataract**

❑ 366.00 **Nonsenile cataract, unspecified**

366.01 **Anterior subcapsular polar cataract**

366.02 **Posterior subcapsular polar cataract**

366.03 **Cortical, lamellar, or zonular cataract**

366.04 **Nuclear cataract**

❑ 366.09 **Other and combined forms of nonsenile cataract**

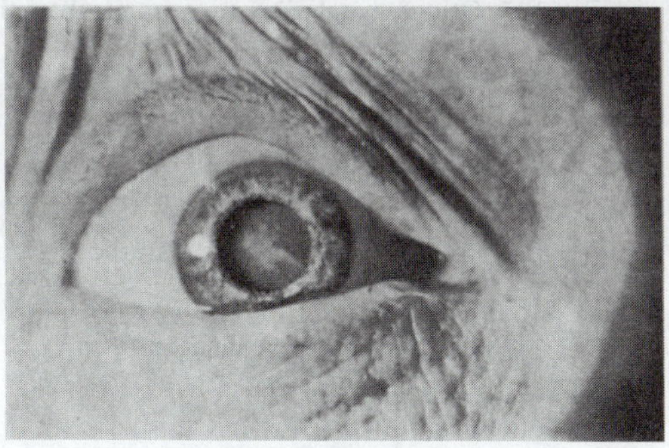

Figure 6–5 Mature cataract with gray fissures. (From Pau H: Differential Diagnosis of Eye Diseases. Philadelphia, WB Saunders, 1978, p 240.)

Item 6–7 Senile cataracts are linked to the aging process. The most common area for the formation of a cataract is the cortical area of the lens. Polar cataracts can be either anterior or posterior. Anterior polar cataracts are more common and are small, white, capsular cataracts located on the anterior portion of the lens.
Total cataracts, also called complete or mature, cause an opacity of all fibers of the lens.
Hypermature describes a mature cataract with a swollen, milky cortex that covers the entire lens.
Immature, also called incipient, cataracts have a clear cortex and are only slightly opaque.

● 366.1 Senile cataract

❑ 366.10 Senile cataract, unspecified

366.11 Pseudoexfoliation of lens capsule

366.12 Incipient cataract
Cataract:
coronary
immature NOS
punctate
Water clefts

366.13 Anterior subcapsular polar senile cataract

366.14 Posterior subcapsular polar senile cataract

366.15 Cortical senile cataract

366.16 Nuclear sclerosis
Cataracta brunescens
Nuclear cataract

366.17 Total or mature cataract

366.18 Hypermature cataract
Morgagni cataract

❑ 366.19 Other and combined forms of senile cataract

● 366.2 Traumatic cataract

❑ 366.20 Traumatic cataract, unspecified

366.21 Localized traumatic opacities
Vossius' ring

366.22 Total traumatic cataract

366.23 Partially resolved traumatic cataract

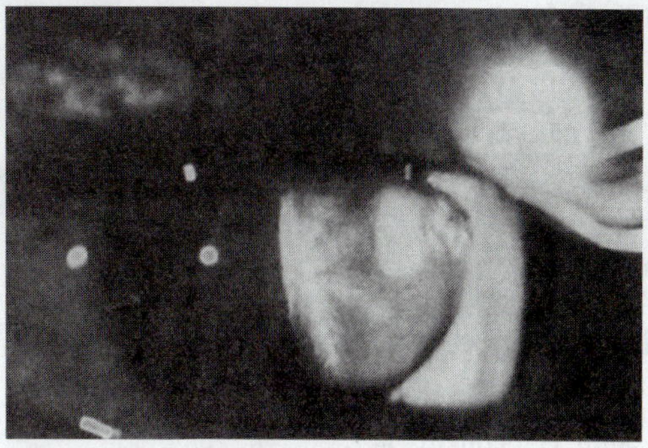

Figure 6–6 Perforation rosette of the lens; feathery opacities along suture lines beneath the posterior capsule. (From Pau H: Differential Diagnosis of Eye Diseases. Philadelphia, WB Saunders, 1978, p 250.)

Item 6–8 Vossius' ring is the result of contusion-type traumatic injury and results in a ring of iris pigment pressed onto the anterior lens capsule.

● 366.3 Cataract secondary to ocular disorders

❑ 366.30 Cataracta complicata, unspecified

366.31 Glaucomatous flecks (subcapsular)

Code first underlying glaucoma (365.0–365.9)

366.32 Cataract in inflammatory disorders

Code first underlying condition, as:
chronic choroiditis (363.0–363.2)

366.33 Cataract with neovascularization

Code first underlying condition, as:
chronic iridocyclitis (364.10)

366.34 Cataract in degenerative disorders
Sunflower cataract

Code first underlying condition, as:
chalcosis (360.24)
degenerative myopia (360.21)
pigmentary retinal dystrophy (362.74)

● 366.4 Cataract associated with other disorders

● *366.41 Diabetic cataract*

Code first diabetes (250.5)

● *366.42 Tetanic cataract*

Code first underlying disease, as:
calcinosis (275.4)
hypoparathyroidism (252.1)

● *366.43 Myotonic cataract*

Code first underlying disorder (359.2)

●❑ *366.44 Cataract associated with other syndromes*

Code first underlying condition, as:
craniofacial dysostosis (756.0)
galactosemia (271.1)

366.45 Toxic cataract
Drug-induced cataract

Use additional E code to identify drug or other toxic substance

❑ 366.46 Cataract associated with radiation and other physical influences

Use additional E code to identify cause

ICD-9-CM 300-399 Vol. 1

366.5 After-cataract

366.50 After-cataract, unspecified
Secondary cataract NOS

366.51 Soemmering's ring

366.52 Other after-cataract, not obscuring vision

366.53 After-cataract, obscuring vision

366.8 Other cataract
Calcification of lens

366.9 Unspecified cataract

367 Disorders of refraction and accommodation

367.0 Hypermetropia
Far-sightedness
Hyperopia

367.1 Myopia
Near-sightedness

367.2 Astigmatism

367.20 Astigmatism, unspecified

367.21 Regular astigmatism

367.22 Irregular astigmatism

367.3 Anisometropia and aniseikonia

367.31 Anisometropia

367.32 Aniseikonia

367.4 Presbyopia

367.5 Disorders of accommodation

367.51 Paresis of accommodation
Cycloplegia

367.52 Total or complete internal ophthalmoplegia

367.53 Spasm of accommodation

367.8 Other disorders of refraction and accommodation

367.81 Transient refractive change

367.89 Other
Drug-induced disorders of refraction and accommodation
Toxic disorders of refraction and accommodation

367.9 Unspecified disorder of refraction and accommodation

368 Visual disturbances

Excludes *electrophysiological disturbances (794.11–794.14)*

368.0 Amblyopia ex anopsia

368.00 Amblyopia, unspecified

368.01 Strabismic amblyopia
Suppression amblyopia

368.02 Deprivation amblyopia

368.03 Refractive amblyopia

368.1 Subjective visual disturbances

368.10 Subjective visual disturbance, unspecified

368.11 Sudden visual loss

368.12 Transient visual loss
Concentric fading
Scintillating scotoma

368.13 Visual discomfort
Asthenopia
Eye strain
Photophobia

368.14 Visual distortions of shape and size
Macropsia
Metamorphopsia
Micropsia

368.15 Other visual distortions and entoptic phenomena
Photopsia
Refractive:
diplopia
polyopia
Visual halos

368.16 Psychophysical visual disturbances
Visual:
agnosia
disorientation syndrome
hallucinations

368.2 Diplopia
Double vision

368.3 Other disorders of binocular vision

368.30 Binocular vision disorder, unspecified

368.31 Suppression of binocular vision

368.32 Simultaneous visual perception without fusion

368.33 Fusion with defective stereopsis

368.34 Abnormal retinal correspondence

368.4 Visual field defects

368.40 Visual field defect, unspecified

368.41 Scotoma involving central area
Scotoma:
central
centrocecal
paracentral

368.42 Scotoma of blind spot area
Enlarged:
angioscotoma
blind spot
Paracecal scotoma

368.43 Sector or arcuate defects
Scotoma:
arcuate
Bjerrum
Seidel

368.44 Other localized visual field defect
Scotoma:
NOS
ring
Visual field defect:
nasal step
peripheral

368.45 Generalized contraction or constriction

368.46 Homonymous bilateral field defects
Hemianopsia (altitudinal) (homonymous)
Quadrant anopia

368.47 Heteronymous bilateral field defects
Hemianopsia:
binasal
bitemporal

368.5 Color vision deficiencies
Color blindness

368.51 Protan defect
Protanomaly
Protanopia

368.52 Deutan defect
Deuteranomaly
Deuteranopia

368.53 Tritan defect
Tritanomaly
Tritanopia

368.54 **Achromatopsia**
Monochromatism (cone) (rod)

368.55 **Acquired color vision deficiencies**

❑368.59 **Other color vision deficiencies**

● 368.6 **Night blindness**
Nyctalopia

❑368.60 **Night blindness, unspecified**

368.61 **Congenital night blindness**
Hereditary night blindness
Oguchi's disease

368.62 **Acquired night blindness**

Excludes *that due to vitamin A deficiency (264.5)*

368.63 **Abnormal dark adaptation curve**
Abnormal threshold of cones or rods
Delayed adaptation of cones or rods

❑368.69 **Other night blindness**

❑368.8 **Other specified visual disturbances**
Blurred vision NOS

❑368.9 **Unspecified visual disturbance**

Classification		**Levels of Visual Impairment**	**Additional Descriptors Which May Be Encountered**
"Legal"	**WHO**	***Visual Acuity and/or Visual Field Limitation (Whichever Is Worse)***	
	(Near-) normal vision	Range of Normal Vision 20/10 20/13 20/16 20/20 20/25 2.0 1.6 1.25 1.0 0.8	
		Near-Normal Vision 20/30 20/40 20/50 20/60 0.7 0.6 0.5 0.4 0.3	
	Low vision	Moderate Visual Impairment 20/70 20/80 20/100 20/125 20/160 0.25 0.20 0.16 0.12	Moderate low vision
Legal Blindness (U.S.A.) both eyes		Severe Visual Impairment 20/200 20/250 20/320 20/400 0.10 0.08 0.06 0.05 Visual field: 20 degrees or less	Severe low vision, "Legal" blindness
	Blindness (WHO) one or both eyes	Profound Visual Impairment 20/500 20/630 20/800 20/1000 0.04 0.03 0.025 0.02 Count fingers at: less than 3 m (10 ft) Visual field: 10 degrees or less	Profound low vision, Moderate blindness
		Near-Total Visual Impairment Visual acuity: less than 0.02 (20/1000) Count fingers: 1 m (3 ft) or less Hand movements: 5 m (15 ft) or less Light projection, light perception Visual field: 5 degrees or less	Severe blindness, Near-total blindness
		Total Visual Impairment No light perception (NLP)	Total blindness

Visual acuity refers to best achievable acuity with correction.
Non-listed Snellen fractions may be classified by converting to the nearest decimal equivalent, e.g., 10/200 = 0.05, 6/30 = 0.20.
CF (count fingers) without designation of distance, may be classified to profound impairment.
HM (hand motion) without designation of distance, may be classified to near-total impairment.
Visual field measurements refer to the largest field diameter for a 1/100 white test object.

● 369 **Blindness and low vision**

Excludes *correctable impaired vision due to refractive errors (367.0–367.9)*

Note: Visual impairment refers to a functional limitation of the eye (e.g., limited visual acuity or visual field). It should be distinguished from visual disability, indicating a limitation of the abilities of the individual (e.g., limited reading skills, vocational skills), and from visual handicap, indicating a limitation of personal and socioeconomic independence (e.g., limited mobility, limited employability).

The levels of impairment defined in the table after 369.9 are based on the recommendations of the WHO Study Group on Prevention of Blindness (Geneva, November 6–10, 1972; WHO Technical Report Series 518), and of the International Council of Ophthalmology (1976).

Note that definitions of blindness vary in different settings.

For international reporting, WHO defines blindness as profound impairment. This definition can be applied to blindness of one eye (369.1, 369.6) and to blindness of the individual (369.0).

For determination of benefits in the U.S.A., the definition of legal blindness as severe impairment is often used. This definition applies to blindness of the individual only.

● 369.0 **Profound impairment, both eyes**

❑369.00 **Impairment level not further specified**
Blindness:
NOS according to WHO definition
both eyes

❑369.01 **Better eye: total impairment; lesser eye: total impairment**

❑369.02 **Better eye: near-total impairment; lesser eye: not further specified**

❑369.03 **Better eye: near-total impairment; lesser eye: total impairment**

❑369.04 **Better eye: near-total impairment; lesser eye: near-total impairment**

❑369.05 **Better eye: profound impairment; lesser eye: not further specified**

❑369.06 **Better eye: profound impairment; lesser eye: total impairment**

❑369.07 **Better eye: profound impairment; lesser eye: near-total impairment**

❑369.08 **Better eye: profound impairment; lesser eye: profound impairment**

● 369.1 **Moderate or severe impairment, better eye, profound impairment, lesser eye**

❑369.10 **Impairment level not further specified**
Blindness, one eye, low vision, other eye

❑369.11 **Better eye: severe impairment; lesser eye: blind, not further specified**

369.12 **Better eye: severe impairment; lesser eye: total impairment**

369.13 **Better eye: severe impairment; lesser eye: near-total impairment**

369.14 **Better eye: severe impairment; lesser eye: profound impairment**

❑369.15 **Better eye: moderate impairment; lesser eye: blind, not further specified**

369.16 **Better eye: moderate impairment; lesser eye: total impairment**

369.17 **Better eye: moderate impairment; lesser eye: near-total impairment**

369.18 **Better eye: moderate impairment; lesser eye: profound impairment**

● 369.2 Moderate or severe impairment, both eyes

❑ 369.20 Impairment level not further specified
Low vision, both eyes NOS

❑ 369.21 Better eye: severe impairment; lesser eye: not further specified

369.22 Better eye: severe impairment; lesser eye: severe impairment

❑ 369.23 Better eye: moderate impairment; lesser eye: not further specified

369.24 Better eye: moderate impairment; lesser eye: severe impairment

369.25 Better eye: moderate impairment; lesser eye: moderate impairment

369.3 Unqualified visual loss, both eyes

Excludes *blindness NOS:*
legal [U.S.A. definition] (369.4)
WHO definition (369.00)

369.4 Legal blindness, as defined in U.S.A.
Blindness NOS according to U.S.A. definition

Excludes *legal blindness with specification of impairment level (369.01–369.08, 369.11–369.14, 369.21–369.22)*

● 369.6 Profound impairment, one eye

❑ 369.60 Impairment level not further specified
Blindness, one eye

❑ 369.61 One eye: total impairment; other eye: not specified

369.62 One eye: total impairment; other eye: near-normal vision

369.63 One eye: total impairment; other eye: normal vision

❑ 369.64 One eye: near-total impairment; other eye: not specified

369.65 One eye: near-total impairment; other eye: near-normal vision

369.66 One eye: near-total impairment; other eye: normal vision

❑ 369.67 One eye: profound impairment; other eye: not specified

369.68 One eye: profound impairment; other eye: near-normal vision

369.69 One eye: profound impairment; other eye: normal vision

● 369.7 Moderate or severe impairment, one eye

❑ 369.70 Impairment level not further specified
Low vision, one eye

❑ 369.71 One eye: severe impairment; other eye: not specified

369.72 One eye: severe impairment; other eye: near-normal vision

369.73 One eye: severe impairment; other eye: normal vision

❑ 369.74 One eye: moderate impairment; other eye: not specified

369.75 One eye: moderate impairment; other eye: near-normal vision

369.76 One eye: moderate impairment; other eye: normal vision

369.8 Unqualified visual loss, one eye

❑ 369.9 Unspecified visual loss

● 370.0 Corneal ulcer

Excludes *that due to vitamin A deficiency (264.3)*

❑ 370.00 Corneal ulcer, unspecified

370.01 Marginal corneal ulcer

370.02 Ring corneal ulcer

370.03 Central corneal ulcer

370.04 Hypopyon ulcer
Serpiginous ulcer

370.05 Mycotic corneal ulcer

370.06 Perforated corneal ulcer

370.07 Mooren's ulcer

● 370.2 Superficial keratitis without conjunctivitis

Excludes *dendritic [herpes simplex] keratitis (054.42)*

❑ 370.20 Superficial keratitis, unspecified

370.21 Punctate keratitis
Thygeson's superficial punctate keratitis

Item 6-9 An infected ulcer is usually called a **serpiginous** or **hypopyon** ulcer which is a pus sac in the anterior chamber of the eye.
Marginal ulcers are usually asymptomatic, not primary, and are often superficial and simple. More severe marginal ulcers spread to form a ring ulcer. **Ring** ulcers can extend around the entire corneal periphery.
Central corneal ulcers develop when there is an abrasion to the epithelium and an infection develops in the eroded area.
The **pyocyaneal** ulcer is the most serious corneal infection, which, if left untreated, can lead to loss of the eye.

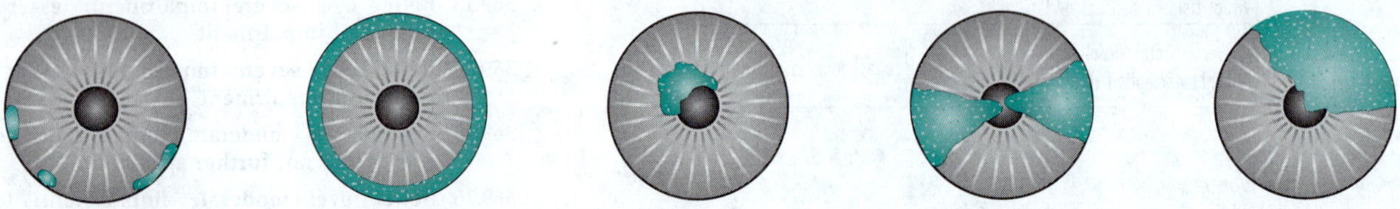

Figure 6-7 Corneal ulcers: marginal, ring, central corneal, rosacea, and Mooren's.

370.22 **Macular keratitis**
Keratitis:
areolar
nummular
stellate
striate

370.23 **Filamentary keratitis**

370.24 **Photokeratitis**
Snow blindness
Welders' keratitis

● 370.3 **Certain types of keratoconjunctivitis**

370.31 **Phlyctenular keratoconjunctivitis**
Phlyctenulosis
Use additional code for any associated tuberculosis (017.3)

370.32 **Limbal and corneal involvement in vernal conjunctivitis**
Use additional code for vernal conjunctivitis (372.13)

❑ 370.33 **Keratoconjunctivitis sicca, not specified as Sjögren's**
Excludes *Sjögren's syndrome (710.2)*

370.34 **Exposure keratoconjunctivitis**

370.35 **Neurotrophic keratoconjunctivitis**

● 370.4 **Other and unspecified keratoconjunctivitis**

❑ 370.40 **Keratoconjunctivitis, unspecified**
Superficial keratitis with conjunctivitis NOS

● *370.44 Keratitis or keratoconjunctivitis in exanthema*
Code first underlying condition (050.0–052.9)
Excludes *herpes simplex (054.43)*
herpes zoster (053.21)
measles (055.71)

❑ 370.49 **Other**
Excludes *epidemic keratoconjunctivitis (077.1)*

● 370.5 **Interstitial and deep keratitis**

❑ 370.50 **Interstitial keratitis, unspecified**

370.52 **Diffuse interstitial keratitis**
Cogan's syndrome

370.54 **Sclerosing keratitis**

370.55 **Corneal abscess**

❑ 370.59 **Other**
Excludes *disciform herpes simplex keratitis (054.43)*
syphilitic keratitis (090.3)

● 370.6 **Corneal neovascularization**

❑ 370.60 **Corneal neovascularization, unspecified**

370.61 **Localized vascularization of cornea**

370.62 **Pannus (corneal)**

370.63 **Deep vascularization of cornea**

370.64 **Ghost vessels (corneal)**

❑ 370.8 **Other forms of keratitis**

❑ 370.9 **Unspecified keratitis**

● 371 **Corneal opacity and other disorders of cornea**

● 371.0 **Corneal scars and opacities**
Excludes *that due to vitamin A deficiency (264.6)*

❑ 371.00 **Corneal opacity, unspecified**
Corneal scar NOS

371.01 **Minor opacity of cornea**
Corneal nebula

371.02 **Peripheral opacity of cornea**
Corneal macula not interfering with central vision

371.03 **Central opacity of cornea**
Corneal:
leucoma interfering with central vision
macula interfering with central vision

371.04 **Adherent leucoma**

● *371.05 Phthisical cornea*
Code first underlying tuberculosis (017.3)

● 371.1 **Corneal pigmentations and deposits**

❑ 371.10 **Corneal deposit, unspecified**

371.11 **Anterior pigmentations**
Stähli's lines

371.12 **Stromal pigmentations**
Hematocornea

371.13 **Posterior pigmentations**
Krukenberg spindle

371.14 **Kayser-Fleischer ring**

❑ 371.15 **Other deposits associated with metabolic disorders**

371.16 **Argentous deposits**

● 371.2 **Corneal edema**

❑ 371.20 **Corneal edema, unspecified**

371.21 **Idiopathic corneal edema**

371.22 **Secondary corneal edema**

371.23 **Bullous keratopathy**

371.24 **Corneal edema due to wearing of contact lenses**

● 371.3 **Changes of corneal membranes**

❑ 371.30 **Corneal membrane change, unspecified**

371.31 **Folds and rupture of Bowman's membrane**

371.32 **Folds in Descemet's membrane**

371.33 **Rupture in Descemet's membrane**

● 371.4 **Corneal degenerations**

❑ 371.40 **Corneal degeneration, unspecified**

371.41 **Senile corneal changes**
Arcus senilis   Hassall-Henle bodies

371.42 **Recurrent erosion of cornea**
Excludes *Mooren's ulcer (370.07)*

371.43 **Band-shaped keratopathy**

❑ 371.44 **Other calcerous degenerations of cornea**

371.45 **Keratomalacia NOS**
Excludes *that due to vitamin A deficiency (264.4)*

371.46 **Nodular degeneration of cornea**
Salzmann's nodular dystrophy

371.48 **Peripheral degenerations of cornea**
Marginal degeneration of cornea [Terrien's]

❑ 371.49 **Other**
Discrete colliquative keratopathy

● 371.5 **Hereditary corneal dystrophies**

❑ 371.50 **Corneal dystrophy, unspecified**

371.51 **Juvenile epithelial corneal dystrophy**

❑ 371.52 **Other anterior corneal dystrophies**
Corneal dystrophy:
microscopic cystic
ring-like

371.53 **Granular corneal dystrophy**

371.54 **Lattice corneal dystrophy**

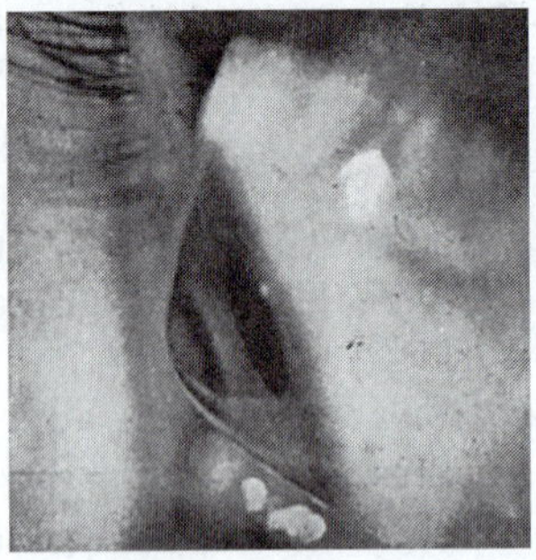

Figure 6–8 Keratoconus. (From Adler FH: Textbook of Ophthalmology, 7th ed. Philadelphia, WB Saunders, 1962, p 223.)

Item 6–10 Keratoconus is corneal degeneration that begins in childhood and gradually forms a cone at the apex of the eye even though the intraocular pressure is normal. The apex of the cornea becomes increasingly thin and can rupture, resulting in scarring.

371.55 **Macular corneal dystrophy**

❑ 371.56 **Other stromal corneal dystrophies**
Crystalline corneal dystrophy

371.57 **Endothelial corneal dystrophy**
Combined corneal dystrophy
Cornea guttata
Fuchs' endothelial dystrophy

❑ 371.58 **Other posterior corneal dystrophies**
Polymorphous corneal dystrophy

● 371.6 **Keratoconus**

❑ 371.60 **Keratoconus, unspecified**

371.61 **Keratoconus, stable condition**

371.62 **Keratoconus, acute hydrops**

● 371.7 **Other corneal deformities**

❑ 371.70 **Corneal deformity, unspecified**

371.71 **Corneal ectasia**

371.72 **Descemetocele**

371.73 **Corneal staphyloma**

● ❑ 371.8 **Other corneal disorders**

371.81 **Corneal anesthesia and hypoesthesia**

371.82 **Corneal disorder due to contact lens**

Excludes *corneal edema due to contact lens (371.24)*

❑ 371.89 **Other**

❑ 371.9 **Unspecified corneal disorder**

● 372 **Disorders of conjunctiva**

Excludes *keratoconjunctivitis (370.3–370.4)*

● 372.0 **Acute conjunctivitis**

❑ 372.00 **Acute conjunctivitis, unspecified**

372.01 **Serous conjunctivitis, except viral**

Excludes *viral conjunctivitis NOS (077.9)*

372.02 **Acute follicular conjunctivitis**
Conjunctival folliculosis NOS

Excludes *conjunctivitis:*
adenoviral (acute follicular) (077.3)
epidemic hemorrhagic (077.4)
inclusion (077.0)
Newcastle (077.8)
epidemic keratoconjunctivitis (077.1)
pharyngoconjunctival fever (077.2)

❑ 372.03 **Other mucopurulent conjunctivitis**
Catarrhal conjunctivitis

Excludes *blennorrhea neonatorum (gonococcal) (098.40)*
neonatal conjunctivitis (771.6)
ophthalmia neonatorum NOS (771.6)

372.04 **Pseudomembranous conjunctivitis**
Membranous conjunctivitis

Excludes *diphtheritic conjunctivitis (032.81)*

372.05 **Acute atopic conjunctivitis**

● 372.1 **Chronic conjunctivitis**

❑ 372.10 **Chronic conjunctivitis, unspecified**

372.11 **Simple chronic conjunctivitis**

372.12 **Chronic follicular conjunctivitis**

372.13 **Vernal conjunctivitis**

❑ 372.14 **Other chronic allergic conjunctivitis**

● *372.15* ***Parasitic conjunctivitis***

Code first underlying disease, as:
filariasis (125.0–125.9)
mucocutaneous leishmaniasis (085.5)

● 372.2 **Blepharoconjunctivitis**

❑ 372.20 **Blepharoconjunctivitis, unspecified**

372.21 **Angular blepharoconjunctivitis**

372.22 **Contact blepharoconjunctivitis**

● 372.3 **Other and unspecified conjunctivitis**

❑ 372.30 **Conjunctivitis, unspecified**

● *372.31* ***Rosacea conjunctivitis***

Code first underlying rosacea dermatitis (695.3)

● *372.33* ***Conjunctivitis in mucocutaneous disease***

Code first underlying disease, as:
erythema multiforme (695.1)
Reiter's disease (099.3)

Excludes *ocular pemphigoid (694.61)*

❑ 372.39 **Other**

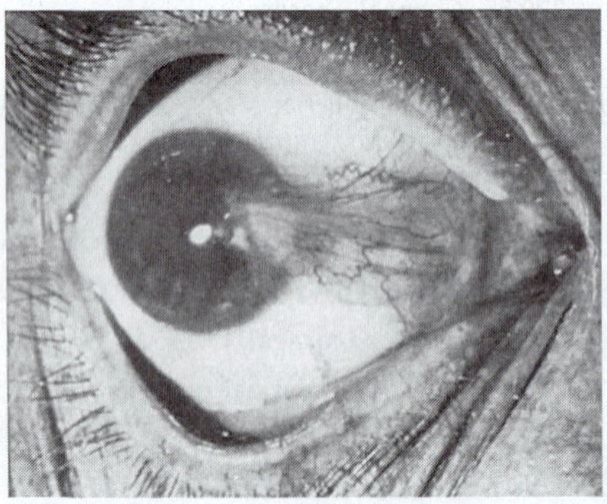

Figure 6–9 Pterygium. (From Adler FH: Textbook of Ophthalmology, 7th ed. Philadelphia, WB Saunders, 1962, p 194.)

Item 6–11 Pterygium is Greek for batlike. The condition is characterized by a membrane that extends from the limbus to the center of the cornea and resembles a wing.

● 372.4 **Pterygium**

Excludes *pseudopterygium (372.52)*

❑ 372.40 **Pterygium, unspecified**

372.41 **Peripheral pterygium, stationary**

372.42 **Peripheral pterygium, progressive**

372.43 **Central pterygium**

372.44 **Double pterygium**

372.45 **Recurrent pterygium**

● 372.5 **Conjunctival degenerations and deposits**

❑ 372.50 **Conjunctival degeneration, unspecified**

372.51 **Pinguecula**

372.52 **Pseudopterygium**

372.53 **Conjunctival xerosis**

Excludes *conjunctival xerosis due to vitamin A deficiency (264.0, 264.1, 264.7)*

372.54 **Conjunctival concretions**

372.55 **Conjunctival pigmentations**
Conjunctival argyrosis

372.56 **Conjunctival deposits**

● 372.6 **Conjunctival scars**

372.61 **Granuloma of conjunctiva**

372.62 **Localized adhesions and strands of conjunctiva**

372.63 **Symblepharon**
Extensive adhesions of conjunctiva

372.64 **Scarring of conjunctiva**
Contraction of eye socket (after enucleation)

● 372.7 **Conjunctival vascular disorders and cysts**

372.71 **Hyperemia of conjunctiva**

372.72 **Conjunctival hemorrhage**
Hyposphagma
Subconjunctival hemorrhage

372.73 **Conjunctival edema**
Chemosis of conjunctiva
Subconjunctival edema

372.74 **Vascular abnormalities of conjunctiva**
Aneurysm(ata) of conjunctiva

372.75 **Conjunctival cysts**

●❑ 372.8 **Other disorders of conjunctiva**

372.81 **Conjunctivochalasis**

❑ 372.89 **Other disorders of conjunctiva**

❑ 372.9 **Unspecified disorder of conjunctiva**

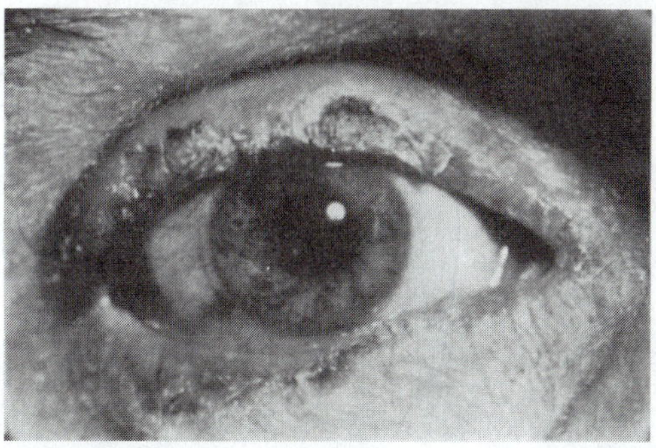

Figure 6–10 Ulcerating blepharitis caused by a staphylococcal infection. (From Pau H: Differential Diagnosis of Eye Diseases. Philadelphia, WB Saunders, 1978, p 106.)

Item 6–12 Blepharitis is a common condition in which the lid is swollen and yellow scaling and conjunctivitis develop. Usually the hair on the scalp and brow is involved.

Item 6–13 Hordeolum is the inflammation of the sebaceous gland of the eyelid.

● 373 **Inflammation of eyelids**

● 373.0 **Blepharitis**

Excludes *blepharoconjunctivitis (372.20–372.22)*

❑ 373.00 **Blepharitis, unspecified**

373.01 **Ulcerative blepharitis**

373.02 **Squamous blepharitis**

● 373.1 **Hordeolum and other deep inflammation of eyelid**

373.11 **Hordeolum externum**
Hordeolum NOS
Stye

373.12 **Hordeolum internum**
Infection of meibomian gland

373.13 **Abscess of eyelid**
Furuncle of eyelid

373.2 **Chalazion**
Meibomian (gland) cyst

Excludes *infected meibomian gland (373.12)*

● 373.3 **Noninfectious dermatoses of eyelid**

373.31 **Eczematous dermatitis of eyelid**

373.32 **Contact and allergic dermatitis of eyelid**

373.33 **Xeroderma of eyelid**

373.34 **Discoid lupus erythematosus of eyelid**

● 373.4 ***Infective dermatitis of eyelid of types resulting in deformity***

Code first underlying disease, as:
leprosy (030.0–030.9)
lupus vulgaris (tuberculous) (017.0)
yaws (102.0–102.9)

●❑ 373.5 ***Other infective dermatitis of eyelid***

Code first underlying disease, as:
actinomycosis (039.3)
impetigo (684)
mycotic dermatitis (110.0–111.9)
vaccinia (051.0)
postvaccination (999.0)

Excludes *herpes:*
simplex (054.41)
zoster (053.20)

● 373.6 ***Parasitic infestation of eyelid***

Code first underlying disease, as:
leishmaniasis (085.0–085.9)
loiasis (125.2)
onchocerciasis (125.3)
pediculosis (132.0)

❑ 373.8 **Other inflammations of eyelids**

❑ 373.9 **Unspecified inflammation of eyelid**

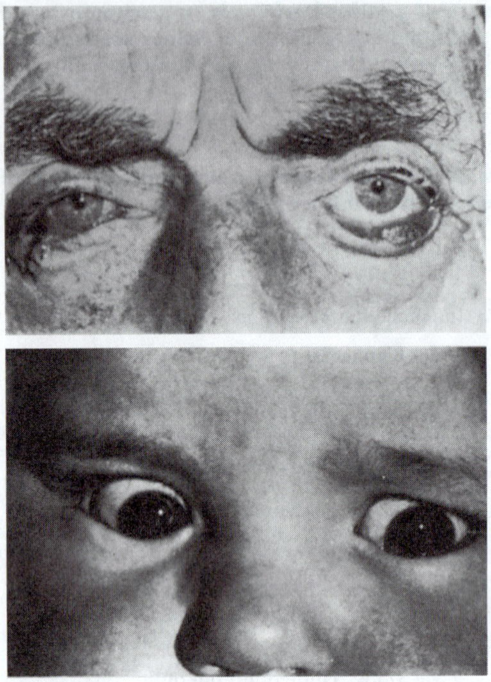

Figure 6–11 **A.** A 72-year-old male with senile ectropion on the left and postsurgical correction on the right. **B.** Entropion in a 6-month-old male infant. (From Pau H: Differential Diagnosis of Eye Diseases. Philadelphia, WB Saunders, 1978, p 90.)

● **374 Other disorders of eyelids**

● **374.0 Entropion and trichiasis of eyelid**

❑ **374.00 Entropion, unspecified**

374.01 Senile entropion

374.02 Mechanical entropion

374.03 Spastic entropion

374.04 Cicatricial entropion

374.05 Trichiasis without entropion

● **374.1 Ectropion**

❑ **374.10 Ectropion, unspecified**

374.11 Senile ectropion

374.12 Mechanical ectropion

374.13 Spastic ectropion

374.14 Cicatricial ectropion

● **374.2 Lagophthalmos**

❑ **374.20 Lagophthalmos, unspecified**

374.21 Paralytic lagophthalmos

374.22 Mechanical lagophthalmos

374.23 Cicatricial lagophthalmos

● **374.3 Ptosis of eyelid**

❑ **374.30 Ptosis of eyelid, unspecified**

374.31 Paralytic ptosis

374.32 Myogenic ptosis

374.33 Mechanical ptosis

374.34 Blepharochalasis
Pseudoptosis

● **374.4 Other disorders affecting eyelid function**

Excludes *blepharoclonus (333.81)*
blepharospasm (333.81)
facial nerve palsy (351.0)
third nerve palsy or paralysis (378.51–378.52)
tic (psychogenic) (307.20–307.23)
organic (333.3)

374.41 Lid retraction or lag

374.43 Abnormal innervation syndrome
Jaw-blinking
Paradoxical facial movements

374.44 Sensory disorders

❑ **374.45 Other sensorimotor disorders**
Deficient blink reflex

374.46 Blepharophimosis
Ankyloblepharon

● **374.5 Degenerative disorders of eyelid and periocular area**

❑ **374.50 Degenerative disorder of eyelid, unspecified**

374.51 Xanthelasma
Xanthoma (planum) (tuberosum) of eyelid
Code first underlying condition (272.0–272.9)

374.52 Hyperpigmentation of eyelid
Chloasma
Dyspigmentation

374.53 Hypopigmentation of eyelid
Vitiligo of eyelid

374.54 Hypertrichosis of eyelid

374.55 Hypotrichosis of eyelid
Madarosis of eyelid

❑ **374.56 Other degenerative disorders of skin affecting eyelid**

● **374.8 Other disorders of eyelid**

374.81 Hemorrhage of eyelid

Excludes *black eye (921.0)*

374.82 Edema of eyelid
Hyperemia of eyelid

374.83 Elephantiasis of eyelid

374.84 Cysts of eyelids
Sebaceous cyst of eyelid

374.85 Vascular anomalies of eyelid

374.86 Retained foreign body of eyelid

374.87 Dermatochalasis

❑ **374.89 Other disorders of eyelid**

❑ **374.9 Unspecified disorder of eyelid**

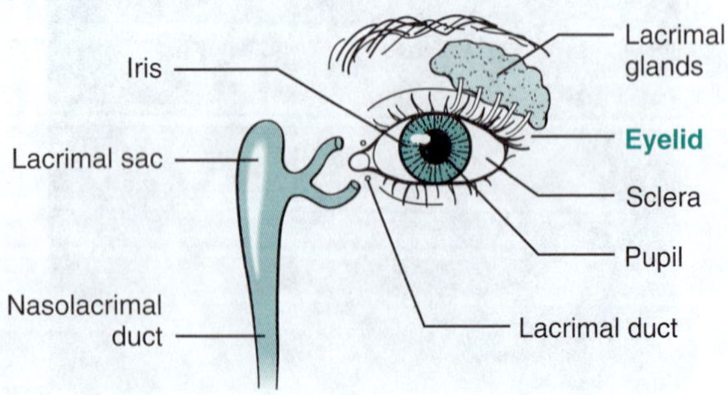

Figure 6–12 Lacrimal apparatus. (From Buck CJ: Step-by-Step Medical Coding, 3rd ed. Philadelphia, WB Saunders, 2000, p. 205.)

● 375 Disorders of lacrimal system

● 375.0 Dacryoadenitis

❑ 375.00 Dacryoadenitis, unspecified

375.01 Acute dacryoadenitis

375.02 Chronic dacryoadenitis

375.03 Chronic enlargement of lacrimal gland

● 375.1 Other disorders of lacrimal gland

❑ 375.11 Dacryops

❑ 375.12 Other lacrimal cysts and cystic degeneration

375.13 Primary lacrimal atrophy

375.14 Secondary lacrimal atrophy

❑ 375.15 Tear film insufficiency, unspecified
Dry eye syndrome

375.16 Dislocation of lacrimal gland

● 375.2 Epiphora

❑ 375.20 Epiphora, unspecified as to cause

375.21 Epiphora due to excess lacrimation

375.22 Epiphora due to insufficient drainage

● 375.3 Acute and unspecified inflammation of lacrimal passages

Excludes *neonatal dacryocystitis (771.6)*

❑ 375.30 Dacryocystitis, unspecified

375.31 Acute canaliculitis, lacrimal

375.32 Acute dacryocystitis
Acute peridacryocystitis

375.33 Phlegmonous dacryocystitis

● 375.4 Chronic inflammation of lacrimal passages

375.41 Chronic canaliculitis

375.42 Chronic dacryocystitis

375.43 Lacrimal mucocele

● 375.5 Stenosis and insufficiency of lacrimal passages

375.51 Eversion of lacrimal punctum

375.52 Stenosis of lacrimal punctum

375.53 Stenosis of lacrimal canaliculi

375.54 Stenosis of lacrimal sac

375.55 Obstruction of nasolacrimal duct, neonatal

Excludes *congenital anomaly of nasolacrimal duct (743.65)*

375.56 Stenosis of nasolacrimal duct, acquired

375.57 Dacryolith

● 375.6 Other changes of lacrimal passages

375.61 Lacrimal fistula

❑ 375.69 Other

● 375.8 Other disorders of lacrimal system

375.81 Granuloma of lacrimal passages

❑ 375.89 Other

❑ 375.9 Unspecified disorder of lacrimal system

● 376 Disorders of the orbit

● 376.0 Acute inflammation of orbit

❑ 376.00 Acute inflammation of orbit, unspecified

376.01 Orbital cellulitis
Abscess of orbit

376.02 Orbital periostitis

376.03 Orbital osteomyelitis

376.04 Tenonitis

● 376.1 Chronic inflammatory disorders of orbit

❑ 376.10 Chronic inflammation of orbit, unspecified

376.11 Orbital granuloma
Pseudotumor (inflammatory) of orbit

376.12 Orbital myositis

● *376.13 Parasitic infestation of orbit*

Code first underlying disease, as:
hydatid infestation of orbit (122.3, 122.6, 122.9)
myiasis of orbit (134.0)

● *376.2 Endocrine exophthalmos*

Code first underlying thyroid disorder (242.0–242.9)

● *376.21 Thyrotoxic exophthalmos*

● *376.22 Exophthalmic ophthalmoplegia*

● 376.3 Other exophthalmic conditions

❑ 376.30 Exophthalmos, unspecified

376.31 Constant exophthalmos

376.32 Orbital hemorrhage

376.33 Orbital edema or congestion

376.34 Intermittent exophthalmos

376.35 Pulsating exophthalmos

376.36 Lateral displacement of globe

● 376.4 Deformity of orbit

❑ 376.40 Deformity of orbit, unspecified

376.41 Hypertelorism of orbit

376.42 Exostosis of orbit

376.43 Local deformities due to bone disease

376.44 Orbital deformities associated with craniofacial deformities

376.45 Atrophy of orbit

376.46 Enlargement of orbit

376.47 Deformity due to trauma or surgery

● 376.5 Enophthalmos

❑ 376.50 Enophthalmos, unspecified as to cause

376.51 Enophthalmos due to atrophy of orbital tissue

376.52 Enophthalmos due to trauma or surgery

376.6 Retained (old) foreign body following penetrating wound of orbit
Retrobulbar foreign body

● 376.8 Other orbital disorders

376.81 Orbital cysts
Encephalocele of orbit

376.82 Myopathy of extraocular muscles

❑ 376.89 Other

❑ 376.9 Unspecified disorder of orbit

● 377 Disorders of optic nerve and visual pathways

● 377.0 Papilledema

❑ 377.00 Papilledema, unspecified

377.01 Papilledema associated with increased intracranial pressure

377.02 Papilledema associated with decreased ocular pressure

377.03 Papilledema associated with retinal disorder

377.04 Foster-Kennedy syndrome

● 377.1 Optic atrophy

❑ 377.10 Optic atrophy, unspecified

377.11 **Primary optic atrophy**

Excludes *neurosyphilitic optic atrophy (094.84)*

377.12 **Postinflammatory optic atrophy**

377.13 **Optic atrophy associated with retinal dystrophies**

377.14 **Glaucomatous atrophy [cupping] of optic disc**

377.15 **Partial optic atrophy**
Temporal pallor of optic disc

377.16 **Hereditary optic atrophy**
Optic atrophy:
dominant hereditary
Leber's

● 377.2 **Other disorders of optic disc**

377.21 **Drusen of optic disc**

377.22 **Crater-like holes of optic disc**

377.23 **Coloboma of optic disc**

377.24 **Pseudopapilledema**

● 377.3 **Optic neuritis**

Excludes *meningococcal optic neuritis (036.81)*

❑ 377.30 **Optic neuritis, unspecified**

377.31 **Optic papillitis**

377.32 **Retrobulbar neuritis (acute)**

Excludes *syphilitic retrobulbar neuritis (094.85)*

377.33 **Nutritional optic neuropathy**

377.34 **Toxic optic neuropathy**
Toxic amblyopia

❑ 377.39 **Other**

Excludes *ischemic optic neuropathy (377.41)*

● 377.4 **Other disorders of optic nerve**

377.41 **Ischemic optic neuropathy**

377.42 **Hemorrhage in optic nerve sheaths**

❑ 377.49 **Other**
Compression of optic nerve

● 377.5 **Disorders of optic chiasm**

377.51 **Associated with pituitary neoplasms and disorders**

❑ 377.52 **Associated with other neoplasms**

377.53 **Associated with vascular disorders**

377.54 **Associated with inflammatory disorders**

● 377.6 **Disorders of other visual pathways**

377.61 **Associated with neoplasms**

377.62 **Associated with vascular disorders**

377.63 **Associated with inflammatory disorders**

● 377.7 **Disorders of visual cortex**

Excludes *visual:*
agnosia (368.16)
hallucinations (368.16)
halos (368.15)

377.71 **Associated with neoplasms**

377.72 **Associated with vascular disorders**

377.73 **Associated with inflammatory disorders**

377.75 **Cortical blindness**

❑ 377.9 **Unspecified disorder of optic nerve and visual pathways**

● 378 **Strabismus and other disorders of binocular eye movements**

Excludes *nystagmus and other irregular eye movements (379.50–379.59)*

● 378.0 **Esotropia**
Convergent concomitant strabismus

Excludes *intermittent esotropia (378.20–378.22)*

❑ 378.00 **Esotropia, unspecified**

378.01 **Monocular esotropia**

378.02 **Monocular esotropia with A pattern**

378.03 **Monocular esotropia with V pattern**

❑ 378.04 **Monocular esotropia with other noncomitancies**
Monocular esotropia with X or Y pattern

378.05 **Alternating esotropia**

378.06 **Alternating esotropia with A pattern**

378.07 **Alternating esotropia with V pattern**

❑ 378.08 **Alternating esotropia with other noncomitancies**
Alternating esotropia with X or Y pattern

● 378.1 **Exotropia**
Divergent concomitant strabismus

Excludes *intermittent exotropia (378.20, 378.23–378.24)*

❑ 378.10 **Exotropia, unspecified**

378.11 **Monocular exotropia**

378.12 **Monocular exotropia with A pattern**

378.13 **Monocular exotropia with V pattern**

❑ 378.14 **Monocular exotropia with other noncomitancies**
Monocular exotropia with X or Y pattern

378.15 **Alternating exotropia**

378.16 **Alternating exotropia with A pattern**

378.17 **Alternating exotropia with V pattern**

❑ 378.18 **Alternating exotropia with other noncomitancies**
Alternating exotropia with X or Y pattern

● 378.2 **Intermittent heterotropia**

Excludes *vertical heterotropia (intermittent) (378.31)*

❑ 378.20 **Intermittent heterotropia, unspecified**
Intermittent:
esotropia NOS
exotropia NOS

378.21 **Intermittent esotropia, monocular**

378.22 **Intermittent esotropia, alternating**

378.23 **Intermittent exotropia, monocular**

378.24 **Intermittent exotropia, alternating**

● 378.3 **Other and unspecified heterotropia**

❑ 378.30 **Heterotropia, unspecified**

378.31 **Hypertropia**
Vertical heterotropia (constant) (intermittent)

378.32 **Hypotropia**

378.33 **Cyclotropia**

378.34 **Monofixation syndrome**
Microtropia

378.35 **Accommodative component in esotropia**

● 378.4 **Heterophoria**

❑ 378.40 **Heterophoria, unspecified**

378.41 **Esophoria**

378.42 **Exophoria**

378.43 **Vertical heterophoria**

378.44 Cyclophoria

378.45 Alternating hyperphoria

● 378.5 Paralytic strabismus

❑ 378.50 Paralytic strabismus, unspecified

378.51 Third or oculomotor nerve palsy, partial

378.52 Third or oculomotor nerve palsy, total

378.53 Fourth or trochlear nerve palsy

378.54 Sixth or abducens nerve palsy

378.55 External ophthalmoplegia

378.56 Total ophthalmoplegia

● 378.6 Mechanical strabismus

❑ 378.60 Mechanical strabismus, unspecified

378.61 Brown's (tendon) sheath syndrome

❑ 378.62 Mechanical strabismus from other musculofascial disorders

❑ 378.63 Limited duction associated with other conditions

● 378.7 Other specified strabismus

378.71 Duane's syndrome

378.72 Progressive external ophthalmoplegia

❑ 378.73 Strabismus in other neuromuscular disorders

● 378.8 Other disorders of binocular eye movements

Excludes *nystagmus (379.50–379.56)*

378.81 Palsy of conjugate gaze

378.82 Spasm of conjugate gaze

378.83 Convergence insufficiency or palsy

378.84 Convergence excess or spasm

378.85 Anomalies of divergence

378.86 Internuclear ophthalmoplegia

❑ 378.87 Other dissociated deviation of eye movements
Skew deviation

❑ 378.9 Unspecified disorder of eye movements
Ophthalmoplegia NOS
Strabismus NOS

● 379 Other disorders of eye

● 379.0 Scleritis and episcleritis

Excludes *syphilitic episcleritis (095.0)*

❑ 379.00 Scleritis, unspecified
Episcleritis NOS

379.01 Episcleritis periodica fugax

379.02 Nodular episcleritis

379.03 Anterior scleritis

379.04 Scleromalacia perforans

379.05 Scleritis with corneal involvement
Scleroperikeratitis

379.06 Brawny scleritis

379.07 Posterior scleritis
Sclerotenonitis

❑ 379.09 Other
Scleral abscess

● 379.1 Other disorders of sclera

Excludes *blue sclera (743.47)*

379.11 Scleral ectasia
Scleral staphyloma NOS

379.12 Staphyloma posticum

379.13 Equatorial staphyloma

379.14 Anterior staphyloma, localized

379.15 Ring staphyloma

❑ 379.16 Other degenerative disorders of sclera

❑ 379.19 Other

● 379.2 Disorders of vitreous body

379.21 Vitreous degeneration
Vitreous:
cavitation
detachment
liquefaction

379.22 Crystalline deposits in vitreous
Asteroid hyalitis
Synchysis scintillans

379.23 Vitreous hemorrhage

❑ 379.24 Other vitreous opacities
Vitreous floaters

379.25 Vitreous membranes and strands

379.26 Vitreous prolapse

❑ 379.29 Other disorders of vitreous

Excludes *vitreous abscess (360.04)*

● 379.3 Aphakia and other disorders of lens

Excludes *after-cataract (366.50–366.53)*

379.31 Aphakia

Excludes *cataract extraction status (V45.61)*

379.32 Subluxation of lens

379.33 Anterior dislocation of lens

379.34 Posterior dislocation of lens

❑ 379.39 Other disorders of lens

● 379.4 Anomalies of pupillary function

❑ 379.40 Abnormal pupillary function, unspecified

379.41 Anisocoria

379.42 Miosis (persistent), not due to miotics

379.43 Mydriasis (persistent), not due to mydriatics

379.45 Argyll Robertson pupil, atypical
Argyll Robertson phenomenon or pupil, nonsyphilitic

Excludes *Argyll Robertson pupil (syphilitic) (094.89)*

379.46 Tonic pupillary reaction
Adie's pupil or syndrome

❑ 379.49 Other
Hippus
Pupillary paralysis

● 379.5 Nystagmus and other irregular eye movements

❑ 379.50 Nystagmus, unspecified

379.51 Congenital nystagmus

379.52 Latent nystagmus

379.53 Visual deprivation nystagmus

379.54 Nystagmus associated with disorders of the vestibular system

379.55 Dissociated nystagmus

❑ 379.56 Other forms of nystagmus

379.57 Deficiencies of saccadic eye movements
Abnormal optokinetic response

379.58 **Deficiencies of smooth pursuit movements**

❑ 379.59 **Other irregularities of eye movements**
Opsoclonus

❑ 379.8 **Other specified disorders of eye and adnexa**

● 379.9 **Unspecified disorder of eye and adnexa**

❑ 379.90 **Disorder of eye, unspecified**

379.91 **Pain in or around eye**

379.92 **Swelling or mass of eye**

379.93 **Redness or discharge of eye**

❑ 379.99 **Other ill-defined disorders of eye**

Excludes *blurred vision NOS (368.8)*

DISEASES OF THE EAR AND MASTOID PROCESS (380–389)

● 380 **Disorders of external ear**

● 380.0 **Perichondritis of pinna**
Perichondritis of auricle

❑ 380.00 **Perichondritis of pinna, unspecified**

380.01 **Acute perichondritis of pinna**

380.02 **Chronic perichondritis of pinna**

● 380.1 **Infective otitis externa**

❑ 380.10 **Infective otitis externa, unspecified**
Otitis externa (acute):
NOS
circumscribed
diffuse
hemorrhagica
infective NOS

380.11 **Acute infection of pinna**

Excludes *furuncular otitis externa (680.0)*

380.12 **Acute swimmers' ear**
Beach ear
Tank ear

●❑ *380.13* ***Other acute infections of external ear***

Code first underlying disease, as:
erysipelas (035)
impetigo (684)
seborrheic dermatitis (690.10–690.18)

Excludes *herpes simplex (054.73)*
herpes zoster (053.71)

380.14 **Malignant otitis externa**

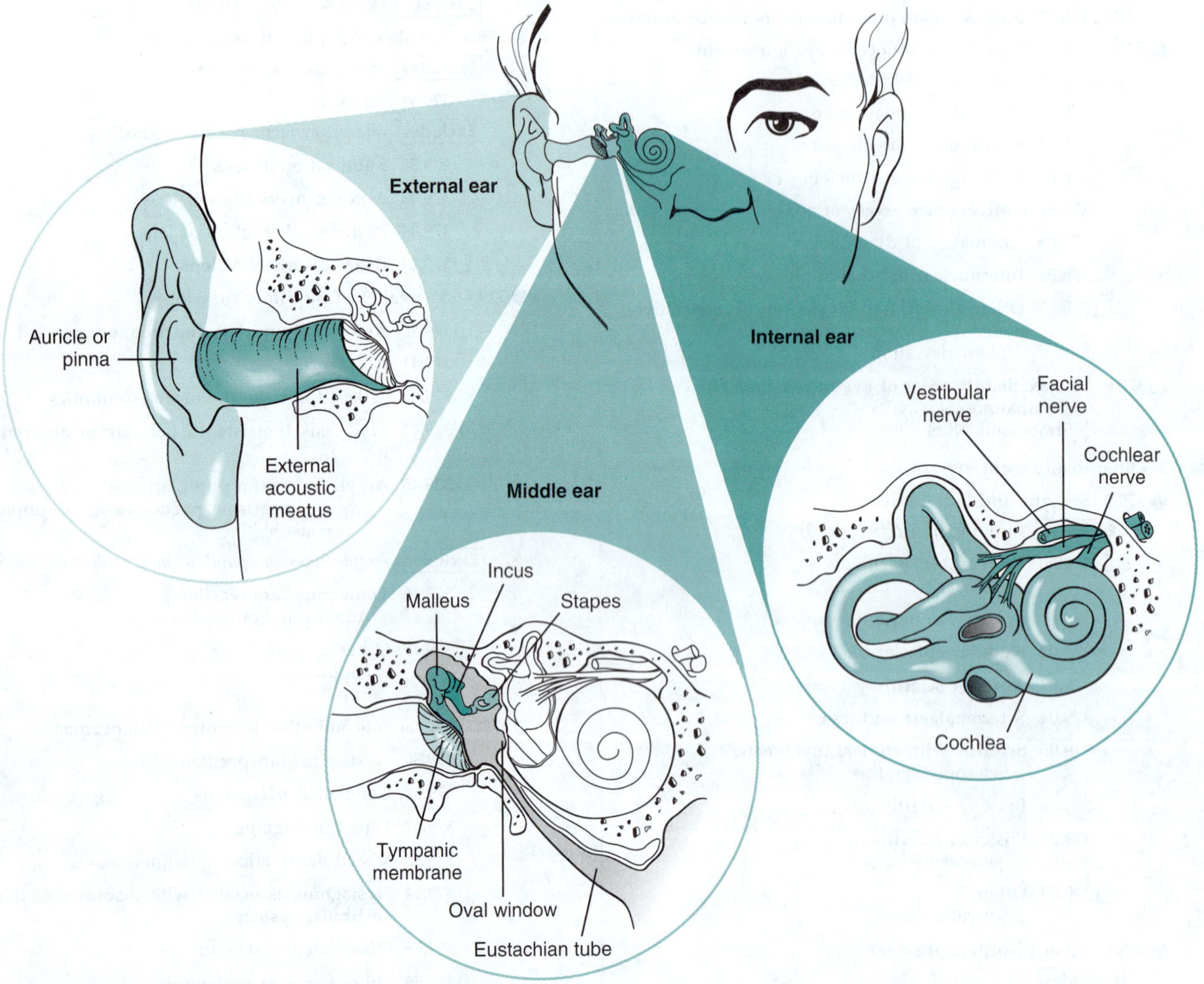

Figure 6–13 Auditory system. (From Buck CJ: Step-by-Step Medical Coding, 3rd ed. Philadelphia, WB Saunders, 2000, p. 208.)

● 380.15 *Chronic mycotic otitis externa*

Code first underlying disease, as:
aspergillosis (117.3)
otomycosis NOS (111.9)

Excludes *candidal otitis externa (112.82)*

❑ **380.16 Other chronic infective otitis externa**
Chronic infective otitis externa NOS

● **380.2 Other otitis externa**

380.21 Cholesteatoma of external ear
Keratosis obturans of external ear (canal)

Excludes *cholesteatoma NOS (385.30–385.35)*
postmastoidectomy (383.32)

❑ **380.22 Other acute otitis externa**
Acute otitis externa:
actinic
chemical
contact
eczematoid
reactive

❑ **380.23 Other chronic otitis externa**
Chronic otitis externa NOS

● **380.3 Noninfectious disorders of pinna**

❑ **380.30 Disorder of pinna, unspecified**

380.31 Hematoma of auricle or pinna

380.32 Acquired deformities of auricle or pinna

Excludes *cauliflower ear (738.7)*

❑ **380.39 Other**

Excludes *gouty tophi of ear (274.81)*

380.4 Impacted cerumen
Wax in ear

● **380.5 Acquired stenosis of external ear canal**
Collapse of external ear canal

❑ **380.50 Acquired stenosis of external ear canal, unspecified as to cause**

380.51 Secondary to trauma

380.52 Secondary to surgery

380.53 Secondary to inflammation

● **380.8 Other disorders of external ear**

380.81 Exostosis of external ear canal

❑ **380.89 Other**

❑ **380.9 Unspecified disorder of external ear**

● **381 Nonsuppurative otitis media and Eustachian tube disorders**

● **381.0 Acute nonsuppurative otitis media**
Acute tubotympanic catarrh
Otitis media, acute or subacute:
catarrhal
exudative
transudative
with effusion

Excludes *otitic barotrauma (993.0)*

❑ **381.00 Acute nonsuppurative otitis media, unspecified**

381.01 Acute serous otitis media
Acute or subacute secretory otitis media

381.02 Acute mucoid otitis media
Acute or subacute seromucinous otitis media
Blue drum syndrome

381.03 Acute sanguinous otitis media

381.04 Acute allergic serous otitis media

381.05 Acute allergic mucoid otitis media

381.06 Acute allergic sanguinous otitis media

● **381.1 Chronic serous otitis media**
Chronic tubotympanic catarrh

381.10 Chronic serous otitis media, simple or unspecified

❑ **381.19 Other**
Serosanguinous chronic otitis media

● **381.2 Chronic mucoid otitis media**
Glue ear

Excludes *adhesive middle ear disease (385.10–385.19)*

381.20 Chronic mucoid otitis media, simple or unspecified

❑ **381.29 Other**
Mucosanguinous chronic otitis media

❑ **381.3 Other and unspecified chronic nonsuppurative otitis media**

Otitis media, chronic:	Otitis media, chronic:
allergic	seromucinous
exudative	transudative
secretory	with effusion

❑ **381.4 Nonsuppurative otitis media, not specified as acute or chronic**

Otitis media:	Otitis media:
allergic	seromucinous
catarrhal	serous
exudative	transudative
mucoid	with effusion
secretory	

● **381.5 Eustachian salpingitis**

❑ **381.50 Eustachian salpingitis, unspecified**

381.51 Acute Eustachian salpingitis

381.52 Chronic Eustachian salpingitis

● **381.6 Obstruction of Eustachian tube**
Stenosis of Eustachian tube
Stricture of Eustachian tube

❑ **381.60 Obstruction of Eustachian tube, unspecified**

381.61 Osseous obstruction of Eustachian tube
Obstruction of Eustachian tube from cholesteatoma, polyp, or other osseous lesion

381.62 Intrinsic cartilaginous obstruction of Eustachian tube

381.63 Extrinsic cartilaginous obstruction of Eustachian tube
Compression of Eustachian tube

381.7 Patulous Eustachian tube

● **381.8 Other disorders of Eustachian tube**

381.81 Dysfunction of Eustachian tube

❑ **381.89 Other**

❑ **381.9 Unspecified Eustachian tube disorder**

● **382 Suppurative and unspecified otitis media**

● **382.0 Acute suppurative otitis media**
Otitis media, acute:
necrotizing NOS
purulent

382.00 Acute suppurative otitis media without spontaneous rupture of ear drum

382.01 Acute suppurative otitis media with spontaneous rupture of ear drum

ICD-9-CM 300-399 Vol. 1

● ❑ 382.02 *Acute suppurative otitis media in diseases classified elsewhere*
Code first underlying disease, as:
influenza (487.8)
scarlet fever (034.1)
Excludes *postmeasles otitis (055.2)*

382.1 **Chronic tubotympanic suppurative otitis media**
Benign chronic suppurative otitis media (with anterior perforation of ear drum)
Chronic tubotympanic disease (with anterior perforation of ear drum)

382.2 **Chronic atticoantral suppurative otitis media**
Chronic atticoantral disease (with posterior or superior marginal perforation of ear drum)
Persistent mucosal disease (with posterior or superior marginal perforation of ear drum)

❑ 382.3 **Unspecified chronic suppurative otitis media**
Chronic purulent otitis media
Excludes *tuberculous otitis media (017.4)*

❑ 382.4 **Unspecified suppurative otitis media**
Purulent otitis media NOS

❑ 382.9 **Unspecified otitis media**
Otitis media:
NOS
acute NOS
chronic NOS

● 383 **Mastoiditis and related conditions**

● 383.0 **Acute mastoiditis**
Abscess of mastoid
Empyema of mastoid

383.00 **Acute mastoiditis without complications**

383.01 **Subperiosteal abscess of mastoid**

❑ 383.02 **Acute mastoiditis with other complications**
Gradenigo's syndrome

383.1 **Chronic mastoiditis**
Caries of mastoid
Fistula of mastoid
Excludes *tuberculous mastoiditis (015.6)*

● 383.2 **Petrositis**
Coalescing osteitis of petrous bone
Inflammation of petrous bone
Osteomyelitis of petrous bone

❑ 383.20 **Petrositis, unspecified**

383.21 **Acute petrositis**

383.22 **Chronic petrositis**

● 383.3 **Complications following mastoidectomy**

❑ 383.30 **Postmastoidectomy complication, unspecified**

383.31 **Mucosal cyst of postmastoidectomy cavity**

383.32 **Recurrent cholesteatoma of postmastoidectomy cavity**

383.33 **Granulations of postmastoidectomy cavity**
Chronic inflammation of postmastoidectomy cavity

● 383.8 **Other disorders of mastoid**

383.81 **Postauricular fistula**

❑ 383.89 **Other**

❑ 383.9 **Unspecified mastoiditis**

● 384 **Other disorders of tympanic membrane**

● 384.0 **Acute myringitis without mention of otitis media**

❑ 384.00 **Acute myringitis, unspecified**
Acute tympanitis NOS

384.01 **Bullous myringitis**
Myringitis bullosa hemorrhagica

❑ 384.09 **Other**

384.1 **Chronic myringitis without mention of otitis media**
Chronic tympanitis

● 384.2 **Perforation of tympanic membrane**
Perforation of ear drum:
NOS
persistent posttraumatic
postinflammatory
Excludes *otitis media with perforation of tympanic membrane (382.00–382.9)*
traumatic perforation [current injury] (872.61)

❑ 384.20 **Perforation of tympanic membrane, unspecified**

384.21 **Central perforation of tympanic membrane**

384.22 **Attic perforation of tympanic membrane**
Pars flaccida

❑ 384.23 **Other marginal perforation of tympanic membrane**

384.24 **Multiple perforations of tympanic membrane**

384.25 **Total perforation of tympanic membrane**

● 384.8 **Other specified disorders of tympanic membrane**

384.81 **Atrophic flaccid tympanic membrane**
Healed perforation of ear drum

384.82 **Atrophic nonflaccid tympanic membrane**

❑ 384.9 **Unspecified disorder of tympanic membrane**

● 385 **Other disorders of middle ear and mastoid**
Excludes *mastoiditis (383.0–383.9)*

● 385.0 **Tympanosclerosis**

❑ 385.00 **Tympanosclerosis, unspecified as to involvement**

385.01 **Tympanosclerosis involving tympanic membrane only**

385.02 **Tympanosclerosis involving tympanic membrane and ear ossicles**

385.03 **Tympanosclerosis involving tympanic membrane, ear ossicles, and middle ear**

❑ 385.09 **Tympanosclerosis involving other combination of structures**

● 385.1 **Adhesive middle ear disease**
Adhesive otitis
Otitis media:
chronic adhesive
fibrotic
Excludes *glue ear (381.20–381.29)*

❑ 385.10 **Adhesive middle ear disease, unspecified as to involvement**

385.11 **Adhesions of drum head to incus**

385.12 **Adhesions of drum head to stapes**

385.13 **Adhesions of drum head to promontorium**

❑ 385.19 **Other adhesions and combinations**

● 385.2 **Other acquired abnormality of ear ossicles**

385.21 **Impaired mobility of malleus**
Ankylosis of malleus

❑ **385.22 Impaired mobility of other ear ossicles**
Ankylosis of ear ossicles, except malleus

385.23 Discontinuity or dislocation of ear ossicles

385.24 Partial loss or necrosis of ear ossicles

● **385.3 Cholesteatoma of middle ear and mastoid**
Cholesterosis of (middle) ear
Epidermosis of (middle) ear
Keratosis of (middle) ear
Polyp of (middle) ear

Excludes *cholesteatoma:*
external ear canal (380.21)
recurrent of postmastoidectomy cavity (383.32)

❑ **385.30 Cholesteatoma, unspecified**

385.31 Cholesteatoma of attic

385.32 Cholesteatoma of middle ear

385.33 Cholesteatoma of middle ear and mastoid

385.35 Diffuse cholesteatosis

● **385.8 Other disorders of middle ear and mastoid**

385.82 Cholesterin granuloma

385.83 Retained foreign body of middle ear

❑ **385.89 Other**

❑ **385.9 Unspecified disorder of middle ear and mastoid**

● **386 Vertiginous syndromes and other disorders of vestibular system**

Excludes *vertigo NOS (780.4)*

● **386.0 Ménière's disease**
Endolymphatic hydrops
Lermoyez's syndrome
Ménière's syndrome or vertigo

❑ **386.00 Ménière's disease, unspecified**
Ménière's disease (active)

386.01 Active Ménière's disease, cochleovestibular

386.02 Active Ménière's disease, cochlear

386.03 Active Ménière's disease, vestibular

386.04 Inactive Ménière's disease
Ménière's disease in remission

● **386.1 Other and unspecified peripheral vertigo**

Excludes *epidemic vertigo (078.81)*

❑ **386.10 Peripheral vertigo, unspecified**

386.11 Benign paroxysmal positional vertigo
Benign paroxysmal positional nystagmus

386.12 Vestibular neuronitis
Acute (and recurrent) peripheral vestibulopathy

❑ **386.19 Other**
Aural vertigo
Otogenic vertigo

386.2 Vertigo of central origin
Central positional nystagmus
Malignant positional vertigo

● **386.3 Labyrinthitis**

❑ **386.30 Labyrinthitis, unspecified**

386.31 Serous labyrinthitis
Diffuse labyrinthitis

386.32 Circumscribed labyrinthitis
Focal labyrinthitis

386.33 Suppurative labyrinthitis
Purulent labyrinthitis

386.34 Toxic labyrinthitis

386.35 Viral labyrinthitis

● **386.4 Labyrinthine fistula**

❑ **386.40 Labyrinthine fistula, unspecified**

386.41 Round window fistula

386.42 Oval window fistula

386.43 Semicircular canal fistula

386.48 Labyrinthine fistula of combined sites

● **386.5 Labyrinthine dysfunction**

❑ **386.50 Labyrinthine dysfunction, unspecified**

386.51 Hyperactive labyrinth, unilateral

386.52 Hyperactive labyrinth, bilateral

386.53 Hypoactive labyrinth, unilateral

386.54 Hypoactive labyrinth, bilateral

386.55 Loss of labyrinthine reactivity, unilateral

386.56 Loss of labyrinthine reactivity, bilateral

❑ **386.58 Other forms and combinations**

❑ **386.8 Other disorders of labyrinth**

❑ **386.9 Unspecified vertiginous syndromes and labyrinthine disorders**

● **387 Otosclerosis**

Includes: otospongiosis

387.0 Otosclerosis involving oval window, nonobliterative

387.1 Otosclerosis involving oval window, obliterative

387.2 Cochlear otosclerosis
Otosclerosis involving:
otic capsule
round window

❑ **387.8 Other otosclerosis**

❑ **387.9 Otosclerosis, unspecified**

● **388 Other disorders of ear**

● **388.0 Degenerative and vascular disorders of ear**

❑ **388.00 Degenerative and vascular disorders, unspecified**

388.01 Presbyacusis

388.02 Transient ischemic deafness

● **388.1 Noise effects on inner ear**

❑ **388.10 Noise effects on inner ear, unspecified**

388.11 Acoustic trauma (explosive) to ear
Otitic blast injury

388.12 Noise-induced hearing loss

❑ **388.2 Sudden hearing loss, unspecified**

● **388.3 Tinnitus**

❑ **388.30 Tinnitus, unspecified**

388.31 Subjective tinnitus

388.32 Objective tinnitus

● **388.4 Other abnormal auditory perception**

❑ **388.40 Abnormal auditory perception, unspecified**

388.41 Diplacusis

388.42 Hyperacusis

388.43 Impairment of auditory discrimination

388.44 Recruitment

388.5 **Disorders of acoustic nerve**
Acoustic neuritis
Degeneration of acoustic or eighth nerve
Disorder of acoustic or eighth nerve
Excludes *acoustic neuroma (225.1)*
syphilitic acoustic neuritis (094.86)

● 388.6 **Otorrhea**
❑ 388.60 **Otorrhea, unspecified**
Discharging ear NOS
388.61 **Cerebrospinal fluid otorrhea**
Excludes *cerebrospinal fluid rhinorrhea (349.81)*
❑ 388.69 **Other**
Otorrhagia

● 388.7 **Otalgia**
❑ 388.70 **Otalgia, unspecified**
Earache NOS
388.71 **Otogenic pain**
388.72 **Referred pain**

❑ 388.8 **Other disorders of ear**

❑ 388.9 **Unspecified disorder of ear**

● 389 **Hearing loss**

● 389.0 **Conductive hearing loss**
Conductive deafness
❑ 389.00 **Conductive hearing loss, unspecified**
389.01 **Conductive hearing loss, external ear**
389.02 **Conductive hearing loss, tympanic membrane**
389.03 **Conductive hearing loss, middle ear**
389.04 **Conductive hearing loss, inner ear**
389.08 **Conductive hearing loss of combined types**

● 389.1 **Sensorineural hearing loss**
Perceptive hearing loss or deafness
Excludes *abnormal auditory perception (388.40–388.44)*
psychogenic deafness (306.7)
❑ 389.10 **Sensorineural hearing loss, unspecified**
389.11 **Sensory hearing loss**
389.12 **Neural hearing loss**
389.14 **Central hearing loss**
389.18 **Sensorineural hearing loss of combined types**

389.2 **Mixed conductive and sensorineural hearing loss**
Deafness or hearing loss of type classifiable to 389.0 with type classifiable to 389.1

389.7 **Deaf mutism, not elsewhere classifiable**
Deaf, nonspeaking

❑ 389.8 **Other specified forms of hearing loss**

❑ 389.9 **Unspecified hearing loss**
Deafness NOS

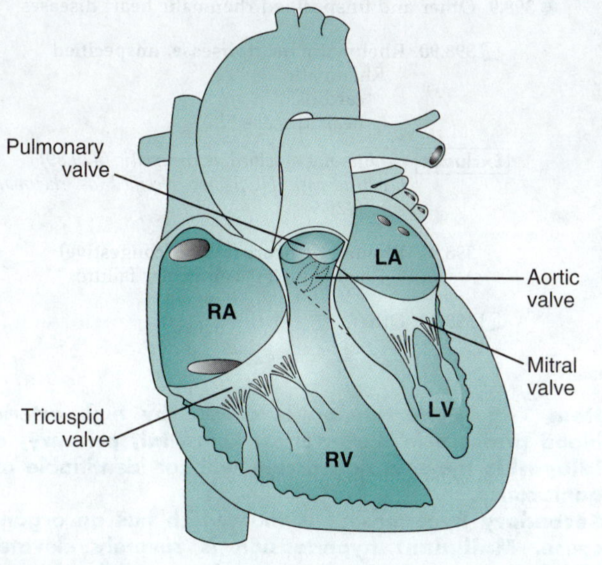

Figure 7–1 Cardiovascular valves.

Item 7–1 Rheumatic fever is the inflammation of the valve(s) of the heart, usually the mitral or aortic, which leads to valve damage. Rheumatic heart inflammations are usually pericarditis (heart), endocarditis (heart cavity), or myocarditis (heart muscle).

Item 7–2 Rheumatic chorea, also called Sydenham's, juvenile, minor, simple, or St. Vitus' dance, is a condition linked with rheumatic fever and is characterized by ceaseless, jerky movements.

7. DISEASES OF THE CIRCULATORY SYSTEM (390–459)

ACUTE RHEUMATIC FEVER (390–392)

390 Rheumatic fever without mention of heart involvement
Arthritis, rheumatic, acute or subacute
Rheumatic fever (active) (acute)
Rheumatism, articular, acute or subacute
Excludes *that with heart involvement (391.0–391.9)*

● **391 Rheumatic fever with heart involvement**
Excludes *chronic heart diseases of rheumatic origin (393.0–398.9) unless rheumatic fever is also present or there is evidence of recrudescence or activity of the rheumatic process*

391.0 Acute rheumatic pericarditis
Rheumatic:
fever (active) (acute) with pericarditis
pericarditis (acute)
Any condition classifiable to 390 with pericarditis
Excludes *that not specified as rheumatic (420.0–420.9)*

391.1 Acute rheumatic endocarditis
Rheumatic:
endocarditis, acute
fever (active) (acute) with endocarditis or valvulitis
valvulitis, acute
Any condition classifiable to 390 with endocarditis or valvulitis

391.2 Acute rheumatic myocarditis
Rheumatic fever (active) (acute) with myocarditis
Any condition classifiable to 390 with myocarditis

❑ **391.8 Other acute rheumatic heart disease**
Rheumatic:
fever (active) (acute) with other or multiple types of heart involvement
pancarditis, acute
Any condition classifiable to 390 with other or multiple types of heart involvement

❑ **391.9 Acute rheumatic heart disease, unspecified**
Rheumatic:
carditis, acute
fever (active) (acute) with unspecified type of heart involvement
heart disease, active or acute
Any condition classifiable to 390 with unspecified type of heart involvement

● **392 Rheumatic chorea**
Includes: Sydenham's chorea
Excludes *chorea:*
NOS (333.5)
Huntington's (333.4)

392.0 With heart involvement
Rheumatic chorea with heart involvement of any type classifiable to 391

392.9 Without mention of heart involvement

CHRONIC RHEUMATIC HEART DISEASE (393–398)

393 Chronic rheumatic pericarditis
Adherent pericardium, rheumatic
Chronic rheumatic:
mediastinopericarditis
myopericarditis
Excludes *pericarditis NOS or not specified as rheumatic (423.0–423.9)*

Item 7–3 Mitral stenosis is the narrowing of the mitral valve. Mitral insufficiency is the improper closure of the mitral valve. These conditions lead to enlargement (hypertrophy) of the left atrium.

● **394 Diseases of mitral valve**
Excludes *that with aortic valve involvement (396.0–396.9)*

394.0 Mitral stenosis
Mitral (valve):
obstruction (rheumatic)
stenosis NOS

394.1 Rheumatic mitral insufficiency
Rheumatic mitral:
incompetence
regurgitation
Excludes *that not specified as rheumatic (424.0)*

394.2 Mitral stenosis with insufficiency
Mitral stenosis with incompetence or regurgitation

❑ **394.9 Other and unspecified mitral valve diseases**
Mitral (valve):
disease (chronic)
failure

Item 7–4 Aortic stenosis is the narrowing of the aortic valve. Aortic insufficiency is the improper closure of the aortic valve. These conditions lead to enlargement (hypertrophy) of the left ventricle.

ICD-9-CM 300-399 Vol. 1

● **395 Diseases of aortic valve**

Excludes *that not specified as rheumatic (424.1)*
that with mitral valve involvement (396.0–396.9)

395.0 Rheumatic aortic stenosis
Rheumatic aortic (valve) obstruction

395.1 Rheumatic aortic insufficiency
Rheumatic aortic:
incompetence
regurgitation

395.2 Rheumatic aortic stenosis with insufficiency
Rheumatic aortic stenosis with incompetence or regurgitation

❑ **395.9 Other and unspecified rheumatic aortic diseases**
Rheumatic aortic (valve) disease

Item 7-5 Mitral and aortic valve stenosis is the narrowing of these valves, which leads to enlargement (hypertrophy) of the left atrium and left ventricle.
Mitral and aortic insufficiency is the improper closure of the mitral and aortic valves, which leads to enlargement (hypertrophy) of the left atrium and left ventricle.

● **396 Diseases of mitral and aortic valves**

Includes: involvement of both mitral and aortic valves, whether specified as rheumatic or not

396.0 Mitral valve stenosis and aortic valve stenosis
Atypical aortic (valve) stenosis
Mitral and aortic (valve) obstruction (rheumatic)

396.1 Mitral valve stenosis and aortic valve insufficiency

396.2 Mitral valve insufficiency and aortic valve stenosis

396.3 Mitral valve insufficiency and aortic valve insufficiency
Mitral and aortic (valve):
incompetence
regurgitation

396.8 Multiple involvement of mitral and aortic valves
Stenosis and insufficiency of mitral or aortic valve with stenosis or insufficiency, or both, of the other valve

❑ **396.9 Mitral and aortic valve diseases, unspecified**

● **397 Diseases of other endocardial structures**

397.0 Diseases of tricuspid valve
Tricuspid (valve) (rheumatic):
disease
insufficiency
obstruction
regurgitation
stenosis

397.1 Rheumatic diseases of pulmonary valve

Excludes *that not specified as rheumatic (424.3)*

❑ **397.9 Rheumatic diseases of endocardium, valve unspecified**
Rheumatic:
endocarditis (chronic)
valvulitis (chronic)

Excludes *that not specified as rheumatic (424.90–424.99)*

● **398 Other rheumatic heart disease**

398.0 Rheumatic myocarditis
Rheumatic degeneration of myocardium

Excludes *myocarditis not specified as rheumatic (429.0)*

● **398.9 Other and unspecified rheumatic heart diseases**

❑ **398.90 Rheumatic heart disease, unspecified**
Rheumatic:
carditis
heart disease NOS

Excludes *carditis not specified as rheumatic (429.89)*
heart disease NOS not specified as rheumatic (429.9)

398.91 Rheumatic heart failure (congestive)
Rheumatic left ventricular failure

❑ **398.99 Other**

Item 7-6 Hypertension is caused by high arterial blood pressure in the arteries. **Essential, primary,** or **idiopathic** hypertension occurs without identifiable organic cause.
Secondary hypertension is that which has an organic cause. **Malignant** hypertension is severely elevated blood pressure. **Benign** hypertension is mildly elevated blood pressure.

HYPERTENSIVE DISEASE (401–405)

Excludes *that complicating pregnancy, childbirth, or the puerperium (642.0–642.9)*
that involving coronary vessels (410.00–414.9)

● **401 Essential hypertension**

Includes: high blood pressure
hyperpiesia
hyperpiesis
hypertension (arterial) (essential) (primary) (systemic)
hypertensive vascular:
degeneration
disease

Excludes *elevated blood pressure without diagnosis of hypertension (796.2)*
pulmonary hypertension (416.0–416.9)
that involving vessels of:
brain (430–438)
eye (362.11)

401.0 Malignant

401.1 Benign

❑ **401.9 Unspecified**

● **402 Hypertensive heart disease**

Includes: hypertensive:
cardiomegaly
cardiopathy
cardiovascular disease
heart (disease) (failure)
any condition classifiable to 428, 429.0–429.3, 429.8, 429.9 due to hypertension

Use additional code to specify type of heart failure (428.0, 428.20–428.23, 428.30–428.33, 428.40–428.43)

● **402.0 Malignant**

402.00 Without heart failure

❑ **402.01 With heart failure**

● **402.1 Benign**

402.10 Without heart failure

402.11 With heart failure

● **402.9 Unspecified**

❑ **402.90 Without heart failure**

❑ **402.91 With heart failure**

● **403 Hypertensive renal disease**

Includes: arteriolar nephritis
arteriosclerosis of:
kidney
renal arterioles
arteriosclerotic nephritis (chronic) (interstitial)
hypertensive:
nephropathy
renal failure
uremia (chronic)
nephrosclerosis
renal sclerosis with hypertension
any condition classifiable to 585, 586, or 587 with any condition classifiable to 401

Excludes *acute renal failure (584.5–584.9)*
renal disease stated as not due to hypertension
renovascular hypertension (405.0–405.9 with fifth-digit 1)

The following fifth-digit subclassification is for use with category 403:
0 without mention of renal failure
1 with renal failure

● **403.0 Malignant**

● **403.1 Benign**

● ❑ **403.9 Unspecified**

● **404 Hypertensive heart and renal disease**

Includes: disease:
cardiorenal
cardiovascular renal
any condition classifiable to 402 with any condition classifiable to 403

Use additional code to specify type of heart failure (428.0, 428.20–428.23, 428.30–428.33, 428.40–428.43)
The following fifth-digit subclassification is for use with category 404:
0 without mention of heart failure or renal failure
1 with heart failure
2 with renal failure
3 with heart failure and renal failure

● **404.0 Malignant**

● **404.1 Benign**

● ❑ **404.9 Unspecified**

● **405 Secondary hypertension**

● **405.0 Malignant**

405.01 Renovascular

❑ **405.09 Other**

● **405.1 Benign**

405.11 Renovascular

❑ **405.19 Other**

● **405.9 Unspecified**

❑ **405.91 Renovascular**

❑ **405.99 Other**

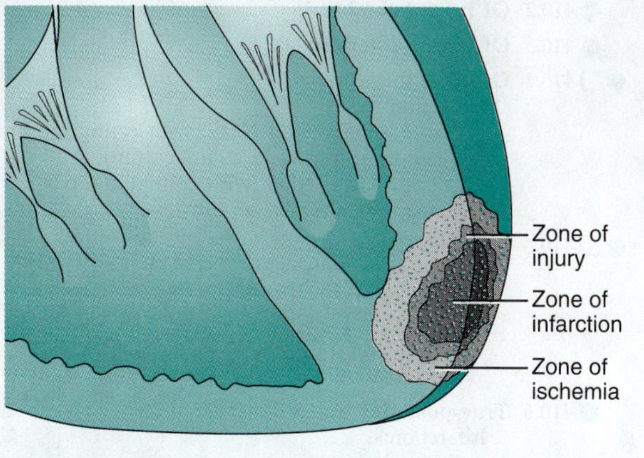

Figure 7–2 Myocardial infarction.

Item 7–7 Myocardial infarction is a sudden decrease in the coronary artery blood flow that results in death of the heart muscle. Classifications are based on the affected heart tissue.

ISCHEMIC HEART DISEASE (410–414)

Includes: that with mention of hypertension

Use additional code to identify presence of hypertension (401.0–405.9)

● **410 Acute myocardial infarction**

Includes: cardiac infarction
coronary (artery):
embolism
occlusion
rupture
thrombosis
infarction of heart, myocardium, or ventricle
rupture of heart, myocardium, or ventricle
any condition classifiable to 414.1–414.9 specified as acute or with a stated duration of 8 weeks or less

The following fifth-digit subclassification is for use with category 410:

❑ **0 episode of care unspecified**
Use when the source document does not contain sufficient information for the assignment of fifth-digit 1 or 2.

1 initial episode of care
Use fifth-digit 1 to designate the first episode of care (regardless of facility site) for a newly diagnosed myocardial infarction. The fifth-digit 1 is assigned regardless of the number of times a patient may be transferred during the initial episode of care.

2 subsequent episode of care
Use fifth-digit 2 to designate an episode of care following the initial episode when the patient is admitted for further observation, evaluation or treatment for a myocardial infarction that has received initial treatment, but is still less than 8 weeks old.

● **410.0 Of anterolateral wall**

● ❑ **410.1 Of other anterior wall**

Infarction:
anterior (wall) NOS (with contiguous portion of intraventricular septum)
anteroapical (with contiguous portion of intraventricular septum)
anteroseptal (with contiguous portion of intraventricular septum)

● 410.2 **Of inferolateral wall**

● 410.3 **Of inferoposterior wall**

● ❑ 410.4 **Of other inferior wall**
Infarction:
diaphragmatic wall NOS (with contiguous portion of intraventricular septum)
inferior (wall) NOS (with contiguous portion of intraventricular septum)

● ❑ 410.5 **Of other lateral wall**
Infarction:
apical-lateral
basal-lateral
high lateral
posterolateral

● 410.6 **True posterior wall infarction**
Infarction:
posterobasal
strictly posterior

● 410.7 **Subendocardial infarction**
Nontransmural infarction

● ❑ 410.8 **Of other specified sites**
Infarction of:
atrium
papillary muscle
septum alone

● ❑ 410.9 **Unspecified site**
Acute myocardial infarction NOS
Coronary occlusion NOS

● 411 **Other acute and subacute forms of ischemic heart disease**

411.0 **Postmyocardial infarction syndrome**
Dressler's syndrome

411.1 **Intermediate coronary syndrome**
Impending infarction
Preinfarction angina
Preinfarction syndrome
Unstable angina

Excludes *angina (pectoris) (413.9)*
decubitus (413.0)

● 411.8 **Other**

411.81 **Acute coronary occlusion without myocardial infarction**
Acute coronary (artery):
embolism without or not resulting in myocardial infarction
obstruction without or not resulting in myocardial infarction
occlusion without or not resulting in myocardial infarction
thrombosis without or not resulting in myocardial infarction

Excludes *obstruction without infarction due to atherosclerosis (414.00–414.07)* ⬅
occlusion without infarction due to atherosclerosis (414.00–414.07) ⬅

❑ 411.89 **Other**
Coronary insufficiency (acute)
Subendocardial ischemia

412 **Old myocardial infarction**
Healed myocardial infarction
Past myocardial infarction diagnosed on ECG [EKG] or other special investigation, but currently presenting no symptoms

● 413 **Angina pectoris**

413.0 **Angina decubitus**
Nocturnal angina

413.1 **Prinzmetal angina**
Variant angina pectoris

❑ 413.9 **Other and unspecified angina pectoris**
Angina:
NOS
cardiac
of effort
Anginal syndrome
Status anginosus
Stenocardia
Syncope anginosa

Excludes *preinfarction angina (411.1)*

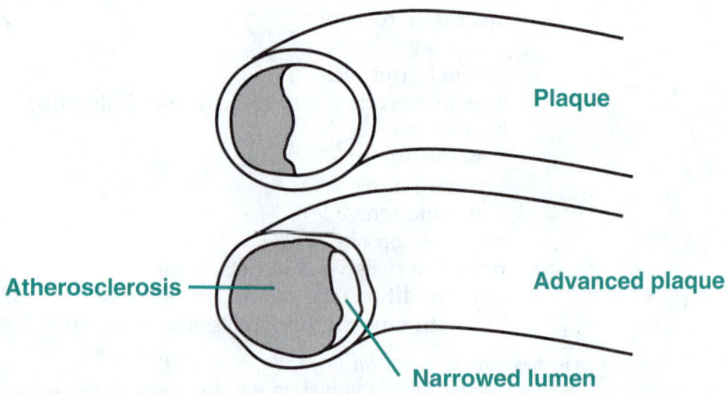

Figure 7–3 Atherosclerosis. (From Buck CJ: Step-by-Step Medical Coding, 3rd ed. Philadelphia, WB Saunders, 2000, p. 164.)

Item 7–8 Classification is based on the location of the atherosclerosis. "Of native coronary artery" indicates the atherosclerosis is within an original heart artery. "Of autologous vein bypass graft" indicates that the atherosclerosis is within a vein graft that was taken from within the patient. "Of nonautologous biological bypass graft" indicates the atherosclerosis is within a vessel grafted from other than the patient. "Of artery bypass graft" indicates the atherosclerosis is within an artery that was grafted from within the patient.

● 414 **Other forms of chronic ischemic heart disease**

Excludes *arteriosclerotic cardiovascular disease [ASCVD] (429.2)*
cardiovascular:
arteriosclerosis or sclerosis (429.2)
degeneration or disease (429.2)

● 414.0 **Coronary atherosclerosis**
Arteriosclerotic heart disease [ASHD]
Atherosclerotic heart disease
Coronary (artery):
arteriosclerosis
arteritis or endarteritis
atheroma
sclerosis
stricture

Excludes *embolism of graft (996.72)*
occlusion NOS of graft (996.72)
thrombus of graft (996.72)

❑ 414.00 **Of unspecified type of vessel, native or graft**

414.01 **Of native coronary artery**

414.02 **Of autologous biological bypass graft**

414.03 **Of nonautologous biological bypass graft**

414.04 **Of artery bypass graft**
Internal mammary artery

414.05 **Of unspecified type of bypass graft**
Bypass graft NOS

414.06 Of native coronary artery of transplanted heart

414.07 Of bypass graft (artery) (vein) of transplanted heart

414.1 Aneurysm and dissection of heart

414.10 Aneurysm of heart (wall)
Aneurysm (arteriovenous):
mural
ventricular

414.11 Aneurysm of coronary vessels
Aneurysm (arteriovenous) of coronary vessels

414.12 Dissection of coronary artery

414.19 Other aneurysm of heart
Arteriovenous fistula, acquired, of heart

414.8 Other specified forms of chronic ischemic heart disease
Chronic coronary insufficiency
Ischemia, myocardial (chronic)
Any condition classifiable to 410 specified as chronic, or presenting with symptoms after 8 weeks from date of infarction

Excludes *coronary insufficiency (acute) (411.89)*

414.9 Chronic ischemic heart disease, unspecified
Ischemic heart disease NOS

DISEASES OF PULMONARY CIRCULATION (415–417)

415 Acute pulmonary heart disease

415.0 Acute cor pulmonale

Excludes *cor pulmonale NOS (416.9)*

415.1 Pulmonary embolism and infarction
Pulmonary (artery) (vein):
apoplexy
embolism
infarction (hemorrhagic)
thrombosis

Excludes *that complicating:*
abortion (634–638 with .6, 639.6)
ectopic or molar pregnancy (639.6)
pregnancy, childbirth, or the puerperium (673.0–673.8)

415.11 Iatrogenic pulmonary embolism and infarction

415.19 Other

416 Chronic pulmonary heart disease

416.0 Primary pulmonary hypertension
Idiopathic pulmonary arteriosclerosis
Pulmonary hypertension (essential) (idiopathic) (primary)

416.1 Kyphoscoliotic heart disease

416.8 Other chronic pulmonary heart diseases
Pulmonary hypertension, secondary

416.9 Chronic pulmonary heart disease, unspecified
Chronic cardiopulmonary disease
Cor pulmonale (chronic) NOS

417 Other diseases of pulmonary circulation

417.0 Arteriovenous fistula of pulmonary vessels

Excludes *congenital arteriovenous fistula (747.3)*

417.1 Aneurysm of pulmonary artery

Excludes *congenital aneurysm (747.3)*

417.8 Other specified diseases of pulmonary circulation
Pulmonary:
arteritis
endarteritis
Rupture of pulmonary vessel
Stricture of pulmonary vessel

417.9 Unspecified disease of pulmonary circulation

OTHER FORMS OF HEART DISEASE (420–429)

420 Acute pericarditis

Includes: acute:
mediastinopericarditis
myopericarditis
pericardial effusion
pleuropericarditis
pneumopericarditis

Excludes *acute rheumatic pericarditis (391.0)*
postmyocardial infarction syndrome [Dressler's] (411.0)

420.0 Acute pericarditis in diseases classified elsewhere

Code first underlying disease, as:
actinomycosis (039.8)
amebiasis (006.8)
nocardiosis (039.8)
tuberculosis (017.9)
uremia (585)

Excludes *pericarditis (acute) (in):*
Coxsackie (virus) (074.21)
gonococcal (098.83)
histoplasmosis (115.0–115.9 with fifth-digit 3)
meningococcal infection (036.41)
syphilitic (093.81)

420.9 Other and unspecified acute pericarditis

420.90 Acute pericarditis, unspecified
Pericarditis (acute):
NOS
infective NOS
sicca

420.91 Acute idiopathic pericarditis
Pericarditis, acute:
benign
nonspecific
viral

420.99 Other
Pericarditis (acute):
pneumococcal
purulent
staphylococcal
streptococcal
suppurative
Pneumopyopericardium
Pyopericardium

Excludes *pericarditis in diseases classified elsewhere (420.0)*

421 Acute and subacute endocarditis

421.0 Acute and subacute bacterial endocarditis
Endocarditis (acute) (chronic) (subacute):
bacterial
infective NOS
lenta
malignant
purulent
septic
ulcerative
vegetative
Infective aneurysm
Subacute bacterial endocarditis [SBE]

Use additional code, if desired, to identify infectious organism [e.g., Streptococcus 041.0, Staphylococcus 041.1]

ICD-9-CM 400-499 Vol. 1

●❑ **421.1** ***Acute and subacute infective endocarditis in diseases classified elsewhere***

Code first underlying disease, as:
blastomycosis (116.0)
Q fever (083.0)
typhoid (fever) (002.0)

Excludes *endocarditis (in):*
Coxsackie (virus) (074.22)
gonococcal (098.84)
histoplasmosis (115.0–115.9 with fifth-digit 4)
meningococcal infection (036.42)
monilial (112.81)

❑ **421.9 Acute endocarditis, unspecified**
Endocarditis, acute or subacute
Myoendocarditis, acute or subacute
Periendocarditis, acute or subacute

Excludes *acute rheumatic endocarditis (391.1)*

● **422 Acute myocarditis**

Excludes *acute rheumatic myocarditis (391.2)*

●❑ **422.0** ***Acute myocarditis in diseases classified elsewhere***

Code first underlying disease, as:
myocarditis (acute):
influenzal (487.8)
tuberculous (017.9)

Excludes *myocarditis (acute) (due to):*
aseptic, of newborn (074.23)
Coxsackie (virus) (074.23)
diphtheritic (032.82)
meningococcal infection (036.43)
syphilitic (093.82)
toxoplasmosis (130.3)

● **422.9 Other and unspecified acute myocarditis**

❑ **422.90 Acute myocarditis, unspecified**
Acute or subacute (interstitial) myocarditis

422.91 Idiopathic myocarditis
Myocarditis (acute or subacute):
Fiedler's
giant cell
isolated (diffuse) (granulomatous)
nonspecific granulomatous

422.92 Septic myocarditis
Myocarditis, acute or subacute:
pneumococcal
staphylococcal

Use additional code to identify infectious organism [e.g., Staphylococcus 041.1]

Excludes *myocarditis, acute or subacute:*
in bacterial diseases classified elsewhere (422.0)
streptococcal (391.2)

422.93 Toxic myocarditis

❑ **422.99 Other**

● **423 Other diseases of pericardium**

Excludes *that specified as rheumatic (393)*

423.0 Hemopericardium

423.1 Adhesive pericarditis
Adherent pericardium
Fibrosis of pericardium
Milk spots
Pericarditis:
adhesive
obliterative
Soldiers' patches

423.2 Constrictive pericarditis
Concato's disease
Pick's disease of heart (and liver)

❑ **423.8 Other specified diseases of pericardium**
Calcification of pericardium
Fistula of pericardium

❑ **423.9 Unspecified disease of pericardium**

● **424 Other diseases of endocardium**

Excludes *bacterial endocarditis (421.0–421.9)*
rheumatic endocarditis (391.1, 394.0–397.9)
syphilitic endocarditis (093.20–093.24)

424.0 Mitral valve disorders
Mitral (valve):
incompetence NOS of specified cause, except rheumatic
insufficiency NOS of specified cause, except rheumatic
regurgitation NOS of specified cause, except rheumatic

Excludes *mitral (valve):*
disease (394.9)
failure (394.9)
stenosis (394.0)
the listed conditions:
specified as rheumatic (394.1)
unspecified as to cause but with mention of:
diseases of aortic valve (396.0–396.9)
mitral stenosis or obstruction (394.2)

424.1 Aortic valve disorders
Aortic (valve):
incompetence NOS of specified cause, except rheumatic
insufficiency NOS of specified cause, except rheumatic
regurgitation NOS of specified cause, except rheumatic
stenosis NOS of specified cause, except rheumatic

Excludes *hypertrophic subaortic stenosis (425.1)*
that specified as rheumatic (395.0–395.9)
that of unspecified cause but with mention of diseases of mitral valve (396.0–396.9)

424.2 Tricuspid valve disorders, specified as nonrheumatic
Tricuspid valve:
incompetence of specified cause, except rheumatic
insufficiency of specified cause, except rheumatic
regurgitation of specified cause, except rheumatic
stenosis of specified cause, except rheumatic

Excludes *rheumatic or of unspecified cause (397.0)*

424.3 Pulmonary valve disorders
Pulmonic:
incompetence NOS
insufficiency NOS
regurgitation NOS
stenosis NOS

Excludes *that specified as rheumatic (397.1)*

● **424.9 Endocarditis, valve unspecified**

❑ **424.90 Endocarditis, valve unspecified, unspecified cause**
Endocarditis (chronic):
NOS
nonbacterial thrombotic
Valvular:
incompetence of unspecified valve, unspecified cause
insufficiency of unspecified valve, unspecified cause
regurgitation of unspecified valve, unspecified cause
stenosis of unspecified valve, unspecified cause
Valvulitis (chronic)

●❑ 424.91 *Endocarditis in diseases classified elsewhere*
Code first underlying disease, as:
atypical verrucous endocarditis [Libman-Sacks] (710.0)
disseminated lupus erythematosus (710.0)
tuberculosis (017.9)
Excludes *syphilitic (093.20–093.24)*

❑ 424.99 **Other**
Any condition classifiable to 424.90 with specified cause, except rheumatic
Excludes *endocardial fibroelastosis (425.3)*
that specified as rheumatic (397.9)

● 425 **Cardiomyopathy**
Includes: myocardiopathy

425.0 **Endomyocardial fibrosis**

425.1 **Hypertrophic obstructive cardiomyopathy**
Hypertrophic subaortic stenosis (idiopathic)

425.2 **Obscure cardiomyopathy of Africa**
Becker's disease
Idiopathic mural endomyocardial disease

425.3 **Endocardial fibroelastosis**
Elastomyofibrosis

❑ 425.4 **Other primary cardiomyopathies**
Cardiomyopathy:
NOS
congestive
constrictive
familial
hypertrophic
idiopathic
nonobstructive
obstructive
restrictive
Cardiovascular collagenosis

425.5 **Alcoholic cardiomyopathy**

● 425.7 *Nutritional and metabolic cardiomyopathy*
Code first underlying disease, as:
amyloidosis (277.3)
beriberi (265.0)
cardiac glycogenosis (271.0)
mucopolysaccharidosis (277.5)
thyrotoxicosis (242.0–242.9)
Excludes *gouty tophi of heart (274.82)*

●❑ 425.8 *Cardiomyopathy in other diseases classified elsewhere*
Code first underlying disease, as:
Friedreich's ataxia (334.0)
myotonia atrophica (359.2)
progressive muscular dystrophy (359.1)
sarcoidosis (135)
Excludes *cardiomyopathy in Chagas' disease (086.0)*

❑ 425.9 **Secondary cardiomyopathy, unspecified**

● 426 **Conduction disorders**

426.0 **Atrioventricular block, complete**
Third degree atrioventricular block

● 426.1 **Atrioventricular block, other and unspecified**

❑ 426.10 **Atrioventricular block, unspecified**
Atrioventricular [AV] block (incomplete) (partial)

426.11 **First degree atrioventricular block**
Incomplete atrioventricular block, first degree
Prolonged P-R interval NOS

426.12 **Mobitz (type) II atrioventricular block**
Incomplete atrioventricular block:
Mobitz (type) II
second degree, Mobitz (type) II

❑ 426.13 **Other second degree atrioventricular block**
Incomplete atrioventricular block:
Mobitz (type) I [Wenckebach's]
second degree:
NOS
Mobitz (type) I
with 2:1 atrioventricular response [block]
Wenckebach's phenomenon

426.2 **Left bundle branch hemiblock**
Block:
left anterior fascicular
left posterior fascicular

❑ 426.3 **Other left bundle branch block**
Left bundle branch block:
NOS
anterior fascicular with posterior fascicular
complete
main stem

426.4 **Right bundle branch block**

● 426.5 **Bundle branch block, other and unspecified**

❑ 426.50 **Bundle branch block, unspecified**

426.51 **Right bundle branch block and left posterior fascicular block**

426.52 **Right bundle branch block and left anterior fascicular block**

❑ 426.53 **Other bilateral bundle branch block**
Bifascicular block NOS
Bilateral bundle branch block NOS
Right bundle branch with left bundle branch block (incomplete) (main stem)

426.54 **Trifascicular block**

❑ 426.6 **Other heart block**
Intraventricular block:
NOS
diffuse
myofibrillar
Sinoatrial block
Sinoauricular block

426.7 **Anomalous atrioventricular excitation**
Atrioventricular conduction:
accelerated
accessory
pre-excitation
Ventricular pre-excitation
Wolff-Parkinson-White syndrome

● 426.8 **Other specified conduction disorders**

426.81 **Lown-Ganong-Levine syndrome**
Syndrome of short P-R interval, normal QRS complexes, and supraventricular tachycardias

❑ 426.89 **Other**
Dissociation:
atrioventricular [AV]
interference
isorhythmic
Nonparoxysmal AV nodal tachycardia

❑ 426.9 **Conduction disorder, unspecified**
Heart block NOS
Stokes-Adams syndrome

● 427 **Cardiac dysrhythmias**
Excludes *that complicating:*
abortion (634–638 with .7, 639.8)
ectopic or molar pregnancy (639.8)
labor or delivery (668.1, 669.4)

ICD-9-CM 400-499 Vol. 1

427.0 Paroxysmal supraventricular tachycardia
Paroxysmal tachycardia:
atrial [PAT]
atrioventricular [AV]
junctional
nodal

427.1 Paroxysmal ventricular tachycardia
Ventricular tachycardia (paroxysmal)

❑**427.2 Paroxysmal tachycardia, unspecified**
Bouveret-Hoffmann syndrome
Paroxysmal tachycardia:
NOS
essential

● **427.3 Atrial fibrillation and flutter**

427.31 Atrial fibrillation

427.32 Atrial flutter

● **427.4 Ventricular fibrillation and flutter**

427.41 Ventricular fibrillation

427.42 Ventricular flutter

❑**427.5 Cardiac arrest**
Cardiorespiratory arrest

● **427.6 Premature beats**

❑**427.60 Premature beats, unspecified**
Ectopic beats
Extrasystoles
Extrasystolic arrhythmia
Premature contractions or systoles NOS

427.61 Supraventricular premature beats
Atrial premature beats, contractions, or systoles

❑**427.69 Other**
Ventricular premature beats, contractions, or systoles

● **427.8 Other specified cardiac dysrhythmias**

427.81 Sinoatrial node dysfunction
Sinus bradycardia:
persistent
severe
Syndrome:
sick sinus
tachycardia-bradycardia

Excludes *sinus bradycardia NOS (427.89)*

❑**427.89 Other**
Rhythm disorder:
coronary sinus
ectopic
nodal
Wandering (atrial) pacemaker

Excludes *carotid sinus syncope (337.0)*
neonatal bradycardia (779.81)
neonatal tachycardia (779.82)
reflex bradycardia (337.0)
tachycardia NOS (785.0)

❑**427.9 Cardiac dysrhythmia, unspecified**
Arrhythmia (cardiac) NOS

● **428 Heart failure**

Excludes *rheumatic (398.91)*
that complicating:
abortion (634–638 with .7, 639.8)
ectopic or molar pregnancy (639.8)
labor or delivery (668.1, 669.4)

Code, if applicable, heart failure due to hypertension first (402.0–402.9, with fifth-digit 1 or 404.0–404.9 with fifth-digit 1 or 3)

❑**428.0 Congestive heart failure, unspecified**
Congestive heart disease
Right heart failure (secondary to left heart failure)

Excludes *fluid overload NOS (276.6)*

428.1 Left heart failure
Acute edema of lung with heart disease NOS or heart failure
Acute pulmonary edema with heart disease NOS or heart failure
Cardiac asthma
Left ventricular failure

● **428.2 Systolic heart failure**

Excludes *combined systolic and diastolic heart failure (428.40–428.43)*

❑**428.20 Unspecified**

428.21 Acute

428.22 Chronic

428.23 Acute on chronic

● **428.3 Diastolic heart failure**

Excludes *combined systolic and diastolic heart failure (428.40–428.43)*

❑**428.30 Unspecified**

428.31 Acute

428.32 Chronic

428.33 Acute on chronic

● **428.4 Combined systolic and diastolic heart failure**

❑**428.40 Unspecified**

428.41 Acute

428.42 Chronic

428.43 Acute on chronic

❑**428.9 Heart failure, unspecified**
Cardiac failure NOS
Heart failure NOS
Myocardial failure NOS
Weak heart

● **429 Ill-defined descriptions and complications of heart disease**

❑**429.0 Myocarditis, unspecified**
Myocarditis (with mention of arteriosclerosis):
NOS (with mention of arteriosclerosis)
chronic (interstitial) (with mention of arteriosclerosis)
fibroid (with mention of arteriosclerosis)
senile (with mention of arteriosclerosis)

Use additional code to identify presence of arteriosclerosis

Excludes *acute or subacute (422.0–422.9)*
rheumatic (398.0)
acute (391.2)
that due to hypertension (402.0–402.9)

429.1 Myocardial degeneration
Degeneration of heart or myocardium (with mention of arteriosclerosis):
fatty (with mention of arteriosclerosis)
mural (with mention of arteriosclerosis)
muscular (with mention of arteriosclerosis)
Myocardial (with mention of arteriosclerosis):
degeneration (with mention of arteriosclerosis)
disease (with mention of arteriosclerosis)

Use additional code to identify presence of arteriosclerosis

Excludes *that due to hypertension (402.0–402.9)*

❑**429.2 Cardiovascular disease, unspecified**
Arteriosclerotic cardiovascular disease [ASCVD]
Cardiovascular arteriosclerosis
Cardiovascular:
degeneration (with mention of arteriosclerosis)
disease (with mention of arteriosclerosis)
sclerosis (with mention of arteriosclerosis)

Use additional code to identify presence of arteriosclerosis

Excludes *that due to hypertension (402.0–402.9)*

429.3 Cardiomegaly
Cardiac:
dilatation
hypertrophy
Ventricular dilatation
Excludes *that due to hypertension (402.0–402.9)*

429.4 Functional disturbances following cardiac surgery
Cardiac insufficiency following cardiac surgery or due to prosthesis
Heart failure following cardiac surgery or due to prosthesis
Postcardiotomy syndrome
Postvalvulotomy syndrome
Excludes *cardiac failure in the immediate postoperative period (997.1)*

429.5 Rupture of chordae tendineae

429.6 Rupture of papillary muscle

● **429.7 Certain sequelae of myocardial infarction, not elsewhere classified**
Use additional code to identify the associated myocardial infarction:
with onset of 8 weeks or less (410.00–410.92)
with onset of more than 8 weeks (414.8)
Excludes *congenital defects of heart (745, 746)*
coronary aneurysm (414.11)
disorders of papillary muscle (429.6, 429.81)
postmyocardial infarction syndrome (411.0)
rupture of chordae tendineae (429.5)

429.71 Acquired cardiac septal defect
Excludes *acute septal infarction (410.00–410.92)*

❑ **429.79 Other**
Mural thrombus (atrial) (ventricular) acquired, following myocardial infarction

● **429.8 Other ill-defined heart diseases**

❑ **429.81 Other disorders of papillary muscle**
Papillary muscle:
atrophy
degeneration
dysfunction
incompetence
incoordination
scarring

429.82 Hyperkinetic heart disease

❑ **429.89 Other**
Carditis
Excludes *that due to hypertension (402.0–402.9)*

❑ **429.9 Heart disease, unspecified**
Heart disease (organic) NOS
Morbus cordis NOS
Excludes *that due to hypertension (402.0–402.9)*

CEREBROVASCULAR DISEASE (430–438)

Includes: with mention of hypertension (conditions classifiable to 401–405)

Use additional code to identify presence of hypertension

Excludes *any condition classifiable to 430–434, 436, 437 occurring during pregnancy, childbirth, or the puerperium, or specified as puerperal (674.0)*
iatrogenic cerebrovascular infarction or hemorrhage (997.02)

430 Subarachnoid hemorrhage
Meningeal hemorrhage
Ruptured:
berry aneurysm
(congenital) cerebral aneurysm NOS
Excludes *syphilitic ruptured cerebral aneurysm (094.87)*

431 Intracerebral hemorrhage
Hemorrhage (of):
basilar
bulbar
cerebellar
cerebral
cerebromeningeal
cortical
Hemorrhage (of):
internal capsule
intrapontine
pontine
subcortical
ventricular
Rupture of blood vessel in brain

● **432 Other and unspecified intracranial hemorrhage**

432.0 Nontraumatic extradural hemorrhage
Nontraumatic epidural hemorrhage

432.1 Subdural hemorrhage
Subdural hematoma, nontraumatic

❑ **432.9 Unspecified intracranial hemorrhage**
Intracranial hemorrhage NOS

● **433 Occlusion and stenosis of precerebral arteries**

The following fifth-digit subclassification is for use with category 433:
0 without mention of cerebral infarction
1 with cerebral infarction

Includes: embolism of basilar, carotid, and vertebral arteries
narrowing of basilar, carotid, and vertebral arteries
obstruction of basilar, carotid, and vertebral arteries
thrombosis of basilar, carotid, and vertebral arteries
Excludes *insufficiency NOS of precerebral arteries (435.0–435.9)*

● **433.0 Basilar artery**

● **433.1 Carotid artery**

● **433.2 Vertebral artery**

● **433.3 Multiple and bilateral**

● ❑ **433.8 Other specified precerebral artery**

● ❑ **433.9 Unspecified precerebral artery**
Precerebral artery NOS

● **434 Occlusion of cerebral arteries**

The following fifth-digit subclassification is for use with category 434:
0 without mention of cerebral infarction
1 with cerebral infarction

● **434.0 Cerebral thrombosis**
Thrombosis of cerebral arteries

● **434.1 Cerebral embolism**

● ❑ **434.9 Cerebral artery occlusion, unspecified**

● **435 Transient cerebral ischemia**

Includes: cerebrovascular insufficiency (acute) with transient focal neurological signs and symptoms
insufficiency of basilar, carotid, and vertebral arteries
spasm of cerebral arteries
Excludes *acute cerebrovascular insufficiency NOS (437.1)*
that due to any condition classifiable to 433 (433.0–433.9)

435.0 **Basilar artery syndrome**

435.1 **Vertebral artery syndrome**

435.2 **Subclavian steal syndrome**

435.3 **Vertebrobasilar artery syndrome**

❑435.8 **Other specified transient cerebral ischemias**

❑435.9 **Unspecified transient cerebral ischemia**
Impending cerebrovascular accident
Intermittent cerebral ischemia
Transient ischemic attack [TIA]

436 **Acute, but ill-defined, cerebrovascular disease**
Apoplexy, apoplectic:
NOS
attack
cerebral
seizure
Cerebral seizure
Cerebrovascular accident [CVA] NOS
Stroke

Excludes *any condition classifiable to categories 430–435*
postoperative cerebrovascular accident (997.02)

●437 **Other and ill-defined cerebrovascular disease**

437.0 **Cerebral atherosclerosis**
Atheroma of cerebral arteries
Cerebral arteriosclerosis

❑437.1 **Other generalized ischemic cerebrovascular disease**
Acute cerebrovascular insufficiency NOS
Cerebral ischemia (chronic)

437.2 **Hypertensive encephalopathy**

437.3 **Cerebral aneurysm, nonruptured**
Internal carotid artery, intracranial portion
Internal carotid artery NOS

Excludes *congenital cerebral aneurysm, nonruptured (747.81)*
internal carotid artery, extracranial portion (442.81)

437.4 **Cerebral arteritis**

437.5 **Moyamoya disease**

437.6 **Nonpyogenic thrombosis of intracranial venous sinus**

Excludes *pyogenic (325)*

437.7 **Transient global amnesia**

❑437.8 **Other**

❑437.9 **Unspecified**
Cerebrovascular disease or lesion NOS

●438 **Late effects of cerebrovascular disease**

Note: This category is to be used to indicate conditions in 430–437 as the cause of late effects. The "late effects" include conditions specified as such, or as sequelae, which may occur at any time after the onset of the causal condition.

438.0 **Cognitive deficits**

●438.1 **Speech and language deficits**

❑438.10 **Speech and language deficit, unspecified**

438.11 **Aphasia**

438.12 **Dysphasia**

❑438.19 **Other speech and language deficits**

●438.2 **Hemiplegia/hemiparesis**

❑438.20 **Hemiplegia affecting unspecified side**

438.21 **Hemiplegia affecting dominant side**

438.22 **Hemiplegia affecting nondominant side**

●438.3 **Monoplegia of upper limb**

❑438.30 **Monoplegia of upper limb affecting unspecified side**

438.31 **Monoplegia of upper limb affecting dominant side**

438.32 **Monoplegia of upper limb affecting nondominant side**

●438.4 **Monoplegia of lower limb**

❑438.40 **Monoplegia of lower limb affecting unspecified side**

438.41 **Monoplegia of lower limb affecting dominant side**

438.42 **Monoplegia of lower limb affecting nondominant side**

●438.5 **Other paralytic syndrome**

Use additional code to identify type of paralytic syndrome, such as:
locked-in state (344.81)
quadriplegia (344.00–344.09)

438.6 **Alterations of sensations**

Use additional code to identify the altered sensation

438.7 **Disturbances of vision**

Use additional code to identify the visual disturbance

Excludes *late effects of cerebrovascular accident with:*
hemiplegia/hemiparesis (438.20–438.22)
monoplegia of lower limb (438.40–438.42)
monoplegia of upper limb (438.30–438.32)

❑438.50 **Other paralytic syndrome affecting unspecified side**

438.51 **Other paralytic syndrome affecting dominant side**

438.52 **Other paralytic syndrome affecting nondominant side**

438.53 **Other paralytic syndrome, bilateral**

●438.8 **Other late effects of cerebrovascular disease**

438.81 **Apraxia**

438.82 **Dysphagia**

438.83 **Facial weakness**
Facial droop

438.84 **Ataxia**

438.85 **Vertigo**

❑438.89 **Other late effects of cerebrovascular disease**

❑438.9 **Unspecified late effects of cerebrovascular disease**
Use additional code to identify the late effect

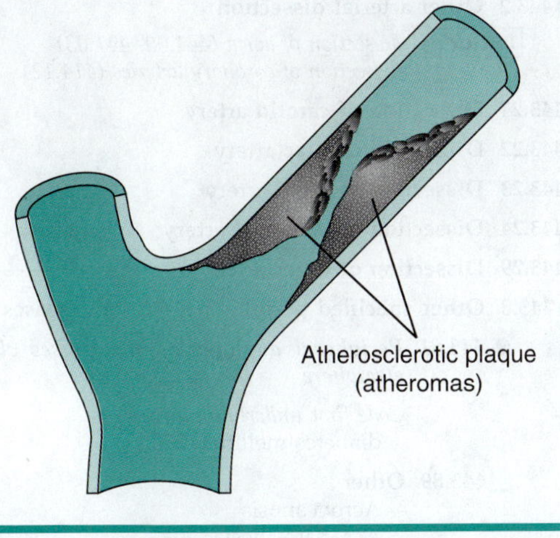

Figure 7–4 Atherosclerotic plaque.

Item 7–9 Classification is based on the location of the atherosclerosis.

DISEASES OF ARTERIES, ARTERIOLES, AND CAPILLARIES (440–448)

● **440 Atherosclerosis**

Includes: arteriolosclerosis
arteriosclerosis (obliterans) (senile)
arteriosclerotic vascular disease
atheroma
degeneration:
arterial
arteriovascular
vascular
endarteritis deformans or obliterans
senile:
arteritis
endarteritis

Excludes *atheroembolism (445.01–445.89)*
atherosclerosis of bypass graft of the extremities (440.30–440.32)

440.0 Of aorta

440.1 Of renal artery

Excludes *atherosclerosis of renal arterioles (403.00–403.91)*

● **440.2 Of native arteries of the extremities**

Excludes *atherosclerosis of bypass graft of the extremities (440.30–440.32)*

❑ **440.20 Atherosclerosis of the extremities, unspecified**

440.21 Atherosclerosis of the extremities with intermittent claudication

440.22 Atherosclerosis of the extremities with rest pain
Includes any condition classifiable to 440.21

440.23 Atherosclerosis of the extremities with ulceration
Includes any condition classifiable to 440.21–440.22
Use additional code for any associated ulceration (707.10–707.9)

440.24 Atherosclerosis of the extremities with gangrene
Includes any condition classifiable to 440.21, 440.22, and 440.23 with ischemic gangrene 785.4

Excludes *gas gangrene (040.0)*

❑ **440.29 Other**

● **440.3 Of bypass graft of the extremities**

Excludes *atherosclerosis of native artery of the extremity (440.21–440.24)*
embolism [occlusion NOS] [thrombus] of graft (996.74)

❑ **440.30 Of unspecified graft**

440.31 Of autologous vein bypass graft

440.32 Of nonautologous vein bypass graft

❑ **440.8 Of other specified arteries**

Excludes *basilar (433.0)*
carotid (433.1)
cerebral (437.0)
coronary (414.00–414.07) ⟸
mesenteric (557.1)
precerebral (433.0–433.9)
pulmonary (416.0)
vertebral (433.2)

❑ **440.9 Generalized and unspecified atherosclerosis**
Arteriosclerotic vascular disease NOS

Excludes *arteriosclerotic cardiovascular disease [ASCVD] (429.2)*

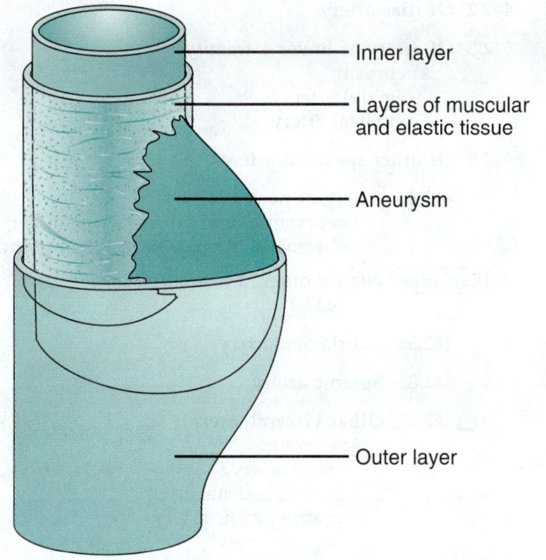

Figure 7–5 An aneurysm is an enclosed swelling on the wall of the vessel.

Item 7–10 Rupture is the tearing of the aneurysm.

● **441 Aortic aneurysm and dissection**

Excludes *syphilitic aortic aneurysm (093.0)*
traumatic aortic aneurysm (901.0, 902.0)

● **441.0 Dissection of aorta**

❑ **441.00 Unspecified site**

441.01 Thoracic

441.02 Abdominal

441.03 Thoracoabdominal

441.1 Thoracic aneurysm, ruptured

441.2 Thoracic aneurysm without mention of rupture

441.3 Abdominal aneurysm, ruptured

441.4 Abdominal aneurysm without mention of rupture

❑ **441.5 Aortic aneurysm of unspecified site, ruptured**
Rupture of aorta NOS

441.6 Thoracoabdominal aneurysm, ruptured

441.7 Thoracoabdominal aneurysm, without mention of rupture

❑ **441.9 Aortic aneurysm of unspecified site without mention of rupture**
Aneurysm
Dilatation of aorta
Hyaline necrosis of aorta

● **442 Other aneurysm**

Includes: aneurysm (ruptured) (cirsoid) (false) (varicose)
aneurysmal varix

Excludes *arteriovenous aneurysm or fistula:*
acquired (447.0)
congenital (747.60–747.69)
traumatic (900.0–904.9)

442.0 Of artery of upper extremity

442.1 Of renal artery

442.2 Of iliac artery

442.3 Of artery of lower extremity
Aneurysm:
femoral artery
popliteal artery

● **442.8 Of other specified artery**

442.81 Artery of neck
Aneurysm of carotid artery (common) (external) (internal, extracranial portion)

Excludes *internal carotid artery, intracranial portion (437.3)*

442.82 Subclavian artery

442.83 Splenic artery

❑ **442.84 Other visceral artery**
Aneurysm:
celiac artery
gastroduodenal artery
gastroepiploic artery
hepatic artery
pancreaticoduodenal artery
superior mesenteric artery

❑ **442.89 Other**
Aneurysm:
mediastinal artery
spinal artery

Excludes *cerebral (nonruptured) (437.3)*
congenital (747.81)
ruptured (430)
coronary (414.11)
heart (414.10)
pulmonary (417.1)

❑ **442.9 Of unspecified site**

● **443 Other peripheral vascular disease**

443.0 Raynaud's syndrome
Raynaud's:
disease
phenomenon (secondary)

Use additional code to identify gangrene (785.4)

443.1 Thromboangiitis obliterans [Buerger's disease]
Presenile gangrene

● **443.2 Other arterial dissection**

Excludes *dissection of aorta (441.00–441.03)*
dissection of coronary arteries (414.12)

443.21 Dissection of carotid artery

443.22 Dissection of iliac artery

443.23 Dissection of renal artery

443.24 Dissection of vertebral artery

❑ **443.29 Dissection of other artery**

● **443.8 Other specified peripheral vascular diseases**

● ***443.81 Peripheral angiopathy in diseases classified elsewhere***

Code first underlying disease, as:
diabetes mellitus (250.7)

❑ **443.89 Other**
Acrocyanosis
Acroparesthesia:
simple [Schultze's type]
vasomotor [Nothnagel's type]
Erythrocyanosis
Erythromelalgia

Excludes *chilblains (991.5)*
frostbite (991.0–991.3)
immersion foot (991.4)

❑ **443.9 Peripheral vascular disease, unspecified**
Intermittent claudication NOS
Peripheral:
angiopathy NOS
vascular disease NOS
Spasm of artery

Excludes *atherosclerosis of the arteries of the extremities (440.20–440.22)*
spasm of cerebral artery (435.0–435.9)

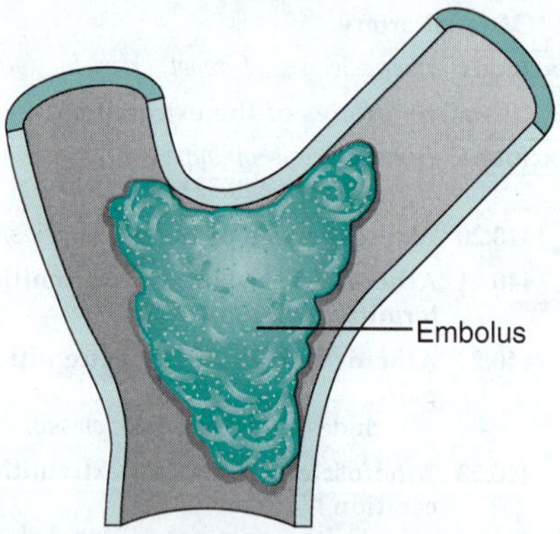

Figure 7–6 An arterial embolism.

Item 7–11 An embolus is a mass of undissolved matter present in the blood that is transported by the blood current. A thrombus is a blood clot that occludes or shuts off a vessel. When a thrombus is dislodged, it becomes an embolus.

● 444 **Arterial embolism and thrombosis**

Includes: infarction:
embolic
thrombotic
occlusion

Excludes *that complicating:*
abortion (634–638 with .6, 639.6)
atheroembolism (445.01–445.89)
ectopic or molar pregnancy (639.6)
pregnancy, childbirth, or the puerperium (673.0–673.8)

444.0 Of abdominal aorta
Aortic bifurcation syndrome
Aortoiliac obstruction
Leriche's syndrome
Saddle embolus

444.1 Of thoracic aorta
Embolism or thrombosis of aorta (thoracic)

● **444.2 Of arteries of the extremities**

444.21 Upper extremity

444.22 Lower extremity
Arterial embolism or thrombosis:
femoral
peripheral NOS
popliteal

Excludes *iliofemoral (444.81)*

● **444.8 Of other specified artery**

444.81 Iliac artery

❑ **444.89 Other**

Excludes *basilar (433.0)*
carotid (433.1)
cerebral (434.0–434.9)
coronary (410.00–410.92)
mesenteric (557.0)
ophthalmic (362.30–362.34)
precerebral (433.0–433.9)
pulmonary (415.19)
renal (593.81)
retinal (362.30–362.34)
vertebral (433.2)

❑ **444.9 Of unspecified artery**

● 445 **Atheroembolism**

Includes: atherothrombotic microembolism
cholesterol embolism

● **445.0 Of extremities**

445.01 Upper extremity

445.02 Lower extremity

● **445.8 Of other sites**

445.81 Kidney

Use additional code for any associated kidney failure (584, 585)

❑ **445.89 Other site**

● 446 **Polyarteritis nodosa and allied conditions**

446.0 Polyarteritis nodosa
Disseminated necrotizing periarteritis
Necrotizing angiitis
Panarteritis (nodosa)
Periarteritis (nodosa)

446.1 Acute febrile mucocutaneous lymph node syndrome [MCLS]
Kawasaki disease

● **446.2 Hypersensitivity angiitis**

Excludes *antiglomerular basement membrane disease without pulmonary hemorrhage (583.89)*

❑ **446.20 Hypersensitivity angiitis, unspecified**

446.21 Goodpasture's syndrome
Antiglomerular basement membrane antibody-mediated nephritis with pulmonary hemorrhage

Use additional code to identify renal disease (583.81)

❑ **446.29 Other specified hypersensitivity angiitis**

446.3 Lethal midline granuloma
Malignant granuloma of face

446.4 Wegener's granulomatosis
Necrotizing respiratory granulomatosis
Wegener's syndrome

446.5 Giant cell arteritis
Cranial arteritis
Horton's disease
Temporal arteritis

446.6 Thrombotic microangiopathy
Moschcowitz's syndrome
Thrombotic thrombocytopenic purpura

446.7 Takayasu's disease
Aortic arch arteritis
Pulseless disease

● 447 **Other disorders of arteries and arterioles**

447.0 Arteriovenous fistula, acquired
Arteriovenous aneurysm, acquired

Excludes *cerebrovascular (437.3)*
coronary (414.19)
pulmonary (417.0)
surgically created arteriovenous shunt or fistula:
complication (996.1, 996.61–996.62)
status or presence (V45.1)
traumatic (900.0–904.9)

447.1 Stricture of artery

447.2 Rupture of artery
Erosion of artery
Fistula, except arteriovenous, of artery
Ulcer of artery

Excludes *traumatic rupture of artery (900.0–904.9)*

447.3 Hyperplasia of renal artery
Fibromuscular hyperplasia of renal artery

447.4 Celiac artery compression syndrome
Celiac axis syndrome
Marable's syndrome

447.5 Necrosis of artery

❑ **447.6 Arteritis, unspecified**
Aortitis NOS
Endarteritis NOS

Excludes *arteritis, endarteritis:*
aortic arch (446.7)
cerebral (437.4)
coronary (414.00–414.07) ⬅
deformans (440.0–440.9)
obliterans (440.0–440.9)
pulmonary (417.8)
senile (440.0–440.9)
polyarteritis NOS (446.0)
syphilitic aortitis (093.1)

❑ **447.8 Other specified disorders of arteries and arterioles**
Fibromuscular hyperplasia of arteries, except renal

❑ **447.9 Unspecified disorders of arteries and arterioles**

● **448 Disease of capillaries**

448.0 Hereditary hemorrhagic telangiectasia
Rendu-Osler-Weber disease

448.1 Nevus, non-neoplastic
Nevus:
araneus
senile
Nevus:
spider
stellar

Excludes *neoplastic (216.0–216.9)*
port wine (757.32)
strawberry (757.32)

❑ **448.9 Other and unspecified capillary diseases**
Capillary:
hemorrhage
hyperpermeability
thrombosis

Excludes *capillary fragility (hereditary) (287.8)*

DISEASES OF VEINS AND LYMPHATICS, AND OTHER DISEASES OF CIRCULATORY SYSTEM (451–459)

● **451 Phlebitis and thrombophlebitis**

Includes: endophlebitis
inflammation, vein
periphlebitis
suppurative phlebitis

Use additional E code to identify drug, if drug-induced

Excludes *that complicating:*
abortion (634–638 with .7, 639.8)
ectopic or molar pregnancy (639.8)
pregnancy, childbirth, or the puerperium (671.0–671.9)
that due to or following:
implant or catheter device (996.61–996.62)
infusion, perfusion, or transfusion (999.2)

451.0 Of superficial vessels of lower extremities
Saphenous vein (greater) (lesser)

● **451.1 Of deep vessels of lower extremities**

451.11 Femoral vein (deep) (superficial)

❑ **451.19 Other**
Femoropopliteal vein
Popliteal vein
Tibial vein

❑ **451.2 Of lower extremities, unspecified**

● **451.8 Of other sites**

Excludes *intracranial venous sinus (325)*
nonpyogenic (437.6)
portal (vein) (572.1)

451.81 Iliac vein

451.82 Of superficial veins of upper extremities
Antecubital vein
Basilic vein
Cephalic vein

451.83 Of deep veins of upper extremities
Brachial vein
Radial vein
Ulnar vein

❑ **451.84 Of upper extremities, unspecified**

❑ **451.89 Other**
Axillary vein
Jugular vein
Subclavian vein
Thrombophlebitis of breast (Mondor's disease)

❑ **451.9 Of unspecified site**

452 Portal vein thrombosis
Portal (vein) obstruction

Excludes *hepatic vein thrombosis (453.0)*
phlebitis of portal vein (572.1)

● **453 Other venous embolism and thrombosis**

Excludes *that complicating:*
abortion (634–638 with .7, 639.8)
ectopic or molar pregnancy (639.8)
pregnancy, childbirth, or the puerperium (671.0–671.9)
that with inflammation, phlebitis, and thrombophlebitis (451.0–451.9)

453.0 Budd-Chiari syndrome
Hepatic vein thrombosis

453.1 Thrombophlebitis migrans

453.2 Of vena cava

453.3 Of renal vein

❑ **453.8 Of other specified veins**

Excludes *cerebral (434.0–434.9)*
coronary (410.00–410.92)
intracranial venous sinus (325)
nonpyogenic (437.6)
mesenteric (557.0)
portal (452)
precerebral (433.0–433.9)
pulmonary (415.19)

❑ **453.9 Of unspecified site**
Embolism of vein
Thrombosis (vein)

● **454 Varicose veins of lower extremities**

Excludes *that complicating pregnancy, childbirth, or the puerperium (671.0)*

454.0 With ulcer
Varicose ulcer (lower extremity, any part)
Varicose veins with ulcer of lower extremity [any part] or of unspecified site
Any condition classifiable to 454.9 with ulcer or specified as ulcerated

454.1 With inflammation
Stasis dermatitis
Varicose veins with inflammation of lower extremity [any part] or of unspecified site
Any condition classifiable to 454.9 with inflammation or specified as inflamed

454.2 With ulcer and inflammation
Varicose veins with ulcer and inflammation of lower extremity [any part] or of unspecified site
Any condition classifiable to 454.9 with ulcer and inflammation

❑ **454.8 With other complications**
Edema
Pain
Swelling

454.9 Asymptomatic varicose veins
Phlebectasia of lower extremity [any part] or of unspecified site
Varicose veins NOS
Varicose veins of lower extremity [any part] or of unspecified site
Varix of lower extremity [any part] or of unspecified site

455 Hemorrhoids

Includes: hemorrhoids (anus) (rectum)
piles
varicose veins, anus or rectum

Excludes *that complicating pregnancy, childbirth, or the puerperium (671.8)*

455.0 Internal hemorrhoids without mention of complication

455.1 Internal thrombosed hemorrhoids

455.2 Internal hemorrhoids with other complication
Internal hemorrhoids:
bleeding
prolapsed
Internal hemorrhoids:
strangulated
ulcerated

455.3 External hemorrhoids without mention of complication

455.4 External thrombosed hemorrhoids

455.5 External hemorrhoids with other complication
External hemorrhoids:
bleeding
prolapsed
strangulated
ulcerated

455.6 Unspecified hemorrhoids without mention of complication
Hemorrhoids NOS

455.7 Unspecified thrombosed hemorrhoids
Thrombosed hemorrhoids, unspecified whether internal or external

455.8 Unspecified hemorrhoids with other complication
Hemorrhoids, unspecified whether internal or external:
bleeding
prolapsed
strangulated
ulcerated

455.9 Residual hemorrhoidal skin tags
Skin tags, anus or rectum

456 Varicose veins of other sites

456.0 Esophageal varices with bleeding

456.1 Esophageal varices without mention of bleeding

456.2 Esophageal varices in diseases classified elsewhere

Code first underlying disease, as:
cirrhosis of liver (571.0–571.9)
portal hypertension (572.3)

456.20 With bleeding

456.21 Without mention of bleeding

456.3 Sublingual varices

456.4 Scrotal varices
Varicocele

456.5 Pelvic varices
Varices of broad ligament

456.6 Vulval varices
Varices of perineum

Excludes *that complicating pregnancy, childbirth, or the puerperium (671.1)*

456.8 Varices of other sites
Varicose veins of nasal septum (with ulcer)

Excludes *placental varices (656.7)*
retinal varices (362.17)
varicose ulcer of unspecified site (454.0)
varicose veins of unspecified site (454.9)

457 Noninfectious disorders of lymphatic channels

457.0 Postmastectomy lymphedema syndrome
Elephantiasis due to mastectomy
Obliteration of lymphatic vessel due to mastectomy

457.1 Other lymphedema
Elephantiasis (nonfilarial) NOS
Lymphangiectasis
Lymphedema:
acquired (chronic)
praecox
Lymphedema:
secondary
Obliteration, lymphatic vessel

Excludes *elephantiasis (nonfilarial):*
congenital (757.0)
eyelid (374.83)
vulva (624.8)

457.2 Lymphangitis
Lymphangitis:
NOS
chronic
subacute

Excludes *acute lymphangitis (682.0–682.9)*

457.8 Other noninfectious disorders of lymphatic channels
Chylocele (nonfilarial)
Chylous:
ascites
cyst
Lymph node or vessel:
fistula
infarction
rupture

Excludes *chylocele:*
filarial (125.0–125.9)
tunica vaginalis (nonfilarial) (608.84)

457.9 Unspecified noninfectious disorder of lymphatic channels

458 Hypotension

Includes: hypopiesis

Excludes *cardiovascular collapse (785.50)*
maternal hypotension syndrome (669.2)
shock (785.50–785.59)
Shy-Drager syndrome (333.0)

458.0 Orthostatic hypotension
Hypotension:
orthostatic (chronic)
postural

458.1 Chronic hypotension
Permanent idiopathic hypotension

458.2 Iatrogenic hypotension

458.21 Hypotension of hemodialysis
Intra-dialytic hypotension

458.29 Other iatrogenic hypodialysis
Postoperative hypotension

458.8 Other specified hypotension

458.9 Hypotension, unspecified
Hypotension (arterial) NOS

459 Other disorders of circulatory system

459.0 Hemorrhage, unspecified
Rupture of blood vessel NOS
Spontaneous hemorrhage NEC

Excludes *hemorrhage:*
gastrointestinal NOS (578.9)
in newborn NOS (772.9)
secondary or recurrent following trauma (958.2)
traumatic rupture of blood vessel (900.0–904.9)

● **459.1 Postphlebitic syndrome**
Chronic venous hypertension due to deep vein thrombosis

Excludes *chronic venous hypertension without deep vein thrombosis (459.30–459.39)*

459.10 Postphlebetic syndrome without complications
Asymptomatic postphlebetic syndrome
Postphlebetic syndrome NOS

459.11 Postphlebetic syndrome with ulcer

459.12 Postphlebetic syndrome with inflammation

459.13 Postphlebetic syndrome with ulcer and inflammation

❑ **459.19 Postphlebetic syndrome with other complication**

459.2 Compression of vein
Stricture of vein
Vena cava syndrome (inferior) (superior)

● **459.3 Chronic venous hypertension (idiopathic)**
Stasis edema

Excludes *chronic venous hypertension due to deep vein thrombosis (459.10–459.19)*
varicose veins (454.0–454.9)

459.30 Chronic venous hypertension without complications
Asymptomatic chronic venous hypertension
Chronic venous hypertension NOS

459.31 Chronic venous hypertension with ulcer

459.32 Chronic venous hypertension with inflammation

459.33 Chronic venous hypertension with ulcer and inflammation

❑ **459.39 Chronic venous hypertension with other complication**

● **459.8 Other specified disorders of circulatory system**

❑ **459.81 Venous (peripheral) insufficiency, unspecified**
Chronic venous insufficiency NOS

Use additional code for any associated ulceration (707.10–707.9)

❑ **459.89 Other**
Collateral circulation (venous), any site
Phlebosclerosis
Venofibrosis

❑ **459.9 Unspecified circulatory system disorder**

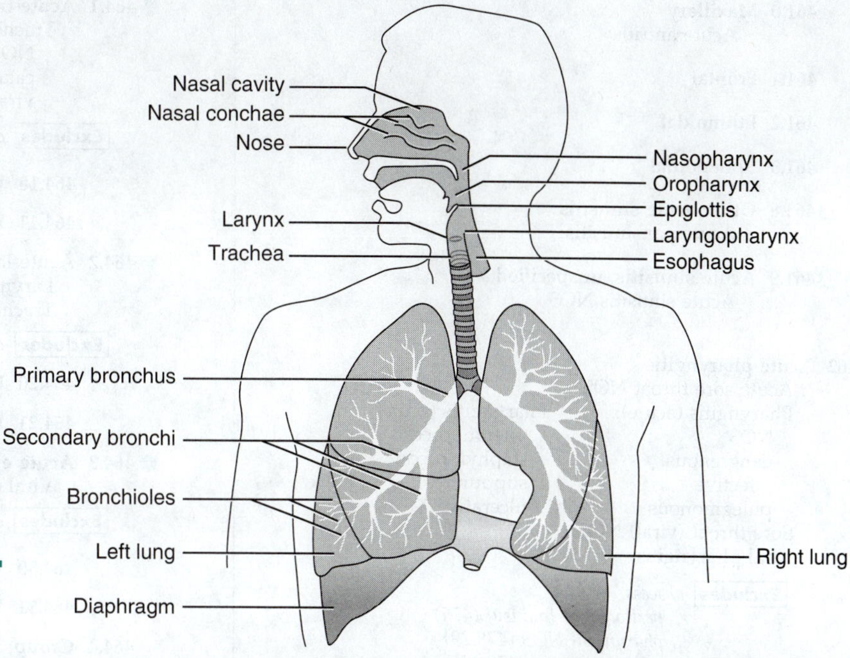

Figure 8–1 Respiratory system. (From Buck CJ: Step-by-Step Medical Coding, 3rd ed. Philadelphia, WB Saunders, 2000, p. 156.)

8. DISEASES OF THE RESPIRATORY SYSTEM (460–519)

Use additional code to identify infectious organism

ACUTE RESPIRATORY INFECTIONS (460–466)

Excludes *pneumonia and influenza (480.0–487.8)*

460 Acute nasopharyngitis [common cold]
Coryza (acute)
Nasal catarrh, acute
Nasopharyngitis:
NOS
acute
infective NOS
Rhinitis:
acute
infective

Excludes *nasopharyngitis, chronic (472.2)*
pharyngitis:
acute or unspecified (462)
chronic (472.1)
rhinitis:
allergic (477.0–477.9)
chronic or unspecified (472.0)
sore throat:
acute or unspecified (462)
chronic (472.1)

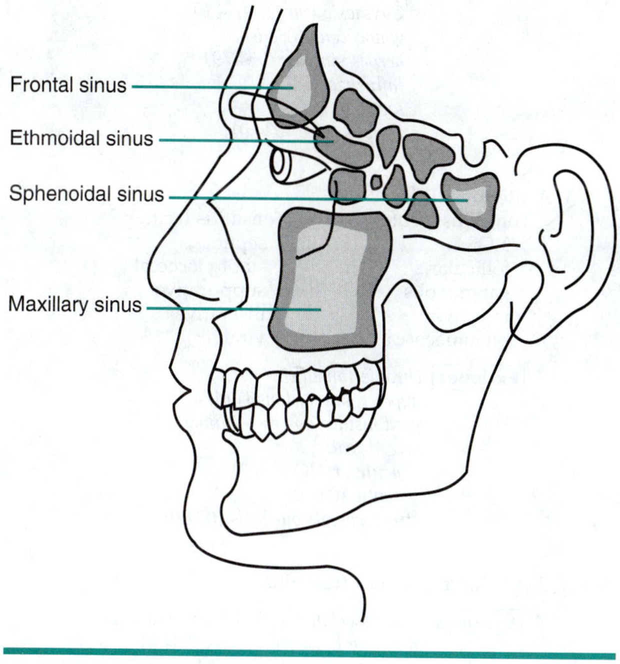

Figure 8–2 Paranasal sinuses. (From Buck CJ: Step-by-Step Medical Coding, 3rd ed. Philadelphia, WB Saunders, 2000, p. 159.)

● **461 Acute sinusitis**

Includes: abscess, acute, of sinus (accessory) (nasal)
empyema, acute, of sinus (accessory) (nasal)
infection, acute, of sinus (accessory) (nasal)
inflammation, acute, of sinus (accessory) (nasal)
suppuration, acute, of sinus (accessory) (nasal)

Excludes *chronic or unspecified sinusitis (473.0–473.9)*

461.0 Maxillary
Acute antritis

461.1 Frontal

461.2 Ethmoidal

461.3 Sphenoidal

❑ **461.8 Other acute sinusitis**
Acute pansinusitis

❑ **461.9 Acute sinusitis, unspecified**
Acute sinusitis NOS

462 Acute pharyngitis
Acute sore throat NOS
Pharyngitis (acute):
NOS
gangrenous
infective
phlegmonous
Pharyngitis (acute):
pneumococcal
staphylococcal
suppurative
ulcerative
Sore throat (viral) NOS
Viral pharyngitis

Excludes *abscess:*
peritonsillar [quinsy] (475)
pharyngeal NOS (478.29)
retropharyngeal (478.24)
chronic pharyngitis (472.1)
infectious mononucleosis (075)
that specified as (due to):
Coxsackie (virus) (074.0)
gonococcus (098.6)
herpes simplex (054.79)
influenza (487.1)
septic (034.0)
streptococcal (034.0)

463 Acute tonsillitis
Tonsillitis (acute):
NOS
follicular
gangrenous
infective
pneumococcal
Tonsillitis (acute):
septic
staphylococcal
suppurative
ulcerative
viral

Excludes *chronic tonsillitis (474.0)*
hypertrophy of tonsils (474.1)
peritonsillar abscess [quinsy] (475)
sore throat:
acute or NOS (462)
septic (034.0)
streptococcal tonsillitis (034.0)

● **464 Acute laryngitis and tracheitis**

Excludes *that associated with influenza (487.1)*
that due to Streptococcus (034.0)

● **464.0 Acute laryngitis**
Laryngitis (acute):
NOS
edematous
Hemophilus influenzae [H. influenzae]
pneumococcal
septic
suppurative
ulcerative

Excludes *chronic laryngitis (476.0–476.1)*
influenzal laryngitis (487.1)

464.00 Without mention of obstruction

464.01 With obstruction

● **464.1 Acute tracheitis**
Tracheitis (acute):
NOS
catarrhal
viral

Excludes *chronic tracheitis (491.8)*

464.10 Without mention of obstruction

464.11 With obstruction

● **464.2 Acute laryngotracheitis**
Laryngotracheitis (acute)
Tracheitis (acute) with laryngitis (acute)

Excludes *chronic laryngotracheitis (476.1)*

464.20 Without mention of obstruction

464.21 With obstruction

● **464.3 Acute epiglottitis**
Viral epiglottitis

Excludes *epiglottitis, chronic (476.1)*

464.30 Without mention of obstruction

464.31 With obstruction

464.4 Croup
Croup syndrome

● **464.5 Supraglottitis, unspecified**

464.50 Without mention of obstruction

464.51 With obstruction

● **465 Acute upper respiratory infections of multiple or unspecified sites**

Excludes *upper respiratory infection due to:*
influenza (487.1)
Streptococcus (034.0)

465.0 Acute laryngopharyngitis

❑ **465.8 Other multiple sites**
Multiple URI

❑ **465.9 Unspecified site**
Acute URI NOS
Upper respiratory infection (acute)

● **466 Acute bronchitis and bronchiolitis**

Includes: that with:
bronchospasm
obstruction

466.0 Acute bronchitis
Bronchitis, acute or subacute:
fibrinous
membranous
pneumococcal
purulent
Bronchitis, acute or subacute:
septic
viral
with tracheitis
Croupous bronchitis
Tracheobronchitis, acute

● **466.1 Acute bronchiolitis**
Bronchiolitis (acute)
Capillary pneumonia

466.11 Acute bronchiolitis due to respiratory syncytial virus (RSV)

❑ **466.19 Acute bronchiolitis due to other infectious organisms**
Use additional code to identify organism

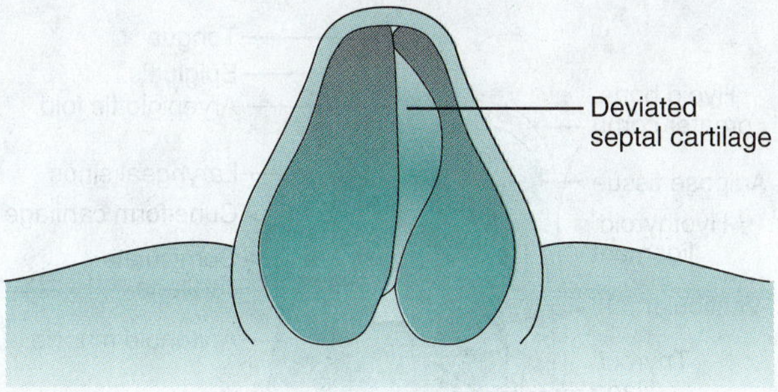

Figure 8–3 Deviated nasal septum.

Item 8-1 A deviated nasal septum is the displacement of the septal cartilage.

OTHER DISEASES OF THE UPPER RESPIRATORY TRACT (470–478)

470 Deviated nasal septum
Deflected septum (nasal) (acquired)
Excludes *congenital (754.0)*

●**471 Nasal polyps**
Excludes *adenomatous polyps (212.0)*

471.0 Polyp of nasal cavity
Polyp:
choanal
nasopharyngeal

471.1 Polypoid sinus degeneration
Woakes' syndrome or ethmoiditis

❑**471.8 Other polyp of sinus**
Polyp of sinus:
accessory
ethmoidal
maxillary
sphenoidal

❑**471.9 Unspecified nasal polyp**
Nasal polyp NOS

●**472 Chronic pharyngitis and nasopharyngitis**

472.0 Chronic rhinitis
Ozena
Rhinitis:
NOS
atrophic
granulomatous
hypertrophic
Rhinitis:
obstructive
purulent
ulcerative
Excludes *allergic rhinitis (477.0–477.9)*

472.1 Chronic pharyngitis
Chronic sore throat
Pharyngitis:
atrophic
granular (chronic)
hypertrophic

472.2 Chronic nasopharyngitis
Excludes *acute or unspecified nasopharyngitis (460)*

●**473 Chronic sinusitis**
Includes: abscess (chronic) of sinus (accessory) (nasal)
empyema (chronic) of sinus (accessory) (nasal)
infection (chronic) of sinus (accessory) (nasal)
suppuration (chronic) of sinus (accessory) (nasal)
Excludes *acute sinusitis (461.0–461.9)*

473.0 Maxillary
Antritis (chronic)

473.1 Frontal

473.2 Ethmoidal
Excludes *Woakes' ethmoiditis (471.1)*

473.3 Sphenoidal

❑**473.8 Other chronic sinusitis**
Pansinusitis (chronic)

❑**473.9 Unspecified sinusitis (chronic)**
Sinusitis (chronic) NOS

●**474 Chronic disease of tonsils and adenoids**

●**474.0 Chronic tonsillitis and adenoiditis**
Excludes *acute or unspecified tonsillitis (463)*

474.00 Chronic tonsillitis

474.01 Chronic adenoiditis

474.02 Chronic tonsillitis and adenoiditis

●**474.1 Hypertrophy of tonsils and adenoids**
Enlargement of tonsils or adenoids
Hyperplasia of tonsils or adenoids
Hypertrophy of tonsils or adenoids
Excludes *that with:*
adenoiditis (474.01)
adenoiditis and tonsillitis (474.02)
tonsillitis (474.00)

474.10 Tonsils with adenoids

474.11 Tonsils alone

474.12 Adenoids alone

474.2 Adenoid vegetations

❑**474.8 Other chronic disease of tonsils and adenoids**
Amygdalolith
Calculus, tonsil
Cicatrix of tonsil (and adenoid)
Tonsillar tag
Ulcer, tonsil

❑**474.9 Unspecified chronic disease of tonsils and adenoids**
Disease (chronic) of tonsils (and adenoids)

475 Peritonsillar abscess
Abscess of tonsil
Peritonsillar cellulitis
Quinsy
Excludes *tonsillitis:*
acute or NOS (463)
chronic (474.0)

●**476 Chronic laryngitis and laryngotracheitis**

476.0 Chronic laryngitis
Laryngitis:
catarrhal
hypertrophic
sicca

ICD-9-CM 400-499 Vol. 1

476.1 **Chronic laryngotracheitis**
Laryngitis, chronic, with tracheitis (chronic)
Tracheitis, chronic, with laryngitis

Excludes *chronic tracheitis (491.8)*
laryngitis and tracheitis, acute or unspecified (464.00–464.51)

● 477 **Allergic rhinitis**

Includes: allergic rhinitis (nonseasonal) (seasonal)
hay fever
spasmodic rhinorrhea

Excludes *allergic rhinitis with asthma (bronchial) (493.0)*

477.0 **Due to pollen**
Pollinosis

477.1 **Due to food**

❑ 477.8 **Due to other allergen**

❑ 477.9 **Cause unspecified**

● 478 **Other diseases of upper respiratory tract**

478.0 **Hypertrophy of nasal turbinates**

❑ 478.1 **Other diseases of nasal cavity and sinuses**
Abscess of nose (septum)
Necrosis of nose (septum)
Ulcer of nose (septum)
Cyst or mucocele of sinus (nasal)
Rhinolith

Excludes *varicose ulcer of nasal septum (456.8)*

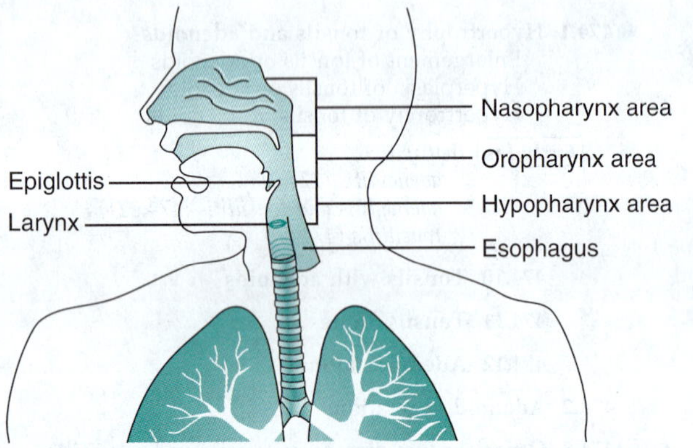

Figure 8–4 The pharynx.

Item 8–2 The pharynx is the passage for both food and air between the mouth and the esophagus and is divided into three areas: nasopharynx, oropharynx, and hypopharynx. The hypopharynx branches into the esophagus and the voice box.

● 478.2 **Other diseases of pharynx, not elsewhere classified**

❑ 478.20 **Unspecified disease of pharynx**

478.21 **Cellulitis of pharynx or nasopharynx**

478.22 **Parapharyngeal abscess**

478.24 **Retropharyngeal abscess**

478.25 **Edema of pharynx or nasopharynx**

478.26 **Cyst of pharynx or nasopharynx**

❑ 478.29 **Other**
Abscess of pharynx or nasopharynx

Excludes *ulcerative pharyngitis (462)*

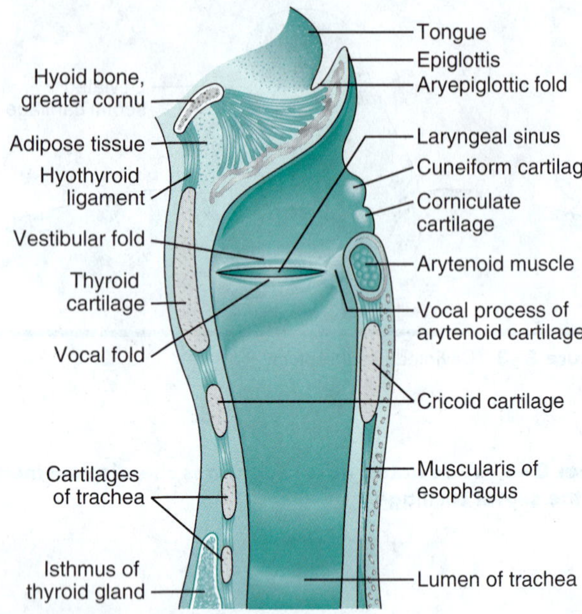

Figure 8–5 Coronal section of the larynx.

Item 8–3 The larynx extends from the tongue to the trachea and is divided into an upper and lower portion separated by folds. The framework of the larynx is cartilage composed of the single cricoid, thyroid, and epiglottic cartilages, and the paired arytenoid, cuneiform, and corniculate cartilages.

● 478.3 **Paralysis of vocal cords or larynx**

❑ 478.30 **Paralysis, unspecified**
Laryngoplegia
Paralysis of glottis

478.31 **Unilateral, partial**

478.32 **Unilateral, complete**

478.33 **Bilateral, partial**

478.34 **Bilateral, complete**

478.4 **Polyp of vocal cord or larynx**

Excludes *adenomatous polyps (212.1)*

❑ 478.5 **Other diseases of vocal cords**
Abscess of vocal cords
Cellulitis of vocal cords
Granuloma of vocal cords
Leukoplakia of vocal cords
Chorditis (fibrinous) (nodosa) (tuberosa)
Singers' nodes

478.6 **Edema of larynx**
Edema (of):
glottis
subglottic
Edema (of):
supraglottic

● 478.7 **Other diseases of larynx, not elsewhere classified**

❑ 478.70 **Unspecified disease of larynx**

478.71 **Cellulitis and perichondritis of larynx**

478.74 **Stenosis of larynx**

478.75 **Laryngeal spasm**
Laryngismus (stridulus)

❑478.79 **Other**
Abscess of larynx
Necrosis of larynx
Obstruction of larynx
Pachyderma of larynx
Ulcer of larynx

Excludes *ulcerative laryngitis (464.00–464.01)*

❑478.8 **Upper respiratory tract hypersensitivity reaction, site unspecified**

Excludes *hypersensitivity reaction of lower respiratory tract, as:*
extrinsic allergic alveolitis (495.0–495.9)
pneumoconiosis (500–505)

❑478.9 **Other and unspecified diseases of upper respiratory tract**
Abscess of trachea   Cicatrix of trachea

PNEUMONIA AND INFLUENZA (480–487)

Excludes *pneumonia:*
allergic or eosinophilic (518.3)
aspiration:
NOS (507.0)
newborn (770.1)
solids and liquids (507.0–507.8)
congenital (770.0)
lipoid (507.1)
passive (514)
rheumatic (390)

● **480 Viral pneumonia**

480.0 Pneumonia due to adenovirus

480.1 Pneumonia due to respiratory syncytial virus

480.2 Pneumonia due to parainfluenza virus

❑480.8 **Pneumonia due to other virus not elsewhere classified**

Excludes *congenital rubella pneumonitis (771.0)*
influenza with pneumonia, any form (487.0)
pneumonia complicating viral diseases classified elsewhere (484.1–484.8)

❑480.9 **Viral pneumonia, unspecified**

481 Pneumococcal pneumonia [Streptococcus pneumoniae pneumonia]
Lobar pneumonia, organism unspecified

● **482 Other bacterial pneumonia**

482.0 Pneumonia due to Klebsiella pneumoniae

482.1 Pneumonia due to Pseudomonas

482.2 Pneumonia due to Haemophilus influenzae [H. influenzae]

● **482.3 Pneumonia due to Streptococcus**

Excludes *Streptococcus pneumoniae pneumonia (481)*

❑482.30 **Streptococcus, unspecified**

482.31 Group A

482.32 Group B

❑482.39 **Other Streptococcus**

● **482.4 Pneumonia due to Staphylococcus**

❑482.40 **Pneumonia due to *Staphylococcus*, unspecified**

482.41 Pneumonia due to *Staphylococcus aureus*

❑482.49 **Other *Staphylococcus* pneumonia**

● **482.8 Pneumonia due to other specified bacteria**

Excludes *pneumonia complicating infectious disease classified elsewhere (484.1–484.8)*

482.81 Anaerobes
Bacteroides (melaninogenicus)
Gram-negative anaerobes

482.82 Escherichia coli [E. coli]

❑482.83 **Other gram-negative bacteria**
Gram-negative pneumonia NOS
Proteus
Serratia marcescens

Excludes *gram-negative anaerobes (482.81)*
Legionnaires' disease (482.84)

482.84 Legionnaires' disease

❑482.89 **Other specified bacteria**

❑482.9 **Bacterial pneumonia unspecified**

● **483 Pneumonia due to other specified organism**

483.0 Mycoplasma pneumoniae
Eaton's agent
Pleuropneumonia-like organisms [PPLO]

483.1 Chlamydia

❑483.8 **Other specified organism**

● **484 Pneumonia in infectious diseases classified elsewhere**

Excludes *influenza with pneumonia, any form (487.0)*

● ***484.1 Pneumonia in cytomegalic inclusion disease***
Code first underlying disease, as: (078.5)

● ***484.3 Pneumonia in whooping cough***
Code first underlying disease, as: (033.0–033.9)

● ***484.5 Pneumonia in anthrax***
Code first underlying disease (022.1)

● ***484.6 Pneumonia in aspergillosis***
Code first underlying disease (117.3)

●❑***484.7 Pneumonia in other systemic mycoses***
Code first underlying disease

Excludes *pneumonia in:*
candidiasis (112.4)
coccidioidomycosis (114.0)
histoplasmosis (115.0–115.9 with fifth-digit 5)

●❑***484.8 Pneumonia in other infectious diseases classified elsewhere***
Code first underlying disease, as:
Q fever (083.0)
typhoid fever (002.0)

Excludes *pneumonia in:*
actinomycosis (039.1)
measles (055.1)
nocardiosis (039.1)
ornithosis (073.0)
Pneumocystis carinii (136.3)
salmonellosis (003.22)
toxoplasmosis (130.4)
tuberculosis (011.6)
tularemia (021.2)
varicella (052.1)

❑485 **Bronchopneumonia, organism unspecified**
Bronchopneumonia:
hemorrhagic
terminal
Pleurobronchopneumonia
Pneumonia:
lobular
segmental

Excludes *bronchiolitis (acute) (466.11- 466.19)*
chronic (491.8)
lipoid pneumonia (507.1)

ICD-9-CM 400–499 Vol. 1

❑ **486 Pneumonia, organism unspecified**

Excludes *hypostatic or passive pneumonia (514)*
influenza with pneumonia, any form (487.0)
inhalation or aspiration pneumonia due to foreign materials (507.0–507.8)
pneumonitis due to fumes and vapors (506.0)

● **487 Influenza**

Excludes *Hemophilus influenzae [H. influenzae]:*
infection NOS (041.5)
laryngitis (464.00–464.01)
meningitis (320.0)
pneumonia (482.2)

487.0 With pneumonia
Influenza with pneumonia, any form
Influenzal:
bronchopneumonia
pneumonia

❑ **487.1 With other respiratory manifestations**
Influenza NOS
Influenzal:
laryngitis
pharyngitis
respiratory infection (upper) (acute)

❑ **487.8 With other manifestations**
Encephalopathy due to influenza
Influenza with involvement of gastrointestinal tract

Excludes *"intestinal flu" [viral gastroenteritis] (008.8)*

CHRONIC OBSTRUCTIVE PULMONARY DISEASE AND ALLIED CONDITIONS (490–496)

Item 8-4 Chronic bronchitis is usually defined as being present in any patient who has persistent cough with sputum production for at least three months in at least two consecutive years. **Simple chronic bronchitis** is marked by a productive cough but no pathological airflow obstruction. **Chronic obstructive pulmonary disease (COPD)** is a group of conditions—bronchitis, emphysema, asthma, bronchiectasis, allergic alveolitis—marked by dyspnea. **Catarrhal** bronchitis is an acute form of bronchitis marked by profuse mucus and pus production (**mucopurulent** discharge). **Croupous** bronchitis, also known as pseudomembranous, fibrinous, plastic, exudative, or membranous, is marked by a violent cough and dyspnea.

❑ **490 Bronchitis, not specified as acute or chronic**
Bronchitis NOS:
catarrhal
with tracheitis NOS
Tracheobronchitis NOS

Excludes *bronchitis:*
allergic NOS (493.9)
asthmatic NOS (493.9)
due to fumes and vapors (506.0)

● **491 Chronic bronchitis**

Excludes *chronic obstructive asthma (493.2)*

491.0 Simple chronic bronchitis
Catarrhal bronchitis, chronic
Smokers' cough

491.1 Mucopurulent chronic bronchitis
Bronchitis (chronic) (recurrent):
fetid
mucopurulent
purulent

● **491.2 Obstructive chronic bronchitis**
Bronchitis:
emphysematous
obstructive (chronic) (diffuse)
Bronchitis with:
chronic airway obstruction
emphysema

Excludes *asthmatic bronchitis (acute) (NOS) 493.9*
chronic obstructive asthma 493.2

491.20 Without exacerbation ⇐
Emphysema with chronic bronchitis

491.21 With (acute) exacerbation ⇐
Acute and chronic obstructive bronchitis
Acute exacerbation of chronic obstructive pulmonary disease [COPD]
Decompensated chronic obstructive pulmonary disease [COPD] ◀
Decompensated chronic obstructive pulmonary disease [COPD] with exacerbation ◀
Emphysema with acute and chronic bronchitis

Excludes *chronic obstructive asthma with acute exacerbation (493.22)*

❑ **491.8 Other chronic bronchitis**
Chronic:
tracheitis
tracheobronchitis

❑ **491.9 Unspecified chronic bronchitis**

● **492 Emphysema**

492.0 Emphysematous bleb
Giant bullous emphysema
Ruptured emphysematous bleb
Tension pneumatocele
Vanishing lung

❑ **492.8 Other emphysema**
Emphysema (lung or pulmonary):
NOS
centriacinar
centrilobular
obstructive
Emphysema (lung or pulmonary):
panacinar
panlobular
unilateral
vesicular
MacLeod's syndrome
Swyer-James syndrome
Unilateral hyperlucent lung

Excludes *emphysema:*
with chronic bronchitis (491.20–491.21) ⇐
compensatory (518.2)
due to fumes and vapors (506.4)
interstitial (518.1)
newborn (770.2)
mediastinal (518.1)
surgical (subcutaneous) (998.81)
traumatic (958.7)
with chronic bronchitis (491.20)

Item 8-5 Asthma is a bronchial condition marked by airway obstruction, hyper-responsiveness, and inflammation. **Extrinsic** asthma, also known as allergic asthma, is characterized by the same symptoms that occur with exposure to allergens and is divided into the following types: **atopic, occupational, and allergic bronchopulmonary aspergillosis. Intrinsic** asthma occurs in patients who have no history of allergy or sensitivities to allergens and is divided into the following types: **nonreaginic and pharmacologic. Status asthmaticus** is the most severe form of asthma attack and can last for days or weeks.

● 493 Asthma

The following fifth-digit subclassification is for use with codes 493.0–493.2, 493.9:

0 unspecified ⬅

1 with status asthmaticus

2 with (acute) exacerbation ⬅

Excludes *wheezing NOS (786.07)*

● 493.0 Extrinsic asthma
Asthma:
allergic with stated cause
atopic
childhood
hay
platinum
Hay fever with asthma

Excludes *asthma:*
allergic NOS (493.9)
detergent (507.8)
miners' (500)
wood (495.8)

● 493.1 Intrinsic asthma
Late-onset asthma

● 493.2 Chronic obstructive asthma
Asthma with chronic obstructive pulmonary disease (COPD)
Chronic asthmatic bronchitis

Excludes *acute bronchitis (466.0)*
chronic obstructive bronchitis (491.2)

● 493.8 Other forms of asthma ◀

493.81 Exercise induced bronchospasm ◀

493.82 Cough variant asthma ◀

● ❑ 493.9 Asthma, unspecified
Asthma (bronchial) (allergic NOS)
Bronchitis:
allergic
asthmatic

● 494 Bronchiectasis
Bronchiectasis (fusiform) (postinfectious) (recurrent)
Bronchiolectasis

Excludes *congenital (748.61)*
tuberculous bronchiectasis (current disease) (011.5)

494.0 Bronchiectasis without acute exacerbation

494.1 Bronchiectasis with acute exacerbation

● 495 Extrinsic allergic alveolitis

Includes: allergic alveolitis and pneumonitis due to inhaled organic dust particles of fungal, thermophilic actinomycete, or other origin

495.0 Farmers' lung

495.1 Bagassosis

495.2 Bird-fanciers' lung
Budgerigar-fanciers' disease or lung
Pigeon-fanciers' disease or lung

495.3 Suberosis
Cork-handlers' disease or lung

495.4 Malt workers' lung
Alveolitis due to Aspergillus clavatus

495.5 Mushroom workers' lung

495.6 Maple bark-strippers' lung
Alveolitis due to Cryptostroma corticale

495.7 "Ventilation" pneumonitis
Allergic alveolitis due to fungal, thermophilic actinomycete, and other organisms growing in ventilation [air conditioning] systems

❑ 495.8 Other specified allergic alveolitis and pneumonitis
Cheese-washers' lung
Coffee workers' lung
Fish-meal workers' lung
Furriers' lung
Grain-handlers' disease or lung
Pituitary snuff-takers' disease
Sequoiosis or red-cedar asthma
Wood asthma

❑ 495.9 Unspecified allergic alveolitis and pneumonitis
Alveolitis, allergic (extrinsic)
Hypersensitivity pneumonitis

❑ 496 Chronic airway obstruction, not elsewhere classified
Chronic:
nonspecific lung disease
obstructive lung disease
obstructive pulmonary disease [COPD] NOS

Note: This code is not to be used with any code from categories 491–493

Excludes *chronic obstructive lung disease [COPD] specified (as) (with):*
allergic alveolitis (495.0–495.9)
asthma (493.2)
bronchiectasis (494.0–494.1)
bronchitis (491.20–491.21) with emphysema (491.20–491.21)
emphysema (492.0–492.8)

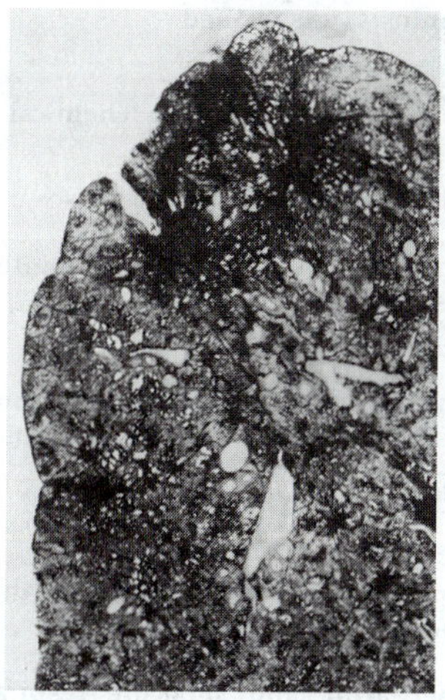

Figure 8–6 Progressive massive fibrosis superimposed on coalworkers' pneumoconiosis. The large, blackened scars are located principally in the upper lobe. Note extensions of scars into surrounding parenchyma and retraction of adjacent pleura. (From Cotran R, Kumar V, Robbins S: Robbins Pathologic Basis of Disease. Philadelphia, WB Saunders, 1994, p 708.)

Item 8–6 Pneumoconiosis refers to a lung condition resulting from exposure to inorganic or organic airborne particles, such as coal dust or moldy hay, as well as chemical fumes and vapors, such as insecticides. In this condition, the lungs retain the airborne particles.

PNEUMOCONIOSES AND OTHER LUNG DISEASES DUE TO EXTERNAL AGENTS (500–508)

500 Coal workers' pneumoconiosis
Anthracosilicosis
Anthracosis
Black lung disease
Coal workers' lung
Miners' asthma

501 Asbestosis

❑ **502 Pneumoconiosis due to other silica or silicates**
Pneumoconiosis due to talc
Silicotic fibrosis (massive) of lung
Silicosis (simple) (complicated)

❑ **503 Pneumoconiosis due to other inorganic dust**
Aluminosis (of lung)
Bauxite fibrosis (of lung)
Berylliosis
Graphite fibrosis (of lung)
Siderosis
Stannosis

❑ **504 Pneumonopathy due to inhalation of other dust**
Byssinosis
Cannabinosis
Flax-dressers' disease

Excludes *allergic alveolitis (495.0–495.9)*
asbestosis (501)
bagassosis (495.1)
farmers' lung (495.0)

❑ **505 Pneumoconiosis, unspecified**

● **506 Respiratory conditions due to chemical fumes and vapors**
Use additional E code to identify cause

506.0 Bronchitis and pneumonitis due to fumes and vapors
Chemical bronchitis (acute)

506.1 Acute pulmonary edema due to fumes and vapors
Chemical pulmonary edema (acute)

Excludes *acute pulmonary edema NOS (518.4)*
chronic or unspecified pulmonary edema (514)

506.2 Upper respiratory inflammation due to fumes and vapors

❑ **506.3 Other acute and subacute respiratory conditions due to fumes and vapors**

506.4 Chronic respiratory conditions due to fumes and vapors
Emphysema (diffuse) (chronic) due to inhalation of chemical fumes and vapors
Obliterative bronchiolitis (chronic) (subacute) due to inhalation of chemical fumes and vapors
Pulmonary fibrosis (chronic) due to inhalation of chemical fumes and vapors

❑ **506.9 Unspecified respiratory conditions due to fumes and vapors**
Silo-fillers' disease

● **507 Pneumonitis due to solids and liquids**

Excludes *fetal aspiration pneumonitis (770.1)*

507.0 Due to inhalation of food or vomitus
Aspiration pneumonia (due to):
NOS
food (regurgitated)
gastric secretions
milk
saliva
vomitus

507.1 Due to inhalation of oils and essences
Lipoid pneumonia (exogenous)

Excludes *endogenous lipoid pneumonia (516.8)*

❑ **507.8 Due to other solids and liquids**
Detergent asthma

● **508 Respiratory conditions due to other and unspecified external agents**
Use additional E code to identify cause

508.0 Acute pulmonary manifestations due to radiation
Radiation pneumonitis

508.1 Chronic and other pulmonary manifestations due to radiation
Fibrosis of lung following radiation

❑ **508.8 Respiratory conditions due to other specified external agents**

❑ **508.9 Respiratory conditions due to unspecified external agent**

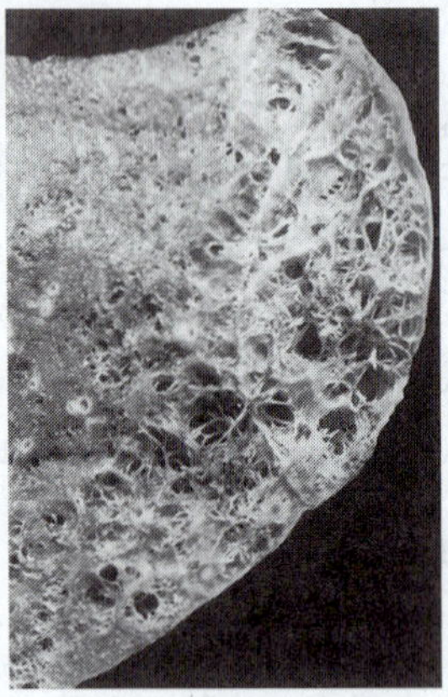

Figure 8–7 The apex of a lung (to the right) in a heavy cigarette smoker with severe emphysema (enlargement and distortion of the airspaces). (From Cotran R, Kumar V, Robbins S: Robbins Pathologic Basis of Disease. Philadelphia, WB Saunders, 1994, p 381.)

Item 8–7 Empyema is a condition in which pus accumulates in a body cavity. Empyema with fistula occurs when the pus passes from one cavity to another organ or structure.

OTHER DISEASES OF RESPIRATORY SYSTEM (510–519)

● **510 Empyema**

Use additional code to identify infectious organism (041.0–041.9)

Excludes *abscess of lung (513.0)*

510.0 With fistula

Fistula:
- bronchocutaneous
- bronchopleural
- hepatopleural

Fistula:
- mediastinal
- pleural
- thoracic

Any condition classifiable to 510.9 with fistula

510.9 Without mention of fistula

Abscess:
- pleura
- thorax

Empyema (chest) (lung) (pleura)
Fibrinopurulent pleurisy
Pleurisy:
- purulent
- septic
- seropurulent
- suppurative

Pyopneumothorax
Pyothorax

● **511 Pleurisy**

Excludes *malignant pleural effusion (197.2)*
pleurisy with mention of tuberculosis, current disease (012.0)

511.0 Without mention of effusion or current tuberculosis

Adhesion, lung or pleura
Calcification of pleura
Pleurisy (acute) (sterile):
- diaphragmatic
- fibrinous
- interlobar

Pleurisy:
- NOS
- pneumococcal
- staphylococcal
- streptococcal

Thickening of pleura

❑ **511.1 With effusion, with mention of a bacterial cause other than tuberculosis**

Pleurisy with effusion (exudative) (serous):
- pneumococcal
- staphylococcal
- streptococcal
- other specified nontuberculous bacterial cause

❑ **511.8 Other specified forms of effusion, except tuberculous**

Encysted pleurisy
Hemopneumothorax
Hemothorax
Hydropneumothorax
Hydrothorax

Excludes *traumatic (860.2–860.5, 862.29, 862.39)*

❑ **511.9 Unspecified pleural effusion**

Pleural effusion NOS
Pleurisy:
- exudative
- serofibrinous
- serous
- with effusion NOS

● **512 Pneumothorax**

512.0 Spontaneous tension pneumothorax

512.1 Iatrogenic pneumothorax

Postoperative pneumothorax

❑ **512.8 Other spontaneous pneumothorax**

Pneumothorax:
- NOS
- acute
- chronic

Excludes *pneumothorax:*
congenital (770.2)
traumatic (860.0–860.1, 860.4–860.5)
tuberculous, current disease (011.7)

● **513 Abscess of lung and mediastinum**

513.0 Abscess of lung

Abscess (multiple) of lung
Gangrenous or necrotic pneumonia
Pulmonary gangrene or necrosis

513.1 Abscess of mediastinum

514 Pulmonary congestion and hypostasis

Hypostatic:
- bronchopneumonia
- pneumonia

Passive pneumonia
Pulmonary congestion (chronic) (passive)
Pulmonary edema:
- NOS
- chronic

Excludes *acute pulmonary edema:*
NOS (518.4)
with mention of heart disease or failure (428.1)

515 Postinflammatory pulmonary fibrosis

Cirrhosis of lung chronic or unspecified
Fibrosis of lung (atrophic) (confluent) (massive) (perialveolar) (peribronchial) chronic or unspecified
Induration of lung chronic or unspecified

● **516 Other alveolar and parietoalveolar pneumonopathy**

516.0 Pulmonary alveolar proteinosis

● ***516.1 Idiopathic pulmonary hemosiderosis***

Essential brown induration of lung
Code first underlying disease (275.0)

516.2 Pulmonary alveolar microlithiasis

516.3 Idiopathic fibrosing alveolitis

Alveolar capillary block
Diffuse (idiopathic) (interstitial) pulmonary fibrosis
Hamman-Rich syndrome

❑ **516.8 Other specified alveolar and parietoalveolar pneumonopathies**

Endogenous lipoid pneumonia
Interstitial pneumonia (desquamative) (lymphoid)

Excludes *lipoid pneumonia, exogenous or unspecified (507.1)*

❑ **516.9 Unspecified alveolar and parietoalveolar pneumonopathy**

● **517 Lung involvement in conditions classified elsewhere**

Excludes *rheumatoid lung (714.81)*

● ***517.1 Rheumatic pneumonia***

Code first underlying disease (390)

● ***517.2 Lung involvement in systemic sclerosis***

Code first underlying disease (710.1)

517.3 Acute chest syndrome ◄

Code first sickle-cell disease in crisis (282.42, 282.62, 282.64, 282.69) ◄

●❑ 517.8 *Lung involvement in other diseases classified elsewhere*

Code first underlying disease, as:
amyloidosis (277.3)
polymyositis (710.4)
sarcoidosis (135)
Sjögren's disease (710.2)
systemic lupus erythematosus (710.0)

Excludes *syphilis (095.1)*

● **518 Other diseases of lung**

518.0 Pulmonary collapse
Atelectasis
Collapse of lung
Middle lobe syndrome

Excludes *atelectasis:*
congenital (partial) (770.5)
primary (770.4)
tuberculous, current disease (011.8)

518.1 Interstitial emphysema
Mediastinal emphysema

Excludes *surgical (subcutaneous) emphysema (998.81)*
that in fetus or newborn (770.2)
traumatic emphysema (958.7)

518.2 Compensatory emphysema

518.3 Pulmonary eosinophilia
Eosinophilic asthma
Löffler's syndrome
Pneumonia:
allergic
eosinophilic
Tropical eosinophilia

❑ **518.4 Acute edema of lung, unspecified**
Acute pulmonary edema NOS
Pulmonary edema, postoperative

Excludes *pulmonary edema:*
acute, with mention of heart disease or failure (428.1)
chronic or unspecified (514)
due to external agents (506.0–508.9)

518.5 Pulmonary insufficiency following trauma and surgery
Adult respiratory distress syndrome
Pulmonary insufficiency following:
shock
surgery
trauma
Shock lung

Excludes *adult respiratory distress syndrome associated with other conditions (518.82)*
pneumonia:
aspiration (507.0)
hypostatic (514)
respiratory failure in other conditions (518.81, 518.83–518.84)

518.6 Allergic bronchopulmonary aspergillosis

● **518.8 Other diseases of lung**

518.81 Acute respiratory failure
Respiratory failure NOS

Excludes *acute and chronic respiratory failure (518.84)*
acute respiratory distress (518.82)
chronic respiratory failure (518.83)
respiratory arrest (799.1)
respiratory failure, newborn (770.84)

❑ **518.82 Other pulmonary insufficiency, not elsewhere classified**
Acute respiratory distress
Acute respiratory insufficiency
Adult respiratory distress syndrome NEC

Excludes *adult respiratory distress syndrome associated with trauma or surgery (518.5)*
pulmonary insufficiency following trauma or surgery (518.5)
respiratory distress:
NOS (786.09)
newborn (770.89)
syndrome, newborn (769)
shock lung (518.5)

518.83 Chronic respiratory failure

518.84 Acute and chronic respiratory failure
Acute on chronic respiratory failure

❑ **518.89 Other diseases of lung, not elsewhere classified**
Broncholithiasis
Calcification of lung
Lung disease NOS
Pulmolithiasis

● **519 Other diseases of respiratory system**

● **519.0 Tracheostomy complications**

❑ **519.00 Tracheostomy complication, unspecified**

519.01 Infection of tracheostomy

Use additional code to identify type of infection, such as:
abscess or cellulitis of neck (682.1)
septicemia (038.0–038.9)

Use additional code to identify organism (041.00–041.9)

519.02 Mechanical complication of tracheostomy
Tracheal stenosis due to tracheostomy

519.09 Other tracheostomy complications
Hemorrhage due to tracheostomy
Tracheoesophageal fistula due to tracheostomy

❑ **519.1 Other diseases of trachea and bronchus, not elsewhere classified**
Calcification of bronchus or trachea
Stenosis of bronchus or trachea
Ulcer of bronchus or trachea

519.2 Mediastinitis

❑ **519.3 Other diseases of mediastinum, not elsewhere classified**
Fibrosis of mediastinum
Hernia of mediastinum
Retraction of mediastinum

519.4 Disorders of diaphragm
Diaphragmitis
Paralysis of diaphragm
Relaxation of diaphragm

Excludes *congenital defect of diaphragm (756.6)*
diaphragmatic hernia (551–553 with .3)
congenital (756.6)

❑ **519.8 Other diseases of respiratory system, not elsewhere classified**

❑ **519.9 Unspecified disease of respiratory system**
Respiratory disease (chronic) NOS

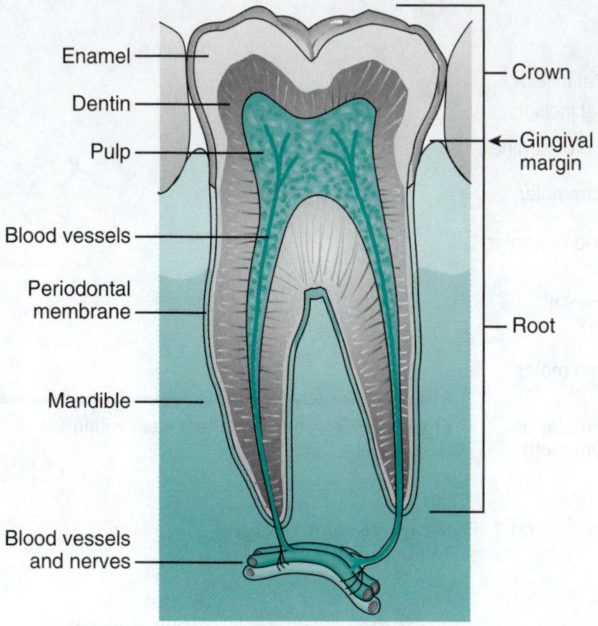

Figure 9–1 Anatomy of a tooth.

Item 9–1 Anodontia is the congenital absence of teeth. Hypodontia is partial anodontia. Oligodontia is the congenital absence of some teeth, whereas supernumerary is having more teeth than the normal number. Mesiodens are small extra teeth that often appear in pairs, although single small teeth are not uncommon.

9. DISEASES OF THE DIGESTIVE SYSTEM (520–579)

DISEASES OF ORAL CAVITY, SALIVARY GLANDS, AND JAWS (520–529)

● **520 Disorders of tooth development and eruption**

520.0 Anodontia
Absence of teeth (complete) (congenital) (partial)
Hypodontia
Oligodontia

Excludes *acquired absence of teeth (525.10–525.19)*

520.1 Supernumerary teeth
Distomolar
Fourth molar
Mesiodens
Paramolar
Supplemental teeth

Excludes *supernumerary roots (520.2)*

520.2 Abnormalities of size and form
Concrescence of teeth
Fusion of teeth
Gemination of teeth
Dens evaginatus
Dens in dente
Dens invaginatus
Enamel pearls
Macrodontia
Microdontia
Peg-shaped [conical] teeth
Supernumerary roots
Taurodontism
Tuberculum paramolare

Excludes *that due to congenital syphilis (090.5)*
tuberculum Carabelli, which is regarded as a normal variation

520.3 Mottled teeth
Dental fluorosis
Mottling of enamel
Nonfluoride enamel opacities

520.4 Disturbances of tooth formation
Aplasia and hypoplasia of cementum
Dilaceration of tooth
Enamel hypoplasia (neonatal) (postnatal) (prenatal)
Horner's teeth
Hypocalcification of teeth
Regional odontodysplasia
Turner's tooth

Excludes *Hutchinson's teeth and mulberry molars in congenital syphilis (090.5)*
mottled teeth (520.3)

520.5 Hereditary disturbances in tooth structure, not elsewhere classified
Amelogenesis imperfecta
Dentinogenesis imperfecta
Odontogenesis imperfecta
Dentinal dysplasia
Shell teeth

520.6 Disturbances in tooth eruption
Teeth:
- embedded
- impacted
- natal
- neonatal
- primary [deciduous]:
  - persistent
  - shedding, premature

Tooth eruption:
- late
- obstructed
- premature

Excludes *exfoliation of teeth (attributable to disease of surrounding tissues) (525.0–525.19)*
impacted or embedded teeth with abnormal position of such teeth or adjacent teeth (524.3)

520.7 Teething syndrome

❑ **520.8 Other specified disorders of tooth development and eruption**
Color changes during tooth formation
Pre-eruptive color changes

Excludes *posteruptive color changes (521.7)*

❑ **520.9 Unspecified disorder of tooth development and eruption**

ICD-9-CM 500–599 Vol. 1

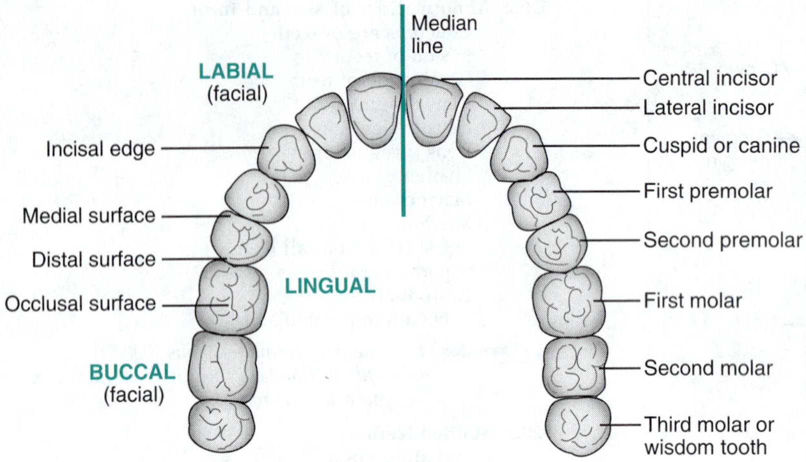

Figure 9–2 The permanent teeth within the dental arch.

Item 9–2 Each dental arch (jaw) normally contains 16 teeth. Tooth decay or dental caries is a disease of the enamel, dentin, and cementum of the tooth and can result in a cavity.

● **521 Diseases of hard tissues of teeth**

● **521.0 Dental caries**

❑ **521.00 Dental caries, unspecified**

521.01 Dental caries limited to enamel
Initial caries
White spot lesion

521.02 Dental caries extending into dentin

521.03 Dental caries extending into pulp

521.04 Arrested dental caries

521.05 Odontoclasia
Infantile melanodontia
Melanodontoclasia

Excludes *internal and external resorption of teeth (521.4)*

❑ **521.09 Other dental caries**

521.1 Excessive attrition
Approximal wear
Occlusal wear

521.2 Abrasion
Abrasion of teeth:
dentifrice
habitual
occupational
Abrasion of teeth:
ritual
traditional
Wedge defect NOS of teeth

521.3 Erosion
Erosion of teeth:
NOS
due to:
medicine
persistent vomiting
idiopathic
occupational

521.4 Pathological resorption
Internal granuloma of pulp
Resorption of tooth or root (external) (internal)

521.5 Hypercementosis
Cementation hyperplasia

521.6 Ankylosis of teeth

521.7 Posteruptive color changes
Staining [discoloration] of teeth:
NOS
due to:
drugs
metals
due to:
pulpal bleeding

Excludes *accretions [deposits] on teeth (523.6)*
pre-eruptive color changes (520.8)

❑ **521.8 Other specified diseases of hard tissues of teeth**
Irradiated enamel
Sensitive dentin

❑ **521.9 Unspecified disease of hard tissues of teeth**

● **522 Diseases of pulp and periapical tissues**

522.0 Pulpitis
Pulpal:
abscess
polyp
Pulpitis:
acute
chronic (hyperplastic) (ulcerative)
suppurative

522.1 Necrosis of the pulp
Pulp gangrene

522.2 Pulp degeneration
Denticles
Pulp calcifications
Pulp stones

522.3 Abnormal hard tissue formation in pulp
Secondary or irregular dentin

522.4 Acute apical periodontitis of pulpal origin

522.5 Periapical abscess without sinus
Abscess:
dental
dentoalveolar

Excludes *periapical abscess with sinus (522.7)*

522.6 Chronic apical periodontitis
Apical or periapical granuloma
Apical periodontitis NOS

522.7 Periapical abscess with sinus
Fistula:
alveolar process
dental

522.8 Radicular cyst
Cyst:
apical (periodontal)
periapical
radiculodental
residual radicular

Excludes *lateral developmental or lateral periodontal cyst (526.0)*

Item 9–3 Acute gingivitis, also known as orilitis or ulitis, is the short-term, severe inflammation of the gums (gingiva) caused by bacteria. Chronic gingivitis is persistent inflammation of the gums. When the gingivitis moves into the periodontium it is called periodontitis, also known as paradentitis.

❑ 522.9 Other and unspecified diseases of pulp and periapical tissues

● 523 Gingival and periodontal diseases

523.0 Acute gingivitis

Excludes *acute necrotizing ulcerative gingivitis (101)*
herpetic gingivostomatitis (054.2)

523.1 Chronic gingivitis
Gingivitis (chronic):
NOS
desquamative
hyperplastic
simple marginal
ulcerative
Gingivostomatitis

Excludes *herpetic gingivostomatitis (054.2)*

523.2 Gingival recession
Gingival recession (generalized) (localized) (postinfective) (postoperative)

523.3 Acute periodontitis
Acute:
pericementitis
pericoronitis
Paradontal abscess
Periodontal abscess

Excludes *acute apical periodontitis (522.4)*
periapical abscess (522.5, 522.7)

523.4 Chronic periodontitis
Alveolar pyorrhea
Chronic pericoronitis
Pericementitis (chronic)
Periodontitis:
NOS
complex
simplex

Excludes *chronic apical periodontitis (522.6)*

523.5 Periodontosis

523.6 Accretions on teeth
Dental calculus:
subgingival
supragingival
Deposits on teeth:
betel
materia alba
soft
tartar
tobacco

❑ 523.8 Other specified periodontal diseases
Giant cell:
epulis
peripheral granuloma
Gingival:
cysts
enlargement NOS
fibromatosis
Gingival polyp
Periodontal lesions due to traumatic occlusion
Peripheral giant cell granuloma

Excludes *leukoplakia of gingiva (528.6)*

❑ 523.9 Unspecified gingival and periodontal disease

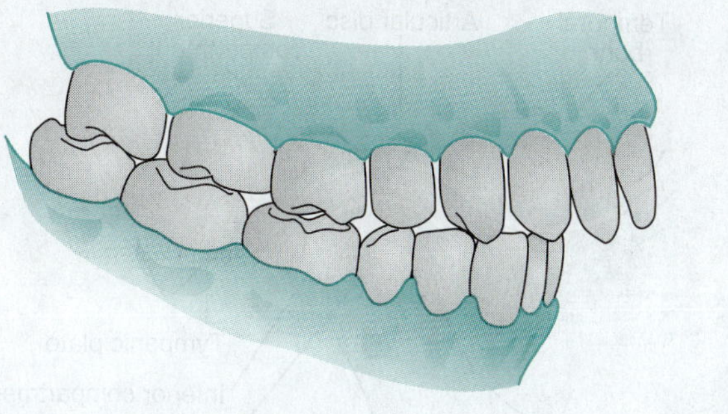

Figure 9–3 Dentofacial malocclusion.

Item 9–4 Hyperplasia is a condition of overdevelopment, whereas hypoplasia is a condition of underdevelopment. Macrogenia is overdevelopment of the chin, whereas microgenia is underdevelopment of the chin.

● 524 Dentofacial anomalies, including malocclusion

● 524.0 Major anomalies of jaw size

Excludes *hemifacial atrophy or hypertrophy (754.0)*
unilateral condylar hyperplasia or hypoplasia of mandible

❑ 524.00 Unspecified anomaly

524.01 Maxillary hyperplasia

524.02 Mandibular hyperplasia

524.03 Maxillary hypoplasia

524.04 Mandibular hypoplasia

524.05 Macrogenia

524.06 Microgenia

❑ 524.09 Other specified anomaly

● 524.1 Anomalies of relationship of jaw to cranial base

❑ 524.10 Unspecified anomaly
Prognathism
Retrognathism

524.11 Maxillary asymmetry

❑ 524.12 Other jaw asymmetry

❑ 524.19 Other specified anomaly

524.2 Anomalies of dental arch relationship
Crossbite (anterior) (posterior)
Disto-occlusion
Mesio-occlusion
Midline deviation
Open bite (anterior) (posterior)
Overbite (excessive):
deep
horizontal
vertical
Overjet
Posterior lingual occlusion of mandibular teeth
Soft tissue impingement

Excludes *hemifacial atrophy or hypertrophy (754.0)*
unilateral condylar hyperplasia or hypoplasia of mandible (526.89)

524.3 Anomalies of tooth position
Crowding of tooth, teeth
Diastema of tooth, teeth
Displacement of tooth, teeth
Rotation of tooth, teeth
Spacing, abnormal, of tooth, teeth
Transposition of tooth, teeth
Impacted or embedded teeth with abnormal position of such teeth or adjacent teeth

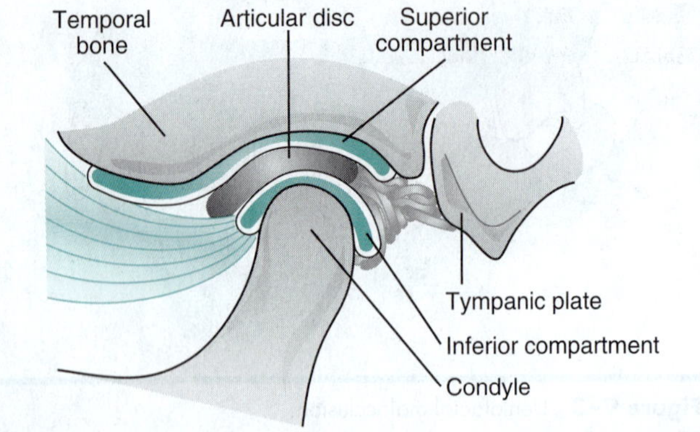

Figure 9–4 Temporomandibular joint.

Item 9–5 Dysfunction of the temporomandibular joint is termed temporomandibular joint (TMJ) syndrome and is characterized by pain and tenderness/spasm of the muscles of mastication, joint noise, and in the later stages, limited mandibular movement.

❑ **524.4 Malocclusion, unspecified**

524.5 Dentofacial functional abnormalities
Abnormal jaw closure
Malocclusion due to:
abnormal swallowing
mouth breathing
tongue, lip, or finger habits

● **524.6 Temporomandibular joint disorders**
Excludes *current temporomandibular joint:*
dislocation (830.0–830.1)
strain (848.1)

❑ **524.60 Temporomandibular joint disorders, unspecified**
Temporomandibular joint-pain-dysfunction syndrome [TMJ]

524.61 Adhesions and ankylosis (bony or fibrous)

524.62 Arthralgia of temporomandibular joint

524.63 Articular disc disorder (reducing or nonreducing)

❑ **524.69 Other specified temporomandibular joint disorders**

● **524.7 Dental alveolar anomalies**

❑ **524.70 Unspecified alveolar anomaly**

524.71 Alveolar maxillary hyperplasia

524.72 Alveolar mandibular hyperplasia

524.73 Alveolar maxillary hypoplasia

524.74 Alveolar mandibular hypoplasia

❑ **524.79 Other specified alveolar anomaly**

❑ **524.8 Other specified dentofacial anomalies**

❑ **524.9 Unspecified dentofacial anomalies**

● **525 Other diseases and conditions of the teeth and supporting structures**

525.0 Exfoliation of teeth due to systemic causes

● **525.1 Loss of teeth due to trauma, extraction, or periodontal disease**

❑ **525.10 Acquired absence of teeth, unspecified**
Edentulism
Tooth extraction status, NOS

525.11 Loss of teeth due to trauma

525.12 Loss of teeth due to periodontal disease

525.13 Loss of teeth due to caries

❑ **525.19 Other loss of teeth**

525.2 Atrophy of edentulous alveolar ridge

525.3 Retained dental root

❑ **525.8 Other specified disorders of the teeth and supporting structures**
Enlargement of alveolar ridge NOS
Irregular alveolar process

❑ **525.9 Unspecified disorder of the teeth and supporting structures**

● **526 Diseases of the jaws**

526.0 Developmental odontogenic cysts
Cyst:
dentigerous
eruption
follicular
lateral developmental
lateral periodontal
primordial
Keratocyst
Excludes *radicular cyst (522.8)*

526.1 Fissural cysts of jaw
Cyst:
globulomaxillary
incisor canal
median anterior maxillary
median palatal
nasopalatine
palatine of papilla
Excludes *cysts of oral soft tissues (528.4)*

❑ **526.2 Other cysts of jaws**
Cyst of jaw:
NOS
aneurysmal
Cyst of jaw:
hemorrhagic
traumatic

526.3 Central giant cell (reparative) granuloma
Excludes *peripheral giant cell granuloma (523.8)*

526.4 Inflammatory conditions
Abscess of jaw (acute) (chronic) (suppurative)
Osteitis of jaw (acute) (chronic) (suppurative)
Osteomyelitis (neonatal) of jaw (acute) (chronic) (suppurative)
Periostitis of jaw (acute) (chronic) (suppurative)
Sequestrum of jaw bone
Excludes *alveolar osteitis (526.5)*

526.5 Alveolitis of jaw
Alveolar osteitis
Dry socket

● **526.8 Other specified diseases of the jaws**

526.81 Exostosis of jaw
Torus mandibularis
Torus palatinus

❑ **526.89 Other**
Cherubism
Fibrous dysplasia of jaw(s)
Latent bone cyst of jaw(s)
Osteoradionecrosis of jaw(s)
Unilateral condylar hyperplasia or hypoplasia of mandible

❑ **526.9 Unspecified disease of the jaws**

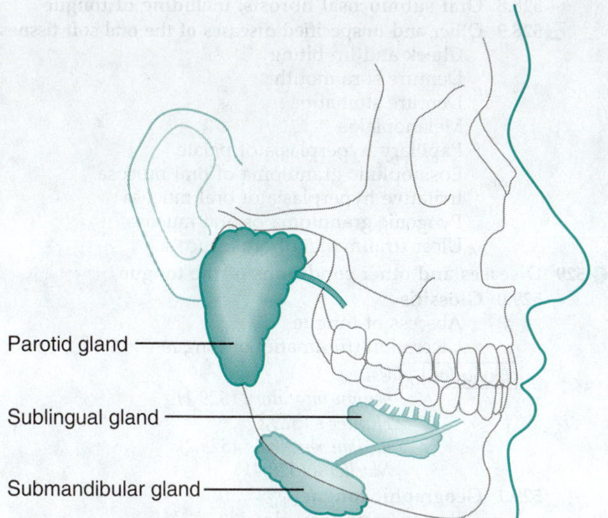

Figure 9–5 Major salivary glands.

Item 9–6 Atrophy is wasting away of a tissue or organ, whereas hypertrophy is overdevelopment or enlargement of a tissue or organ. Sialoadenitis is salivary gland inflammation. Parotitis is the inflammation of the parotid gland. In the epidemic form, parotitis is also known as mumps. Sialolithiasis is the formation of calculus within a salivary gland. Mucocele is a polyp composed of mucus.

● 527 **Diseases of the salivary glands**

527.0 **Atrophy**

527.1 **Hypertrophy**

527.2 **Sialoadenitis**
Parotitis:
NOS
allergic
toxic
Sialoangitis
Sialodochitis

Excludes *epidemic or infectious parotitis (072.0–072.9)*
uveoparotid fever (135)

527.3 **Abscess**

527.4 **Fistula**

Excludes *congenital fistula of salivary gland (750.24)*

527.5 **Sialolithiasis**
Calculus of salivary gland or duct
Stone of salivary gland or duct
Sialodocholithiasis

527.6 **Mucocele**
Mucous:
extravasation cyst of salivary gland
retention cyst of salivary gland
Ranula

527.7 **Disturbance of salivary secretion**
Hyposecretion
Ptyalism
Sialorrhea
Xerostomia

❑ 527.8 **Other specified diseases of the salivary glands**
Benign lymphoepithelial lesion of salivary gland
Sialectasia
Sialosis
Stenosis of salivary duct
Stricture of salivary duct

❑ 527.9 **Unspecified disease of the salivary glands**

Item 9–7 Stomatitis is the inflammation of the oral mucosa. Cancrum oris, also known as noma or gangrenous stomatitis, begins as an ulcer of the gingiva and results in a progressive gangrenous process.

● 528 **Diseases of the oral soft tissues, excluding lesions specific for gingiva and tongue**

528.0 **Stomatitis**
Stomatitis:
NOS
ulcerative
Vesicular stomatitis

Excludes *stomatitis:*
acute necrotizing ulcerative (101)
aphthous (528.2)
gangrenous (528.1)
herpetic (054.2)
Vincent's (101)

528.1 **Cancrum oris**
Gangrenous stomatitis
Noma

528.2 **Oral aphthae**
Aphthous stomatitis
Canker sore
Periadenitis mucosa necrotica recurrens
Recurrent aphthous ulcer
Stomatitis herpetiformis

Excludes *herpetic stomatitis (054.2)*

528.3 **Cellulitis and abscess**
Cellulitis of mouth (floor)
Ludwig's angina
Oral fistula

Excludes *abscess of tongue (529.0)*
cellulitis or abscess of lip (528.5)
fistula (of):
dental (522.7)
lip (528.5)
gingivitis (523.0–523.1)

528.4 **Cysts**
Dermoid cyst of mouth
Epidermoid cyst of mouth
Epstein's pearl of mouth
Lymphoepithelial cyst of mouth
Nasoalveolar cyst of mouth
Nasolabial cyst of mouth

Excludes *cyst:*
gingiva (523.8)
tongue (529.8)

528.5 **Diseases of lips**
Abscess of lip(s)
Cellulitis of lip(s)
Fistula of lip(s)
Hypertrophy of lip(s)
Cheilitis:
NOS
angular
Cheilodynia
Cheilosis

Excludes *actinic cheilitis (692.79)*
congenital fistula of lip (750.25)
leukoplakia of lips (528.6)

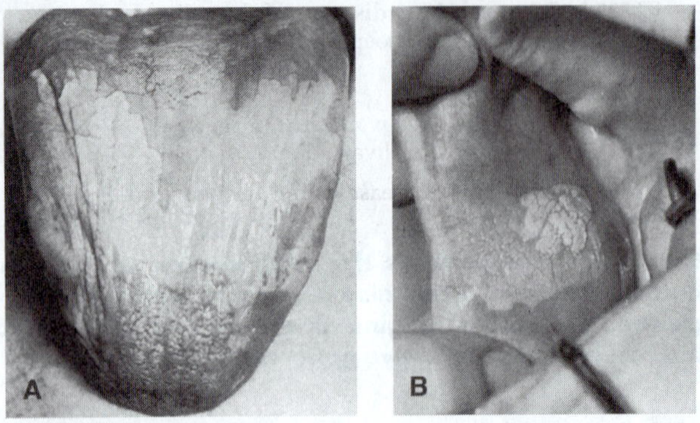

Figure 9–6 **A.** Lingual leukoplakia. **B.** Buccal leukoplakia. (From Pindborg JJ: In Jones JH, Mason DK (eds): Oral Manifestations of Systemic Disease. Philadelphia, WB Saunders, 1980, p 322.)

528.6 Leukoplakia of oral mucosa, including tongue
Leukokeratosis of oral mucosa
Leukoplakia of:
gingiva
lips
tongue

Excludes *carcinoma in situ (230.0, 232.0)*
leukokeratosis nicotina palati (528.7)

❑ **528.7 Other disturbances of oral epithelium, including tongue**
Erythroplakia of mouth or tongue
Focal epithelial hyperplasia of mouth or tongue
Leukoedema of mouth or tongue
Leukokeratosis nicotina palati

Excludes *carcinoma in situ (230.0, 232.0)*
leukokeratosis NOS (702)

528.8 Oral submucosal fibrosis, including of tongue

❑ **528.9 Other and unspecified diseases of the oral soft tissues**
Cheek and lip biting
Denture sore mouth
Denture stomatitis
Melanoplakia
Papillary hyperplasia of palate
Eosinophilic granuloma of oral mucosa
Irritative hyperplasia of oral mucosa
Pyogenic granuloma of oral mucosa
Ulcer (traumatic) of oral mucosa

● **529 Diseases and other conditions of the tongue**

529.0 Glossitis
Abscess of tongue
Ulceration (traumatic) of tongue

Excludes *glossitis:*
benign migratory (529.1)
Hunter's (529.4)
median rhomboid (529.2)
Moeller's (529.4)

529.1 Geographic tongue
Benign migratory glossitis
Glossitis areata exfoliativa

529.2 Median rhomboid glossitis

529.3 Hypertrophy of tongue papillae
Black hairy tongue
Coated tongue
Hypertrophy of foliate papillae
Lingua villosa nigra

529.4 Atrophy of tongue papillae
Bald tongue
Glazed tongue
Glossitis:
Hunter's
Moeller's
Glossodynia exfoliativa
Smooth atrophic tongue

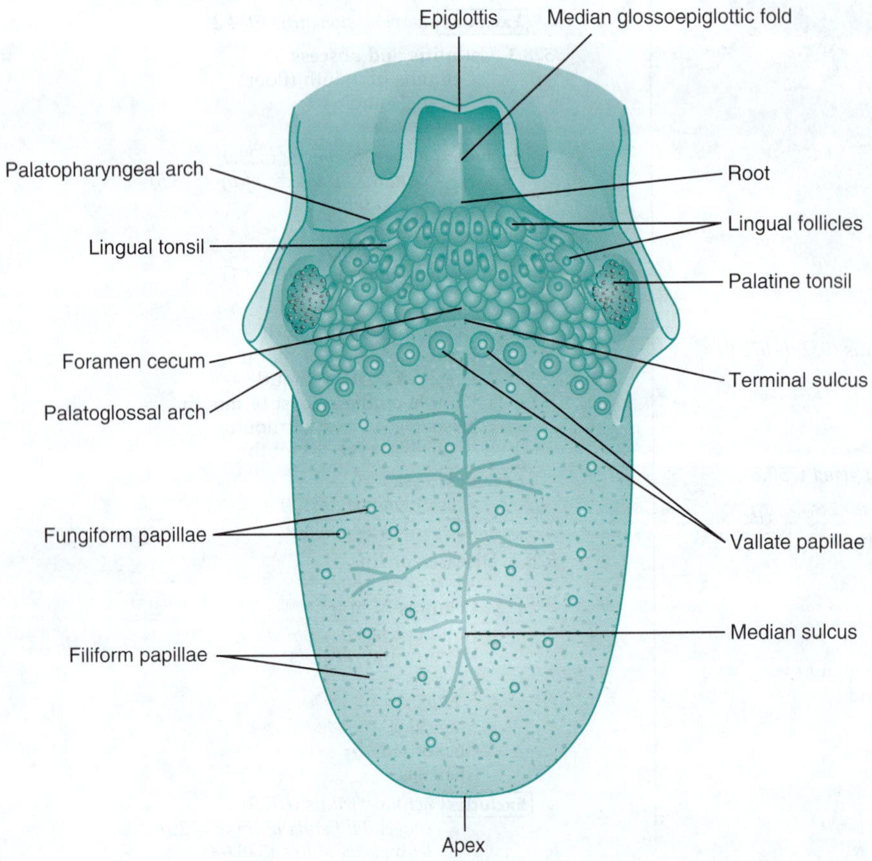

Figure 9–7 Structure of the tongue.

529.5 **Plicated tongue**
Fissured tongue
Furrowed tongue
Scrotal tongue
Excludes *fissure of tongue, congenital (750.13)*

529.6 **Glossodynia**
Glossopyrosis
Painful tongue
Excludes *glossodynia exfoliativa (529.4)*

❑ 529.8 **Other specified conditions of the tongue**
Atrophy (of) tongue
Crenated (of) tongue
Enlargement (of) tongue
Hypertrophy (of) tongue
Glossocele
Glossoptosis
Excludes *erythroplasia of tongue (528.7)*
leukoplakia of tongue (528.6)
macroglossia (congenital) (750.15)
microglossia (congenital) (750.16)
oral submucosal fibrosis (528.8)

❑ 529.9 **Unspecified condition of the tongue**

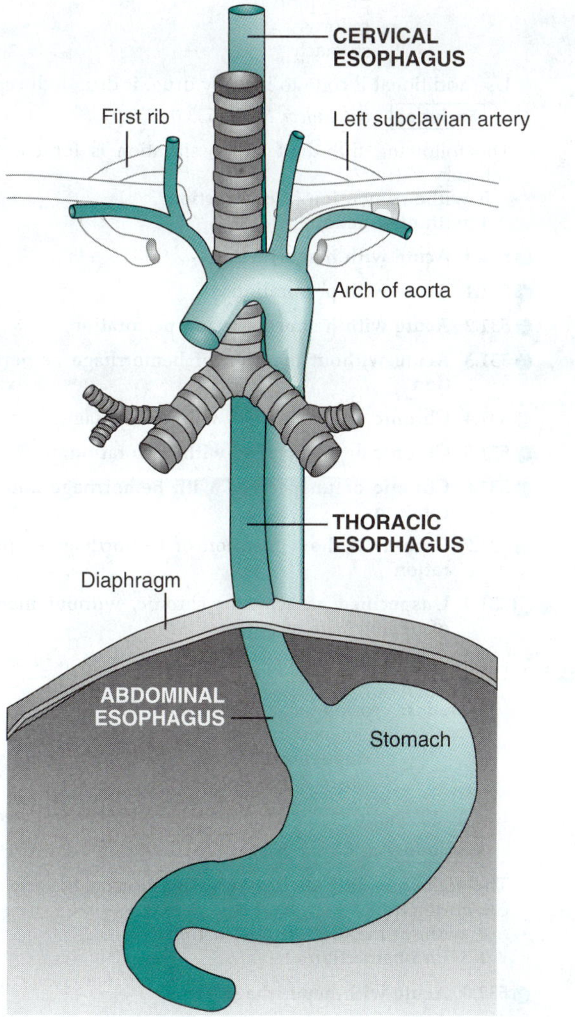

Figure 9–8 The esophagus is the muscular tube that connects the pharynx and the stomach. The 10 inch (25 cm) long esophagus is divided into three parts: **cervical, thoracic,** and **abdominal.**

Item 9–8 Achalasia is a condition in which the smooth muscle fibers of the esophagus do not relax. Most frequently, this condition occurs at the esophagogastric sphincter. Cardiospasm, also known as megaesophagus, is achalasia of the thoracic esophagus.

Item 9–9 Dyskinesia is difficulty in moving, and diverticulum is a sac or pouch.

DISEASES OF ESOPHAGUS, STOMACH, AND DUODENUM (530–537)

● 530 **Diseases of esophagus**
Excludes *esophageal varices (456.0–456.2)*

530.0 **Achalasia and cardiospasm**
Achalasia (of cardia)
Aperistalsis of esophagus
Megaesophagus
Excludes *congenital cardiospasm (750.7)*

● 530.1 **Esophagitis**
Abscess of esophagus
Esophagitis:
NOS
chemical
peptic
Esophagitis:
postoperative
regurgitant

Use additional E code to identify cause, if induced by chemical
Excludes *tuberculous esophagitis (017.8)*

❑ 530.10 **Esophagitis, unspecified**

530.11 **Reflux esophagitis**

530.12 **Acute esophagitis**

❑ 530.19 **Other esophagitis**

● 530.2 **Ulcer of esophagus**
Ulcer of esophagus
fungal
peptic
Ulcer of esophagus due to ingestion of:
aspirin
chemicals
medicines

Use additional E code to identify cause, if induced by chemical or drug

530.20 **Ulcer of esophagus without bleeding** ◀
Ulcer of esophagus NOS ◀

530.21 **Ulcer of esophagus with bleeding** ◀
Excludes *bleeding esophageal varices (456.0, 456.20)* ◀

530.3 **Stricture and stenosis of esophagus**
Compression of esophagus
Obstruction of esophagus
Excludes *congenital stricture of esophagus (750.3)*

530.4 **Perforation of esophagus**
Rupture of esophagus
Excludes *traumatic perforation of esophagus (862.22, 862.32, 874.4–874.5)*

530.5 **Dyskinesia of esophagus**
Corkscrew esophagus
Curling esophagus
Esophagospasm
Spasm of esophagus
Excludes *cardiospasm (530.0)*

530.6 **Diverticulum of esophagus, acquired**
Diverticulum, acquired:
epiphrenic
pharyngoesophageal
pulsion
subdiaphragmatic
traction
Zenker's (hypopharyngeal)
Esophageal pouch, acquired
Esophagocele, acquired

Excludes *congenital diverticulum of esophagus (750.4)*

530.7 **Gastroesophageal laceration-hemorrhage syndrome**
Mallory-Weiss syndrome

● 530.8 **Other specified disorders of esophagus**

530.81 **Esophageal reflux**
Gastroesophageal reflux

Excludes *reflux esophagitis (530.11)*

530.82 **Esophageal hemorrhage**

Excludes *hemorrhage due to esophageal varices (456.0–456.2)*

530.83 **Esophageal leukoplakia**

530.84 **Tracheoesophageal fistula**

Excludes *congenital tracheoesophageal fistula (750.3)*

530.85 **Barrett's esophagus** ◀

❑ 530.89 **Other**

Excludes *Paterson-Kelly syndrome (280.8)*

❑ 530.9 **Unspecified disorder of esophagus**

Item 9-10 Esophageal reflux is the return flow of the contents of the stomach to the esophagus. **Gastroesophageal reflux** is the return flow of the contents of the stomach and duodenum to the esophagus. **Esophageal leukoplakia** are white areas on the mucous membrane of the esophagus for which no specific cause can be identified.

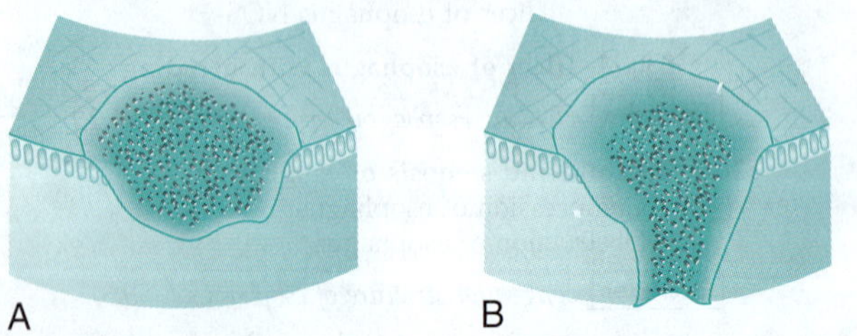

Figure 9-9 A. Ulcer. **B.** Perforated ulcer.

Item 9-11 Gastric ulcers are lesions of the stomach that result in the death of the tissue and a defect of the surface. **Perforated ulcers** are those in which the lesion penetrates the gastric wall, leaving a hole. **Peptic ulcers** are lesions of the stomach or the duodenum. **Peptic** refers to the gastric juice, pepsin.

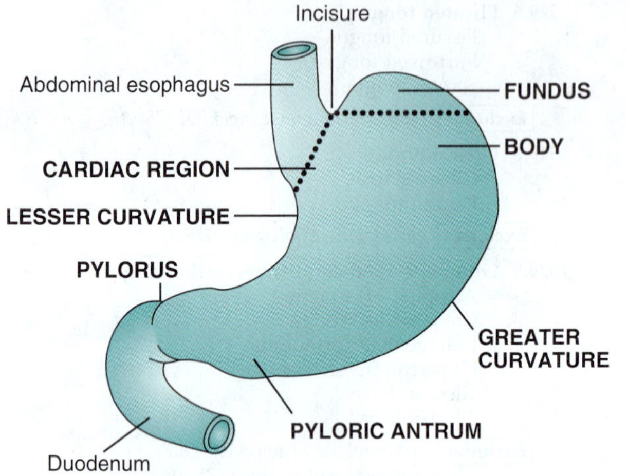

Figure 9-10 Parts of the stomach.

● 531 **Gastric ulcer**

Includes: ulcer (peptic):
prepyloric
pylorus
stomach

Use additional E code to identify drug, if drug-induced

Excludes *peptic ulcer NOS (533.0–533.9)*

The following fifth-digit subclassification is for use with category 531:
0 **without mention of obstruction**
1 **with obstruction**

● 531.0 **Acute with hemorrhage**

● 531.1 **Acute with perforation**

● 531.2 **Acute with hemorrhage and perforation**

● 531.3 **Acute without mention of hemorrhage or perforation**

● 531.4 **Chronic or unspecified with hemorrhage**

● 531.5 **Chronic or unspecified with perforation**

● 531.6 **Chronic or unspecified with hemorrhage and perforation**

● 531.7 **Chronic without mention of hemorrhage or perforation**

● ❑ 531.9 **Unspecified as acute or chronic, without mention of hemorrhage or perforation**

● 532 **Duodenal ulcer**

Includes: erosion (acute) of duodenum
ulcer (peptic):
duodenum
postpyloric

Use additional E code to identify drug, if drug-induced

Excludes *peptic ulcer NOS (533.0–533.9)*

The following fifth-digit subclassification is for use with category 532:
0 **without mention of obstruction**
1 **with obstruction**

● 532.0 **Acute with hemorrhage**

● 532.1 **Acute with perforation**

● 532.2 **Acute with hemorrhage and perforation**

● 532.3 **Acute without mention of hemorrhage or perforation**

532.4 Chronic or unspecified with hemorrhage

532.5 Chronic or unspecified with perforation

532.6 Chronic or unspecified with hemorrhage and perforation

532.7 Chronic without mention of hemorrhage or perforation

532.9 Unspecified as acute or chronic, without mention of hemorrhage or perforation

533 Peptic ulcer, site unspecified

Includes: gastroduodenal ulcer NOS
peptic ulcer NOS
stress ulcer NOS

Use additional E code to identify drug, if drug-induced

Excludes *peptic ulcer:*
duodenal (532.0–532.9)
gastric (531.0–531.9)

The following fifth-digit subclassification is for use with category 533:
0 without mention of obstruction
1 with obstruction

533.0 Acute with hemorrhage

533.1 Acute with perforation

533.2 Acute with hemorrhage and perforation

533.3 Acute without mention of hemorrhage and perforation

533.4 Chronic or unspecified with hemorrhage

533.5 Chronic or unspecified with perforation

533.6 Chronic or unspecified with hemorrhage and perforation

533.7 Chronic without mention of hemorrhage or perforation

533.9 Unspecified as acute or chronic, without mention of hemorrhage or perforation

534 Gastrojejunal ulcer

Includes: ulcer (peptic) or erosion:
anastomotic
gastrocolic
gastrointestinal
gastrojejunal
jejunal
marginal
stomal

Excludes *primary ulcer of small intestine (569.82)*

The following fifth-digit subclassification is for use with category 534:
0 without mention of obstruction
1 with obstruction

534.0 Acute with hemorrhage

534.1 Acute with perforation

534.2 Acute with hemorrhage and perforation

534.3 Acute without mention of hemorrhage or perforation

534.4 Chronic or unspecified with hemorrhage

534.5 Chronic or unspecified with perforation

534.6 Chronic or unspecified with hemorrhage and perforation

534.7 Chronic without mention of hemorrhage or perforation

534.9 Unspecified as acute or chronic, without mention of hemorrhage or perforation

Item 9-12 Gastritis is a severe inflammation of the stomach. Atrophic gastritis is a chronic inflammation of the stomach that results in destruction of the cells of the mucosa of the stomach.

535 Gastritis and duodenitis

The following fifth-digit subclassification is for use with category 535:
0 without mention of hemorrhage
1 with hemorrhage

535.0 Acute gastritis

535.1 Atrophic gastritis
Gastritis:
atrophic-hyperplastic
chronic (atrophic)

535.2 Gastric mucosal hypertrophy
Hypertrophic gastritis

535.3 Alcoholic gastritis

535.4 Other specified gastritis
Gastritis:
allergic
bile induced
irritant
superficial
toxic

535.5 Unspecified gastritis and gastroduodenitis

535.6 Duodenitis

Item 9-13 Achlorhydria, also known as gastric anacidity, is the absence of gastric acid. Gastroparesis is paralysis of the stomach.

536 Disorders of function of stomach

Excludes *functional disorders of stomach specified as psychogenic (306.4)*

536.0 Achlorhydria

536.1 Acute dilatation of stomach
Acute distention of stomach

536.2 Persistent vomiting
Habit vomiting
Persistent vomiting [not of pregnancy]
Uncontrollable vomiting

Excludes *excessive vomiting in pregnancy (643.0–643.9)*
vomiting NOS (787.0)

536.3 Gastroparesis

536.4 Gastrostomy complications

536.40 Gastrostomy complication, unspecified

536.41 Infection of gastrostomy

Use additional code to specify type of infection, such as:
abscess or cellulitis of abdomen (682.2)
septicemia (038.0–038.9)

Use additional code to identify organism (041.00–041.9)

536.42 Mechanical complication of gastrostomy

536.49 Other gastrostomy complications

536.8 Dyspepsia and other specified disorders of function of stomach
Achylia gastrica
Hourglass contraction of stomach
Hyperacidity
Hyperchlorhydria
Hypochlorhydria
Indigestion

Excludes *achlorhydria (536.0)*
heartburn (787.1)

ICD-9-CM 500-599 Vol. 1

❑536.9 **Unspecified functional disorder of stomach**
Functional gastrointestinal:
disorder
disturbance
irritation

● 537 **Other disorders of stomach and duodenum**

537.0 **Acquired hypertrophic pyloric stenosis**
Constriction of pylorus, acquired or adult
Obstruction of pylorus, acquired or adult
Stricture of pylorus, acquired or adult

Excludes *congenital or infantile pyloric stenosis (750.5)*

537.1 **Gastric diverticulum**

Excludes *congenital diverticulum of stomach (750.7)*

537.2 **Chronic duodenal ileus**

❑537.3 **Other obstruction of duodenum**
Cicatrix of duodenum
Stenosis of duodenum
Stricture of duodenum
Volvulus of duodenum

Excludes *congenital obstruction of duodenum (751.1)*

537.4 **Fistula of stomach or duodenum**
Gastrocolic fistula
Gastrojejunocolic fistula

537.5 **Gastroptosis**

537.6 **Hourglass stricture or stenosis of stomach**
Cascade stomach

Excludes *congenital hourglass stomach (750.7)*
hourglass contraction of stomach (536.8)

● 537.8 **Other specified disorders of stomach and duodenum**

537.81 **Pylorospasm**

Excludes *congenital pylorospasm (750.5)*

537.82 **Angiodysplasia of stomach and duodenum without mention of hemorrhage**

537.83 **Angiodysplasia of stomach and duodenum with hemorrhage**

537.84 **Dieulafoy lesion (hemorrhagic) of stomach and duodenum**

❑537.89 **Other**
Gastric or duodenal:
prolapse
rupture
Intestinal metaplasia of gastric mucosa
Passive congestion of stomach

Excludes *diverticula of duodenum (562.00–562.01)*
gastrointestinal hemorrhage (578.0–578.9)

❑537.9 **Unspecified disorder of stomach and duodenum**

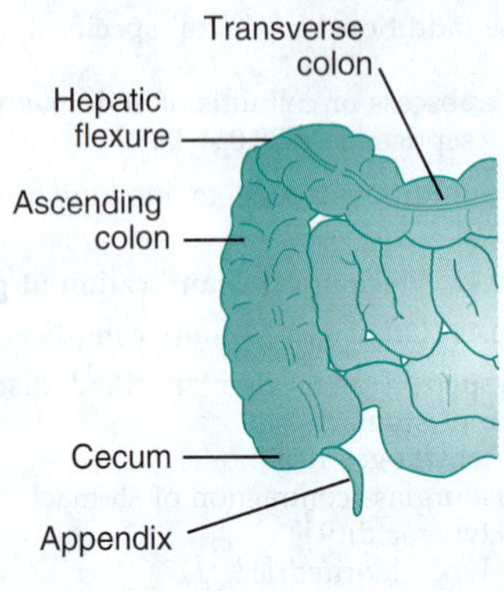

Figure 9–11 Acute appendicitis is the inflammation of the appendix, usually associated with obstruction. Most often this is a disease of adolescents and young adults.

APPENDICITIS (540–543)

● 540 **Acute appendicitis**

540.0 **With generalized peritonitis**
Appendicitis (acute) with: perforation, peritonitis (generalized), rupture:
fulminating
gangrenous
obstructive
Cecitis (acute) with: perforation, peritonitis (generalized), rupture
Rupture of appendix

Excludes *acute appendicitis with peritoneal abscess (540.1)*

540.1 **With peritoneal abscess**
Abscess of appendix
With generalized peritonitis

540.9 **Without mention of peritonitis**
Acute:
appendicitis without mention of perforation, peritonitis, or rupture:
fulminating
gangrenous
inflamed
obstructive
cecitis without mention of perforation, peritonitis, or rupture

❑541 **Appendicitis, unqualified**

❑542 **Other appendicitis**
Appendicitis:
chronic
recurrent
Appendicitis:
relapsing
subacute

Excludes *hyperplasia (lymphoid) of appendix (543.0)*

● 543 **Other diseases of appendix**

543.0 **Hyperplasia of appendix (lymphoid)**

❑543.9 **Other and unspecified diseases of appendix**
Appendicular or appendiceal:
colic
concretion
fistula
Diverticulum of appendix
Fecalith of appendix
Intussusception of appendix
Mucocele of appendix
Stercolith of appendix

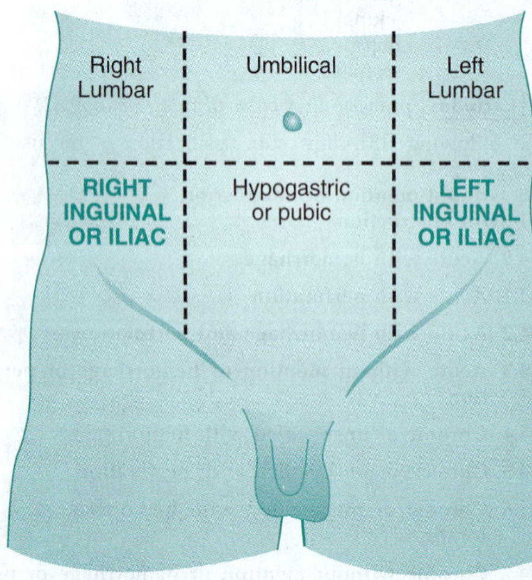

Figure 9–12 Inguinal hernias are those that are located in the inguinal or iliac areas of the abdomen.

Item 9-14 **Hernias of the groin are the most common type, accounting for 80 percent of all hernias. There are two major types of inguinal hernias: indirect (oblique) and direct. Indirect inguinal hernias result when the intestines emerge through the abdominal wall in an indirect fashion through the inguinal canal. Direct inguinal hernias penetrate through the abdominal wall in a direct fashion.**
Femoral hernias occur at the femoral ring where the femoral vessels enter the thigh.
Classification is based on location of the hernia and whether there is obstruction or gangrene.

HERNIA OF ABDOMINAL CAVITY (550–553)

Includes: hernia:
acquired
congenital, except diaphragmatic or hiatal

● **550 Inguinal hernia**

Includes: bubonocele
inguinal hernia (direct) (double) (indirect) (oblique) (sliding)
scrotal hernia

The following fifth-digit subclassification is for use with category 550:
❑ **0 unilateral or unspecified (not specified as recurrent)**
Unilateral NOS
1 unilateral or unspecified, recurrent
2 bilateral (not specified as recurrent)
Bilateral NOS
3 bilateral, recurrent

● **550.0 Inguinal hernia, with gangrene**
Inguinal hernia with gangrene (and obstruction)

● **550.1 Inguinal hernia, with obstruction, without mention of gangrene**
Inguinal hernia with mention of incarceration, irreducibility, or strangulation

● **550.9 Inguinal hernia, without mention of obstruction or gangrene**
Inguinal hernia NOS

● **551 Other hernia of abdominal cavity, with gangrene**

Includes: that with gangrene (and obstruction)

● **551.0 Femoral hernia with gangrene**

❑ **551.00 Unilateral or unspecified (not specified as recurrent)**
Femoral hernia NOS with gangrene

551.01 Unilateral or unspecified, recurrent

551.02 Bilateral (not specified as recurrent)

551.03 Bilateral, recurrent

551.1 Umbilical hernia with gangrene
Parumbilical hernia specified as gangrenous

● **551.2 Ventral hernia with gangrene**

❑ **551.20 Ventral, unspecified, with gangrene**

551.21 Incisional, with gangrene
Hernia:
postoperative specified as gangrenous
recurrent, ventral specified as gangrenous

❑ **551.29 Other**
Epigastric hernia specified as gangrenous

551.3 Diaphragmatic hernia with gangrene
Hernia:
hiatal (esophageal) (sliding) specified as gangrenous
paraesophageal specified as gangrenous
Thoracic stomach specified as gangrenous

Excludes *congenital diaphragmatic hernia (756.6)*

❑ **551.8 Hernia of other specified sites, with gangrene**
Any condition classifiable to 553.8 if specified as gangrenous

❑ **551.9 Hernia of unspecified site, with gangrene**
Any condition classifiable to 553.9 if specified as gangrenous

● **552 Other hernia of abdominal cavity, with obstruction, but without mention of gangrene**

Excludes *that with mention of gangrene (551.0–551.9)*

● **552.0 Femoral hernia with obstruction**
Femoral hernia specified as incarcerated, irreducible, strangulated, or causing obstruction

❑ **552.00 Unilateral or unspecified (not specified as recurrent)**

552.01 Unilateral or unspecified, recurrent

552.02 Bilateral (not specified as recurrent)

552.03 Bilateral, recurrent

552.1 Umbilical hernia with obstruction
Parumbilical hernia specified as incarcerated, irreducible, strangulated, or causing obstruction

● **552.2 Ventral hernia with obstruction**
Ventral hernia specified as incarcerated, irreducible, strangulated, or causing obstruction

❑ **552.20 Ventral, unspecified, with obstruction**

552.21 Incisional, with obstruction
Hernia:
postoperative specified as incarcerated, irreducible, strangulated, or causing obstruction
recurrent, ventral specified as incarcerated, irreducible, strangulated, or causing obstruction

❑ **552.29 Other**
Epigastric hernia specified as incarcerated, irreducible, strangulated, or causing obstruction

552.3 Diaphragmatic hernia with obstruction
Hernia:
hiatal (esophageal) (sliding) specified as incarcerated, irreducible, strangulated, or causing obstruction
paraesophageal specified as incarcerated, irreducible, strangulated, or causing obstruction
Thoracic stomach specified as incarcerated, irreducible, strangulated, or causing obstruction

Excludes *congenital diaphragmatic hernia (756.6)*

❑ **552.8 Hernia of other specified sites, with obstruction**
Any condition classifiable to 553.8 if specified as incarcerated, irreducible, strangulated, or causing obstruction

❑ 552.9 **Hernia of unspecified site, with obstruction**
Any condition classifiable to 553.9 if specified as incarcerated, irreducible, strangulated, or causing obstruction

● 553 **Other hernia of abdominal cavity without mention of obstruction or gangrene**
Excludes *the listed conditions with mention of:*
gangrene (and obstruction) (551.0–551.9)
obstruction (552.0–552.9)

● 553.0 **Femoral hernia**

❑ 553.00 **Unilateral or unspecified (not specified as recurrent)**
Femoral hernia NOS

553.01 **Unilateral or unspecified, recurrent**

553.02 **Bilateral (not specified as recurrent)**

553.03 **Bilateral, recurrent**

553.1 **Umbilical hernia**
Parumbilical hernia

● 553.2 **Ventral hernia**

❑ 553.20 **Ventral, unspecified**

553.21 **Incisional**
Hernia:
postoperative
recurrent, ventral

❑ 553.29 **Other**
Hernia:
epigastric
spigelian

553.3 **Diaphragmatic hernia**
Hernia:
hiatal (esophageal) (sliding)
paraesophageal
Thoracic stomach
Excludes *congenital:*
diaphragmatic hernia (756.6)
hiatal hernia (750.6)
esophagocele (530.6)

❑ 553.8 **Hernia of other specified sites**
Hernia:
ischiatic
ischiorectal
lumbar
obturator
pudendal
retroperitoneal
sciatic
Other abdominal hernia of specified site
Excludes *vaginal enterocele (618.6)*

❑ 553.9 **Hernia of unspecified site**
Enterocele
Epiplocele
Hernia:
NOS
interstitial
intestinal
intra-abdominal
Rupture (nontraumatic)
Sarcoepiplocele

NONINFECTIOUS ENTERITIS AND COLITIS (555–558)

● 555 **Regional enteritis**
Includes: Crohn's disease
Granulomatous enteritis
Excludes *ulcerative colitis (556)*

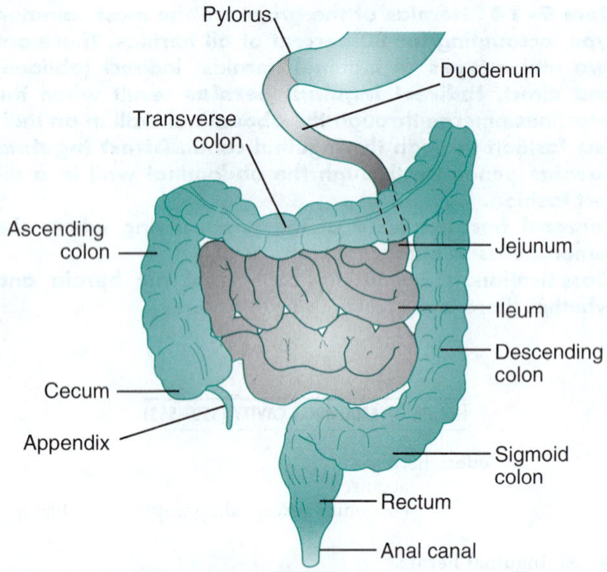

Figure 9–13 Small and large intestines.

Item 9–15 Crohn's disease, also known as regional enteritis, is a chronic inflammatory disease of the intestines. Classification is based on location in the small (duodenum, ileum, jejunum) or large (cecum, colon, rectum, anal canal) intestine.

555.0 **Small intestine**
Ileitis:
regional
segmental
terminal
Regional enteritis or Crohn's disease of:
duodenum
ileum
jejunum

555.1 **Large intestine**
Colitis:
granulomatous
regional
transmural
Regional enteritis or Crohn's disease of:
colon
large bowel
rectum

555.2 **Small intestine with large intestine**
Regional ileocolitis

❑ 555.9 **Unspecified site**
Crohn's disease NOS
Regional enteritis NOS

● 556 **Ulcerative colitis**

556.0 **Ulcerative (chronic) enterocolitis**

556.1 **Ulcerative (chronic) ileocolitis**

556.2 **Ulcerative (chronic) proctitis**

Item 9–16 Ulcerative colitis attacks the colonic mucosa and forms abscesses. The disease involves the intestines.
Classification is based on the location:
enterocolitis: large and small intestine
ileocolitis: ileum and colon
proctitis: rectum
proctosigmoiditis: sigmoid colon and rectum

556.3 Ulcerative (chronic) proctosigmoiditis

556.4 Pseudopolyposis of colon

556.5 Left-sided ulcerative (chronic) colitis

556.6 Universal ulcerative (chronic) colitis
Pancolitis

❑ **556.8 Other ulcerative colitis**

❑ **556.9 Ulcerative colitis, unspecified**
Ulcerative enteritis NOS

● **557 Vascular insufficiency of intestine**

Excludes *necrotizing enterocolitis of the newborn (777.5)*

557.0 Acute vascular insufficiency of intestine
Acute:
- hemorrhagic enterocolitis
- ischemic colitis, enteritis, or enterocolitis
- massive necrosis of intestine

Bowel infarction
Embolism of mesenteric artery
Fulminant enterocolitis
Hemorrhagic necrosis of intestine
Infarction of appendices epiploicae
Intestinal gangrene
Intestinal infarction (acute) (agnogenic) (hemorrhagic) (nonocclusive)
Mesenteric infarction (embolic) (thrombotic)
Necrosis of intestine
Terminal hemorrhagic enteropathy
Thrombosis of mesenteric artery

557.1 Chronic vascular insufficiency of intestine
Angina, abdominal
Chronic ischemic colitis, enteritis, or enterocolitis
Ischemic stricture of intestine
Mesenteric:
- angina
- artery syndrome (superior)
- vascular insufficiency

❑ **557.9 Unspecified vascular insufficiency of intestine**
Alimentary pain due to vascular insufficiency
Ischemic colitis, enteritis, or enterocolitis NOS

● **558 Other and unspecified noninfectious gastroenteritis and colitis**

Excludes *infectious:*
colitis, enteritis, or gastroenteritis (009.0–009.1)
diarrhea (009.2–009.3)

558.1 Gastroenteritis and colitis due to radiation
Radiation enterocolitis

558.2 Toxic gastroenteritis and colitis
Use additional E code to identify cause

558.3 Allergic gastroenteritis and colitis
Use additional code to identify type of food allergy (V15.01–V15.05) ◀

❑ **558.9 Other and unspecified noninfectious gastroenteritis and colitis**
Colitis, NOS, dietetic, or noninfectious
Enteritis, NOS, dietetic, or noninfectious
Gastroenteritis, NOS, dietetic, or noninfectious
Ileitis, NOS, dietetic, or noninfectious
Jejunitis, NOS, dietetic, or noninfectious
Sigmoiditis, NOS, dietetic, or noninfectious

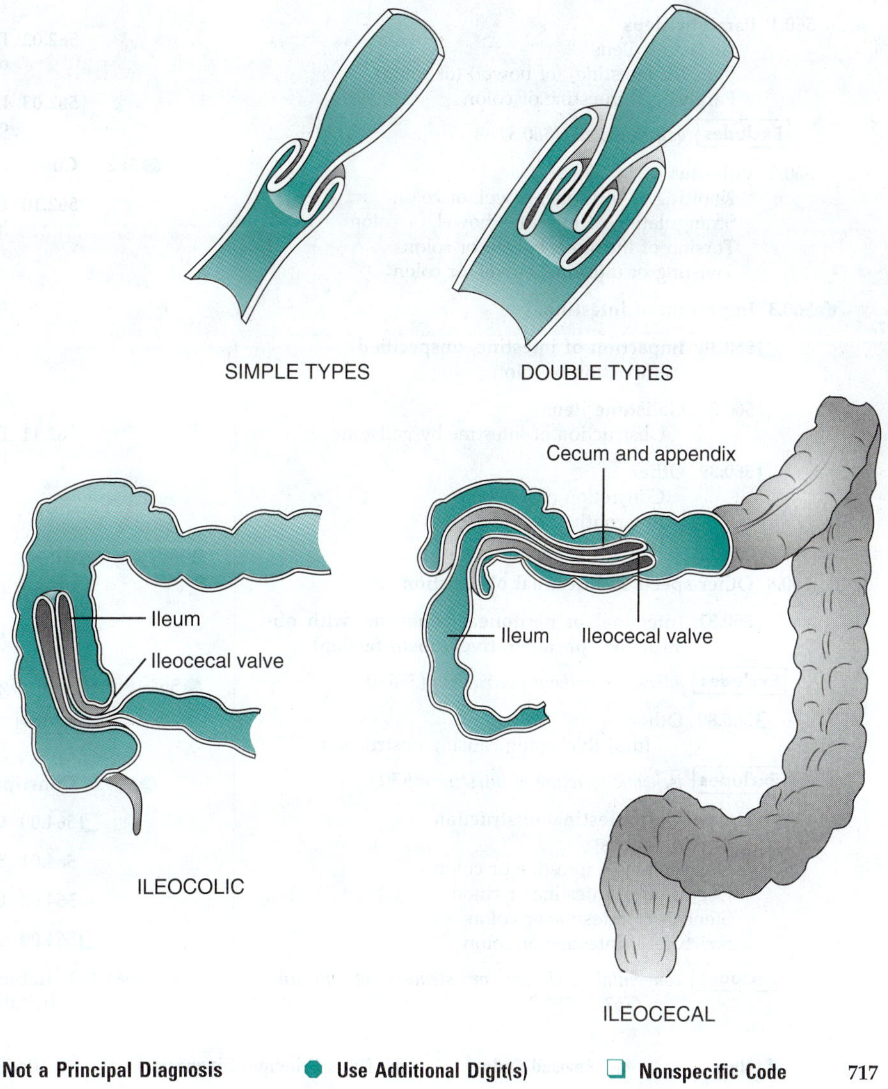

Figure 9–14 Types of intussusception.

Item 9-17 Intussusception is the prolapse of a part of the intestine into another adjacent part of the intestine. Intussusception may be enteric (ileoileal, jejunoileal, jejunojejunal), colic (colocolic), or intracolic (ileocecal, ileocolic).

Item 9-18 Volvulus is the twisting of a segment of the intestine, resulting in obstruction.

OTHER DISEASES OF INTESTINES AND PERITONEUM (560–569)

● **560 Intestinal obstruction without mention of hernia**

Excludes *duodenum (537.2–537.3)*
inguinal hernia with obstruction (550.1)
intestinal obstruction complicating hernia (552.0–552.9)
mesenteric:
embolism (557.0)
infarction (557.0)
thrombosis (557.0)
neonatal intestinal obstruction (277.01, 777.1–777.2, 777.4)

560.0 Intussusception
Intussusception (colon) (intestine) (rectum)
Invagination of intestine or colon

Excludes *intussusception of appendix (543.9)*

560.1 Paralytic ileus
Adynamic ileus
Ileus (of intestine) (of bowel) (of colon)
Paralysis of intestine or colon

Excludes *gallstone ileus (560.31)*

560.2 Volvulus
Knotting of intestine, bowel, or colon
Strangulation of intestine, bowel, or colon
Torsion of intestine, bowel, or colon
Twisting of intestine, bowel, or colon

● **560.3 Impaction of intestine**

❑ **560.30 Impaction of intestine, unspecified**
Impaction of colon

560.31 Gallstone ileus
Obstruction of intestine by gallstone

❑ **560.39 Other**
Concretion of intestine
Enterolith
Fecal impaction

● **560.8 Other specified intestinal obstruction**

560.81 Intestinal or peritoneal adhesions with obstruction (postoperative) (postinfection)

Excludes *adhesions without obstruction (568.0)*

❑ **560.89 Other**
Mural thickening causing obstruction

Excludes *ischemic stricture of intestine (557.1)*

❑ **560.9 Unspecified intestinal obstruction**
Enterostenosis
Obstruction of intestine or colon
Occlusion of intestine or colon
Stenosis of intestine or colon
Stricture of intestine or colon

Excludes *congenital stricture or stenosis of intestine (751.1–751.2)*

Item 9-19 Diverticula of the intestines are acquired herniations of the mucosa.
Classification is based on location (small intestine or colon) and whether it occurs with or without hemorrhage.

● **562 Diverticula of intestine**

Use additional code to identify any associated:
peritonitis (567.0–567.9)

Excludes *congenital diverticulum of colon (751.5)*
diverticulum of appendix (543.9)
Meckel's diverticulum (751.0)

● **562.0 Small intestine**

562.00 Diverticulosis of small intestine (without mention of hemorrhage)
Diverticulosis:
duodenum without mention of diverticulitis
ileum without mention of diverticulitis
jejunum without mention of diverticulitis

562.01 Diverticulitis of small intestine (without mention of hemorrhage)
Diverticulitis (with diverticulosis):
duodenum
ileum
jejunum
small intestine

562.02 Diverticulosis of small intestine with hemorrhage

562.03 Diverticulitis of small intestine with hemorrhage

● **562.1 Colon**

562.10 Diverticulosis of colon (without mention of hemorrhage)
Diverticulosis without mention of diverticulitis:
NOS
intestine (large) without mention of diverticulitis
Diverticular disease (colon) without mention of diverticulitis

562.11 Diverticulitis of colon without mention of hemorrhage
Diverticulitis (with diverticulosis):
NOS
colon
intestine (large)

562.12 Diverticulosis of colon with hemorrhage

562.13 Diverticulitis of colon with hemorrhage

● **564 Functional digestive disorders, not elsewhere classified**

Excludes *functional disorders of stomach (536.0–536.9)*
those specified as psychogenic (306.4)

● **564.0 Constipation**

❑ **564.00 Constipation, unspecified**

564.01 Slow transit constipation

564.02 Outlet dysfunction constipation

❑ **564.09 Other constipation**

564.1 Irritable bowel syndrome
Irritable colon

564.2 Postgastric surgery syndromes
Dumping syndrome
Jejunal syndrome
Postgastrectomy syndrome
Postvagotomy syndrome
Excludes *malnutrition following gastrointestinal surgery (579.3)*
postgastrojejunostomy ulcer (534.0–534.9)

564.3 Vomiting following gastrointestinal surgery
Vomiting (bilious) following gastrointestinal surgery

❑ **564.4 Other postoperative functional disorders**
Diarrhea following gastrointestinal surgery
Excludes *colostomy and enterostomy complications (569.60–569.69)*

564.5 Functional diarrhea
Excludes *diarrhea:*
NOS (787.91)
psychogenic (306.4)

564.6 Anal spasm
Proctalgia fugax

564.7 Megacolon, other than Hirschsprung's
Dilatation of colon
Excludes *megacolon:*
congenital [Hirschsprung's] (751.3)
toxic (556)

● **564.8 Other specified functional disorders of intestine**
Excludes *malabsorption (579.0–579.9)*

564.81 Neurogenic bowel

❑ **564.89 Other functional disorders of intestine**
Atony of colon

❑ **564.9 Unspecified functional disorder of intestine**

Item 9-20 A fissure is a groove in the surface, whereas a fistula is an abnormal passage.

● **565 Anal fissure and fistula**

565.0 Anal fissure
Tear of anus, nontraumatic
Excludes *traumatic (863.89, 863.99)*

565.1 Anal fistula
Fistula:
anorectal
rectal
rectum to skin
Excludes *fistula of rectum to internal organs - see Alphabetic Index*
ischiorectal fistula (566)
rectovaginal fistula (619.1)

566 Abscess of anal and rectal regions
Abscess:
ischiorectal
perianal
perirectal
Cellulitis:
anal
perirectal
rectal
Ischiorectal fistula

● **567 Peritonitis**
Excludes *peritonitis:*
benign paroxysmal (277.3)
pelvic, female (614.5, 614.7)
periodic familial (277.3)
puerperal (670)
with or following:
abortion (634–638 with .0, 639.0)
appendicitis (540.0–540.1)
ectopic or molar pregnancy (639.0)

● ***567.0 Peritonitis in infectious diseases classified elsewhere***
Code first underlying disease
Excludes *peritonitis:*
gonococcal (098.86)
syphilitic (095.2)
tuberculous (014.0)

567.1 Pneumococcal peritonitis

❑ **567.2 Other suppurative peritonitis**
Abscess (of):
abdominopelvic
mesenteric
omentum
peritoneum
retrocecal
retroperitoneal
subdiaphragmatic
subhepatic
subphrenic
Peritonitis (acute):
general
pelvic, male
subphrenic
suppurative

❑ **567.8 Other specified peritonitis**
Chronic proliferative peritonitis
Fat necrosis of peritoneum
Mesenteric saponification
Peritonitis due to:
bile
urine

❑ **567.9 Unspecified peritonitis**
Peritonitis:
NOS
of unspecified cause

● **568 Other disorders of peritoneum**

568.0 Peritoneal adhesions (postoperative) (postinfection)
Adhesions (of):
abdominal (wall)
diaphragm
intestine
male pelvis
mesenteric
omentum
stomach
Adhesive bands
Excludes *adhesions:*
pelvic, female (614.6)
with obstruction:
duodenum (537.3)
intestine (560.81)

● **568.8 Other specified disorders of peritoneum**

568.81 Hemoperitoneum (nontraumatic)

568.82 Peritoneal effusion (chronic)
Excludes *ascites NOS (789.5)*

❑ **568.89 Other**
Peritoneal:
cyst
granuloma

❑ **568.9 Unspecified disorder of peritoneum**

● **569 Other disorders of intestine**

569.0 Anal and rectal polyp
Anal and rectal polyp NOS
Excludes *adenomatous anal and rectal polyp (211.4)*

569.1 Rectal prolapse
Procidentia:
anus (sphincter)
rectum (sphincter)
Proctoptosis
Prolapse:
anal canal
rectal mucosa
Excludes *prolapsed hemorrhoids (455.2, 455.5)*

569.2 Stenosis of rectum and anus
Stricture of anus (sphincter)

569.3 Hemorrhage of rectum and anus

Excludes *gastrointestinal bleeding NOS (578.9)*
melena (578.1)

569.4 Other specified disorders of rectum and anus

569.41 Ulcer of anus and rectum
Solitary ulcer of anus (sphincter) or rectum (sphincter)
Stercoral ulcer of anus (sphincter) or rectum (sphincter)

569.42 Anal or rectal pain

569.49 Other
Granuloma of rectum (sphincter)
Rupture of rectum (sphincter)
Hypertrophy of anal papillae
Proctitis NOS

Excludes *fistula of rectum to:*
internal organs - see Alphabetic Index
skin (565.1)
hemorrhoids (455.0–455.9)
incontinence of sphincter ani (787.6)

569.5 Abscess of intestine

Excludes *appendiceal abscess (540.1)*

569.6 Colostomy and enterostomy complications

569.60 Colostomy and enterostomy complication, unspecified

569.61 Infection of colostomy or enterostomy
Use additional code to identify organism (041.00–041.9)
Use additional code to specify type of infection, such as:
abscess or cellulitis of abdomen (682.2)
septicemia (038.0–038.9)

569.62 Mechanical complication of colostomy and enterostomy
Malfunction of colostomy and enterostomy

569.69 Other complication
Fistula
Hernia
Prolapse

569.8 Other specified disorders of intestine

569.81 Fistula of intestine, excluding rectum and anus
Fistula:
abdominal wall
enterocolic
enteroenteric
ileorectal

Excludes *fistula of intestine to internal organs-see Alphabetic Index*
persistent postoperative fistula (998.6)

569.82 Ulceration of intestine
Primary ulcer of intestine
Ulceration of colon

Excludes *that with perforation (569.83)*

569.83 Perforation of intestine

569.84 Angiodysplasia of intestine (without mention of hemorrhage)

569.85 Angiodysplasia of intestine with hemorrhage

569.86 Dieulafoy lesion (hemorrhagic) of intestine

569.89 Other
Enteroptosis
Granuloma of intestine
Prolapse of intestine
Pericolitis
Perisigmoiditis
Visceroptosis

Excludes *gangrene of intestine, mesentery, or omentum (557.0)*
hemorrhage of intestine NOS (578.9)
obstruction of intestine (560.0–560.9)

569.9 Unspecified disorder of intestine

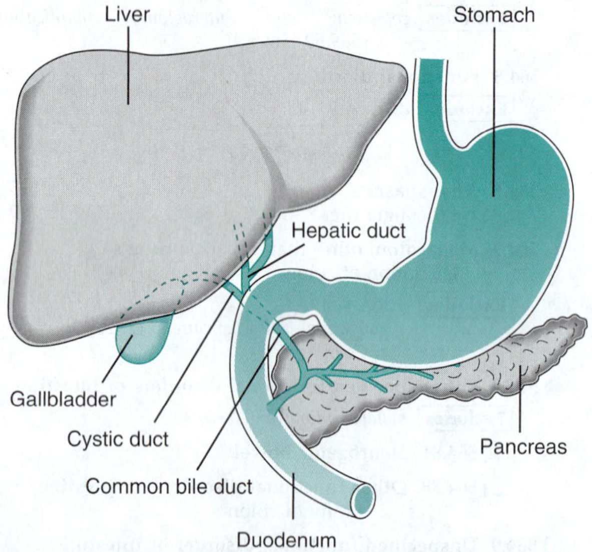

Figure 9–15 Liver and bile ducts.

Item 9–21 Cirrhosis is the progressive fibrosis of the liver resulting in loss of liver function. The main causes of cirrhosis of the liver are alcohol abuse, chronic hepatitis (inflammation of the liver), biliary disease, and excessive amounts of iron. Alcoholic cirrhosis of the liver is also called portal, Laënnec's, or fatty nutritional cirrhosis.

OTHER DISEASES OF DIGESTIVE SYSTEM (570–579)

570 Acute and subacute necrosis of liver
Acute hepatic failure
Acute or subacute hepatitis, not specified as infective
Necrosis of liver (acute) (diffuse) (massive) (subacute)
Parenchymatous degeneration of liver
Yellow atrophy (liver) (acute) (subacute)

Excludes *icterus gravis of newborn (773.0–773.2)*
serum hepatitis (070.2–070.3)
that with:
abortion (634–638 with .7, 639.8)
ectopic or molar pregnancy (639.8)
pregnancy, childbirth, or the puerperium (646.7)
viral hepatitis (070.0–070.9)

571 Chronic liver disease and cirrhosis

571.0 Alcoholic fatty liver

571.1 Acute alcoholic hepatitis
Acute alcoholic liver disease

571.2 **Alcoholic cirrhosis of liver**
Florid cirrhosis
Laënnec's cirrhosis (alcoholic)

❑ 571.3 **Alcoholic liver damage, unspecified**

● 571.4 **Chronic hepatitis**
Excludes *viral hepatitis (acute) (chronic) (070.0–070.9)*

❑ 571.40 **Chronic hepatitis, unspecified**

571.41 **Chronic persistent hepatitis**

❑ 571.49 **Other**
Chronic hepatitis:
active
aggressive
Recurrent hepatitis

571.5 **Cirrhosis of liver without mention of alcohol**
Cirrhosis of liver:
NOS
cryptogenic
macronodular
micronodular
posthepatitic
postnecrotic
Healed yellow atrophy (liver)
Portal cirrhosis

571.6 **Biliary cirrhosis**
Chronic nonsuppurative destructive cholangitis
Cirrhosis:
cholangitic
cholestatic

❑ 571.8 **Other chronic nonalcoholic liver disease**
Chronic yellow atrophy (liver)
Fatty liver, without mention of alcohol

❑ 571.9 **Unspecified chronic liver disease without mention of alcohol**

● 572 **Liver abscess and sequelae of chronic liver disease**

572.0 **Abscess of liver**
Excludes *amebic liver abscess (006.3)*

572.1 **Portal pyemia**
Phlebitis of portal vein
Portal thrombophlebitis
Pylephlebitis
Pylethrombophlebitis

572.2 **Hepatic coma**
Hepatic encephalopathy
Hepatocerebral intoxication
Portal-systemic encephalopathy

572.3 **Portal hypertension**

572.4 **Hepatorenal syndrome**
Excludes *that following delivery (674.8)*

❑ 572.8 **Other sequelae of chronic liver disease**

● 573 **Other disorders of liver**
Excludes *amyloid or lardaceous degeneration of liver (277.3)*
congenital cystic disease of liver (751.62)
glycogen infiltration of liver (271.0)
hepatomegaly NOS (789.1)
portal vein obstruction (452)

573.0 **Chronic passive congestion of liver**

● 573.1 ***Hepatitis in viral diseases classified elsewhere***
Code first underlying disease, as:
Coxsackie virus disease (074.8)
cytomegalic inclusion virus disease (078.5)
infectious mononucleosis (075)
Excludes *hepatitis (in):*
mumps (072.71)
viral (070.0–070.9)
yellow fever (060.0–060.9)

●❑ 573.2 ***Hepatitis in other infectious diseases classified elsewhere***
Code first underlying disease, as:
malaria (084.9)
Excludes *hepatitis in:*
late syphilis (095.3)
secondary syphilis (091.62)
toxoplasmosis (130.5)

❑ 573.3 **Hepatitis, unspecified**
Toxic (noninfectious) hepatitis
Use additional E code to identify cause

573.4 **Hepatic infarction**

❑ 573.8 **Other specified disorders of liver**
Hepatoptosis

❑ 573.9 **Unspecified disorder of liver**

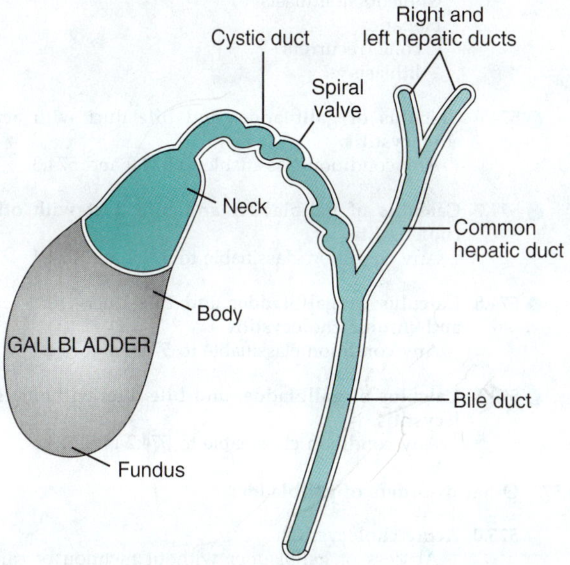

Figure 9–16 Gallbladder and bile ducts.

● 574 **Cholelithiasis**
The following fifth-digit subclassification is for use with category 574:
0 without mention of obstruction
1 with obstruction

● 574.0 **Calculus of gallbladder with acute cholecystitis**
Biliary calculus with acute cholecystitis
Calculus of cystic duct with acute cholecystitis
Cholelithiasis with acute cholecystitis
Any condition classifiable to 574.2 with acute cholecystitis

●❑ 574.1 **Calculus of gallbladder with other cholecystitis**
Biliary calculus with cholecystitis
Calculus of cystic duct with cholecystitis
Cholelithiasis with cholecystitis
Cholecystitis with cholelithiasis NOS
Any condition classifiable to 574.2 with cholecystitis (chronic)

● 574.2 **Calculus of gallbladder without mention of cholecystitis**
Biliary:
calculus NOS
colic NOS
Calculus of cystic duct
Cholelithiasis NOS
Colic (recurrent) of gallbladder
Gallstone (impacted)

ICD-9-CM 500–599 Vol. 1

● 574.3 **Calculus of bile duct with acute cholecystitis**
Calculus of bile duct [any] with acute cholecystitis
Choledocholithiasis with acute cholecystitis
Any condition classifiable to 574.5 with acute cholecystitis

● ❑ 574.4 **Calculus of bile duct with other cholecystitis**
Calculus of bile duct [any] with cholecystitis (chronic)
Choledocholithiasis with cholecystitis (chronic)
Any condition classifiable to 574.5 with cholecystitis (chronic)

● 574.5 **Calculus of bile duct without mention of cholecystitis**
Calculus of:
bile duct [any]
common duct
hepatic duct
Choledocholithiasis
Hepatic:
colic (recurrent)
lithiasis

● 574.6 **Calculus of gallbladder and bile duct with acute cholecystitis**
Any condition classifiable to 574.0 and 574.3

● 574.7 **Calculus of gallbladder and bile duct with other cholecystitis**
Any condition classifiable to 574.1 and 574.4

● 574.8 **Calculus of gallbladder and bile duct with acute and chronic cholecystitis**
Any condition classifiable to 574.6 and 574.7

● 574.9 **Calculus of gallbladder and bile duct without cholecystitis**
Any condition classifiable to 574.2 and 574.5

● 575 **Other disorders of gallbladder**

575.0 **Acute cholecystitis**
Abscess of gallbladder without mention of calculus
Angiocholecystitis without mention of calculus
Cholecystitis without mention of calculus:
emphysematous (acute)
gangrenous
suppurative
Empyema of gallbladder without mention of calculus
Gangrene of gallbladder without mention of calculus

Excludes *that with:*
acute and chronic cholecystitis (575.12)
choledocholithiasis (574.3)
choledocholithiasis and cholelithiasis (574.6)
cholelithiasis (574.0)

● 575.1 **Other cholecystitis**
Cholecystitis without mention of calculus:
NOS without mention of calculus
chronic without mention of calculus

Excludes *that with:*
choledocholithiasis (574.4)
choledocholithiasis and cholelithiasis (574.8)
cholelithiasis (574.1)

❑ 575.10 **Cholecystitis, unspecified**
Cholecystitis NOS

575.11 **Chronic cholecystitis**

575.12 **Acute and chronic cholecystitis**

575.2 **Obstruction of gallbladder**
Occlusion of cystic duct or gallbladder without mention of calculus
Stenosis of cystic duct or gallbladder without mention of calculus
Stricture of cystic duct or gallbladder without mention of calculus

Excludes *that with calculus (574.0–574.2 with fifth digit 1)*

575.3 **Hydrops of gallbladder**
Mucocele of gallbladder

575.4 **Perforation of gallbladder**
Rupture of cystic duct or gallbladder

575.5 **Fistula of gallbladder**
Fistula:
cholecystoduodenal
cholecystoenteric

575.6 **Cholesterolosis of gallbladder**
Strawberry gallbladder

❑ 575.8 **Other specified disorders of gallbladder**
Adhesions (of) cystic duct gallbladder
Atrophy (of) cystic duct gallbladder
Cyst (of) cystic duct gallbladder
Hypertrophy (of) cystic duct gallbladder
Nonfunctioning (of) cystic duct gallbladder
Ulcer (of) cystic duct gallbladder
Biliary dyskinesia

Excludes *Hartmann's pouch of intestine (V44.3)*
nonvisualization of gallbladder (793.3)

❑ 575.9 **Unspecified disorder of gallbladder**

● 576 **Other disorders of biliary tract**

Excludes *that involving the:*
cystic duct (575.0–575.9)
gallbladder (575.0–575.9)

576.0 **Postcholecystectomy syndrome**

576.1 **Cholangitis**

Cholangitis:	Cholangitis:
NOS	recurrent
acute	sclerosing
ascending	secondary
chronic	stenosing
primary	suppurative

576.2 **Obstruction of bile duct**
Occlusion of bile duct, except cystic duct, without mention of calculus
Stenosis of bile duct, except cystic duct, without mention of calculus
Stricture of bile duct, except cystic duct, without mention of calculus

Excludes *congenital (751.61)*
that with calculus (574.3–574.5 with fifth-digit 1)

576.3 **Perforation of bile duct**
Rupture of bile duct, except cystic duct

576.4 **Fistula of bile duct**
Choledochoduodenal fistula

576.5 **Spasm of sphincter of Oddi**

❑ 576.8 **Other specified disorders of biliary tract**
Adhesions of bile duct [any]
Atrophy of bile duct [any]
Cyst of bile duct [any]
Hypertrophy of bile duct [any]
Stasis of bile duct [any]
Ulcer of bile duct [any]

Excludes *congenital choledochal cyst (751.69)*

❑ 576.9 **Unspecified disorder of biliary tract**

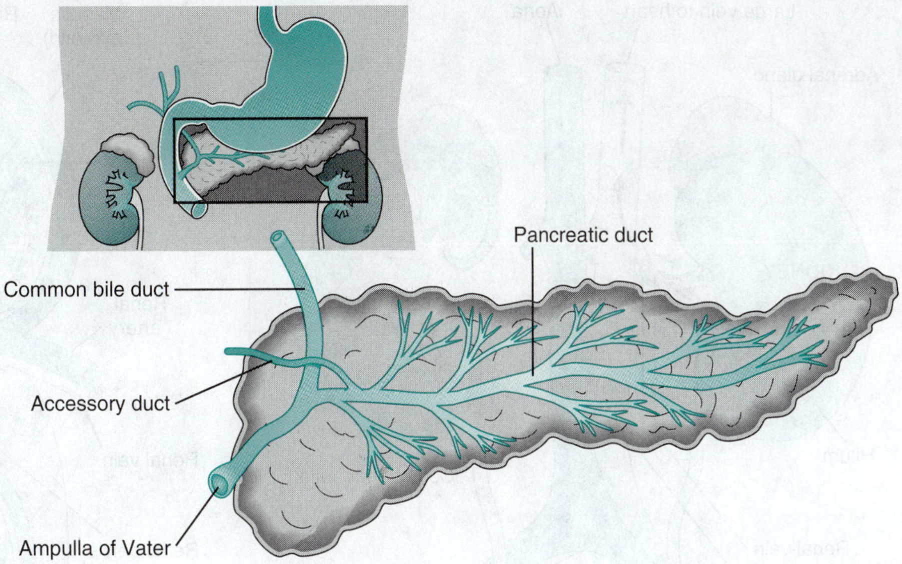

Figure 9–17 Pancreas.

● 577 **Diseases of pancreas**

577.0 **Acute pancreatitis**

Abscess of pancreas
Necrosis of pancreas:
acute
infective
Pancreatitis:
NOS
acute (recurrent)
apoplectic
Pancreatitis:
hemorrhagic
subacute
suppurative

Excludes *mumps pancreatitis (072.3)*

577.1 **Chronic pancreatitis**

Chronic pancreatitis:
NOS
infectious
interstitial
Pancreatitis:
painless
recurrent
relapsing

577.2 **Cyst and pseudocyst of pancreas**

❏ 577.8 **Other specified diseases of pancreas**

Atrophy of pancreas
Calculus of pancreas
Cirrhosis of pancreas
Fibrosis of pancreas
Pancreatic:
infantilism
necrosis:
NOS
aseptic
fat
Pancreatolithiasis

Excludes *fibrocystic disease of pancreas (277.00–277.09)*
islet cell tumor of pancreas (211.7)
pancreatic steatorrhea (579.4)

❏ 577.9 **Unspecified disease of pancreas**

● 578 **Gastrointestinal hemorrhage**

Excludes *that with mention of:*
angiodysplasia of stomach and duodenum (537.83)
angiodysplasia of intestine (569.85)
diverticulitis, intestine:
large (562.13)
small (562.03)
diverticulosis, intestine:
large (562.12)
small (562.02)
gastritis and duodenitis (535.0–535.6)
ulcer:
duodenal, gastric, gastrojejunal, or peptic (531.00–534.91)

578.0 **Hematemesis**

Vomiting of blood

578.1 **Blood in stool**

Melena

Excludes *melena of the newborn (772.4, 777.3)*
occult blood (792.1)

❏ 578.9 **Hemorrhage of gastrointestinal tract, unspecified**

Gastric hemorrhage
Intestinal hemorrhage

● 579 **Intestinal malabsorption**

579.0 **Celiac disease**

Celiac:
crisis
infantilism
rickets
Gee (-Herter) disease
Gluten enteropathy
Idiopathic steatorrhea
Nontropical sprue

579.1 **Tropical sprue**

Sprue:
NOS
tropical
Tropical steatorrhea

579.2 **Blind loop syndrome**

Postoperative blind loop syndrome

❏ 579.3 **Other and unspecified postsurgical nonabsorption**

Hypoglycemia following gastrointestinal surgery
Malnutrition following gastrointestinal surgery

579.4 **Pancreatic steatorrhea**

❏ 579.8 **Other specified intestinal malabsorption**

Enteropathy:
exudative
protein-losing
Steatorrhea (chronic)

❏ 579.9 **Unspecified intestinal malabsorption**

Malabsorption syndrome NOS

ICD-9-CM 500–599 Vol. 1

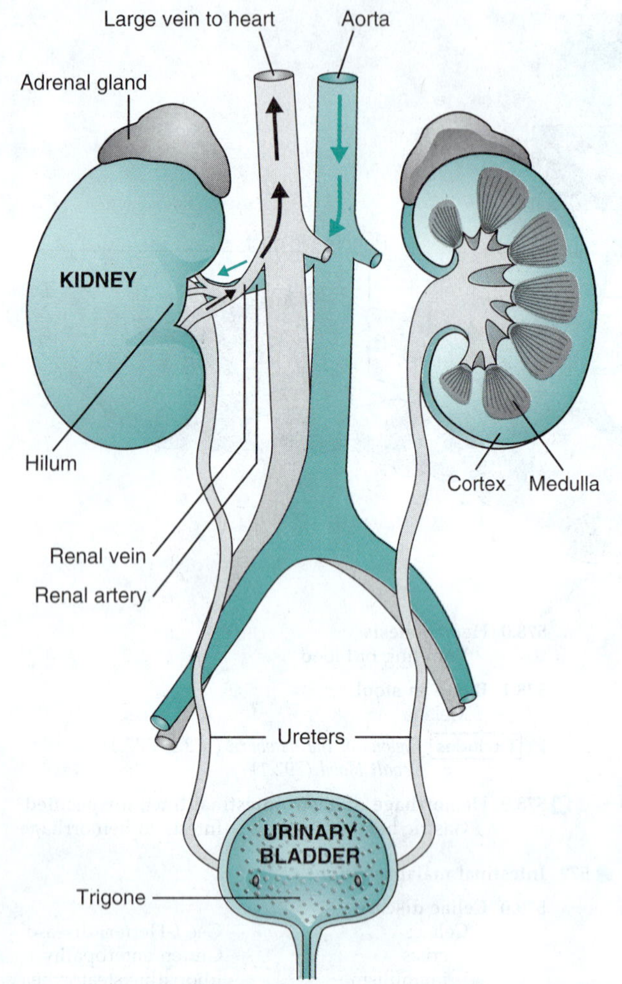

Figure 10–1 Kidneys within the urinary system.

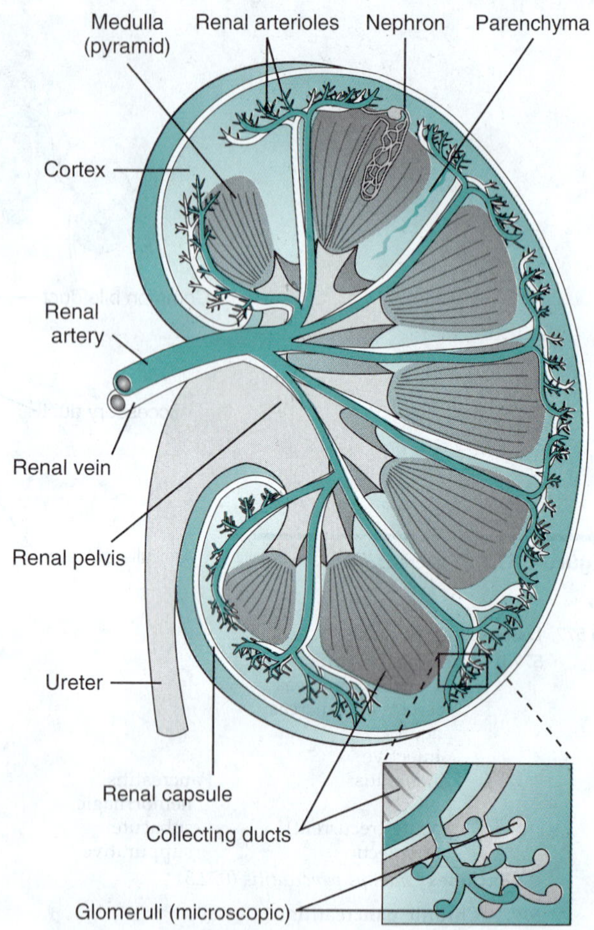

Figure 10–2 Kidney.

Item 10–1 Glomerulonephritis is nephritis accompanied by inflammation of the glomeruli of the kidney, resulting in the degeneration of the glomeruli and the nephrons.
Acute glomerulonephritis primarily affects children and young adults and is usually a result of a streptococcal infection.
Proliferative glomerulonephritis is the acute form of the disease resulting from a streptococcal infection.
Rapidly progressive glomerulonephritis, also known as crescentic or malignant glomerulonephritis, is the acute form of the disease, which leads quickly to rapid and progressive decline in renal function.

10. DISEASES OF THE GENITOURINARY SYSTEM (580–629)

NEPHRITIS, NEPHROTIC SYNDROME, AND NEPHROSIS (580–589)

Excludes *hypertensive renal disease (403.00–403.91)*

● **580 Acute glomerulonephritis**

Includes: acute nephritis

580.0 **With lesion of proliferative glomerulonephritis**
Acute (diffuse) proliferative glomerulonephritis
Acute poststreptococcal glomerulonephritis

580.4 **With lesion of rapidly progressive glomerulonephritis**
Acute nephritis with lesion of necrotizing glomerulitis

● 580.8 **With other specified pathological lesion in kidney**

● *580.81 Acute glomerulonephritis in diseases classified elsewhere*

Code first underlying disease, as:
infectious hepatitis (070.0–070.9)
mumps (072.79)
subacute bacterial endocarditis (421.0)
typhoid fever (002.0)

❑ 580.89 **Other**
Glomerulonephritis, acute, with lesion of:
exudative nephritis
interstitial (diffuse) (focal) nephritis

❑ 580.9 **Acute glomerulonephritis with unspecified pathological lesion in kidney**
Glomerulonephritis: specified as acute
NOS specified as acute
hemorrhagic specified as acute
Nephritis specified as acute
Nephropathy specified as acute

Item 10-2 Nephrotic syndrome (NS) is marked by massive proteinuria (protein in the urine) and water retention. Patients with NS are particularly vulnerable to staphylococcal and pneumococcal infections.
NS with lesion of proliferative glomerulonephritis results from a streptococcal infection.
NS with lesion of membranous glomerulonephritis results in thickening of the capillary walls.
NS with lesion of minimal change glomerulonephritis is usually a benign disorder that occurs mostly in children and requires electron microscopy to verify changes in the glomeruli.

● 581 Nephrotic syndrome

581.0 With lesion of proliferative glomerulonephritis

581.1 With lesion of membranous glomerulonephritis
Epimembranous nephritis
Idiopathic membranous glomerular disease
Nephrotic syndrome with lesion of:
focal glomerulosclerosis
sclerosing membranous glomerulonephritis
segmental hyalinosis

581.2 With lesion of membranoproliferative glomerulonephritis
Nephrotic syndrome with lesion (of):
endothelial glomerulonephritis
hypocomplementemic glomerulonephritis
persistent glomerulonephritis
lobular glomerulonephritis
mesangiocapillary glomerulonephritis
mixed membranous and proliferative glomerulonephritis

581.3 With lesion of minimal change glomerulonephritis
Foot process disease
Lipoid nephrosis
Minimal change:
glomerular disease
glomerulitis
nephrotic syndrome

● 581.8 With other specified pathological lesion in kidney

● *581.81 Nephrotic syndrome in diseases classified elsewhere*
Code first underlying disease, as:
amyloidosis (277.3)
diabetes mellitus (250.4)
malaria (084.9)
polyarteritis (446.0)
systemic lupus erythematosus (710.0)

Excludes *nephrosis in epidemic hemorrhagic fever (078.6)*

❑ 581.89 Other
Glomerulonephritis with edema and lesion of:
exudative nephritis
interstitial (diffuse) (focal) nephritis

❑ 581.9 Nephrotic syndrome with unspecified pathological lesion in kidney
Glomerulonephritis with edema NOS
Nephritis:
nephrotic NOS
with edema NOS
Nephrosis NOS
Renal disease with edema NOS

Item 10-3 Chronic glomerulonephritis (GN) persists over a period of years, with remissions and exacerbation.
Chronic GN with lesion of proliferative glomerulonephritis results from a streptococcal infection.
Chronic GN with lesion of membranous glomerulonephritis, also known as membranous nephropathy, is characterized by deposits along the epithelial side of the basement membrane.
Chronic GN with lesion of membranoproliferative glomerulonephritis (MPGN) is a group of disorders characterized by alterations in the basement membranes of the kidney and the glomerular cells.
Chronic GN with lesion of rapidly progressive glomerulonephritis is characterized by necrosis, endothelial proliferation, and mesangial proliferation. The condition is marked by rapid and progressive decline in renal function.

● 582 Chronic glomerulonephritis

Includes: chronic nephritis

582.0 With lesion of proliferative glomerulonephritis
Chronic (diffuse) proliferative glomerulonephritis

582.1 With lesion of membranous glomerulonephritis
Chronic glomerulonephritis:
membranous
sclerosing
Focal glomerulosclerosis
Segmental hyalinosis

582.2 With lesion of membranoproliferative glomerulonephritis
Chronic glomerulonephritis:
endothelial
hypocomplementemic persistent
lobular
membranoproliferative
mesangiocapillary
mixed membranous and proliferative

582.4 With lesion of rapidly progressive glomerulonephritis
Chronic nephritis with lesion of necrotizing glomerulitis

● 582.8 With other specified pathological lesion in kidney

● *582.81 Chronic glomerulonephritis in diseases classified elsewhere*
Code first underlying disease, as:
amyloidosis (277.3)
systemic lupus erythematosus (710.0)

❑ 582.89 Other
Chronic glomerulonephritis with lesion of:
exudative nephritis
interstitial (diffuse) (focal) nephritis

❑ 582.9 Chronic glomerulonephritis with unspecified pathological lesion in kidney
Glomerulonephritis: specified as chronic
NOS specified as chronic
hemorrhagic specified as chronic
Nephritis specified as chronic
Nephropathy specified as chronic

Item 10-4 Nephritis (inflammation) or **nephropathy** (disease) **with lesion of proliferative glomerulonephritis** results from a streptococcal infection. **Nephritis** (inflammation) or **nephropathy** (disease) **with lesion of membranous glomerulonephritis** is characterized by deposits along the epithelial side of the basement membrane. **Nephritis** (inflammation) or **nephropathy** (disease) **with lesion of membranoproliferative glomerulonephritis** is characterized by alterations in the basement membranes of the kidney and the glomerular cells. **Nephritis** (inflammation) or **nephropathy** (disease) **with lesion of rapidly progressive glomerulonephritis** is characterized by rapid and progressive decline in renal function. **Nephritis** (inflammation) or **nephropathy** (disease) **with lesion of renal cortical necrosis** is characterized by death of the cortical tissues. **Nephritis** (inflammation) or **nephropathy** (disease) **with lesion of renal medullary necrosis** is characterized by death of the tissues that collect urine.

● **583 Nephritis and nephropathy, not specified as acute or chronic**

Includes: "renal disease" so stated, not specified as acute or chronic but with stated pathology or cause

583.0 With lesion of proliferative glomerulonephritis
Proliferative:
glomerulonephritis (diffuse) NOS
nephritis NOS
nephropathy NOS

583.1 With lesion of membranous glomerulonephritis
Membranous:
glomerulonephritis NOS
nephritis NOS
Membranous nephropathy NOS

583.2 With lesion of membranoproliferative glomerulonephritis
Membranoproliferative:
glomerulonephritis NOS
nephritis NOS
nephropathy NOS
Nephritis NOS, with lesion of:
hypocomplementemic persistent glomerulonephritis
lobular glomerulonephritis
mesangiocapillary glomerulonephritis
mixed membranous and proliferative glomerulonephritis

583.4 With lesion of rapidly progressive glomerulonephritis
Necrotizing or rapidly progressive:
glomerulitis NOS
glomerulonephritis NOS
nephritis NOS
nephropathy NOS
Nephritis, unspecified, with lesion of necrotizing glomerulitis

583.6 With lesion of renal cortical necrosis
Nephritis NOS with (renal) cortical necrosis
Nephropathy NOS with (renal) cortical necrosis
Renal cortical necrosis NOS

583.7 With lesion of renal medullary necrosis
Nephritis NOS with (renal) medullary [papillary] necrosis
Nephropathy NOS with (renal) medullary [papillary] necrosis

● **583.8 With other specified pathological lesion in kidney**

● *583.81 Nephritis and nephropathy, not specified as acute or chronic, in diseases classified elsewhere*

Code first underlying disease, as:
amyloidosis (277.3)
diabetes mellitus (250.4)
gonococcal infection (098.19)
Goodpasture's syndrome (446.21)
systemic lupus erythematosus (710.0)
tuberculosis (016.0)

Excludes *gouty nephropathy (274.10)*
syphilitic nephritis (095.4)

❑ **583.89 Other**
Glomerulitis with lesion of:
exudative nephritis
interstitial nephritis
Glomerulonephritis with lesion of:
exudative nephritis
interstitial nephritis
Nephritis with lesion of:
exudative nephritis
interstitial nephritis
Nephropathy with lesion of:
exudative nephritis
interstitial nephritis
Renal disease with lesion of:
exudative nephritis
interstitial nephritis

❑ **583.9 With unspecified pathological lesion in kidney**
Glomerulitis NOS
Glomerulonephritis NOS
Nephritis NOS
Nephropathy NOS

Excludes *nephropathy complicating pregnancy, labor, or the puerperium (642.0–642.9, 646.2)*
renal disease NOS with no stated cause (593.9)

Item 10-5 Decreased blood flow is the usual cause of acute renal failure that offers a good prognosis for recovery. Chronic renal failure is usually the result of long-standing kidney disease and is a very serious condition that generally results in death.

● **584 Acute renal failure**

Excludes *following labor and delivery (669.3)*
posttraumatic (958.5)
that complicating:
abortion (634–638 with .3, 639.3)
ectopic or molar pregnancy (639.3)

584.5 With lesion of tubular necrosis
Lower nephron nephrosis
Renal failure with (acute) tubular necrosis
Tubular necrosis:
NOS
acute

584.6 With lesion of renal cortical necrosis

584.7 With lesion of renal medullary [papillary] necrosis
Necrotizing renal papillitis

❑ **584.8 With other specified pathological lesion in kidney**

❑ **584.9 Acute renal failure, unspecified**

585 Chronic renal failure
Chronic uremia

Use additional code to identify manifestation as:
uremic:
neuropathy (357.4)
pericarditis (420.0)

Excludes *that with any condition classifiable to 401 (403.0–403.9 with fifth-digit 1)*

❑ **586 Renal failure, unspecified**
Uremia NOS
Excludes *following labor and delivery (669.3)*
posttraumatic renal failure (958.5)
that complicating:
abortion (634–638 with .3, 639.3)
ectopic or molar pregnancy (639.3)
uremia:
extrarenal (788.9)
prerenal (788.9)
with any condition classifiable to 401 (403.0–403.9 with fifth-digit 1)

❑ **587 Renal sclerosis, unspecified**
Atrophy of kidney
Contracted kidney
Renal:
cirrhosis
fibrosis
Excludes *nephrosclerosis (arteriolar) (arteriosclerotic) (403.00–403.92)*
with hypertension (403.00–403.92)

● **588 Disorders resulting from impaired renal function**

588.0 Renal osteodystrophy
Azotemic osteodystrophy
Phosphate-losing tubular disorders
Renal:
dwarfism
infantilism
rickets

588.1 Nephrogenic diabetes insipidus
Excludes *diabetes insipidus NOS (253.5)*

❑ **588.8 Other specified disorders resulting from impaired renal function**
Hypokalemic nephropathy
Secondary hyperparathyroidism (of renal origin)
Excludes *secondary hypertension (405.0–405.9)*

❑ **588.9 Unspecified disorder resulting from impaired renal function**

● **589 Small kidney of unknown cause**

589.0 Unilateral small kidney

589.1 Bilateral small kidneys

❑ **589.9 Small kidney, unspecified**

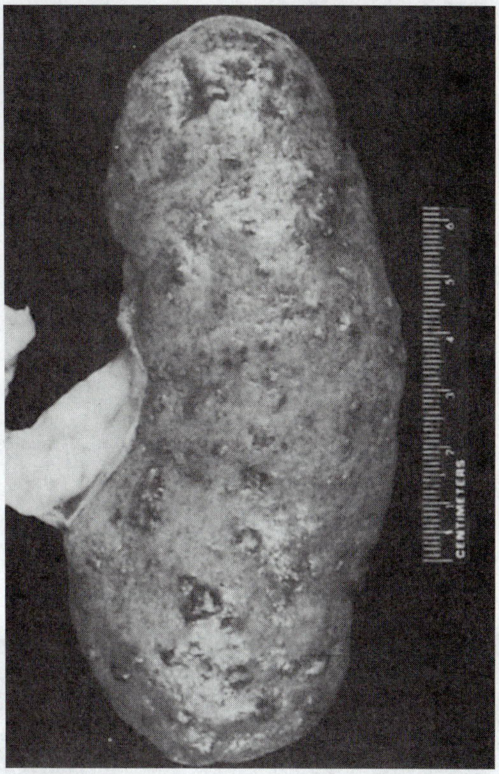

Figure 10–3 Acute pyelonephritis. Cortical surface is dotted with abscesses. (From Cotran R, Kumar V, Robbins S: Robbins Pathologic Basis of Disease. Philadelphia, WB Saunders, 1994, p 969.)

OTHER DISEASES OF URINARY SYSTEM (590–599)

● **590 Infections of kidney**
Use additional code to identify organism, such as Escherichia coli [E. coli] (041.4)

● **590.0 Chronic pyelonephritis**
Chronic pyelitis
Chronic pyonephrosis
Code, if applicable, any causal condition first

590.00 Without lesion of renal medullary necrosis

590.01 With lesion of renal medullary necrosis

● **590.1 Acute pyelonephritis**
Acute pyelitis
Acute pyonephrosis

590.10 Without lesion of renal medullary necrosis

590.11 With lesion of renal medullary necrosis

590.2 Renal and perinephric abscess
Abscess:
kidney
nephritic
perirenal
Carbuncle of kidney

590.3 Pyeloureteritis cystica
Infection of renal pelvis and ureter
Ureteritis cystica

● 590.8 **Other pyelonephritis or pyonephrosis, not specified as acute or chronic**

❑ 590.80 **Pyelonephritis, unspecified**
Pyelitis NOS
Pyelonephritis NOS

● ***590.81 Pyelitis or pyelonephritis in diseases classified elsewhere***

Code first underlying disease, as:
tuberculosis (016.0)

❑ 590.9 **Infection of kidney, unspecified**

Excludes *urinary tract infection NOS (599.0)*

591 **Hydronephrosis**
Hydrocalycosis
Hydronephrosis
Hydroureteronephrosis

Excludes *congenital hydronephrosis (753.29)*
hydroureter (593.5)

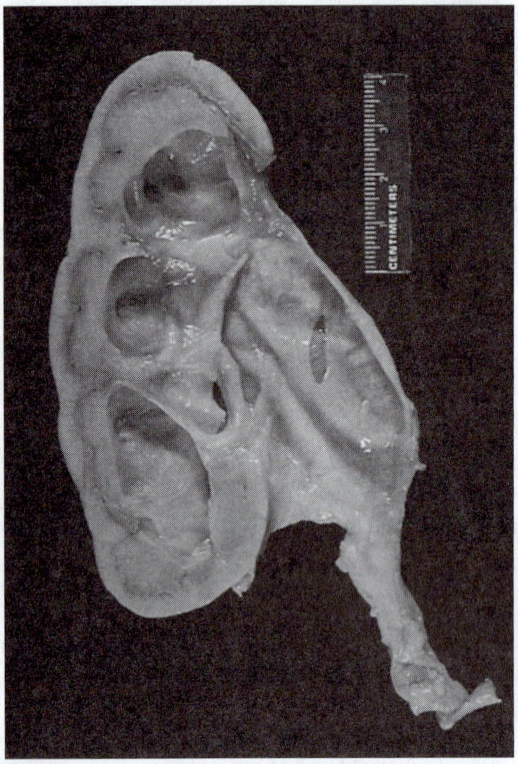

Figure 10–4 Hydronephrosis of the kidney, with marked dilatation of pelvis and calyces and thinning of renal parenchyma. (From Cotran R, Kumar V, Robbins S: Robbins Pathologic Basis of Disease. Philadelphia, WB Saunders, 1994, p 983.)

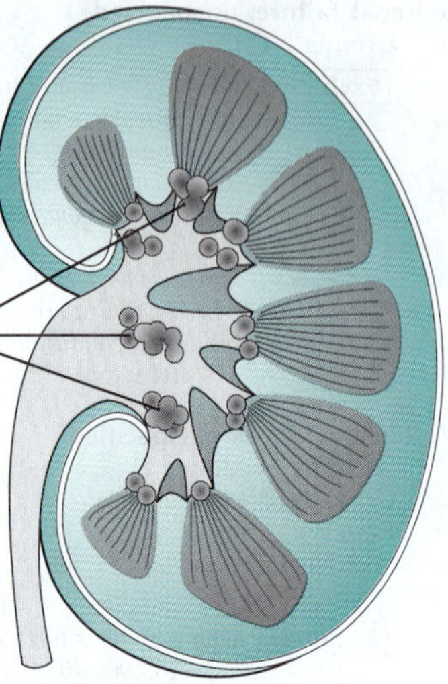

Figure 10–5 Multiple urinary calculi.

● 592 **Calculus of kidney and ureter**

Excludes *nephrocalcinosis (275.4)*

592.0 **Calculus of kidney**
Nephrolithiasis NOS
Renal calculus or stone
Staghorn calculus
Stone in kidney

Excludes *uric acid nephrolithiasis (274.11)*

592.1 **Calculus of ureter**
Ureteric stone
Ureterolithiasis

❑ 592.9 **Urinary calculus, unspecified**

● 593 **Other disorders of kidney and ureter**

593.0 **Nephroptosis**
Floating kidney   Mobile kidney

593.1 **Hypertrophy of kidney**

593.2 **Cyst of kidney, acquired**
Cyst (multiple) (solitary) of kidney, not congenital
Peripelvic (lymphatic) cyst

Excludes *calyceal or pyelogenic cyst of kidney (591)*
congenital cyst of kidney (753.1)
polycystic (disease of) kidney (753.1)

593.3 **Stricture or kinking of ureter**
Angulation of ureter (postoperative)
Constriction of ureter (postoperative)
Stricture of pelviureteric junction

❑ 593.4 **Other ureteric obstruction**
Idiopathic retroperitoneal fibrosis
Occlusion NOS of ureter

Excludes *that due to calculus (592.1)*

593.5 **Hydroureter**

Excludes *congenital hydroureter (753.22)*
hydroureteronephrosis (591)

593.6 **Postural proteinuria**
Benign postural proteinuria
Orthostatic proteinuria

Excludes *proteinuria NOS (791.0)*

Item 10-6 Vesicoureteral reflux occurs when urine flows from the bladder back into the ureters, often resulting in urinary tract infection.

● **593.7 Vesicoureteral reflux**

❑ **593.70 Unspecified or without reflux nephropathy**

593.71 With reflux nephropathy, unilateral

593.72 With reflux nephropathy, bilateral

❑ **593.73 With reflux nephropathy NOS**

● **593.8 Other specified disorders of kidney and ureter**

593.81 Vascular disorders of kidney
Renal (artery):
embolism
hemorrhage
thrombosis
Renal infarction

593.82 Ureteral fistula
Intestinoureteral fistula

Excludes *fistula between ureter and female genital tract (619.0)*

❑ **593.89 Other**
Adhesions, kidney or ureter
Periureteritis
Polyp of ureter
Pyelectasia
Ureterocele

Excludes *tuberculosis of ureter (016.2)*
ureteritis cystica (590.3)

❑ **593.9 Unspecified disorder of kidney and ureter**
Renal disease (chronic) NOS
Renal insufficiency (acute) (chronic)
Salt-losing nephritis or syndrome

Excludes *cystic kidney disease (753.1)*
nephropathy, so stated (583.0–583.9)
renal disease:
acute (580.0–580.9)
arising in pregnancy or the puerperium (642.1–642.2, 642.4–642.7, 646.2)
chronic (582.0–582.9)
not specified as acute or chronic, but with stated pathology or cause (583.0–583.9)

● **594 Calculus of lower urinary tract**

594.0 Calculus in diverticulum of bladder

❑ **594.1 Other calculus in bladder**
Urinary bladder stone

Excludes *staghorn calculus (592.0)*

594.2 Calculus in urethra

❑ **594.8 Other lower urinary tract calculus**

❑ **594.9 Calculus of lower urinary tract, unspecified**

Excludes *calculus of urinary tract NOS (592.9)*

● **595 Cystitis**

Excludes *prostatocystitis (601.3)*

Use additional code to identify organism, such as Escherichia coli [E. coli] (041.4)

595.0 Acute cystitis

Excludes *trigonitis (595.3)*

595.1 Chronic interstitial cystitis
Hunner's ulcer
Panmural fibrosis of bladder
Submucous cystitis

❑ **595.2 Other chronic cystitis**
Chronic cystitis NOS
Subacute cystitis

Excludes *trigonitis (595.3)*

595.3 Trigonitis
Follicular cystitis
Trigonitis (acute) (chronic)
Urethrotrigonitis

● ***595.4 Cystitis in diseases classified elsewhere***

Code first underlying disease, as:
actinomycosis (039.8)
amebiasis (006.8)
bilharziasis (120.0–120.9)
Echinococcus infestation (122.3, 122.6)

Excludes *cystitis:*
diphtheritic (032.84)
gonococcal (098.11, 098.31)
monilial (112.2)
trichomonal (131.09)
tuberculous (016.1)

● **595.8 Other specified types of cystitis**

595.81 Cystitis cystica

595.82 Irradiation cystitis
Use additional E code to identify cause

❑ **595.89 Other**
Abscess of bladder
Cystitis:
bullous
emphysematous
glandularis

❑ **595.9 Cystitis, unspecified**

Item 10-7 Intestinovesical fistula is a passage between the bladder and the intestine. Diverticulum of the bladder is the formation of a sac from a herniation of the wall of the bladder through a deviation. Atony of the bladder is diminished tone of the bladder muscle.

● **596 Other disorders of bladder**

Use additional code to identify urinary incontinence (625.6, 788.30–788.39)

596.0 Bladder neck obstruction
Contracture (acquired) of bladder neck or vesicourethral orifice
Obstruction (acquired) of bladder neck or vesicourethral orifice
Stenosis (acquired) of bladder neck or vesicourethral orifice

Excludes *congenital (753.6)*

596.1 Intestinovesical fistula
Fistula:
enterovesical
vesicocolic
Fistula:
vesicoenteric
vesicorectal

596.2 Vesical fistula, not elsewhere classified
Fistula:
bladder NOS
urethrovesical
Fistula:
vesicocutaneous
vesicoperineal

Excludes *fistula between bladder and female genital tract (619.0)*

596.3 Diverticulum of bladder
Diverticulitis of bladder
Diverticulum (acquired) (false) of bladder

Excludes *that with calculus in diverticulum of bladder (594.0)*

596.4 Atony of bladder
High compliance bladder
Hypotonicity of bladder
Inertia of bladder

Excludes *neurogenic bladder (596.54)*

● **596.5 Other functional disorders of bladder**

Excludes *cauda equina syndrome with neurogenic bladder (344.61)*

596.51 Hypertonicity of bladder
Hyperactivity
Overactive bladder

596.52 Low bladder compliance

596.53 Paralysis of bladder

596.54 Neurogenic bladder NOS

596.55 Detrusor sphincter dyssynergia

❑ **596.59 Other functional disorder of bladder**
Detrusor instability

596.6 Rupture of bladder, nontraumatic

596.7 Hemorrhage into bladder wall
Hyperemia of bladder

Excludes *acute hemorrhagic cystitis (595.0)*

❑ **596.8 Other specified disorders of bladder**
calcified
contracted
hemorrhage
hypertrophy

Excludes *cystocele, female (618.0, 618.2–618.4)*
hernia or prolapse of bladder, female (618.0, 618.2–618.4)

❑ **596.9 Unspecified disorder of bladder**

● **597 Urethritis, not sexually transmitted, and urethral syndrome**

Excludes *nonspecific urethritis, so stated (099.4)*

597.0 Urethral abscess
Abscess of:
bulbourethral gland
Cowper's gland
Littré's gland
Abscess:
periurethral
urethral (gland)
Periurethral cellulitis

Excludes *urethral caruncle (599.3)*

● **597.8 Other urethritis**

❑ **597.80 Urethritis, unspecified**

597.81 Urethral syndrome NOS

❑ **597.89 Other**
Adenitis, Skene's glands
Cowperitis
Meatitis, urethral
Ulcer, urethra (meatus)
Verumontanitis

Excludes *trichomonal (131.02)*

● **598 Urethral stricture**

Includes: pinhole meatus
stricture of urinary meatus

Use additional code to identify urinary incontinence (625.6, 788.30–788.39)

Excludes *congenital stricture of urethra and urinary meatus (753.6)*

● **598.0 Urethral stricture due to infection**

❑ **598.00 Due to unspecified infection**

● *598.01 Due to infective diseases classified elsewhere*

Code first underlying disease, as:
gonococcal infection (098.2)
schistosomiasis (120.0–120.9)
syphilis (095.8)

598.1 Traumatic urethral stricture
Stricture of urethra:
late effect of injury
postobstetric

Excludes *postoperative following surgery on genitourinary tract (598.2)*

598.2 Postoperative urethral stricture
Postcatheterization stricture of urethra

❑ **598.8 Other specified causes of urethral stricture**

❑ **598.9 Urethral stricture, unspecified**

● **599 Other disorders of urethra and urinary tract**

❑ **599.0 Urinary tract infection, site not specified**

Excludes *Candidiasis of urinary tract (112.2)*
urinary tract infection of newborn (771.82)

Use additional code to identify organism, such as Escherichia coli [E. coli] (041.4)

599.1 Urethral fistula
Fistula:
urethroperineal
urethrorectal
Urinary fistula NOS

Excludes *fistula:*
urethroscrotal (608.89)
urethrovaginal (619.0)
urethrovesicovaginal (619.0)

599.2 Urethral diverticulum

599.3 Urethral caruncle
Polyp of urethra

599.4 Urethral false passage

599.5 Prolapsed urethral mucosa
Prolapse of urethra
Urethrocele

Excludes *urethrocele, female (618.0, 618.2–618.4)*

❑ **599.6 Urinary obstruction, unspecified**
Obstructive uropathy NOS
Urinary (tract) obstruction NOS

Use additional code to identify urinary incontinence (625.6, 788.30–788.39)

Excludes *obstructive nephropathy NOS (593.89)*

599.7 Hematuria
Hematuria (benign) (essential)

Excludes *hemoglobinuria (791.2)*

● **599.8 Other specified disorders of urethra and urinary tract**

Use additional code to identify urinary incontinence (625.6, 788.30–788.39)

Excludes *symptoms and other conditions classifiable to 788.0–788.2, 788.4–788.9, 791.0–791.9*

599.81 Urethral hypermobility

599.82 Intrinsic (urethral) sphincter deficiency [ISD]

599.83 Urethral instability

❑ **599.84 Other specified disorders of urethra**
Rupture of urethra (nontraumatic)
Urethral:
cyst
granuloma

❑ **599.89 Other specified disorders of urinary tract**

❑ **599.9 Unspecified disorder of urethra and urinary tract**

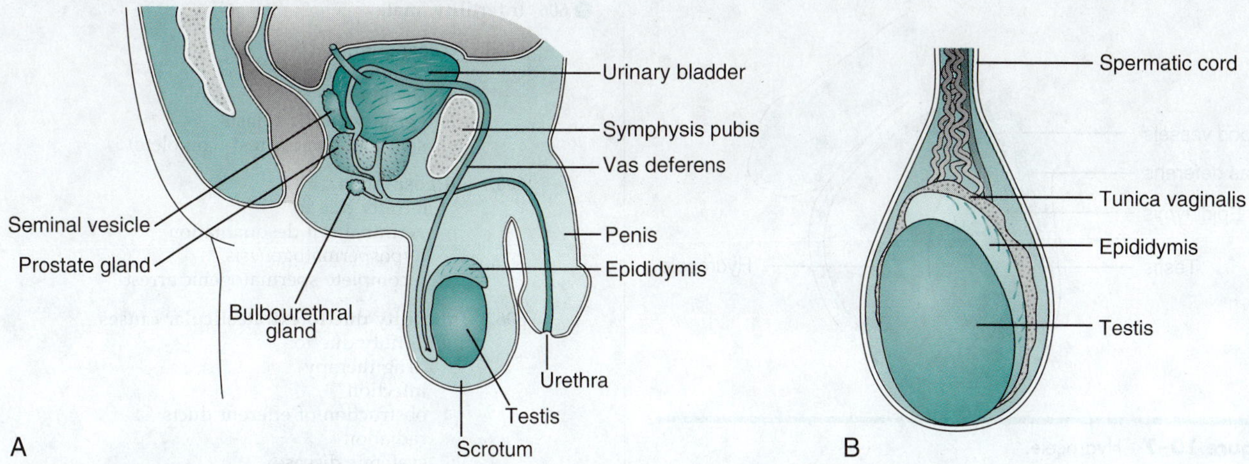

Figure 10–6 **A.** Male genital system. **B.** Testis.

DISEASES OF MALE GENITAL ORGANS (600–608)

● **600 Hyperplasia of prostate**

Use additional code to identify urinary incontinence (788.30–788.39)

● **600.0 Hypertrophy (benign) of prostate**

Benign prostatic hypertrophy
Enlargement of prostate
Smooth enlarged prostate
Soft enlarged prostate

600.00 Hypertropy (benign) of prostate without urinary obstruction ◀

Hypertrophy (benign) of prostate NOS ◀

600.01 Hypertrophy (benign) of prostate with urinary obstruction ◀

Hypertrophy (benign) of prostate with urinary retention ◀

● **600.1 Nodular prostate**

Hard, firm prostate
Multinodular prostate

Excludes *malignant neoplasm of prostate (185)*

600.10 Nodular prostate without urinary obstruction ◀

Nodular prostate NOS ◀

600.11 Nodular prostate with urinary obstruction ◀

Nodular prostate with urinary retention ◀

● **600.2 Benign localized hyperplasia of prostate**

Adenofibromatous hypertrophy of prostate
Adenoma of prostate
Fibroadenoma of prostate
Fibroma of prostate
Myoma of prostate
Polyp of prostate

Excludes *benign neoplasms of prostate (222.2)*
hypertrophy of prostate (600.00–600.01) ⬅
malignant neoplasm of prostate (185)

600.20 Benign localized hyperplasia of prostate without urinary obstruction ◀

Benign localized hyperplasia of prostate NOS ◀

600.21 Benign localized hyperplasia of prostate with urinary obstruction ◀

Benign localized hyperplasia of prostate with urinary retention ◀

600.3 Cyst of prostate

● **600.9 Hyperplasia of prostate, unspecified**

Median bar
Prostatic obstruction NOS

❑ **600.90 Hyperplasia of prostate, unspecified, without urinary obstruction** ◀

Hyperplasia of prostate NOS ◀

❑ **600.91 Hyperplasia of prostate, unspecified, with urinary obstruction** ◀

Hyperplasia of prostate, unspecified, with urinary retention ◀

● **601 Inflammatory diseases of prostate**

Use additional code to identify organism, such as Staphylococcus (041.1), or Streptococcus (041.0)

601.0 Acute prostatitis

601.1 Chronic prostatitis

601.2 Abscess of prostate

601.3 Prostatocystitis

● ***601.4 Prostatitis in diseases classified elsewhere***

Code first underlying disease, as:
actinomycosis (039.8)
blastomycosis (116.0)
syphilis (095.8)
tuberculosis (016.5)

Excludes *prostatitis:*
gonococcal (098.12, 098.32)
monilial (112.2)
trichomonal (131.03)

❑ **601.8 Other specified inflammatory diseases of prostate**

Prostatitis:
cavitary
diverticular
granulomatous

❑ **601.9 Prostatitis, unspecified**

Prostatitis NOS

● **602 Other disorders of prostate**

602.0 Calculus of prostate

Prostatic stone

602.1 Congestion or hemorrhage of prostate

602.2 Atrophy of prostate

602.3 Dysplasia of prostate

Prostatic intraepithelial neoplasia I (PIN I)
Prostatic intraepithelial neoplasia II (PIN II)

Excludes *Prostatic intraepithelial neoplasia III (PIN III) (233.4)*

❑ **602.8 Other specified disorders of prostate**

Fistula of prostate
Infarction of prostate
Stricture of prostate
Periprostatic adhesions

❑ **602.9 Unspecified disorder of prostate**

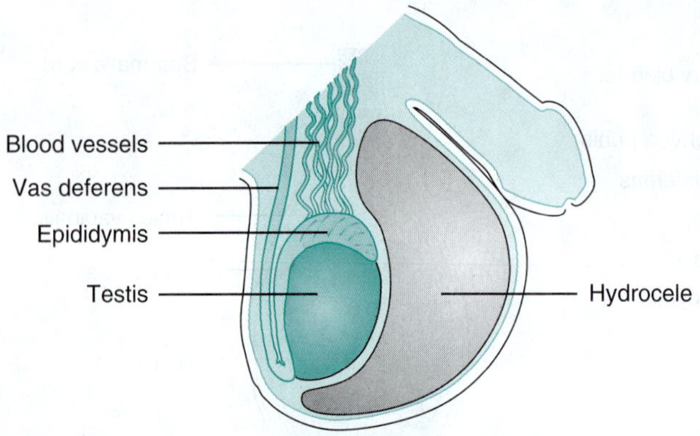

Figure 10–7 Hydrocele.

Item 10–8 Hydrocele is a sac of fluid in the testes membrane.

● 603 **Hydrocele**

Includes: hydrocele of spermatic cord, testis, or tunica vaginalis

Excludes *congenital (778.6)*

603.0 **Encysted hydrocele**

603.1 **Infected hydrocele**
Use additional code to identify organism

❑ 603.8 **Other specified types of hydrocele**

❑ 603.9 **Hydrocele, unspecified**

● 604 **Orchitis and epididymitis**

Use additional code to identify organism, such as Escherichia coli [E. coli] (041.4), Staphylococcus (041.1), or Streptococcus (041.0)

604.0 **Orchitis, epididymitis, and epididymo-orchitis, with abscess**
Abscess of epididymis or testis

● 604.9 **Other orchitis, epididymitis, and epididymo-orchitis, without mention of abscess**

❑ 604.90 **Orchitis and epididymitis, unspecified**

● *604.91* ***Orchitis and epididymitis in diseases classified elsewhere***

Code first underlying disease, as:
diphtheria (032.89)
filariasis (125.0–125.9)
syphilis (095.8)

Excludes *orchitis:*
gonococcal (098.13, 098.33)
mumps (072.0)
tuberculous (016.5)
tuberculous epididymitis (016.4)

❑ 604.99 **Other**

605 **Redundant prepuce and phimosis**
Adherent prepuce
Paraphimosis
Phimosis (congenital)
Tight foreskin

● 606 **Infertility, male**

606.0 **Azoospermia**
Absolute infertility
Infertility due to:
germinal (cell) aplasia
spermatogenic arrest (complete)

606.1 **Oligospermia**
Infertility due to:
germinal cell desquamation
hypospermatogenesis
incomplete spermatogenic arrest

606.8 **Infertility due to extratesticular causes**
Infertility due to:
drug therapy
infection
obstruction of efferent ducts
radiation
systemic disease

❑ 606.9 **Male infertility, unspecified**

● 607 **Disorders of penis**

Excludes *phimosis (605)*

607.0 **Leukoplakia of penis**
Kraurosis of penis

Excludes *carcinoma in situ of penis (233.5)*
erythroplasia of Queyrat (233.5)

607.1 **Balanoposthitis**
Balanitis

Use additional code to identify organism

❑ 607.2 **Other inflammatory disorders of penis**
Abscess of corpus cavernosum or penis
Boil of corpus cavernosum or penis
Carbuncle of corpus cavernosum or penis
Cellulitis of corpus cavernosum or penis
Cavernitis (penis)

Use additional code to identify organism

Excludes *herpetic infection (054.13)*

607.3 **Priapism**
Painful erection

● 607.8 **Other specified disorders of penis**

607.81 **Balanitis xerotica obliterans**
Induratio penis plastica

607.82 **Vascular disorders of penis**
Embolism of corpus cavernosum or penis
Hematoma (nontraumatic) of corpus cavernosum or penis
Hemorrhage of corpus cavernosum or penis
Thrombosis of corpus cavernosum or penis

607.83 **Edema of penis**

607.84 **Impotence of organic origin**

Excludes *nonorganic or unspecified (302.72)*

607.85 **Peyronie's disease** ◀

❑ 607.89 **Other**
Atrophy of corpus cavernosum or penis
Fibrosis of corpus cavernosum or penis
Hypertrophy of corpus cavernosum or penis
Ulcer (chronic) of corpus cavernosum or penis

❑ 607.9 **Unspecified disorder of penis**

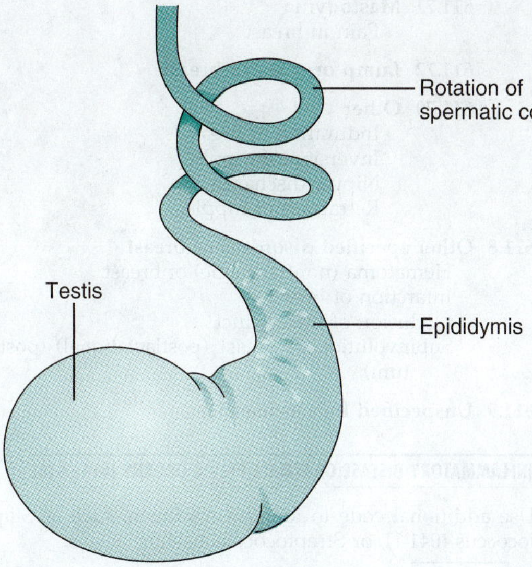

Figure 10-8 Torsion of testis.

Item 10-9 Rotation of the spermatic cord causes strangulation and infarction of the testis.

● **608 Other disorders of male genital organs**

608.0 Seminal vesiculitis
Abscess of seminal vesicle
Cellulitis of seminal vesicle
Vesiculitis (seminal)

Use additional code to identify organism

Excludes *gonococcal infection (098.14, 098.34)*

608.1 Spermatocele

608.2 Torsion of testis
Torsion of:
epididymis
spermatic cord
testicle

608.3 Atrophy of testis

❑ **608.4 Other inflammatory disorders of male genital organs**
Abscess of scrotum, spermatic cord, testis [except abscess], tunica vaginalis, or vas deferens
Boil of scrotum, spermatic cord, testis [except abscess], tunica vaginalis, or vas deferens
Carbuncle of scrotum, spermatic cord, testis [except abscess], tunica vaginalis, or vas deferens
Cellulitis of scrotum, spermatic cord, testis [except abscess], tunica vaginalis, or vas deferens
Vasitis

Use additional code to identify organism

Excludes *abscess of testis (604.0)*

● **608.8 Other specified disorders of male genital organs**

● ***608.81 Disorders of male genital organs in diseases classified elsewhere***

Code first underlying disease, as:
filariasis (125.0–125.9)
tuberculosis (016.5)

608.82 Hematospermia

608.87 Retrograde ejaculation

608.83 Vascular disorders
Hematoma (nontraumatic) of seminal vesicle, spermatic cord, testis, scrotum, tunica vaginalis, or vas deferens
Hemorrhage of seminal vesicle, spermatic cord, testis, scrotum, tunica vaginalis, or vas deferens
Thrombosis of seminal vesicle, spermatic cord, testis, scrotum, tunica vaginalis, or vas deferens
Hematocele NOS, male

608.84 Chylocele of tunica vaginalis

608.85 Stricture
Stricture of:
spermatic cord
tunica vaginalis
vas deferens

608.86 Edema

❑ **608.89 Other**
Atrophy of seminal vesicle, spermatic cord, testis, scrotum, tunica vaginalis, or vas deferens
Fibrosis of seminal vesicle, spermatic cord, testis, scrotum, tunica vaginalis, or vas deferens
Hypertrophy of seminal vesicle, spermatic cord, testis, scrotum, tunica vaginalis, or vas deferens
Ulcer of seminal vesicle, spermatic cord, testis, scrotum, tunica vaginalis, or vas deferens

Excludes *atrophy of testis (608.3)*

❑ **608.9 Unspecified disorder of male genital organs**

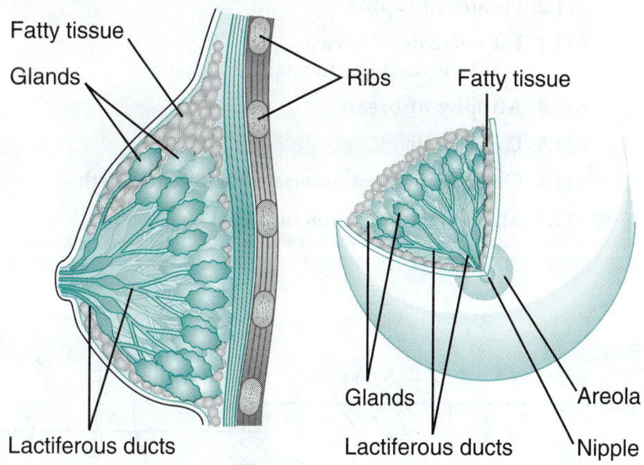

Figure 10-9 Breast.

DISORDERS OF BREAST (610–611)

● **610 Benign mammary dysplasias**

610.0 Solitary cyst of breast
Cyst (solitary) of breast

610.1 Diffuse cystic mastopathy
Chronic cystic mastitis
Cystic breast
Fibrocystic disease of breast

610.2 Fibroadenosis of breast
Fibroadenosis of breast:
NOS
chronic
cystic
Fibroadenosis of breast:
diffuse
periodic
segmental

ICD-9-CM 600-699 Vol. 1

610.3 **Fibrosclerosis of breast**

610.4 **Mammary duct ectasia**
Comedomastitis
Duct ectasia
Mastitis:
periductal
plasma cell

❑ 610.8 **Other specified benign mammary dysplasias**
Mazoplasia
Sebaceous cyst of breast

❑ 610.9 **Benign mammary dysplasia, unspecified**

● 611 **Other disorders of breast**
Excludes *that associated with lactation or the puerperium (675.0–676.9)*

611.0 **Inflammatory disease of breast**
Abscess (acute) (chronic) (nonpuerperal) of:
areola
breast
Mammillary fistula
Mastitis (acute) (subacute) (nonpuerperal):
NOS
infective
retromammary
submammary
Excludes *carbuncle of breast (680.2)*
chronic cystic mastitis (610.1)
neonatal infective mastitis (771.5)
thrombophlebitis of breast [Mondor's disease] (451.89)

611.1 **Hypertrophy of breast**
Gynecomastia
Hypertrophy of breast:
NOS
massive pubertal

611.2 **Fissure of nipple**

611.3 **Fat necrosis of breast**
Fat necrosis (segmental) of breast

611.4 **Atrophy of breast**

611.5 **Galactocele**

611.6 **Galactorrhea not associated with childbirth**

● 611.7 **Signs and symptoms in breast**

611.71 **Mastodynia**
Pain in breast

611.72 **Lump or mass in breast**

❑ 611.79 **Other**
Induration of breast
Inversion of nipple
Nipple discharge
Retraction of nipple

❑ 611.8 **Other specified disorders of breast**
Hematoma (nontraumatic) of breast
Infarction of breast
Occlusion of breast duct
Subinvolution of breast (postlactational) (postpartum)

❑ 611.9 **Unspecified breast disorder**

INFLAMMATORY DISEASE OF FEMALE PELVIC ORGANS (614–616)

Use additional code to identify organism, such as Staphylococcus (041.1), or Streptococcus (041.0)

Excludes *that associated with pregnancy, abortion, childbirth, or the puerperium (630–676.9)*

● 614 **Inflammatory disease of ovary, fallopian tube, pelvic cellular tissue, and peritoneum**
Excludes *endometritis (615.0–615.9)*
major infection following delivery (670)
that complicating:
abortion (634–638 with .0, 639.0)
ectopic or molar pregnancy (639.0)
pregnancy or labor (646.6)

614.0 **Acute salpingitis and oophoritis**
Any condition classifiable to 614.2, specified as acute or subacute

614.1 **Chronic salpingitis and oophoritis**
Hydrosalpinx
Salpingitis:
follicularis
isthmica nodosa
Any condition classifiable to 614.2, specified as chronic

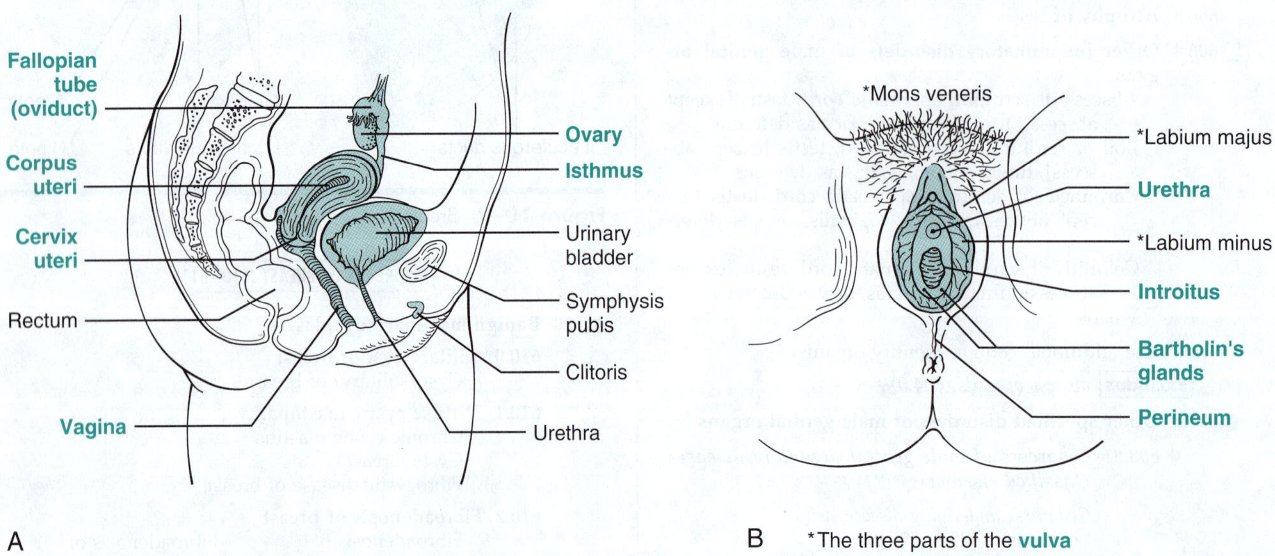

Figure 10–10 **A.** Female genital system. **B.** External female genital system. (From Buck CJ: Step-by-Step Medical Coding, 3rd ed. Philadelphia, WB Saunders, 2000, p. 193.)

❑614.2 **Salpingitis and oophoritis not specified as acute, subacute, or chronic**

Abscess (of):
- fallopian tube
- ovary
- tubo-ovarian

Oophoritis
Tubo-ovarian inflammatory disease
Perioophoritis
Perisalpingitis
Pyosalpinx
Salpingitis
Salpingo-oophoritis

Excludes *gonococcal infection (chronic) (098.37)*
acute (098.17)
tuberculous (016.6)

614.3 **Acute parametritis and pelvic cellulitis**

Acute inflammatory pelvic disease
Any condition classifiable to 614.4, specified as acute

614.4 **Chronic or unspecified parametritis and pelvic cellulitis**

Abscess (of):
- broad ligament chronic or NOS
- parametrium chronic or NOS
- pelvis, female chronic or NOS
- pouch of Douglas chronic or NOS

Chronic inflammatory pelvic disease
Pelvic cellulitis, female

Excludes *tuberculous (016.7)*

614.5 **Acute or unspecified pelvic peritonitis, female**

614.6 **Pelvic peritoneal adhesions, female (postoperative) (postinfection)**

Adhesions:
- peritubal
- tubo-ovarian

Use additional code to identify any associated infertility (628.2)

❑614.7 **Other chronic pelvic peritonitis, female**

Excludes *tuberculous (016.7)*

❑614.8 **Other specified inflammatory disease of female pelvic organs and tissues**

❑614.9 **Unspecified inflammatory disease of female pelvic organs and tissues**

Pelvic infection or inflammation, female NOS
Pelvic inflammatory disease [PID]

● 615 **Inflammatory diseases of uterus, except cervix**

Excludes *following delivery (670)*
hyperplastic endometritis (621.3)
that complicating:
abortion (634–638 with .0, 639.0)
ectopic or molar pregnancy (639.0)
pregnancy or labor (646.6)

615.0 **Acute**

Any condition classifiable to 615.9, specified as acute or subacute

615.1 **Chronic**

Any condition classifiable to 615.9, specified as chronic

❑615.9 **Unspecified inflammatory disease of uterus**

Endometritis
Endomyometritis
Metritis
Myometritis
Perimetritis
Pyometra
Uterine abscess

● 616 **Inflammatory disease of cervix, vagina, and vulva**

Excludes *that complicating:*
abortion (634–638 with .0, 639.0)
ectopic or molar pregnancy (639.0)
pregnancy, childbirth, or the puerperium (646.6)

616.0 **Cervicitis and endocervicitis**

Cervicitis with or without mention of erosion or ectropion
Endocervicitis with or without mention of erosion or ectropion
Nabothian (gland) cyst or follicle

Excludes *erosion or ectropion without mention of cervicitis (622.0)*

● 616.1 **Vaginitis and vulvovaginitis**

❑616.10 **Vaginitis and vulvovaginitis, unspecified**

Vaginitis:
- NOS
- postirradiation

Vulvitis NOS
Vulvovaginitis NOS

Use additional code to identify organism, such as Escherichia coli [E. coli] (041.4), Staphylococcus (041.1), or Streptococcus (041.0)

Excludes *noninfective leukorrhea (623.5)*
postmenopausal or senile vaginitis (627.3)

● 616.11 ***Vaginitis and vulvovaginitis in diseases classified elsewhere***

Code first underlying disease, as:
pinworm vaginitis (127.4)

Excludes *herpetic vulvovaginitis (054.11)*
monilial vulvovaginitis (112.1)
trichomonal vaginitis or vulvovaginitis (131.01)

616.2 **Cyst of Bartholin's gland**

Bartholin's duct cyst

616.3 **Abscess of Bartholin's gland**

Vulvovaginal gland abscess

❑616.4 **Other abscess of vulva**

Abscess of vulva
Carbuncle of vulva
Furuncle of vulva

● 616.5 **Ulceration of vulva**

❑616.50 **Ulceration of vulva, unspecified**

Ulcer NOS of vulva

● 616.51 ***Ulceration of vulva in diseases classified elsewhere***

Code first underlying disease, as:
Behçet's syndrome (136.1)
tuberculosis (016.7)

Excludes *vulvar ulcer (in):*
gonococcal (098.0)
herpes simplex (054.12)
syphilitic (091.0)

❑616.8 **Other specified inflammatory diseases of cervix, vagina, and vulva**

Caruncle, vagina or labium
Ulcer, vagina

Excludes *noninflammatory disorders of:*
cervix (622.0–622.9)
vagina (623.0–623.9)
vulva (624.0–624.9)

❑616.9 **Unspecified inflammatory disease of cervix, vagina, and vulva**

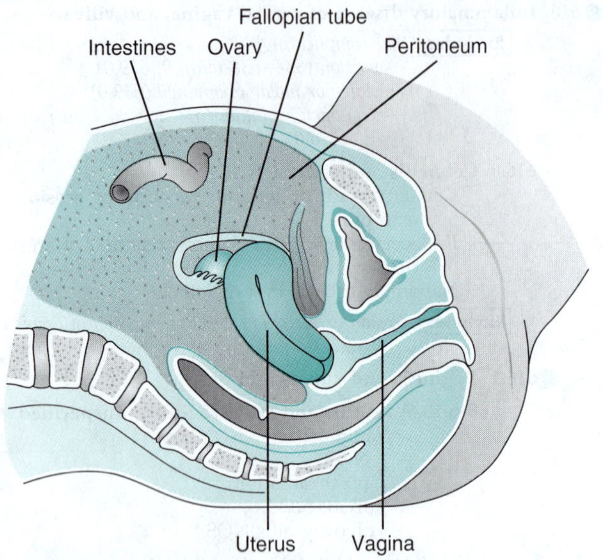

Figure 10–11 Sites of potential endometrial implants.

Item 10–10 Endometriosis is a condition for which no clear cause has been identified. Endometrial tissue is expelled from the uterus into the body and can implant onto a variety of organs. Classification is based on the site of implant of the endometrial tissue.

OTHER DISORDERS OF FEMALE GENITAL TRACT (617–629)

● **617 Endometriosis**

617.0 Endometriosis of uterus
Adenomyosis
Endometriosis:
cervix
internal
Endometriosis:
myometrium

Excludes *stromal endometriosis (236.0)*

617.1 Endometriosis of ovary
Chocolate cyst of ovary
Endometrial cystoma of ovary

617.2 Endometriosis of fallopian tube

617.3 Endometriosis of pelvic peritoneum
Endometriosis:
broad ligament
cul-de-sac (Douglas')
parametrium
round ligament

617.4 Endometriosis of rectovaginal septum and vagina

617.5 Endometriosis of intestine
Endometriosis:
appendix
colon
rectum

617.6 Endometriosis in scar of skin

❑ **617.8 Endometriosis of other specified sites**
Endometriosis:
bladder
lung
umbilicus
vulva

❑ **617.9 Endometriosis, site unspecified**

● **618 Genital prolapse**

Use additional code to identify urinary incontinence (625.6, 788.31, 788.33–788.39)

Excludes *that complicating pregnancy, labor, or delivery (654.4)*

618.0 Prolapse of vaginal walls without mention of uterine prolapse
Cystocele
Cystourethrocele
Proctocele, female, without mention of uterine prolapse
Rectocele, without mention of uterine prolapse
Urethrocele, female, without mention of uterine prolapse
Vaginal prolapse, without mention of uterine prolapse

Excludes *that with uterine prolapse (618.2–618.4)*
enterocele (618.6)
vaginal vault prolapse following hysterectomy (618.5)

618.1 Uterine prolapse without mention of vaginal wall prolapse
Descensus uteri
Uterine prolapse:
NOS
complete
first degree
second degree
third degree

Excludes *that with mention of cystocele, urethrocele, or rectocele (618.2–618.4)*

618.2 Uterovaginal prolapse, incomplete

618.3 Uterovaginal prolapse, complete

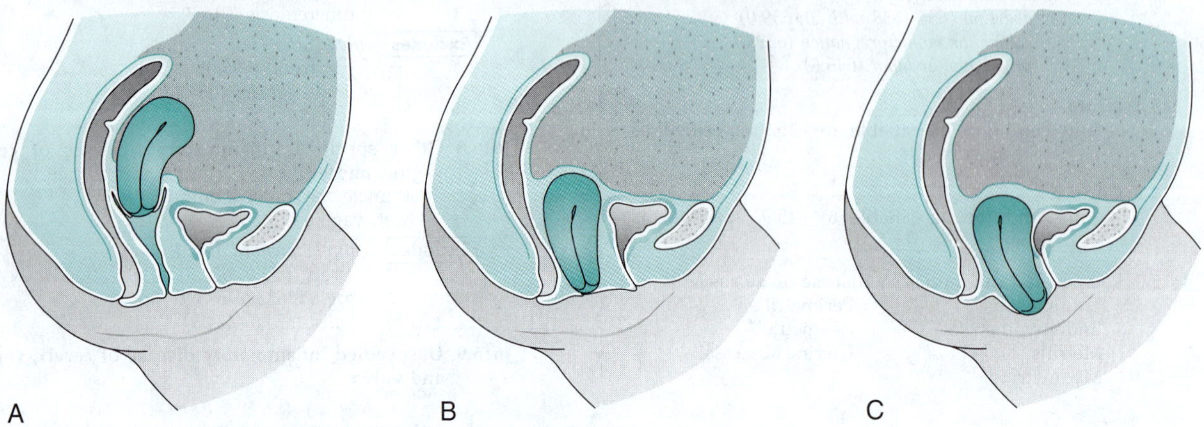

Figure 10–12 Three stages of uterine prolapse. **A.** Uterus is prolapsed. **B.** Vagina and uterus are prolapsed (incomplete uterovaginal prolapse). **C.** Vagina and uterus are completely prolapsed and are exposed through the external genitalia (complete uterovaginal prolapse).

❑618.4 **Uterovaginal prolapse, unspecified**

618.5 **Prolapse of vaginal vault after hysterectomy**

618.6 **Vaginal enterocele, congenital or acquired**
Pelvic enterocele, congenital or acquired

618.7 **Old laceration of muscles of pelvic floor**

❑618.8 **Other specified genital prolapse**
Incompetence or weakening of pelvic fundus
Relaxation of vaginal outlet or pelvis

❑618.9 **Unspecified genital prolapse**

● 619 **Fistula involving female genital tract**

Excludes *vesicorectal and intestinovesical fistula (596.1)*

619.0 **Urinary-genital tract fistula, female**
Fistula:
cervicovesical
ureterovaginal
urethrovaginal
urethrovesicovaginal
uteroureteric
uterovesical
vesicocervicovaginal
vesicovaginal

619.1 **Digestive-genital tract fistula, female**
Fistula:
intestinouterine
intestinovaginal
rectovaginal
Fistula:
rectovulval
sigmoidovaginal
uterorectal

619.2 **Genital tract-skin fistula, female**
Fistula:
uterus to abdominal wall
vaginoperineal

❑619.8 **Other specified fistulas involving female genital tract**
Fistula:
cervix
cul-de-sac (Douglas')
uterus
vagina

❑619.9 **Unspecified fistula involving female genital tract**

● 620 **Noninflammatory disorders of ovary, fallopian tube, and broad ligament**

Excludes *hydrosalpinx (614.1)*

620.0 **Follicular cyst of ovary**
Cyst of graafian follicle

620.1 **Corpus luteum cyst or hematoma**
Corpus luteum hemorrhage or rupture
Lutein cyst

❑620.2 **Other and unspecified ovarian cyst**
Cyst of ovary:
NOS
corpus albicans
retention NOS
Cyst of ovary:
serous
theca-lutein
Simple cystoma of ovary

Excludes *cystadenoma (benign) (serous) (220)*
developmental cysts (752.0)
neoplastic cysts (220)
polycystic ovaries (256.4)
Stein-Leventhal syndrome (256.4)

620.3 **Acquired atrophy of ovary and fallopian tube**
Senile involution of ovary

620.4 **Prolapse or hernia of ovary and fallopian tube**
Displacement of ovary and fallopian tube
Salpingocele

620.5 **Torsion of ovary, ovarian pedicle, or fallopian tube**
Torsion:
accessory tube
hydatid of Morgagni

620.6 **Broad ligament laceration syndrome**
Masters-Allen syndrome

620.7 **Hematoma of broad ligament**
Hematocele, broad ligament

❑620.8 **Other noninflammatory disorders of ovary, fallopian tube, and broad ligament**
Cyst of broad ligament or fallopian tube
Polyp of broad ligament or fallopian tube
Infarction of ovary or fallopian tube
Rupture of ovary or fallopian tube
Hematosalpinx of ovary or fallopian tube

Excludes *hematosalpinx in ectopic pregnancy (639.2)*
peritubal adhesions (614.6)
torsion of ovary, ovarian pedicle, or fallopian tube (620.5)

❑620.9 **Unspecified noninflammatory disorder of ovary, fallopian tube, and broad ligament**

● 621 **Disorders of uterus, not elsewhere classified**

621.0 **Polyp of corpus uteri**
Polyp:
endometrium
uterus NOS

Excludes *cervical polyp NOS (622.7)*

621.1 **Chronic subinvolution of uterus**

Excludes *puerperal (674.8)*

621.2 **Hypertrophy of uterus**
Bulky or enlarged uterus

Excludes *puerperal (674.8)*

621.3 **Endometrial cystic hyperplasia**
Hyperplasia (adenomatous) (cystic) (glandular) of endometrium
Hyperplastic endometritis

621.4 **Hematometra**
Hemometra

Excludes *that in congenital anomaly (752.2–752.3)*

621.5 **Intrauterine synechiae**
Adhesions of uterus
Band(s) of uterus

621.6 **Malposition of uterus**
Anteversion of uterus
Retroflexion of uterus
Retroversion of uterus

Excludes *malposition complicating pregnancy, labor, or delivery (654.3–654.4)*
prolapse of uterus (618.1–618.4)

621.7 **Chronic inversion of uterus**

Excludes *current obstetrical trauma (665.2)*
prolapse of uterus (618.1–618.4)

❑621.8 **Other specified disorders of uterus, not elsewhere classified**
Atrophy, acquired of uterus
Cyst of uterus
Fibrosis NOS of uterus
Old laceration (postpartum) of uterus
Ulcer of uterus

Excludes *bilharzial fibrosis (120.0–120.9)*
endometriosis (617.0)
fistulas (619.0–619.8)
inflammatory diseases (615.0–615.9)

❑621.9 **Unspecified disorder of uterus**

● 622 **Noninflammatory disorders of cervix**

Excludes *abnormality of cervix complicating pregnancy, labor, or delivery (654.5–654.6)*
fistula (619.0–619.8)

622.0 **Erosion and ectropion of cervix**
Eversion of cervix
Ulcer of cervix

Excludes *that in chronic cervicitis (616.0)*

622.1 Dysplasia of cervix (uteri)
Anaplasia of cervix
Cervical atypism
Cervical intraepithelial neoplasia I (CIN I)
Cervical intraepithelial neoplasia II (CIN II)
High grade squamous intraepithelial dysplasia (HGSIL)
Low grade squamous intraepithelial dysplasia (LGSIL)
Excludes *carcinoma in situ of cervix (233.1)*
cervical intraepithelial neoplasia III [CIN III] (233.1)

622.2 Leukoplakia of cervix (uteri)
Excludes *carcinoma in situ of cervix (233.1)*

622.3 Old laceration of cervix
Adhesions of cervix
Band(s) of cervix
Cicatrix (postpartum) of cervix
Excludes *current obstetrical trauma (665.3)*

622.4 Stricture and stenosis of cervix
Atresia (acquired) of cervix
Contracture of cervix
Occlusion of cervix
Pinpoint os uteri
Excludes *congenital (752.49)*
that complicating labor (654.6)

622.5 Incompetence of cervix
Excludes *complicating pregnancy (654.5)*
that affecting fetus or newborn (761.0)

622.6 Hypertrophic elongation of cervix

622.7 Mucous polyp of cervix
Polyp NOS of cervix
Excludes *adenomatous polyp of cervix (219.0)*

❑ **622.8 Other specified noninflammatory disorders of cervix**
Atrophy (senile) of cervix
Cyst of cervix
Fibrosis of cervix
Hemorrhage of cervix
Excludes *endometriosis (617.0)*
fistula (619.0–619.8)
inflammatory diseases (616.0)

❑ **622.9 Unspecified noninflammatory disorder of cervix**

● **623 Noninflammatory disorders of vagina**
Excludes *abnormality of vagina complicating pregnancy, labor, or delivery (654.7)*
congenital absence of vagina (752.49)
congenital diaphragm or bands (752.49)
fistulas involving vagina (619.0–619.8)

623.0 Dysplasia of vagina
Excludes *carcinoma in situ of vagina (233.3)*

623.1 Leukoplakia of vagina

623.2 Stricture or atresia of vagina
Adhesions (postoperative) (postradiation) of vagina
Occlusion of vagina
Stenosis, vagina
Use additional E code to identify any external cause
Excludes *congenital atresia or stricture (752.49)*

623.3 Tight hymenal ring
Rigid hymen acquired or congenital
Tight hymenal ring acquired or congenital
Tight introitus acquired or congenital
Excludes *imperforate hymen (752.42)*

623.4 Old vaginal laceration
Excludes *old laceration involving muscles of pelvic floor (618.7)*

623.5 Leukorrhea, not specified as infective
Leukorrhea NOS of vagina
Vaginal discharge NOS
Excludes *trichomonal (131.00)*

623.6 Vaginal hematoma
Excludes *current obstetrical trauma (665.7)*

623.7 Polyp of vagina

❑ **623.8 Other specified noninflammatory disorders of vagina**
Cyst of vagina
Hemorrhage of vagina

❑ **623.9 Unspecified noninflammatory disorder of vagina**

● **624 Noninflammatory disorders of vulva and perineum**
Excludes *abnormality of vulva and perineum complicating pregnancy, labor, or delivery (654.8)*
condyloma acuminatum (078.1)
fistulas involving:
perineum-see Alphabetic Index
vulva (619.0–619.8)
vulval varices (456.6)
vulvar involvement in skin conditions (690–709.9)

624.0 Dystrophy of vulva
Kraurosis of vulva
Leukoplakia of vulva
Excludes *carcinoma in situ of vulva (233.3)*

624.1 Atrophy of vulva

624.2 Hypertrophy of clitoris
Excludes *that in endocrine disorders (255.2, 256.1)*

624.3 Hypertrophy of labia
Hypertrophy of vulva NOS

624.4 Old laceration or scarring of vulva

624.5 Hematoma of vulva
Excludes *that complicating delivery (664.5)*

624.6 Polyp of labia and vulva

❑ **624.8 Other specified noninflammatory disorders of vulva and perineum**
Cyst of vulva
Edema of vulva
Stricture of vulva

❑ **624.9 Unspecified noninflammatory disorder of vulva and perineum**

● **625 Pain and other symptoms associated with female genital organs**

625.0 Dyspareunia
Excludes *psychogenic dyspareunia (302.76)*

625.1 Vaginismus
Colpospasm
Vulvismus
Excludes *psychogenic vaginismus (306.51)*

625.2 Mittelschmerz
Intermenstrual pain
Ovulation pain

625.3 Dysmenorrhea
Painful menstruation
Excludes *psychogenic dysmenorrhea (306.52)*

625.4 Premenstrual tension syndrome
Menstrual:
migraine
molimen
Premenstrual dysphoric disorder ◀
Premenstrual syndrome
Premenstrual tension NOS

625.5 **Pelvic congestion syndrome**
Congestion-fibrosis syndrome
Taylor's syndrome

625.6 **Stress incontinence, female**
Excludes *mixed incontinence (788.33)*
stress incontinence, male (788.32)

❑625.8 **Other specified symptoms associated with female genital organs**

❑625.9 **Unspecified symptoms associated with female genital organs**

● 626 **Disorders of menstruation and other abnormal bleeding from female genital tract**
Excludes *menopausal and premenopausal bleeding (627.0)*
pain and other symptoms associated with menstrual cycle (625.2–625.4)
postmenopausal bleeding (627.1)

626.0 **Absence of menstruation**
Amenorrhea (primary) (secondary)

626.1 **Scanty or infrequent menstruation**
Hypomenorrhea
Oligomenorrhea

626.2 **Excessive or frequent menstruation**
Heavy periods
Menometrorrhagia
Menorrhagia
Polymenorrhea
Excludes *premenopausal (627.0)*
that in puberty (626.3)

626.3 **Puberty bleeding**
Excessive bleeding associated with onset of menstrual periods
Pubertal menorrhagia

626.4 **Irregular menstrual cycle**
Irregular:
bleeding NOS
menstruation
periods

626.5 **Ovulation bleeding**
Regular intermenstrual bleeding

626.6 **Metrorrhagia**
Bleeding unrelated to menstrual cycle
Irregular intermenstrual bleeding

626.7 **Postcoital bleeding**

❑626.8 **Other**
Dysfunctional or functional uterine hemorrhage NOS
Menstruation:
retained
suppression of

❑626.9 **Unspecified**

● 627 **Menopausal and postmenopausal disorders**
Excludes *asymptomatic age-related (natural) postmenopausal status (V49.81)*

627.0 **Premenopausal menorrhagia**
Excessive bleeding associated with onset of menopause
Menorrhagia:
climacteric
menopausal
preclimacteric

627.1 **Postmenopausal bleeding**

627.2 **Symptomatic or female climacteric states**
Symptoms, such as flushing, sleeplessness, headache, lack of concentration, associated with the menopause

627.3 **Postmenopausal atrophic vaginitis**
Senile (atrophic) vaginitis

627.4 **Symptomatic states associated with artificial menopause**
Postartificial menopause syndromes
Any condition classifiable to 627.1, 627.2, or 627.3 which follows induced menopause

❑627.8 **Other specified menopausal and postmenopausal disorders**
Excludes *premature menopause NOS (256.31)*

❑627.9 **Unspecified menopausal and postmenopausal disorder**

● 628 **Infertility, female**
Includes: primary and secondary sterility

628.0 **Associated with anovulation**
Anovulatory cycle
Use additional code for any associated Stein-Leventhal syndrome (256.4)

● 628.1 ***Of pituitary-hypothalamic origin***
Code first underlying disease, as:
adiposogenital dystrophy (253.8)
anterior pituitary disorder (253.0–253.4)

628.2 **Of tubal origin**
Infertility associated with congenital anomaly of tube
Tubal:
block
occlusion
stenosis
Use additional code for any associated peritubal adhesions (614.6)

628.3 **Of uterine origin**
Infertility associated with congenital anomaly of uterus
Nonimplantation
Use additional code for any associated tuberculous endometritis (016.7)

628.4 **Of cervical or vaginal origin**
Infertility associated with:
anomaly or cervical mucus
congenital structural anomaly
dysmucorrhea

❑628.8 **Of other specified origin**

❑628.9 **Of unspecified origin**

● 629 **Other disorders of female genital organs**

629.0 **Hematocele, female, not elsewhere classified**
Excludes *hematocele or hematoma:*
broad ligament (620.7)
fallopian tube (620.8)
that associated with ectopic pregnancy (633.00–633.91)
uterus (621.4)
vagina (623.6)
vulva (624.5)

629.1 **Hydrocele, canal of Nuck**
Cyst of canal of Nuck (acquired)
Excludes *congenital (752.41)*

❑629.8 **Other specified disorders of female genital organs**

❑629.9 **Unspecified disorder of female genital organs**
Habitual aborter without current pregnancy

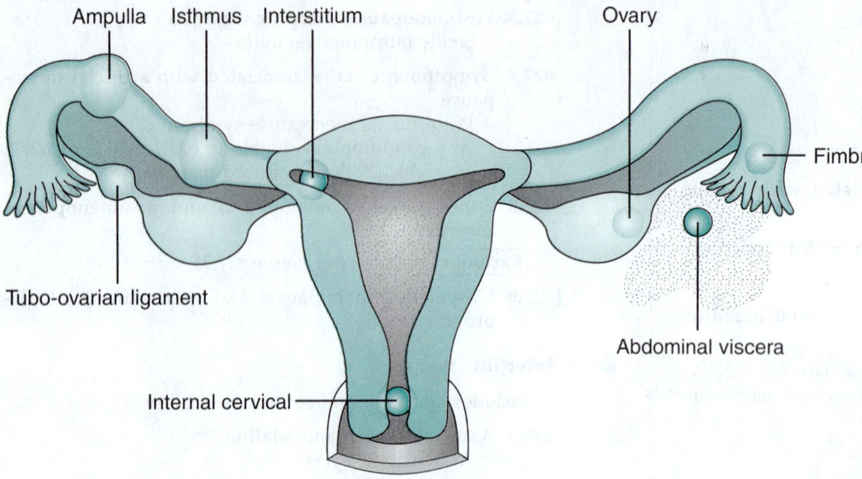

Figure 11–1 Implantation sites of ectopic pregnancy.

Item 11–1 A hydatidiform mole is a benign tumor of the placenta. The tumor secretes a hormone, chorionic gonadotropic hormone (CGH), that indicates a positive pregnancy test.

Item 11–2 Ectopic pregnancy most often occurs in the fallopian tube. Pregnancy outside the uterus may end in a life-threatening rupture.

11. COMPLICATIONS OF PREGNANCY, CHILDBIRTH, AND THE PUERPERIUM (630–677)

ECTOPIC AND MOLAR PREGNANCY (630–633)

Use additional code from category 639 to identify any complications

630 Hydatidiform mole
Trophoblastic disease NOS
Vesicular mole
Excludes *chorioadenoma (destruens) (236.1)*
chorioepithelioma (181)
malignant hydatidiform mole (236.1)

❑ **631 Other abnormal product of conception**
Blighted ovum
Mole: NOS, carneous
Mole: fleshy, stone

632 Missed abortion
Early fetal death before completion of 22 weeks' gestation with retention of dead fetus
Retained products of conception, not following spontaneous or induced abortion or delivery
Excludes *failed induced abortion (638.0–638.9)*
fetal death (intrauterine) (late) (656.4)
missed delivery (656.4)
that with abnormal product of conception (630, 631)

● **633 Ectopic pregnancy**
Includes: ruptured ectopic pregnancy

● **633.0 Abdominal pregnancy**
Intraperitoneal pregnancy
633.00 Abdominal pregnancy without intrauterine pregnancy
633.01 Abdominal pregnancy with intrauterine pregnancy

● **633.1 Tubal pregnancy**
Fallopian pregnancy
Rupture of (fallopian) tube due to pregnancy
Tubal abortion
633.10 Tubal pregnancy without intrauterine pregnancy
633.11 Tubal pregnancy with intrauterine pregnancy

● **633.2 Ovarian pregnancy**
633.20 Ovarian pregnancy without intrauterine pregnancy
633.21 Ovarian pregnancy with intrauterine pregnancy

● ❑ **633.8 Other ectopic pregnancy**
Pregnancy: cervical, combined, cornual
Pregnancy: intraligamentous, mesometric, mural
633.80 Other ectopic pregnancy without intrauterine pregnancy
633.81 Other ectopic pregnancy with intrauterine pregnancy

● ❑ **633.9 Unspecified ectopic pregnancy**
633.90 Unspecified ectopic pregnancy without intrauterine pregnancy
633.91 Unspecified ectopic pregnancy with intrauterine pregnancy

OTHER PREGNANCY WITH ABORTIVE OUTCOME (634–639)

The following fourth digit subdivisions are for use with categories 634–638:

.0 Complicated by genital tract and pelvic infection
Endometritis
Salpingo-oophoritis
Sepsis NOS
Septicemia NOS
Any condition classifiable to 639.0, with condition classifiable to 634–638
Excludes *urinary tract infection (634–638 with .7)*

.1 Complicated by delayed or excessive hemorrhage
Afibrinogenemia
Defibrination syndrome
Intravascular hemolysis
Any condition classifiable to 639.1, with condition classifiable to 634–638

.2 Complicated by damage to pelvic organs and tissues
Laceration, perforation, or tear of: bladder, uterus
Any condition classifiable to 639.2, with condition classifiable to 634–638

.3 Complicated by renal failure
Oliguria
Uremia
Any condition classifiable to 639.3, with condition classifiable to 634–638

.4 Complicated by metabolic disorder
Electrolyte imbalance with conditions classifiable to 634–638
.5 Complicated by shock
Circulatory collapse
Shock (postoperative) (septic)
Any condition classifiable to 639.5, with condition classifiable to 634–638
.6 Complicated by embolism
Embolism:
NOS
amniotic fluid
Embolism:
pulmonary
Any condition classifiable to 639.6, with condition classifiable to 634–638
.7 With other specified complications
Cardiac arrest or failure
Urinary tract infection
Any condition classifiable to 639.8, with condition classifiable to 634–638
.8 With unspecified complications
.9 Without mention of complication

634 Spontaneous abortion

Requires fifth digit to identify stage:
0 unspecified
1 incomplete
2 complete

Includes: miscarriage
spontaneous abortion

634.0 Complicated by genital tract and pelvic infection
634.1 Complicated by delayed or excessive hemorrhage
634.2 Complicated by damage to pelvic organs or tissues
634.3 Complicated by renal failure
634.4 Complicated by metabolic disorder
634.5 Complicated by shock
634.6 Complicated by embolism
634.7 With other specified complications
634.8 With unspecified complication
634.9 Without mention of complication

635 Legally induced abortion

Requires fifth digit to identify stage:
0 unspecified
1 incomplete
2 complete

Includes: abortion or termination of pregnancy:
elective
legal
therapeutic

Excludes *menstrual extraction or regulation (V25.3)*

635.0 Complicated by genital tract and pelvic infection
635.1 Complicated by delayed or excessive hemorrhage
635.2 Complicated by damage to pelvic organs or tissues
635.3 Complicated by renal failure
635.4 Complicated by metabolic disorder
635.5 Complicated by shock
635.6 Complicated by embolism
635.7 With other specified complications
635.8 With unspecified complication
635.9 Without mention of complication

636 Illegally induced abortion

Requires fifth digit to identify stage:
0 unspecified
1 incomplete
2 complete

Includes: abortion:
criminal
illegal
self-induced

636.0 Complicated by genital tract and pelvic infection
636.1 Complicated by delayed or excessive hemorrhage
636.2 Complicated by damage to pelvic organs or tissues
636.3 Complicated by renal failure
636.4 Complicated by metabolic disorder
636.5 Complicated by shock
636.6 Complicated by embolism
636.7 With other specified complications
636.8 With unspecified complication
636.9 Without mention of complication

637 Unspecified abortion

Requires following fifth digit to identify stage:
0 unspecified
1 incomplete
2 complete

Includes: abortion NOS
retained products of conception following abortion, not classifiable elsewhere

637.0 Complicated by genital tract and pelvic infection
637.1 Complicated by delayed or excessive hemorrhage
637.2 Complicated by damage to pelvic organs or tissues
637.3 Complicated by renal failure
637.4 Complicated by metabolic disorder
637.5 Complicated by shock
637.6 Complicated by embolism
637.7 With other specified complications
637.8 With unspecified complication
637.9 Without mention of complication

638 Failed attempted abortion

Includes: failure of attempted induction of (legal) abortion
Excludes *incomplete abortion (634.0–637.9)*

638.0 Complicated by genital tract and pelvic infection
638.1 Complicated by delayed or excessive hemorrhage
638.2 Complicated by damage to pelvic organs or tissues
638.3 Complicated by renal failure
638.4 Complicated by metabolic disorder
638.5 Complicated by shock
638.6 Complicated by embolism
638.7 With other specified complications
638.8 With unspecified complication
638.9 Without mention of complication

639 Complications following abortion and ectopic and molar pregnancies

Note: This category is provided for use when it is required to classify separately the complications classifiable to the fourth digit level in categories 634–638; for example:
a) when the complication itself was responsible for an episode of medical care, the abortion, ectopic or molar pregnancy itself having been dealt with at a previous episode
b) when these conditions are immediate complications of ectopic or molar pregnancies classifiable to 630–633 where they cannot be identified at fourth digit level.

639.0 Genital tract and pelvic infection
Endometritis following conditions classifiable to 630–638
Parametritis following conditions classifiable to 630–638
Pelvic peritonitis following conditions classifiable to 630–638
Salpingitis following conditions classifiable to 630–638
Salpingo-oophoritis following conditions classifiable to 630–638
Sepsis NOS following conditions classifiable to 630–638
Septicemia NOS following conditions classifiable to 630–638

Excludes *urinary tract infection (639.8)*

639.1 Delayed or excessive hemorrhage
Afibrinogenemia following conditions classifiable to 630–638
Defibrination syndrome following conditions classifiable to 630–638
Intravascular hemolysis following conditions classifiable to 630–638

639.2 Damage to pelvic organs and tissues
Laceration, perforation, or tear of:
bladder following conditions classifiable to 630–638
bowel following conditions classifiable to 630–638
broad ligament following conditions classifiable to 630–638
cervix following conditions classifiable to 630–638
periurethral tissue following conditions classifiable to 630–638
uterus following conditions classifiable to 630–638
vagina following conditions classifiable to 630–638

639.3 Renal failure
Oliguria following conditions classifiable to 630–638
Renal:
failure (acute) following conditions classifiable to 630–638
shutdown following conditions classifiable to 630–638
tubular necrosis following conditions classifiable to 630–638
Uremia following conditions classifiable to 630–638

639.4 Metabolic disorders
Electrolyte imbalance following conditions classifiable to 630–638

639.5 Shock
Circulatory collapse following conditions classifiable to 630–638
Shock (postoperative) (septic) following conditions classifiable to 630–638

639.6 Embolism
Embolism:
NOS following conditions classifiable to 630–638
air following conditions classifiable to 630–638
amniotic fluid following conditions classifiable to 630–638
blood-clot following conditions classifiable to 630–638
fat following conditions classifiable to 630–638
pulmonary following conditions classifiable to 630–638
pyemic following conditions classifiable to 630–638
septic following conditions classifiable to 630–638
septic following conditions classifiable to 630–638
soap following conditions classifiable to 630–638

❑ **639.8 Other specified complications following abortion or ectopic and molar pregnancy**
Acute yellow atrophy or necrosis of liver following conditions classifiable to 630–638
Cardiac arrest or failure following conditions classifiable to 630–638
Cerebral anoxia following conditions classifiable to 630–638
Urinary tract infection following conditions classifiable to 630–638

❑ **639.9 Unspecified complication following abortion or ectopic and molar pregnancy**
Complication(s) not further specified following conditions classifiable to 630–638

COMPLICATIONS MAINLY RELATED TO PREGNANCY (640–648)

Includes: the listed conditions even if they arose or were present during labor, delivery, or the puerperium

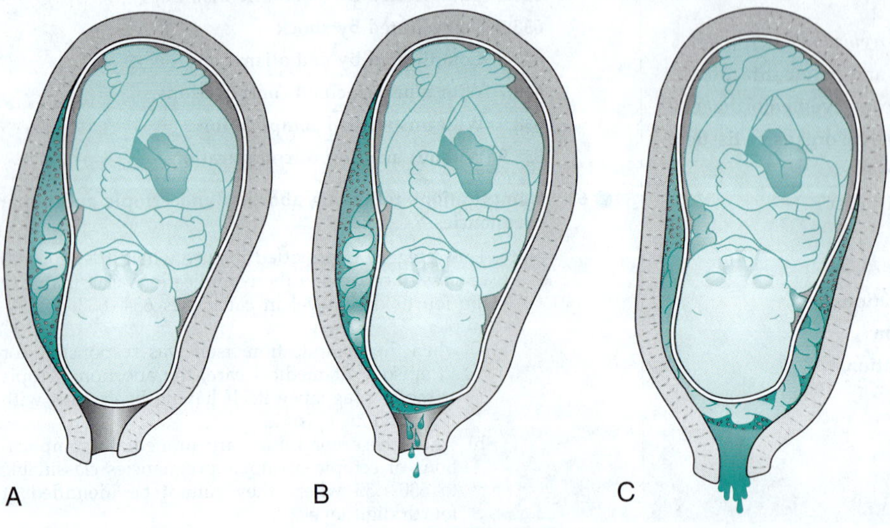

Figure 11–2 A. Marginal placenta previa. **B.** Partial placenta previa. **C.** Total placenta previa.

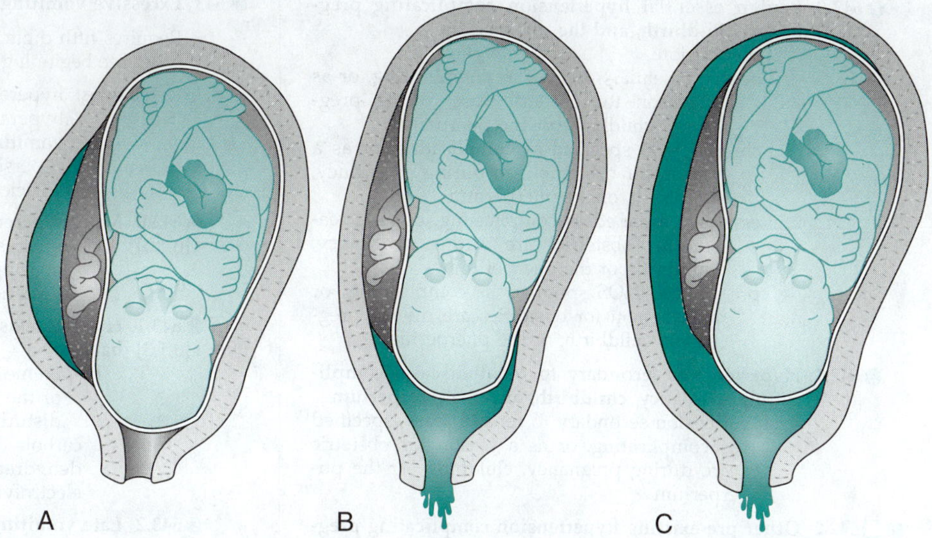

Figure 11-3 Abruptio placentae is classified according to the grade of separation of the placenta from the uterine wall. **A.** Mild separation in which hemorrhage is internal. **B.** Moderate separation in which there is external hemorrhage. **C.** Severe separation in which there is external hemorrhage and extreme separation.

Item 11-3 Placenta previa is a condition in which the opening of the cervix is obstructed by the displaced placenta. The three types, marginal, partial, and total, are varying degrees of placenta displacement.

The following fifth-digit subclassification is for use with categories 640–648 to denote the current episode of care:

❑ **0 unspecified as to episode of care or not applicable**
1 delivered, with or without mention of antepartum condition
Antepartum condition with delivery
Delivery NOS (with mention of antepartum complication during current episode of care)
Intrapartum
obstetric condition (with mention of antepartum complication during current episode of care)
Pregnancy, delivered (with mention of antepartum complication during current episode of care)
2 delivered, with mention of postpartum complication
Delivery with mention of puerperal complication during current episode of care
3 antepartum condition or complication
Antepartum obstetric condition, not delivered during the current episode of care
4 postpartum condition or complication
Postpartum or puerperal obstetric condition or complication following delivery that occurred:
during previous episode of care
outside hospital, with subsequent admission for observation or care

● **640 Hemorrhage in early pregnancy**

Requires fifth digit; valid digits are in [brackets] under each code. See beginning of section 640–648 for definitions.

Includes: hemorrhage before completion of 22 weeks' gestation

● **640.0 Threatened abortion**
[0,1,3]

● ❑ **640.8 Other specified hemorrhage in early pregnancy**
[0,1,3]

● ❑ **640.9 Unspecified hemorrhage in early pregnancy**
[0,1,3]

● **641 Antepartum hemorrhage, abruptio placentae, and placenta previa**

Requires fifth digit; valid digits are in [brackets] under each code. See beginning of section 640–648 for definitions.

● **641.0 Placenta previa without hemorrhage**
[0,1,3] Low implantation of placenta without hemorrhage
Placenta previa noted:
during pregnancy without hemorrhage
before labor (and delivered by cesarean delivery) without hemorrhage

● **641.1 Hemorrhage from placenta previa**
[0,1,3] Low-lying placenta NOS or with hemorrhage (intrapartum)
Placenta previa:
incomplete NOS or with hemorrhage (intrapartum)
marginal NOS or with hemorrhage (intrapartum)
partial NOS or with hemorrhage (intrapartum)
total NOS or with hemorrhage (intrapartum)

Excludes *hemorrhage from vasa previa (663.5)*

● **641.2 Premature separation of placenta**
[0,1,3] Ablatio placentae
Abruptio placentae
Accidental antepartum hemorrhage
Couvelaire uterus
Detachment of placenta (premature)
Premature separation of normally implanted placenta

● **641.3 Antepartum hemorrhage associated with coagulation defects**
[0,1,3] Antepartum or intrapartum hemorrhage associated with:
afibrinogenemia
hyperfibrinolysis
hypofibrinogenemia

● ❑ **641.8 Other antepartum hemorrhage**
[0,1,3] Antepartum or intrapartum hemorrhage associated with:
trauma
uterine leiomyoma

● ❑ **641.9 Unspecified antepartum hemorrhage**
[0,1,3] Hemorrhage:
antepartum NOS
intrapartum NOS
of pregnancy NOS

● **642 Hypertension complicating pregnancy, childbirth, and the puerperium**

Requires fifth digit; valid digits are in [brackets] under each code. See beginning of section 640–648 for definitions.

● **642.0 Benign essential hypertension complicating pregnancy, childbirth, and the puerperium**
[0–4]
Hypertension:
benign essential specified as complicating, or as a reason for obstetric care during pregnancy, childbirth, or the puerperium
chronic NOS specified as complicating, or as a reason for obstetric care during pregnancy, childbirth, or the puerperium
essential specified as complicating, or as a reason for obstetric care during pregnancy, childbirth, or the puerperium
pre-existing NOS specified as complicating, or as a reason for obstetric care during pregnancy, childbirth, or the puerperium

● **642.1 Hypertension secondary to renal disease, complicating pregnancy, childbirth, and the puerperium**
[0–4]
Hypertension secondary to renal disease, specified as complicating, or as a reason for obstetric care during pregnancy, childbirth, or the puerperium

● ❑ **642.2 Other pre-existing hypertension complicating pregnancy, childbirth, and the puerperium**
[0–4]
Hypertensive:
heart and renal disease specified as complicating, or as a reason for obstetric care during pregnancy, childbirth, or the puerperium
heart disease specified as complicating, or as a reason for obstetric care during pregnancy, childbirth, or the puerperium
renal disease specified as complicating, or as a reason for obstetric care during pregnancy, childbirth, or the puerperium
Malignant hypertension specified as complicating, or as a reason for obstetric care during pregnancy, childbirth, or the puerperium

● **642.3 Transient hypertension of pregnancy**
[0–4]
Gestational hypertension
Transient hypertension, so described, in pregnancy, childbirth, or the puerperium

● **642.4 Mild or unspecified pre-eclampsia**
[0–4]
Hypertension in pregnancy, childbirth, or the puerperium, not specified as pre-existing, with either albuminuria or edema, or both; mild or unspecified

Pre-eclampsia:	Toxemia (pre-eclamptic):
NOS	NOS
mild	mild

Excludes *albuminuria in pregnancy, without mention of hypertension (646.2)*
edema in pregnancy, without mention of hypertension (646.1)

● **642.5 Severe pre-eclampsia**
[0–4]
Hypertension in pregnancy, childbirth, or the puerperium, not specified as pre-existing, with either albuminuria or edema, or both; specified as severe
Pre-eclampsia, severe
Toxemia (pre-eclamptic), severe

● **642.6 Eclampsia**
[0–4]

Toxemia:	Toxemia:
eclamptic	with convulsions

● **642.7 Pre-eclampsia or eclampsia superimposed on pre-existing hypertension**
[0–4]
Conditions classifiable to 642.4–642.6, with conditions classifiable to 642.0–642.2

● ❑ **642.9 Unspecified hypertension complicating pregnancy, childbirth, or the puerperium**
[0–4]
Hypertension NOS, without mention of albuminuria or edema, complicating pregnancy, childbirth, or the puerperium

● **643 Excessive vomiting in pregnancy**

Requires fifth digit; valid digits are in [brackets] under each code. See beginning of section 640–648 for definitions.

Includes: hyperemesis arising during pregnancy
hyperemesis gravidarum
vomiting:
persistent arising during pregnancy
vicious arising during pregnancy

● **643.0 Mild hyperemesis gravidarum**
[0,1,3]
Hyperemesis gravidarum, mild or unspecified, starting before the end of the 22nd week of gestation

● **643.1 Hyperemesis gravidarum with metabolic disturbance**
[0,1,3]
Hyperemesis gravidarum, starting before the end of the 22nd week of gestation, with metabolic disturbance, such as:
carbohydrate depletion
dehydration
electrolyte imbalance

● **643.2 Late vomiting of pregnancy**
[0,1,3]
Excessive vomiting starting after 22 completed weeks of gestation

● ❑ **643.8 Other vomiting complicating pregnancy**
[0,1,3]
Vomiting due to organic disease or other cause, specified as complicating pregnancy, or as a reason for obstetric care during pregnancy

Use additional code to specify cause

● ❑ **643.9 Unspecified vomiting of pregnancy**
[0,1,3]
Vomiting as a reason for care during pregnancy, length of gestation unspecified

● **644 Early or threatened labor**

Requires fifth digit; valid digits are in [brackets] under each code. See beginning of section 640–648 for definitions.

● **644.0 Threatened premature labor**
[0,3]
Premature labor after 22 weeks, but before 37 completed weeks of gestation without delivery

Excludes *that occurring before 22 completed weeks of gestation (640.0)*

● ❑ **644.1 Other threatened labor**
[0,3]
False labor:
NOS without delivery
after 37 completed weeks of gestation without delivery
Threatened labor NOS without delivery

● **644.2 Early onset of delivery**
[0–1]
Onset (spontaneous) of delivery before 37 completed weeks of gestation
Premature labor with onset of delivery before 37 completed weeks of gestation

● **645 Late pregnancy**

Requires fifth digit; valid digits are in [brackets] under each code. See beginning of section 640–648 for definitions.

645.1 Post term pregnancy
[0,1,3]
Pregnancy over 40 completed weeks to 42 completed weeks gestation

645.2 Prolonged pregnancy
[0,1,3]
Pregnancy which has advanced beyond 42 completed weeks of gestation

● **646 Other complications of pregnancy, not elsewhere classified**

Use additional code(s) to further specify complication

Requires fifth digit; valid digits are in [brackets] under each code. See beginning of section 640–648 for definitions.

646.0 Papyraceous fetus
[0,1,3]

646.1 Edema or excessive weight gain in pregnancy, without mention of hypertension
[0–4]
Gestational edema
Maternal obesity syndrome

Excludes *that with mention of hypertension (642.0–642.9)*

646.2 Unspecified renal disease in pregnancy, without mention of hypertension
[0–4]
Albuminuria in pregnancy or the puerperium, without mention of hypertension
Nephropathy NOS in pregnancy or the puerperium, without mention of hypertension
Renal disease NOS in pregnancy or the puerperium, without mention of hypertension
Uremia in pregnancy or the puerperium, without mention of hypertension
Gestational proteinuria in pregnancy or the puerperium, without mention of hypertension

Excludes *that with mention of hypertension (642.0–642.9)*

646.3 Habitual aborter
[0–1,3]

Excludes *with current abortion (634.0–634.9)*
without current pregnancy (629.9)

646.4 Peripheral neuritis in pregnancy
[0–4]

646.5 Asymptomatic bacteriuria in pregnancy
[0–4]

646.6 Infections of genitourinary tract in pregnancy
[0–4]
Conditions classifiable to 590, 595, 597, 599.0, 616 complicating pregnancy, childbirth, or the puerperium
Conditions classifiable to 614.0–614.5, 614.7–614.9, 615

Excludes *major puerperal infection (670)*

646.7 Liver disorders in pregnancy
[0,1,3]
Acute yellow atrophy of liver (obstetric) (true) of pregnancy
Icterus gravis of pregnancy
Necrosis of liver of pregnancy

Excludes *hepatorenal syndrome following delivery (674.8)*
viral hepatitis (647.6)

646.8 Other specified complications of pregnancy
[0–4]
Fatigue during pregnancy
Herpes gestationis
Insufficient weight gain of pregnancy
Uterine size-date discrepancy

646.9 Unspecified complication of pregnancy
[0,1,3]

647 Infectious and parasitic conditions in the mother classifiable elsewhere, but complicating pregnancy, childbirth, or the puerperium

Use additional code(s) to further specify complication

Requires fifth digit; valid digits are in [brackets] under each code. See beginning of section 640–648 for definitions.

Includes: the listed conditions when complicating the pregnant state, aggravated by the pregnancy, or when a main reason for obstetric care

Excludes *those conditions in the mother known or suspected to have affected the fetus (655.0–655.9)*

647.0 Syphilis
[0–4]
Conditions classifiable to 090–097

647.1 Gonorrhea
[0–4]
Conditions classifiable to 098

647.2 Other venereal diseases
[0–4]
Conditions classifiable to 099

647.3 Tuberculosis
[0–4]
Conditions classifiable to 010–018

647.4 Malaria
[0–4]
Conditions classifiable to 084

647.5 Rubella
[0–4]
Conditions classifiable to 056

647.6 Other viral diseases
[0–4]
Conditions classifiable to 042 and 050–079, except 056

647.8 Other specified infectious and parasitic diseases
[0–4]

647.9 Unspecified infection or infestation
[0–4]

648 Other current conditions in the mother classifiable elsewhere, but complicating pregnancy, childbirth, or the puerperium

Use additional code(s) to identify the condition

Requires fifth digit; valid digits are in [brackets] under each code. See beginning of section 640–648 for definitions.

Includes: the listed conditions when complicating the pregnant state, aggravated by the pregnancy, or when a main reason for obstetric care

Excludes *those conditions in the mother known or suspected to have affected the fetus (655.0–665.9)*

648.0 Diabetes mellitus
[0–4]
Conditions classifiable to 250

Excludes *gestational diabetes (648.8)*

648.1 Thyroid dysfunction
[0–4]
Conditions classifiable to 240–246

648.2 Anemia
[0–4]
Conditions classifiable to 280–285

648.3 Drug dependence
[0–4]
Conditions classifiable to 304

648.4 Mental disorders
[0–4]
Conditions classifiable to 290–303, 305–316, 317–319

648.5 Congenital cardiovascular disorders
[0–4]
Conditions classifiable to 745–747

648.6 Other cardiovascular diseases
[0–4]
Conditions classifiable to 390–398, 410–429

Excludes *cerebrovascular disorders in the puerperium (674.0)*
venous complications (671.0–671.9)

648.7 Bone and joint disorders of back, pelvis, and lower limbs
[0–4]
Conditions classifiable to 720–724, and those classifiable to 711–719 or 725–738, specified as affecting the lower limbs

648.8 Abnormal glucose tolerance
[0–4]
Conditions classifiable to 790.2
Gestational diabetes

648.9 Other current conditions classifiable elsewhere
[0–4]
Conditions classifiable to 440–459
Nutritional deficiencies [conditions classifiable to 260–269]

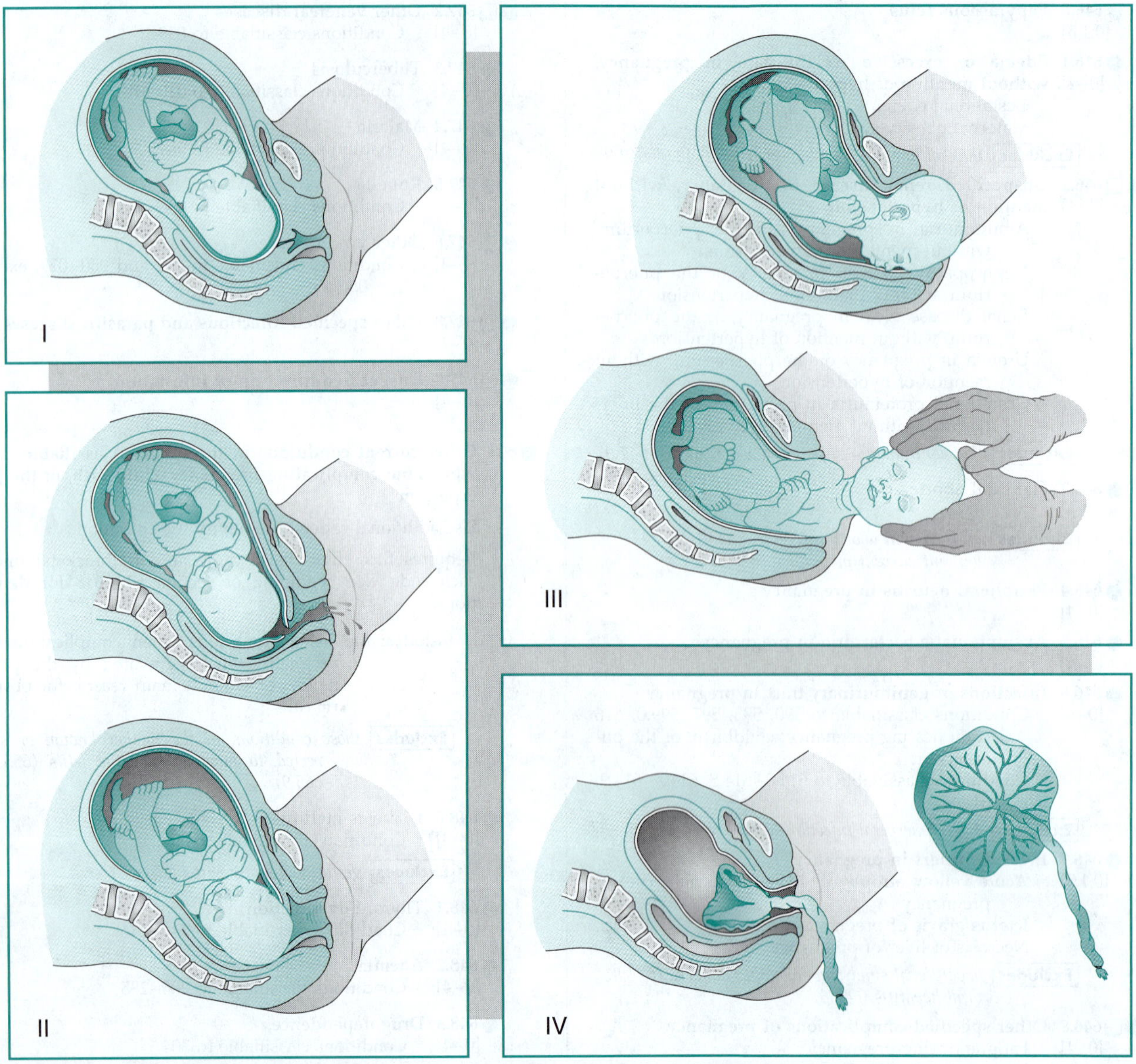

Figure 11–4 The four stages of normal delivery: **I.** Lightening, which occurs 2 to 4 weeks before birth, at which time the fetus turns with head toward the vagina. **II.** Regular contractions begin, the amniotic sac ruptures, and dilation is complete. **III.** Delivery of the head and rotation. **IV.** Recovery of the mother to full homeostasis.

NORMAL DELIVERY, AND OTHER INDICATIONS FOR CARE IN PREGNANCY, LABOR, AND DELIVERY (650–659)

The following fifth-digit subclassification is for use with categories 651–659 to denote the current episode of care:

❑ **0 unspecified as to episode of care or not applicable**
1 delivered, with or without mention of antepartum condition
2 delivered, with mention of postpartum complication
3 antepartum condition or complication
4 postpartum condition or complication

650 Normal delivery

Delivery requiring minimal or no assistance, with or without episiotomy, without fetal manipulation [e.g., rotation version] or instrumentation [forceps] of a spontaneous, cephalic, vaginal, full-term, single, live-born infant. This code is for use as a single diagnosis code and is not to be used with any other code in the range 630–676.

Use additional code to indicate outcome of delivery (V27.0)

Excludes *breech delivery (assisted) (spontaneous) NOS (652.2)*
delivery by vacuum extractor, forceps, cesarean section, or breech extraction, without specified complication (669.5–669.7)

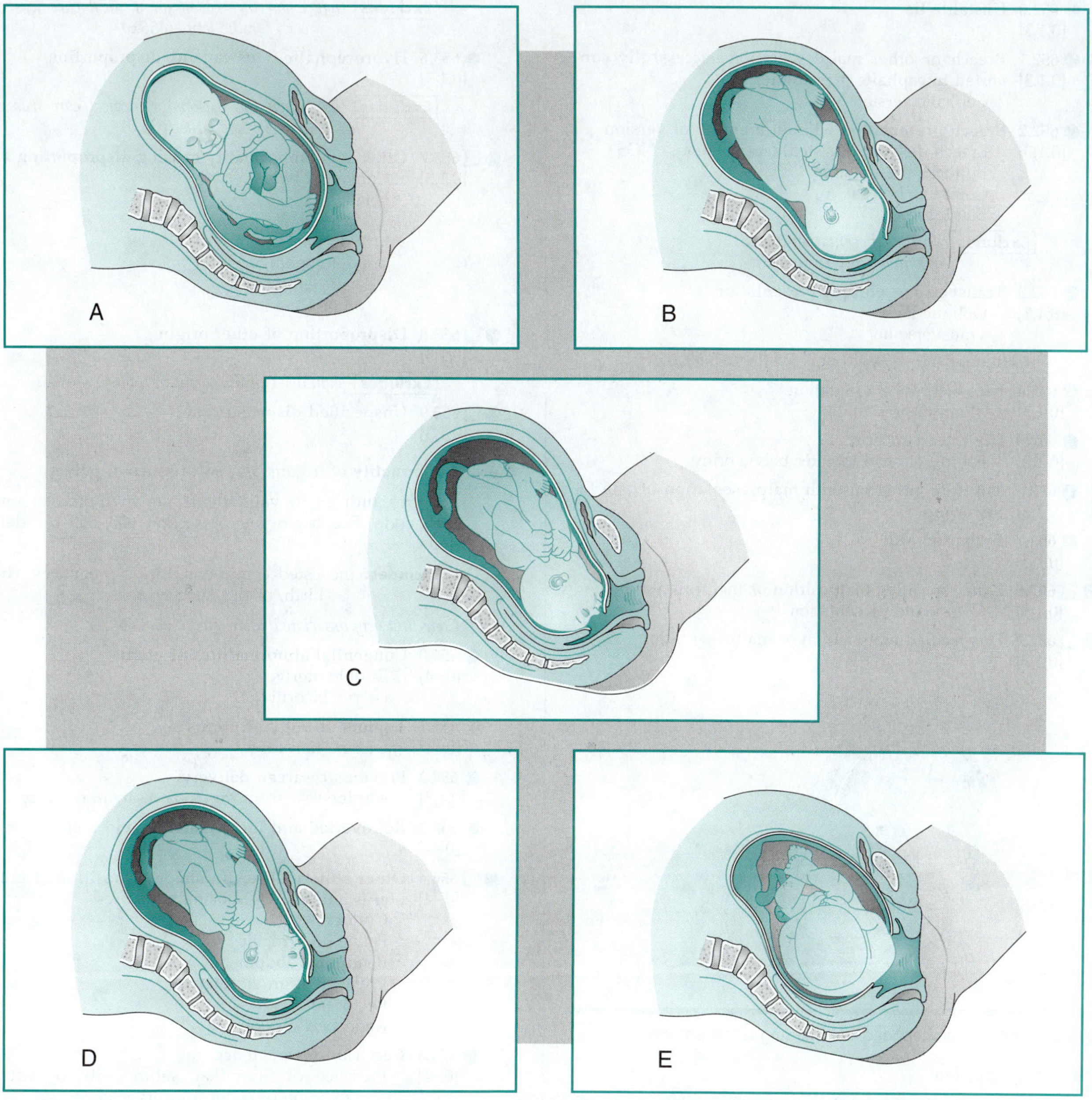

Figure 11–5 Five types of malposition and malpresentation of the fetus: **A.** Breech. **B.** Vertex. **C.** Face. **D.** Brow. **E.** Shoulder.

● **651 Multiple gestation**

Requires fifth digit; valid digits are in [brackets] under each code. See beginning of section 650–659 for definitions.

● **651.0 Twin pregnancy**
[0,1,3]

● **651.1 Triplet pregnancy**
[0,1,3]

● **651.2 Quadruplet pregnancy**
[0,1,3]

● **651.3 Twin pregnancy with fetal loss and retention of one fetus**
[0,1,3]

● **651.4 Triplet pregnancy with fetal loss and retention of one or more fetus(es)**
[0,1,3]

● **651.5 Quadruplet pregnancy with fetal loss and retention of one or more fetus(es)**
[0,1,3]

● ❑ **651.6 Other multiple pregnancy with fetal loss and retention of one or more fetus(es)**
[0,1,3]

● ❑ **651.8 Other specified multiple gestation**
[0,1,3]

● ❑ **651.9 Unspecified multiple gestation**
[0,1,3]

● **652 Malposition and malpresentation of fetus**

Requires fifth digit; valid digits are in [brackets] under each code. See beginning of section 650–659 for definitions.

Code first any associated obstructed labor (660.0)

● **652.0 Unstable lie**
[0,1,3]

● **652.1 Breech or other malpresentation successfully converted to cephalic presentation**
[0,1,3]
Cephalic version NOS

● **652.2 Breech presentation without mention of version**
[0,1,3]
Breech delivery (assisted) (spontaneous) NOS
Buttocks presentation
Complete breech
Frank breech

Excludes *footling presentation (652.8)*
incomplete breech (652.8)

● **652.3 Transverse or oblique presentation**
[0,1,3]
Oblique lie
Transverse lie

Excludes *transverse arrest of fetal head (660.3)*

● **652.4 Face or brow presentation**
[0,1,3]
Mentum presentation

● **652.5 High head at term**
[0,1,3]
Failure of head to enter pelvic brim

● **652.6 Multiple gestation with malpresentation of one fetus or more**
[0,1,3]

● **652.7 Prolapsed arm**
[0,1,3]

● ❑ **652.8 Other specified malposition or malpresentation**
[0,1,3]
Compound presentation

● ❑ **652.9 Unspecified malposition or malpresentation**
[0,1,3]

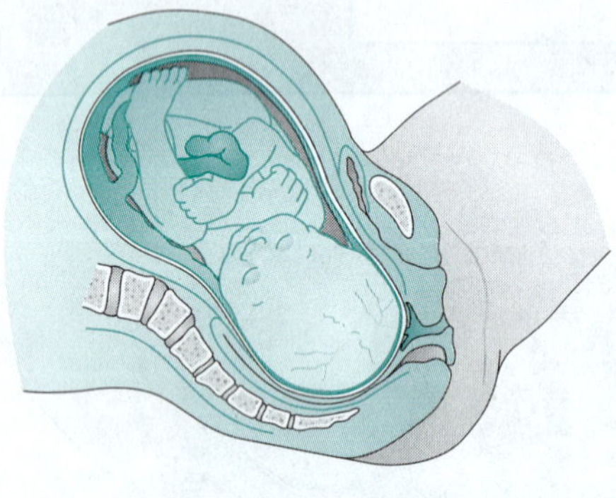

Figure 11–6 Hydrocephalic fetus causing disproportion.

● **653 Disproportion**

Requires fifth digit; valid digits are in [brackets] under each code. See beginning of section 650–659 for definitions.

Code first any associated obstructed labor (660.1)

● **653.0 Major abnormality of bony pelvis, not further specified**
[0,1,3]
Pelvic deformity NOS

● **653.1 Generally contracted pelvis**
[0,1,3]
Contracted pelvis NOS

● **653.2 Inlet contraction of pelvis**
[0,1,3]
Inlet contraction (pelvis)

● **653.3 Outlet contraction of pelvis**
[0,1,3]
Outlet contraction (pelvis)

● **653.4 Fetopelvic disproportion**
[0,1,3]
Cephalopelvic disproportion NOS
Disproportion of mixed maternal and fetal origin, with normally formed fetus

● **653.5 Unusually large fetus causing disproportion**
[0,1,3]
Disproportion of fetal origin with normally formed fetus
Fetal disproportion NOS

Excludes *that when the reason for medical care was concern for the fetus (656.6)*

● **653.6 Hydrocephalic fetus causing disproportion**
[0,1,3]

Excludes *that when the reason for medical care was concern for the fetus (655.0)*

● ❑ **653.7 Other fetal abnormality causing disproportion**
[0,1,3]
Conjoined twins
Fetal:
ascites
hydrops
myelomeningocele
sacral teratoma
tumor

● ❑ **653.8 Disproportion of other origin**
[0,1,3]

Excludes *shoulder (girdle) dystocia (660.4)*

● ❑ **653.9 Unspecified disproportion**
[0,1,3]

● **654 Abnormality of organs and soft tissues of pelvis**

Requires fifth digit; valid digits are in [brackets] under each code. See beginning of section 650–659 for definitions.

Includes: the listed conditions during pregnancy, childbirth, or the puerperium

Code first any associated obstructed labor (660.2)

● **654.0 Congenital abnormalities of uterus**
[0–4]
Double uterus
Uterus bicornis

● **654.1 Tumors of body of uterus**
[0–4]
Uterine fibroids

● **654.2 Previous cesarean delivery**
[0,1,3]
Uterine scar from previous cesarean delivery

● **654.3 Retroverted and incarcerated gravid uterus**
[0–4]

● ❑ **654.4 Other abnormalities in shape or position of gravid uterus and of neighboring structures**
[0–4]
Cystocele
Pelvic floor repair
Pendulous abdomen
Prolapse of gravid uterus
Rectocele
Rigid pelvic floor

● **654.5 Cervical incompetence**
[0–4]
Presence of Shirodkar suture with or without mention of cervical incompetence

● ❑ **654.6 Other congenital or acquired abnormality of cervix**
[0–4]
Cicatricial cervix
Polyp of cervix
Previous surgery to cervix
Rigid cervix (uteri)
Stenosis or stricture of cervix
Tumor of cervix

● **654.7 Congenital or acquired abnormality of vagina**
[0–4]
Previous surgery to vagina
Septate vagina
Stenosis of vagina (acquired) (congenital)
Stricture of vagina
Tumor of vagina

● **654.8 Congenital or acquired abnormality of vulva**
[0–4]
Fibrosis of perineum
Persistent hymen
Previous surgery to perineum or vulva
Rigid perineum
Tumor of vulva

Excludes *varicose veins of vulva (671.1)*

● ❑ **654.9 Other and unspecified**
[0–4] Uterine scar NEC

● **655 Known or suspected fetal abnormality affecting management of mother**

Requires fifth digit; valid digits are in [brackets] under each code. See beginning of section 650–659 for definitions.

Includes: the listed conditions in the fetus as a reason for observation or obstetrical care of the mother, or for termination of pregnancy

● **655.0 Central nervous system malformation in fetus**
[0,1,3] Fetal or suspected fetal:
anencephaly
hydrocephalus
spina bifida (with myelomeningocele)

● **655.1 Chromosomal abnormality in fetus**
[0,1,3]

● **655.2 Hereditary disease in family possibly affecting fetus**
[0,1,3]

● **655.3 Suspected damage to fetus from viral disease in the mother**
[0,1,3] Suspected damage to fetus from maternal rubella

● ❑ **655.4 Suspected damage to fetus from other disease in the mother**
[0,1,3] Suspected damage to fetus from maternal:
alcohol addiction
listeriosis
toxoplasmosis

● **655.5 Suspected damage to fetus from drugs**
[0,1,3]

● **655.6 Suspected damage to fetus from radiation**
[0,1,3]

● **655.7 Decreased fetal movements**
[0,1,3]

● ❑ **655.8 Other known or suspected fetal abnormality, not elsewhere classified**
[0,1,3] Suspected damage to fetus from:
environmental toxins
intrauterine contraceptive device

● ❑ **655.9 Unspecified**
[0,1,3]

● **656 Other fetal and placental problems affecting management of mother**

Requires fifth digit; valid digits are in [brackets] under each code. See beginning of section 650–659 for definitions.

● **656.0 Fetal-maternal hemorrhage**
[0,1,3] Leakage (microscopic) of fetal blood into maternal circulation

● **656.1 Rhesus isoimmunization**
[0,1,3] Anti-D [Rh] antibodies
Rh incompatibility

● ❑ **656.2 Isoimmunization from other and unspecified blood-group incompatibility**
[0,1,3] ABO isoimmunization

● **656.3 Fetal distress**
[0,1,3] Fetal metabolic acidemia

Excludes *abnormal fetal acid-base balance (656.8)*
abnormality in fetal heart rate or rhythm (659.7)
fetal bradycardia (659.7)
fetal tachycardia (659.7)
meconium in liquor (656.8)

● **656.4 Intrauterine death**
[0,1,3] Fetal death:
NOS
after completion of 22 weeks' gestation
late
Missed delivery

Excludes *missed abortion (632)*

● **656.5 Poor fetal growth**
[0,1,3] "Light-for-dates"
"Placental insufficiency"
"Small-for-dates"

● **656.6 Excessive fetal growth**
[0,1,3] "Large-for-dates"

● ❑ **656.7 Other placental conditions**
[0,1,3] Abnormal placenta
Placental infarct

Excludes *placental polyp (674.4)*
placentitis (658.4)

● ❑ **656.8 Other specified fetal and placental problems**
[0,1,3] Abnormal acid-base balance
Intrauterine acidosis
Lithopedian
Meconium in liquor

● ❑ **656.9 Unspecified fetal and placental problem**
[0,1,3]

● **657 Polyhydramnios**
[0,1,3] Hydramnios

Requires fifth digit; valid digits are in [brackets] under each code. See beginning of section 650–659 for definitions.

Use 0 as fourth digit for category 657

● **658 Other problems associated with amniotic cavity and membranes**

Requires fifth digit; valid digits are in [brackets] under each code. See beginning of section 650–659 for definitions.

Excludes *amniotic fluid embolism (673.1)*

● **658.0 Oligohydramnios**
[0,1,3] Oligohydramnios without mention of rupture of membranes

● **658.1 Premature rupture of membranes**
[0,1,3] Rupture of amniotic sac less than 24 hours prior to the onset of labor

● **658.2 Delayed delivery after spontaneous or unspecified rupture of membranes**
[0,1,3] Prolonged rupture of membranes NOS
Rupture of amniotic sac 24 hours or more prior to the onset of labor

● **658.3 Delayed delivery after artificial rupture of membranes**
[0,1,3]

● **658.4 Infection of amniotic cavity**
[0,1,3] Amnionitis
Chorioamnionitis
Membranitis
Placentitis

● ❑ **658.8 Other**
[0,1,3] Amnion nodosum
Amniotic cyst

● ❑ **658.9 Unspecified**
[0,1,3]

● **659 Other indications for care or intervention related to labor and delivery, not elsewhere classified**

Requires fifth digit; valid digits are in [brackets] under each code. See beginning of section 650–659 for definitions.

● **659.0 Failed mechanical induction**
[0,1,3] Failure of induction of labor by surgical or other instrumental methods

● 659.1 **Failed medical or unspecified induction**
[0,1,3] Failed induction NOS
Failure of induction of labor by medical methods, such as oxytocic drugs

● ❑ 659.2 **Maternal pyrexia during labor, unspecified**
[0,1,3]

● 659.3 **Generalized infection during labor**
[0,1,3] Septicemia during labor

● 659.4 **Grand multiparity**
[0,1,3]
Excludes *supervision only, in pregnancy (V23.3)*
without current pregnancy (V61.5)

● 659.5 **Elderly primigravida**
[0,1,3] First pregnancy in a woman who will be 35 years of age or older at expected date of delivery
Excludes *supervision only, in pregnancy (V23.81)*

● ❑ 659.6 **Elderly multigravida**
[0,1,3] Second or more pregnancy in a woman who will be 35 years of age or older at expected date of delivery
Excludes *elderly primigravida (659.5)*

● ❑ 659.7 **Abnormality in fetal heart rate or rhythm**
[0,1,3] Depressed fetal heart tones
Fetal:
bradycardia
tachycardia
Fetal heart rate decelerations
Non-reassuring fetal heart rate or rhythm

● ❑ 659.8 **Other specified indications for care or intervention related to labor and delivery**
[0,1,3] Pregnancy in a female less than 16 years old at expected date of delivery
Very young maternal age

● ❑ 659.9 **Unspecified indication for care or intervention related to labor and delivery**
[0,1,3]

COMPLICATIONS OCCURRING MAINLY IN THE COURSE OF LABOR AND DELIVERY (660–669)

The following fifth-digit subclassification is for use with categories 660–669 to denote the current episode of care:

❑ **0 unspecified as to episode of care or not applicable**
1 delivered, with or without mention of antepartum condition
2 delivered, with mention of postpartum complication
3 antepartum condition or complication
4 postpartum condition or complication

● **660 Obstructed labor**

Requires fifth digit; valid digits are in [brackets] under each code. See beginning of section 660–669 for definitions.

● 660.0 **Obstruction caused by malposition of fetus at onset of labor**
[0,1,3] Any condition classifiable to 652, causing obstruction during labor

Use additional code from 652.0–652.9 to identify condition

● 660.1 **Obstruction by bony pelvis**
[0,1,3] Any condition classifiable to 653, causing obstruction during labor

Use additional code from 653.0–653.9 to identify condition

● 660.2 **Obstruction by abnormal pelvic soft tissues**
[0,1,3] Prolapse of anterior lip of cervix
Any condition classifiable to 654, causing obstruction during labor

Use additional code from 654.0–654.9 to identify condition

● 660.3 **Deep transverse arrest and persistent occipitoposterior position**
[0,1,3]

● 660.4 **Shoulder (girdle) dystocia**
[0,1,3] Impacted shoulders

● 660.5 **Locked twins**
[0,1,3]

● ❑ 660.6 **Failed trial of labor, unspecified**
[0,1,3] Failed trial of labor, without mention of condition or suspected condition

● ❑ 660.7 **Failed forceps or vacuum extractor, unspecified**
[0,1,3] Application of ventouse or forceps, without mention of condition

● ❑ 660.8 **Other causes of obstructed labor**
[0,1,3]

● ❑ 660.9 **Unspecified obstructed labor**
[0,1,3] Dystocia:
NOS
fetal NOS
maternal NOS

● **661 Abnormality of forces of labor**

Requires fifth digit; valid digits are in [brackets] under each code. See beginning of section 660–669 for definitions.

● 661.0 **Primary uterine inertia**
[0,1,3] Failure of cervical dilation
Hypotonic uterine dysfunction, primary
Prolonged latent phase of labor

● 661.1 **Secondary uterine inertia**
[0,1,3] Arrested active phase of labor
Hypotonic uterine dysfunction, secondary

● ❑ 661.2 **Other and unspecified uterine inertia**
[0,1,3] Desultory labor
Irregular labor
Poor contractions
Slow slope active phase of labor

● 661.3 **Precipitate labor**
[0,1,3]

● 661.4 **Hypertonic, incoordinate, or prolonged uterine contractions**
[0,1,3] Cervical spasm
Contraction ring (dystocia)
Dyscoordinate labor
Hourglass contraction of uterus
Hypertonic uterine dysfunction
Incoordinate uterine action
Retraction ring (Bandl's) (pathological)
Tetanic contractions
Uterine dystocia NOS
Uterine spasm

● ❑ 661.9 **Unspecified abnormality of labor**
[0,1,3]

● **662 Long labor**

Requires fifth digit; valid digits are in [brackets] under each code. See beginning of section 660–669 for definitions.

● 662.0 **Prolonged first stage**
[0,1,3]

● ❑ 662.1 **Prolonged labor, unspecified**
[0,1,3]

● 662.2 **Prolonged second stage**
[0,1,3]

● 662.3 **Delayed delivery of second twin, triplet, etc.**
[0,1,3]

● **663 Umbilical cord complications**

Requires fifth digit; valid digits are in [brackets] under each code. See beginning of section 660–669 for definitions.

● 663.0 **Prolapse of cord**
[0,1,3] Presentation of cord

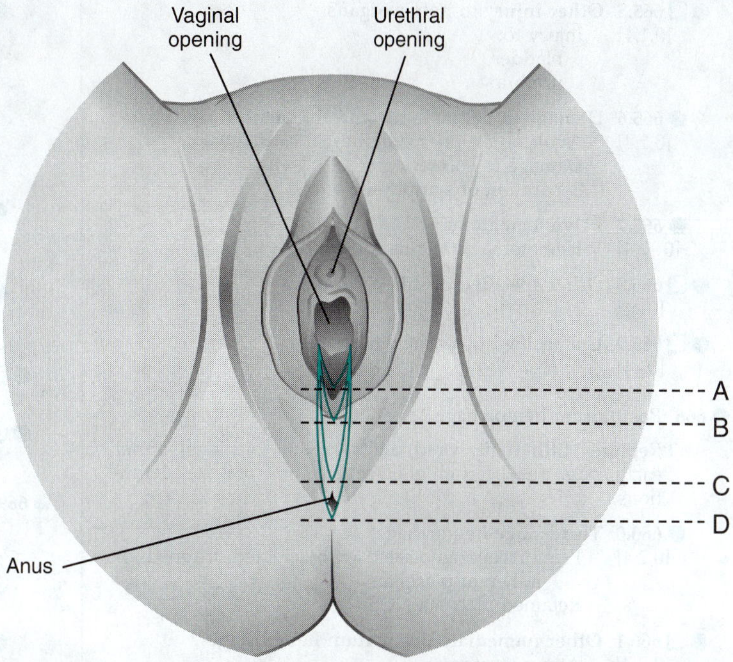

Figure 11–7 Perineal lacerations: **A.** First-degree is laceration of superficial tissues. **B.** Second-degree is limited to the pelvic floor and may involve the perineal or vaginal muscles. **C.** Third-degree involves the anal sphincter. **D.** Fourth-degree involves anal or rectal mucosa.

● **663.1 Cord around neck, with compression**
[0,1,3] Cord tightly around neck

● ❑ **663.2 Other and unspecified cord entanglement, with compression**
[0,1,3] Entanglement of cords of twins in mono-amniotic sac
Knot in cord (with compression)

● ❑ **663.3 Other and unspecified cord entanglement, without mention of compression**
[0,1,3]

● **663.4 Short cord**
[0,1,3]

● **663.5 Vasa previa**
[0,1,3]

● **663.6 Vascular lesions of cord**
[0,1,3] Bruising of cord
Hematoma of cord
Thrombosis of vessels of cord

● ❑ **663.8 Other umbilical cord complications**
[0,1,3] Velamentous insertion of umbilical cord

● ❑ **663.9 Unspecified umbilical cord complication**
[0,1,3]

● **664 Trauma to perineum and vulva during delivery**

Requires fifth digit; valid digits are in [brackets] under each code. See beginning of section 660–669 for definitions.

Includes: damage from instruments
that from extension of episiotomy

● **664.0 First-degree perineal laceration**
[0,1,4] Perineal laceration, rupture, or tear involving:
fourchette
hymen
labia
skin
vagina
vulva

● **664.1 Second-degree perineal laceration**
[0,1,4] Perineal laceration, rupture, or tear (following episiotomy) involving:
pelvic floor
perineal muscles
vaginal muscles

Excludes *that involving anal sphincter (664.2)*

● **664.2 Third-degree perineal laceration**
[0,1,4] Perineal laceration, rupture, or tear (following episiotomy) involving:
anal sphincter
rectovaginal septum
sphincter NOS

Excludes *that with anal or rectal mucosal laceration (664.3)*

● **664.3 Fourth-degree perineal laceration**
[0,1,4] Perineal laceration, rupture, or tear as classifiable to 664.2 and involving also:
anal mucosa
rectal mucosa

● ❑ **664.4 Unspecified perineal laceration**
[0,1,4] Central laceration

● **664.5 Vulval and perineal hematoma**
[0,1,4]

● ❑ **664.8 Other specified trauma to perineum and vulva**
[0,1,4]

● ❑ **664.9 Unspecified trauma to perineum and vulva**
[0,1,4]

● **665 Other obstetrical trauma**

Requires fifth digit; valid digits are in [brackets] under each code. See beginning of section 660–669 for definitions.

Includes: damage from instruments

● **665.0 Rupture of uterus before onset of labor**
[0,1,3]

● **665.1 Rupture of uterus during labor**
[0,1] Rupture of uterus NOS

● **665.2 Inversion of uterus**
[0,2,4]

● **665.3 Laceration of cervix**
[0,1,4]

● **665.4 High vaginal laceration**
[0,1,4] Laceration of vaginal wall or sulcus without mention of perineal laceration

● ❑ **665.5 Other injury to pelvic organs**
[0,1,4] Injury to:
bladder
urethra

● **665.6 Damage to pelvic joints and ligaments**
[0,1,4] Avulsion of inner symphyseal cartilage
Damage to coccyx
Separation of symphysis (pubis)

● **665.7 Pelvic hematoma**
[0–2,4] Hematoma of vagina

● ❑ **665.8 Other specified obstetrical trauma**
[0–4]

● ❑ **665.9 Unspecified obstetrical trauma**
[0–4]

● **666 Postpartum hemorrhage**

Requires fifth digit; valid digits are in [brackets] under each code. See beginning of section 660–669 for definitions.

● **666.0 Third-stage hemorrhage**
[0,2,4] Hemorrhage associated with retained, trapped, or adherent placenta
Retained placenta NOS

● ❑ **666.1 Other immediate postpartum hemorrhage**
[0,2,4] Atony of uterus
Hemorrhage within the first 24 hours following delivery of placenta
Postpartum hemorrhage (atonic) NOS

● **666.2 Delayed and secondary postpartum hemorrhage**
[0,2,4] Hemorrhage:
after the first 24 hours following delivery
associated with retained portions of placenta or membranes
Postpartum hemorrhage specified as delayed or secondary
Retained products of conception NOS, following delivery

● **666.3 Postpartum coagulation defects**
[0,2,4] Postpartum:
afibrinogenemia
fibrinolysis

● **667 Retained placenta without hemorrhage**

Requires fifth digit; valid digits are in [brackets] under each code. See beginning of section 660–669 for definitions.

● **667.0 Retained placenta without hemorrhage**
[0,2,4] Placenta accreta without hemorrhage
Retained placenta:
NOS without hemorrhage
total without hemorrhage

● **667.1 Retained portions of placenta or membranes, without hemorrhage**
[0,2,4] Retained products of conception following delivery, without hemorrhage

● **668 Complications of the administration of anesthetic or other sedation in labor and delivery**

Use additional code(s) to further specify complication

Requires fifth digit; valid digits are in [brackets] under each code. See beginning of section 660–669 for definitions.

Includes: complications arising from the administration of a general or local anesthetic, analgesic, or other sedation in labor and delivery

Excludes *reaction to spinal or lumbar puncture (349.0)*
spinal headache (349.0)

● **668.0 Pulmonary complications**
[0–4] Inhalation [aspiration] of stomach contents or secretions following anesthesia or other sedation in labor or delivery
Mendelson's syndrome following anesthesia or other sedation in labor or delivery
Pressure collapse of lung following anesthesia or other sedation in labor or delivery

● **668.1 Cardiac complications**
[0–4] Cardiac arrest or failure following anesthesia or other sedation in labor and delivery

● **668.2 Central nervous system complications**
[0–4] Cerebral anoxia following anesthesia or other sedation in labor and delivery

● ❑ **668.8 Other complications of anesthesia or other sedation in labor and delivery**
[0–4]

● ❑ **668.9 Unspecified complication of anesthesia and other sedation**
[0–4]

● **669 Other complications of labor and delivery, not elsewhere classified**

Requires fifth digit; valid digits are in [brackets] under each code. See beginning of section 660–669 for definitions.

● **669.0 Maternal distress**
[0–4] Metabolic disturbance in labor and delivery

● **669.1 Shock during or following labor and delivery**
[0–4] Obstetric shock

● **669.2 Maternal hypotension syndrome**
[0–4]

● **669.3 Acute renal failure following labor and delivery**
[0,2,4]

● ❑ **669.4 Other complications of obstetrical surgery and procedures**
[0–4] Cardiac:
arrest following cesarean or other obstetrical surgery or procedure, including delivery NOS
failure following cesarean or other obstetrical surgery or procedure, including delivery NOS
Cerebral anoxia following cesarean or other obstetrical surgery or procedure, including delivery NOS

Excludes *complications of obstetrical surgical wounds (674.1–674.3)*

● **669.5 Forceps or vacuum extractor delivery without mention of indication**
[0,1] Delivery by ventouse, without mention of indication

● **669.6 Breech extraction, without mention of indication**
[0,1]

Excludes *breech delivery NOS (652.2)*

● **669.7 Cesarean delivery, without mention of indication**
[0,1]

● ❑ **669.8 Other complications of labor and delivery**
[0–4]

● ❑ **669.9 Unspecified complication of labor and delivery**
[0–4]

COMPLICATIONS OF THE PUERPERIUM (670–677)

Note: Categories 671 and 673–676 include the listed conditions even if they occur during pregnancy or childbirth.

The following fifth-digit subclassification is for use with categories 670–676 to denote the current episode of care:

❑ **0 unspecified as to episode of care or not applicable**
1 delivered, with or without mention of antepartum condition
2 delivered, with mention of postpartum complication
3 antepartum condition or complication
4 postpartum condition or complication

● **670 Major puerperal infection**
[0,2,4]
Requires fifth digit; valid digits are in [brackets] under each code. See beginning of section 670–676 for definitions.

Use 0 as fourth digit for category 670
Puerperal:
endometritis
fever (septic)
pelvic:
cellulitis
sepsis
peritonitis
pyemia
salpingitis
septicemia

Excludes *infection following abortion (639.0)*
minor genital tract infection following delivery (646.6)
puerperal fever NOS (672)
puerperal pyrexia NOS (672)
puerperal pyrexia of unknown origin (672)
urinary tract infection following delivery (646.6)

● **671 Venous complications in pregnancy and the puerperium**

Requires fifth digit; valid digits are in [brackets] under each code. See beginning of section 670–676 for definitions.

● **671.0 Varicose veins of legs**
[0–4] Varicose veins NOS

● **671.1 Varicose veins of vulva and perineum**
[0–4]

● **671.2 Superficial thrombophlebitis**
[0–4] Thrombophlebitis (superficial)

● **671.3 Deep phlebothrombosis, antepartum**
[0,1,3] Deep-vein thrombosis, antepartum

● **671.4 Deep phlebothrombosis, postpartum**
[0,2,4] Deep-vein thrombosis, postpartum
Pelvic thrombophlebitis, postpartum
Phlegmasia alba dolens (puerperal)

● ❑ **671.5 Other phlebitis and thrombosis**
[0–4] Cerebral venous thrombosis
Thrombosis of intracranial venous sinus

● ❑ **671.8 Other venous complications**
[0–4] Hemorrhoids

● ❑ **671.9 Unspecified venous complication**
[0–4] Phlebitis NOS
Thrombosis NOS

● **672 Pyrexia of unknown origin during the puerperium**
[0,2,4] Postpartum fever NOS
Puerperal fever NOS
Puerperal pyrexia NOS

Requires fifth digit; valid digits are in [brackets] under each code. See beginning of section 670–676 for definitions.

Use 0 as fourth digit for category 672

● **673 Obstetrical pulmonary embolism**

Requires fifth digit; valid digits are in [brackets] under each code. See beginning of section 670–676 for definitions.

Includes: pulmonary emboli in pregnancy, childbirth, or the puerperium, or specified as puerperal

Excludes *embolism following abortion (639.6)*

● **673.0 Obstetrical air embolism**
[0–4]

● **673.1 Amniotic fluid embolism**
[0–4]

● **673.2 Obstetrical blood-clot embolism**
[0–4] Puerperal pulmonary embolism NOS

● **673.3 Obstetrical pyemic and septic embolism**
[0–4]

● ❑ **673.8 Other pulmonary embolism**
[0–4] Fat embolism

● **674 Other and unspecified complications of the puerperium, not elsewhere classified**

Requires fifth digit; valid digits are in [brackets] under each code. See beginning of section 670–676 for definitions.

● **674.0 Cerebrovascular disorders in the puerperium**
[0–4] Any condition classifiable to 430–434, 436–437 occurring during pregnancy, childbirth, or the puerperium, or specified as puerperal

Excludes *intracranial venous sinus thrombosis (671.5)*

● **674.1 Disruption of cesarean wound**
[0,2,4] Dehiscence or disruption of uterine wound

Excludes *uterine rupture before onset of labor (665.0)*
uterine rupture during labor (665.1)

● **674.2 Disruption of perineal wound**
[0,2,4] Breakdown of perineum
Disruption of wound of:
episiotomy
perineal laceration
Secondary perineal tear

● ❑ **674.3 Other complications of obstetrical surgical wounds**
[0,2,4] Hematoma of cesarean section or perineal wound
Hemorrhage of cesarean section or perineal wound
Infection of cesarean section or perineal wound

Excludes *damage from instruments in delivery (664.0–665.9)*

● **674.4 Placental polyp**
[0,2,4]

674.5 Peripartum cardiomyopathy
[0–4] Postpartum cardiomyopathy

● ❑ **674.8 Other**
[0,2,4] Hepatorenal syndrome, following delivery
Postpartum:
subinvolution of uterus
uterine hypertrophy

● ❑ **674.9 Unspecified**
[0,2,4] Sudden death of unknown cause during the puerperium

● **675 Infections of the breast and nipple associated with childbirth**

Requires fifth digit; valid digits are in [brackets] under each code. See beginning of section 670–676 for definitions.

Includes: the listed conditions during pregnancy, childbirth, or the puerperium

● **675.0 Infections of nipple**
[0–4] Abscess of nipple

● **675.1 Abscess of breast**
[0–4] Abscess:
mammary
subareolar
submammary
Mastitis:
purulent
retromammary
submammary

● **675.2 Nonpurulent mastitis**
[0–4] Lymphangitis of breast
Mastitis:
NOS
interstitial
parenchymatous

● ❑ **675.8 Other specified infections of the breast and nipple**
[0–4]

● ❑ **675.9 Unspecified infection of the breast and nipple**
[0–4]

● **676 Other disorders of the breast associated with childbirth and disorders of lactation**

Requires fifth digit; valid digits are in [brackets] under each code. See beginning of section 670–676 for definitions.

Includes: the listed conditions during pregnancy, the puerperium, or lactation

● **676.0 Retracted nipple**
[0–4]

● **676.1 Cracked nipple**
[0–4] Fissure of nipple

● **676.2 Engorgement of breasts**
[0–4]

● ❑ **676.3 Other and unspecified disorder of breast**
[0–4]

● **676.4 Failure of lactation**
[0–4] Agalactia

● **676.5 Suppressed lactation**
[0–4]

● **676.6 Galactorrhea**
[0–4]

Excludes *galactorrhea not associated with childbirth (611.6)*

● ❑ **676.8 Other disorders of lactation**
[0–4] Galactocele

● ❑ **676.9 Unspecified disorder of lactation**
[0–4]

❑ **677 Late effect of complication of pregnancy, childbirth, and the puerperium**

Note: This category is to be used to indicate conditions in 632–648.9 and 651–676.9 as the cause of the late effect, themselves classifiable elsewhere. The "late effects " include conditions specified as such, or as sequelae, which may occur at any time after the puerperium.

Code first any sequelae

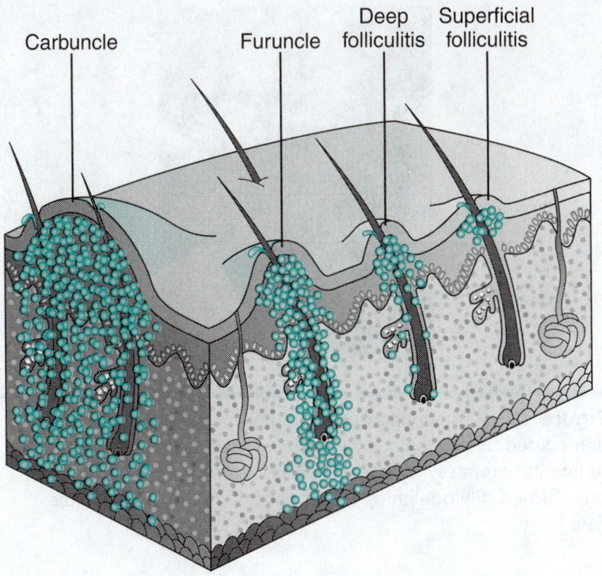

Figure 12–1 Furuncle, also known as a boil, is a staphylococcal infection. The organism enters the body through a hair follicle and so furuncles usually appear in hairy areas of the body. A cluster of furuncles is known as a carbuncle and involves infection into the deep subcutaneous fascia. These usually appear on the back and neck.

12. DISEASES OF THE SKIN AND SUBCUTANEOUS TISSUE (680–709)

INFECTIONS OF SKIN AND SUBCUTANEOUS TISSUE (680–686)

Excludes *certain infections of skin classified under "Infectious and Parasitic Diseases," such as:*
erysipelas (035)
erysipeloid of Rosenbach (027.1)
herpes:
simplex (054.0–054.9)
zoster (053.0–053.9)
molluscum contagiosum (078.0)
viral warts (078.1)

680 Carbuncle and furuncle

Includes: boil
furunculosis

680.0 Face
Ear [any part] — Nose (septum)
Face [any part, except eye] — Temple (region)

Excludes *eyelid (373.13)*
lacrimal apparatus (375.31)
orbit (376.01)

680.1 Neck

680.2 Trunk
Abdominal wall
Back [any part, except buttocks]
Breast
Chest wall
Flank
Groin
Pectoral region
Perineum
Umbilicus

Excludes *buttocks (680.5)*
external genital organs:
female (616.4)
male (607.2, 608.4)

680.3 Upper arm and forearm
Arm [any part, except hand]
Axilla
Shoulder

680.4 Hand
Finger [any] — Wrist
Thumb

680.5 Buttock
Anus — Gluteal region

680.6 Leg, except foot
Ankle — Knee
Hip — Thigh

680.7 Foot
Heel — Toe

680.8 Other specified sites
Head [any part, except face]
Scalp

Excludes *external genital organs:*
female (616.4)
male (607.2, 608.4)

680.9 Unspecified site
Boil NOS — Furuncle NOS
Carbuncle NOS

681 Cellulitis and abscess of finger and toe

Includes: that with lymphangitis

Use additional code to identify organism, such as Staphylococcus (041.1)

681.0 Finger

681.00 Cellulitis and abscess, unspecified

681.01 Felon
Pulp abscess — Whitlow

Excludes *herpetic whitlow (054.6)*

681.02 Onychia and paronychia of finger
Panaritium of finger
Perionychia of finger

681.1 Toe

681.10 Cellulitis and abscess, unspecified

681.11 Onychia and paronychia of toe
Panaritium of toe
Perionychia of toe

681.9 Cellulitis and abscess of unspecified digit
Infection of nail NOS

682 Other cellulitis and abscess

Includes: abscess (acute) (with lymphangitis) except of finger or toe
cellulitis (diffuse) (with lymphangitis) except of finger or toe
lymphangitis, acute (with lymphangitis) except of finger or toe

Use additional code to identify organism, such as Staphylococcus (041.1)

Excludes *lymphangitis (chronic) (subacute) (457.2)*

682.0 Face
Cheek, external — Nose, external
Chin — Submandibular
Forehead — Temple (region)

Excludes *ear [any part] (380.10–380.16)*
eyelid (373.13)
lacrimal apparatus (375.31)
lip (528.5)
mouth (528.3)
nose (internal) (478.1)
orbit (376.01)

682.1 Neck

682.2 Trunk
Abdominal wall
Back [any part, except buttocks]
Chest wall
Flank
Groin
Pectoral region
Perineum
Umbilicus, except newborn

Excludes *anal and rectal regions (566)*
breast:
NOS (611.0)
puerperal (675.1)
external genital organs:
female (616.3–616.4)
male (604.0, 607.2, 608.4)
umbilicus, newborn (771.4)

682.3 Upper arm and forearm
Arm [any part, except hand]
Axilla
Shoulder

Excludes *hand (682.4)*

682.4 Hand, except fingers and thumb
Wrist

Excludes *fingers and thumb (681.00–681.02)*

682.5 Buttocks
Gluteal region

Excludes *anal and rectal regions (566)*

682.6 Leg, except foot
Ankle
Hip
Knee
Thigh

682.7 Foot, except toes
Heel

Excludes *toe (681.10–681.11)*

❑682.8 Other specified sites
Head [except face]
Scalp

Excludes *face (682.0)*

❑682.9 Unspecified site
Abscess NOS
Cellulitis NOS
Lymphangitis, acute NOS

Excludes *lymphangitis NOS (457.2)*

683 Acute lymphadenitis
Abscess (acute) lymph gland or node, except mesenteric
Adenitis, acute lymph gland or node, except mesenteric
Lymphadenitis, acute lymph gland or node, except mesenteric

Use additional code to identify organism such as Staphylococcus (041.1)

Excludes *enlarged glands NOS (785.6)*
lymphadenitis:
chronic or subacute, except mesenteric (289.1)
mesenteric (acute) (chronic) (subacute) (289.2)
unspecified (289.3)

684 Impetigo
Impetiginization of other dermatoses
Impetigo (contagiosa) [any site] [any organism]:
bullous
circinate
neonatorum
simplex
Pemphigus neonatorum

Excludes *impetigo herpetiformis (694.3)l*

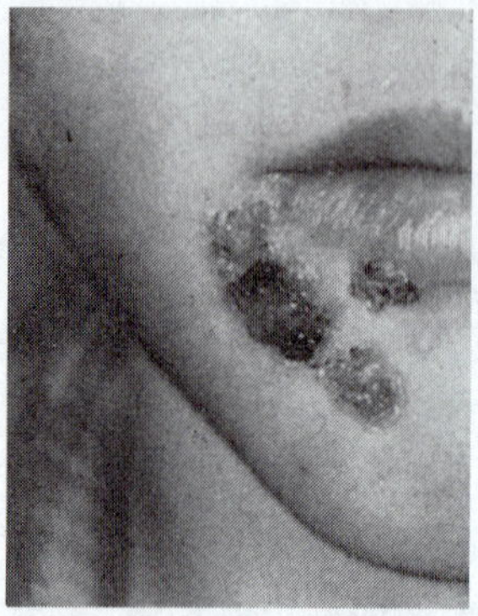

Figure 12–2 Impetigo is a contagious, superficial skin infection caused by *Staphylococcus aureus*. It appears most frequently in infants. (From Lewis GM, Wheeler CE, Jr: Practical Dermatology, 3rd ed. Philadelphia, WB Saunders, 1967, p 234, Plate 79B.)

Item 12–1 Pilonidal cyst, also called a coccygeal cyst, is the result of a disorder called pilonidal disease. The cyst usually contains hair and pus.

● 685 Pilonidal cyst

Includes: fistula, coccygeal or pilonidal
sinus, coccygeal or pilonidal

685.0 With abscess

685.1 Without mention of abscess

● 686 Other local infections of skin and subcutaneous tissue

Use additional code to identify any infectious organism (041.0–041.8)

● 686.0 Pyoderma
Dermatitis:
purulent
septic
suppurative

❑686.00 Pyoderma, unspecified

686.01 Pyoderma gangrenosum

❑686.09 Other pyoderma

686.1 Pyogenic granuloma
Granuloma:
septic
suppurative
telangiectaticum

Excludes *pyogenic granuloma of oral mucosa (528.9)*

❑686.8 Other specified local infections of skin and subcutaneous tissue
Bacterid (pustular)
Dermatitis vegetans
Ecthyma
Perlèche

Excludes *dermatitis infectiosa eczematoides (690.8)*
panniculitis (729.30–729.39)

❑686.9 Unspecified local infection of skin and subcutaneous tissue
Fistula of skin NOS
Skin infection NOS

Excludes *fistula to skin from internal organs—see Alphabetic Index*

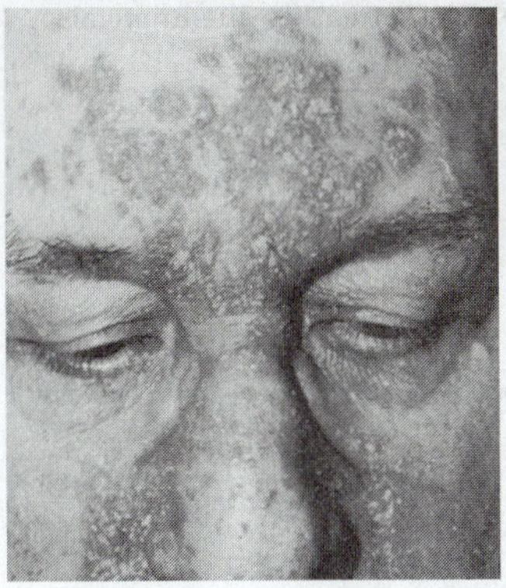

Figure 12-3 Severe seborrheic dermatitis. (From Arnold HL, Odom RB, James WD: Andrews' Diseases of the Skin, Clinical Dermatology, 8th ed. Philadelphia, WB Saunders, 1990, p 195.)

Item 12-2 Seborrheic dermatitis is characterized by greasy, scaly, red patches and is associated with oily skin and scalp.

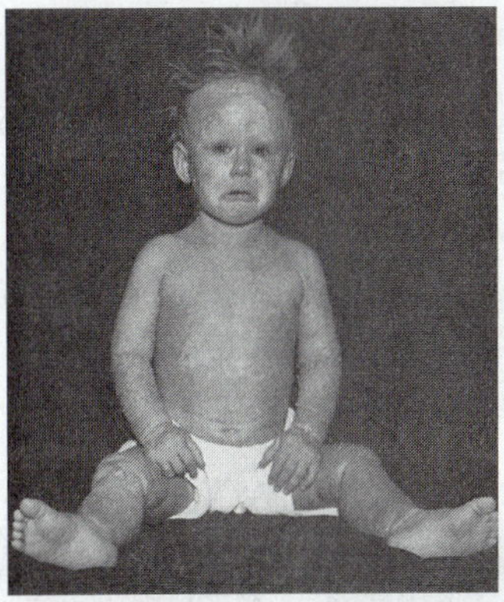

Figure 12-4 Atopic dermatitis. (From Moschella SL, Hurley HJ: Dermatology, 2nd ed. Philadelphia, WB Saunders, 1985, p 336.)

Item 12-3 Atopic dermatitis, also known as atopic eczema, infantile eczema, disseminated neurodermatitis, flexural eczema, and *prurigo diathesique* (Besnier), is characterized by intense itching and is often hereditary.

OTHER INFLAMMATORY CONDITIONS OF SKIN AND SUBCUTANEOUS TISSUE (690–698)

Excludes *panniculitis (729.30–729.39)*

● **690 Erythematosquamous dermatosis**

Excludes *eczematous dermatitis of eyelid (373.31)*
parakeratosis variegata (696.2)
psoriasis (696.0–696.1)
seborrheic keratosis (702.11–702.19)

● **690.1 Seborrheic dermatitis**

❑ **690.10 Seborrheic dermatitis, unspecified**
Seborrheic dermatitis NOS

690.11 Seborrhea capitis
Cradle cap

690.12 Seborrheic infantile dermatitis

❑ **690.18 Other seborrheic dermatitis**

❑ **690.8 Other erythematosquamous dermatosis**

● **691 Atopic dermatitis and related conditions**

691.0 Diaper or napkin rash
Ammonia dermatitis
Diaper or napkin:
- dermatitis
- erythema
- rash

Psoriasiform napkin eruption

❑ **691.8 Other atopic dermatitis and related conditions**
Atopic dermatitis
Besnier's prurigo
Eczema:
- atopic
- flexural
- intrinsic (allergic)

Neurodermatitis:
- atopic
- diffuse (of Brocq)

● **692 Contact dermatitis and other eczema**

Includes: dermatitis:
- NOS
- contact
- occupational
- venenata

eczema (acute) (chronic):
- NOS
- allergic
- erythematous
- occupational

Excludes *allergy NOS (995.3)*
contact dermatitis of eyelids (373.32)
dermatitis due to substances taken internally (693.0–693.9)
eczema of external ear (380.22)
perioral dermatitis (695.3)
urticarial reactions (708.0–708.9, 995.1)

692.0 Due to detergents

692.1 Due to oils and greases

692.2 Due to solvents
Dermatitis due to solvents of:
- chlorocompound group
- cyclohexane group
- ester group
- glycol group
- hydrocarbon group
- ketone group

692.3 Due to drugs and medicines in contact with skin
Dermatitis (allergic) (contact) due to:
- arnica
- fungicides
- iodine
- keratolytics
- mercurials
- neomycin
- pediculocides
- phenols
- scabicides
- any drug applied to skin

Dermatitis medicamentosa due to drug applied to skin

Use additional E code to identify drug

Excludes *allergy NOS due to drugs (995.2)*
dermatitis due to ingested drugs (693.0)
dermatitis medicamentosa NOS (693.0)

❑ **692.4 Due to other chemical products**
Dermatitis due to:
- acids
- adhesive plaster
- alkalis
- caustics
- dichromate

Dermatitis due to:
- insecticide
- nylon
- plastic
- rubber

ICD-9-CM 600-699 Vol. 1

692.5 Due to food in contact with skin
Dermatitis, contact, due to:
cereals
fish
flour
fruit
meat
milk
Excludes *dermatitis due to:*
dyes (692.89)
ingested foods (693.1)
preservatives (692.89)

692.6 Due to plants [except food]
Dermatitis due to:
lacquer tree [Rhus verniciflua]
poison:
ivy [Rhus toxicodendron]
oak [Rhus diversiloba]
sumac [Rhus venenata]
vine [Rhus radicans]
primrose [Primula]
ragweed [Senecio jacobae]
other plants in contact with the skin
Excludes *allergy NOS due to pollen (477.0)*
nettle rash (708.8)

● **692.7 Due to solar radiation**
Excludes *sunburn due to other ultraviolet radiation exposure (692.82)*

❑ **692.70 Unspecified dermatitis due to sun**

692.71 Sunburn
First degree sunburn
Sunburn NOS

692.72 Acute dermatitis due to solar radiation
Berloque dermatitis
Photoallergic response
Phototoxic response
Polymorphous light eruption
Acute solar skin damage NOS
Excludes *sunburn (692.71, 692.76–692.77)*
Use additional E code to identify drug, if drug induced

692.73 Actinic reticuloid and actinic granuloma

❑ **692.74 Other chronic dermatitis due to solar radiation**
Chronic solar skin damage NOS
Solar elastosis
Excludes *actinic [solar] keratosis (702.0)*

692.75 Disseminated superficial actinic porokeratosis (DSAP)

692.76 Sunburn of second degree

692.77 Sunburn of third degree

❑ **692.79 Other dermatitis due to solar radiation**
Hydroa aestivale
Photodermatitis (due to sun)
Photosensitiveness (due to sun)
Solar skin damage NOS

● **692.8 Due to other specified agents**

692.81 Dermatitis due to cosmetics

❑ **692.82 Dermatitis due to other radiation**
Infrared rays
Light, except from sun
Radiation NOS
Tanning bed
Ultraviolet rays, except from sun
X-rays
Excludes *that due to solar radiation (692.70–692.79)*

692.83 Dermatitis due to metals
Jewelry

❑ **692.89 Other**
Dermatitis due to:
cold weather
dyes
furs
hot weather
preservatives
Excludes *allergy NOS due to animal hair, dander (animal), or dust (477.8)*
sunburn (692.71, 692.76–692.77)

❑ **692.9 Unspecified cause**
Dermatitis:
NOS
contact NOS
venenata NOS
Eczema NOS

● **693 Dermatitis due to substances taken internally**
Excludes *adverse effect NOS of drugs and medicines (995.2)*
allergy NOS (995.3)
contact dermatitis (692.0–692.9)
urticarial reactions (708.0–708.9, 995.1)

693.0 Due to drugs and medicines
Dermatitis medicamentosa NOS
Use additional E code to identify drug
Excludes *that due to drugs in contact with skin (692.3)*

693.1 Due to food

❑ **693.8 Due to other specified substances taken internally**

❑ **693.9 Due to unspecified substance taken internally**
Excludes *dermatitis NOS (692.9)*

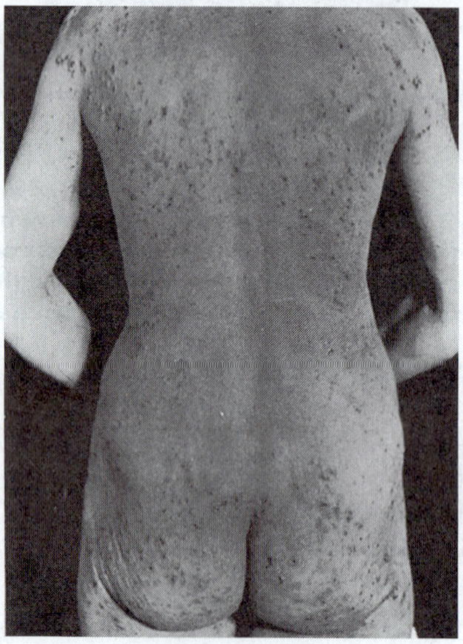

Figure 12–5 Dermatitis herpetiformis. (From Arnold HL, Odom RB, James WD: Andrews' Diseases of the Skin, Clinical Dermatology, 8th ed. Philadelphia, WB Saunders, 1990, p 553.)

Item 12–4 Dermatitis herpetiformis, also known as Duhring's disease, is a systemic disease characterized by small blisters (3 to 5 mm) and occasionally large bullae (+5 mm).

● 694 **Bullous dermatoses**

694.0 **Dermatitis herpetiformis**
Dermatosis herpetiformis
Duhring's disease
Hydroa herpetiformis

Excludes *herpes gestationis (646.8)*
dermatitis herpetiformis:
juvenile (694.2)
senile (694.5)

694.1 **Subcorneal pustular dermatosis**
Sneddon-Wilkinson disease or syndrome

694.2 **Juvenile dermatitis herpetiformis**
Juvenile pemphigoid

694.3 **Impetigo herpetiformis**

694.4 **Pemphigus**
Pemphigus:
NOS
erythematosus
foliaceus
malignant
vegetans
vulgaris

Excludes *pemphigus neonatorum (684)*

694.5 **Pemphigoid**
Benign pemphigus NOS
Bullous pemphigoid
Herpes circinatus bullosus
Senile dermatitis herpetiformis

● 694.6 **Benign mucous membrane pemphigoid**
Cicatricial pemphigoid
Mucosynechial atrophic bullous dermatitis

694.60 **Without mention of ocular involvement**

694.61 **With ocular involvement**
Ocular pemphigus

❑ 694.8 **Other specified bullous dermatoses**

Excludes *herpes gestationis (646.8)*

❑ 694.9 **Unspecified bullous dermatoses**

● 695 **Erythematous conditions**

695.0 **Toxic erythema**
Erythema venenatum

695.1 **Erythema multiforme**
Erythema iris
Herpes iris
Lyell's syndrome
Scalded skin syndrome
Stevens-Johnson syndrome
Toxic epidermal necrolysis

695.2 **Erythema nodosum**

Excludes *tuberculous erythema nodosum (017.1)*

695.3 **Rosacea**
Acne:
erythematosa
rosacea
Perioral dermatitis
Rhinophyma

695.4 **Lupus erythematosus**
Lupus:
erythematodes (discoid)
erythematosus (discoid), not disseminated

Excludes *lupus (vulgaris) NOS (017.0)*
systemic [disseminated] lupus erythematosus (710.0)

● 695.8 **Other specified erythematous conditions**

695.81 **Ritter's disease**
Dermatitis exfoliativa neonatorum

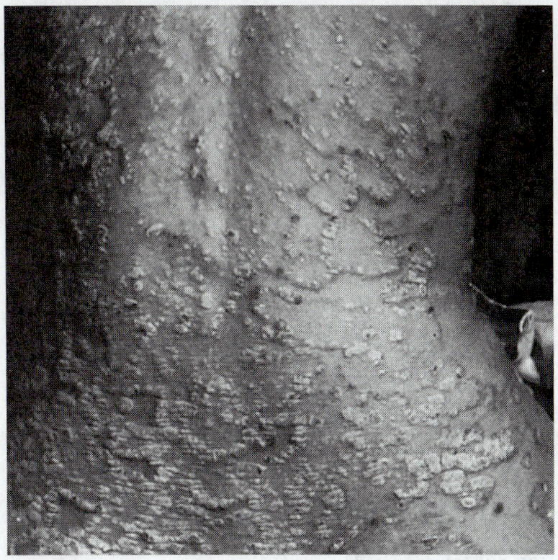

Figure 12-6 Psoriasis. (From Moschella SL, Hurley HJ: Dermatology, 2nd ed. Philadelphia, WB Saunders, 1985, p 512.)

Item 12-5 Psoriasis is a chronic, recurrent inflammatory skin disease characterized by small patches covered with thick silvery scales. Parapsoriasis is a treatment-resistant erythroderma. Pityriasis rosea is characterized by a herald patch that is a single large lesion and that usually appears on the trunk and is followed by scattered, smaller lesions.

❑ 695.89 **Other**
Erythema intertrigo
Intertrigo
Pityriasis rubra (Hebra)

Excludes *mycotic intertrigo (111.0–111.9)*

❑ 695.9 **Unspecified erythematous condition**
Erythema NOS
Erythroderma (secondary)

● 696 **Psoriasis and similar disorders**

696.0 **Psoriatic arthropathy**

❑ 696.1 **Other psoriasis**
Acrodermatitis continua
Dermatitis repens
Psoriasis:
NOS
any type, except arthropathic

Excludes *psoriatic arthropathy (696.0)*

696.2 **Parapsoriasis**
Parakeratosis variegata
Parapsoriasis lichenoides chronica
Pityriasis lichenoides et varioliformis

696.3 **Pityriasis rosea**
Pityriasis circinata (et maculata)

696.4 **Pityriasis rubra pilaris**
Devergie's disease
Lichen ruber acuminatus

Excludes *pityriasis rubra (Hebra) (695.89)*

❑ 696.5 **Other and unspecified pityriasis**
Pityriasis:
NOS
alba
streptogenes

Excludes *pityriasis:*
simplex (690.18)
versicolor (111.0)

❑ **696.8 Other**

● **697 Lichen**

Excludes *lichen:*
obtusus corneus (698.3)
pilaris (congenital) (757.39)
ruber acuminatus (696.4)
sclerosus et atrophicus (701.0)
scrofulosus (017.0)
simplex chronicus (698.3)
spinulosus (congenital) (757.39)
urticatus (698.2)

697.0 Lichen planus
Lichen:
planopilaris
ruber planus

697.1 Lichen nitidus
Pinkus' disease

❑ **697.8 Other lichen, not elsewhere classified**
Lichen:
ruber moniliforme
striata

❑ **697.9 Lichen, unspecified**

● **698 Pruritus and related conditions**

Excludes *pruritus specified as psychogenic (306.3)*

698.0 Pruritus ani
Perianal itch

698.1 Pruritus of genital organs

698.2 Prurigo
Lichen urticatus
Prurigo:
NOS
Hebra's
mitis
simplex
Urticaria papulosa (Hebra)

Excludes *prurigo nodularis (698.3)*

698.3 Lichenification and lichen simplex chronicus
Hyde's disease
Neurodermatitis (circumscripta) (local)
Prurigo nodularis

Excludes *neurodermatitis, diffuse (of Brocq) (691.8)*

698.4 Dermatitis factitia [artefacta]
Dermatitis ficta
Neurotic excoriation

Use additional code to identify any associated mental disorder

❑ **698.8 Other specified pruritic conditions**
Pruritus:
hiemalis
senilis
Winter itch

❑ **698.9 Unspecified pruritic disorder**
Itch NOS
Pruritus NOS

Item 12-6 Keratoderma is characterized by firm horny papules that have a cobblestone appearance. Keratoderma climactericum, also known as endocrine keratoderma, is hyperkeratosis located on the palms and soles.

OTHER DISEASES OF SKIN AND SUBCUTANEOUS TISSUE (700–709)

Excludes *conditions confined to eyelids (373.0–374.9)*
congenital conditions of skin, hair, and nails (757.0–757.9)

700 Corns and callosities
Callus
Clavus

● **701 Other hypertrophic and atrophic conditions of skin**

Excludes *dermatomyositis (710.3)*
hereditary edema of legs (757.0)
scleroderma (generalized) (710.1)

701.0 Circumscribed scleroderma
Addison's keloid
Dermatosclerosis, localized
Lichen sclerosus et atrophicus
Morphea
Scleroderma, circumscribed or localized

701.1 Keratoderma, acquired
Acquired:
ichthyosis
keratoderma palmaris et plantaris
Elastosis perforans serpiginosa
Hyperkeratosis:
NOS
follicularis in cutem penetrans
palmoplantaris climacterica
Keratoderma:
climactericum
tylodes, progressive
Keratosis (blennorrhagica)

Excludes *Darier's disease [keratosis follicularis] (congenital) (757.39)*
keratosis:
arsenical (692.4)
gonococcal (098.81)

701.2 Acquired acanthosis nigricans
Keratosis nigricans

701.3 Striae atrophicae
Atrophic spots of skin
Atrophoderma maculatum
Atrophy blanche (of Milian)
Degenerative colloid atrophy
Senile degenerative atrophy
Striae distensae

701.4 Keloid scar
Cheloid
Hypertrophic scar
Keloid

❑ **701.5 Other abnormal granulation tissue**
Excessive granulation

❑ **701.8 Other specified hypertrophic and atrophic conditions of skin**
Acrodermatitis atrophicans chronica
Atrophia cutis senilis
Atrophoderma neuriticum
Confluent and reticulate papillomatosis
Cutis laxa senilis
Elastosis senilis
Folliculitis ulerythematosa reticulata
Gougerot-Carteaud syndrome or disease

❑ **701.9 Unspecified hypertrophic and atrophic conditions of skin**
Atrophoderma

● **702 Other dermatoses**

Excludes *carcinoma in situ (232.0–232.9)*

702.0 Actinic keratosis

● 702.1 Seborrheic keratosis

702.11 Inflamed seborrheic keratosis

❏ 702.19 Other seborrheic keratosis
Seborrheic keratosis NOS

❏ 702.8 Other specified dermatoses

● 703 Diseases of nail

Excludes *congenital anomalies (757.5)*
onychia and paronychia (681.02, 681.11)

703.0 Ingrowing nail
Ingrowing nail with infection
Unguis incarnatus

Excludes *infection, nail NOS (681.9)*

❏ 703.8 Other specified diseases of nail
Dystrophia unguium
Hypertrophy of nail
Koilonychia
Leukonychia (punctata) (striata)
Onychauxis
Onychogryposis
Onycholysis

❏ 703.9 Unspecified disease of nail

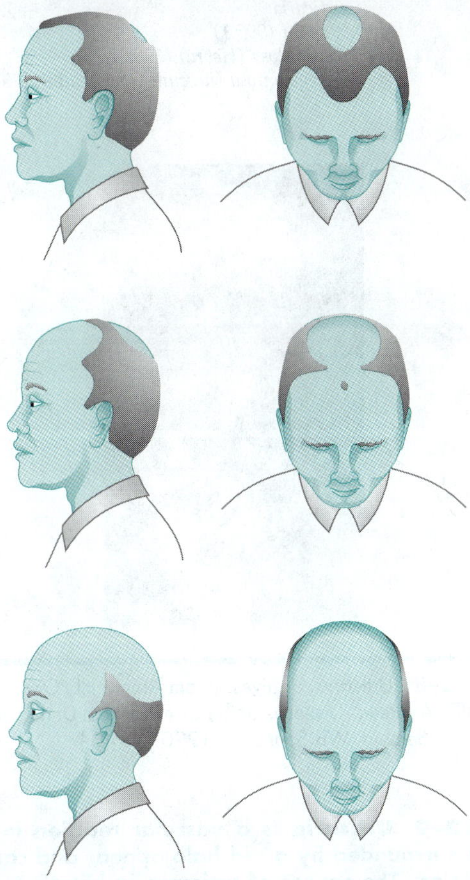

Figure 12–7 Male pattern alopecia.

Item 12-7 Alopecia is lack of hair and takes many forms. The most common is male pattern alopecia, also known as androgenetic alopecia. Telogen effluvium is early and excessive loss of hair resulting from a trauma to the hair (fever, drugs, surgery, etc.).

● 704 Diseases of hair and hair follicles

Excludes *congenital anomalies (757.4)*

● 704.0 Alopecia

Excludes *madarosis (374.55)*
syphilitic alopecia (091.82)

❏ 704.00 Alopecia, unspecified
Baldness
Loss of hair

704.01 Alopecia areata
Ophiasis

704.02 Telogen effluvium

❏ 704.09 Other
Folliculitis decalvans
Hypotrichosis:
NOS
postinfectional NOS
Pseudopelade

Item 12-8 Hirsutism is excessive growth of hair.

704.1 Hirsutism
Hypertrichosis:
NOS
lanuginosa, acquired
Polytrichia

Excludes *hypertrichosis of eyelid (374.54)*

704.2 Abnormalities of the hair
Atrophic hair
Clastothrix
Fragilitas crinium
Trichiasis:
NOS
cicatrical
Trichorrhexis (nodosa)

Excludes *trichiasis of eyelid (374.05)*

704.3 Variations in hair color
Canities (premature)
Grayness, hair (premature)
Heterochromia of hair
Poliosis:
NOS
circumscripta, acquired

❏ 704.8 Other specified diseases of hair and hair follicles
Folliculitis:
NOS
abscedens et suffodiens
pustular
Perifolliculitis:
NOS
capitis abscedens et suffodiens
scalp
Sycosis:
NOS
barbae [not parasitic]
lupoid
vulgaris

❏ 704.9 Unspecified disease of hair and hair follicles

● 705 Disorders of sweat glands

705.0 Anhidrosis
Hypohidrosis
Oligohidrosis

705.1 Prickly heat
Heat rash
Miliaria rubra (tropicalis)
Sudamina

● 705.8 Other specified disorders of sweat glands

705.81 Dyshidrosis
Cheiropompholyx
Pompholyx

705.82 **Fox-Fordyce disease**

705.83 **Hidradenitis**
Hidradenitis suppurativa

❑705.89 **Other**
Bromhidrosis
Chromhidrosis
Granulosis rubra nasi
Urhidrosis

Excludes *hidrocystoma (216.0–216.9)*
hyperhidrosis (780.8)

❑705.9 **Unspecified disorder of sweat glands**
Disorder of sweat glands NOS

● 706 **Diseases of sebaceous glands**

706.0 **Acne varioliformis**
Acne:
frontalis
Acne:
necrotica

❑706.1 **Other acne**
Acne:
NOS
conglobata
cystic
pustular
vulgaris
Blackhead
Comedo

Excludes *acne rosacea (695.3)*

706.2 **Sebaceous cyst**
Atheroma, skin
Wen
Keratin cyst

706.3 **Seborrhea**

Excludes *seborrhea:*
capitis (690.11)
sicca (690.18)
seborrheic:
dermatitis (690.10)
keratosis (702.11–702.19)

❑706.8 **Other specified diseases of sebaceous glands**
Asteatosis (cutis)
Xerosis cutis

❑706.9 **Unspecified disease of sebaceous glands**

● 707 **Chronic ulcer of skin**

Includes: non-infected sinus of skin
non-healing ulcer

Excludes *specific infections classified under "Infectious and Parasitic Diseases" (001.0–136.9)*
varicose ulcer (454.0, 454.2)

707.0 **Decubitus ulcer**
Bed sore
Decubitus ulcer [any site]
Plaster ulcer
Pressure ulcer

707.1 **Ulcer of lower limbs, except decubitus**
Ulcer, chronic, of lower limb:
neurogenic of lower limb
trophic of lower limb

Code if applicable, any causal condition first:
atherosclerosis of the extremities with ulceration (440.23)
chronic venous hypertension with ulcer (459.31)
chronic venous hypertension with ulcer and inflammation (459.33)
diabetes mellitus (250.80–250.83)
postphlebetic syndrome with ulcer (459.11)
postphlebetic syndrome with ulcer and inflammation (459.13)

707.10 **Ulcer of lower limb, unspecified**

707.11 **Ulcer of thigh**

707.12 **Ulcer of calf**

707.13 **Ulcer of ankle**

707.14 **Ulcer of heel and midfoot**
Plantar surface of midfoot

707.15 **Ulcer of other part of foot**
Toes

707.19 **Ulcer of other part of lower limb**

❑707.8 **Chronic ulcer of other specified sites**
Ulcer, chronic, of other specified sites:
neurogenic of other specified sites
trophic of other specified sites

❑707.9 **Chronic ulcer of unspecified site**
Chronic ulcer NOS
Trophic ulcer NOS
Tropical ulcer NOS
Ulcer of skin NOS

● 708 **Urticaria**

Excludes *edema:*
angioneurotic (995.1)
Quincke's (995.1)
hereditary angioedema (277.6)
urticaria:
giant (995.1)
papulosa (Hebra) (698.2)
pigmentosa (juvenile) (congenital) (757.33)

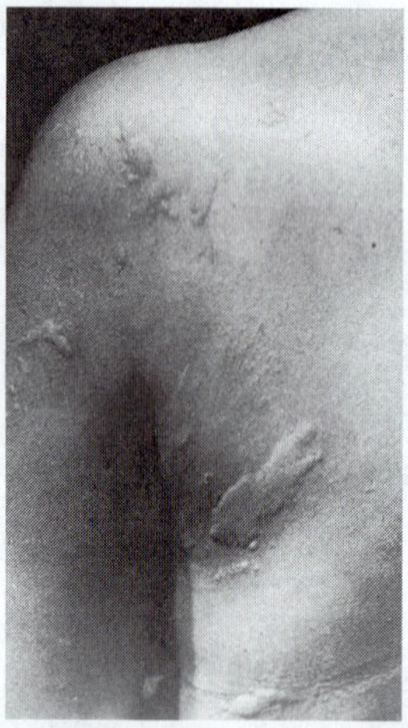

Figure 12–8 Urticaria, or hives. (From Arnold HL, Odom RB, James WD: Andrews' Diseases of the Skin, Clinical Dermatology, 8th ed. Philadelphia, WB Saunders, 1990, p 148.)

Item 12–9 Urticaria is a vascular reaction in which wheals surrounded by a red halo appear and cause severe itching. The causes of urticaria or hives are extensive and varied (e.g., food, heat, cold, drugs, stress, infections).

708.0 Allergic urticaria

708.1 Idiopathic urticaria

708.2 Urticaria due to cold and heat
Thermal urticaria

708.3 Dermatographic urticaria
Dermatographia
Factitial urticaria

708.4 Vibratory urticaria

708.5 Cholinergic urticaria

❑ **708.8 Other specified urticaria**
Nettle rash
Urticaria:
chronic
recurrent periodic

❑ **708.9 Urticaria, unspecified**
Hives NOS

● **709 Other disorders of skin and subcutaneous tissue**

● **709.0 Dyschromia**

Excludes *albinism (270.2)*
pigmented nevus (216.0–216.9)
that of eyelid (374.52–374.53)

❑ **709.00 Dyschromia, unspecified**

709.01 Vitiligo

❑ **709.09 Other**

709.1 Vascular disorders of skin
Angioma serpiginosum
Purpura (primary) annularis telangiectodes

709.2 Scar conditions and fibrosis of skin
Adherent scar (skin)
Cicatrix
Disfigurement (due to scar)
Fibrosis, skin NOS
Scar NOS

Excludes *keloid scar (701.4)*

709.3 Degenerative skin disorders
Calcinosis:
circumscripta
cutis
Colloid milium
Degeneration, skin
Deposits, skin
Senile dermatosis NOS
Subcutaneous calcification

709.4 Foreign body granuloma of skin and subcutaneous tissue

Excludes *residual foreign body without granuloma of skin and subcutaneous tissue (729.6)*
that of muscle (728.82)

❑ **709.8 Other specified disorders of skin**
Epithelial hyperplasia
Menstrual dermatosis
Vesicular eruption

❑ **709.9 Unspecified disorder of skin and subcutaneous tissue**
Dermatosis NOS

13. DISEASES OF THE MUSCULOSKELETAL SYSTEM AND CONNECTIVE TISSUE (710–739)

The following fifth-digit subclassification is for use with categories 711–712, 715–716, 718–719, and 730:

❑ **0 site unspecified**
1 shoulder region
Acromioclavicular joint(s)
Clavicle
Glenohumeral joint(s)
Scapula
Sternoclavicular joint(s)
2 upper arm
Elbow joint
Humerus
3 forearm
Radius
Ulna
Wrist joint
4 hand
Carpus
Metacarpus
Phalanges [fingers]
5 pelvic region and thigh
Buttock
Femur
Hip (joint)
6 lower leg
Fibula
Knee joint
Patella
Tibia
7 ankle and foot
Ankle joint
Digits [toes]
Metatarsus
Phalanges, foot
Tarsus
Other joints in foot
❑ **8 other specified sites**
Head
Neck
Ribs
Skull
Trunk
Vertebral column
❑ **9 multiple sites**

ARTHROPATHIES AND RELATED DISORDERS (710–719)

Excludes *disorders of spine (720.0–724.9)*

● **710 Diffuse diseases of connective tissue**

Includes: all collagen diseases whose effects are not mainly confined to a single system

Excludes *those affecting mainly the cardiovascular system, i.e., polyarteritis nodosa and allied conditions (446.0–446.7)*

710.0 Systemic lupus erythematosus
Disseminated lupus erythematosus
Libman-Sacks disease

Use additional code to identify manifestation, as:
endocarditis (424.91)
nephritis (583.81)
chronic (582.81)
nephrotic syndrome (581.81)

Excludes *lupus erythematosus (discoid) NOS (695.4)*

710.1 Systemic sclerosis
Acrosclerosis
CRST syndrome
Progressive systemic sclerosis
Scleroderma

Use additional code to identify manifestations, as:
lung involvement (517.2) ⇐
myopathy (359.6)

Excludes *circumscribed scleroderma (701.0)*

710.2 Sicca syndrome
Keratoconjunctivitis sicca
Sjögren's disease

710.3 Dermatomyositis
Poikilodermatomyositis
Polymyositis with skin involvement

710.4 Polymyositis

710.5 Eosinophilia myalgia syndrome
Toxic oil syndrome

Use additional E code to identify drug, if drug induced

❑ **710.8 Other specified diffuse diseases of connective tissue**
Multifocal fibrosclerosis (idiopathic) NEC
Systemic fibrosclerosing syndrome

❑ **710.9 Unspecified diffuse connective tissue disease**
Collagen disease NOS

● **711 Arthropathy associated with infections**

Includes: arthritis associated with conditions classifiable below
arthropathy associated with conditions classifiable below
polyarthritis associated with conditions classifiable below
polyarthropathy associated with conditions classifiable below

Excludes *rheumatic fever (390)*

The following fifth-digit subclassification is for use with category 711; valid digits are in [brackets] under each code. See list at beginning of chapter for definitions:

❑ **0 site unspecified**
1 shoulder region
2 upper arm
3 forearm
4 hand
5 pelvic region and thigh
6 lower leg
7 ankle and foot
❑ **8 other specified sites**
❑ **9 multiple sites**

● **711.0 Pyogenic arthritis**
[0–9] Arthritis or polyarthritis (due to):
coliform [*Escherichia coli*]
Hemophilus influenzae [H. influenzae]
pneumococcal
Pseudomonas
staphylococcal
streptococcal
Pyarthrosis

Use additional code to identify infectious organism (041.0–041.8)

●● *711.1* ***Arthropathy associated with Reiter's disease and***
[0–9] ***nonspecific urethritis***

Code first underlying disease, as:
nonspecific urethritis (099.4)
Reiter's disease (099.3)

●● *711.2* ***Arthropathy in Behçet's syndrome***
[0–9] *Code first underlying disease (136.1)*

●● *711.3 Postdysentericarthropathy*
[0–9]
Code first underlying disease, as:
dysentery (009.0)
enteritis, infectious (008.0–009.3)
paratyphoid fever (002.1–002.9)
typhoid fever (002.0)
Excludes *salmonella arthritis (003.23)*

●●❑ *711.4 Arthropathy associated with other bacterial diseases*
[0–9]
Code first underlying disease, as:
diseases classifiable to 010–040, 090–099, except as in 711.1, 711.3, and 713.5
leprosy (030.0–030.9)
tuberculosis (015.0–015.9)
Excludes *gonococcal arthritis (098.50)*
meningococcal arthritis (036.82)

●●❑ *711.5 Arthropathy associated with other viral diseases*
[0–9]
Code first underlying disease, as:
diseases classifiable to 045–049, 050–079, 480, 487
O'nyong-nyong (066.3)
Excludes *that due to rubella (056.71)*

●● *711.6 Arthropathy associated with mycoses*
[0–9]
Code first underlying disease (110.0–118)

●● *711.7 Arthropathy associated with helminthiasis*
[0–9]
Code first underlying disease, as:
filariasis (125.0–125.9)

●●❑ *711.8 Arthropathy associated with other infectious and parasitic diseases*
[0–9]
Code first underlying disease, as:
diseases classifiable to 080–088, 100–104, 130–136
Excludes *arthropathy associated with sarcoidosis (713.7)*

●❑ **711.9 Unspecified infective arthritis**
[0–9]
Infective arthritis or polyarthritis (acute) (chronic) (subacute) NOS

● **712 Crystal arthropathies**

Includes: crystal-induced arthritis and synovitis
Excludes *gouty arthropathy (274.0)*

The following fifth-digit subclassification is for use with category 712; valid digits are in [brackets] under each code. See list at beginning of chapter for definitions:
❑ **0 site unspecified**
1 shoulder region
2 upper arm
3 forearm
4 hand
5 pelvic region and thigh
6 lower leg
7 ankle and foot
❑ **8 other specified sites**
❑ **9 multiple sites**

●● *712.1 Chondrocalcinosis due to dicalcium phosphate crystals*
[0–9]
Chondrocalcinosis due to dicalcium phosphate crystals (with other crystals)
Code first underlying disease (275.4)

●● *712.2 Chondrocalcinosis due to pyrophosphate crystals*
[0–9]
Code first underlying disease (275.4)

●●❑ *712.3 Chondrocalcinosis, unspecified*
[0–9]
Code first underlying disease (275.4)

●❑ *712.8 Other specified crystal arthropathies*
[0–9]

●❑ **712.9 Unspecified crystal arthropathy**
[0–9]

● **713 Arthropathy associated with other disorders classified elsewhere**

Includes: arthritis associated with conditions classifiable below
arthropathy associated with conditions classifiable below
polyarthritis associated with conditions classifiable below
polyarthropathy associated with conditions classifiable below

●❑ *713.0 Arthropathy associated with other endocrine and metabolic disorders*
Code first underlying disease, as:
acromegaly (253.0)
hemochromatosis (275.0)
hyperparathyroidism (252.0)
hypogammaglobulinemia (279.00–279.09)
hypothyroidism (243–244.9)
lipoid metabolism disorder (272.0–272.9)
ochronosis (270.2)
Excludes *arthropathy associated with:*
amyloidosis (713.7)
crystal deposition disorders, except gout (712.1–712.9)
diabetic neuropathy (713.5)
gouty arthropathy (274.0)

● *713.1 Arthropathy associated with gastrointestinal conditions other than infections*
Code first underlying disease, as:
regional enteritis (555.0–555.9)
ulcerative colitis (556)

● *713.2 Arthropathy associated with hematological disorders*
Code first underlying disease, as:
hemoglobinopathy (282.4–282.7)
hemophilia (286.0–286.2)
leukemia (204.0–208.9)
malignant reticulosis (202.3)
multiple myelomatosis (203.0)
Excludes *arthropathy associated with Henoch-Schönlein purpura (713.6)*

● *713.3 Arthropathy associated with dermatological disorders*
Code first underlying disease, as:
erythema multiforme (695.1)
erythema nodosum (695.2)
Excludes *psoriatic arthropathy (696.0)*

● *713.4 Arthropathy associated with respiratory disorders*
Code first underlying disease, as:
diseases classifiable to 490–519
Excludes *arthropathy associated with respiratory infections (711.0, 711.4–711.8)*

● *713.5 Arthropathy associated with neurological disorders*
Charcot's arthropathy associated with diseases classifiable elsewhere
Neuropathic arthritis associated with diseases classifiable elsewhere
Code first underlying disease, as:
neuropathic joint disease [Charcot's joints]:
NOS (094.0)
diabetic (250.6)
syringomyelic (336.0)
tabetic [syphilitic] (094.0)

● *713.6 Arthropathy associated with hypersensitivity reaction*

Code first underlying disease, as:
Henoch (-Schönlein) purpura (287.0)
serum sickness (999.5)

Excludes *allergic arthritis NOS (716.2)*

●❑ *713.7 Other general diseases with articular involvement*

Code first underlying disease, as:
amyloidosis (277.3)
familial Mediterranean fever (277.3)
sarcoidosis (135)

●❑ *713.8 Arthropathy associated with other conditions classifiable elsewhere*

Code first underlying disease, as:
conditions classifiable elsewhere except as in 711.1–711.8, 712, and 713.0–713.7

● **714 Rheumatoid arthritis and other inflammatory polyarthropathies**

Excludes *rheumatic fever (390)*
rheumatoid arthritis of spine NOS (720.0)

714.0 Rheumatoid arthritis
Arthritis or polyarthritis:
atrophic
rheumatic (chronic)

Use additional code to identify manifestation, as:
myopathy (359.6)
polyneuropathy (357.1)

Excludes *juvenile rheumatoid arthritis NOS (714.30)*

714.1 Felty's syndrome
Rheumatoid arthritis with splenoadenomegaly and leukopenia

❑ **714.2 Other rheumatoid arthritis with visceral or systemic involvement**
Rheumatoid carditis

● **714.3 Juvenile chronic polyarthritis**

❑ **714.30 Polyarticular juvenile rheumatoid arthritis, chronic or unspecified**
Juvenile rheumatoid arthritis NOS
Still's disease

714.31 Polyarticular juvenile rheumatoid arthritis, acute

714.32 Pauciarticular juvenile rheumatoid arthritis

714.33 Monoarticular juvenile rheumatoid arthritis

714.4 Chronic postrheumatic arthropathy
Chronic rheumatoid nodular fibrositis
Jaccoud's syndrome

● **714.8 Other specified inflammatory polyarthropathies**

714.81 Rheumatoid lung
Caplan's syndrome
Diffuse interstitial rheumatoid disease of lung
Fibrosing alveolitis, rheumatoid

❑ **714.89 Other**

❑ **714.9 Unspecified inflammatory polyarthropathy**
Inflammatory polyarthropathy or polyarthritis NOS

Excludes *polyarthropathy NOS (716.5)*

● **715 Osteoarthrosis and allied disorders**

Note: Localized, in the subcategories below, includes bilateral involvement of the same site.

Includes: arthritis or polyarthritis:
degenerative
hypertrophic
degenerative joint disease
osteoarthritis

Excludes *Marie-Strümpell spondylitis (720.0)*
osteoarthrosis [osteoarthritis] of spine (721.0–721.9)

The following fifth-digit subclassification is for use with category 715; valid digits are in [brackets] under each code. See list at beginning of chapter for definitions:

❑ **0 site unspecified**
1 shoulder region
2 upper arm
3 forearm
4 hand
5 pelvic region and thigh
6 lower leg
7 ankle and foot
❑ **8 other specified sites**
❑ **9 multiple sites**

● **715.0 Osteoarthrosis, generalized**
[0,4,9] Degenerative joint disease, involving multiple joints
Primary generalized hypertrophic osteoarthrosis

● **715.1 Osteoarthrosis, localized, primary**
[0–8] Localized osteoarthropathy, idiopathic

● **715.2 Osteoarthrosis, localized, secondary**
[0–8] Coxae malum senilis

●❑ **715.3 Osteoarthrosis, localized, not specified whether primary or secondary**
[0–8] Otto's pelvis

●❑ **715.8 Osteoarthrosis involving, or with mention of more than one site, but not specified as generalized**
[0,9]

●❑ **715.9 Osteoarthrosis, unspecified whether generalized or localized**
[0–8]

● **716 Other and unspecified arthropathies**

Excludes *cricoarytenoid arthropathy (478.79)*

The following fifth-digit subclassification is for use with category 716; valid digits are in [brackets] under each code. See list at beginning of chapter for definitions:

❑ **0 site unspecified**
1 shoulder region
2 upper arm
3 forearm
4 hand
5 pelvic region and thigh
6 lower leg
7 ankle and foot
❑ **8 other specified sites**
❑ **9 multiple sites**

● **716.0 Kaschin-Beck disease**
[0–9] Endemic polyarthritis

● **716.1 Traumatic arthropathy**
[0–9]

● **716.2 Allergic arthritis**
[0–9]

Excludes *arthritis associated with Henoch-Schönlein purpura or serum sickness (713.6)*

● **716.3 Climacteric arthritis**
[0–9] Menopausal arthritis

● **716.4 Transient arthropathy**
[0–9]

Excludes *palindromic rheumatism (719.3)*

● ❑ 716.5 **Unspecified polyarthropathy or polyarthritis**
[0–9]

● ❑ 716.6 **Unspecified monoarthritis**
[0–8] Coxitis

● ❑ 716.8 **Other specified arthropathy**
[0–9]

● ❑ 716.9 **Arthropathy, unspecified**
[0–9] Arthritis (acute) (chronic) (subacute)
Arthropathy (acute) (chronic) (subacute)
Articular rheumatism (chronic)
Inflammation of joint NOS

● **717 Internal derangement of knee**

Includes: degeneration of articular cartilage or meniscus of knee
rupture, old of articular cartilage or meniscus of knee
tear, old of articular cartilage or meniscus of knee

Excludes *acute derangement of knee (836.0–836.6)*
ankylosis (718.5)
contracture (718.4)
current injury (836.0–836.6)
deformity (736.4–736.6)
recurrent dislocation (718.3)

717.0 **Old bucket handle tear of medial meniscus**
Old bucket handle tear of unspecified cartilage

717.1 **Derangement of anterior horn of medial meniscus**

717.2 **Derangement of posterior horn of medial meniscus**

❑ 717.3 **Other and unspecified derangement of medial meniscus**
Degeneration of internal semilunar cartilage

● 717.4 **Derangement of lateral meniscus**

❑ 717.40 **Derangement of lateral meniscus, unspecified**

717.41 **Bucket handle tear of lateral meniscus**

717.42 **Derangement of anterior horn of lateral meniscus**

717.43 **Derangement of posterior horn of lateral meniscus**

❑ 717.49 **Other**

717.5 **Derangement of meniscus, not elsewhere classified**
Congenital discoid meniscus
Cyst of semilunar cartilage
Derangement of semilunar cartilage NOS

717.6 **Loose body in knee**
Joint mice, knee
Rice bodies, knee (joint)

717.7 **Chondromalacia of patella**
Chondromalacia patellae
Degeneration [softening] of articular cartilage of patella

● 717.8 **Other internal derangement of knee**

717.81 **Old disruption of lateral collateral ligament**

717.82 **Old disruption of medial collateral ligament**

717.83 **Old disruption of anterior cruciate ligament**

717.84 **Old disruption of posterior cruciate ligament**

❑ 717.85 **Old disruption of other ligaments of knee**
Capsular ligament of knee

❑ 717.89 **Other**
Old disruption of ligaments of knee NOS

❑ 717.9 **Unspecified internal derangement of knee**
Derangement NOS of knee

● **718 Other derangement of joint**

Excludes *current injury (830.0–848.9)*
jaw (524.6)

The following fifth-digit subclassification is for use with category 718; valid digits are in [brackets] under each code. See list at beginning of chapter for definitions:

❑ **0 site unspecified**
1 shoulder region
2 upper arm
3 forearm
4 hand
5 pelvic region and thigh
6 lower leg
7 ankle and foot
❑ **8 other specified sites**
❑ **9 multiple sites**

● 718.0 **Articular cartilage disorder**
[0–5,7–9] Meniscus:
disorder
rupture, old
tear, old
Old rupture of ligament(s) of joint NOS

Excludes *articular cartilage disorder:*
in ochronosis (270.2)
knee (717.0–717.9)
chondrocalcinosis (275.4)
metastatic calcification (275.4)

● 718.1 **Loose body in joint**
[0–5,7–9] Joint mice

Excludes *knee (717.6)*

● 718.2 **Pathological dislocation**
[0–9] Dislocation or displacement of joint, not recurrent and not current

● 718.3 **Recurrent dislocation of joint**
[0–9]

● 718.4 **Contracture of joint**
[0–9]

● 718.5 **Ankylosis of joint**
[0–9] Ankylosis of joint (fibrous) (osseous)

Excludes *spine (724.9)*
stiffness of joint without mention of ankylosis (719.5)

● ❑ 718.6 **Unspecified intrapelvic protrusion of acetabulum**
[0,5] Protrusio acetabuli, unspecified

● 718.7 **Developmental dislocation of joint**
[0–9]

Excludes *congenital dislocation of joint (754.0–755.8)*
traumatic dislocation of joint (830–839)

● ❑ 718.8 **Other joint derangement, not elsewhere classified**
[0–9] Flail joint (paralytic)
Instability of joint

Excludes *deformities classifiable to 736 (736.0–736.9)*

● ❑ 718.9 **Unspecified derangement of joint**
[0–5,7–9]

Excludes *knee (717.9)*

● **719 Other and unspecified disorders of joint**

Excludes *jaw (524.6)*

The following fifth-digit subclassification is for use with codes 719.0–719.6, 719.8–719.9; valid digits are in [brackets] under each code. See list at beginning of chapter for definitions: ⬅

❑ **0 site unspecified**
1 shoulder region
2 upper arm

ICD-9-CM 700-799 Vol. 1

3 forearm
4 hand
5 pelvic region and thigh
6 lower leg
7 ankle and foot
❑ 8 other specified sites
❑ 9 multiple sites

● **719.0 Effusion of joint**
[0–9] Hydrarthrosis
Swelling of joint, with or without pain
Excludes *intermittent hydrarthrosis (719.3)*

● **719.1 Hemarthrosis**
[0–9]
Excludes *current injury (840.0–848.9)*

● **719.2 Villonodular synovitis**
[0–9]

● **719.3 Palindromic rheumatism**
[0–9] Hench-Rosenberg syndrome
Intermittent hydrarthrosis

● **719.4 Pain in joint**
[0–9] Arthralgia

● **719.5 Stiffness of joint, not elsewhere classified**
[0–9]

● ❑ **719.6 Other symptoms referable to joint**
[0–9] Joint crepitus
Snapping hip

719.7 Difficulty in walking ⬅
Excludes *abnormality of gait (781.2)*

● ❑ **719.8 Other specified disorders of joint**
[0–9] Calcification of joint
Fistula of joint
Excludes *temporomandibular joint-pain-dysfunction syndrome [Costen's syndrome] (524.6)*

● ❑ **719.9 Unspecified disorder of joint**
[0–9]

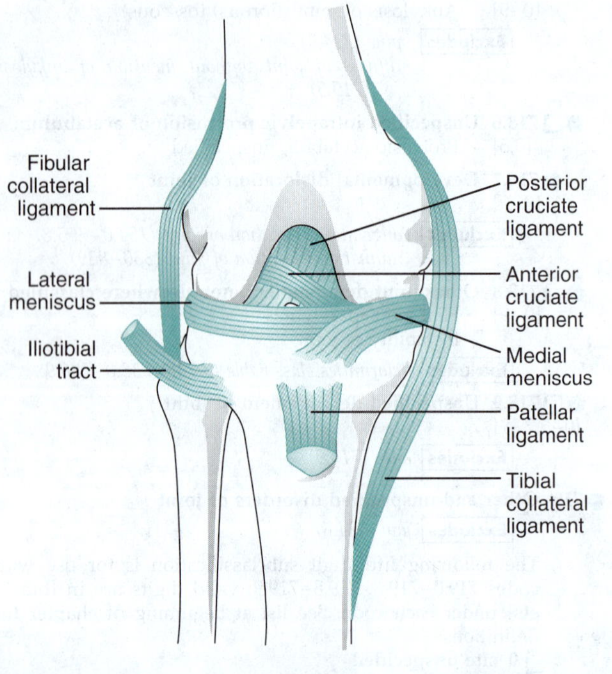

Figure 13–1 Anterior aspect of the right knee joint.

DORSOPATHIES (720–724)

Excludes *curvature of spine (737.0–737.9)*
osteochondrosis of spine (juvenile) (732.0) adult (732.8)

● **720 Ankylosing spondylitis and other inflammatory spondylopathies**

720.0 Ankylosing spondylitis
Rheumatoid arthritis of spine NOS
Spondylitis:
Marie-Strümpell
Spondylitis:
rheumatoid

720.1 Spinal enthesopathy
Disorder of peripheral ligamentous or muscular attachments of spine
Romanus lesion

720.2 Sacroiliitis, not elsewhere classified
Inflammation of sacroiliac joint NOS

● **720.8 Other inflammatory spondylopathies**

● *720.81 Inflammatory spondylopathies in diseases classified elsewhere*
Code first underlying disease, as:
tuberculosis (015.0)

❑ **720.89 Other**

❑ **720.9 Unspecified inflammatory spondylopathy**
Spondylitis NOS

● **721 Spondylosis and allied disorders**

721.0 Cervical spondylosis without myelopathy
Cervical or cervicodorsal:
arthritis
osteoarthritis
spondylarthritis

721.1 Cervical spondylosis with myelopathy
Anterior spinal artery compression syndrome
Spondylogenic compression of cervical spinal cord
Vertebral artery compression syndrome

721.2 Thoracic spondylosis without myelopathy
Thoracic:
arthritis
osteoarthritis
spondylarthritis

721.3 Lumbosacral spondylosis without myelopathy
Lumbar or lumbosacral:
arthritis
osteoarthritis
spondylarthritis

● **721.4 Thoracic or lumbar spondylosis with myelopathy**

721.41 Thoracic region
Spondylogenic compression of thoracic spinal cord

721.42 Lumbar region
Spondylogenic compression of lumbar spinal cord

721.5 Kissing spine
Baastrup's syndrome

721.6 Ankylosing vertebral hyperostosis

721.7 Traumatic spondylopathy
Kümmell's disease or spondylitis

❑ **721.8 Other allied disorders of spine**

● **721.9 Spondylosis of unspecified site**

721.90 Without mention of myelopathy
Spinal:
arthritis (deformans) (degenerative) (hypertrophic)
osteoarthritis NOS
Spondylarthrosis NOS

721.91 **With myelopathy**
Spondylogenic compression of spinal cord NOS

● **722 Intervertebral disc disorders**

722.0 **Displacement of cervical intervertebral disc without myelopathy**
Neuritis (brachial) or radiculitis due to displacement or rupture of cervical intervertebral disc
Any condition classifiable to 722.2 of the cervical or cervicothoracic intervertebral disc

● 722.1 **Displacement of thoracic or lumbar intervertebral disc without myelopathy**

722.10 **Lumbar intervertebral disc without myelopathy**
Lumbago or sciatica due to displacement of intervertebral disc
Neuritis or radiculitis due to displacement or rupture of lumbar intervertebral disc
Any condition classifiable to 722.2 of the lumbar or lumbosacral intervertebral disc

722.11 **Thoracic intervertebral disc without myelopathy**
Any condition classifiable to 722.2 of thoracic intervertebral disc

❑ 722.2 **Displacement of intervertebral disc, site unspecified, without myelopathy**
Discogenic syndrome NOS
Herniation of nucleus pulposus NOS
Intervertebral disc NOS:
- extrusion
- prolapse
- protrusion
- rupture

Neuritis or radiculitis due to displacement or rupture of intervertebral disc

● 722.3 **Schmorl's nodes**

❑ 722.30 **Unspecified region**

722.31 **Thoracic region**

722.32 **Lumbar region**

❑ 722.39 **Other**

722.4 **Degeneration of cervical intervertebral disc**
Degeneration of cervicothoracic intervertebral disc

● 722.5 **Degeneration of thoracic or lumbar intervertebral disc**

722.51 **Thoracic or thoracolumbar intervertebral disc**

722.52 **Lumbar or lumbosacral intervertebral disc**

❑ 722.6 **Degeneration of intervertebral disc, site unspecified**
Degenerative disc disease NOS
Narrowing of intervertebral disc or space NOS

● 722.7 **Intervertebral disc disorder with myelopathy**

❑ 722.70 **Unspecified region**

722.71 **Cervical region**

722.72 **Thoracic region**

722.73 **Lumbar region**

● 722.8 **Postlaminectomy syndrome**

❑ 722.80 **Unspecified region**

722.81 **Cervical region**

722.82 **Thoracic region**

722.83 **Lumbar region**

● 722.9 **Other and unspecified disc disorder**
Calcification of intervertebral cartilage or disc Discitis

❑ 722.90 **Unspecified region**

722.91 **Cervical region**

722.92 **Thoracic region**

722.93 **Lumbar region**

● **723 Other disorders of cervical region**

Excludes *conditions due to:*
intervertebral disc disorders (722.0–722.9)
spondylosis (721.0–721.9)

723.0 **Spinal stenosis of cervical region**

723.1 **Cervicalgia**
Pain in neck

723.2 **Cervicocranial syndrome**
Barré-Liéou syndrome
Posterior cervical sympathetic syndrome

723.3 **Cervicobrachial syndrome (diffuse)**

723.4 **Brachia neuritis or radiculitis NOS**
Cervical radiculitis
Radicular syndrome of upper limbs

❑ 723.5 **Torticollis, unspecified**
Contracture of neck

Excludes *congenital (754.1)*
due to birth injury (767.8)
hysterical (300.11)
ocular torticollis (781.93)
psychogenic (306.0)
spasmodic (333.83)
traumatic, current (847.0)

723.6 **Panniculitis specified as affecting neck**

723.7 **Ossification of posterior longitudinal ligament in cervical region**

❑ 723.8 **Other syndromes affecting cervical region**
Cervical syndrome NEC
Klippel's disease
Occipital neuralgia

❑ 723.9 **Unspecified musculoskeletal disorders and symptoms referable to neck**
Cervical (region) disorder NOS

● **724 Other and unspecified disorders of back**

Excludes *collapsed vertebra (code to cause, e.g., osteoporosis, 733.00–733.09)*
conditions due to:
intervertebral disc disorders (722.0–722.9)
spondylosis (721.0–721.9)

● 724.0 **Spinal stenosis, other than cervical**

❑ 724.00 **Spinal stenosis, unspecified region**

724.01 **Thoracic region**

724.02 **Lumbar region**

❑ 724.09 **Other**

724.1 **Pain in thoracic spine**

724.2 **Lumbago**
Low back pain
Low back syndrome
Lumbalgia

724.3 **Sciatica**
Neuralgia or neuritis of sciatic nerve

Excludes *specified lesion of sciatic nerve (355.0)*

❑ 724.4 **Thoracic or lumbosacral neuritis or radiculitis, unspecified**
Radicular syndrome of lower limbs

❑ 724.5 Backache, unspecified
Vertebrogenic (pain) syndrome NOS

724.6 Disorders of sacrum
Ankylosis, lumbosacral or sacroiliac (joint)
Instability, lumbosacral or sacroiliac (joint)

● 724.7 Disorders of coccyx

❑ 724.70 Unspecified disorder of coccyx

724.71 Hypermobility of coccyx

❑ 724.79 Other
Coccygodynia

❑ 724.8 Other symptoms referable to back
Ossification of posterior longitudinal ligament NOS
Panniculitis specified as sacral or affecting back

❑ 724.9 Other unspecified back disorders
Ankylosis of spine NOS
Compression of spinal nerve root NEC
Spinal disorder NOS

Excludes *sacroiliitis (720.2)*

Item 13-1 Polymyalgia rheumatica is a syndrome characterized by aching and morning stiffness and is related to aging and hereditary predisposition.

RHEUMATISM, EXCLUDING THE BACK (725–729)

Includes: disorders of muscles and tendons and their attachments, and of other soft tissues

725 Polymyalgia rheumatica

● 726 Peripheral enthesopathies and allied syndromes

Note: Enthesopathies are disorders of peripheral ligamentous or muscular attachments.

Excludes *spinal enthesopathy (720.1)*

726.0 Adhesive capsulitis of shoulder

● 726.1 Rotator cuff syndrome of shoulder and allied disorders

❑ 726.10 Disorders of bursae and tendons in shoulder region, unspecified
Rotator cuff syndrome NOS
Supraspinatus syndrome NOS

726.11 Calcifying tendinitis of shoulder

726.12 Bicipital tenosynovitis

❑ 726.19 Other specified disorders

Excludes *complete rupture of rotator cuff, nontraumatic (727.61)*

❑ 726.2 Other affections of shoulder region, not elsewhere classified
Periarthritis of shoulder
Scapulohumeral fibrositis

● 726.3 Enthesopathy of elbow region

❑ 726.30 Enthesopathy of elbow, unspecified

726.31 Medial epicondylitis

726.32 Lateral epicondylitis
Epicondylitis NOS
Golfers'elbow
Tennis elbow

726.33 Olecranon bursitis
Bursitis of elbow

❑ 726.39 Other

726.4 Enthesopathy of wrist and carpus
Bursitis of hand or wrist
Periarthritis of wrist

726.5 Enthesopathy of hip region
Bursitis of hip
Gluteal tendinitis
Iliac crest spur
Psoas tendinitis
Trochanteric tendinitis

● 726.6 Enthesopathy of knee

❑ 726.60 Enthesopathy of knee, unspecified
Bursitis of knee NOS

726.61 Pes anserinus tendinitis or bursitis

726.62 Tibial collateral ligament bursitis
Pellegrini-Stieda syndrome

726.63 Fibular collateral ligament bursitis

726.64 Patellar tendinitis

726.65 Prepatellar bursitis

❑ 726.69 Other
Bursitis:
infrapatellar
subpatellar

● 726.7 Enthesopathy of ankle and tarsus

❑ 726.70 Enthesopathy of ankle and tarsus, unspecified
Metatarsalgia NOS

Excludes *Morton's metatarsalgia (355.6)*

726.71 Achilles bursitis or tendinitis

726.72 Tibialis tendinitis
Tibialis (anterior) (posterior) tendinitis

726.73 Calcaneal spur

❑ 726.79 Other
Peroneal tendinitis

❑ 726.8 Other peripheral enthesopathies

● 726.9 Unspecified enthesopathy

❑ 726.90 Enthesopathy of unspecified site
Capsulitis NOS
Periarthritis NOS
Tendinitis NOS

❑ 726.91 Exostosis of unspecified site
Bone spur NOS

● 727 Other disorders of synovium, tendon, and bursa

● 727.0 Synovitis and tenosynovitis

❑ 727.00 Synovitis and tenosynovitis, unspecified
Synovitis NOS
Tenosynovitis NOS

● 727.01 *Synovitis and tenosynovitis in diseases classified elsewhere*
Code first underlying disease, as:
tuberculosis (015.0–015.9)

Excludes *crystal-induced (275.4)*
gonococcal (098.51)
gouty (274.0)
syphilitic (095.7)

727.02 Giant cell tumor of tendon sheath

727.03 Trigger finger (acquired)

727.04 Radial styloid tenosynovitis
de Quervain's disease

❑ 727.05 Other tenosynovitis of hand and wrist

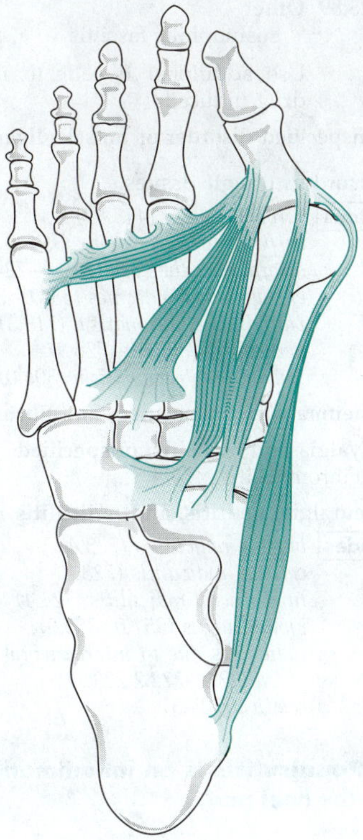

Figure 13–2 Hallux valgus or bunion.

Item 13–2 Hallux valgus, or bunion, is a bursa usually found along the medial aspect of the big toe. It is most often attributed to heredity or poorly fitted shoes.

727.06 **Tenosynovitis of foot and ankle**

❑727.09 **Other**

727.1 **Bunion**

❑727.2 **Specific bursitides often of occupational origin**
Beat:
elbow
hand
knee
Chronic crepitant synovitis of wrist
Miners':
elbow
knee

❑727.3 **Other bursitis**
Bursitis NOS

Excludes *bursitis:*
gonococcal (098.52)
subacromial (726.19)
subcoracoid (726.19)
subdeltoid (726.19)
syphilitic (095.7)
"frozen shoulder" (726.0)

● 727.4 **Ganglion and cyst of synovium, tendon, and bursa**

❑727.40 **Synovial cyst, unspecified**

Excludes *that of popliteal space (727.51)*

727.41 **Ganglion of joint**

727.42 **Ganglion of tendon sheath**

❑727.43 **Ganglion, unspecified**

❑727.49 **Other**
Cyst of bursa

● 727.5 **Rupture of synovium**

❑727.50 **Rupture of synovium, unspecified**

727.51 **Synovial cyst of popliteal space**
Baker's cyst (knee)

❑727.59 **Other**

● 727.6 **Rupture of tendon, nontraumatic**

❑727.60 **Nontraumatic rupture of unspecified tendon**

727.61 **Complete rupture of rotator cuff**

727.62 **Tendons of biceps (long head)**

727.63 **Extensor tendons of hand and wrist**

727.64 **Flexor tendons of hand and wrist**

727.65 **Quadriceps tendon**

727.66 **Patellar tendon**

727.67 **Achilles tendon**

❑727.68 **Other tendons of foot and ankle**

❑727.69 **Other**

● 727.8 **Other disorders of synovium, tendon, and bursa**

727.81 **Contracture of tendon (sheath)**
Short Achilles tendon (acquired)

727.82 **Calcium deposits in tendon and bursa**
Calcification of tendon NOS
Calcific tendinitis NOS

Excludes *peripheral ligamentous or muscular attachments (726.0–726.9)*

727.83 **Plica syndrome**
Plica knee

❑727.89 **Other**
Abscess of bursa or tendon

Excludes *xanthomatosis localized to tendons (272.7)*

❑727.9 **Unspecified disorder of synovium, tendon, and bursa**

● 728 **Disorders of muscle, ligament, and fascia**

Excludes *enthesopathies (726.0–726.9)*
muscular dystrophies (359.0–359.1)
myoneural disorders (358.00–358.9) ⬅
myopathies (359.2–359.9)
old disruption of ligaments of knee (717.81–717.89)

728.0 **Infective myositis**
Myositis:
purulent
suppurative

Excludes *myositis:*
epidemic (074.1)
interstitial (728.81)
syphilitic (095.6)
tropical (040.81)

● 728.1 **Muscular calcification and ossification**

❑728.10 **Calcification and ossification, unspecified**
Massive calcification (paraplegic)

728.11 **Progressive myositis ossificans**

728.12 **Traumatic myositis ossificans**
Myositis ossificans (circumscripta)

728.13 **Postoperative heterotopic calcification**

❑728.19 **Other**
Polymyositis ossificans

728.2 **Muscular wasting and disuse atrophy, not elsewhere classified**
Amyotrophia NOS
Myofibrosis

Excludes *neuralgic amyotrophy (353.5)*
progressive muscular atrophy (335.0–335.9)

❑ **728.3 Other specific muscle disorders**
Arthrogryposis
Immobility syndrome (paraplegic)

Excludes *arthrogryposis multiplex congenita (754.89)*
stiff-man syndrome (333.91)

728.4 Laxity of ligament

728.5 Hypermobility syndrome

728.6 Contracture of palmar fascia
Dupuytren's contracture

● **728.7 Other fibromatoses**

728.71 Plantar fascial fibromatosis
Contracture of plantar fascia
Plantar fasciitis (traumatic)

❑ **728.79 Other**
Garrod's or knuckle pads
Nodular fasciitis
Pseudosarcomatous fibromatosis (proliferative) (subcutaneous)

● **728.8 Other disorders of muscle, ligament, and fascia**

728.81 Interstitial myositis

728.82 Foreign body granuloma of muscle
Talc granuloma of muscle

728.83 Rupture of muscle, nontraumatic

728.84 Diastasis of muscle
Diastasis recti (abdomen)

Excludes *diastasis recti complicating pregnancy, labor, and delivery (665.8)*

728.85 Spasm of muscle

728.86 Necrotizing fasciitis
Use additional code to identify:
infectious organism (041.00–041.89)
gangrene (785.4), if applicable

728.87 Muscle weakness ◄

Excludes *generalized weakness (780.79)* ◄

728.88 Rhabdomyolysis ◄

❑ **728.89 Other**
Eosinophilic fasciitis

Use additional E code to identify drug, if drug induced

❑ **728.9 Unspecified disorder of muscle, ligament, and fascia**

● **729 Other disorders of soft tissues**

Excludes *acroparesthesia (443.89)*
carpal tunnel syndrome (354.0)
disorders of the back (720.0–724.9)
entrapment syndromes (354.0–355.9)
palindromic rheumatism (719.3)
periarthritis (726.0–726.9)
psychogenic rheumatism (306.0)

❑ **729.0 Rheumatism, unspecified, and fibrositis**

❑ **729.1 Myalgia and myositis, unspecified**
Fibromyositis NOS

❑ **729.2 Neuralgia, neuritis, and radiculitis, unspecified**

Excludes *brachia radiculitis (723.4)*
cervical radiculitis (723.4)
lumbosacral radiculitis (724.4)
mononeuritis (354.0–355.9)
radiculitis due to intervertebral disc involvement (722.0–722.2,722.7)
sciatica (724.3)

Item 13-3 Panniculitis is an inflammation of the adipose tissue of the heel pad.

● **729.3 Panniculitis, unspecified**

❑ **729.30 Panniculitis, unspecified site**
Weber-Christian disease

729.31 Hypertrophy of fat pad, knee
Hypertrophy of infrapatellar fat pad

❑ **729.39 Other site**

Excludes *panniculitis specified as (affecting):*
back (724.8)
neck (723.6)
sacral (724.8)

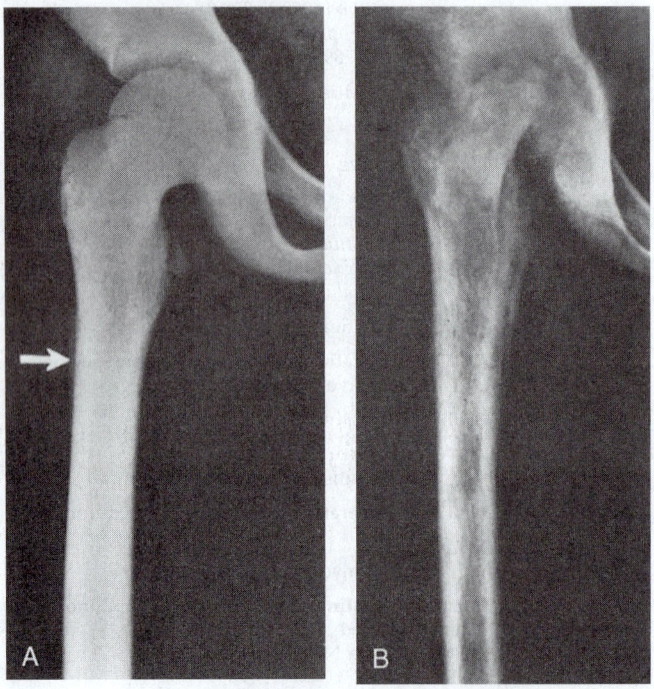

Figure 13-3 Suppurative osteomyelitis. The initial radiograph **(A)** shows only minimal periosteal reaction along the lateral aspect of the proximal femur *(arrow)*. Eight months after onset **(B)** there is gross destruction of the joint and the proximal femur. (From Aegerter E, Kirkpatrick J Jr: Orthopedic Diseases, 4th ed. Philadelphia, WB Saunders, 1975, p 257.)

❑ 729.4 Fasciitis, unspecified
Excludes *necrotizing fasciitis (728.86)*
nodular fasciitis (728.79)

729.5 Pain in limb

729.6 Residual foreign body in soft tissue
Excludes *foreign body granuloma:*
muscle (728.82)
skin and subcutaneous tissue (709.4)

● 729.8 Other musculoskeletal symptoms referable to limbs
729.81 Swelling of limb
729.82 Cramp
❑ 729.89 Other
Excludes *abnormality of gait (781.2)*
tetany (781.7)
transient paralysis of limb (781.4)

❑ 729.9 Other and unspecified disorders of soft tissue
Polyalgia

Item 13-4 Osteomyelitis is an inflammation of the bone. Acute osteomyelitis is a rapidly destructive, pus-producing infection capable of causing severe bone destruction. Chronic osteomyelitis can remain long after the initial acute episode has passed and may lead to a recurrence of the acute phase. Brodie's abscess is an encapsulated focal abscess that must be surgically drained.

OSTEOPATHIES, CHONDROPATHIES, AND ACQUIRED MUSCULOSKELETAL DEFORMITIES (730–739)

● 730 Osteomyelitis, periostitis, and other infections involving bone
Excludes *jaw (526.4–526.5)*
petrous bone (383.2)

Use additional code to identify organism, such as Staphylococcus (041.1)

The following fifth-digit subclassification is for use with category 730; valid digits are in [brackets] under each code. See list at beginning of chapter for definitions:
❑ 0 site unspecified
1 shoulder region
2 upper arm
3 forearm
4 hand
5 pelvic region and thigh
6 lower leg
7 ankle and foot
❑ 8 other specified sites
❑ 9 multiple sites

● 730.0 Acute osteomyelitis
[0–9] Abscess of any bone except accessory sinus, jaw, or mastoid
Acute or subacute osteomyelitis, with or without mention of periostitis

● 730.1 Chronic osteomyelitis
[0–9] Brodie's abscess
Chronic or old osteomyelitis, with or without mention of periostitis
Sequestrum
Sclerosing osteomyelitis of Garré
Excludes *aseptic necrosis of bone (733.40–733.49)*

● ❑ 730.2 Unspecified osteomyelitis
[0–9] Osteitis or osteomyelitis NOS, with or without mention of periostitis

● 730.3 Periostitis without mention of osteomyelitis
[0–9] Abscess of periosteum, without mention of osteomyelitis
Periostosis, without mention of osteomyelitis
Excludes *that in secondary syphilis (091.61)*

● ● *730.7 Osteopathy resulting from poliomyelitis*
[0–9] *Code first underlying disease* (045.0–045.9)

● ● ❑ *730.8 Other infections involving bone in disease classified elsewhere*
[0–9]
Code first underlying disease, as:
tuberculosis (015.0–015.9)
typhoid fever (002.0)
Excludes *syphilitis of bone NOS (095.5)*

● ❑ 730.9 Unspecified infection of bone
[0–9]

● 731 Osteitis deformans and osteopathies associated with other disorders classified elsewhere
731.0 Osteitis deformans without mention of bone tumor
Paget's disease of bone

● *731.1 Osteitis deformans in diseases classified elsewhere*
Code first underlying disease, as:
malignant neoplasm of bone (170.0–170.9)

731.2 Hypertrophic pulmonary osteoarthropathy
Bamberger-Marie disease

● ❑ *731.8 Other bone involvement in diseases classified elsewhere*
Code first underlying disease, as:
diabetes mellitus (250.8)

Use additional code to specify bone condition, such as:
acute osteomyelitis (730.00–730.09)

● 732 Osteochondropathies
732.0 Juvenile osteochondrosis of spine
Juvenile osteochondrosis (of):
marginal or vertebral ephiphysis (of Scheuermann) spine NOS
Vertebral epiphysitis
Excludes *adolescent postural kyphosis (737.0)*

732.1 Juvenile osteochondrosis of hip and pelvis
Coxa plana
Ischiopubic synchondrosis (of van Neck)
Osteochondrosis (juvenile) of:
acetabulum
head of femur (of Legg-Calvé-Perthes)
iliac crest (of Buchanan)
symphysis pubis (of Pierson)
Pseudocoxalgia

732.2 Nontraumatic slipped upper femoral epiphysis
Slipped upper femoral epiphysis NOS

732.3 Juvenile osteochondrosis of upper extremity
Osteochondrosis (juvenile) of:
capitulum of humerus (of Panner)
carpal lunate (of Kienbock)
hand NOS
head of humerus (of Haas)
heads of metacarpals (of Mauclaire)
lower ulna (of Burns)
radial head (of Brailsford)
upper extremity NOS

732.4 Juvenile osteochondrosis of lower extremity, excluding foot
Osteochondrosis (juvenile) of:
lower extremity NOS
primary patellar center (of Köhler)
proximal tibia (of Blount)
secondary patellar center (of Sinding-Larsen)
tibial tubercle (of Osgood-Schlatter)
Tibia vara

732.5 **Juvenile osteochondrosis of foot**
Calcaneal apophysitis
Epiphysitis, os calcis
Osteochondrosis (juvenile) of:
astragalus (of Diaz)
calcaneum (of Sever)
foot NOS
metatarsal:
second (of Freiberg)
fifth (of Iselin)
os tibiale externum (of Haglund)
tarsal navicular (of Köhler)

❑732.6 **Other juvenile osteochondrosis**
Apophysitis specified as juvenile, of other site, or site NOS
Epiphysitis specified as juvenile, of other site, or site NOS
Osteochondritis specified as juvenile, of other site, or site NOS
Osteochondrosis specified as juvenile, of other site, or site NOS

732.7 **Osteochondritis dissecans**

❑732.8 **Other specified forms of osteochondropathy**
Adult osteochondrosis of spine

❑732.9 **Unspecified osteochondropathy**
Apophysitis
NOS
not specified as adult or juvenile, of unspecified site
Epiphysitis
NOS
not specified as adult or juvenile, of unspecified site
Osteochondritis
NOS
not specified as adult or juvenile, of unspecified site
Osteochondrosis
NOS
not specified as adult or juvenile, of unspecified site

● 733 **Other disorders of bone and cartilage**

Excludes *bone spur (726.91)*
cartilage of, or loose body in, joint (717.0–717.9, 718.0–718.9)
giant cell granuloma of jaw (526.3)
osteitis fibrosa cystica generalisata (252.0)
osteomalacia (268.2)
polyostotic fibrous dysplasia of bone (756.54)
prognathism, retrognathism (524.1)
xanthomatosis localized to bone (272.7)

● 733.0 **Osteoporosis**

❑733.00 **Osteoporosis, unspecified**
Wedging of vertebra NOS

733.01 **Senile osteoporosis**
Postmenopausal osteoporosis

733.02 **Idiopathic osteoporosis**

733.03 **Disuse osteoporosis**

❑733.09 **Other**
Drug-induced osteoporosis

Use additional E code to identify drug

● 733.1 **Pathologic fracture**
Spontaneous fracture

Excludes *stress fracture (733.93–733.95)*
traumatic fractures (800–829)

❑733.10 **Pathologic fracture, unspecified site**

733.11 **Pathologic fracture of humerus**

733.12 **Pathologic fracture of distal radius and ulna**
Wrist NOS

733.13 **Pathologic fracture of vertebrae**
Collapse of vertebra NOS

733.14 **Pathologic fracture of neck of femur**
Femur NOS
Hip NOS

❑733.15 **Pathologic fracture of other specified part of femur**

733.16 **Pathologic fracture of tibia and fibula**
Ankle NOS

❑733.19 **Pathologic fracture of other specified site**

● 733.2 **Cyst of bone**

❑733.20 **Cyst of bone (localized), unspecified**

733.21 **Solitary bone cyst**
Unicameral bone cyst

733.22 **Aneurysmal bone cyst**

❑733.29 **Other**
Fibrous dysplasia (monostotic)

Excludes *cyst of jaw (526.0–526.2, 526.89)*
osteitis fibrosa cystica (252.0)
polyostotic fibrous dysplasia of bone (756.54)

733.3 **Hyperostosis of skull**
Hyperostosis interna frontalis
Leontiasis ossium

● 733.4 **Aseptic necrosis of bone**

Excludes *osteochondropathies (732.0–732.9)*

❑733.40 **Aseptic necrosis of bone, site unspecified**

733.41 **Head of humerus**

733.42 **Head and neck of femur**
Femur NOS

Excludes *Legg-Calvé-Perthes disease (732.1)*

733.43 **Medial femoral condyle**

733.44 **Talus**

❑733.49 **Other**

733.5 **Osteitis condensans**
Piriform sclerosis of ilium

733.6 **Tietze's disease**
Costochondral junction syndrome
Costochondritis

733.7 **Algoneurodystrophy**
Disuse atrophy of bone
Sudeck's atrophy

● 733.8 **Malunion and nonunion of fracture**

733.81 **Malunion of fracture**

733.82 **Nonunion of fracture**
Pseudoarthrosis (bone)

● 733.9 **Other and unspecified disorders of bone and cartilage**

❑733.90 **Disorder of bone and cartilage, unspecified**

733.91 **Arrest of bone development or growth**
Epiphyseal arrest

733.92 **Chondromalacia**
Chondromalacia:
NOS
localized, except patella
systemic
tibial plateau

Excludes *chondromalacia of patella (717.7)*

733.93 Stress fracture of tibia or fibula
Stress reaction of tibia or fibula

733.94 Stress fracture of the metatarsals
Stress reaction of metatarsals

❑ 733.95 Stress fracture of other bone
Stress reaction of other bone

❑ 733.99 Other
Diaphysitis
Hypertrophy of bone
Relapsing polychondritis

734 Flat foot
Pes planus (acquired)
Talipes planus (acquired)

Excludes *congenital (754.61)*
rigid flat foot (754.61)
spastic (everted) flat foot (754.61)

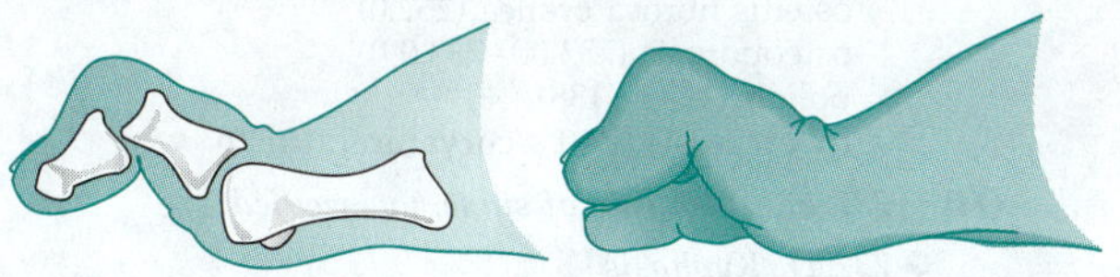

Figure 13-4 Claw toe.

Item 13-5 Claw toe is caused by a contraction of the flexor tendon producing a flexion deformity characterized by hyperextension of the big toe.

● 735 Acquired deformities of toe

Excludes *congenital (754.60–754.69, 755.65–755.66)*

735.0 Hallux valgus (acquired)

735.1 Hallux varus (acquired)

735.2 Hallux rigidus

735.3 Hallux malleus

❑ 735.4 Other hammer toe (acquired)

735.5 Claw toe (acquired)

❑ 735.8 Other acquired deformities of toe

❑ 735.9 Unspecified acquired deformity of toe

● 736 Other acquired deformities of limbs

Excludes *congenital (754.3–755.9)*

● 736.0 Acquired deformities of forearm, excluding fingers

❑ 736.00 Unspecified deformity
Deformity of elbow, forearm, hand, or wrist (acquired) NOS

736.01 Cubitus valgus (acquired)

736.02 Cubitus varus (acquired)

736.03 Valgus deformity of wrist (acquired)

736.04 Varus deformity of wrist (acquired)

736.05 Wrist drop (acquired)

736.06 Claw hand (acquired)

736.07 Club hand (acquired)

❑ 736.09 Other

736.1 Mallet finger

● 736.2 Other acquired deformities of finger

❑ 736.20 Unspecified deformity
Deformity of finger (acquired) NOS

736.21 Boutonniere deformity

736.22 Swan-neck deformity

❑ 736.29 Other

Excludes *trigger finger (727.03)*

● 736.3 Acquired deformities of hip

❑ 736.30 Unspecified deformity
Deformity of hip (acquired) NOS

736.31 Coxa valga (acquired)

736.32 Coxa vara (acquired)

❑ 736.39 Other

● 736.4 Genu valgum or varum (acquired)

736.41 Genu valgum (acquired)

736.42 Genu varum (acquired)

736.5 Genu recurvatum (acquired)

❑ 736.6 Other acquired deformities of knee
Deformity of knee (acquired) NOS

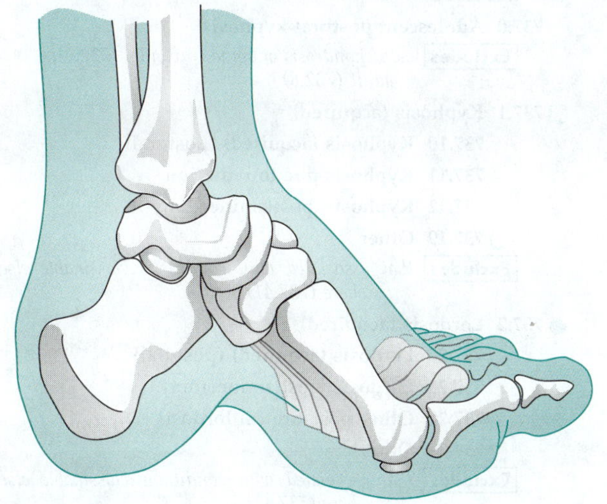

Figure 13-5 Pes cavovarus, meaning "foot with high arch."

Item 13-6 Equinus foot is a term referring to the hoof of a horse. The deformity is usually congenital or spastic.

● 736.7 Other acquired deformities of ankle and foot

Excludes *deformities of toe (acquired) (735.0–735.9)*
pes planus (acquired) (734)

❑ 736.70 Unspecified deformity of ankle and foot, acquired

736.71 Acquired equinovarus deformity
Clubfoot, acquired

Excludes *clubfoot not specified as acquired (754.5–754.7)*

736.72 Equinus deformity of foot, acquired

736.73 Cavus deformity of foot

Excludes *that with claw foot (736.74)*

736.74 Claw foot, acquired

736.75 Cavovarus deformity of foot, acquired

❑ 736.76 Other calcaneus deformity

❑ 736.79 Other
Acquired:
pes not elsewhere classified
talipes not elsewhere classified

● 736.8 Acquired deformities of other parts of limbs

736.81 Unequal leg length (acquired)

❑ 736.89 Other

Deformity (acquired):
arm or leg, not elsewhere classified
shoulder

❑ 736.9 Acquired deformity of limb, site unspecified

Item 13-7 Kyphosis is an abnormal curvature of the spine. **Senile kyphosis** is a result of disc degeneration causing ossification (turning to bone). **Adolescent or juvenile kyphosis** is also known as **Scheuermann's disease,** a condition in which the discs of the lower thoracic spine herniate, causing the disc space to narrow and the spine to tilt forward. This condition is attributed to poor posture.

Item 13-8 Spondylolisthesis is a condition caused by the slipping forward of one disc over another.

● 737 Curvature of spine

Excludes *congenital (754.2)*

737.0 Adolescent postural kyphosis

Excludes *osteochondrosis of spine (juvenile) (732.0)*
adult (732.8)

❑ 737.1 Kyphosis (acquired)

737.10 Kyphosis (acquired) (postural)

737.11 Kyphosis due to radiation

737.12 Kyphosis, postlaminectomy

❑ 737.19 Other

Excludes *that associated with conditions classifiable elsewhere (737.41)*

● 737.2 Lordosis (acquired)

737.20 Lordosis (acquired) (postural)

737.21 Lordosis, postlaminectomy

737.22 Other postsurgical lordosis

❑ 737.29 Other

Excludes *that associated with conditions classifiable elsewhere (737.42)*

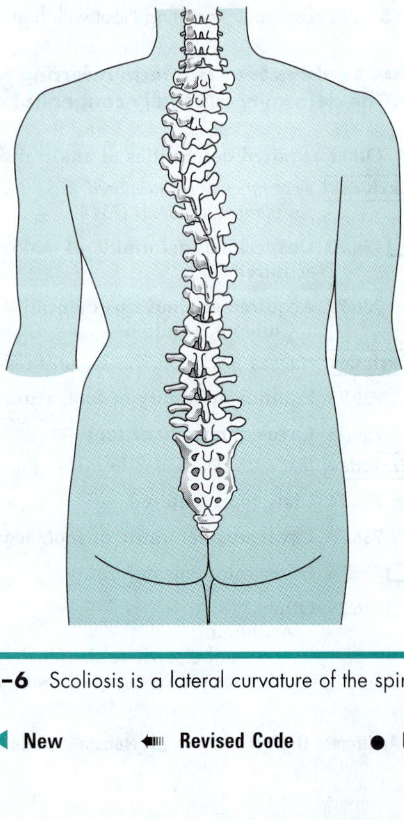

Figure 13-6 Scoliosis is a lateral curvature of the spine.

● 737.3 Kyphoscoliosis and scoliosis

737.30 Scoliosis [and kyphoscoliosis], idiopathic

737.31 Resolving infantile idiopathic scoliosis

737.32 Progressive infantile idiopathic scoliosis

737.33 Scoliosis due to radiation

737.34 Thoracogenic scoliosis

❑ 737.39 Other

Excludes *that associated with conditions classifiable elsewhere (737.43)*
that in kyphoscoliotic heart disease (416.1)

●● *737.4 Curvature of spine associated with other conditions*

Code first associated condition, as:
Charcot-Marie-Tooth disease (356.1)
mucopolysaccharidosis (277.5)
neurofibromatosis (237.7)
osteitis deformans (731.0)
osteitis fibrosa cystica (252.0)
osteoporosis (733.00–733.09)
poliomyelitis (138)
tuberculosis [Pott's curvature] (015.0)

●●❑ *737.40 Curvature of spine, unspecified*

● *737.41 Kyphosis*

● *737.42 Lordosis*

● *737.43 Scoliosis*

❑ 737.8 Other curvatures of spine

❑ 737.9 Unspecified curvature of spine

Curvature of spine (acquired) (idiopathic) NOS
Hunchback, acquired

Excludes *deformity of spine NOS (738.5)*

● 738 Other acquired deformity

Excludes *congenital (754.0–756.9, 758.0–759.9)*
dentofacial anomalies (524.0–524.9)

738.0 Acquired deformity of nose

Deformity of nose (acquired)
Overdevelopment of nasal bones

Excludes *deflected or deviated nasal septum (470)*

● 738.1 Other acquired deformity of head

❑ 738.10 Unspecified deformity

738.11 Zygomatic hyperplasia

738.12 Zygomatic hypoplasia

❑ 738.19 Other specified deformity

738.2 Acquired deformity of neck

738.3 Acquired deformity of chest and rib

Deformity:
chest (acquired)
rib (acquired)
Pectus:
carinatum, acquired
excavatum, acquired

738.4 Acquired spondylolisthesis

Degenerative spondylolisthesis
Spondylolysis, acquired

Excludes *congenital (756.12)*

❑ 738.5 Other acquired deformity of back or spine

Deformity of spine NOS

Excludes *curvature of spine (737.0–737.9)*

738.6 Acquired deformity of pelvis

Pelvic obliquity

Excludes *intrapelvic protrusion of acetabulum (718.6)*
that in relation to labor and delivery (653.0–653.4, 653.8–653.9)

738.7 **Cauliflower ear**

❑ 738.8 **Acquired deformity of other specified site**
Deformity of clavicle

❑ 738.9 **Acquired deformity of unspecified site**

● 739 **Nonallopathic lesions, not elsewhere classified**

Includes: segmental dysfunction
somatic dysfunction

739.0 **Head region**
Occipitocervical region

739.1 **Cervical region**
Cervicothoracic region

739.2 **Thoracic region**
Thoracolumbar region

739.3 **Lumbar region**
Lumbosacral region

739.4 **Sacral region**
Sacrococcygeal region
Sacroiliac region

739.5 **Pelvic region**
Hip region
Pubic region

739.6 **Lower extremities**

739.7 **Upper extremities**
Acromioclavicular region
Sternoclavicular region

739.8 **Rib cage**
Costochondral region
Costovertebral region
Sternochondral region

739.9 **Abdomen and other**

ICD-9-CM 700-799 Vol. 1

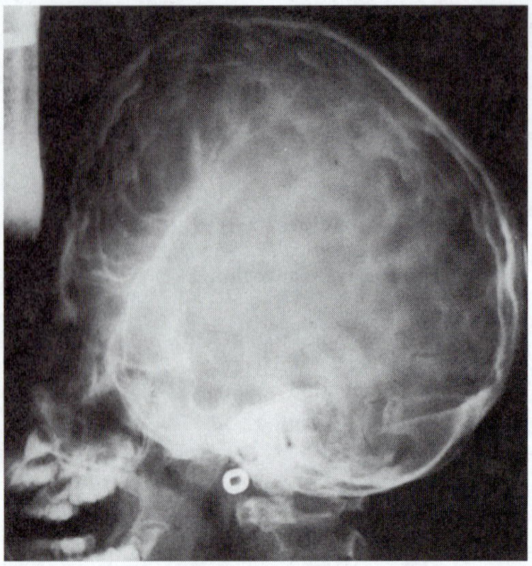

Figure 14–1 Generalized craniosynostosis in a 4-year-old girl without symptoms or signs of increased intracranial pressure. The child was referred for medical evaluation because of abnormal facial characteristics, features similar to those of her mother and aunt. Her fronto-occipital head circumference was found to be 47 cm. (From Bell WE, McCormick WF: Increased Intracranial Pressure in Children, 2nd ed. Philadelphia, WB Saunders, 1978, p 116.)

Item 14–1 Anencephalus is a congenital deformity of the cranial vault. Craniosynostosis, also known as craniostenosis and stenocephaly, signifies any form of congenital deformity of the skull that results from the premature closing of the sutures of the skull. Iniencephaly is a deformity in which the head and neck are flexed backward to a great extent and the head is very large in comparison to the shortened body.

14. CONGENITAL ANOMALIES (740–759)

● **740 Anencephalus and similar anomalies**

740.0 Anencephalus
Acrania
Amyelencephalus
Hemianencephaly
Hemicephaly

740.1 Craniorachischisis

740.2 Iniencephaly

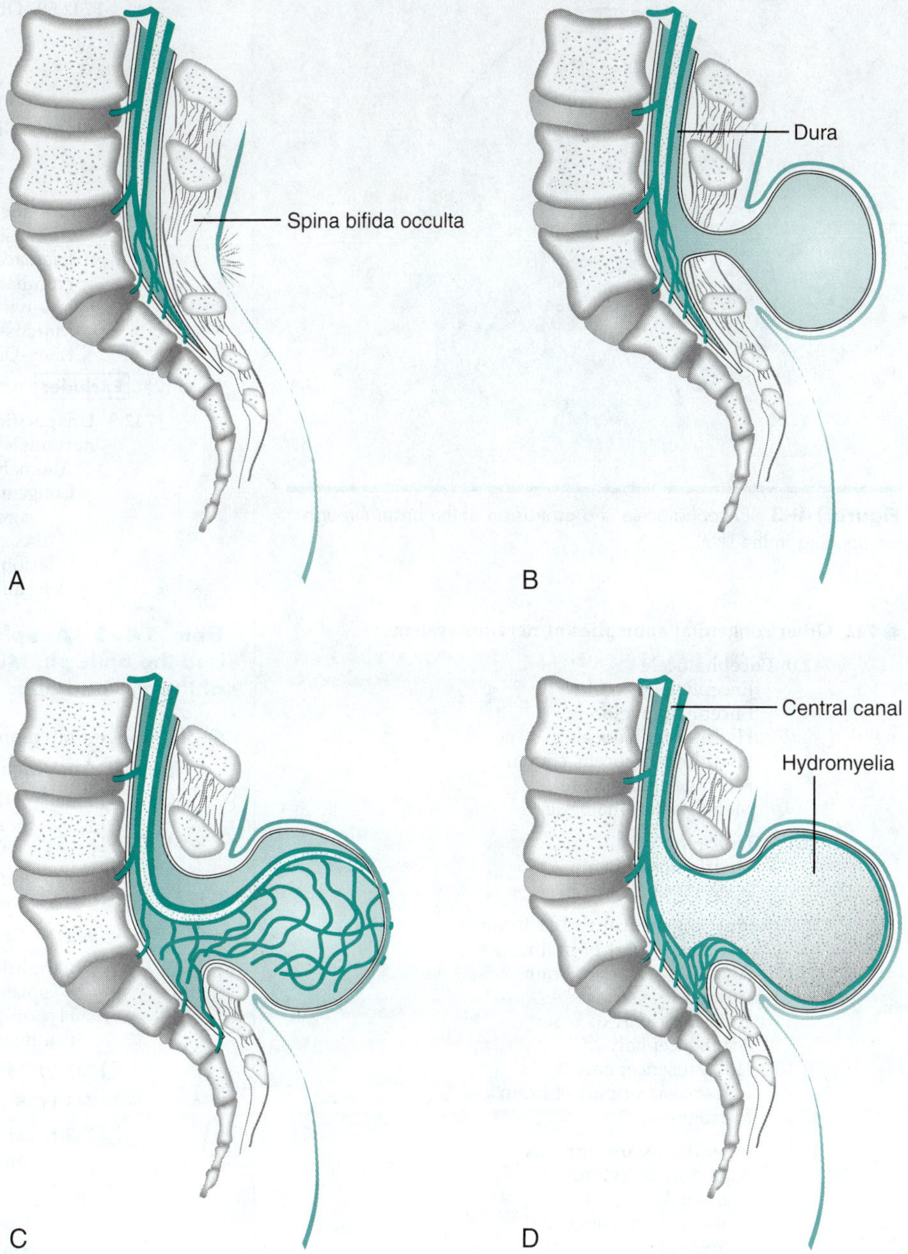

Figure 14–2 **A.** Spina bifida occulta. **B.** Meningocele. **C.** Myelomeningocele. **D.** Myelocystocele (syringomyelocele) or hydromyelia.

Item 14–2 Spina bifida is a midline spinal defect in which one or more vertebrae fail to fuse, leaving an opening in the vertebral canal. When the defect is not visible, it is called spina bifida occulta, and when it is visible, it is called spina bifida cystica.

● **741 Spina bifida**

Excludes *spina bifida occulta (756.17)*

The following fifth-digit subclassification is for use with category 741:

❑ **0 unspecified region**
1 cervical region
2 dorsal (thoracic) region
3 lumbar region

● **741.0 With hydrocephalus**

Arnold-Chiari syndrome, type II
Any condition classifiable to 741.9 with any condition classifiable to 742.3
Chiari malformation, type II

● **741.9 Without mention of hydrocephalus**

Hydromeningocele (spinal)
Hydromyelocele
Meningocele (spinal)
Meningomyelocele
Myelocele
Myelocystocele
Rachischisis
Spina bifida (aperta)
Syringomyelocele

ICD-9-CM 700-799 Vol. 1

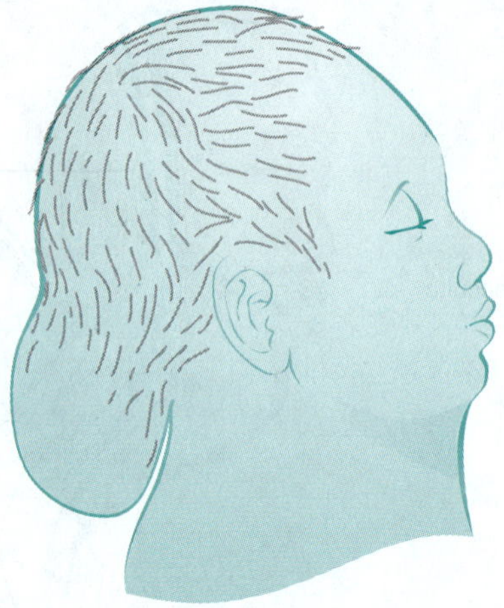

Figure 14–3 Encephalocele is a protrusion of the brain through an opening in the skull.

● 742 **Other congenital anomalies of nervous system**

742.0 **Encephalocele**
Encephalocystocele
Encephalomyelocele
Hydroencephalocele
Hydromeningocele, cranial
Meningocele, cerebral
Meningoencephalocele

742.1 **Microcephalus**
Hydromicrocephaly
Micrencephaly

742.2 **Reduction deformities of brain**
Absence of part of brain
Agenesis of part of brain
Agyria
Aplasia of part of brain
Arhinencephaly
Holoprosencephaly
Hypoplasia of part of brain
Microgyria

742.3 **Congenital hydrocephalus**
Aqueduct of Sylvius:
anomaly
obstruction, congenital
stenosis
Atresia of foramina of Magendie and Luschka
Hydrocephalus in newborn

Excludes *hydrocephalus:*
acquired (331.3–331.4)
due to congenital toxoplasmosis (771.2)
with any condition classifiable to 741.9 (741.0)

❑ 742.4 **Other specified anomalies of brain**
Congenital cerebral cyst
Macroencephaly
Macrogyria
Megalencephaly
Multiple anomalies of brain NOS
Porencephaly
Ulegyria

● 742.5 **Other specified anomalies of spinal cord**

742.51 **Diastematomyelia**

742.53 **Hydromyelia**
Hydrorhachis

❑ 742.59 **Other**
Amyelia
Atelomyelia
Congenital anomaly of spinal meninges
Defective development of cauda equina
Hypoplasia of spinal cord
Myelatelia
Myelodysplasia

❑ 742.8 **Other specified anomalies of nervous system**
Agenesis of nerve
Displacement of brachial plexus
Familial dysautonomia
Jaw-winking syndrome
Marcus-Gunn syndrome
Riley-Day syndrome

Excludes *neurofibromatosis (237.7)*

❑ 742.9 **Unspecified anomaly of brain, spinal cord, and nervous system**
Anomaly of brain, nervous system, and spinal cord
Congenital, of brain, nervous system, and spinal cord:
disease of brain, nervous system, and spinal cord
lesion of brain, nervous system, and spinal cord
Deformity of brain, nervous system, and spinal cord

Item 14–3 Anophthalmia is the absence of the eye and the optic pit. Microphthalmia is the partial absence of the eye and optic pit.

● 743 **Congenital anomalies of eye**

● 743.0 **Anophthalmos**

❑ 743.00 **Clinical anophthalmos, unspecified**
Agenesis
Congenital absence of eye
Anophthalmos NOS

743.03 **Cystic eyeball, congenital**

743.06 **Cryptophthalmos**

● 743.1 **Microphthalmos**
Dysplasia of eye
Hypoplasia of eye
Rudimentary eye

❑ 743.10 **Microphthalmos, unspecified**

743.11 **Simple microphthalmos**

❑ 743.12 **Microphthalmos associated with other anomalies of eye and adnexa**

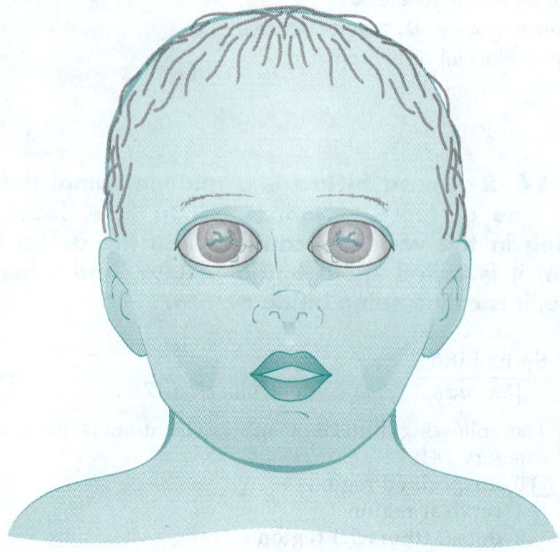

Figure 14–4 Bilateral congenital hydrophthalmia, in which the eyes are very large in comparison to the other facial features.

● 743.2 **Buphthalmos**
Glaucoma:
congenital
newborn
Hydrophthalmos
Excludes *glaucoma of childhood (365.14)*
traumatic glaucoma due to birth injury (767.8)

❑ 743.20 **Buphthalmos, unspecified**

743.21 **Simple buphthalmos**

❑ 743.22 **Buphthalmos associated with other ocular anomalies**
Keratoglobus, congenital, associated with buphthalmos
Megalocornea associated with buphthalmos

● 743.3 **Congenital cataract and lens anomalies**
Excludes *infantile cataract (366.00–366.09)*

❑ 743.30 **Congenital cataract, unspecified**

743.31 **Capsular and subcapsular cataract**

743.32 **Cortical and zonular cataract**

743.33 **Nuclear cataract**

743.34 **Total and subtotal cataract, congenital**

743.35 **Congenital aphakia**
Congenital absence of lens

743.36 **Anomalies of lens shape**
Microphakia
Spherophakia

743.37 **Congenital ectopic lens**

❑ 743.39 **Other**

● 743.4 **Coloboma and other anomalies of anterior segment**

743.41 **Anomalies of corneal size and shape**
Microcornea
Excludes *that associated with buphthalmos (743.22)*

743.42 **Corneal opacities, interfering with vision, congenital**

❑ 743.43 **Other corneal opacities, congenital**

❑ 743.44 **Specified anomalies of anterior chamber, chamber angle, and related structures**
Anomaly:
Axenfeld's
Peters'
Rieger's

743.45 **Aniridia**

❑ 743.46 **Other specified anomalies of iris and ciliary body**
Anisocoria, congenital
Atresia of pupil
Coloboma of iris
Corectopia

❑ 743.47 **Specified anomalies of sclera**

❑ 743.48 **Multiple and combined anomalies of anterior segment**

❑ 743.49 **Other**

● 743.5 **Congenital anomalies of posterior segment**

743.51 **Vitreous anomalies**
Congenital vitreous opacity

743.52 **Fundus coloboma**

743.53 **Chorioretinal degeneration, congenital**

743.54 **Congenital folds and cysts of posterior segment**

743.55 **Congenital macular changes**

❑ 743.56 **Other retinal changes, congenital**

❑ 743.57 **Specified anomalies of optic disc**
Coloboma of optic disc (congenital)

743.58 **Vascular anomalies**
Congenital retinal aneurysm

❑ 743.59 **Other**

● 743.6 **Congenital anomalies of eyelids, lacrimal system, and orbit**

743.61 **Congenital ptosis**

743.62 **Congenital deformities of eyelids**
Ablepharon
Absence of eyelid
Accessory eyelid
Congenital:
ectropion
entropion

❑ 743.63 **Other specified congenital anomalies of eyelid**
Absence, agenesis, of cilia

❑ 743.64 **Specified congenital anomalies of lacrimal gland**

❑ 743.65 **Specified congenital anomalies of lacrimal passages**
Absence, agenesis, of:
lacrimal apparatus
punctum lacrimale
Accessory lacrimal canal

❑ 743.66 **Specified congenital anomalies of orbit**

❑ 743.69 **Other**
Accessory eye muscles

❑ 743.8 **Other specified anomalies of eye**
Excludes *congenital nystagmus (379.51)*
ocular albinism (270.2)
retinitis pigmentosa (362.74)

❑ 743.9 **Unspecified anomaly of eye**
Congenital:
anomaly NOS of eye [any part]
deformity NOS of eye [any part]

● 744 **Congenital anomalies of ear, face, and neck**
Excludes *anomaly of:*
cervical spine (754.2, 756.10–756.19)
larynx (748.2–748.3)
nose (748.0–748.1)
parathyroid gland (759.2)
thyroid gland (759.2)
cleft lip (749.10–749.25)

● ❑ 744.0 **Anomalies of ear causing impairment of hearing**
Excludes *congenital deafness without mention of cause (380.0–389.9)*

❑ 744.00 **Unspecified anomaly of ear with impairment of hearing**

744.01 **Absence of external ear**
Absence of:
auditory canal (external)
auricle (ear) (with stenosis or atresia of auditory canal)

❑ 744.02 **Other anomalies of external ear with impairment of hearing**
Atresia or stricture of auditory canal (external)

744.03 **Anomaly of middle ear, except ossicles**
Atresia or stricture of osseous meatus (ear)

744.04 **Anomalies of ear ossicles**
Fusion of ear ossicles

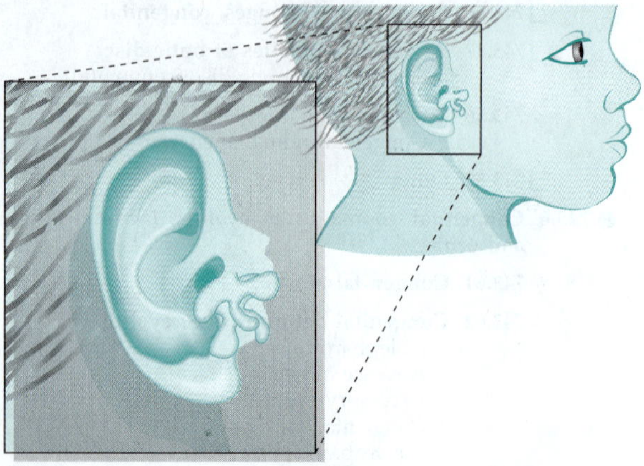

Figure 14–5 Multiple auricular appendage.

744.05 **Anomalies of inner ear**
Congenital anomaly of:
membranous labyrinth
organ of Corti

❑ 744.09 **Other**
Absence of ear, congenital

744.1 **Accessory auricle**
Accessory tragus
Polyotia
Preauricular appendage
Supernumerary:
ear
lobule

● 744.2 **Other specified anomalies of ear**
Excludes *that with impairment of hearing (744.00–744.09)*

744.21 **Absence of ear lobe, congenital**

744.22 **Macrotia**

744.23 **Microtia**

❑ 744.24 **Specified anomalies of Eustachian tube**
Absence of Eustachian tube

❑ 744.29 **Other**
Bat ear
Darwin's tubercle
Pointed ear
Prominence of auricle
Ridge ear

Excludes *preauricular sinus (744.46)*

❑ 744.3 **Unspecified anomaly of ear**
Congenital:
anomaly NOS of ear, NEC
deformity NOS of ear, NEC

● 744.4 **Branchial cleft cyst or fistula; preauricular sinus**

744.41 **Branchial cleft sinus or fistula**
Branchial:
sinus (external) (internal)
vestige

744.42 **Branchial cleft cyst**

744.43 **Cervical auricle**

744.46 **Preauricular sinus or fistula**

744.47 **Preauricular cyst**

❑ 744.49 **Other**
Fistula (of):
auricle, congenital
cervicoaural

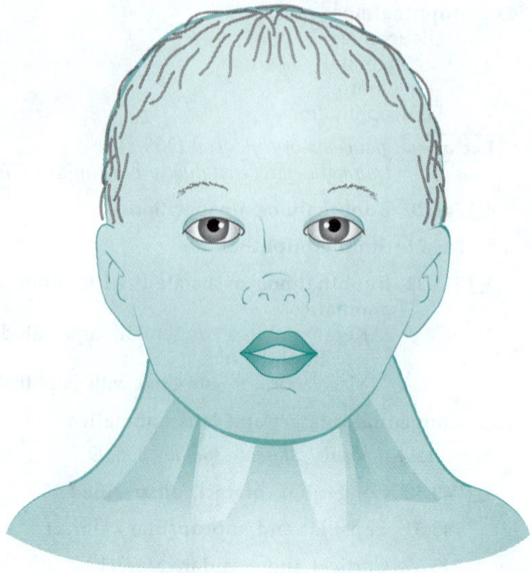

Figure 14–6 Webbing of the neck.

744.5 **Webbing of neck**
Pterygium colli

● 744.8 **Other specified anomalies of face and neck**

744.81 **Macrocheilia**
Hypertrophy of lip, congenital

744.82 **Microcheilia**

744.83 **Macrostomia**

744.84 **Microstomia**

❑ 744.89 **Other**

Excludes *congenital fistula of lip (750.25)*
musculoskeletal anomalies (754.0–754.1, 756.0)

❑ 744.9 **Unspecified anomalies of face and neck**
Congenital:
anomaly NOS of face [any part] or neck [any part]
deformity NOS of face [any part] or neck [any part]

● 745 **Bulbus cordis anomalies and anomalies of cardiac septal closure**

745.0 **Common truncus**
Absent septum between aorta and pulmonary artery
Communication (abnormal) between aorta and pulmonary artery
Aortic septal defect
Common aortopulmonary trunk
Persistent truncus arteriosus

● 745.1 **Transposition of great vessels**

745.10 **Complete transposition of great vessels**
Transposition of great vessels:
NOS
classical

745.11 **Double outlet right ventricle**
Dextrotransposition of aorta
Incomplete transposition of great vessels
Origin of both great vessels from right ventricle
Taussig-Bing syndrome or defect

745.12 **Corrected transposition of great vessels**

❑ 745.19 **Other**

745.2 **Tetralogy of Fallot**
Fallot's pentalogy
Ventricular septal defect with pulmonary stenosis or atresia, dextroposition of aorta, and hypertrophy of right ventricle
Excludes *Fallot's triad (746.09)*

745.3 **Common ventricle**
Cor triloculare biatriatum
Single ventricle

745.4 **Ventricular septal defect**
Eisenmenger's defect or complex
Gerbode defect
Interventricular septal defect
Left ventricular-right atrial communication
Roger's disease
Excludes *common atrioventricular canal type (745.69)*
single ventricle (745.3)

745.5 **Ostium secundum type atrial septal defect**
Defect:
atrium secundum
fossa ovalis
Lutembacher's syndrome
Patent or persistent:
foramen ovale
ostium secundum

● 745.6 **Endocardial cushion defects**

❑ 745.60 **Endocardial cushion defect, unspecified type**

745.61 **Ostium primum defect**
Persistent ostium primum

❑ 745.69 **Other**
Absence of atrial septum
Atrioventricular canal type ventricular septal defect
Common atrioventricular canal
Common atrium

745.7 **Cor biloculare**
Absence of atrial and ventricular septa

❑ 745.8 **Other**

❑ 745.9 **Unspecified defect of septal closure**
Septal defect NOS

● 746 **Other congenital anomalies of heart**
Excludes *endocardial fibroelastosis (425.3)*

● 746.0 **Anomalies of pulmonary valve**
Excludes *infundibular or subvalvular pulmonic stenosis (746.83)*
tetralogy of Fallot (745.2)

❑ 746.00 **Pulmonary valve anomaly, unspecified**

746.01 **Atresia, congenital**
Congenital absence of pulmonary valve

746.02 **Stenosis, congenital**

❑ 746.09 **Other**
Congenital insufficiency of pulmonary valve
Fallot's triad or trilogy

746.1 **Tricuspid atresia and stenosis, congenital**
Absence of tricuspid valve

746.2 **Ebstein's anomaly**

746.3 **Congenital stenosis of aortic valve**
Congenital aortic stenosis
Excludes *congenital:*
subaortic stenosis (746.81)
supravalvular aortic stenosis (747.22)

746.4 **Congenital insufficiency of aortic valve**
Bicuspid aortic valve
Congenital aortic insufficiency

746.5 **Congenital mitral stenosis**
Fused commissure of mitral valve
Parachute deformity of mitral valve
Supernumerary cusps of mitral valve

746.6 **Congenital mitral insufficiency**

746.7 **Hypoplastic left heart syndrome**
Atresia, or marked hypoplasia, of aortic orifice or valve, with hypoplasia of ascending aorta and defective development of left ventricle (with mitral valve atresia)

● 746.8 **Other specified anomalies of heart**

746.81 **Subaortic stenosis**

746.82 **Cor triatriatum**

746.83 **Infundibular pulmonic stenosis**
Subvalvular pulmonic stenosis

746.84 **Obstructive anomalies of heart, NEC**
Uhl's disease

746.85 **Coronary artery anomaly**
Anomalous origin or communication of coronary artery
Arteriovenous malformation of coronary artery
Coronary artery:
absence
arising from aorta or pulmonary trunk
single

746.86 **Congenital heart block**
Complete or incomplete atrioventricular [AV] block

746.87 **Malposition of heart and cardiac apex**
Abdominal heart
Dextrocardia
Ectopia cordis
Levocardia (isolated)
Mesocardia
Excludes *dextrocardia with complete transposition of viscera (759.3)*

❑ 746.89 **Other**
Atresia of cardiac vein
Hypoplasia of cardiac vein
Congenital:
cardiomegaly
diverticulum, left ventricle
pericardial defect

❑ 746.9 **Unspecified anomaly of heart**
Congenital:
anomaly of heart NOS
heart disease NOS

● 747 **Other congenital anomalies of circulatory system**

747.0 **Patent ductus arteriosus**
Patent ductus Botalli
Persistent ductus arteriosus

● 747.1 **Coarctation of aorta**

747.10 **Coarctation of aorta (preductal) (postductal)**
Hypoplasia of aortic arch

747.11 **Interruption of aortic arch**

● 747.2 **Other anomalies of aorta**

❑ 747.20 **Anomaly of aorta, unspecified**

747.21 Anomalies of aortic arch
Anomalous origin, right subclavian artery
Dextroposition of aorta
Double aortic arch
Kommerell's diverticulum
Overriding aorta
Persistent:
convolutions, aortic arch
right aortic arch
Vascular ring

Excludes *hypoplasia of aortic arch (747.10)*

747.22 Atresia and stenosis of aorta
Absence of aorta
Aplasia of aorta
Hypoplasia of aorta
Stricture of aorta
Supra (valvular)-aortic stenosis

Excludes *congenital aortic (valvular) stenosis or stricture, so stated (746.3)*
hypoplasia of aorta in hypoplastic left heart syndrome (746.7)

❑ **747.29 Other**
Aneurysm of sinus of Valsalva
Congenital:
aneurysm of aorta
dilation of aorta

747.3 Anomalies of pulmonary artery
Agenesis of pulmonary artery
Anomaly of pulmonary artery
Atresia of pulmonary artery
Coarctation of pulmonary artery
Hypoplasia of pulmonary artery
Stenosis of pulmonary artery
Pulmonary arteriovenous aneurysm

● **747.4 Anomalies of great veins**

❑ **747.40 Anomaly of great veins, unspecified**
Anomaly NOS of:
pulmonary veins
vena cava

747.41 Total anomalous pulmonary venous connection
Total anomalous pulmonary venous return [TAPVR]:
subdiaphragmatic
supradiaphragmatic

747.42 Partial anomalous pulmonary venous connection
Partial anomalous pulmonary venous return

❑ **747.49 Other anomalies of great veins**
Absence of vena cava (inferior) (superior)
Congenital stenosis of vena cava (inferior) (superior)
Persistent:
left posterior cardinal vein
left superior vena cava
Scimitar syndrome
Transposition of pulmonary veins NOS

747.5 Absence or hypoplasia of umbilical artery
Single umbilical artery

● **747.6 Other anomalies of peripheral vascular system**
Absence of artery or vein, NEC
Anomaly of artery or vein, NEC
Atresia of artery or vein, NEC
Arteriovenous aneurysm (peripheral)
Arteriovenous malformation of the peripheral vascular system
Congenital:
aneurysm (peripheral)
phlebectasia
stricture, artery
varix
Multiple renal arteries

Excludes *anomalies of:*
cerebral vessels (747.81)
pulmonary artery (747.3)
congenital retinal aneurysm (743.58)
hemangioma (228.00–228.09)
lymphangioma (228.1)

❑ **747.60 Anomaly of the peripheral vascular system, unspecified site**

747.61 Gastrointestinal vessel anomaly

747.62 Renal vessel anomaly

747.63 Upper limb vessel anomaly

747.64 Lower limb vessel anomaly

❑ **747.69 Anomalies of other specified sites of peripheral vascular system**

● **747.8 Other specified anomalies of circulatory system**

747.81 Anomalies of cerebrovascular system
Arteriovenous malformation of brain
Cerebral arteriovenous aneurysm, congenital
Congenital anomalies of cerebral vessels

Excludes *ruptured cerebral (arteriovenous) aneurysm (430)*

747.82 Spinal vessel anomaly
Arteriovenous malformation of spinal vessel

747.83 Persistent fetal circulation
Persistent pulmonary hypertension
Primary pulmonary hypertension of newborn

❑ **747.89 Other**
Aneurysm, congenital, specified site not elsewhere classified

Excludes *congenital aneurysm:*
coronary (746.85)
peripheral (747.6)
pulmonary (747.3)
retinal (743.58)

❑ **747.9 Unspecified anomaly of circulatory system**

● **748 Congenital anomalies of respiratory system**

Excludes *congenital defect of diaphragm (756.6)*

748.0 Choanal atresia
Atresia of nares (anterior) (posterior)
Congenital stenosis of nares (anterior) (posterior)

❑ **748.1 Other anomalies of nose**
Absent nose
Accessory nose
Cleft nose
Deformity of wall of nasal sinus
Congenital:
deformity of nose
notching of tip of nose
perforation of wall of nasal sinus

Excludes *congenital deviation of nasal septum (754.0)*

748.2 Web of larynx
Web of larynx:
NOS
glottic
subglottic

❑**748.3 Other anomalies of larynx, trachea, and bronchus**
Absence or agenesis of:
bronchus
larynx
trachea
Anomaly (of):
cricoid cartilage
epiglottis
thyroid cartilage
tracheal cartilage
Atresia (of):
epiglottis
glottis
larynx
trachea
Cleft thyroid, cartilage, congenital
Congenital:
dilation, trachea
stenosis:
larynx
trachea
tracheocele
Diverticulum:
bronchus
trachea
Fissure of epiglottis
Laryngocele
Posterior cleft of cricoid cartilage (congenital)
Rudimentary tracheal bronchus
Stridor, laryngeal, congenital

748.4 Congenital cystic lung
Disease, lung:
cystic, congenital
polycystic, congenital
Honeycomb lung, congenital
Excludes *acquired or unspecified cystic lung (518.89)*

748.5 Agenesis, hypoplasia, and dysplasia of lung
Absence of lung (fissures) (lobe)
Aplasia of lung
Hypoplasia of lung (lobe)
Sequestration of lung

● **748.6 Other anomalies of lung**

❑**748.60 Anomaly of lung, unspecified**

748.61 Congenital bronchiectasis

❑**748.69 Other**
Accessory lung (lobe)
Azygos lobe (fissure), lung

❑**748.8 Other specified anomalies of respiratory system**
Abnormal communication between pericardial and pleural sacs
Anomaly, pleural folds
Atresia of nasopharynx
Congenital cyst of mediastinum

❑**748.9 Unspecified anomaly of respiratory system**
Anomaly of respiratory system NOS

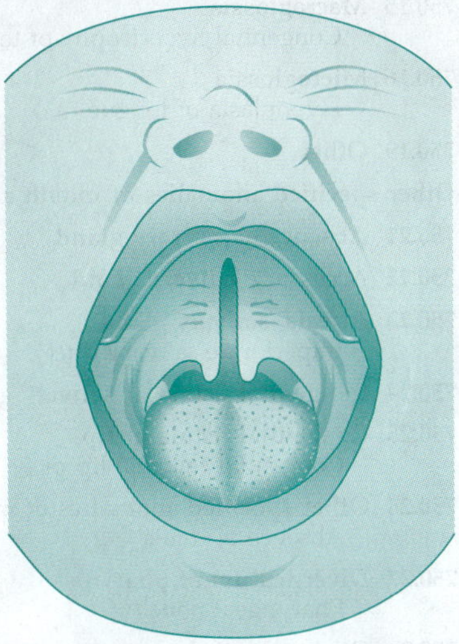

Figure 14-7 Cleft palate.

● **749 Cleft palate and cleft lip**

● **749.0 Cleft palate**

❑**749.00 Cleft palate, unspecified**

749.01 Unilateral, complete

749.02 Unilateral, incomplete
Cleft uvula

749.03 Bilateral, complete

749.04 Bilateral, incomplete

● **749.1 Cleft lip**
Cheiloschisis
Congenital fissure of lip
Harelip
Labium leporinum

❑**749.10 Cleft lip, unspecified**

749.11 Unilateral, complete

749.12 Unilateral, incomplete

749.13 Bilateral, complete

749.14 Bilateral, incomplete

● **749.2 Cleft palate with cleft lip**
Cheilopalatoschisis

❑**749.20 Cleft palate with cleft lip, unspecified**

749.21 Unilateral, complete

749.22 Unilateral, incomplete

749.23 Bilateral, complete

749.24 Bilateral, incomplete

❑**749.25 Other combinations**

● **750 Other congenital anomalies of upper alimentary tract**
Excludes *dentofacial anomalies (524.0–524.9)*

750.0 Tongue tie
Ankyloglossia

● **750.1 Other anomalies of tongue**

❑**750.10 Anomaly of tongue, unspecified**

750.11 Aglossia

750.12 Congenital adhesions of tongue

750.13 Fissure of tongue
Bifid tongue
Double tongue

750.15 **Macroglossia**
Congenital hypertrophy of tongue

750.16 **Microglossia**
Hypoplasia of tongue

❑ 750.19 **Other**

● 750.2 **Other specified anomalies of mouth and pharynx**

750.21 **Absence of salivary gland**

750.22 **Accessory salivary gland**

750.23 **Atresia, salivary gland**
Imperforate salivary duct

750.24 **Congenital fistula of salivary gland**

750.25 **Congenital fistula of lip**
Congenital (mucus) lip pits

❑ 750.26 **Other specified anomalies of mouth**
Absence of uvula

750.27 **Diverticulum of pharynx**
Pharyngeal pouch

❑ 750.29 **Other specified anomalies of pharynx**
Imperforate pharynx

750.3 **Tracheoesophageal fistula, esophageal atresia and stenosis**
Absent esophagus
Atresia of esophagus
Congenital:
esophageal ring
stenosis of esophagus
stricture of esophagus
Congenital fistula:
esophagobronchial
esophagotracheal
Imperforate esophagus
Webbed esophagus

❑ 750.4 **Other specified anomalies of esophagus**
Dilatation, congenital, of esophagus
Displacement, congenital, of esophagus
Diverticulum of esophagus
Duplication of esophagus
Esophageal pouch
Giant esophagus
Excludes *congenital hiatus hernia (750.6)*

750.5 **Congenital hypertrophic pyloric stenosis**
Congenital or infantile:
constriction of pylorus
hypertrophy of pylorus
spasm of pylorus
stenosis of pylorus
stricture of pylorus

750.6 **Congenital hiatus hernia**
Displacement of cardia through esophageal hiatus
Excludes *congenital diaphragmatic hernia (756.6)*

❑ 750.7 **Other specified anomalies of stomach**
Congenital:
cardiospasm
hourglass stomach
Displacement of stomach
Diverticulum of stomach, congenital
Duplication of stomach
Megalogastria
Microgastria
Transposition of stomach

❑ 750.8 **Other specified anomalies of upper alimentary tract**

❑ 750.9 **Unspecified anomaly of upper alimentary tract**
Congenital:
anomaly NOS of upper alimentary tract [any part, except tongue]
deformity NOS of upper alimentary tract [any part, except tongue]

● 751 **Other congenital anomalies of digestive system**

751.0 **Meckel's diverticulum**
Meckel's diverticulum (displaced) (hypertrophic)
Persistent:
omphalomesenteric duct
vitelline duct

751.1 **Atresia and stenosis of small intestine**
Atresia of:
duodenum
ileum
intestine NOS
Congenital:
absence of small intestine or intestine NOS
obstruction of small intestine or intestine NOS
stenosis of small intestine or intestine NOS
stricture of small intestine or intestine NOS
Imperforate jejunum

751.2 **Atresia and stenosis of large intestine, rectum, and anal canal**
Absence:
anus (congenital)
appendix, congenital
large instestine, congenital
rectum
Atresia of:
anus
colon
rectum
Congenital or infantile:
obstruction of large intestine
occlusion of anus
stricture of anus
Imperforate:
anus
rectum
Stricture of rectum, congenital

❑ 751.3 **Hirschsprung's disease and other congenital functional disorders of colon**
Aganglionosis
Congenital dilation of colon
Congenital megacolon
Macrocolon

751.4 **Anomalies of intestinal fixation**
Congenital adhesions:
omental, anomalous
peritoneal
Jackson's membrane
Malrotation of colon
Rotation of cecum or colon:
failure of
incomplete
insufficient
Universal mesentery

❑ 751.5 **Other anomalies of intestine**
Congenital diverticulum, colon
Dolichocolon
Duplication of:
anus
appendix
cecum
intestine
Ectopic anus
Megaloappendix
Megaloduodenum
Microcolon
Persistent cloaca
Transposition of:
appendix
colon
intestine

● 751.6 **Anomalies of gallbladder, bile ducts, and liver**

❑ 751.60 **Unspecified anomaly of gallbladder, bile ducts, and liver**

751.61 **Biliary atresia**
Congenital:
absence of bile duct (common) or passage
hypoplasia of bile duct (common) or passage
obstruction of bile duct (common) or passage
stricture of bile duct (common) or passage

751.62 Congenital cystic disease of liver
Congenital polycystic disease of liver
Fibrocystic disease of liver

❑ **751.69 Other anomalies of gallbladder, bile ducts, and liver**
Absence of:
gallbladder, congenital
liver (lobe)
Accessory:
hepatic ducts
liver
Congenital:
choledochal cyst
hepatomegaly
Duplication of:
biliary duct
cystic duct
gallbladder
liver
Floating:
gallbladder
liver
Intrahepatic gallbladder

751.7 Anomalies of pancreas
Absence of pancreas
Accessory pancreas
Agenesis of pancreas
Annular pancreas
Ectopic pancreatic tissue
Hypoplasia of pancreas
Pancreatic heterotopia
Excludes *diabetes mellitus:*
congenital (250.0–250.9)
neonatal (775.1)
fibrocystic disease of pancreas (277.00–277.09)

❑ **751.8 Other specified anomalies of digestive system**
Absence (complete) (partial) of alimentary tract NOS
Duplication of digestive organs NOS
Malposition, congenital, of digestive organs NOS
Excludes *congenital diaphragmatic hernia (756.6)*
congenital hiatus hernia (750.6)

❑ **751.9 Unspecified anomaly of digestive system**
Congenital:
anomaly NOS of digestive system NOS
deformity NOS of digestive system NOS

● **752 Congenital anomalies of genital organs**
Excludes *syndromes associated with anomalies in the number and form of chromosomes (758.0–758.9)*
testicular feminization syndrome (257.8)

752.0 Anomalies of ovaries
Absence, congenital, of ovary
Accessory ovary
Ectopic ovary
Streak of ovary

● **752.1 Anomalies of fallopian tubes and broad ligaments**

❑ **752.10 Unspecified anomaly of fallopian tubes and broad ligaments**

752.11 Embryonic cyst of fallopian tubes and broad ligaments
Cyst:
epoöphoron
fimbrial
Gartner's duct
parovarian

❑ **752.19 Other**
Absence of fallopian tube or broad ligament
Accessory fallopian tube or broad ligament
Atresia of fallopian tube or broad ligament

752.2 Doubling of uterus
Didelphic uterus
Doubling of uterus [any degree] (associated with doubling of cervix and vagina)

❑ **752.3 Other anomalies of uterus**
Absence, congenital, of uterus
Agenesis of uterus
Aplasia of uterus
Bicornuate uterus
Uterus unicornis
Uterus with only one functioning horn

● **752.4 Anomalies of cervix, vagina, and external female genitalia**

❑ **752.40 Unspecified anomaly of cervix, vagina, and external female genitalia**

752.41 Embryonic cyst of cervix, vagina, and external female genitalia
Cyst of:
canal of Nuck, congenital
vagina, embryonal
vulva, congenital

752.42 Imperforate hymen

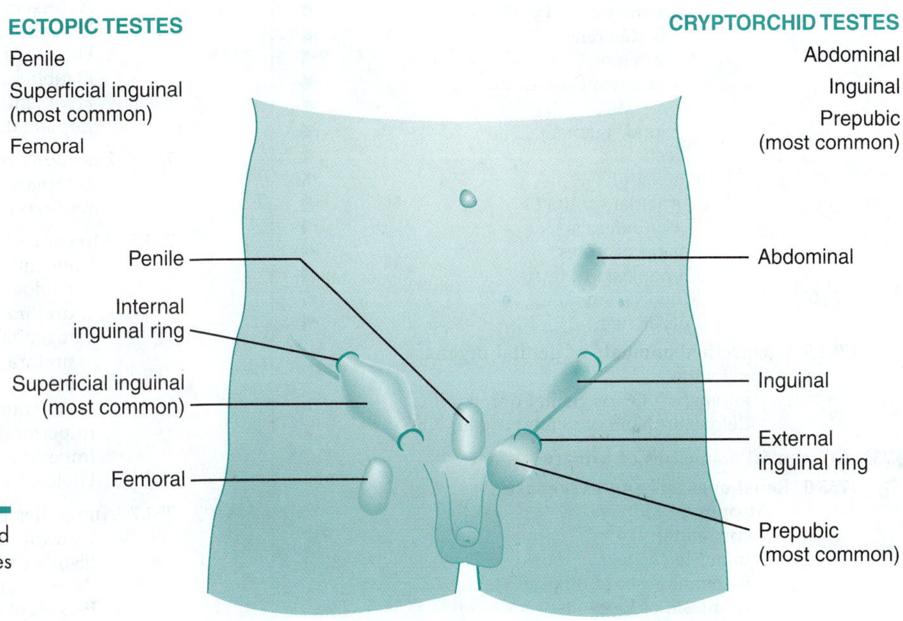

Figure 14–6 Undescended testes and the positions of the testes in various types of cryptorchidism or abnormal paths of descent.

ICD-9-CM 700–799 Vol. 1

❑752.49 **Other anomalies of cervix, vagina, and external female genitalia**
Absence of cervix, clitoris, vagina, or vulva
Agenesis of cervix, clitoris, vagina, or vulva
Congenital stenosis or stricture of:
cervical canal
vagina
Excludes *double vagina associated with total duplication (752.2)*

● 752.5 **Undescended and retractile testicle**
752.51 **Undescended testis**
Cryptorchism
Ectopic testis
752.52 **Retractile testis**

● 752.6 **Hypospadias and epispadias and other penile anomalies**
752.61 **Hypospadias**
752.62 **Epispadias**
Anaspadias
752.63 **Congenital chordee**
752.64 **Micropenis**
752.65 **Hidden penis**
❑752.69 **Other penile anomalies**

752.7 **Indeterminate sex and pseudohermaphroditism**
Gynandrism
Hermaphroditism
Ovotestis
Pseudohermaphroditism (male) (female)
Pure gonadal dysgenesis
Excludes *pseudohermaphroditism:*
female, with adrenocortical disorder (255.2)
male, with gonadal disorder (257.8)
with specified chromosomal anomaly (758.0–758.9)
testicular feminization syndrome (257.8)

● 752.8 **Other specified anomalies of genital organs**
Excludes *congenital hydrocele (778.6)*
penile anomalies (752.61–752.69)
phimosis or paraphimosis (605)
752.81 **Scrotal transposition** ◄
❑752.89 **Other specified anomalies of genital organs** ◄
Absence of: ◄
prostate ◄
spermatic cord ◄
vas deferens ◄
Anorchism ◄
Aplasia (congenital) of: ◄
prostate ◄
round ligament ◄
testicle ◄
Atresia of: ◄
ejaculatory duct ◄
vas deferens ◄
Fusion of testes ◄
Hypoplasia of testis ◄
Monorchism ◄
Polyorchism ◄

❑752.9 **Unspecified anomaly of genital organs**
Congenital:
anomaly NOS of genital organ, NEC
deformity NOS of genital organ, NEC

● 753 **Congenital anomalies of urinary system**
753.0 **Renal agenesis and dysgenesis**
Atrophy of kidney:
congenital
infantile
Congenital absence of kidney(s)
Hypoplasia of kidney(s)

● 753.1 **Cystic kidney disease**
Excludes *acquired cyst of kidney (593.2)*
❑753.10 **Cystic kidney disease, unspecified**
753.11 **Congenital single renal cyst**
❑753.12 **Polycystic kidney, unspecified type**
753.13 **Polycystic kidney, autosomal dominant**
753.14 **Polycystic kidney, autosomal recessive**
753.15 **Renal dysplasia**
753.16 **Medullary cystic kidney**
Nephronophthisis
753.17 **Medullary sponge kidney**
❑753.19 **Other specified cystic kidney disease**
Multicystic kidney

● 753.2 **Obstructive defects of renal pelvis and ureter**
❑753.20 **Unspecified obstructive defect of renal pelvis and ureter**
753.21 **Congenital obstruction of ureteropelvic junction**
753.22 **Congenital obstruction of ureterovesical junction**
Adynamic ureter
Congenital hydroureter
753.23 **Congenital ureterocele**
❑753.29 **Other**

❑753.3 **Other specified anomalies of kidney**
Accessory kidney
Congenital:
calculus of kidney
displaced kidney
Discoid kidney
Double kidney with double pelvis
Ectopic kidney
Fusion of kidneys
Giant kidney
Horseshoe kidney
Hyperplasia of kidney
Lobulation of kidney
Malrotation of kidney
Trifid kidney (pelvis)

❑753.4 **Other specified anomalies of ureter**
Absent ureter
Accessory ureter
Deviaton of ureter
Displaced ureteric orifice
Double ureter
Ectopic ureter
Implantation, anomalous, of ureter

753.5 **Exstrophy of urinary bladder**
Ectopia vesicae
Extroversion of bladder

753.6 **Atresia and stenosis of urethra and bladder neck**
Congenital obstruction:
bladder neck
urethra
Congenital stricture of:
urethra (valvular)
urinary meatus
vesicourethral orifice
Imperforate urinary meatus
Impervious urethra
Urethral valve formation

753.7 **Anomalies of urachus**
Cyst (of) urachus
Fistula (of) urachus
Patent (of) urachus
Persistent umbilical sinus

❑753.8 **Other specified anomalies of bladder and urethra**
Absence, congenital, of:
bladder
urethra
Accessory:
bladder
urethra
Congenital:
diverticulum of bladder
hernia of bladder
Congenital urethrorectal fistula
Congenital prolapse of:
bladder (mucosa)
urethra
Double:
urethra
urinary meatus

❑753.9 **Unspecified anomaly of urinary system**
Congenital:
anomaly NOS of urinary system [any part, except urachus]
deformity NOS of urinary system [any part, except urachus]

● 754 **Certain congenital musculoskeletal deformities**
Includes: nonteratogenic deformities which are considered to be due to intrauterine malposition and pressure

754.0 **Of skull, face, and jaw**
Asymmetry of face
Compression facies
Depressions in skull
Deviation of nasal septum, congenital
Dolichocephaly
Plagiocephaly
Potter's facies
Squashed or bent nose, congenital
Excludes *dentofacial anomalies (524.0–524.9)*
syphilitic saddle nose (090.5)

754.1 **Of sternocleidomastoid muscle**
Congenital sternomastoid torticollis
Congenital wryneck
Contracture of sternocleidomastoid (muscle)
Sternomastoid tumor

754.2 **Of spine**
Congenital postural:
lordosis
scoliosis

● 754.3 **Congenital dislocation of hip**
754.30 **Congenital dislocation of hip, unilateral**
Congenital dislocation of hip NOS

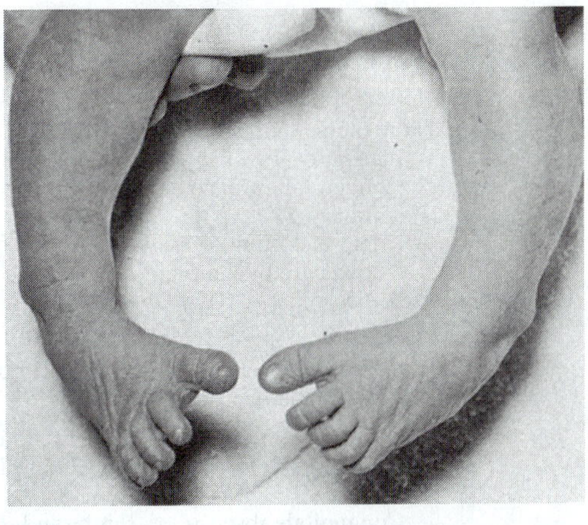

Figure 14–9 Mild to moderate inbowing of the lower leg. (From Jones KL: Smith's Recognizable Patterns of Human Malformation, 4th ed. Philadelphia, WB Saunders, 1988, p 671.)

754.31 **Congenital dislocation of hip, bilateral**
754.32 **Congenital subluxation of hip, unilateral**
Congenital flexion deformity, hip or thigh
Predislocation status of hip at birth
Preluxation of hip, congenital
754.33 **Congenital subluxation of hip, bilateral**
754.35 **Congenital dislocation of one hip with subluxation of other hip**

● 754.4 **Congenital genu recurvatum and bowing of long bones of leg**
754.40 **Genu recurvatum**
754.41 **Congenital dislocation of knee (with genu recurvatum)**
754.42 **Congenital bowing of femur**
754.43 **Congenital bowing of tibia and fibula**
❑754.44 **Congenital bowing of unspecified long bones of leg**

● 754.5 **Varus deformities of feet**
Excludes *acquired (736.71, 736.75, 736.79)*
754.50 **Talipes varus**
Congenital varus deformity of foot, unspecified
Pes varus
754.51 **Talipes equinovarus**
Equinovarus (congenital)
754.52 **Metatarsus primus varus**
754.53 **Metatarsus varus**
❑754.59 **Other**
Talipes calcaneovarus

● 754.6 **Valgus deformities of feet**
Excludes *valgus deformity of foot (acquired) (736.79)*
754.60 **Talipes valgus**
Congenital valgus deformity of foot, unspecified
754.61 **Congenital pes planus**
Congenital rocker bottom flat foot
Flat foot, congenital
Excludes *pes planus (acquired) (734)*
754.62 **Talipes calcaneovalgus**
❑754.69 **Other**
Talipes:
equinovalgus
planovalgus

● 754.7 **Other deformities of feet**
Excludes *acquired (736.70–736.79)*
❑754.70 **Talipes, unspecified**
Congenital deformity of foot NOS
754.71 **Talipes cavus**
Cavus foot (congenital)
❑754.79 **Other**
Asymmetric talipes
Talipes:
calcaneus
equinus

● 754.8 **Other specified nonteratogenic anomalies**
754.81 **Pectus excavatum**
Congenital funnel chest
754.82 **Pectus carinatum**
Congenital pigeon chest [breast]
❑754.89 **Other**
Club hand (congenital)
Congenital:
deformity of chest wall
dislocation of elbow
Generalized flexion contractures of lower limb joints, congenital
Spade-like hand (congenital)

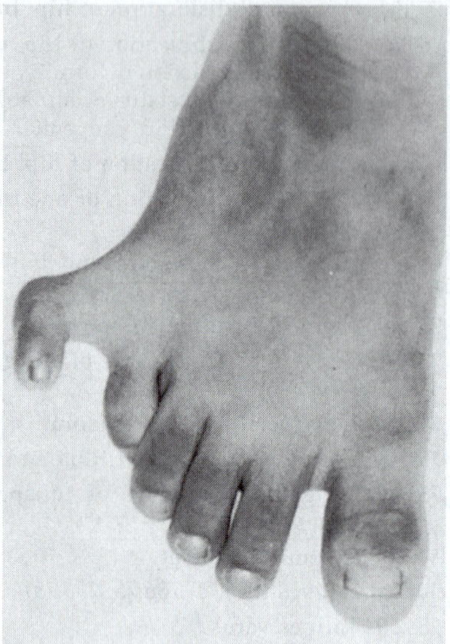

Figure 14–10 Polydactyly. (From Tachdjian MO: Pediatric Orthopedics, 2nd ed, Vol 4. Philadelphia, WB Saunders, 1990, p 2644.)

● 755 **Other congenital anomalies of limbs**

Excludes *those deformities classifiable to 754.0–754.8*

● 755.0 **Polydactyly**

❑ 755.00 **Polydactyly, unspecified digits**
Supernumerary digits

755.01 **Of fingers**
Accessory fingers

755.02 **Of toes**
Accessory toes

● 755.1 **Syndactyly**
Symphalangy
Webbing of digits

❑ 755.10 **Of multiple and unspecified sites**

755.11 **Of fingers without fusion of bone**

755.12 **Of fingers with fusion of bone**

755.13 **Of toes without fusion of bone**

755.14 **Of toes with fusion of bone**

● 755.2 **Reduction deformities of upper limb**

❑ 755.20 **Unspecified reduction deformity of upper limb**
Ectromelia NOS of upper limb
Hemimelia NOS of upper limb
Shortening of arm, congenital

755.21 **Transverse deficiency of upper limb**
Amelia of upper limb
Congenital absence of:
fingers, all (complete or partial)
forearm, including hand and fingers
upper limb, complete
Congenital amputation of upper limb
Transverse hemimelia of upper limb

755.22 **Longitudinal deficiency of upper limb, NEC**
Phocomelia NOS of upper limb
Rudimentary arm

755.23 **Longitudinal deficiency, combined, involving humerus, radius, and ulna (complete or incomplete)**
Congenital absence of arm and forearm (complete or incomplete) with or without metacarpal deficiency and/or phalangeal deficiency, incomplete
Phocomelia, complete, of upper limb

755.24 **Longitudinal deficiency, humeral, complete or partial (with or without distal deficiencies, incomplete)**
Congenital absence of humerus (with or without absence of some [but not all] distal elements)
Proximal phocomelia of upper limb

755.25 **Longitudinal deficiency, radioulnar, complete or partial (with or without distal deficiencies, incomplete)**
Congenital absence of radius and ulna (with or without absence of some [but not all] distal elements)
Distal phocomelia of upper limb

755.26 **Longitudinal deficiency, radial, complete or partial (with or without distal deficiencies, incomplete)**
Agenesis of radius
Congenital absence of radius (with or without absence of some [but not all] distal elements)

755.27 **Longitudinal deficiency, ulnar, complete or partial (with or without distal deficiencies, incomplete)**
Agenesis of ulna
Congenital absence of ulna (with or without absence of some [but not all] distal elements)

755.28 **Longitudinal deficiency, carpals or metacarpals, complete or partial (with or without incomplete phalangeal deficiency)**

755.29 **Longitudinal deficiency, phalanges, complete or partial**
Absence of finger, congenital
Aphalangia of upper limb, terminal, complete or partial

Excludes *terminal deficiency of all five digits (755.21)*
transverse deficiency of phalanges (755.21)

● 755.3 **Reduction deformities of lower limb**

❑ 755.30 **Unspecified reduction deformity of lower limb**
Ectromelia NOS of lower limb
Hemimelia NOS of lower limb
Shortening of leg, congenital

755.31 **Transverse deficiency of lower limb**
Amelia of lower limb
Congenital absence of:
foot
leg, including foot and toes
lower limb, complete
toes, all, complete
Transverse hemimelia of lower limb

755.32 **Longitudinal deficiency of lower limb, NEC**
Phocomelia NOS of lower limb

755.33 **Longitudinal deficiency, combined, involving femur, tibia, and fibula (complete or incomplete)**
Congenital absence of thigh and (lower) leg (complete or incomplete) with or without metacarpal deficiency and/or phalangeal deficiency, incomplete
Phocomelia, complete, of lower limb

755.34 **Longitudinal deficiency, femoral, complete or partial (with or without distal deficiencies, incomplete)**
Congenital absence of femur (with or without absence of some [but not all] distal elements)
Proximal phocomelia of lower limb

755.35 **Longitudinal deficiency, tibiofibular, complete or partial (with or without distal deficiencies, incomplete)**
Congenital absence of tibia and fibula (with or without absence of some [but not all] distal elements)
Distal phocomelia of lower limb

755.36 **Longitudinal deficiency, tibia, complete or partial (with or without distal deficiencies, incomplete)**
Agenesis of tibia
Congenital absence of tibia (with or without absence of some [but not all] distal elements)

755.37 **Longitudinal deficiency, fibular, complete or partial (with or without distal deficiencies, incomplete)**
Agenesis of fibula
Congenital absence of fibula (with or without absence of some [but not all] distal elements)

755.38 **Longitudinal deficiency, tarsals or metatarsals, complete or partial (with or without incomplete phalangeal deficiency)**

755.39 **Longitudinal deficiency, phalanges, complete or partial**
Absence of toe, congenital
Aphalangia of lower limb, terminal, complete or partial

Excludes *terminal deficiency of all five digits (755.31)*
transverse deficiency of phalanges (755.31)

❑755.4 **Reduction deformities, unspecified limb**
Absence, congenital (complete or partial) of limb NOS
Amelia of unspecified limb
Ectromelia of unspecified limb
Hemimelia of unspecified limb
Phocomelia of unspecified limb

● 755.5 **Other anomalies of upper limb, including shoulder girdle**

❑755.50 **Unspecified anomaly of upper limb**

755.51 **Congenital deformity of clavicle**

755.52 **Congenital elevation of scapula**
Sprengel's deformity

755.53 **Radioulnar synostosis**

755.54 **Madelung's deformity**

755.55 **Acrocephalosyndactyly**
Apert's syndrome

755.56 **Accessory carpal bones**

755.57 **Macrodactylia (fingers)**

755.58 **Cleft hand, congenital**
Lobster-claw hand

❑755.59 **Other**
Cleidocranial dysostosis
Cubitus:
valgus, congenital
varus, congenital

Excludes *club hand (congenital) (754.89)*
congenital dislocation of elbow (754.89)

● 755.6 **Other anomalies of lower limb, including pelvic girdle**

❑755.60 **Unspecified anomaly of lower limb**

755.61 **Coxa valga, congenital**

755.62 **Coxa vara, congenital**

❑755.63 **Other congenital deformity of hip (joint)**
Congenital anteversion of femur (neck)

Excludes *congenital dislocation of hip (754.30–754.35)*

755.64 **Congenital deformity of knee (joint)**
Congenital:
absence of patella
genu valgum [knock-knee]
genu varum [bowleg]
Rudimentary patella

755.65 **Macrodactylia of toes**

❑755.66 **Other anomalies of toes**
Congenital:
hallux valgus
hallux varus
hammer toe

755.67 **Anomalies of foot, NEC**
Astragaloscaphoid synostosis
Calcaneonavicular bar
Coalition of calcaneus
Talonavicular synostosis
Tarsal coalitions

❑755.69 **Other**
Congenital:
angulation of tibia
deformity (of):
ankle (joint)
sacroiliac (joint)
fusion of sacroiliac joint

❑755.8 **Other specified anomalies of unspecified limb**

❑755.9 **Unspecified anomaly of unspecified limb**
Congenital:
anomaly NOS of unspecified limb
deformity NOS of unspecified limb

Excludes *reduction deformity of unspecified limb (755.4)*

● 756 **Other congenital musculoskeletal anomalies**

Excludes *those deformities classifiable to 754.0–754.8*

756.0 **Anomalies of skull and face bones**
Absence of skull bones
Acrocephaly
Congenital deformity of forehead
Craniosynostosis
Crouzon's disease
Hypertelorism
Imperfect fusion of skull
Oxycephaly
Platybasia
Premature closure of cranial sutures
Tower skull
Trigonocephaly

Excludes *acrocephalosyndactyly [Apert's syndrome] (755.55)*
dentofacial anomalies (524.0–524.9)
skull defects associated with brain anomalies, such as:
anencephalus (740.0)
encephalocele (742.0)
hydrocephalus (742.3)
microcephalus (742.1)

● 756.1 **Anomalies of spine**

❑756.10 **Anomaly of spine, unspecified**

756.11 **Spondylolysis, lumbosacral region**
Prespondylolisthesis (lumbosacral)

756.12 **Spondylolisthesis**

756.13 **Absence of vertebra, congenital**

756.14 **Hemivertebra**

756.15 **Fusion of spine [vertebral], congenital**

756.16 **Klippel-Feil syndrome**

756.17 **Spina bifida occulta**

Excludes *spina bifida (aperta) (741.0–741.9)*

❑756.19 **Other**
Platyspondylia
Supernumerary vertebra

756.2 **Cervical rib**
Supernumerary rib in the cervical region

❑756.3 **Other anomalies of ribs and sternum**
Congenital absence of:
rib
sternum
Congenital:
fissure of sternum
fusion of ribs
Sternum bifidum

Excludes *nonteratogenic deformity of chest wall (754.81–754.89)*

756.4 **Chondrodystrophy**
Achondroplasia
Chondrodystrophia (fetalis)
Dyschondroplasia
Enchondromatosis
Ollier's disease

Excludes *lipochondrodystrophy [Hurler's syndrome] (277.5)*
Morquio's disease (277.5)

● 756.5 **Osteodystrophies**

❑756.50 **Osteodystrophy, unspecified**

756.51 **Osteogenesis imperfecta**
Fragilitas ossium
Osteopsathyrosis

756.52 **Osteopetrosis**

756.53 **Osteopoikilosis**

756.54 **Polyostotic fibrous dysplasia of bone**

756.55 **Chondroectodermal dysplasia**
Ellis-van Creveld syndrome

756.56 **Multiple epiphyseal dysplasia**

❑756.59 **Other**
Albright (-McCune)-Sternberg syndrome

756.6 **Anomalies of diaphragm**
Absence of diaphragm
Congenital hernia:
diaphragmatic
foramen of Morgagni
Eventration of diaphragm

Excludes *congenital hiatus hernia (750.6)*

● 756.7 **Anomalies of abdominal wall**

❑756.70 **Anomaly of abdominal wall, unspecified**

756.71 **Prune belly syndrome**
Eagle-Barrett syndrome
Prolapse of bladder mucosa

❑756.79 **Other congenital anomalies of abdominal wall**
Exomphalos
Gastroschisis
Omphalocele

Excludes *umbilical hernia (551–553 with .1)*

● 756.8 **Other specified anomalies of muscle, tendon, fascia, and connective tissue**

756.81 **Absence of muscle and tendon**
Absence of muscle (pectoral)

756.82 **Accessory muscle**

756.83 **Ehlers-Danlos syndrome**

❑756.89 **Other**
Amyotrophia congenita
Congenital shortening of tendon

❑756.9 **Other and unspecified anomalies of musculoskeletal system**
Congenital:
anomaly NOS of musculoskeletal system, NEC
deformity NOS of musculoskeletal system, NEC

● 757 **Congenital anomalies of the integument**

Includes: anomalies of skin, subcutaneous tissue, hair, nails, and breast

Excludes *hemangioma (228.00–228.09)*
pigmented nevus (216.0–216.9)

757.0 **Hereditary edema of legs**
Congenital lymphedema
Hereditary trophedema
Milroy's disease

757.1 **Ichthyosis congenita**
Congenital ichthyosis
Harlequin fetus
Ichthyosiform erythroderma

757.2 **Dermatoglyphic anomalies**
Abnormal palmar creases

● 757.3 **Other specified anomalies of skin**

757.31 **Congenital ectodermal dysplasia**

757.32 **Vascular hamartomas**
Birthmarks
Port-wine stain
Strawberry nevus

757.33 **Congenital pigmentary anomalies of skin**
Congenital poikiloderma
Urticaria pigmentosa
Xeroderma pigmentosum

Excludes *albinism (270.2)*

❑757.39 **Other**
Accessory skin tags, congenital
Congenital scar
Epidermolysis bullosa
Keratoderma (congenital)

Excludes *pilonidal cyst (685.0–685.1)*

❑757.4 **Specified anomalies of hair**
Congenital:
alopecia
atrichosis
beaded hair
hypertrichosis
monilethrix
Persistent lanugo

❑757.5 **Specified anomalies of nails**
Anonychia
Congenital:
clubnail
koilonychia
leukonychia
onychauxis
pachyonychia

❑757.6 **Specified anomalies of breast**
Absent breast or nipple
Accessory breast or nipple
Supernumerary breast or nipple
Hypoplasia of breast
Excludes *absence of pectoral muscle (756.81)*

❑757.8 **Other specified anomalies of the integument**

❑757.9 **Unspecified anomaly of the integument**
Congenital:
anomaly NOS of integument
deformity NOS of integument

● 758 **Chromosomal anomalies**

Includes: syndromes associated with anomalies in the number and form of chromosomes

758.0 **Down's syndrome**
Mongolism
Translocation Down's syndrome
Trisomy:
21 or 22
G

758.1 **Patau's syndrome**
Trisomy:
13
D_1

758.2 **Edwards's syndrome**
Trisomy:
18
E_3

758.3 **Autosomal deletion syndromes**
Antimongolism syndrome
Cri-du-chat syndrome

758.4 **Balanced autosomal translocation in normal individual**

❑758.5 **Other conditions due to autosomal anomalies**
Accessory autosomes, NEC

758.6 **Gonadal dysgenesis**
Ovarian dysgenesis
Turner's syndrome
XO syndrome
Excludes *pure gonadal dysgenesis (752.7)*

758.7 **Klinefelter's syndrome**
XXY syndrome

● 758.8 **Other conditions due to chromosome anomalies**

❑758.81 **Other conditions due to sex chromosome anomalies**

❑758.89 **Other**

❑758.9 **Conditions due to anomaly of unspecified chromosome**

● 759 **Other and unspecified congenital anomalies**

759.0 **Anomalies of spleen**
Aberrant spleen
Absent spleen
Accessory spleen
Congenital splenomegaly
Ectopic spleen
Lobulation of spleen

759.1 **Anomalies of adrenal gland**
Aberrant adrenal gland
Absent adrenal gland
Accessory adrenal gland
Excludes *adrenogenital disorders (255.2)*
congenital disorders of steroid metabolism (255.2)

❑759.2 **Anomalies of other endocrine glands**
Absent parathyroid gland
Accessory thyroid gland
Persistent thyroglossal or thyrolingual duct
Thyroglossal (duct) cyst
Excludes *congenital:*
goiter (246.1)
hypothyroidism (243)

759.3 **Situs inversus**
Situs inversus or transversus:
abdominalis
thoracis
Transposition of viscera:
abdominal
thoracic
Excludes *dextrocardia without mention of complete transposition (746.87)*

759.4 **Conjoined twins**
Craniopagus
Dicephalus
Pygopagus
Thoracopagus
Xiphopagus

759.5 **Tuberous sclerosis**
Bourneville's disease
Epiloia

❑759.6 **Other hamartoses, NEC**
Syndrome:
Peutz-Jeghers
Sturge-Weber (-Dimitri)
von Hippel-Lindau
Excludes *neurofibromatosis (237.7)*

759.7 **Multiple congenital anomalies, so described**
Congenital:
anomaly, multiple NOS
deformity, multiple NOS

● 759.8 **Other specified anomalies**

759.81 **Prader-Willi syndrome**

759.82 **Marfan syndrome**

759.83 **Fragile X syndrome**

❑759.89 **Other**
Congenital malformation syndromes affecting multiple systems, NEC
Laurence-Moon-Biedl syndrome

❑759.9 **Congenital anomaly, unspecified**

15. CERTAIN CONDITIONS ORIGINATING IN THE PERINATAL PERIOD (760–779)

Includes: conditions which have their origin in the perinatal period even though death or morbidity occurs later

Use additional code(s) to further specify condition

MATERNAL CAUSES OF PERINATAL MORBIDITY AND MORTALITY (760–763)

● **760 Fetus or newborn affected by maternal conditions which may be unrelated to present pregnancy**

Includes: the listed maternal conditions only when specified as a cause of mortality or morbidity of the fetus or newborn

Excludes *maternal endocrine and metabolic disorders affecting fetus or newborn (775.0–775.9)*

760.0 Maternal hypertensive disorders
Fetus or newborn affected by maternal conditions classifiable to 642

760.1 Maternal renal and urinary tract diseases
Fetus or newborn affected by maternal conditions classifiable to 580–599

760.2 Maternal infections
Fetus or newborn affected by maternal infectious disease classifiable to 001–136 and 487, but fetus or newborn not manifesting that disease

Excludes *congenital infectious diseases (771.0–771.8)*
maternal genital tract and other localized infections (760.8)

❑ **760.3 Other chronic maternal circulatory and respiratory diseases**
Fetus or newborn affected by chronic maternal conditions classifiable to 390–459, 490–519, 745–748

760.4 Maternal nutritional disorders
Fetus or newborn affected by:
maternal disorders classifiable to 260–269
maternal malnutrition NOS

Excludes *fetal malnutrition (764.10–764.29)*

760.5 Maternal injury
Fetus or newborn affected by maternal conditions classifiable to 800–995

760.6 Surgical operation on mother

Excludes *cesarean section for present delivery (763.4)*
damage to placenta from amniocentesis, cesarean section, or surgical induction (762.1)
previous surgery to uterus or pelvic organs (763.89)

● **760.7 Noxious influences affecting fetus via placenta or breast milk**
Fetus or newborn affected by noxious substance transmitted via placenta or breast milk

Excludes *anesthetic and analgesic drugs administered during labor and delivery (763.5)*
drug withdrawal syndrome in newborn (779.5)

❑ **760.70 Unspecified noxious substance**
Fetus or newborn affected by:
Drug, NEC

760.71 Alcohol
Fetal alcohol syndrome

760.72 Narcotics

760.73 Hallucinogenic agents

760.74 Anti-infectives
Antibiotics

760.75 Cocaine

760.76 Diethylstilbestrol [DES]

❑ **760.79 Other**
Fetus or newborn affected by:
immune sera transmitted via placenta or breast milk
medicinal agents, NEC, transmitted via placenta or breast milk
toxic substance, NEC, transmitted via placenta or breast milk

❑ **760.8 Other specified maternal conditions affecting fetus or newborn**
Maternal genital tract and other localized infection affecting fetus or newborn, but fetus or newborn not manifesting that disease

Excludes *maternal urinary tract infection affecting fetus or newborn (760.1)*

❑ **760.9 Unspecified maternal condition affecting fetus or newborn**

● **761 Fetus or newborn affected by maternal complications of pregnancy**

Includes: the listed maternal conditions only when specified as a cause of mortality or morbidity of the fetus or newborn

761.0 Incompetent cervix

761.1 Premature rupture of membranes

761.2 Oligohydramnios

Excludes *that due to premature rupture of membranes (761.1)*

761.3 Polyhydramnios
Hydramnios (acute) (chronic)

761.4 Ectopic pregnancy
Pregnancy:
abdominal
intraperitoneal
tubal

761.5 Multiple pregnancy
Triplet (pregnancy)
Twin (pregnancy)

761.6 Maternal death

761.7 Malpresentation before labor
Breech presentation before labor
External version before labor
Oblique lie before labor
Transverse lie before labor
Unstable lie before labor

❑ **761.8 Other specified maternal complications of pregnancy affecting fetus or newborn**
Spontaneous abortion, fetus

❑ **761.9 Unspecified maternal complication of pregnancy affecting fetus or newborn**

● **762 Fetus or newborn affected by complications of placenta, cord, and membranes**

Includes: the listed maternal conditions only when specified as a cause of mortality or morbidity in the fetus or newborn

762.0 Placenta previa

❑ **762.1 Other forms of placental separation and hemorrhage**
Abruptio placentae
Antepartum hemorrhage
Damage to placenta from amniocentesis, cesarean section, or surgical induction
Maternal blood loss
Premature separation of placenta
Rupture of marginal sinus

❑ **762.2 Other and unspecified morphological and functional abnormalities of placenta**
Placental:
dysfunction
infarction
insufficiency

762.3 Placental transfusion syndromes
Placental and cord abnormality resulting in twin-to-twin or other transplacental transfusion

Use additional code to indicate resultant condition in fetus or newborn:
fetal blood loss (772.0)
polycythemia neonatorum (776.4)

762.4 Prolapsed cord
Cord presentation

❑ **762.5 Other compression of umbilical cord**
Cord around neck
Entanglement of cord
Knot in cord
Torsion of cord

❑ **762.6 Other and unspecified conditions of umbilical cord**
Short cord
Thrombosis of umbilical cord
Varices of umbilical cord
Velamentous insertion of umbilical cord
Vasa previa

Excludes *infection of umbilical cord (771.4)*
single umbilical artery (747.5)

762.7 Chorioamnionitis
Amnionitis
Membranitis
Placentitis

❑ **762.8 Other specified abnormalities of chorion and amnion**

❑ **762.9 Unspecified abnormality of chorion and amnion**

● **763 Fetus or newborn affected by other complications of labor and delivery**

Includes: the listed conditions only when specified as a cause of mortality or morbidity in the fetus or newborn

763.0 Breech delivery and extraction

❑ **763.1 Other malpresentation, malposition, and disproportion during labor and delivery**
Fetus or newborn affected by:
abnormality of bony pelvis
contracted pelvis
persistent occipitoposterior position
shoulder presentation
transverse lie
conditions classifiable to 652, 653, and 660

763.2 Forceps delivery
Fetus or newborn affected by forceps extraction

763.3 Delivery by vacuum extractor

763.4 Cesarean delivery

Excludes *placental separation or hemorrhage from cesarean section (762.1)*

763.5 Maternal anesthesia and analgesia
Reactions and intoxications from maternal opiates and tranquilizers during labor and delivery

Excludes *drug withdrawal syndrome in newborn (779.5)*

763.6 Precipitate delivery
Rapid second stage

763.7 Abnormal uterine contractions
Fetus or newborn affected by:
contraction ring
hypertonic labor
hypotonic uterine dysfunction
uterine inertia or dysfunction
conditions classifiable to 661, except 661.3

● **763.8 Other specified complications of labor and delivery affecting fetus or newborn**

763.81 Abnormality in fetal heart rate or rhythm before the onset of labor

763.82 Abnormality in fetal heart rate or rhythm during labor

❑ **763.83 Abnormality in fetal heart rate or rhythm, unspecified as to time of onset**

❑ **763.89 Other specified complications of labor and delivery affecting fetus or newborn**
Fetus or newborn affected by:
abnormality of maternal soft tissues
destructive operation on live fetus to facilitate delivery
induction of labor (medical)
previous surgery to uterus or pelvic organs
other conditions classifiable to 650–669
other procedures used in labor and delivery

❑ **763.9 Unspecified complication of labor and delivery affecting fetus or newborn**

OTHER CONDITIONS ORIGINATING IN THE PERINATAL PERIOD (764–779)

The following fifth-digit subclassification is for use with category 764 and codes 765.0 and 765.1 to denote birthweight:
❑ **0 unspecified [weight]**
1 less than 500 grams
2 500–749 grams
3 750–999 grams
4 1,000–1,249 grams
5 1,250–1,499 grams
6 1,500–1,749 grams
7 1,750–1,999 grams
8 2,000–2,499 grams
9 2,500 grams and over

● **764 Slow fetal growth and fetal malnutrition**

Requires fifth digit. See beginning of section 764–779 for codes and definitions.

● **764.0 "Light-for-dates" without mention of fetal malnutrition**
Infants underweight for gestational age
"Small-for-dates"

● **764.1 "Light-for-dates" with signs of fetal malnutrition**
Infants "light-for-dates" classifiable to 764.0, who in addition show signs of fetal malnutrition, such as dry peeling skin and loss of subcutaneous tissue

● **764.2 Fetal malnutrition without mention of "light-for-dates"**
Infants, not underweight for gestational age, showing signs of fetal malnutrition, such as dry peeling skin and loss of subcutaneous tissue
Intrauterine malnutrition

● ❑ **764.9 Fetal growth retardation, unspecified**
Intrauterine growth retardation

● **765 Disorders relating to short gestation and low birthweight**

Requires fifth digit. See beginning of section 764–779 for codes and definitions.

Includes: the listed conditions, without further specification, as causes of mortality, morbidity, or additional care, in fetus or newborn

● **765.0 Extreme immaturity**

Note: Usually implies a birthweight of less than 1,000 grams

Use additional code for weeks of gestation (765.20–765.29)

● ❑ **765.1 Other preterm infants**

Note: Usually implies birthweight of 1,000–2,499 grams

Prematurity NOS

Prematurity or small size, not classifiable to 765.0 or as "light-for-dates" in 764

Use additional code for weeks of gestation (765.20–765.29)

● **765.2 Weeks of gestation**

❑ **765.20 Unspecified weeks of gestation**

765.21 Less than 24 completed weeks of gestation

765.22 24 completed weeks of gestation

765.23 25–26 completed weeks of gestation

765.24 27–28 completed weeks of gestation

765.25 29–30 completed weeks of gestation

765.26 31–32 completed weeks of gestation

765.27 33–34 completed weeks of gestation

765.28 35–36 completed weeks of gestation

765.29 37 or more completed weeks of gestation

● **766 Disorders relating to long gestation and high birthweight**

Includes: the listed conditions, without further specification, as causes of mortality, morbidity, or additional care, in fetus or newborn

766.0 Exceptionally large baby

Note: Usually implies a birthweight of 4,500 grams or more.

❑ **766.1 Other "heavy-for-dates" infants**

Other fetus or infant "heavy-" or "large-for-dates" regardless of period of gestation

● **766.2 Late infant, not "heavy-for-dates"** ⬅

766.21 Post-term infant ◀

Infant with gestation period over 40 completed weeks to 42 completed weeks ◀

766.22 Prolonged gestation of infant ◀

Infant with gestation period over 42 completed weeks ◀

Postmaturity NOS ◀

● **767 Birth trauma**

767.0 Subdural and cerebral hemorrhage

Subdural and cerebral hemorrhage, whether described as due to birth trauma or to intrapartum anoxia or hypoxia

Subdural hematoma (localized)

Tentorial tear

Use additional code to identify cause

Excludes *intraventricular hemorrhage (772.10–772.14)*
subarachnoid hemorrhage (772.2)

● **767.1 Injuries to scalp**

767.11 Epicranial subaponeurotic hemorrhage (massive) ◀

Subgaleal hemorrhage ◀

❑ **767.19 Other injuries to scalp** ◀

Caput succedaneum ◀

Cephalhematoma ◀

Chignon (from vacuum extraction) ◀

767.2 Fracture of clavicle

❑ **767.3 Other injuries to skeleton**

Fracture of:
- long bones
- skull

Excludes *congenital dislocation of hip (754.30–754.35)*
fracture of spine, congenital (767.4)

767.4 Injury to spine and spinal cord

Dislocation of spine or spinal cord due to birth trauma

Fracture of spine or spinal cord due to birth trauma

Laceration of spine or spinal cord due to birth trauma

Rupture of spine or spinal cord due to birth trauma

767.5 Facial nerve injury

Facial palsy

767.6 Injury to brachial plexus

Palsy or paralysis:
- brachial
- Erb (-Duchenne)
- Klumpke (-Déjérine)

❑ **767.7 Other cranial and peripheral nerve injuries**

Phrenic nerve paralysis

❑ **767.8 Other specified birth trauma**

Eye damage

Hematoma of:
- liver (subcapsular)
- testes
- vulva

Rupture of:
- liver
- spleen

Scalpel wound

Traumatic glaucoma

Excludes *hemorrhage classifiable to 772.0–772.9*

❑ **767.9 Birth trauma, unspecified**

Birth injury NOS

● **768 Intrauterine hypoxia and birth asphyxia**

Use only when associated with newborn morbidity classifiable elsewhere

❑ **768.0 Fetal death from asphyxia or anoxia before onset of labor or at unspecified time**

768.1 Fetal death from asphyxia or anoxia during labor

768.2 Fetal distress before onset of labor, in liveborn infant

Fetal metabolic acidemia before onset of labor, in liveborn infant

768.3 Fetal distress first noted during labor, in liveborn infant

Fetal metabolic acidemia first noted during labor, in liveborn infant

❑ **768.4 Fetal distress, unspecified as to time of onset, in liveborn infant**

Fetal metabolic acidemia unspecified as to time of onset, in liveborn infant

768.5 **Severe birth asphyxia**
Birth asphyxia with neurologic involvement

768.6 **Mild or moderate birth asphyxia**
Other specified birth asphyxia (without mention of neurologic involvement)

❑768.9 **Unspecified birth asphyxia in liveborn infant**
Anoxia NOS, in liveborn infant
Asphyxia NOS, in liveborn infant
Hypoxia NOS, in liveborn infant

769 **Respiratory distress syndrome**
Cardiorespiratory distress syndrome of newborn
Hyaline membrane disease (pulmonary)
Idiopathic respiratory distress syndrome [IRDS or RDS] of newborn
Pulmonary hypoperfusion syndrome

Excludes *transient tachypnea of newborn (770.6)*

● 770 **Other respiratory conditions of fetus and newborn**

770.0 **Congenital pneumonia**
Infective pneumonia acquired prenatally

Excludes *pneumonia from infection acquired after birth (480.0–486)*

770.1 **Meconium aspiration syndrome**
Aspiration of contents of birth canal NOS
Meconium aspiration below vocal cords
Pneumonitis:
fetal aspiration
meconium

770.2 **Interstitial emphysema and related conditions**
Pneumomediastinum originating in the perinatal period
Pneumopericardium originating in the perinatal period
Pneumothorax originating in the perinatal period

770.3 **Pulmonary hemorrhage**
Hemorrhage:
alveolar (lung) originating in the perinatal period
intra-alveolar (lung) originating in the perinatal period
massive pulmonary originating in the perinatal period

770.4 **Primary atelectasis**
Pulmonary immaturity NOS

❑770.5 **Other and unspecified atelectasis**
Atelectasis:
NOS originating in the perinatal period
partial originating in the perinatal period
secondary originating in the perinatal period
Pulmonary collapse originating in the perinatal period

770.6 **Transitory tachypnea of newborn**
Idiopathic tachypnea of newborn
Wet lung syndrome

Excludes *respiratory distress syndrome (769)*

770.7 **Chronic respiratory disease arising in the perinatal period**
Bronchopulmonary dysplasia
Interstitial pulmonary fibrosis of prematurity
Wilson-Mikity syndrome

● ❑770.8 **Other respiratory problems after birth**

770.81 **Primary apnea of newborn**
Apneic spells of newborn NOS
Essential apnea of newborn
Sleep apnea of newborn

770.82 **Other apnea of newborn**
Obstructive apnea of newborn

770.83 **Cyanotic attacks of newborn**

770.84 **Respiratory failure of newborn**

Excludes *respiratory distress syndrome (769)*

❑770.89 **Other respiratory problems after birth**

❑770.9 **Unspecified respiratory condition of fetus and newborn**

● 771 **Infections specific to the perinatal period**

Includes: infections acquired before or during birth or via the umbilicus

Excludes *congenital pneumonia (770.0)*
congenital syphilis (090.0–090.9)
maternal infectious disease as a cause of mortality or morbidity in fetus or newborn, but fetus or newborn not manifesting the disease (760.2)
ophthalmia neonatorum due to gonococcus (098.40)
other infections not specifically classified to this category

771.0 **Congenital rubella**
Congenital rubella pneumonitis

771.1 **Congenital cytomegalovirus infection**
Congenital cytomegalic inclusion disease

❑771.2 **Other congenital infections**
Congenital:
herpes simplex
listeriosis
malaria
toxoplasmosis
tuberculosis

771.3 **Tetanus neonatorum**
Tetanus omphalitis

Excludes *hypocalcemic tetany (775.4)*

771.4 **Omphalitis of the newborn**
Infection:
navel cord
umbilical stump

Excludes *tetanus omphalitis (771.3)*

771.5 **Neonatal infective mastitis**

Excludes *noninfective neonatal mastitis (778.7)*

771.6 **Neonatal conjunctivitis and dacryocystitis**
Ophthalmia neonatorum NOS

Excludes *ophthalmia neonatorum due to gonococcus (098.40)*

771.7 **Neonatal Candida infection**
Neonatal moniliasis
Thrush in newborn

● ❑771.8 **Other infections specific to the perinatal period**
Use additional code to identify organism

771.81 **Septicemia [sepsis] of newborn**

771.82 **Urinary tract infection of newborn**

771.83 **Bacteremia of newborn**

❑771.89 **Other infections specific to the perinatal period**
Intra-amniotic infection of fetus NOS
Infection of newborn NOS

● 772 **Fetal and neonatal hemorrhage**

Excludes *hematological disorders of fetus and newborn (776.0–776.9)*

772.0 **Fetal blood loss**
Fetal blood loss from:
cut end of co-twin's cord
placenta
ruptured cord
vasa previa
Fetal exsanguination
Fetal hemorrhage into:
co-twin
mother's circulation

● 772.1 **Intraventricular hemorrhage**
Intraventricular hemorrhage from any perinatal cause

❑ 772.10 **Unspecified grade**

772.11 **Grade I**
Bleeding into germinal matrix

772.12 **Grade II**
Bleeding into ventricle

772.13 **Grade III**
Bleeding with enlargement of ventricle

772.14 **Grade IV**
Bleeding into cerebral cortex

772.2 **Subarachnoid hemorrhage**
Subarachnoid hemorrhage from any perinatal cause

Excludes *subdural and cerebral hemorrhage (767.0)*

772.3 **Umbilical hemorrhage after birth**
Slipped umbilical ligature

772.4 **Gastrointestinal hemorrhage**

Excludes *swallowed maternal blood (777.3)*

772.5 **Adrenal hemorrhage**

772.6 **Cutaneous hemorrhage**
Bruising in fetus or newborn
Ecchymoses in fetus or newborn
Petechiae in fetus or newborn
Superficial hematoma in fetus or newborn

❑ 772.8 **Other specified hemorrhage of fetus or newborn**

Excludes *hemorrhagic disease of newborn (776.0)*
pulmonary hemorrhage (770.3)

❑ 772.9 **Unspecified hemorrhage of newborn**

● 773 **Hemolytic disease of fetus or newborn, due to isoimmunization**

773.0 **Hemolytic disease due to Rh isoimmunization**
Anemia due to RH:
- antibodies
- isoimmunization
- maternal/fetal incompatibility

Erythroblastosis (fetalis) due to RH:
- antibodies
- isoimmunization
- maternal/fetal incompatibility

Hemolytic disease (fetus) (newborn) due to RH:
- antibodies
- isoimmunization
- maternal/fetal incompatibility

Jaundice due to RH:
- antibodies
- isoimmunization
- maternal/fetal incompatibility

Rh hemolytic disease
Rh isoimmunization

773.1 **Hemolytic disease due to ABO isoimmunization**
ABO hemolytic disease
ABO isoimmunization
Anemia due to ABO:
- antibodies
- isoimmunization
- maternal/fetal incompatibility

Erythroblastosis (fetalis) due to ABO:
- antibodies
- isoimmunization
- maternal/fetal incompatibility

Hemolytic disease (fetus) (newborn) due to ABO:
- antibodies
- isoimmunization
- maternal/fetal incompatibility

Jaundice due to ABO:
- antibodies
- isoimmunization
- maternal/fetal incompatibility

❑ 773.2 **Hemolytic disease due to other and unspecified isoimmunization**
Erythroblastosis (fetalis) (neonatorum) NOS
Hemolytic disease (fetus) (newborn) NOS
Jaundice or anemia due to other and unspecified blood-group incompatibility

773.3 **Hydrops fetalis due to isoimmunization**

Use additional code , if desired, to identify type of isoimmunization (773.0–773.2)

773.4 **Kernicterus due to isoimmunization**

Use additional code , if desired, to identify type of isoimmunization (773.0–773.2)

773.5 **Late anemia due to isoimmunization**

● 774 **Other perinatal jaundice**

● *774.0 Perinatal jaundice from hereditary hemolytic anemias*

Code first underlying disease (282.0–282.9)

❑ 774.1 **Perinatal jaundice from other excessive hemolysis**
Fetal or neonatal jaundice from:
- bruising
- drugs or toxins transmitted from mother
- infection
- polycythemia
- swallowed maternal blood

Use additional code to identify cause

Excludes *jaundice due to isoimmunization (773.0–773.2)*

774.2 **Neonatal jaundice associated with preterm delivery**
Hyperbilirubinemia of prematurity
Jaundice due to delayed conjugation associated with preterm delivery

● 774.3 **Neonatal jaundice due to delayed conjugation from other causes**

❑ 774.30 **Neonatal jaundice due to delayed conjugation, cause unspecified**

● *774.31 Neonatal jaundice due to delayed conjugation in diseases classified elsewhere*

Code first underlying diseases, as:
- congenital hypothyroidism (243)
- Crigler-Najjar syndrome (277.4)
- Gilbert's syndrome (277.4)

❑ 774.39 **Other**
Jaundice due to delayed conjugation from causes, such as:
- breast milk inhibitors
- delayed development of conjugating system

774.4 **Perinatal jaundice due to hepatocellular damage**
Fetal or neonatal hepatitis
Giant cell hepatitis
Inspissated bile syndrome

●❑ *774.5 Perinatal jaundice from other causes*

Code first underlying cause, as:
- congenital obstruction of bile duct (751.61)
- galactosemia (271.1)
- mucoviscidosis (277.00–277.09)

❑ 774.6 **Unspecified fetal and neonatal jaundice**
Icterus neonatorum
Neonatal hyperbilirubinemia (transient)
Physiologic jaundice NOS in newborn

Excludes *that in preterm infants (774.2)*

774.7 Kernicterus not due to isoimmunization
Bilirubin encephalopathy
Kernicterus of newborn NOS

Excludes *kernicterus due to isoimmunization (773.4)*

● **775 Endocrine and metabolic disturbances specific to the fetus and newborn**

Includes: transitory endocrine and metabolic disturbances caused by the infant's response to maternal endocrine and metabolic factors, its removal from them, or its adjustment to extrauterine existence

775.0 Syndrome of "infant of a diabetic mother"
Maternal diabetes mellitus affecting fetus or newborn (with hypoglycemia)

775.1 Neonatal diabetes mellitus
Diabetes mellitus syndrome in newborn infant

775.2 Neonatal myasthenia gravis

775.3 Neonatal thyrotoxicosis
Neonatal hyperthyroidism (transient)

775.4 Hypocalcemia and hypomagnesemia of newborn
Cow's milk hypocalcemia
Hypocalcemic tetany, neonatal
Neonatal hypoparathyroidism
Phosphate-loading hypocalcemia

❑ **775.5 Other transitory neonatal electrolyte disturbances**
Dehydration, neonatal

775.6 Neonatal hypoglycemia

Excludes *infant of mother with diabetes mellitus (775.0)*

775.7 Late metabolic acidosis of newborn

❑ **775.8 Other transitory neonatal endocrine and metabolic disturbances**
Amino-acid metabolic disorders described as transitory

❑ **775.9 Unspecified endocrine and metabolic disturbances specific to the fetus and newborn**

● **776 Hematological disorders of fetus and newborn**

Includes: disorders specific to the fetus or newborn

776.0 Hemorrhagic disease of newborn
Hemorrhagic diathesis of newborn
Vitamin K deficiency of newborn

Excludes *fetal or neonatal hemorrhage (772.0–772.9)*

776.1 Transient neonatal thrombocytopenia
Neonatal thrombocytopenia due to:
exchange transfusion
idiopathic maternal thrombocytopenia
isoimmunization

776.2 Disseminated intravascular coagulation in newborn

❑ **776.3 Other transient neonatal disorders of coagulation**
Transient coagulation defect, newborn

776.4 Polycythemia neonatorum
Plethora of newborn
Polycythemia due to:
donor twin transfusion
maternal-fetal transfusion

776.5 Congenital anemia
Anemia following fetal blood loss

Excludes *anemia due to isoimmunization (773.0–773.2, 773.5)*
hereditary hemolytic anemias (282.0–282.9)

776.6 Anemia of prematurity

776.7 Transient neonatal neutropenia
Isoimmune neutropenia
Maternal transfer neutropenia

Excludes *congenital neutropenia (nontransient) (288.0)*

❑ **776.8 Other specified transient hematological disorders**

❑ **776.9 Unspecified hematological disorder specific to fetus or newborn**

● **777 Perinatal disorders of digestive system**

Includes: disorders specific to the fetus and newborn

Excludes *intestinal obstruction classifiable to 560.0–560.9*

777.1 Meconium obstruction
Congenital fecaliths
Delayed passage of meconium
Meconium ileus NOS
Meconium plug syndrome

Excludes *meconium ileus in cystic fibrosis (277.01)*

777.2 Intestinal obstruction due to inspissated milk

777.3 Hematemesis and melena due to swallowed maternal blood
Swallowed blood syndrome in newborn

Excludes *that not due to swallowed maternal blood (772.4)*

777.4 Transitory ileus of newborn

Excludes *Hirschsprung's disease (751.3)*

777.5 Necrotizing enterocolitis in fetus or newborn
Pseudomembranous enterocolitis in newborn

777.6 Perinatal intestinal perforation
Meconium peritonitis

❑ **777.8 Other specified perinatal disorders of digestive system**

❑ **777.9 Unspecified perinatal disorder of digestive system**

● **778 Conditions involving the integument and temperature regulation of fetus and newborn**

778.0 Hydrops fetalis not due to isoimmunization
Idiopathic hydrops

Excludes *hydrops fetalis due to isoimmunization (773.3)*

778.1 Sclerema neonatorum

778.2 Cold injury syndrome of newborn

❑ **778.3 Other hypothermia of newborn**

❑ **778.4 Other disturbances of temperature regulation of newborn**
Dehydration fever in newborn
Environmentally induced pyrexia
Hyperthermia in newborn
Transitory fever of newborn

❑ **778.5 Other and unspecified edema of newborn**
Edema neonatorum

778.6 Congenital hydrocele
Congenital hydrocele of tunica vaginalis

778.7 Breast engorgement in newborn
Noninfective mastitis of newborn

Excludes *infective mastitis of newborn (771.5)*

❑ **778.8 Other specified conditions involving the integument of fetus and newborn**
Urticaria neonatorum

Excludes *impetigo neonatorum (684)*
pemphigus neonatorum (684)

❑ **778.9 Unspecified condition involving the integument and temperature regulation of fetus and newborn**

● 779 **Other and ill-defined conditions originating in the perinatal period**

779.0 **Convulsions in newborn**
Fits in newborn
Seizures in newborn

❑ 779.1 **Other and unspecified cerebral irritability in newborn**

779.2 **Cerebral depression, coma, and other abnormal cerebral signs**
CNS dysfunction in newborn NOS

779.3 **Feeding problems in newborn**
Regurgitation of food in newborn
Slow feeding in newborn
Vomiting in newborn

779.4 **Drug reactions and intoxications specific to newborn**
Gray syndrome from chloramphenicol administration in newborn

Excludes *fetal alcohol syndrome (760.71)*
reactions and intoxications from maternal opiates and tranquilizers (763.5)

779.5 **Drug withdrawal syndrome in newborn**
Drug withdrawal syndrome in infant of dependent mother

Excludes *fetal alcohol syndrome (760.71)*

779.6 **Termination of pregnancy (fetus)**
Fetal death due to:
induced abortion
termination of pregnancy

Excludes *spontaneous abortion (fetus) (761.8)*

779.7 **Periventricular leukomalacia**

● ❑ 779.8 **Other specified conditions originating in the perinatal period**

779.81 **Neonatal bradycardia**

Excludes *abnormality in fetal heart rate or rhythm complicating labor and delivery (763.81–763.83)*
bradycardia due to birth asphyxia (768.5–768.9)

779.82 **Neonatal tachycardia**

Excludes *abnormality in fetal heart rate or rhythm complicating labor and delivery (763.81–763.83)*

779.83 **Delayed separation of umbilical cord** ◀

❑ 779.89 **Other specified conditions originating in the perinatal period**

❑ 779.9 **Unspecified condition originating in the perinatal period**
Congenital debility NOS
Stillbirth, NEC

16. SYMPTOMS, SIGNS, AND ILL-DEFINED CONDITIONS (780–799)

This section includes symptoms, signs, abnormal results of laboratory or other investigative procedures, and ill-defined conditions regarding which no diagnosis classifiable elsewhere is recorded.

Signs and symptoms that point rather definitely to a given diagnosis are assigned to some category in the preceding part of the classification. In general, categories 780–796 include the more ill-defined conditions and symptoms that point with perhaps equal suspicion to two or more diseases or to two or more systems of the body, and without the necessary study of the case to make a final diagnosis. Practically all categories in this group could be designated as "not otherwise specified," or as "unknown etiology," or as "transient." The Alphabetic Index should be consulted to determine which symptoms and signs are to be allocated here and which to more specific sections of the classification; the residual subcategories numbered .9 are provided for other relevant symptoms which cannot be allocated elsewhere in the classification.

The conditions and signs or symptoms included in categories 780–796 consist of: (a) cases for which no more specific diagnosis can be made even after all facts bearing on the case have been investigated; (b) signs or symptoms existing at the time of initial encounter that proved to be transient and whose causes could not be determined; (c) provisional diagnoses in a patient who failed to return for further investigation or care; (d) cases referred elsewhere for investigation or treatment before the diagnosis was made; (e) cases in which a more precise diagnosis was not available for any other reason; (f) certain symptoms which represent important problems in medical care and which it might be desired to classify in addition to a known cause.

SYMPTOMS (780–789)

● **780 General symptoms**

● **780.0 Alteration of consciousness**

Excludes *coma:*
diabetic (250.2–250.3)
hepatic (572.2)
originating in the perinatal period (779.2)

780.01 Coma

780.02 Transient alteration of awareness

780.03 Persistent vegetative state

❑ **780.09 Other**
Drowsiness
Semicoma
Somnolence
Stupor
Unconsciousness

780.1 Hallucinations
Hallucinations:
NOS
auditory
gustatory
olfactory
tactile

Excludes *those associated with mental disorders, as functional psychoses (295.0–298.9)*
organic brain syndromes (290.0–294.9, 310.0–310.9)
visual hallucinations (368.16)

780.2 Syncope and collapse
Blackout
Fainting
(Near) (Pre)syncope
Vasovagal attack

Excludes *carotid sinus syncope (337.0)*
heat syncope (992.1)
neurocirculatory asthenia (306.2)
orthostatic hypotension (458.0)
shock NOS (785.50)

● **780.3 Convulsions**

Excludes *convulsions:*
epileptic (345.10–345.91)
in newborn (779.0)

780.31 Febrile convulsions
Febrile seizures

❑ **780.39 Other convulsions**
Convulsive disorder NOS
Fits NOS
Seizures NOS

780.4 Dizziness and giddiness
Light-headedness
Vertigo NOS

Excludes *Ménière's disease and other specified vertiginous syndromes (386.0–386.9)*

● **780.5 Sleep disturbances**

Excludes *that of nonorganic origin (307.40–307.49)*

❑ **780.50 Sleep disturbance, unspecified**

780.51 Insomnia with sleep apnea

❑ **780.52 Other insomnia**
Insomnia NOS

780.53 Hypersomnia with sleep apnea

❑ **780.54 Other hypersomnia**
Hypersomnia NOS

780.55 Disruptions of 24-hour sleep-wake cycle
Inversion of sleep rhythm
Irregular sleep-wake rhythm NOS
Non-24-hour sleep-wake rhythm

780.56 Dysfunctions associated with sleep stages or arousal from sleep

❑ **780.57 Other and unspecified sleep apnea**

❑ **780.59 Other**

780.6 Fever
Chills with fever
Fever NOS
Fever of unknown origin (FUO)
Hyperpyrexia NOS
Pyrexia NOS
Pyrexia of unknown origin

Excludes *pyrexia of unknown origin (during):*
in newborn (778.4)
labor (659.2)
the puerperium (672)

● **780.7 Malaise and fatigue**

Excludes *debility, unspecified (799.3)*
fatigue (during):
combat (308.0–308.9)
heat (992.6)
pregnancy (646.8)
neurasthenia (300.5)
senile asthenia (797)

780.71 Chronic fatigue syndrome

❑ **780.79 Other malaise and fatigue**
Asthenia NOS
Lethargy
Postviral (asthenic) syndrome
Tiredness

780.8 Hyperhidrosis
Diaphoresis
Excessive sweating

● **780.9 Other general symptoms**

Excludes *hypothermia:*
NOS (accidental) (991.6)
due to anesthesia (995.89)
memory disturbance as part of a pattern of mental disorder
of newborn (778.2–778.3)

780.91 Fussy infant (baby)

780.92 Excessive crying of infant (baby)

780.93 Memory loss ◀
Amnesia (retrograde) ◀
Memory loss NOS ◀

Excludes *mild memory disturbance due to organic brain damage (310.1)* ◀
transient global amnesia (437.7) ◀

780.94 Early satiety ◀

780.99 Other general symptoms
Chill(s) NOS
Generalized pain
Hypothermia, not associated with low environmental temperature

● **781 Symptoms involving nervous and musculoskeletal systems**

Excludes *depression NOS (311)*
disorders specifically relating to:
back (724.0–724.9)
hearing (388.0–389.9)
joint (718.0–719.9)
limb (729.0–729.9)
neck (723.0–723.9)
vision (368.0–369.9)
pain in limb (729.5)

781.0 Abnormal involuntary movements
Abnormal head movements
Fasciculation
Spasms NOS
Tremor NOS

Excludes *abnormal reflex (796.1)*
chorea NOS (333.5)
infantile spasms (345.60–345.61)
spastic paralysis (342.1, 343.0–344.9)
specified movement disorders classifiable to 333 (333.0–333.9)
that of nonorganic origin (307.2–307.3)

781.1 Disturbances of sensation of smell and taste
Anosmia
Parageusia
Parosmia

781.2 Abnormality of gait
Gait:
ataxic
paralytic
spastic
staggering

Excludes *ataxia:*
NOS (781.3)
locomotor (progressive) (094.0)
difficulty in walking (719.7)

781.3 Lack of coordination
Ataxia NOS
Muscular incoordination

Excludes *ataxic gait (781.2)*
cerebellar ataxia (334.0–334.9)
difficulty in walking (719.7)
vertigo NOS (780.4)

781.4 Transient paralysis of limb
Monoplegia, transient NOS

Excludes *paralysis (342.0–344.9)*

781.5 Clubbing of fingers

781.6 Meningismus
Dupré's syndrome
Meningism

781.7 Tetany
Carpopedal spasm

Excludes *tetanus neonatorum (771.3)*
tetany:
hysterical (300.11)
newborn (hypocalcemic) (775.4)
parathyroid (252.1)
psychogenic (306.0)

781.8 Neurologic neglect syndrome
Asomatognosia
Hemi-akinesia
Hemi-inattention
Hemispatial neglect
Left-sided neglect
Sensory extinction
Sensory neglect
Visuospatial neglect

● **781.9 Other symptoms involving nervous and musculoskeletal systems**

781.91 Loss of height

Excludes *osteoporosis (733.00–733.09)*

781.92 Abnormal posture

781.93 Ocular torticollis

781.94 Facial weakness ◀
Facial droop ◀

Excludes *facial weakness due to late effect of cerebrovascular accident (438.83)* ◀

781.99 Other symptoms involving nervous and musculoskeletal system

● **782 Symptoms involving skin and other integumentary tissue**

Excludes *symptoms relating to breast (611.71–611.79)*

782.0 Disturbance of skin sensation
Anesthesia of skin
Burning or prickling sensation
Hyperesthesia
Hypoesthesia
Numbness
Paresthesia
Tingling

❑ **782.1 Rash and other nonspecific skin eruption**
Exanthem

Excludes *vesicular eruption (709.8)*

782.2 Localized superficial swelling, mass, or lump
Subcutaneous nodules

Excludes *localized adiposity (278.1)*

782.3 Edema
Anasarca
Dropsy
Localized edema NOS

Excludes *ascites (789.5)*
edema of:
newborn NOS (778.5)
pregnancy (642.0–642.9, 646.1)
fluid retention (276.6)
hydrops fetalis (773.3, 778.0)
hydrothorax (511.8)
nutritional edema (260, 262)

❑782.4 **Jaundice, unspecified, not of newborn**
Cholemia NOS
Icterus NOS
Excludes *due to isoimmunization (773.0–773.2, 773.4)*
jaundice in newborn (774.0–774.7)

782.5 **Cyanosis**
Excludes *newborn (770.83)*

●782.6 **Pallor and flushing**

❑782.61 **Pallor**

❑782.62 **Flushing**
Excessive blushing

782.7 **Spontaneous ecchymoses**
Petechiae
Excludes *ecchymosis in fetus or newborn (772.6)*
purpura (287.0–287.9)

782.8 **Changes in skin texture**
Induration of skin
Thickening of skin

❑782.9 **Other symptoms involving skin and integumentary tissues**

●783 **Symptoms concerning nutrition, metabolism, and development**

783.0 **Anorexia**
Loss of appetite
Excludes *anorexia nervosa (307.1)*
loss of appetite of nonorganic origin (307.59)

783.1 **Abnormal weight gain**
Excludes *excessive weight gain in pregnancy (646.1)*
obesity (278.00)
morbid (278.01)

●783.2 **Abnormal loss of weight and underweight**

783.21 **Loss of weight**

783.22 **Underweight**

783.3 **Feeding difficulties and mismanagement**
Feeding problem (elderly) (infant)
Excludes *feeding disturbance or problems:*
in newborn (779.3)
of nonorganic origin (307.50–307.59)

●783.4 **Lack of expected normal physiological development in childhood**
Excludes *delay in sexual development and puberty (259.0)*
gonadal dysgenesis (758.6)
pituitary dwarfism (253.3)
slow fetal growth and fetal malnutrition (764.00–764.99)
specific delays in mental development (315.0–315.9)

❑783.40 **Lack of normal physiological development, unspecified**
Inadequate development
Lack of development

783.41 **Failure to thrive**
Failure to gain weight

783.42 **Delayed milestones**
Late talker
Late walker

783.43 **Short stature**
Growth failure
Growth retardation
Lack of growth
Physical retardation

783.5 **Polydipsia**
Excessive thirst

783.6 **Polyphagia**
Excessive eating
Hyperalimentation NOS
Excludes *disorders of eating of nonorganic origin (307.50–307.59)*

783.7 **Adult failure to thrive**

❑783.9 **Other symptoms concerning nutrition, metabolism, and development**
Hypometabolism
Excludes *abnormal basal metabolic rate (794.7)*
dehydration (276.5)
other disorders of fluid, electrolyte, and acid-base balance (276.0–276.9)

●784 **Symptoms involving head and neck**
Excludes *encephalopathy NOS (348.30)*
specific symptoms involving neck classifiable to 723 (723.0–723.9)

784.0 **Headache**
Facial pain
Pain in head NOS
Excludes *atypical face pain (350.2)*
migraine (346.0–346.9)
tension headache (307.81)

784.1 **Throat pain**
Excludes *dysphagia (787.2)*
neck pain (723.1)
sore throat (462)
chronic (472.1)

784.2 **Swelling, mass, or lump in head and neck**
Space-occupying lesion, intracranial NOS

784.3 **Aphasia**
Excludes *developmental aphasia (315.31)*

●784.4 **Voice disturbance**

❑784.40 **Voice disturbance, unspecified**

784.41 **Aphonia**
Loss of voice

❑784.49 **Other**
Change in voice
Dysphonia
Hoarseness
Hypernasality
Hyponasality

❑784.5 **Other speech disturbance**
Dysarthria
Dysphasia
Slurred speech
Excludes *stammering and stuttering (307.0)*
that of nonorganic origin (307.0, 307.9)

●784.6 **Other symbolic dysfunction**
Excludes *developmental learning delays (315.0–315.9)*

❑784.60 **Symbolic dysfunction, unspecified**

784.61 **Alexia and dyslexia**
Alexia (with agraphia)

❑784.69 **Other**
Acalculia
Agnosia
Agraphia NOS
Apraxia

784.7 **Epistaxis**
Hemorrhage from nose
Nosebleed

784.8 **Hemorrhage from throat**
Excludes *hemoptysis (786.3)*

❑ 784.9 **Other symptoms involving head and neck**
Choking sensation
Halitosis
Mouth breathing
Sneezing

● 785 **Symptoms involving cardiovascular system**
Excludes *heart failure NOS (428.9)*

❑ 785.0 **Tachycardia, unspecified**
Rapid heart beat
Excludes *neonatal tachycardia (779.82)*
paroxysmal tachycardia (427.0–427.2)

785.1 **Palpitations**
Awareness of heart beat
Excludes *specified dysrhythmias (427.0–427.9)*

785.2 **Undiagnosed cardiac murmurs**
Heart murmur NOS

❑ 785.3 **Other abnormal heart sounds**
Cardiac dullness, increased or decreased
Friction fremitus, cardiac
Precordial friction

785.4 **Gangrene**
Gangrene:
NOS
spreading cutaneous
Gangrenous cellulitis
Phagedena
Code first any associated underlying condition
diabetes
Raynaud's syndrome (443.0)
Excludes *gangrene of certain sites—see Alphabetic Index*
gangrene with atherosclerosis of the extremities (440.24)
gas gangrene (040.0)

● 785.5 **Shock without mention of trauma**

❑ 785.50 **Shock, unspecified**
Failure of peripheral circulation

785.51 **Cardiogenic shock**

785.52 **Septic shock** ◄
Code first systemic inflammatory response syndrome due to infectious process with organ dysfunction (995.92) ◄

❑ 785.59 **Other**
Shock:
endotoxic
gram-negative
hypovolemic
Excludes *shock (due to):*
anesthetic (995.4)
anaphylactic (995.0)
due to serum (999.4)
electric (994.8)
following abortion (639.5)
lightning (994.0)
obstetrical (669.1)
postoperative (998.0)
traumatic (958.4)

785.6 **Enlargement of lymph nodes**
Lymphadenopathy
"Swollen glands"
Excludes *lymphadenitis (chronic) (289.1–289.3)*
acute (683)

❑ 785.9 **Other symptoms involving cardiovascular system**
Bruit (arterial)
Weak pulse

● 786 **Symptoms involving respiratory system and other chest symptoms**

● 786.0 **Dyspnea and respiratory abnormalities**

❑ 786.00 **Respiratory abnormality, unspecified**

786.01 **Hyperventilation**
Excludes *hyperventilation, psychogenic (306.1)*

786.02 **Orthopnea**

786.03 **Apnea**
Excludes *apnea of newborn (770.81, 770.82)*
sleep apnea (780.51, 780.53, 780.57)

786.04 **Cheyne-Stokes respiration**

786.05 **Shortness of breath**

786.06 **Tachypnea**
Excludes *transitory tachypnea of newborn (770.6)*

786.07 **Wheezing**
Excludes *asthma (493.00–493.92)*

❑ 786.09 **Other**
Respiratory:
distress
insufficiency
Excludes *respiratory distress:*
following trauma and surgery (518.5)
newborn (770.89)
respiratory failure (518.81, 518.83–518.84)
newborn (770.84)
syndrome (newborn) (769)
adult (518.5)

786.1 **Stridor**
Excludes *congenital laryngeal stridor (748.3)*

786.2 **Cough**
Excludes *cough:*
psychogenic (306.1)
smokers' (491.0)
with hemorrhage (786.3)

786.3 **Hemoptysis**
Cough with hemorrhage
Pulmonary hemorrhage NOS
Excludes *pulmonary hemorrhage of newborn (770.3)*

786.4 **Abnormal sputum**
Abnormal:
amount of sputum
color of sputum
odor of sputum
Excessive sputum

● 786.5 **Chest pain**

❑ 786.50 **Chest pain, unspecified**

786.51 **Precordial pain**

786.52 **Painful respiration**
Pain:
anterior chest wall
pleuritic
pleurodynia
Excludes *epidemic pleurodynia (074.1)*

❑ 786.59 **Other**
Discomfort in chest
Pressure in chest
Tightness in chest
Excludes *pain in breast (611.71)*

786.6 Swelling, mass, or lump in chest

Excludes *lump in breast (611.72)*

786.7 Abnormal chest sounds

Abnormal percussion, chest
Friction sounds, chest
Rales
Tympany, chest

Excludes *wheezing (786.07)*

786.8 Hiccough

Excludes *psychogenic hiccough (306.1)*

❑ **786.9 Other symptoms involving respiratory system and chest**

Breath-holding spell

● **787 Symptoms involving digestive system**

Excludes *constipation (564.00–564.09)*
pylorospasm (537.81)
congenital (750.5)

● **787.0 Nausea and vomiting**

Emesis

Excludes *hematemesis NOS (578.0)*
vomiting:
bilious, following gastrointestinal surgery (564.3)
cyclical (536.2)
psychogenic (306.4)
excessive, in pregnancy (643.0–643.9)
habit (536.2)
of newborn (779.3)
psychogenic NOS (307.54)

787.01 Nausea with vomiting

787.02 Nausea alone

787.03 Vomiting alone

787.1 Heartburn

Pyrosis
Waterbrash

Excludes *dyspepsia or indigestion (536.8)*

787.2 Dysphagia

Difficulty in swallowing

787.3 Flatulence, eructation, and gas pain

Abdominal distention (gaseous)
Bloating
Tympanites (abdominal) (intestinal)

Excludes *aerophagy (306.4)*

787.4 Visible peristalsis

Hyperperistalsis

787.5 Abnormal bowel sounds

Absent bowel sounds
Hyperactive bowel sounds

787.6 Incontinence of feces

Encopresis NOS
Incontinence of sphincter ani

Excludes *that of nonorganic origin (307.7)*

787.7 Abnormal feces

Bulky stools

Excludes *abnormal stool content (792.1)*
melena:
NOS (578.1)
newborn (772.4, 777.3)

● **787.9 Other symptoms involving digestive system**

Excludes *gastrointestinal hemorrhage (578.0–578.9)*
intestinal obstruction (560.0–560.9)
specific functional digestive disorders:
esophagus (530.0–530.9)
stomach and duodenum (536.0–536.9)
those not elsewhere classified (564.00–564.9)

787.91 Diarrhea

Diarrhea NOS

787.99 Other

Change in bowel habits
Tenesmus (rectal)

● **788 Symptoms involving urinary system**

Excludes *hematuria (599.7)*
nonspecific findings on examination of the urine (791.0–791.9)
small kidney of unknown cause (589.0–589.9)
uremia NOS (586)

788.0 Renal colic

Colic (recurrent) of:
kidney
ureter

788.1 Dysuria

Painful urination
Strangury

● **788.2 Retention of urine**

❑ **788.20 Retention of urine, unspecified**

788.21 Incomplete bladder emptying

❑ **788.29 Other specified retention of urine**

● **788.3 Incontinence of urine**

Excludes *that of nonorganic origin (307.6)*

Code, if applicable, any causal condition first, such as:
congenital ureterocele (753.23)
genital prolapse (618.0–618.9)

❑ **788.30 Urinary incontinence, unspecified**

Enuresis NOS

788.31 Urge incontinence

788.32 Stress incontinence, male

Excludes *stress incontinence, female (625.6)*

788.33 Mixed incontinence (female) (male)

Urge and stress

788.34 Incontinence without sensory awareness

788.35 Post-void dribbling

788.36 Nocturnal enuresis

788.37 Continuous leakage

❑ **788.39 Other urinary incontinence**

● **788.4 Frequency of urination and polyuria**

788.41 Urinary frequency

Frequency of micturition

788.42 Polyuria

788.43 Nocturia

788.5 Oliguria and anuria

Deficient secretion of urine
Suppression of urinary secretion

Excludes *that complicating:*
abortion (634–638 with .3, 639.3)
ectopic or molar pregnancy (639.3)
pregnancy, childbirth, or the puerperium (642.0–642.9, 646.2)

● **788.6 Other abnormality of urination**

788.61 Splitting of urinary stream

Intermittent urinary stream

788.62 Slowing of urinary stream

Weak stream

788.63 Urgency of urination ◀

Excludes *urge incontinence (788.31, 788.33)*

❑ **788.69 Other**

788.7 **Urethral discharge**
Penile discharge
Urethrorrhea

788.8 **Extravasation of urine**

❑ 788.9 **Other symptoms involving urinary system**
Extrarenal uremia
Vesical:
pain
tenesmus

● 789 **Other symptoms involving abdomen and pelvis**

The following fifth-digit subclassification is to be used for codes 789.0, 789.3, 789.4, 789.6

❑ 0 **unspecified site**
1 **right upper quadrant**
2 **left upper quadrant**
3 **right lower quadrant**
4 **left lower quadrant**
5 **periumbilic**
6 **epigastric**
❑ 7 **generalized**
❑ 9 **other specified site**
multiple sites

Excludes *symptoms referable to genital organs:*
female (625.0–625.9)
male (607.0–608.9)
psychogenic (302.70–302.79)

● 789.0 **Abdominal pain**
Colic:
NOS
infantile
Cramps, abdominal

Excludes *renal colic (788.0)*

789.1 **Hepatomegaly**
Enlargement of liver

789.2 **Splenomegaly**
Enlargement of spleen

● 789.3 **Abdominal or pelvic swelling, mass, or lump**
Diffuse or generalized swelling or mass:
abdominal NOS
umbilical

Excludes *abdominal distention (gaseous) (787.3)*
ascites (789.5)

● 789.4 **Abdominal rigidity**

789.5 **Ascites**
Fluid in peritoneal cavity

● 789.6 **Abdominal tenderness**
Rebound tenderness

❑ 789.9 **Other symptoms involving abdomen and pelvis**
Umbilical:
bleeding
discharge

NONSPECIFIC ABNORMAL FINDINGS (790–796)

● 790 **Nonspecific findings on examination of blood**

Excludes *abnormality of:*
platelets (287.0–287.9)
thrombocytes (287.0–287.9)
white blood cells (288.0–288.9)

● 790.0 **Abnormality of red blood cells**

Excludes *anemia:*
congenital (776.5)
newborn, due to isoimmunization (773.0–773.2, 773.5)
of premature infant (776.6)
other specified types (280.0–285.9)
hemoglobin disorders (282.5–282.7)
polycythemia:
familial (289.6)
neonatorum (776.4)
secondary (289.0)
vera (238.4)

790.01 **Precipitous drop in hematocrit**
Drop in hematocrit

❑ 790.09 **Other abnormality of red blood cells**
Abnormal red cell morphology NOS
Abnormal red cell volume NOS
Anisocytosis
Poikilocytosis

❑ 790.1 **Elevated sedimentation rate**

● 790.2 **Abnormal glucose** ⇐

Excludes *diabetes mellitus (250.00–250.93)* ◄
dysmetabolic syndrome X (277.7) ◄
gestational diabetes (648.8) ◄
glycosuria (791.5) ◄
hypoglycemia (251.2) ◄
that complicating pregnancy, childbirth or the puerperium (648.8)

790.21 **Impaired fasting glucose** ◄
Elevated fasting glucose ◄

790.22 **Impaired glucose tolerance test (oral)** ◄
Elevated glucose tolerance test ◄

790.29 **Other abnormal glucose** ◄
Abnormal glucose NOS ◄
Abnormal non-fasting glucose ◄
Pre-diabetes NOS ◄

790.3 **Excessive blood level of alcohol**
Elevated blood-alcohol

❑ 790.4 **Nonspecific elevation of levels of transaminase or lactic acid dehydrogenase [LDH]**

❑ 790.5 **Other nonspecific abnormal serum enzyme levels**
Abnormal serum level of:
acid phosphatase
alkaline phosphatase
amylase
lipase

Excludes *deficiency of circulating enzymes (277.6)*

❑ 790.6 **Other abnormal blood chemistry**
Abnormal blood levels of:
cobalt
copper
iron
lithium
magnesium
mineral
zinc

Excludes *abnormality of electrolyte or acid-base balance (276.0–276.9)*
hypoglycemia NOS (251.2)
specific finding indicating abnormality of:
amino-acid transport and metabolism (270.0–270.9)
carbohydrate transport and metabolism (271.0–271.9)
lipid metabolism (272.0–272.9)
uremia NOS (586)

790.7 **Bacteremia**

Excludes *bacteremia of newborn (771.83)*
septicemia (038)

Use additional code to identify organism (041)

❑ 790.8 **Viremia, unspecified**

● 790.9 **Other nonspecific findings on examination of blood**

❑ 790.91 **Abnormal arterial blood gases**

❑ 790.92 **Abnormal coagulation profile**
Abnormal or prolonged:
bleeding time
coagulation time
partial thromboplastin time [PTT]
prothrombin time [PT]
Excludes *coagulation (hemorrhagic) disorders (286.0–286.9)*

790.93 **Elevated prostate specific antigen [PSA]**

790.94 **Euthyroid sick syndrome**

❑ 790.99 **Other**

● 791 **Nonspecific findings on examination of urine**
Excludes *hematuria NOS (599.7)*
specific findings indicating abnormality of:
amino-acid transport and metabolism (270.0–270.9)
carbohydrate transport and metabolism (271.0–271.9)

791.0 **Proteinuria**
Albuminuria
Bence-Jones proteinuria
Excludes *postural proteinuria (593.6)*
that arising during pregnancy or the puerperium (642.0–642.9, 646.2)

791.1 **Chyluria**
Excludes *filarial (125.0–125.9)*

791.2 **Hemoglobinuria**

791.3 **Myoglobinuria**

791.4 **Biliuria**

791.5 **Glycosuria**
Excludes *renal glycosuria (271.4)*

791.6 **Acetonuria**
Ketonuria

❑ 791.7 **Other cells and casts in urine**

● ❑ 791.9 **Other nonspecific findings on examination of urine**
Crystalluria
Elevated urine levels of:
17-ketosteroids
catecholamines
indolacetic acid
vanillylmandelic acid [VMA]
Melanuria

● 792 **Nonspecific abnormal findings in other body substances**
Excludes *that in chromosomal analysis (795.2)*

792.0 **Cerebrospinal fluid**

792.1 **Stool contents**
Abnormal stool color
Fat in stool
Mucus in stool
Occult blood
Pus in stool
Excludes *blood in stool [melena] (578.1)*
newborn (772.4, 777.3)

792.2 **Semen**
Abnormal spermatozoa
Excludes *azoospermia (606.0)*
oligospermia (606.1)

792.3 **Amniotic fluid**

792.4 **Saliva**
Excludes *that in chromosomal analysis (795.2)*

792.5 **Cloudy (hemodialysis) (peritoneal) dialysis effluent**

❑ 792.9 **Other nonspecific abnormal findings in body substances**
Peritoneal fluid
Pleural fluid
Synovial fluid
Vaginal fluids

● 793 **Nonspecific abnormal findings on radiological and other examination of body structure**
Includes: nonspecific abnormal findings of:
thermography
ultrasound examination [echogram]
x-ray examination
Excludes *abnormal results of function studies and radioisotope scans (794.0–794.9)*

793.0 **Skull and head**
Excludes *nonspecific abnormal echoencephalogram (794.01)*

793.1 **Lung field**
Coin lesion lung
Shadow, lung

❑ 793.2 **Other intrathoracic organ**
Abnormal:
echocardiogram
heart shadow
ultrasound cardiogram
Mediastinal shift

793.3 **Biliary tract**
Nonvisualization of gallbladder

793.4 **Gastrointestinal tract**

793.5 **Genitourinary organs**
Filling defect:
bladder
kidney
ureter

793.6 **Abdominal area, including retroperitoneum**

793.7 **Musculoskeletal system**

● 793.8 **Breast**

❑ 793.80 **Abnormal mammogram, unspecified**

793.81 **Mammographic microcalcification**

❑ 793.89 **Other abnormal findings on radiological examination of breast**

❑ 793.9 **Other**
Abnormal:
placental finding by x-ray or ultrasound method
radiological findings in skin and subcutaneous tissue
Excludes *abnormal finding by radioisotope localization of placenta (794.9)*

● 794 **Nonspecific abnormal results of function studies**
Includes: radioisotope:
scans
uptake studies
scintiphotography

● 794.0 **Brain and central nervous system**

❑ 794.00 **Abnormal function study, unspecified**

794.01 **Abnormal echoencephalogram**

794.02 **Abnormal electroencephalogram [EEG]**

❑ 794.09 **Other**
Abnormal brain scan

● 794.1 **Peripheral nervous system and special senses**

❑ 794.10 **Abnormal response to nerve stimulation, unspecified**

794.11 **Abnormal retinal function studies**
Abnormal electroretinogram [ERG]

794.12 **Abnormal electro-oculogram [EOG]**

794.13 **Abnormal visually evoked potential**

794.14 **Abnormal oculomotor studies**

794.15 **Abnormal auditory function studies**

794.16 **Abnormal vestibular function studies**

794.17 **Abnormal electromyogram [EMG]**

Excludes *that of eye (794.14)*

❑ 794.19 **Other**

794.2 **Pulmonary**
Abnormal lung scan
Reduced:
ventilatory capacity
vital capacity

● 794.3 **Cardiovascular**

❑ 794.30 **Abnormal function study, unspecified**

794.31 **Abnormal electrocardiogram [ECG] [EKG]**

❑ 794.39 **Other**
Abnormal:
ballistocardiogram
phonocardiogram
vectorcardiogram

794.4 **Kidney**
Abnormal renal function test

794.5 **Thyroid**
Abnormal thyroid:
scan
uptake

❑ 794.6 **Other endocrine function study**

794.7 **Basal metabolism**
Abnormal basal metabolic rate [BMR]

794.8 **Liver**
Abnormal liver scan

❑ 794.9 **Other**
Bladder
Pancreas
Placenta
Spleen

● 795 **Nonspecific abnormal histological and immunological findings**

Excludes *nonspecific abnormalities of red blood cells (790.01–790.09)*

● ❑ 795.0 **Nonspecific abnormal Papanicolaou smear of cervix**

Excludes *carcinoma in-situ of cervix (233.1)*
cervical intraepithelial neoplasia I (CIN I) (622.1)
cervical intraepithelial neoplasia II (CIN II) (622.1)
cervical intraepithelial neoplasia III (CIN III) (233.1)
dysplasia of cervix (uteri) (622.1)
high grade squamous intraepithelial dysplasia (HGSIL) (622.1)
low grade squamous intraepithelial dysplasia (LGSIL) (622.1)

❑ 795.00 **Nonspecific abnormal Papanicolaou smear of cervix unspecified**

795.01 **Atypical squamous cell changes of undetermined significance favor benign (ASCUS favor benign)**
Atypical glandular cell changes of undetermined significance favor benign (AGCUS favor benign)

795.02 **Atypical squamous cell changes of undetermined significance favor dysplasia (ASCUS) favor dysplasia)**
Atypical glandular cell changes of undetermined signifance favor dysplasia (AGCUS favor dysplasia)

❑ 795.09 **Other nonspecific abnormal Papanicolaou smear of cervix**
Benign cellular changes
Unsatisfactory smear

❑ 795.1 **Nonspecific abnormal Papanicolaou smear of other site**

❑ 795.2 **Nonspecific abnormal findings on chromosomal analysis**
Abnormal karyotype

● ❑ 795.3 **Nonspecific positive culture findings**
Positive culture findings in:
nose
sputum
throat
wound

Excludes *that of:*
blood (790.7–790.8)
urine (791.9)

795.31 **Nonspecific positive findings for anthrax**
Positive findings by nasal swab

❑ 795.39 **Other nonspecific positive culture findings**

❑ 795.4 **Other nonspecific abnormal histological findings**

❑ 795.5 **Nonspecific reaction to tuberculin skin test without active tuberculosis**
Abnormal result of Mantoux test
PPD positive
Tuberculin (skin test):
positive
reactor

795.6 **False positive serological test for syphilis**
False positive Wassermann reaction

● 795.7 **Other nonspecific immunological findings**

Excludes *isoimmunization, in pregnancy (656.1–656.2)*
affecting fetus or newborn (773.0–773.2)

❑ 795.71 **Nonspecific serologic evidence of human immunodeficiency virus [HIV]**
Inconclusive human immunodeficiency virus [HIV] test (adult) (infant)

Note: This code is ONLY to be used when a test finding is reported as nonspecific. Asymptomatic positive findings are coded to V08. If any HIV infection symptom or condition is present, see code 042. Negative findings are not coded.

Excludes *acquired immunodeficiency syndrome [AIDS] (042)*
asymptomatic human immunodeficiency virus [HIV] infection status (V08)
HIV infection, symptomatic (042)
human immunodeficiency virus [HIV] disease (042)
positive (status) NOS (V08)

❑ 795.79 **Other and unspecified nonspecific immunological findings**
Raised antibody titer
Raised level of immunoglobulins

● 796 **Other nonspecific abnormal findings**

❑ 796.0 **Nonspecific abnormal toxicological findings**
Abnormal levels of heavy metals or drugs in blood, urine, or other tissue

Excludes *excessive blood level of alcohol (790.3)*

796.1 **Abnormal reflex**

796.2 **Elevated blood pressure reading without diagnosis of hypertension**

Note: This category is to be used to record an episode of elevated blood pressure in a patient in whom no formal diagnosis of hypertension has been made, or as an incidental finding.

❑ **796.3 Nonspecific low blood pressure reading**

❑ **796.4 Other abnormal clinical findings**

❑ **796.5 Abnormal finding on antenatal screening**

❑ **796.9 Other**

ILL-DEFINED AND UNKNOWN CAUSES OF MORBIDITY AND MORTALITY (797–799)

797 Senility without mention of psychosis

Old age
Senescence
Senile asthenia
Senile:
debility
exhaustion

Excludes *senile psychoses (290.0–290.9)*

● **798 Sudden death, cause unknown**

798.0 Sudden infant death syndrome

Cot death
Crib death
Sudden death of nonspecific cause in infancy

● **798.1 Instantaneous death**

● **798.2 Death occurring in less than 24 hours from onset of symptoms, not otherwise explained**

Death known not to be violent or instantaneous, for which no cause could be discovered
Died without sign of disease

● **798.9 Unattended death**

Death in circumstances where the body of the deceased was found and no cause could be discovered
Found dead

● **799 Other ill-defined and unknown causes of morbidity and mortality**

799.0 Asphyxia

Excludes *asphyxia (due to):*
carbon monoxide (986)
inhalation of food or foreign body (932–934.9)
newborn (768.0–768.9)
traumatic (994.7)

799.1 Respiratory arrest

Cardiorespiratory failure

Excludes *cardiac arrest (427.5)*
failure of peripheral circulation (785.50)
respiratory distress:
NOS (786.09)
acute (518.82)
following trauma or surgery (518.5)
newborn (770.89)
syndrome (newborn) (769)
adult (following trauma or surgery) (518.5)
other (518.82)
respiratory failure (518.81, 518.83–518.84)
newborn (770.84)
respiratory insufficiency (786.09)
acute (518.82)

799.2 Nervousness

"Nerves"

❑ **799.3 Debility, unspecified**

Excludes *asthenia (780.79)*
nervous debility (300.5)
neurasthenia (300.5)
senile asthenia (797)

799.4 Cachexia

Wasting disease

Excludes *nutritional marasmus (261)*

● **799.8 Other ill-defined conditions**

799.81 Decreased libido ◀

Decreased sexual desire ◀

Excludes *psychosexual dysfunction with inhibited sexual desire (302.71)* ◀

❑ **799.89 Other ill-defined conditions** ◀

❑ **799.9 Other unknown and unspecified cause**

Undiagnosed disease, not specified as to site or system involved
Unknown cause of morbidity or mortality

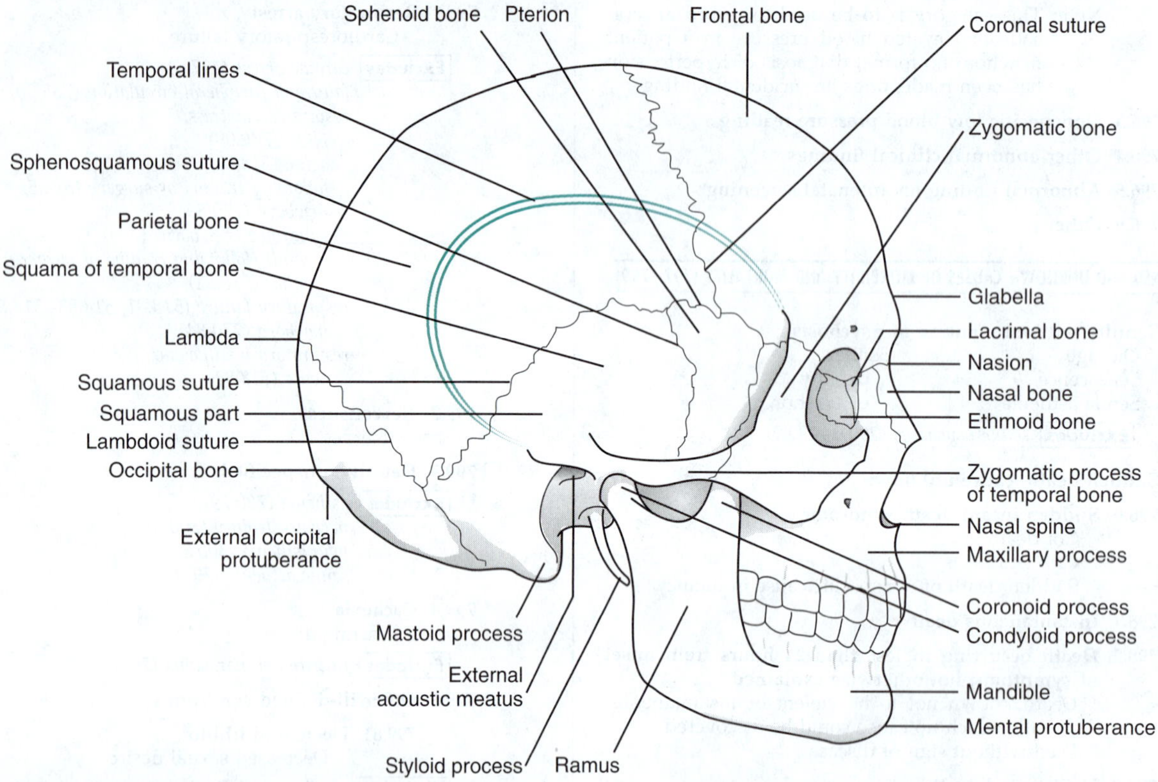

Figure 17–1 Lateral view of skull.

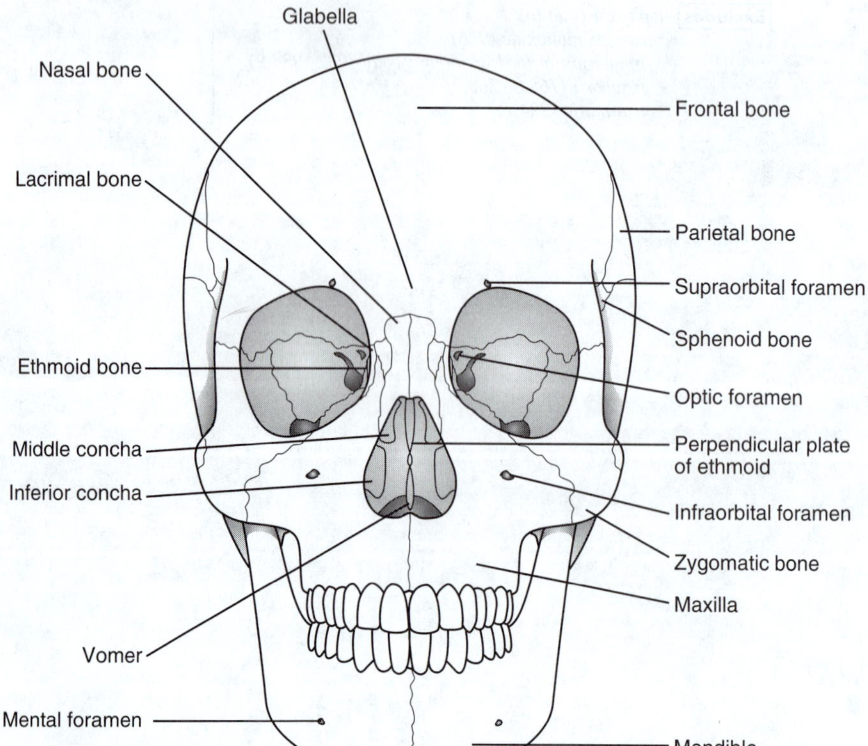

Figure 17–2 Frontal view of skull.

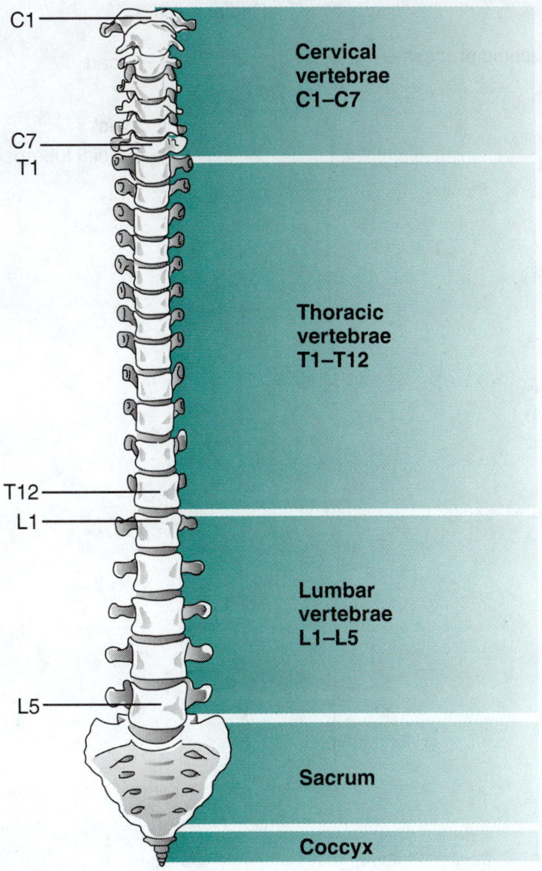

Figure 17–3 Anterior view of vertebral column.

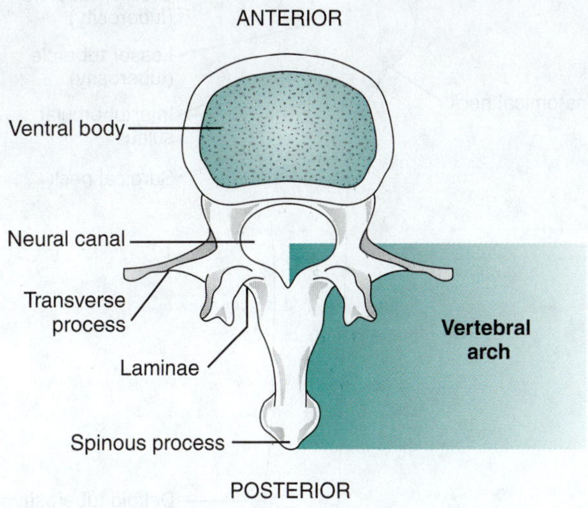

Figure 17–4 Vertebra viewed from above.

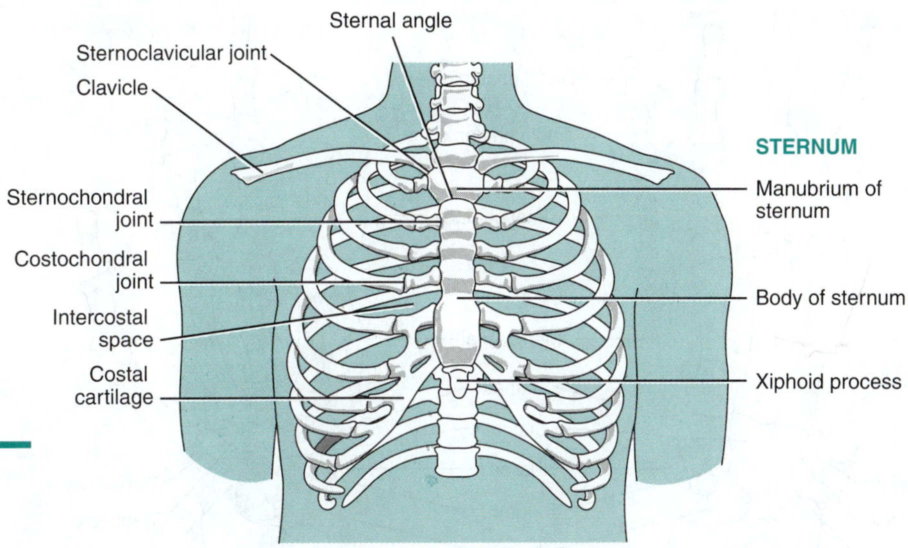

Figure 17–5 Anterior view of rib cage.

ICD-9-CM
800-899
Vol. 1

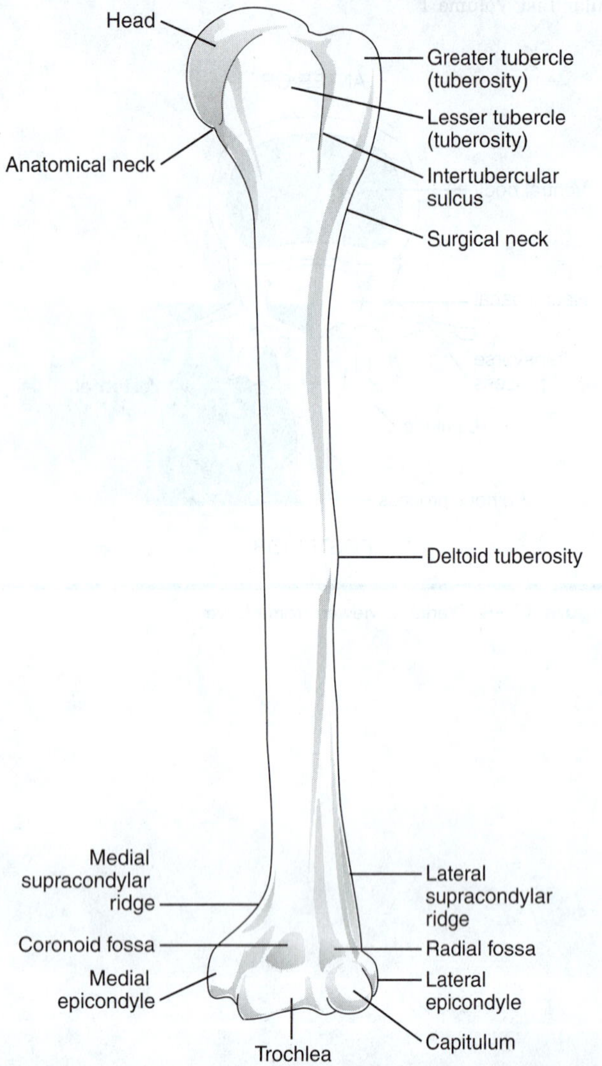

Figure 17–6 Anterior aspect of left humerus.

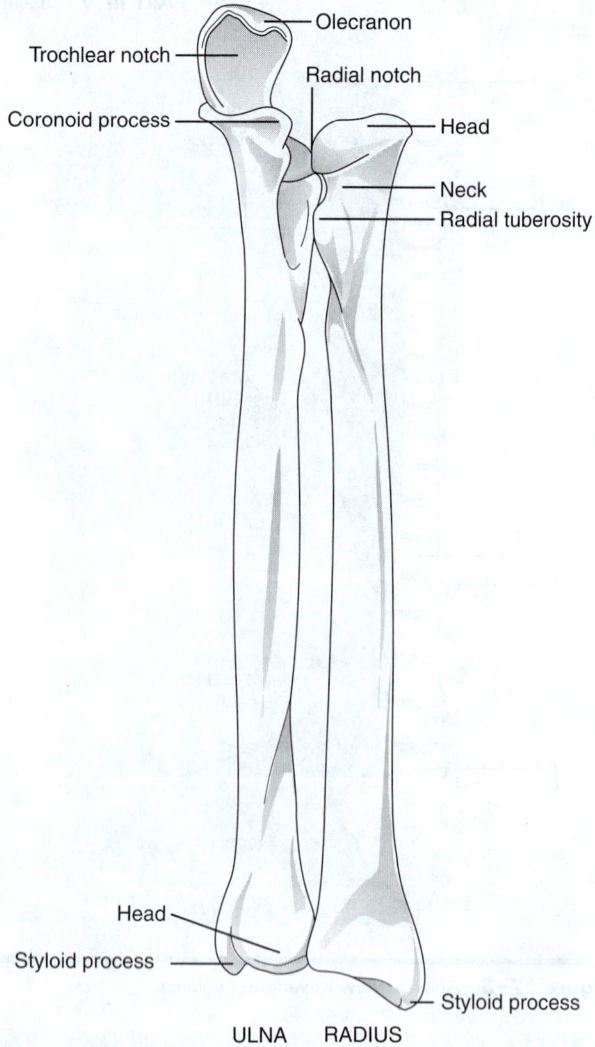

Figure 17–7 Anterior aspect of left radius and ulna.

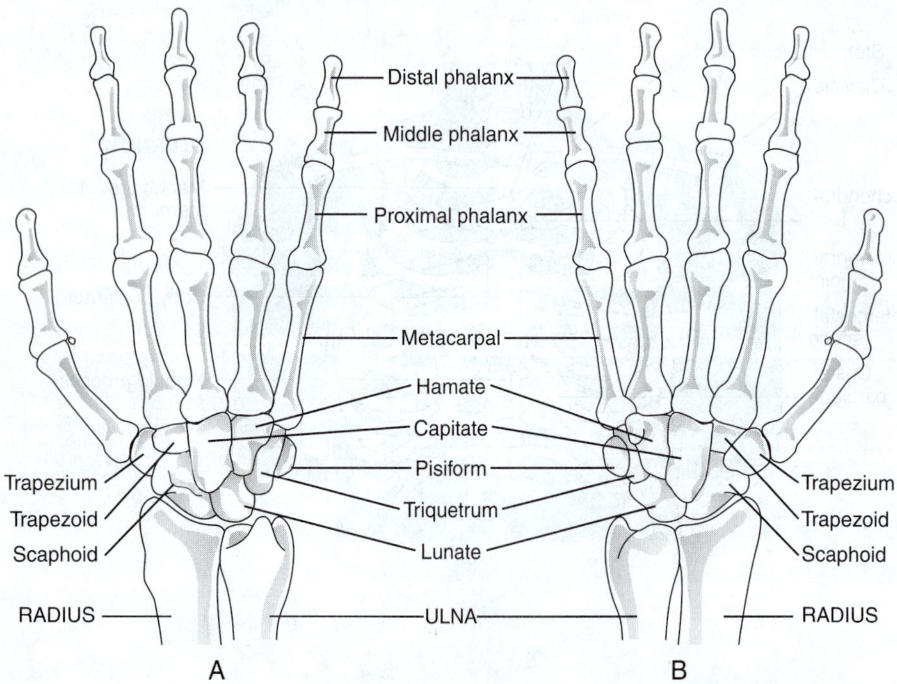

Figure 17–8 Right hand and wrist: **A.** Dorsal surface. **B.** Palmar surface.

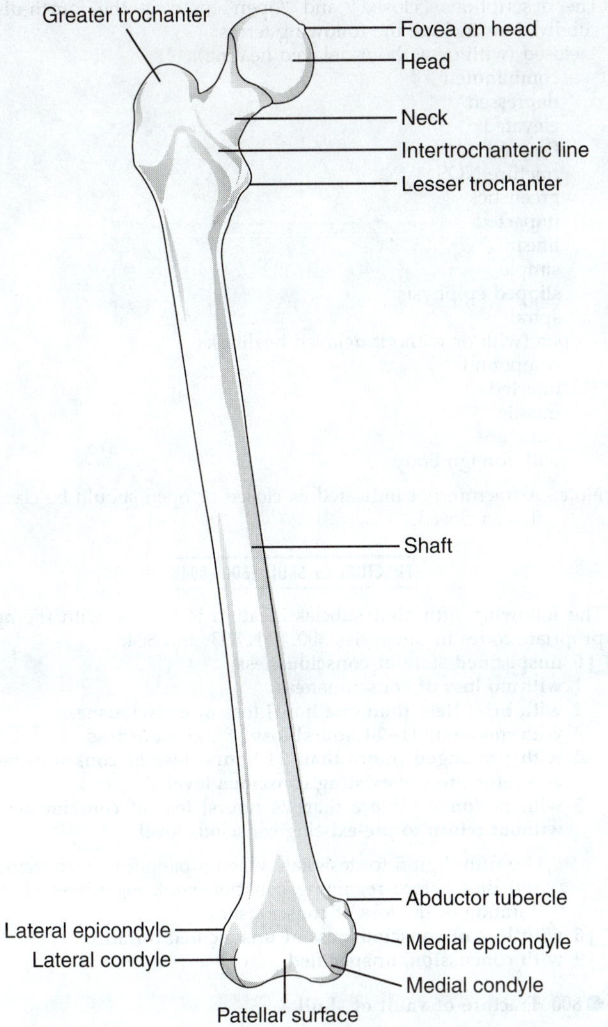

Figure 17–9 Anterior aspect of right femur.

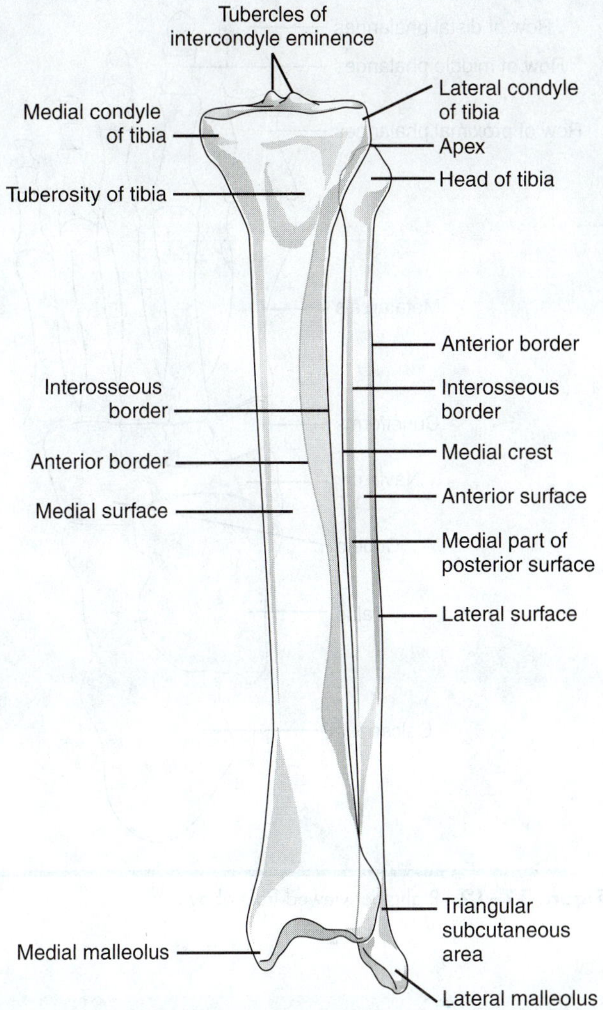

Figure 17–10 Anterior aspect of left tibia and fibula.

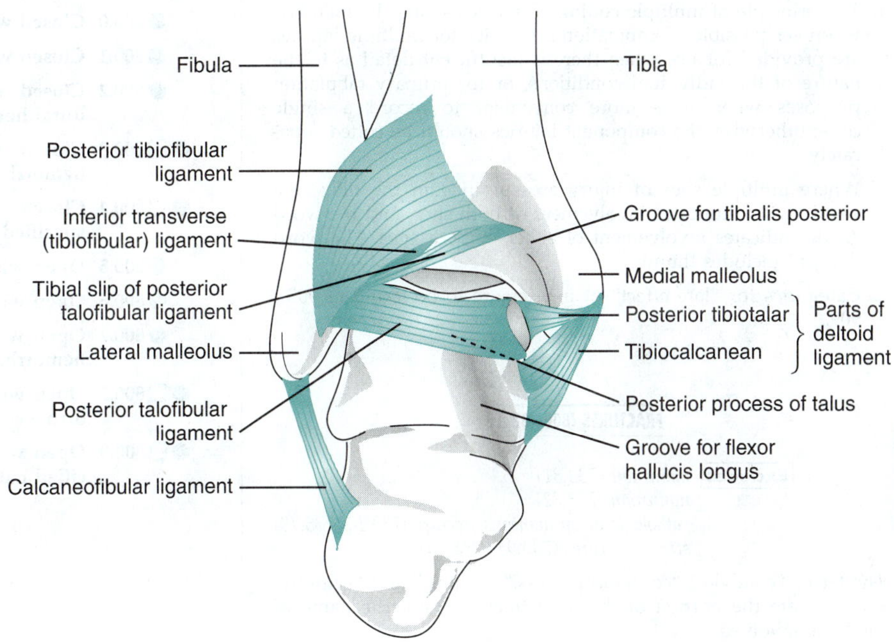

Figure 17–11 Posterior aspect of the left ankle joint.

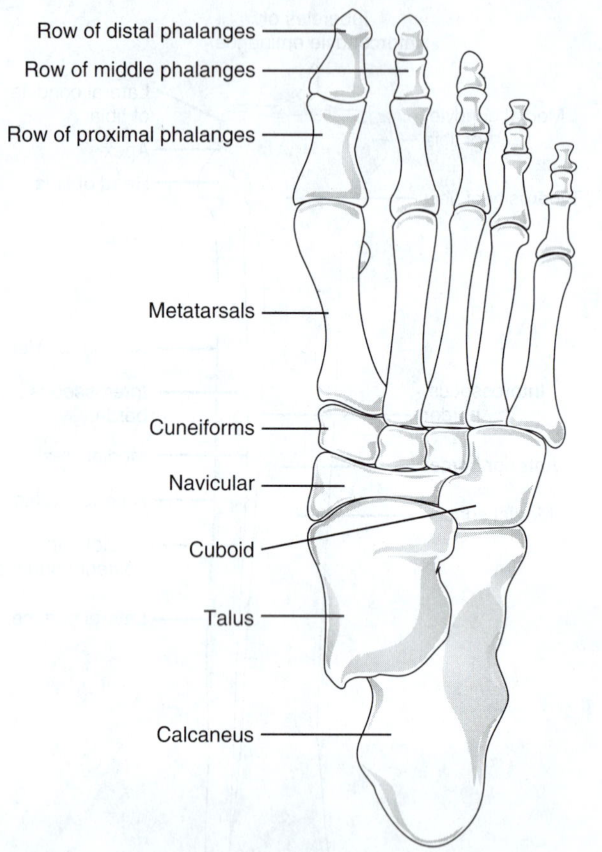

Figure 17–12 Right foot viewed from above.

17. INJURY AND POISONING (800–999)

Use E code(s) to identify the cause and intent of the injury or poisoning (E800-E999)

Note:

1. The principle of multiple coding of injuries should be followed wherever possible. Combination categories for multiple injuries are provided for use when there is insufficient detail as to the nature of the individual conditions, or for primary tabulation purposes when it is more convenient to record a single code; otherwise, the component injuries should be coded separately.

   Where multiple sites of injury are specified in the titles, the word "with" indicates involvement of both sites, and the word "and" indicates involvement of either or both sites. The word "finger" includes thumb.

2. Categories for "late effect" of injuries are to be found at 905–909.

FRACTURES (800–829)

Excludes *malunion (733.81)*
nonunion (733.82)
pathologic or spontaneous fracture (733.10–733.19)
stress fractures (733.93–733.95)

The terms "condyle," "coronoid process," "ramus," and "symphysis" indicate the portion of the bone fractured, not the name of the bone involved.

The descriptions "closed" and "open" used in the fourth-digit subdivisions include the following terms:

closed (with or without delayed healing):
- comminuted
- depressed
- elevated
- fissured
- fracture NOS
- greenstick
- impacted
- linear
- simple
- slipped epiphysis
- spiral

open (with or without delayed healing):
- compound
- infected
- missile
- puncture
- with foreign body

Note: A fracture not indicated as closed or open should be classified as closed.

FRACTURE OF SKULL (800–804)

The following fifth-digit subclassification is for use with the appropriate codes in categories 800, 801, 803, and 804:

❑ **0 unspecified state of consciousness**
1 with no loss of consciousness
2 with brief [less than one hour] loss of consciousness
3 with moderate [1–24 hours] loss of consciousness
4 with prolonged [more than 24 hours] loss of consciousness and return to pre-existing conscious level
5 with prolonged [more than 24 hours] loss of consciousness, without return to pre-existing conscious level

Use fifth-digit 5 to designate when a patient is unconscious and dies before regaining consciousness, regardless of the duration of the loss of consciousness

❑ **6 with loss of consciousness of unspecified duration**
❑ **9 with concussion, unspecified**

● **800 Fracture of vault of skull**

Requires fifth digit. See beginning of section 800–804 for codes and definitions.

Includes: frontal bone
parietal bone

● **800.0 Closed without mention of intracranial injury**
● **800.1 Closed with cerebral laceration and contusion**
● **800.2 Closed with subarachnoid, subdural, and extradural hemorrhage**
● ❑ **800.3 Closed with other and unspecified intracranial hemorrhage**
● ❑ **800.4 Closed with intracranial injury of other and unspecified nature**
● **800.5 Open without mention of intracranial injury**
● **800.6 Open with cerebral laceration and contusion**
● **800.7 Open with subarachnoid, subdural, and extradural hemorrhage**
● ❑ **800.8 Open with other and unspecified intracranial hemorrhage**
● ❑ **800.9 Open with intracranial injury of other and unspecified nature**

● **801 Fracture of base of skull**

Requires fifth digit. See beginning of section 800–804 for codes and definitions.

Includes: fossa:
anterior
middle
posterior
occiput bone
orbital roof
sinus:
ethmoid
frontal
sphenoid bone
temporal bone

● **801.0 Closed without mention of intracranial injury**

● **801.1 Closed with cerebral laceration and contusion**

● **801.2 Closed with subarachnoid, subdural, and extradural hemorrhage**

● ❑ **801.3 Closed with other and unspecified intracranial hemorrhage**

● ❑ **801.4 Closed with intracranial injury of other and unspecified nature**

● **801.5 Open without mention of intracranial injury**

● **801.6 Open with cerebral laceration and contusion**

● **801.7 Open with subarachnoid, subdural, and extradural hemorrhage**

● ❑ **801.8 Open with other and unspecified intracranial hemorrhage**

● ❑ **801.9 Open with intracranial injury of other and unspecified nature**

● **802 Fracture of face bones**

802.0 Nasal bones, closed

802.1 Nasal bones, open

● **802.2 Mandible, closed**
Inferior maxilla
Lower jaw (bone)

❑ **802.20 Unspecified site**

802.21 Condylar process

802.22 Subcondylar

802.23 Coronoid process

❑ **802.24 Ramus, unspecified**

802.25 Angle of jaw

802.26 Symphysis of body

802.27 Alveolar border of body

❑ **802.28 Body, other and unspecified**

❑ **802.29 Multiple sites**

● **802.3 Mandible, open**

❑ **802.30 Unspecified site**

802.31 Condylar process

802.32 Subcondylar

802.33 Coronoid process

❑ **802.34 Ramus, unspecified**

802.35 Angle of jaw

802.36 Symphysis of body

802.37 Alveolar border of body

❑ **802.38 Body, other and unspecified**

❑ **802.39 Multiple sites**

802.4 Malar and maxillary bones, closed
Superior maxilla
Upper jaw (bone)
Zygoma
Zygomatic arch

802.5 Malar and maxillary bones, open

802.6 Orbital floor (blow-out), closed

802.7 Orbital floor (blow-out), open

❑ **802.8 Other facial bones, closed**
Alveolus
Orbit:
NOS
part other than roof or floor
Palate

Excludes *orbital:*
floor (802.6)
roof (801.0–801.9)

❑ **802.9 Other facial bones, open**

● **803 Other and unqualified skull fractures**

Requires fifth digit. See beginning of section 800–804 for codes and definitions.

Includes: skull NOS
skull multiple NOS

● **803.0 Closed without mention of intracranial injury**

● **803.1 Closed with cerebral laceration and contusion**

● **803.2 Closed with subarachnoid, subdural, and extradural hemorrhage**

● ❑ **803.3 Closed with other and unspecified intracranial hemorrhage**

● ❑ **803.4 Closed with intracranial injury of other and unspecified nature**

● **803.5 Open without mention of intracranial injury**

● **803.6 Open with cerebral laceration and contusion**

● **803.7 Open with subarachnoid, subdural, and extradural hemorrhage**

● ❑ **803.8 Open with other and unspecified intracranial hemorrhage**

● ❑ **803.9 Open with intracranial injury of other and unspecified nature**

● **804 Multiple fractures involving skull or face with other bones**

Requires fifth digit. See beginning of section 800–804 for codes and definitions.

● **804.0 Closed without mention of intracranial injury**

● **804.1 Closed with cerebral laceration and contusion**

● **804.2 Closed with subarachnoid, subdural, and extradural hemorrhage**

● ❑ **804.3 Closed with other and unspecified intracranial hemorrhage**

● ❑ **804.4 Closed with intracranial injury of other and unspecified nature**

● **804.5 Open without mention of intracranial injury**

● **804.6 Open with cerebral laceration and contusion**

● **804.7 Open with subarachnoid, subdural, and extradural hemorrhage**

● ❑ **804.8 Open with other and unspecified intracranial hemorrhage**

● ❑ **804.9 Open with intracranial injury of other and unspecified nature**

FRACTURE OF NECK AND TRUNK (805–809)

● 805 Fracture of vertebral column without mention of spinal cord injury

Includes: neural arch
spine
spinous process
transverse process
vertebra

The following fifth-digit subclassification is for use with codes 805.0–805.1:
❑ 0 cervical vertebra, unspecified level
1 first cervical vertebra
2 second cervical vertebra
3 third cervical vertebra
4 fourth cervical vertebra
5 fifth cervical vertebra
6 sixth cervical vertebra
7 seventh cervical vertebra
❑ 8 multiple cervical vertebrae

● 805.0 Cervical, closed
Atlas
Axis

● 805.1 Cervical, open

805.2 Dorsal [thoracic], closed

805.3 Dorsal [thoracic], open

805.4 Lumbar, closed

805.5 Lumbar, open

805.6 Sacrum and coccyx, closed

805.7 Sacrum and coccyx, open

❑ 805.8 Unspecified, closed

❑ 805.9 Unspecified, open

● 806 Fracture of vertebral column with spinal cord injury

Includes: any condition classifiable to 805 with:
complete or incomplete transverse lesion (of cord)
hematomyelia
injury to:
cauda equina
nerve
paralysis
paraplegia
quadriplegia
spinal concussion

● 806.0 Cervical, closed

❑ 806.00 C_1-C_4 level with unspecified spinal cord injury
Cervical region NOS with spinal cord injury NOS

806.01 C_1-C_4 level with complete lesion of cord

806.02 C_1-C_4 level with anterior cord syndrome

806.03 C_1-C_4 level with central cord syndrome

❑ 806.04 C_1-C_4 level with other specified spinal cord injury
C_1-C_4 level with:
incomplete spinal cord lesion NOS
posterior cord syndrome

❑ 806.05 C_5-C_7 level with unspecified spinal cord injury

806.06 C_5-C_7 level with complete lesion of cord

806.07 C_5-C_7 level with anterior cord syndrome

806.08 C_5-C_7 level with central cord syndrome

❑ 806.09 C_5-C_7 level with other specified spinal cord injury
C_5-C_7 level with:
incomplete spinal cord lesion NOS
posterior cord syndrome

● 806.1 Cervical, open

❑ 806.10 C_1-C_4 level with unspecified spinal cord injury

806.11 C_1-C_4 level with complete lesion of cord

806.12 C_1-C_4 level with anterior cord syndrome

806.13 C_1-C_4 level with central cord syndrome

❑ 806.14 C_1-C_4 level with other specified spinal cord injury
C_1-C_4 level with:
incomplete spinal cord lesion NOS
posterior cord syndrome

❑ 806.15 C_5-C_7 level with unspecified spinal cord injury

806.16 C_5-C_7 level with complete lesion of cord

806.17 C_5-C_7 level with anterior cord syndrome

806.18 C_5-C_7 level with central cord syndrome

❑ 806.19 C_5-C_7 level with other specified spinal cord injury
C_5-C_7 level with:
incomplete spinal cord lesion NOS
posterior cord syndrome

● 806.2 Dorsal [thoracic], closed

❑ 806.20 T_1-T_6 level with unspecified spinal cord injury
Thoracic region NOS with spinal cord injury NOS

806.21 T_1-T_6 level with complete lesion of cord

806.22 T_1-T_6 level with anterior cord syndrome

806.23 T_1-T_6 level with central cord syndrome

❑ 806.24 T_1-T_6 level with other specified spinal cord injury
T_1-T_6 level with:
incomplete spinal cord lesion NOS
posterior cord syndrome

❑ 806.25 T_7-T_{12} level with unspecified spinal cord injury

806.26 T_7-T_{12} level with complete lesion of cord

806.27 T_7-T_{12} level with anterior cord syndrome

806.28 T_7-T_{12} level with central cord syndrome

❑ 806.29 T_7-T_{12} level with other specified spinal cord injury
T_7-T_{12} level with:
incomplete spinal cord lesion NOS
posterior cord syndrome

● 806.3 Dorsal [thoracic], open

❑ 806.30 T_1-T_6 level with unspecified spinal cord injury

806.31 T_1-T_6 level with complete lesion of cord

806.32 T_1-T_6 level with anterior cord syndrome

806.33 T_1-T_6 level with central cord syndrome

❑ 806.34 T_1-T_6 level with other specified spinal cord injury
T_1-T_6 level with:
incomplete spinal cord lesion NOS
posterior cord syndrome

❑ 806.35 T_7-T_{12} level with unspecified spinal cord injury

806.36 T_7-T_{12} level with complete lesion of cord

806.37 T_7-T_{12} level with anterior cord syndrome

806.38 T_7-T_{12} level with central cord syndrome

❑806.39 T_7-T_{12} level with other specified spinal cord injury
T_7-T_{12} level with:
incomplete spinal cord lesion NOS
posterior cord syndrome

806.4 Lumbar, closed

806.5 Lumbar, open

● 806.6 Sacrum and coccyx, closed

❑806.60 With unspecified spinal cord injury

806.61 With complete cauda equina lesion

❑806.62 With other cauda equina injury

❑806.69 With other spinal cord injury

● 806.7 Sacrum and coccyx, open

❑806.70 With unspecified spinal cord injury

806.71 With complete cauda equina lesion

❑806.72 With other cauda equina injury

❑806.79 With other spinal cord injury

❑806.8 Unspecified, closed

❑806.9 Unspecified, open

● 807 Fracture of rib(s), sternum, larynx, and trachea

The following fifth-digit subclassification is for use with codes 807.0–807.1:

❑0 rib(s), unspecified
1 one rib
2 two ribs
3 three ribs
4 four ribs
5 five ribs
6 six ribs
7 seven ribs
8 eight or more ribs
❑9 multiple ribs, unspecified

● 807.0 Rib(s), closed

● 807.1 Rib(s), open

807.2 Sternum, closed

807.3 Sternum, open

807.4 Flail chest

807.5 Larynx and trachea, closed
Hyoid bone
Thyroid cartilage
Trachea

807.6 Larynx and trachea, open

● 808 Fracture of pelvis

808.0 Acetabulum, closed

808.1 Acetabulum, open

808.2 Pubis, closed

808.3 Pubis, open

● 808.4 Other specified part, closed

808.41 Ilium

808.42 Ischium

❑808.43 Multiple pelvic fractures with disruption of pelvic circle

❑808.49 Other
Innominate bone
Pelvic rim

● 808.5 Other specified part, open

808.51 Ilium

808.52 Ischium

❑808.53 Multiple pelvic fractures with disruption of pelvic circle

❑808.59 Other

❑808.8 Unspecified, closed

❑808.9 Unspecified, open

● 809 Ill-defined fractures of bones of trunk

Includes: bones of trunk with other bones except those of skull and face
multiple bones of trunk

Excludes *multiple fractures of:*
pelvic bones alone (808.0–808.9)
ribs alone (807.0–807.1, 807.4)
ribs or sternum with limb bones (819.0–819.1, 828.0–828.1)
skull or face with other bones (804.0–804.9)

809.0 Fracture of bones of trunk, closed

809.1 Fracture of bones of trunk, open

FRACTURE OF UPPER LIMB (810–819)

● 810 Fracture of clavicle

Includes: collar bone
interligamentous part of clavicle

The following fifth-digit subclassification is for use with category 810:

❑0 unspecified part
clavicle NOS
1 sternal end of clavicle
2 shaft of clavicle
3 acromial end of clavicle

● 810.0 Closed

● 810.1 Open

● 811 Fracture of scapula

Includes: shoulder blade

The following fifth-digit subclassification is for use with category 811:

❑0 unspecified part
1 acromial process
acromion (process)
2 coracoid process
3 glenoid cavity and neck of scapula
❑9 other

● 811.0 Closed

● 811.1 Open

● 812 Fracture of humerus

● 812.0 Upper end, closed

❑812.00 Upper end, unspecified part
Proximal end
Shoulder

812.01 Surgical neck
Neck of humerus NOS

812.02 Anatomical neck

812.03 Greater tuberosity

❑812.09 Other
Head
Upper epiphysis

● 812.1 Upper end, open

❑812.10 Upper end, unspecified part

812.11 Surgical neck

812.12 Anatomical neck

812.13 Greater tuberosity

❑ 812.19 Other

● 812.2 Shaft or unspecified part, closed

❑ 812.20 Unspecified part of humerus
Humerus NOS
Upper arm NOS

812.21 Shaft of humerus

● 812.3 Shaft or unspecified part, open

❑ 812.30 Unspecified part of humerus

812.31 Shaft of humerus

● 812.4 Lower end, closed
Distal end of humerus
Elbow

❑ 812.40 Lower end, unspecified part

812.41 Supracondylar fracture of humerus

812.42 Lateral condyle
External condyle

812.43 Medial condyle
Internal epicondyle

❑ 812.44 Condyle(s), unspecified
Articular process NOS
Lower epiphysis

❑ 812.49 Other
Multiple fractures of lower end
Trochlea

● 812.5 Lower end, open

❑ 812.50 Lower end, unspecified part

812.51 Supracondylar fracture of humerus

812.52 Lateral condyle

812.53 Medial condyle

❑ 812.54 Condyle(s), unspecified

❑ 812.59 Other

● 813 Fracture of radius and ulna

● 813.0 Upper end, closed
Proximal end

❑ 813.00 Upper end of forearm, unspecified

813.01 Olecranon process of ulna

813.02 Coronoid process of ulna

813.03 Monteggia's fracture

❑ 813.04 Other and unspecified fractures of proximal end of ulna (alone)
Multiple fractures of ulna, upper end

813.05 Head of radius

813.06 Neck of radius

❑ 813.07 Other and unspecified fractures of proximal end of radius (alone)
Multiple fractures of radius, upper end

813.08 Radius with ulna, upper end [any part]

● 813.1 Upper end, open

❑ 813.10 Upper end of forearm, unspecified

813.11 Olecranon process of ulna

813.12 Coronoid process of ulna

813.13 Monteggia's fracture

❑ 813.14 Other and unspecified fractures of proximal end of ulna (alone)

813.15 Head of radius

813.16 Neck of radius

❑ 813.17 Other and unspecified fractures of proximal end of radius (alone)

813.18 Radius with ulna, upper end [any part]

● 813.2 Shaft, closed

❑ 813.20 Shaft, unspecified

813.21 Radius (alone)

813.22 Ulna (alone)

813.23 Radius with ulna

● 813.3 Shaft, open

❑ 813.30 Shaft, unspecified

813.31 Radius (alone)

813.32 Ulna (alone)

813.33 Radius with ulna

● 813.4 Lower end, closed
Distal end

❑ 813.40 Lower end of forearm, unspecified

813.41 Colles' fracture
Smith's fracture

❑ 813.42 Other fractures of distal end of radius (alone)
Dupuytren's fracture, radius
Radius, lower end

813.43 Distal end of ulna (alone)
Ulna:
head
lower end
lower epiphysis
styloid process

813.44 Radius with ulna, lower end

813.45 Torus fracture of radius

● 813.5 Lower end, open

❑ 813.50 Lower end of forearm, unspecified

813.51 Colles' fracture

❑ 813.52 Other fractures of distal end of radius (alone)

813.53 Distal end of ulna (alone)

813.54 Radius with ulna, lower end

● 813.8 Unspecified part, closed

❑ 813.80 Forearm, unspecified

❑ 813.81 Radius (alone)

❑ 813.82 Ulna (alone)

❑ 813.83 Radius with ulna

● 813.9 Unspecified part, open

❑ 813.90 Forearm, unspecified

❑ 813.91 Radius (alone)

❑ 813.92 Ulna (alone)

❑ 813.93 Radius with ulna

● **814 Fracture of carpal bone(s)**

The following fifth-digit subclassification is for use with category 814:

❑ **0 carpal bone, unspecified**
Wrist NOS
1 navicular [scaphoid] of wrist
2 lunate [semilunar] bone of wrist
3 triquetral [cuneiform] bone of wrist
4 pisiform
5 trapezium bone [larger multangular]
6 trapezoid bone [smaller multangular]
7 capitate bone [os magnum]
8 hamate [unciform] bone
❑ **9 other**

● **814.0 Closed**

● **814.1 Open**

● **815 Fracture of metacarpal bone(s)**

Includes: hand [except finger]
metacarpus

The following fifth-digit subclassification is for use with category 815:

❑ **0 metacarpal bone(s), site unspecified**
1 base of thumb [first] metacarpal
Bennett's fracture
2 base of other metacarpal bone(s)
3 shaft of metacarpal bone(s)
4 neck of metacarpal bone(s)
❑ **9 multiple sites of metacarpus**

● **815.0 Closed**

● **815.1 Open**

● **816 Fracture of one or more phalanges of hand**

Includes: finger(s)
thumb

The following fifth-digit subclassification is for use with category 816:

❑ **0 phalanx or phalanges, unspecified**
1 middle or proximal phalanx or phalanges
2 distal phalanx or phalanges
❑ **3 multiple sites**

● **816.0 Closed**

● **816.1 Open**

● **817 Multiple fractures of hand bones**

Includes: metacarpal bone(s) with phalanx or phalanges of same hand

817.0 Closed

817.1 Open

● **818 Ill-defined fractures of upper limb**

Includes: arm NOS
multiple bones of same upper limb

Excludes *multiple fractures of:*
metacarpal bone(s) with phalanx or phalanges (817.0–817.1)
phalanges of hand alone (816.0–816.1)
radius with ulna (813.0–813.9)

❑ **818.0 Closed**

❑ **818.1 Open**

● **819 Multiple fractures involving both upper limbs, and upper limb with rib(s) and sternum**

Includes: arm(s) with rib(s) or sternum
both arms [any bones]

819.0 Closed

819.1 Open

FRACTURE OF LOWER LIMB (820–829)

● **820 Fracture of neck of femur**

● **820.0 Transcervical fracture, closed**

❑ **820.00 Intracapsular section, unspecified**

820.01 Epiphysis (separation) (upper)
Transepiphyseal

820.02 Midcervical section
Transcervical NOS

820.03 Base of neck
Cervicotrochanteric section

❑ **820.09 Other**
Head of femur
Subcapital

● **820.1 Transcervical fracture, open**

❑ **820.10 Intracapsular section, unspecified**

820.11 Epiphysis (separation) (upper)

820.12 Midcervical section

820.13 Base of neck

❑ **820.19 Other**

● **820.2 Pertrochanteric fracture, closed**

❑ **820.20 Trochanteric section, unspecified**
Trochanter:
NOS
greater
lesser

820.21 Intertrochanteric section

820.22 Subtrochanteric section

● **820.3 Pertrochanteric fracture, open**

❑ **820.30 Trochanteric section, unspecified**

820.31 Intertrochanteric section

820.32 Subtrochanteric section

❑ **820.8 Unspecified part of neck of femur, closed**
Hip NOS
Neck of femur NOS

❑ **820.9 Unspecified part of neck of femur, open**

● **821 Fracture of other and unspecified parts of femur**

● **821.0 Shaft or unspecified part, closed**

❑ **821.00 Unspecified part of femur**
Thigh
Upper leg

Excludes *hip NOS (820.8)*

821.01 Shaft

● **821.1 Shaft or unspecified part, open**

❑ **821.10 Unspecified part of femur**

821.11 Shaft

● **821.2 Lower end, closed**
Distal end

❑ **821.20 Lower end, unspecified part**

821.21 Condyle, femoral

821.22 Epiphysis, lower (separation)

821.23 Supracondylar fracture of femur

❑ **821.29 Other**
Multiple fractures of lower end

● **821.3 Lower end, open**

❑ **821.30 Lower end, unspecified part**

ICD-9-CM 800-899 Vol. 1

821.31 **Condyle, femoral**

821.32 **Epiphysis, lower (separation)**

821.33 **Supracondylar fracture of femur**

❑821.39 **Other**

● 822 **Fracture of patella**

822.0 **Closed**

822.1 **Open**

● 823 **Fracture of tibia and fibula**

Excludes *Dupuytren's fracture (824.4–824.5)*
ankle (824.4–824.5)
radius (813.42, 813.52)
Pott's fracture (824.4–824.5)
that involving ankle (824.0–824.9)

The following fifth-digit subclassification is for use with category 823:

0 tibia alone
1 fibula alone
2 fibula with tibia

● 823.0 **Upper end, closed**
Head
Proximal end
Tibia:
condyles
tuberosity

● 823.1 **Upper end, open**

● 823.2 **Shaft, closed**

● 823.3 **Shaft, open**

● 823.4 **Torus fracture**

● ❑823.8 **Unspecified part, closed**
Lower leg NOS

● ❑823.9 **Unspecified part, open**

● 824 **Fracture of ankle**

824.0 **Medial malleolus, closed**
Tibia involving:
ankle
malleolus

824.1 **Medial malleolus, open**

824.2 **Lateral malleolus, closed**
Fibula involving:
ankle
malleolus

824.3 **Lateral malleolus, open**

824.4 **Bimalleolar, closed**
Dupuytren's fracture, fibula
Pott's fracture

824.5 **Bimalleolar, open**

824.6 **Trimalleolar, closed**
Lateral and medial malleolus with anterior or posterior lip of tibia

824.7 **Trimalleolar, open**

❑824.8 **Unspecified, closed**
Ankle NOS

❑824.9 **Unspecified, open**

● 825 **Fracture of one or more tarsal and metatarsal bones**

❑825.0 **Fracture of calcaneus, closed**
Heel bone
Os calcis

825.1 **Fracture of calcaneus, open**

● 825.2 **Fracture of other tarsal and metatarsal bones, closed**

❑825.20 **Unspecified bone(s) of foot [except toes]**
Instep

825.21 **Astragalus**
Talus

825.22 **Navicular [scaphoid], foot**

825.23 **Cuboid**

825.24 **Cuneiform, foot**

825.25 **Metatarsal bone(s)**

❑825.29 **Other**
Tarsal with metatarsal bone(s) only

Excludes *calcaneus (825.0)*

● 825.3 **Fracture of other tarsal and metatarsal bones, open**

❑825.30 **Unspecified bone(s) of foot [except toes]**

825.31 **Astragalus**

825.32 **Navicular [scaphoid], foot**

825.33 **Cuboid**

825.34 **Cuneiform, foot**

825.35 **Metatarsal bone(s)**

❑825.39 **Other**

● 826 **Fracture of one or more phalanges of foot**

Includes: toe(s)

826.0 **Closed**

826.1 **Open**

● 827 **Other, multiple, and ill-defined fractures of lower limb**

Includes: leg NOS
multiple bones of same lower limb

Excludes *multiple fractures of:*
ankle bones alone (824.4–824.9)
phalanges of foot alone (826.0–826.1)
tarsal with metatarsal bones (825.29, 825.39)
tibia with fibula (823.0–823.9 with fifth-digit 2)

827.0 **Closed**

827.1 **Open**

● 828 **Multiple fractures involving both lower limbs, lower with upper limb, and lower limb(s) with rib(s) and sternum**

Includes: arm(s) with leg(s) [any bones]
both legs [any bones]
leg(s) with rib(s) or sternum

828.0 **Closed**

828.1 **Open**

● 829 **Fracture of unspecified bones**

❑829.0 **Unspecified bone, closed**

❑829.1 **Unspecified bone, open**

DISLOCATION (830–839)

Includes: displacement
subluxation

Excludes *congenital dislocation (754.0–755.8)*
pathological dislocation (718.2)
recurrent dislocation (718.3)

The descriptions "closed" and "open," used in the fourth-digit subdivisions, include the following terms:
closed:
complete
dislocation NOS
partial
simple
uncomplicated
open:
compound
infected
with foreign body

Note: A dislocation not indicated as closed or open should be classified as closed.

● **830 Dislocation of jaw**

Includes: jaw (cartilage) (meniscus)
mandible
maxilla (inferior)
temporomandibular (joint)

830.0 Closed dislocation

830.1 Open dislocation

● **831 Dislocation of shoulder**

Excludes *sternoclavicular joint (839.61, 839.71)*
sternum (839.61, 839.71)

The following fifth-digit subclassification is for use with category 831:
❑ **0 shoulder, unspecified**
humerus NOS
1 anterior dislocation of humerus
2 posterior dislocation of humerus
3 inferior dislocation of humerus
4 acromioclavicular (joint)
clavicle
❑ **9 other**
Scapula

● **831.0 Closed dislocation**

● **831.1 Open dislocation**

● **832 Dislocation of elbow**

The following fifth-digit subclassification is for use with category 832:
❑ **0 elbow unspecified**
1 anterior dislocation of elbow
2 posterior dislocation of elbow
3 medial dislocation of elbow
4 lateral dislocation of elbow
❑ **9 other**

● **832.0 Closed dislocation**

● **832.1 Open dislocation**

● **833 Dislocation of wrist**

The following fifth-digit subclassification is for use with category 833:
❑ **0 wrist, unspecified part**
carpal (bone)
radius, distal end
1 radioulnar (joint), distal
2 radiocarpal (joint)
3 midcarpal (joint)
4 carpometacarpal (joint)
5 metacarpal (bone), proximal end
❑ **9 other**
ulna, distal end

● **833.0 Closed dislocation**

● **833.1 Open dislocation**

● **834 Dislocation of finger**

Includes: finger(s)
phalanx of hand
thumb

The following fifth-digit subclassification is for use with category 834:
❑ **0 finger, unspecified part**
1 metacarpophalangeal (joint)
metacarpal (bone), distal end
2 interphalangeal (joint), hand

● **834.0 Closed dislocation**

● **834.1 Open dislocation**

● **835 Dislocation of hip**

The following fifth-digit subclassification is for use with category 835:
❑ **0 dislocation of hip, unspecified**
1 posterior dislocation
2 obturator dislocation
❑ **3 other anterior dislocation**

● **835.0 Closed dislocation**

● **835.1 Open dislocation**

● **836 Dislocation of knee**

Excludes *dislocation of knee:*
old or pathological (718.2)
recurrent (718.3)
internal derangement of knee joint (717.0–717.5, 717.8–717.9)
old tear of cartilage or meniscus of knee (717.0–717.5, 717.8–717.9)

836.0 Tear of medial cartilage or meniscus of knee, current
Bucket handle tear:
NOS current injury
medial meniscus current injury

836.1 Tear of lateral cartilage or meniscus of knee, current

❑ **836.2 Other tear of cartilage or meniscus of knee, current**
Tear of:
cartilage (semilunar) current injury, not specified as medial or lateral
meniscus current injury, not specified as medial or lateral

836.3 Dislocation of patella, closed

836.4 Dislocation of patella, open

● **836.5 Other dislocation of knee, closed**

❑ **836.50 Dislocation of knee, unspecified**

836.51 Anterior dislocation of tibia, proximal end
Posterior dislocation of femur, distal end

836.52 Posterior dislocation of tibia, proximal end
Anterior dislocation of femur, distal end

836.53 Medial dislocation of tibia, proximal end

836.54 Lateral dislocation of tibia, proximal end

❑ **836.59 Other**

● **836.6 Other dislocation of knee, open**

❑ **836.60 Dislocation of knee, unspecified**

836.61 Anterior dislocation of tibia, proximal end

836.62 Posterior dislocation of tibia, proximal end

836.63 Medial dislocation of tibia, proximal end

836.64 Lateral dislocation of tibia, proximal end

❑ **836.69 Other**

● 837 Dislocation of ankle

Includes: astragalus
fibula, distal end
navicular, foot
scaphoid, foot
tibia, distal end

837.0 Closed dislocation

837.1 Open dislocation

● 838 Dislocation of foot

The following fifth-digit subclassification is for use with category 838:

❑ 0 foot, unspecified
1 tarsal (bone), joint unspecified
2 midtarsal (joint)
3 tarsometatarsal (joint)
4 metatarsal (bone), joint unspecified
5 metatarsophalangeal (joint)
6 interphalangeal (joint), foot
❑ 9 other
phalanx of foot
toe(s)

● 838.0 Closed dislocation

● 838.1 Open dislocation

● 839 Other, multiple, and ill-defined dislocations

● 839.0 Cervical vertebra, closed
Cervical spine
Neck

❑ 839.00 Cervical vertebra, unspecified

839.01 First cervical vertebra

839.02 Second cervical vertebra

839.03 Third cervical vertebra

839.04 Fourth cervical vertebra

839.05 Fifth cervical vertebra

839.06 Sixth cervical vertebra

839.07 Seventh cervical vertebra

❑ 839.08 Multiple cervical vertebrae

● 839.1 Cervical vertebra, open

❑ 839.10 Cervical vertebra, unspecified

839.11 First cervical vertebra

839.12 Second cervical vertebra

839.13 Third cervical vertebra

839.14 Fourth cervical vertebra

839.15 Fifth cervical vertebra

839.16 Sixth cervical vertebra

839.17 Seventh cervical vertebra

❑ 839.18 Multiple cervical vertebrae

● 839.2 Thoracic and lumbar vertebra, closed

839.20 Lumbar vertebra

839.21 Thoracic vertebra
Dorsal [thoracic] vertebra

● 839.3 Thoracic and lumbar vertebra, open

839.30 Lumbar vertebra

839.31 Thoracic vertebra

● 839.4 Other vertebra, closed

❑ 839.40 Vertebra, unspecified site
Spine NOS

839.41 Coccyx

839.42 Sacrum
Sacroiliac (joint)

❑ 839.49 Other

● 839.5 Other vertebra, open

❑ 839.50 Vertebra, unspecified site

839.51 Coccyx

839.52 Sacrum

❑ 839.59 Other

● 839.6 Other location, closed

839.61 Sternum
Sternoclavicular joint

❑ 839.69 Other
Pelvis

● 839.7 Other location, open

839.71 Sternum

❑ 839.79 Other

❑ 839.8 Multiple and ill-defined, closed
Arm
Back
Hand
Multiple locations, except fingers or toes alone
Other ill-defined locations
Unspecified location

❑ 839.9 Multiple and ill-defined, open

SPRAINS AND STRAINS OF JOINTS AND ADJACENT MUSCLES (840–848)

Includes: avulsion of joint capsule, ligament, muscle, tendon
hemarthrosis of joint capsule, ligament, muscle, tendon
laceration of joint capsule, ligament, muscle, tendon
rupture of joint capsule, ligament, muscle, tendon
sprain of joint capsule, ligament, muscle, tendon
strain of joint capsule, ligament, muscle, tendon
tear of joint capsule, ligament, muscle, tendon

Excludes *laceration of tendon in open wounds (880–884 and 890–894 with .2)*

● 840 Sprains and strains of shoulder and upper arm

840.0 Acromioclavicular (joint) (ligament)

840.1 Coracoclavicular (ligament)

840.2 Coracohumeral (ligament)

840.3 Infraspinatus (muscle) (tendon)

840.4 Rotator cuff (capsule)

Excludes *complete rupture of rotator cuff, nontraumatic (727.61)*

840.5 Subscapularis (muscle)

840.6 Supraspinatus (muscle) (tendon)

840.7 Superior glenoid labrum lesion
SLAP lesion

❑ 840.8 Other specified sites of shoulder and upper arm

❑ 840.9 Unspecified site of shoulder and upper arm
Arm NOS
Shoulder NOS

● 841 Sprains and strains of elbow and forearm

841.0 Radial collateral ligament

841.1 Ulnar collateral ligament

841.2 Radiohumeral (joint)

841.3 Ulnohumeral (joint)

❑ 841.8 Other specified sites of elbow and forearm

❑841.9 **Unspecified site of elbow and forearm**
Elbow NOS

● **842 Sprains and strains of wrist and hand**

● **842.0 Wrist**

❑842.00 **Unspecified site**

842.01 **Carpal (joint)**

842.02 **Radiocarpal (joint) (ligament)**

❑842.09 **Other**
Radioulnar joint, distal

● **842.1 Hand**

❑842.10 **Unspecified site**

842.11 **Carpometacarpal (joint)**

842.12 **Metacarpophalangeal (joint)**

842.13 **Interphalangeal (joint)**

❑842.19 **Other**
Midcarpal (joint)

● **843 Sprains and strains of hip and thigh**

843.0 **Iliofemoral (ligament)**

843.1 **Ischiocapsular (ligament)**

❑843.8 **Other specified sites of hip and thigh**

❑843.9 **Unspecified site of hip and thigh**
Hip NOS
Thigh NOS

● **844 Sprains and strains of knee and leg**

844.0 **Lateral collateral ligament of knee**

844.1 **Medial collateral ligament of knee**

844.2 **Cruciate ligament of knee**

844.3 **Tibiofibular (joint) (ligament), superior**

❑844.8 **Other specified sites of knee and leg**

❑844.9 **Unspecified site of knee and leg**
Knee NOS
Leg NOS

● **845 Sprains and strains of ankle and foot**

● **845.0 Ankle**

❑845.00 **Unspecified site**

845.01 **Deltoid (ligament), ankle**
Internal collateral (ligament), ankle

845.02 **Calcaneofibular (ligament)**

845.03 **Tibiofibular (ligament), distal**

❑845.09 **Other**
Achilles tendon

● **845.1 Foot**

❑845.10 **Unspecified site**

845.11 **Tarsometatarsal (joint) (ligament)**

845.12 **Metatarsophalangeal (joint)**

845.13 **Interphalangeal (joint), toe**

❑845.19 **Other**

● **846 Sprains and strains of sacroiliac region**

846.0 **Lumbosacral (joint) (ligament)**

846.1 **Sacroiliac ligament**

846.2 **Sacrospinatus (ligament)**

846.3 **Sacrotuberous (ligament)**

❑846.8 **Other specified sites of sacroiliac region**

❑846.9 **Unspecified site of sacroiliac region**

● **847 Sprains and strains of other and unspecified parts of back**

Excludes *lumbosacral (846.0)*

847.0 **Neck**
Anterior longitudinal (ligament), cervical
Atlanto-axial (joints)
Atlanto-occipital (joints)
Whiplash injury

Excludes *neck injury NOS (959.09)*
thyroid region (848.2)

847.1 **Thoracic**

847.2 **Lumbar**

847.3 **Sacrum**
Sacrococcygeal (ligament)

847.4 **Coccyx**

❑847.9 **Unspecified site of back**
Back NOS

● **848 Other and ill-defined sprains and strains**

848.0 **Septal cartilage of nose**

848.1 **Jaw**
Temporomandibular (joint) (ligament)

848.2 **Thyroid region**
Cricoarytenoid (joint) (ligament)
Cricothyroid (joint) (ligament)
Thyroid cartilage

848.3 **Ribs**
Chondrocostal (joint) without mention of injury to sternum
Costal cartilage without mention of injury to sternum

● **848.4 Sternum**

❑848.40 **Unspecified site**

848.41 **Sternoclavicular (joint) (ligament)**

848.42 **Chondrosternal (joint)**

❑848.49 **Other**
Xiphoid cartilage

848.5 **Pelvis**
Symphysis pubis

Excludes *that in childbirth (665.6)*

❑848.8 **Other specified sites of sprains and strains**

❑848.9 **Unspecified site of sprain and strain**

INTRACRANIAL INJURY, EXCLUDING THOSE WITH SKULL FRACTURE (850–854)

Excludes *intracranial injury with skull fracture (800–801 and 803–804, except .0 and .5)*
open wound of head without intracranial injury (870.0–873.9)
skull fracture alone (800–801 and 803–804 with .0, .5)

Note: The description "with open intracranial wound," used in the fourth-digit subdivisions, includes those specified as open or with mention of infection or foreign body.

The following fifth-digit subclassification is for use with categories 851–854:

- ❑ **0 unspecified state of consciousness**
- **1 with no loss of consciousness**
- **2 with brief [less than one hour] loss of consciousness**
- **3 with moderate [1–24 hours] loss of consciousness**
- **4 with prolonged [more than 24 hours] loss of consciousness and return to pre-existing conscious level**
- **5 with prolonged [more than 24 hours] loss of consciousness without return to pre-existing conscious level**

  Use fifth-digit 5 to designate when a patient is unconscious and dies before regaining consciousness, regardless of the duration of the loss of consciousness
- ❑ **6 with loss of consciousness of unspecified duration**
- ❑ **9 with concussion, unspecified**

● **850 Concussion**

Includes: commotio cerebri

Excludes *concussion with:*
cerebral laceration or contusion (851.0–851.9)
cerebral hemorrhage (852–853)
head injury NOS (959.01)

850.0 With no loss of consciousness
Concussion with mental confusion or disorientation, without loss of consciousness

● **850.1 With brief loss of consciousness**
Loss of consciousness for less than one hour

850.11 with loss of consciousness less than 30 minutes ◀

850.12 with loss of consciousness from 31 to 59 minutes ◀

850.2 With moderate loss of consciousness
Loss of consciousness for 1–24 hours

850.3 With prolonged loss of consciousness and return to pre-existing conscious level
Loss of consciousness for more than 24 hours with complete recovery

850.4 With prolonged loss of consciousness, without return to pre-existing conscious level

❑ **850.5 With loss of consciousness of unspecified duration**

❑ **850.9 Concussion, unspecified**

● **851 Cerebral laceration and contusion**

Requires fifth digit. See beginning of section 850–854 for codes and definitions.

● **851.0 Cortex (cerebral) contusion without mention of open intracranial wound**

● **851.1 Cortex (cerebral) contusion with open intracranial wound**

● **851.2 Cortex (cerebral) laceration without mention of open intracranial wound**

● **851.3 Cortex (cerebral) laceration with open intracranial wound**

● **851.4 Cerebellar or brain stem contusion without mention of open intracranial wound**

● **851.5 Cerebellar or brain stem contusion with open intracranial wound**

● **851.6 Cerebellar or brain stem laceration without mention of open intracranial wound**

● **851.7 Cerebellar or brain stem laceration with open intracranial wound**

● ❑ **851.8 Other and unspecified cerebral laceration and contusion, without mention of open intracranial wound**
Brain (membrane) NOS

● ❑ **851.9 Other and unspecified cerebral laceration and contusion, with open intracranial wound**

● **852 Subarachnoid, subdural, and extradural hemorrhage, following injury**

Requires fifth digit. See beginning of section 850–854 for codes and definitions.

Excludes *cerebral contusion or laceration (with hemorrhage) (851.0–851.9)*

● **852.0 Subarachnoid hemorrhage following injury without mention of open intracranial wound**
Middle meningeal hemorrhage following injury

● **852.1 Subarachnoid hemorrhage following injury with open intracranial wound**

● **852.2 Subdural hemorrhage following injury without mention of open intracranial wound**

● **852.3 Subdural hemorrhage following injury with open intracranial wound**

● **852.4 Extradural hemorrhage following injury without mention of open intracranial wound**
Epidural hematoma following injury

● **852.5 Extradural hemorrhage following injury with open intracranial wound**

● **853 Other and unspecified intracranial hemorrhage following injury**

Requires fifth digit. See beginning of section 850–854 for codes and definitions.

● ❑ **853.0 Without mention of open intracranial wound**
Cerebral compression due to injury
Intracranial hematoma following injury
Traumatic cerebral hemorrhage

● ❑ **853.1 With open intracranial wound**

● **854 Intracranial injury of other and unspecified nature**

Includes: injury:
brain NOS
cavernous sinus
intracranial

Excludes *any condition classifiable to 850–853*
head injury NOS (959.01)

● ❑ **854.0 Without mention of open intracranial wound**

● ❑ **854.1 With open intracranial wound**

INTERNAL INJURY OF THORAX, ABDOMEN, AND PELVIS (860–869)

Includes: blast injuries of internal organs
blunt trauma of internal organs
bruise of internal organs
concussion injuries (except cerebral) of internal organs
crushing of internal organs
hematoma of internal organs
laceration of internal organs
puncture of internal organs
tear of internal organs
traumatic rupture of internal organs

Excludes *concussion NOS (850.0–850.9)*
flail chest (807.4)
foreign body entering through orifice (930.0–939.9)
injury to blood vessels (901.0–902.9)

Note: The description "with open wound," used in the fourth-digit subdivisions, includes those with mention of infection or foreign body.

● **860 Traumatic pneumothorax and hemothorax**

860.0 Pneumothorax without mention of open wound into thorax

860.1 Pneumothorax with open wound into thorax

860.2 Hemothorax without mention of open wound into thorax

860.3 Hemothorax with open wound into thorax

860.4 Pneumohemothorax without mention of open wound into thorax

860.5 Pneumohemothorax with open wound into thorax

● **861 Injury to heart and lung**

Excludes *injury to blood vessels of thorax (901.0–901.9)*

● **861.0 Heart, without mention of open wound into thorax**

❑ **861.00 Unspecified injury**

861.01 Contusion
Cardiac contusion
Myocardial contusion

861.02 Laceration without penetration of heart chambers

861.03 Laceration with penetration of heart chambers

● **861.1 Heart, with open wound into thorax**

❑ **861.10 Unspecified injury**

861.11 Contusion

861.12 Laceration without penetration of heart chambers

861.13 Laceration with penetration of heart chambers

● **861.2 Lung, without mention of open wound into thorax**

❑ **861.20 Unspecified injury**

861.21 Contusion

861.22 Laceration

● **861.3 Lung, with open wound into thorax**

❑ **861.30 Unspecified injury**

861.31 Contusion

861.32 Laceration

● **862 Injury to other and unspecified intrathoracic organs**

Excludes *injury to blood vessels of thorax (901.0–901.9)*

862.0 Diaphragm, without mention of open wound into cavity

862.1 Diaphragm, with open wound into cavity

● **862.2 Other specified intrathoracic organs, without mention of open wound into cavity**

862.21 Bronchus

862.22 Esophagus

❑ **862.29 Other**
Pleura
Thymus gland

● **862.3 Other specified intrathoracic organs, with open wound into cavity**

862.31 Bronchus

862.32 Esophagus

❑ **862.39 Other**

❑ **862.8 Multiple and unspecified intrathoracic organs, without mention of open wound into cavity**
Crushed chest
Multiple intrathoracic organs

❑ **862.9 Multiple and unspecified intrathoracic organs, with open wound into cavity**

● **863 Injury to gastrointestinal tract**

Excludes *anal sphincter laceration during delivery (664.2)*
bile duct (868.0–868.1 with fifth-digit 2)
gallbladder (868.0–868.1 with fifth-digit 2)

863.0 Stomach, without mention of open wound into cavity

863.1 Stomach, with open wound into cavity

● **863.2 Small intestine, without mention of open wound into cavity**

❑ **863.20 Small intestine, unspecified site**

863.21 Duodenum

❑ **863.29 Other**

● **863.3 Small intestine, with open wound into cavity**

❑ **863.30 Small intestine, unspecified site**

863.31 Duodenum

❑ **863.39 Other**

● **863.4 Colon or rectum, without mention of open wound into cavity**

❑ **863.40 Colon, unspecified site**

863.41 Ascending [right] colon

863.42 Transverse colon

863.43 Descending [left] colon

863.44 Sigmoid colon

863.45 Rectum

❑ **863.46 Multiple sites in colon and rectum**

❑ **863.49 Other**

● **863.5 Colon or rectum, with open wound into cavity**

❑ **863.50 Colon, unspecified site**

863.51 Ascending [right] colon

863.52 Transverse colon

863.53 Descending [left] colon

863.54 Sigmoid colon

863.55 Rectum

❑ **863.56 Multiple sites in colon and rectum**

❑ **863.59 Other**

● **863.8 Other and unspecified gastrointestinal sites, without mention of open wound into cavity**

❑ **863.80 Gastrointestinal tract, unspecified site**

863.81 Pancreas, head

863.82 Pancreas, body

863.83 Pancreas, tail

❑ **863.84 Pancreas, multiple and unspecified sites**

863.85 Appendix

❑ **863.89 Other**

Intestine NOS

● **863.9 Other and unspecified gastrointestinal sites, with open wound into cavity**

❑ **863.90 Gastrointestinal tract, unspecified site**

863.91 Pancreas, head

863.92 Pancreas, body

863.93 Pancreas, tail

❑ **863.94 Pancreas, multiple and unspecified sites**

863.95 Appendix

❑ **863.99 Other**

● **864 Injury to liver**

The following fifth-digit subclassification is for use with category 864:

❑ **0 unspecified injury**
1 hematoma and contusion
2 laceration, minor
Laceration involving capsule only, or without significant involvement of hepatic parenchyma [i.e., less than 1 cm deep]
3 laceration, moderate
Laceration involving parenchyma but without major disruption of parenchyma [i.e., less than 10 cm long and less than 3 cm deep]
4 laceration, major
Laceration with significant disruption of hepatic parenchyma [i.e., 10 cm long and 3 cm deep]
Multiple moderate lacerations, with or without hematoma
Stellate lacerations of liver
❑ **5 laceration, unspecified**
❑ **9 other**

● **864.0 Without mention of open wound into cavity**

● **864.1 With open wound into cavity**

● **865 Injury to spleen**

The following fifth-digit subclassification is for use with category 865:

❑ **0 unspecified injury**
1 hematoma without rupture of capsule
2 capsular tears, without major disruption of parenchyma
3 laceration extending into parenchyma
4 massive parenchymal disruption
❑ **9 other**

● **865.0 Without mention of open wound into cavity**

● **865.1 With open wound into cavity**

● **866 Injury to kidney**

The following fifth-digit subclassification is for use with category 866:

❑ **0 unspecified injury**
1 hematoma without rupture of capsule
2 laceration
3 complete disruption of kidney parenchyma

● **866.0 Without mention of open wound into cavity**

● **866.1 With open wound into cavity**

● **867 Injury to pelvic organs**

Excludes *injury during delivery (664.0–665.9)*

867.0 Bladder and urethra, without mention of open wound into cavity

867.1 Bladder and urethra, with open wound into cavity

867.2 Ureter, without mention of open wound into cavity

867.3 Ureter, with open wound into cavity

867.4 Uterus, without mention of open wound into cavity

867.5 Uterus, with open wound into cavity

❑ **867.6 Other specified pelvic organs, without mention of open wound into cavity**

Fallopian tube
Ovary
Prostate
Seminal vesicle
Vas deferens

❑ **867.7 Other specified pelvic organs, with open wound into cavity**

❑ **867.8 Unspecified pelvic organ, without mention of open wound into cavity**

❑ **867.9 Unspecified pelvic organ, with open wound into cavity**

● **868 Injury to other intra-abdominal organs**

The following fifth-digit subclassification is for use with category 868:

❑ **0 unspecified intra-abdominal organ**
1 adrenal gland
2 bile duct and gallbladder
3 peritoneum
4 retroperitoneum
❑ **9 other and multiple intra-abdominal organs**

● **868.0 Without mention of open wound into cavity**

● **868.1 With open wound into cavity**

● **869 Internal injury to unspecified or ill-defined organs**

Includes: internal injury NOS
multiple internal injury NOS

❑ **869.0 Without mention of open wound into cavity**

❑ **869.1 With open wound into cavity**

OPEN WOUNDS (870–897)

Note: The description "complicated" used in the fourth-digit subdivisions includes those with mention of delayed healing, delayed treatment, foreign body, or infection.

Includes: animal bite
avulsion
cut
laceration
puncture wound
traumatic amputation

Excludes *burn (940.0–949.5)*
crushing (925–929.9)
puncture of internal organs (860.0–869.1)
superficial injury (910.0–919.9)
that incidental to:
dislocation (830.0–839.9)
fracture (800.0–829.1)
internal injury (860.0–869.1)
intracranial injury (851.0–854.1)

Use additional code to identify infection

OPEN WOUND OF HEAD, NECK, AND TRUNK (870–879)

● 870 Open wound of ocular adnexa

870.0 Laceration of skin of eyelid and periocular area

870.1 Laceration of eyelid, full-thickness, not involving lacrimal passages

870.2 Laceration of eyelid involving lacrimal passages

870.3 Penetrating wound of orbit, without mention of foreign body

870.4 Penetrating wound of orbit with foreign body

Excludes *retained (old) foreign body in orbit (376.6)*

❑ 870.8 Other specified open wounds of ocular adnexa

❑ 870.9 Unspecified open wound of ocular adnexa

● 871 Open wound of eyeball

Excludes *2nd cranial nerve [optic] injury (950.0–950.9)*
3rd cranial nerve [oculomotor] injury (951.0)

871.0 Ocular laceration without prolapse of intraocular tissue

871.1 Ocular laceration with prolapse or exposure of intraocular tissue

871.2 Rupture of eye with partial loss of intraocular tissue

871.3 Avulsion of eye
Traumatic enucleation

❑ 871.4 Unspecified laceration of eye

871.5 Penetration of eyeball with magnetic foreign body

Excludes *retained (old) magnetic foreign body in globe (360.50–360.59)*

871.6 Penetration of eyeball with (nonmagnetic) foreign body

Excludes *retained (old) (nonmagnetic) foreign body in globe (360.60–360.69)*

❑ 871.7 Unspecified ocular penetration

❑ 871.9 Unspecified open wound of eyeball

● 872 Open wound of ear

● 872.0 External ear, without mention of complication

❑ 872.00 External ear, unspecified site

872.01 Auricle, ear
Pinna

872.02 Auditory canal

● 872.1 External ear, complicated

❑ 872.10 External ear, unspecified site

872.11 Auricle, ear

872.12 Auditory canal

● 872.6 Other specified parts of ear, without mention of complication

872.61 Ear drum
Drumhead
Tympanic membrane

872.62 Ossicles

872.63 Eustachian tube

872.64 Cochlea

❑ 872.69 Other and multiple sites

● 872.7 Other specified parts of ear, complicated

872.71 Ear drum

872.72 Ossicles

872.73 Eustachian tube

872.74 Cochlea

❑ 872.79 Other and multiple sites

❑ 872.8 Ear, part unspecified, without mention of complication
Ear NOS

❑ 872.9 Ear, part unspecified, complicated

● 873 Other open wound of head

873.0 Scalp, without mention of complication

873.1 Scalp, complicated

● 873.2 Nose, without mention of complication

❑ 873.20 Nose, unspecified site

873.21 Nasal septum

873.22 Nasal cavity

873.23 Nasal sinus

❑ 873.29 Multiple sites

● 873.3 Nose, complicated

❑ 873.30 Nose, unspecified site

873.31 Nasal septum

873.32 Nasal cavity

873.33 Nasal sinus

❑ 873.39 Multiple sites

● 873.4 Face, without mention of complication

❑ 873.40 Face, unspecified site

873.41 Cheek

873.42 Forehead
Eyebrow

873.43 Lip

873.44 Jaw

❑ 873.49 Other and multiple sites

● 873.5 Face, complicated

❑ 873.50 Face, unspecified site

873.51 Cheek

873.52 Forehead

873.53 Lip

873.54 Jaw

❑ 873.59 Other and multiple sites

● 873.6 Internal structures of mouth, without mention of complication

❑ 873.60 Mouth, unspecified site

873.61 Buccal mucosa

873.62 Gum (alveolar process)

873.63 Tooth (broken)

873.64 Tongue and floor of mouth

873.65 Palate

❑ 873.69 Other and multiple sites

● 873.7 Internal structures of mouth, complicated

❑ 873.70 Mouth, unspecified site

873.71 Buccal mucosa

873.72 Gum (alveolar process)

873.73 Tooth (broken)

873.74 Tongue and floor of mouth

873.75 Palate

❑ 873.79 Other and multiple sites

❑ 873.8 Other and unspecified open wound of head without mention of complication
Head NOS

❑ 873.9 Other and unspecified open wound of head, complicated

● 874 Open wound of neck

● 874.0 Larynx and trachea, without mention of complication

874.00 Larynx with trachea

874.01 Larynx

874.02 Trachea

● 874.1 Larynx and trachea, complicated

874.10 Larynx with trachea

874.11 Larynx

874.12 Trachea

874.2 Thyroid gland, without mention of complication

874.3 Thyroid gland, complicated

874.4 Pharynx, without mention of complication
Cervical esophagus

874.5 Pharynx, complicated

❑ 874.8 Other and unspecified parts, without mention of complication
Nape of neck
Supraclavicular region
Throat NOS

❑ 874.9 Other and unspecified parts, complicated

● 875 Open wound of chest (wall)

Excludes *open wound into thoracic cavity (860.0–862.9)*
traumatic pneumothorax and hemothorax (860.1, 860.3, 860.5)

875.0 Without mention of complication

875.1 Complicated

● 876 Open wound of back

Includes: loin
lumbar region

Excludes *open wound into thoracic cavity (860.0–862.9)*
traumatic pneumothorax and hemothorax (860.1, 860.3, 860.5)

876.0 Without mention of complication

876.1 Complicated

● 877 Open wound of buttock

Includes: sacroiliac region

877.0 Without mention of complication

877.1 Complicated

● 878 Open wound of genital organs (external), including traumatic amputation

Excludes *injury during delivery (664.0–665.9)*
internal genital organs (867.0–867.9)

878.0 Penis, without mention of complication

878.1 Penis, complicated

878.2 Scrotum and testes, without mention of complication

878.3 Scrotum and testes, complicated

878.4 Vulva, without mention of complication
Labium (majus) (minus)

878.5 Vulva, complicated

878.6 Vagina, without mention of complication

878.7 Vagina, complicated

❑ 878.8 Other and unspecified parts, without mention of complication

❑ 878.9 Other and unspecified parts, complicated

● 879 Open wound of other and unspecified sites, except limbs

879.0 Breast, without mention of complication

879.1 Breast, complicated

879.2 Abdominal wall, anterior, without mention of complication
Abdominal wall NOS
Epigastric region
Hypogastric region
Pubic region
Umbilical region

879.3 Abdominal wall, anterior, complicated

879.4 Abdominal wall, lateral, without mention of complication
Flank
Groin
Hypochondrium
Iliac (region)
Inguinal region

879.5 Abdominal wall, lateral, complicated

❑ 879.6 Other and unspecified parts of trunk, without mention of complication
Pelvic region
Perineum
Trunk NOS

❑ 879.7 Other and unspecified parts of trunk, complicated

❑ 879.8 Open wound(s) (multiple) of unspecified site(s), without mention of complication
Multiple open wounds NOS
Open wound NOS

❑ 879.9 Open wound(s) (multiple) of unspecified site(s), complicated

OPEN WOUND OF UPPER LIMB (880–887)

● 880 Open wound of shoulder and upper arm

The following fifth-digit subclassification is for use with category 880:
0 shoulder region
1 scapular region
2 axillary region
3 upper arm
❑ 9 multiple sites

● 880.0 Without mention of complication

● 880.1 Complicated

● 880.2 With tendon involvement

● 881 Open wound of elbow, forearm, and wrist

The following fifth-digit subclassification is for use with category 881:
0 forearm
1 elbow
2 wrist

● 881.0 Without mention of complication

● 881.1 Complicated

● 881.2 With tendon involvement

● 882 Open wound of hand except finger(s) alone

882.0 Without mention of complication

882.1 Complicated

882.2 With tendon involvement

● 883 **Open wound of finger(s)**

Includes: fingernail
thumb (nail)

883.0 **Without mention of complication**

883.1 **Complicated**

883.2 **With tendon involvement**

● 884 **Multiple and unspecified open wound of upper limb**

Includes: arm NOS
multiple sites of one upper limb
upper limb NOS

❑ 884.0 **Without mention of complication**

❑ 884.1 **Complicated**

❑ 884.2 **With tendon involvement**

● 885 **Traumatic amputation of thumb (complete) (partial)**

Includes: thumb(s) (with finger(s) of either hand)

885.0 **Without mention of complication**

885.1 **Complicated**

● 886 **Traumatic amputation of other finger(s) (complete) (partial)**

Includes: finger(s) of one or both hands, without mention of thumb(s)

886.0 **Without mention of complication**

886.1 **Complicated**

● 887 **Traumatic amputation of arm and hand (complete) (partial)**

887.0 **Unilateral, below elbow, without mention of complication**

887.1 **Unilateral, below elbow, complicated**

887.2 **Unilateral, at or above elbow, without mention of complication**

887.3 **Unilateral, at or above elbow, complicated**

❑ 887.4 **Unilateral, level not specified, without mention of complication**

❑ 887.5 **Unilateral, level not specified, complicated**

887.6 **Bilateral [any level], without mention of complication**
One hand and other arm

887.7 **Bilateral [any level], complicated**

OPEN WOUND OF LOWER LIMB (890–897)

● 890 **Open wound of hip and thigh**

890.0 **Without mention of complication**

890.1 **Complicated**

890.2 **With tendon involvement**

● 891 **Open wound of knee, leg [except thigh], and ankle**

Includes: leg NOS
multiple sites of leg, except thigh

Excludes *that of thigh (890.0–890.2)*
with multiple sites of lower limb (894.0–894.2)

891.0 **Without mention of complication**

891.1 **Complicated**

891.2 **With tendon involvement**

● 892 **Open wound of foot except toe(s) alone**

Includes: heel

892.0 **Without mention of complication**

892.1 **Complicated**

892.2 **With tendon involvement**

● 893 **Open wound of toe(s)**

Includes: toenail

893.0 **Without mention of complication**

893.1 **Complicated**

893.2 **With tendon involvement**

● 894 **Multiple and unspecified open wound of lower limb**

Includes: lower limb NOS
multiple sites of one lower limb, with thigh

❑ 894.0 **Without mention of complication**

❑ 894.1 **Complicated**

❑ 894.2 **With tendon involvement**

● 895 **Traumatic amputation of toe(s) (complete) (partial)**

Includes: toe(s) of one or both feet

895.0 **Without mention of complication**

895.1 **Complicated**

● 896 **Traumatic amputation of foot (complete) (partial)**

896.0 **Unilateral, without mention of complication**

896.1 **Unilateral, complicated**

896.2 **Bilateral, without mention of complication**

Excludes *one foot and other leg (897.6–897.7)*

896.3 **Bilateral, complicated**

● 897 **Traumatic amputation of leg(s) (complete) (partial)**

897.0 **Unilateral, below knee, without mention of complication**

897.1 **Unilateral, below knee, complicated**

897.2 **Unilateral, at or above knee, without mention of complication**

897.3 **Unilateral, at or above knee, complicated**

❑ 897.4 **Unilateral, level not specified, without mention of complication**

❑ 897.5 **Unilateral, level not specified, complicated**

897.6 **Bilateral [any level], without mention of complication**
One foot and other leg

897.7 **Bilateral [any level], complicated**

INJURY TO BLOOD VESSELS (900–904)

Includes: arterial hematoma of blood vessel, secondary to other injuries, e.g., fracture or open wound
avulsion of blood vessel, secondary to other injuries, e.g., fracture or open wound
cut of blood vessel, secondary to other injuries, e.g., fracture or open wound
laceration of blood vessel, secondary to other injuries, e.g., fracture or open wound
rupture of blood vessel, secondary to other injuries, e.g., fracture or open wound
traumatic aneurysm or fistula (arteriovenous) of blood vessel, secondary to other injuries, e.g., fracture or open wound

Excludes *accidental puncture or laceration during medical procedure (998.2)*
intracranial hemorrhage following injury (851.0–854.1)

- 900 Injury to blood vessels of head and neck
  - 900.0 Carotid artery
    - 900.00 Carotid artery, unspecified
    - 900.01 Common carotid artery
    - 900.02 External carotid artery
    - 900.03 Internal carotid artery
  - 900.1 Internal jugular vein
  - 900.8 Other specified blood vessels of head and neck
    - 900.81 External jugular vein
      Jugular vein NOS
    - 900.82 Multiple blood vessels of head and neck
    - 900.89 Other
  - 900.9 Unspecified blood vessel of head and neck

- 901 Injury to blood vessels of thorax
  Excludes *traumatic hemothorax (860.2–860.5)*
  - 901.0 Thoracic aorta
  - 901.1 Innominate and subclavian arteries
  - 901.2 Superior vena cava
  - 901.3 Innominate and subclavian veins
  - 901.4 Pulmonary blood vessels
    - 901.40 Pulmonary vessel(s), unspecified
    - 901.41 Pulmonary artery
    - 901.42 Pulmonary vein
  - 901.8 Other specified blood vessels of thorax
    - 901.81 Intercostal artery or vein
    - 901.82 Internal mammary artery or vein
    - 901.83 Multiple blood vessels of thorax
    - 901.89 Other
      Azygos vein
      Hemiazygos vein
  - 901.9 Unspecified blood vessel of thorax

- 902 Injury to blood vessels of abdomen and pelvis
  - 902.0 Abdominal aorta
  - 902.1 Inferior vena cava
    - 902.10 Inferior vena cava, unspecified
    - 902.11 Hepatic veins
    - 902.19 Other
  - 902.2 Celiac and mesenteric arteries
    - 902.20 Celiac and mesenteric arteries, unspecified
    - 902.21 Gastric artery
    - 902.22 Hepatic artery
    - 902.23 Splenic artery
    - 902.24 Other specified branches of celiac axis
    - 902.25 Superior mesenteric artery (trunk)
    - 902.26 Primary branches of superior mesenteric artery
      Ileo-colic artery
    - 902.27 Inferior mesenteric artery
    - 902.29 Other
  - 902.3 Portal and splenic veins
    - 902.31 Superior mesenteric vein and primary subdivisions
      Ileo-colic vein
    - 902.32 Inferior mesenteric vein
    - 902.33 Portal vein
    - 902.34 Splenic vein
    - 902.39 Other
      Cystic vein
      Gastric vein
  - 902.4 Renal blood vessels
    - 902.40 Renal vessel(s), unspecified
    - 902.41 Renal artery
    - 902.42 Renal vein
    - 902.49 Other
      Suprarenal arteries
  - 902.5 Iliac blood vessels
    - 902.50 Iliac vessel(s), unspecified
    - 902.51 Hypogastric artery
    - 902.52 Hypogastric vein
    - 902.53 Iliac artery
    - 902.54 Iliac vein
    - 902.55 Uterine artery
    - 902.56 Uterine vein
    - 902.59 Other
  - 902.8 Other specified blood vessels of abdomen and pelvis
    - 902.81 Ovarian artery
    - 902.82 Ovarian vein
    - 902.87 Multiple blood vessels of abdomen and pelvis
    - 902.89 Other
  - 902.9 Unspecified blood vessel of abdomen and pelvis

- 903 Injury to blood vessels of upper extremity
  - 903.0 Axillary blood vessels
    - 903.00 Axillary vessel(s), unspecified
    - 903.01 Axillary artery
    - 903.02 Axillary vein
  - 903.1 Brachial blood vessels
  - 903.2 Radial blood vessels
  - 903.3 Ulnar blood vessels
  - 903.4 Palmar artery
  - 903.5 Digital blood vessels
  - 903.8 Other specified blood vessels of upper extremity
    Multiple blood vessels of upper extremity
  - 903.9 Unspecified blood vessel of upper extremity

- 904 Injury to blood vessels of lower extremity and unspecified sites
  - 904.0 Common femoral artery
    Femoral artery above profunda origin
  - 904.1 Superficial femoral artery
  - 904.2 Femoral veins
  - 904.3 Saphenous veins
    Saphenous vein (greater) (lesser)
  - 904.4 Popliteal blood vessels
    - 904.40 Popliteal vessel(s), unspecified
    - 904.41 Popliteal artery
    - 904.42 Popliteal vein

● 904.5 Tibial blood vessels

❑ 904.50 Tibial vessel(s), unspecified

904.51 Anterior tibial artery

904.52 Anterior tibial vein

904.53 Posterior tibial artery

904.54 Posterior tibial vein

904.6 Deep plantar blood vessels

❑ 904.7 Other specified blood vessels of lower extremity
Multiple blood vessels of lower extremity

❑ 904.8 Unspecified blood vessel of lower extremity

❑ 904.9 Unspecified site
Injury to blood vessel NOS

LATE EFFECTS OF INJURIES, POISONINGS, TOXIC EFFECTS, AND OTHER EXTERNAL CAUSES (905–909)

Note: These categories are to be used to indicate conditions classifiable to 800–999 as the cause of late effects, which are themselves classified elsewhere. The "late effects" include those specified as such, or as sequelae, which may occur at any time after the acute injury.

● 905 Late effects of musculoskeletal and connective tissue injuries

❑ 905.0 Late effect of fracture of skull and face bones
Late effect of injury classifiable to 800–804

❑ 905.1 Late effect of fracture of spine and trunk without mention of spinal cord lesion
Late effect of injury classifiable to 805, 807–809

❑ 905.2 Late effect of fracture of upper extremities
Late effect of injury classifiable to 810–819

❑ 905.3 Late effect of fracture of neck of femur
Late effect of injury classifiable to 820

❑ 905.4 Late effect of fracture of lower extremities
Late effect of injury classifiable to 821–827

❑ 905.5 Late effect of fracture of multiple and unspecified bones
Late effect of injury classifiable to 828–829

❑ 905.6 Late effect of dislocation
Late effect of injury classifiable to 830–839

❑ 905.7 Late effect of sprain and strain without mention of tendon injury
Late effect of injury classifiable to 840–848, except tendon injury

❑ 905.8 Late effect of tendon injury
Late effect of tendon injury due to:
open wound [injury classifiable to 880–884 with .2, 890–894 with .2]
sprain and strain [injury classifiable to 840–848]

❑ 905.9 Late effect of traumatic amputation
Late effect of injury classifiable to 885–887, 895–897

Excludes *late amputation stump complication (997.60–997.69)*

● 906 Late effects of injuries to skin and subcutaneous tissues

❑ 906.0 Late effect of open wound of head, neck, and trunk
Late effect of injury classifiable to 870–879

❑ 906.1 Late effect of open wound of extremities without mention of tendon injury
Late effect of injury classifiable to 880–884, 890–894 except .2

❑ 906.2 Late effect of superficial injury
Late effect of injury classifiable to 910–919

❑ 906.3 Late effect of contusion
Late effect of injury classifiable to 920–924

❑ 906.4 Late effect of crushing
Late effect of injury classifiable to 925–929

❑ 906.5 Late effect of burn of eye, face, head, and neck
Late effect of injury classifiable to 940–941

❑ 906.6 Late effect of burn of wrist and hand
Late effect of injury classifiable to 944

❑ 906.7 Late effect of burn of other extremities
Late effect of injury classifiable to 943 or 945

❑ 906.8 Late effect of burns of other specified sites
Late effect of injury classifiable to 942, 946–947

❑ 906.9 Late effect of burn of unspecified site
Late effect of injury classifiable to 948–949

● 907 Late effects of injuries to the nervous system

❑ 907.0 Late effect of intracranial injury without mention of skull fracture
Late effect of injury classifiable to 850–854

❑ 907.1 Late effect of injury to cranial nerve
Late effect of injury classifiable to 950–951

❑ 907.2 Late effect of spinal cord injury
Late effect of injury classifiable to 806, 952

❑ 907.3 Late effect of injury to nerve root(s), spinal plexus(es), and other nerves of trunk
Late effect of injury classifiable to 953–954

❑ 907.4 Late effect of injury to peripheral nerve of shoulder girdle and upper limb
Late effect of injury classifiable to 955

❑ 907.5 Late effect of injury to peripheral nerve of pelvic girdle and lower limb
Late effect of injury classifiable to 956

❑ 907.9 Late effect of injury to other and unspecified nerve
Late effect of injury classifiable to 957

● 908 Late effects of other and unspecified injuries

❑ 908.0 Late effect of internal injury to chest
Late effect of injury classifiable to 860–862

❑ 908.1 Late effect of internal injury to intra-abdominal organs
Late effect of injury classifiable to 863–866, 868

❑ 908.2 Late effect of internal injury to other internal organs
Late effect of injury classifiable to 867 or 869

❑ 908.3 Late effect of injury to blood vessel of head, neck, and extremities
Late effect of injury classifiable to 900, 903–904

❑ 908.4 Late effect of injury to blood vessel of thorax, abdomen, and pelvis
Late effect of injury classifiable to 901–902

❑ 908.5 Late effect of foreign body in orifice
Late effect of injury classifiable to 930–939

❑ 908.6 Late effect of certain complications of trauma
Late effect of complications classifiable to 958

❑ 908.9 Late effect of unspecified injury
Late effect of injury classifiable to 959

● 909 Late effects of other and unspecified external causes

❑ 909.0 Late effect of poisoning due to drug, medicinal or biological substance
Late effect of conditions classifiable to 960–979

Excludes *Late effect of adverse effect of drug, medicinal or biological substance (909.5)*

❑ 909.1 Late effect of toxic effects of nonmedical substances
Late effect of conditions classifiable to 980–989

❑ **909.2 Late effect of radiation**
Late effect of conditions classifiable to 990

❑ **909.3 Late effect of complications of surgical and medical care**
Late effect of conditions classifiable to 996–999

❑ **909.4 Late effect of certain other external causes**
Late effect of conditions classifiable to 991–994

❑ **909.5 Late effect of adverse effect of drug, medicinal or biological substance**

Excludes *late effect of poisoning due to drug, medicinal or biological substances (909.0)*

❑ **909.9 Late effect of other and unspecified external causes**

SUPERFICIAL INJURY (910–919)

Excludes *burn (blisters) (940.0–949.5)*
contusion (920–924.9)
foreign body:
granuloma (728.82)
inadvertently left in operative wound (998.4)
residual, in soft tissue (729.6)
insect bite, venomous (989.5)
open wound with incidental foreign body (870.0–897.7)

● **910 Superficial injury of face, neck, and scalp except eye**

Includes: cheek, ear, gum, lip, nose, throat

Excludes *eye and adnexa (918.0–918.9)*

910.0 Abrasion or friction burn without mention of infection

910.1 Abrasion or friction burn, infected

910.2 Blister without mention of infection

910.3 Blister, infected

910.4 Insect bite, nonvenomous, without mention of infection

910.5 Insect bite, nonvenomous, infected

910.6 Superficial foreign body (splinter) without major open wound and without mention of infection

910.7 Superficial foreign body (splinter) without major open wound, infected

❑ **910.8 Other and unspecified superficial injury of face, neck, and scalp without mention of infection**

❑ **910.9 Other and unspecified superficial injury of face, neck, and scalp, infected**

● **911 Superficial injury of trunk**

Includes: abdominal wall
anus
back
breast
buttock
chest wall
flank
groin
interscapular region
labium (majus) (minus)
penis
perineum
scrotum
testis
vagina
vulva

Excludes *hip (916.0–916.9)*
scapular region (912.0–912.9)

911.0 Abrasion or friction burn without mention of infection

911.1 Abrasion or friction burn, infected

911.2 Blister without mention of infection

911.3 Blister, infected

911.4 Insect bite, nonvenomous, without mention of infection

911.5 Insect bite, nonvenomous, infected

911.6 Superficial foreign body (splinter) without major open wound and without mention of infection

911.7 Superficial foreign body (splinter) without major open wound, infected

❑ **911.8 Other and unspecified superficial injury of trunk without mention of infection**

❑ **911.9 Other and unspecified superficial injury of trunk, infected**

● **912 Superficial injury of shoulder and upper arm**

Includes: axilla
scapular region

912.0 Abrasion or friction burn without mention of infection

912.1 Abrasion or friction burn, infected

912.2 Blister without mention of infection

912.3 Blister, infected

912.4 Insect bite, nonvenomous, without mention of infection

912.5 Insect bite, nonvenomous, infected

912.6 Superficial foreign body (splinter) without major open wound and without mention of infection

912.7 Superficial foreign body (splinter) without major open wound, infected

❑ **912.8 Other and unspecified superficial injury of shoulder and upper arm without mention of infection**

❑ **912.9 Other and unspecified superficial injury of shoulder and upper arm, infected**

● **913 Superficial injury of elbow, forearm, and wrist**

913.0 Abrasion or friction burn without mention of infection

913.1 Abrasion or friction burn, infected

913.2 Blister without mention of infection

913.3 Blister, infected

913.4 Insect bite, nonvenomous, without mention of infection

913.5 Insect bite, nonvenomous, infected

913.6 Superficial foreign body (splinter) without major open wound and without mention of infection

913.7 Superficial foreign body (splinter) without major open wound, infected

❑ **913.8 Other and unspecified superficial injury of elbow, forearm, and wrist without mention of infection**

❑ **913.9 Other and unspecified superficial injury of elbow, forearm, and wrist, infected**

● **914 Superficial injury of hand(s) except finger(s) alone**

914.0 Abrasion or friction burn without mention of infection

914.1 Abrasion or friction burn, infected

914.2 Blister without mention of infection

914.3 Blister, infected

914.4 **Insect bite, nonvenomous, without mention of infection**

914.5 **Insect bite, nonvenomous, infected**

914.6 **Superficial foreign body (splinter) without major open wound and without mention of infection**

914.7 **Superficial foreign body (splinter) without major open wound, infected**

❑ **914.8** **Other and unspecified superficial injury of hand without mention of infection**

❑ **914.9** **Other and unspecified superficial injury of hand, infected**

● **915** **Superficial injury of finger(s)**

Includes: fingernail
thumb (nail)

915.0 **Abrasion or friction burn without mention of infection**

915.1 **Abrasion or friction burn, infected**

915.2 **Blister without mention of infection**

915.3 **Blister, infected**

915.4 **Insect bite, nonvenomous, without mention of infection**

915.5 **Insect bite, nonvenomous, infected**

915.6 **Superficial foreign body (splinter) without major open wound and without mention of infection**

915.7 **Superficial foreign body (splinter) without major open wound, infected**

❑ **915.8** **Other and unspecified superficial injury of fingers without mention of infection**

❑ **915.9** **Other and unspecified superficial injury of fingers, infected**

● **916** **Superficial injury of hip, thigh, leg, and ankle**

916.0 **Abrasion or friction burn without mention of infection**

916.1 **Abrasion or friction burn, infected**

916.2 **Blister without mention of infection**

916.3 **Blister, infected**

916.4 **Insect bite, nonvenomous, without mention of infection**

916.5 **Insect bite, nonvenomous, infected**

916.6 **Superficial foreign body (splinter) without major open wound and without mention of infection**

916.7 **Superficial foreign body (splinter) without major open wound, infected**

❑ **916.8** **Other and unspecified superficial injury of hip, thigh, leg, and ankle without mention of infection**

❑ **916.9** **Other and unspecified superficial injury of hip, thigh, leg, and ankle, infected**

● **917** **Superficial injury of foot and toe(s)**

Includes: heel
toenail

917.0 **Abrasion or friction burn without mention of infection**

917.1 **Abrasion or friction burn, infected**

917.2 **Blister without mention of infection**

917.3 **Blister, infected**

917.4 **Insect bite, nonvenomous, without mention of infection**

917.5 **Insect bite, nonvenomous, infected**

917.6 **Superficial foreign body (splinter) without major open wound and without mention of infection**

917.7 **Superficial foreign body (splinter) without major open wound, infected**

❑ **917.8** **Other and unspecified superficial injury of foot and toes without mention of infection**

❑ **917.9** **Other and unspecified superficial injury of foot and toes, infected**

● **918** **Superficial injury of eye and adnexa**

Excludes *burn (940.0–940.9)*
foreign body on external eye (930.0–930.9)

918.0 **Eyelids and periocular area**
Abrasion
Insect bite
Superficial foreign body (splinter)

918.1 **Cornea**
Corneal abrasion
Superficial laceration

Excludes *corneal injury due to contact lens (371.82)*

918.2 **Conjunctiva**

❑ **918.9** **Other and unspecified superficial injuries of eye**
Eye (ball) NOS

● **919** **Superficial injury of other, multiple, and unspecified sites**

Excludes *multiple sites classifiable to the same three-digit category (910.0–918.9)*

❑ **919.0** **Abrasion or friction burn without mention of infection**

❑ **919.1** **Abrasion or friction burn, infected**

❑ **919.2** **Blister without mention of infection**

❑ **919.3** **Blister, infected**

❑ **919.4** **Insect bite, nonvenomous, without mention of infection**

❑ **919.5** **Insect bite, nonvenomous, infected**

❑ **919.6** **Superficial foreign body (splinter) without major open wound and without mention of infection**

❑ **919.7** **Superficial foreign body (splinter) without major open wound, infected**

❑ **919.8** **Other and unspecified superficial injury without mention of infection**

❑ **919.9** **Other and unspecified superficial injury, infected**

CONTUSION WITH INTACT SKIN SURFACE (920–924)

Includes: bruise without fracture or open wound
hematoma without fracture or open wound

Excludes *concussion (850.0–850.9)*
hemarthrosis (840.0–848.9)
internal organs (860.0–869.1)
that incidental to:
crushing injury (925–929.9)
dislocation (830.0–839.9)
fracture (800.0–829.1)
internal injury (860.0–869.1)
intracranial injury (850.0–854.1)
nerve injury (950.0–957.9)
open wound (870.0–897.7)

920 **Contusion of face, scalp, and neck except eye(s)**
Cheek
Ear (auricle)
Gum
Lip
Mandibular joint area
Nose
Throat

● 921 Contusion of eye and adnexa

❑ 921.0 Black eye, NOS

921.1 Contusion of eyelids and periocular area

921.2 Contusion of orbital tissues

921.3 Contusion of eyeball

❑ 921.9 Unspecified contusion of eye
Injury of eye NOS

● 922 Contusion of trunk

922.0 Breast

922.1 Chest wall

922.2 Abdominal wall
Flank
Groin

● 922.3 Back

922.31 Back

Excludes *interscapular region (922.33)*

922.32 Buttock

922.33 Interscapular region

Excludes *scapular region (923.01)*

922.4 Genital organs
Labium (majus) (minus)
Penis
Perineum
Scrotum
Testis
Vagina
Vulva

❑ 922.8 Multiple sites of trunk

❑ 922.9 Unspecified part
Trunk NOS

● 923 Contusion of upper limb

● 923.0 Shoulder and upper arm

923.00 Shoulder region

923.01 Scapular region

923.02 Axillary region

923.03 Upper arm

❑ 923.09 Multiple sites

● 923.1 Elbow and forearm

923.10 Forearm

923.11 Elbow

● 923.2 Wrist and hand(s), except finger(s) alone

923.20 Hand(s)

923.21 Wrist

923.3 Finger
Fingernail
Thumb (nail)

❑ 923.8 Multiple sites of upper limb

❑ 923.9 Unspecified part of upper limb
Arm NOS

● 924 Contusion of lower limb and of other and unspecified sites

● 924.0 Hip and thigh

924.00 Thigh

924.01 Hip

● 924.1 Knee and lower leg

924.10 Lower leg

924.11 Knee

● 924.2 Ankle and foot, excluding toe(s)

924.20 Foot
Heel

924.21 Ankle

924.3 Toe
Toenail

❑ 924.4 Multiple sites of lower limb

❑ 924.5 Unspecified part of lower limb
Leg NOS

❑ 924.8 Multiple sites, not elsewhere classified

❑ 924.9 Unspecified site

CRUSHING INJURY (925–929)

Use additional code to identify any associated injuries, such as: ◀
fractures (800–829) ◀
internal organs (860.0–869.1) ◀
intracranial injury (850.0–854.1) ◀

● 925 Crushing injury of face, scalp, and neck
Cheek
Ear
Larynx
Pharynx
Throat

925.1 Crushing injury of face and scalp
Cheek
Ear

925.2 Crushing injury of neck
Larynx
Throat
Pharynx

● 926 Crushing injury of trunk

926.0 External genitalia
Labium (majus) (minus)
Penis
Scrotum
Testis
Vulva

● 926.1 Other specified sites

926.11 Back

926.12 Buttock

❑ 926.19 Other
Breast

❑ 926.8 Multiple sites of trunk

❑ 926.9 Unspecified site
Trunk NOS

● 927 Crushing injury of upper limb

● 927.0 Shoulder and upper arm

927.00 Shoulder region

927.01 Scapular region

927.02 Axillary region

927.03 Upper arm

❑ 927.09 Multiple sites

● 927.1 Elbow and forearm

927.10 Forearm

927.11 Elbow

● 927.2 Wrist and hand(s), except finger(s) alone

927.20 Hand(s)

927.21 Wrist

927.3 Finger(s)

❑ 927.8 Multiple sites of upper limb

❑ 927.9 Unspecified site
Arm NOS

● 928 Crushing injury of lower limb

● 928.0 Hip and thigh

928.00 Thigh

928.01 Hip

● 928.1 Knee and lower leg

928.10 Lower leg

928.11 Knee

● 928.2 Ankle and foot, excluding toe(s) alone

928.20 Foot
Heel

928.21 Ankle

928.3 Toe(s)

❑ 928.8 Multiple sites of lower limb

❑ 928.9 Unspecified site
Leg NOS

● 929 Crushing injury of multiple and unspecified sites

❑ 929.0 Multiple sites, not elsewhere classified

❑ 929.9 Unspecified site

EFFECTS OF FOREIGN BODY ENTERING THROUGH ORIFICE (930–939)

Excludes *foreign body:*
granuloma (728.82)
inadvertently left in operative wound (998.4, 998.7)
in open wound (800–839, 851–897)
residual, in soft tissues (729.6)
superficial without major open wound (910–919 with .6 or .7)

● 930 Foreign body on external eye

Excludes *foreign body in penetrating wound of:*
eyeball (871.5–871.6)
retained (old) (360.5–360.6)
ocular adnexa (870.4)
retained (old) (376.6)

930.0 Corneal foreign body

930.1 Foreign body in conjunctival sac

930.2 Foreign body in lacrimal punctum

❑ 930.8 Other and combined sites

❑ 930.9 Unspecified site
External eye NOS

931 Foreign body in ear
Auditory canal
Auricle

932 Foreign body in nose
Nasal sinus
Nostril

● 933 Foreign body in pharynx and larynx

933.0 Pharynx
Nasopharynx
Throat NOS

933.1 Larynx
Asphyxia due to foreign body
Choking due to:
food (regurgitated)
phlegm

● 934 Foreign body in trachea, bronchus, and lung

934.0 Trachea

934.1 Main bronchus

❑ 934.8 Other specified parts
Bronchioles
Lung

❑ 934.9 Respiratory tree, unspecified
Inhalation of liquid or vomitus, lower respiratory tract NOS

● 935 Foreign body in mouth, esophagus, and stomach

935.0 Mouth

935.1 Esophagus

935.2 Stomach

936 Foreign body in intestine and colon

937 Foreign body in anus and rectum
Rectosigmoid (junction)

❑ 938 Foreign body in digestive system, unspecified
Alimentary tract NOS
Swallowed foreign body

● 939 Foreign body in genitourinary tract

939.0 Bladder and urethra

939.1 Uterus, any part

Excludes *intrauterine contraceptive device:*
complications from (996.32, 996.65)
presence of (V45.51)

939.2 Vulva and vagina

939.3 Penis

❑ 939.9 Unspecified site

BURNS (940–949)

Includes: burns from:
electrical heating appliance
electricity
flame
hot object
lightning
radiation
chemical burns (external) (internal)
scalds

Excludes *friction burns (910–919 with .0, .1)*
sunburn (692.71, 692.76–692.77)

● 940 Burn confined to eye and adnexa

940.0 Chemical burn of eyelids and periocular area

❑ 940.1 Other burns of eyelids and periocular area

940.2 Alkaline chemical burn of cornea and conjunctival sac

940.3 Acid chemical burn of cornea and conjunctival sac

❑ 940.4 Other burn of cornea and conjunctival sac

940.5 Burn with resulting rupture and destruction of eyeball

❑ 940.9 Unspecified burn of eye and adnexa

● 941 Burn of face, head, and neck

Excludes *mouth (947.0)*

The following fifth-digit subclassification is for use with category 941:

❑ 0 face and head, unspecified site
1 ear [any part]
2 eye (with other parts of face, head, and neck)
3 lip(s)
4 chin
5 nose (septum)
6 scalp [any part]
temple (region)
7 forehead and cheek
8 neck
❑ 9 multiple sites [except with eye] of face, head, and neck

● ❑ 941.0 Unspecified degree

● 941.1 Erythema [first degree]

● 941.2 Blisters, epidermal loss [second degree]

● 941.3 Full-thickness skin loss [third degree NOS]

● 941.4 Deep necrosis of underlying tissues [deep third degree] without mention of loss of a body part

● 941.5 Deep necrosis of underlying tissues [deep third degree] with loss of a body part

● 942 Burn of trunk

Excludes *scapular region (943.0–943.5 with fifth-digit 6)*

The following fifth-digit subclassification is for use with category 942:

❑ 0 trunk, unspecified site
1 breast
2 chest wall, excluding breast and nipple
3 abdominal wall
flank
groin
4 back [any part]
buttock
interscapular region
5 genitalia
labium (majus) (minus)
penis
perineum
scrotum
testis
vulva
❑ 9 other and multiple sites of trunk

● ❑ 942.0 Unspecified degree

● 942.1 Erythema [first degree]

● 942.2 Blisters, epidermal loss [second degree]

● 942.3 Full-thickness skin loss [third degree NOS]

● 942.4 Deep necrosis of underlying tissues [deep third degree] without mention of loss of a body part

● 942.5 Deep necrosis of underlying tissues [deep third degree] with loss of a body part

● 943 Burn of upper limb, except wrist and hand

The following fifth-digit subclassification is for use with category 943:

❑ 0 upper limb, unspecified site
1 forearm
2 elbow
3 upper arm
4 axilla
5 shoulder
6 scapular region
❑ 9 multiple sites of upper limb, except wrist and hand

● ❑ 943.0 Unspecified degree

● 943.1 Erythema [first degree]

● 943.2 Blisters, epidermal loss [second degree]

● 943.3 Full-thickness skin loss [third degree NOS]

● 943.4 Deep necrosis of underlying tissues [deep third degree] without mention of loss of a body part

● 943.5 Deep necrosis of underlying tissues [deep third degree] with loss of a body part

● 944 Burn of wrist(s) and hand(s)

The following fifth-digit subclassification is for use with category 944:

❑ 0 hand, unspecified site
1 single digit [finger (nail)] other than thumb
2 thumb (nail)
3 two or more digits, not including thumb
4 two or more digits including thumb
5 palm
6 back of hand
7 wrist
❑ 8 multiple sites of wrist(s) and hand(s)

● ❑ 944.0 Unspecified degree

● 944.1 Erythema [first degree]

● 944.2 Blisters, epidermal loss [second degree]

● 944.3 Full-thickness skin loss [third degree NOS]

● 944.4 Deep necrosis of underlying tissues [deep third degree] without mention of loss of a body part

● 944.5 Deep necrosis of underlying tissues [deep third degree] with loss of a body part

● 945 Burn of lower limb(s)

The following fifth-digit subclassification is for use with category 945:

❑ 0 lower limb [leg], unspecified site
1 toe(s) (nail)
2 foot
3 ankle
4 lower leg
5 knee
6 thigh [any part]
❑ 9 multiple sites of lower limb(s)

● ❑ 945.0 Unspecified degree

● 945.1 Erythema [first degree]

● 945.2 Blisters, epidermal loss [second degree]

● 945.3 Full-thickness skin loss [third degree NOS]

● 945.4 Deep necrosis of underlying tissues [deep third degree] without mention of loss of a body part

● 945.5 Deep necrosis of underlying tissues [deep third degree] with loss of a body part

● 946 Burns of multiple specified sites

Includes: burns of sites classifiable to more than one three-digit category in 940–945

Excludes *multiple burns NOS (949.0–949.5)*

❑ **946.0 Unspecified degree**

946.1 Erythema [first degree]

946.2 Blisters, epidermal loss [second degree]

946.3 Full-thickness skin loss [third degree NOS]

946.4 Deep necrosis of underlying tissues [deep third degree] without mention of loss of a body part

946.5 Deep necrosis of underlying tissues [deep third degree] with loss of a body part

● **947 Burn of internal organs**

Includes: burns from chemical agents (ingested)

947.0 Mouth and pharynx
Gum
Tongue

947.1 Larynx, trachea, and lung

947.2 Esophagus

947.3 Gastrointestinal tract
Colon
Rectum
Small intestine
Stomach

947.4 Vagina and uterus

❑ **947.8 Other specified sites**

❑ **947.9 Unspecified site**

● **948 Burns classified according to extent of body surface involved**

Note: This category is to be used when the site of the burn is unspecified, or with categories 940–947 when the site is specified.

Excludes *sunburn (692.71, 692.76–692.77)*

The following fifth-digit subclassification is for use with category 948 to indicate the percent of body surface with third degree burn; valid digits are in [brackets] under each code:

0 less than 10 percent or unspecified
1 10–19%
2 20–29%
3 30–39%
4 40–49%
5 50–59%
6 60–69%
7 70–79%
8 80–89%
9 90% or more of body surface

● **948.0 Burn [any degree] involving less than 10 percent of body surface**
[0]

● **948.1 10–19 percent of body surface**
[0–1]

● **948.2 20–29 percent of body surface**
[0–2]

● **948.3 30–39 percent of body surface**
[0–3]

● **948.4 40–49 percent of body surface**
[0–4]

● **948.5 50–59 percent of body surface**
[0–5]

● **948.6 60–69 percent of body surface**
[0–6]

● **948.7 70–79 percent of body surface**
[0–7]

● **948.8 80–89 percent of body surface**
[0–8]

● **948.9 90 percent or more of body surface**
[0–9]

● **949 Burn, unspecified**

Includes: burn NOS
multiple burns NOS

Excludes *burn of unspecified site but with statement of the extent of body surface involved (948.0–948.9)*

❑ **949.0 Unspecified degree**

❑ **949.1 Erythema [first degree]**

❑ **949.2 Blisters, epidermal loss [second degree]**

❑ **949.3 Full-thickness skin loss [third degree NOS]**

❑ **949.4 Deep necrosis of underlying tissues [deep third degree] without mention of loss of a body part**

❑ **949.5 Deep necrosis of underlying tissues [deep third degree] with loss of a body part**

INJURY TO NERVES AND SPINAL CORD (950–957)

Includes: division of nerve
lesion in continuity (with open wound)
traumatic neuroma (with open wound)
traumatic transient paralysis (with open wound)

Excludes *accidental puncture or laceration during medical procedure (998.2)*

● **950 Injury to optic nerve and pathways**

950.0 Optic nerve injury
Second cranial nerve

950.1 Injury to optic chiasm

950.2 Injury to optic pathways

950.3 Injury to visual cortex

❑ **950.9 Unspecified**
Traumatic blindness NOS

● **951 Injury to other cranial nerve(s)**

951.0 Injury to oculomotor nerve
Third cranial nerve

951.1 Injury to trochlear nerve
Fourth cranial nerve

951.2 Injury to trigeminal nerve
Fifth cranial nerve

951.3 Injury to abducens nerve
Sixth cranial nerve

951.4 Injury to facial nerve
Seventh cranial nerve

951.5 Injury to acoustic nerve
Auditory nerve
Eighth cranial nerve
Traumatic deafness NOS

951.6 Injury to accessory nerve
Eleventh cranial nerve

951.7 Injury to hypoglossal nerve
Twelfth cranial nerve

❑ **951.8 Injury to other specified cranial nerves**
Glossopharyngeal [9th cranial] nerve
Olfactory [1st cranial] nerve
Pneumogastric [10th cranial] nerve
Traumatic anosmia NOS
Vagus [10th cranial] nerve

❑ **951.9 Injury to unspecified cranial nerve**

● 952 Spinal cord injury without evidence of spinal bone injury

● 952.0 Cervical

❑ 952.00 C_1-C_4 level with unspecified spinal cord injury
Spinal cord injury, cervical region NOS

952.01 C_1-C_4 level with complete lesion of spinal cord

952.02 C_1-C_4 level with anterior cord syndrome

952.03 C_1-C_4 level with central cord syndrome

❑ 952.04 C_1-C_4 level with other specified spinal cord injury
Incomplete spinal cord lesion at C_1-C_4 level:
NOS
with posterior cord syndrome

❑ 952.05 C_5-C_7 level with unspecified spinal cord injury

952.06 C_5-C_7 level with complete lesion of spinal cord

952.07 C_5-C_7 level with anterior cord syndrome

952.08 C_5-C_7 level with central cord syndrome

❑ 952.09 C_5-C_7 level with other specified spinal cord injury
Incomplete spinal cord lesion at C_5-C_7 level:
NOS
with posterior cord syndrome

● 952.1 Dorsal [thoracic]

❑ 952.10 T_1-T_6 level with unspecified spinal cord injury
Spinal cord injury, thoracic region NOS

952.11 T_1-T_6 level with complete lesion of spinal cord

952.12 T_1-T_6 level with anterior cord syndrome

952.13 T_1-T_6 level with central cord syndrome

❑ 952.14 T_1-T_6 level with other specified spinal cord injury
Incomplete spinal cord lesion at T_1-T_6 level:
NOS
with posterior cord syndrome

❑ 952.15 T_7-T_{12} level with unspecified spinal cord injury

952.16 T_7-T_{12} level with complete lesion of spinal cord

952.17 T_7-T_{12} level with anterior cord syndrome

952.18 T_7-T_{12} level with central cord syndrome

❑ 952.19 T_7-T_{12} level with other specified spinal cord injury
Incomplete spinal cord lesion at T_7-T_{12} level:
NOS
with posterior cord syndrome

952.2 Lumbar

952.3 Sacral

952.4 Cauda equina

❑ 952.8 Multiple sites of spinal cord

❑ 952.9 Unspecified site of spinal cord

● 953 Injury to nerve roots and spinal plexus

953.0 Cervical root

953.1 Dorsal root

953.2 Lumbar root

953.3 Sacral root

953.4 Brachial plexus

953.5 Lumbosacral plexus

❑ 953.8 Multiple sites

❑ 953.9 Unspecified site

● 954 Injury to other nerve(s) of trunk, excluding shoulder and pelvic girdles

954.0 Cervical sympathetic

❑ 954.1 Other sympathetic
Celiac ganglion or plexus
Inferior mesenteric plexus
Splanchnic nerve(s)
Stellate ganglion

❑ 954.8 Other specified nerve(s) of trunk

❑ 954.9 Unspecified nerve of trunk

● 955 Injury to peripheral nerve(s) of shoulder girdle and upper limb

955.0 Axillary nerve

955.1 Median nerve

955.2 Ulnar nerve

955.3 Radial nerve

955.4 Musculocutaneous nerve

955.5 Cutaneous sensory nerve, upper limb

955.6 Digital nerve

❑ 955.7 Other specified nerve(s) of shoulder girdle and upper limb

❑ 955.8 Multiple nerves of shoulder girdle and upper limb

❑ 955.9 Unspecified nerve of shoulder girdle and upper limb

● 956 Injury to peripheral nerve(s) of pelvic girdle and lower limb

956.0 Sciatic nerve

956.1 Femoral nerve

956.2 Posterior tibial nerve

956.3 Peroneal nerve

956.4 Cutaneous sensory nerve, lower limb

❑ 956.5 Other specified nerve(s) of pelvic girdle and lower limb

❑ 956.8 Multiple nerves of pelvic girdle and lower limb

❑ 956.9 Unspecified nerve of pelvic girdle and lower limb

● 957 Injury to other and unspecified nerves

957.0 Superficial nerves of head and neck

❑ 957.1 Other specified nerve(s)

❑ 957.8 Multiple nerves in several parts
Multiple nerve injury NOS

❑ 957.9 Unspecified site
Nerve injury NOS

CERTAIN TRAUMATIC COMPLICATIONS AND UNSPECIFIED INJURIES (958–959)

● 958 Certain early complications of trauma

Excludes *adult respiratory distress syndrome (518.5)*
flail chest (807.4)
shock lung (518.5)
that occurring during or following medical procedures (996.0–999.9)

958.0 Air embolism
Pneumathemia

Excludes *that complicating:*
abortion (634–638 with .6, 639.6)
ectopic or molar pregnancy (639.6)
pregnancy, childbirth, or the puerperium (673.0)

958.1 Fat embolism

Excludes *that complicating:*
abortion (634–638 with .6, 639.6)
pregnancy, childbirth, or the puerperium (673.8)

958.2 Secondary and recurrent hemorrhage

958.3 Posttraumatic wound infection, not elsewhere classified

Excludes *infected open wounds—code to complicated open wound of site*

958.4 Traumatic shock
Shock (immediate) (delayed) following injury

Excludes *shock:*
anaphylactic (995.0)
due to serum (999.4)
anesthetic (995.4)
electric (994.8)
following abortion (639.5)
lightning (994.0)
nontraumatic NOS (785.50)
obstetric (669.1)
postoperative (998.0)

958.5 Traumatic anuria
Crush syndrome
Renal failure following crushing

Excludes *that due to a medical procedure (997.5)*

958.6 Volkmann's ischemic contracture
Posttraumatic muscle contracture

958.7 Traumatic subcutaneous emphysema

Excludes *subcutaneous emphysema resulting from a procedure (998.81)*

❑ **958.8 Other early complications of trauma**

● **959 Injury, other and unspecified**

Includes: injury NOS

Excludes *injury NOS of:*
blood vessels (900.0–904.9)
eye (921.0–921.9)
internal organs (860.0–869.1)
intracranial sites (854.0–854.1)
nerves (950.0–951.9, 953.0–957.9)
spinal cord (952.0–952.9)

● **959.0 Head, face and neck**

❑ **959.01 Head injury, unspecified**

Excludes *concussion (850.1–850.9)*
with head injury NOS (850.1–850.5)
head injury NOS with loss of consciousness (850.1–850.5)
specified intracranial injuries (850.0–854.1)

959.09 Injury of face and neck

● **959.1 Trunk**

❑ **959.11 Other injury of chest wall** ◀

❑ **959.12 Other injury of abdomen** ◀

959.13 Fracture of corpus cavernosum penis ◀

959.14 Other injury of external genitals ◀

❑ **959.19 Other injury of other sites of trunk** ◀
Injury of trunk NOS ◀

Excludes *scapular region (959.2)*

959.2 Shoulder and upper arm
Axilla
Scapular region

959.3 Elbow, forearm, and wrist

959.4 Hand, except finger

959.5 Finger
Fingernail
Thumb (nail)

959.6 Hip and thigh
Upper leg

959.7 Knee, leg, ankle, and foot

❑ **959.8 Other specified sites, including multiple**

Excludes *multiple sites classifiable to the same four-digit category (959.0–959.7)*

❑ **959.9 Unspecified site**

POISONING BY DRUGS, MEDICINAL AND BIOLOGICAL SUBSTANCES (960–979)

Includes: overdose of these substances
wrong substance given or taken in error

Excludes *adverse effects ["hypersensitivity," "reaction," etc.] of correct substance properly administered. Such cases are to be classified according to the nature of the adverse effect, such as:*
adverse effect NOS (995.2)
allergic lymphadenitis (289.3)
aspirin gastritis (535.4)
blood disorders (280.0–289.9)
dermatitis:
contact (692.0–692.9)
due to ingestion (693.0–693.9)
nephropathy (583.9)
[The drug giving rise to the adverse effect may be identified by use of categories E930–E949.]
drug dependence (304.0–304.9)
drug reaction and poisoning affecting the newborn (760.0–779.9)
nondependent abuse of drugs (305.0–305.9)
pathological drug intoxication (292.2)

Use additional code to specify the effects of the poisoning

● **960 Poisoning by antibiotics**

Excludes *antibiotics:*
ear, nose, and throat (976.6)
eye (976.5)
local (976.0)

960.0 Penicillins
Ampicillin
Carbenicillin
Cloxacillin
Penicillin G

960.1 Antifungal antibiotics
Amphotericin B
Griseofulvin
Nystatin
Trichomycin

Excludes *preparations intended for topical use (976.0–976.9)*

960.2 Chloramphenicol group
Chloramphenicol
Thiamphenicol

960.3 Erythromycin and other macrolides
Oleandomycin
Spiramycin

960.4 **Tetracycline group**
Doxycycline
Minocycline
Oxytetracycline

960.5 **Cephalosporin group**
Cephalexin
Cephaloglycin
Cephaloridine
Cephalothin

960.6 **Antimycobacterial antibiotics**
Cycloserine
Kanamycin
Rifampin
Streptomycin

960.7 **Antineoplastic antibiotics**
Actinomycin such as:
Bleomycin
Cactinomycin
Dactinomycin
Daunorubicin
Mitomycin

❑ 960.8 **Other specified antibiotics**

❑ 960.9 **Unspecified antibiotic**

● 961 **Poisoning by other anti-infectives**

Excludes *anti-infectives:*
ear, nose, and throat (976.6)
eye (976.5)
local (976.0)

961.0 **Sulfonamides**
Sulfadiazine
Sulfafurazole
Sulfamethoxazole

961.1 **Arsenical anti-infectives**

961.2 **Heavy metal anti-infectives**
Compounds of:
antimony
bismuth
Compounds of:
lead
mercury

Excludes *mercurial diuretics (974.0)*

961.3 **Quinoline and hydroxyquinoline derivatives**
Chiniofon
Diiodohydroxyquin

Excludes *antimalarial drugs (961.4)*

961.4 **Antimalarials and drugs acting on other blood protozoa**
Chloroquine
Cycloguanil
Primaquine
Proguanil [chloroguanide]
Pyrimethamine
Quinine

❑ 961.5 **Other antiprotozoal drugs**
Emetine

961.6 **Anthelmintics**
Hexylresorcinol
Piperazine
Thiabendazole

961.7 **Antiviral drugs**
Methisazone

Excludes *amantadine (966.4)*
cytarabine (963.1)
idoxuridine (976.5)

❑ 961.8 **Other antimycobacterial drugs**
Ethambutol
Ethionamide
Isoniazid
Para-aminosalicylic acid derivatives
Sulfones

❑ 961.9 **Other and unspecified anti-infectives**
Flucytosine
Nitrofuran derivatives

● 962 **Poisoning by hormones and synthetic substitutes**

Excludes *oxytocic hormones (975.0)*

962.0 **Adrenal cortical steroids**
Cortisone derivatives
Desoxycorticosterone derivatives
Fluorinated corticosteroids

962.1 **Androgens and anabolic congeners**
Methandriol
Nandrolone
Oxymetholone
Testosterone

962.2 **Ovarian hormones and synthetic substitutes**
Contraceptives, oral
Estrogens
Estrogens and progestogens, combined
Progestogens

962.3 **Insulins and antidiabetic agents**
Acetohexamide
Biguanide derivatives, oral
Chlorpropamide
Glucagon
Insulin
Phenformin
Sulfonylurea derivatives, oral
Tolbutamide

962.4 **Anterior pituitary hormones**
Corticotropin
Gonadotropin
Somatotropin [growth hormone]

962.5 **Posterior pituitary hormones**
Vasopressin

Excludes *oxytocic hormones (975.0)*

962.6 **Parathyroid and parathyroid derivatives**

962.7 **Thyroid and thyroid derivatives**
Dextrothyroxin
Levothyroxine sodium
Liothyronine
Thyroglobulin

962.8 **Antithyroid agents**
Iodides
Thiouracil
Thiourea

❑ 962.9 **Other and unspecified hormones and synthetic substitutes**

● 963 **Poisoning by primarily systemic agents**

963.0 **Antiallergic and antiemetic drugs**
Antihistamines
Chlorpheniramine
Diphenhydramine
Diphenylpyraline
Thonzylamine
Tripelennamine

Excludes *phenothiazine-based tranquilizers (969.1)*

963.1 **Antineoplastic and immunosuppressive drugs**
Azathioprine
Busulfan
Chlorambucil
Cyclophosphamide
Cytarabine
Fluorouracil
Mercaptopurine
thio-TEPA

Excludes *antineoplastic antibiotics (960.7)*

963.2 **Acidifying agents**

963.3 **Alkalizing agents**

963.4 Enzymes, not elsewhere classified
Penicillinase

963.5 Vitamins, not elsewhere classified
Vitamin A
Vitamin D
Excludes *nicotinic acid (972.2)*
vitamin K (964.3)

❑ 963.8 Other specified systemic agents
Heavy metal antagonists

❑ 963.9 Unspecified systemic agent

● 964 Poisoning by agents primarily affecting blood constituents

964.0 Iron and its compounds
Ferric salts
Ferrous sulfate and other ferrous salts

964.1 Liver preparations and other antianemic agents
Folic acid

964.2 Anticoagulants
Coumarin
Heparin
Phenindione
Warfarin sodium

964.3 Vitamin K [phytonadione]

964.4 Fibrinolysis-affecting drugs
Aminocaproic acid
Streptodornase
Streptokinase
Urokinase

964.5 Anticoagulant antagonists and other coagulants
Hexadimethrine
Protamine sulfate

964.6 Gamma globulin

964.7 Natural blood and blood products
Blood plasma
Human fibrinogen
Packed red cells
Whole blood
Excludes *transfusion reactions (999.4–999.8)*

❑ 964.8 Other specified agents affecting blood constituents
Macromolecular blood substitutes
Plasma expanders

❑ 964.9 Unspecified agents affecting blood constituents

● 965 Poisoning by analgesics, antipyretics, and antirheumatics
Excludes *drug dependence (304.0–304.9)*
nondependent abuse (305.0–305.9)

● 965.0 Opiates and related narcotics

❑ 965.00 Opium (alkaloids), unspecified

965.01 Heroin
Diacetylmorphine

965.02 Methadone

❑ 965.09 Other
Codeine [methylmorphine]
Meperidine [pethidine]
Morphine

965.1 Salicylates
Acetylsalicylic acid [aspirin]
Salicylic acid salts

965.4 Aromatic analgesics, not elsewhere classified
Acetanilid
Paracetamol [acetaminophen]
Phenacetin [acetophenetidin]

965.5 Pyrazole derivatives
Aminophenazone [aminopyrine]
Phenylbutazone

● 965.6 Antirheumatics [antiphlogistics]
Excludes *salicylates (965.1)*
steroids (962.0–962.9)

965.61 Propionic acid derivatives
Fenoprofen
Flurbiprofen
Ibuprofen
Ketoprofen
Naproxen
Oxaprozin

❑ 965.69 Other antirheumatics
Gold salts
Indomethacin

❑ 965.7 Other non-narcotic analgesics
Pyrabital

❑ 965.8 Other specified analgesics and antipyretics
Pentazocine

❑ 965.9 Unspecified analgesic and antipyretic

● 966 Poisoning by anticonvulsants and anti-Parkinsonism drugs

966.0 Oxazolidine derivatives
Paramethadione
Trimethadione

966.1 Hydantoin derivatives
Phenytoin

966.2 Succinimides
Ethosuximide
Phensuximide

❑ 966.3 Other and unspecified anticonvulsants
Primidone
Excludes *barbiturates (967.0)*
sulfonamides (961.0)

966.4 Anti-Parkinsonism drugs
Amantadine
Ethopropazine [profenamine]
Levodopa [L-dopa]

● 967 Poisoning by sedatives and hypnotics
Excludes *drug dependence (304.0–304.9)*
nondependent abuse (305.0–305.9)

967.0 Barbiturates
Amobarbital [amylobarbitone]
Barbital [barbitone]
Butabarbital [butabarbitone]
Pentobarbital [pentobarbitone]
Phenobarbital [phenobarbitone]
Secobarbital [quinalbarbitone]
Excludes *thiobarbiturate anesthetics (968.3)*

967.1 Chloral hydrate group

967.2 Paraldehyde

967.3 Bromine compounds
Bromide
Carbromal (derivatives)

967.4 Methaqualone compounds

967.5 Glutethimide group

967.6 Mixed sedatives, not elsewhere classified

❑ 967.8 Other sedatives and hypnotics

❑ 967.9 Unspecified sedative or hypnotic
Sleeping:
drug NOS
pill NOS
tablet NOS

● 968 **Poisoning by other central nervous system depressants and anesthetics**

Excludes *drug dependence (304.0–304.9)*
nondependent abuse (305.0–305.9)

968.0 **Central nervous system muscle-tone depressants**
Chlorphenesin (carbamate)
Mephenesin
Methocarbamol

968.1 **Halothane**

❑ 968.2 **Other gaseous anesthetics**
Ether
Halogenated hydrocarbon derivatives, except halothane
Nitrous oxide

968.3 **Intravenous anesthetics**
Ketamine
Methohexital [methohexitone]
Thiobarbiturates, such as thiopental sodium

❑ 968.4 **Other and unspecified general anesthetics**

968.5 **Surface [topical] and infiltration anesthetics**
Cocaine
Lidocaine [lignocaine]
Procaine
Tetracaine

968.6 **Peripheral nerve- and plexus-blocking anesthetics**

968.7 **Spinal anesthetics**

❑ 968.9 **Other and unspecified local anesthetics**

● 969 **Poisoning by psychotropic agents**

Excludes *drug dependence (304.0–304.9)*
nondependent abuse (305.0–305.9)

969.0 **Antidepressants**
Amitriptyline
Imipramine
Monoamine oxidase [MAO] inhibitors

969.1 **Phenothiazine-based tranquilizers**
Chlorpromazine
Fluphenazine
Prochlorperazine
Promazine

969.2 **Butyrophenone-based tranquilizers**
Haloperidol
Spiperone
Trifluperidol

❑ 969.3 **Other antipsychotics, neuroleptics, and major tranquilizers**

969.4 **Benzodiazepine-based tranquilizers**
Chlordiazepoxide
Diazepam
Flurazepam
Lorazepam
Medazepam
Nitrazepam

❑ 969.5 **Other tranquilizers**
Hydroxyzine
Meprobamate

969.6 **Psychodysleptics [hallucinogens]**
Cannabis (derivatives)
Lysergide [LSD]
Marijuana (derivatives)
Mescaline
Psilocin
Psilocybin

969.7 **Psychostimulants**
Amphetamine
Caffeine

Excludes *central appetite depressants (977.0)*

❑ 969.8 **Other specified psychotropic agents**

❑ 969.9 **Unspecified psychotropic agent**

● 970 **Poisoning by central nervous system stimulants**

970.0 **Analeptics**
Lobeline
Nikethamide

970.1 **Opiate antagonists**
Levallorphan
Nalorphine
Naloxone

❑ 970.8 **Other specified central nervous system stimulants**

❑ 970.9 **Unspecified central nervous system stimulant**

● 971 **Poisoning by drugs primarily affecting the autonomic nervous system**

971.0 **Parasympathomimetics [cholinergics]**
Acetylcholine
Anticholinesterase:
organophosphorus
reversible
Pilocarpine

971.1 **Parasympatholytics [anticholinergics and antimuscarinics] and spasmolytics**
Atropine
Homatropine
Hyoscine [scopolamine]
Quaternary ammonium derivatives

Excludes *papaverine (972.5)*

971.2 **Sympathomimetics [adrenergics]**
Epinephrine [adrenalin]
Levarterenol [noradrenalin]

971.3 **Sympatholytics [antiadrenergics]**
Phenoxybenzamine
Tolazoline hydrochloride

❑ 971.9 **Unspecified drug primarily affecting autonomic nervous system**

● 972 **Poisoning by agents primarily affecting the cardiovascular system**

972.0 **Cardiac rhythm regulators**
Practolol
Procainamide
Propranolol
Quinidine

Excludes *lidocaine (968.5)*

972.1 **Cardiotonic glycosides and drugs of similar action**
Digitalis glycosides
Digoxin
Strophanthins

972.2 **Antilipemic and antiarteriosclerotic drugs**
Clofibrate
Nicotinic acid derivatives

972.3 **Ganglion-blocking agents**
Pentamethonium bromide

972.4 **Coronary vasodilators**
Dipyridamole
Nitrates [nitroglycerin]
Nitrites

❑ 972.5 **Other vasodilators**
Cyclandelate
Diazoxide
Papaverine

Excludes *nicotinic acid (972.2)*

❑ 972.6 **Other antihypertensive agents**
Clonidine
Guanethidine
Rauwolfia alkaloids
Reserpine

972.7 Antivaricose drugs, including sclerosing agents
Sodium morrhuate
Zinc salts

972.8 Capillary-active drugs
Adrenochrome derivatives
Metaraminol

❑ **972.9 Other and unspecified agents primarily affecting the cardiovascular system**

● **973 Poisoning by agents primarily affecting the gastrointestinal system**

973.0 Antacids and antigastric secretion drugs
Aluminum hydroxide
Magnesium trisilicate

973.1 Irritant cathartics
Bisacodyl
Castor oil
Phenolphthalein

973.2 Emollient cathartics
Dioctyl sulfosuccinates

❑ **973.3 Other cathartics, including intestinal atonia drugs**
Magnesium sulfate

973.4 Digestants
Pancreatin
Papain
Pepsin

973.5 Antidiarrheal drugs
Kaolin
Pectin

Excludes *anti-infectives (960.0–961.9)*

973.6 Emetics

❑ **973.8 Other specified agents primarily affecting the gastrointestinal system**

❑ **973.9 Unspecified agent primarily affecting the gastrointestinal system**

● **974 Poisoning by water, mineral, and uric acid metabolism drugs**

974.0 Mercurial diuretics
Chlormerodrin
Mercaptomerin
Mersalyl

974.1 Purine derivative diuretics
Theobromine
Theophylline

Excludes *aminophylline [theophylline ethylenediamine] (975.7)*
caffeine (969.7)

974.2 Carbonic acid anhydrase inhibitors
Acetazolamide

974.3 Saluretics
Benzothiadiazides
Chlorothiazide group

❑ **974.4 Other diuretics**
Ethacrynic acid
Furosemide

974.5 Electrolytic, caloric, and water-balance agents

❑ **974.6 Other mineral salts, not elsewhere classified**

974.7 Uric acid metabolism drugs
Allopurinol
Colchicine
Probenecid

● **975 Poisoning by agents primarily acting on the smooth and skeletal muscles and respiratory system**

975.0 Oxytocic agents
Ergot alkaloids
Oxytocin
Prostaglandins

975.1 Smooth muscle relaxants
Adiphenine
Metaproterenol [orciprenaline]

Excludes *papaverine (972.5)*

975.2 Skeletal muscle relaxants

❑ **975.3 Other and unspecified drugs acting on muscles**

975.4 Antitussives
Dextromethorphan
Pipazethate

975.5 Expectorants
Acetylcysteine
Guaifenesin
Terpin hydrate

975.6 Anti-common cold drugs

975.7 Antiasthmatics
Aminophylline [theophylline ethylenediamine]

❑ **975.8 Other and unspecified respiratory drugs**

● **976 Poisoning by agents primarily affecting skin and mucous membrane, ophthalmological, otorhinolaryngological, and dental drugs**

976.0 Local anti-infectives and anti-inflammatory drugs

976.1 Antipruritics

976.2 Local astringents and local detergents

976.3 Emollients, demulcents, and protectants

976.4 Keratolytics, keratoplastics, other hair treatment drugs and preparations

976.5 Eye anti-infectives and other eye drugs
Idoxuridine

976.6 Anti-infectives and other drugs and preparations for ear, nose, and throat

976.7 Dental drugs topically applied

Excludes *anti-infectives (976.0)*
local anesthetics (968.5)

❑ **976.8 Other agents primarily affecting skin and mucous membrane**
Spermicides [vaginal contraceptives]

❑ **976.9 Unspecified agent primarily affecting skin and mucous membrane**

● **977 Poisoning by other and unspecified drugs and medicinal substances**

977.0 Dietetics
Central appetite depressants

977.1 Lipotropic drugs

977.2 Antidotes and chelating agents, not elsewhere classified

977.3 Alcohol deterrents

977.4 Pharmaceutical excipients
Pharmaceutical adjuncts

❑ **977.8 Other specified drugs and medicinal substances**
Contrast media used for diagnostic x-ray procedures
Diagnostic agents and kits

❑ **977.9 Unspecified drug or medicinal substance**

● **978 Poisoning by bacterial vaccines**

978.0 BCG

978.1 **Typhoid and paratyphoid**

978.2 **Cholera**

978.3 **Plague**

978.4 **Tetanus**

978.5 **Diphtheria**

978.6 **Pertussis vaccine, including combinations with a pertussis component**

❑978.8 **Other and unspecified bacterial vaccines**

978.9 **Mixed bacterial vaccines, except combinations with a pertussis component**

● 979 **Poisoning by other vaccines and biological substances**

Excludes *gamma globulin (964.6)*

979.0 **Smallpox vaccine**

979.1 **Rabies vaccine**

979.2 **Typhus vaccine**

979.3 **Yellow fever vaccine**

979.4 **Measles vaccine**

979.5 **Poliomyelitis vaccine**

❑979.6 **Other and unspecified viral and rickettsial vaccines**
Mumps vaccine

979.7 **Mixed viral-rickettsial and bacterial vaccines, except combinations with a pertussis component**

Excludes *combinations with a pertussis component (978.6)*

❑979.9 **Other and unspecified vaccines and biological substances**

TOXIC EFFECTS OF SUBSTANCES CHIEFLY NONMEDICINAL AS TO SOURCE (980–989)

Excludes *burns from chemical agents (ingested) (947.0–947.9)*
localized toxic effects indexed elsewhere (001.0–799.9)
respiratory conditions due to external agents (506.0–508.9)

Use additional code to specify the nature of the toxic effect

● 980 **Toxic effect of alcohol**

980.0 **Ethyl alcohol**
Denatured alcohol
Ethanol
Grain alcohol

Use additional code to identify any associated:
acute alcohol intoxication (305.0)
in alcoholism (303.0)
drunkenness (simple) (305.0)
pathological (291.4)

980.1 **Methyl alcohol**
Methanol
Wood alcohol

980.2 **Isopropyl alcohol**
Dimethyl carbinol
Isopropanol
Rubbing alcohol

980.3 **Fusel oil**
Alcohol:
amyl
butyl
propyl

❑980.8 **Other specified alcohols**

❑980.9 **Unspecified alcohol**

981 **Toxic effect of petroleum products**
Benzine
Gasoline
Kerosene
Paraffin wax
Petroleum:
ether
naphtha
spirit

● 982 **Toxic effect of solvents other than petroleum based**

982.0 **Benzene and homologues**

982.1 **Carbon tetrachloride**

982.2 **Carbon disulfide**
Carbon bisulfide

❑982.3 **Other chlorinated hydrocarbon solvents**
Tetrachloroethylene
Trichloroethylene

Excludes *chlorinated hydrocarbon preparations other than solvents (989.2)*

982.4 **Nitroglycol**

❑982.8 **Other nonpetroleum-based solvents**
Acetone

● 983 **Toxic effect of corrosive aromatics, acids, and caustic alkalis**

983.0 **Corrosive aromatics**
Carbolic acid or phenol
Cresol

983.1 **Acids**
Acid:
hydrochloric
nitric
sulfuric

983.2 **Caustic alkalis**
Lye
Potassium hydroxide
Sodium hydroxide

❑983.9 **Caustic, unspecified**

● 984 **Toxic effect of lead and its compounds (including fumes)**

Includes: that from all sources except medicinal substances

984.0 **Inorganic lead compounds**
Lead dioxide
Lead salts

984.1 **Organic lead compounds**
Lead acetate
Tetraethyl lead

❑984.8 **Other lead compounds**

❑984.9 **Unspecified lead compound**

● 985 **Toxic effect of other metals**

Includes: that from all sources except medicinal substances

985.0 **Mercury and its compounds**
Minamata disease

985.1 **Arsenic and its compounds**

985.2 **Manganese and its compounds**

985.3 **Beryllium and its compounds**

985.4 **Antimony and its compounds**

985.5 **Cadmium and its compounds**

985.6 **Chromium**

❑985.8 **Other specified metals**
Brass fumes
Copper salts
Iron compounds
Nickel compounds

❑985.9 **Unspecified metal**

986 Toxic effect of carbon monoxide

● **987 Toxic effect of other gases, fumes, or vapors**

987.0 Liquefied petroleum gases
Butane
Propane

❑ **987.1 Other hydrocarbon gas**

987.2 Nitrogen oxides
Nitrogen dioxide
Nitrous fumes

987.3 Sulfur dioxide

987.4 Freon
Dichloromonofluoromethane

987.5 Lacrimogenic gas
Bromobenzyl cyanide
Chloroacetophenone
Ethyliodoacetate

987.6 Chlorine gas

987.7 Hydrocyanic acid gas

❑ **987.8 Other specified gases, fumes, or vapors**
Phosgene
Polyester fumes

❑ **987.9 Unspecified gas, fume, or vapor**

● **988 Toxic effect of noxious substances eaten as food**

Excludes *allergic reaction to food, such as:*
gastroenteritis (558.3)
rash (692.5, 693.1)
food poisoning (bacterial) (005.0–005.9)
toxic effects of food contaminants, such as:
aflatoxin and other mycotoxin (989.7)
mercury (985.0)

988.0 Fish and shellfish

988.1 Mushrooms

988.2 Berries and other plants

❑ **988.8 Other specified noxious substances eaten as food**

❑ **988.9 Unspecified noxious substance eaten as food**

● **989 Toxic effect of other substances, chiefly nonmedicinal as to source**

989.0 Hydrocyanic acid and cyanides
Potassium cyanide
Sodium cyanide

Excludes *gas and fumes (987.7)*

989.1 Strychnine and salts

989.2 Chlorinated hydrocarbons
Aldrin
Chlordane
DDT
Dieldrin

Excludes *chlorinated hydrocarbon solvents (982.0–982.3)*

989.3 Organophosphate and carbamate
Carbaryl
Dichlorvos
Malathion
Parathion
Phorate
Phosdrin

❑ **989.4 Other pesticides, not elsewhere classified**
Mixtures of insecticides

989.5 Venom
Bites of venomous snakes, lizards, and spiders
Tick paralysis

989.6 Soaps and detergents

989.7 Aflatoxin and other mycotoxin [food contaminants]

● **989.8 Other substances, chiefly nonmedicinal as to source**

989.81 Asbestos

Excludes *asbestosis (501)*
exposure to asbestos (V15.84)

989.82 Latex

989.83 Silicone

Excludes *silicone used in medical devices, implants and grafts (996.00–996.79)*

989.84 Tobacco

❑ **989.89 Other**

❑ **989.9 Unspecified substance, chiefly nonmedicinal as to source**

OTHER AND UNSPECIFIED EFFECTS OF EXTERNAL CAUSES (990–995)

❑ **990 Effects of radiation, unspecified**
Complication of:
phototherapy
radiation therapy
Radiation sickness

Excludes *specified adverse effects of radiation. Such conditions are to be classified according to the nature of the adverse effect, as:*
burns (940.0–949.5)
dermatitis (692.7–692.8)
leukemia (204.0–208.9)
pneumonia (508.0)
sunburn (692.71, 692.76–692.77)
[The type of radiation giving rise to the adverse effect may be identified by use of the E codes.]

● **991 Effects of reduced temperature**

991.0 Frostbite of face

991.1 Frostbite of hand

991.2 Frostbite of foot

❑ **991.3 Frostbite of other and unspecified sites**

991.4 Immersion foot
Trench foot

991.5 Chilblains
Erythema pernio
Perniosis

991.6 Hypothermia
Hypothermia (accidental)

Excludes *hypothermia following anesthesia (995.89)*
hypothermia not associated with low environmental temperature (780.99)

❑ **991.8 Other specified effects of reduced temperature**

❑ **991.9 Unspecified effect of reduced temperature**
Effects of freezing or excessive cold NOS

● **992 Effects of heat and light**

Excludes *burns (940.0–949.5)*
diseases of sweat glands due to heat (705.0–705.9)
malignant hyperpyrexia following anesthesia (995.86)
sunburn (692.71, 692.76–692.77)

992.0 Heat stroke and sunstroke
Heat apoplexy
Heat pyrexia
Ictus solaris
Siriasis
Thermoplegia

992.1 Heat syncope
Heat collapse

992.2 **Heat cramps**

992.3 **Heat exhaustion, anhydrotic**
Heat prostration due to water depletion
Excludes *that associated with salt depletion (992.4)*

992.4 **Heat exhaustion due to salt depletion**
Heat prostration due to salt (and water) depletion

❑992.5 **Heat exhaustion, unspecified**
Heat prostration NOS

992.6 **Heat fatigue, transient**

992.7 **Heat edema**

❑992.8 **Other specified heat effects**

❑992.9 **Unspecified**

● 993 **Effects of air pressure**

993.0 **Barotrauma, otitic**
Aero-otitis media
Effects of high altitude on ears

993.1 **Barotrauma, sinus**
Aerosinusitis
Effects of high altitude on sinuses

❑993.2 **Other and unspecified effects of high altitude**
Alpine sickness
Andes disease
Anoxia due to high altitude
Hypobaropathy
Mountain sickness

993.3 **Caisson disease**
Bends
Compressed-air disease
Decompression sickness
Divers' palsy or paralysis

993.4 **Effects of air pressure caused by explosion**

❑993.8 **Other specified effects of air pressure**

❑993.9 **Unspecified effect of air pressure**

● 994 **Effects of other external causes**
Excludes *certain adverse effects not elsewhere classified (995.0–995.8)*

994.0 **Effects of lightning**
Shock from lightning
Struck by lightning NOS
Excludes *burns (940.0–949.5)*

994.1 **Drowning and nonfatal submersion**
Bathing cramp
Immersion

994.2 **Effects of hunger**
Deprivation of food
Starvation

994.3 **Effects of thirst**
Deprivation of water

994.4 **Exhaustion due to exposure**

994.5 **Exhaustion due to excessive exertion**
Overexertion

994.6 **Motion sickness**
Air sickness
Seasickness
Travel sickness

994.7 **Asphyxiation and strangulation**
Suffocation (by):
bedclothes
cave-in
constriction
mechanical
Suffocation (by):
plastic bag
pressure
strangulation
Excludes *asphyxia from:*
carbon monoxide (986)
inhalation of food or foreign body (932–934.9)
other gases, fumes, and vapors (987.0–987.9)

994.8 **Electrocution and nonfatal effects of electric current**
Shock from electric current
Excludes *electric burns (940.0–949.5)*

❑994.9 **Other effects of external causes**
Effects of:
abnormal gravitational [G] forces or states
weightlessness

● 995 **Certain adverse effects not elsewhere classified**
Excludes *complications of surgical and medical care (996.0–999.9)*

❑995.0 **Other anaphylactic shock**
Allergic shock NOS or due to adverse effect of correct medicinal substance properly administered
Anaphylactic reaction NOS or due to adverse effect of correct medicinal substance properly administered
Anaphylaxis NOS or due to adverse effect of correct medicinal substance properly administered
Excludes *anaphylactic reaction to serum (999.4)*
anaphylactic shock due to adverse food reaction (995.60–995.69)

Use additional E code to identify external cause, such as:
adverse effects of correct medicinal substance properly administered [E930-E949]

995.1 **Angioneurotic edema**
Giant urticaria
Excludes *urticaria:*
due to serum (999.5)
other specified (698.2, 708.0–708.9, 757.33)

❑995.2 **Unspecified adverse effect of drug, medicinal and biological substance (due) to correct medicinal substance properly administered**
Adverse effect to correct medicinal substance properly administered
Allergic reaction to correct medicinal substance properly administered
Hypersensitivity to correct medicinal substance properly administered
Idiosyncrasy due to correct medicinal substance properly administered
Drug:
hypersensitivity NOS
reaction NOS
Excludes *pathological drug intoxication (292.2)*

❑995.3 **Allergy, unspecified**
Allergic reaction NOS
Hypersensitivity NOS
Idiosyncrasy NOS
Excludes *allergic reaction NOS to correct medicinal substance properly administered (995.2)*
specific types of allergic reaction, such as:
allergic diarrhea (558.3)
dermatitis (691.0–693.9)
hayfever (477.0–477.9)

995.4 **Shock due to anesthesia**
Shock due to anesthesia in which the correct substance was properly administered
Excludes *complications of anesthesia in labor or delivery (668.0–668.9)*
overdose or wrong substance given (968.0–969.9)
postoperative shock NOS (998.0)
specified adverse effects of anesthesia classified elsewhere, such as:
anoxic brain damage (348.1)
hepatitis (070.0–070.9), etc.
unspecified adverse effect of anesthesia (995.2)

● 995.5 **Child maltreatment syndrome**

Use additional code(s), if applicable, to identify any associated injuries

Use additional E code to identify:
nature of abuse (E960-E968)
perpetrator (E967.0-E967.9)

❑995.50 **Child abuse, unspecified**

995.51 **Child emotional/psychological abuse**

995.52 **Child neglect (nutritional)**

995.53 **Child sexual abuse**

995.54 **Child physical abuse**
Battered baby or child syndrome

Excludes *Shaken infant syndrome (995.55)*

995.55 **Shaken infant syndrome**
Use additional code(s) to identify any associated injuries

❑995.59 **Other child abuse and neglect**
Multiple forms of abuse

● 995.6 **Anaphylactic shock due to adverse food reaction**
Anaphylactic shock due to nonpoisonous foods

❑995.60 **Due to unspecified food**

995.61 **Due to peanuts**

995.62 **Due to crustaceans**

995.63 **Due to fruits and vegetables**

995.64 **Due to tree nuts and seeds**

995.65 **Due to fish**

995.66 **Due to food additives**

995.67 **Due to milk products**

995.68 **Due to eggs**

❑995.69 **Due to other specified food**

995.7 **Other adverse food reactions, not elsewhere classified**
Use additional code to identify the type of reaction, such as:
hives (708.0)
wheezing (786.07)

Excludes *anaphylactic shock due to adverse food reaction (995.60–995.69)*
asthma (493.0, 493.9)
dermatitis due to food (693.1)
in contact with the skin (692.5)
gastroenteritis and colitis due to food (558.3)
rhinitis due to food (477.1)

● 995.8 **Other specified adverse effects, not elsewhere classified**

❑995.80 **Adult maltreatment, unspecified**
Abused person NOS
Use additional code to identify:
any associated injury
perpetrator (E967.0-E967.9)

995.81 **Adult physical abuse**
Battered:
person syndrome, NEC
man
spouse
woman
Use additional code to identify:
any associated injury
nature of abuse (E960-E968)
perpetrator (E967.0-E967.9)

995.82 **Adult emotional/psychological abuse**
Use additional E code to identify perpetrator (E967.0-E967.9)

995.83 **Adult sexual abuse**
Use additional code to identify:
any associated injury
perpetrator (E967.0-E967.9)

995.84 **Adult neglect (nutritional)**
Use additional code to identify:
intent of neglect (E904.0-E968.4)
perpetrator (E967.0-E967.9)

❑995.85 **Other adult abuse and neglect**
Multiple forms of abuse and neglect
Use additional code to identify any associated injury
intent of neglect (E904.0, E968.4)
nature of abuse (E960-E968)
perpetrator (E967.0-E967.9)

995.86 **Malignant hyperthermia**
Malignant hyperpyrexia due to anesthesia

❑995.89 **Other**
Hypothermia due to anesthesia

● 995.9 **Systemic inflammatory response syndrome (SIRS)**
Code first underlying condition ◄

❑995.90 **Systemic inflammatory response syndrome, unspecified SIRS NOS**

995.91 **Systemic inflammatory response syndrome due to infectious process without organ dysfunction**
Sepsis ◄

995.92 **Systemic inflammatory response syndrome due to infectious process with organ dysfunction**
Severe sepsis
Use additional code to specify organ dysfunction, such as:
acute renal failure (584.5–584.9) ◄
acute respiratory failure (518.81) ◄
critical illness myopathy (359.81) ◄
critial illness polyneuropathy (357.82) ◄
encephalopathy (348.31) ⇐
hepatic failure (570) ◄
kidney failure (584.5–584.9, 585, 586)
septic shock (785.52) ◄

995.93 **Systemic inflammatory response syndrome due to noninfectious process without organ dysfunction**

995.94 **Systemic inflammatory response syndrome due to noninfectious process with organ dysfunction**
Use additional code to specify organ dysfunction, such as:
acute renal failure (584.5–584.9) ◄
acute respiratory failure (518.81) ◄
critical illness myopathy (359.81) ◄
critial illness polyneuropathy (357.82) ◄
encephalopathy (348.31) ⇐
hepatic failure (570) ◄
kidney failure (584.5–584.9, 585, 586)
septic shock (785.52) ◄

COMPLICATIONS OF SURGICAL AND MEDICAL CARE, NOT ELSEWHERE CLASSIFIED (996–999)

Excludes *adverse effects of medicinal agents (001.0–799.9, 995.0–995.8)*
burns from local applications and irradiation (940.0–949.5)
complications of:
conditions for which the procedure was performed
surgical procedures during abortion, labor, and delivery (630–676.9)
poisoning and toxic effects of drugs and chemicals (960.0–989.9)
postoperative conditions in which no complications are present, such as:
artificial opening status (V44.0–V44.9)
closure of external stoma (V55.0–V55.9)
fitting of prosthetic device (V52.0–V52.9)
specified complications classified elsewhere:
anesthetic shock (995.4)
electrolyte imbalance (276.0–276.9)
postlaminectomy syndrome (722.80–722.83)

postmastectomy lymphedema syndrome (457.0)
postoperative psychosis (293.0–293.9)
any other condition classified elsewhere in the Alphabetic Index when described as due to a procedure

● **996 Complications peculiar to certain specified procedures**

Includes: complications, not elsewhere classified, in the use of artificial substitutes [e.g., Dacron, metal, Silastic, Teflon] or natural sources [e.g., bone] involving:
anastomosis (internal)
graft (bypass) (patch)
implant
internal device:
catheter
electronic
fixation
prosthetic
reimplant
transplant

Excludes *accidental puncture or laceration during procedure (998.2)*
complications of internal anastomosis of:
gastrointestinal tract (997.4)
urinary tract (997.5)
other specified complications classified elsewhere, such as:
hemolytic anemia (283.1)
functional cardiac disturbances (429.4)
serum hepatitis (070.2–070.3)

● **996.0 Mechanical complication of cardiac device, implant, and graft**
Breakdown (mechanical)
Displacement
Leakage
Obstruction, mechanical
Perforation
Protrusion

❑ **996.00 Unspecified device, implant, and graft**

996.01 Due to cardiac pacemaker (electrode)

996.02 Due to heart valve prosthesis

996.03 Due to coronary bypass graft

Excludes *atherosclerosis of graft (414.02, 414.03)*
embolism [occlusion NOS] [thrombus] of graft (996.72)

996.04 Due to automatic implantable cardiac defibrillator

❑ **996.09 Other**

❑ **996.1 Mechanical complication of other vascular device, implant, and graft**
Mechanical complications involving:
aortic (bifurcation) graft (replacement)
arteriovenous:
dialysis catheter
fistula surgically created
shunt surgically created
balloon (counterpulsation) device, intra-aortic
carotid artery bypass graft
femoral-popliteal bypass graft
umbrella device, vena cava

Excludes *atherosclerosis of biological graft (440.30–440.32)*
embolism [occlusion NOS] [thrombus] of (biological) (synthetic) graft (996.74)
peritoneal dialysis catheter (996.56)

996.2 Mechanical complication of nervous system device, implant, and graft
Mechanical complications involving:
dorsal column stimulator
electrodes implanted in brain [brain "pacemaker"]
peripheral nerve graft
ventricular (communicating) shunt

● **996.3 Mechanical complication of genitourinary device, implant, and graft**

❑ **996.30 Unspecified device, implant, and graft**

996.31 Due to urethral [indwelling] catheter

996.32 Due to intrauterine contraceptive device

❑ **996.39 Other**
Cystostomy catheter
Prosthetic reconstruction of vas deferens
Repair (graft) of ureter without mention of resection

Excludes *complications due to:*
external stoma of urinary tract (997.5)
internal anastomosis of urinary tract (997.5)

996.4 Mechanical complication of internal orthopedic device, implant, and graft
Mechanical complications involving:
external (fixation) device utilizing internal screw(s), pin(s) or other methods of fixation
grafts of bone, cartilage, muscle, or tendon
internal (fixation) device such as nail, plate, rod, etc.

Excludes *complications of external orthopedic device, such as:*
pressure ulcer due to cast (707.0)

● **996.5 Mechanical complication of other specified prosthetic device, implant, and graft**
Mechanical complications involving:
prosthetic implant in:
bile duct
breast
chin
orbit of eye
nonabsorbable surgical material NOS
other graft, implant, and internal device, not elsewhere classified

996.51 Due to corneal graft

❑ **996.52 Due to graft of other tissue, not elsewhere classified**
Skin graft failure or rejection

Excludes *failure of artificial skin graft (996.55)*
failure of decellularized allodermis (996.55)
sloughing of temporary skin allografts or xenografts (pigskin)-omit code

996.53 Due to ocular lens prosthesis

Excludes *contact lenses—code to condition*

996.54 Due to breast prosthesis
Breast capsule (prosthesis)
Mammary implant

996.55 Due to artificial skin graft and decellularized allodermis
Dislodgement
Displacement
Failure
Non-adherence
Poor incorporation
Shearing

996.56 Due to peritoneal dialysis catheter

Excludes *mechanical complication of arteriovenous dialysis catheter (996.1)*

996.57 Due to insulin pump ◀

❑ **996.59 Due to other implant and internal device, not elsewhere classified**
Nonabsorbable surgical material NOS
Prosthetic implant in:
bile duct
chin
orbit of eye

● 996.6 **Infection and inflammatory reaction due to internal prosthetic device, implant, and graft**
Infection (causing obstruction) due to (presence of) any device, implant, and graft classifiable to 996.0–996.5
Inflammation due to (presence of) any device, implant, and graft classifiable to 996.0–996.5

Use additional code to identify specified infections

❑ 996.60 **Due to unspecified device, implant and graft**

996.61 **Due to cardiac device, implant and graft**
Cardiac pacemaker or defibrillator:
electrode(s), lead(s)
pulse generator
subcutaneous pocket
Coronary artery bypass graft
Heart valve prosthesis

❑ 996.62 **Due to vascular device, implant and graft**
Arterial graft
Arteriovenous fistula or shunt
Infusion pump
Vascular catheter (arterial) (dialysis) (venous)

996.63 **Due to nervous system device, implant and graft**
Electrodes implanted in brain
Peripheral nerve graft
Spinal canal catheter
Ventricular (communicating) shunt (catheter)

996.64 **Due to indwelling urinary catheter**
Use additional code to identify specified infections, such as:
Cystitis (595.0–595.9)
Sepsis (038.0–038.9)

❑ 996.65 **Due to other genitourinary device, implant and graft**
Intrauterine contraceptive device

996.66 **Due to internal joint prosthesis**

❑ 996.67 **Due to other internal orthopedic device, implant and graft**
Bone growth stimulator (electrode)
Internal fixation device (pin) (rod) (screw)

996.68 **Due to peritoneal dialysis catheter**
Exit-site infection or inflammation

❑ 996.69 **Due to other internal prosthetic device, implant, and graft**
Breast prosthesis
Ocular lens prosthesis
Prosthetic orbital implant

● 996.7 **Other complications of internal (biological) (synthetic) prosthetic device, implant, and graft**
Complication NOS due to (presence of) any device, implant, and graft classifiable to 996.0–996.5
occlusion NOS
Embolism due to (presence of) any device, implant, and graft classifiable to 996.0–996.5
Fibrosis due to (presence of) any device, implant, and graft classifiable to 996.0–996.5
Hemorrhage due to (presence of) any device, implant, and graft classifiable to 996.0–996.5
Pain due to (presence of) any device, implant, and graft classifiable to 996.0–996.5
Stenosis due to (presence of) any device, implant, and graft classifiable to 996.0–996.5
Thrombus due to (presence of) any device, implant, and graft classifiable to 996.0–996.5

Excludes *transplant rejection (996.8)*

❑ 996.70 **Due to unspecified device, implant, and graft**

996.71 **Due to heart valve prosthesis**

996.72 **Due to other cardiac device, implant, and graft**
Cardiac pacemaker or defibrillator:
electrode(s), lead(s)
subcutaneous pocket
Coronary artery bypass (graft)

Excludes *occlusion due to atherosclerosis (414.00–414.06)*

996.73 **Due to renal dialysis device, implant, and graft**

❑ 996.74 **Due to vascular device, implant, and graft**

Excludes *occlusion of biological graft due to atherosclerosis (440.30–440.32)*

996.75 **Due to nervous system device, implant, and graft**

996.76 **Due to genitourinary device, implant, and graft**

996.77 **Due to internal joint prosthesis**

❑ 996.78 **Due to other internal orthopedic device, implant, and graft**

❑ 996.79 **Due to other internal prosthetic device, implant, and graft**

● 996.8 **Complications of transplanted organ**
Transplant failure or rejection

Use additional code to identify nature of complication, such as:
Cytomegalovirus [CMV] infection (078.5)

❑ 996.80 **Transplanted organ, unspecified**

996.81 **Kidney**

996.82 **Liver**

996.83 **Heart**

996.84 **Lung**

996.85 **Bone marrow**
Graft-versus-host disease (acute) (chronic)

996.86 **Pancreas**

996.87 **Intestine**

❑ 996.89 **Other specified transplanted organ**

● 996.9 **Complications of reattached extremity or body part**

❑ 996.90 **Unspecified extremity**

996.91 **Forearm**

996.92 **Hand**

996.93 **Finger(s)**

❑ 996.94 **Upper extremity, other and unspecified**

996.95 **Foot and toe(s)**

❑ 996.96 **Lower extremity, other and unspecified**

❑ 996.99 **Other specified body part**

● 997 **Complications affecting specified body systems, not elsewhere classified**

Use additional code to identify complication

Excludes *the listed conditions when specified as:*
causing shock (998.0)
complications of:
anesthesia:
adverse effect (001.0–799.9, 995.0–995.8)
in labor or delivery (668.0–668.9)
poisoning (968.0–969.9)
implanted device or graft (996.0–996.9)
obstetrical procedures (669.0–669.4)
reattached extremity (996.90–996.96)
transplanted organ (996.80–996.89)

● 997.0 **Nervous system complications**

❑ 997.00 **Nervous system complication, unspecified**

997.01 **Central nervous system complication**
Anoxic brain damage
Cerebral hypoxia

Excludes *Cerebrovascular hemorrhage or infarction (997.02)*

997.02 **Iatrogenic cerebrovascular infarction or hemorrhage**
Postoperative stroke

❑ 997.09 **Other nervous system complications**

997.1 **Cardiac complications**
Cardiac:
arrest during or resulting from a procedure
insufficiency during or resulting from a procedure
Cardiorespiratory failure during or resulting from a procedure
Heart failure during or resulting from a procedure

Excludes *the listed conditions as long-term effects of cardiac surgery or due to the presence of cardiac prosthetic device (429.4)*

997.2 **Peripheral vascular complications**
Phlebitis or thrombophlebitis during or resulting from a procedure

Excludes *the listed conditions due to:*
implant or catheter device (996.62)
infusion, perfusion, or transfusion (999.2)
complications affecting blood vessels (997.71–997.79)

997.3 **Respiratory complications**
Mendelson's syndrome resulting from a procedure
Pneumonia (aspiration) resulting from a procedure

Excludes *iatrogenic [postoperative] pneumothorax (512.1)*
iatrogenic pulmonary embolism (415.11)
Mendelson's syndrome in labor and delivery (668.0)
specified complications classified elsewhere, such as:
adult respiratory distress syndrome (518.5)
pulmonary edema, postoperative (518.4)
respiratory insufficiency, acute, postoperative (518.5)
shock lung (518.5)
tracheostomy complication (519.00–519.09)

997.4 **Digestive system complications**
Complications of:
Intestinal (internal) anastomosis and bypass, not elsewhere classified, except that involving urinary tract
Hepatic failure specified as due to a procedure
Hepatorenal syndrome specified as due to a procedure
Intestinal obstruction NOS specified as due to a procedure

Excludes *specified gastrointestinal complications classified elsewhere, such as:*
blind loop syndrome (579.2)
colostomy or enterostomy complications (569.60–569.69)
gastrojejunal ulcer (534.0–534.9)
gastrostomy complications (536.40–536.49)
infection of external stoma (569.61)
pelvic peritoneal adhesions, female (614.6)
peritoneal adhesions (568.0)
peritoneal adhesions with obstruction (560.81)
postcholecystectomy syndrome (576.0)
postgastric surgery syndromes (564.2)
vomiting following gastrointestinal surgery (564.3) ◀

997.5 **Urinary complications**
Complications of:
external stoma of urinary tract
internal anastomosis and bypass of urinary tract, including that involving intestinal tract
Oliguria or anuria specified as due to procedure
Renal:
failure (acute) specified as due to procedure
insufficiency (acute) specified as due to procedure
Tubular necrosis (acute) specified as due to procedure

Excludes *specified complications classified elsewhere, such as:*
postoperative stricture of:
ureter (593.3)
urethra (598.2)

● 997.6 **Amputation stump complication**

Excludes *admission for treatment for a current traumatic amputation—code to complicated traumatic amptutation*
phantom limb (syndrome) (353.6)

❑ 997.60 **Unspecified complication**

997.61 **Neuroma of amputation stump**

997.62 **Infection (chronic)**
Use additional code to identify the organism

❑ 997.69 **Other**

● 997.7 **Vascular complications of other vessels**

Excludes *peripheral vascular complications (997.2)*

997.71 **Vascular complications of mesenteric artery**

997.72 **Vascular complications of renal artery**

❑ 997.79 **Vascular complications of other vessels**

● 997.9 **Complications affecting other specified body systems, not elsewhere classified**

Excludes *specified complications classified elsewhere, such as:*
broad ligament laceration syndrome (620.6)
postartificial menopause syndrome (627.4)
postoperative stricture of vagina (623.2)

997.91 **Hypertension**

Excludes *Essential hypertension (401.0–401.9)*

❑ 997.99 **Other**
Vitreous touch syndrome

● 998 **Other complications of procedures, NEC**

998.0 **Postoperative shock**
Collapse NOS during or resulting from a surgical procedure
Shock (endotoxic) (hypovolemic) (septic) during or resulting from a surgical procedure

Excludes *shock:*
anaphylactic due to serum (999.4)
anesthetic (995.4)
electric (994.8)
following abortion (639.5)
obstetric (669.1)
traumatic (958.4)

● 998.1 **Hemorrhage or hematoma or seroma complicating a procedure**

Excludes *hemorrhage, hematoma or seroma:*
complicating cesarean section or puerperal perineal wound (674.3)

998.11 **Hemorrhage complicating a procedure**

998.12 **Hematoma complicating a procedure**

998.13 **Seroma complicating a procedure**

998.2 Accidental puncture or laceration during a procedure
Accidental perforation by catheter or other instrument during a procedure on:
blood vessel
nerve
organ

Excludes *iatrogenic [postoperative] pneumothorax (512.1)*
puncture or laceration caused by implanted device intentionally left in operation wound (996.0–996.5)
specified complications classified elsewhere, such as:
broad ligament laceration syndrome (620.6)
trauma from instruments during delivery (664.0–665.9)

● **998.3 Disruption of operation wound**
Dehiscence of operation wound
Rupture of operation wound

Excludes *disruption of:*
cesarean wound (674.1)
perineal wound, puerperal (674.2)

998.31 Disruption of internal operation wound

998.32 Disruption of external operation wound
Disruption of operation wound NOS

998.4 Foreign body accidentally left during a procedure
Adhesions due to foreign body accidentally left in operative wound or body cavity during a procedure
Obstruction due to foreign body accidentally left in operative wound or body cavity during a procedure
Perforation due to foreign body accidentally left in operative wound or body cavity during a procedure

Excludes *obstruction or perforation caused by implanted device intentionally left in body (996.0–996.5)*

● **998.5 Postoperative infection**

Excludes *infection due to:*
implanted device (996.60–996.69)
infusion, perfusion, or transfusion (999.3)
postoperative obstetrical wound infection (674.3)

998.51 Infected postoperative seroma
Use additional code to identify organism

❑ **998.59 Other postoperative infection**
Abscess: postoperative
intra-abdominal postoperative
stitch postoperative
subphrenic postoperative
wound postoperative
Septicemia postoperative

Use additional code to identify infection

998.6 Persistent postoperative fistula

998.7 Acute reaction to foreign substance accidentally left during a procedure
Peritonitis:
aseptic
chemical

● **998.8 Other specified complications of procedures, not elsewhere classified**

998.81 Emphysema (subcutaneous) (surgical) resulting from a procedure

998.82 Cataract fragments in eye following cataract surgery

998.83 Non-healing surgical wound

❑ **998.89 Other specified complications**

❑ **998.9 Unspecified complication of procedure, not elsewhere classified**
Postoperative complication NOS

Excludes *complication NOS of obstetrical surgery or procedure (669.4)*

● **999 Complications of medical care, not elsewhere classified**

Includes: complications, not elsewhere classified, of:
dialysis (hemodialysis) (peritoneal) (renal)
extracorporeal circulation
hyperalimentation therapy
immunization
infusion
inhalation therapy
injection
inoculation
perfusion
transfusion
vaccination
ventilation therapy

Excludes *specified complications classified elsewhere such as:*
complications of implanted device (996.0–996.9)
contact dermatitis due to drugs (692.3)
dementia dialysis (294.8)
transient (293.9)
dialysis disequilibrium syndrome (276.0–276.9)
poisoning and toxic effects of drugs and chemicals (960.0–989.9)
postvaccinal encephalitis (323.5)
water and electrolyte imbalance (276.0–276.9)

999.0 Generalized vaccinia

999.1 Air embolism
Air embolism to any site following infusion, perfusion, or transfusion

Excludes *embolism specified as:*
complicating:
abortion (634–638 with .6, 639.6)
ectopic or molar pregnancy (639.6)
pregnancy, childbirth, or the puerperium (673.0)
due to implanted device (996.7)
traumatic (958.0)

❑ **999.2 Other vascular complications**
Phlebitis following infusion, perfusion, or transfusion
Thromboembolism following infusion, perfusion, or transfusion
Thrombophlebitis following infusion, perfusion, or transfusion

Excludes *the listed conditions when specified as:*
due to implanted device (996.61–996.62, 996.72–996.74)
postoperative NOS (997.2, 997.71–997.79)

❑ **999.3 Other infection**
Infection following infusion, injection, transfusion, or vaccination
Sepsis following infusion, injection, transfusion, or vaccination
Septicemia following infusion, injection, transfusion, or vaccination

Excludes *the listed conditions when specified as:*
due to implanted device (996.60–996.69)
postoperative NOS (998.51–998.59)

999.4 Anaphylactic shock due to serum

Excludes *shock:*
allergic NOS (995.0)
anaphylactic:
NOS (995.0)
due to drugs and chemicals (995.0)

❑ **999.5 Other serum reaction**
Intoxication by serum
Protein sickness
Serum rash
Serum sickness
Urticaria due to serum

Excludes *serum hepatitis (070.2–070.3)*

999.6 ABO incompatibility reaction
Incompatible blood transfusion
Reaction to blood group incompatibility in infusion or transfusion

999.7 Rh incompatibility reaction
Reactions due to Rh factor in infusion or transfusion

❑ **999.8 Other transfusion reaction**
Septic shock due to transfusion
Transfusion reaction NOS

Excludes *postoperative shock (998.0)*

❑ **999.9 Other and unspecified complications of medical care, not elsewhere classified**
Complications, not elsewhere classified, of:
electroshock therapy
inhalation therapy
ultrasound therapy
ventilation therapy
Unspecified misadventure of medical care

Excludes *unspecified complication of:*
phototherapy (990)
radiation therapy (990)

V-Codes—SUPPLEMENTARY CLASSIFICATION OF FACTORS INFLUENCING HEALTH STATUS AND CONTACT WITH HEALTH SERVICES (V01–V83)

This classification is provided to deal with occasions when circumstances other than a disease or injury classifiable to categories 001–999 (the main part of ICD) are recorded as "diagnoses" or "problems." This can arise mainly in three ways:

a) When a person who is not currently sick encounters the health services for some specific purpose, such as to act as a donor of an organ or tissue, to receive prophylactic vaccination, or to discuss a problem which is in itself not a disease or injury. This will be a fairly rare occurrence among hospital inpatients, but will be relatively more common among hospital outpatients and patients of family practitioners, health clinics, etc.

b) When a person with a known disease or injury, whether it is current or resolving, encounters the health care system for a specific treatment of that disease or injury (e.g., dialysis for renal disease; chemotherapy for malignancy; cast change).

c) When some circumstance or problem is present which influences the person's health status but is not in itself a current illness or injury. Such factors may be elicited during population surveys, when the person may or may not be currently sick, or be recorded as an additional factor to be borne in mind when the person is receiving care for some current illness or injury classifiable to categories 001–999.

In the latter circumstances the V code should be used only as a supplementary code and should not be the one selected for use in primary, single cause tabulations. Examples of these circumstances are a personal history of certain diseases, or a person with an artificial heart valve in situ.

PERSONS WITH POTENTIAL HEALTH HAZARDS RELATED TO COMMUNICABLE DISEASES (V01–V06)

Excludes *family history of infectious and parasitic diseases (V18.8)*
personal history of infectious and parasitic diseases (V12.0)

● **V01 Contact with or exposure to communicable diseases**
- ● **V01.0 Cholera**
  Conditions classifiable to 001
- ● **V01.1 Tuberculosis**
  Conditions classifiable to 010–018
- ● **V01.2 Poliomyelitis**
  Conditions classifiable to 045
- ● **V01.3 Smallpox**
  Conditions classifiable to 050
- ● **V01.4 Rubella**
  Conditions classifiable to 056
- ● **V01.5 Rabies**
  Conditions classifiable to 071
- ● **V01.6 Venereal diseases**
  Conditions classifiable to 090–099
- ●❑ **V01.7 Other viral diseases**
  Conditions classifiable to 042–078, and V08, except as above
- ●❑ **V01.8 Other communicable diseases**
  Conditions classifiable to 001–136, except as above
  - ● **V01.81 Anthrax**
  - ●❑ **V01.89 Other communicable diseases**
- ●❑ **V01.9 Unspecified communicable disease**

● **V02 Carrier or suspected carrier of infectious diseases**
- ● **V02.0 Cholera**
- ● **V02.1 Typhoid**
- ● **V02.2 Amebiasis**
- ●❑ **V02.3 Other gastrointestinal pathogens**
- ● **V02.4 Diphtheria**
- ● **V02.5 Other specified bacterial diseases**
  - **V02.51 Group B streptococcus**
  - ●❑ **V02.52 Other streptococcus**
  - ●❑ **V02.59 Other specified bacterial diseases**
    Meningococcal
    Staphylococcal
- ● **V02.6 Viral hepatitis**
  - ●❑ **V02.60 Viral hepatitis carrier, unspecified**
  - ● **V02.61 Hepatitis B carrier**
  - ● **V02.62 Hepatitis C carrier**
  - ●❑ **V02.69 Other viral hepatitis carrier**
- ● **V02.7 Gonorrhea**
- ●❑ **V02.8 Other venereal diseases**
- ●❑ **V02.9 Other specified infectious organism**

● **V03 Need for prophylactic vaccination and inoculation against bacterial diseases**

Excludes *vaccination not carried out because of contraindication (V64.0)*
vaccines against combinations of diseases (V06.0–V06.9)

- ● **V03.0 Cholera alone**
- ● **V03.1 Typhoid-paratyphoid alone [TAB]**
- ● **V03.2 Tuberculosis [BCG]**
- ● **V03.3 Plague**
- ● **V03.4 Tularemia**
- ● **V03.5 Diphtheria alone**
- ● **V03.6 Pertussis alone**
- ● **V03.7 Tetanus toxoid alone**
- ● **V03.8 Other specified vaccinations against single bacterial diseases**
  - ● **V03.81 Haemophilus influenzae, type B [Hib]**
  - ● **V03.82 Streptococcus pneumoniae [pneumococcus]**
  - ●❑ **V03.89 Other specified vaccination**
- ●❑ **V03.9 Unspecified single bacterial disease**

● **V04 Need for prophylactic vaccination and inoculation against certain diseases**

Excludes *vaccines against combinations of diseases (V06.0–V06.9)*

- ● **V04.0 Poliomyelitis**
- ● **V04.1 Smallpox**
- ● **V04.2 Measles alone**
- ● **V04.3 Rubella alone**
- ● **V04.4 Yellow fever**
- ● **V04.5 Rabies**
- ● **V04.6 Mumps alone**
- ● **V04.7 Common cold**
- ● **V04.8 Other viral diseases** ⇐
  - ● **V04.81 Influenza** ◀
  - ● **V04.82 Respiratory syncytial virus (RSV)** ◀
  - ●❑ **V04.89 Other viral disease** ◀

● **V05 Need for prophylactic vaccination and inoculation against single diseases**

Excludes *vaccines against combinations of diseases (V06.0–V06.9)*

- ● **V05.0 Arthropod-borne viral encephalitis**
- ●❑ **V05.1 Other arthropod-borne viral diseases**
- ● **V05.2 Leishmaniasis**
- ● **V05.3 Viral hepatitis**
- ● **V05.4 Varicella**
  Chicken pox
- ●❑ **V05.8 Other specified disease**
- ●❑ **V05.9 Unspecified single disease**

● **V06 Need for prophylactic vaccination and inoculation against combinations of diseases**

Note: Use additional single vaccination codes from categories V03–V05 to identify any vaccinations not included in a combination code.

- ● **V06.0 Cholera with typhoid-paratyphoid [cholera TAB]**
- ● **V06.1 Diphtheria-tetanus-pertussis, combined [DTP] [DTaP]** ◀ (Revised Code)
- ● **V06.2 Diphtheria-tetanus-pertussis with typhoid-paratyphoid [DTP TAB]**
- ● **V06.3 Diphtheria-tetanus-pertussis with poliomyelitis [DTP+polio]**
- ● **V06.4 Measles-mumps-rubella [MMR]**
- ● **V06.5 Tetanus-diphtheria [Td] [DT]** ◀ (Revised Code)
- ● **V06.6 Streptococcus pneumoniae [pneumococcus] and influenza**
- ●❑ **V06.8 Other combinations**

  Excludes *multiple single vaccination codes (V03.0–V05.9)*
- ●❑ **V06.9 Unspecified combined vaccine**

PERSONS WITH NEED FOR ISOLATION, OTHER POTENTIAL HEALTH HAZARDS AND PROPHYLACTIC MEASURES (V07–V09)

● **V07 Need for isolation and other prophylactic measures**

Excludes *prophylactic organ removal (V50.41–V50.49)*

- **V07.0 Isolation**
  Admission to protect the individual from his surroundings or for isolation of individual after contact with infectious diseases
- ● **V07.1 Desensitization to allergens**
- ● **V07.2 Prophylactic immunotherapy**
  Administration of:
  antivenin
  immune sera [gamma globulin]
  RhoGAM
  tetanus antitoxin
- ● **V07.3 Other prophylactic chemotherapy**
  - ● **V07.31 Prophylactic fluoride administration**
  - ❑ **V07.39 Other prophylactic chemotherapy**

  Excludes *maintenance chemotherapy following disease (V58.1)*
- ● **V07.4 Postmenopausal hormone replacement therapy**
- ❑ **V07.8 Other specified prophylactic measure**
- ●❑ **V07.9 Unspecified prophylactic measure**

● **V08 Asymptomatic human immunodeficiency virus [HIV] infection status**
HIV positive NOS

Note: This code is ONLY to be used when NO HIV infection symptoms or conditions are present. If any HIV infection symptoms or conditions are present, see code 042.

Excludes *AIDS (042)*
human immunodeficiency virus [HIV] disease (042)
exposure to HIV (V01.7)
nonspecific serologic evidence of HIV (795.71)
symptomatic human immunodeficiency virus [HIV] infection (042)

● **V09 Infection with drug-resistant microorganisms**

Note: This category is intended for use as an additional code for infectious conditions classified elsewhere to indicate the presence of drug-resistance of the infectious organism.

- ● **V09.0 Infection with microorganisms resistant to penicillins**
- ● **V09.1 Infection with microorganisms resistant to cephalosporins and other B-lactam antibiotics**
- ● **V09.2 Infection with microorganisms resistant to macrolides**
- ● **V09.3 Infection with microorganisms resistant to tetracyclines**
- ● **V09.4 Infection with microorganisms resistant to aminoglycosides**
- ● **V09.5 Infection with microorganisms resistant to quinolones and fluoroquinolones**
  - ● **V09.50 Without mention of resistance to multiple quinolones and fluoroquinols**
  - ● **V09.51 With resistance to multiple quinolones and fluoroquinols**
- ● **V09.6 Infection with microorganisms resistant to sulfonamides**
- ● **V09.7 Infection with microorganisms resistant to other specified antimycobacterial agents**

  Excludes *amikacin (V09.4)*
  kanamycin (V09.4)
  streptomycin [SM] (V09.4)
  - ●❑ **V09.70 Without mention of resistance to multiple antimycobacterial agents**
  - ●❑ **V09.71 With resistance to multiple antimycobacterial agents**
- ● **V09.8 Infection with microorganisms resistant to other specified drugs**
  - ●❑ **V09.80 Without mention of resistance to multiple drugs**
  - ●❑ **V09.81 With resistance to multiple drugs**
- ● **V09.9 Infection with drug-resistant microorganisms, unspecified**
  Drug resistance NOS
  - ●❑ **V09.90 Without mention of multiple drug resistance**
  - ●❑ **V09.91 With multiple drug resistance**
    Multiple drug resistance NOS

PERSONS WITH POTENTIAL HEALTH HAZARDS RELATED TO PERSONAL AND FAMILY HISTORY (V10–V19)

Excludes *obstetric patients where the possibility that the fetus might be affected is the reason for observation or management during pregnancy (655.0–655.9)*

● **V10 Personal history of malignant neoplasm**

● **V10.0 Gastrointestinal tract**
History of conditions classifiable to 140–159

●❑ **V10.00 Gastrointestinal tract, unspecified**
● **V10.01 Tongue**
●❑ **V10.02 Other and unspecified oral cavity and pharynx**
● **V10.03 Esophagus**
● **V10.04 Stomach**
● **V10.05 Large intestine**
● **V10.06 Rectum, rectosigmoid junction, and anus**
● **V10.07 Liver**
●❑ **V10.09 Other**

● **V10.1 Trachea, bronchus, and lung**
History of conditions classifiable to 162

● **V10.11 Bronchus and lung**
● **V10.12 Trachea**

● **V10.2 Other respiratory and intrathoracic organs**
History of conditions classifiable to 160, 161, 163–165

●❑ **V10.20 Respiratory organ, unspecified**
● **V10.21 Larynx**
● **V10.22 Nasal cavities, middle ear, and accessory sinuses**
●❑ **V10.29 Other**

● **V10.3 Breast**
History of conditions classifiable to 174 and 175

● **V10.4 Genital organs**
History of conditions classifiable to 179–187

●❑ **V10.40 Female genital organ, unspecified**
● **V10.41 Cervix uteri**
●❑ **V10.42 Other parts of uterus**
● **V10.43 Ovary**
●❑ **V10.44 Other female genital organs**
●❑ **V10.45 Male genital organ, unspecified**
● **V10.46 Prostate**
● **V10.47 Testis**
● **V10.48 Epididymis**
●❑ **V10.49 Other male genital organs**

● **V10.5 Urinary organs**
History of conditions classifiable to 188 and 189

●❑ **V10.50 Urinary organ, unspecified**
● **V10.51 Bladder**
● **V10.52 Kidney**

Excludes *renal pelvis (V10.53)*

● **V10.53 Renal pelvis**
●❑ **V10.59 Other**

● **V10.6 Leukemia**
Conditions classifiable to 204–208

Excludes *leukemia in remission (204–208)*

●❑ **V10.60 Leukemia, unspecified**
● **V10.61 Lymphoid leukemia**
● **V10.62 Myeloid leukemia**
● **V10.63 Monocytic leukemia**
●❑ **V10.69 Other**

● **V10.7 Other lymphatic and hematopoietic neoplasms**
Conditions classifiable to 200–203

Excludes *listed conditions in 200–203 in remission*

● **V10.71 Lymphosarcoma and reticulosarcoma**
● **V10.72 Hodgkin's disease**
●❑ **V10.79 Other**

● **V10.8 Personal history of malignant neoplasm of other sites**
History of conditions classifiable to 170–173, 190–195

● **V10.81 Bone**
● **V10.82 Malignant melanoma of skin**
●❑ **V10.83 Other malignant neoplasm of skin**
● **V10.84 Eye**
● **V10.85 Brain**
●❑ **V10.86 Other parts of nervous system**

Excludes *peripheral, sympathetic, and parasympathetic nerves (V10.89)*

● **V10.87 Thyroid**
●❑ **V10.88 Other endocrine glands and related structures**
●❑ **V10.89 Other**

●❑ **V10.9 Unspecified personal history of malignant neoplasm**

● **V11 Personal history of mental disorder**

● **V11.0 Schizophrenia**

Excludes *that in remission (295.0–295.9 with fifth-digit 5)*

● **V11.1 Affective disorders**
Personal history of manic-depressive psychosis

Excludes *that in remission (296.0–296.6 with fifth-digit 5, 6)*

● **V11.2 Neurosis**
● **V11.3 Alcoholism**
●❑ **V11.8 Other mental disorders**
●❑ **V11.9 Unspecified mental disorder**

● **V12 Personal history of certain other diseases**

● **V12.0 Infectious and parasitic diseases**

●❑ **V12.00 Unspecified infectious and parasitic disease**
● **V12.01 Tuberculosis**
● **V12.02 Poliomyelitis**
● **V12.03 Malaria**
●❑ **V12.09 Other**

● **V12.1 Nutritional deficiency**
● **V12.2 Endocrine, metabolic, and immunity disorders**

Excludes *history of allergy (V14.0–V14.9, V15.01–V15.09)*

● **V12.3 Diseases of blood and blood-forming organs**
● **V12.4 Disorders of nervous system and sense organs**

●❑ **V12.40 Unspecified disorder of nervous system and sense organs**

● V12.41 Benign neoplasm of the brain

●❑ V12.49 Other disorders of nervous system and sense organs

● V12.5 Diseases of circulatory system

Excludes *old myocardial infarction (412)*
postmyocardial infarction syndrome (411.0)

●❑ V12.50 Unspecified circulatory disease

● V12.51 Venous thrombosis and embolism
Pulmonary embolism

● V12.52 Thrombophlebitis

●❑ V12.59 Other

● V12.6 Diseases of respiratory system

● V12.7 Diseases of digestive system

●❑ V12.70 Unspecified digestive disease

● V12.71 Peptic ulcer disease

● V12.72 Colonic polyps

●❑ V12.79 Other

● V13 Personal history of other diseases

● V13.0 Disorders of urinary system

●❑ V13.00 Unspecified urinary disorder

● V13.01 Urinary calculi

●❑ V13.09 Other

● V13.1 Trophoblastic disease

Excludes *supervision during a current pregnancy (V23.1)*

●❑ V13.2 Other genital system and obstetric disorders

Excludes *supervision during a current pregnancy of a woman with poor obstetric history (V23.0–V23.9)*
habitual aborter (646.3)
without current pregnancy (629.9)

● V13.21 Personal history of pre-term labor

Excludes *current pregnancy with history of pre-term labor (V23.41)*

●❑ V13.29 Other genital system and obstetric disorders

● V13.3 Diseases of skin and subcutaneous tissue

● V13.4 Arthritis

●❑ V13.5 Other musculoskeletal disorders

● V13.6 Congenital malformations

● V13.61 Hypospadias

●❑ V13.69 Other congenital malformations

● V13.7 Perinatal problems

Excludes *low birth weight status (V21.30–V21.35)*

●❑ V13.8 Other specified diseases

●❑ V13.9 Unspecified disease

● V14 Personal history of allergy to medicinal agents

● V14.0 Penicillin

●❑ V14.1 Other antibiotic agent

● V14.2 Sulfonamides

●❑ V14.3 Other anti-infective agent

● V14.4 Anesthetic agent

● V14.5 Narcotic agent

● V14.6 Analgesic agent

● V14.7 Serum or vaccine

●❑ V14.8 Other specified medicinal agents

●❑ V14.9 Unspecified medicinal agent

● V15 Other personal history presenting hazards to health

●❑ V15.0 Allergy, other than to medicinal agents

Excludes *allergy to food substance used as base for medicinal agent (V14.0–V14.9)*

● V15.01 Allergy to peanuts

● V15.02 Allergy to milk products

Excludes *lactose intolerance (271.3)*

● V15.03 Allergy to eggs

● V15.04 Allergy to seafood
Seafood (octopus) (squid) ink
Shellfish

● V15.05 Allergy to other foods
Food additives
Nuts other than peanuts

● V15.06 Allergy to insects
Bugs
Insect bites and stings
Spiders

● V15.07 Allergy to latex
Latex sensitivity

● V15.08 Allergy to radiographic dye
Contrast media used for diagnostic x-ray procedures

● V15.09 Other allergy, other than to medicinal agents

● V15.1 Surgery to heart and great vessels

Excludes *replacement by transplant or other means (V42.1–V42.2, V43.2–V43.4)*

●❑ V15.2 Surgery to other major organs

Excludes *replacement by transplant or other means (V42.0–V43.8)*

● V15.3 Irradiation
Previous exposure to therapeutic or other ionizing radiation

● V15.4 Psychological trauma

Excludes *history of condition classifiable to 290–316 (V11.0–V11.9)*

● V15.41 History of physical abuse
Rape

● V15.42 History of emotional abuse
Neglect

●❑ V15.49 Other

● V15.5 Injury

● V15.6 Poisoning

● V15.7 Contraception

Excludes *current contraceptive management (V25.0–V25.4)*
presence of intrauterine contraceptive device as incidental finding (V45.5)

● V15.8 Other specified personal history presenting hazards to health

● V15.81 Noncompliance with medical treatment

● V15.82 History of tobacco use

Excludes *tobacco dependence (305.1)*

● V15.84 Exposure to asbestos

● V15.85 Exposure to potentially hazardous body fluids

● V15.86 Exposure to lead

● V15.87 History of Extracorporeal Membrane Oxygenation [ECMO] ◀

●❑ V15.89 Other

●❑ V15.9 Unspecified personal history presenting hazards to health

V16 Family history of malignant neoplasm

V16.0 Gastrointestinal tract
Family history of condition classifiable to 140–159

V16.1 Trachea, bronchus, and lung
Family history of condition classifiable to 162

V16.2 Other respiratory and intrathoracic organs
Family history of condition classifiable to 160–161, 163–165

V16.3 Breast
Family history of condition classifiable to 174

V16.4 Genital organs
Family history of condition classifiable to 179–187

V16.40 Genital organ, unspecified

V16.41 Ovary

V16.42 Prostate

V16.43 Testis

V16.49 Other

V16.5 Urinary organs
Family history of condition classifiable to 189

V16.51 Kidney

V16.59 Other

V16.6 Leukemia
Family history of condition classifiable to 204–208

V16.7 Other lymphatic and hematopoietic neoplasms
Family history of condition classifiable to 200–203

V16.8 Other specified malignant neoplasm
Family history of other condition classifiable to 140–199

V16.9 Unspecified malignant neoplasm

V17 Family history of certain chronic disabling diseases

V17.0 Psychiatric condition
Excludes *family history of mental retardation (V18.4)*

V17.1 Stroke (cerebrovascular)

V17.2 Other neurological diseases
Epilepsy
Huntington's chorea

V17.3 Ischemic heart disease

V17.4 Other cardiovascular diseases

V17.5 Asthma

V17.6 Other chronic respiratory conditions

V17.7 Arthritis

V17.8 Other musculoskeletal diseases

V18 Family history of certain other specific conditions

V18.0 Diabetes mellitus

V18.1 Other endocrine and metabolic diseases

V18.2 Anemia

V18.3 Other blood disorders

V18.4 Mental retardation

V18.5 Digestive disorders

V18.6 Kidney diseases

V18.61 Polycystic kidney

V18.69 Other kidney diseases

V18.7 Other genitourinary diseases

V18.8 Infectious and parasitic diseases

V19 Family history of other conditions

V19.0 Blindness or visual loss

V19.1 Other eye disorders

V19.2 Deafness or hearing loss

V19.3 Other ear disorders

V19.4 Skin conditions

V19.5 Congenital anomalies

V19.6 Allergic disorders

V19.7 Consanguinity

V19.8 Other condition

PERSONS ENCOUNTERING HEALTH SERVICES IN CIRCUMSTANCES RELATED TO REPRODUCTION AND DEVELOPMENT (V20–V29)

V20 Health supervision of infant or child

V20.0 Foundling

V20.1 Other healthy infant or child receiving care
Medical or nursing care supervision of healthy infant in cases of:
maternal illness, physical or psychiatric
socioeconomic adverse condition at home
too many children at home preventing or interfering with normal care

V20.2 Routine infant or child health check
Developmental testing of infant or child
Immunizations appropriate for age
Routine vision and hearing testing
Excludes *special screening for developmental handicaps (V79.3)*

Use additional code(s) to identify:
Special screening examination(s) performed (V73.0–V82.9)

V21 Constitutional states in development

V21.0 Period of rapid growth in childhood

V21.1 Puberty

V21.2 Other adolescence

V21.3 Low birth weight status
Excludes *history of perinatal problems (V13.7)*

V21.30 Low birth weight status, unspecified

V21.31 Low birth weight status, less than 500 grams

V21.32 Low birth weight status, 500–999 grams

V21.33 Low birth weight status, 1000–1499 grams

V21.34 Low birth weight status, 1500–1999 grams

V21.35 Low birth weight status, 2000–2500 grams

V21.8 Other specified constitutional states in development

V21.9 Unspecified constitutional state in development

V22 Normal pregnancy
Excludes *pregnancy examination or test, pregnancy unconfirmed (V72.4)*

V22.0 Supervision of normal first pregnancy

V22.1 Supervision of other normal pregnancy

V22.2 Pregnant state, incidental
Pregnant state NOS

● V23 **Supervision of high-risk pregnancy**

● V23.0 **Pregnancy with history of infertility**

● V23.1 **Pregnancy with history of trophoblastic disease**
Pregnancy with history of:
hydatidiform mole
vesicular mole

Excludes *that without current pregnancy (V13.1)*

● V23.2 **Pregnancy with history of abortion**
Pregnancy with history of conditions classifiable to 634–638

Excludes *habitual aborter:*
care during pregnancy (646.3)
that without current pregnancy (629.9)

● V23.3 **Grand multiparity**

Excludes *care in relation to labor and delivery (659.4)*
that without current pregnancy (V61.5)

● ❑ V23.4 **Pregnancy with other poor obstetric history**
Pregnancy with history of other conditions classifiable to 630–676

● V23.41 **Pregnancy with history of pre-term labor**

● ❑ V23.49 **Pregnancy with other poor obstetric history**

● ❑ V23.5 **Pregnancy with other poor reproductive history**
Pregnancy with history of stillbirth or neonatal death

● V23.7 **Insufficient prenatal care**
History of little or no prenatal care

● V23.8 **Other high-risk pregnancy**

● V23.81 **Elderly primigravida**
First pregnancy in a woman who will be 35 years of age or older at expected date of delivery

Excludes *elderly primigravida complcating pregnancy (659.5)*

● V23.82 **Elderly multigravida**
Second or more pregnancy in a woman who will be 35 years of age or older at expected date of delivery

Excludes *elderly multigravida complicating pregnancy (659.6)*

● V23.83 **Young primigravida**
First pregnancy in a female less than 16 years old at expected date of delivery

Excludes *young primigravida complicating pregnancy (659.8)*

● V23.84 **Young multigravida**
Second or more pregnancy in a female less than 16 years old at expected date of delivery

Excludes *young multigravida complicating pregnancy (659.8)*

● ❑ V23.89 **Other high-risk pregnancy**

● ❑ V23.9 **Unspecified high-risk pregnancy**

● V24 **Postpartum care and examination**

V24.0 **Immediately after delivery**
Care and observation in uncomplicated cases

● V24.1 **Lactating mother**
Supervision of lactation

● V24.2 **Routine postpartum follow-up**

● V25 **Encounter for contraceptive management**

● V25.0 **General counseling and advice**

● V25.01 **Prescription of oral contraceptives**

● ❑ V25.02 **Initiation of other contraceptive measures**
Fitting of diaphragm
Prescription of foams, creams, or other agents

● V25.03 **Encounter for emergency contraceptive counseling and prescription** ◄
Encounter for postcoital contraceptive counseling and prescription

● ❑ V25.09 **Other**
Family planning advice

● V25.1 **Insertion of intrauterine contraceptive device**

V25.2 **Sterilization**
Admission for interruption of fallopian tubes or vas deferens

V25.3 **Menstrual extraction**
Menstrual regulation

● V25.4 **Surveillance of previously prescribed contraceptive methods**
Checking, reinsertion, or removal of contraceptive device
Repeat prescription for contraceptive method
Routine examination in connection with contraceptive maintenance

Excludes *presence of intrauterine contraceptive device as incidental finding (V45.5)*

● ❑ V25.40 **Contraceptive surveillance, unspecified**

● V25.41 **Contraceptive pill**

● V25.42 **Intrauterine contraceptive device**
Checking, reinsertion, or removal of intrauterine device

● V25.43 **Implantable subdermal contraceptive**

● ❑ V25.49 **Other contraceptive method**

● V25.5 **Insertion of implantable subdermal contraceptive**

● ❑ V25.8 **Other specified contraceptive management**
Postvasectomy sperm count

Excludes *sperm count following sterilization reversal (V26.22)*
sperm count for fertility testing (V26.21)

● ❑ V25.9 **Unspecified contraceptive management**

● V26 **Procreative management**

V26.0 **Tuboplasty or vasoplasty after previous sterilization**

● V26.1 **Artificial insemination**

● V26.2 **Investigation and testing**

Excludes *postvasectomy sperm count (V25.8)*

● V26.21 **Fertility testing**
Fallopian insufflation
Sperm count for fertility testing

Excludes *Genetic counseling and testing (V26.3)*

● V26.22 **Aftercare following sterilization reversal**
Fallopian insufflation following sterilization reversal
Sperm count following sterilization reversal

● V26.29 **Other investigation and testing**

● V26.3 Genetic counseling and testing

Excludes *fertility testing (V26.21)*

● V26.4 General counseling and advice

● V26.5 Sterilization status

V26.51 Tubal ligation status

Excludes *infertility not due to previous tubal ligation (628.0–628.9)*

V26.52 Vasectomy status

● ❑ V26.8 Other specified procreative management

● ❑ V26.9 Unspecified procreative management

● V27 Outcome of delivery

Note: This category is intended for the coding of the outcome of delivery on the mother 's record.

● V27.0 Single liveborn

● V27.1 Single stillborn

● V27.2 Twins, both liveborn

● V27.3 Twins, one liveborn and one stillborn

● V27.4 Twins, both stillborn

● ❑ V27.5 Other multiple birth, all liveborn

● ❑ V27.6 Other multiple birth, some liveborn

● ❑ V27.7 Other multiple birth, all stillborn

● ❑ V27.9 Unspecified outcome of delivery
single birth, outcome to infant unspecified
multiple birth, outcome to infant unspecified

● V28 Antenatal screening

Excludes *abnormal findings on screening—code to findings*
routine prenatal care (V22.0–V23.9)

● V28.0 Screening for chromosomal anomalies by amniocentesis

● V28.1 Screening for raised alpha-fetoprotein levels in amniotic fluid

● ❑ V28.2 Other screening based on amniocentesis

● V28.3 Screening for malformation using ultrasonics

● V28.4 Screening for fetal growth retardation using ultrasonics

● V28.5 Screening for isoimmunization

● V28.6 Screening for Streptococcus B

● ❑ V28.8 Other specified antenatal screening

● ❑ V28.9 Unspecified antenatal screening

● V29 Observation and evaluation of newborns for suspected condition not found

Note: This category is to be used for newborns, within the neonatal period (the first 28 days of life), who are suspected of having an abnormal condition resulting from exposure from the mother or the birth process, but without signs or symptoms, and which, after examination and observation, is found not to exist.

V29.0 Observation for suspected infectious condition

V29.1 Observation for suspected neurological condition

V29.2 Observation for suspected respiratory condition

● V29.3 Observation for suspected genetic or metabolic condition

❑ V29.8 Observation for other specified suspected condition

● ❑ V29.9 Observation for unspecified suspected condition

LIVEBORN INFANTS ACCORDING TO TYPE OF BIRTH (V30–V39)

Note: These categories are intended for the coding of liveborn infants who are consuming health care [e.g., crib or bassinet occupancy].

The following fourth-digit subdivisions are for use with categories V30–V39:

.0 Born in hospital
.1 Born before admission to hospital
● .2 Born outside hospital and not hospitalized

The following two fifth-digits are for use with the fourth-digit .0, born in hospital:

0 delivered without mention of cesarean delivery
1 delivered by cesarean delivery

● V30 Single liveborn

● V31 Twin, mate liveborn

● V32 Twin, mate stillborn

● ❑ V33 Twin, unspecified

● ❑ V34 Other multiple, mates all liveborn

● ❑ V35 Other multiple, mates all stillborn

● ❑ V36 Other multiple, mates live- and stillborn

● ❑ V37 Other multiple, unspecified

● ❑ V39 Unspecified

PERSONS WITH A CONDITION INFLUENCING THEIR HEALTH STATUS (V40–V49)

Note: These categories are intended for use when these conditions are recorded as "diagnoses" or "problems."

● V40 Mental and behavioral problems

● V40.0 Problems with learning

● V40.1 Problems with communication [including speech]

● ❑ V40.2 Other mental problems

● ❑ V40.3 Other behavioral problems

● ❑ V40.9 Unspecified mental or behavioral problem

● V41 Problems with special senses and other special functions

● V41.0 Problems with sight

● ❑ V41.1 Other eye problems

● V41.2 Problems with hearing

● ❑ V41.3 Other ear problems

● V41.4 Problems with voice production

● V41.5 Problems with smell and taste

● V41.6 Problems with swallowing and mastication

● V41.7 Problems with sexual function

Excludes *marital problems (V61.10)*
psychosexual disorders (302.0–302.9)

● V41.8 Other problems with special functions

● V41.9 Unspecified problem with special functions

● V42 Organ or tissue replaced by transplant

Includes: homologous or heterologous (animal) (human) transplant organ status

● V42.0 Kidney
● V42.1 Heart
● V42.2 Heart valve
● V42.3 Skin
● V42.4 Bone
● V42.5 Cornea
● V42.6 Lung
● V42.7 Liver
● V42.8 Other specified organ or tissue
● V42.81 Bone marrow
● V42.82 Peripheral stem cells
● V42.83 Pancreas
● V42.84 Intestines
●❑ V42.89 Other
●❑ V42.9 Unspecified organ or tissue

● V43 Organ or tissue replaced by other means

Includes: organ or tissue assisted by other means
replacement of organ by:
artificial device
mechanical device
prosthesis

Excludes *cardiac pacemaker in situ (V45.01)*
fitting and adjustment of prosthetic device (V52.0–V52.9)
renal dialysis status (V45.1)

● V43.0 Eye globe
● V43.1 Lens
Pseudophakos
●● V43.2 Heart (Revised)
V43.21 Heart assist device (New)
V43.22 Fully implantable artificial heart (New)
● V43.3 Heart valve
● V43.4 Blood vessel
● V43.5 Bladder
● V43.6 Joint
●❑ V43.60 Unspecified joint
● V43.61 Shoulder
● V43.62 Elbow
● V43.63 Wrist
● V43.64 Hip
● V43.65 Knee
● V43.66 Ankle
●❑ V43.69 Other
● V43.7 Limb
● V43.8 Other organ or tissue
● V43.81 Larynx
● V43.82 Breast
● V43.83 Artificial skin
●❑ V43.89 Other

● V44 Artificial opening status

Excludes *artificial openings requiring attention or management (V55.0–V55.9)*

● V44.0 Tracheostomy
● V44.1 Gastrostomy
● V44.2 Ileostomy
● V44.3 Colostomy
●❑ V44.4 Other artificial opening of gastrointestinal tract
● V44.5 Cystostomy
●❑ V44.50 Cystostomy, unspecified
● V44.51 Cutaneous-vesicostomy
● V44.52 Appendico-vesicostomy
●❑ V44.59 Other cystostomy
●❑ V44.6 Other artificial opening of urinary tract
Nephrostomy
Ureterostomy
Urethrostomy
● V44.7 Artificial vagina
●❑ V44.8 Other artificial opening status
●❑ V44.9 Unspecified artificial opening status

● V45 Other postprocedural states (Revised)

Excludes *aftercare management (V51–V58.9)*
malfunction or other complication—code to condition

● V45.0 Cardiac device in situ

Excludes *artificial heart (V43.22)* (New)
heart assist device (V43.21) (New)

●❑ V45.00 Unspecified cardiac device
● V45.01 Cardiac pacemaker
● V45.02 Automatic implantable cardiac defibrillator
●❑ V45.09 Other specified cardiac device
Carotid sinus pacemaker in situ
● V45.1 Renal dialysis status
Patient requiring intermittent renal dialysis
Presence of arterial-venous shunt (for dialysis)

Excludes *admission for dialysis treatment or session (V56.0)*

● V45.2 Presence of cerebrospinal fluid drainage device
Cerebral ventricle (communicating) shunt, valve, or device in situ

Excludes *malfunction (996.2)*

● V45.3 Intestinal bypass or anastomosis status
● V45.4 Arthrodesis status
● V45.5 Presence of contraceptive device

Excludes *checking, reinsertion, or removal of device (V25.42)*
complication from device (996.32)
insertion of device (V25.1)

● V45.51 Intrauterine contraceptive device
● V45.52 Subdermal contraceptive implant
●❑ V45.59 Other
● V45.6 States following surgery of eye and adnexa

Excludes *aphakia (379.31)*
artificial:
eye globe (V43.0)

● V45.61 Cataract extraction status
Use additional code for associated artificial lens status (V43.1)
●❑ V45.69 Other states following surgery of eye and adnexa

● V45.7 Acquired absence of organ

● V45.71 Acquired absence of breast

● V45.72 Acquired absence of intestine (large) (small)

● V45.73 Acquired absence of kidney

● V45.74 Other parts of urinary tract
Bladder

● V45.75 Stomach

● V45.76 Lung

● V45.77 Genital organs

● V45.78 Eye

● V45.79 Other acquired absence of organ

● V45.8 Other postprocedural status

● V45.81 Aortocoronary bypass status

● V45.82 Percutaneous transluminal coronary angioplasty status

● V45.83 Breast implant removal status

● V45.84 Dental restoration status
Dental crowns status
Dental fillings status

● V45.85 Insulin pump status

●❑ V45.89 Other
Presence of neuropacemaker or other electronic device

Excludes *artificial heart valve in situ (V43.3)*
vascular prosthesis in situ (V43.4)

● V46 Other dependence on machines

● V46.0 Aspirator

● V46.1 Respirator
Iron lung

● V46.2 Supplemental oxygen
Long-term oxygen therapy

●❑ V46.8 Other enabling machines
Hyperbaric chamber
Possum [Patient-Operated-Selector-Mechanism]

Excludes *cardiac pacemaker (V45.0)*
kidney dialysis machine (V45.1)

●❑ V46.9 Unspecified machine dependence

● V47 Other problems with internal organs

● V47.0 Deficiencies of internal organs

● V47.1 Mechanical and motor problems with internal organs

●❑ V47.2 Other cardiorespiratory problems
Cardiovascular exercise intolerance with pain (with):
at rest
less than ordinary activity
ordinary activity

●❑ V47.3 Other digestive problems

●❑ V47.4 Other urinary problems

●❑ V47.5 Other genital problems

●❑ V47.9 Unspecified

● V48 Problems with head, neck, and trunk

● V48.0 Deficiencies of head

Excludes *deficiencies of ears, eyelids, and nose (V48.8)*

● V48.1 Deficiencies of neck and trunk

● V48.2 Mechanical and motor problems with head

● V48.3 Mechanical and motor problems with neck and trunk

● V48.4 Sensory problem with head

● V48.5 Sensory problem with neck and trunk

● V48.6 Disfigurements of head

● V48.7 Disfigurements of neck and trunk

●❑ V48.8 Other problems with head, neck, and trunk

●❑ V48.9 Unspecified problem with head, neck, or trunk

● V49 Other conditions influencing health status

● V49.0 Deficiencies of limbs

● V49.1 Mechanical problems with limbs

● V49.2 Motor problems with limbs

● V49.3 Sensory problems with limbs

● V49.4 Disfigurements of limbs

●❑ V49.5 Other problems of limbs

● V49.6 Upper limb amputation status

●❑ V49.60 Unspecified level

● V49.61 Thumb

●❑ V49.62 Other finger(s)

● V49.63 Hand

● V49.64 Wrist
Disarticulation of wrist

● V49.65 Below elbow

● V49.66 Above elbow
Disarticulation of elbow

● V49.67 Shoulder
Disarticulation of shoulder

● V49.7 Lower limb amputation status

●❑ V49.70 Unspecified level

● V49.71 Great toe

●❑ V49.72 Other toe(s)

● V49.73 Foot

● V49.74 Ankle
Disarticulation of ankle

● V49.75 Below knee

● V49.76 Above knee
Disarticulation of knee

● V49.77 Hip
Disarticulation of hip

● V49.8 Other specified conditions influencing health status

● V49.81 Asymptomatic postmenopausal status (age-related) (natural)

Excludes *menopausal and premenopausal disorders (627.0–627.9)*
postsurgical menopause (256.2)
premature menopause (256.31)
symptomatic menopause (627.0–627.9)

● V49.82 Dental sealant status

● V49.89 Other specified conditions influencing health status

●❑ V49.9 Unspecified

ICD-9-CM V01-V99 Vol. 1

PERSONS ENCOUNTERING HEALTH SERVICES FOR SPECIFIC PROCEDURES AND AFTERCARE (V50–V59)

Note: Categories V51–V58 are intended for use to indicate a reason for care in patients who may have already been treated for some disease or injury not now present, or who are receiving care to consolidate the treatment, to deal with residual states, or to prevent recurrence.

Excludes *follow-up examination for medical surveillance following treatment (V67.0–V67.9)*

● **V50 Elective surgery for purposes other than remedying health states**

V50.0 Hair transplant

❑ **V50.1 Other plastic surgery for unacceptable cosmetic appearance**
Breast augmentation or reduction
Face-lift

Excludes *plastic surgery following healed injury or operation (V51)*

V50.2 Routine or ritual circumcision
Circumcision in the absence of significant medical indication

● **V50.3 Ear piercing**

● **V50.4 Prophylactic organ removal**

Excludes *organ donations (V59.0–V59.9)*
therapeutic organ removal—code to condition

V50.41 Breast

V50.42 Ovary

❑ **V50.49 Other**

●❑ **V50.8 Other**

●❑ **V50.9 Unspecified**

V51 Aftercare involving the use of plastic surgery
Plastic surgery following healed injury or operation

Excludes *cosmetic plastic surgery (V50.1)*
plastic surgery as treatment for current injury—code to condition
repair of scar tissue—code to scar

● **V52 Fitting and adjustment of prosthetic device and implant**

Includes: removal of device

Excludes *malfunction or complication of prosthetic device (996.0–996.7)*
status only, without need for care (V43.0–V43.8)

V52.0 Artificial arm (complete) (partial)

V52.1 Artificial leg (complete) (partial)

V52.2 Artificial eye

V52.3 Dental prosthetic device

V52.4 Breast prosthesis and implant

Excludes *admission for breast implant insertion (V50.1)*

❑ **V52.8 Other specified prosthetic device**

❑ **V52.9 Unspecified prosthetic device**

● **V53 Fitting and adjustment of other device**

Includes: removal of device
replacement of device

Excludes *status only, without need for care (V45.0–V45.8)*

● **V53.0 Devices related to nervous system and special senses**

V53.01 Fitting and adjustment of cerebral ventricle (communicating) shunt

V53.02 Neuropacemaker (brain) (peripheral nerve) (spinal cord)

V53.09 Fitting and adjustment of other devices related to nervous system and special senses
Auditory substitution device
Visual substitution device

V53.1 Spectacles and contact lenses

V53.2 Hearing aid

● **V53.3 Cardiac device**
Reprogramming

V53.31 Cardiac pacemaker

Excludes *mechanical complication of cardiac pacemaker (996.01)*

V53.32 Automatic implantable cardiac defibrillator

❑ **V53.39 Other cardiac device**

V53.4 Orthodontic devices

V53.5 Other intestinal appliance

Excludes *colostomy (V55.3)*
ileostomy (V55.2)
other artifical opening of digestive tract (V55.4)

V53.6 Urinary devices
Urinary catheter

Excludes *cystostomy (V55.5)*
nephrostomy (V55.6)
ureterostomy (V55.6)
urethrostomy (V55.6)

V53.7 Orthopedic devices
Orthopedic:
brace
cast
corset
shoes

Excludes *other orthopedic aftercare (V54)*

V53.8 Wheelchair

● **V53.9 Other and unspecified device**

❑ **V53.90 Unspecified device** ◄

V53.91 Fiting and adjustment of insulin pump ◄
Insulin pump titration ◄

❑ **V53.99 Other device** ◄

● **V54 Other orthopedic aftercare**

Excludes *fitting and adjustment of orthopedic devices (V53.7)*
malfunction of internal orthopedic device (996.4)
other complication of nonmechanical nature (996.60–996.79)

● V54.0 Aftercare involving internal fixation device

Excludes *removal of external fixation device (V54.89)*

V54.01 Encounter for removal of internal fixation device ◀

V54.02 Encounter for lengthening/adjustment of growth rod ◀

❑ V54.09 Other aftercare involving internal fixation device ◀

● V54.1 Aftercare for healing traumatic fracture

❑ V54.10 Aftercare for healing traumatic fracture of arm, unspecified

V54.11 Aftercare for healing traumatic fracture of upper arm

V54.12 Aftercare for healing traumatic fracture of lower arm

V54.13 Aftercare for healing traumatic fracture of hip

❑ V54.14 Aftercare for healing traumatic fracture of leg, unspecified

V54.15 Aftercare for healing traumatic fracture of upper leg

Excludes *aftercare for healing traumatic fracture of hip (V54.13)*

V54.16 Aftercare for healing traumatic fracture of lower leg

V54.17 Aftercare for healing traumatic fracture of vertebrae

❑ V54.19 Aftercare for healing traumatic fracture of other bone

● V54.2 Aftercare for healing pathologic fracture

❑ V54.20 Aftercare for healing pathologic fracture of arm, unspecified

V54.21 Aftercare for healing pathologic fracture of upper arm

V54.22 Aftercare for healing pathologic fracture of lower arm

V54.23 Aftercare for healing pathologic fracture of hip

❑ V54.24 Aftercare for healing pathologic fracture of leg, unspecified

V54.25 Aftercare for healing pathologic fracture of upper leg

Excludes *aftercare for healing pathologic fracture of hip (V54.23)*

V54.26 Aftercare for healing pathologic fracture of lower leg

V54.27 Aftercare for healing pathologic fracture of vertebrae

❑ V54.29 Aftercare for healing pathologic fracture of other bone

● ❑ V54.8 Other orthopedic aftercare

V54.81 Aftercare following joint replacement

Use additional code to identify joint replacement site (V43.60–V43.69)

❑ V54.89 Other orthopedic aftercare

Aftercare for healing fracture NOS

❑ V54.9 Unspecified orthopedic aftercare

● V55 Attention to artificial openings

Includes: adjustment or repositioning of catheter
closure
passage of sounds or bougies
reforming
removal or replacement of catheter
toilet or cleansing

Excludes *complications of external stoma (519.00–519.09, 569.60–569.69, 997.4, 997.5)*
status only, without need for care (V44.0–V44.9)

V55.0 Tracheostomy

V55.1 Gastrostomy

V55.2 Ileostomy

V55.3 Colostomy

❑ V55.4 Other artificial opening of digestive tract

V55.5 Cystostomy

❑ V55.6 Other artificial opening of urinary tract

Nephrostomy
Ureterostomy
Urethrostomy

V55.7 Artificial vagina

❑ V55.8 Other specified artificial opening

❑ V55.9 Unspecified artificial opening

● V56 Encounter for dialysis and dialysis catheter care

Use additional code to identify the associated condition

Excludes *dialysis preparation—code to condition*

V56.0 Extracorporeal dialysis

Dialysis (renal) NOS

Excludes *dialysis status (V45.1)*

V56.1 Fitting and adjustment of extracoporeal dialysis catheter

Removal or replacement of catheter
Toilet or cleansing

Use additional code for any concurrent extracorporeal dialysis (V56.0)

V56.2 Fitting and adjustment of peritoneal dialysis catheter

Use additional code for any concurrent peritoneal dialysis (V56.8)

● V56.3 Encounter for adequacy testing for dialysis

● V56.31 Encounter for adequacy testing for hemodialysis

● V56.32 Encounter for adequacy testing for peritoneal dialysis

Peritoneal equilibration test

❑ V56.8 Other dialysis

Peritoneal dialysis

● V57 **Care involving use of rehabilitation procedures**
Use additional code to identify underlying condition

V57.0 **Breathing exercises**

❑ V57.1 **Other physical therapy**
Therapeutic and remedial exercises, except breathing

● V57.2 **Occupational therapy and vocational rehabilitation**

V57.21 **Encounter for occupational therapy**

V57.22 **Encounter for vocational therapy**

V57.3 **Speech therapy**

V57.4 **Orthoptic training**

● V57.8 **Other specified rehabilitation procedure**

V57.81 **Orthotic training**
Gait training in the use of artificial limbs

❑ V57.89 **Other**
Multiple training or therapy

❑ V57.9 **Unspecified rehabilitation procedure**

● V58 **Encounter for other and unspecified procedures and aftercare**

Excludes *convalescence and palliative care (V66.0–V66.9)*

V58.0 **Radiotherapy**
Encounter or admission for radiotherapy

Excludes *encounter for radioactive implant—code to condition*
radioactive iodine therapy—code to condition

V58.1 **Chemotherapy**
Encounter or admission for chemotherapy

Excludes *prophylactic chemotherapy against disease which has never been present (V03.0–V07.9)*

V58.2 **Blood transfusion, without reported diagnosis**

V58.3 **Attention to surgical dressings and sutures**
Change of dressings
Removal of sutures

● V58.4 **Other aftercare following surgery**

Note: Codes from this subcategory should be used in conjunction with other after care codes to fully identify the reason for the aftercare encounter.

Excludes *aftercare following sterilization reversal surgery (V26.22)*
attention to artificial openings (V55.0–V55.9)
orthopedic aftercare (V54.0–V54.9)

V58.41 **Encounter for planned post-operative wound closure**

Excludes *disruption of operative wound (998.3)*

V58.42 **Aftercare following surgery for neoplasm**
Conditions classifiable to 140–239

V58.43 **Aftercare following surgery for injury and trauma**
Conditions classifiable to 800–999

Excludes *aftercare for healing traumatic fracture (V54.10–V54.19)*

❑ V58.49 **Other specified aftercare following surgery**

V58.5 **Orthodontics**

Excludes *fitting and adjustment of orthodontic device (V53.4)*

● V58.6 **Long-term (current) drug use**

Excludes *drug abuse (305.00–305.93)*
drug dependence (304.00–304.93)

V58.61 **Long-term (current) use of anticoagulants**

V58.62 **Long-term (current) use of antibiotics**

V58.63 **Long-term (current) use of antiplatelet/antithrombotic** ◀

V58.64 **Long-term (current) use of non-steroidal anti-inflammatories (NSAID)** ◀

V58.65 **Long-term (current) use of steroids** ◀

❑ V58.69 **Long-term (current) use of other medications**
High-risk medications

● V58.7 **Aftercare following surgery to specified body systems, not elsewhere classified**

Note: Codes from this subcategory should be used in conjunction with other aftercare codes to fully identify the reason for the aftercare encounter

V58.71 **Aftercare following surgery of the sense organs, NEC**
Conditions classifiable to 360–379, 380–389

V58.72 **Aftercare following surgery of the nervous system, NEC**
Conditions classifiable to 320–359

Excludes *aftercare following surgery of the sense organs, NEC (V58.71)*

V58.73 **Aftercare following surgery of the circulatory system, NEC**
Conditions classifiable to 390–459

V58.74 **Aftercare following surgery of the respiratory system, NEC**
Conditions classifiable to 460–519

V58.75 **Aftercare following surgery of the teeth, oral cavity and digestive system, NEC**
Conditions classifiable to 520–579

V58.76 **Aftercare following surgery of the genitourinary system, NEC**
Conditions classifiable to 580–629

Excludes *aftercare following sterilization reversal (V26.22)*

V58.77 **Aftercare following surgery of the skin and subcutaneous tissue, NEC**
Conditions classifiable to 680–709

V58.78 **Aftercare following surgery of the musculoskeletal system, NEC**
Conditions classifiable to 710–739

● V58.8 Other specified procedures and aftercare

V58.81 Fitting and adjustment of vascular catheter
Removal or replacement of catheter
Toilet or cleansing

Excludes *complications of renal dialysis (996.73)*
complications of vascular catheter (996.74)
dialysis preparation—code to condition
encounter for dialysis (V56.0–V56.8)
fitting and adjustment of dialysis catheter (V56.2)

V58.82 Fitting and adjustment of non-vascular catheter, NEC
Removal or replacement of catheter
Toilet or cleansing

Excludes *fitting and adjustment of peritoneal dialysis catheter (V56.2)*
fitting and adjustment of urinary catheter (V53.6)

V58.83 Encounter for therapeutic drug monitoring

Use additional code for any associated long-term (current) drug use (V58.61–V58.69)

Excludes *blood-drug testing for medicolegal reasons (V70.4)*

❏ V58.89 Other specified aftercare

❏ V58.9 Unspecified aftercare

● V59 Donors

Excludes *examination of potential donor (V70.8)*
self-donation of organ or tissue—code to condition

● V59.0 Blood

V59.01 Whole blood

V59.02 Stem cells

❏ V59.09 Other

V59.1 Skin

V59.2 Bone

V59.3 Bone marrow

V59.4 Kidney

V59.5 Cornea

V59.6 Liver

V59.8 Other specified organ or tissue

V59.9 Unspecified organ or tissue

PERSONS ENCOUNTERING HEALTH SERVICES IN OTHER CIRCUMSTANCES (V60–V68)

● V60 Housing, household, and economic circumstances

V60.0 Lack of housing
Hobos
Social migrants
Tramps
Transients
Vagabonds

● V60.1 Inadequate housing
Lack of heating
Restriction of space
Technical defects in home preventing adequate care

● V60.2 Inadequate material resources
Economic problem
Poverty NOS

● V60.3 Person living alone

● V60.4 No other household member able to render care
Person requiring care (has) (is):
family member too handicapped, ill, or otherwise unsuited to render care
partner temporarily away from home
temporarily away from usual place of abode

Excludes *holiday relief care (V60.5)*

● V60.5 Holiday relief care
Provision of health care facilities to a person normally cared for at home, to enable relatives to take a vacation

● V60.6 Person living in residential institution
Boarding school resident

● ❏ V60.8 Other specified housing or economic circumstances

● ❏ V60.9 Unspecified housing or economic circumstance

● V61 Other family circumstances

Includes: when these circumstances or fear of them, affecting the person directly involved or others, are mentioned as the reason, justified or not, for seeking or receiving medical advice or care

● V61.0 Family disruption
Divorce
Estrangement

● V61.1 Counseling for marital and partner problems

Excludes *problems related to:*
psychosexual disorders (302.0–302.9)
sexual function (V41.7)

● V61.10 Counseling for marital and partner problems, unspecified
Marital conflict
Partner conflict

● V61.11 Counseling for victim of spousal and partner abuse

Excludes *encounter for treatment of current injuries due to abuse (995.80–995.85)*

● V61.12 Counseling for perpetrator of spousal and partner abuse

● **V61.2 Parent-child problems**

●❑ **V61.20 Counseling for parent-child problem, unspecified**
Concern about behavior of child
Parent-child conflict

● **V61.21 Counseling for victim of child abuse**
Child battering
Child neglect

Excludes *current injuries due to abuse (995.50–995.59)*

● **V61.22 Counseling for perpetrator of parental child abuse**

Excludes *counseling for non-parental abuser (V62.83)*

●❑ **V61.29 Other**
Problem concerning adopted or foster child

● **V61.3 Problems with aged parents or in-laws**

● **V61.4 Health problems within family**

● **V61.41 Alcoholism in family**

●❑ **V61.49 Other**
Care of sick or handicapped person in family or household
Presence of sick or handicapped person in family or household

● **V61.5 Multiparity**

● **V61.6 Illegitimacy or illegitimate pregnancy**

●❑ **V61.7 Other unwanted pregnancy**

●❑ **V61.8 Other specified family circumstances**
Problems with family members, NEC

●❑ **V61.9 Unspecified family circumstance**

● **V62 Other psychosocial circumstances**

Includes: those circumstances or fear of them, affecting the person directly involved or others, mentioned as the reason, justified or not, for seeking or receiving medical advice or care

Excludes *previous psychological trauma (V15.41–V15.49)*

● **V62.0 Unemployment**

Excludes *circumstances when main problem is economic inadequacy or poverty (V60.2)*

● **V62.1 Adverse effects of work environment**

●❑ **V62.2 Other occupational circumstances or maladjustment**
Career choice problem
Dissatisfaction with employment

● **V62.3 Educational circumstances**
Dissatisfaction with school environment
Educational handicap

● **V62.4 Social maladjustment**
Cultural deprivation
Political, religious, or sex discrimination
Social:
isolation
persecution

● **V62.5 Legal circumstances**
Imprisonment
Legal investigation
Litigation
Prosecution

● **V62.6 Refusal of treatment for reasons of religion or conscience**

● **V62.8 Other psychological or physical stress, not elsewhere classified**

● **V62.81 Interpersonal problems, not elsewhere classified**

● **V62.82 Bereavement, uncomplicated**

Excludes *bereavement as adjustment reaction (309.0)*

● **V62.83 Counseling for perpetrator of physical/sexual abuse**

Excludes *counseling for perpetrator of parental child abuse (V61.22)*
counseling for perpetrator of spousal and partner abuse (V61.12)

●❑ **V62.89 Other**
Life circumstance problems
Phase of life problems

●❑ **V62.9 Unspecified psychosocial circumstance**

● **V63 Unavailability of other medical facilities for care**

● **V63.0 Residence remote from hospital or other health care facility**

● **V63.1 Medical services in home not available**

Excludes *no other household member able to render care (V60.4)*

● **V63.2 Person awaiting admission to adequate facility elsewhere**

●❑ **V63.8 Other specified reasons for unavailability of medical facilities**
Person on waiting list undergoing social agency investigation

●❑ **V63.9 Unspecified reason for unavailability of medical facilities**

● **V64 Persons encountering health services for specific procedures, not carried out**

● **V64.0 Vaccination not carried out because of contraindication**

● **V64.1 Surgical or other procedure not carried out because of contraindication**

● **V64.2 Surgical or other procedure not carried out because of patient's decision**

●❑ **V64.3 Procedure not carried out for other reasons**

● **V64.4 Closed surgical procedure converted to open procedure** ⟸

● **V64.41 Laparoscopic surgical procedure converted to open procedure** ◀

● **V64.42 Thoracoscopic surgical procedure converted to open procedure** ◀

● **V64.43 Arthroscopic surgical procedure converted to open procedure** ◀

● **V65 Other persons seeking consultation** ⟸

V65.0 Healthy person accompanying sick person
Boarder

● **V65.1 Person consulting on behalf of another person**
Advice or treatment for nonattending third party

Excludes *concern (normal) about sick person in family (V61.41–V61.49)*

● **V65.11 Pediatric pre-birth visit for expectant mother** ◀

● **V65.19 Other person consulting on behalf of another person** ◀

V65.2 Person feigning illness
Malingerer
Peregrinating patient

● **V65.3 Dietary surveillance and counseling**
Dietary surveillance and counseling (in):
NOS
colitis
diabetes mellitus
food allergies or intolerance
gastritis
hypercholesterolemia
hypoglycemia
obesity

● V65.4 Other counseling, not elsewhere classified
Health:
advice
education
instruction

Excludes *counseling (for):*
contraception (V25.40–V25.49)
genetic (V26.3)
on behalf of third party (V65.11–V65.19)
procreative management (V26.4)

● V65.40 Counseling NOS

● V65.41 Exercise counseling

● V65.42 Counseling on substance use and abuse

● V65.43 Counseling on injury prevention

● V65.44 Human immunodeficiency virus [HIV] counseling

●❑ V65.45 Counseling on other sexually transmitted diseases

● V65.46 Encounter for insulin pump training

●❑ V65.49 Other specified counseling

● V65.5 Person with feared complaint in whom no diagnosis was made
Feared condition not demonstrated
Problem was normal state
"Worried well"

●❑ V65.8 Other reasons for seeking consultation

Excludes *specified symptoms*

●❑ V65.9 Unspecified reason for consultation

● V66 Convalescence and palliative care

V66.0 Following surgery

V66.1 Following radiotherapy

V66.2 Following chemotherapy

V66.3 Following psychotherapy and other treatment for mental disorder

V66.4 Following treatment of fracture

●❑ V66.5 Following other treatment

❑ V66.6 Following combined treatment

● V66.7 Encounter for palliative care
End-of-life care
Hospice care
Terminal care

Code first underlying disease

●❑ V66.9 Unspecified convalescence

● V67 Follow-up examination

Includes: surveillance only following completed treatment

Excludes *surveillance of contraception (V25.40–V25.49)*

● V67.0 Following surgery

V67.00 Following surgery, unspecified

V67.01 Follow-up vaginal pap smear
Vaginal pap smear, status-post hysterectomy for malignant condition

Use additional code to identify:
acquired absence of uterus (V45.77)
personal history of malignant neoplasm (V10.40–V10.44)

Excludes *vaginal pap smear status-post hysterectomy for non-malignant condition (V76.47)*

V67.09 Following other surgery

Excludes *sperm count following sterilization reversal (V26.22)*
sperm count for fertility testing (V26.21)

V67.1 Following radiotherapy

V67.2 Following chemotherapy
Cancer chemotherapy follow-up

V67.3 Following psychotherapy and other treatment for mental disorder

V67.4 Following treatment of healed fracture

Excludes *current (healing) fracture aftercare (V54.0–V54.9)*

● V67.5 Following other treatment

V67.51 Following completed treatment with high-risk medication, not elsewhere classified

Excludes *Long-term (current) drug use (V58.61–V58.69)*

❑ V67.59 Other

❑ V67.6 Following combined treatment

●❑ V67.9 Unspecified follow-up examination

● V68 Encounters for administrative purposes

● V68.0 Issue of medical certificates
Issue of medical certificate of:
cause of death
fitness
incapacity

Excludes *encounter for general medical examination (V70.0–V70.9)*

● V68.1 Issue of repeat prescriptions
Issue of repeat prescription for:
appliance
glasses
medications

Excludes *repeat prescription for contraceptives (V25.41–V25.49)*

● V68.2 Request for expert evidence

● V68.8 Other specified administrative purpose

● V68.81 Referral of patient without examination or treatment

●❑ V68.89 Other

●❑ V68.9 Unspecified administrative purpose

● V69 Problems related to lifestyle

● V69.0 Lack of physical exercise

● V69.1 Inappropriate diet and eating habits

Excludes *anorexia nervosa (307.1)*
bulimia (783.6)
malnutrition and other nutritional deficiencies (260–269.9)
other and unspecified eating disorders (307.50–307.59)

● V69.2 High-risk sexual behavior

● V69.3 Gambling and betting

Excludes *pathological gambling (312.31)*

●❑ V69.8 Other problems related to lifestyle
Self-damaging behavior

●❑ V69.9 Problem related to lifestyle, unspecified

PERSONS WITHOUT REPORTED DIAGNOSIS ENCOUNTERED DURING EXAMINATION AND INVESTIGATION OF INDIVIDUALS AND POPULATIONS (V70–V83)

Note: Nonspecific abnormal findings disclosed at the time of these examinations are classifiable to categories 790–796.

● **V70 General medical examination**

Use additional code(s) to identify any special screening examination(s) performed (V73.0–V82.9)

● **V70.0 Routine general medical examination at a health care facility**
Health checkup

Excludes *health checkup of infant or child (V20.2)*

V70.1 General psychiatric examination, requested by the authority

●❑ **V70.2 General psychiatric examination, other and unspecified**

●❑ **V70.3 Other medical examination for administrative purposes**
General medical examination for:
admission to old age home
adoption
camp
driving license
immigration and naturalization
insurance certification
marriage
prison
school admission
sports competition

Excludes *attendance for issue of medical certificates (V68.0)*
pre-employment screening (V70.5)

V70.4 Examination for medicolegal reasons
Blood-alcohol tests
Blood-drug tests
Paternity testing

Excludes *examination and observation following:*
accidents (V71.3, V71.4)
assault (V71.6)
rape (V71.5)

V70.5 Health examination of defined subpopulations
Armed forces personnel
Inhabitants of institutions
Occupational health examinations
Pre-employment screening
Preschool children
Prisoners
Prostitutes
Refugees
School children
Students

● **V70.6 Health examination in population surveys**

Excludes *special screening (V73.0–V82.9)*

V70.7 Examination of participant in clinical trial
Examination of participant or control in clinical research

●❑ **V70.8 Other specified general medical examinations**
Examination of potential donor of organ or tissue

●❑ **V70.9 Unspecified general medical examination**

● **V71 Observation and evaluation for suspected conditions not found**

Note: This category is to be used when persons without a diagnosis are suspected of having an abnormal condition, without signs or symptoms, which requires study, but after examination and observation, is found not to exist. This category is also for use for administrative and legal observation status.

● **V71.0 Observation for suspected mental condition**

V71.01 Adult antisocial behavior
Dyssocial behavior or gang activity in adult without manifest psychiatric disorder

V71.02 Childhood or adolescent antisocial behavior
Dyssocial behavior or gang activity in child or adolescent without manifest psychiatric disorder

❑ **V71.09 Other suspected mental condition**

V71.1 Observation for suspected malignant neoplasm

V71.2 Observation for suspected tuberculosis

V71.3 Observation following accident at work

❑ **V71.4 Observation following other accident**
Examination of individual involved in motor vehicle traffic accident

V71.5 Observation following alleged rape or seduction
Examination of victim or culprit

❑ **V71.6 Observation following other inflicted injury**
Examination of victim or culprit

V71.7 Observation for suspected cardiovascular disease

●❑ **V71.8 Observation and evaluation for other specified suspected conditions**

V71.81 Abuse and neglect

V71.82 Observation and evaluation for suspected exposure to anthrax

❑ **V71.83 Observation and evaluation for suspected exposure to other biological agent**

Excludes *adult abuse and neglect (995.80–995.85)*
child abuse and neglect (995.50–995.59)

V71.89 Other specified suspected conditions

●❑ **V71.9 Observation for unspecified suspected condition**

● **V72 Special investigations and examinations**

Includes: routine examination of specific system

Excludes *general medical examination (V70.0–70.4)*
general screening examination of defined population groups (V70.5, V70.6, V70.7)
routine examination of infant or child (V20.2)

Use additional code(s) to identify any special screening examination(s) performed (V73.0–V82.9)

V72.0 Examination of eyes and vision

● **V72.1 Examination of ears and hearing**

● **V72.2 Dental examination**

V72.3 Gynecological examination
Papanicolaou cervical smear as part of general gynecological examination
Pelvic examination (annual) (periodic)

Excludes *cervical Papanicolaou smear without general gynecological examination (V76.2)*
routine examination in contraceptive management (V25.40–V25.49)

Use additional code to identify routine vaginal Papanicolaou smear (V76.47)

V72.4 Pregnancy examination or test, pregnancy unconfirmed
Possible pregnancy, not (yet) confirmed

Excludes *pregnancy examination with immediate confirmation (V22.0–V22.1)*

● **V72.5 Radiological examination, not elsewhere classified**
Routine chest x-ray

Excludes *examination for suspected tuberculosis (V71.2)*

● **V72.6 Laboratory examination**

Excludes *that for suspected disorder (V71.0–V71.9)*

● **V72.7 Diagnostic skin and sensitization tests**
Allergy tests
Skin tests for hypersensitivity

Excludes *diagnostic skin tests for bacterial diseases (V74.0–V74.9)*

● **V72.8 Other specified examinations**

V72.81 Preoperative cardiovascular examination

V72.82 Preoperative respiratory examination

❑ **V72.83 Other specified preoperative examination**

●❑ **V72.84 Preoperative examination, unspecified**

●❑ **V72.85 Other specified examination**

●❑ **V72.9 Unspecified examination**

● **V73 Special screening examination for viral and chlamydial diseases**

● **V73.0 Poliomyelitis**

● **V73.1 Smallpox**

● **V73.2 Measles**

● **V73.3 Rubella**

● **V73.4 Yellow fever**

●❑ **V73.5 Other arthropod-borne viral diseases**
Dengue fever
Hemorrhagic fever
Viral encephalitis:
mosquito-borne
tick-borne

● **V73.6 Trachoma**

● **V73.8 Other specified viral and chlamydial diseases**

●❑ **V73.88 Other specified chlamydial diseases**

●❑ **V73.89 Other specified viral diseases**

● **V73.9 Unspecified viral and chlamydial disease**

●❑ **V73.98 Unspecified chlamydial disease**

●❑ **V73.99 Unspecified viral disease**

● **V74 Special screening examination for bacterial and spirochetal diseases**

Includes: diagnostic skin tests for these diseases

● **V74.0 Cholera**

● **V74.1 Pulmonary tuberculosis**

● **V74.2 Leprosy [Hansen's disease]**

● **V74.3 Diphtheria**

● **V74.4 Bacterial conjunctivitis**

● **V74.5 Venereal disease**

● **V74.6 Yaws**

●❑ **V74.8 Other specified bacterial and spirochetal diseases**
Brucellosis
Leptospirosis
Plague
Tetanus
Whooping cough

●❑ **V74.9 Unspecified bacterial and spirochetal disease**

● **V75 Special screening examination for other infectious diseases**

● **V75.0 Rickettsial diseases**

● **V75.1 Malaria**

● **V75.2 Leishmaniasis**

● **V75.3 Trypanosomiasis**
Chagas' disease
Sleeping sickness

● **V75.4 Mycotic infections**

● **V75.5 Schistosomiasis**

● **V75.6 Filariasis**

● **V75.7 Intestinal helminthiasis**

●❑ **V75.8 Other specified parasitic infections**

●❑ **V75.9 Unspecified infectious disease**

● **V76 Special screening for malignant neoplasms**

● **V76.0 Respiratory organs**

● **V76.1 Breast**

●❑ **V76.10 Breast screening, unspecified**

● **V76.11 Screening mammogram for high-risk patient**

● **V76.12 Other screening mammogram**

●❑ **V76.19 Other screening breast examination**

● **V76.2 Cervix**
Routine cervical Papanicolaou smear

Excludes *that as part of a general gynecological examination (V72.3)*

● **V76.3 Bladder**

● **V76.4 Other sites**

● **V76.41 Rectum**

● **V76.42 Oral cavity**

● **V76.43 Skin**

V76.44 Prostate

● **V76.45 Testis**

● **V76.46 Ovary**

● V76.47 Vagina
Vaginal pap smear status-post hysterectomy for nonmalignant condition

Use additional code to identify acquired absence of uterus (V45.77)

Excludes *vaginal pap smear status-post hysterectomy for malignant condition (V67.01)*

●❑ V76.49 Other sites

● V76.5 Intestine

● V76.50 Intestine, unspecified

● V76.51 Colon

Excludes *rectum (V76.41)*

● V76.52 Small intestine

●❑ V76.8 Other neoplasm

● V76.81 Nervous system

● V76.89 Other neoplasm

❑ V76.9 Unspecified

● **V77 Special screening for endocrine, nutritional, metabolic, and immunity disorders**

● V77.0 Thyroid disorders

● V77.1 Diabetes mellitus

● V77.2 Malnutrition

● V77.3 Phenylketonuria [PKU]

● V77.4 Galactosemia

● V77.5 Gout

● V77.6 Cystic fibrosis
Screening for mucoviscidosis

●❑ V77.7 Other inborn errors of metabolism

● V77.8 Obesity

● V77.9 Other and unspecified endocrine, nutritional, metabolic, and immunity disorders

● V77.91 Screening for lipoid disorders
Screening cholesterol level
Screening for hypercholesterolemia
Screening for hyperlipidemia

● V77.99 Other and unspecified endocrine, nutritional, metabolic, and immunity disorders

● **V78 Special screening for disorders of blood and blood-forming organs**

● V78.0 Iron deficiency anemia

●❑ V78.1 Other and unspecified deficiency anemia

● V78.2 Sickle-cell disease or trait

●❑ V78.3 Other hemoglobinopathies

●❑ V78.8 Other disorders of blood and blood-forming organs

●❑ V78.9 Unspecified disorder of blood and blood-forming organs

● **V79 Special screening for mental disorders and developmental handicaps**

● V79.0 Depression

● V79.1 Alcoholism

● V79.2 Mental retardation

● V79.3 Developmental handicaps in early childhood

●❑ V79.8 Other specified mental disorders and developmental handicaps

●❑ V79.9 Unspecified mental disorder and developmental handicap

● **V80 Special screening for neurological, eye, and ear diseases**

● V80.0 Neurological conditions

● V80.1 Glaucoma

●❑ V80.2 Other eye conditions
Screening for:
cataract
congenital anomaly of eye
senile macular lesions

Excludes *general vision examination (V72.0)*

● V80.3 Ear diseases

Excludes *general hearing examination (V72.1)*

● **V81 Special screening for cardiovascular, respiratory, and genitourinary diseases**

● V81.0 Ischemic heart disease

● V81.1 Hypertension

●❑ V81.2 Other and unspecified cardiovascular conditions

● V81.3 Chronic bronchitis and emphysema

●❑ V81.4 Other and unspecified respiratory conditions

Excludes *screening for:*
lung neoplasm (V76.0)
pulmonary tuberculosis (V74.1)

● V81.5 Nephropathy
Screening for asymptomatic bacteriuria

●❑ V81.6 Other and unspecified genitourinary conditions

● **V82 Special screening for other conditions**

● V82.0 Skin conditions

● V82.1 Rheumatoid arthritis

●❑ V82.2 Other rheumatic disorders

● V82.3 Congenital dislocation of hip

● V82.4 Maternal screening for chromosomal anomalies

Excludes *antenatal screening by amniocentesis (V28.0)*

● V82.5 Chemical poisoning and other contamination
Screening for:
heavy metal poisoning
ingestion of radioactive substance
poisoning from contaminated water supply
radiation exposure

● V82.6 Multiphasic screening

● V82.8 Other specified conditions

● V82.81 Osteoporosis

Use additional code to identify:
postmenopausal hormone replacement therapy status (V07.4)
postmenopausal (natural) status (V49.81)

● V82.89 Other specified conditions

●❑ V82.9 Unspecified condition

● **V83 Generic carrier status**

● V83.0 Hemophilia A carrier

● V83.01 Asymptomatic hemophilia A carrier

● V83.02 Symptomatic hemophilia A carrier

●❑ V83.8 Other genetic carrier status

● V83.81 Cystic fibrosis gene carrier

●❑ V83.89 Other genetic carrier status

E-Codes—SUPPLEMENTARY CLASSIFICATION OF EXTERNAL CAUSES OF INJURY AND POISONING (E800-E999)

This section is provided to permit the classification of environmental events, circumstances, and conditions as the cause of injury, poisoning, and other adverse effects. Where a code from this section is applicable, it is intended that it shall be used in addition to a code from one of the main chapters of ICD-9-CM, indicating the nature of the condition. Certain other conditions which may be stated to be due to external causes are classified in Chapters 1 to 16 of ICD-9-CM. For these, the "E" code classification should be used as an additional code for more detailed analysis.

Machinery accidents [other than those connected with transport] are classifiable to category E919, in which the fourth digit allows a broad classification of the type of machinery involved. If a more detailed classification of type of machinery is required, it is suggested that the "Classification of Industrial Accidents according to Agency," prepared by the International Labor Office, be used in addition; it is included in this publication.

Categories for "late effects" of accidents and other external causes are to be found at E929, E959, E969, E977, E989, and E999.

Definitions and examples related to transport accidents:

(a) A transport accident (E800-E848) is any accident involving a device designed primarily for, or being used at the time primarily for, conveying persons or goods from one place to another.

Includes: accidents involving:
- aircraft and spacecraft (E840-E845)
- watercraft (E830-E838)
- motor vehicle (E810-E825)
- railway (E800-E807)
- other road vehicles (E826-E829)

In classifying accidents which involve more than one kind of transport, the above order of precedence of transport accidents should be used.

Accidents involving agricultural and construction machines, such as tractors, cranes, and bulldozers, are regarded as transport accidents only when these vehicles are under their own power on a highway [otherwise the vehicles are regarded as machinery]. Vehicles which can travel on land or water, such as hovercraft and other amphibious vehicles, are regarded as watercraft when on the water, as motor vehicles when on the highway, and as off-road motor vehicles when on land, but off the highway.

Excludes *accidents:*
- *in sports which involve the use of transport but where the transport vehicle itself was not involved in the accident*
- *involving vehicles which are part of industrial equipment used entirely on industrial premises*
- *occurring during transportation but unrelated to the hazards associated with the means of transportation [e.g., injuries received in a fight on board ship; transport vehicle involved in a cataclysm such as an earthquake]*
- *to persons engaged in the maintenance or repair of transport equipment or vehicle not in motion, unless injured by another vehicle in motion*

(b) A railway accident is a transport accident involving a railway train or other railway vehicle operated on rails, whether in motion or not.

Excludes *accidents:*
- *in repair shops*
- *in roundhouse or on turntable*
- *on railway premises but not involving a train or other railway vehicle*

(c) A railway train or railway vehicle is any device with or without cars coupled to it, designed for traffic on a railway.

Includes: interurban:
- electric car (operated chiefly on its own right-of-way, not open to other traffic)
- streetcar (operated chiefly on its own right-of-way, not open to other traffic)

railway train, any power [diesel] [electric] [steam]
- funicular
- monorail or two-rail
- subterranean or elevated

other vehicle designed to run on a railway track

Excludes *interurban electric cars [streetcars] specified to be operating on a right-of-way that forms part of the public street or highway [definition (n)]*

(d) A railway or railroad is a right-of-way designed for traffic on rails, which is used by carriages or wagons transporting passengers or freight, and by other rolling stock, and which is not open to other public vehicular traffic

(e) A motor vehicle accident is a transport accident involving a motor vehicle. It is defined as a motor vehicle traffic accident or as a motor vehicle nontraffic accident according to whether the accident occurs on a public highway or elsewhere.

Excludes *injury or damage due to cataclysm*
injury or damage while a motor vehicle, not under its own power, is being loaded on, or unloaded from, another conveyance

(f) A motor vehicle traffic accident is any motor vehicle accident occurring on a public highway [i.e., originating, terminating, or involving a vehicle partially on the highway]. A motor vehicle accident is assumed to have occurred on the highway unless another place is specified, except in the case of accidents involving only off-road motor vehicles which are classified as nontraffic accidents unless the contrary is stated.

(g) A motor vehicle nontraffic accident is any motor vehicle accident which occurs entirely in any place other than a public highway.

(h) A public highway [trafficway] or street is the entire width between property lines [or other boundary lines] of every way or place, of which any part is open to the use of the public for purposes of vehicular traffic as a matter of right or custom. A roadway is that part of the public highway designed, improved, and ordinarily used, for vehicular travel.

Includes: approaches (public) to:
- docks
- public building
- station

Excludes *driveway (private)*
parking lot
ramp
roads in:
- *airfield*
- *farm*
- *industrial premises*
- *mine*
- *private grounds*
- *quarry*

(i) A motor vehicle is any mechanically or electrically powered device, not operated on rails, upon which any person or property may be transported or drawn upon a highway. Any object such as a trailer, coaster, sled, or wagon being towed by a motor vehicle is considered a part of the motor vehicle.

Includes: automobile [any type]
bus
construction machinery, farm and industrial machinery, steam roller, tractor, army tank, highway grader, or similar vehicle on wheels or treads, while in transport under own power
fire engine (motorized)
motorcycle
motorized bicycle [moped] or scooter
trolley bus not operating on rails
truck
van

Excludes *devices used solely to move persons or materials within the confines of a building and its premises, such as:*
building elevator
coal car in mine
electric baggage or mail truck used solely within a railroad station
electric truck used solely within an industrial plant
moving overhead crane

(j) A motorcycle is a two-wheeled motor vehicle having one or two riding saddles and sometimes having a third wheel for the support of a sidecar. The sidecar is considered part of the motorcycle.

Includes: motorized:
bicycle [moped]
scooter
tricycle

(k) An off-road motor vehicle is a motor vehicle of special design, to enable it to negotiate rough or soft terrain or snow. Examples of special design are high construction, special wheels and tires, driven by treads, or support on a cushion of air.

Includes: all terrain vehicle [ATV]
army tank
hovercraft, on land or swamp
snowmobile

(l) A driver of a motor vehicle is the occupant of the motor vehicle operating it or intending to operate it. A motorcyclist is the driver of a motorcycle. Other authorized occupants of a motor vehicle are passengers.

(m) An other road vehicle is any device, except a motor vehicle, in, on, or by which any person or property may be transported on a highway.

Includes: animal carrying a person or goods
animal-drawn vehicle
animal harnessed to conveyance
bicycle [pedal cycle]
streetcar
tricycle (pedal)

Excludes *pedestrian conveyance [definition (q)]*

(n) A streetcar is a device designed and used primarily for transporting persons within a municipality, running on rails, usually subject to normal traffic control signals, and operated principally on a right-of-way that forms part of the traffic way. A trailer being towed by a streetcar is considered a part of the streetcar.

Includes: interurban or intraurban electric or streetcar, when specified to be operating on a street or public highway
tram (car)
trolley (car)

(o) A pedal cycle is any road transport vehicle operated solely by pedals.

Includes: bicycle
pedal cycle
tricycle

Excludes *motorized bicycle [definition (i)]*

(p) A pedal cyclist is any person riding on a pedal cycle or in a sidecar attached to such a vehicle.

(q) A pedestrian conveyance is any human powered device by which a pedestrian may move other than by walking or by which a walking person may move another pedestrian.

Includes: baby carriage
coaster wagon
ice skates
perambulator
pushcart
pushchair
roller skates
scooter
skateboard
skis
sled
wheelchair

(r) A pedestrian is any person involved in an accident who was not at the time of the accident riding in or on a motor vehicle, railroad train, streetcar, animal-drawn or other vehicle, or on a bicycle or animal.

Includes: person:
changing tire of vehicle
in or operating a pedestrian conveyance
making adjustment to motor of vehicle
on foot

(s) A watercraft is any device for transporting passengers or goods on the water.

(t) A small boat is any watercraft propelled by paddle, oars, or small motor, with a passenger capacity of less than ten.

Includes: boat NOS
canoe
coble
dinghy
punt
raft
rowboat
rowing shell
scull
skiff
small motorboat

Excludes *barge*
lifeboat (used after abandoning ship)
raft (anchored) being used as a diving platform
yacht

(u) An aircraft is any device for transporting passengers or goods in the air.

Includes: airplane [any type]
balloon
bomber
dirigible
glider (hang)
military aircraft
parachute

(v) A commercial transport aircraft is any device for collective passenger or freight transportation by air, whether run on commercial lines for profit or by government authorities, with the exception of military craft.

RAILWAY ACCIDENTS (E800-E807)

Note: For definitions of railway accident and related terms see definitions (a) to (d).

Excludes *accidents involving railway train and:*
aircraft (E840.0-E845.9)
motor vehicle (E810.0-E825.9)
watercraft (E830.0-E838.9)

The following fourth-digit subdivisions are for use with categories E800-E807 to identify the injured person:

.0 Railway employee
Any person who by virtue of his employment in connection with a railway, whether by the railway company or not, is at increased risk of involvement in a railway accident, such as:
catering staff of train
driver
guard
porter
postal staff on train
railway fireman
shunter
sleeping car attendant

.1 Passenger on railway
Any authorized person traveling on a train, except a railway employee.

Excludes *intending passenger waiting at station (8)*
unauthorized rider on railway vehicle (8)

.2 Pedestrian
See definition (r)

.3 Pedal cyclist
See definition (p)

❑ **.8 Other specified person**
Intending passenger or bystander waiting at station
Unauthorized rider on railway vehicle

❑ **.9 Unspecified person**

● **E800 Railway accident involving collision with rolling stock**
Requires fourth digit. See beginning of section E800-E845 for codes and definitions.

Includes: collision between railway trains or railway vehicles, any kind
collision NOS on railway
derailment with antecedent collision with rolling stock or NOS

●❑ **E801 Railway accident involving collision with other object**
Requires fourth digit. See beginning of section E800-E845 for codes and definitions.

Includes: collision of railway train with:
buffers
fallen tree on railway
gates
platform
rock on railway
streetcar
other nonmotor vehicle
other object

Excludes *collision with:*
aircraft (E840.0-E842.9)
motor vehicle (E810.0-E810.9, E820.0-E822.9)

● **E802 Railway accident involving derailment without antecedent collision**

Requires fourth digit. See beginning of section E800-E845 for codes and definitions.

● **E803 Railway accident involving explosion, fire, or burning**
Requires fourth digit. See beginning of section E800-E845 for codes and definitions.

Excludes *explosion or fire, with antecedent derailment (E802.0-E802.9)*
explosion or fire, with mention of antecedent collision (E800.0-E801.9)

● **E804 Fall in, on, or from railway train**
Requires fourth digit. See beginning of section E800-E845 for codes and definitions.

Includes: fall while alighting from or boarding railway train

Excludes *fall related to collision, derailment, or explosion of railway train (E800.0-E803.9)*

● **E805 Hit by rolling stock**
Requires fourth digit. See beginning of section E800-E845 for codes and definitions.

Includes: crushed by railway train or part
injured by railway train or part
killed by railway train or part
knocked down by railway train or part
run over by railway train or part

Excludes *pedestrian hit by object set in motion by railway train (E806.0-E806.9)*

●❑ **E806 Other specified railway accident**
Requires fourth digit. See beginning of section E800-E845 for codes and definitions.

Includes: hit by object falling in railway train
injured by door or window on railway train
nonmotor road vehicle or pedestrian hit by object set in motion by railway train
railway train hit by falling:
earth NOS
rock
tree
other object

Excludes *railway accident due to cataclysm (E908-E909)*

●❑ **E807 Railway accident of unspecified nature**
Requires fourth digit. See beginning of section E800-E845 for codes and definitions.

Includes: found dead on railway right-of-way NOS
injured on railway right-of-way NOS
railway accident NOS

MOTOR VEHICLE TRAFFIC ACCIDENTS (E810-E819)

Note: For definitions of motor vehicle traffic accident, and related terms, see definitions (e) to (k).

Excludes *accidents involving motor vehicle and aircraft (E840.0-E845.9)*

The following fourth-digit subdivisions are for use with categories E810-E819 to identify the injured person:

.0 **Driver of motor vehicle other than motorcycle**
See definition (l)

.1 **Passenger in motor vehicle other than motorcycle**
See definition (l)

.2 **Motorcyclist**
See definition (l)

.3 **Passenger on motorcycle**
See definition (l)

.4 **Occupant of streetcar**

.5 **Rider of animal; occupant of animal-drawn vehicle**

.6 **Pedal cyclist**
See definition (p)

.7 **Pedestrian**
See definition (r)

❑ .8 **Other specified person**
Occupant of vehicle other than above
Person in railway train involved in accident
Unauthorized rider of motor vehicle

❑ .9 **Unspecified person**

● **E810 Motor vehicle traffic accident involving collision with train**

Requires fourth digit. See beginning of section E800-E845 for codes and definitions.

Excludes *motor vehicle collision with object set in motion by railway train (E815.0-E815.9)*
railway train hit by object set in motion by motor vehicle (E818.0-E818.9)

● **E811 Motor vehicle traffic accident involving re-entrant collision with another motor vehicle**

Requires fourth digit. See beginning of section E800-E845 for codes and definitions.

Includes: collision between motor vehicle which accidentally leaves the roadway then re-enters the same roadway, or the opposite roadway on a divided highway, and another motor vehicle

Excludes *collision on the same roadway when none of the motor vehicles involved have left and re-entered the roadway (E812.0-E812.9)*

●❑ **E812 Other motor vehicle traffic accident involving collision with motor vehicle**

Requires fourth digit. See beginning of section E800-E845 for codes and definitions.

Includes: collision with another motor vehicle parked, stopped, stalled, disabled, or abandoned on the highway
motor vehicle collision NOS

Excludes *collision with object set in motion by another motor vehicle (E815.0-E815.9)*
re-entrant collision with another motor vehicle (E811.0-E811.9)

●❑ **E813 Motor vehicle traffic accident involving collision with other vehicle**

Requires fourth digit. See beginning of section E800-E845 for codes and definitions.

Includes: collision between motor vehicle, any kind, and:
other road (nonmotor transport) vehicle, such as:
animal carrying a person
animal-drawn vehicle
pedal cycle
streetcar

Excludes *collision with:*
object set in motion by nonmotor road vehicle (E815.0-E815.9)
pedestrian (E814.0-E814.9)
nonmotor road vehicle hit by object set in motion by motor vehicle (E818.0-E818.9)

● **E814 Motor vehicle traffic accident involving collision with pedestrian**

Requires fourth digit. See beginning of section E800-E845 for codes and definitions.

Includes: collision between motor vehicle, any kind, and pedestrian
pedestrian dragged, hit, or run over by motor vehicle, any kind

Excludes *pedestrian hit by object set in motion by motor vehicle (E818.0-E818.9)*

●❑ **E815 Other motor vehicle traffic accident involving collision on the highway**

Requires fourth digit. See beginning of section E800-E845 for codes and definitions.

Includes: collision (due to loss of control) (on highway) between motor vehicle, any kind, and:
abutment (bridge) (overpass)
animal (herded) (unattended)
fallen stone, traffic sign, tree, utility pole
guard rail or boundary fence
interhighway divider
landslide (not moving)
object set in motion by railway train or road vehicle (motor) (nonmotor)
object thrown in front of motor vehicle
safety island
temporary traffic sign or marker
wall of cut made for road
other object, fixed, movable, or moving

Excludes *collision with:*
any object off the highway (resulting from loss of control) (E816.0-E816.9)
any object which normally would have been off the highway and is not stated to have been on it (E816.0-E816.9)
motor vehicle parked, stopped, stalled, disabled, or abandoned on highway (E812.0-E812.9)
moving landslide (E909.2)
motor vehicle hit by object:
set in motion by railway train or road vehicle (motor) (nonmotor) (E818.0-E818.9)
thrown into or on vehicle (E818.0-E818.9)

● E816 Motor vehicle traffic accident due to loss of control, without collision on the highway

Requires fourth digit. See beginning of section E800-E845 for codes and definitions.

Includes: motor vehicle:
- failing to make curve and:
  - colliding with object off the highway
  - overturning
  - stopping abruptly off the highway
- going out of control (due to)
  - blowout and:
    - colliding with object off the highway
    - overturning
    - stopping abruptly off the highway
  - burst tire and:
    - colliding with object off the highway
    - overturning
    - stopping abruptly off the highway
  - driver falling asleep and:
    - colliding with object off the highway
    - overturning
    - stopping abruptly off the highway
  - driver inattention and:
    - colliding with object off the highway
    - overturning
    - stopping abruptly off the highway
  - excessive speed and:
    - colliding with object off the highway
    - overturning
    - stopping abruptly off the highway
  - failure of mechanical part and:
    - colliding with object off the highway
    - overturning
    - stopping abruptly off the highway

Excludes *collision on highway following loss of control (E810.0-E815.9)*
loss of control of motor vehicle following collision on the highway (E810.0-E815.9)

● E817 Noncollision motor vehicle traffic accident while boarding or alighting

Requires fourth digit. See beginning of section E800-E845 for codes and definitions.

Includes: fall down stairs of motor bus while boarding or alighting
fall from car in street while boarding or alighting
injured by moving part of the vehicle while boarding or alighting
trapped by door of motor bus while boarding or alighting

● ❑ E818 Other noncollision motor vehicle traffic accident

Requires fourth digit. See beginning of section E800-E845 for codes and definitions.

Includes: accidental poisoning from exhaust gas generated by motor vehicle while in motion
breakage of any part of motor vehicle while in motion
explosion of any part of motor vehicle while in motion
fall, jump, or being accidentally pushed from motor vehicle while in motion
fire starting in motor vehicle while in motion
hit by object thrown into or on motor vehicle while in motion
injured by being thrown against some part of, or object in, motor vehicle while in motion
injury from moving part of motor vehicle while in motion
object falling in or on motor vehicle while in motion
object thrown on motor vehicle while in motion
collision of railway train or road vehicle except motor vehicle, with object set in motion by motor vehicle
motor vehicle hit by object set in motion by railway train or road vehicle (motor) (nonmotor)
pedestrian, railway train, or road vehicle (motor) (nonmotor) hit by object set in motion by motor vehicle

Excludes *collision between motor vehicle and:*
- *object set in motion by railway train or road vehicle (motor) (nonmotor) (E815.0-E815.9)*
- *object thrown towards the motor vehicle (E815.0-E815.9)*

person overcome by carbon monoxide generated by stationary motor vehicle off the roadway with motor running (E868.2)

● ❑ E819 Motor vehicle traffic accident of unspecified nature

Requires fourth digit. See beginning of section E800-E845 for codes and definitions.

Includes: motor vehicle traffic accident NOS
traffic accident NOS

ICD-9-CM E800-E899 Vol. 1

MOTOR VEHICLE NONTRAFFIC ACCIDENTS (E820-E825)

Note: For definitions of motor vehicle nontraffic accident and related terms see definitions (a) to (k).

Includes: accidents involving motor vehicles being used in recreational or sporting activities off the highway
collision and noncollision motor vehicle accidents occurring entirely off the highway

Excludes *accidents involving motor vehicle and:*
aircraft (E840.0-E845.9)
watercraft (E830.0-E838.9)
accidents, not on the public highway, involving agricultural and construction machinery but not involving another motor vehicle (E919.0, E919.2, E919.7)

The following fourth-digit subdivisions are for use with categories E820-E825 to identify the injured person:

.0 Driver of motor vehicle other than motorcycle
See definition (l)

.1 Passenger in motor vehicle other than motorcycle
See definition (l)

.2 Motorcyclist
See definition (l)

.3 Passenger on motorcycle
See definition (l)

.4 Occupant of streetcar

.5 Rider of animal; occupant of animal-drawn vehicle

.6 Pedal cyclist
See definition (p)

.7 Pedestrian
See definition (r)

❑ **.8 Other specified person**
Occupant of vehicle other than above
Person on railway train involved in accident
Unauthorized rider of motor vehicle

❑ **.9 Unspecified person**

● **E820 Nontraffic accident involving motor-driven snow vehicle**

Requires fourth digit. See beginning of section E800-E845 for codes and definitions.

Includes: breakage of part of motor-driven snow vehicle (not on public highway)
fall from motor-driven snow vehicle (not on public highway)
hit by motor-driven snow vehicle (not on public highway)
overturning of motor-driven snow vehicle (not on public highway)
run over or dragged by motor-driven snow vehicle (not on public highway)
collision of motor-driven snow vehicle with:
animal (being ridden) (-drawn vehicle)
another off-road motor vehicle
other motor vehicle, not on public highway
railway train
other object, fixed or movable
injury caused by rough landing of motor-driven snow vehicle (after leaving ground on rough terrain)

Excludes *accident on the public highway involving motor driven snow vehicle (E810.0-E819.9)*

● ❑ **E821 Nontraffic accident involving other off-road motor vehicle**

Requires fourth digit. See beginning of section E800-E845 for codes and definitions.

Includes: breakage of part of off-road motor vehicle, except snow vehicle (not on public highway)
fall from off-road motor vehicle, except snow vehicle (not on public highway)
hit by off-road motor vehicle, except snow vehicle (not on public highway)
overturning of off-road motor vehicle, except snow vehicle (not on public highway)
run over or dragged by off-road motor vehicle, except snow vehicle (not on public highway)
thrown against some part of or object in off-road motor vehicle, except snow vehicle (not on public highway)
collision with:
animal (being ridden) (-drawn vehicle)
another off-road motor vehicle, except snow vehicle
other motor vehicle, not on public highway
other object, fixed or movable

Excludes *accident on public highway involving off-road motor vehicle (E810.0-E819.9)*
collision between motor driven snow vehicle and other off-road motor vehicle (E820.0-E820.9)
hovercraft accident on water (E830.0-E838.9)

● ❑ **E822 Other motor vehicle nontraffic accident involving collision with moving object**

Requires fourth digit. See beginning of section E800-E845 for codes and definitions.

Includes: collision, not on public highway, between motor vehicle, except off-road motor vehicle and:
animal
nonmotor vehicle
other motor vehicle, except off-road motor vehicle
pedestrian
railway train
other moving object

Excludes *collision with:*
motor-driven snow vehicle (E820.0-E820.9)
other off-road motor vehicle (E821.0-E821.9)

● ❑ **E823 Other motor vehicle nontraffic accident involving collision with stationary object**

Requires fourth digit. See beginning of section E800-E845 for codes and definitions.

Includes: collision, not on public highway, between motor vehicle, except off-road motor vehicle, and any object, fixed or movable, but not in motion

● ❑ **E824 Other motor vehicle nontraffic accident while boarding and alighting**

Requires fourth digit. See beginning of section E800-E845 for codes and definitions.

Includes: fall while boarding or alighting from motor vehicle except off-road motor vehicle, not on public highway
injury from moving part of motor vehicle while boarding or alighting from motor vehicle except off-road motor vehicle, not on public highway
trapped by door of motor vehicle while boarding or alighting from motor vehicle except off-road motor vehicle, not on public highway

●❑E825 Other motor vehicle nontraffic accident of other and unspecified nature

Requires fourth digit. See beginning of section E800-E845 for codes and definitions.

Includes: accidental poisoning from carbon monoxide generated by motor vehicle while in motion, not on public highway
breakage of any part of motor vehicle while in motion, not on public highway
explosion of any part of motor vehicle while in motion, not on public highway
fall, jump, or being accidentally pushed from motor vehicle while in motion, not on public highway
fire starting in motor vehicle while in motion, not on public highway
hit by object thrown into, towards, or on motor vehicle while in motion, not on public highway
injured by being thrown against some part of, or object in, motor vehicle while in motion, not on public highway
injury from moving part of motor vehicle while in motion, not on public highway
object falling in or on motor vehicle while in motion, not on public highway
motor vehicle nontraffic accident NOS

Excludes *fall from or in stationary motor vehicle (E884.9, E885.9)*
overcome by carbon monoxide or exhaust gas generated by stationary motor vehicle off the roadway with motor running (E868.2)
struck by falling object from or in stationary motor vehicle (E916)

OTHER ROAD VEHICLE ACCIDENTS (E826-E829)

Note: Other road vehicle accidents are transport accidents involving road vehicles other than motor vehicles. For definitions of other road vehicle and related terms see definitions (m) to (o).

Includes: accidents involving other road vehicles being used in recreational or sporting activities

Excludes *collision of other road vehicle [any] with:*
aircraft (E840.0-E845.9)
motor vehicle (E813.0-E813.9, E820.0-E822.9)
railway train (E801.0-E801.9)

The following fourth-digit subdivisions are for use with categories E826-E829 to identify the injured person:

.0 Pedestrian
See definition (r)
.1 Pedal cyclist
See definition (p)
.2 Rider of animal
.3 Occupant of animal-drawn vehicle
.4 Occupant of streetcar
❑ **.8 Other specified person**
❑ **.9 Unspecified person**

●E826 Pedal cycle accident
[0–9]

Requires fourth digit. See beginning of section E800-E845 for codes and definitions.

Includes: breakage of any part of pedal cycle
collision between pedal cycle and:
animal (being ridden) (herded) (unattended)
another pedal cycle
nonmotor road vehicle, any
pedestrian
other object, fixed, movable, or moving, not set in motion by motor vehicle, railway train, or aircraft
entanglement in wheel of pedal cycle
fall from pedal cycle
hit by object falling or thrown on the pedal cycle
pedal cycle accident NOS
pedal cycle overturned

●E827 Animal-drawn vehicle accident
[0,2–4,8,9]

Requires fourth digit. See beginning of section E800-E845 for codes and definitions.

Includes: breakage of any part of vehicle
collision between animal-drawn vehicle and:
animal (being ridden) (herded) (unattended)
nonmotor road vehicle, except pedal cycle
pedestrian, pedestrian conveyance, or pedestrian vehicle
other object, fixed, movable, or moving, not set in motion by motor vehicle, railway train, or aircraft
fall from animal-drawn vehicle
knocked down by animal-drawn vehicle
overturning of animal-drawn vehicle
run over by animal-drawn vehicle
thrown from animal-drawn vehicle

Excludes *collision of animal-drawn vehicle with pedal cycle (E826.0-E826.9)*

● E828 Accident involving animal being ridden
[0,2,4,8,9]

Requires fourth digit. See beginning of section E800-E845 for codes and definitions.

Includes: collision between animal being ridden and:
another animal
nonmotor road vehicle, except pedal cycle, and animal-drawn vehicle
pedestrian, pedestrian conveyance, or pedestrian vehicle
other object, fixed, movable, or moving, not set in motion by motor vehicle, railway train, or aircraft
fall from animal being ridden
knocked down by animal being ridden
thrown from animal being ridden
trampled by animal being ridden
ridden animal stumbled and fell

Excludes *collision of animal being ridden with:*
animal-drawn vehicle (E827.0-E827.9)
pedal cycle (E826.0-E826.9)

● ❑ E829 Other road vehicle accidents
[0,4,8,9]

Requires fourth digit. See beginning of section E800-E845 for codes and definitions.

Includes: accident while boarding or alighting from
streetcar
nonmotor road vehicle not classifiable to E826-E828
blow from object in
streetcar
nonmotor road vehicle not classifiable to E826-E828
breakage of any part of
streetcar
nonmotor road vehicle not classifiable to E826-E828
caught in door of
streetcar
nonmotor road vehicle not classifiable to E826-E828
derailment of
streetcar
nonmotor road vehicle not classifiable to E826-E828
fall in, on, or from
streetcar
nonmotor road vehicle not classifiable to E826-E828
fire in
streetcar
nonmotor road vehicle not classifiable to E826-E828
collision between streetcar or nonmotor road vehicle, except as in E826-E828, and:
animal (not being ridden)
another nonmotor road vehicle not classifiable to E826-E828
pedestrian
other object, fixed, movable, or moving, not set in motion by motor vehicle, railway train, or aircraft
nonmotor road vehicle accident NOS
streetcar accident NOS

Excludes *collision with:*
animal being ridden (E828.0-E828.9)
animal-drawn vehicle (E827.0-E827.9)
pedal cycle (E826.0-E826.9)

WATER TRANSPORT ACCIDENTS (E830-E838)

Note: For definitions of water transport accident and related terms see definitions (a), (s), and (t).

Includes: watercraft accidents in the course of recreational activities

Excludes *accidents involving both aircraft, including objects set in motion by aircraft, and watercraft (E840.0-E845.9)*

The following fourth-digit subdivisions are for use with categories E830-E838 to identify the injured person:

.0 Occupant of small boat, unpowered
.1 Occupant of small boat, powered
See definition (t)

Excludes *water skier (4)*

❑ .2 Occupant of other watercraft-crew
Persons:
engaged in operation of watercraft
providing passenger services [cabin attendants, ship's physician, catering personnel]
working on ship during voyage in other capacity [musician in band, operators of shops and beauty parlors]

❑ .3 Occupant of other watercraft -- other than crew
Passenger
Occupant of lifeboat, other than crew, after abandoning ship

.4 Water skier
.5 Swimmer
.6 Dockers, stevedores
Longshoreman employed on the dock in loading and unloading ships

❑ .8 Other specified person
Immigration and customs officials on board ship
Person:
accompanying passenger or member of crew visiting boat
Pilot (guiding ship into port)

❑ .9 Unspecified person

● E830 Accident to watercraft causing submersion

Requires fourth digit. See beginning of section E800-E845 for codes and definitions.

Includes: submersion and drowning due to:
boat overturning
boat submerging
falling or jumping from burning ship
falling or jumping from crushed watercraft
ship sinking
other accident to watercraft

● ❑ E831 Accident to watercraft causing other injury

Requires fourth digit. See beginning of section E800-E845 for codes and definitions.

Includes: any injury, except submersion and drowning, as a result of an accident to watercraft
burned while ship on fire
crushed between ships in collision
crushed by lifeboat after abandoning ship
fall due to collision or other accident to watercraft
hit by falling object due to accident to watercraft
injured in watercraft accident involving collision
struck by boat or part thereof after fall or jump from damaged boat

Excludes *burns from localized fire or explosion on board ship (E837.0-E837.9)*

● ❑ E832 **Other accidental submersion or drowning in water transport accident**

Requires fourth digit. See beginning of section E800-E845 for codes and definitions.

Includes: submersion or drowning as a result of an accident other than accident to the watercraft, such as:
fall:
from gangplank
from ship
overboard
thrown overboard by motion of ship
washed overboard

Excludes *submersion or drowning of swimmer or diver who voluntarily jumps from boat not involved in an accident (E910.0-E910.9)*

● E833 **Fall on stairs or ladders in water transport**

Requires fourth digit. See beginning of section E800-E845 for codes and definitions.

Excludes *fall due to accident to watercraft (E831.0-E831.9)*

● ❑ E834 **Other fall from one level to another in water transport**

Requires fourth digit. See beginning of section E800-E845 for codes and definitions.

Excludes *fall due to accident to watercraft (E831.0-E831.9)*

● ❑ E835 **Other and unspecified fall in water transport**

Requires fourth digit. See beginning of section E800-E845 for codes and definitions.

Excludes *fall due to accident to watercraft (E831.0-E831.9)*

● E836 **Machinery accident in water transport**

Requires fourth digit. See beginning of section E800-E845 for codes and definitions.

Includes: injuries in water transport caused by:
deck machinery
engine room machinery
galley machinery
laundry machinery
loading machinery

● E837 **Explosion, fire, or burning in watercraft**

Requires fourth digit. See beginning of section E800-E845 for codes and definitions.

Includes: explosion of boiler on steamship
localized fire on ship

Excludes *burning ship (due to collision or explosion) resulting in:*
submersion or drowning (E830.0-E830.9)
other injury (E831.0-E831.9)

● ❑ E838 **Other and unspecified water transport accident**

Requires fourth digit. See beginning of section E800-E845 for codes and definitions.

Includes: accidental poisoning by gases or fumes on ship
atomic power plant malfunction in watercraft
crushed between ship and stationary object [wharf]
crushed between ships without accident to watercraft
crushed by falling object on ship or while loading or unloading
hit by boat while water skiing
struck by boat or part thereof (after fall from boat)
watercraft accident NOS

AIR AND SPACE TRANSPORT ACCIDENTS (E840-E845)

Note: For definition of aircraft and related terms see definitions (u) and (v).

The following fourth-digit subdivisions are for use with categories E840-E845 to identify the injured person:

.0 Occupant of spacecraft

.1 Occupant of military aircraft, any
Crew in military aircraft [air force] [army] [national guard] [navy]
Passenger (civilian) (military) in military aircraft [air force] [army] [national guard] [navy]
Troops in military aircraft [air force] [army] [national guard] [navy]

Excludes *occupants of aircraft operated under jurisdiction of police departments (5)*
parachutist (7)

.2 Crew of commercial aircraft (powered) in surface-to-surface transport

❑ **.3 Other occupant of commercial aircraft (powered) in surface-to-surface transport**
Flight personnel:
not part of crew
on familiarization flight
Passenger on aircraft (powered) NOS

.4 Occupant of commercial aircraft (powered) in surface-to-air transport
Occupant [crew] [passenger] of aircraft (powered) engaged in activities, such as:
aerial spraying (crops) (fire retardants)
air drops of emergency supplies
air drops of parachutists, except from military craft
crop dusting
lowering of construction material [bridge or telephone pole]
sky writing

❑ **.5 Occupant of other powered aircraft**
Occupant [crew] [passenger] of aircraft [powered] engaged in activities, such as:
aerobatic flying
aircraft racing
rescue operation
storm surveillance
traffic surveillance
Occupant of private plane NOS

.6 Occupant of unpowered aircraft, except parachutist
Occupant of aircraft classifiable to E842

.7 Parachutist (military) (other)
Person making voluntary descent

Excludes *person making descent after accident to aircraft (.1-.6)*

.8 Ground crew, airline employee
Persons employed at airfields (civil) (military) or launching pads, not occupants of aircraft

❑ **.9 Other person**

● E840 **Accident to powered aircraft at takeoff or landing**

Requires fourth digit. See beginning of section E800-E845 for codes and definitions.

Includes: collision of aircraft with any object, fixed, movable, or moving while taking off or landing
crash while taking off or landing
explosion on aircraft while taking off or landing
fire on aircraft while taking off or landing
forced landing

●❑E841 Accident to powered aircraft, other and unspecified

Requires fourth digit. See beginning of section E800-E845 for codes and definitions.

Includes: aircraft accident NOS
aircraft crash or wreck NOS
any accident to powered aircraft while in transit or when not specified whether in transit, taking off, or landing
collision of aircraft with another aircraft, bird, or any object, while in transit
explosion on aircraft while in transit
fire on aircraft while in transit

●E842 Accident to unpowered aircraft
[6–9]

Requires fourth digit. See beginning of section E800-E845 for codes and definitions.

Includes: any accident, except collision with powered aircraft, to:
balloon
glider
hang glider
kite carrying a person
hit by object falling from unpowered aircraft

●E843 Fall in, on, or from aircraft
[0–9]

Requires fourth digit. See beginning of section E800-E845 for codes and definitions.

Includes: accident in boarding or alighting from aircraft, any kind
fall in, on, or from aircraft [any kind], while in transit, taking off, or landing, except when as a result of an accident to aircraft

●❑E844 Other specified air transport accidents
[0–9]

Requires fourth digit. See beginning of section E800-E845 for codes and definitions.

Includes: hit by aircraft without accident to aircraft
hit by object falling from aircraft without accident to aircraft
injury by or from machinery on aircraft without accident to aircraft
injury by or from rotating propeller without accident to aircraft
injury by or from voluntary parachute descent without accident to aircraft
poisoning by carbon monoxide from aircraft while in transit without accident to aircraft
sucked into jet without accident to aircraft
any accident involving other transport vehicle (motor) (nonmotor) due to being hit by object set in motion by aircraft (powered)

Excludes *air sickness (E903)*
effects of:
high altitude (E902.0-E902.1)
pressure change (E902.0-E902.1)
injury in parachute descent due to accident to aircraft (E840.0-E842.9)

●E845 Accident involving spacecraft
[0,8,9]

Requires fourth digit. See beginning of section E800-E845 for codes and definitions.

Includes: launching pad accident

Excludes *effects of weightlessness in spacecraft (E928.0)*

VEHICLE ACCIDENTS NOT ELSEWHERE CLASSIFIABLE (E846-E848)

E846 Accidents involving powered vehicles used solely within the buildings and premises of industrial or commercial establishment

Accident to, on, or involving:
battery-powered airport passenger vehicle
battery-powered trucks (baggage) (mail)
coal car in mine
logging car
self-propelled truck, industrial
station baggage truck (powered)
tram, truck, or tub (powered) in mine or quarry
Breakage of any part of vehicle
Collision with:
pedestrian
other vehicle or object within premises
Explosion of powered vehicle, industrial or commercial
Fall from powered vehicle, industrial or commercial
Overturning of powered vehicle, industrial or commercial
Struck by powered vehicle, industrial or commercial

Excludes *accidental poisoning by exhaust gas from vehicle not elsewhere classifiable (E868.2)*
injury by crane, lift (fork), or elevator (E919.2)

E847 Accidents involving cable cars not running on rails

Accident to, on, or involving:
cable car, not on rails
ski chair-lift
ski-lift with gondola
teleferique
Breakage of cable
Caught or dragged by cable car, not on rails
Fall or jump from cable car, not on rails
Object thrown from or in cable car not on rails

❑E848 Accidents involving other vehicles, not elsewhere classifiable

Accident to, on, or involving:
ice yacht
land yacht
nonmotor, nonroad vehicle NOS

●*E849 Place of occurrence*

Note: The following category is for use to denote the place where the injury or poisoning occurred.

E849.0 Home

Apartment
Boarding house
Farm house
Home premises
House (residential)
Noninstitutional place of residence
Private:
driveway
garage
garden
home
walk
Swimming pool in private house or garden
Yard of home

Excludes *home under construction but not yet occupied (E849.3)*
institutional place of residence (E849.7)

E849.1 Farm

buildings
land under cultivation

Excludes *farm house and home premises of farm (E849.0)*

E849.2 Mine and quarry
Gravel pit
Sand pit
Tunnel under construction

E849.3 Industrial place and premises
Building under construction
Dockyard
Dry dock
Factory
building
premises
Garage (place of work)
Industrial yard
Loading platform (factory) (store)
Plant, industrial
Railway yard
Shop (place of work)
Warehouse
Workhouse

E849.4 Place for recreation and sport

Amusement park	*Playground, including school playground*
Baseball field	*Public park*
Basketball court	*Racecourse*
Beach resort	*Resort NOS*
Cricket ground	*Riding school*
Fives court	*Rifle range*
Football field	*Seashore resort*
Golf course	*Skating rink*
Gymnasium	*Sports palace*
Hockey field	*Stadium*
Holiday camp	*Swimming pool, public*
Ice palace	*Tennis court*
Lake resort	*Vacation resort*
Mountain resort	

Excludes *that in private house or garden (E849.0)*

E849.5 Street and highway

E849.6 Public building
Building (including adjacent grounds) used by the general public or by a particular group of the public, such as:
airport
bank
cafe
casino
church
cinema
clubhouse
courthouse
dance hall
garage building (for car storage)
hotel
market (grocery or other commodity)
movie house
music hall
nightclub
office
office building
opera house
post office
public hall
radio broadcasting station
restaurant
school (state) (public) (private)
shop, commercial
station (bus) (railway)
store
theater

Excludes *home garage (E849.0)*
industrial building or workplace (E849.3)

E849.7 Residential institution
Children's home
Dormitory
Hospital
Jail
Old people's home
Orphanage
Prison
Reform school

❑*E849.8 Other specified places*
Beach NOS
Canal
Caravan site NOS
Derelict house
Desert
Dock
Forest
Harbor
Hill
Lake NOS
Mountain
Parking lot
Parking place
Pond or pool (natural)
Prairie
Public place NOS
Railway line
Reservoir
River
Sea
Seashore NOS
Stream
Swamp
Trailer court
Woods

❑*E849.9 Unspecified place*

ACCIDENTAL POISONING BY DRUGS, MEDICINAL SUBSTANCES, AND BIOLOGICALS (E850-E858)

Includes: accidental overdose of drug, wrong drug given or taken in error, and drug taken inadvertently
accidents in the use of drugs and biologicals in medical and surgical procedures

Excludes *administration with suicidal or homicidal intent or intent to harm, or in circumstances classifiable to E980-E989 (E950.0-E950.5, E962.0, E980.0-E980.5)*
correct drug properly administered in therapeutic or prophylactic dosage, as the cause of adverse effect (E930.0-E949.9)

Note: See Alphabetic Index for more complete list of specific drugs to be classified under the fourth-digit subdivisions. The American Hospital Formulary numbers can be used to classify new drugs listed by the American Hospital Formulary Service (AHFS). See appendix C.

●**E850 Accidental poisoning by analgesics, antipyretics, and antirheumatics**

E850.0 Heroin
Diacetylmorphine

E850.1 Methadone

❑**E850.2 Other opiates and related narcotics**
Codeine [methylmorphine]
Meperidine [pethidine]
Morphine
Opium (alkaloids)

E850.3 **Salicylates**
Acetylsalicylic acid [aspirin]
Amino derivatives of salicylic acid
Salicylic acid salts

E850.4 **Aromatic analgesics, not elsewhere classified**
Acetanilid
Paracetamol [acetaminophen]
Phenacetin [acetophenetidin]

E850.5 **Pyrazole derivatives**
Aminophenazone [amidopyrine]
Phenylbutazone

E850.6 **Antirheumatics [antiphlogistics]**
Gold salts
Indomethacin

Excludes *salicylates (E850.3)*
steroids (E858.0)

❑ E850.7 **Other non-narcotic analgesics**
Pyrabital

❑ E850.8 **Other specified analgesics and antipyretics**
Pentazocine

❑ E850.9 **Unspecified analgesic or antipyretic**

E851 **Accidental poisoning by barbiturates**
Amobarbital [amylobarbitone]
Barbital [barbitone]
Butabarbital [butabarbitone]
Pentobarbital [pentobarbitone]
Phenobarbital [phenobarbitone]
Secobarbital [quinalbarbitone]

Excludes *thiobarbiturates (E855.1)*

● E852 **Accidental poisoning by other sedatives and hypnotics**

E852.0 **Chloral hydrate group**

E852.1 **Paraldehyde**

E852.2 **Bromine compounds**
Bromides
Carbromal (derivatives)

E852.3 **Methaqualone compounds**

E852.4 **Glutethimide group**

E852.5 **Mixed sedatives, not elsewhere classified**

❑ E852.8 **Other specified sedatives and hypnotics**

❑ E852.9 **Unspecified sedative or hypnotic**
Sleeping:
drug NOS
pill NOS
tablet NOS

● E853 **Accidental poisoning by tranquilizers**

E853.0 **Phenothiazine-based tranquilizers**
Chlorpromazine
Fluphenazine
Prochlorperazine
Promazine

E853.1 **Butyrophenone-based tranquilizers**
Haloperidol
Spiperone
Trifluperidol

E853.2 **Benzodiazepine-based tranquilizers**
Chlordiazepoxide
Diazepam
Flurazepam
Lorazepam
Medazepam
Nitrazepam

❑ E853.8 **Other specified tranquilizers**
Hydroxyzine
Meprobamate

❑ E853.9 **Unspecified tranquilizer**

● E854 **Accidental poisoning by other psychotropic agents**

E854.0 **Antidepressants**
Amitriptyline
Imipramine
Monoamine oxidase [MAO] inhibitors

E854.1 **Psychodysleptics [hallucinogens]**
Cannabis derivatives
Lysergide [LSD]
Marihuana (derivatives)
Mescaline
Psilocin
Psilocybin

E854.2 **Psychostimulants**
Amphetamine
Caffeine

Excludes *central appetite depressants (E858.8)*

E854.3 **Central nervous system stimulants**
Analeptics
Opiate antagonists

E854.8 **Other psychotropic agents**

● E855 **Accidental poisoning by other drugs acting on central and autonomic nervous system**

E855.0 **Anticonvulsant and anti-Parkinsonism drugs**
Amantadine
Hydantoin derivatives
Levodopa [L-dopa]
Oxazolidine derivatives [paramethadione] [trimethadione]
Succinimides

❑ E855.1 **Other central nervous system depressants**
Ether
Gaseous anesthetics
Halogenated hydrocarbon derivatives
Intravenous anesthetics
Thiobarbiturates, such as thiopental sodium

E855.2 **Local anesthetics**
Cocaine
Lidocaine [lignocaine]
Procaine
Tetracaine

E855.3 **Parasympathomimetics [cholinergics]**
Acetylcholine
Anticholinesterase:
organophosphorus
reversible
Pilocarpine

E855.4 **Parasympatholytics [anticholinergics and antimuscarinics] and spasmolytics**
Atropine
Homatropine
Hyoscine [scopolamine]
Quaternary ammonium derivatives

E855.5 **Sympathomimetics [adrenergics]**
Epinephrine [adrenalin]
Levarterenol [noradrenalin]

E855.6 **Sympatholytics [antiadrenergics]**
Phenoxybenzamine
Tolazoline hydrochloride

❑ E855.8 **Other specified drugs acting on central and autonomic nervous systems**

❑ E855.9 **Unspecified drug acting on central and autonomic nervous systems**

E856 **Accidental poisoning by antibiotics**

❑ E857 **Accidental poisoning by other anti-infectives**

● **E858 Accidental poisoning by other drugs**

E858.0 Hormones and synthetic substitutes

E858.1 Primarily systemic agents

E858.2 Agents primarily affecting blood constituents

E858.3 Agents primarily affecting cardiovascular system

E858.4 Agents primarily affecting gastrointestinal system

E858.5 Water, mineral, and uric acid metabolism drugs

E858.6 Agents primarily acting on the smooth and skeletal muscles and respiratory system

E858.7 Agents primarily affecting skin and mucous membrane, ophthalmological, otorhinolaryngological, and dental drugs

❑ **E858.8 Other specified drugs**
Central appetite depressants

❑ **E858.9 Unspecified drug**

ACCIDENTAL POISONING BY OTHER SOLID AND LIQUID SUBSTANCES, GASES, AND VAPORS (E860-E869)

Note: Categories in this section are intended primarily to indicate the external cause of poisoning states classifiable to 980–989. They may also be used to indicate external causes of localized effects classifiable to 001–799.

● **E860 Accidental poisoning by alcohol, not elsewhere classified**

E860.0 Alcoholic beverages
Alcohol in preparations intended for consumption

❑ **E860.1 Other and unspecified ethyl alcohol and its products**
Denatured alcohol
Ethanol NOS
Grain alcohol NOS
Methylated spirit

E860.2 Methyl alcohol
Methanol
Wood alcohol

E860.3 Isopropyl alcohol
Dimethyl carbinol
Isopropanol
Rubbing alcohol substitute
Secondary propyl alcohol

E860.4 Fusel oil
Alcohol:
amyl
butyl
propyl

❑ **E860.8 Other specified alcohols**

❑ **E860.9 Unspecified alcohol**

● **E861 Accidental poisoning by cleansing and polishing agents, disinfectants, paints, and varnishes**

E861.0 Synthetic detergents and shampoos

E861.1 Soap products

E861.2 Polishes

❑ **E861.3 Other cleansing and polishing agents**
Scouring powders

E861.4 Disinfectants
Household and other disinfectants not ordinarily used on the person

Excludes *carbolic acid or phenol (E864.0)*

E861.5 Lead paints

❑ **E861.6 Other paints and varnishes**
Lacquers
Oil colors
Paints, other than lead
Whitewashes

❑ **E861.9 Unspecified**

● **E862 Accidental poisoning by petroleum products, other solvents and their vapors, not elsewhere classified**

E862.0 Petroleum solvents
Petroleum:
ether
benzine
naphtha

E862.1 Petroleum fuels and cleaners
Antiknock additives to petroleum fuels
Gas oils
Gasoline or petrol
Kerosene

Excludes *kerosene insecticides (E863.4)*

E862.2 Lubricating oils

E862.3 Petroleum solids
Paraffin wax

❑ **E862.4 Other specified solvents**
Benzene

❑ **E862.9 Unspecified solvent**

● **E863 Accidental poisoning by agricultural and horticultural chemical and pharmaceutical preparations other than plant foods and fertilizers**

Excludes *plant foods and fertilizers (E866.5)*

E863.0 Insecticides of organochlorine compounds
Benzene hexachloride
Chlordane
DDT
Dieldrin
Endrine
Toxaphene

E863.1 Insecticides of organophosphorus compounds
Demeton
Diazinon
Dichlorvos
Malathion
Methyl parathion
Parathion
Phenylsulphthion
Phorate
Phosdrin

E863.2 Carbamates
Aldicarb
Carbaryl
Propoxur

E863.3 Mixtures of insecticides

❑ **E863.4 Other and unspecified insecticides**
Kerosene insecticides

E863.5 Herbicides
2,4-Dichlorophenoxyacetic acid [2, 4-D]
2,4,5-Trichlorophenoxyacetic acid [2, 4, 5-T]
Chlorates
Diquat
Mixtures of plant foods and fertilizers with herbicides
Paraquat

E863.6 Fungicides
Organic mercurials (used in seed dressing)
Pentachlorophenols

E863.7 Rodenticides
Fluoroacetates
Squill and derivatives
Thallium
Warfarin
Zinc phosphide

E863.8 Fumigants
Cyanides
Methyl bromide
Phosphine

❑ **E863.9 Other and unspecified**

● **E864 Accidental poisoning by corrosives and caustics, not elsewhere classified**

Excludes *those as components of disinfectants (E861.4)*

E864.0 Corrosive aromatics
Carbolic acid or phenol

E864.1 Acids
Acid:
hydrochloric
nitric
sulfuric

E864.2 Caustic alkalis
Lye

❑ **E864.3 Other specified corrosives and caustics**

❑ **E864.4 Unspecified corrosives and caustics**

● **E865 Accidental poisoning from poisonous foodstuffs and poisonous plants**

Includes: any meat, fish, or shellfish
plants, berries, and fungi eaten as, or in mistake for food, or by a child

Excludes *anaphlyactic shock due to adverse food reaction (995.60–995.69)*
food poisoning (bacterial) (005.0–005.9)
poisoning and toxic reactions to venomous plants (E905.6-E905.7)

E865.0 Meat

E865.1 Shellfish

❑ **E865.2 Other fish**

E865.3 Berries and seeds

❑ **E865.4 Other specified plants**

E865.5 Mushrooms and other fungi

❑ **E865.8 Other specified foods**

❑ **E865.9 Unspecified foodstuff or poisonous plant**

● **E866 Accidental poisoning by other and unspecified solid and liquid substances**

Excludes *these substances as a component of:*
medicines (E850.0-E858.9)
paints (E861.5-E861.6)
pesticides (E863.0-E863.9)
petroleum fuels (E862.1)

E866.0 Lead and its compounds and fumes

E866.1 Mercury and its compounds and fumes

E866.2 Antimony and its compounds and fumes

E866.3 Arsenic and its compounds and fumes

❑ **E866.4 Other metals and their compounds and fumes**
Beryllium (compounds)
Brass fumes
Cadmium (compounds)
Copper salts
Iron (compounds)
Manganese (compounds)
Nickel (compounds)
Thallium (compounds)

E866.5 Plant foods and fertilizers

Excludes *mixtures with herbicides (E863.5)*

E866.6 Glues and adhesives

E866.7 Cosmetics

❑ **E866.8 Other specified solid or liquid substances**

❑ **E866.9 Unspecified solid or liquid substance**

E867 Accidental poisoning by gas distributed by pipeline
Carbon monoxide from incomplete combustion of piped gas
Coal gas NOS
Liquefied petroleum gas distributed through pipes (pure or mixed with air)
Piped gas (natural) (manufactured)

● **E868 Accidental poisoning by other utility gas and other carbon monoxide**

E868.0 Liquefied petroleum gas distributed in mobile containers
Butane or carbon monoxide from incomplete combustion of these gases
Liquefied hydrocarbon gas NOS or carbon monoxide from incomplete combustion of these gases
Propane or carbon monoxide from incomplete combustion of these gases

❑ **E868.1 Other and unspecified utility gas**
Acetylene or carbon monoxide from incomplete combustion of these gases
Gas NOS used for lighting, heating, or cooking or carbon monoxide from incomplete combustion of these gases
Water gas or carbon monoxide from incomplete combustion of these gases

E868.2 Motor vehicle exhaust gas
Exhaust gas from:
farm tractor, not in transit
gas engine
motor pump
motor vehicle, not in transit
any type of combustion engine not in watercraft

Excludes *poisoning by carbon monoxide from:*
aircraft while in transit (E844.0-E844.9)
motor vehicle while in transit (E818.0-E818.9)
watercraft whether or not in transit (E838.0-E838.9)

❑ **E868.3 Carbon monoxide from incomplete combustion of other domestic fuels**
Carbon monoxide from incomplete combustion of:
coal in domestic stove or fireplace
coke in domestic stove or fireplace
kerosene in domestic stove or fireplace
wood in domestic stove or fireplace

Excludes *carbon monoxide from smoke and fumes due to conflagration (E890.0-E893.9)*

❑ **E868.8 Carbon monoxide from other sources**
Carbon monoxide from:
blast furnace gas
incomplete combustion of fuels in industrial use
kiln vapor

❑ **E868.9 Unspecified carbon monoxide**

● E869 Accidental poisoning by other gases and vapors

Excludes *effects of gases used as anesthetics (E855.1, E938.2)*
fumes from heavy metals (E866.0-E866.4)
smoke and fumes due to conflagration or explosion (E890.0-E899)

E869.0 Nitrogen oxides

E869.1 Sulfur dioxide

E869.2 Freon

E869.3 Lacrimogenic gas [tear gas]
Bromobenzyl cyanide
Chloroacetophenone
Ethyliodoacetate

E869.4 Second-hand tobacco smoke

❑ **E869.8 Other specified gases and vapors**
Chlorine
Hydrocyanic acid gas

❑ **E869.9 Unspecified gases and vapors**

MISADVENTURES TO PATIENTS DURING SURGICAL AND MEDICAL CARE (E870-E876)

Excludes *accidental overdose of drug and wrong drug given in error (E850.0-E858.9)*
surgical and medical procedures as the cause of abnormal reaction by the patient, without mention of misadventure at the time of procedure (E878.0-E879.9)

● **E870 Accidental cut, puncture, perforation, or hemorrhage during medical care**

E870.0 Surgical operation

E870.1 Infusion or transfusion

E870.2 Kidney dialysis or other perfusion

E870.3 Injection or vaccination

E870.4 Endoscopic examination

E870.5 Aspiration of fluid or tissue, puncture, and catheterization
Abdominal paracentesis
Aspirating needle biopsy
Blood sampling
Lumbar puncture
Thoracentesis

Excludes *heart catheterization (E870.6)*

E870.6 Heart catheterization

E870.7 Administration of enema

❑ **E870.8 Other specified medical care**

❑ **E870.9 Unspecified medical care**

● **E871 Foreign object left in body during procedure**

E871.0 Surgical operation

E871.1 Infusion or transfusion

E871.2 Kidney dialysis or other perfusion

E871.3 Injection or vaccination

E871.4 Endoscopic examination

E871.5 Aspiration of fluid or tissue, puncture, and catheterization
Abdominal paracentesis
Aspiration needle biopsy
Blood sampling
Lumbar puncture
Thoracentesis

Excludes *heart catheterization (E871.6)*

E871.6 Heart catheterization

E871.7 Removal of catheter or packing

❑ **E871.8 Other specified procedures**

❑ **E871.9 Unspecified procedure**

● **E872 Failure of sterile precautions during procedure**

E872.0 Surgical operation

E872.1 Infusion or transfusion

E872.2 Kidney dialysis and other perfusion

E872.3 Injection or vaccination

E872.4 Endoscopic examination

E872.5 Aspiration of fluid or tissue, puncture, and catheterization
Abdominal paracentesis
Aspirating needle biopsy
Blood sampling
Lumbar puncture
Thoracentesis

Excludes *heart catheterization (E872.6)*

E872.6 Heart catheterization

❑ **E872.8 Other specified procedures**

❑ **E872.9 Unspecified procedure**

● **E873 Failure in dosage**

Excludes *accidental overdose of drug, medicinal or biological substance (E850.0-E858.9)*

❑ **E873.0 Excessive amount of blood or other fluid during transfusion or infusion**

E873.1 Incorrect dilution of fluid during infusion

E873.2 Overdose of radiation in therapy

E873.3 Inadvertent exposure of patient to radiation during medical care

E873.4 Failure in dosage in electroshock or insulin-shock therapy

E873.5 Inappropriate [too hot or too cold] temperature in local application and packing

E873.6 Nonadministration of necessary drug or medicinal substance

❑ **E873.8 Other specified failure in dosage**

❑ **E873.9 Unspecified failure in dosage**

● **E874 Mechanical failure of instrument or apparatus during procedure**

E874.0 Surgical operation

E874.1 Infusion and transfusion
Air in system

E874.2 Kidney dialysis and other perfusion

E874.3 Endoscopic examination

E874.4 Aspiration of fluid or tissue, puncture, and catheterization
Abdominal paracentesis
Aspirating needle biopsy
Blood sampling
Lumbar puncture
Thoracentesis

Excludes *heart catheterization (E874.5)*

E874.5 Heart catheterization

❑ **E874.8 Other specified procedures**

❑ **E874.9 Unspecified procedure**

● E875 **Contaminated or infected blood, other fluid, drug, or biological substance**

Includes: presence of:
bacterial pyrogens
endotoxin-producing bacteria
serum hepatitis-producing agent

E875.0 **Contaminated substance transfused or infused**

E875.1 **Contaminated substance injected or used for vaccination**

❑ E875.2 **Contaminated drug or biological substance administered by other means**

❑ E875.8 **Other**

❑ E875.9 **Unspecified**

● E876 **Other and unspecified misadventures during medical care**

E876.0 **Mismatched blood in transfusion**

E876.1 **Wrong fluid in infusion**

E876.2 **Failure in suture and ligature during surgical operation**

E876.3 **Endotracheal tube wrongly placed during anesthetic procedure**

❑ E876.4 **Failure to introduce or to remove other tube or instrument**

Excludes *foreign object left in body during procedure (E871.0-E871.9)*

E876.5 **Performance of inappropriate operation**

❑ E876.8 **Other specified misadventures during medical care**
Performance of inappropriate treatment, NEC

❑ E876.9 **Unspecified misadventure during medical care**

SURGICAL AND MEDICAL PROCEDURES AS THE CAUSE OF ABNORMAL REACTION OF PATIENT OR LATER COMPLICATION, WITHOUT MENTION OF MISADVENTURE AT THE TIME OF PROCEDURE (E878-E879)

Includes: procedures as the cause of abnormal reaction, such as:
displacement or malfunction of prosthetic device
hepatorenal failure, postoperative
malfunction of external stoma
postoperative intestinal obstruction
rejection of transplanted organ

Excludes *anesthetic management properly carried out as the cause of adverse effect (E937.0-E938.9)*
infusion and transfusion, without mention of misadventure in the technique of procedure (E930.0-E949.9)

● E878 **Surgical operation and other surgical procedures as the cause of abnormal reaction of patient, or of later complication, without mention of misadventure at the time of operation**

E878.0 **Surgical operation with transplant of whole organ**
Transplantation of:
heart
kidney
liver

E878.1 **Surgical operation with implant of artificial internal device**
Cardiac pacemaker
Electrodes implanted in brain
Heart valve prosthesis
Internal orthopedic device

E878.2 **Surgical operation with anastomosis, bypass, or graft, with natural or artificial tissues used as implant**
Anastomosis:
arteriovenous
gastrojejunal
Graft of blood vessel, tendon, or skin

Excludes *external stoma (E878.3)*

E878.3 **Surgical operation with formation of external stoma**
Colostomy
Cystostomy
Duodenostomy
Gastrostomy
Ureterostomy

❑ E878.4 **Other restorative surgery**

E878.5 **Amputation of limb(s)**

❑ E878.6 **Removal of other organ (partial) (total)**

❑ E878.8 **Other specified surgical operations and procedures**

❑ E878.9 **Unspecified surgical operations and procedures**

● E879 **Other procedures, without mention of misadventure at the time of procedure, as the cause of abnormal reaction of patient, or of later complication**

E879.0 **Cardiac catheterization**

E879.1 **Kidney dialysis**

E879.2 **Radiological procedure and radiotherapy**

Excludes *radio-opaque dyes for diagnostic x-ray procedures (E947.8)*

E879.3 **Shock therapy**
Electroshock therapy
Insulin-shock therapy

E879.4 **Aspiration of fluid**
Lumbar puncture
Thoracentesis

E879.5 **Insertion of gastric or duodenal sound**

E879.6 **Urinary catheterization**

E879.7 **Blood sampling**

❑ E879.8 **Other specified procedures**
Blood transfusion

❑ E879.9 **Unspecified procedure**

ACCIDENTAL FALLS (E880-E888)

Excludes *falls (in or from):*
burning building (E890.8, E891.8)
into fire (E890.0-E899)
into water (with submersion or drowning) (E910.0-E910.9)
machinery (in operation) (E919.0-E919.9)
on edged, pointed, or sharp object (E920.0-E920.9)
transport vehicle (E800.0-E845.9)
vehicle not elsewhere classifiable (E846-E848)

● E880 **Fall on or from stairs or steps**

E880.0 **Escalator**

E880.1 **Fall on or from sidewalk curb**

Excludes *fall from moving sidewalk (E885.9)*

❑ E880.9 **Other stairs or steps**

● E881 **Fall on or from ladders or scaffolding**

E881.0 **Fall from ladder**

E881.1 **Fall from scaffolding**

❑ **E882 Fall from or out of building or other structure**
Fall from:
balcony
bridge
building
flagpole
tower
turret
viaduct
wall
window
Fall through roof

Excludes *collapse of a building or structure (E916)*
fall or jump from burning building (E890.8, E891.8)

● **E883 Fall into hole or other opening in surface**

Includes: fall into:
cavity
dock
hole
pit
quarry
shaft
swimming pool
tank
well

Excludes *fall into water NOS (E910.9)*
that resulting in drowning or submersion without mention of injury (E910.0-E910.9)

E883.0 Accident from diving or jumping into water [swimming pool]
Strike or hit:
against bottom when jumping or diving into water
wall or board of swimming pool
water surface

Excludes *diving with insufficient air supply (E913.2)*
effects of air pressure from diving (E902.2)

E883.1 Accidental fall into well

E883.2 Accidental fall into storm drain or manhole

❑ **E883.9 Fall into other hole or other opening in surface**

● **E884 Other fall from one level to another**

E884.0 Fall from playground equipment

Excludes *recreational machinery (E919.8)*

E884.1 Fall from cliff

E884.2 Fall from chair

E884.3 Fall from wheelchair

E884.4 Fall from bed

E884.5 Fall from other furniture

E884.6 Fall from commode
Toilet

❑ **E884.9 Other fall from one level to another**
Fall from:
embankment
haystack
stationary vehicle
tree

● **E885 Fall on same level from slipping, tripping, or stumbling**

E885.0 Fall from (nonmotorized) scooter

E885.1 Fall from roller skates
In-line skates

E885.2 Fall from skateboard

E885.3 Fall from skis

E885.4 Fall from snowboard

E885.9 Fall from other slipping, tripping, or stumbling
Fall on moving sidewalk

● **E886 Fall on same level from collision, pushing, or shoving, by or with other person**

Excludes *crushed or pushed by a crowd or human stampede (E917.1, E917.6)*

E886.0 In sports
Tackles in sports

Excludes *kicked, stepped on, struck by object, in sports (E917.0, E917.5)*

❑ **E886.9 Other and unspecified**
Fall from collision of pedestrian (conveyance) with another pedestrian (conveyance)

❑ **E887 Fracture, cause unspecified**

● **E888 Other and unspecified fall**
Accidental fall NOS

E888.0 Fall resulting in striking against sharp object
Use additional external cause code to identify object (E920)

E888.1 Fall resulting in striking against other object

E888.8 Other fall

E888.9 Unspecified fall
Fall NOS

ACCIDENTS CAUSED BY FIRE AND FLAMES (E890-E899)

Includes: asphyxia or poisoning due to conflagration or ignition
burning by fire
secondary fires resulting from explosion

Excludes *arson (E968.0)*
fire in or on:
machinery (in operation) (E919.0-E919.9)
transport vehicle other than stationary vehicle (E800.0-E845.9)
vehicle not elsewhere classifiable (E846-E848)

● **E890 Conflagration in private dwelling**

Includes: conflagration in:
apartment
boarding house
camping place
caravan
farmhouse
house
lodging house
mobile home
private garage
rooming house
tenement
conflagration originating from sources classifiable to E893-E898 in the above buildings

E890.0 Explosion caused by conflagration

E890.1 Fumes from combustion of polyvinylchloride [PVC] and similar material in conflagration

❑ **E890.2 Other smoke and fumes from conflagration**
Carbon monoxide from conflagration in private building
Fumes NOS from conflagration in private building
Smoke NOS from conflagration in private building

E890.3 Burning caused by conflagration

ICD-9-CM E800-E899 Vol. 1

❑**E890.8 Other accident resulting from conflagration**
Collapse of burning private building
Fall from burning private building
Hit by object falling from burning private building
Jump from burning private building

❑**E890.9 Unspecified accident resulting from conflagration in private dwelling**

●**E891 Conflagration in other and unspecified building or structure**
Conflagration in:
barn
church
convalescent and other residential home
dormitory of educational institution
factory
farm outbuildings
hospital
hotel
school
store
theater
Conflagration originating from sources classifiable to E893-E898, in the above buildings

E891.0 Explosion caused by conflagration

E891.1 Fumes from combustion of polyvinylchloride [PVC] and similar material in conflagration

❑**E891.2 Other smoke and fumes from conflagration**
Carbon monoxide from conflagration in building or structure
Fumes NOS from conflagration in building or structure
Smoke NOS from conflagration in building or structure

E891.3 Burning caused by conflagration

❑**E891.8 Other accident resulting from conflagration**
Collapse of burning building or structure
Fall from burning building or structure
Hit by object falling from burning building or structure
Jump from burning building or structure

❑**E891.9 Unspecified accident resulting from conflagration of other and unspecified building or structure**

E892 Conflagration not in building or structure
Fire (uncontrolled) (in) (of):
forest
grass
hay
lumber
mine
prairie
transport vehicle [any], except while in transit
tunnel

●**E893 Accident caused by ignition of clothing**

Excludes *ignition of clothing:*
from highly inflammable material (E894)
with conflagration (E890.0-E892)

E893.0 From controlled fire in private dwelling
Ignition of clothing from:
normal fire (charcoal) (coal) (electric) (gas) (wood) in:
brazier in private dwelling (as listed in E890)
fireplace in private dwelling (as listed in E890)
furnace in private dwelling (as listed in E890)
stove in private dwelling (as listed in E890)

❑**E893.1 From controlled fire in other building or structure**
Ignition of clothing from:
normal fire (charcoal) (coal) (electric) (gas) (wood) in:
brazier in other building or structure (as listed in E891)
fireplace in other building or structure (as listed in E891)
furnace in other building or structure (as listed in E891)
stove in other building or structure (as listed in E891)

E893.2 From controlled fire not in building or structure
Ignition of clothing from:
bonfire (controlled)
brazier fire (controlled), not in building or structure
trash fire (controlled)

Excludes *conflagration not in building (E892)*
trash fire out of control (E892)

❑**E893.8 From other specified sources**
Ignition of clothing from:
blowlamp
blowtorch
burning bedspread
candle
cigar
cigarette
lighter
matches
pipe
welding torch

❑**E893.9 Unspecified source**
Ignition of clothing (from controlled fire NOS) (in building NOS) NOS

E894 Ignition of highly inflammable material
Ignition of:
benzine (with ignition of clothing)
gasoline (with ignition of clothing)
fat (with ignition of clothing)
kerosene (with ignition of clothing)
paraffin (with ignition of clothing)
petrol (with ignition of clothing)

Excludes *ignition of highly inflammable material with:*
conflagration (E890.0-E892)
explosion (E923.0-E923.9)

E895 Accident caused by controlled fire in private dwelling
Burning by (flame of) normal fire (charcoal) (coal) (electric) (gas) (wood) in:
brazier in private dwelling (as listed in E890)
fireplace in private dwelling (as listed in E890)
furnace in private dwelling (as listed in E890)
stove in private dwelling (as listed in E890)

Excludes *burning by hot objects not producing fire or flames (E924.0-E924.9)*
ignition of clothing from these sources (E893.0)
poisoning by carbon monoxide from incomplete combustion of fuel (E867-E868.9)
that with conflagration (E890.0-E890.9)

❑E896 **Accident caused by controlled fire in other and unspecified building or structure**
Burning by (flame of) normal fire (charcoal) (coal) (electric) (gas) (wood) in:
brazier in other building or structure (as listed in E891)
fireplace in other building or structure (as listed in E891)
furnace in other building or structure (as listed in E891)
stove in other building or structure (as listed in E891)

Excludes *burning by hot objects not producing fire or flames (E924.0-E924.9)*
ignition of clothing from these sources (E893.1)
poisoning by carbon monoxide from incomplete combustion of fuel (E867-E868.9)
that with conflagration (E891.0-E891.9)

E897 **Accident caused by controlled fire not in building or structure**
Burns from flame of:
bonfire (controlled)
brazier fire (controlled), not in building or structure
trash fire (controlled)

Excludes *ignition of clothing from these sources (E893.2)*
trash fire out of control (E892)
that with conflagration (E892)

●E898 **Accident caused by other specified fire and flames**

Excludes *conflagration (E890.0-E892)*
that with ignition of:
clothing (E893.0-E893.9)
highly inflammable material (E894)

E898.0 **Burning bedclothes**
Bed set on fire NOS

❑E898.1 **Other**
Burning by:
blowlamp
blowtorch
candle
cigar
cigarette
fire in room NOS
lamp
lighter
matches
pipe
welding torch

❑E899 **Accident caused by unspecified fire**
Burning NOS

ACCIDENTS DUE TO NATURAL AND ENVIRONMENTAL FACTORS (E900-E909)

●E900 **Excessive heat**

E900.0 **Due to weather conditions**
Excessive heat as the external cause of:
ictus solaris
siriasis
sunstroke

E900.1 **Of man-made origin**
Heat (in):
boiler room
drying room
factory
furnace room
generated in transport vehicle
kitchen

❑E900.9 **Of unspecified origin**

●E901 **Excessive cold**

E901.0 **Due to weather conditions**
Excessive cold as the cause of:
chilblains NOS
immersion foot

E901.1 **Of man-made origin**
Contact with or inhalation of:
dry ice
liquid air
liquid hydrogen
liquid nitrogen
Prolonged exposure in:
deep freeze unit
refrigerator

❑E901.8 **Other specified origin**

❑E901.9 **Of unspecified origin**

●E902 **High and low air pressure and changes in air pressure**

E902.0 **Residence or prolonged visit at high altitude**
Residence or prolonged visit at high altitude as the cause of:
Acosta syndrome
Alpine sickness
altitude sickness
Andes disease
anoxia, hypoxia
barotitis, barodontalgia, barosinusitis, otitic barotrauma
hypobarism, hypobaropathy
mountain sickness
range disease

E902.1 **In aircraft**
Sudden change in air pressure in aircraft during ascent or descent as the cause of:
aeroneurosis
aviators' disease

E902.2 **Due to diving**
High air pressure from rapid descent in water as the cause of:
caisson disease
divers' disease
divers' palsy or paralysis
Reduction in atmospheric pressure while surfacing from deep water diving as the cause of:
caisson disease
divers' disease
divers' palsy or paralysis

❑E902.8 **Due to other specified causes**
Reduction in atmospheric pressure while surfacing from under ground

❑E902.9 **Unspecified cause**

E903 **Travel and motion**

●E904 **Hunger, thirst, exposure, and neglect**

Excludes *any condition resulting from homicidal intent (E968.0-E968.9)*
hunger, thirst, and exposure resulting from accidents connected with transport (E800.0-E848)

E904.0 **Abandonment or neglect of infants and helpless persons**
Exposure to weather conditions resulting from abandonment or neglect
Hunger or thirst resulting from abandonment or neglect
Desertion of newborn
Inattention at or after birth
Lack of care (helpless person) (infant)

Excludes *criminal [purposeful] neglect (E968.4)*

ICD-9-CM E800-E899 Vol. 1

E904.1 Lack of food
Lack of food as the cause of:
inanition
insufficient nourishment
starvation

Excludes *hunger resulting from abandonment or neglect (E904.0)*

E904.2 Lack of water
Lack of water as the cause of:
dehydration
inanition

Excludes *dehydration due to acute fluid loss (276.5)*

E904.3 Exposure (to weather conditions), not elsewhere classifiable
Exposure NOS
Humidity
Struck by hailstones

Excludes *struck by lightning (E907)*

E904.9 Privation, unqualified
Destitution

● **E905 Venomous animals and plants as the cause of poisoning and toxic reactions**

Includes: chemical released by animal
insects
release of venom through fangs, hairs, spines, tentacles, and other venom apparatus

Excludes *eating of poisonous animals or plants (E865.0-E865.9)*

E905.0 Venomous snakes and lizards

Cobra	Mamba
Copperhead snake	Rattlesnake
Coral snake	Sea snake
Fer de lance	Snake (venomous)
Gila monster	Viper
Krait	Water moccasin

Excludes *bites of snakes and lizards known to be nonvenomous (E906.2)*

E905.1 Venomous spiders
Black widow spider
Brown recluse spider
Tarantula (venomous)

E905.2 Scorpion

E905.3 Hornets, wasps, and bees
Yellow jacket

E905.4 Centipede and venomous millipede (tropical)

❑ **E905.5 Other venomous arthropods**
Sting of:
ant
caterpillar

E905.6 Venomous marine animals and plants
Puncture by sea urchin spine
Sting of:
coral
jelly fish
nematocysts
sea anemone
sea cucumber
other marine animal or plant

Excludes *bites and other injuries caused by nonvenomous marine animal (E906.2-E906.8)*
bite of sea snake (venomous) (E905.0)

❑ **E905.7 Poisoning and toxic reactions caused by other plants**
Injection of poisons or toxins into or through skin by plant thorns, spines, or other mechanisms

Excludes *puncture wound NOS by plant thorns or spines (E920.8)*

❑ **E905.8 Other specified**

❑ **E905.9 Unspecified**
Sting NOS
Venomous bite NOS

● **E906 Other injury caused by animals**

Excludes *poisoning and toxic reactions caused by venomous animals and insects (E905.0-E905.9)*
road vehicle accident involving animals (E827.0-E828.9)
tripping or falling over an animal (E885.9)

E906.0 Dog bite

E906.1 Rat bite

E906.2 Bite of nonvenomous snakes and lizards

❑ **E906.3 Bite of other animal except arthropod**

Cats	Rodents, except rats
Moray eel	Shark

E906.4 Bite of nonvenomous arthropod
Insect bite NOS

E906.5 Bite by unspecified animal
Animal bite NOS

❑ **E906.8 Other specified injury caused by animal**
Butted by animal
Fallen on by horse or other animal, not being ridden
Gored by animal
Implantation of quills of porcupine
Pecked by bird
Run over by animal, not being ridden
Stepped on by animal, not being ridden

Excludes *injury by animal being ridden (E828.0-E828.9)*

❑ **E906.9 Unspecified injury caused by animal**

E907 Lightning

Excludes *injury from:*
fall of tree or other object caused by lightning (E916)
fire caused by lightning (E890.0-E892)

● **E908 Cataclysmic storms, and floods resulting from storms**

Excludes *collapse of dam or man-made structure causing flood (E909.3)*

E908.0 Hurricane
Storm surge
"Tidal wave" caused by storm action
Typhoon

E908.1 Tornado
Cyclone
Twisters

E908.2 Floods
Torrential rainfall
Flash flood

Excludes *collapse of dam or man-made structure causing flood (E909.3)*

E908.3 Blizzard (snow) (ice)

E908.4 Dust storm

E908.8 Other cataclysmic storms

E908.9 Unspecified cataclysmic storms, and floods resulting from storms
Storm NOS

E909 Cataclysmic earth surface movements and eruptions

E909.0 Earthquakes

E909.1 Volcanic eruptions
Burns from lava
Ash inhalation

E909.2 Avalanche, landslide, or mudslide

E909.3 Collapse of dam or man-made structure

E909.4 Tidal wave caused by earthquake
Tidal wave NOS
Tsunami

Excludes *tidal wave caused by tropical storm (E908.0)*

E909.8 Other cataclysmic earth surface movements and eruptions

E909.9 Unspecified cataclysmic earth surface movements and eruptions

ACCIDENTS CAUSED BY SUBMERSION, SUFFOCATION, AND FOREIGN BODIES (E910-E915)

●**E910 Accidental drowning and submersion**

Includes: immersion
swimmers' cramp

Excludes *diving accident (NOS) (resulting in injury except drowning) (E883.0)*
diving with insufficient air supply (E913.2)
drowning and submersion due to:
cataclysm (E908-E909)
machinery accident (E919.0-E919.9)
transport accident (E800.0-E845.9)
effect of high and low air pressure (E902.2)
injury from striking against objects while in running water (E917.2)

E910.0 While water-skiing
Fall from water skis with submersion or drowning

Excludes *accident to water-skier involving a watercraft and resulting in submersion or other injury (E830.4, E831.4)*

❑**E910.1 While engaged in other sport or recreational activity with diving equipment**
Scuba diving NOS
Skin diving NOS
Underwater spear fishing NOS

❑**E910.2 While engaged in other sport or recreational activity without diving equipment**
Fishing or hunting, except from boat or with diving equipment
Ice skating
Playing in water
Surfboarding
Swimming NOS
Voluntarily jumping from boat, not involved in accident, for swim NOS
Wading in water

Excludes *jumping into water to rescue another person (E910.3)*

E910.3 While swimming or diving for purposes other than recreation or sport
Marine salvage (with diving equipment)
Pearl diving (with diving equipment)
Placement of fishing nets (with diving equipment)
Rescue (attempt) of another person (with diving equipment)
Underwater construction or repairs (with diving equipment)

E910.4 In bathtub

❑**E910.8 Other accidental drowning or submersion**
Drowning in:
quenching tank
swimming pool

❑**E910.9 Unspecified accidental drowning or submersion**
Accidental fall into water NOS
Drowning NOS

E911 Inhalation and ingestion of food causing obstruction of respiratory tract or suffocation
Aspiration and inhalation of food [any] (into respiratory tract) NOS
Asphyxia by food [including bone, seed in food, regurgitated food]
Choked on food [including bone, seed in food, regurgitated food]
Suffocation by food [including bone, seed in food, regurgitated food]
Compression of trachea by food lodged in esophagus
Interruption of respiration by food lodged in esophagus
Obstruction of respiration by food lodged in esophagus
Obstruction of pharynx by food (bolus)

Excludes *injury, except asphyxia and obstruction of respiratory passage, caused by food (E915)*
obstruction of esophagus by food without mention of asphyxia or obstruction of respiratory passage (E915)

❑**E912 Inhalation and ingestion of other object causing obstruction of respiratory tract or suffocation**
Aspiration and inhalation of foreign body except food (into respiratory tract) NOS
Foreign object [bean] [marble] in nose
Obstruction of pharynx by foreign body
Compression by foreign body in esophagus
Interruption of respiration by foreign body in esophagus
Obstruction of respiration by foreign body in esophagus

Excludes *injury, except asphyxia and obstruction of respiratory passage, caused by foreign body (E915)*
obstruction of esophagus by foreign body without mention of asphyxia or obstruction in respiratory passage (E915)

●**E913 Accidental mechanical suffocation**

Excludes *mechanical suffocation from or by:*
accidental inhalation or ingestion of:
food (E911)
foreign object (E912)
cataclysm (E908-E909)
explosion (E921.0-E921.9, E923.0-E923.9)
machinery accident (E919.0-E919.9)

E913.0 In bed or cradle

Excludes *suffocation by plastic bag (E913.1)*

E913.1 By plastic bag

E913.2 Due to lack of air (in closed place)
Accidentally closed up in refrigerator or other airtight enclosed space
Diving with insufficient air supply

Excludes *suffocation by plastic bag (E913.1)*

E913.3 By falling earth or other substance
Cave-in NOS

Excludes *cave-in caused by cataclysmic earth surface movements and eruptions (E909.8)*
struck by cave-in without asphyxiation or suffocation (E916)

❑ **E913.8 Other specified means**
Accidental hanging, except in bed or cradle

❑ **E913.9 Unspecified means**
Asphyxia, mechanical NOS
Strangulation NOS
Suffocation NOS

E914 Foreign body accidentally entering eye and adnexa
Excludes *corrosive liquid (E924.1)*

❑ **E915 Foreign body accidentally entering other orifice**
Excludes *aspiration and inhalation of foreign body, any, (into respiratory tract) NOS (E911-E912)*

OTHER ACCIDENTS (E916-E928)

E916 Struck accidentally by falling object
Collapse of building, except on fire
Falling:
rock
snowslide NOS
stone
tree
Object falling from:
machine, not in operation
stationary vehicle

Code first: collapse of building on fire (E890.0-E891.9)
falling object in:
cataclysm (E908-E909)
machinery accidents (E919.0-E919.9)
transport accidents (E800.0-E845.9)
vehicle accidents not elsewhere classifiable (E846-E848)
object set in motion by:
explosion (E921.0-E921.9, E923.0-E923.9)
firearm (E922.0-E922.9)
projected object (E917.0-E917.9)

● **E917 Striking against or struck accidentally by objects or persons**
Includes: bumping into or against
object (moving) (projected) (stationary)
pedestrian conveyance
person
colliding with
object (moving) (projected) (stationary)
pedestrian conveyance
person
kicking against
object (moving) (projected) (stationary)
pedestrian conveyance
person
stepping on
object (moving) (projected) (stationary)
pedestrian conveyance
person
struck by
object (moving) (projected) (stationary)
pedestrian conveyance
person
Excludes *fall from:*
collision with another person, except when caused by a crowd (E886.0-E886.9)
stumbling over object (E885.9)
fall resulting in striking against object (E888.0, E888.1)
injury caused by:
assault (E960.0-E960.1, E967.0-E967.9)
cutting or piercing instrument (E920.0-E920.9)
explosion (E921.0-E921.9, E923.0-E923.9)
firearm (E922.0-E922.9)
machinery (E919.0-E919.9)
transport vehicle (E800.0-E845.9)
vehicle not elsewhere classifiable (E846-E848)

E917.0 In sports without subsequent fall
Kicked or stepped on during game (football) (rugby)
Struck by hit or thrown ball
Struck by hockey stick or puck

E917.1 Caused by a crowd, by collective fear or panic without subsequent fall
Crushed by crowd or human stampede
Pushed by crowd or human stampede
Stepped on by crowd or human stampede

E917.2 In running water without subsequent fall
Excludes *drowning or submersion (E910.0-E910.9) that in sports (E917.0, E917.5)*

E917.3 Furniture without subsequent fall
Excludes *fall from furniture (E884.2, E884.4–E884.5)*

E917.4 Other stationary object without subsequent fall
Bath tub
Fence
Lamp-post

E917.5 Object in sports with subsequent fall
Knocked down while boxing

E917.6 Caused by a crowd, by collective fear or panic with subsequent fall

E917.7 Furniture with subsequent fall
Excludes *fall from furniture (E884.2, E884.4–E884.5)*

❑ **E917.8 Other stationary object with subsequent fall**
Bath tub
Fence
Lamp-post

❑ **E917.9 Other striking against with or without subsequent fall**

E918 Caught accidentally in or between objects
Caught, crushed, jammed, or pinched in or between moving or stationary objects, such as:
escalator
folding object
hand tools, appliances, or implements
sliding door and door frame
under packing crate
washing machine wringer
Excludes *injury caused by:*
cutting or piercing instrument (E920.0-E920.9)
machinery (E919.0-E919.9)
transport vehicle (E800.0-E845.9)
vehicle not elsewhere classifiable (E846-E848)
struck accidentally by:
falling object (E916)
object (moving) (projected) (E917.0-E917.9)

● **E919 Accidents caused by machinery**
Includes: burned by machinery (accident)
caught in (moving parts of) machinery (accident)
collapse of machinery (accident)
crushed by machinery (accident)
cut or pierced by machinery (accident)
drowning or submersion caused by machinery (accident)
explosion of, on, in machinery (accident)
fall from or into moving part of machinery (accident)
fire starting in or on machinery (accident)
mechanical suffocation caused by machinery (accident)
object falling from, on, in motion by machinery (accident)
overturning of machinery (accident)
pinned under machinery (accident)
run over by machinery (accident)
struck by machinery (accident)
thrown from machinery (accident)
caught between machinery and other object
machinery accident NOS

Excludes *accidents involving machinery, not in operation (E884.9, E916-E918)*
injury caused by:
electric current in connection with machinery (E925.0-E925.9)
escalator (E880.0, E918)
explosion of pressure vessel in connection with machinery (E921.0-E921.9)
moving sidewalk (E885.9)
powered hand tools, appliances, and implements (E916-E918, E920.0-E921.9, E923.0-E926.9)
transport vehicle accidents involving machinery (E800.0-E848.9)
poisoning by carbon monoxide generated by machine (E868.8)

E919.0 Agricultural machines
Animal-powered agricultural machine
Combine
Derrick, hay
Farm machinery NOS
Farm tractor
Harvester
Hay mower or rake
Reaper
Thresher

Excludes *that in transport under own power on the highway (E810.0-E819.9)*
that being towed by another vehicle on the highway (E810.0-E819.9, E827.0-E827.9, E829.0-E829.9)
that involved in accident classifiable to E820-E829 (E820.0-E829.9)

E919.1 Mining and earth-drilling machinery
Bore or drill (land) (seabed)
Shaft hoist
Shaft lift
Under-cutter

Excludes *coal car, tram, truck, and tub in mine (E846)*

E919.2 Lifting machines and appliances
Chain hoist except in agricultural or mining operations
Crane except in agricultural or mining operations
Derrick except in agricultural or mining operations
Elevator (building) (grain) except in agricultural or mining operations
Forklift truck except in agricultural or mining operations
Lift except in agricultural or mining operations
Pulley block except in agricultural or mining operations
Winch except in agricultural or mining operations

Excludes *that being towed by another vehicle on the highway (E810.0-E819.9, E827.0-E827.9, E829.0-E829.9)*
that in transport under own power on the highway (E810.0-E819.9)
that involved in accident classifiable to E820-E829 (E820.0-E829.9)

E919.3 Metalworking machines
Abrasive wheel
Forging machine
Lathe
Mechanical shears
Metal:
drilling machine
Metal:
milling machine
power press
rolling-mill
sawing machine

E919.4 Woodworking and forming machines
Band saw
Bench saw
Circular saw
Molding machine
Overhead plane
Powered saw
Radial saw
Sander

Excludes *hand saw (E920.1)*

E919.5 Prime movers, except electrical motors
Gas turbine
Internal combustion engine
Steam engine
Water driven turbine

Excludes *that being towed by other vehicle on the highway (E810.0-E819.9, E827.0-E827.9, E829.0-E829.9)*
that in transport under own power on the highway (E810.0-E819.9)

E919.6 Transmission machinery
Transmission:
belt
cable
chain
gear
Transmission:
pinion
pulley
shaft

E919.7 Earth moving, scraping, and other excavating machines
Bulldozer
Road scraper
Steam shovel

Excludes *that being towed by other vehicle on the highway (E810.0-E819.9)*
that in transport under own power on the highway (E810.0-E819.9)

❑ **E919.8 Other specified machinery**
Machines for manufacture of:
clothing
foodstuffs and beverages
paper
Printing machine
Recreational machinery
Spinning, weaving, and textile machines

❑ **E919.9 Unspecified machinery**

● **E920 Accidents caused by cutting and piercing instruments or objects**

Includes: accidental injury (by) object:
edged
pointed
sharp

E920.0 Powered lawn mower

❑ **E920.1 Other powered hand tools**
Any powered hand tool [compressed air] [electric] [explosive cartridge] [hydraulic power], such as:
drill
hand saw
hedge clipper
rivet gun
snow blower
staple gun

Excludes *band saw (E919.4)*
bench saw (E919.4)

E920.2 Powered household appliances and implements
Blender
Electric:
beater or mixer
can opener
fan
knife
sewing machine
Garbage disposal appliance

E920.3 Knives, swords, and daggers

❑ **E920.4 Other hand tools and implements**
Axe
Can opener NOS
Chisel
Fork
Hand saw

ICD-9-CM E900-E999 Vol. 1

Hoe
Ice pick
Needle (sewing)
Paper cutter
Pitchfork
Rake
Scissors
Screwdriver
Sewing machine, not powered
Shovel

E920.5 Hypodermic needle
Contaminated needle
Needle stick

❑ **E920.8 Other specified cutting and piercing instruments or objects**
Arrow
Broken glass
Dart
Edge of stiff paper
Lathe turnings
Nail
Plant thorn
Splinter
Tin can lid

Excludes *animal spines or quills (E906.8)*
flying glass due to explosion (E921.0-E923.9)

❑ **E920.9 Unspecified cutting and piercing instrument or object**

● **E921 Accident caused by explosion of pressure vessel**

Includes: accidental explosion of pressure vessels, whether or not part of machinery

Excludes *explosion of pressure vessel on transport vehicle (E800.0-E845.9)*

E921.0 Boilers

E921.1 Gas cylinders
Air tank
Pressure gas tank

❑ **E921.8 Other specified pressure vessels**
Aerosol can
Automobile tire
Pressure cooker

❑ **E921.9 Unspecified pressure vessel**

● **E922 Accident caused by firearm and air gun missile**

E922.0 Handgun
Pistol
Revolver

Excludes *Very pistol (E922.8)*

E922.1 Shotgun (automatic)

E922.2 Hunting rifle

E922.3 Military firearms
Army rifle
Machine gun

E922.4 Air gun
BB gun
Pellet gun

E922.5 Paintball gun

❑ **E922.8 Other specified firearm missile**
Very pistol [flare]

❑ **E922.9 Unspecified firearm missile**
Gunshot wound NOS
Shot NOS

● **E923 Accident caused by explosive material**

Includes: flash burns and other injuries resulting from explosion of explosive material
ignition of highly explosive material with explosion

Excludes *explosion:*
in or on machinery (E919.0-E919.9)
on any transport vehicle, except stationary motor vehicle (E800.0-E848)
with conflagration (E890.0, E891.0, E892)
secondary fires resulting from explosion (E890.0-E899)

E923.0 Fireworks

E923.1 Blasting materials
Blasting cap
Detonator
Dynamite
Explosive [any] used in blasting operations

E923.2 Explosive gases
Acetylene
Butane
Coal gas
Explosion in mine NOS
Fire damp
Gasoline fumes
Methane
Propane

❑ **E923.8 Other explosive materials**
Bomb
Explosive missile
Grenade
Mine
Shell
Torpedo
Explosion in munitions:
dump
factory

❑ **E923.9 Unspecified explosive material**
Explosion NOS

● **E924 Accident caused by hot substance or object, caustic or corrosive material, and steam**

Excludes *burning NOS (E899)*
chemical burn resulting from swallowing a corrosive substance (E860.0-E864.4)
fire caused by these substances and objects (E890.0-E894)
radiation burns (E926.0-E926.9)
therapeutic misadventures (E870.0-E876.9)

E924.0 Hot liquids and vapors, including steam
Burning or scalding by:
boiling water
hot or boiling liquids not primarily caustic or corrosive
liquid metal
steam
other hot vapor

Excludes *hot (boiling) tap water (E924.2)*

E924.1 Caustic and corrosive substances
Burning by:
acid [any kind]
ammonia
caustic oven cleaner or other substance
corrosive substance
lye
vitriol

E924.2 Hot (boiling) tap water

❑ **E924.8 Other**
Burning by:
heat from electric heating appliance
hot object NOS
light bulb
steam pipe

❑ **E924.9 Unspecified**

● **E925 Accident caused by electric current**

Includes: electric current from exposed wire, faulty appliance, high voltage cable, live rail, or open electric socket as the cause of:
burn
cardiac fibrillation
convulsion
electric shock
electrocution
puncture wound
respiratory paralysis

Excludes *burn by heat from electrical appliance (E924.8)*
lightning (E907)

E925.0 Domestic wiring and appliances

E925.1 Electric power generating plants, distribution stations, transmission lines
Broken power line

E925.2 Industrial wiring, appliances, and electrical machinery
Conductors
Control apparatus
Electrical equipment and machinery
Transformers

❑ **E925.8 Other electric current**
Wiring and appliances in or on:
farm [not farmhouse]
outdoors
public building
residential institutions
schools

❑ **E925.9 Unspecified electric current**
Burns or other injury from electric current NOS
Electric shock NOS
Electrocution NOS

● **E926 Exposure to radiation**

Excludes *abnormal reaction to or complication of treatment without mention of misadventure (E879.2)*
atomic power plant malfunction in water transport (E838.0-E838.9)
misadventure to patient in surgical and medical procedures (E873.2-E873.3)
use of radiation in war operations (E996-E997.9)

E926.0 Radiofrequency radiation
Overexposure to:
microwave radiation from:
high-powered radio and television transmitters
industrial radiofrequency induction heaters
radar installations
radar radiation from:
high-powered radio and television transmitters
industrial radiofrequency induction heaters
radar installations
radiofrequency from:
high-powered radio and television transmitters
industrial radiofrequency induction heaters
radar installations
radiofrequency radiation [any] from:
high-powered radio and television transmitters
industrial radiofrequency induction heaters
radar installations

E926.1 Infra-red heaters and lamps
Exposure to infra-red radiation from heaters and lamps as the cause of:
blistering
burning
charring
inflammatory change

Excludes *physical contact with heater or lamp (E924.8)*

E926.2 Visible and ultraviolet light sources
Arc lamps
Black light sources
Electrical welding arc
Oxygas welding torch
Sun rays
Tanning bed

Excludes *excessive heat from these sources (E900.1-E900.9)*

E926.3 X-rays and other electromagnetic ionizing radiation
Gamma rays
X-rays (hard) (soft)

E926.4 Lasers

E926.5 Radioactive isotopes
Radiobiologicals
Radiopharmaceuticals

❑ **E926.8 Other specified radiation**
Artificially accelerated beams of ionized particles generated by:
betatrons
synchrotrons

❑ **E926.9 Unspecified radiation**
Radiation NOS

E927 Overexertion and strenuous movements
Excessive physical exercise
Overexertion (from):
lifting
pulling
pushing
Strenuous movements in:
recreational activities
other activities

● **E928 Other and unspecified environmental and accidental causes**

E928.0 Prolonged stay in weightless environment
Weightlessness in spacecraft (simulator)

E928.1 Exposure to noise
Noise (pollution)
Sound waves
Supersonic waves

E928.2 Vibration

E928.3 Human bite

E928.4 External constriction caused by hair ◀

E928.5 External constriction caused by other object ◀

❑ **E928.8 Other**

❑ **E928.9 Unspecified accident**
Accident NOS stated as accidentally inflicted
Blow NOS stated as accidentally inflicted
Casualty (not due to war) stated as accidentally inflicted
Decapitation stated as accidentally inflicted
Injury [any part of body, or unspecified] stated as accidentally inflicted, but not otherwise specified
Killed stated as accidentally inflicted, but not otherwise specified
Knocked down stated as accidentally inflicted, but not otherwise specified
Mangled stated as accidentally inflicted, but not otherwise specified
Wound stated as accidentally inflicted, but not otherwise specified

Excludes *fracture, cause unspecified (E887)*
injuries undetermined whether accidentally or purposely inflicted (E980.0-E989)

LATE EFFECTS OF ACCIDENTAL INJURY (E929)

Note: This category is to be used to indicate accidental injury as the cause of death or disability from late effects, which are themselves classifiable elsewhere. The "late effects" include conditions reported as such or as sequelae, which may occur at any time after the acute accidental injury.

● **E929 Late effects of accidental injury**

Excludes *late effects of:*
surgical and medical procedures (E870.0-E879.9)
therapeutic use of drugs and medicines (E930.0-E949.9)

E929.0 Late effects of motor vehicle accident
Late effects of accidents classifiable to E810-E825

❑ **E929.1 Late effects of other transport accident**
Late effects of accidents classifiable to E800-E807, E826-E838, E840-E848

E929.2 Late effects of accidental poisoning
Late effects of accidents classifiable to E850-E858, E860-E869

E929.3 Late effects of accidental fall
Late effects of accidents classifiable to E880-E888

E929.4 Late effects of accident caused by fire
Late effects of accidents classifiable to E890-E899

E929.5 Late effects of accident due to natural and environmental factors
Late effects of accidents classifiable to E900-E909

❑ **E929.8 Late effects of other accidents**
Late effects of accidents classifiable to E910-E928.8

❑ **E929.9 Late effects of unspecified accident**
Late effects of accidents classifiable to E928.9

DRUGS, MEDICINAL AND BIOLOGICAL SUBSTANCES CAUSING ADVERSE EFFECTS IN THERAPEUTIC USE (E930-E949)

Includes: correct drug properly administered in therapeutic or prophylactic dosage, as the cause of any adverse effect including allergic or hypersensitivity reactions

Excludes *accidental overdose of drug and wrong drug given or taken in error (E850.0-E858.9)*
accidents in the technique of administration of drug or biological substance such as accidental puncture during injection, or contamination of drug (E870.0-E876.9)
administration with suicidal or homicidal intent or intent to harm, or in circumstances classifiable to E980-E989 (E950.0-E950.5, E962.0, E980.0-E980.5)
See Alphabetic Index for more complete list of specific drugs to be classified under the fourth-digit subdivisions. The American Hospital Formulary numbers can be used to classify new drugs listed by the American Hospital Formulary Service (AHFS). See appendix C.

● **E930 Antibiotics**

Excludes *that used as eye, ear, nose, and throat [ENT], and local anti-infectives (E946.0-E946.9)*

E930.0 Penicillins
Natural
Synthetic
Semisynthetic, such as:
ampicillin
cloxacillin
nafcillin
oxacillin

E930.1 Antifungal antibiotics
Amphotericin B
Griseofulvin
Hachimycin [trichomycin]
Nystatin

E930.2 Chloramphenicol group
Chloramphenicol
Thiamphenicol

E930.3 Erythromycin and other macrolides
Oleandomycin
Spiramycin

E930.4 Tetracycline group
Doxycycline
Minocycline
Oxytetracycline

E930.5 Cephalosporin group
Cephalexin
Cephaloglycin
Cephaloridine
Cephalothin

E930.6 Antimycobacterial antibiotics
Cycloserine
Kanamycin
Rifampin
Streptomycin

E930.7 Antineoplastic antibiotics
Actinomycins, such as:
Bleomycin
Cactinomycin
Dactinomycin
Daunorubicin
Mitomycin

Excludes *other antineoplastic drugs (E933.1)*

❑ E930.8 **Other specified antibiotics**

❑ E930.9 **Unspecified antibiotic**

● E931 **Other anti-infectives**

Excludes *ENT, and local anti-infectives (E946.0-E946.9)*

E931.0 **Sulfonamides**
Sulfadiazine
Sulfafurazole
Sulfamethoxazole

E931.1 **Arsenical anti-infectives**

E931.2 **Heavy metal anti-infectives**
Compounds of:
antimony
bismuth
lead
mercury

Excludes *mercurial diuretics (E944.0)*

E931.3 **Quinoline and hydroxyquinoline derivatives**
Chiniofon
Diiodohydroxyquin

Excludes *antimalarial drugs (E931.4)*

E931.4 **Antimalarials and drugs acting on other blood protozoa**
Chloroquine phosphate
Cycloguanil
Primaquine
Proguanil [chloroguanide]
Pyrimethamine
Quinine (sulphate)

❑ E931.5 **Other antiprotozoal drugs**
Emetine

E931.6 **Anthelmintics**
Hexylresorcinol
Male fern oleoresin
Piperazine
Thiabendazole

E931.7 **Antiviral drugs**
Methisazone

Excludes *amantadine (E936.4)*
cytarabine (E933.1)
idoxuridine (E946.5)

❑ E931.8 **Other antimycobacterial drugs**
Ethambutol
Ethionamide
Isoniazid
Para-aminosalicylic acid derivatives
Sulfones

❑ E931.9 **Other and unspecified anti-infectives**
Flucytosine
Nitrofuran derivatives

● E932 **Hormones and synthetic substitutes**

E932.0 **Adrenal cortical steroids**
Cortisone derivatives
Desoxycorticosterone derivatives
Fluorinated corticosteroids

E932.1 **Androgens and anabolic congeners**
Nandrolone phenpropionate
Oxymetholone
Testosterone and preparations

E932.2 **Ovarian hormones and synthetic substitutes**
Contraceptives, oral
Estrogens
Estrogens and progestogens combined
Progestogens

E932.3 **Insulins and antidiabetic agents**
Acetohexamide
Biguanide derivatives, oral
Chlorpropamide
Glucagon
Insulin
Phenformin
Sulfonylurea derivatives, oral
Tolbutamide

Excludes *adverse effect of insulin administered for shock therapy (E879.3)*

E932.4 **Anterior pituitary hormones**
Corticotropin
Gonadotropin
Somatotropin [growth hormone]

E932.5 **Posterior pituitary hormones**
Vasopressin

Excludes *oxytocic agents (E945.0)*

E932.6 **Parathyroid and parathyroid derivatives**

E932.7 **Thyroid and thyroid derivatives**
Dextrothyroxine
Levothyroxine sodium
Liothyronine
Thyroglobulin

E932.8 **Antithyroid agents**
Iodides
Thiouracil
Thiourea

❑ E932.9 **Other and unspecified hormones and synthetic substitutes**

● E933 **Primarily systemic agents**

E933.0 **Antiallergic and antiemetic drugs**
Antihistamines
Chlorpheniramine
Diphenhydramine
Diphenylpyraline
Thonzylamine
Tripelennamine

Excludes *phenothiazine-based tranquilizers (E939.1)*

E933.1 **Antineoplastic and immunosuppressive drugs**
Azathioprine
Busulfan
Chlorambucil
Cyclophosphamide
Cytarabine
Fluorouracil
Mechlorethamine hydrochloride
Mercaptopurine
Triethylenethiophosphoramide [thio-TEPA]

Excludes *antineoplastic antibiotics (E930.7)*

E933.2 **Acidifying agents**

E933.3 **Alkalizing agents**

E933.4 **Enzymes, not elsewhere classified**
Penicillinase

E933.5 **Vitamins, not elsewhere classified**
Vitamin A
Vitamin D

Excludes *nicotinic acid (E942.2)*
vitamin K (E934.3)

❑ E933.8 **Other systemic agents, not elsewhere classified**
Heavy metal antagonists

❑ E933.9 **Unspecified systemic agent**

ICD-9-CM E900-E999 Vol. 1

● **E934 Agents primarily affecting blood constituents**

E934.0 Iron and its compounds
Ferric salts
Ferrous sulphate and other ferrous salts

❑ **E934.1 Liver preparations and other antianemic agents**
Folic acid

E934.2 Anticoagulants
Coumarin
Heparin
Phenindione
Prothrombin synthesis inhibitor
Warfarin sodium

E934.3 Vitamin K [phytonadione]

E934.4 Fibrinolysis-affecting drugs
Aminocaproic acid
Streptodornase
Streptokinase
Urokinase

❑ **E934.5 Anticoagulant antagonists and other coagulants**
Hexadimethrine bromide
Protamine sulfate

E934.6 Gamma globulin

E934.7 Natural blood and blood products
Blood plasma
Human fibrinogen
Packed red cells
Whole blood

❑ **E934.8 Other agents affecting blood constituents**
Macromolecular blood substitutes

❑ **E934.9 Unspecified agent affecting blood constituents**

● **E935 Analgesics, antipyretics, and antirheumatics**

E935.0 Heroin
Diacetylmorphine

E935.1 Methadone

❑ **E935.2 Other opiates and related narcotics**
Codeine [methylmorphine]
Morphine
Opium (alkaloids)
Meperidine [pethidine]

E935.3 Salicylates
Acetylsalicylic acid [aspirin]
Amino derivatives of salicylic acid
Salicylic acid salts

E935.4 Aromatic analgesics, not elsewhere classified
Acetanilid
Paracetamol [acetaminophen]
Phenacetin [acetophenetidin]

E935.5 Pyrazole derivatives
Aminophenazone [aminopyrine]
Phenylbutazone

E935.6 Antirheumatics [antiphlogistics]
Gold salts
Indomethacin

Excludes *salicylates (E935.3)*
steroids (E932.0)

❑ **E935.7 Other non-narcotic analgesics**
Pyrabital

❑ **E935.8 Other specified analgesics and antipyretics**
Pentazocine

❑ **E935.9 Unspecified analgesic and antipyretic**

● **E936 Anticonvulsants and anti-Parkinsonism drugs**

E936.0 Oxazolidine derivatives
Paramethadione
Trimethadione

E936.1 Hydantoin derivatives
Phenytoin

E936.2 Succinimides
Ethosuximide
Phensuximide

❑ **E936.3 Other and unspecified anticonvulsants**
Beclamide
Primidone

E936.4 Anti-Parkinsonism drugs
Amantadine
Ethopropazine [profenamine]
Levodopa [L-dopa]

● **E937 Sedatives and hypnotics**

E937.0 Barbiturates
Amobarbital [amylobarbitone]
Barbital [barbitone]
Butabarbital [butabarbitone]
Pentobarbital [pentobarbitone]
Phenobarbital [phenobarbitone]
Secobarbital [quinalbarbitone]

Excludes *thiobarbiturates (E938.3)*

E937.1 Chloral hydrate group

E937.2 Paraldehyde

E937.3 Bromine compounds
Bromide
Carbromal (derivatives)

E937.4 Methaqualone compounds

E937.5 Glutethimide group

E937.6 Mixed sedatives, not elsewhere classified

❑ **E937.8 Other sedatives and hypnotics**

❑ **E937.9 Unspecified**
Sleeping:
drug NOS
pill NOS
tablet NOS

● **E938 Other central nervous system depressants and anesthetics**

E938.0 Central nervous system muscle-tone depressants
Chlorphenesin (carbamate)
Mephenesin
Methocarbamol

E938.1 Halothane

❑ **E938.2 Other gaseous anesthetics**
Ether
Halogenated hydrocarbon derivatives, except halothane
Nitrous oxide

E938.3 Intravenous anesthetics
Ketamine
Methohexital [methohexitone]
Thiobarbiturates, such as thiopental sodium

❑ **E938.4 Other and unspecified general anesthetics**

E938.5 Surface and infiltration anesthetics
Cocaine
Lidocaine [lignocaine]
Procaine
Tetracaine

E938.6 Peripheral nerve- and plexus-blocking anesthetics

E938.7 Spinal anesthetics

❑ **E938.9 Other and unspecified local anesthetics**

● **E939 Psychotropic agents**

E939.0 Antidepressants
Amitriptyline
Imipramine
Monoamine oxidase [MAO] inhibitors

E939.1 Phenothiazine-based tranquilizers
Chlorpromazine
Fluphenazine
Phenothiazine
Prochlorperazine
Promazine

E939.2 Butyrophenone-based tranquilizers
Haloperidol
Spiperone
Trifluperidol

❑ **E939.3 Other antipsychotics, neuroleptics, and major tranquilizers**

E939.4 Benzodiazepine-based tranquilizers
Chlordiazepoxide
Diazepam
Flurazepam
Lorazepam
Medazepam
Nitrazepam

❑ **E939.5 Other tranquilizers**
Hydroxyzine
Meprobamate

E939.6 Psychodysleptics [hallucinogens]
Cannabis (derivatives)
Lysergide [LSD]
Marihuana (derivatives)
Mescaline
Psilocin
Psilocybin

E939.7 Psychostimulants
Amphetamine
Caffeine

Excludes *central appetite depressants (E947.0)*

❑ **E939.8 Other psychotropic agents**

❑ **E939.9 Unspecified psychotropic agent**

● **E940 Central nervous system stimulants**

E940.0 Analeptics
Lobeline
Nikethamide

E940.1 Opiate antagonists
Levallorphan
Nalorphine
Naloxone

❑ **E940.8 Other specified central nervous system stimulants**

❑ **E940.9 Unspecified central nervous system stimulant**

● **E941 Drugs primarily affecting the autonomic nervous system**

E941.0 Parasympathomimetics [cholinergics]
Acetylcholine
Anticholinesterase:
organophosphorus
reversible
Pilocarpine

E941.1 Parasympatholytics [anticholinergics and antimuscarinics] and spasmolytics
Atropine
Homatropine
Hyoscine [scopolamine]
Quaternary ammonium derivatives

Excludes *papaverine (E942.5)*

E941.2 Sympathomimetics [adrenergics]
Epinephrine [adrenalin]
Levarterenol [noradrenalin]

E941.3 Sympatholytics [antiadrenergics]
Phenoxybenzamine
Tolazoline hydrochloride

❑ **E941.9 Unspecified drug primarily affecting the autonomic nervous system**

● **E942 Agents primarily affecting the cardiovascular system**

E942.0 Cardiac rhythm regulators
Practolol
Procainamide
Propranolol
Quinidine

E942.1 Cardiotonic glycosides and drugs of similar action
Digitalis glycosides
Digoxin
Strophanthins

E942.2 Antilipemic and antiarteriosclerotic drugs
Cholestyramine
Clofibrate
Nicotinic acid derivatives
Sitosterols

Excludes *dextrothyroxine (E932.7)*

E942.3 Ganglion-blocking agents
Pentamethonium bromide

E942.4 Coronary vasodilators
Dipyridamole
Nitrates [nitroglycerin]
Nitrites
Prenylamine

❑ **E942.5 Other vasodilators**
Cyclandelate
Diazoxide
Hydralazine
Papaverine

❑ **E942.6 Other antihypertensive agents**
Clonidine
Guanethidine
Rauwolfia alkaloids
Reserpine

E942.7 Antivaricose drugs, including sclerosing agents
Monoethanolamine
Zinc salts

ICD-9-CM E900-E999 Vol. 1

E942.8 **Capillary-active drugs**
Adrenochrome derivatives
Bioflavonoids
Metaraminol

❑ E942.9 **Other and unspecified agents primarily affecting the cardiovascular system**

● E943 **Agents primarily affecting gastrointestinal system**

E943.0 **Antacids and antigastric secretion drugs**
Aluminum hydroxide
Magnesium trisilicate

E943.1 **Irritant cathartics**
Bisacodyl
Castor oil
Phenolphthalein

E943.2 **Emollient cathartics**
Sodium dioctyl sulfosuccinate

❑ E943.3 **Other cathartics, including intestinal atonia drugs**
Magnesium sulfate

E943.4 **Digestants**
Pancreatin
Papain
Pepsin

E943.5 **Antidiarrheal drugs**
Bismuth subcarbonate
Kaolin
Pectin

Excludes *anti-infectives (E930.0-E931.9)*

E943.6 **Emetics**

❑ E943.8 **Other specified agents primarily affecting the gastrointestinal system**

❑ E943.9 **Unspecified agent primarily affecting the gastrointestinal system**

● E944 **Water, mineral, and uric acid metabolism drugs**

E944.0 **Mercurial diuretics**
Chlormerodrin
Mercaptomerin
Mercurophylline
Mersalyl

E944.1 **Purine derivative diuretics**
Theobromine
Theophylline

Excludes *aminophylline [theophylline ethylenediamine] (E945.7)*

E944.2 **Carbonic acid anhydrase inhibitors**
Acetazolamide

E944.3 **Saluretics**
Benzothiadiazides
Chlorothiazide group

❑ E944.4 **Other diuretics**
Ethacrynic acid
Furosemide

E944.5 **Electrolytic, caloric, and water-balance agents**

❑ E944.6 **Other mineral salts, not elsewhere classified**

E944.7 **Uric acid metabolism drugs**
Cinchophen and congeners
Colchicine
Phenoquin
Probenecid

● E945 **Agents primarily acting on the smooth and skeletal muscles and respiratory system**

E945.0 **Oxytocic agents**
Ergot alkaloids
Prostaglandins

E945.1 **Smooth muscle relaxants**
Adiphenine
Metaproterenol [orciprenaline]

Excludes *papaverine (E942.5)*

E945.2 **Skeletal muscle relaxants**
Alcuronium chloride
Suxamethonium chloride

❑ E945.3 **Other and unspecified drugs acting on muscles**

E945.4 **Antitussives**
Dextromethorphan
Pipazethate hydrochloride

E945.5 **Expectorants**
Acetylcysteine
Cocillana
Guaifenesin [glyceryl guaiacolate]
Ipecacuanha
Terpin hydrate

E945.6 **Anti-common cold drugs**

E945.7 **Antiasthmatics**
Aminophylline [theophylline ethylenediamine]

❑ E945.8 **Other and unspecified respiratory drugs**

● E946 **Agents primarily affecting skin and mucous membrane, ophthalmological, otorhinolaryngological, and dental drugs**

E946.0 **Local anti-infectives and anti-inflammatory drugs**

E946.1 **Antipruritics**

E946.2 **Local astringents and local detergents**

E946.3 **Emollients, demulcents, and protectants**

E946.4 **Keratolytics, keratoplastics, other hair treatment drugs and preparations**

E946.5 **Eye anti-infectives and other eye drugs**
Idoxuridine

E946.6 **Anti-infectives and other drugs and preparations for ear, nose, and throat**

E946.7 **Dental drugs topically applied**

❑ E946.8 **Other agents primarily affecting skin and mucous membrane**
Spermicides

❑ E946.9 **Unspecified agent primarily affecting skin and mucous membrane**

● E947 **Other and unspecified drugs and medicinal substances**

E947.0 **Dietetics**

E947.1 **Lipotropic drugs**

E947.2 **Antidotes and chelating agents, not elsewhere classified**

E947.3 **Alcohol deterrents**

E947.4 **Pharmaceutical excipients**

❑ **E947.8 Other drugs and medicinal substances**
Contrast media used for diagnostic x-ray procedures
Diagnostic agents and kits

❑ **E947.9 Unspecified drug or medicinal substance**

● **E948 Bacterial vaccines**

E948.0 BCG vaccine

E948.1 Typhoid and paratyphoid

E948.2 Cholera

E948.3 Plague

E948.4 Tetanus

E948.5 Diphtheria

E948.6 Pertussis vaccine, including combinations with a pertussis component

❑ **E948.8 Other and unspecified bacterial vaccines**

E948.9 Mixed bacterial vaccines, except combinations with a pertussis component

● **E949 Other vaccines and biological substances**

Excludes *gamma globulin (E934.6)*

E949.0 Smallpox vaccine

E949.1 Rabies vaccine

E949.2 Typhus vaccine

E949.3 Yellow fever vaccine

E949.4 Measles vaccine

E949.5 Poliomyelitis vaccine

❑ **E949.6 Other and unspecified viral and rickettsial vaccines**
Mumps vaccine

E949.7 Mixed viral-rickettsial and bacterial vaccines, except combinations with a pertussis component

Excludes *combinations with a pertussis component (E948.6)*

❑ **E949.9 Other and unspecified vaccines and biological substances**

SUICIDE AND SELF-INFLICTED INJURY (E950-E959)

Includes: injuries in suicide and attempted suicide
self-inflicted injuries specified as intentional

● **E950 Suicide and self-inflicted poisoning by solid or liquid substances**

E950.0 Analgesics, antipyretics, and antirheumatics

E950.1 Barbiturates

❑ **E950.2 Other sedatives and hypnotics**

E950.3 Tranquilizers and other psychotropic agents

❑ **E950.4 Other specified drugs and medicinal substances**

❑ **E950.5 Unspecified drug or medicinal substance**

E950.6 Agricultural and horticultural chemical and pharmaceutical preparations other than plant foods and fertilizers

E950.7 Corrosive and caustic substances
Suicide and self-inflicted poisoning by substances classifiable to E864

E950.8 Arsenic and its compounds

❑ **E950.9 Other and unspecified solid and liquid substances**

● **E951 Suicide and self-inflicted poisoning by gases in domestic use**

E951.0 Gas distributed by pipeline

E951.1 Liquefied petroleum gas distributed in mobile containers

❑ **E951.8 Other utility gas**

● **E952 Suicide and self-inflicted poisoning by other gases and vapors**

E952.0 Motor vehicle exhaust gas

❑ **E952.1 Other carbon monoxide**

❑ **E952.8 Other specified gases and vapors**

❑ **E952.9 Unspecified gases and vapors**

● **E953 Suicide and self-inflicted injury by hanging, strangulation, and suffocation**

E953.0 Hanging

E953.1 Suffocation by plastic bag

❑ **E953.8 Other specified means**

❑ **E953.9 Unspecified means**

E954 Suicide and self-inflicted injury by submersion [drowning]

● **E955 Suicide and self-inflicted injury by firearms, air guns and explosives**

E955.0 Handgun

E955.1 Shotgun

E955.2 Hunting rifle

E955.3 Military firearms

❑ **E955.4 Other and unspecified firearm**
Gunshot NOS
Shot NOS

E955.5 Explosives

E955.6 Air gun
BB gun
Pellet gun

E955.7 Paintball gun

❑ **E955.9 Unspecified**

E956 Suicide and self-inflicted injury by cutting and piercing instrument

● **E957 Suicide and self-inflicted injuries by jumping from high place**

E957.0 Residential premises

❑ **E957.1 Other man-made structures**

E957.2 Natural sites

❑ **E957.9 Unspecified**

● **E958 Suicide and self-inflicted injury by other and unspecified means**

E958.0 Jumping or lying before moving object

E958.1 Burns, fire

E958.2 Scald

E958.3 Extremes of cold

E958.4 Electrocution

E958.5 Crashing of motor vehicle

E958.6 Crashing of aircraft

E958.7 Caustic substances, except poisoning

Excludes *poisoning by caustic substance (E950.7)*

❑E958.8 Other specified means

❑E958.9 Unspecified means

E959 Late effects of self-inflicted injury

Note: This category is to be used to indicate circumstances classifiable to E950-E958 as the cause of death or disability from late effects, which are themselves classifiable elsewhere. The "late effects" include conditions reported as such or as sequelae which may occur at any time after the attempted suicide or self-inflicted injury.

HOMICIDE AND INJURY PURPOSELY INFLICTED BY OTHER PERSONS (E960-E969)

Includes: injuries inflicted by another person with intent to injure or kill, by any means

Excludes *injuries due to:*
legal intervention (E970-E978)
operations of war (E990-E999)
terrorism (E979)

●**E960 Fight, brawl, rape**

E960.0 Unarmed fight or brawl
Beatings NOS
Brawl or fight with hands, fists, feet
Injured or killed in fight NOS

Excludes *homicidal:*
injury by weapons (E965.0-E966, E969)
strangulation (E963)
submersion (E964)

E960.1 Rape

E961 Assault by corrosive or caustic substance, except poisoning
Injury or death purposely caused by corrosive or caustic substance, such as:
acid [any]
corrosive substance
vitriol

Excludes *burns from hot liquid (E968.3)*
chemical burns from swallowing a corrosive substance (E962.0-E962.9)

●**E962 Assault by poisoning**

E962.0 Drugs and medicinal substances
Homicidal poisoning by any drug or medicinal substance

❑**E962.1 Other solid and liquid substances**

❑**E962.2 Other gases and vapors**

❑**E962.9 Unspecified poisoning**

E963 Assault by hanging and strangulation
Homicidal (attempt):
garrotting or ligature
hanging
strangulation
suffocation

E964 Assault by submersion [drowning]

●**E965 Assault by firearms and explosives**

E965.0 Handgun
Pistol
Revolver

E965.1 Shotgun

E965.2 Hunting rifle

E965.3 Military firearms

❑**E965.4 Other and unspecified firearm**

E965.5 Antipersonnel bomb

E965.6 Gasoline bomb

E965.7 Letter bomb

❑**E965.8 Other specified explosive**
Bomb NOS (placed in):
car
house
Dynamite

❑**E965.9 Unspecified explosive**

E966 Assault by cutting and piercing instrument
Assassination (attempt), homicide (attempt) by any instrument classifiable under E920
Homicidal:
cut any part of body
puncture any part of body
stab any part of body
Stabbed any part of body

●**E967 Perpetrator of child and adult abuse**

Note: selection of the correct perpetrator code is based on the relationship between the perpetrator and the victim

E967.0 By father, stepfather, or boyfriend
Male partner of child's parent or guardian

❑**E967.1 By other specified person**

E967.2 By mother, stepmother, or girlfriend
Female partner of child's parent or guardian

E967.3 By spouse or partner
Abuse of spouse or partner by ex-spouse or ex-partner

E967.4 By child

E967.5 By sibling

E967.6 By grandparent

❑**E967.7 By other relative**

❑**E967.8 By non-related caregiver**

❑**E967.9 By unspecified person**

●**E968 Assault by other and unspecified means**

E968.0 Fire
Arson
Homicidal burns NOS

Excludes *burns from hot liquid (E968.3)*

E968.1 Pushing from a high place

E968.2 Striking by blunt or thrown object

E968.3 Hot liquid
Homicidal burns by scalding

E968.4 Criminal neglect
Abandonment of child, infant, or other helpless person with intent to injure or kill

E968.5 Transport vehicle
Being struck by other vehicle or run down with intent to injure
Pushed in front of, thrown from, or dragged by moving vehicle with intent to injure

E968.6 Air gun
BB gun
Pellet gun

E968.7 Human bite

❑**E968.8 Other specified means**

❑ **E968.9 Unspecified means**
Assassination (attempt) NOS
Homicidal (attempt):
injury NOS
wound NOS
Manslaughter (nonaccidental)
Murder (attempt) NOS
Violence, non-accidental

E969 Late effects of injury purposely inflicted by other person

Note: This category is to be used to indicate circumstances classifiable to E960-E968 as the cause of death or disability from late effects, which are themselves classifiable elsewhere. The "late effects" include conditions reported as such, or as sequelae which may occur at any time after the injury purposely inflicted by another person.

LEGAL INTERVENTION (E970-E978)

Includes: injuries inflicted by the police or other law-enforcing agents, including military on duty, in the course of arresting or attempting to arrest lawbreakers, suppressing disturbances, maintaining order, and other legal action
legal execution

Excludes *injuries caused by civil insurrections (E990.0-E999)*

E970 Injury due to legal intervention by firearms
Gunshot wound
Injury by:
machine gun
revolver
rifle pellet or rubber bullet
shot NOS

E971 Injury due to legal intervention by explosives
Injury by:
dynamite
explosive shell
grenade
motor bomb

E972 Injury due to legal intervention by gas
Asphyxiation by gas
Injury by tear gas
Poisoning by gas

E973 Injury due to legal intervention by blunt object
Hit, struck by:
baton (nightstick)
blunt object
stave

E974 Injury due to legal intervention by cutting and piercing instrument
Cut
Incised wound
Injured by bayonet
Stab wound

❑ **E975 Injury due to legal intervention by other specified means**
Blow
Manhandling

❑ **E976 Injury due to legal intervention by unspecified means**

E977 Late effects of injuries due to legal intervention

Note: This category is to be used to indicate circumstances classifiable to E970-E976 as the cause of death or disability from late effects, which are themselves classifiable elsewhere. The "late effects" include conditions reported as such, or as sequelae which may occur at any time after the injury due to legal intervention.

E978 Legal execution
All executions performed at the behest of the judiciary or ruling authority [whether permanent or temporary] as:
asphyxiation by gas
beheading, decapitation (by guillotine)
capital punishment
electrocution
hanging
poisoning
shooting
other specified means

TERRORISM (E979) ◀

● **E979 Terrorism**

Includes: injuries resulting from the unlawful use of force or violence against persons or property to intimidate or coerce a Government, the civilian population, or any segment thereof, in furtherance of political or social objective

E979.0 Terrorism involving explosion of marine weapons
Depth-charge
Marine mine
mine NOS, at sea or in harbour
Sea-based artillery shell
Torpedo
Underwater blast

E979.1 Terrorism involving destruction of aircraft
Aircraft used as a weapon
Aircraft:
burned
exploded
shot down
Crushed by falling aircraft

❑ **E979.2 Terrorism involving other explosions and fragments**
Antipersonnel bomb (fragments)
Blast NOS
Explosion (of):
artillery shell
breech-block
cannon block
mortar bomb
munitions being used in terrorism
NOS
Fragments from:
artillery shell
bomb
grenade
guided missile
land-mine
rocket
shell
shrapnel
Mine NOS

E979.3 Terrorism involving fires, conflagration and hot substances
Burning building or structure
collapse of
fall from
hit by falling object in
jump from
Conflagration NOS
Fire (causing)
Asphyxia
Burns
NOS
Other injury
Melting of fittings and furniture in burning
Petrol bomb
Smouldering building or structure

E979.4 Terrorism involving firearms
Bullet:
carbine
machine gun
pistol
rifle
rubber (rifle)
Pellets (shotgun)

E979.5 Terrorism involving nuclear weapons
Blast effects
Exposure to ionizing radiation from nuclear weapon
Fireball effects
Heat from nuclear weapon
Other direct and secondary effects of nuclear weapons

E979.6 Terrorism involving biological weapons
Anthrax
Cholera
Smallpox

E979.7 Terrorism involving chemical weapons
Gases, fumes, chemicals
Hydrogen cyanide
Phosgene
Sarin

❑ **E979.8 Terrorism involving other means**
Drowning and submersion
Lasers
Piercing or stabbing instruments
Terrorism NOS

❑ **E979.9 Terrorism secondary effects**

Note: This code is for use to identify conditions occurring subsequent to a terrorist attack not those that are due to the initial terrorist act.

Excludes *late effect of terrorist attack (E999.1)*

INJURY UNDETERMINED WHETHER ACCIDENTALLY OR PURPOSELY INFLICTED (E980-E989)

Note: Categories E980-E989 are for use when it is unspecified or it cannot be determined whether the injuries are accidental (unintentional), suicide (attempted), or assault.

● **E980 Poisoning by solid or liquid substances, undetermined whether accidentally or purposely inflicted**

E980.0 Analgesics, antipyretics, and antirheumatics

E980.1 Barbiturates

❑ **E980.2 Other sedatives and hypnotics**

E980.3 Tranquilizers and other psychotropic agents

❑ **E980.4 Other specified drugs and medicinal substances**

❑ **E980.5 Unspecified drug or medicinal substance**

E980.6 Corrosive and caustic substances
Poisoning, undetermined whether accidental or purposeful, by substances classifiable to E864

E980.7 Agricultural and horticultural chemical and pharmaceutical preparations other than plant foods and fertilizers

E980.8 Arsenic and its compounds

❑ **E980.9 Other and unspecified solid and liquid substances**

● **E981 Poisoning by gases in domestic use, undetermined whether accidentally or purposely inflicted**

E981.0 Gas distributed by pipeline

E981.1 Liquefied petroleum gas distributed in mobile containers

❑ **E981.8 Other utility gas**

● **E982 Poisoning by other gases, undetermined whether accidentally or purposely inflicted**

E982.0 Motor vehicle exhaust gas

❑ **E982.1 Other carbon monoxide**

❑ **E982.8 Other specified gases and vapors**

❑ **E982.9 Unspecified gases and vapors**

● **E983 Hanging, strangulation, or suffocation, undetermined whether accidentally or purposely inflicted**

E983.0 Hanging

E983.1 Suffocation by plastic bag

❑ **E983.8 Other specified means**

❑ **E983.9 Unspecified means**

E984 Submersion [drowning], undetermined whether accidentally or purposely inflicted

● **E985 Injury by firearms, air guns and explosives, undetermined whether accidentally or purposely inflicted**

E985.0 Handgun

E985.1 Shotgun

E985.2 Hunting rifle

E985.3 Military firearms

❑ **E985.4 Other and unspecified firearm**

E985.5 Explosives

E985.6 Air gun
BB gun
Pellet gun

E985.7 Paintball gun

E986 Injury by cutting and piercing instruments, undetermined whether accidentally or purposely inflicted

● **E987 Falling from high place, undetermined whether accidentally or purposely inflicted**

E987.0 Residential premises

❑ **E987.1 Other man-made structures**

E987.2 Natural sites

❑ **E987.9 Unspecified site**

● **E988 Injury by other and unspecified means, undetermined whether accidentally or purposely inflicted**

E988.0 Jumping or lying before moving object

E988.1 Burns, fire

E988.2 Scald

E988.3 Extremes of cold

E988.4 Electrocution

E988.5 Crashing of motor vehicle

E988.6 Crashing of aircraft

E988.7 Caustic substances, except poisoning

❑ **E988.8 Other specified means**

❑ **E988.9 Unspecified means**

E989 Late effects of injury, undetermined whether accidentally or purposely inflicted

Note: This category is to be used to indicate circumstances classifiable to E980-E988 as the cause of death or disability from late effects, which are themselves classifiable elsewhere. The "late effects" include conditions reported as such or as sequelae which may occur at any time after injury, undetermined whether accidentally or purposely inflicted.

INJURY RESULTING FROM OPERATIONS OF WAR (E990-E999)

Includes: injuries to military personnel and civilians caused by war and civil insurrections and occurring during the time of war and insurrection

Excludes *accidents during training of military personnel, manufacture of war material and transport, unless attributable to enemy action*

● **E990 Injury due to war operations by fires and conflagrations**

Includes: asphyxia, burns, or other injury originating from fire caused by a fire-producing device or indirectly by any conventional weapon

E990.0 From gasoline bomb

❏ **E990.9 From other and unspecified source**

● **E991 Injury due to war operations by bullets and fragments**

E991.0 Rubber bullets (rifle)

E991.1 Pellets (rifle)

❏ **E991.2 Other bullets**

Bullet [any, except rubber bullets and pellets]
- carbine
- machine gun
- pistol
- rifle
- shotgun

E991.3 Antipersonnel bomb (fragments)

❏ **E991.9 Other and unspecified fragments**

Fragments from:
- artillery shell
- bombs, except antipersonnel
- grenade
- guided missile
- land mine
- rockets
- shell

Shrapnel

E992 Injury due to war operations by explosion of marine weapons

Depth charge
Marine mines
Mine NOS, at sea or in harbor
Sea-based artillery shell
Torpedo
Underwater blast

❏ **E993 Injury due to war operations by other explosion**

Accidental explosion of munitions being used in war
Accidental explosion of own weapons
Air blast NOS
Blast NOS
Explosion NOS
Explosion of:
- artillery shell
- breech block
- cannon block
- mortar bomb

Injury by weapon burst

E994 Injury due to war operations by destruction of aircraft

Airplane:
- burned
- exploded
- shot down

Crushed by falling airplane

❏ **E995 Injury due to war operations by other and unspecified forms of conventional warfare**

Battle wounds
Bayonet injury
Drowned in war operations

E996 Injury due to war operations by nuclear weapons

Blast effects
Exposure to ionizing radiation from nuclear weapons
Fireball effects
Heat
Other direct and secondary effects of nuclear weapons

● **E997 Injury due to war operations by other forms of unconventional warfare**

E997.0 Lasers

E997.1 Biological warfare

E997.2 Gases, fumes, and chemicals

❏ **E997.8 Other specified forms of unconventional warfare**

❏ **E997.9 Unspecified form of unconventional warfare**

E998 Injury due to war operations but occurring after cessation of hostilities

Injuries due to operations of war but occurring after cessation of hostilities by any means classifiable under E990-E997

Injuries by explosion of bombs or mines placed in the course of operations of war, if the explosion occurred after cessation of hostilities

● **E999 Late effect of injury due to war operations and terrorism**

Note: This category is to be used to indicate circumstances classifiable to E979, E990-E998 as the cause of death or disability from late effects, which are themselves classifiable elsewhere. The "late effects" include conditions reported as such or as sequelae which may occur at any time after injury resulting from operations of war or terrorism.

E999.0 Late effect of injury due to war operations

E999.1 Late effect of injury due to terrorism

APPENDIX A

MORPHOLOGY OF NEOPLASMS

The World Health Organization has published an adaptation of the International Classification of Diseases for Oncology (ICD-O). It contains a coded nomenclature for the morphology of neoplasms, which is reproduced here for those who wish to use it in conjunction with Chapter 2 of the International Classification of Diseases, 9th Revision, Clinical Modification.

The morphology code numbers consist of five digits; the first four identify the histological type of the neoplasm and the fifth indicates its behavior. The one-digit behavior code is as follows:

/0 Benign
/1 Uncertain whether benign or malignant
  Borderline malignancy
/2 Carcinoma in situ
  Intraepithelial
  Noninfiltrating
  Noninvasive
/3 Malignant, primary site
/6 Malignant, metastatic site
  Secondary site
/9 Malignant, uncertain whether primary or metastatic site

In the nomenclature below, the morphology code numbers include the behavior code appropriate to the histological type of neoplasm, but this behavior code should be changed if other reported information makes this necessary. For example, "chordoma (M9370/3)" is assumed to be malignant; the term "benign chordoma" should be coded M9370/0. Similarly, "superficial spreading adenocarcinoma (M8143/3)" described as "noninvasive" should be coded M8143/2 and "melanoma (M8720/3)" described as "secondary" should be coded M8720/6.

The following table shows the correspondence between the morphology code and the different sections of Chapter 2:

Morphology Code Histology/Behavior		ICD-9-CM Chapter 2	
Any	0	210-229	Benign neoplasms
M800-M8004	1	239	Neoplasms of unspecified nature
M8010+	1	235-238	Neoplasms of uncertain behavior
Any	2	230-234	Carcinoma in situ
Any	3	140-195 200-208	Malignant neoplasms, stated or presumed to be primary
Any	6	196-198	Malignant neoplasms, stated or presumed to be secondary

The ICD-O behavior digit/9 is inapplicable in an ICD context, since all malignant neoplasms are presumed to be primary (/3) or secondary (/6) according to other information on the medical record.

Only the first-listed term of the full ICD-O morphology nomenclature appears against each code number in the list below. The ICD-9-CM Alphabetical Index (Volume 2), however, includes all the ICD-O synonyms as well as a number of other morphological names still likely to be encountered on medical records but omitted from ICD-O as outdated or otherwise undesirable.

A coding difficulty sometimes arises where a morphological diagnosis contains two qualifying adjectives that have different code numbers. An example is "transitional cell epidermoid carcinomas." "Transitional cell carcinoma NOS" is M8120/3 and "epidermoid carcinoma NOS" is M8070/3. In such circumstances, the higher number (M8120/3 in this example) should be used, as it is usually more specific.

CODED NOMENCLATURE FOR MORPHOLOGY OF NEOPLASMS

M800 **Neoplasms NOS**
M8000/0 *Neoplasm, benign*
M8000/1 *Neoplasm, uncertain whether benign or malignant*
M8000/3 *Neoplasm, malignant*
M8000/6 *Neoplasm, metastatic*
M8000/9 *Neoplasm, malignant, uncertain whether primary or metastatic*
M8001/0 *Tumor cells, benign*
M8001/1 *Tumor cells, uncertain whether benign or malignant*
M8001/3 *Tumor cells, malignant*
M8002/3 *Malignant tumor, small cell type*
M8003/3 *Malignant tumor, giant cell type*
M8004/3 *Malignant tumor, fusiform cell type*

M801-M804 **Epithelial neoplasms NOS**
M8010/0 *Epithelial tumor, benign*
M8010/2 *Carcinoma in situ NOS*
M8010/3 *Carcinoma NOS*
M8010/6 *Carcinoma, metastatic NOS*
M8010/9 *Carcinomatosis*
M8011/0 *Epithelioma, benign*
M8011/3 *Epithelioma, malignant*
M8012/3 *Large cell carcinoma NOS*
M8020/3 *Carcinoma, undifferentiated type NOS*
M8021/3 *Carcinoma, anaplastic type NOS*
M8022/3 *Pleomorphic carcinoma*
M8030/3 *Giant cell and spindle cell carcinoma*
M8031/3 *Giant cell carcinoma*
M8032/3 *Spindle cell carcinoma*
M8033/3 *Pseudosarcomatous carcinoma*
M8034/3 *Polygonal cell carcinoma*
M8035/3 *Spheroidal cell carcinoma*
M8040/1 *Tumorlet*
M8041/3 *Small cell carcinoma NOS*
M8042/3 *Oat cell carcinoma*
M8043/3 *Small cell carcinoma, fusiform cell type*

M805-M808 **Papillary and squamous cell neoplasms**
M8050/0 *Papilloma NOS (except Papilloma of urinary bladder M8120/1)*
M8050/2 *Papillary carcinoma in situ*
M8050/3 *Papillary carcinoma NOS*
M8051/0 *Verrucous papilloma*
M8051/3 *Verrucous carcinoma NOS*
M8052/0 *Squamous cell papilloma*
M8052/3 *Papillary squamous cell carcinoma*
M8053/0 *Inverted papilloma*
M8060/0 *Papillomatosis NOS*
M8070/2 *Squamous cell carcinoma in situ NOS*
M8070/3 *Squamous cell carcinoma NOS*
M8070/6 *Squamous cell carcinoma, metastatic NOS*
M8071/3 *Squamous cell carcinoma, keratinizing type NOS*
M8072/3 *Squamous cell carcinoma, large cell, nonkeratinizing type*
M8073/3 *Squamous cell carcinoma, small cell, nonkeratinizing type*
M8074/3 *Squamous cell carcinoma, spindle cell type*
M8075/3 *Adenoid squamous cell carcinoma*
M8076/2 *Squamous cell carcinoma in situ with questionable stromal invasion*
M8076/3 *Squamous cell carcinoma, microinvasive*
M8080/2 *Queyrat's erythroplasia*
M8081/2 *Bowen's disease*
M8082/3 *Lymphoepithelial carcinoma*

M809-M811 **Basal cell neoplasms**
M8090/1 *Basal cell tumor*
M8090/3 *Basal cell carcinoma NOS*
M8091/3 *Multicentric basal cell carcinoma*
M8092/3 *Basal cell carcinoma, morphea type*
M8093/3 *Basal cell carcinoma, fibroepithelial type*
M8094/3 *Basosquamous carcinoma*
M8095/3 *Metatypical carcinoma*
M8096/0 *Intraepidermal epithelioma of Jadassohn*
M8100/0 *Trichoepithelioma*
M8101/0 *Trichofolliculoma*
M8102/0 *Tricholemmoma*

M8110/0 *Pilomatrixoma*

M812-M813 Transitional cell papillomas and carcinomas

M8120/0 *Transitional cell papilloma NOS*
M8120/1 *Urothelial papilloma*
M8120/2 *Transitional cell carcinoma in situ*
M8120/3 *Transitional cell carcinoma NOS*
M8121/0 *Schneiderian papilloma*
M8121/1 *Transitional cell papilloma, inverted type*
M8121/3 *Schneiderian carcinoma*
M8122/3 *Transitional cell carcinoma, spindle cell type*
M8123/3 *Basaloid carcinoma*
M8124/3 *Cloacogenic carcinoma*
M8130/3 *Papillary transitional cell carcinoma*

M814-M838 Adenomas and adenocarcinomas

M8140/0 *Adenoma NOS*
M8140/1 *Bronchial adenoma NOS*
M8140/2 *Adenocarcinoma in situ*
M8140/3 *Adenocarcinoma NOS*
M8140/6 *Adenocarcinoma, metastatic NOS*
M8141/3 *Scirrhous adenocarcinoma*
M8142/3 *Linitis plastica*
M8143/3 *Superficial spreading adenocarcinoma*
M8144/3 *Adenocarcinoma, intestinal type*
M8145/3 *Carcinoma, diffuse type*
M8146/0 *Monomorphic adenoma*
M8147/0 *Basal cell adenoma*
M8150/0 *Islet cell adenoma*
M8150/3 *Islet cell carcinoma*
M8151/0 *Insulinoma NOS*
M8151/3 *Insulinoma, malignant*
M8152/0 *Glucagonoma NOS*
M8152/3 *Glucagonoma, malignant*
M8153/1 *Gastrinoma NOS*
M8153/3 *Gastrinoma, malignant*
M8154/3 *Mixed islet cell and exocrine adenocarcinoma*
M8160/0 *Bile duct adenoma*
M8160/3 *Cholangiocarcinoma*
M8161/0 *Bile duct cystadenoma*
M8161/3 *Bile duct cystadenocarcinoma*
M8170/0 *Liver cell adenoma*
M8170/3 *Hepatocellular carcinoma NOS*
M8180/0 *Hepatocholangioma, benign*
M8180/3 *Combined hepatocellular carcinoma and cholangiocarcinoma*
M8190/0 *Trabecular adenoma*
M8190/3 *Trabecular adenocarcinoma*
M8191/0 *Embryonal adenoma*
M8200/0 *Eccrine dermal cylindroma*
M8200/3 *Adenoid cystic carcinoma*
M8201/3 *Cribriform carcinoma*
M8210/0 *Adenomatous polyp NOS*
M8210/3 *Adenocarcinoma in adenomatous polyp*
M8211/0 *Tubular adenoma NOS*
M8211/3 *Tubular adenocarcinoma*
M8220/0 *Adenomatous polyposis coli*
M8220/3 *Adenocarcinoma in adenomatous polyposis coli*
M8221/0 *Multiple adenomatous polyps*
M8230/3 *Solid carcinoma NOS*
M8231/3 *Carcinoma simplex*
M8240/1 *Carcinoid tumor NOS*
M8240/3 *Carcinoid tumor, malignant*
M8241/1 *Carcinoid tumor, argentaffin NOS*
M8241/3 *Carcinoid tumor, argentaffin, malignant*
M8242/1 *Carcinoid tumor, nonargentaffin NOS*
M8242/3 *Carcinoid tumor, nonargentaffin, malignant*
M8243/3 *Mucocarcinoid tumor, malignant*
M8244/3 *Composite carcinoid*
M8250/1 *Pulmonary adenomatosis*
M8250/3 *Bronchiolo-alveolar adenocarcinoma*
M8251/0 *Alveolar adenoma*
M8251/3 *Alveolar adenocarcinoma*
M8260/0 *Papillary adenoma NOS*
M8260/3 *Papillary adenocarcinoma NOS*
M8261/1 *Villous adenoma NOS*
M8261/3 *Adenocarcinoma in villous adenoma*
M8262/3 *Villous adenocarcinoma*
M8263/0 *Tubulovillous adenoma*
M8270/0 *Chromophobe adenoma*
M8270/3 *Chromophobe carcinoma*
M8280/0 *Acidophil adenoma*
M8280/3 *Acidophil carcinoma*
M8281/0 *Mixed acidophil-basophil adenoma*
M8281/3 *Mixed acidophil-basophil carcinoma*
M8290/0 *Oxyphilic adenoma*
M8290/3 *Oxyphilic adenocarcinoma*
M8300/0 *Basophil adenoma*
M8300/3 *Basophil carcinoma*
M8310/0 *Clear cell adenoma*
M8310/3 *Clear cell adenocarcinoma NOS*
M8311/1 *Hypernephroid tumor*
M8312/3 *Renal cell carcinoma*
M8313/0 *Clear cell adenofibroma*
M8320/3 *Granular cell carcinoma*
M8321/0 *Chief cell adenoma*
M8322/0 *Water-clear cell adenoma*
M8322/3 *Water-clear cell adenocarcinoma*
M8323/0 *Mixed cell adenoma*
M8323/3 *Mixed cell adenocarcinoma*
M8324/0 *Lipoadenoma*
M8330/0 *Follicular adenoma*
M8330/3 *Follicular adenocarcinoma NOS*
M8331/3 *Follicular adenocarcinoma, well differentiated type*
M8332/3 *Follicular adenocarcinoma, trabecular type*
M8333/0 *Microfollicular adenoma*
M8334/0 *Macrofollicular adenoma*
M8340/3 *Papillary and follicular adenocarcinoma*
M8350/3 *Nonencapsulated sclerosing carcinoma*
M8360/1 *Multiple endocrine adenomas*
M8361/1 *Juxtaglomerular tumor*
M8370/0 *Adrenal cortical adenoma NOS*
M8370/3 *Adrenal cortical carcinoma*
M8371/0 *Adrenal cortical adenoma, compact cell type*
M8372/0 *Adrenal cortical adenoma, heavily pigmented variant*
M8373/0 *Adrenal cortical adenoma, clear cell type*
M8374/0 *Adrenal cortical adenoma, glomerulosa cell type*
M8375/0 *Adrenal cortical adenoma, mixed cell type*
M8380/0 *Endometrioid adenoma NOS*
M8380/1 *Endometrioid adenoma, borderline malignancy*
M8380/3 *Endometrioid carcinoma*
M8381/0 *Endometrioid adenofibroma NOS*
M8381/1 *Endometrioid adenofibroma, borderline malignancy*
M8381/3 *Endometrioid adenofibroma, malignant*

M839-M842 Adnexal and skin appendage neoplasms

M8390/0 *Skin appendage adenoma*
M8390/3 *Skin appendage carcinoma*
M8400/0 *Sweat gland adenoma*
M8400/1 *Sweat gland tumor NOS*
M8400/3 *Sweat gland adenocarcinoma*
M8401/0 *Apocrine adenoma*
M8401/3 *Apocrine adenocarcinoma*
M8402/0 *Eccrine acrospiroma*
M8403/0 *Eccrine spiradenoma*
M8404/0 *Hidrocystoma*
M8405/0 *Papillary hydradenoma*
M8406/0 *Papillary syringadenoma*
M8407/0 *Syringoma NOS*
M8410/0 *Sebaceous adenoma*
M8410/3 *Sebaceous adenocarcinoma*
M8420/0 *Ceruminous adenoma*
M8420/3 *Ceruminous adenocarcinoma*

M843 Mucoepidermoid neoplasms

M8430/1 *Mucoepidermoid tumor*
M8430/3 *Mucoepidermoid carcinoma*

M844-M849 Cystic, mucinous, and serous neoplasms

M8440/0 *Cystadenoma NOS*
M8440/3 *Cystadenocarcinoma NOS*

M8441/0 *Serous cystadenoma NOS*
M8441/1 *Serous cystadenoma, borderline malignancy*
M8441/3 *Serous cystadenocarcinoma NOS*
M8450/0 *Papillary cystadenoma NOS*
M8450/1 *Papillary cystadenoma, borderline malignancy*
M8450/3 *Papillary cystadenocarcinoma NOS*
M8460/0 *Papillary serous cystadenoma NOS*
M8460/1 *Papillary serous cystadenoma, borderline malignancy*
M8460/3 *Papillary serous cystadenocarcinoma*
M8461/0 *Serous surface papilloma NOS*
M8461/1 *Serous surface papilloma, borderline malignancy*
M8461/3 *Serous surface papillary carcinoma*
M8470/0 *Mucinous cystadenoma NOS*
M8470/1 *Mucinous cystadenoma, borderline malignancy*
M8470/3 *Mucinous cystadenocarcinoma NOS*
M8471/0 *Papillary mucinous cystadenoma NOS*
M8471/1 *Papillary mucinous cystadenoma, borderline malignancy*
M8471/3 *Papillary mucinous cystadenocarcinoma*
M8480/0 *Mucinous adenoma*
M8480/3 *Mucinous adenocarcinoma*
M8480/6 *Pseudomyxoma peritonei*
M8481/3 *Mucin-producing adenocarcinoma*
M8490/3 *Signet ring cell carcinoma*
M8490/6 *Metastatic signet ring cell carcinoma*

M850-M854 Ductal, lobular, and medullary neoplasms
M8500/2 *Intraductal carcinoma, noninfiltrating NOS*
M8500/3 *Infiltrating duct carcinoma*
M8501/2 *Comedocarcinoma, noninfiltrating*
M8501/3 *Comedocarcinoma NOS*
M8502/3 *Juvenile carcinoma of the breast*
M8503/0 *Intraductal papilloma*
M8503/2 *Noninfiltrating intraductal papillary adenocarcinoma*
M8504/0 *Intracystic papillary adenoma*
M8504/2 *Noninfiltrating intracystic carcinoma*
M8505/0 *Intraductal papillomatosis NOS*
M8506/0 *Subareolar duct papillomatosis*
M8510/3 *Medullary carcinoma NOS*
M8511/3 *Medullary carcinoma with amyloid stroma*
M8512/3 *Medullary carcinoma with lymphoid stroma*
M8520/2 *Lobular carcinoma in situ*
M8520/3 *Lobular carcinoma NOS*
M8521/3 *Infiltrating ductular carcinoma*
M8530/3 *Inflammatory carcinoma*
M8540/3 *Paget's disease, mammary*
M8541/3 *Paget's disease and infiltrating duct carcinoma of breast*
M8542/3 *Paget's disease, extramammary (except Paget's disease of bone)*

M855 Acinar cell neoplasms
M8550/0 *Acinar cell adenoma*
M8550/1 *Acinar cell tumor*
M8550/3 *Acinar cell carcinoma*

M856-M858 Complex epithelial neoplasms
M8560/3 *Adenosquamous carcinoma*
M8561/0 *Adenolymphoma*
M8570/3 *Adenocarcinoma with squamous metaplasia*
M8571/3 *Adenocarcinoma with cartilaginous and osseous metaplasia*
M8572/3 *Adenocarcinoma with spindle cell metaplasia*
M8573/3 *Adenocarcinoma with apocrine metaplasia*
M8580/0 *Thymoma, benign*
M8580/3 *Thymoma, malignant*

M859-M867 Specialized gonadal neoplasms
M8590/1 *Sex cord-stromal tumor*
M8600/0 *Thecoma NOS*
M8600/3 *Theca cell carcinoma*
M8610/0 *Luteoma NOS*
M8620/1 *Granulosa cell tumor NOS*
M8620/3 *Granulosa cell tumor, malignant*
M8621/1 *Granulosa cell-theca cell tumor*
M8630/0 *Androblastoma, benign*
M8630/1 *Androblastoma NOS*
M8630/3 *Androblastoma, malignant*
M8631/0 *Sertoli-Leydig cell tumor*
M8632/1 *Gynandroblastoma*
M8640/0 *Tubular androblastoma NOS*
M8640/3 *Sertoli cell carcinoma*
M8641/0 *Tubular androblastoma with lipid storage*
M8650/0 *Leydig cell tumor, benign*
M8650/1 *Leydig cell tumor NOS*
M8650/3 *Leydig cell tumor, malignant*
M8660/0 *Hilar cell tumor*
M8670/0 *Lipid cell tumor of ovary*
M8671/0 *Adrenal rest tumor*

M868-M871 Paragangliomas and glomus tumors
M8680/1 *Paraganglioma NOS*
M8680/3 *Paraganglioma, malignant*
M8681/1 *Sympathetic paraganglioma*
M8682/1 *Parasympathetic paraganglioma*
M8690/1 *Glomus jugulare tumor*
M8691/1 *Aortic body tumor*
M8692/1 *Carotid body tumor*
M8693/1 *Extra-adrenal paraganglioma NOS*
M8693/3 *Extra-adrenal paraganglioma, malignant*
M8700/0 *Pheochromocytoma NOS*
M8700/3 *Pheochromocytoma, malignant*
M8710/3 *Glomangiosarcoma*
M8711/0 *Glomus tumor*
M8712/0 *Glomangioma*

M872-M879 Nevi and melanomas
M8720/0 *Pigmented nevus NOS*
M8720/3 *Malignant melanoma NOS*
M8721/3 *Nodular melanoma*
M8722/0 *Balloon cell nevus*
M8722/3 *Balloon cell melanoma*
M8723/0 *Halo nevus*
M8724/0 *Fibrous papule of the nose*
M8725/0 *Neuronevus*
M8726/0 *Magnocellular nevus*
M8730/0 *Nonpigmented nevus*
M8730/3 *Amelanotic melanoma*
M8740/0 *Junctional nevus*
M8740/3 *Malignant melanoma in junctional nevus*
M8741/2 *Precancerous melanosis NOS*
M8741/3 *Malignant melanoma in precancerous melanosis*
M8742/2 *Hutchinson's melanotic freckle*
M8742/3 *Malignant melanoma in Hutchinson's melanotic freckle*
M8743/3 *Superficial spreading melanoma*
M8750/0 *Intradermal nevus*
M8760/0 *Compound nevus*
M8761/1 *Giant pigmented nevus*
M8761/3 *Malignant melanoma in giant pigmented nevus*
M8770/0 *Epithelioid and spindle cell nevus*
M8771/3 *Epithelioid cell melanoma*
M8772/3 *Spindle cell melanoma NOS*
M8773/3 *Spindle cell melanoma, type A*
M8774/3 *Spindle cell melanoma, type B*
M8775/3 *Mixed epithelioid and spindle cell melanoma*
M8780/0 *Blue nevus NOS*
M8780/3 *Blue nevus, malignant*
M8790/0 *Cellular blue nevus*

M880 Soft tissue tumors and sarcomas NOS
M8800/0 *Soft tissue tumor, benign*
M8800/3 *Sarcoma NOS*
M8800/9 *Sarcomatosis NOS*
M8801/3 *Spindle cell sarcoma*
M8802/3 *Giant cell sarcoma (except of bone M9250/3)*
M8803/3 *Small cell sarcoma*
M8804/3 *Epithelioid cell sarcoma*

M881-M883 Fibromatous neoplasms
M8810/0 *Fibroma NOS*
M8810/3 *Fibrosarcoma NOS*
M8811/0 *Fibromyxoma*
M8811/3 *Fibromyxosarcoma*

M8812/0 *Periosteal fibroma*
M8812/3 *Periosteal fibrosarcoma*
M8813/0 *Fascial fibroma*
M8813/3 *Fascial fibrosarcoma*
M8814/3 *Infantile fibrosarcoma*
M8820/0 *Elastofibroma*
M8821/1 *Aggressive fibromatosis*
M8822/1 *Abdominal fibromatosis*
M8823/1 *Desmoplastic fibroma*
M8830/0 *Fibrous histiocytoma NOS*
M8830/1 *Atypical fibrous histiocytoma*
M8830/3 *Fibrous histiocytoma, malignant*
M8831/0 *Fibroxanthoma NOS*
M8831/1 *Atypical fibroxanthoma*
M8831/3 *Fibroxanthoma, malignant*
M8832/0 *Dermatofibroma NOS*
M8832/1 *Dermatofibroma protuberans*
M8832/3 *Dermatofibrosarcoma NOS*

M884 Myxomatous neoplasms
M8840/0 *Myxoma NOS*
M8840/3 *Myxosarcoma*

M885-M888 Lipomatous neoplasms
M8850/0 *Lipoma NOS*
M8850/3 *Liposarcoma NOS*
M8851/0 *Fibrolipoma*
M8851/3 *Liposarcoma, well differentiated type*
M8852/0 *Fibromyxolipoma*
M8852/3 *Myxoid liposarcoma*
M8853/3 *Round cell liposarcoma*
M8854/3 *Pleomorphic liposarcoma*
M8855/3 *Mixed type liposarcoma*
M8856/0 *Intramuscular lipoma*
M8857/0 *Spindle cell lipoma*
M8860/0 *Angiomyolipoma*
M8860/3 *Angiomyoliposarcoma*
M8861/0 *Angiolipoma NOS*
M8861/1 *Angiolipoma, infiltrating*
M8870/0 *Myelolipoma*
M8880/0 *Hibernoma*
M8881/0 *Lipoblastomatosis*

M889-M892 Myomatous neoplasms
M8890/0 *Leiomyoma NOS*
M8890/1 *Intravascular leiomyomatosis*
M8890/3 *Leiomyosarcoma NOS*
M8891/1 *Epithelioid leiomyoma*
M8891/3 *Epithelioid leiomyosarcoma*
M8892/1 *Cellular leiomyoma*
M8893/0 *Bizarre leiomyoma*
M8894/0 *Angiomyoma*
M8894/3 *Angiomyosarcoma*
M8895/0 *Myoma*
M8895/3 *Myosarcoma*
M8900/0 *Rhabdomyoma NOS*
M8900/3 *Rhabdomyosarcoma NOS*
M8901/3 *Pleomorphic rhabdomyosarcoma*
M8902/3 *Mixed type rhabdomyosarcoma*
M8903/0 *Fetal rhabdomyoma*
M8904/0 *Adult rhabdomyoma*
M8910/3 *Embryonal rhabdomyosarcoma*
M8920/3 *Alveolar rhabdomyosarcoma*

M893-M899 Complex mixed and stromal neoplasms
M8930/3 *Endometrial stromal sarcoma*
M8931/1 *Endolymphatic stromal myosis*
M8932/0 *Adenomyoma*
M8940/0 *Pleomorphic adenoma*
M8940/3 *Mixed tumor, malignant NOS*
M8950/3 *Mullerian mixed tumor*
M8951/3 *Mesodermal mixed tumor*
M8960/1 *Mesoblastic nephroma*
M8960/3 *Nephroblastoma NOS*
M8961/3 *Epithelial nephroblastoma*
M8962/3 *Mesenchymal nephroblastoma*
M8970/3 *Hepatoblastoma*
M8980/3 *Carcinosarcoma NOS*
M8981/3 *Carcinosarcoma, embryonal type*
M8982/0 *Myoepithelioma*
M8990/0 *Mesenchymoma, benign*
M8990/1 *Mesenchymoma NOS*
M8990/3 *Mesenchymoma, malignant*
M8991/3 *Embryonal sarcoma*

M900-M903 Fibroepithelial neoplasms
M9000/0 *Brenner tumor NOS*
M9000/1 *Brenner tumor, borderline malignancy*
M9000/3 *Brenner tumor, malignant*
M9010/0 *Fibroadenoma NOS*
M9011/0 *Intracanalicular fibroadenoma NOS*
M9012/0 *Pericanalicular fibroadenoma*
M9013/0 *Adenofibroma NOS*
M9014/0 *Serous adenofibroma*
M9015/0 *Mucinous adenofibroma*
M9020/0 *Cellular intracanalicular fibroadenoma*
M9020/1 *Cystosarcoma phyllodes NOS*
M9020/3 *Cystosarcoma phyllodes, malignant*
M9030/0 *Juvenile fibroadenoma*

M904 Synovial neoplasms
M9040/0 *Synovioma, benign*
M9040/3 *Synovial sarcoma NOS*
M9041/3 *Synovial sarcoma, spindle cell type*
M9042/3 *Synovial sarcoma, epithelioid cell type*
M9043/3 *Synovial sarcoma, biphasic type*
M9044/3 *Clear cell sarcoma of tendons and aponeuroses*

M905 Mesothelial neoplasms
M9050/0 *Mesothelioma, benign*
M9050/3 *Mesothelioma, malignant*
M9051/0 *Fibrous mesothelioma, benign*
M9051/3 *Fibrous mesothelioma, malignant*
M9052/0 *Epithelioid mesothelioma, benign*
M9052/3 *Epithelioid mesothelioma, malignant*
M9053/0 *Mesothelioma, biphasic type, benign*
M9053/3 *Mesothelioma, biphasic type, malignant*
M9054/0 *Adenomatoid tumor NOS*

M906-M909 Germ cell neoplasms
M9060/3 *Dysgerminoma*
M9061/3 *Seminoma NOS*
M9062/3 *Seminoma, anaplastic type*
M9063/3 *Spermatocytic seminoma*
M9064/3 *Germinoma*
M9070/3 *Embryonal carcinoma NOS*
M9071/3 *Endodermal sinus tumor*
M9072/3 *Polyembryoma*
M9073/1 *Gonadoblastoma*
M9080/0 *Teratoma, benign*
M9080/1 *Teratoma NOS*
M9080/3 *Teratoma, malignant NOS*
M9081/3 *Teratocarcinoma*
M9082/3 *Malignant teratoma, undifferentiated type*
M9083/3 *Malignant teratoma, intermediate type*
M9084/0 *Dermoid cyst*
M9084/3 *Dermoid cyst with malignant transformation*
M9090/0 *Struma ovarii NOS*
M9090/3 *Struma ovarii, malignant*
M9091/1 *Strumal carcinoid*

M910 Trophoblastic neoplasms
M9100/0 *Hydatidiform mole NOS*
M9100/1 *Invasive hydatidiform mole*
M9100/3 *Choriocarcinoma*
M9101/3 *Choriocarcinoma combined with teratoma*
M9102/3 *Malignant teratoma, trophoblastic*

M911 Mesonephromas
M9110/0 *Mesonephroma, benign*
M9110/1 *Mesonephric tumor*
M9110/3 *Mesonephroma, malignant*
M9111/1 *Endosalpingioma*

M912-M916	**Blood vessel tumors**
M9120/0	*Hemangioma NOS*
M9120/3	*Hemangiosarcoma*
M9121/0	*Cavernous hemangioma*
M9122/0	*Venous hemangioma*
M9123/0	*Racemose hemangioma*
M9124/3	*Kupffer cell sarcoma*
M9130/0	*Hemangioendothelioma, benign*
M9130/1	*Hemangioendothelioma NOS*
M9130/3	*Hemangioendothelioma, malignant*
M9131/0	*Capillary hemangioma*
M9132/0	*Intramuscular hemangioma*
M9140/3	*Kaposi's sarcoma*
M9141/0	*Angiokeratoma*
M9142/0	*Verrucous keratotic hemangioma*
M9150/0	*Hemangiopericytoma, benign*
M9150/1	*Hemangiopericytoma NOS*
M9150/3	*Hemangiopericytoma, malignant*
M9160/0	*Angiofibroma NOS*
M9161/1	*Hemangioblastoma*
M917	**Lymphatic vessel tumors**
M9170/0	*Lymphangioma NOS*
M9170/3	*Lymphangiosarcoma*
M9171/0	*Capillary lymphangioma*
M9172/0	*Cavernous lymphangioma*
M9173/0	*Cystic lymphangioma*
M9174/0	*Lymphangiomyoma*
M9174/1	*Lymphangiomyomatosis*
M9175/0	*Hemolymphangioma*
M918-M920	**Osteomas and osteosarcomas**
M9180/0	*Osteoma NOS*
M9180/3	*Osteosarcoma NOS*
M9181/3	*Chondroblastic osteosarcoma*
M9182/3	*Fibroblastic osteosarcoma*
M9183/3	*Telangiectatic osteosarcoma*
M9184/3	*Osteosarcoma in Paget's disease of bone*
M9190/3	*Juxtacortical osteosarcoma*
M9191/0	*Osteoid osteoma NOS*
M9200/0	*Osteoblastoma*
M921-M924	**Chondromatous neoplasms**
M9210/0	*Osteochondroma*
M9210/1	*Osteochondromatosis NOS*
M9220/0	*Chondroma NOS*
M9220/1	*Chondromatosis NOS*
M9220/3	*Chondrosarcoma NOS*
M9221/0	*Juxtacortical chondroma*
M9221/3	*Juxtacortical chondrosarcoma*
M9230/0	*Chondroblastoma NOS*
M9230/3	*Chondroblastoma, malignant*
M9240/3	*Mesenchymal chondrosarcoma*
M9241/0	*Chondromyxoid fibroma*
M925	**Giant cell tumors**
M9250/1	*Giant cell tumor of bone NOS*
M9250/3	*Giant cell tumor of bone, malignant*
M9251/1	*Giant cell tumor of soft parts NOS*
M9251/3	*Malignant giant cell tumor of soft parts*
M926	**Miscellaneous bone tumors**
M9260/3	*Ewing's sarcoma*
M9261/3	*Adamantinoma of long bones*
M9262/0	*Ossifying fibroma*
M927-M934	**Odontogenic tumors**
M9270/0	*Odontogenic tumor, benign*
M9270/1	*Odontogenic tumor NOS*
M9270/3	*Odontogenic tumor, malignant*
M9271/0	*Dentinoma*
M9272/0	*Cementoma NOS*
M9273/0	*Cementoblastoma, benign*
M9274/0	*Cementifying fibroma*
M9275/0	*Gigantiform cementoma*
M9280/0	*Odontoma NOS*
M9281/0	*Compound odontoma*
M9282/0	*Complex odontoma*
M9290/0	*Ameloblastic fibro-odontoma*
M9290/3	*Ameloblastic odontosarcoma*
M9300/0	*Adenomatoid odontogenic tumor*
M9301/0	*Calcifying odontogenic cyst*
M9310/0	*Ameloblastoma NOS*
M9310/3	*Ameloblastoma, malignant*
M9311/0	*Odontoameloblastoma*
M9312/0	*Squamous odontogenic tumor*
M9320/0	*Odontogenic myxoma*
M9321/0	*Odontogenic fibroma NOS*
M9330/0	*Ameloblastic fibroma*
M9330/3	*Ameloblastic fibrosarcoma*
M9340/0	*Calcifying epithelial odontogenic tumor*
M935-M937	**Miscellaneous tumors**
M9350/1	*Craniopharyngioma*
M9360/1	*Pinealoma*
M9361/1	*Pineocytoma*
M9362/3	*Pineoblastoma*
M9363/0	*Melanotic neuroectodermal tumor*
M9370/3	*Chordoma*
M938-M948	**Gliomas**
M9380/3	*Glioma, malignant*
M9381/3	*Gliomatosis cerebri*
M9382/3	*Mixed glioma*
M9383/1	*Subependymal glioma*
M9384/1	*Subependymal giant cell astrocytoma*
M9390/0	*Choroid plexus papilloma NOS*
M9390/3	*Choroid plexus papilloma, malignant*
M9391/3	*Ependymoma NOS*
M9392/3	*Ependymoma, anaplastic type*
M9393/1	*Papillary ependymoma*
M9394/1	*Myxopapillary ependymoma*
M9400/3	*Astrocytoma NOS*
M9401/3	*Astrocytoma, anaplastic type*
M9410/3	*Protoplasmic astrocytoma*
M9411/3	*Gemistocytic astrocytoma*
M9420/3	*Fibrillary astrocytoma*
M9421/3	*Pilocytic astrocytoma*
M9422/3	*Spongioblastoma NOS*
M9423/3	*Spongioblastoma polare*
M9430/3	*Astroblastoma*
M9440/3	*Glioblastoma NOS*
M9441/3	*Giant cell glioblastoma*
M9442/3	*Glioblastoma with sarcomatous component*
M9443/3	*Primitive polar spongioblastoma*
M9450/3	*Oligodendroglioma NOS*
M9451/3	*Oligodendroglioma, anaplastic type*
M9460/3	*Oligodendroblastoma*
M9470/3	*Medulloblastoma NOS*
M9471/3	*Desmoplastic medulloblastoma*
M9472/3	*Medullomyoblastoma*
M9480/3	*Cerebellar sarcoma NOS*
M9481/3	*Monstrocellular sarcoma*
M949-M952	**Neuroepitheliomatous neoplasms**
M9490/0	*Ganglioneuroma*
M9490/3	*Ganglioneuroblastoma*
M9491/0	*Ganglioneuromatosis*
M9500/3	*Neuroblastoma NOS*
M9501/3	*Medulloepithelioma NOS*
M9502/3	*Teratoid medulloepithelioma*
M9503/3	*Neuroepithelioma NOS*
M9504/3	*Spongioneuroblastoma*
M9505/1	*Ganglioglioma*
M9506/0	*Neurocytoma*
M9507/0	*Pacinian tumor*
M9510/3	*Retinoblastoma NOS*
M9511/3	*Retinoblastoma, differentiated type*
M9512/3	*Retinoblastoma, undifferentiated type*
M9520/3	*Olfactory neurogenic tumor*
M9521/3	*Esthesioneurocytoma*
M9522/3	*Esthesioneuroblastoma*
M9523/3	*Esthesioneuroepithelioma*

M953 **Meningiomas**
M9530/0 *Meningioma NOS*
M9530/1 *Meningiomatosis NOS*
M9530/3 *Meningioma, malignant*
M9531/0 *Meningotheliomatous meningioma*
M9532/0 *Fibrous meningioma*
M9533/0 *Psammomatous meningioma*
M9534/0 *Angiomatous meningioma*
M9535/0 *Hemangioblastic meningioma*
M9536/0 *Hemangiopericytic meningioma*
M9537/0 *Transitional meningioma*
M9538/1 *Papillary meningioma*
M9539/3 *Meningeal sarcomatosis*

M954-M957 **Nerve sheath tumor**
M9540/0 *Neurofibroma NOS*
M9540/1 *Neurofibromatosis NOS*
M9540/3 *Neurofibrosarcoma*
M9541/0 *Melanotic neurofibroma*
M9550/0 *Plexiform neurofibroma*
M9560/0 *Neurilemmoma NOS*
M9560/1 *Neurinomatosis*
M9560/3 *Neurilemmoma, malignant*
M9570/0 *Neuroma NOS*

M958 **Granular cell tumors and alveolar soft part sarcoma**
M9580/0 *Granular cell tumor NOS*
M9580/3 *Granular cell tumor, malignant*
M9581/3 *Alveolar soft part sarcoma*

M959-M963 **Lymphomas, NOS or diffuse**
M9590/0 *Lymphomatous tumor, benign*
M9590/3 *Malignant lymphoma NOS*
M9591/3 *Malignant lymphoma, non Hodgkin's type*
M9600/3 *Malignant lymphoma, undifferentiated cell type NOS*
M9601/3 *Malignant lymphoma, stem cell type*
M9602/3 *Malignant lymphoma, convoluted cell type NOS*
M9610/3 *Lymphosarcoma NOS*
M9611/3 *Malignant lymphoma, lymphoplasmacytoid type*
M9612/3 *Malignant lymphoma, immunoblastic type*
M9613/3 *Malignant lymphoma, mixed lymphocytic-histiocytic NOS*
M9614/3 *Malignant lymphoma, centroblastic-centrocytic, diffuse*
M9615/3 *Malignant lymphoma, follicular center cell NOS*
M9620/3 *Malignant lymphoma, lymphocytic, well differentiated NOS*
M9621/3 *Malignant lymphoma, lymphocytic, intermediate differentiation NOS*
M9622/3 *Malignant lymphoma, centrocytic*
M9623/3 *Malignant lymphoma, follicular center cell, cleaved NOS*
M9630/3 *Malignant lymphoma, lymphocytic, poorly differentiated NOS*
M9631/3 *Prolymphocytic lymphosarcoma*
M9632/3 *Malignant lymphoma, centroblastic type NOS*
M9633/3 *Malignant lymphoma, follicular center cell, noncleaved NOS*

M964 **Reticulosarcomas**
M9640/3 *Reticulosarcoma NOS*
M9641/3 *Reticulosarcoma, pleomorphic cell type*
M9642/3 *Reticulosarcoma, nodular*

M965-M966 **Hodgkin's disease**
M9650/3 *Hodgkin's disease NOS*
M9651/3 *Hodgkin's disease, lymphocytic predominance*
M9652/3 *Hodgkin's disease, mixed cellularity*
M9653/3 *Hodgkin's disease, lymphocytic depletion NOS*
M9654/3 *Hodgkin's disease, lymphocytic depletion, diffuse fibrosis*
M9655/3 *Hodgkin's disease, lymphocytic depletion, reticular type*
M9656/3 *Hodgkin's disease, nodular sclerosis NOS*
M9657/3 *Hodgkin's disease, nodular sclerosis, cellular phase*
M9660/3 *Hodgkin's paragranuloma*
M9661/3 *Hodgkin's granuloma*
M9662/3 *Hodgkin's sarcoma*

M969 **Lymphomas, nodular or follicular**
M9690/3 *Malignant lymphoma, nodular NOS*
M9691/3 *Malignant lymphoma, mixed lymphocytic-histiocytic, nodular*
M9692/3 *Malignant lymphoma, centroblastic-centrocytic, follicular*
M9693/3 *Malignant lymphoma, lymphocytic, well differentiated, nodular*
M9694/3 *Malignant lymphoma, lymphocytic, intermediate differentiation, nodular*
M9695/3 *Malignant lymphoma, follicular center cell, cleaved, follicular*
M9696/3 *Malignant lymphoma, lymphocytic, poorly differentiated, nodular*
M9697/3 *Malignant lymphoma, centroblastic type, follicular*
M9698/3 *Malignant lymphoma, follicular center cell, noncleaved, follicular*

M970 **Mycosis fungoides**
M9700/3 *Mycosis fungoides*
M9701/3 *Sezary's disease*

M971-M972 **Miscellaneous reticuloendothelial neoplasms**
M9710/3 *Microglioma*
M9720/3 *Malignant histiocytosis*
M9721/3 *Histiocytic medullary reticulosis*
M9722/3 *Letterer-Siwe's disease*

M973 **Plasma cell tumors**
M9730/3 *Plasma cell myeloma*
M9731/0 *Plasma cell tumor, benign*
M9731/1 *Plasmacytoma NOS*
M9731/3 *Plasma cell tumor, malignant*

M974 **Mast cell tumors**
M9740/1 *Mastocytoma NOS*
M9740/3 *Mast cell sarcoma*
M9741/3 *Malignant mastocytosis*

M975 **Burkitt's tumor**
M9750/3 *Burkitt's tumor*

M980-M994 **Leukemias**

M980 **Leukemias NOS**
M9800/3 *Leukemia NOS*
M9801/3 *Acute leukemia NOS*
M9802/3 *Subacute leukemia NOS*
M9803/3 *Chronic leukemia NOS*
M9804/3 *Aleukemic leukemia NOS*

M981 **Compound leukemias**
M9810/3 *Compound leukemia*

M982 **Lymphoid leukemias**
M9820/3 *Lymphoid leukemia NOS*
M9821/3 *Acute lymphoid leukemia*
M9822/3 *Subacute lymphoid leukemia*
M9823/3 *Chronic lymphoid leukemia*
M9824/3 *Aleukemic lymphoid leukemia*
M9825/3 *Prolymphocytic leukemia*

M983 **Plasma cell leukemias**
M9830/3 *Plasma cell leukemia*

M984 **Erythroleukemias**
M9840/3 *Erythroleukemia*
M9841/3 *Acute erythremia*
M9842/3 *Chronic erythremia*

M985 **Lymphosarcoma cell leukemias**
M9850/3 *Lymphosarcoma cell leukemia*

M986 **Myeloid leukemias**
M9860/3 *Myeloid leukemia NOS*
M9861/3 *Acute myeloid leukemia*
M9862/3 *Subacute myeloid leukemia*

M9863/3	*Chronic myeloid leukemia*
M9864/3	*Aleukemic myeloid leukemia*
M9865/3	*Neutrophilic leukemia*
M9866/3	*Acute promyelocytic leukemia*
M987	**Basophilic leukemias**
M9870/3	*Basophilic leukemia*
M988	**Eosinophilic leukemias**
M9880/3	*Eosinophilic leukemia*
M989	**Monocytic leukemias**
M9890/3	*Monocytic leukemia NOS*
M9891/3	*Acute monocytic leukemia*
M9892/3	*Subacute monocytic leukemia*
M9893/3	*Chronic monocytic leukemia*
M9894/3	*Aleukemic monocytic leukemia*
M990-M994	**Miscellaneous leukemias**
M9900/3	*Mast cell leukemia*
M9910/3	*Megakaryocytic leukemia*
M9920/3	*Megakaryocytic myelosis*
M9930/3	*Myeloid sarcoma*
M9940/3	*Hairy cell leukemia*
M995-M997	**Miscellaneous myeloproliferative and lymphoproliferative disorders**
M9950/1	*Polycythemia vera*
M9951/1	*Acute panmyelosis*
M9960/1	*Chronic myeloproliferative disease*
M9961/1	*Myelosclerosis with myeloid metaplasia*
M9962/1	*Idiopathic thrombocythemia*
M9970/1	*Chronic lymphoproliferative disease*

APPENDIX B

GLOSSARY OF MENTAL DISORDERS

The psychiatric terms which appear in Chapter 5, "Mental Disorders," are listed here in alphabetic sequence. Many of the glossary descriptions originally appeared in the section on Mental Disorders in the International Classification of Diseases, 9th Revision,[1] and others are included to define the psychiatric conditions added to ICD-9-CM. The additional definitions are based on material furnished by the American Psychiatric Association's Task Force on Nomenclature and Statistics[2] and from A Psychiatric Glossary.[3] In a few instances definitions were obtained from Dorland's Illustrated Medical Dictionary[4] and from Stedman's Medical Dictionary, Illustrated.[5]

1. Manual of the International Classification of Diseases, Injuries, and Causes of Death, 9th Revision. World Health Organization, Geneva, Switzerland, 1975.
2. American Psychiatric Association, Task Force on Nomenclature and Statistics, Robert L. Spitzer, Chairman.
3. A Psychiatric Glossary. Fourth Edition, American Psychiatric Association, Washington, D.C., 1975.
4. Dorland's Illustrated Medical Dictionary. Twenty-fifth Edition, W. B. Saunders Company, Philadelphia, 1974.
5. Stedman's Medical Dictionary, Illustrated. Twenty-third Edition, the Williams and Wilkins Company, Baltimore, 1976.

Academic underachievement disorder: Failure to achieve in most school tasks despite adequate intellectual capacity, a supportive and encouraging social environment, and apparent effort. The failure occurs in the absence of a demonstrable specific learning disability and is caused by emotional conflict not clearly associated with any other mental disorder.[2]

Adaptation reaction—*see* Adjustment reaction

Adjustment reaction or disorder: Mild or transient disorders lasting longer than acute stress reactions which occur in individuals of any age without any apparent pre-existing mental disorder. Such disorders are often relatively circumscribed or situation-specific, are generally reversible, and usually last only a few months. They are usually closely related in time and content to stresses such as bereavement, migration, or other experiences. Reactions to major stress that last longer than a few days are also included. In children such disorders are associated with no significant distortion of development.[1]

conduct disturbance: Mild or transient disorders in which the main disturbance predominantly involves a disturbance of conduct (e.g., an adolescent grief reaction resulting in aggressive or antisocial disorder).[1]

depressive reaction: States of depression, not specifiable as manic-depressive, psychotic, or neurotic.[1]

brief: Generally transient, in which the depressive symptoms are usually closely related in time and content to some stressful event.[1]

prolonged: Generally long-lasting, usually developing in association with prolonged exposure to a stressful situation.[1]

emotional disturbance: An adjustment disorder in which the main symptoms are emotional in type (e.g., anxiety, fear, worry) but not specifically depressive.[1]

mixed conduct and emotional disturbance: An adjustment reaction in which both emotional disturbance and disturbance of conduct are prominent features.[1]

Affective psychoses: Mental disorders, usually recurrent, in which there is a severe disturbance of mood (mostly compounded of depression and anxiety but also manifested as elation, and excitement) which is accompanied by one or more of the following: delusions, perplexity, disturbed attitude to self, disorder of perception and behavior; these are all in keeping with the individual's prevailing mood (as are hallucinations when they occur). There is a strong tendency to suicide. For practical reasons, mild disorders of mood may also be included here if the symptoms match closely the descriptions given; this applies particularly to mild hypomania.[1]

bipolar: A manic-depressive psychosis which has appeared in both the depressive and manic form, either alternating or separated by an interval of normality.[1]

atypical: An episode of affective psychosis with some, but not all, of the features of the one form of the disorder in individuals who have had a previous episode of the other form of the disorder.[2]

depressed: A manic-depressive psychosis, circular type, in which the depressive form is currently present.[1]

manic: A manic-depressive psychosis, circular type, in which the manic form is currently present.[1]

mixed: A manic-depressive psychosis, circular type, in which both manic and depressive symptoms are present at the same time.[1]

depressed type: A manic-depressive psychosis in which there is a widespread depressed mood of gloom and wretchedness with some degree of anxiety. There is often reduced activity but there may be restlessness and agitation. There is marked tendency to recurrence; in a few cases this may be at regular intervals.[1]

atypical: An affective depressive disorder that cannot be classified as a manic-depressive psychosis, depressed type, or chronic depressive personality disorder, or as an adjustment disorder.[2]

manic type: A manic-depressive psychosis characterized by states of elation or excitement out of keeping with the individual's circumstances and varying from enhanced liveliness (hypomania) to violent, almost uncontrollable, excitement. Aggression and anger, flight of ideas, distractibility, impaired judgment, and grandiose ideas are common.[1]

mixed type: Manic-depressive psychosis syndromes corresponding to both the manic and depressed types, but which for other reasons cannot be classified more specifically.[1]

Aggressive personality—*see* Personality disorder, explosive type

Agoraphobia—*see* agoraphobia under Phobia

Alcohol dependence syndrome: A state, psychic and usually also physical, resulting from taking alcohol, characterized by behavioral and other responses that always include a compulsion to take alcohol on a continuous or periodic basis in order to experience its psychic effects, and sometimes to avoid the discomfort of its absence; tolerance may or may not be present. A person may be dependent on alcohol and other drugs; if so, also record the diagnosis of drug dependence to identify the agent. If alcohol dependence is associated with alcoholic psychosis or with physical complications, both diagnoses should be recorded.[1]

Alcohol intoxication

acute: A psychic and physical state resulting from alcohol ingestion characterized by slurred speech, unsteady gait, poor coordination, flushed facies, nystagmus, sluggish reflexes, fetor alcoholica, loud speech, emotional instability (e.g., jollity followed by lugubriousness), excessive conviviality, loquacity, and poorly inhibited sexual and aggressive behavior.[2]

idiosyncratic: Acute psychotic episodes induced by relatively small amounts of alcohol. These are regarded as individual idiosyncratic reactions to alcohol, not due to excessive consumption and without conspicuous neurological signs of intoxication.[1]

pathological—*see* Alcohol intoxication, idiosyncratic

Alcoholic psychoses: Organic psychotic states due mainly to excessive consumption of alcohol; defects of nutrition are thought to play an important role.[1]

alcohol abstinence syndrome—*see* alcohol withdrawal syndrome below

alcohol amnestic syndrome: A syndrome of prominent and lasting reduction of memory span, including striking loss of recent memory, disordered time appreciation and confabulation, occurring in alcoholics as the sequel to an acute alcoholic psychosis (especially delirium tremens) or, more rarely, in the course of chronic alcoholism. It is usually accompanied by peripheral neuritis and may be associated with Wernicke's encephalopathy.[1]

alcohol withdrawal delirium [delirium tremens]: Acute or subacute organic psychotic states in alcoholics, characterized by clouded consciousness, disorientation, fear, illusions, delusions, hallucinations of any kind, notably visual and tactile, and restlessness, tremor and sometimes fever.[1]

alcohol withdrawal hallucinosis: A psychosis usually of less than six months' duration, with slight or no clouding of consciousness and much anxious restlessness in which auditory hallucinations, mostly of voices uttering insults and threats, predominate.[1]

alcohol withdrawal syndrome: Tremor of hands, tongue, and eyelids following cessation of prolonged heavy drinking of alcohol. Nausea and vomiting, dry mouth, headache, heavy perspiration, fitful sleep, acute anxiety attacks, mood depression, feelings of guilt and remorse, and irritability are associated features.[2]

alcohol delirium—*see* alcohol withdrawal delirium above

alcoholic dementia: Nonhallucinatory dementias occurring in association with alcoholism, but not characterized by the features of either alcohol withdrawal delirium [delirium tremens] or alcohol amnestic syndrome [Korsakoff's alcoholic psychosis].[1]

alcoholic hallucinosis—*see* alcohol withdrawal hallucinosis above

alcoholic jealousy: Chronic paranoid psychosis characterized by delusional jealousy and associated with alcoholism.

alcoholic paranoia—*see* alcoholic jealousy

alcoholic polyneuritic psychosis—*see* alcohol amnestic syndrome above

Alcoholism

acute—*see* Alcohol intoxication, acute

chronic—*see* Alcohol dependence syndrome

Alexia: Loss of a previously possessed reading facility that cannot be explained by defective visual acuity.[3]

Amnesia, psychogenic: A form of dissociative hysteria in which there is a temporary disturbance in the ability to recall important personal information which has already been registered and stored in memory. The sudden onset of this disturbance in the absence of an underlying organic mental disorder, and the extent of the disturbance being too great to be explained by ordinary forgetfulness, are the essential features.[2]

Amnestic syndrome: A syndrome of prominent and lasting reduction of memory span, including striking loss of recent memory, disordered time appreciation, and confabulation. The commonest causes are chronic alcoholism [alcohol amnestic syndrome; Korsakoff's alcoholic psychosis], chronic barbiturate dependence, and malnutrition. An amnestic syndrome may be the predominating disturbance in the early states of presenile and senile dementia, arteriosclerotic dementia, and in encephalitis and other inflammatory and degenerative diseases in which there is particular bilateral involvement of the temporal lobes, and certain temporal lobe tumors.[2]

alcoholic—*see* alcohol amnestic syndrome under Alcoholic psychoses

Amoral personality—*see* Personality disorder, antisocial type

Anancastic [anankastic] neurosis—*see* Neurotic disorder, obsessive-compulsive

Anancastic [anankastic] personality—*see* Personality disorder, compulsive type

Anorexia nervosa: A disorder in which the main features are persistent active refusal to eat and marked loss of weight. The level of activity and alertness is characteristically high in relation to the degree of emaciation. Typically the disorder begins in teenage girls but it may sometimes begin before puberty and rarely it occurs in males. Amenorrhea is usual and there may be a variety of other physiological changes including slow pulse and respiration, low body temperature, and dependent edema. Unusual eating habits and attitudes toward food are typical and sometimes starvation follows or alternates with periods of overeating. The accompanying psychiatric symptoms are diverse.[1]

Anxiety hysteria—*see* phobia under Neurotic disorders

Anxiety state (neurotic): Apprehension, tension, or uneasiness that stems from the anticipation of danger, the source of which is largely unknown or unrecognized.[3]

atypical: An anxiety disorder that does not fulfill the criteria of generalized or panic attack anxiety. An example might be an individual with a single morbid fear.[2]

generalized: A disorder of at least six months' duration in which the predominant feature is limited to diffuse and persistent anxiety without the specific symptoms that characterize phobic disorders, panic disorder, or obsessive-compulsive disorder.[2]

panic attack: An episodic and often chronic, recurrent disorder in which the predominant features are anxiety attacks and nervousness. The anxiety attacks are manifested by discrete periods of sudden onset of intense apprehension, fearfulness, or terror often associated with feelings of impending doom.[2]

Aphasia, developmental: A delay in the production of spoken language. Rarely, there is also a developmental delay in the comprehension of speech sounds.[1]

Arteriosclerotic dementia: Dementia attributable, because of physical signs (on examination of the central nervous system), to degenerative arterial disease of the brain. Symptoms suggesting a focal lesion in the brain are common. There may be a fluctuating or patchy intellectual defect with insight, and an intermittent course is common. Clinical differentiation from senile or presenile dementia, which may coexist with it, may be very difficult or impossible. The diagnosis of cerebral atherosclerosis should also be recorded.[1]

Asocial personality—*see* Personality disorder, antisocial type

Astasia-abasia, hysterical: A form of conversion hysteria in which the individual is unable to stand or walk although the legs are otherwise under control.[4]

Asthenia, psychogenic—*see* neurasthenia under Neurotic disorders

Asthenic personality—*see* Personality disorder, dependent type

Attention deficit disorder—*see* attention deficit disorder under Hyperkinetic syndrome of childhood

Autism, infantile: A syndrome present from birth or beginning almost invariably in the first 30 months. Responses to auditory and sometimes to visual stimuli are abnormal, and there are usually severe problems in the understanding of spoken language. Speech is delayed and, if it develops, is characterized by echolalia, the reversal of pronouns, immature grammatical structure, and inability to use abstract terms. There is generally an impairment in the social use of both verbal and gestural language. Problems in social relationships are most severe before the age of five years and include an impairment in the development of eye-to-eye gaze, social attachments, and cooperative play. Ritualistic behavior is usual and may include abnormal routines, resistance to change, attachment to odd objects, and stereotyped patterns of play. The capacity for abstract or symbolic thought and for imaginative play is diminished. Intelligence ranges from severely subnormal to normal or above. Performance is usually better on tasks involving rote memory or visuospatial skills than on those requiring symbolic or linguistic skills.[1]

Avoidant personality—*see* Personality disorder, avoidant type

"Bad trips": Acute intoxication from hallucinogen abuse, manifested by hallucinatory states lasting only a few days or less.[1]

Barbiturate abuse: Cases where an individual has taken the drug to the detriment of his health or social functioning, in doses above or for periods beyond those normally regarded as therapeutic.[1]

Bestiality—*see* Zoophilia

Bipolar disorder—*see* Affective psychosis, bipolar

atypical—*see* Affective psychosis, bipolar, atypical

Body-rocking—*see* Stereotyped repetitive movements

Borderline personality—*see* Personality disorder, borderline type

Borderline psychosis of childhood—*see* Psychosis, atypical childhood

Borderline schizophrenia—*see* Schizophrenia, latent

Bouffée délirante—*see* Paranoid reaction, acute

Briquet's disorder—*see* somatization disorder under Neurotic disorders

Bulimia: An episodic pattern of overeating [binge eating] accompanied by an awareness of the disordered eating pattern with a fear of not being able to stop eating voluntarily. Depressive moods and self-deprecating thoughts follow the episodes of binge eating.[2]

Catalepsy schizophrenia—*see* Schizophrenia, catatonic type
Catastrophic stress—*see* Gross stress reaction
Catatonia (schizophrenic)—*see* Schizophrenia, catatonic type
Character neurosis—*see* Personality disorders
Childhood autism—*see* Autism, infantile
Childhood type schizophrenia—*see* Psychosis, child
Chronic alcoholic brain syndrome—*see* alcoholic dementia under Alcoholic psychoses
Clay-eating—*see* Pica
Clumsiness syndrome—*see* coordination disorder under Developmental delay disorders, specific
Combat fatigue—*see* Posttraumatic disorder, acute
Compensation neurosis—*see* compensation neurosis under Neurotic disorders
Compulsive conduct disorder—*see* impulse control disorders under Conduct disorders
Compulsive neurosis—*see* Neurotic disorder, obsessive-compulsive
Compulsive personality—*see* Personality disorder, compulsive type
Concentration camp syndrome—*see* Posttraumatic stress disorder, prolonged

Conduct disorders: Disorders mainly involving aggressive and destructive behavior and disorders involving delinquency. It should be used for abnormal behavior, in individuals of any age, which gives rise to social disapproval but which is not part of any other psychiatric condition. Minor emotional disturbances may also be present. To be included, the behavior, as judged by its frequency, severity, and type of associations with other symptoms, must be abnormal in its context. Disturbances of conduct are distinguished from an adjustment reaction by a longer duration and by a lack of close relationship in time and content to some stress. They differ from a personality disorder by the absence of deeply ingrained maladaptive patterns of behavior present from adolescence or earlier.[1]

impulse control disorders: A failure to resist an impulse, drive, or temptation to perform some action which is harmful to the individual or to others. The impulse may or may not be consciously resisted, and the act may or may not be premeditated or planned. Prior to committing the act, there is an increasing sense of tension, and at the time of committing the act, there is an experience of either pleasure, gratification, or release. Immediately following the act, there may or may not be genuine regret, self-reproach, or guilt.[2] See also Intermittent explosive disorder, Isolated explosive disorder, Kleptomania, Pathological gambling, and Pyromania.

mixed disturbance of conduct and emotions: A disorder characterized by features of undersocialized and socialized disturbance of conduct, but in which there is also considerable emotional disturbance as shown, for example, by anxiety, misery, or obsessive manifestations.[1]

socialized conduct disorder: Conduct disorders in individuals who have acquired the values or behavior of a delinquent peer group to whom they are loyal and with whom they characteristically steal, play truant, and stay out late at night. There may also be sexual promiscuity.[1]

undersocialized conduct disturbance

aggressive type: A disorder characterized by a persistent pattern of disrespect for the feelings and well-being of others (bullying, physical aggression, cruel behavior, hostility, verbal abusiveness, impudence, defiance, negativism), aggressive antisocial behavior (destructiveness, stealing, persistent lying, frequent truancy, and vandalism), and failure to develop close and stable relationships with others.[2]

unaggressive type: A disorder in which there is a lack of concern for the rights and feelings of others to a degree which indicates a failure to establish a normal degree of affection, empathy, or bond with others. There are two patterns of behavior found. In one, the child is fearful and timid, lacking self-assertiveness, resorts to self-protective and manipulative lying, indulges in whining demandingness and temper tantrums, feels rejected and unfairly treated, and is mistrustful of others. In the other pattern of the disorder, the child approaches others strictly for his own gains and acts exclusively because of exploitative and extractive goals. The child lies brazenly and steals, appearing to feel no guilt, and forms no social bonds to other individuals.[2]

Confusion, psychogenic—*see* Psychosis, reactive confusion
Confusion, reactive—*see* Psychosis, reactive confusion
Confusional state
acute—*see* Delirium, acute
epileptic—*see* Delirium, acute
subacute—*see* Delirium, subacute
Conversion hysteria—*see* hysteria, conversion type under Neurotic disorders
Coordination disorder—*see* coordination disorder under Developmental delay disorders, specific

Culture shock: A form of stress reaction associated with an individual's assimilation into a new culture which is vastly different from that in which he was raised.[5]

Cyclic schizophrenia—*see* Schizophrenia, schizo-affective type
Cyclothymic personality or disorder—*see* Personality disorder, cyclothymic type

Delirium: Transient organic psychotic conditions with a short course in which there is a rapidly developing onset of disorganization of higher mental processes manifested by some degree of impairment of information processing, impaired or abnormal attention, perception, memory, and thinking. Clouded consciousness, confusion, disorientation, delusions, illusions, and often vivid hallucinations predominate in the clinical picture.[1,2]

acute: short-lived states, lasting hours or days, of the above type.[1]

subacute: states of the above type in which the symptoms, usually less florid, last for several weeks or longer, during which they may show marked fluctuations in intensity.[1]

Delirium tremens—*see* alcohol withdrawal delirium under Alcoholic psychoses
Delusions, systematized—*see* Paranoia

Dementia: A decrement in intellectual functioning of sufficient severity to interfere with occupational or social performance, or both. There is impairment of memory and abstract thinking, the ability to learn new skills, problem solving, and judgment. There is often also personality change or impairment in impulse control. Dementia in organic psychoses may be of a chronic or progressive nature, which if untreated is usually irreversible and terminal.[1,2]

alcoholic—*see* alcoholic dementia under Alcoholic psychoses
arteriosclerotic—*see* Arteriosclerotic dementia
multi-infarct—*see* Arteriosclerotic dementia
presenile—*see* Presenile dementia
repeated infarct—*see* Arteriosclerotic dementia
senile—*see* Senile dementia

Depersonalization syndrome—*see* depersonalization syndrome under Neurotic disorders

Depression: States of depression, usually of moderate but occasionally of marked intensity, which have no specifically manic-depressive or other psychotic depressive features, and which do not appear to be associated with stressful events or other features specified under neurotic depressions.[1]

anxiety—*see* depression under Neurotic disorders
endogenous—*see* Affective psychosis, depressed type
monopolar—*see* Affective psychosis, depressed type
neurotic—*see* depression under Neurotic disorders
psychotic—*see* Affective psychosis, depressed type
psychotic reactive—*see* Psychosis, depressive
reactive—*see* depression under Neurotic disorders
reactive psychotic—*see* Psychosis, depressive

Depressive personality or character—*see* Personality disorder, chronic depressive type
Depressive reaction—*see* depressive reaction under Adjustment reaction
Depressive psychosis—*see* Affective psychosis, depressed type
Derealization (neurotic)—*see* depersonalization syndrome under Neurotic disorders

Developmental delay disorders, specific: A group of disorders in which a specific delay in development is the main feature. For many the delay is not explicable in terms of general intellectual retardation or of inadequate schooling. In each case development is related to biological maturation, but it is also influenced by nonbiological factors. A diagnosis of a specific developmental delay carries no etiological implications. A diagnosis of specific delay in development should not be made if it is due to a known neurological disorder.[1]

arithmetical disorder: Disorders in which the main feature is a serious impairment in the development of arithmetical skills.[1]

articulation disorder: A delay in the development of normal word-sound production resulting in defects of articulation. Omissions or substitutions of consonants are most frequent.[1]

coordination disorder: Disorders in which the main feature is a serious impairment in the development of motor coordination which is not explicable in terms of general intellectual retardation. The clumsiness is commonly associated with perceptual difficulties.[1]

mixed development disorder: A delay in the development of one specific skill (e.g., reading, arithmetic, speech, or coordination) is frequently associated with lesser delays in other skills. When this occurs the diagnosis should be made according to the skill most seriously impaired. The mixed category should be used only where the mixture of delayed skills is such that no one skill is preponderantly affected.[1]

motor retardation—*see* coordination disorder above

reading disorder or retardation: Disorders in which the main feature is a serious impairment in the development of reading or spelling skills which is not explicable in terms of general intellectual retardation or of inadequate schooling. Speech or language difficulties, impaired right-left differentiation, perceptuo-motor problems, and coding difficulties are frequently associated. Similar problems are often present in other members of the family. Adverse psychosocial factors may be present.[1]

speech or language disorder: Disorders in which the main feature is a serious impairment in the development of speech or language (syntax or semantic) which is not explicable in terms of general intellectual retardation. Most commonly there is a delay in the development of normal word-sound production resulting in defects of articulation. Omissions or substitutions of consonants are most frequent. There may also be a delay in the production of spoken language. Rarely, there is also a developmental delay in the comprehension of sounds. Includes cases in which delay is largely due to environmental privation.[1]

Dipsomania—*see* Alcohol dependence syndrome

Disorganized schizophrenia—*see* Schizophrenia, disorganized type

Dissociative hysteria—*see* hysteria, dissociative type under Neurotic disorders

Drug abuse: Includes cases where an individual, for whom no other diagnosis is possible, has come under medical care because of the maladaptive effect of a drug on which he is not dependent (*see* Drug dependence) and that he has taken on his own initiative to the detriment of his health or social functioning. When drug abuse is secondary to a psychiatric disorder, record the disorder as an additional diagnosis.[1]

Drug dependence: A state, psychic and sometimes also physical, resulting from taking a drug, characterized by behavioral and other responses that always include a compulsion to take a drug on a continuous or periodic basis in order to experience its psychic effects, and sometimes to avoid the discomfort of its absence. Tolerance may or may not be present. A person may be dependent on more than one drug.[1]

Drug psychoses: Organic mental syndromes which are due to consumption of drugs (notably amphetamines, barbiturates, and opiate and LSD groups) and solvents. Some of the syndromes in this group are not as severe as most conditions labeled "psychotic," but they are included here for practical reasons. The drug should be identified, and also a diagnosis of drug dependence should be recorded, if present.[1]

drug-induced hallucinosis: Hallucinatory states of more than a few days, but not more than a few months' duration, associated with large or prolonged intake of drugs, notably of the amphetamine and LSD groups. Auditory hallucinations usually predominate and there may be anxiety or restlessness. States following LSD or other hallucinogens lasting only a few days or less ["bad trips"] are not included.[1]

drug-induced organic delusional syndrome: Paranoid states of more than a few days, but not more than a few months' duration, associated with large or prolonged intake of drugs, notably of the amphetamine and LSD groups.[1]

drug withdrawal syndrome: States associated with drug withdrawal ranging from severe, as specified for alcohol withdrawal delirium [delirium tremens], to less severe states characterized by one or more symptoms such as convulsions, tremor, anxiety, restlessness, gastrointestinal and muscular complaints, and mild disorientation and memory disturbance.[1]

Drunkenness:

acute—*see* Alcohol intoxication, acute

pathologic—*see* Alcohol intoxication, idiosyncratic

simple: A state of inebriation due to alcohol consumption without conspicuous neurological signs of intoxications.[2]

sleep: An inability to fully arouse from the sleep state characterized by failure to attain full consciousness after arousal.[2]

Dyscalculia—*see* arithmetical disorder under Developmental delay disorders, specific

Dyslalia—*see* articulation disorder under Developmental delay disorders, specific

Dyslexia, developmental: A disorder in which the main feature is a serious impairment of reading skills which is not explicable in terms of general intellectual retardation or of inadequate schooling. Word-blindness and strephosymbolia (tendency to reverse letters and words in reading) are included.[1,3]

Dysmenorrhea, psychogenic: Painful menstruation due to disturbance of psychic control.[4]

Dyspareunia, functional—*see* functional dyspareunia under Psychosexual dysfunctions

Dyspraxia syndrome—*see* coordination disorder under Developmental delay disorders, specific

Dyssocial personality—*see* Personality disorder, antisocial type

Dysuria, psychogenic: Difficulty in passing urine due to psychic factors.[4]

Eating disorders: A group of disorders characterized by a conspicuous disturbance in eating behavior.[2] See also Bulimia, Pica, and Rumination, psychogenic.

Eccentric personality—*see* Personality disorder, eccentric type

Elective mutism: A pervasive and persistent refusal to speak in situations not attributable to a mental disorder. In some cases the behavior may manifest a form of withdrawal reaction to a specific stressful situation, or as a predominant feature in children exhibiting shyness or social withdrawal disorders.[2]

Emancipation disorder: An adjustment reaction in adolescents or young adults in which there is symptomatic expression (e.g., difficulty in making independent decisions, increased dependence on parental advice, adoption of values deliberately oppositional to parents) of a conflict over independence following the recent assumption of a status in which the individual is more independent of parental control or supervision.[2]

Emotional disturbances specific to childhood and adolescence: Less well-differentiated emotional disorders characteristic of the childhood period. When the emotional disorder takes the form of a neurosis, the appropriate diagnosis should be made. These disorders differ from adjustment reactions in terms of longer duration and by the lack of close relationship in time and content to some stress.[1] See also Academic underachievement disorder, Elective mutism, Identity disorder, Introverted disorder of childhood, Misery and unhappiness disorder, Oppositional disorder, Overanxious disorder, and Shyness disorder of childhood.

Encopresis: A disorder in which the main manifestation is the persistent voluntary or involuntary passage of formed stools of normal or near-normal consistency into places not intended for that purpose in the individual's own sociocultural setting. Sometimes the child has failed to gain bowel control, and sometimes he has gained control but then later again became encopretic. There may be a variety of associated psychiatric symptoms and there may be smearing of feces. The condition would not usually be diagnosed under the age of four years.[1]

Endogenous depression—*see* Affective psychosis, depressed type

Enuresis: A disorder in which the main manifestation is a persistent involuntary voiding of urine by day or night which is considered abnormal for the age of the individual. Sometimes the child will have failed to gain bladder control and in other cases he will have gained control and then lost it. Episodic or fluctuating enuresis should be included. The disorder would not usually be diagnosed under the age of four years.[1]

Epileptic confusional or twilight state—*see* Delirium, acute

Excitation

catatonic—*see* Schizophrenia, catatonic type

psychogenic—*see* Psychosis, excitative type

reactive—*see* Psychosis, excitative type

Exhaustion delirium—*see* Stress reaction, acute

Exhibitionism: Sexual deviation in which the main sexual pleasure and gratification is derived from exposure of the genitals to a person of the opposite sex.[1]

Explosive personality disorder—*see* Personality disorder, explosive type

Factitious illness: A form of hysterical neurosis in which there are physical or psychological symptoms that are not real, genuine, or natural, which are produced by the individual and are under his voluntary control.[2]

physical symptom type: The presentation of physical symptoms that may be total fabrication, self-inflicted, an exaggeration or exacerbation of a pre-existing physical condition, or any combination or variation of these.[2]

psychological symptom type: The voluntary production of symptoms suggestive of a mental disorder. Behavior may mimic psychosis or, rather, the individual's idea of psychosis.[2]

Fanatic personality—*see* Personality disorder, paranoid type

Fatigue neurosis—*see* neurasthenia under Neurotic disorders

Feeble-minded—*see* Mental retardation, mild

Fetishism: A sexual deviation in which nonliving objects are utilized as a preferred or exclusive method of stimulating erotic arousal.[2]

Finger-flicking—*see* Stereotyped repetitive movements

Folie à deux—*see* Shared paranoid disorder

Frigidity: A psychosexual dysfunction in which there is partial or complete failure to attain or maintain the lubrication-swelling response of sexual excitement until completion of the sexual act.[2]

Frontal lobe syndrome: Changes in behavior following damage to the frontal areas of the brain or following interference with the connections of those areas. There is a general diminution of self-control, foresight, creativity, and spontaneity, which may be manifest as increased irritability, selfishness, restlessness and lack of concern for others. Conscientiousness and powers of concentration are often diminished, but measurable deterioration of intellect or memory is not necessarily present. The overall picture is often one of emotional dullness, lack of drive, and slowness; but, particularly in persons previously with energetic, restless, or aggressive characteristics, there may be a change towards impulsiveness, boastfulness, temper outbursts, silly fatuous humor, and the development of unrealistic ambitions; the direction of change usually depends upon the previous personality. A considerable degree of recovery is possible and may continue over the course of several years.[1]

Fugue, psychogenic: A form of dissociative hysteria characterized by an episode of wandering with inability to recall one's prior identity. Both onset and recovery are rapid. Following recovery there is no recollection of events which took place during the fugue state.[2]

Ganser's syndrome (hysterical): A form of factitious illness in which the patient voluntarily produces symptoms suggestive of a mental disorder.[2]

Gender identity disorder—*see* gender identity disorder under Psychosexual identity disorders

Gilles de la Tourette's disorder or syndrome—*see* Gilles de la Tourette's disorder under Tics

Grief reaction—*see* depressive reaction, brief under Adjustment reaction

Gross stress reaction—*see* Stress reaction, acute

Group delinquency—*see* socialized conduct disorder under Conduct disorders

Habit spasm—*see* chronic motor tic disorder under Tics

Hangover (alcohol)—*see* Drunkenness, simple

Head-banging—*see* Stereotyped repetitive movements

Hebephrenia—*see* Schizophrenia, disorganized type

Heller's syndrome—*see* Psychosis, disintegrative

High grade defect—*see* Mental retardation, mild

Homosexuality: Exclusive or predominant sexual attraction for persons of the same sex with or without physical relationship. Record homosexuality as a diagnosis whether or not it is considered as a mental disorder.[1]

Hospital addiction syndrome—*see* Munchausen syndrome

Hospital hoboes—*see* Munchausen syndrome

Hospitalism: A mild or transient adjustment reaction characterized by withdrawal seen in hospitalized patients. In young children this may be manifested by elective mutism.[1]

Hyperkinetic syndrome of childhood: Disorders in which the essential features are short attention span and distractibility. In early childhood the most striking symptom is disinhibited, poorly organized and poorly regulated extreme overactivity but in adolescence this may be replaced by underactivity. Impulsiveness, marked mood fluctuations, and aggression are also common symptoms. Delays in the development of specific skills are often present and disturbed, poor relationships are common. If the hyperkinesis is symptomatic of an underlying disorder, the diagnosis of the underlying disorder is recorded instead.[1]

attention deficit disorder: Cases of hyperkinetic syndrome in which short attention span, distractibility, and overactivity are the main manifestations without significant disturbance of conduct or delay in specific skills.[1]

hyperkinesis with developmental delay: Cases in which the hyperkinetic syndrome is associated with speech delay, clumsiness, reading difficulties, or other delays of specific skills.[1]

hyperkinetic conduct disorder: Cases in which the hyperkinetic syndrome is associated with marked conduct disturbance but not developmental delay.[1]

Hypersomnia: A disorder of initiating arousal from sleep or maintaining wakefulness.[2]

persistent: Chronic difficulty in initiating arousal from sleep or maintaining wakefulness associated with major or minor depressive mental disorders.[2]

transient: Episodes of difficulty in arousal from sleep or maintaining wakefulness associated with acute or intermittent emotional reactions or conflicts.[2]

Hypochondriasis—*see* hypochondriasis under Neurotic disorders

Hypomania—*see* Affective psychosis, manic type

Hypomanic personality—*see* Personality disorder, chronic hypomanic type

Hyposomnia—*see* Insomnia

Hysteria—*see* hysteria under Neurotic disorders

anxiety—*see* phobia under Neurotic disorders

psychosis—*see* Psychosis, reactive

acute—*see* Psychosis, excitative type

Hysterical personality—*see* Personality disorder, histrionic type

Identity disorder: An emotional disorder caused by distress over the inability to reconcile aspects of the self into a relatively coherent and acceptable sense of self, not secondary to another mental disorder. The disturbance is manifested by intense subjective distress regarding uncertainty about a variety of issues relating to identity, including long-term goals, career choice, friendship patterns, values, and loyalties.[2]

Idiocy—*see* Mental retardation, profound

Imbecile—*see* Mental retardation, moderate

Impotence: A psychosexual dysfunction in which there is partial or complete failure to attain or maintain erection until completion of the sexual act.[2]

Impulse control disorder—*see* impulse control disorders under Conduct disorders

Inadequate personality—*see* Personality disorder, dependent type

Induced paranoid disorder—*see* Shared paranoid disorder

Inebriety—*see* Drunkenness, simple
Infantile autism—*see* Autism, infantile
Insomnia: A disorder of initiating or maintaining sleep.[2]
persistent: A chronic state of sleeplessness associated with chronic anxiety, major or minor depressive disorders, or psychoses.[2]
transient: Episodes of sleeplessness associated with acute or intermittent emotional reactions or conflicts.[2]
Intermittent explosive disorder: Recurrent episodes of sudden and significant loss of control of aggressive impulses, not accounted for by any other mental disorder, which results in serious assault or destruction of property. The magnitude of the behavior during an episode is grossly out of proportion to any psychosocial stressors which may have played a role in eliciting the episode of lack of control. Following each episode there is genuine regret or self-reproach at the consequences of the action and the inability to control the aggressive impulse.[2]
Introverted disorder of childhood: An emotional disturbance in children chiefly manifested by a lack of interest in social relationships and indifference to social praise or criticism.[2]
Introverted personality—*see* Personality disorder, introverted type
Involutional melancholia—*see* Affective psychosis, depressed type
Involutional paranoid state—*see* Paraphrenia
Isolated explosive disorder: A disorder of impulse control in which there is a single discrete episode characterized by failure to resist an impulse which leads to a single, violent externally-directed act, which has a catastrophic impact on others, and for which the available information does not justify the diagnosis of another mental disorder.[2]
Isolated phobia—*see* simple phobia under Phobia
Jet lag syndrome: A phase-shift disruption of the 24-hour sleep-wake cycle due to rapid time-zone changes experienced in long-distance travel.[2]
Kanner's syndrome—*see* Autism, infantile
Kleptomania: A disorder of impulse control characterized by a recurrent failure to resist impulses to steal objects not for immediate use or their monetary value. An increasing sense of tension is experienced prior to committing the act, with an intense experience of gratification at the time of committing the theft.[2]
Korsakoff's psychosis:
alcoholic—*see* alcohol amnestic syndrome under Alcoholic psychoses
nonalcoholic—*see* Amnestic syndrome
Latent schizophrenia—*see* Schizophrenia, latent
Lesbianism—*see* Homosexuality
Lobotomy syndrome—*see* Frontal lobe syndrome
LSD reaction: Acute intoxication from hallucinogen abuse, manifested by hallucinatory states lasting only a few days or less.[1]
Major depressive disorder—*see* Affective psychosis, depressed type
Malingering: A clinical picture in which the predominant feature is the presentation of fake or grossly exaggerated physical or psychiatric illness apparently under voluntary control. In contrast to factitious illness, the symptoms produced in malingering are in pursuit of a goal which, when known, is recognizable and obviously understandable in light of knowledge of the individual's circumstances. Examples of understandable goals include, but are not limited to, becoming a "patient" in order to avoid conscription or military duty, avoid work, obtain financial compensation, evade criminal prosecution, and obtain drugs.[2]
Mania (monopolar)—*see* Affective psychosis, manic type
Manic-depressive psychosis
circular type—*see* Affective psychosis, bipolar
depressed type—*see* Affective psychosis, depressed type
manic type—*see* Affective psychosis, manic type
mixed type—*see* Affective psychosis, mixed type
Manic disorder—*see* Affective psychosis, manic type
atypical—*see* Affective psychosis, manic type, atypical
Masochistic personality—*see* Personality disorder, masochistic type
Melancholia—*see* Affective psychoses
involutional—*see* Affective psychosis, depressed type
Mental retardation: A condition of arrested or incomplete development of mind which is especially characterized by subnormality of intelligence. The coding should be made on the individual's current level of functioning without regard to its nature or causation, such as psychosis, cultural deprivation, Down's syndrome, etc. Where there is a specific cognitive handicap—such as in speech—the diagnosis of mental retardation should be based on assessments of cognition outside the area of specific handicap. The assessment of intellectual level should be based on whatever information is available, including clinical evidence, adaptive behavior, and psychometric findings. The IQ levels given are based on a test with a mean of 100 and a standard deviation of 15, such as the Wechsler scales. They are provided only as a guide and should not be applied rigidly. Mental retardation often involves psychiatric disturbances and may often develop as a result of some physical disease or injury. In these cases, an additional diagnosis should be recorded to identify any associated condition, psychiatric or physical.[1]
mild mental retardation: IQ criteria 50–70. Individuals with this level of retardation are usually educable. During the preschool period they can develop social and communication skills, have minimal retardation in sensorimotor areas, and often are not distinguished from normal children until a later age. During the school age period they can learn academic skills up to approximately the sixth-grade level. During the adult years, they can usually achieve social and vocational skills adequate for minimum self-support, but may need guidance and assistance when under social or economic stress.[2]
moderate mental retardation: IQ criteria 35–49. Individuals with this level of retardation are usually trainable. During the pre-school period they can talk or learn to communicate. They have poor social awareness and fair motor development. During the school age period they can profit from training in social and occupational skills, but they are unlikely to progress beyond the second-grade level in academic subjects. During their adult years they may achieve self-maintenance in unskilled or semi-skilled work under sheltered conditions. They need supervision and guidance when under mild social or economic stress.[2]
severe mental retardation: IQ criteria 20–34. Individuals with this level of retardation evidence poor motor development, minimal speech, and are generally unable to profit from training and self-help during the pre-school period. During the school age period they can talk or learn to communicate, can be trained in elementary health habits, and may profit from systematic habit training. During the adult years they may contribute partially to self-maintenance under complete supervision.[2]
profound mental retardation: IQ criteria under 20. Individuals with this level of retardation evidence minimal capacity for sensorimotor functioning and need nursing care during the pre-school period. During the school age period some further motor development may occur, and they may respond to minimal or limited training in self-help. During the adult years some motor and speech development may occur, and they may achieve very limited self-care and need nursing care.[2]
Merycism—*see* Rumination, psychogenic
Minimal brain dysfunction [MBD]—*see* Hyperkinetic syndrome of childhood
Misery and unhappiness disorder: An emotional disorder characteristic of childhood in which the main symptoms involve misery and unhappiness. There may also be eating and sleep disturbances.[1]
Mood swings (brief compensatory) (rebound): Mild disorders of mood (depression and anxiety or elation and excitement, occurring alternatingly or episodically) seen in affective psychosis.[1]
Motor tic disorders—*see* Tics
Motor-verbal tic disorder—*see* Gilles de la Tourette's disorder under Tics

Multi-infarct dementia or psychosis—*see* Arteriosclerotic dementia

Multiple operations syndrome—*see* Munchausen syndrome

Multiple personality: A form of dissociative hysteria in which there is the domination of the individual at any one time by one of two or more distinct personalities. Each personality is a fully-integrated and complex unit with memories, behavior patterns, and social friendships which determine the nature of the individual's acts when uppermost in consciousness.[2]

Munchausen syndrome: A chronic form of factitious illness in which the individual demonstrates a plausible presentation of voluntarily produced physical symptomatology of such a degree that he is able to obtain and sustain multiple hospitalizations.[2]

Narcissistic personality—*see* Personality disorder, narcissistic type

Nervous debility—*see* neurasthenia under Neurotic disorders

Neurasthenia—*see* neurasthenia under Neurotic disorders

Neurotic delinquency—*see* mixed disturbance of conduct and emotions under Conduct disorders

Neurotic disorders: Neurotic disorders are mental disorders without any demonstrable organic basis in which the individual may have considerable insight and has unimpaired reality testing, in that he usually does not confuse his morbid subjective experiences and fantasies with external reality. Behavior may be greatly affected although usually remaining within socially acceptable limits, but personality is not disorganized. The principal manifestations include excessive anxiety, hysterical symptoms, phobias, obsessional and compulsive symptoms, and depression.[1]

anxiety states: Various combinations of physical and mental manifestations of anxiety, not attributable to real danger and occurring either in attacks [*see* Anxiety state, panic attacks] or as a persisting state [*see* Anxiety state, generalized]. The anxiety is usually diffuse and may extend to panic. Other neurotic features such as obsessional or hysterical symptoms may be present but do not dominate the clinical picture.[1]

compensation neurosis: Certain unconscious neurotic reactions in which features of secondary gain, such as a situational or financial advantage, are prominent.[3]

depersonalization: A neurotic disorder with an unpleasant state of disturbed perception in which external objects or parts of one's own body are experienced as changed in their quality, unreal, remote, or automatized. The patient is aware of the subjective nature of the change he experiences. If depersonalization occurs as a feature of anxiety, schizophrenia, or other mental disorder, the condition is classified according to the major psychiatric disorder.[1]

depression: A neurotic disorder characterized by disproportionate depression which has usually recognizably ensued on a distressing experience; it does not include among its features delusions or hallucinations, and there is often preoccupation with the psychic trauma which preceded the illness, e.g., loss of a cherished person or possession. Anxiety is also frequently present and mixed states of anxiety and depression should be included here. The distinction between depressive neurosis and psychosis should be made not only upon the degree of depression but also on the presence or absence of other neurotic and psychotic characteristics, and upon the degree of disturbance of the individual's behavior.[1]

hypochondriasis: A neurotic disorder in which the conspicuous features are excessive concern with one's health in general or the integrity and functioning of some part of one's body, or less frequently, one's mind. It is usually associated with anxiety and depression. It may occur as a feature of some other severe mental disorder (e.g., manic-depressive psychosis, depressed type, schizophrenia, hysteria) and in that case should be classified according to the corresponding major disorder.[1]

hysteria: A neurotic mental disorder in which motives, of which the patient seems unaware, produce either a restriction of the field of consciousness or disturbances of motor or sensory function which may seem to have psychological advantage or symbolic value.[1] There are three subtypes:

conversion type: The chief or only symptoms of the hysterical neurosis consist of psychogenic disturbance of function in some part of the body, e.g., paralysis, tremor, blindness, deafness, seizures.[1]

dissociative type: The most prominent feature of the hysterical neurosis is a narrowing of the field of consciousness which seems to serve an unconscious purpose and is commonly accompanied or followed by a selective amnesia. There may be dramatic but essentially superficial changes of personality [multiple personality], or sometimes the patient enters into a wandering state [fugue].[1]

factitious illness: Physical or psychological symptoms that are not real, genuine, or natural, which are produced by the individual and are under his voluntary control.[2]

neurasthenia: A neurotic disorder characterized by fatigue, irritability, headache, depression, insomnia, difficulty in concentration, and lack of capacity for enjoyment [anhedonia]. It may follow or accompany an infection or exhaustion, or arise from continued emotional stress. If neurasthenia is associated with a physical disorder, the latter should also be recorded as a diagnosis.[1]

obsessive-compulsive: States in which the outstanding symptom is a feeling of subjective compulsion, which must be resisted, to carry out some action, to dwell on an idea, to recall an experience, or to ruminate on an abstract topic. Unwanted thoughts which intrude, the insistency of words or ideas, ruminations or trains of thought are perceived by the individual to be inappropriate or nonsensical. The obsessional urge or idea is recognized as alien to the personality but as coming from within the self. Obsessional actions may be quasi-ritual performances designed to relieve anxiety, e.g., washing the hands to cope with contamination. Attempts to dispel the unwelcome thoughts or urges may lead to a severe inner struggle, with intense anxiety.[1]

occupational: A neurosis characterized by a functional disorder of a group of muscles used chiefly in one's occupation, marked by the occurrence of spasm, paresis, or incoordination on attempt to repeat the habitual movements (e.g., writers' cramp).[5]

phobic disorders: Neurotic states with abnormally intense dread of certain objects or specific situations which would not normally have that effect. If the anxiety tends to spread from a specified situation or object to a wider range of circumstances, it becomes akin to or identical with anxiety state and should be classified as such.[1] See also Phobia.

somatization disorder: A chronic, but fluctuating, neurotic disorder which begins early in life and is characterized by recurrent and multiple somatic complaints for which medical attention is sought but which are not apparently due to any physical illness. Complaints are presented in a dramatic, vague, or exaggerated way, or are part of a complicated medical history in which often many specific diagnoses have allegedly been made by other physicians. Complaints invariably refer to many organ systems (headache, fatigue, palpitations, fainting, nausea and vomiting, abdominal pains, bowel trouble, allergies, menstrual and sexual difficulties), and the individual frequently receives medical care from a number of physicians, sometimes simultaneously.[2]

Neurosis—*see* Neurotic disorders

Nightmares: Anxiety attacks occurring in dreams during REM sleep.[2]

Night terrors: A pathology of arousal from stage 4 sleep in which the individual experiences excessive terror and extreme panic (screaming, verbalizations), symptoms of autonomic activity, confusion, and poor recall for event.[2]

Nymphomania: Abnormal and excessive need or desire in the woman for sexual intercourse.[3]

Obsessional personality—*see* Personality disorder, compulsive type

Occupational neurosis—*see* Neurotic disorder, occupational

Oneirophrenia—*see* Schizophrenia, acute episode

Oppositional disorder of childhood or adolescence: A disorder characterized by pervasive opposition to all in authority regardless of self-interest, a continuous argumentativeness, and an unwillingness to respond to reasonable persuasion, not accounted for by a conduct disorder, adjustment disorder, or a psychosis of childhood. The oppositional behavior in this disorder is evoked by any demand, rule, suggestion, request, or admonishment placed on the individual.[2]

Organic affective syndrome: A clinical picture in which the predominating symptoms closely resemble those seen in either the depressive or manic affective disorders, occurring in the presence of evidence or history of a specific organic factor which is etiologically related to the disturbance, such as head trauma, endocranial tumors, and exocranial tumors secreting neurotoxic diatheses (e.g., pancreatic carcinoma). Excessive use of steroids, Cushing's syndrome, and other endocrine disorders may lead to an organic affective syndrome.[2]

Organic personality syndrome: Chronic, mild states of memory disturbance and intellectual deterioration, of nonpsychotic nature, often accompanied by increased irritability, querulousness, lassitude, and complaints of physical weakness. These states are often associated with old age, and may precede more severe states due to brain damage classifiable under senile or presenile dementia, dementia associated with other chronic organic psychotic brain syndromes, or delirium, delusions, hallucinosis, and depression in transient organic psychotic conditions.[1]

Organic psychosyndrome, focal (partial): A nonpsychotic organic mental disorder resembling the postconcussion syndrome associated with localized diseases of the brain or surrounding tissues.[1]

Organic psychotic conditions: Syndromes in which there is impairment of orientation, memory, comprehension, calculation, learning capacity, and judgment. These are the essential features but there may also be shallowness or lability of affect, or a more persistent disturbance of mood, lowering of ethical standards and exaggeration or emergence of personality traits, and diminished capacity for independent decision.[1] See also Alcohol psychoses, Arteriosclerotic dementia, Drug psychoses, Presenile dementia, and Senile dementia.

- **mixed paranoid and affective:** Organic psychosis in which depressive and paranoid symptoms are the main features.[1]
- **transient:** States characterized by clouded consciousness, confusion, disorientation, illusions, and often vivid hallucinations. They are usually due to some intra- or extracerebral toxic, infectious, metabolic or other systemic disturbance and are generally reversible. Depressive and paranoid symptoms may also be present but are not the main feature. The diagnosis of the associated physical or neurological condition should also be recorded.[1]
  - **acute delirium:** Short-lived states, lasting hours or days, of the above type.[1]
  - **subacute delirium:** States of the above type in which the symptoms, usually less florid, last for several weeks or longer during which they may show marked fluctuations in intensity.[1]

Organic reaction—*see* Organic psychotic conditions, transient

Overanxious disorder: An ill-defined emotional disorder characteristic of childhood in which the main symptoms involve anxiety and fearfulness.[1]

Panic disorder—*see* panic attack under Anxiety state

Paranoia: A rare chronic psychosis in which logically constructed systematized delusions have developed gradually without concomitant hallucinations or the schizophrenic type of disordered thinking. The delusions are mostly of grandeur (the paranoiac prophet or inventor), persecution, or somatic abnormality.[1]

- **alcoholic**—*see* alcoholic jealousy under Alcoholic psychoses
- **querulans:** A paranoid state which, though in many ways akin to schizophrenic or affective states, differs from other paranoid states and psychogenic paranoid psychosis.[1]
- **senile**—*see* Paraphrenia

Paranoid personality—*see* Personality disorder, paranoid type

Paranoid reaction, acute: Paranoid states apparently provoked by some emotional stress. The stress is often misconstrued as an attack or threat. Such states are particularly prone to occur in prisoners or as acute reactions to a strange and threatening environment, e.g., in immigrants.[1]

Paranoid schizophrenia—*see* Schizophrenia, paranoid type

Paranoid state

- **involutional**—*see* Paraphrenia
- **senile**—*see* Paraphrenia
- **simple:** A psychosis, acute or chronic, not classifiable as schizophrenia or affective psychosis, in which delusions, especially of being influenced, persecuted, or treated in some special way, are the main symptoms. The delusions are of a fairly fixed, elaborate, and systematized kind.[1]

Paranoid traits—*see* Personality disorder, paranoid type

Paraphilia—*see* Sexual deviations

Paraphrenia: Paranoid psychosis in which there are conspicuous hallucinations, often in several modalities. Affective symptoms and disordered thinking, if present, do not dominate the clinical picture, and the personality is well preserved.[1]

Paraphrenic schizophrenia—*see* Schizophrenia, paranoid type

Passive-aggressive personality—*see* Personality disorder, passive-aggressive type

Passive personality—*see* Personality disorder, dependent type

Pathological

- **alcohol intoxication**—*see* Alcohol intoxication, idiosyncratic
- **drug intoxication:** Individual idiosyncratic reactions to comparatively small quantities of a drug, which take the form of acute, brief psychotic states of any type.[1]
- **drunkenness**—*see* Alcohol intoxication, idiosyncratic
- **gambling:** A disorder of impulse control characterized by a chronic and progressive preoccupation with gambling and urge to gamble, with subsequent gambling behavior that compromises, disrupts, or damages personal, family, and vocational pursuits.[2]
- **personality**—*see* Personality disorder

Pedophilia: Sexual deviations in which an adult engages in sexual activity with a child of the same or opposite sex.[1]

Peregrinating patient—*see* Malingering

Personality disorders: Deeply ingrained maladaptive patterns of behavior generally recognizable by the time of adolescence or earlier and continuing throughout most of adult life, although often becoming less obvious in middle or old age. The personality is abnormal either in the balance of its components, their quality and expression, or in its total aspect. Because of this deviation or psychopathy the patient suffers or others have to suffer, and there is an adverse effect upon the individual or on society. It includes what is sometimes called psychopathic personality, but if this is determined primarily by malfunctioning of the brain, it should be classified as one of the nonpsychotic organic brain syndromes. When the patient exhibits an anomaly of personality directly related to his neurosis or psychosis, e.g., schizoid personality and schizophrenia or anancastic personality and obsessive compulsive neurosis, the relevant neurosis or psychosis which is in evidence should be diagnosed in addition.[1]

- **affective type:** A chronic personality disorder characterized by lifelong predominance of a pronounced mood. The illness does not have a clear onset, and there may be intermittent periods of disturbed mood separated by periods of normal mood.[1]
- **anancastic [anankastic] type**—*see* Personality disorder, compulsive type
- **antisocial type:** A personality disorder characterized by disregard for social obligations, lack of feeling for others, and impetuous violence or callous unconcern. There is a gross disparity between behavior and the prevailing social norms. Behavior is not readily modifiable by experience, including punishment. People with this personality are often affectively cold, and may be abnormally aggressive or irresponsible. Their tolerance to frustration is low; they blame others or offer plausible rationalizations for the behavior which brings them into conflict with society.[1]
- **asthenic type**—*see* Personality disorder, dependent type
- **avoidant type:** Individuals with this disorder exhibit excessive social inhibitions and shyness, a tendency to withdraw from opportunities for developing close relationships, and a fearful expectation that they will be belittled and humiliated. Desires for affection and acceptance are strong, but they are unwilling to enter relationships unless given unusually strong guarantees that they will be uncritically accepted. Therefore, they

have few close relationships and suffer from feelings of loneliness and isolation.[2]

borderline type: Individuals with this disorder are characterized by instability in a variety of areas, including interpersonal relationships, behavior, mood, and self image. Interpersonal relationships are often intense and unstable with marked shifts of attitude over time. Frequently there is impulsive and unpredictable behavior which is potentially physically self-damaging. There may be problems tolerating being alone, and chronic feelings of emptiness or boredom.[2]

chronic depressive type: An affective personality disorder characterized by lifelong predominance of a chronic nonpsychotic disturbance involving either intermittent or sustained periods of depressed mood (marked by worry, pessimism, low output of energy, and a sense of futility).[2]

chronic hypomanic type: An affective personality disorder characterized by lifelong predominance of a chronic nonpsychotic disturbance involving either intermittent or sustained periods of abnormally elevated mood (unshakable optimism and an enhanced zest for life and activity).[2]

compulsive type: A personality disorder characterized by feelings of personal insecurity, doubt, and incompleteness leading to excessive conscientiousness, checking, stubbornness, and caution. There may be insistent and unwelcome thoughts or impulses which do not attain the severity of an obsessional neurosis. There is perfectionism and meticulous accuracy and a need to check repeatedly in an attempt to ensure this. Rigidity and excessive doubt may be conspicuous.[1]

cyclothymic type: A chronic nonpsychotic disturbance involving depressed and elevated mood, lasting at least two years, separated by periods of normal mood.[2]

dependent type: A personality disorder characterized by passive compliance with the wishes of elders and others and a weak inadequate response to the demands of daily life. Lack of vigor may show itself in the intellectual or emotional spheres; there is little capacity for enjoyment.[1]

eccentric type: A personality disorder characterized by oddities of behavior which do not conform to the clinical syndromes of personality disorders described elsewhere.[2]

explosive type: A personality disorder characterized by instability of mood with liability to intemperate outbursts of anger, hate, violence, or affection. Aggression may be expressed in words or in physical violence. The outbursts cannot readily be controlled by the affected persons, who are not otherwise prone to antisocial behavioral.[1]

histrionic type: A personality disorder characterized by shallow, labile affectivity, dependence on others, craving for appreciation and attention, suggestibility, and theatricality. There is often sexual immaturity, e.g., frigidity and over-responsiveness to stimuli. Under stress hysterical symptoms [neurosis] may develop.[1]

hysterical type—*see* Personality disorder, histrionic type

inadequate type—*see* Personality disorder, dependent type

introverted type: A form of schizoid personality in which the essential features are a profound defect in the ability to form social relationships and to respond to the usual forms of social reinforcements. Such patients are characteristically "loners " who do not appear distressed by their social distance and are not interested in greater social involvement.[2]

masochistic type: A personality disorder in which the individual appears to arrange life situations so as to be defeated and humiliated.[2]

narcissistic type: A personality disorder in which interpersonal difficulties are caused by an inflated sense of self-worth, and indifference to the welfare of others. Achievement deficits and social irresponsibilities are justified and sustained by a boastful arrogance, expansive fantasies, facile rationalization, and frank prevarication.[2]

paranoid type: A personality disorder in which there is excessive sensitiveness to setbacks or to what are taken to be humiliations and rebuffs, a tendency to distort experience by misconstruing the neutral or friendly actions of others as hostile or contemptuous, and a combative and tenacious sense of personal rights. There may be a proneness to jealousy or excessive self-importance. Such persons may feel helplessly humiliated and put upon; others, likewise excessively sensitive, are aggressive and insistent. In all cases there is excessive self-reference.[1]

passive-aggressive type: A personality disorder characterized by aggressive behavior manifested in passive ways, such as obstructionism, pouting, procrastination, intentional inefficiency, or stubbornness. The aggression often arises from resentment at failing to find gratification in a relationship with an individual or institution upon which the individual is overdependent.[3]

passive type—*see* Personality disorder, dependent type

schizoid type: A personality disorder in which there is withdrawal from affectional, social, and other contacts with autistic preference for fantasy and introspective reserve. Behavior may be slightly eccentric or indicate avoidance of competitive situations. Apparent coolness and detachment may mask an incapacity to express feeling.[1]

schizotypal type: A form of schizoid personality in which individuals with this disorder manifest various oddities of thinking, perception, communication, and behavior. The disturbance in thinking may be expressed as magical thinking, ideas of reference, or paranoid ideation. Perceptual disturbances may include recurrent illusions and derealization [depersonalization]. Frequently, but not invariably, the behavioral manifestations include social isolation and constricted or inappropriate affect which interferes with rapport in face-to-face interaction without any of the frank psychotic features which characterize schizophrenia.[2]

Phobia: Neurotic states with abnormally intense dread of certain objects or specific situations which would not normally have that effect. If the anxiety tends to spread from a specified situation or object to a wider range of circumstances, it becomes akin to or identical with anxiety state, and should be classified as such.[1]

acrophobia: Fear of heights[3]

agoraphobia: Fear of leaving the familiar setting of the home, and is almost always preceded by a phase during which there are recurrent panic attacks. Because of the anticipatory fear of helplessness when having a panic attack, the patient is reluctant or refuses to be alone, travel or walk alone, or to be in situations where there is no ready access to help, such as in crowds, closed or open spaces, or crowded stores.[2]

ailurophobia: Fear of cats[3]

algophobia: Fear of pain[3]

claustrophobia: Fear of closed spaces[3]

isolated phobia—*see* simple phobia below

mysophobia: Fear of dirt or germs[3]

obsessional—*see* Neurotic disorder, obsessive-compulsive

panphobia: Fear of everything

simple phobia: Fear of a discrete object or situation which is neither fear of leaving the familiar setting of the home [agoraphobia], or of being observed by others in certain situations [social phobia]. Examples of simple phobia are fear of animals, acrophobia, and claustrophobia.[2]

social phobia: Fear of situations in which the subject is exposed to possible scrutiny by others, and the possibility exists that he may act in a fashion that will be considered shameful. The most common social phobias are fears of public speaking, blushing, eating in public, writing in front of others, or using public lavatories.[2]

xenophobia: Fear of strangers[3]

Pica: Perverted appetite of nonorganic origin in which there is persistent eating of non-nutritional substances. Typically, infants ingest paint, plaster, string, hair, or cloth. Older children may have access to animal droppings, sand, bugs, leaves, or pebbles. In the adult, eating of starch or clay-earth has been observed.[2]

Postconcussion syndrome: States occurring after generalized contusion of the brain, in which the symptom picture may resemble that of the frontal lobe syndrome or that of any of the neurotic disorders, but in which in addition, headache, giddiness, fatigue, insomnia, and a subjective feeling of impaired intellectual ability are usually prominent. Mood may fluctuate, and quite ordinary stress may produce exaggerated fear and apprehension. There may be marked intolerance of mental and physical exertion, undue sensitivity to noise, and hypochondriacal preoccupation. The symptoms are more common in persons who have previously suffered from neurotic or personality disorders, or when there is a possibility of compensation. This syndrome is particularly associated with the closed type of head injury when signs of localized brain damage are slight or absent, but it may also occur in other conditions.[1]

Postcontusion syndrome or encephalopathy—*see* Postconcussion syndrome

Postencephalitic syndrome: A nonpsychotic organic mental disorder resembling the postconcussion syndrome associated with central nervous system infections.[1]

Postleucotomy syndrome—*see* Frontal lobe syndrome

Posttraumatic brain syndrome, nonpsychotic—*see* Postconcussion syndrome

Posttraumatic organic psychosis—*see* Organic psychotic conditions, transient

Posttraumatic stress disorder: The development of characteristic symptoms (re-experiencing the traumatic event, numbing of responsiveness to or involvement with the external world, and a variety of other autonomic, dysphoric, or cognitive symptoms) after experiencing a psychologically traumatic event or events outside the normal range of human experience (e.g., rape or assault, military combat, natural catastrophes such as flood or earthquake, or other disaster, such as airplane crash, fires, bombings).[2]

- **acute:** Brief, episodic, or recurrent disorders lasting less than six months' duration after the onset of trauma.[2]
- **prolonged:** Chronic disorders of the above type lasting six months or more following the trauma.[2]

Premature ejaculation—*see* premature ejaculation under Psychosexual dysfunctions

Prepsychotic schizophrenia—*see* Schizophrenia, latent

Presbyophrenia—*see* Organic personality syndrome

Presenile dementia: Dementia occurring usually before the age of 65 in patients with the relatively rare forms of diffuse or lobar cerebral atrophy. The associated neurological condition (e.g., Alzheimer's disease, Pick's disease, Jakob-Creutzfeldt disease) should also be recorded as a diagnosis.[1]

Prodromal schizophrenia—*see* Schizophrenia, latent

Pseudoneurotic schizophrenia—*see* Schizophrenia, latent

Psychalgia: Pains of mental origin, e.g., headache or backache, for which a more precise medical or psychiatric diagnosis cannot be made.[1]

Psychasthenia: A functional neurosis marked by stages of pathological fear or anxiety, obsessions, fixed ideas, tics, feelings of inadequacy, self-accusation, and peculiar feelings of strangeness, unreality, and depersonalization.[4]

Psychic shock: A sudden disturbance of mental equilibrium produced by strong emotion in response to physical or mental stress.[4]

Psychic factors associated with physical diseases: Mental disturbances or psychic factors of any type thought to have played a major part in the etiology of physical conditions, usually involving tissue damage, classified elsewhere. The mental disturbance is usually mild and nonspecific, and the psychic factors (worry, fear, conflict, etc.) may be present without any overt psychiatric disorder. Examples of these conditions are asthma, dermatitis, eczema, duodenal ulcer, ulcerative colitis, and urticaria, specified as due to psychogenic factors.

Use an additional diagnosis to identify the physical condition. In the rare instance that an overt psychiatric disorder is thought to have caused the physical condition, the psychiatric diagnosis should be recorded in addition.[1]

Psychoneurosis—*see* Neurotic disorders

Psycho-organic syndrome—*see* Organic psychotic conditions, transient

Psychopathic constitutional state—*see* Personality disorders

Psychopathic personality—*see* Personality disorders

Psychophysiological disorders: A variety of physical symptoms or types of physiological malfunctions of mental origin, not involving tissue damage, and usually mediated through the autonomic nervous system. The disorders are classified according to the body system involved. If the physical symptom is secondary to a psychiatric disorder classifiable elsewhere, the physical symptom is not classified as a psychophysiological disorder. If tissue damage is involved, then the diagnosis is classified as a psychic factor associated with diseases classified elsewhere.[1]

Psychosexual dysfunctions: A group of disorders in which there is recurrent and persistent dysfunction encountered during sexual activity. The dysfunction may be lifelong or acquired, generalized or situational, and total or partial.[2]

- **functional dyspareunia:** Recurrent and persistent genital pain associated with coitus.[2]
- **functional vaginismus:** A history of recurrent and persistent involuntary spasm of the musculature of the outer one-third of the vagina that interferes with sexual activity.[2]
- **inhibited female orgasm:** Recurrent and persistent inhibition of the female orgasm as manifested by a delay or absence of orgasm following a normal sexual excitement phase during sexual activity.[2]
- **inhibited male orgasm:** Recurrent and persistent inhibition of the male orgasm as manifested by a delay or absence of either the emission or ejaculation phases, or more usually, both following an adequate phase of sexual excitement.[2]
- **inhibited sexual desire:** Persistent inhibition of desire for engaging in a particular form of sexual activity.[2]
- **inhibited sexual excitement:** Recurrent and persistent inhibition of sexual excitement during sexual activity, manifested either by partial or complete failure to attain or maintain erection until completion of the sexual act [impotence], or partial or complete failure to attain or maintain the lubrication-swelling response of sexual excitement until completion of the sexual act [frigidity].[2]
- **premature ejaculation:** Ejaculation occurs before the individual wishes it, because of recurrent and persistent absence of reasonable voluntary control of ejaculation and orgasm during sexual activity.[2]

Psychosexual gender identity disorders: Behavior occurring in preadolescents of immature psychosexuality, or in adults, in which there is an incongruence between the individual's anatomic sex and gender identity.[2]

- **gender identity disorder:** In children or in adults a condition in which the individual would prefer to be of the other sex, and strongly prefers the clothes, toys, activities, and companionship of the other sex. Cross-dressing is intermittent, although it may be frequent. In children the commonest form is feminism in boys.[2]
- **trans-sexualism:** A psychosexual identity disorder centered around fixed beliefs that the overt bodily sex is wrong. The resulting behavior is directed towards either changing the sexual organs by operation, or completely concealing the bodily sex by adopting both the dress and behavior of the opposite sex.[1]

Psychosomatic disorders—*see* Psychophysiological disorders

Psychosis: Mental disorders in which impairment of mental function has developed to a degree that interferes grossly with insight, ability to meet some ordinary demands of life or to maintain adequate contact with reality. It is not an exact or well defined term. Mental retardation is excluded.[1]

- **affective**—*see* Affective psychoses
- **alcoholic**—*see* Alcoholic psychoses
- **atypical childhood:** A variety of atypical infantile psychoses which may show some, but not all, of the features of infantile autism. Symptoms may include stereotyped repetitive movements, hyperkinesis, self-injury, retarded speech development, echolalia, and impaired social relationships. Such disorders may occur in children of any level of intelligence but are particularly common in those with mental retardation.[1]
- **borderline, of childhood**—*see* Psychosis, atypical childhood
- **child:** A group of disorders in children, characterized by distortions in the timing, rate, and sequence of many psychological functions involving language development and social relations in which the severe qualitative abnormalities are not

normal for any stage of development.[2] See also Autism, infantile, Psychosis, disintegrative, Psychosis, atypical childhood.

depressive—*see* Affective psychosis, depressed type

depressive type: A depressive psychosis which can be similar in its symptoms to manic-depressive psychosis, depressed type but is apparently provoked by saddening stress such as a bereavement, or a severe disappointment or frustration. There may be less diurnal variation of symptoms than in manic-depressive psychosis, depressed type, and the delusions are more often understandable in the context of the life experiences. There is usually a serious disturbance of behavior, e.g., major suicidal attempt.[1]

disintegrative: A disorder in which normal or near-normal development for the first few years is followed by a loss of social skills and of speech, together with a severe disorder of emotions, behavior, and relationships. Usually this loss of speech and of social competence takes place over a period of a few months and is accompanied by the emergence of overactivity and of stereotypies. In most cases there is intellectual impairment, but this is not a necessary part of the disorder. The condition may follow overt brain disease, such as measles encephalitis, but it may also occur in the absence of any known organic brain disease or damage. Any associated neurological disorder should also be recorded.[1]

epileptic: An organic psychotic condition associated with epilepsy.[1]

excitative type: An affective psychosis similar in its symptoms to manic-depressive psychosis, manic type, but apparently provoked by emotional stress.[1]

hypomanic—*see* Affective psychosis, manic type

hysterical—*see* Psychosis, reactive

  acute—*see* Psychosis, excitative type

induced—*see* Shared paranoid disorder

infantile—*see* Autism, infantile

infective—*see* Organic psychotic conditions, transient

Korsakoff's:

  alcoholic—*see* alcohol amnestic syndrome under Alcoholic psychoses

  nonalcoholic—*see* Amnestic syndrome

manic-depressive—*see* Affective psychoses

multi-infarct—*see* Arteriosclerotic dementia

paranoid

  chronic—*see* Paranoia

  protracted reactive—*see* Psychosis, paranoid, psychogenic

  psychogenic: Psychogenic or reactive paranoid psychosis of any type which is more protracted than the reactions described under Paranoid reaction, acute.[1]

    acute—*see* Paranoid reaction, acute

postpartum—*see* Psychosis, puerperal

psychogenic—*see* Psychosis, reactive

  depressive—*see* Psychosis, depressive type

puerperal: Any psychosis occurring within a fixed period (approximately 90 days) after childbirth.[3] The diagnosis should be classified according to the predominant symptoms or characteristics, such as schizophrenia, affective psychosis, paranoid states, or other specified psychosis.

reactive: A psychotic condition which is largely or entirely attributable to a recent life experience. This diagnosis is not used for the wider range of psychoses in which environmental factors play some, but not the major, part in etiology.[1]

  brief: A florid psychosis of at least a few hours' duration but lasting no more than two weeks, with sudden onset immediately following a severe environmental stress and eventually terminating in complete recovery to the pre-psychotic state.[2]

  confusion: Mental disorders with clouded consciousness, disorientation (though less marked than in organic confusion), and diminished accessibility often accompanied by excessive activity and apparently provoked by emotional stress.[1]

  depressive—*see* Psychosis, depressive type

schizo-affective—*see* Schizophrenia, schizo-affective type

schizophrenic—*see* Schizophrenia

schizophreniform—*see* Schizophrenia

  affective type —*see* Schizophrenia, schizo-affective type

  confusional type —*see* Schizophrenia, acute episode

senile—*see* Senile dementia, delusional type

Pyromania: A disorder of impulse control characterized by a recurrent failure to resist impulses to set fires without regard for the consequences, or with deliberate destructive intent. Invariably there is intense fascination with the setting of fires, seeing fires burn, and a satisfaction with the resultant destruction.[2]

Relationship problems of childhood: Emotional disorders characteristic of childhood in which the main symptoms involve relationship problems.[1]

Repeated infarct dementia—*see* Arteriosclerotic dementia

Residual schizophrenia—*see* Schizophrenia, residual type

Restzustand (schizophrenia)—*see* Schizophrenia, residual type

Rumination:

  obsessional: The constant preoccupation with certain thoughts, with inability to dismiss them from the mind.[4] See Neurotic disorder, obsessive-compulsive.

  psychogenic: In children the regurgitation of food, with failure to thrive or weight loss developing after a period of normal functioning. Food is brought up without nausea, retching, or disgust. The food is then ejected from the mouth, or chewed and reswallowed.[2]

Sander's disease—*see* Paranoia

Satyriasis: Pathologic or exaggerated sexual desire or excitement in the man.[3]

Schizoid personality disorder—*see* Personality disorder, schizoid type

Schizophrenia: A group of psychoses in which there is a fundamental disturbance of personality, a characteristic distortion of thinking, often a sense of being controlled by alien forces, delusions which may be bizarre, disturbed perception, abnormal affect out of keeping with the real situation, and autism. Nevertheless, clear consciousness and intellectual capacity are usually maintained. The disturbance of personality involves its most basic functions which give the normal person his feeling of individuality, uniqueness, and self-direction. The most intimate thoughts, feelings, and acts are often felt to be known to or shared by others and explanatory delusions may develop, to the effect that natural or supernatural forces are at work to influence the schizophrenic person's thoughts and actions in ways that are often bizarre. He may see himself as the pivot of all that happens. Hallucinations, especially of hearing, are common and may comment on the patient or address him. Perception is frequently disturbed in other ways; there may be perplexity, irrelevant features may become all-important and accompanied by passivity feelings, and may lead the patient to believe that everyday objects and situations possess a special, usually sinister, meaning intended for him. In the characteristic schizophrenic disturbance of thinking, peripheral and irrelevant features of a total concept, which are inhibited in normal directed mental activity, are brought to the forefront and utilized in place of the elements relevant and appropriate to the situation. Thus, thinking becomes vague, elliptical and obscure, and its expression in speech sometimes incomprehensible. Breaks and interpolations in the flow of consecutive thought are frequent, and the patient may be convinced that his thoughts are being withdrawn by some outside agency. Mood may be shallow, capricious, or incongruous. Ambivalence and disturbance of volition may appear as inertia, negativism, or stupor. Catatonia may be present. The diagnosis "schizophrenia " should not be made unless there is, or has been evident during the same illness, characteristic disturbance of thought, perception, mood, conduct, or personality—preferably in at least two of these areas. The diagnosis should not be restricted to conditions running a protracted, deteriorating, or chronic course. In addition to making the diagnosis on the criteria just given, effort should be made to specify one of the following subtypes of schizophrenia, according to the predominant symptoms.[1]

  acute (undifferentiated): Schizophrenia of florid nature which cannot be classified as simple, catatonic, hebephrenic, paranoid, or any other types.[1]

  acute episode: Schizophrenic disorders, other than simple, hebephrenic, catatonic, and paranoid, in which there is a dream-like state with slight clouding of consciousness and perplexity. External things, people, and events may become charged with personal significance for the patient. There may be ideas of reference and emotional turmoil. In many such cases remission occurs within a few weeks or months, even without treatment.[1]

atypical—*see* Schizophrenia, acute (undifferentiated)

borderline—*see* Schizophrenia, latent

catatonic type: Includes as an essential feature prominent psychomotor disturbances often alternating between extremes such as hyperkinesis and stupor, or automatic obedience and negativism. Constrained attitudes may be maintained for long periods: if the patient's limbs are put in some unnatural position they may be held there for some time after the external force has been removed. Severe excitement may be a striking feature of the condition. Depressive or hypomanic concomitants may be present.[1]

cenesthopathic—*see* Schizophrenia, acute (undifferentiated)

childhood type—*see* Psychosis, child

chronic undifferentiated—*see* Schizophrenia, residual

cyclic—*see* Schizophrenia, schizo-affective type

disorganized type: A form of schizophrenia in which affective changes are prominent, delusions and hallucinations fleeting and fragmentary, behavior irresponsible and unpredictable, and mannerisms common. The mood is shallow and inappropriate, accompanied by giggling or self-satisfied, self-absorbed smiling, or by a lofty manner, grimaces, mannerisms, pranks, hypochondriacal complaints, and reiterated phrases. Thought is disorganized. There is a tendency to remain solitary, and behavior seems empty of purpose and feeling. This form of schizophrenia usually starts between the ages of 15 and 25 years.[1]

hebephrenic type—*see* Schizophrenia, disorganized type

latent: It has not been possible to produce a generally acceptable description for this condition. It is not recommended for general use, but a description is provided for those who believe it to be useful: a condition of eccentric or inconsequent behavior and anomalies of affect which give the impression of schizophrenia though no definite and characteristic schizophrenic anomalies, present or past, have been manifest.[1]

paranoid type: The form of schizophrenia in which relatively stable delusions, which may be accompanied by hallucinations, dominate the clinical picture. The delusions are frequently of persecution, but may take other forms (for example, of jealousy, exalted birth, Messianic mission, or bodily change). Hallucinations and erratic behavior may occur; in some cases conduct is seriously disturbed from the outset, thought disorder may be gross, and affective flattening with fragmentary delusions and hallucinations may develop.[1]

prepsychotic—*see* Schizophrenia, latent

prodromal—*see* Schizophrenia, latent

pseudoneurotic—*see* Schizophrenia, latent

pseudopsychopathic—*see* Schizophrenia, latent

residual: A chronic form of schizophrenia in which the symptoms that persist from the acute phase have mostly lost their sharpness. Emotional response is blunted and thought disorder, even when gross, does not prevent the accomplishment of routine work.[1]

schizo-affective type: A psychosis in which pronounced manic or depressive features are intermingled with schizophrenic features and which tends towards remission without permanent defect, but which is prone to recur. The diagnosis should be made only when both the affective and schizophrenic symptoms are pronounced.[1]

simple type: A psychosis in which there is insidious development of oddities of conduct, inability to meet the demands of society, and decline in total performance. Delusions and hallucinations are not in evidence and the condition is less obviously psychotic than are the hebephrenic, catatonic, and paranoid types of schizophrenia. With increasing social impoverishment vagrancy may ensue and the patient becomes self-absorbed, idle, and aimless. Because the schizophrenic symptoms are not clear-cut, diagnosis of this form should be made sparingly, if at all.[1]

simplex—*see* Schizophrenia, simple type

Schizophrenic syndrome of childhood—*see* Psychosis, child

Schizophreniform

attack—*see* Schizophrenia, acute episode

disorder—*see* Schizophrenia, acute episode

psychosis—*see* Schizophrenia

affective type—*see* Schizophrenia, schizo-affective type

confusional type—*see* Schizophrenia, acute episode

Schizotypal personality—*see* Personality disorder, schizotypal type

Senile dementia: Dementia occurring usually after the age of 65 in which any cerebral pathology other than that of senile atrophic change can be reasonably excluded.[1]

delirium: Senile dementia with a superimposed reversible episode of acute confusional state.[1]

delusional type: A type of senile dementia characterized by development in advanced old age, progressive in nature, in which delusions, varying from simple poorly formed paranoid delusions to highly formed paranoid delusional states, and hallucinations are also present.[1,2]

depressed type: A type of senile dementia characterized by development in advanced old age, progressive in nature, in which depressive features, ranging from mild to severe forms of manic-depressive affective psychosis, are also present. Disturbance of the sleep-waking cycle and preoccupation with dead people are often particularly prominent.[1,2]

paranoid type—*see* Senile dementia, delusional type

simple type—*see* Senile dementia

Sensitiver Beziehungswahn: A paranoid state which, though in many ways akin to schizophrenic or affective states, differs from paranoia, simple paranoid state, shared paranoid disorder, or psychogenic psychosis.[1]

Sensitivity reaction of childhood or adolescence—*see* Shyness disorder of childhood

Separation anxiety disorder: A clinical disorder in children in which the predominant disturbance is exaggerated distress at separation from parents, home, or other familial surroundings. When separation is instituted, the child may experience anxiety to the point of panic. In adults a similar disorder is seen in agoraphobic reactions.[2]

Sexual deviations: Abnormal sexual inclinations or behavior which are part of a referral problem. The limits and features of normal sexual behavior have not been stated absolutely in different societies and cultures, but are broadly such as serve approved social and biological purposes. The sexual activity of affected persons is directed primarily either towards people not of the opposite sex, or towards sexual acts not associated with coitus normally, or towards coitus performed under abnormal circumstances. If the anomalous behavior becomes manifest only during psychosis or other mental illness the condition should be classified under the major illness. It is common for more than one anomaly to occur together in the same individual; in that case the predominant deviation is classified. It is preferable not to diagnose sexual deviation in individuals who perform deviant sexual acts when normal sexual outlets are not available to them.[1] See also Exhibitionism, Fetishism, Homosexuality, Nymphomania, Pedophilia, Satyriasis, Sexual masochism, Sexual sadism, Transvestism, Voyeurism, and Zoophilia.

Gender identity disorder and trans-sexualism are considered to be psychosexual gender identity disorders and are not included here.

Sexual masochism: A sexual deviation in which sexual arousal and pleasure is produced in an individual by his own physical or psychological suffering, and in which there are insistent and persistent fantasies wherein sexual excitement is produced as a result of suffering.[2]

Sexual sadism: A sexual deviation in which physical or psychological suffering inflicted on another person is utilized as a method of stimulating erotic excitement and orgasm, and in which there are insistent and persistent fantasies wherein sexual excitement is produced as a result of suffering inflicted on the partner.[2]

Shared paranoid disorder: Mainly delusional psychosis, usually chronic and often without florid features, which appears to have developed as a,result of a close, if not dependent, relationship with another person who already has an established similar psychosis. The delusions are at least partly shared. The rare cases in which several persons are affected should also be included here.[1]

Shifting sleep-work schedule: A sleep disorder in which the phase-shift disruption of the 24-hour sleep-wake cycle occurs due to rapid changes in the individual's work schedule.[2]

Short sleeper: Individuals who typically need only 4-6 hours of sleep within the 24-hour cycle.[2]

Shyness disorder of childhood: A persistent and excessive shrinking from familiarity or contact with all strangers of sufficient severity as to interfere with peer functioning, yet there are warm and satisfying relationships with family members. A critical feature of this disorder is that the avoidant behavior with strangers persists even after prolonged exposure or contact.[2]

Sibling jealousy or rivalry: An emotional disorder related to competition between siblings for the love of a parent or for other recognition or gain.[3]

Simple phobia—*see* simple phobia under Phobia

Situational disturbance, acute—*see* Stress reaction, acute

Social phobia—*see* social phobia under Phobia

Social withdrawal of childhood—*see* Introverted disorder of childhood

Socialized conduct disorder—*see* socialized conduct disorder under Conduct disorders

Somatization disorder—*see* somatization disorder under Neurotic disorders

Somatoform disorder, atypical—*see* hypochondriasis under Neurotic disorders

Spasmus nutans—*see* Stereotyped repetitive movements

Specific academic or work inhibition: An adjustment reaction in which a specific academic or work inhibition occurs in an individual whose intellectual capacity, skills, and previous academic or work performance have been at least adequate, and in which the inhibition occurs despite apparent effort and is not due to any other mental disorder.[2]

Stammering—*see* Stuttering

Starch-eating—*see* Pica

Status postcommotio cerebri—*see* Postconcussion syndrome

Stereotyped repetitive movements: Disorders in which voluntary repetitive stereotyped movements, which are not due to any psychiatric or neurological condition, constitute the main feature. Includes head-banging, spasmus nutans, rocking, twirling, finger-flicking mannerisms, and eye poking. Such movements are particularly common in cases of mental retardation with sensory impairment or with environmental monotony.[1]

Stereotypies—*see* Stereotyped repetitive movements

Stress reaction

acute: Acute transient disorders of any severity and nature of emotions, consciousness, and psychomotor states (singly or in combination) which occur in individuals, without any apparent pre-existing mental disorder, in response to exceptional physical or mental stress, such as natural catastrophe or battle, and which usually subside within hours or days.[1]

chronic—*see* Adjustment reaction

Stupor

catatonic—*see* Schizophrenia, catatonic type

psychogenic—*see* Psychosis, reactive

Stuttering: Disorders in the rhythm of speech, in which the individual knows precisely what he wishes to say, but at the time is unable to say it because of an involuntary, repetitive prolongation or cessation of a sound.[1]

Subjective insomnia complaint: A complaint of insomnia made by the individual, which has not been investigated or proven.[2]

Tension headache: Headache of mental origin for which a more precise medical or psychiatric diagnosis cannot be made.[1]

Systematized delusions—*see* Paranoia

Tics: Disorders of no known organic origin in which the outstanding feature consists of quick, involuntary, apparently purposeless, and frequently repeated movements which are not due to any neurological condition. Any part of the body may be involved but the face is most frequently affected. Only one form of tic may be present, or there may be a combination of tics which are carried out simultaneously, alternatively, or consecutively.[1]

chronic motor tic disorder: A tic disorder starting in childhood and persisting into adult life. The tic is limited to no more than three motor areas, and rarely has a verbal component.[2]

Gilles de la Tourette's disorder [motor-verbal tic disorder]: A rare disorder occurring in individuals of any level of intelligence in which facial tics and tic-like throat noises become more marked and more generalized, and in which later whole words or short sentences (often with obscene content) are ejaculated spasmodically and involuntarily. There is some overlap with other varieties of tic.[1]

transient tic disorder of childhood: Facial or other tics beginning in childhood, but limited to one year in duration.[2]

Tobacco use disorder: Cases in which tobacco is used to the detriment of a person's health or social functioning or in which there is tobacco dependence. Dependence is included here rather than under drug dependence because tobacco differs from other drugs of dependence in its psychotoxic effects.[1]

Tranquilizer abuse: Cases where an individual has taken the drug to the detriment of his health or social functioning, in doses above or for periods beyond those normally regarded as therapeutic.[1]

Transient organic psychotic condition—*see* Organic psychotic conditions, transient

Trans-sexualism—*see* trans-sexualism under Psychosexual identity disorders

Transvestism: Sexual deviation in which there is recurrent and persistent dressing in clothes of the opposite sex, and initially in the early stage of the illness, for the purpose of sexual arousal.[2]

Twilight state

confusional—*see* Delirium, acute

psychogenic—*see* Psychosis, reactive confusion

Undersocialized conduct disorder—*see* undersocialized conduct disorder under Conduct disorders

Unsocialized aggressive disorder—*see* undersocialized conduct disorder, aggressive type under Conduct disorders

Vaginismus, functional—*see* functional vaginismus under Psychosexual dysfunctions

Vorbeireden: The symptom of the approximate answer or talking past the point, seen in the Ganser syndrome, a form of factitious illness.[2]

Voyeurism: A sexual deviation in which the individual repetitively seeks out situations in which he engages in looking at unsuspecting women who are either naked, in the act of disrobing, or engaging in sexual activity. The act of looking is accompanied by sexual excitement, frequently with orgasm. In its severe form, the act of peeping constitutes the preferred or exclusive sexual activity of the individual.[2]

Wernicke-Korsakoff syndrome—*see* alcohol amnestic syndrome under Alcoholic psychoses

Withdrawal reaction of childhood or adolescence—*see* Introverted disorder of childhood

Word-deafness: A developmental delay in the comprehension of speech sounds.[1]

Zoophilia: Sexual or anal intercourse with animals.[1]

APPENDIX C

CLASSIFICATION OF DRUGS BY AMERICAN HOSPITAL FORMULARY SERVICES LIST NUMBER AND THEIR ICD-9-CM EQUIVALENTS

The coding of adverse effects of drugs is keyed to the continually revised Hospital Formulary of the American Hospital Formulary Service (AHFS) published under the direction of the American Society of Hospital Pharmacists.

The following section gives the ICD-9-CM diagnosis code for each AHFS list.

AHFS List		ICD-9-CM Diagnosis Code
4:00	**ANTIHISTAMINE DRUGS**	**963.0**
8:00	**ANTI-INFECTIVE AGENTS**	
8:04	Amebicides	961.5
	hydroxyquinoline derivatives	961.3
	arsenical anti-infectives	961.1
8:08	Anthelmintics	961.6
	quinoline derivatives	961.3
8:12.04	Antifungal Antibiotics	960.1
	nonantibiotics	961.9
8:12.06	Cephalosporins	960.5
8:12.08	Chloramphenicol	960.2
8:12.12	The Erythromycins	960.3
8:12.16	The Penicillins	960.0
8:12.20	The Streptomycins	960.6
8:12.24	The Tetracyclines	960.4
8:12.28	Other Antibiotics	960.8
	antimycobacterial antibiotics	960.6
	macrolides	960.3
8:16	Antituberculars	961.8
	antibiotics	960.6
8:18	Antivirals	961.7
8:20	Plasmodicides (antimalarials)	961.4
8:24	Sulfonamides	961.0
8:26	The Sulfones	961.8
8:28	Treponemicides	961.2
8:32	Trichomonacides	961.5
	hydroxyquinoline derivatives	961.3
	nitrofuran derivatives	961.9
8:36	Urinary Germicides	961.9
	quinoline derivatives	961.3
8:40	Other Anti-Infectives	961.9
10:00	**ANTINEOPLASTIC AGENTS**	**963.1**
	antibiotics	960.7
	progestogens	962.2
12:00	**AUTONOMIC DRUGS**	
12:04	Parasympathomimetic (Cholinergic) Agents	971.0
12:08	Parasympatholytic (Cholinergic Blocking) Agents	971.1
12:12	Sympathomimetic (Adrenergic) Agents	971.2
12:16	Sympatholytic (Adrenergic Blocking) Agents	971.3
12:20	Skeletal Muscle Relaxants	975.2
	central nervous system muscle-tone depressants	968.0
16:00	**BLOOD DERIVATIVES**	**964.7**
20:00	**BLOOD FORMATION AND COAGULATION**	
20:04	Antianemia Drugs	964.1
20:04.04	Iron Preparations	964.0
20:04.08	Liver and Stomach Preparations	964.1
20:12.04	Anticoagulants	964.2
20:12.08	Antiheparin agents	964.5
20:12.12	Coagulants	964.5
20.12.16	Hemostatics	964.5
	capillary-active drugs	972.8
	fibrinolysis-affecting agents	964.4
	natural products	964.7
24:00	**CARDIOVASCULAR DRUGS**	
24:04	Cardiac Drugs	972.9
	cardiotonic agents	972.1
	rhythm regulators	972.0
24:06	Antilipemic Agents	972.2
	thyroid derivatives	962.7
24:08	Hypotensive Agents	972.6
	adrenergic blocking agents	971.3
	ganglion-blocking agents	972.3
	vasodilators	972.5
24:12	Vasodilating Agents	972.5
	coronary	972.4
	nicotinic acid derivatives	972.2
24:16	Sclerosing Agents	972.7
28:00	**CENTRAL NERVOUS SYSTEM DRUGS**	
28:04	General Anesthetics	968.4
	gaseous anesthetics	968.2
	halothane	968.1
	intravenous anesthetics	968.3
28:08	Analgesics and Antipyretics	965.9
	antirheumatics	965.6
	aromatic analgesics	965.4
	non-narcotics NEC	965.7
	opium alkaloids	965.00
	heroin	965.01
	methadone	965.02
	specified type NEC	965.09
	pyrazole derivatives	965.5
	salicylates	965.1
	specified type NEC	965.8
28:10	Narcotic Antagonists	970.1
28:12	Anticonvulsants	966.3
	barbiturates	967.0
	benzodiazepine-based tranquilizers	969.4
	bromides	967.3
	hydantoin derivatives	966.1
	oxazolidine derivative	966.0
	succinamides	966.2
28:16.04	Antidepressants	969.0
28:16.08	Tranquilizers	969.5
	benzodiazepine-based	969.4
	butyrophenone-based	969.2
	major NEC	969.3
	phenothiazine-based	969.1
28:16.12	Other Psychotherapeutic Agents	969.8
28:20	Respiratory and Cerebral Stimulants	970.9
	analeptics	970.0
	anorexigenic agents	977.0
	psychostimulants	969.7
	specified type NEC	970.8
28:24	Sedatives and Hypnotics	967.9
	barbiturates	967.0
	benzodiazepine-based tranquilizers	969.4
	chloral hydrate group	967.1
	glutethimide group	967.5
	intravenous anesthetics	968.3
	methaqualone	967.4
	paraldehyde	967.2
	phenothiazine-based tranquilizers	969.1
	specified type NEC	967.8
	thiobarbiturates	968.3
	tranquilizer NEC	969.5
36:00	**DIAGNOSTIC AGENTS**	**977.8**
40:00	**ELECTROLYTE, CALORIC, AND WATER BALANCE AGENTS NEC**	**974.5**

40:04	Acidifying Agents	963.2
40:08	Alkalinizing Agents	963.3
40:10	Ammonia Detoxicants	974.5
40:12	Replacement Solutions NEC	974.5
	plasma volume expanders	964.8
40:16	Sodium-Removing Resins	974.5
40:18	Potassium-Removing Resins	974.5
40:20	Caloric Agents	974.5
40:24	Salt and Sugar Substitutes	974.5
40:28	Diuretics NEC	974.4
	carbonic acid anhydrase inhibitors	974.2
	mercurials	974.0
	purine derivatives	974.1
	saluretics	974.3
40:36	Irrigating Solutions	974.5
40:40	Uricosuric Agents	974.7
44:00	**ENZYMES NEC**	**963.4**
	fibrinolysis-affecting agents	964.4
	gastric agents	973.4
48:00	**EXPECTORANTS AND COUGH PREPARATIONS**	
	antihistamine agents	963.0
	antitussives	975.4
	codeine derivatives	965.09
	expectorants	975.5
	narcotic agents NEC	965.09
52:00	**EYE, EAR, NOSE, AND THROAT PREPARATIONS**	
52:04	Anti-Infectives	
	ENT	976.6
	ophthalmic	976.5
52:04.04	Antibiotics	
	ENT	976.6
	ophthalmic	976.5
52:04.06	Antivirals	
	ENT	976.6
	ophthalmic	976.5
52:04.08	Sulfonamides	
	ENT	976.6
	ophthalmic	976.5
52:04.12	Miscellaneous Anti-Infectives	
	ENT	976.6
	ophthalmic	976.5
52:08	Anti-Inflammatory Agents	
	ENT	976.6
	ophthalmic	976.5
52:10	Carbonic Anhydrase Inhibitors	974.2
52:12	Contact Lens Solutions	976.5
52:16	Local Anesthetics	968.5
52:20	Miotics	971.0
52:24	Mydriatics	
	adrenergics	971.2
	anticholinergics	971.1
	antimuscarinics	971.1
	parasympatholytics	971.1
	spasmolytics	971.1
	sympathomimetics	971.2
52:28	Mouth Washes and Gargles	976.6
52:32	Vasoconstrictors	971.2
52:36	Unclassified Agents	
	ENT	976.6
	ophthalmic	976.5
56:00	**GASTROINTESTINAL DRUGS**	
56:04	Antacids and Absorbents	973.0
56:08	Anti-Diarrhea Agents	973.5
56:10	Antiflatulents	973.8
56:12	Cathartics NEC	973.3
	emollients	973.2
	irritants	973.1
56:16	Digestants	973.4
56:20	Emetics and Antiemetics	
	antiemetics	963.0
	emetics	973.6
56:24	Lipotropic Agents	977.1
60:00	**GOLD COMPOUNDS**	**965.6**
64:00	**HEAVY METAL ANTAGONISTS**	**963.8**
68:00	**HORMONES AND SYNTHETIC SUBSTITUTES**	
68:04	Adrenals	962.0
68:08	Androgens	962.1
68:12	Contraceptives	962.2
68:16	Estrogens	962.2
68:18	Gonadotropins	962.4
68:20	Insulins and Antidiabetic Agents	962.3
68:20.08	Insulins	962.3
68:24	Parathyroid	962.6
68:28	Pituitary	
	anterior	962.4
	posterior	962.5
68:32	Progestogens	962.2
68:34	Other Corpus Luteum Hormones	962.2
68:36	Thyroid and Antithyroid	
	antithyroid	962.8
	thyroid	962.7
72:00	**LOCAL ANESTHETICS NEC**	**968.9**
	topical (surface) agents	968.5
	infiltrating agents (intradermal) (subcutaneous) (submucosal)	968.5
	nerve blocking agents (peripheral) (plexus) (regional)	968.6
	spinal	968.7
76:00	**OXYTOCICS**	**975.0**
78:00	**RADIOACTIVE AGENTS**	**990**
80:00	**SERUMS, TOXOIDS, AND VACCINE**	
80:04	Serums	979.9
	immune globulin (gamma) (human)	964.6
80:08	Toxoids NEC	978.8
	diphtheria	978.5
	and tetanus	978.9
	with pertussis component	978.6
	tetanus	978.4
	and diphtheria	978.9
	with pertussis component	978.6
80:12	Vaccines NEC	979.9
	bacterial NEC	978.8
	with	
	other bacterial component	978.9
	pertussis component	978.6
	viral and rickettsial component	979.7
	rickettsial NEC	979.6
	with	
	bacterial component	979.7
	pertussis component	978.6
	viral component	979.7
	viral NEC	979.6
	with	
	bacterial component	979.7
	pertussis component	978.6
	rickettsial component	979.7
84:00	**SKIN AND MUCOUS MEMBRANE PREPARATIONS**	
84:04	Anti-Infectives	976.0
84:04.04	Antibiotics	976.0
84:04.08	Fungicides	976.0
84:04.12	Scabicides and Pediculicides	976.0
84:04.16	Miscellaneous Local Anti-Infectives	976.0
84:06	Anti-Inflammatory Agents	976.0
84:08	Antipruritics and Local Anesthetics	
	antipruritics	976.1
	local anesthetics	968.5

84:12	Astringents	976.2
84:16	Cell Stimulants and Proliferants	976.8
84:20	Detergents	976.2
84:24	Emollients, Demulcents, and Protectants	976.3
84:28	Keratolytic Agents	976.4
84:32	Keratoplastic Agents	976.4
84:36	Miscellaneous Agents	976.8
86:00	**SPASMOLYTIC AGENTS**	**975.1**
	antiasthmatics	975.7
	papaverine	972.5
	theophylline	974.1
88:00	**VITAMINS**	
88:04	Vitamin A	963.5
88:08	Vitamin B Complex	963.5
	hematopoietic vitamin	964.1
	nicotinic acid derivatives	972.2
88:12	Vitamin C	963.5
88:16	Vitamin D	963.5
88:20	Vitamin E	963.5
88:24	Vitamin K Activity	964.3
88:28	Multivitamin Preparations	963.5
92:00	**UNCLASSIFIED THERAPEUTIC AGENTS**	**977.8**

APPENDIX D

CLASSIFICATION OF INDUSTRIAL ACCIDENTS ACCORDING TO AGENCY

Annex B to the Resolution concerning Statistics of Employment Injuries adopted by the Tenth International Conference of Labor Statisticians on 12 October 1962

1 MACHINES

11 **Prime-Movers, except Electrical Motors**
- 111 *Steam engines*
- 112 *Internal combustion engines*
- 119 *Others*

12 **Transmission Machinery**
- 121 *Transmission shafts*
- 122 *Transmission belts, cables, pulleys, pinions, chains, gears*
- 129 *Others*

13 **Metalworking Machines**
- 131 *Power presses*
- 132 *Lathes*
- 133 *Milling machines*
- 134 *Abrasive wheels*
- 135 *Mechanical shears*
- 136 *Forging machines*
- 137 *Rolling-mills*
- 139 *Others*

14 **Wood and Assimilated Machines**
- 141 *Circular saws*
- 142 *Other saws*
- 143 *Molding machines*
- 144 *Overhand planes*
- 149 *Others*

15 **Agricultural Machines**
- 151 *Reapers (including combine reapers)*
- 152 *Threshers*
- 159 *Others*

16 **Mining Machinery**
- 161 *Under-cutters*
- 169 *Others*

19 **Other Machines Not Elsewhere Classified**
- 191 *Earth-moving machines, excavating and scraping machines, except means of transport*
- 192 *Spinning, weaving and other textile machines*
- 193 *Machines for the manufacture of foodstuffs and beverages*
- 194 *Machines for the manufacture of paper*
- 195 *Printing machines*
- 199 *Others*

2 MEANS OF TRANSPORT AND LIFTING EQUIPMENT

21 **Lifting Machines and Appliances**
- 211 *Cranes*
- 212 *Lifts and elevators*
- 213 *Winches*
- 214 *Pulley blocks*
- 219 *Others*

22 **Means of Rail Transport**
- 221 *Inter-urban railways*
- 222 *Rail transport in mines, tunnels, quarries, industrial establishments, docks, etc.*
- 229 *Others*

23 **Other Wheeled Means of Transport, Excluding Rail Transport**
- 231 *Tractors*
- 232 *Lorries*
- 233 *Trucks*
- 234 *Motor vehicles, not elsewhere classified*
- 235 *Animal-drawn vehicles*
- 236 *Hand-drawn vehicles*
- 239 *Others*

24 **Means of Air Transport**

25 **Means of Water Transport**
- 251 *Motorized means of water transport*
- 252 *Non-motorized means of water transport*

26 **Other Means of Transport**
- 261 *Cable-cars*
- 262 *Mechanical conveyors, except cable-cars*
- 269 *Others*

3 OTHER EQUIPMENT

31 **Pressure Vessels**
- 311 *Boilers*
- 312 *Pressurized containers*
- 313 *Pressurized piping and accessories*
- 314 *Gas cylinders*
- 315 *Caissons, diving equipment*
- 319 *Others*

32 **Furnaces, Ovens, Kilns**
- 321 *Blast furnaces*
- 322 *Refining furnaces*
- 323 *Other furnaces*
- 324 *Kilns*
- 325 *Ovens*

33 **Refrigerating Plants**

34 **Electrical Installations, Including Electric Motors, but Excluding Electric Hand Tools**
- 341 *Rotating machines*
- 342 *Conductors*
- 343 *Transformers*
- 344 *Control apparatus*
- 349 *Others*

35 **Electric Hand Tools**

36 **Tools, Implements, and Appliances, Except Electric Hand Tools**
- 361 *Power-driven hand tools, except electric hand tools*
- 362 *Hand tools, not power-driven*
- 369 *Others*

37 **Ladders, Mobile Ramps**

38 **Scaffolding**

39 **Other Equipment, Not Elsewhere Classified**

4 MATERIALS, SUBSTANCES, AND RADIATIONS

41 **Explosives**

42 **Dusts, Gases, Liquids and Chemicals, Excluding Explosives**
- 421 *Dusts*
- 422 *Gases, vapors, fumes*
- 423 *Liquids, not elsewhere classified*
- 424 *Chemicals, not elsewhere classified*

43 **Flying Fragments**

44 **Radiations**
- 441 *Ionizing radiations*
- 449 *Others*

49 Other Materials and Substances Not Elsewhere Classified

5 WORKING ENVIRONMENT

51 Outdoor
511 *Weather*
512 *Traffic and working surfaces*
513 *Water*
519 *Others*

52 Indoor
521 *Floors*
522 *Confined quarters*
523 *Stairs*
524 *Other traffic and working surfaces*
525 *Floor openings and wall openings*
526 *Environmental factors (lighting, ventilation, temperature, noise, etc.)*
529 *Others*

53 Underground
531 *Roofs and faces of mine roads and tunnels, etc.*
532 *Floors of mine roads and tunnels, etc.*
533 *Working-faces of mines, tunnels, etc.*
534 *Mine shafts*
535 *Fire*
536 *Water*
539 *Others*

6 OTHER AGENCIES, NOT ELSEWHERE CLASSIFIED

61 Animals
611 *Live animals*
612 *Animals products*

69 Other Agencies, Not Elsewhere Classified

7 AGENCIES NOT CLASSIFIED FOR LACK OF SUFFICIENT DATA

APPENDIX E

LIST OF THREE-DIGIT CATEGORIES

1. INFECTIOUS AND PARASITIC DISEASES

Intestinal infectious diseases (001–009)
001 Cholera
002 Typhoid and paratyphoid fevers
003 Other salmonella infections
004 Shigellosis
005 Other food poisoning (bacterial)
006 Amebiasis
007 Other protozoal intestinal diseases
008 Intestinal infections due to other organisms
009 Ill-defined intestinal infections

Tuberculosis (010–018)
010 Primary tuberculous infection
011 Pulmonary tuberculosis
012 Other respiratory tuberculosis
013 Tuberculosis of meninges and central nervous system
014 Tuberculosis of intestines, peritoneum, and mesenteric glands
015 Tuberculosis of bones and joints
016 Tuberculosis of genitourinary system
017 Tuberculosis of other organs
018 Miliary tuberculosis

Zoonotic bacterial diseases (020–027)
020 Plague
021 Tularemia
022 Anthrax
023 Brucellosis
024 Glanders
025 Melioidosis
026 Rat-bite fever
027 Other zoonotic bacterial diseases

Other bacterial diseases (030–041)
030 Leprosy
031 Diseases due to other mycobacteria
032 Diphtheria
033 Whooping cough
034 Streptococcal sore throat and scarlet fever
035 Erysipelas
036 Meningococcal infection
037 Tetanus
038 Septicemia
039 Actinomycotic infections
040 Other bacterial diseases
041 Bacterial infection in conditions classified elsewhere and of unspecified site

Human immunodeficiency virus (042)
042 Human immunodeficiency virus [HIV] disease

Poliomyelitis and other non-arthropod-borne viral diseases of central nervous system (045–049)
045 Acute poliomyelitis
046 Slow virus infection of central nervous system
047 Meningitis due to enterovirus
048 Other enterovirus diseases of central nervous system
049 Other non-arthropod-borne viral diseases of central nervous system

Viral diseases accompanied by exanthem (050–057)
050 Smallpox
051 Cowpox and paravaccinia
052 Chickenpox
053 Herpes zoster
054 Herpes simplex
055 Measles
056 Rubella
057 Other viral exanthemata

Arthropod-borne viral diseases (060–066)
060 Yellow fever
061 Dengue
062 Mosquito-borne viral encephalitis
063 Tick-borne viral encephalitis
064 Viral encephalitis transmitted by other and unspecified arthropods
065 Arthropod-borne hemorrhagic fever
066 Other arthropod-borne viral diseases

Other diseases due to viruses and Chlamydiae (070–079)
070 Viral hepatitis
071 Rabies
072 Mumps
073 Ornithosis
074 Specific diseases due to Coxsackie virus
075 Infectious mononucleosis
076 Trachoma
077 Other diseases of conjunctiva due to viruses and Chlamydiae
078 Other diseases due to viruses and Chlamydiae
079 Viral infection in conditions classified elsewhere and of unspecified site

Rickettsioses and other arthropod-borne diseases (080–088)
080 Louse-borne [epidemic] typhus
081 Other typhus
082 Tick-borne rickettsioses
083 Other rickettsioses
084 Malaria
085 Leishmaniasis
086 Trypanosomiasis
087 Relapsing fever
088 Other arthropod-borne diseases

Syphilis and other venereal diseases (090–099)
090 Congenital syphilis
091 Early syphilis, symptomatic
092 Early syphilis, latent
093 Cardiovascular syphilis
094 Neurosyphilis
095 Other forms of late syphilis, with symptoms
096 Late syphilis, latent
097 Other and unspecified syphilis
098 Gonococcal infections
099 Other venereal diseases

Other spirochetal diseases (100–104)
100 Leptospirosis
101 Vincent's angina
102 Yaws
103 Pinta
104 Other spirochetal infection

Mycoses (110–118)
110 Dermatophytosis
111 Dermatomycosis, other and unspecified
112 Candidiasis
114 Coccidioidomycosis
115 Histoplasmosis
116 Blastomycotic infection
117 Other mycoses
118 Opportunistic mycoses

Helminthiases (120–129)
120 Schistosomiasis [bilharziasis]
121 Other trematode infections
122 Echinococcosis
123 Other cestode infection
124 Trichinosis
125 Filarial infection and dracontiasis
126 Ancylostomiasis and necatoriasis
127 Other intestinal helminthiases
128 Other and unspecified helminthiases
129 Intestinal parasitism, unspecified

Other infectious and parasitic diseases (130–136)
130 Toxoplasmosis
131 Trichomoniasis
132 Pediculosis and phthirus infestation
133 Acariasis
134 Other infestation
135 Sarcoidosis
136 Other and unspecified infectious and parasitic diseases

Late effects of infectious and parasitic diseases (137–139)
137 Late effects of tuberculosis
138 Late effects of acute poliomyelitis
139 Late effects of other infectious and parasitic diseases

2. NEOPLASMS

Malignant neoplasm of lip, oral cavity, and pharynx (140–149)
140 Malignant neoplasm of lip
141 Malignant neoplasm of tongue
142 Malignant neoplasm of major salivary glands
143 Malignant neoplasm of gum
144 Malignant neoplasm of floor of mouth
145 Malignant neoplasm of other and unspecified parts of mouth
146 Malignant neoplasm of oropharynx
147 Malignant neoplasm of nasopharynx
148 Malignant neoplasm of hypopharynx
149 Malignant neoplasm of other and ill-defined sites within the lip, oral cavity, and pharynx

Malignant neoplasm of digestive organs and peritoneum (150–159)
150 Malignant neoplasm of esophagus
151 Malignant neoplasm of stomach
152 Malignant neoplasm of small intestine, including duodenum
153 Malignant neoplasm of colon
154 Malignant neoplasm of rectum, rectosigmoid junction, and anus
155 Malignant neoplasm of liver and intrahepatic bile ducts
156 Malignant neoplasm of gallbladder and extrahepatic bile ducts
157 Malignant neoplasm of pancreas
158 Malignant neoplasm of retroperitoneum and peritoneum
159 Malignant neoplasm of other and ill-defined sites within the digestive organs and peritoneum

Malignant neoplasm of respiratory and intrathoracic organs (160–165)
160 Malignant neoplasm of nasal cavities, middle ear, and accessory sinuses
161 Malignant neoplasm of larynx
162 Malignant neoplasm of trachea, bronchus, and lung
163 Malignant neoplasm of pleura
164 Malignant neoplasm of thymus, heart, and mediastinum
165 Malignant neoplasm of other and ill-defined sites within the respiratory system and intrathoracic organs

Malignant neoplasm of bone, connective tissue, skin, and breast (170–176)
170 Malignant neoplasm of bone and articular cartilage
171 Malignant neoplasm of connective and other soft tissue
172 Malignant melanoma of skin
173 Other malignant neoplasm of skin
174 Malignant neoplasm of female breast
175 Malignant neoplasm of male breast

Kaposi's sarcoma (176)
176 Kaposi's sarcoma

Malignant neoplasm of genitourinary organs (179–189)
179 Malignant neoplasm of uterus, part unspecified
180 Malignant neoplasm of cervix uteri
181 Malignant neoplasm of placenta
182 Malignant neoplasm of body of uterus
183 Malignant neoplasm of ovary and other uterine adnexa
184 Malignant neoplasm of other and unspecified female genital organs
185 Malignant neoplasm of prostate
186 Malignant neoplasm of testis
187 Malignant neoplasm of penis and other male genital organs
188 Malignant neoplasm of bladder
189 Malignant neoplasm of kidney and other and unspecified urinary organs

Malignant neoplasm of other and unspecified sites (190–199)
190 Malignant neoplasm of eye
191 Malignant neoplasm of brain
192 Malignant neoplasm of other and unspecified parts of nervous system
193 Malignant neoplasm of thyroid gland
194 Malignant neoplasm of other endocrine glands and related structures
195 Malignant neoplasm of other and ill-defined sites
196 Secondary and unspecified malignant neoplasm of lymph nodes
197 Secondary malignant neoplasm of respiratory and digestive systems
198 Secondary malignant neoplasm of other specified sites
199 Malignant neoplasm without specification of site

Malignant neoplasm of lymphatic and hematopoietic tissue (200–208)
200 Lymphosarcoma and reticulosarcoma
201 Hodgkin's disease
202 Other malignant neoplasm of lymphoid and histiocytic tissue
203 Multiple myeloma and immunoproliferative neoplasms
204 Lymphoid leukemia
205 Myeloid leukemia
206 Monocytic leukemia
207 Other specified leukemia
208 Leukemia of unspecified cell type

Benign neoplasms (210–229)
210 Benign neoplasm of lip, oral cavity, and pharynx
211 Benign neoplasm of other parts of digestive system
212 Benign neoplasm of respiratory and intrathoracic organs
213 Benign neoplasm of bone and articular cartilage
214 Lipoma
215 Other benign neoplasm of connective and other soft tissue
216 Benign neoplasm of skin
217 Benign neoplasm of breast
218 Uterine leiomyoma
219 Other benign neoplasm of uterus
220 Benign neoplasm of ovary
221 Benign neoplasm of other female genital organs
222 Benign neoplasm of male genital organs
223 Benign neoplasm of kidney and other urinary organs
224 Benign neoplasm of eye
225 Benign neoplasm of brain and other parts of nervous system
226 Benign neoplasm of thyroid gland
227 Benign neoplasm of other endocrine glands and related structures
228 Hemangioma and lymphangioma, any site
229 Benign neoplasm of other and unspecified sites

Carcinoma in situ (230–234)
230 Carcinoma in situ of digestive organs
231 Carcinoma in situ of respiratory system
232 Carcinoma in situ of skin
233 Carcinoma in situ of breast and genitourinary system
234 Carcinoma in situ of other and unspecified sites

Neoplasms of uncertain behavior (235–238)
235 Neoplasm of uncertain behavior of digestive and respiratory systems
236 Neoplasm of uncertain behavior of genitourinary organs
237 Neoplasm of uncertain behavior of endocrine glands and nervous system
238 Neoplasm of uncertain behavior of other and unspecified sites and tissues

Neoplasms of unspecified nature (239)
239 Neoplasm of unspecified nature

3. ENDOCRINE, NUTRITIONAL AND METABOLIC DISEASES, AND IMMUNITY DISORDERS

Disorders of thyroid gland (240–246)
240 Simple and unspecified goiter
241 Nontoxic nodular goiter
242 Thyrotoxicosis with or without goiter
243 Congenital hypothyroidism
244 Acquired hypothyroidism
245 Thyroiditis
246 Other disorders of thyroid

Diseases of other endocrine glands (250–259)
250 Diabetes mellitus
251 Other disorders of pancreatic internal secretion
252 Disorders of parathyroid gland
253 Disorders of the pituitary gland and its hypothalamic control
254 Diseases of thymus gland
255 Disorders of adrenal glands
256 Ovarian dysfunction
257 Testicular dysfunction
258 Polyglandular dysfunction and related disorders
259 Other endocrine disorders

Nutritional deficiencies (260–269)
260 Kwashiorkor
261 Nutritional marasmus
262 Other severe protein-calorie malnutrition
263 Other and unspecified protein-calorie malnutrition
264 Vitamin A deficiency
265 Thiamine and niacin deficiency states
266 Deficiency of B-complex components
267 Ascorbic acid deficiency
268 Vitamin D deficiency
269 Other nutritional deficiencies

Other metabolic disorders and immunity disorders (270–279)
270 Disorders of amino-acid transport and metabolism
271 Disorders of carbohydrate transport and metabolism
272 Disorders of lipid metabolism
273 Disorders of plasma protein metabolism
274 Gout
275 Disorders of mineral metabolism
276 Disorders of fluid, electrolyte, and acid-base balance
277 Other and unspecified disorders of metabolism
278 Obesity and other hyperalimentation
279 Disorders involving the immune mechanism

4. DISEASES OF BLOOD AND BLOOD-FORMING ORGANS

Diseases of the blood and blood-forming organs (280–289)
280 Iron deficiency anemias
281 Other deficiency anemias
282 Hereditary hemolytic anemias
283 Acquired hemolytic anemias
284 Aplastic anemia
285 Other and unspecified anemias
286 Coagulation defects
287 Purpura and other hemorrhagic conditions
288 Diseases of white blood cells
289 Other diseases of blood and blood-forming organs

5. MENTAL DISORDERS

Organic psychotic conditions (290–294)
290 Senile and presenile organic psychotic conditions
291 Alcoholic psychoses
292 Drug psychoses
293 Transient organic psychotic conditions
294 Other organic psychotic conditions (chronic)

Other psychoses (295–299)
295 Schizophrenic psychoses
296 Affective psychoses
297 Paranoid states
298 Other nonorganic psychoses
299 Psychoses with origin specific to childhood

Neurotic disorders, personality disorders, and other nonpsychotic mental disorders (300–316)
300 Neurotic disorders
301 Personality disorders
302 Sexual deviations and disorders
303 Alcohol dependence syndrome
304 Drug dependence
305 Nondependent abuse of drugs
306 Physiological malfunction arising from mental factors
307 Special symptoms or syndromes, not elsewhere classified
308 Acute reaction to stress
309 Adjustment reaction
310 Specific nonpsychotic mental disorders following organic brain damage
311 Depressive disorder, not elsewhere classified
312 Disturbance of conduct, not elsewhere classified
313 Disturbance of emotions specific to childhood and adolescence
314 Hyperkinetic syndrome of childhood
315 Specific delays in development
316 Psychic factors associated with diseases classified elsewhere

Mental retardation (317–319)
317 Mild mental retardation
318 Other specified mental retardation
319 Unspecified mental retardation

6. DISEASES OF THE NERVOUS SYSTEM AND SENSE ORGANS

Inflammatory diseases of the central nervous system (320–326)
320 Bacterial meningitis
321 Meningitis due to other organisms
322 Meningitis of unspecified cause
323 Encephalitis, myelitis, and encephalomyelitis
324 Intracranial and intraspinal abscess
325 Phlebitis and thrombophlebitis of intracranial venous sinuses
326 Late effects of intracranial abscess or pyogenic infection

Hereditary and degenerative diseases of the central nervous system (330–337)
330 Cerebral degenerations usually manifest in childhood
331 Other cerebral degenerations
332 Parkinson's disease
333 Other extrapyramidal disease and abnormal movement disorders
334 Spinocerebellar disease
335 Anterior horn cell disease
336 Other diseases of spinal cord
337 Disorders of the autonomic nervous system

Other disorders of the central nervous system (340–349)
340 Multiple sclerosis
341 Other demyelinating diseases of central nervous system
342 Hemiplegia and hemiparesis
343 Infantile cerebral palsy
344 Other paralytic syndromes
345 Epilepsy
346 Migraine
347 Cataplexy and narcolepsy
348 Other conditions of brain
349 Other and unspecified disorders of the nervous system

Disorders of the peripheral nervous system (350–359)
350 Trigeminal nerve disorders
351 Facial nerve disorders
352 Disorders of other cranial nerves
353 Nerve root and plexus disorders
354 Mononeuritis of upper limb and mononeuritis multiplex
355 Mononeuritis of lower limb

356 Hereditary and idiopathic peripheral neuropathy
357 Inflammatory and toxic neuropathy
358 Myoneural disorders
359 Muscular dystrophies and other myopathies

Disorders of the eye and adnexa (360–379)
360 Disorders of the globe
361 Retinal detachments and defects
362 Other retinal disorders
363 Chorioretinal inflammations and scars and other disorders of choroid
364 Disorders of iris and ciliary body
365 Glaucoma
366 Cataract
367 Disorders of refraction and accommodation
368 Visual disturbances
369 Blindness and low vision
370 Keratitis
371 Corneal opacity and other disorders of cornea
372 Disorders of conjunctiva
373 Inflammation of eyelids
374 Other disorders of eyelids
375 Disorders of lacrimal system
376 Disorders of the orbit
377 Disorders of optic nerve and visual pathways
378 Strabismus and other disorders of binocular eye movements
379 Other disorders of eye

Diseases of the ear and mastoid process (380–389)
380 Disorders of external ear
381 Nonsuppurative otitis media and eustachian tube disorders
382 Suppurative and unspecified otitis media
383 Mastoiditis and related conditions
384 Other disorders of tympanic membrane
385 Other disorders of middle ear and mastoid
386 Vertiginous syndromes and other disorders of vestibular system
387 Otosclerosis
388 Other disorders of ear
389 Hearing loss

7. DISEASES OF THE CIRCULATORY SYSTEM

Acute rheumatic fever (390–392)
390 Rheumatic fever without mention of heart involvement
391 Rheumatic fever with heart involvement
392 Rheumatic chorea

Chronic rheumatic heart disease (393–398)
393 Chronic rheumatic pericarditis
394 Diseases of mitral valve
395 Diseases of aortic valve
396 Diseases of mitral and aortic valves
397 Diseases of other endocardial structures
398 Other rheumatic heart disease

Hypertensive disease (401–405)
401 Essential hypertension
402 Hypertensive heart disease
403 Hypertensive renal disease
404 Hypertensive heart and renal disease
405 Secondary hypertension

Ischemic heart disease (410–414)
410 Acute myocardial infarction
411 Other acute and subacute form of ischemic heart disease
412 Old myocardial infarction
413 Angina pectoris
414 Other forms of chronic ischemic heart disease

Diseases of pulmonary circulation (415–417)
415 Acute pulmonary heart disease
416 Chronic pulmonary heart disease
417 Other diseases of pulmonary circulation

Other forms of heart disease (420–429)
420 Acute pericarditis
421 Acute and subacute endocarditis
422 Acute myocarditis
423 Other diseases of pericardium
424 Other diseases of endocardium
425 Cardiomyopathy
426 Conduction disorders
427 Cardiac dysrhythmias
428 Heart failure
429 Ill-defined descriptions and complications of heart disease

Cerebrovascular disease (430–438)
430 Subarachnoid hemorrhage
431 Intracerebral hemorrhage
432 Other and unspecified intracranial hemorrhage
433 Occlusion and stenosis of precerebral arteries
434 Occlusion of cerebral arteries
435 Transcient cerebral ischemia
436 Acute but ill-defined cerebrovascular disease
437 Other and ill-defined cerebrovascular disease
438 Late effects of cerebrovascular disease

Diseases of arteries, arterioles, and capillaries (440–448)
440 Atherosclerosis
441 Aortic aneurysm and dissection
442 Other aneurysm
443 Other peripheral vascular disease
444 Arterial embolism and thrombosis
446 Polyarteritis nodosa and allied conditions
447 Other disorders of arteries and arterioles
448 Diseases of capillaries

Diseases of veins and lymphatics, and other diseases of circulatory system (451–459)
451 Phlebitis and thrombophlebitis
452 Portal vein thrombosis
453 Other venous embolism and thrombosis
454 Varicose veins of lower extremities
455 Hemorrhoids
456 Varicose veins of other sites
457 Noninfective disorders of lymphatic channels
458 Hypotension
459 Other disorders of circulatory system

8. DISEASES OF THE RESPIRATORY SYSTEM

Acute respiratory infections (460–466)
460 Acute nasopharyngitis [common cold]
461 Acute sinusitis
462 Acute pharyngitis
463 Acute tonsillitis
464 Acute laryngitis and tracheitis
465 Acute upper respiratory infections of multiple or unspecified sites
466 Acute bronchitis and bronchiolitis

Other diseases of upper respiratory tract (470–478)
470 Deviated nasal septum
471 Nasal polyps
472 Chronic pharyngitis and nasopharyngitis
473 Chronic sinusitis
474 Chronic disease of tonsils and adenoids
475 Peritonsillar abscess
476 Chronic laryngitis and laryngotracheitis
477 Allergic rhinitis
478 Other diseases of upper respiratory tract

Pneumonia and influenza (480–487)
480 Viral pneumonia
481 Pneumococcal pneumonia [*Streptococcus pneumoniae* pneumonia]
482 Other bacterial pneumonia
483 Pneumonia due to other specified organism
484 Pneumonia in infectious diseases classified elsewhere
485 Bronchopneumonia, organism unspecified

486 Pneumonia, organism unspecified
487 Influenza

Chronic obstructive pulmonary disease and allied conditions (490–496)
490 Bronchitis, not specified as acute or chronic
491 Chronic bronchitis
492 Emphysema
493 Asthma
494 Bronchiectasis
495 Extrinsic allergic alveolitis
496 Chronic airways obstruction, not elsewhere classified

Pneumoconioses and other lung diseases due to external agents (500–508)
500 Coalworkers' pneumoconiosis
501 Asbestosis
502 Pneumoconiosis due to other silica or silicates
503 Pneumoconiosis due to other inorganic dust
504 Pneumopathy due to inhalation of other dust
505 Pneumoconiosis, unspecified
506 Respiratory conditions due to chemical fumes and vapors
507 Pneumonitis due to solids and liquids
508 Respiratory conditions due to other and unspecified external agents

Other diseases of respiratory system (510–519)
510 Empyema
511 Pleurisy
512 Pneumothorax
513 Abscess of lung and mediastinum
514 Pulmonary congestion and hypostasis
515 Postinflammatory pulmonary fibrosis
516 Other alveolar and parietoalveolar pneumopathy
517 Lung involvement in conditions classified elsewhere
518 Other diseases of lung
519 Other diseases of respiratory system

9. DISEASES OF THE DIGESTIVE SYSTEM

Diseases of oral cavity, salivary glands, and jaws (520–529)
520 Disorders of tooth development and eruption
521 Diseases of hard tissues of teeth
522 Diseases of pulp and periapical tissues
523 Gingival and periodontal diseases
524 Dentofacial anomalies, including malocclusion
525 Other diseases and conditions of the teeth and supporting structures
526 Diseases of the jaws
527 Diseases of the salivary glands
528 Diseases of the oral soft tissues, excluding lesions specific for gingiva and tongue
529 Diseases and other conditions of the tongue

Diseases of esophagus, stomach, and duodenum (530–537)
530 Diseases of esophagus
531 Gastric ulcer
532 Duodenal ulcer
533 Peptic ulcer, site unspecified
534 Gastrojejunal ulcer
535 Gastritis and duodenitis
536 Disorders of function of stomach
537 Other disorders of stomach and duodenum

Appendicitis (540–543)
540 Acute appendicitis
541 Appendicitis, unqualified
542 Other appendicitis
543 Other diseases of appendix

Hernia of abdominal cavity (550–553)
550 Inguinal hernia
551 Other hernia of abdominal cavity, with gangrene
552 Other hernia of abdominal cavity, with obstruction, but without mention of gangrene
553 Other hernia of abdominal cavity without mention of obstruction or gangrene

Noninfective enteritis and colitis (555–558)
555 Regional enteritis
556 Ulcerative colitis
557 Vascular insufficiency of intestine
558 Other noninfective gastroenteritis and colitis

Other diseases of intestines and peritoneum (560–569)
560 Intestinal obstruction without mention of hernia
562 Diverticula of intestine
564 Functional digestive disorders, not elsewhere classified
565 Anal fissure and fistula
566 Abscess of anal and rectal regions
567 Peritonitis
568 Other disorders of peritoneum
569 Other disorders of intestine

Other diseases of digestive system (570–579)
570 Acute and subacute necrosis of liver
571 Chronic liver disease and cirrhosis
572 Liver abscess and sequelae of chronic liver disease
573 Other disorders of liver
574 Cholelithiasis
575 Other disorders of gallbladder
576 Other disorders of biliary tract
577 Diseases of pancreas
578 Gastrointestinal hemorrhage
579 Intestinal malabsorption

10. DISEASES OF THE GENITOURINARY SYSTEM

Nephritis, nephrotic syndrome, and nephrosis (580–589)
580 Acute glomerulonephritis
581 Nephrotic syndrome
582 Chronic glomerulonephritis
583 Nephritis and nephropathy, not specified as acute or chronic
584 Acute renal failure
585 Chronic renal failure
586 Renal failure, unspecified
587 Renal sclerosis, unspecified
588 Disorders resulting from impaired renal function
589 Small kidney of unknown cause

Other diseases of urinary system (590–599)
590 Infections of kidney
591 Hydronephrosis
592 Calculus of kidney and ureter
593 Other disorders of kidney and ureter
594 Calculus of lower urinary tract
595 Cystitis
596 Other disorders of bladder
597 Urethritis, not sexually transmitted, and urethral syndrome
598 Urethral stricture
599 Other disorders of urethra and urinary tract

Diseases of male genital organs (600–608)
600 Hyperplasia of prostate
601 Inflammatory diseases of prostate
602 Other disorders of prostate
603 Hydrocele
604 Orchitis and epididymitis
605 Redundant prepuce and phimosis
606 Infertility, male
607 Disorders of penis
608 Other disorders of male genital organs

Disorders of breast (610–611)
610 Benign mammary dysplasias
611 Other disorders of breast

Inflammatory disease of female pelvic organs (614–616)
614 Inflammatory disease of ovary, fallopian tube, pelvic cellular tissue, and peritoneum
615 Inflammatory diseases of uterus, except cervix
616 Inflammatory disease of cervix, vagina, and vulva

Other disorders of female genital tract (617–629)
617 Endometriosis
618 Genital prolapse
619 Fistula involving female genital tract
620 Noninflammatory disorders of ovary, fallopian tube, and broad ligament
621 Disorders of uterus, not elsewhere classified
622 Noninflammatory disorders of cervix
623 Noninflammatory disorders of vagina
624 Noninflammatory disorders of vulva and perineum
625 Pain and other symptoms associated with female genital organs
626 Disorders of menstruation and other abnormal bleeding from female genital tract
627 Menopausal and postmenopausal disorders
628 Infertility, female
629 Other disorders of female genital organs

11. COMPLICATIONS OF PREGNANCY, CHILDBIRTH, AND THE PUERPERIUM

Ectopic and molar pregnancy and other pregnancy with abortive outcome (630–639)
630 Hydatidiform mole
631 Other abnormal product of conception
632 Missed abortion
633 Ectopic pregnancy
634 Spontaneous abortion
635 Legally induced abortion
636 Illegally induced abortion
637 Unspecified abortion
638 Failed attempted abortion
639 Complications following abortion and ectopic and molar pregnancies

Complications mainly related to pregnancy (640–648)
640 Hemorrhage in early pregnancy
641 Antepartum hemorrhage, abruptio placentae, and placenta previa
642 Hypertension complicating pregnancy, childbirth, and the puerperium
643 Excessive vomiting in pregnancy
644 Early or threatened labor
645 Prolonged pregnancy
646 Other complications of pregnancy, not elsewhere classified
647 Infective and parasitic conditions in the mother classifiable elsewhere but complicating pregnancy, childbirth, and the puerperium
648 Other current conditions in the mother classifiable elsewhere but complicating pregnancy, childbirth, and the puerperium

Normal delivery, and other indications for care in pregnancy, labor, and delivery (650–659)
650 Normal delivery
651 Multiple gestation
652 Malposition and malpresentation of fetus
653 Disproportion
654 Abnormality of organs and soft tissues of pelvis
655 Known or suspected fetal abnormality affecting management of mother
656 Other fetal and placental problems affecting management of mother
657 Polyhydramnios
658 Other problems associated with amniotic cavity and membranes
659 Other indications for care or intervention related to labor and delivery and not elsewhere classified

Complications occurring mainly in the course of labor and delivery (660–669)
660 Obstructed labor
661 Abnormality of forces of labor
662 Long labor
663 Umbilical cord complications
664 Trauma to perineum and vulva during delivery
665 Other obstetrical trauma
666 Postpartum hemorrhage
667 Retained placenta or membranes, without hemorrhage
668 Complications of the administration of anesthetic or other sedation in labor and delivery
669 Other complications of labor and delivery, not elsewhere classified

Complications of the puerperium (670–677)
670 Major puerperal infection
671 Venous complications in pregnancy and the puerperium
672 Pyrexia of unknown origin during the puerperium
673 Obstetrical pulmonary embolism
674 Other and unspecified complications of the puerperium, not elsewhere classified
675 Infections of the breast and nipple associated with childbirth
676 Other disorders of the breast associated with childbirth, and disorders of lactation
677 Late effect of complication of pregnancy, childbirth, and the puerperium

12. DISEASES OF THE SKIN AND SUBCUTANEOUS TISSUE

Infections of skin and subcutaneous tissue (680–686)
680 Carbuncle and furuncle
681 Cellulitis and abscess of finger and toe
682 Other cellulitis and abscess
683 Acute lymphadenitis
684 Impetigo
685 Pilonidal cyst
686 Other local infections of skin and subcutaneous tissue

Other inflammatory conditions of skin and subcutaneous tissue (690–698)
690 Erythematosquamous dermatosis
691 Atopic dermatitis and related conditions
692 Contact dermatitis and other eczema
693 Dermatitis due to substances taken internally
694 Bullous dermatoses
695 Erythematous conditions
696 Psoriasis and similar disorders
697 Lichen
698 Pruritus and related conditions

Other diseases of skin and subcutaneous tissue (700–709)
700 Corns and callosities
701 Other hypertrophic and atrophic conditions of skin
702 Other dermatoses
703 Diseases of nail
704 Diseases of hair and hair follicles
705 Disorders of sweat glands
706 Diseases of sebaceous glands
707 Chronic ulcer of skin
708 Urticaria
709 Other disorders of skin and subcutaneous tissue

13. DISEASES OF THE MUSCULOSKELETAL SYSTEM AND CONNECTIVE TISSUE

Arthropathies and related disorders (710–719)
710 Diffuse diseases of connective tissue
711 Arthropathy associated with infections
712 Crystal arthropathies
713 Arthropathy associated with other disorders classified elsewhere
714 Rheumatoid arthritis and other inflammatory polyarthropathies
715 Osteoarthrosis and allied disorders
716 Other and unspecified arthropathies
717 Internal derangement of knee
718 Other derangement of joint
719 Other and unspecified disorder of joint

Dorsopathies (720–724)
720 Ankylosing spondylitis and other inflammatory spondylopathies
721 Spondylosis and allied disorders
722 Intervertebral disc disorders
723 Other disorders of cervical region
724 Other and unspecified disorders of back

Rheumatism, excluding the back (725–729)
725 Polymyalgia rheumatica
726 Peripheral enthesopathies and allied syndromes
727 Other disorders of synovium, tendon, and bursa
728 Disorders of muscle, ligament, and fascia
729 Other disorders of soft tissues

Osteopathies, chondropathies, and acquired musculoskeletal deformities (730–739)
730 Osteomyelitis, periostitis, and other infections involving bone
731 Osteitis deformans and osteopathies associated with other disorders classified elsewhere
732 Osteochondropathies
733 Other disorders of bone and cartilage
734 Flat foot
735 Acquired deformities of toe
736 Other acquired deformities of limbs
737 Curvature of spine
738 Other acquired deformity
739 Nonallopathic lesions, not elsewhere classified

14. CONGENITAL ANOMALIES

Congential anomalies (740–759)
740 Anencephalus and similar anomalies
741 Spina bifida
742 Other congenital anomalies of nervous system
743 Congenital anomalies of eye
744 Congenital anomalies of ear, face, and neck
745 Bulbus cordis anomalies and anomalies of cardiac septal closure
746 Other congenital anomalies of heart
747 Other congenital anomalies of circulatory system
748 Congenital anomalies of respiratory system
749 Cleft palate and cleft lip
750 Other congenital anomalies of upper alimentary tract
751 Other congenital anomalies of digestive system
752 Congenital anomalies of genital organs
753 Congenital anomalies of urinary system
754 Certain congenital musculoskeletal deformities
755 Other congenital anomalies of limbs
756 Other congenital musculoskeletal anomalies
757 Congenital anomalies of the integument
758 Chromosomal anomalies
759 Other and unspecified congenital anomalies

15. CERTAIN CONDITIONS ORIGINATING IN THE PERINATAL PERIOD

Maternal causes of perinatal morbidity and mortality (760–763)
760 Fetus or newborn affected by maternal conditions which may be unrelated to present pregnancy
761 Fetus or newborn affected by maternal complications of pregnancy
762 Fetus or newborn affected by complications of placenta, cord, and membranes
763 Fetus or newborn affected by other complications of labor and delivery

Other conditions originating in the perinatal period (764–779)
764 Slow fetal growth and fetal malnutrition
765 Disorders relating to short gestation and unspecified low birthweight
766 Disorders relating to long gestation and high birthweight
767 Birth trauma
768 Intrauterine hypoxia and birth asphyxia
769 Respiratory distress syndrome
770 Other respiratory conditions of fetus and newborn
771 Infections specific to the perinatal period
772 Fetal and neonatal hemorrhage
773 Hemolytic disease of fetus or newborn, due to isoimmunization
774 Other perinatal jaundice
775 Endocrine and metabolic disturbances specific to the fetus and newborn
776 Hematological disorders of fetus and newborn
777 Perinatal disorders of digestive system
778 Conditions involving the integument and temperature regulation of fetus and newborn
779 Other and ill-defined conditions originating in the perinatal period

16. SYMPTOMS, SIGNS, AND ILL-DEFINED CONDITIONS

Symptoms (780–789)
780 General symptoms
781 Symptoms involving nervous and musculoskeletal systems
782 Symptoms involving skin and other integumentary tissue
783 Symptoms concerning nutrition, metabolism, and development
784 Symptoms involving head and neck
785 Symptoms involving cardiovascular system
786 Symptoms involving respiratory system and other chest symptoms
787 Symptoms involving digestive system
788 Symptoms involving urinary system
789 Other symptoms involving abdomen and pelvis

Nonspecific abnormal findings (790–796)
790 Nonspecific findings on examination of blood
791 Nonspecific findings on examination of urine
792 Nonspecific abnormal findings in other body substances
793 Nonspecific abnormal findings on radiological and other examination of body structure
794 Nonspecific abnormal results of function studies
795 Nonspecific abnormal histological and immunological findings
796 Other nonspecific abnormal findings

Ill-defined and unknown causes of morbidity and mortality (797–799)
797 Senility without mention of psychosis
798 Sudden death, cause unknown
799 Other ill-defined and unknown causes of morbidity and mortality

17. INJURY AND POISONING

Fracture of skull (800–804)
800 Fracture of vault of skull
801 Fracture of base of skull
802 Fracture of face bones
803 Other and unqualified skull fractures
804 Multiple fractures involving skull or face with other bones

Fracture of spine and trunk (805–809)
805 Fracture of vertebral column without mention of spinal cord lesion
806 Fracture of vertebral column with spinal cord lesion
807 Fracture of rib(s), sternum, larynx, and trachea
808 Fracture of pelvis
809 Ill-defined fractures of bones of trunk

Fracture of upper limb (810–819)
810 Fracture of clavicle
811 Fracture of scapula
812 Fracture of humerus
813 Fracture of radius and ulna
814 Fracture of carpal bone(s)
815 Fracture of metacarpal bone(s)
816 Fracture of one or more phalanges of hand
817 Multiple fractures of hand bones

818 Ill-defined fractures of upper limb
819 Multiple fractures involving both upper limbs, and upper limb with rib(s) and sternum

Fracture of lower limb (820–829)
820 Fracture of neck of femur
821 Fracture of other and unspecified parts of femur
822 Fracture of patella
823 Fracture of tibia and fibula
824 Fracture of ankle
825 Fracture of one or more tarsal and metatarsal bones
826 Fracture of one or more phalanges of foot
827 Other, multiple, and ill-defined fractures of lower limb
828 Multiple fractures involving both lower limbs, lower with upper limb, and lower limb(s) with rib(s) and sternum
829 Fracture of unspecified bones

Dislocation (830–839)
830 Dislocation of jaw
831 Dislocation of shoulder
832 Dislocation of elbow
833 Dislocation of wrist
834 Dislocation of finger
835 Dislocation of hip
836 Dislocation of knee
837 Dislocation of ankle
838 Dislocation of foot
839 Other, multiple, and ill-defined dislocations

Sprains and strains of joints and adjacent muscles (840–848)
840 Sprains and strains of shoulder and upper arm
841 Sprains and strains of elbow and forearm
842 Sprains and strains of wrist and hand
843 Sprains and strains of hip and thigh
844 Sprains and strains of knee and leg
845 Sprains and strains of ankle and foot
846 Sprains and strains of sacroiliac region
847 Sprains and strains of other and unspecified parts of back
848 Other and ill-defined sprains and strains

Intracranial injury, excluding those with skull fracture (850–854)
850 Concussion
851 Cerebral laceration and contusion
852 Subarachnoid, subdural, and extradural hemorrhage, following injury
853 Other and unspecified intracranial hemorrhage following injury
854 Intracranial injury of other and unspecified nature

Internal injury of chest, abdomen, and pelvis (860–869)
860 Traumatic pneumothorax and hemothorax
861 Injury to heart and lung
862 Injury to other and unspecified intrathoracic organs
863 Injury to gastrointestinal tract
864 Injury to liver
865 Injury to spleen
866 Injury to kidney
867 Injury to pelvic organs
868 Injury to other intra-abdominal organs
869 Internal injury to unspecified or ill-defined organs

Open wound of head, neck, and trunk (870–879)
870 Open wound of ocular adnexa
871 Open wound of eyeball
872 Open wound of ear
873 Other open wound of head
874 Open wound of neck
875 Open wound of chest (wall)
876 Open wound of back
877 Open wound of buttock
878 Open wound of genital organs (external), including traumatic amputation
879 Open wound of other and unspecified sites, except limbs

Open wound of upper limb (880–887)
880 Open wound of shoulder and upper arm
881 Open wound of elbow, forearm, and wrist
882 Open wound of hand except finger(s) alone
883 Open wound of finger(s)
884 Multiple and unspecified open wound of upper limb
885 Traumatic amputation of thumb (complete) (partial)
886 Traumatic amputation of other finger(s) (complete) (partial)
887 Traumatic amputation of arm and hand (complete) (partial)

Open wound of lower limb (890–897)
890 Open wound of hip and thigh
891 Open wound of knee, leg [except thigh], and ankle
892 Open wound of foot except toe(s) alone
893 Open wound of toe(s)
894 Multiple and unspecified open wound of lower limb
895 Traumatic amputation of toe(s) (complete) (partial)
896 Traumatic amputation of foot (complete) (partial)
897 Traumatic amputation of leg(s) (complete) (partial)

Injury to blood vessels (900–904)
900 Injury to blood vessels of head and neck
901 Injury to blood vessels of thorax
902 Injury to blood vessels of abdomen and pelvis
903 Injury to blood vessels of upper extremity
904 Injury to blood vessels of lower extremity and unspecified sites

Late effects of injuries, poisonings, toxic effects, and other external causes (905–909)
905 Late effects of musculoskeletal and connective tissue injuries
906 Late effects of injuries to skin and subcutaneous tissues
907 Late effects of injuries to the nervous system
908 Late effects of other and unspecified injuries
909 Late effects of other and unspecified external causes

Superficial injury (910–919)
910 Superficial injury of face, neck, and scalp except eye
911 Superficial injury of trunk
912 Superficial injury of shoulder and upper arm
913 Superficial injury of elbow, forearm, and wrist
914 Superficial injury of hand(s) except finger(s) alone
915 Superficial injury of finger(s)
916 Superficial injury of hip, thigh, leg, and ankle
917 Superficial injury of foot and toe(s)
918 Superficial injury of eye and adnexa
919 Superficial injury of other, multiple, and unspecified sites

Contusion with intact skin surface (920–924)
920 Contusion of face, scalp, and neck except eye(s)
921 Contusion of eye and adnexa
922 Contusion of trunk
923 Contusion of upper limb
924 Contusion of lower limb and of other and unspecified sites

Crushing injury (925–929)
925 Crushing injury of face, scalp, and neck
926 Crushing injury of trunk
927 Crushing injury of upper limb
928 Crushing injury of lower limb
929 Crushing injury of multiple and unspecified sites

Effects of foreign body entering through orifice (930–939)
930 Foreign body on external eye
931 Foreign body in ear
932 Foreign body in nose
933 Foreign body in pharynx and larynx
934 Foreign body in trachea, bronchus, and lung
935 Foreign body in mouth, esophagus, and stomach
936 Foreign body in intestine and colon
937 Foreign body in anus and rectum
938 Foreign body in digestive system, unspecified
939 Foreign body in genitourinary tract

Burns (940–949)
940 Burn confined to eye and adnexa
941 Burn of face, head, and neck

942 Burn of trunk
943 Burn of upper limb, except wrist and hand
944 Burn of wrist(s) and hand(s)
945 Burn of lower limb(s)
946 Burns of multiple specified sites
947 Burn of internal organs
948 Burns classified according to extent of body surface involved
949 Burn, unspecified

Injury to nerves and spinal cord (950–957)

950 Injury to optic nerve and pathways
951 Injury to other cranial nerve(s)
952 Spinal cord injury without evidence of spinal bone injury
953 Injury to nerve roots and spinal plexus
954 Injury to other nerve(s) of trunk excluding shoulder and pelvic girdles
955 Injury to peripheral nerve(s) of shoulder girdle and upper limb
956 Injury to peripheral nerve(s) of pelvic girdle and lower limb
957 Injury to other and unspecified nerves

Certain traumatic complications and unspecified injuries (958–959)

958 Certain early complications of trauma
959 Injury, other and unspecified

Poisoning by drugs, medicinals and biological substances (960–979)

960 Poisoning by antibiotics
961 Poisoning by other anti-infectives
962 Poisoning by hormones and synthetic substitutes
963 Poisoning by primarily systemic agents
964 Poisoning by agents primarily affecting blood constituents
965 Poisoning by analgesics, antipyretics, and antirheumatics
966 Poisoning by anticonvulsants and anti-parkinsonism drugs
967 Poisoning by sedatives and hypnotics
968 Poisoning by other central nervous system depressants and anesthetics
969 Poisoning by psychotropic agents
970 Poisoning by central nervous system stimulants
971 Poisoning by drugs primarily affecting the autonomic nervous system
972 Poisoning by agents primarily affecting the cardiovascular system
973 Poisoning by agents primarily affecting the gastrointestinal system
974 Poisoning by water, mineral, and uric acid metabolism drugs
975 Poisoning by agents primarily acting on the smooth and skeletal muscles and respiratory system
976 Poisoning by agents primarily affecting skin and mucous membrane, ophthalmological, otorhinolaryngological, and dental drugs
977 Poisoning by other and unspecified drugs and medicinals
978 Poisoning by bacterial vaccines
979 Poisoning by other vaccines and biological substances

Toxic effects of substances chiefly nonmedicinal as to source (980–989)

980 Toxic effect of alcohol
981 Toxic effect of petroleum products
982 Toxic effect of solvents other than petroleum-based
983 Toxic effect of corrosive aromatics, acids, and caustic alkalis
984 Toxic effect of lead and its compounds (including fumes)
985 Toxic effect of other metals
986 Toxic effect of carbon monoxide
987 Toxic effect of other gases, fumes, or vapors
988 Toxic effect of noxious substances eaten as food
989 Toxic effect of other substances, chiefly nonmedicinal as to source

Other and unspecified effects of external causes (990–995)

990 Effects of radiation, unspecified
991 Effects of reduced temperature
992 Effects of heat and light
993 Effects of air pressure
994 Effects of other external causes
995 Certain adverse effects, not elsewhere classified

Complications of surgical and medical care, not elsewhere classified (996–999)

996 Complications peculiar to certain specified procedures
997 Complications affecting specified body systems, not elsewhere classified
998 Other complications of procedures, not elsewhere classified
999 Complications of medical care, not elsewhere classified

SUPPLEMENTARY CLASSIFICATION OF FACTORS INFLUENCING HEALTH STATUS AND CONTACT WITH HEALTH SERVICES

Persons with potential health hazards related to communicable diseases (V01–V09)

V01 Contact with or exposure to communicable diseases
V02 Carrier or suspected carrier of infectious diseases
V03 Need for prophylactic vaccination and inoculation against bacterial diseases
V04 Need for prophylactic vaccination and inoculation against certain viral diseases
V05 Need for other prophylactic vaccination and inoculation against single diseases
V06 Need for prophylactic vaccination and inoculation against combinations of diseases
V07 Need for isolation and other prophylactic measures
V08 Asymptomatic human immunodeficiency virus [HIV] infection status
V09 Infection with drug-resistant microorganisms

Persons with potential health hazards related to personal and family history (V10–V19)

V10 Personal history of malignant neoplasm
V11 Personal history of mental disorder
V12 Personal history of certain other diseases
V13 Personal history of other diseases
V14 Personal history of allergy to medicinal agents
V15 Other personal history presenting hazards to health
V16 Family history of malignant neoplasm
V17 Family history of certain chronic disabling diseases
V18 Family history of certain other specific conditions
V19 Family history of other conditions

Persons encountering health services in circumstances related to reproduction and development (V20–V29)

V20 Health supervision of infant or child
V21 Constitutional states in development
V22 Normal pregnancy
V23 Supervision of high-risk pregnancy
V24 Postpartum care and examination
V25 Encounter for contraceptive management
V26 Procreative management
V27 Outcome of delivery
V28 Antenatal screening
V29 Observation and evaluation of newborns and infants for suspected condition not found

Liveborn infants according to type of birth (V30–V39)

V30 Single liveborn
V31 Twin, mate liveborn
V32 Twin, mate stillborn
V33 Twin, unspecified
V34 Other multiple, mates all liveborn
V35 Other multiple, mates all stillborn
V36 Other multiple, mates live- and stillborn
V37 Other multiple, unspecified
V39 Unspecified

Persons with a condition influencing their health status (V40–V49)

V40 Mental and behavioral problems

V41 Problems with special senses and other special functions
V42 Organ or tissue replaced by transplant
V43 Organ or tissue replaced by other means
V44 Artificial opening status
V45 Other postsurgical states
V46 Other dependence on machines
V47 Other problems with internal organs
V48 Problems with head, neck, and trunk
V49 Problems with limbs and other problems

Persons encountering health services for specific procedures and aftercare (V50–V59)
V50 Elective surgery for purposes other than remedying health states
V51 Aftercare involving the use of plastic surgery
V52 Fitting and adjustment of prosthetic device
V53 Fitting and adjustment of other device
V54 Other orthopedic aftercare
V55 Attention to artificial openings
V56 Encounter for dialysis and dialysis catheter care
V57 Care involving use of rehabilitation procedures
V58 Other and unspecified aftercare
V59 Donors

Persons encountering health services in other circumstances (V60–V69)
V60 Housing, household, and economic circumstances
V61 Other family circumstances
V62 Other psychosocial circumstances
V63 Unavailability of other medical facilities for care
V64 Persons encountering health services for specific procedures, not carried out
V65 Other persons seeking consultation without complaint or sickness
V66 Convalescence and palliative care
V67 Follow-up examination
V68 Encounters for administrative purposes
V69 Problems related to lifestyle

Persons without reported diagnosis encountered during examination and investigation of individuals and populations (V70–V82)
V70 General medical examination
V71 Observation and evaluation for suspected conditions
V72 Special investigations and examinations
V73 Special screening examination for viral and chlamydial diseases
V74 Special screening examination for bacterial and spirochetal diseases
V75 Special screening examination for other infectious diseases
V76 Special screening for malignant neoplasms
V77 Special screening for endocrine, nutritional, metabolic, and immunity disorders
V78 Special screening for disorders of blood and blood-forming organs
V79 Special screening for mental disorders and developmental handicaps
V80 Special screening for neurological, eye, and ear diseases
V81 Special screening for cardiovascular, respiratory, and genitourinary diseases
V82 Special screening for other conditions

SUPPLEMENTARY CLASSIFICATION OF EXTERNAL CAUSES OF INJURY AND POISONING

Railway accidents (E800–E807)
E800 Railway accident involving collision with rolling stock
E801 Railway accident involving collision with other object
E802 Railway accident involving derailment without antecedent collision
E803 Railway accident involving explosion, fire, or burning
E804 Fall in, on, or from railway train
E805 Hit by rolling stock
E806 Other specified railway accident
E807 Railway accident of unspecified nature

Motor vehicle traffic accidents (E810–E819)
E810 Motor vehicle traffic accident involving collision with train
E811 Motor vehicle traffic accident involving re-entrant collision with another motor vehicle
E812 Other motor vehicle traffic accident involving collision with another motor vehicle
E813 Motor vehicle traffic accident involving collision with other vehicle
E814 Motor vehicle traffic accident involving collision with pedestrian
E815 Other motor vehicle traffic accident involving collision on the highway
E816 Motor vehicle traffic accident due to loss of control, without collision on the highway
E817 Noncollision motor vehicle traffic accident while boarding or alighting
E818 Other noncollision motor vehicle traffic accident
E819 Motor vehicle traffic accident of unspecified nature

Motor vehicle nontraffic accidents (E820–E825)
E820 Nontraffic accident involving motor-driven snow vehicle
E821 Nontraffic accident involving other off-road motor vehicle
E822 Other motor vehicle nontraffic accident involving collision with moving object
E823 Other motor vehicle nontraffic accident involving collision with stationary object
E824 Other motor vehicle nontraffic accident while boarding and alighting
E825 Other motor vehicle nontraffic accident of other and unspecified nature

Other road vehicle accidents (E826–E829)
E826 Pedal cycle accident
E827 Animal-drawn vehicle accident
E828 Accident involving animal being ridden
E829 Other road vehicle accidents

Water transport accidents (E830–E838)
E830 Accident to watercraft causing submersion
E831 Accident to watercraft causing other injury
E832 Other accidental submersion or drowning in water transport accident
E833 Fall on stairs or ladders in water transport
E834 Other fall from one level to another in water transport
E835 Other and unspecified fall in water transport
E836 Machinery accident in water transport
E837 Explosion, fire, or burning in watercraft
E838 Other and unspecified water transport accident

Air and space transport accidents (E840–E845)
E840 Accident to powered aircraft at takeoff or landing
E841 Accident to powered aircraft, other and unspecified
E842 Accident to unpowered aircraft
E843 Fall in, on, or from aircraft
E844 Other specified air transport accidents
E845 Accident involving spacecraft

Vehicle accidents, not elsewhere classifiable (E846–E849)
E846 Accidents involving powered vehicles used solely within the buildings and premises of an industrial or commercial establishment
E847 Accidents involving cable cars not running on rails
E848 Accidents involving other vehicles, not elsewhere classifiable
E849 Place of occurrence

Accidental poisoning by drugs, medicinal substances, and biologicals (E850–E858)
E850 Accidental poisoning by analgesics, antipyretics, and antirheumatics
E851 Accidental poisoning by barbiturates
E852 Accidental poisoning by other sedatives and hypnotics
E853 Accidental poisoning by tranquilizers
E854 Accidental poisoning by other psychotropic agents

E855 Accidental poisoning by other drugs acting on central and autonomic nervous systems
E856 Accidental poisoning by antibiotics
E857 Accidental poisoning by anti-infectives
E858 Accidental poisoning by other drugs

Accidental poisoning by other solid and liquid substances, gases, and vapors (E860–E869)
E860 Accidental poisoning by alcohol, not elsewhere classified
E861 Accidental poisoning by cleansing and polishing agents, disinfectants, paints, and varnishes
E862 Accidental poisoning by petroleum products, other solvents and their vapors, not elsewhere classified
E863 Accidental poisoning by agricultural and horticultural chemical and pharmaceutical preparations other than plant foods and fertilizers
E864 Accidental poisoning by corrosives and caustics, not elsewhere classified
E865 Accidental poisoning from poisonous foodstuffs and poisonous plants
E866 Accidental poisoning by other and unspecified solid and liquid substances
E867 Accidental poisoning by gas distributed by pipeline
E868 Accidental poisoning by other utility gas and other carbon monoxide
E869 Accidental poisoning by other gases and vapors

Misadventures to patients during surgical and medical care (E870–E876)
E870 Accidental cut, puncture, perforation, or hemorrhage during medical care
E871 Foreign object left in body during procedure
E872 Failure of sterile precautions during procedure
E873 Failure in dosage
E874 Mechanical failure of instrument or apparatus during procedure
E875 Contaminated or infected blood, other fluid, drug, or biological substance
E876 Other and unspecified misadventures during medical care

Surgical and medical procedures as the cause of abnormal reaction of patient or later complication, without mention of misadventure at the time of procedure (E878–E879)
E878 Surgical operation and other surgical procedures as the cause of abnormal reaction of patient, or of later complication, without mention of misadventure at the time of operation
E879 Other procedures, without mention of misadventure at the time of procedure, as the cause of abnormal reaction of patient, or of later complication

Accidental falls (E880–E888)
E880 Fall on or from stairs or steps
E881 Fall on or from ladders or scaffolding
E882 Fall from or out of building or other structure
E883 Fall into hole or other opening in surface
E884 Other fall from one level to another
E885 Fall on same level from slipping, tripping, or stumbling
E886 Fall on same level from collision, pushing or shoving, by or with other person
E887 Fracture, cause unspecified
E888 Other and unspecified fall

Accidents caused by fire and flames (E890–E899)
E890 Conflagration in private dwelling
E891 Conflagration in other and unspecified building or structure
E892 Conflagration not in building or structure
E893 Accident caused by ignition of clothing
E894 Ignition of highly inflammable material
E895 Accident caused by controlled fire in private dwelling
E896 Accident caused by controlled fire in other and unspecified building or structure
E897 Accident caused by controlled fire not in building or structure
E898 Accident caused by other specified fire and flames
E899 Accident caused by unspecified fire

Accidents due to natural and environmental factors (E900–E909)
E900 Excessive heat
E901 Excessive cold
E902 High and low air pressure and changes in air pressure
E903 Travel and motion
E904 Hunger, thirst, exposure, and neglect
E905 Venomous animals and plants as the cause of poisoning and toxic reactions
E906 Other injury caused by animals
E907 Lightning
E908 Cataclysmic storms, and floods resulting from storms
E909 Cataclysmic earth surface movements and eruptions

Accidents caused by submersion, suffocation, and foreign bodies (E910–E915)
E910 Accidental drowning and submersion
E911 Inhalation and ingestion of food causing obstruction of respiratory tract or suffocation
E912 Inhalation and ingestion of other object causing obstruction of respiratory tract or suffocation
E913 Accidental mechanical suffocation
E914 Foreign body accidentally entering eye and adnexa
E915 Foreign body accidentally entering other orifice

Other accidents (E916–E928)
E916 Struck accidentally by falling object
E917 Striking against or struck accidentally by objects or persons
E918 Caught accidentally in or between objects
E919 Accidents caused by machinery
E920 Accidents caused by cutting and piercing instruments or objects
E921 Accident caused by explosion of pressure vessel
E922 Accident caused by firearm missile
E923 Accident caused by explosive material
E924 Accident caused by hot substance or object, caustic or corrosive material, and steam
E925 Accident caused by electric current
E926 Exposure to radiation
E927 Overexertion and strenuous movements
E928 Other and unspecified environmental and accidental causes

Late effects of accidental injury (E929)
E929 Late effects of accidental injury

Drugs, medicinal and biological substances causing adverse effects in therapeutic use (E930–E949)
E930 Antibiotics
E931 Other anti-infectives
E932 Hormones and synthetic substitutes
E933 Primarily systemic agents
E934 Agents primarily affecting blood constituents
E935 Analgesics, antipyretics, and antirheumatics
E936 Anticonvulsants and anti-parkinsonism drugs
E937 Sedatives and hypnotics
E938 Other central nervous system depressants and anesthetics
E939 Psychotropic agents
E940 Central nervous system stimulants
E941 Drugs primarily affecting the autonomic nervous system
E942 Agents primarily affecting the cardiovascular system
E943 Agents primarily affecting gastrointestinal system
E944 Water, mineral, and uric acid metabolism drugs
E945 Agents primarily acting on the smooth and skeletal muscles and respiratory system
E946 Agents primarily affecting skin and mucous membrane, ophthalmological, otorhinolaryngological, and dental drugs
E947 Other and unspecified drugs and medicinal substances
E948 Bacterial vaccines
E949 Other vaccines and biological substances

Suicide and self-inflicted injury (E950–E959)

E950 Suicide and self-inflicted poisoning by solid or liquid substances
E951 Suicide and self-inflicted poisoning by gases in domestic use
E952 Suicide and self-inflicted poisoning by other gases and vapors
E953 Suicide and self-inflicted injury by hanging, strangulation, and suffocation
E954 Suicide and self-inflicted injury by submersion [drowning]
E955 Suicide and self-inflicted injury by firearms and explosives
E956 Suicide and self-inflicted injury by cutting and piercing instruments
E957 Suicide and self-inflicted injuries by jumping from high place
E958 Suicide and self-inflicted injury by other and unspecified means
E959 Late effects of self-inflicted injury

Homicide and injury purposely inflicted by other persons (E960–E969)

E960 Fight, brawl, and rape
E961 Assault by corrosive or caustic substance, except poisoning
E962 Assault by poisoning
E963 Assault by hanging and strangulation
E964 Assault by submersion [drowning]
E965 Assault by firearms and explosives
E966 Assault by cutting and piercing instrument
E967 Child and adult battering and other maltreatment
E968 Assault by other and unspecified means
E969 Late effects of injury purposely inflicted by other person

Legal intervention (E970–E978)

E970 Injury due to legal intervention by firearms
E971 Injury due to legal intervention by explosives
E972 Injury due to legal intervention by gas
E973 Injury due to legal intervention by blunt object
E974 Injury due to legal intervention by cutting and piercing instruments
E975 Injury due to legal intervention by other specified means
E976 Injury due to legal intervention by unspecified means
E977 Late effects of injuries due to legal intervention
E978 Legal execution

Injury undetermined whether accidentally or purposely inflicted (E980–E989)

E980 Poisoning by solid or liquid substances, undetermined whether accidentally or purposely inflicted
E981 Poisoning by gases in domestic use, undetermined whether accidentally or purposely inflicted
E982 Poisoning by other gases, undetermined whether accidentally or purposely inflicted
E983 Hanging, strangulation, or suffocation, undetermined whether accidentally or purposely inflicted
E984 Submersion [drowning], undetermined whether accidentally or purposely inflicted
E985 Injury by firearms and explosives, undetermined whether accidentally or purposely inflicted
E986 Injury by cutting and piercing instruments, undetermined whether accidentally or purposely inflicted
E987 Falling from high place, undetermined whether accidentally or purposely inflicted
E988 Injury by other and unspecified means, undetermined whether accidentally or purposely inflicted
E989 Late effects of injury, undetermined whether accidentally or purposely inflicted

Injury resulting from operations of war (E990–E999)

E990 Injury due to war operations by fires and conflagrations
E991 Injury due to war operations by bullets and fragments
E992 Injury due to war operations by explosion of marine weapons
E993 Injury due to war operations by other explosion
E994 Injury due to war operations by destruction of aircraft
E995 Injury due to war operations by other and unspecified forms of conventional warfare
E996 Injury due to war operations by nuclear weapons
E997 Injury due to war operations by other forms of unconventional warfare
E998 Injury due to war operations but occurring after cessation of hostilities
E999 Late effects of injury due to war operations

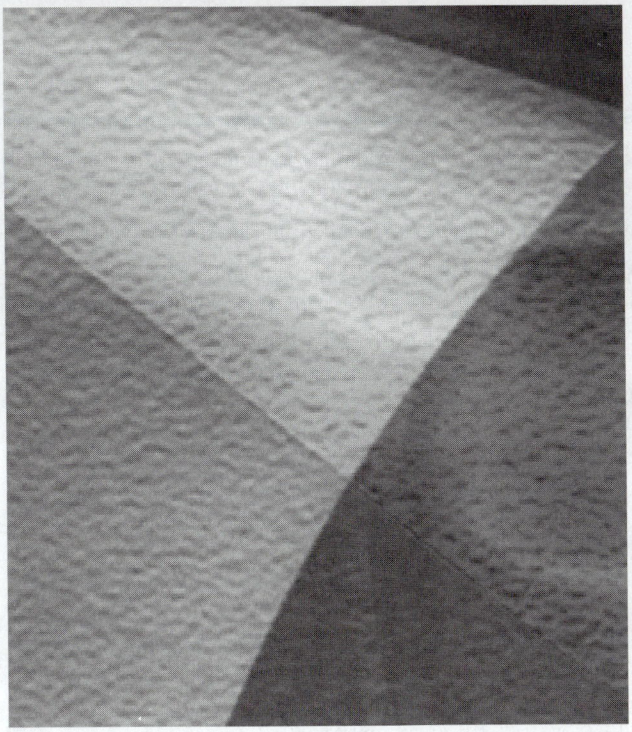

PART IV

Procedures Volume 3

INDEX TO PROCEDURES

A

◀ New ⬅ Revised Code

B

C

ICD-9-CM
C
Vol. 3

D

D

ICD-9-CM
D
Vol. 3

E

> Note Use the following fourth-digit subclassification with categories 90-91 to identify type of examination:
>
> 1 bacterial smear
> 2 culture
> 3 culture and sensitivity
> 4 parasitology
> 5 toxicology
> 6 cell block and Papanicolaou smear
> 9 other microscopic examination

ICD-9-CM
E
Vol. 3

F

ICD-9-CM F Vol. 3

G

H

ICD-9-CM

H

Vol. 3

I

◀ **New** ⬅ **Revised Code**

ICD-9-CM – Vol. 3

J

K

L

◀ **New** ⬅ **Revised Code**

ICD-9-CM
L
Vol. 3

◀ New ⟸ Revised Code

M

N

O

◀ **New** ⇐ **Revised Code**

P

ICD-9-CM
P, Q
Vol. 3

R

ICD-9-CM
R
Vol. 3

◄ **New** ⬅ **Revised Code**

ICD-9-CM
R
Vol. 3

◀ **New** ⟸ **Revised Code**

ICD-9-CM
R
Vol. 3

ICD-9-CM R Vol. 3

S

ICD-9-CM

S

Vol. 3

T

ICD-9-CM
T
Vol. 3

ICD-9-CM
T
Vol. 3

U

V

ICD-9-CM
V–Z
Vol. 3

TABULAR LIST OF PROCEDURES

00 PROCEDURES AND INTERVENTIONS, NOT ELSEWHERE CLASSIFIED (00)

● **00.0 Therapeutic ultrasound**

00.01 Therapeutic ultrasound of vessels of head and neck
Anti-restenotic ultrasound
Intravascular non-ablative ultrasound

Excludes *diagnostic ultrasound of:*
eye (95.13)
head and neck (88.71)
that of inner ear (20.79)
ultrasonic:
angioplasty of non-coronary vessel (39.50)
embolectomy (38.01, 38.02)
endarterectomy (38.11, 38.12)
thrombectomy (38.01, 38.02)

00.02 Therapeutic ultrasound of heart
Anti-restenotic ultrasound
Intravascular non-ablative ultrasound

Excludes *diagnostic ultrasound of heart (88.72)*
ultrasonic ablation of heart lesion (37.34)
ultrasonic angioplasty of coronary vessels (36.01, 36.02, 36.05, 36.09)

00.03 Therapeutic ultrasound of peripheral vascular vessels
Anti-restenotic ultrasound
Intravascular non-ablative ultrasound

Excludes *diagnostic ultrasound of peripheral vascular system (88.77)*
ultrasonic angioplasty of:
non-coronary vessel (39.50)

00.09 Other therapeutic ultrasound

Excludes *ultrasonic:*
fragmentation of urinary stones (59.95)
percutaneous nephrostomy with fragmentation (55.04)
physical therapy (93.35)
transurethral guided laster induced prostatectomy (TULIP) (60.21)

● **00.1 Pharmaceuticals**

00.10 Implantation of chemotherapeutic agent
Brain wafer chemotherapy
Interstitial/intracavitary

Excludes *injection or infusion of cancer chemotherapeutic substance (99.25)*

00.11 Infusion of drotrecogin alfa (activated)
Infusion of recombinant protein

00.12 Administration of inhaled nitric oxide
Nitric oxide therapy

00.13 Injection or infusion of nesiritide
Human B-type natriuretic peptide (hBNP)

00.14 Injection or infusion of oxazolidinone class of antibiotics
Linezolid injection

00.15 High-dose infusion interleukin-2 (Il-2) ◀
Infusion (IV bolus, CIV) interleukin ◀
Infusion aldesleukin ◀

Excludes *low-dose infusion interleukin-2 (99.28)* ◀

● **00.5 Other cardiovascular procedures**

✖ **00.50 Implantation of cardiac resynchronization pacemaker without mention of defibrillation, total system [CRT-P]**
Biventricular pacing without internal cardiac defibrillator
Implantation of cardiac resynchronization (biventricular) pulse generator pacing device, formation of pocket, transvenous leads including placement of lead into left ventricular coronary venous system, and intraoperative procedures for evaluation of lead signals.

Excludes *implantation of cardiac resynchronization defibrillator, total system [CRT-D] (00.51)*
insertion or replacement of any type pacemaker device (37.80–37.87)
replacement of cardiac resynchronization defibrillator pulse generator only [CRT-D] (00.54)
replacement of cardiac resynchronization pacemaker pulse generator only [CRT-P] (00.53)

✖ **00.51 Implantation of cardiac resynchronization defibrillator, total system [CRT-D]**
Biventricular pacing with internal cardiac defibrillator
Implantation of a cardiac resynchronization (biventricular) pulse generator with defibrillator [AICD], formation of pocket, transvenous leads, including placement of lead into left ventricular coronary venous system, intraoperative procedures for evaluation of lead signals, and obtaining defibrillator threshold measurements.

Excludes *implantation of cardiac resynchronization pacemaker, total system [CRT-P] (00.50)*
implantation or replacement of automatic cardioverter/defibrillator, total system [AICD] (37.94)
replacement of cardiac resynchronization defibrillator pulse generator, only [CRT-D] (00.54)

✖ **00.52 Implantation or replacement of transvenous lead [electrode] into left ventricular coronary venous system**

Excludes *implantation of cardiac resynchronization defibrillator, total system [CRT-D] (00.51)*
implantation of cardiac resynchronization pacemaker, total system [CRT-P] (00.50)
initial insertion of transvenous lead [electrode] (37.70–37.72)
replacement of transvenous atrial and/or ventricular lead(s) [electrodes] (37.76)

✖ **00.53 Implantation or replacement of cardiac resynchronization pacemaker pulse generator only [CRT-P]**
Implantation of CRT-P device with removal of any existing CRT-P or other pacemaker device

Excludes *implantation of cardiac resynchronization pacemaker, total system [CRT-P] (00.50)*
implantation or replacement of cardiac resynchronization defibrillator pulse generator only [CRT-D] (00.54)
insertion or replacement of any type pacemaker device (37.80–37.87)

✖ **00.54 Implantation or replacement of cardiac resynchronization defibrillator pulse generator device only [CRT-D]**

Implantation of CRT-D device with removal of any existing CRT-D, CRT-P, pacemaker, or defibrillator device

Excludes *implantation of automatic cardioverter/defibrillator pulse generator only (37.96)*
implantation of cardiac resynchronization defibrillator, total system [CRT-D] (00.51)
implantation or replacement of cardiac resynchronization pacemaker pulse generator only [CRT-P] (00.53)

00.55 Insertion of drug-eluting non-coronary artery stent(s)

Endograft(s)
Endovascular graft(s)
Stent grafts

Code also any non-coronary angioplasty or atherectomy (39.50)

Excludes *drug-coated stents, e.g., heparin costed (39.90)*
insertion of drug-eluting coronary artery stent (36.07)
insertion of non-drug-eluting stent(s):
coronary artery (36.06)
non-coronary artery (39.90)
that for aneurysm repair (39.71–39.79)

1. OPERATIONS ON THE NERVOUS SYSTEM (01–05)

● 01 **Incision and excision of skull, brain, and cerebral meninges**

● 01.0 **Cranial puncture**

01.01 **Cisternal puncture**
Cisternal tap

Excludes *pneumocisternogram (87.02)*

01.02 **Ventriculopuncture through previously implanted catheter**
Puncture of ventricular shunt tubing

01.09 **Other cranial puncture**
Aspiration of:
subarachnoid space
subdural space
Cranial aspiration NOS
Puncture of anterior fontanel
Subdural tap (through fontanel)

● 01.1 **Diagnostic procedures on skull, brain, and cerebral meninges**

01.11 **Closed [percutaneous] [needle] biopsy of cerebral meninges**
Burr hole approach

✖ 01.12 **Open biopsy of cerebral meninges**

01.13 **Closed [percutaneous] [needle] biopsy of brain**
Burr hole approach
Stereotactic method

✖ 01.14 **Open biopsy of brain**

✖ 01.15 **Biopsy of skull**

✖ 01.18 **Other diagnostic procedures on brain and cerebral meninges**

Excludes *cerebral:*
arteriography (88.41)
thermography (88.81)
contrast radiogram of brain (87.01–87.02)
echoencephalogram (88.71)
electroencephalogram (89.14)
microscopic examination of specimen from nervous system and of spinal fluid (90.01–90.09)
neurologic examination (89.13)
phlebography of head and neck (88.61)
pneumoencephalogram (87.01)
radioisotope scan:
cerebral (92.11)
head NEC (92.12)
tomography of head:
C.A.T. scan (87.03)
other (87.04)

✖ 01.19 **Other diagnostic procedures on skull**

Excludes *transillumination of skull (89.16)*
x-ray of skull (87.17)

● 01.2 **Craniotomy and craniectomy**

Excludes *decompression of skull fracture (02.02)*
exploration of orbit (16.01–16.09)
that as operative approach—omit code

✖ 01.21 **Incision and drainage of cranial sinus**

✖ 01.22 **Removal of intracranial neurostimulator**

Excludes *removal with synchronous replacement (02.93)*

✖ 01.23 **Reopening of craniotomy site**

✖ 01.24 **Other craniotomy**
Cranial:
decompression
exploration
trephination
Craniotomy NOS
Craniotomy with removal of:
epidural abscess
extradural hematoma
foreign body of skull

Excludes *removal of foreign body with incision into brain (01.39)*

✖ 01.25 **Other craniectomy**
Debridement of skull NOS
Sequestrectomy of skull

Excludes *debridement of compound fracture of skull (02.02)*
strip craniectomy (02.01)

● 01.3 **Incision of brain and cerebral meninges**

✖ 01.31 **Incision of cerebral meninges**
Drainage of:
intracranial hygroma
subarachnoid abscess (cerebral)
subdural empyema

✖ 01.32 **Lobotomy and tractotomy**
Division of:
brain tissue
cerebral tracts
Percutaneous (radiofrequency) cingulotomy

✖ 01.39 **Other incision of brain**
Amygdalohippocampotomy
Drainage of intracerebral hematoma
Incision of brain NOS

Excludes *division of cortical adhesions (02.91)*

● 01.4 **Operations on thalamus and globus pallidus**

✖ 01.41 **Operations on thalamus**
Chemothalamectomy
Thalamotomy

Excludes *that by stereotactic radiosurgery (92.30–92.39)*

✖ 01.42 **Operations on globus pallidus**
Pallidoansectomy
Pallidotomy

Excludes *that by stereotactic radiosurgery (92.30–92.39)*

● 01.5 **Other excision or destruction of brain and meninges**

✖ 01.51 **Excision of lesion or tissue of cerebral meninges**
Decortication of (cerebral) meninges
Resection of (cerebral) meninges
Stripping of subdural membrane of (cerebral) meninges

Excludes *biopsy of cerebral meninges (01.11–01.12)*

✖ 01.52 **Hemispherectomy**

✖ 01.53 **Lobectomy of brain**

✖ 01.59 **Other excision or destruction of lesion or tissue of brain**
Curettage of brain
Debridement of brain
Marsupialization of brain cyst
Transtemporal (mastoid) excision of brain tumor

Excludes *biopsy of brain (01.13–01.14)*
that by stereotactic radiosurgery (92.30–92.39)

✖ 01.6 **Excision of lesion of skull**
Removal of granulation tissue of cranium
Excludes *biopsy of skull (01.15)*
sequestrectomy (01.25)

● 02 **Other operations on skull, brain, and cerebral meninges**

● 02.0 **Cranioplasty**
Excludes *that with synchronous repair of encephalocele (02.12)*

✖ 02.01 **Opening of cranial suture**
Linear craniectomy
Strip craniectomy

✖ 02.02 **Elevation of skull fracture fragments**
Debridement of compound fracture of skull
Decompression of skull fracture
Reduction of skull fracture
Code also any synchronous debridement of brain (01.59)
Excludes *debridement of skull NOS (01.25)*
removal of granulation tissue of cranium (01.6)

✖ 02.03 **Formation of cranial bone flap**
Repair of skull with flap

✖ 02.04 **Bone graft to skull**
Pericranial graft (autogenous) (heterogenous)

✖ 02.05 **Insertion of skull plate**
Replacement of skull plate

✖ 02.06 **Other cranial osteoplasty**
Repair of skull NOS
Revision of bone flap of skull

✖ 02.07 **Removal of skull plate**
Excludes *removal with synchronous replacement (02.05)*

● 02.1 **Repair of cerebral meninges**
Excludes *marsupialization of cerebral lesion (01.59)*

✖ 02.11 **Simple suture of dura mater of brain**

✖ 02.12 **Other repair of cerebral meninges**
Closure of fistula of cerebrospinal fluid
Dural graft
Repair of encephalocele including synchronous cranioplasty
Repair of meninges NOS
Subdural patch

✖ 02.13 **Ligation of meningeal vessel**
Ligation of:
longitudinal sinus
middle meningeal artery

✖ 02.14 **Choroid plexectomy**
Cauterization of choroid plexus

✖ 02.2 **Ventriculostomy**
Anastomosis of ventricle to:
cervical subarachnoid space
cisterna magna
Insertion of Holter valve
Ventriculocisternal intubation

● 02.3 **Extracranial ventricular shunt**
Includes: that with insertion of valve

✖ 02.31 **Ventricular shunt to structure in head and neck**
Ventricle to nasopharynx shunt
Ventriculomastoid anastomosis

✖ 02.32 **Ventricular shunt to circulatory system**
Ventriculoatrial anastomosis
Ventriculocaval shunt

✖ 02.33 **Ventricular shunt to thoracic cavity**
Ventriculopleural anastomosis

✖ 02.34 **Ventricular shunt to abdominal cavity and organs**
Ventriculocholecystostomy
Ventriculoperitoneostomy

✖ 02.35 **Ventricular shunt to urinary system**
Ventricle to ureter shunt

✖ 02.39 **Other operations to establish drainage of ventricle**
Ventricle to bone marrow shunt
Ventricular shunt to extracranial site NEC

● 02.4 **Revision, removal, and irrigation of ventricular shunt**
Excludes *revision of distal catheter of ventricular shunt (54.95)*

02.41 **Irrigation and exploration of ventricular shunt**
Exploration of ventriculoperitoneal shunt at ventricular site
Re-programming of ventriculoperitoneal shunt ◀

✖ 02.42 **Replacement of ventricular shunt**
Reinsertion of Holter valve
Replacement of ventricular catheter
Revision of ventriculoperitoneal shunt at ventricular site

✖ 02.43 **Removal of ventricular shunt**

● 02.9 **Other operations on skull, brain, and cerebral meninges**
Excludes *operations on:*
pineal gland (07.17, 07.51–07.59)
pituitary gland [hypophysis] (07.13–07.15, 07.61–07.79)

✖ 02.91 **Lysis of cortical adhesions**

✖ 02.92 **Repair of brain**

✖ 02.93 **Implantation of intracranial neurostimulator**
Implantation, insertion, placement, or replacement of intracranial:
brain pacemaker [neuropacemaker]
depth electrodes
epidural pegs
electroencephalographic receiver
foramen ovale electrodes
intracranial electrostimulator
subdural grids
subdural strips

✖ 02.94 **Insertion or replacement of skull tongs or halo traction device**

02.95 **Removal of skull tongs or halo traction device**

02.96 **Insertion of sphenoidal electrodes**

✖ 02.99 **Other**
Excludes *chemical shock therapy (94.24)*
electroshock therapy:
subconvulsive (94.26)
other (94.27)

● 03 **Operations on spinal cord and spinal canal structures**
Code also any application or administration of an adhesion barrier substance (99.77)

● 03.0 **Exploration and decompression of spinal canal structures**

✖ 03.01 **Removal of foreign body from spinal canal**

✖ 03.02 **Reopening of laminectomy site**

✖ 03.09 **Other exploration and decompression of spinal canal**
Decompression:
laminectomy
laminotomy
Expansile laminoplasty
Exploration of spinal nerve root
Foraminotomy

Excludes *drainage of spinal fluid by anastomosis (03.71–03.79)*
laminectomy with excision of intervertebral disc (80.51)
spinal tap (03.31)
that as operative approach—omit code

✖ **03.1 Division of intraspinal nerve root**
Rhizotomy

● **03.2 Chordotomy**

✖ **03.21 Percutaneous chordotomy**
Stereotactic chordotomy

✖ **03.29 Other chordotomy**
Chordotomy NOS
Tractotomy (one-stage) (two-stage) of spinal cord
Transection of spinal cord tracts

● **03.3 Diagnostic procedures on spinal cord and spinal canal structures**

03.31 Spinal tap
Lumbar puncture for removal of dye

Excludes *lumbar puncture for injection of dye [myelogram] (87.21)*

✖ **03.32 Biopsy of spinal cord or spinal meninges**

✖ **03.39 Other diagnostic procedures on spinal cord and spinal canal structures**

Excludes *microscopic examination of specimen from nervous system or of spinal fluid (90.01–90.09)*
x-ray of spine (87.21–87.29)

✖ **03.4 Excision or destruction of lesion of spinal cord or spinal meninges**
Curettage of spinal cord or spinal meninges
Debridement of spinal cord or spinal meninges
Marsupialization of cyst of spinal cord or spinal meninges
Resection of spinal cord or spinal meninges

Excludes *biopsy of spinal cord or meninges (03.32)*

● **03.5 Plastic operations on spinal cord structures**

✖ **03.51 Repair of spinal meningocele**
Repair of meningocele NOS

✖ **03.52 Repair of spinal myelomeningocele**

✖ **03.53 Repair of vertebral fracture**
Elevation of spinal bone fragments
Reduction of fracture of vertebrae
Removal of bony spicules from spinal canal

Excludes *kyphoplasty (78.49)* ◀
vertebroplasty (78.49) ◀

✖ **03.59 Other repair and plastic operations on spinal cord structures**
Repair of:
diastematomyelia
spina bifida NOS
spinal cord NOS
spinal meninges NOS
vertebral arch defect

✖ **03.6 Lysis of adhesions of spinal cord and nerve roots**

● **03.7 Shunt of spinal theca**

Includes: that with valve

✖ **03.71 Spinal subarachnoid-peritoneal shunt**

✖ **03.72 Spinal subarachnoid-ureteral shunt**

✖ **03.79 Other shunt of spinal theca**
Lumbar-subarachnoid shunt NOS
Pleurothecal anastomosis
Salpingothecal anastomosis

03.8 Injection of destructive agent into spinal canal

● **03.9 Other operations on spinal cord and spinal canal structures**

03.90 Insertion of catheter into spinal canal for infusion of therapeutic or palliative substances
Insertion of catheter into epidural, subarachnoid, or subdural space of spine with intermittent or continuous infusion of drug (with creation of any reservoir)

Code also any implantation of infusion pump (86.06)

03.91 Injection of anesthetic into spinal canal for analgesia

Excludes *that for operative anesthesia—omit code*

03.92 Injection of other agent into spinal canal
Intrathecal injection of steroid
Subarachnoid perfusion of refrigerated saline

Excludes *injection of:*
contrast material for myelogram (87.21)
destructive agent into spinal canal (03.8)

✖ **03.93 Insertion or replacement of spinal neurostimulator**

✖ **03.94 Removal of spinal neurostimulator**

03.95 Spinal blood patch

03.96 Percutaneous denervation of facet

✖ **03.97 Revision of spinal thecal shunt**

✖ **03.98 Removal of spinal thecal shunt**

✖ **03.99 Other**

● **04 Operations on cranial and peripheral nerves**

● **04.0 Incision, division, and excision of cranial and peripheral nerves**

Excludes *opticociliary neurectomy (12.79)*
sympathetic ganglionectomy (05.21–05.29)

✖ **04.01 Excision of acoustic neuroma**
That by craniotomy

Excludes *that by stereotactic radiosurgery (92.3)*

✖ **04.02 Division of trigeminal nerve**
Retrogasserian neurotomy

✖ **04.03 Division or crushing of other cranial and peripheral nerves**

Excludes *that of:*
glossopharyngeal nerve (29.92)
laryngeal nerve (31.91)
nerves to adrenal glands (07.42)
phrenic nerve for collapse of lung (33.31)
vagus nerve (44.00–44.03)

✖ **04.04 Other incision of cranial and peripheral nerves**

✖ **04.05 Gasserian ganglionectomy**

✖ **04.06 Other cranial or peripheral ganglionectomy**

Excludes *sympathetic ganglionectomy (05.21–05.29)*

✖ **04.07 Other excision or avulsion of cranial and peripheral nerves**
Curettage of peripheral nerve
Debridement of peripheral nerve
Resection of peripheral nerve
Excision of peripheral neuroma [Morton's]

Excludes *biopsy of cranial or peripheral nerve (04.11–04.12)*

● **04.1 Diagnostic procedures on peripheral nervous system**

04.11 Closed [percutaneous] [needle] biopsy of cranial or peripheral nerve or ganglion

✖ **04.12 Open biopsy of cranial or peripheral nerve or ganglion**

✖04.19 **Other diagnostic procedures on cranial and peripheral nerves and ganglia**

Excludes *microscopic examination of specimen from nervous system (90.01–90.09)*
neurologic examination (89.13)

04.2 **Destruction of cranial and peripheral nerves**
Destruction of cranial or peripheral nerves by:
cryoanalgesia
injection of neurolytic agent
radiofrequency
Radiofrequency ablation

✖04.3 **Suture of cranial and peripheral nerves**

● 04.4 **Lysis of adhesions and decompression of cranial and peripheral nerves**

✖04.41 **Decompression of trigeminal nerve root**

✖04.42 **Other cranial nerve decompression**

✖04.43 **Release of carpal tunnel**

✖04.44 **Release of tarsal tunnel**

✖04.49 **Other peripheral nerve or ganglion decompression or lysis of adhesions**
Peripheral nerve neurolysis NOS

✖04.5 **Cranial or peripheral nerve graft**

✖04.6 **Transposition of cranial and peripheral nerves**
Nerve transplantation

● 04.7 **Other cranial or peripheral neuroplasty**

✖04.71 **Hypoglossal-facial anastomosis**

✖04.72 **Accessory-facial anastomosis**

✖04.73 **Accessory-hypoglossal anastomosis**

✖04.74 **Other anastomosis of cranial or peripheral nerve**

✖04.75 **Revision of previous repair of cranial and peripheral nerves**

✖04.76 **Repair of old traumatic injury of cranial and peripheral nerves**

✖04.79 **Other neuroplasty**

● 04.8 **Injection into peripheral nerve**

Excludes *destruction of nerve (by injection of neurolytic agent) (04.2)*

04.80 **Peripheral nerve injection, not otherwise specified**

04.81 **Injection of anesthetic into peripheral nerve for analgesia**

Excludes *that for operative anesthesia—omit code*

04.89 **Injection of other agent, except neurolytic**

Excludes *injection of neurolytic agent (04.2)*

● 04.9 **Other operations on cranial and peripheral nerves**

✖04.91 **Neurectasis**

✖04.92 **Implantation or replacement of peripheral neurostimulator**

✖04.93 **Removal of peripheral neurostimulator**

✖04.99 **Other**

● 05 **Operations on sympathetic nerves or ganglia**

Excludes *paracervical uterine denervation (69.3)*

✖05.0 **Division of sympathetic nerve or ganglion**

Excludes *that of nerves to adrenal glands (07.42)*

● 05.1 **Diagnostic procedures on sympathetic nerves or ganglia**

✖05.11 **Biopsy of sympathetic nerve or ganglion**

✖05.19 **Other diagnostic procedures on sympathetic nerves or ganglia**

● 05.2 **Sympathectomy**

✖05.21 **Sphenopalatine ganglionectomy**

✖05.22 **Cervical sympathectomy**

✖05.23 **Lumbar sympathectomy**

✖05.24 **Presacral sympathectomy**

✖05.25 **Periarterial sympathectomy**

✖05.29 **Other sympathectomy and ganglionectomy**
Excision or avulsion of sympathetic nerve NOS
Sympathetic ganglionectomy NOS

Excludes *biopsy of sympathetic nerve or ganglion (05.11)*
opticociliary neurectomy (12.79)
periarterial sympathectomy (05.25)
tympanosympathectomy (20.91)

● 05.3 **Injection into sympathetic nerve or ganglion**

Excludes *injection of ciliary sympathetic ganglion (12.79)*

05.31 **Injection of anesthetic into sympathetic nerve for analgesia**

05.32 **Injection of neurolytic agent into sympathetic nerve**

05.39 **Other injection into sympathetic nerve or ganglion**

● 05.8 **Other operations on sympathetic nerves or ganglia**

✖05.81 **Repair of sympathetic nerve or ganglion**

✖05.89 **Other**

✖05.9 **Other operations on nervous system**

2. OPERATIONS ON THE ENDOCRINE SYSTEM (06–07)

● **06 Operations on thyroid and parathyroid glands**

Includes: incidental resection of hyoid bone

06.0 Incision of thyroid field

Excludes *division of isthmus (06.91)*

06.01 Aspiration of thyroid field

Percutaneous or needle drainage of thyroid field

Excludes *aspiration biopsy of thyroid (06.11)*
drainage by incision (06.09)
postoperative aspiration of field (06.02)

✖**06.02 Reopening of wound of thyroid field**

Reopening of wound of thyroid field for:
control of (postoperative) hemorrhage
examination
exploration
removal of hematoma

✖**06.09 Other incision of thyroid field**

Drainage of hematoma by incision
Drainage of thyroglossal tract by incision
Exploration:
neck by incision
thyroid (field) by incision
Removal of foreign body by incision
Thyroidotomy NOS by incision

Excludes *postoperative exploration (06.02)*
removal of hematoma by aspiration (06.01)

● **06.1 Diagnostic procedures on thyroid and parathyroid glands**

06.11 Closed [percutaneous] [needle] biopsy of thyroid gland

Aspiration biopsy of thyroid

✖**06.12 Open biopsy of thyroid gland**

✖**06.13 Biopsy of parathyroid gland**

✖**06.19 Other diagnostic procedures on thyroid and parathyroid glands**

Excludes *radioisotope scan of:*
parathyroid (92.13)
thyroid (92.01)
soft tissue x-ray of thyroid field (87.09)

✖**06.2 Unilateral thyroid lobectomy**

Complete removal of one lobe of thyroid (with removal of isthmus or portion of other lobe)
Hemithyroidectomy

Excludes *partial substernal thyroidectomy (06.51)*

● **06.3 Other partial thyroidectomy**

✖**06.31 Excision of lesion of thyroid**

Excludes *biopsy of thyroid (06.11–06.12)*

✖**06.39 Other**

Isthmectomy
Partial thyroidectomy NOS

Excludes *partial substernal thyroidectomy (06.51)*

✖**06.4 Complete thyroidectomy**

Excludes *complete substernal thyroidectomy (06.52)*
that with laryngectomy (30.3–30.4)

● **06.5 Substernal thyroidectomy**

✖**06.50 Substernal thyroidectomy, not otherwise specified**

✖**06.51 Partial substernal thyroidectomy**

✖**06.52 Complete substernal thyroidectomy**

✖**06.6 Excision of lingual thyroid**

Excision of thyroid by:
submental route
transoral route

✖**06.7 Excision of thyroglossal duct or tract**

● **06.8 Parathyroidectomy**

✖**06.81 Complete parathyroidectomy**

✖**06.89 Other parathyroidectomy**

Parathyroidectomy NOS
Partial parathyroidectomy

Excludes *biopsy of parathyroid (06.13)*

● **06.9 Other operations on thyroid (region) and parathyroid**

✖**06.91 Division of thyroid isthmus**

Transection of thyroid isthmus

✖**06.92 Ligation of thyroid vessels**

✖**06.93 Suture of thyroid gland**

✖**06.94 Thyroid tissue reimplantation**

Autotransplantation of thyroid tissue

✖**06.95 Parathyroid tissue reimplantation**

Autotransplantation of parathyroid tissue

✖**06.98 Other operations on thyroid glands**

✖**06.99 Other operations on parathyroid glands**

● **07 Operations on other endocrine glands**

Includes: operations on:
adrenal glands
pineal gland
pituitary gland
thymus

Excludes *operations on:*
aortic and carotid bodies (39.8)
ovaries (65.0–65.99)
pancreas (52.01–52.99)
testes (62.0–62.99)

● **07.0 Exploration of adrenal field**

Excludes *incision of adrenal (gland) (07.41)*

✖**07.00 Exploration of adrenal field, not otherwise specified**

✖**07.01 Unilateral exploration of adrenal field**

✖**07.02 Bilateral exploration of adrenal field**

● **07.1 Diagnostic procedures on adrenal glands, pituitary gland, pineal gland, and thymus**

07.11 Closed [percutaneous] [needle] biopsy of adrenal gland

✖**07.12 Open biopsy of adrenal gland**

✖**07.13 Biopsy of pituitary gland, transfrontal approach**

✖**07.14 Biopsy of pituitary gland, transsphenoidal approach**

✖**07.15 Biopsy of pituitary gland, unspecified approach**

✖**07.16 Biopsy of thymus**

✖**07.17 Biopsy of pineal gland**

✖**07.19 Other diagnostic procedures on adrenal glands, pituitary gland, pineal gland, and thymus**

Excludes *microscopic examination of specimen from endocrine gland (90.11–90.19)*
radioisotope scan of pituitary gland (92.11)

● **07.2 Partial adrenalectomy**

✖**07.21 Excision of lesion of adrenal gland**

Excludes *biopsy of adrenal gland (07.11–07.12)*

✖ 07.22 Unilateral adrenalectomy
Adrenalectomy NOS

Excludes *excision of remaining adrenal gland (07.3)*

✖ 07.29 Other partial adrenalectomy
Partial adrenalectomy NOS

✖ 07.3 Bilateral adrenalectomy
Excision of remaining adrenal gland

Excludes *bilateral partial adrenalectomy (07.29)*

● 07.4 Other operations on adrenal glands, nerves, and vessels

✖ 07.41 Incision of adrenal gland
Adrenalotomy (with drainage)

✖ 07.42 Division of nerves to adrenal glands

✖ 07.43 Ligation of adrenal vessels

✖ 07.44 Repair of adrenal gland

✖ 07.45 Reimplantation of adrenal tissue
Autotransplantation of adrenal tissue

✖ 07.49 Other

● 07.5 Operations on pineal gland

✖ 07.51 Exploration of pineal field

Excludes *that with incision of pineal gland (07.52)*

✖ 07.52 Incision of pineal gland

✖ 07.53 Partial excision of pineal gland

Excludes *biopsy of pineal gland (07.17)*

✖ 07.54 Total excision of pineal gland
Pinealectomy (complete) (total)

✖ 07.59 Other operations on pineal gland

● 07.6 Hypophysectomy

✖ 07.61 Partial excision of pituitary gland, transfrontal approach
Cryohypophysectomy, partial transfrontal approach
Division of hypophyseal stalk transfrontal approach
Excision of lesion of pituitary [hypophysis] transfrontal approach
Hypophysectomy, subtotal transfrontal approach
Infundibulectomy, hypophyseal transfrontal approach

Excludes *biopsy of pituitary gland, transfrontal approach (07.13)*

✖ 07.62 Partial excision of pituitary gland, transsphenoidal approach

Excludes *biopsy of pituitary gland, transsphenoidal approach (07.14)*

✖ 07.63 Partial excision of pituitary gland, unspecified approach

Excludes *biopsy of pituitary gland NOS (07.15)*

✖ 07.64 Total excision of pituitary gland, transfrontal approach
Ablation of pituitary by implantation (strontium-yttrium) (Y) transfrontal approach
Cryohypophysectomy, complete transfrontal approach

✖ 07.65 Total excision of pituitary gland, transsphenoidal approach

✖ 07.68 Total excision of pituitary gland, other specified approach

✖ 07.69 Total excision of pituitary gland, unspecified approach
Hypophysectomy NOS
Pituitectomy NOS

● 07.7 Other operations on hypophysis

✖ 07.71 Exploration of pituitary fossa

Excludes *exploration with incision of pituitary gland (07.72)*

✖ 07.72 Incision of pituitary gland
Aspiration of:
craniobuccal pouch
craniopharyngioma
hypophysis
pituitary gland
Rathke's pouch

✖ 07.79 Other
Insertion of pack into sella turcica

● 07.8 Thymectomy

✖ 07.80 Thymectomy, not otherwise specified

✖ 07.81 Partial excision of thymus

Excludes *biopsy of thymus (07.16)*

✖ 07.82 Total excision of thymus

● 07.9 Other operations on thymus

✖ 07.91 Exploration of thymus field

Excludes *exploration with incision of thymus (07.92)*

✖ 07.92 Incision of thymus

✖ 07.93 Repair of thymus

✖ 07.94 Transplantation of thymus

✖ 07.99 Other
Thymopexy

3. OPERATIONS ON THE EYE (08–16)

● **08 Operations on eyelids**

Includes: operations on the eyebrow

● **08.0 Incision of eyelid**

08.01 Incision of lid margin

08.02 Severing of blepharorrhaphy

08.09 Other incision of eyelid

● **08.1 Diagnostic procedures on eyelid**

✖**08.11 Biopsy of eyelid**

08.19 Other diagnostic procedures on eyelid

● **08.2 Excision or destruction of lesion or tissue of eyelid**

Code also any synchronous reconstruction (08.61–08.74)

Excludes *biopsy of eyelid (08.11)*

✖**08.20 Removal of lesion of eyelid, not otherwise specified**
Removal of meibomian gland NOS

✖**08.21 Excision of chalazion**

✖**08.22 Excision of other minor lesion of eyelid**
Excision of:
verucca
wart

✖**08.23 Excision of major lesion of eyelid, partial-thickness**
Excision involving one-fourth or more of lid margin, partial-thickness

✖**08.24 Excision of major lesion of eyelid, full-thickness**
Excision involving one-fourth or more of lid margin, full-thickness
Wedge resection of eyelid

✖**08.25 Destruction of lesion of eyelid**

● **08.3 Repair of blepharoptosis and lid retraction**

✖**08.31 Repair of blepharoptosis by frontalis muscle technique with suture**

✖**08.32 Repair of blepharoptosis by frontalis muscle technique with fascial sling**

✖**08.33 Repair of blepharoptosis by resection or advancement of levator muscle or aponeurosis**

✖**08.34 Repair of blepharoptosis by other levator muscle techniques**

✖**08.35 Repair of blepharoptosis by tarsal technique**

✖**08.36 Repair of blepharoptosis by other techniques**
Correction of eyelid ptosis NOS
Orbicularis oculi muscle sling for correction of blepharoptosis

✖**08.37 Reduction of overcorrection of ptosis**

✖**08.38 Correction of lid retraction**

● **08.4 Repair of entropion or ectropion**

✖**08.41 Repair of entropion or ectropion by thermocauterization**

✖**08.42 Repair of entropion or ectropion by suture technique**

✖**08.43 Repair of entropion or ectropion with wedge resection**

✖**08.44 Repair of entropion or ectropion with lid reconstruction**

✖**08.49 Other repair of entropion or ectropion**

● **08.5 Other adjustment of lid position**

✖**08.51 Canthotomy**
Enlargement of palpebral fissure

✖**08.52 Blepharorrhaphy**
Canthorrhaphy
Tarsorrhaphy

✖**08.59 Other**
Canthoplasty NOS
Repair of epicanthal fold

● **08.6 Reconstruction of eyelid with flaps or grafts**

Excludes *that associated with repair of entropion and ectropion (08.44)*

✖**08.61 Reconstruction of eyelid with skin flap or graft**

✖**08.62 Reconstruction of eyelid with mucous membrane flap or graft**

✖**08.63 Reconstruction of eyelid with hair follicle graft**

✖**08.64 Reconstruction of eyelid with tarsoconjunctival flap**
Transfer of tarsoconjunctival flap from opposing lid

✖**08.69 Other reconstruction of eyelid with flaps or grafts**

● **08.7 Other reconstruction of eyelid**

Excludes *that associated with repair of entropion and ectropion (08.44)*

✖**08.70 Reconstruction of eyelid, not otherwise specified**

✖**08.71 Reconstruction of eyelid involving lid margin, partial-thickness**

✖**08.72 Other reconstruction of eyelid, partial-thickness**

✖**08.73 Reconstruction of eyelid involving lid margin, full-thickness**

✖**08.74 Other reconstruction of eyelid, full-thickness**

● **08.8 Other repair of eyelid**

08.81 Linear repair of laceration of eyelid or eyebrow

08.82 Repair of laceration involving lid margin, partial-thickness

08.83 Other repair of laceration of eyelid, partial-thickness

08.84 Repair of laceration involving lid margin, full-thickness

08.85 Other repair of laceration of eyelid, full-thickness

08.86 Lower eyelid rhytidectomy

08.87 Upper eyelid rhytidectomy

08.89 Other eyelid repair

● **08.9 Other operations on eyelids**

✖**08.91 Electrosurgical epilation of eyelid**

✖**08.92 Cryosurgical epilation of eyelid**

✖**08.93 Other epilation of eyelid**

✖**08.99 Other**

● **09 Operations on lacrimal system**

✖**09.0 Incision of lacrimal gland**
Incision of lacrimal cyst (with drainage)

● **09.1 Diagnostic procedures on lacrimal system**

✖**09.11 Biopsy of lacrimal gland**

✖**09.12 Biopsy of lacrimal sac**

✖**09.19 Other diagnostic procedures on lacrimal system**

Excludes *contrast dacryocystogram (87.05)*
soft tissue x-ray of nasolacrimal duct (87.09)

● 09.2 Excision of lesion or tissue of lacrimal gland

✖ 09.20 Excision of lacrimal gland, not otherwise specified

✖ 09.21 Excision of lesion of lacrimal gland

Excludes *biopsy of lacrimal gland (09.11)*

✖ 09.22 Other partial dacryoadenectomy

Excludes *biopsy of lacrimal gland (09.11)*

✖ 09.23 Total dacryoadenectomy

✖ 09.3 Other operations on lacrimal gland

● 09.4 Manipulation of lacrimal passage

Includes: removal of calculus
that with dilation

Excludes *contrast dacryocystogram (87.05)*

✖ 09.41 Probing of lacrimal punctum

✖ 09.42 Probing of lacrimal canaliculi

✖ 09.43 Probing of nasolacrimal duct

Excludes *that with insertion of tube or stent (09.44)*

✖ 09.44 Intubation of nasolacrimal duct

Insertion of stent into nasolacrimal duct

✖ 09.49 Other manipulation of lacrimal passage

● 09.5 Incision of lacrimal sac and passages

✖ 09.51 Incision of lacrimal punctum

✖ 09.52 Incision of lacrimal canaliculi

✖ 09.53 Incision of lacrimal sac

✖ 09.59 Other incision of lacrimal passages

Incision (and drainage) of nasolacrimal duct NOS

✖ 09.6 Excision of lacrimal sac and passage

Excludes *biopsy of lacrimal sac (09.12)*

● 09.7 Repair of canaliculus and punctum

Excludes *repair of eyelid (08.81–08.89)*

✖ 09.71 Correction of everted punctum

✖ 09.72 Other repair of punctum

✖ 09.73 Repair of canaliculus

● 09.8 Fistulization of lacrimal tract to nasal cavity

✖ 09.81 Dacryocystorhinostomy [DCR]

✖ 09.82 Conjunctivocystorhinostomy

Conjunctivodacryocystorhinostomy [CDCR]

Excludes *that with insertion of tube or stent (09.83)*

✖ 09.83 Conjunctivorhinostomy with insertion of tube or stent

● 09.9 Other operations on lacrimal system

✖ 09.91 Obliteration of lacrimal punctum

✖ 09.99 Other

● 10 Operations on conjunctiva

✖ 10.0 Removal of embedded foreign body from conjunctiva by incision

Excludes *removal of:*
embedded foreign body without incision (98.22)
superficial foreign body (98.21)

✖ 10.1 Other incision of conjunctiva

● 10.2 Diagnostic procedures on conjunctiva

✖ 10.21 Biopsy of conjunctiva

✖ 10.29 Other diagnostic procedures on conjunctiva

● 10.3 Excision or destruction of lesion or tissue of conjunctiva

✖ 10.31 Excision of lesion or tissue of conjunctiva

Excision of ring of conjunctiva around cornea

Excludes *biopsy of conjunctiva (10.21)*

✖ 10.32 Destruction of lesion of conjunctiva

Excludes *excision of lesion (10.31)*
thermocauterization for entropion (08.41)

✖ 10.33 Other destructive procedures on conjunctiva

Removal of trachoma follicles

● 10.4 Conjunctivoplasty

✖ 10.41 Repair of symblepharon with free graft

✖ 10.42 Reconstruction of conjunctival cul-de-sac with free graft

Excludes *revision of enucleation socket with graft (16.63)*

✖ 10.43 Other reconstruction of conjunctival cul-de-sac

Excludes *revision of enucleation socket (16.64)*

✖ 10.44 Other free graft to conjunctiva

✖ 10.49 Other conjunctivoplasty

Excludes *repair of cornea with conjunctival flap (11.53)*

✖ 10.5 Lysis of adhesions of conjunctiva and eyelid

Division of symblepharon (with insertion of conformer)

✖ 10.6 Repair of laceration of conjunctiva

Excludes *that with repair of sclera (12.81)*

● 10.9 Other operations on conjunctiva

✖ 10.91 Subconjunctival injection

✖ 10.99 Other

● 11 Operations on cornea

✖ 11.0 Magnetic removal of embedded foreign body from cornea

Excludes *that with incision (11.1)*

✖ 11.1 Incision of cornea

Incision of cornea for removal of foreign body

● 11.2 Diagnostic procedures on cornea

✖ 11.21 Scraping of cornea for smear or culture

✖ 11.22 Biopsy of cornea

✖ 11.29 Other diagnostic procedures on cornea

● 11.3 Excision of pterygium

✖ 11.31 Transposition of pterygium

✖ 11.32 Excision of pterygium with corneal graft

✖ 11.39 Other excision of pterygium

● 11.4 Excision or destruction of tissue or other lesion of cornea

✖ 11.41 Mechanical removal of corneal epithelium

That by chemocauterization

Excludes *that for smear or culture (11.21)*

✖ 11.42 Thermocauterization of corneal lesion

✖ 11.43 Cryotherapy of corneal lesion

✖ 11.49 Other removal or destruction of corneal lesion

Excision of cornea NOS

Excludes *biopsy of cornea (11.22)*

● 11.5 Repair of cornea

✖ 11.51 Suture of corneal laceration

✖ 11.52 Repair of postoperative wound dehiscence of cornea

✖ 11.53 Repair of corneal laceration or wound with conjunctival flap

✖ 11.59 Other repair of cornea

● 11.6 **Corneal transplant**
Excludes *excision of pterygium with corneal graft (11.32)*

✖ 11.60 **Corneal transplant, not otherwise specified**
Keratoplasty NOS

✖ 11.61 **Lamellar keratoplasty with autograft**

✖ 11.62 **Other lamellar keratoplasty**

✖ 11.63 **Penetrating keratoplasty with autograft**
Perforating keratoplasty with autograft

✖ 11.64 **Other penetrating keratoplasty**
Perforating keratoplasty (with homograft)

✖ 11.69 **Other corneal transplant**

● 11.7 **Other reconstructive and refractive surgery on cornea**

✖ 11.71 **Keratomileusis**

✖ 11.72 **Keratophakia**

✖ 11.73 **Keratoprosthesis**

✖ 11.74 **Thermokeratoplasty**

✖ 11.75 **Radial keratotomy**

✖ 11.76 **Epikeratophakia**

✖ 11.79 **Other**

● 11.9 **Other operations on cornea**

✖ 11.91 **Tattooing of cornea**

✖ 11.92 **Removal of artificial implant from cornea**

✖ 11.99 **Other**

● 12 **Operations on iris, ciliary body, sclera, and anterior chamber**
Excludes *operations on cornea (11.0–11.99)*

● 12.0 **Removal of intraocular foreign body from anterior segment of eye**

✖ 12.00 **Removal of intraocular foreign body from anterior segment of eye, not otherwise specified**

✖ 12.01 **Removal of intraocular foreign body from anterior segment of eye with use of magnet**

✖ 12.02 **Removal of intraocular foreign body from anterior segment of eye without use of magnet**

● 12.1 **Iridotomy and simple iridectomy**
Excludes *iridectomy associated with:*
cataract extraction (13.11–13.69)
removal of lesion (12.41–12.42)
scleral fistulization (12.61–12.69)

✖ 12.11 **Iridotomy with transfixion**

✖ 12.12 **Other iridotomy**
Corectomy
Discission of iris
Iridotomy NOS

✖ 12.13 **Excision of prolapsed iris**

✖ 12.14 **Other iridectomy**
Iridectomy (basal) (peripheral) (total)

● 12.2 **Diagnostic procedures on iris, ciliary body, sclera, and anterior chamber**

✖ 12.21 **Diagnostic aspiration of anterior chamber of eye**

✖ 12.22 **Biopsy of iris**

✖ 12.29 **Other diagnostic procedures on iris, ciliary body, sclera, and anterior chamber**

● 12.3 **Iridoplasty and coreoplasty**

✖ 12.31 **Lysis of goniosynechiae**
Lysis of goniosynechiae by injection of air or liquid

✖ 12.32 **Lysis of other anterior synechiae**
Lysis of anterior synechiae:
NOS
by injection of air or liquid

✖ 12.33 **Lysis of posterior synechiae**
Lysis of iris adhesions NOS

✖ 12.34 **Lysis of corneovitreal adhesions**

✖ 12.35 **Coreoplasty**
Needling of pupillary membrane

✖ 12.39 **Other iridoplasty**

● 12.4 **Excision or destruction of lesion of iris and ciliary body**

✖ 12.40 **Removal of lesion of anterior segment of eye, not otherwise specified**

✖ 12.41 **Destruction of lesion of iris, nonexcisional**
Destruction of lesion of iris by:
cauterization
cryotherapy
photocoagulation

✖ 12.42 **Excision of lesion of iris**
Excludes *biopsy of iris (12.22)*

✖ 12.43 **Destruction of lesion of ciliary body, nonexcisional**

✖ 12.44 **Excision of lesion of ciliary body**

● 12.5 **Facilitation of intraocular circulation**

✖ 12.51 **Goniopuncture without goniotomy**

✖ 12.52 **Goniotomy without goniopuncture**

✖ 12.53 **Goniotomy with goniopuncture**

✖ 12.54 **Trabeculotomy ab externo**

✖ 12.55 **Cyclodialysis**

✖ 12.59 **Other facilitation of intraocular circulation**

● 12.6 **Scleral fistulization**
Excludes *exploratory sclerotomy (12.89)*

✖ 12.61 **Trephination of sclera with iridectomy**

✖ 12.62 **Thermocauterization of sclera with iridectomy**

✖ 12.63 **Iridencleisis and iridotasis**

✖ 12.64 **Trabeculectomy ab externo**

✖ 12.65 **Other scleral fistulization with iridectomy**

✖ 12.66 **Postoperative revision of scleral fistulization procedure**
Revision of filtering bleb
Excludes *repair of fistula (12.82)*

✖ 12.69 **Other fistulizing procedure**

● 12.7 **Other procedures for relief of elevated intraocular pressure**

✖ 12.71 **Cyclodiathermy**

✖ 12.72 **Cyclocryotherapy**

✖ 12.73 **Cyclophotocoagulation**

✖ 12.74 **Diminution of ciliary body, not otherwise specified**

✖ 12.79 **Other glaucoma procedures**

● 12.8 **Operations on sclera**
Excludes *those associated with:*
retinal reattachment (14.41–14.59)
scleral fistulization (12.61–12.69)

✖ 12.81 **Suture of laceration of sclera**
Suture of sclera with synchronous repair of conjunctiva

✖12.82 **Repair of scleral fistula**

Excludes *postoperative revision of scleral fistulization procedure (12.66)*

✖12.83 **Revision of operative wound of anterior segment, not elsewhere classified**

Excludes *postoperative revision of scleral fistulization procedure (12.66)*

✖12.84 **Excision or destruction of lesion of sclera**

✖12.85 **Repair of scleral staphyloma with graft**

✖12.86 **Other repair of scleral staphyloma**

✖12.87 **Scleral reinforcement with graft**

✖12.88 **Other scleral reinforcement**

✖12.89 **Other operations on sclera**
Exploratory sclerotomy

●12.9 **Other operations on iris, ciliary body, and anterior chamber**

✖12.91 **Therapeutic evacuation of anterior chamber**
Paracentesis of anterior chamber

Excludes *diagnostic aspiration (12.21)*

✖12.92 **Injection into anterior chamber**
Injection of:
air into anterior chamber
liquid into anterior chamber
medication into anterior chamber

✖12.93 **Removal or destruction of epithelial downgrowth from anterior chamber**

Excludes *that with iridectomy (12.41–12.42)*

✖12.97 **Other operations on iris**

✖12.98 **Other operations on ciliary body**

✖12.99 **Other operations on anterior chamber**

●13 **Operations on lens**

●13.0 **Removal of foreign body from lens**

Excludes *removal of pseudophakos (13.8)*

✖13.00 **Removal of foreign body from lens, not otherwise specified**

✖13.01 **Removal of foreign body from lens with use of magnet**

✖13.02 **Removal of foreign body from lens without use of magnet**

●13.1 **Intracapsular extraction of lens**

Code also any synchronous insertion of pseudophakos (13.71)

✖13.11 **Intracapsular extraction of lens by temporal inferior route**

✖13.19 **Other intracapsular extraction of lens**
Cataract extraction NOS
Cryoextraction of lens
Erysiphake extraction of cataract
Extraction of lens NOS

✖13.2 **Extracapsular extraction of lens by linear extraction technique**

✖13.3 **Extracapsular extraction of lens by simple aspiration (and irrigation) technique**
Irrigation of traumatic cataract

●13.4 **Extracapsular extraction of lens by fragmentation and aspiration technique**

✖13.41 **Phacoemulsification and aspiration of cataract**

✖13.42 **Mechanical phacofragmentation and aspiration of cataract by posterior route**

Code also any synchronous vitrectomy (14.74)

✖13.43 **Mechanical phacofragmentation and other aspiration of cataract**

●13.5 **Other extracapsular extraction of lens**

Code also any synchronous insertion of pseudophakos (13.71)

✖13.51 **Extracapsular extraction of lens by temporal inferior route**

✖13.59 **Other extracapsular extraction of lens**

●13.6 **Other cataract extraction**

Code also any synchronous insertion of pseudophakos (13.71)

✖13.64 **Discission of secondary membrane [after cataract]**

✖13.65 **Excision of secondary membrane [after cataract]**
Capsulectomy

✖13.66 **Mechanical fragmentation of secondary membrane [after cataract]**

✖13.69 **Other cataract extraction**

●13.7 **Insertion of prosthetic lens [pseudophakos]**

✖13.70 **Insertion of pseudophakos, not otherwise specified**

✖13.71 **Insertion of intraocular lens prosthesis at time of cataract extraction, one-stage**

Code also synchronous extraction of cataract (13.11–13.69)

✖13.72 **Secondary insertion of intraocular lens prosthesis**

✖13.8 **Removal of implanted lens**
Removal of pseudophakos

✖13.9 **Other operations on lens**

●14 **Operations on retina, choroid, vitreous, and posterior chamber**

●14.0 **Removal of foreign body from posterior segment of eye**

Excludes *removal of surgically implanted material (14.6)*

✖14.00 **Removal of foreign body from posterior segment of eye, not otherwise specified**

✖14.01 **Removal of foreign body from posterior segment of eye with use of magnet**

✖14.02 **Removal of foreign body from posterior segment of eye without use of magnet**

●14.1 **Diagnostic procedures on retina, choroid, vitreous, and posterior chamber**

✖14.11 **Diagnostic aspiration of vitreous**

✖14.19 **Other diagnostic procedures on retina, choroid, vitreous, and posterior chamber**

●14.2 **Destruction of lesion of retina and choroid**

Includes: destruction of chorioretinopathy or isolated chorioretinal lesion

Excludes *that for repair of retina (14.31–14.59)*

✖14.21 **Destruction of chorioretinal lesion by diathermy**

✖14.22 **Destruction of chorioretinal lesion by cryotherapy**

14.23 **Destruction of chorioretinal lesion by xenon arc photocoagulation**

14.24 **Destruction of chorioretinal lesion by laser photocoagulation**

14.25 Destruction of chorioretinal lesion by photocoagulation of unspecified type

✖14.26 Destruction of chorioretinal lesion by radiation therapy

✖14.27 Destruction of chorioretinal lesion by implantation of radiation source

✖14.29 Other destruction of chorioretinal lesion
Destruction of lesion of retina and choroid NOS

●14.3 Repair of retinal tear

Includes: repair of retinal defect

Excludes *repair of retinal detachment (14.41–14.59)*

✖14.31 Repair of retinal tear by diathermy

✖14.32 Repair of retinal tear by cryotherapy

14.33 Repair of retinal tear by xenon arc photocoagulation

14.34 Repair of retinal tear by laser photocoagulation

14.35 Repair of retinal tear by photocoagulation of unspecified type

✖14.39 Other repair of retinal tear

●14.4 Repair of retinal detachment with scleral buckling and implant

✖14.41 Scleral buckling with implant

✖14.49 Other scleral buckling
Scleral buckling with:
air tamponade
resection of sclera
vitrectomy

●14.5 Other repair of retinal detachment

Includes: that with drainage

✖14.51 Repair of retinal detachment with diathermy

✖14.52 Repair of retinal detachment with cryotherapy

✖14.53 Repair of retinal detachment with xenon arc photocoagulation

✖14.54 Repair of retinal detachment with laser photocoagulation

✖14.55 Repair of retinal detachment with photocoagulation of unspecified type

✖14.59 Other

✖14.6 Removal of surgically implanted material from posterior segment of eye

●14.7 Operations on vitreous

✖14.71 Removal of vitreous, anterior approach
Open sky technique
Removal of vitreous, anterior approach (with replacement)

✖14.72 Other removal of vitreous
Aspiration of vitreous by posterior sclerotomy

✖14.73 Mechanical vitrectomy by anterior approach

✖14.74 Other mechanical vitrectomy

✖14.75 Injection of vitreous substitute

Excludes *that associated with removal (14.71–14.72)*

✖14.79 Other operations on vitreous

✖14.9 Other operations on retina, choroid, and posterior chamber

●15 Operations on extraocular muscles

●15.0 Diagnostic procedures on extraocular muscles or tendons

✖15.01 Biopsy of extraocular muscle or tendon

✖15.09 Other diagnostic procedures on extraocular muscles and tendons

●15.1 Operations on one extraocular muscle involving temporary detachment from globe

✖15.11 Recession of one extraocular muscle

✖15.12 Advancement of one extraocular muscle

✖15.13 Resection of one extraocular muscle

✖15.19 Other operations on one extraocular muscle involving temporary detachment from globe

Excludes *transposition of muscle (15.5)*

●15.2 Other operations on one extraocular muscle

✖15.21 Lengthening procedure on one extraocular muscle

✖15.22 Shortening procedure on one extraocular muscle

✖15.29 Other

✖15.3 Operations on two or more extraocular muscles involving temporary detachment from globe, one or both eyes

✖15.4 Other operations on two or more extraocular muscles, one or both eyes

✖15.5 Transposition of extraocular muscles

Excludes *that for correction of ptosis (08.31–08.36)*

✖15.6 Revision of extraocular muscle surgery

✖15.7 Repair of injury of extraocular muscle
Freeing of entrapped extraocular muscle
Lysis of adhesions of extraocular muscle
Repair of laceration of extraocular muscle, tendon, or Tenon's capsule

✖15.9 Other operations on extraocular muscles and tendons

●16 Operations on orbit and eyeball

Excludes *reduction of fracture of orbit (76.78–76.79)*

●16.0 Orbitotomy

✖16.01 Orbitotomy with bone flap
Orbitotomy with lateral approach

✖16.02 Orbitotomy with insertion of orbital implant

Excludes *that with bone flap (16.01)*

✖16.09 Other orbitotomy

✖16.1 Removal of penetrating foreign body from eye, not otherwise specified

Excludes *removal of nonpenetrating foreign body (98.21)*

●16.2 Diagnostic procedures on orbit and eyeball

16.21 Ophthalmoscopy

✖16.22 Diagnostic aspiration of orbit

✖16.23 Biopsy of eyeball and orbit

✖16.29 Other diagnostic procedures on orbit and eyeball

Excludes *examination of form and structure of eye (95.11–95.16)*
general and subjective eye examination (95.01–95.09)
microscopic examination of specimen from eye (90.21–90.29)
objective functional tests of eye (95.21–95.26)
ocular thermography (88.82)
tonometry (89.11)
x-ray of orbit (87.14, 87.16)

●16.3 Evisceration of eyeball

✖16.31 **Removal of ocular contents with synchronous implant into scleral shell**

✖16.39 **Other evisceration of eyeball**

● 16.4 **Enucleation of eyeball**

✖16.41 **Enucleation of eyeball with synchronous implant into Tenon's capsule with attachment of muscles**
Integrated implant of eyeball

✖16.42 **Enucleation of eyeball with other synchronous implant**

✖16.49 **Other enucleation of eyeball**
Removal of eyeball NOS

● 16.5 **Exenteration of orbital contents**

✖16.51 **Exenteration of orbit with removal of adjacent structures**
Radical orbitomaxillectomy

✖16.52 **Exenteration of orbit with therapeutic removal of orbital bone**

✖16.59 **Other exenteration of orbit**
Evisceration of orbit NOS
Exenteration of orbit with temporalis muscle transplant

● 16.6 **Secondary procedures after removal of eyeball**
Excludes *that with synchronous:*
enucleation of eyeball (16.41–16.42)
evisceration of eyeball (16.31)

✖16.61 **Secondary insertion of ocular implant**

✖16.62 **Revision and reinsertion of ocular implant**

✖16.63 **Revision of enucleation socket with graft**

✖16.64 **Other revision of enucleation socket**

✖16.65 **Secondary graft to exenteration cavity**

✖16.66 **Other revision of exenteration cavity**

✖16.69 **Other secondary procedures after removal of eyeball**

● 16.7 **Removal of ocular or orbital implant**

✖16.71 **Removal of ocular implant**

✖16.72 **Removal of orbital implant**

● 16.8 **Repair of injury of eyeball and orbit**

✖16.81 **Repair of wound of orbit**
Excludes *reduction of orbital fracture (76.78–76.79)*
repair of extraocular muscles (15.7)

✖16.82 **Repair of rupture of eyeball**
Repair of multiple structures of eye
Excludes *repair of laceration of:*
cornea (11.51–11.59)
sclera (12.81)

✖16.89 **Other repair of injury of eyeball or orbit**

● 16.9 **Other operations on orbit and eyeball**
Excludes *irrigation of eye (96.51)*
prescription and fitting of low vision aids (95.31–95.33)
removal of:
eye prosthesis NEC (97.31)
nonpenetrating foreign body from eye without incision (98.21)

16.91 **Retrobulbar injection of therapeutic agent**
Excludes *injection of radiographic contrast material (87.14)*
opticociliary injection (12.79)

✖16.92 **Excision of lesion of orbit**
Excludes *biopsy of orbit (16.23)*

✖16.93 **Excision of lesion of eye, unspecified structure**
Excludes *biopsy of eye NOS (16.23)*

✖16.98 **Other operations on orbit**

✖16.99 **Other operations on eyeball**

4. OPERATIONS ON THE EAR (18–20)

● **18 Operations on external ear**

Includes: operations on:
external auditory canal
skin and cartilage of:
auricle
meatus

● **18.0 Incision of external ear**

Excludes *removal of intraluminal foreign body (98.11)*

18.01 Piercing of ear lobe
Piercing of pinna

18.02 Incision of external auditory canal

18.09 Other incision of external ear

● **18.1 Diagnostic procedures on external ear**

18.11 Otoscopy

18.12 Biopsy of external ear

18.19 Other diagnostic procedures on external ear

Excludes *microscopic examination of specimen from ear (90.31–90.39)*

● **18.2 Excision or destruction of lesion of external ear**

✖ **18.21 Excision of preauricular sinus**
Radical excision of preauricular sinus or cyst

Excludes *excision of preauricular remnant [appendage] (18.29)*

18.29 Excision or destruction of other lesion of external ear
Cauterization of external ear
Coagulation of external ear
Cryosurgery of external ear
Curettage of external ear
Electrocoagulation of external ear
Enucleation of external ear
Excision of:
exostosis of external auditory canal
preauricular remnant [appendage]
Partial excision of ear

Excludes *biopsy of external ear (18.12)*
radical excision of lesion (18.31)
removal of cerumen (96.52)

● **18.3 Other excision of external ear**

Excludes *biopsy of external ear (18.12)*

✖ **18.31 Radical excision of lesion of external ear**

Excludes *radical excision of preauricular sinus (18.21)*

✖ **18.39 Other**
Amputation of external ear

Excludes *excision of lesion (18.21–18.29, 18.31)*

18.4 Suture of laceration of external ear

✖ **18.5 Surgical correction of prominent ear**
Ear:
pinning
setback

✖ **18.6 Reconstruction of external auditory canal**
Canaloplasty of external auditory meatus
Construction [reconstruction] of external meatus of ear:
osseous portion
skin-lined portion (with skin graft)

● **18.7 Other plastic repair of external ear**

✖ **18.71 Construction of auricle of ear**
Prosthetic appliance for absent ear
Reconstruction:
auricle
ear

✖ **18.72 Reattachment of amputated ear**

✖ **18.79 Other plastic repair of external ear**
Otoplasty NOS
Postauricular skin graft
Repair of lop ear

✖ **18.9 Other operations on external ear**

Excludes *irrigation of ear (96.52)*
packing of external auditory canal (96.11)
removal of:
cerumen (96.52)
foreign body (without incision) (98.11)

● **19 Reconstructive operations on middle ear**

✖ **19.0 Stapes mobilization**
Division, otosclerotic:
material
process
Remobilization of stapes
Stapediolysis
Transcrural stapes mobilization

Excludes *that with synchronous stapedectomy (19.11–19.19)*

● **19.1 Stapedectomy**

Excludes *revision of previous stapedectomy (19.21–19.29)*
stapes mobilization only (19.0)

✖ **19.11 Stapedectomy with incus replacement**
Stapedectomy with incus:
homograft
prosthesis

✖ **19.19 Other stapedectomy**

● **19.2 Revision of stapedectomy**

✖ **19.21 Revision of stapedectomy with incus replacement**

✖ **19.29 Other revision of stapedectomy**

✖ **19.3 Other operations on ossicular chain**
Incudectomy NOS
Ossiculectomy NOS
Reconstruction of ossicles, second stage

✖ **19.4 Myringoplasty**
Epitympanic, type I
Myringoplasty by:
cauterization
graft
Tympanoplasty (type I)

● **19.5 Other tympanoplasty**

✖ **19.52 Type II tympanoplasty**
Closure of perforation with graft against incus or malleus

✖ **19.53 Type III tympanoplasty**
Graft placed in contact with mobile and intact stapes

✖ **19.54 Type IV tympanoplasty**
Mobile footplate left exposed with air pocket between round window and graft

✖ **19.55 Type V tympanoplasty**
Fenestra in horizontal semicircular canal covered by graft

✖ **19.6 Revision of tympanoplasty**

✖ **19.9 Other repair of middle ear**
Closure of mastoid fistula
Mastoid myoplasty
Obliteration of tympanomastoid cavity

● **20 Other operations on middle and inner ear**

● **20.0 Myringotomy**

✖ 20.01 **Myringotomy with insertion of tube**
Myringostomy

✖ 20.09 **Other myringotomy**
Aspiration of middle ear NOS

20.1 **Removal of tympanostomy tube**

● 20.2 **Incision of mastoid and middle ear**

✖ 20.21 **Incision of mastoid**

✖ 20.22 **Incision of petrous pyramid air cells**

✖ 20.23 **Incision of middle ear**
Atticotomy
Division of tympanum
Lysis of adhesions of middle ear

Excludes *division of otosclerotic process (19.0)*
stapediolysis (19.0)
that with stapedectomy (19.11–19.19)

● 20.3 **Diagnostic procedures on middle and inner ear**

20.31 **Electrocochleography**

✖ 20.32 **Biopsy of middle and inner ear**

✖ 20.39 **Other diagnostic procedures on middle and inner ear**

Excludes *auditory and vestibular function tests (89.13, 95.41–95.49)*
microscopic examination of specimen from ear (90.31–90.39)

● 20.4 **Mastoidectomy**

Code also any:
skin graft (18.79)
tympanoplasty (19.4–19.55)

Excludes *that with implantation of cochlear prosthetic device (20.96–20.98)*

✖ 20.41 **Simple mastoidectomy**

✖ 20.42 **Radical mastoidectomy**

✖ 20.49 **Other mastoidectomy**
Atticoantrostomy
Mastoidectomy:
NOS
modified radical

● 20.5 **Other excision of middle ear**

Excludes *that with synchronous mastoidectomy (20.41–20.49)*

✖ 20.51 **Excision of lesion of middle ear**

Excludes *biopsy of middle ear (20.32)*

✖ 20.59 **Other**
Apicectomy of petrous pyramid
Tympanectomy

● 20.6 **Fenestration of inner ear**

✖ 20.61 **Fenestration of inner ear (initial)**
Fenestration of:
labyrinth with graft (skin) (vein)
semicircular canals with graft (skin) (vein)
vestibule with graft (skin) (vein)

Excludes *that with tympanoplasty, type V (19.55)*

✖ 20.62 **Revision of fenestration of inner ear**

● 20.7 **Incision, excision, and destruction of inner ear**

✖ 20.71 **Endolymphatic shunt**

✖ 20.72 **Injection into inner ear**
Destruction by injection (alcohol):
inner ear
semicircular canals
vestibule

✖ 20.79 **Other incision, excision, and destruction of inner ear**
Decompression of labyrinth
Drainage of inner ear
Fistulization:
endolymphatic sac
labyrinth
Incision of endolymphatic sac
Labyrinthectomy (transtympanic)
Opening of bony labyrinth
Perilymphatic tap

Excludes *biopsy of inner ear (20.32)*

20.8 **Operations on Eustachian tube**
Catheterization of eustachian tube
Inflation of eustachian tube
Injection (Teflon paste) of eustachian tube
Insufflation (boric acid-salicylic acid)
Intubation of eustachian tube
Politzerization of eustachian tube

● 20.9 **Other operations on inner and middle ear**

✖ 20.91 **Tympanosympathectomy**

✖ 20.92 **Revision of mastoidectomy**

✖ 20.93 **Repair of oval and round windows**
Closure of fistula:
oval window
perilymph
round window

20.94 **Injection of tympanum**

✖ 20.95 **Implantation of electromagnetic hearing device**
Bone conduction hearing device

Excludes *cochlear prosthetic device (20.96–20.98)*

✖ 20.96 **Implantation or replacement of cochlear prosthetic device, not otherwise specified**
Implantation of receiver (within skull) and insertion of electrode(s) in the cochlea

Includes: mastoidectomy

Excludes *electromagnetic hearing device (20.95)*

✖ 20.97 **Implantation or replacement of cochlear prosthetic device, single channel**
Implantation of receiver (within skull) and insertion of electrode in the cochlea

Includes: mastoidectomy

Excludes *electromagnetic hearing device (20.95)*

✖ 20.98 **Implantation or replacement of cochlear prosthetic device, multiple channel**
Implantation of receiver (within skull) and insertion of electrodes in the cochlea

Includes: mastoidectomy

Excludes *electromagnetic hearing device (20.95)*

✖ 20.99 **Other operations on middle and inner ear**
Repair or removal of cochlear prosthetic device (receiver) (electrode)

Excludes *adjustment (external components) of cochlear prosthetic device (95.49)*
fitting of hearing aid (95.48)

5. OPERATIONS ON THE NOSE, MOUTH, AND PHARYNX (21–29)

● 21 Operations on nose

Includes: operations on:
bone of nose
skin of nose

● 21.0 Control of epistaxis

21.00 Control of epistaxis, not otherwise specified

21.01 Control of epistaxis by anterior nasal packing

21.02 Control of epistaxis by posterior (and anterior) packing

21.03 Control of epistaxis by cauterization (and packing)

✖ 21.04 Control of epistaxis by ligation of ethmoidal arteries

✖ 21.05 Control of epistaxis by (transantral) ligation of the maxillary artery

✖ 21.06 Control of epistaxis by ligation of the external carotid artery

✖ 21.07 Control of epistaxis by excision of nasal mucosa and skin grafting of septum and lateral nasal wall

✖ 21.09 Control of epistaxis by other means

21.1 Incision of nose
Chondrotomy
Incision of skin of nose
Nasal septotomy

● 21.2 Diagnostic procedures on nose

21.21 Rhinoscopy

21.22 Biopsy of nose

21.29 Other diagnostic procedures on nose

Excludes *microscopic examination of specimen from nose (90.31–90.39)*
nasal:
function study (89.12)
x-ray (87.16)
rhinomanometry (89.12)

● 21.3 Local excision or destruction of lesion of nose

Excludes *biopsy of nose (21.22)*
nasal fistulectomy (21.82)

21.30 Excision or destruction of lesion of nose, not otherwise specified

21.31 Local excision or destruction of intranasal lesion
Nasal polypectomy

21.32 Local excision or destruction of other lesion of nose

✖ 21.4 Resection of nose
Amputation of nose

✖ 21.5 Submucous resection of nasal septum

● 21.6 Turbinectomy

✖ 21.61 Turbinectomy by diathermy or cryosurgery

✖ 21.62 Fracture of the turbinates

✖ 21.69 Other turbinectomy

Excludes *turbinectomy associated with sinusectomy (22.31–22.39, 22.42, 22.60–22.64)*

● 21.7 Reduction of nasal fracture

21.71 Closed reduction of nasal fracture

✖ 21.72 Open reduction of nasal fracture

● 21.8 Repair and plastic operations on the nose

21.81 Suture of laceration of nose

✖ 21.82 Closure of nasal fistula
Nasolabial fistulectomy
Nasopharyngeal fistulectomy
Oronasal fistulectomy

✖ 21.83 Total nasal reconstruction
Reconstruction of nose with:
arm flap
forehead flap

✖ 21.84 Revision rhinoplasty
Rhinoseptoplasty
Twisted nose rhinoplasty

✖ 21.85 Augmentation rhinoplasty
Augmentation rhinoplasty with:
graft
synthetic implant

✖ 21.86 Limited rhinoplasty
Plastic repair of nasolabial flaps
Tip rhinoplasty

✖ 21.87 Other rhinoplasty
Rhinoplasty NOS

✖ 21.88 Other septoplasty
Crushing of nasal septum
Repair of septal perforation

Excludes *septoplasty associated with submucous resection of septum (21.5)*

✖ 21.89 Other repair and plastic operations on nose
Reattachment of amputated nose

● 21.9 Other operations on nose

21.91 Lysis of adhesions of nose
Posterior nasal scrub

✖ 21.99 Other

Excludes *dilation of frontonasal duct (96.21)*
irrigation of nasal passages (96.53)
removal of:
intraluminal foreign body without incision (98.12)
nasal packing (97.32)
replacement of nasal packing (97.21)

● 22 Operations on nasal sinuses

● 22.0 Aspiration and lavage of nasal sinus

22.00 Aspiration and lavage of nasal sinus, not otherwise specified

22.01 Puncture of nasal sinus for aspiration or lavage

22.02 Aspiration or lavage of nasal sinus through natural ostium

● 22.1 Diagnostic procedures on nasal sinus

22.11 Closed [endoscopic] [needle] biopsy of nasal sinus

✖ 22.12 Open biopsy of nasal sinus

22.19 Other diagnostic procedures on nasal sinuses
Endoscopy without biopsy

Excludes *transillumination of sinus (89.35)*
x-ray of sinus (87.15–87.16)

22.2 Intranasal antrotomy

Excludes *antrotomy with external approach (22.31–22.39)*

● 22.3 External maxillary antrotomy

✖ 22.31 Radical maxillary antrotomy
Removal of lining membrane of maxillary sinus using Caldwell-Luc approach

✖22.39 **Other external maxillary antrotomy**
Exploration of maxillary antrum with Caldwell-Luc approach

● 22.4 **Frontal sinusotomy and sinusectomy**

✖22.41 **Frontal sinusotomy**

✖22.42 **Frontal sinusectomy**
Excision of lesion of frontal sinus
Obliteration of frontal sinus (with fat)

Excludes *biopsy of nasal sinus (22.11–22.12)*

● 22.5 **Other nasal sinusotomy**

✖22.50 **Sinusotomy, not otherwise specified**

✖22.51 **Ethmoidotomy**

✖22.52 **Sphenoidotomy**

✖22.53 **Incision of multiple nasal sinuses**

● 22.6 **Other nasal sinusectomy**

Includes: that with incidental turbinectomy

Excludes *biopsy of nasal sinus (22.11–22.12)*

✖22.60 **Sinusectomy, not otherwise specified**

✖22.61 **Excision of lesion of maxillary sinus with Caldwell-Luc approach**

✖22.62 **Excision of lesion of maxillary sinus with other approach**

✖22.63 **Ethmoidectomy**

✖22.64 **Sphenoidectomy**

● 22.7 **Repair of nasal sinus**

✖22.71 **Closure of nasal sinus fistula**
Repair of oro-antral fistula

✖22.79 **Other repair of nasal sinus**
Reconstruction of frontonasal duct
Repair of bone of accessory sinus

✖22.9 **Other operations on nasal sinuses**
Exteriorization of maxillary sinus
Fistulization of sinus

Excludes *dilation of frontonasal duct (96.21)*

● 23 **Removal and restoration of teeth**

● 23.0 **Forceps extraction of tooth**

23.01 **Extraction of deciduous tooth**

23.09 **Extraction of other tooth**
Extraction of tooth NOS

● 23.1 **Surgical removal of tooth**

23.11 **Removal of residual root**

23.19 **Other surgical extraction of tooth**
Odontectomy NOS
Removal of impacted tooth
Tooth extraction with elevation of mucoperiosteal flap

23.2 **Restoration of tooth by filling**

23.3 **Restoration of tooth by inlay**

● 23.4 **Other dental restoration**

23.41 **Application of crown**

23.42 **Insertion of fixed bridge**

23.43 **Insertion of removable bridge**

23.49 **Other**

23.5 **Implantation of tooth**

23.6 **Prosthetic dental implant**
Endosseous dental implant

● 23.7 **Apicoectomy and root canal therapy**

23.70 **Root canal, not otherwise specified**

23.71 **Root canal therapy with irrigation**

23.72 **Root canal therapy with apicoectomy**

23.73 **Apicoectomy**

● 24 **Other operations on teeth, gums, and alveoli**

24.0 **Incision of gum or alveolar bone**
Apical alveolotomy

● 24.1 **Diagnostic procedures on teeth, gums, and alveoli**

24.11 **Biopsy of gum**

24.12 **Biopsy of alveolus**

24.19 **Other diagnostic procedures on teeth, gums, and alveoli**

Excludes *dental:*
examination (89.31)
x-ray:
full-mouth (87.11)
other (87.12)
microscopic examination of dental specimen (90.81–90.89)

✖24.2 **Gingivoplasty**
Gingivoplasty with bone or soft tissue graft

● 24.3 **Other operations on gum**

24.31 **Excision of lesion or tissue of gum**

Excludes *biopsy of gum (24.11)*
excision of odontogenic lesion (24.4)

24.32 **Suture of laceration of gum**

24.39 **Other**

✖24.4 **Excision of dental lesion of jaw**
Excision of odontogenic lesion

✖24.5 **Alveoloplasty**
Alveolectomy (interradicular) (intraseptal) (radical) (simple) (with graft or implant)

Excludes *biopsy of alveolus (24.12)*
en bloc resection of alveolar process and palate (27.32)

24.6 **Exposure of tooth**

24.7 **Application of orthodontic appliance**
Application, insertion, or fitting of:
arch bars
orthodontic obturator
orthodontic wiring
periodontal splint

Excludes *nonorthodontic dental wiring (93.55)*

24.8 **Other orthodontic operation**
Closure of diastema (alveolar) (dental)
Occlusal adjustment
Removal of arch bars
Repair of dental arch

Excludes *removal of nonorthodontic wiring (97.33)*

● 24.9 **Other dental operations**

24.91 **Extension or deepening of buccolabial or lingual sulcus**

24.99 Other

Excludes *dental:*
debridement (96.54)
examination (89.31)
prophylaxis (96.54)
scaling and polishing (96.54)
wiring (93.55)
fitting of dental appliance [denture] (99.97)
microscopic examination of dental specimen (90.81–90.89)
removal of dental:
packing (97.34)
prosthesis (97.35)
wiring (97.33)
replacement of dental packing (97.22)

● 25 Operations on tongue

● 25.0 Diagnostic procedures on tongue

25.01 Closed [needle] biopsy of tongue

✖ 25.02 Open biopsy of tongue
Wedge biopsy

25.09 Other diagnostic procedures on tongue

✖ 25.1 Excision or destruction of lesion or tissue of tongue

Excludes *biopsy of tongue (25.01–25.02)*
frenumectomy:
labial (27.41)
lingual (25.92)

✖ 25.2 Partial glossectomy

✖ 25.3 Complete glossectomy
Glossectomy NOS
Code also any neck dissection (40.40–40.42)

✖ 25.4 Radical glossectomy
Code also any:
neck dissection (40.40–40.42)
tracheostomy (31.1–31.29)

● 25.5 Repair of tongue and glossoplasty

25.51 Suture of laceration of tongue

✖ 25.59 Other repair and plastic operations on tongue
Fascial sling of tongue
Fusion of tongue (to lip)
Graft of mucosa or skin to tongue

Excludes *lysis of adhesions of tongue (25.93)*

● 25.9 Other operations on tongue

25.91 Lingual frenotomy

Excludes *labial frenotomy (27.91)*

25.92 Lingual frenectomy

Excludes *labial frenectomy (27.41)*

25.93 Lysis of adhesions of tongue

✖ 25.94 Other glossotomy

✖ 25.99 Other

● 26 Operations on salivary glands and ducts

Includes: operations on:
lesser salivary gland and duct
parotid gland and duct
sublingual gland and duct
submaxillary gland and duct

Code also any neck dissection (40.40–40.42)

26.0 Incision of salivary gland or duct

● 26.1 Diagnostic procedures on salivary glands and ducts

26.11 Closed [needle] biopsy of salivary gland or duct

✖ 26.12 Open biopsy of salivary gland or duct

26.19 Other diagnostic procedures on salivary glands and ducts

Excludes *x-ray of salivary gland (87.09)*

● 26.2 Excision of lesion of salivary gland

✖ 26.21 Marsupialization of salivary gland cyst

✖ 26.29 Other excision of salivary gland lesion

Excludes *biopsy of salivary gland (26.11–26.12)*
salivary fistulectomy (26.42)

● 26.3 Sialoadenectomy

✖ 26.30 Sialoadenectomy, not otherwise specified

✖ 26.31 Partial sialoadenectomy

✖ 26.32 Complete sialoadenectomy
En bloc excision of salivary gland lesion
Radical sialoadenectomy

● 26.4 Repair of salivary gland or duct

✖ 26.41 Suture of laceration of salivary gland

✖ 26.42 Closure of salivary fistula

✖ 26.49 Other repair and plastic operations on salivary gland or duct
Fistulization of salivary gland
Plastic repair of salivary gland or duct NOS
Transplantation of salivary duct opening

● 26.9 Other operations on salivary gland or duct

26.91 Probing of salivary duct

✖ 26.99 Other

● 27 Other operations on mouth and face

Includes: operations on:
lips
palate
soft tissue of face and mouth, except tongue and gingiva

Excludes *operations on:*
gingiva (24.0–24.99)
tongue (25.01–25.99)

✖ 27.0 Drainage of face and floor of mouth
Drainage of:
facial region (abscess)
fascial compartment of face
Ludwig's angina

Excludes *drainage of thyroglossal tract (06.09)*

✖ 27.1 Incision of palate

● 27.2 Diagnostic procedures on oral cavity

✖ 27.21 Biopsy of bony palate

✖ 27.22 Biopsy of uvula and soft palate

27.23 Biopsy of lip

27.24 Biopsy of mouth, unspecified structure

27.29 Other diagnostic procedures on oral cavity

Excludes *soft tissue x-ray (87.09)*

● 27.3 Excision of lesion or tissue of bony palate

✖ 27.31 Local excision or destruction of lesion or tissue of bony palate
Local excision or destruction of palate by:
cautery
chemotherapy
cryotherapy

Excludes *biopsy of bony palate (27.21)*

✖ 27.32 Wide excision or destruction of lesion or tissue of bony palate
En bloc resection of alveolar process and palate

● 27.4 Excision of other parts of mouth

27.41 Labial frenectomy

Excludes *division of labial frenum (27.91)*

✖ 27.42 Wide excision of lesion of lip

✖ 27.43 Other excision of lesion or tissue of lip

✖ 27.49 Other excision of mouth

Excludes *biopsy of mouth NOS (27.24)*
excision of lesion of:
palate (27.31–27.32)
tongue (25.1)
uvula (27.72)
fistulectomy of mouth (27.53)
frenectomy of:
lip (27.41)
tongue (25.92)

● 27.5 Plastic repair of mouth

Excludes *palatoplasty (27.61–27.69)*

27.51 Suture of laceration of lip

27.52 Suture of laceration of other part of mouth

✖ 27.53 Closure of fistula of mouth

Excludes *fistulectomy:*
nasolabial (21.82)
oro-antral (22.71)
oronasal (21.82)

✖ 27.54 Repair of cleft lip

✖ 27.55 Full-thickness skin graft to lip and mouth

✖ 27.56 Other skin graft to lip and mouth

✖ 27.57 Attachment of pedicle or flap graft to lip and mouth

✖ 27.59 Other plastic repair of mouth

● 27.6 Palatoplasty

✖ 27.61 Suture of laceration of palate

✖ 27.62 Correction of cleft palate

Correction of cleft palate by push-back operation

Excludes *revision of cleft palate repair (27.63)*

✖ 27.63 Revision of cleft palate repair

Secondary:
attachment of pharyngeal flap
lengthening of palate

✖ 27.69 Other plastic repair of palate

Excludes *fistulectomy of mouth (27.53)*

● 27.7 Operations on uvula

✖ 27.71 Incision of uvula

✖ 27.72 Excision of uvula

Excludes *biopsy of uvula (27.22)*

✖ 27.73 Repair of uvula

Excludes *that with synchronous cleft palate repair (27.62)*
uranostaphylorrhaphy (27.62)

✖ 27.79 Other operations on uvula

● 27.9 Other operations on mouth and face

27.91 Labial frenotomy

Division of labial frenum

Excludes *lingual frenotomy (25.91)*

✖ 27.92 Incision of mouth, unspecified structure

Excludes *incision of:*
gum (24.0)
palate (27.1)
salivary gland or duct (26.0)
tongue (25.94)
uvula (27.71)

✖ 27.99 Other operations on oral cavity

Graft of buccal sulcus

Excludes *removal of:*
intraluminal foreign body (98.01)
penetrating foreign body from mouth without incision (98.22)

● 28 Operations on tonsils and adenoids

28.0 Incision and drainage of tonsil and peritonsillar structures

Drainage (oral) (transcervical) of:
parapharyngeal abscess
peritonsillar abscess
retropharyngeal abscess
tonsillar abscess

● 28.1 Diagnostic procedures on tonsils and adenoids

✖ 28.11 Biopsy of tonsils and adenoids

✖ 28.19 Other diagnostic procedures on tonsils and adenoids

Excludes *soft tissue x-ray (87.09)*

✖ 28.2 Tonsillectomy without adenoidectomy

✖ 28.3 Tonsillectomy with adenoidectomy

✖ 28.4 Excision of tonsil tag

✖ 28.5 Excision of lingual tonsil

✖ 28.6 Adenoidectomy without tonsillectomy

Excision of adenoid tag

✖ 28.7 Control of hemorrhage after tonsillectomy and adenoidectomy

● 28.9 Other operations on tonsils and adenoids

✖ 28.91 Removal of foreign body from tonsil and adenoid by incision

Excludes *that without incision (98.13)*

✖ 28.92 Excision of lesion of tonsil and adenoid

Excludes *biopsy of tonsil and adenoid (28.11)*

✖ 28.99 Other

● 29 Operations on pharynx

Includes: operations on:
hypopharynx
nasopharynx
oropharynx
pharyngeal pouch
pyriform sinus

✖ 29.0 Pharyngotomy

Drainage of pharyngeal bursa

Excludes *incision and drainage of retropharyngeal abscess (28.0)*
removal of foreign body (without incision) (98.13)

● 29.1 Diagnostic procedures on pharynx

29.11 Pharyngoscopy

29.12 Pharyngeal biopsy

Biopsy of supraglottic mass

29.19 Other diagnostic procedures on pharynx

Excludes *x-ray of nasopharynx:*
contrast (87.06)
other (87.09)

✖ 29.2 Excision of branchial cleft cyst or vestige

Excludes *branchial cleft fistulectomy (29.52)*

● 29.3 Excision or destruction of lesion or tissue of pharynx

✖ 29.31 Cricopharyngeal myotomy

Excludes *that with pharyngeal diverticulectomy (29.32)*

✖ 29.32 Pharyngeal diverticulectomy

✖29.33 Pharyngectomy (partial)
Excludes *laryngopharyngectomy (30.3)*

✖29.39 Other excision or destruction of lesion or tissue of pharynx

✖29.4 Plastic operation on pharynx
Correction of nasopharyngeal atresia
Excludes *pharyngoplasty associated with cleft palate repair (27.62–27.63)*

● 29.5 Other repair of pharynx

✖29.51 Suture of laceration of pharynx

✖29.52 Closure of branchial cleft fistula

✖29.53 Closure of other fistula of pharynx
Pharyngoesophageal fistulectomy

✖29.54 Lysis of pharyngeal adhesions

✖29.59 Other

● 29.9 Other operations on pharynx

29.91 Dilation of pharynx
Dilation of nasopharynx

✖29.92 Division of glossopharyngeal nerve

✖29.99 Other
Excludes *insertion of radium into pharynx and nasopharynx (92.27)*
removal of intraluminal foreign body (98.13)

6. OPERATIONS ON THE RESPIRATORY SYSTEM (30–34)

● **30 Excision of larynx**

● **30.0 Excision or destruction of lesion or tissue of larynx**

✖ **30.01 Marsupialization of laryngeal cyst**

✖ **30.09 Other excision or destruction of lesion or tissue of larynx**

Stripping of vocal cords

Excludes *biopsy of larynx (31.43)*
laryngeal fistulectomy (31.62)
laryngotracheal fistulectomy (31.62)

✖ **30.1 Hemilaryngectomy**

● **30.2 Other partial laryngectomy**

✖ **30.21 Epiglottidectomy**

✖ **30.22 Vocal cordectomy**

Excision of vocal cords

✖ **30.29 Other partial laryngectomy**

Excision of laryngeal cartilage

✖ **30.3 Complete laryngectomy**

Block dissection of larynx (with thyroidectomy) (with synchronous tracheostomy)
Laryngopharyngectomy

Excludes *that with radical neck dissection (30.4)*

✖ **30.4 Radical laryngectomy**

Complete [total] laryngectomy with radical neck dissection (with thyroidectomy) (with synchronous tracheostomy)

● **31 Other operations on larynx and trachea**

31.0 Injection of larynx

Injection of inert material into larynx or vocal cords

31.1 Temporary tracheostomy

Tracheotomy for assistance in breathing

● **31.2 Permanent tracheostomy**

✖ **31.21 Mediastinal tracheostomy**

✖ **31.29 Other permanent tracheostomy**

Excludes *that with laryngectomy (30.3–30.4)*

✖ **31.3 Other incision of larynx or trachea**

Excludes *that for assistance in breathing (31.1–31.29)*

● **31.4 Diagnostic procedures on larynx and trachea**

31.41 Tracheoscopy through artificial stoma

Excludes *that with biopsy (31.43–31.44)*

31.42 Laryngoscopy and other tracheoscopy

Excludes *that with biopsy (31.43–31.44)*

31.43 Closed [endoscopic] biopsy of larynx

31.44 Closed [endoscopic] biopsy of trachea

✖ **31.45 Open biopsy of larynx or trachea**

31.48 Other diagnostic procedures on larynx

Excludes *contrast laryngogram (87.07)*
microscopic examination of specimen from larynx (90.31–90.39)
soft tissue x-ray of larynx NEC (87.09)

31.49 Other diagnostic procedures on trachea

Excludes *microscopic examination of specimen from trachea (90.41–90.49)*
x-ray of trachea (87.49)

✖ **31.5 Local excision or destruction of lesion or tissue of trachea**

Excludes *biopsy of trachea (31.44–31.45)*
laryngotracheal fistulectomy (31.62)
tracheoesophageal fistulectomy (31.73)

● **31.6 Repair of larynx**

✖ **31.61 Suture of laceration of larynx**

✖ **31.62 Closure of fistula of larynx**

Laryngotracheal fistulectomy
Take-down of laryngostomy

✖ **31.63 Revision of laryngostomy**

✖ **31.64 Repair of laryngeal fracture**

✖ **31.69 Other repair of larynx**

Arytenoidopexy
Graft of larynx
Transposition of vocal cords

Excludes *construction of artificial larynx (31.75)*

● **31.7 Repair and plastic operations on trachea**

✖ **31.71 Suture of laceration of trachea**

✖ **31.72 Closure of external fistula of trachea**

Closure of tracheotomy

✖ **31.73 Closure of other fistula of trachea**

Tracheoesophageal fistulectomy

Excludes *laryngotracheal fistulectomy (31.62)*

✖ **31.74 Revision of tracheostomy**

✖ **31.75 Reconstruction of trachea and construction of artificial larynx**

Tracheoplasty with artificial larynx

✖ **31.79 Other repair and plastic operations on trachea**

● **31.9 Other operations on larynx and trachea**

✖ **31.91 Division of laryngeal nerve**

✖ **31.92 Lysis of adhesions of trachea or larynx**

31.93 Replacement of laryngeal or tracheal stent

31.94 Injection of locally-acting therapeutic substance into trachea

31.95 Tracheoesophageal fistulization

✖ **31.98 Other operations on larynx**

Dilation of larynx
Division of congenital web of larynx
Removal of keel or stent of larynx

Excludes *removal of intraluminal foreign body from larynx without incision (98.14)*

✖ **31.99 Other operations on trachea**

Excludes *removal of:*
intraluminal foreign body from trachea without incision (98.15)
tracheostomy tube (97.37)
replacement of tracheostomy tube (97.23)
tracheostomy toilette (96.55)

● **32 Excision of lung and bronchus**

Includes: rib resection as operative approach
sternotomy as operative approach
sternum-splitting incision as operative approach
thoracotomy as operative approach

Code also any synchronous bronchoplasty (33.48)

● **32.0 Local excision or destruction of lesion or tissue of bronchus**

Excludes *biopsy of bronchus (33.24–33.25)*
bronchial fistulectomy (33.42)

32.01 Endoscopic excision or destruction of lesion or tissue of bronchus

✖ **32.09 Other local excision or destruction of lesion or tissue of bronchus**

Excludes *that by endoscopic approach (32.01)*

✖ **32.1 Other excision of bronchus**
Resection (wide sleeve) of bronchus

Excludes *radical dissection [excision] of bronchus (32.6)*

● **32.2 Local excision or destruction of lesion or tissue of lung**

✖ **32.21 Plication of emphysematous bleb**

✖ **32.22 Lung volume reduction surgery**

32.28 Endoscopic excision or destruction of lesion or tissue of lung

Excludes *biopsy of lung (33.26–33.27)*

✖ **32.29 Other local excision or destruction of lesion or tissue of lung**
Resection of lung:
NOS
wedge

Excludes *biopsy of lung (33.26–33.27)*
that by endoscopic approach (32.28)
wide excision of lesion of lung (32.3)

✖ **32.3 Segmental resection of lung**
Partial lobectomy

✖ **32.4 Lobectomy of lung**
Lobectomy with segmental resection of adjacent lobes of lung

Excludes *that with radical dissection [excision] of thoracic structures (32.6)*

✖ **32.5 Complete pneumonectomy**
Excision of lung NOS
Pneumonectomy (with mediastinal dissection)

✖ **32.6 Radical dissection of thoracic structures**
Block [en bloc] dissection of bronchus, lobe of lung, brachial plexus, intercostal structure, ribs (transverse process), and sympathetic nerves

✖ **32.9 Other excision of lung**

Excludes *biopsy of lung and bronchus (33.24–33.27)*
pulmonary decortication (34.51)

● **33 Other operations on lung and bronchus**

Includes: rib resection as operative approach
sternotomy as operative approach
sternum-splitting incision as operative approach
thoracotomy as operative approach

✖ **33.0 Incision of bronchus**

✖ **33.1 Incision of lung**

Excludes *puncture of lung (33.93)*

● **33.2 Diagnostic procedures on lung and bronchus**

33.21 Bronchoscopy through artificial stoma

Excludes *that with biopsy (33.24, 33.27)*

33.22 Fiber-optic bronchoscopy

Excludes *that with biopsy (33.24, 33.27)*

33.23 Other bronchoscopy

Excludes *that for:*
aspiration (96.05)
biopsy (33.24, 33.27)

✖ **33.24 Closed [endoscopic] biopsy of bronchus**
Bronchoscopy (fiberoptic) (rigid) with:
brush biopsy of "lung"
brushing or washing for specimen collection
excision (bite) biopsy
Diagnostic bronchoalveolar lavage (BAL)

Excludes *closed biopsy of lung, other than brush biopsy of "lung" (33.26, 33.27)*
whole lung lavage (33.99)

✖ **33.25 Open biopsy of bronchus**

Excludes *open biopsy of lung (33.28)*

33.26 Closed [percutaneous] [needle] biopsy of lung

Excludes *endoscopic biopsy of lung (33.27)*

✖ **33.27 Closed endoscopic biopsy of lung**
Fiber-optic (flexible) bronchoscopy with fluoroscopic guidance with biopsy
Transbronchial lung biopsy

Excludes *brush biopsy of "lung" (33.24)*
percutaneous biopsy of lung (33.26)

✖ **33.28 Open biopsy of lung**

✖ **33.29 Other diagnostic procedures on lung and bronchus**

Excludes *contrast bronchogram:*
endotracheal (87.31)
other (87.32)
lung scan (92.15)
magnetic resonance imaging (88.92)
microscopic examination of specimen from bronchus or lung (90.41–90.49)
routine chest x-ray (87.44)
ultrasonography of lung (88.73)
vital capacity determination (89.37)
x-ray of bronchus or lung NOS (87.49)

● **33.3 Surgical collapse of lung**

33.31 Destruction of phrenic nerve for collapse of lung

33.32 Artificial pneumothorax for collapse of lung
Thoracotomy for collapse of lung

33.33 Pneumoperitoneum for collapse of lung

✖ **33.34 Thoracoplasty**

✖ **33.39 Other surgical collapse of lung**
Collapse of lung NOS

● **33.4 Repair and plastic operation on lung and bronchus**

✖ **33.41 Suture of laceration of bronchus**

✖ **33.42 Closure of bronchial fistula**
Closure of bronchostomy
Fistulectomy:
bronchocutaneous
bronchoesophageal
bronchovisceral

Excludes *closure of fistula:*
bronchomediastinal (34.73)
bronchopleural (34.73)
bronchopleuromediastinal (34.73)

✖ **33.43 Closure of laceration of lung**

✖ **33.48 Other repair and plastic operations on bronchus**

✖ **33.49 Other repair and plastic operations on lung**

Excludes *closure of pleural fistula (34.73)*

✖ **33.5 Lung transplant**

Excludes *combined heart-lung transplantation (33.6)*

Code also cardiopulmonary bypass [extracorporeal circulation] [heart-lung machine] (39.61)

✖ **33.50 Lung transplantation, not otherwise specified**

✖33.51 **Unilateral lung transplantation**

✖33.52 **Bilateral lung transplantation**
Double-lung transplantation
En bloc transplantation

Code also cardiopulmonary bypass [extracorporeal circulation] [heart-lung machine] (39.61)

✖33.6 **Combined heart-lung transplantation**

Code also cardiopulmonary bypass [extracorporeal circulation] [heart-lung machine] (39.61)

● 33.9 **Other operations on lung and bronchus**

33.91 **Bronchial dilation**

✖33.92 **Ligation of bronchus**

✖33.93 **Puncture of lung**

Excludes *needle biopsy (33.26)*

✖33.98 **Other operations on bronchus**

Excludes *bronchial lavage (96.56)*
removal of intraluminal foreign body from bronchus without incision (98.15)

✖33.99 **Other operations on lung**
Whole lung lavage

Excludes *other continuous mechanical ventilation (96.70–96.72)*
respiratory therapy (93.90–93.99)

● 34 **Operations on chest wall, pleura, mediastinum, and diaphragm**

Excludes *operations on breast (85.0–85.99)*

● 34.0 **Incision of chest wall and pleura**

Excludes *that as operative approach—omit code*

34.01 **Incision of chest wall**
Extrapleural drainage

Excludes *incision of pleura (34.09)*

✖34.02 **Exploratory thoracotomy**

✖34.03 **Reopening of recent thoracotomy site**

34.04 **Insertion of intercostal catheter for drainage**
Chest tube
Closed chest drainage
Revision of intercostal catheter (chest tube) (with lysis of adhesions)

34.05 **Creation of pleuroperitoneal shunt**

34.09 **Other incision of pleura**
Creation of pleural window for drainage
Intercostal stab
Open chest drainage

Excludes *thoracoscopy (34.21)*
thoracotomy for collapse of lung (33.32)

✖34.1 **Incision of mediastinum**

Excludes *mediastinoscopy (34.22)*
mediastinotomy associated with pneumonectomy (32.5)

● 34.2 **Diagnostic procedures on chest wall, pleura, mediastinum, and diaphragm**

✖34.21 **Transpleural thoracoscopy**

✖34.22 **Mediastinoscopy**

Code also any lymph node biopsy (40.11)

34.23 **Biopsy of chest wall**

34.24 **Pleural biopsy**

34.25 **Closed [percutaneous] [needle] biopsy of mediastinum**

✖34.26 **Open mediastinal biopsy**

✖34.27 **Biopsy of diaphragm**

✖34.28 **Other diagnostic procedures on chest wall, pleura, and diaphragm**

Excludes *angiocardiography (88.50–88.58)*
aortography (88.42)
arteriography of:
intrathoracic vessels NEC (88.44)
pulmonary arteries (88.43)
microscopic examination of specimen from chest wall, pleura, and diaphragm (90.41–90.49)
phlebography of:
intrathoracic vessels NEC (88.63)
pulmonary veins (88.62)
radiological examinations of thorax:
C.A.T. scan (87.41)
diaphragmatic x-ray (87.49)
intrathoracic lymphangiogram (87.34)
routine chest x-ray (87.44)
sinogram of chest wall (87.38)
soft tissue x-ray of chest wall NEC (87.39)
tomogram of thorax NEC (87.42)
ultrasonography of thorax 88.73)

✖34.29 **Other diagnostic procedures on mediastinum**

Excludes *mediastinal:*
pneumogram (87.33)
x-ray NEC (87.49)

✖34.3 **Excision or destruction of lesion or tissue of mediastinum**

Excludes *biopsy of mediastinum (34.25–34.26)*
mediastinal fistulectomy (34.73)

✖34.4 **Excision or destruction of lesion of chest wall**
Excision of lesion of chest wall NOS (with excision of ribs)

Excludes *biopsy of chest wall (34.23)*
costectomy not incidental to thoracic procedure (77.91)
excision of lesion of:
breast (85.20–85.25)
cartilage (80.89)
skin (86.2–86.3)
fistulectomy (34.73)

● 34.5 **Pleurectomy**

✖34.51 **Decortication of lung**

✖34.59 **Other excision of pleura**
Excision of pleural lesion

Excludes *biopsy of pleura (34.24)*
pleural fistulectomy (34.73)

✖34.6 **Scarification of pleura**
Pleurosclerosis

Excludes *injection of sclerosing agent (34.92)*

● 34.7 **Repair of chest wall**

34.71 **Suture of laceration of chest wall**

Excludes *suture of skin and subcutaneous tissue alone (86.59)*

34.72 **Closure of thoracostomy**

✖34.73 **Closure of other fistula of thorax**
Closure of:
bronchopleural fistula
bronchopleurocutaneous fistula
bronchopleuromediastinal fistula

✖34.74 **Repair of pectus deformity**
Repair of:
pectus carinatum (with implant)
pectus excavatum (with implant)

✖34.79 **Other repair of chest wall**
Repair of chest wall NOS

● 34.8 **Operations on diaphragm**

✖ **34.81 Excision of lesion or tissue of diaphragm**

Excludes *biopsy of diaphragm (34.27)*

✖ **34.82 Suture of laceration of diaphragm**

✖ **34.83 Closure of fistula of diaphragm**

Thoracicoabdominal fistulectomy
Thoracicogastric fistulectomy
Thoracicointestinal fistulectomy

✖ **34.84 Other repair of diaphragm**

Excludes *repair of diaphragmatic hernia (53.7–53.82)*

✖ **34.85 Implantation of diaphragmatic pacemaker**

✖ **34.89 Other operations on diaphragm**

● **34.9 Other operations on thorax**

34.91 Thoracentesis

34.92 Injection into thoracic cavity

Chemical pleurodesis
Injection of cytotoxic agent or tetracycline
Requires additional code for any cancer chemotherapeutic substance (99.25)

Excludes *that for collapse of lung (33.32)*

✖ **34.93 Repair of pleura**

✖ **34.99 Other**

Excludes *removal of:*
mediastinal drain (97.42)
sutures (97.43)
thoracotomy tube (97.41)

7. OPERATIONS ON THE CARDIOVASCULAR SYSTEM (35–39)

● **35 Operations on valves and septa of heart**

Includes: sternotomy (median) (transverse) as operative approach
thoracotomy as operative approach

Code also cardiopulmonary bypass [extracorporeal circulation] [heart-lung machine] (39.61)

● **35.0 Closed heart valvotomy**

Excludes *percutaneous (balloon) valvuloplasty (35.96)*

✖ **35.00 Closed heart valvotomy, unspecified valve**

✖ **35.01 Closed heart valvotomy, aortic valve**

✖ **35.02 Closed heart valvotomy, mitral valve**

✖ **35.03 Closed heart valvotomy, pulmonary valve**

✖ **35.04 Closed heart valvotomy, tricuspid valve**

● **35.1 Open heart valvuloplasty without replacement**

Includes: open heart valvotomy

Excludes *that associated with repair of:*
endocardial cushion defect (35.54, 35.63, 35.73)
percutaneous (balloon) valvuloplasty (35.96)
valvular defect associated with atrial and ventricular septal defects (35.54, 35.63, 35.73)

Code also cardiopulmonary bypass if performed [extracorporeal circulation] [heart-lung machine] (39.61)

✖ **35.10 Open heart valvuloplasty without replacement, unspecified valve**

✖ **35.11 Open heart valvuloplasty of aortic valve without replacement**

✖ **35.12 Open heart valvuloplasty of mitral valve without replacement**

✖ **35.13 Open heart valvuloplasty of pulmonary valve without replacement**

✖ **35.14 Open heart valvuloplasty of tricuspid valve without replacement**

● **35.2 Replacement of heart valve**

Includes: excision of heart valve with replacement

Code also cardiopulmonary bypass [extracorporeal circulation] [heart-lung machine] (39.61)

Excludes *that associated with repair of:*
endocardial cushion defect (35.54, 35.63, 35.73)
valvular defect associated with atrial and ventricular septal defects (35.54, 35.63, 35.73)

✖ **35.20 Replacement of unspecified heart valve**
Repair of unspecified heart valve with tissue graft or prosthetic implant

✖ **35.21 Replacement of aortic valve with tissue graft**
Repair of aortic valve with tissue graft (autograft) (heterograft) (homograft)

✖ **35.22 Other replacement of aortic valve**
Repair of aortic valve with replacement:
NOS
prosthetic (partial) (synthetic) (total)

✖ **35.23 Replacement of mitral valve with tissue graft**
Repair of mitral valve with tissue graft (autograft) (heterograft) (homograft)

✖ **35.24 Other replacement of mitral valve**
Repair of mitral valve with replacement:
NOS
prosthetic (partial) (synthetic) (total)

✖ **35.25 Replacement of pulmonary valve with tissue graft**
Repair of pulmonary valve with tissue graft (autograft) (heterograft) (homograft)

✖ **35.26 Other replacement of pulmonary valve**
Repair of pulmonary valve with replacement:
NOS
prosthetic (partial) (synthetic) (total)

✖ **35.27 Replacement of tricuspid valve with tissue graft**
Repair of tricuspid valve with tissue graft (autograft) (heterograft) (homograft)

✖ **35.28 Other replacement of tricuspid valve**
Repair of tricuspid valve with replacement:
NOS
prosthetic (partial) (synthetic) (total)

● **35.3 Operations on structures adjacent to heart valves**

Code also cardiopulmonary bypass [extracorporeal circulation] [heart-lung machine] (39.61)

✖ **35.31 Operations on papillary muscle**
Division of papillary muscle
Reattachment of papillary muscle
Repair of papillary muscle

✖ **35.32 Operations on chordae tendineae**
Division of chordae tendineae
Repair of chordae tendineae

✖ **35.33 Annuloplasty**
Plication of annulus

✖ **35.34 Infundibulectomy**
Right ventricular infundibulectomy

✖ **35.35 Operations on trabeculae carneae cordis**
Division of trabeculae carneae cordis
Excision of trabeculae carneae cordis
Excision of aortic subvalvular ring

✖ **35.39 Operations on other structures adjacent to valves of heart**
Repair of sinus of Valsalva (aneurysm)

● **35.4 Production of septal defect in heart**

35.41 Enlargement of existing atrial septal defect
Rashkind procedure
Septostomy (atrial) (balloon)

✖ **35.42 Creation of septal defect in heart**
Blalock-Hanlon operation

● **35.5 Repair of atrial and ventricular septa with prosthesis**

Includes: repair of septa with synthetic implant or patch

Code also cardiopulmonary bypass [extracorporeal circulation] [heart-lung machine] (39.61)

✖ **35.50 Repair of unspecified septal defect of heart with prosthesis**

Excludes *that associated with repair of:*
endocardial cushion defect (35.54)
septal defect associated with valvular defect (35.54)

✖ **35.51 Repair of atrial septal defect with prosthesis, open technique**
Atrioseptoplasty with prosthesis
Correction of atrial septal defect with prosthesis
Repair:
foramen ovale (patent)
with prosthesis ostium secundum defect with prosthesis

Excludes *that associated with repair of:*
atrial septal defect associated with valvular and ventricular septal defects (35.54)
endocardial cushion defect (35.54)

✖35.52 Repair of atrial septal defect with prosthesis, closed technique
Insertion of atrial septal umbrella [King-Mills]

✖35.53 Repair of ventricular septal defect with prosthesis
Correction of ventricular septal defect with prosthesis
Repair of supracristal defect with prosthesis

Excludes *that associated with repair of:*
endocardial cushion defect (35.54)
ventricular defect associated with valvular and atrial septal defects (35.54)

✖35.54 Repair of endocardial cushion defect with prosthesis
Repair:
atrioventricular canal with prosthesis (grafted to septa)
ostium primum defect with prosthesis (grafted to septa)
valvular defect associated with atrial and ventricular septal defects with prosthesis (grafted to septa)

Excludes *repair of isolated:*
atrial septal defect (35.51–35.52)
valvular defect (35.20, 35.22, 35.24, 35.26, 35.28)
ventricular septal defect (35.53)

● 35.6 Repair of atrial and ventricular septa with tissue graft

Code also cardiopulmonary bypass [extracorporeal circulation] [heart-lung machine] (39.61)

✖35.60 Repair of unspecified septal defect of heart with tissue graft

Excludes *that associated with repair of:*
endocardial cushion defect (35.63)
septal defect associated withvalvular defect (35.63)

✖35.61 Repair of atrial septal defect with tissue graft
Atrioseptoplasty with tissue graft
Correction of atrial septal defect with tissue graft
Repair:
foramen ovale (patent) with tissue graft
ostium secundum defect with tissue graft

Excludes *that associated with repair of:*
atrial septal defect associated with valvular and ventricular septal defects (35.63)
endocardial cushion defect (35.63)

✖35.62 Repair of ventricular septal defect with tissue graft
Correction of ventricular septal defect with tissue graft
Repair of supracristal defect with tissue graft

Excludes *that associated with repair of:*
endocardial cushion defect(35.63)
ventricular defect associate with valvular and atrial septal defects (35.63)

✖35.63 Repair of endocardial cushion defect with tissue graft
Repair of:
atrioventricular canal with tissue graft
ostium primum defect with tissue graft
valvular defect associated with atrial and ventricular septal defects with tissue graft

Excludes *repair of isolated:*
atrial septal defect (35.61)
valvular defect (35.20–35.21, 35.23, 35.25, 35.27)
ventricular septal defect (35.62)

● 35.7 Other and unspecified repair of atrial and ventricular septa

Code also cardiopulmonary bypass [extracorporeal circulation] [heart-lung machine] (39.61)

✖35.70 Other and unspecified repair of unspecified septal defect of heart
Repair of septal defect NOS

Excludes *that associated with repair of:*
endocardial cushion defect (35.73)
septal defect associated with valvular defect (35.73)

✖35.71 Other and unspecified repair of atrial septal defect
Repair NOS:
atrial septum
foramen ovale (patent)
ostium secundum defect

Excludes *that associated with repair of:*
atrial septal defect associated with valvular ventricular septal defects (35.73)
endocardial cushion defect (35.73)

✖35.72 Other and unspecified repair of ventricular septal defect
Repair NOS:
supracristal defect
ventricular septum

Excludes *that associated with repair of:*
endocardial cushion defect (35.73)
ventricular septal defect associated with valvular and atrial septal defects (35.73)

✖35.73 Other and unspecified repair of endocardial cushion defect
Repair NOS:
atrioventricular canal
ostium primum defect
valvular defect associated with atrial and ventricular septal defects

Excludes *repair of isolated:*
atrial septal defect (35.71)
valvular defect (35.20, 35.22, 35.24, 35.26, 35.28)
ventricular septal defect (35.72)

● 35.8 Total repair of certain congenital cardiac anomalies

Note: For partial repair of defect [e.g. repair of atrial septal defect in tetralogy of Fallot]—code to specific procedure

✖35.81 Total repair of tetralogy of Fallot
One-stage total correction of tetralogy of Fallot with or without:
commissurotomy of pulmonary valve
infundibulectomy
outflow tract prosthesis
patch graft of outflow tract
prosthetic tube for pulmonary artery
repair of ventricular septal defect (with prosthesis)
take-down of previous systemic-pulmonary artery anastomosis

✖**35.82 Total repair of total anomalous pulmonary venous connection**

One-stage total correction of total anomalous pulmonary venous connection with or without:
- anastomosis between (horizontal) common pulmonary trunk and posterior wall of left atrium (side-to-side)
- enlargement of foramen ovale
- incision [excision] of common wall between posterior left atrium and coronary sinus and roofing of resultant defect with patch graft (synthetic)
- ligation of venous connection (descending anomalous vein) (to left innominate vein) (to superior vena cava)
- repair of atrial septal defect (with prosthesis)

✖**35.83 Total repair of truncus arteriosus**

One-stage total correction of truncus arteriosus with or without:
- construction (with aortic homograft) (with prosthesis) of a pulmonary artery placed from right ventricle to arteries supplying the lung
- ligation of connections between aorta and pulmonary artery
- repair of ventricular septal defect (with prosthesis)

✖**35.84 Total correction of transposition of great vessels, not elsewhere classified**

Arterial switch operation [Jatene]

Total correction of transposition of great arteries at the arterial level by switching the great arteries, including the left or both coronary arteries, implanted in the wall of the pulmonary artery

Excludes *baffle operation [Mustard] [Senning] (35.91)*
creation of shunt between right ventricle and pulmonary artery [Rastelli] (35.92)

●**35.9 Other operations on valves and septa of heart**

Code also cardiopulmonary bypass, if performed [extracorporeal circulation] [heart-lung machine] (39.61)

✖**35.91 Interatrial transposition of venous return**

Baffle:
- atrial
- interatrial

Mustard's operation

Resection of atrial septum and insertion of patch to direct systemic venous return to tricuspid valve and pulmonary venous return to mitral valve

✖**35.92 Creation of conduit between right ventricle and pulmonary artery**

Creation of shunt between right ventricle and (distal) pulmonary artery

Excludes *that associated with total repair of truncus arteriosus (35.83)*

✖**35.93 Creation of conduit between left ventricle and aorta**

Creation of apicoaortic shunt

Shunt between apex of left ventricle and aorta

✖**35.94 Creation of conduit between atrium and pulmonary artery**

Fontan procedure

✖**35.95 Revision of corrective procedure on heart**

Replacement of prosthetic heart valve poppet

Resuture of prosthesis of:
- septum
- valve

Excludes *complete revision—code to specific procedure*
replacement of prosthesis or graft of:
septum (35.50–35.63)
valve (35.20–35.28)

✖**35.96 Percutaneous valvuloplasty**

Percutaneous balloon valvuloplasty

✖**35.98 Other operations on septa of heart**

✖**35.99 Other operations on valves of heart**

●**36 Operations on vessels of heart**

Includes: sternotomy (median) (transverse) as operative approach
thoracotomy as operative approach

Code also cardiopulmonary bypass, if performed [extracorporeal circulation] [heart-lung machine] (39.61)

Code also any injection or infusion of platelet inhibitor (99.20)

●**36.0 Removal of coronary artery obstruction and insertion of stent(s)**

✖**36.01 Single vessel percutaneous transluminal coronary angioplasty [PTCA] or coronary atherectomy without mention of thrombolytic agent**

Balloon angioplasty of coronary artery

Coronary atherectomy

Percutaneous coronary angioplasty NOS

PTCA NOS

Excludes *multiple vessel percutaneous transluminal coronary angioplasty [PTCA] or coronary atherectomy performed during the same operation (36.05)*

Code also any insertion of coronary stent(s)(36.06)

✖**36.02 Single vessel percutaneous transluminal coronary angioplasty [PTCA] or coronary atherectomy with mention of thrombolytic agent**

Balloon angioplasty of coronary artery with infusion of thrombolytic agent [streptokinase]

Coronary atherectomy

Excludes *multiple vessel percutaneous transluminal coronary angioplasty [PTCA] or coronary atherectomy performed during the same operation (36.05)*
single vessel PTCA or coronary atherectomy without mention of thrombolytic agent (36.01)

Code also any insertion of coronary stent(s) (36.06)

✖**36.03 Open chest coronary artery angioplasty**

Coronary (artery):
- endarterectomy (with patch graft)
- thromboendarterectomy (with patch graft)

Open surgery for direct relief of coronary artery obstruction

Excludes *that with coronary artery bypass graft (36.10–36.19)*

Code also any insertion of coronary stent(s) (36.06)

36.04 Intracoronary artery thrombolytic infusion

That by direct coronary artery injection, infusion, or catheterization
- enzyme infusion
- platelet inhibitor

Excludes *infusion of platelet inhibitor (99.20)*
infusion of thrombolytic agent (99.10)

✖ **36.05 Multiple vessel percutaneous transluminal coronary angioplasty [PTCA] or coronary atherectomy performed during the same operation, with or without mention of thrombolytic agent**
Balloon angioplasty of multiple coronary arteries
Coronary atherectomy
Code also any:
intracoronary artery thrombolytic infusion (36.04)
insertion of coronary stent(s) (36.06)

Excludes *single vessel PTCA or coronary atherectomy without mention of thrombolytic agent (36.01)*
with mention of thrombolytic agent (36.02)

✖ **36.06 Insertion of non-drug-eluting coronary artery stent(s)**
Bare stent(s)
Bonded stent(s)
Drug-coated stent(s), i.e., heparin coated
Endograft(s)
Endovascular graft(s)
Stent graft(s)
Code also any:
open chest coronary artery angioplasty (36.03)
percutaneous transluminal coronary angioplasty [PTCA] or coronary atherectomy (36.01, 36.02, 36.05)

Excludes *insertion of drug-eluting coronary artery stent(s) (36.07)*

36.07 Insertion of drug-eluting coronary artery stent(s)
Endograft(s)
Endovascular graft(s)
Stent graft(s)
Code also any:
open chest coronary artery angioplasty (36.03)
percutaneous transluminal coronary angioplasty [PCTA] or coronary atherectomy (36.01, 36.02, 36.05)

Excludes *drug-coated stents, e.g., heparin coated (36.06)*
insertion of non-drug-eluting coronary artery stent(s) (36.06)

✖ **36.09 Other removal of coronary artery obstruction**
Coronary angioplasty NOS

Excludes *that by open angioplasty (36.03)*
that by percutaneous transluminal coronary angioplasty [PTCA] or coronary atherectomy (36.01–36.02, 36.05)

● **36.1 Bypass anastomosis for heart revascularization**
Code also cardiopulmonary bypass [extracorporeal circulation] [heart-lung machine] (39.61)

✖ **36.10 Aortocoronary bypass for heart revascularization, not otherwise specified**
Direct revascularization:
cardiac with catheter stent, prosthesis, or vein graft
coronary with catheter stent, prosthesis, or vein graft
heart muscle with catheter stent, prosthesis, or vein graft
myocardial with catheter stent, prosthesis, or vein graft
Heart revascularization NOS

✖ **36.11 Aortocoronary bypass of one coronary artery**

✖ **36.12 Aortocoronary bypass of two coronary arteries**

✖ **36.13 Aortocoronary bypass of three coronary arteries**

✖ **36.14 Aortocoronary bypass of four or more coronary arteries**

✖ **36.15 Single internal mammary-coronary artery bypass**
Anastomosis (single):
mammary artery to coronary artery
thoracic artery to coronary artery

✖ **36.16 Double internal mammary-coronary artery bypass**
Anastomosis, double:
mammary artery to coronary artery
thoracic artery to coronary artery

✖ **36.17 Abdominal-coronary artery bypass**
Anastomosis:
Gastroepiploic-coronary artery

✖ **36.19 Other bypass anastomosis for heart revascularization**

✖ **36.2 Heart revascularization by arterial implant**
Implantation of:
aortic branches [ascending aortic branches] into heart muscle
blood vessels into myocardium
internal mammary artery [internal thoracic artery] into:
heart muscle
myocardium
ventricle
ventricular wall
indirect heart revascularization NOS

● **36.3 Other heart revascularization**

✖ **36.31 Open chest transmyocardial revascularization**

✖ **36.32 Other transmyocardial revascularization**
Percutaneous transmyocardial revascularization
Thoracoscopic transmyocardial revascularization

✖ **36.39 Other heart revascularization**
Abrasion of epicardium
Cardio-omentopexy
Intrapericardial poudrage
Myocardial graft:
mediastinal fat
omentum
pectoral muscles

● **36.9 Other operations on vessels of heart**
Code also cardiopulmonary bypass [extracorporeal circulation] [heart-lung machine] (39.61)

✖ **36.91 Repair of aneurysm of coronary vessel**

✖ **36.99 Other operations on vessels of heart**
Exploration of coronary artery
Incision of coronary artery
Ligation of coronary artery
Repair of arteriovenous fistula

● **37 Other operations on heart and pericardium**
Code also any injection or infusion of platelet inhibitor (99.20)

37.0 Pericardiocentesis

● **37.1 Cardiotomy and pericardiotomy**
Code also cardiopulmonary bypass [extracorporeal circulation] [heart-lung machine] (39.61)

✖ **37.10 Incision of heart, not otherwise specified**
Cardiolysis NOS

✖37.11 **Cardiotomy**
Incision of:
atrium
endocardium
myocardium
ventricle

✖37.12 **Pericardiotomy**
Pericardial window operation
Pericardiolysis
Pericardiotomy

● 37.2 **Diagnostic procedures on heart and pericardium**

37.21 **Right heart cardiac catheterization**
Cardiac catheterization NOS
Excludes *that with catheterization of left heart (37.23)*

37.22 **Left heart cardiac catheterization**
Excludes *that with catheterization of right heart (37.23)*

37.23 **Combined right and left heart cardiac catheterization**

✖37.24 **Biopsy of pericardium**

37.25 **Biopsy of heart**

37.26 **Cardiac electrophysiologic stimulation and recording studies**
Electrophysiologic studies [EPS]
Non-invasive programmed electrical stimulation (NIPS)
Programmed electrical stimulation
Code also any concomitant procedure
Excludes *His bundle recording (37.29)*

37.27 **Cardiac mapping**
Code also any concomitant procedure
Excludes *electrocardiogram (89.52)*
His bundle recording (37.29)

37.28 **Intracardiac echocardiography**
ICE
Code also any synchronous Doppler flow mapping (88.72)

37.29 **Other diagnostic procedures on heart and pericardium**
Excludes *angiocardiography (88.50–88.58)*
cardiac function tests (89.41–89.69)
cardiovascular radioisotopic scan and function study (92.05)
coronary arteriography (88.55–88.57)
diagnostic pericardiocentesis (37.0)
diagnostic ultrasound of heart (88.72)
x-ray of heart (87.49)

● 37.3 **Pericardiectomy and excision of lesion of heart**
Code also cardiopulmonary bypass [extracorporeal circulation] [heart-lung machine] (39.61)

✖37.31 **Pericardiectomy**
Excision of:
adhesions of pericardium
constricting scar of:
epicardium
pericardium

✖37.32 **Excision of aneurysm of heart**
Repair of aneurysm of heart

✖37.33 **Excision or destruction of other lesion or tissue of heart, open approach** ⬅
Ablation of heart tissue (cryoablation) (electrocurrent) (laser) (microwave) (radiofrequency) (resection), open chest approach ◀
Cox-maze procedure ◀
Maze procedure ◀
Modified maze procedure, trans-thoracic approach ◀

Excludes *ablation, excision or destruction of lesion or tissue of heart, endovascular approach (37.34)* ⬅

✖37.34 **Excision or destruction of other lesion or tissue of heart, other approach** ⬅
Ablation of heart tissue (cryoablation) (electrocurrent) (laser) (microwave) (radiofrequency) (resection), via peripherally inserted catheter ◀
Modified maze procedure, endovascular approach ◀

✖37.35 **Partial ventriculectomy**
Ventricular reduction surgery
Ventricular remodeling
Code also any synchronous:
mitral valve repair (35.02, 35.12)
mitral valve replacement (35.23–35.24)

✖37.4 **Repair of heart and pericardium**

● 37.5 **Heart replacement procedures** ⬅
Excludes *combined heart-lung transplantation (33.6)* ◀

✖37.51 **Heart transplantation** ◀
Excludes *combined heart-lung transplantation (33.6)* ◀

✖37.52 **Implantation of total replacement heart system** ◀
Artificial heart ◀
Implantation of fully implantable total replacement heart system, including ventriculectomy ◀
Excludes *implantation of heart assist system (37.62, 37.65, 37.66)* ◀

✖37.53 **Replacement or repair of thoracic unit of total replacement heart system** ◀
Excludes *replacement and repair of heart assist system (37.63)* ◀

✖37.54 **Replacement or repair of other implantable component of total replacement heart system** ◀
Implantable battery ◀
Implantable controller ◀
Transcutaneous energy transfer (TET) device ◀
Excludes *replacement and repair of heart assist system (37.63)* ◀
replacement or repair of thoracic unit of total replacement heart system (37.53) ◀

● 37.6 **Implantation of heart assist system**

✖37.61 **Implant of pulsation balloon**

✖37.62 **Implant of other heart assist system**
Insertion of centrifugal pump
Insertion of heart assist system, NOS
Insertion of heart assist system, not specified as pulsatile
Insertion of heart pump
Excludes *implantation of total replacement heart system (37.52)* ◀

✖37.63 **Replacement and repair of heart assist system**
Excludes *replacement or repair of other implantable component of total replacement heart system (37.54)* ◀
replacement or repair of thoracic unit of total replacement heart system (37.53) ◀

✖37.64 **Removal of heart assist system**
Excludes *nonoperative removal of heart assist system (97.44)*
that with replacement of implant (37.63)

✖37.65 **Implant of external, pulsatile heart assist system**
Note: Device not implantable (outside the body but connected to heart) with external circulation and pump.

Excludes *implant of pulsation balloon (37.61)*
implantation of total replacement heart system (37.52) ◀

✖**37.66 Implant of an implantable, pulsatile heart assist system**

Note: Device directly connected to the heart and implanted in the upper left quadrant of peritoneal cavity.

Transportable, implantable heart assist system.

Excludes *implant of pulsation balloon (37.61)*
implantation of total replacement heart system (37.52) ◀

✖**37.67 Implantation of cardiomyostimulation system**

Note: Two-step open procedure consisting of transfer of one end of the latissimus dorsi muscle; wrapping it around the heart; rib resection; implantation of epicardial cardiac pacing leads into the right ventricle; tunneling and pocket creation for the cardiomyostimulator.

● **37.7 Insertion, revision, replacement, and removal of pacemaker leads; insertion of temporary pacemaker system; or revision of pocket**

Code also any insertion and replacement of pacemaker device (37.80–37.87)

Excludes *implantation or replacement of transvenous lead [electrode] into left ventricular cardiac venous system (00.52)*

37.70 Initial insertion of lead [electrode], not otherwise specified

Excludes *insertion of temporary transvenous pacemaker system (37.78)*
replacement of atrial and/or ventricular lead(s) (37.76)

37.71 Initial insertion of transvenous lead [electrode] into ventricle

Excludes *insertion of temporary transvenous pacemaker system (37.78)*
replacement of atrial and/or ventricular lead(s) (37.76)

37.72 Initial insertion of transvenous leads [electrodes] into atrium and ventricle

Excludes *insertion of temporary transvenous pacemaker system (37.78)*
replacement of atrial and/or ventricular lead(s) (37.76)

37.73 Initial insertion of transvenous lead [electrode] into atrium

Excludes *insertion of temporary transvenous pacemaker system (37.78)*
replacement of atrial and/or ventricular lead(s) (37.76)

✖**37.74 Insertion or replacement of epicardial lead [electrode] into epicardium**

Insertion or replacement of epicardial by:
sternotomy
thoracotomy

Excludes *replacement of atrial and/or ventricular lead(s) (37.76)*

✖**37.75 Revision of lead [electrode]**

Repair of electrode [removal with re-insertion]
Repositioning of lead [electrode]
Revision of lead NOS

Excludes *repositioning of temporary transvenous pacemaker system—omit code*

✖**37.76 Replacement of transvenous atrial and/or ventricular lead(s) [electrode]**

Removal or abandonment of existing transvenous or epicardial lead(s) with transvenous lead(s) replacement

Excludes *replacement of epicardial lead [electrode] (37.74)*

✖**37.77 Removal of lead(s) [electrode] without replacement**

Removal:
epicardial lead (transthoracic approach)
transvenous lead(s)

Excludes *removal of temporary transvenous pacemaker system—omit code*
that with replacement of:
atrial and/or ventricular lead(s) [electrode] (37.76)
epicardial lead [electrode] (37.74)

37.78 Insertion of temporary transvenous pacemaker system

Excludes *intraoperative cardiac pacemaker (39.64)*

✖**37.79 Revision or relocation of pacemaker pocket**

Debridement and reforming pocket (skin and subcutaneous tissue)

Relocation of pocket [creation of new pocket] pacemaker or CRT-P

● **37.8 Insertion, replacement, removal, and revision of pacemaker device**

Code also any lead insertion, lead replacement, lead removal and/or lead revision (37.70–37.77)

Excludes *implantation of cardiac resynchronization pacemaker [CRT-P] (00.50)*
implantation or replacement of cardiac resynchronization pacemaker pulse generator only [CRT-P] (00.53)

✖**37.80 Insertion of permanent pacemaker, initial or replacement, type of device not specified**

37.81 Initial insertion of single-chamber device, not specified as rate responsive

Excludes *replacement of existing pacemaker device (37.85-37.87)*

37.82 Initial insertion of single-chamber device, rate responsive

Rate responsive to physiologic stimuli other than atrial rate

Excludes *replacement of existing pacemaker device (37.85-37.87)*

37.83 Initial insertion of dual-chamber device

Atrial ventricular sequential device

Excludes *replacement of existing pacemaker device (37.85-37.87)*

✖**37.85 Replacement of any type pacemaker device with single-chamber device, not specified as rate responsive**

✖**37.86 Replacement of any type of pacemaker device with single-chamber device, rate responsive**

Rate responsive to physiologic stimuli other than atrial rate

✖**37.87 Replacement of any type pacemaker device with dual-chamber device**

Atrial ventricular sequential device

✖**37.89 Revision or removal of pacemaker device**

Removal without replacement of cardiac resynchronization pacemaker device [CRT-P]

Repair of pacemaker device

Excludes *removal of temporary transvenous pacemaker system—omit code*
replacement of existing pacemaker device (37.85–37.87)
replacement of existing pacemaker device with CRT-P pacemaker device (00.53)

● **37.9 Other operations on heart and pericardium**

✖**37.91 Open chest cardiac massage**

Excludes *closed chest cardiac massage (99.63)*

37.92 Injection of therapeutic substance into heart

37.93 Injection of therapeutic substance into pericardium

✖**37.94 Implantation or replacement of automatic cardioverter/defibrillator, total system [AICD]**

Implantation of defibrillator with leads (epicardial patches), formation of pocket (abdominal fascia) (subcutaneous), any transvenous leads, intraoperative procedures for evaluation of lead signals, and obtaining defibrillator threshold measurements (electrophysiologic studies [EPS]) ⬅

Techniques:
lateral thoracotomy
medial sternotomy
subxiphoid procedure

Code also extracorporeal circulation, if performed (39.61)

Code also any concomitant procedure [e.g., coronary bypass] (36.00–36.19)

Excludes *implantation of cardiac resynchronization defibrillator, total system [CRT-D] (00.51)*

✖**37.95 Implantation of automatic cardioverter/defibrillator lead(s) only**

✖**37.96 Implantation of automatic cardioverter/defibrillator pulse generator only**

Excludes *implantation or replacement of cardiac resynchronization defibrillator, pulse generator device only [CRT-D] (00.54)*

✖**37.97 Replacement of automatic cardioverter/defibrillator lead(s) only**

✖**37.98 Replacement of automatic cardioverter/defibrillator pulse generator only**

Excludes *replacement of cardiac resynchronization defibrillator, pulse generator device only [CRT-D] (00.54)*

✖**37.99 Other**

Removal of cardioverter/defibrillator pulse generator only without replacement
Removal without replacement of cardiac resynchronization defibrillator device [CRT-D]
Repositioning of lead(s) (sensing) (pacing) [electrode]
Repositioning of pulse generator
Revision of cardioverter/defibrillator (automatic) pocket
Revision or relocation of CRT-D pocket

Excludes *cardiac retraining (93.36)*
conversion of cardiac rhythm (99.60–99.69)
maze procedure (Cox-maze), open (37.33) ◀
maze procedure, endovascular approach (37.34) ◀

● **38 Incision, excision, and occlusion of vessels**

Code also any application or administration of an adhesion barrier substance (99.77)

Code also cardiopulmonary bypass [extracorporeal circulation] [heart-lung machine] (39.61)

Excludes *that of coronary vessels (36.01–36.99)*

The following fourth-digit subclassification is for use with appropriate categories in section 38.0, 38.1, 38.3, 38.5, 38.6, 38.8, and 38.9 according to site. Valid fourth-digits are in [brackets] at the end of each code/description.

0 unspecified site

1 intracranial vessels
Cerebral (anterior) (middle)
Circle of Willis
Posterior communicating artery

2 other vessels of head and neck
Carotid artery (common) (external) (internal)
Jugular vein (external) (internal)

3 upper limb vessels
Axillary
Brachial
Radial
Ulnar

4 aorta

5 other thoracic vessels
Innominate
Pulmonary (artery) (vein)
Subclavian
Vena cava, superior

6 abdominal arteries
Celiac
Gastric
Hepatic
Iliac
Mesenteric
Renal
Splenic
Umbilical

Excludes *abdominal aorta (4)*

7 abdominal veins
Iliac
Portal
Renal
Splenic
Vena cava (inferior)

8 lower limb arteries
Femoral (common) (superficial)
Popliteal
Tibial

9 lower limb veins
Femoral
Popliteal
Saphenous
Tibial

✖● **38.0 Incision of vessel**
[0–9] Embolectomy
Thrombectomy

Excludes *puncture or catheterization of any:*
artery (38.91, 38.98)
vein (38.92–38.95, 38.99)

✖● **38.1 Endarterectomy**
[0–6, 8] Endarterectomy with:
embolectomy
patch graft
temporary bypass during procedure
thrombectomy

● **38.2 Diagnostic procedures on blood vessels**

✖**38.21 Biopsy of blood vessel**

38.22 Percutaneous angioscopy

Excludes *angioscopy of eye (95.12)*

✖**38.29 Other diagnostic procedures on blood vessels**

Excludes *blood vessel thermography (88.86)*
circulatory monitoring (89.61–89.69)
contrast:
angiocardiography (88.50–88.58)
arteriography (88.40–88.49)
phlebography (88.60–88.67)
impedance phlebography (88.68)
peripheral vascular ultrasonography (88.77)
plethysmogram (89.58)

✖● **38.3 Resection of vessel with anastomosis**
[0–9] Angiectomy
Excision of:
aneurysm (arteriovenous) with anastomosis
blood vessel (lesion) with anastomosis

✖● **38.4 Resection of vessel with replacement**
[0–9] Angiectomy
Excision of:
aneurysm (arteriovenous) or blood vessel (lesion) with replacement

Excludes *endovascular repair of aneurysm (39.71–39.79)*

Requires the use of one of the following fourth-digit subclassifications to identify site:

0 unspecified site

1 intracranial vessels
Cerebral (anterior) (middle)
Circle of Willis
Posterior communicating artery

2 other vessels of head and neck
Carotid artery (common) (external) (internal)
Jugular vein (external) (internal)

3 upper limb vessels
Axillary
Brachial
Radial
Ulnar

4 aorta, abdominal
Code also any thoracic vessel involvement (thoracoabdominal procedure) (38.45)

5 thoracic vessels
Aorta (thoracic)
Innominate
Pulmonary (artery) (vein)
Subclavian
Vena cava, superior
Code also any abdominal aorta involvement (thoracoabdominal procedure) (38.44)

6 abdominal arteries
Celiac
Gastric
Hepatic
Iliac
Mesenteric
Renal
Splenic
Umbilical

Excludes *abdominal aorta (4)*

7 abdominal veins
Iliac
Portal
Renal
Splenic
Vena cava (inferior)

8 lower limb arteries
Femoral (common) (superficial)
Popliteal
Tibial

9 lower limb veins
Femoral
Popliteal
Saphenous
Tibial

✖● **38.5 Ligation and stripping of varicose veins**
[0–3, 5, 7, 9]

Excludes *ligation of varices:*
esophageal (42.91)
gastric (44.91)

✖● **38.6 Other excision of vessel**
[0–9] Excision of blood vessel (lesion) NOS

Excludes *excision of vessel for aortocoronary bypass (36.10–36.14)*
excision with:
anastomosis (38.30–38.39)
graft replacement (38.40–38.49)
implant (38.40–38.49)

38.7 Interruption of the vena cava
Insertion of implant or sieve in vena cava
Ligation of vena cava (inferior) (superior)
Plication of vena cava

✖● **38.8 Other surgical occlusion of vessels**
[0–9] Clamping of blood vessel
Division of blood vessel
Ligation of blood vessel
Occlusion of blood vessel

Excludes *adrenal vessels (07.43)*
esophageal varices (42.91)
gastric or duodenal vessel for ulcer (44.40–44.49)
gastric varices (44.91)
meningeal vessel (02.13)
percutaneous transcatheter infusion embolization (99.29)
spermatic vein for varicocele (63.1)
surgical occlusion of vena cava (38.7)
that for chemoembolization (99.25)
that for control of (postoperative) hemorrhage:
anus (49.95)
bladder (57.93)
following vascular procedure (39.41)
nose (21.00–21.09)
prostate (60.94)
tonsil (28.7)
thyroid vessel (06.92)
transcatheter (infusion) (99.29

● **38.9 Puncture of vessel**

Excludes *that for circulatory monitoring (89.60–89.69)*

38.91 Arterial catheterization

38.92 Umbilical vein catheterization

38.93 Venous catheterization, not elsewhere classified

Excludes *that for cardiac catheterization (37.21–37.23)*
that for renal dialysis (38.95)

38.94 Venous cutdown

38.95 Venous catheterization for renal dialysis

Excludes *insertion of totally implantable vascular access device [VAD] (86.07)*

38.98 Other puncture of artery

Excludes *that for:*
arteriography (88.40–88.49)
coronary arteriography (88.55–88.57)

38.99 Other puncture of vein
Phlebotomy

Excludes *that for:*
angiography (88.60–88.69)
extracorporeal circulation (39.61, 50.92)
injection or infusion of:
sclerosing solution (39.92)
therapeutic or prophylactic substance (99.11–99.29)
perfusion (39.96–39.97)
phlebography (88.60–88.69)
transfusion (99.01–99.09)

● **39 Other operations on vessels**

Excludes *those on coronary vessels (36.00–36.99)*

✖ **39.0 Systemic to pulmonary artery shunt**

Descending aorta-pulmonary artery anastomosis (graft)
Left to right anastomosis (graft)
Subclavian-pulmonary anastomosis (graft)

Code also cardiopulmonary bypass [extracorporeal circulation] [heart-lung machine] (39.61)

✖ **39.1 Intra-abdominal venous shunt**

Anastomosis:
- mesocaval
- portacaval
- portal vein to inferior vena cava
- splenic and renal veins
- transjugular intrahepatic portosystemic shunt (TIPS)

Excludes *peritoneovenous shunt (54.94)*

● **39.2 Other shunt or vascular bypass**

✖ **39.21 Caval-pulmonary artery anastomosis**

Code also cardiopulmonary bypass (39.61)

✖ **39.22 Aorta-subclavian-carotid bypass**

Bypass (arterial):
- aorta to carotid and brachial
- aorta to subclavian and carotid
- carotid to subclavian

✖ **39.23 Other intrathoracic vascular shunt or bypass**

Intrathoracic (arterial) bypass graft NOS

Excludes *coronary artery bypass (36.10–36.19)*

✖ **39.24 Aorta-renal bypass**

✖ **39.25 Aorta-iliac-femoral bypass**

Bypass:
- aortofemoral
- aortoiliac
- aortoiliac to popliteal
- aortopopliteal
- iliofemoral [iliac-femoral]

✖ **39.26 Other intra-abdominal vascular shunt or bypass**

Bypass:
- aortoceliac
- aortic-superior mesenteric
- common hepatic-common iliac-renal

Intra-abdominal arterial bypass graft NOS

Excludes *peritoneovenous shunt (54.94)*

✖ **39.27 Arteriovenostomy for renal dialysis**

Anastomosis for renal dialysis
Formation of (peripheral) arteriovenous fistula for renal [kidney] dialysis

Code also any renal dialysis (39.95)

✖ **39.28 Extracranial-intracranial (EC-IC) vascular bypass**

✖ **39.29 Other (peripheral) vascular shunt or bypass**

Bypass (graft):
- axillary-brachial
- axillary-femoral [axillofemoral] (superficial)
- brachial
- femoral-femoral
- femoroperoneal
- femoropopliteal (arteries)
- femorotibial (anterior) (posterior)
- popliteal
- vascular NOS

Excludes *peritoneovenous shunt (54.94)*

● **39.3 Suture of vessel**

Repair of laceration of blood vessel

Excludes *any other vascular puncture closure device-omit code*
suture of aneurysm (39.52)
that for control of hemorrhage (postoperative):
- *anus (49.95)*
- *bladder (57.93)*
- *following vascular procedure (39.41)*
- *nose (21.00–21.09)*
- *prostate (60.94)*
- *tonsil (28.7)*

✖ **39.30 Suture of unspecified blood vessel**

✖ **39.31 Suture of artery**

✖ **39.32 Suture of vein**

● **39.4 Revision of vascular procedure**

✖ **39.41 Control of hemorrhage following vascular surgery**

Excludes *that for control of hemorrhage (post operative):*
- *anus (49.95)*
- *bladder (57.93)*
- *nose (21.00–21.09)*
- *prostate (60.94)*
- *tonsil (28.7)*

✖ **39.42 Revision of arteriovenous shunt for renal dialysis**

Conversion of renal dialysis:
- end-to-end anastomosis to end-to-side
- end-to-side anastomosis to end-to-end
- vessel-to-vessel cannula to arteriovenous shunt

Removal of old arteriovenous shunt and creation of new shunt

Excludes *replacement of vessel-to-vessel cannula (39.94)*

✖ **39.43 Removal of arteriovenous shunt for renal dialysis**

Excludes *that with replacement [revision] of shunt (39.42)*

✖ **39.49 Other revision of vascular procedure**

Declotting (graft)
Revision of:
- anastomosis of blood vessel
- vascular procedure (previous)

● **39.5 Other repair of vessels**

✖ **39.50 Angioplasty or atherectomy of non-coronary vessel**

Percutaneous transluminal angioplasty (PTA) of non-coronary vessels:
- Head and neck arteries:
  - basilar
  - carotid
  - vertebral
- Lower extremity vessels
- Mesenteric artery
- Renal artery
- Upper extremity vessels

Code also any:
- injection or infusion of thrombolytic agent (99.10)
- insertion of non-coronary stent(s) or stent grafts(s) (39.90)

✖ **39.51 Clipping of aneurysm**

Excludes *clipping of arteriovenous fistula (39.53)*

✖ **39.52 Other repair of aneurysm**

Repair of aneurysm by:
- coagulation
- electrocoagulation
- filipuncture
- methyl methacrylate
- suture
- wiring
- wrapping

Excludes *endovascular repair of aneurysm (39.71–39.79)*
re-entry operation (aorta) (39.54)
that with:
graft replacement (38.40–38.49)
resection (38.30–38.49, 38.60–38.69)

✖ **39.53 Repair of arteriovenous fistula**
Embolization of carotid cavernous fistula
Repair of arteriovenous fistula by:
clipping
coagulation
ligation and division

Excludes *repair of:*
arteriovenous shunt for renal dialysis (39.42)
head and neck vessels, endovascular approach (39.72)
that with:
graft replacement (38.40–38.49)
resection (38.30–38.49, 38.60–38.69)

✖ **39.54 Re-entry operation (aorta)**
Fenestration of dissecting aneurysm of thoracic aorta

Code also cardiopulmonary bypass [extracorporeal circulation] [heart-lung machine] (39.61)

✖ **39.55 Reimplantation of aberrant renal vessel**

✖ **39.56 Repair of blood vessel with tissue patch graft**

Excludes *that with resection (38.40–38.49)*

✖ **39.57 Repair of blood vessel with synthetic patch graft**

Excludes *that with resection (38.40–38.49)*

✖ **39.58 Repair of blood vessel with unspecified type of patch graft**

Excludes *that with resection (38.40–38.49)*

✖ **39.59 Other repair of vessel**
Aorticopulmonary window operation
Arterioplasty NOS
Construction of venous valves (peripheral)
Plication of vein (peripheral)
Reimplantation of artery

Code also cardiopulmonary bypass [extracorporeal circulation] [heart-lung machine] (39.61)

Excludes *interruption of the vena cava (38.7)*
reimplantation of renal artery (39.55)
that with:
graft (39.56–39.58)
resection (38.30–38.49, 38.60–38.69)

● **39.6 Extracorporeal circulation and procedures auxiliary to heart surgery**

39.61 Extracorporeal circulation auxiliary to open heart surgery
Artificial heart and lung
Cardiopulmonary bypass
Pump oxygenator

Excludes *extracorporeal hepatic assistance (50.92)*
extracorporeal membrane oxygenation [ECMO] (39.65)
hemodialysis (39.95)
percutaneous cardiopulmonary bypass (39.66)

39.62 Hypothermia (systemic) incidental to open heart surgery

39.63 Cardioplegia
Arrest:
anoxic
circulatory

39.64 Intraoperative cardiac pacemaker
Temporary pacemaker used during and immediately following cardiac surgery

39.65 Extracorporeal membrane oxygenation [ECMO]

Excludes *extracorporeal circulation auxiliary to open heart surgery (39.61)*
percutaneous cardiopulmonary bypass (39.66)

39.66 Percutaneous cardiopulmonary bypass
Closed chest

Excludes *extracorporeal circulation auxiliary to open heart surgery (39.61)*
extracorporeal hepatic assistance (50.92)
extracorporeal membrane oxygenation [ECMO] (39.65)
hemodialysis (39.95)

● **39.7 Endovascular repair of vessel**
Endoluminal repair

Excludes *angioplasty or atherectomy of non-coronary vessel (39.50)*
insertion of non-coronary stent or stents (39.90)
other repair of aneurysm (39.52)
resection of abdominal aorta with replacement (38.44)
resection of lower limb arteries with replacement (38.48)
resection of thoracic aorta with replacement (38.45)
resection of upper limb vessels with replacement (38.43)

✖ **39.71 Endovascular implantation of graft in abdominal aorta**
Endovascular repair of abdominal aortic aneurysm with graft
Stent graft(s)

✖ **39.72 Endovascular repair or occlusion of head and neck vessels**
Coil embolization or occlusion
Endograft(s)
Endovascular graft(s)
Liquid tissue adhesive (glue) embolization or occlusion
Other implant or substance for repair, embolization or occlusion
That for repair of aneurysm, arteriovenous malformation [AVM] or fistula

✖ **39.79 Other endovascular repair (of aneurysm) of other vessels** ⬅
Coil embolization or occlusion
Endograft(s)
Endovascular graft(s)
Liquid tissue adhesive (glue) embolization or occlusion
Other implant or substance for repair, embolization or occlusion

Excludes *endovascular repair or occlusion of head and neck vessels (39.72)*
insertion of drug-eluting non-coronary artery stent(s) (00.55)
insertion of non-coronary artery stent(s) for other than aneurysm repair (39.90)
non-endovascular repair of arteriovenous fistula (39.53)
other surgical occlusion of vessels - see category *38.8*
percutaneous transcatheter infusion (99.29)
transcatheter embolization for gastric or duodenal bleeding (44.44)

✖ **39.8 Operations on carotid body and other vascular bodies**
Chemodectomy
Denervation of:
aortic body
carotid body
Glomectomy, carotid
Implantation into carotid body:
electronic stimulator
pacemaker

Excludes *excision of glomus jugulare (20.51)*

● **39.9 Other operations on vessels**

39.90 Insertion of non-drug-eluting, non-coronary artery stent(s)
Bare stent(s)
Bonded stent(s)
Drug-coated stent(s), i.e., heparin coated
Endograft(s)
Endovascular graft(s)

Excludes *insertion of drug-eluting, noncoronary artery stent(s) (00.55)*
that for aneurysm repair (39.71–39.79)
Endovascular recanalization techniques
Stent graft(s)

Code also any non-coronary angioplasty or atherectomy (39.50)

✖ **39.91 Freeing of vessel**
Dissection and freeing of adherent tissue:
artery-vein-nerve bundle
vascular bundle

✖ **39.92 Injection of sclerosing agent into vein**

Excludes *injection:*
esophageal varices (42.33)
hemorrhoids (49.42)

✖ **39.93 Insertion of vessel-to-vessel cannula**
Formation of:
arteriovenous:
fistula by external cannula
shunt by external cannula

Code also any renal dialysis (39.95)

✖ **39.94 Replacement of vessel-to-vessel cannula**
Revision of vessel-to-vessel cannula

39.95 Hemodialysis
Artificial kidney
Hemodiafiltration
Hemofiltration
Renal dialysis

Excludes *peritoneal dialysis (54.98)*

39.96 Total body perfusion
Code also substance perfused (99.21–99.29)

39.97 Other perfusion
Perfusion NOS
Perfusion, local [regional] of:
carotid artery
coronary artery
head
lower limb
neck
upper limb

Code also substance perfused (99.21–99.29)

Excludes *perfusion of:*
kidney (55.95)
large intestine (46.96)
liver (50.93)
small intestine (46.95)

✖ **39.98 Control of hemorrhage, not otherwise specified**
Angiotripsy
Control of postoperative hemorrhage NOS
Venotripsy

Excludes *control of hemorrhage (postoperative):*
anus (49.95)
bladder (57.93)
following vascular procedure (39.41)
nose (21.00–21.09)
prostate (60.94)
tonsil (28.7)
that by:
ligation (38.80–38.89)
suture (39.30–39.32)

✖ **39.99 Other operations on vessels**

Excludes *injection or infusion of therapeutic or prophylactic substance (99.11–99.29)*
transfusion of blood and blood components (99.01–99.09)

8. OPERATIONS ON THE HEMIC AND LYMPHATIC SYSTEM (40–41)

● **40 Operations on lymphatic system**

✖ **40.0 Incision of lymphatic structures**

● **40.1 Diagnostic procedures on lymphatic structures**

✖ **40.11 Biopsy of lymphatic structure**

✖ **40.19 Other diagnostic procedures on lymphatic structures**

Excludes *lymphangiogram:*
abdominal (88.04)
cervical (87.08)
intrathoracic (87.34)
lower limb (88.36)
upper limb (88.34)
microscopic examination of specimen (90.71–90.79)
radioisotope scan (92.16)
thermography (88.89)

● **40.2 Simple excision of lymphatic structure**

Excludes *biopsy of lymphatic structure (40.11)*

✖ **40.21 Excision of deep cervical lymph node**

✖ **40.22 Excision of internal mammary lymph node**

✖ **40.23 Excision of axillary lymph node**

✖ **40.24 Excision of inguinal lymph node**

✖ **40.29 Simple excision of other lymphatic structure**
Excision of:
cystic hygroma
lymphangioma
Simple lymphadenectomy

✖ **40.3 Regional lymph node excision**
Extended regional lymph node excision
Regional lymph node excision with excision of lymphatic drainage area including skin, subcutaneous tissue, and fat

● **40.4 Radical excision of cervical lymph nodes**
Resection of cervical lymph nodes down to muscle and deep fascia

Excludes *that associated with radical laryngectomy (30.4)*

✖ **40.40 Radical neck dissection, not otherwise specified**

✖ **40.41 Radical neck dissection, unilateral**

✖ **40.42 Radical neck dissection, bilateral**

● **40.5 Radical excision of other lymph nodes**

Excludes *that associated with radical mastectomy (85.45–85.48)*

✖ **40.50 Radical excision of lymph nodes, not otherwise specified**
Radical (lymph) node dissection NOS

✖ **40.51 Radical excision of axillary lymph nodes**

✖ **40.52 Radical excision of periaortic lymph nodes**

✖ **40.53 Radical excision of iliac lymph nodes**

✖ **40.54 Radical groin dissection**

✖ **40.59 Radical excision of other lymph nodes**

Excludes *radical neck dissection (40.40–40.42)*

● **40.6 Operations on thoracic duct**

✖ **40.61 Cannulation of thoracic duct**

✖ **40.62 Fistulization of thoracic duct**

✖ **40.63 Closure of fistula of thoracic duct**

✖ **40.64 Ligation of thoracic duct**

✖ **40.69 Other operations on thoracic duct**

✖ **40.9 Other operations on lymphatic structures**
Anastomosis of peripheral lymphatics
Dilation of peripheral lymphatics
Ligation of peripheral lymphatics
Obliteration of peripheral lymphatics
Reconstruction of peripheral lymphatics
Repair of peripheral lymphatics
Transplantation of peripheral lymphatics
Correction of lymphedema of limb, NOS

Excludes *reduction of elephantiasis of scrotum (61.3)*

● **41 Operations on bone marrow and spleen**

● **41.0 Bone marrow or hematopoietic stem cell transplant**

Excludes *aspiration of bone marrow from donor (41.91)*

✖ **41.00 Bone marrow transplant, not otherwise specified**

✖ **41.01 Autologous bone marrow transplant without purging**

Excludes *that with purging (41.09)*

✖ **41.02 Allogeneic bone marrow transplant with purging**
Allograft of bone marrow with in vitro removal (purging) of T-cells

✖ **41.03 Allogeneic bone marrow transplant without purging**
Allograft of bone marrow NOS

✖ **41.04 Autologous hematopoietic stem cell transplant without purging**

Excludes *that with purging (41.07)*

✖ **41.05 Allogeneic hematopoietic stem cell transplant without purging**

Excludes *that with purging (41.08)*

✖ **41.06 Cord blood stem cell transplant**

✖ **41.07 Autologous hematopoietic stem cell transplant with purging**
Cell depletion

✖ **41.08 Allogeneic hematopoietic stem cell transplant with purging**
Cell depletion

✖ **41.09 Autologous bone marrow transplant with purging**
with extracorporeal purging of malignant cells from marrow
Cell depletion

41.1 Puncture of spleen

Excludes *aspiration biopsy of spleen (41.32)*

✖ **41.2 Splenotomy**

● **41.3 Diagnostic procedures on bone marrow and spleen**

41.31 Biopsy of bone marrow

41.32 Closed [aspiration] [percutaneous] biopsy of spleen

✖ **41.33 Open biopsy of spleen**

41.38 Other diagnostic procedures on bone marrow

Excludes *microscopic examination of specimen from bone marrow (90.61–90.69)*
radioisotope scan (92.05)

41.39 Other diagnostic procedures on spleen

Excludes *microscopic examination of specimen from spleen (90.61–90.69)*
radioisotope scan (92.05)

● **41.4 Excision or destruction of lesion or tissue of spleen**

Excludes *excision of accessory spleen (41.93)*

Code also any application or administration of an adhesion barrier substance (99.77)

✖ **41.41 Marsupialization of splenic cyst**

✖ **41.42 Excision of lesion or tissue of spleen**

Excludes *biopsy of spleen (41.32–41.33)*

✖ **41.43 Partial splenectomy**

✖ **41.5 Total splenectomy**

Splenectomy NOS

Code also any application or administration of an adhesion barrier substance (99.77)

● **41.9 Other operations on spleen and bone marrow**

Code also any application or administration of an adhesion barrier substance (99.77)

41.91 Aspiration of bone marrow from donor for transplant

Excludes *biopsy of bone marrow (41.31)*

41.92 Injection into bone marrow

Excludes *bone marrow transplant (41.00–41.03)*

✖ **41.93 Excision of accessory spleen**

✖ **41.94 Transplantation of spleen**

✖ **41.95 Repair and plastic operations on spleen**

41.98 Other operations on bone marrow

✖ **41.99 Other operations on spleen**

9. OPERATIONS ON THE DIGESTIVE SYSTEM (42–54)

● 42 Operations on esophagus

● 42.0 Esophagotomy

✖ 42.01 Incision of esophageal web

✖ 42.09 Other incision of esophagus
Esophagotomy NOS

Excludes *esophagomyotomy (42.7)*
esophagostomy (42.10–42.19)

● 42.1 Esophagostomy

✖ 42.10 Esophagostomy, not otherwise specified

✖ 42.11 Cervical esophagostomy

✖ 42.12 Exteriorization of esophageal pouch

✖ 42.19 Other external fistulization of esophagus
Thoracic esophagostomy

Code also any resection (42.40–42.42)

● 42.2 Diagnostic procedures on esophagus

✖ 42.21 Operative esophagoscopy by incision

42.22 Esophagoscopy through artificial stoma

Excludes *that with biopsy (42.24)*

42.23 Other esophagoscopy

Excludes *that with biopsy (42.24)*

42.24 Closed [endoscopic] biopsy of esophagus
Brushing or washing for specimen collection
Esophagoscopy with biopsy
Suction biopsy of the esophagus

Excludes *esophagogastroduodenoscopy [EGD] with closed biopsy (45.16)*

✖ 42.25 Open biopsy of esophagus

42.29 Other diagnostic procedures on esophagus

Excludes *barium swallow (87.61)*
esophageal manometry (89.32)
microscopic examination of specimen from esophagus (90.81–90.89)

● 42.3 Local excision or destruction of lesion or tissue of esophagus

✖ 42.31 Local excision of esophageal diverticulum

✖ 42.32 Local excision of other lesion or tissue of esophagus

Excludes *biopsy of esophagus (42.24–42.25)*
esophageal fistulectomy (42.84)

42.33 Endoscopic excision or destruction of lesion or tissue of esophagus
Ablation of esophageal neoplasm by endoscopic approach
Control of esophageal bleeding by endoscopic approach
Esophageal polypectomy by endoscopic approach
Esophageal varices by endoscopic approach
Injection of esophageal varices by endoscopic approach

Excludes *biopsy of esophagus (42.24–42.25)*
fistulectomy (42.84)
open ligation of esophageal varices (42.91)

✖ 42.39 Other destruction of lesion or tissue of esophagus

Excludes *that by endoscopic approach (42.33)*

● 42.4 Excision of esophagus

Excludes *esophagogastrectomy NOS (43.99)*

✖ 42.40 Esophagectomy, not otherwise specified

✖ 42.41 Partial esophagectomy
Code also any synchronous:
anastomosis other than end-to-end (42.51–42.69)
esophagostomy (42.10–42.19)
gastrostomy (43.11–43.19)

✖ 42.42 Total esophagectomy
Code also any synchronous:
gastrostomy (43.11–43.19)
interposition or anastomosis other than end-to-end (42.51–42.69)

Excludes *esophagogastrectomy (43.99)*

● 42.5 Intrathoracic anastomosis of esophagus
Code also any synchronous:
esophagectomy (42.40–42.42)
gastrostomy (43.1)

✖ 42.51 Intrathoracic esophagoesophagostomy

✖ 42.52 Intrathoracic esophagogastrostomy

✖ 42.53 Intrathoracic esophageal anastomosis with interposition of small bowel

✖ 42.54 Other intrathoracic esophagoenterostomy
Anastomosis of esophagus to intestinal segment NOS

✖ 42.55 Intrathoracic esophageal anastomosis with interposition of colon

✖ 42.56 Other intrathoracic esophagocolostomy
Esophagocolostomy NOS

✖ 42.58 Intrathoracic esophageal anastomosis with other interposition
Construction of artificial esophagus
Retrosternal formation of reversed gastric tube

✖ 42.59 Other intrathoracic anastomosis of esophagus

● 42.6 Antesternal anastomosis of esophagus
Code also any synchronous:
esophagectomy (42.40–42.42)
gastrostomy (43.1)

✖ 42.61 Antesternal esophagoesophagostomy

✖ 42.62 Antesternal esophagogastrostomy

✖ 42.63 Antesternal esophageal anastomosis with interposition of small bowel

✖ 42.64 Other antesternal esophagoenterostomy
Antethoracic:
esophagoenterostomy
esophagoileostomy
esophagojejunostomy

✖ 42.65 Antesternal esophageal anastomosis with interposition of colon

✖ 42.66 Other antesternal esophagocolostomy
Antethoracic esophagocolostomy

✖ 42.68 Other antesternal esophageal anastomosis with interposition

✖ 42.69 Other antesternal anastomosis of esophagus

✖ 42.7 Esophagomyotomy

● 42.8 Other repair of esophagus

42.81 Insertion of permanent tube into esophagus

✖ 42.82 Suture of laceration of esophagus

✖ 42.83 Closure of esophagostomy

✖ **42.84 Repair of esophageal fistula, not elsewhere classified**

Excludes *repair of fistula:*
bronchoesophageal (33.42)
esophagopleurocutaneous (34.73)
pharyngoesophageal (29.53)
tracheoesophageal (31.73)

✖ **42.85 Repair of esophageal stricture**

✖ **42.86 Production of subcutaneous tunnel without esophageal anastomosis**

✖ **42.87 Other graft of esophagus**

Excludes *antesternal esophageal anastomosis with interposition of:*
colon (42.65)
small bowel (42.63)
antesternal esophageal anastomosis with other interposition (42.68)
intrathoracic esophageal anastomosis with interposition of:
colon (42.55)
small bowel (42.53)
intrathoracic esophageal anastomosis with other interposition (42.58)

✖ **42.89 Other repair of esophagus**

● **42.9 Other operations on esophagus**

✖ **42.91 Ligation of esophageal varices**

Excludes *that by endoscopic approach (42.33)*

42.92 Dilation of esophagus
Dilation of cardiac sphincter

Excludes *intubation of esophagus (96.03, 96.06–96.08)*

42.99 Other

Excludes *insertion of Sengstaken tube (96.06)*
intubation of esophagus (96.03, 96.06–96.08)
removal of intraluminal foreign body from esophagus without incision (98.02)
tamponade of esophagus (96.06)

● **43 Incision and excision of stomach**

Code also any application or administration of an adhesion barrier substance (99.77)

✖ **43.0 Gastrotomy**

Excludes *gastrostomy (43.11–43.19)*
that for control of hemorrhage (44.49)

● **43.1 Gastrostomy**

43.11 Percutaneous [endoscopic] gastrostomy [PEG]
Percutaneous transabdominal gastrostomy

43.19 Other gastrostomy

Excludes *percutaneous [endoscopic] gastrostomy [PEG] (43.11)*

✖ **43.3 Pyloromyotomy**

● **43.4 Local excision or destruction of lesion or tissue of stomach**

43.41 Endoscopic excision or destruction of lesion or tissue of stomach
Gastric polypectomy by endoscopic approach
Gastric varices by endoscopic approach

Excludes *biopsy of stomach (44.14–44.15)*
control of hemorrhage (44.43)
open ligation of gastric varices (44.91)

✖ **43.42 Local excision of other lesion or tissue of stomach**

Excludes *biopsy of stomach (44.14–44.15)*
gastric fistulectomy (44.62–44.63)
partial gastrectomy (43.5–43.89)

✖ **43.49 Other destruction of lesion or tissue of stomach**

Excludes *that by endoscopic approach (43.41)*

✖ **43.5 Partial gastrectomy with anastomosis to esophagus**
Proximal gastrectomy

✖ **43.6 Partial gastrectomy with anastomosis to duodenum**
Billroth I operation
Distal gastrectomy
Gastropylorectomy

✖ **43.7 Partial gastrectomy with anastomosis to jejunum**
Billroth II operation

● **43.8 Other partial gastrectomy**

✖ **43.81 Partial gastrectomy with jejunal transposition**
Henley jejunal transposition operation

Code also any synchronous intestinal resection (45.51)

✖ **43.89 Other**
Partial gastrectomy with bypass gastrogastrostomy
Sleeve resection of stomach

● **43.9 Total gastrectomy**

✖ **43.91 Total gastrectomy with intestinal interposition**

✖ **43.99 Other total gastrectomy**
Complete gastroduodenectomy
Esophagoduodenostomy with complete gastrectomy
Esophagogastrectomy NOS
Esophagojejunostomy with complete gastrectomy
Radical gastrectomy

● **44 Other operations on stomach**

Code also any application or administration of an adhesion barrier substance (99.77)

● **44.0 Vagotomy**

✖ **44.00 Vagotomy, not otherwise specified**
Division of vagus nerve NOS

✖ **44.01 Truncal vagotomy**

✖ **44.02 Highly selective vagotomy**
Parietal cell vagotomy
Selective proximal vagotomy

✖ **44.03 Other selective vagotomy**

● **44.1 Diagnostic procedures on stomach**

✖ **44.11 Transabdominal gastroscopy**
Intraoperative gastroscopy

Excludes *that with biopsy (44.14)*

44.12 Gastroscopy through artificial stoma

Excludes *that with biopsy (44.14)*

44.13 Other gastroscopy

Excludes *that with biopsy (44.14)*

44.14 Closed [endoscopic] biopsy of stomach
Brushing or washing for specimen collection

Excludes *esophagogastroduodenoscopy [EGD] with closed biopsy (45.16)*

✖ **44.15 Open biopsy of stomach**

44.19 Other diagnostic procedures on stomach

Excludes *gastric lavage (96.33)*
microscopic examination of specimen from stomach (90.81–90.89)
upper GI series (87.62)

● **44.2 Pyloroplasty**

✖ **44.21 Dilation of pylorus by incision**

44.22 Endoscopic dilation of pylorus
Dilation with balloon endoscope
Endoscopic dilation of gastrojejunostomy site

✖ **44.29 Other pyloroplasty**
Pyloroplasty NOS
Revision of pylorus

● **44.3 Gastroenterostomy without gastrectomy**

✖ **44.31 High gastric bypass**
Printen and Mason gastric bypass

✖ **44.32 Percutaneous [endoscopic] gastrojejunostomy**
Endoscopic conversion of gastrostomy or jejunostomy

✖ **44.39 Other gastroenterostomy**
Bypass:
gastroduodenostomy
gastroenterostomy
gastrogastrostomy
Gastrojejunostomy without gastrectomy NOS

● **44.4 Control of hemorrhage and suture of ulcer of stomach or duodenum**

✖ **44.40 Suture of peptic ulcer, not otherwise specified**

✖ **44.41 Suture of gastric ulcer site**
Excludes *ligation of gastric varices (44.91)*

✖ **44.42 Suture of duodenal ulcer site**

44.43 Endoscopic control of gastric or duodenal bleeding

44.44 Transcatheter embolization for gastric or duodenal bleeding
Excludes *surgical occlusion of abdominal vessels (38.86–38.87)*

44.49 Other control of hemorrhage of stomach or duodenum
That with gastrotomy

✖ **44.5 Revision of gastric anastomosis**
Closure of:
gastric anastomosis
gastroduodenostomy
gastrojejunostomy
Pantaloon operation

● **44.6 Other repair of stomach**

✖ **44.61 Suture of laceration of stomach**
Excludes *that of ulcer site (44.41)*

44.62 Closure of gastrostomy

✖ **44.63 Closure of other gastric fistula**
Closure of:
gastrocolic fistula
gastrojejunocolic fistula

✖ **44.64 Gastropexy**

✖ **44.65 Esophagogastroplasty**
Belsey operation
Esophagus and stomach cardioplasty

✖ **44.66 Other procedures for creation of esophagogastric sphincteric competence**
Fundoplication
Gastric cardioplasty
Nissen's fundoplication
Restoration of cardio-esophageal angle

✖ **44.69 Other**
Inversion of gastric diverticulum
Repair of stomach NOS

● **44.9 Other operations on stomach**

✖ **44.91 Ligation of gastric varices**
Excludes *that by endoscopic approach (43.41)*

✖ **44.92 Intraoperative manipulation of stomach**
Reduction of gastric volvulus

44.93 Insertion of gastric bubble (balloon)

44.94 Removal of gastric bubble (balloon)

✖ **44.99 Other**
Excludes *change of gastrostomy tube (97.02)*
dilation of cardiac sphincter (42.92)
gastric:
cooling (96.31)
freezing (96.32)
gavage (96.35)
hypothermia (96.31)
lavage (96.33)
insertion of nasogastric tube (96.07)
irrigation of gastrostomy (96.36)
irrigation of nasogastric tube (96.34)
removal of:
gastrostomy tube (97.51)
intraluminal foreign body from stomach without incision (98.03)
replacement of:
gastrostomy tube (97.02)
(naso-)gastric tube (97.01)

● **45 Incision, excision, and anastomosis of intestine**

Code also any application or administration of an adhesion barrier substance (99.77)

● **45.0 Enterotomy**
Excludes *duodenocholedochotomy (51.41–51.42, 51.51)*
that for destruction of lesion (45.30–45.34)
that of exteriorized intestine (46.14, 46.24, 46.31)

✖ **45.00 Incision of intestine, not otherwise specified**

✖ **45.01 Incision of duodenum**

✖ **45.02 Other incision of small intestine**

✖ **45.03 Incision of large intestine**
Excludes *proctotomy (48.0)*

● **45.1 Diagnostic procedures on small intestine**

Code also any laparotomy (54.11–54.19)

✖ **45.11 Transabdominal endoscopy of small intestine**
Intraoperative endoscopy of small intestine
Excludes *that with biopsy (45.14)*

45.12 Endoscopy of small intestine through artificial stoma
Excludes *that with biopsy (45.14)*

45.13 Other endoscopy of small intestine
Esophagogastroduodenoscopy [EGD]
Excludes *that with biopsy (45.14, 45.16)*

45.14 Closed [endoscopic] biopsy of small intestine
Brushing or washing for specimen collection
Excludes *esophagogastroduodenoscopy [EGD] with closed biopsy (45.16)*

✖ **45.15 Open biopsy of small intestine**

45.16 Esophagogastroduodenoscopy [EGD] with closed biopsy
Biopsy of one or more sites involving esophagus, stomach, and/or duodenum

45.19 Other diagnostic procedures on small intestine

Excludes *microscopic examination of specimen from small intestine (90.91–90.99)*
radioisotope scan (92.04)
ultrasonography (88.74)
x-ray (87.61–87.69)

● **45.2 Diagnostic procedures on large intestine**

Code also any laparotomy (54.11–54.19)

✖ **45.21 Transabdominal endoscopy of large intestine**
Intraoperative endoscopy of large intestine

Excludes *that with biopsy (45.25)*

45.22 Endoscopy of large intestine through artificial stoma

Excludes *that with biopsy (45.25)*

45.23 Colonoscopy
Flexible fiberoptic colonoscopy

Excludes *endoscopy of large intestine through artificial stoma (45.22)*
flexible sigmoidoscopy (45.24)
rigid proctosigmoidoscopy (48.23)
transabdominal endoscopy of large intestine (45.21)

45.24 Flexible sigmoidoscopy
Endoscopy of descending colon

Excludes *rigid proctosigmoidoscopy (48.23)*

45.25 Closed [endoscopic] biopsy of large intestine
Biopsy, closed, of unspecified intestinal site
Brushing or washing for specimen collection
Colonoscopy with biopsy

Excludes *proctosigmoidoscopy with biopsy (48.24)*

✖ **45.26 Open biopsy of large intestine**

45.27 Intestinal biopsy, site unspecified

45.28 Other diagnostic procedures on large intestine

45.29 Other diagnostic procedures on intestine, site unspecified

Excludes *microscopic examination of specimen (90.91–90.99)*
scan and radioisotope function study (92.04)
ultrasonography (88.74)
x-ray (87.61–87.69)

● **45.3 Local excision or destruction of lesion or tissue of small intestine**

45.30 Endoscopic excision or destruction of lesion of duodenum

Excludes *biopsy of duodenum (45.14–45.15)*
control of hemorrhage (44.43)
fistulectomy (46.72)

✖ **45.31 Other local excision of lesion of duodenum**

Excludes *biopsy of duodenum (45.14–45.15)*
fistulectomy (46.72)
multiple segmental resection (45.61)
that by endoscopic approach (45.30)

✖ **45.32 Other destruction of lesion of duodenum**

Excludes *that by endoscopic approach (45.30)*

✖ **45.33 Local excision of lesion or tissue of small intestine, except duodenum**
Excision of redundant mucosa of ileostomy

Excludes *biopsy of small intestine (45.14–45.15)*
fistulectomy (46.74)
multiple segmental resection (45.61)

✖ **45.34 Other destruction of lesion of small intestine, except duodenum**

● **45.4 Local excision or destruction of lesion or tissue of large intestine**

✖ **45.41 Excision of lesion or tissue of large intestine**
Excision of redundant mucosa of colostomy

Excludes *biopsy of large intestine (45.25–45.27)*
endoscopic polypectomy of large intestine (45.42)
fistulectomy (46.76)
multiple segmental resection (45.71)
that by endoscopic approach (45.42–45.43)

45.42 Endoscopic polypectomy of large intestine

Excludes *that by open approach (45.41)*

45.43 Endoscopic destruction of other lesion or tissue of large intestine
Endoscopic ablation of tumor of large intestine
Endoscopic control of colonic bleeding

Excludes *endoscopic polypectomy of large intestine (45.42)*

✖ **45.49 Other destruction of lesion of large intestine**

Excludes *that by endoscopic approach (45.43)*

● **45.5 Isolation of intestinal segment**

Code also any synchronous:
anastomosis other than end-to-end (45.90–45.94)
enterostomy (46.10–46.39)

✖ **45.50 Isolation of intestinal segment, not otherwise specified**
Isolation of intestinal pedicle flap
Reversal of intestinal segment

✖ **45.51 Isolation of segment of small intestine**
Isolation of ileal loop
Resection of small intestine for interposition

✖ **45.52 Isolation of segment of large intestine**
Resection of colon for interposition

● **45.6 Other excision of small intestine**

Code also any synchronous:
anastomosis other than end-to-end (45.90–45.93, 45.95)
colostomy (46.10–46.13)
enterostomy (46.10–46.39)

Excludes *cecectomy (45.72)*
enterocolectomy (45.79)
gastroduodenectomy (43.6–43.99)
ileocolectomy (45.73)
pancreatoduodenectomy (52.51–52.7)

✖ **45.61 Multiple segmental resection of small intestine**
Segmental resection for multiple traumatic lesions of small intestine

✖ **45.62 Other partial resection of small intestine**
Duodenectomy
Ileectomy
Jejunectomy

Excludes *duodenectomy with synchronous pancreatectomy (52.51–52.7)*
resection of cecum and terminal ileum (45.72)

✖ **45.63 Total removal of small intestine**

● **45.7 Partial excision of large intestine**

Code also any synchronous:
anastomosis other than end-to-end (45.92–45.94)
enterostomy (46.10–46.39)

✖ **45.71 Multiple segmental resection of large intestine**
Segmental resection for multiple traumatic lesions of large intestine

✖ **45.72 Cecectomy**
Resection of cecum and terminal ileum

✖ **45.73 Right hemicolectomy**
Ileocolectomy
Right radical colectomy

✖ **45.74 Resection of transverse colon**

✖ **45.75 Left hemicolectomy**

Excludes *proctosigmoidectomy (48.41–48.69)*
second stage Mikulicz operation (46.04)

✖ **45.76 Sigmoidectomy**

✖ **45.79 Other partial excision of large intestine**
Enterocolectomy NEC

✖ **45.8 Total intra-abdominal colectomy**
Excision of cecum, colon, and sigmoid

Excludes *coloproctectomy (48.41–48.69)*

● **45.9 Intestinal anastomosis**

Code also any synchronous resection (45.31–45.8, 48.41–48.69)

Excludes *end-to-end anastomosis—omit code*

✖ **45.90 Intestinal anastomosis, not otherwise specified**

✖ **45.91 Small-to-small intestinal anastomosis**

✖ **45.92 Anastomosis of small intestine to rectal stump**
Hampton procedure

✖ **45.93 Other small-to-large intestinal anastomosis**

✖ **45.94 Large-to-large intestinal anastomosis**

Excludes *rectorectostomy (48.74)*

✖ **45.95 Anastomosis to anus**
Formation of endorectal ileal pouch (H-pouch) (J-pouch) (S-pouch) with anastomosis of small intestine to anus

● **46 Other operations on intestine**

Code also any application or administration of an adhesion barrier substance (99.77)

● **46.0 Exteriorization of intestine**

Includes: loop enterostomy
multiple stage resection of intestine

✖ **46.01 Exteriorization of small intestine**
Loop ileostomy

✖ **46.02 Resection of exteriorized segment of small intestine**

✖ **46.03 Exteriorization of large intestine**
Exteriorization of intestine NOS
First stage Mikulicz exteriorization of intestine
Loop colostomy

✖ **46.04 Resection of exteriorized segment of large intestine**
Resection of exteriorized segment of intestine NOS
Second stage Mikulicz operation

● **46.1 Colostomy**

Code also any synchronous resection (45.49, 45.71–45.79, 45.8)

Excludes *loop colostomy (46.03)*
that with abdominoperineal resection of rectum (48.5)
that with synchronous anterior rectal resection (48.62)

✖ **46.10 Colostomy, not otherwise specified**

✖ **46.11 Temporary colostomy**

✖ **46.13 Permanent colostomy**

46.14 Delayed opening of colostomy

● **46.2 Ileostomy**

Code also any synchronous resection (45.34, 45.61–45.63)

Excludes *loop ileostomy (46.01)*

✖ **46.20 Ileostomy, not otherwise specified**

✖ **46.21 Temporary ileostomy**

✖ **46.22 Continent ileostomy**

✖ **46.23 Other permanent ileostomy**

46.24 Delayed opening of ileostomy

● **46.3 Other enterostomy**

Code also any synchronous resection (45.61–45.8)

46.31 Delayed opening of other enterostomy

46.32 Percutaneous (endoscopic) jejunostomy [PEJ]

46.39 Other
Duodenostomy
Feeding enterostomy

● **46.4 Revision of intestinal stoma**

✖ **46.40 Revision of intestinal stoma, not otherwise specified**
Plastic enlargement of intestinal stoma
Reconstruction of stoma of intestine
Release of scar tissue of intestinal stoma

Excludes *excision of redundant mucosa (45.41)*

✖ **46.41 Revision of stoma of small intestine**

Excludes *excision of redundant mucosa (45.33)*

✖ **46.42 Repair of pericolostomy hernia**

✖ **46.43 Other revision of stoma of large intestine**

Excludes *excision of redundant mucosa (45.41)*

● **46.5 Closure of intestinal stoma**

Code also any synchronous resection (45.34, 45.49, 45.61–45.8)

✖ **46.50 Closure of intestinal stoma, not otherwise specified**

✖ **46.51 Closure of stoma of small intestine**

✖ **46.52 Closure of stoma of large intestine**
Closure or take-down of:
cecostomy
colostomy
sigmoidostomy

● **46.6 Fixation of intestine**

✖ **46.60 Fixation of intestine, not otherwise specified**
Fixation of intestine to abdominal wall

✖ **46.61 Fixation of small intestine to abdominal wall**
Ileopexy

✖ **46.62 Other fixation of small intestine**
Noble plication of small intestine
Plication of jejunum

✖ **46.63 Fixation of large intestine to abdominal wall**
Cecocoloplicopexy
Sigmoidopexy (Moschowitz)

✖ **46.64 Other fixation of large intestine**
Cecofixation
Colofixation

● **46.7 Other repair of intestine**

Excludes *closure of:*
ulcer of duodenum (44.42)
vesicoenteric fistula (57.83)

✖ **46.71 Suture of laceration of duodenum**

✖ **46.72 Closure of fistula of duodenum**

✖46.73 **Suture of laceration of small intestine, except duodenum**

✖46.74 **Closure of fistula of small intestine, except duodenum**

Excludes *closure of:*
artificial stoma (46.51)
vaginal fistula (70.74)
repair of gastrojejunocolic fistula (44.63)

✖46.75 **Suture of laceration of large intestine**

✖46.76 **Closure of fistula of large intestine**

Excludes *closure of:*
gastrocolic fistula (44.63)
rectal fistula (48.73)
sigmoidovesical fistula (57.83)
stoma (46.52)
vaginal fistula (70.72–70.73)
vesicocolic fistula (57.83)
vesicosigmoidovaginal fistula (57.83)

✖46.79 **Other repair of intestine**
Duodenoplasty

● 46.8 **Dilation and manipulation of intestine**

✖46.80 **Intra-abdominal manipulation of intestine, not otherwise specified**
Correction of intestinal malrotation
Reduction of:
intestinal torsion
intestinal volvulus
intussusception

Excludes *reduction of intussusception with:*
fluoroscopy (96.29)
ionizing radiation enema (96.29)
ultrasonography guidance (96.29)

✖46.81 **Intra-abdominal manipulation of small intestine**

✖46.82 **Intra-abdominal manipulation of large intestine**

46.85 **Dilation of intestine**
Dilation (balloon) of duodenum
Dilation (balloon) of jejunum
Endoscopic dilation (balloon) of large intestine
That through rectum or colostomy

● 46.9 **Other operations on intestines**

✖46.91 **Myotomy of sigmoid colon**

✖46.92 **Myotomy of other parts of colon**

✖46.93 **Revision of anastomosis of small intestine**

✖46.94 **Revision of anastomosis of large intestine**

46.95 **Local perfusion of small intestine**
Code also substance perfused (99.21–99.29)

46.96 **Local perfusion of large intestine**
Code also substance perfused (99.21–99.29)

46.97 **Transplant of intestine**

✖46.99 **Other**
Ileoentectropy

Excludes *diagnostic procedures on intestine (45.11–45.29)*
dilation of enterostomy stoma (96.24)
intestinal intubation (96.08)
removal of:
intraluminal foreign body from large intestine without incision (98.04)
intraluminal foreign body from small intestine without incision (98.03)
tube from large intestine (97.53)
tube from small intestine (97.52)
replacement of:
large intestine tube or enterostomy device (97.04)
small intestine tube or enterostomy device (97.03)

● 47 **Operations on appendix**

Code also any application or administration of an adhesion barrier substance (99.77)

Includes: appendiceal stump

✖47.0 **Appendectomy**

Excludes *incidental appendectomy, so described*
laparoscopic (47.11)
other (47.19)

✖47.01 **Laparoscopic appendectomy**

✖47.09 **Other appendectomy**

● 47.1 **Incidental appendectomy**

✖47.11 **Laparoscopic incidental appendectomy**

✖47.19 **Other incidental appendectomy**

✖47.2 **Drainage of appendiceal abscess**

Excludes *that with appendectomy (47.0)*

● 47.9 **Other operations on appendix**

✖47.91 **Appendicostomy**

✖47.92 **Closure of appendiceal fistula**

✖47.99 **Other**
Anastomosis of appendix

Excludes *diagnostic procedures on appendix (45.21–45.29)*

● 48 **Operations on rectum, rectosigmoid and perirectal tissue**

Code also any application or administration of an adhesion barrier substance (99.77)

✖48.0 **Proctotomy**
Decompression of imperforate anus
Panas' operation [linear proctotomy]

Excludes *incision of perirectal tissue (48.81)*

✖48.1 **Proctostomy**

● 48.2 **Diagnostic procedures on rectum, rectosigmoid and perirectal tissue**

✖48.21 **Transabdominal proctosigmoidoscopy**
Intraoperative proctosigmoidoscopy

Excludes *that with biopsy (48.24)*

48.22 **Proctosigmoidoscopy through artificial stoma**

Excludes *that with biopsy (48.24)*

48.23 **Rigid proctosigmoidoscopy**

Excludes *flexible sigmoidoscopy (45.24)*

48.24 **Closed [endoscopic] biopsy of rectum**
Brushing or washing for specimen collection
Proctosigmoidoscopy with biopsy

✖48.25 **Open biopsy of rectum**

48.26 **Biopsy of perirectal tissue**

48.29 **Other diagnostic procedures on rectum, rectosigmoid and perirectal tissue**

Excludes *digital examination of rectum (89.34)*
lower GI series (87.64)
microscopic examination of specimen from rectum (90.91–90.99)

● 48.3 **Local excision or destruction of lesion or tissue of rectum**

48.31 **Radical electrocoagulation of rectal lesion or tissue**

48.32 **Other electrocoagulation of rectal lesion or tissue**

48.33 **Destruction of rectal lesion or tissue by laser**

48.34 **Destruction of rectal lesion or tissue by cryosurgery**

✖48.35 **Local excision of rectal lesion or tissue**

Excludes *biopsy of rectum (48.24–48.25)*
excision of perirectal tissue (48.82)
hemorrhoidectomy (49.46)
[endoscopic] polypectomy of rectum (48.36)
rectal fistulectomy (48.73)

48.36 **[Endoscopic] polypectomy of rectum**

● 48.4 **Pull-through resection of rectum**

Code also any synchronous anastomosis other than end-to-end (45.90, 45.92–45.95)

✖48.41 **Save submucosal resection of rectum**
Endorectal pull-through operation

✖48.49 **Other pull-through resection of rectum**
Abdominoperineal pull-through
Altemeier operation
Swenson proctectomy

Excludes *Duhamel abdominoperineal pull-through (48.65)*

✖48.5 **Abdominoperineal resection of rectum**

Includes: with synchronous colostomy
Combined abdominoendorectal resection
Complete proctectomy

Code also any synchronous anastomosis other than end-to-end (45.90, 45.92–45.95)

Excludes *Duhamel abdominoperineal pull-through (48.65)*
that as part of pelvic exenteration (68.8)

● 48.6 **Other resection of rectum**

Code also any synchronous anastomosis other than end-to-end (45.90, 45.92–45.95)

✖48.61 **Transsacral rectosigmoidectomy**

✖48.62 **Anterior resection of rectum with synchronous colostomy**

✖48.63 **Other anterior resection of rectum**

Excludes *that with synchronous colostomy (48.62)*

✖48.64 **Posterior resection of rectum**

✖48.65 **Duhamel resection of rectum**
Duhamel abdominoperineal pull-through

✖48.69 **Other**
Partial proctectomy
Rectal resection NOS

● 48.7 **Repair of rectum**

Excludes *repair of:*
current obstetric laceration (75.62)
vaginal rectocele (70.50, 70.52)

✖48.71 **Suture of laceration of rectum**

✖48.72 **Closure of proctostomy**

✖48.73 **Closure of other rectal fistula**

Excludes *fistulectomy:*
perirectal (48.93)
rectourethral (58.43)
rectovaginal (70.73)
rectovesical (57.83)
rectovesicovaginal (57.83)

✖48.74 **Rectorectostomy**
Rectal anastomosis NOS

✖48.75 **Abdominal proctopexy**
Frickman procedure
Ripstein repair of rectal prolapse

✖48.76 **Other proctopexy**
Delorme repair of prolapsed rectum
Proctosigmoidopexy
Puborectalis sling operation

Excludes *manual reduction of rectal prolapse (96.26)*

✖48.79 **Other repair of rectum**
Repair of old obstetric laceration of rectum

Excludes *anastomosis to:*
large intestine (45.94)
small intestine (45.92–45.93)
repair of:
current obstetric laceration (75.62)
vaginal rectocele (70.50, 70.52)

● 48.8 **Incision or excision of perirectal tissue or lesion**

Includes: pelvirectal tissue
rectovaginal septum

✖48.81 **Incision of perirectal tissue**
Incision of rectovaginal septum

✖48.82 **Excision of perirectal tissue**

Excludes *perirectal biopsy (48.26)*
perirectofistulectomy (48.93)
rectal fistulectomy (48.73)

● 48.9 **Other operations on rectum and perirectal tissue**

✖48.91 **Incision of rectal stricture**

✖48.92 **Anorectal myectomy**

✖48.93 **Repair of perirectal fistula**

Excludes *that opening into rectum (48.73)*

✖48.99 **Other**

Excludes *digital examination of rectum (89.34)*
dilation of rectum (96.22)
insertion of rectal tube (96.09)
irrigation of rectum (96.38–96.39)
manual reduction of rectal prolapse (96.26)
proctoclysis (96.37)
rectal massage (99.93)
rectal packing (96.19)
removal of:
impacted feces (96.38)
intraluminal foreign body from rectum without incision (98.05)
rectal packing (97.59)
transanal enema (96.39)

● 49 **Operations on anus**

Code also any application or administration of an adhesion barrier substance (99.77)

● 49.0 **Incision or excision of perianal tissue**

✖49.01 **Incision of perianal abscess**

✖49.02 **Other incision of perianal tissue**
Undercutting of perianal tissue

Excludes *anal fistulotomy (49.11)*

49.03 Excision of perianal skin tags

✖49.04 Other excision of perianal tissue

Excludes *anal fistulectomy (49.12)*
biopsy of perianal tissue (49.22)

● 49.1 Incision or excision of anal fistula

Excludes *closure of anal fistula (49.73)*

✖49.11 Anal fistulotomy

✖49.12 Anal fistulectomy

● 49.2 Diagnostic procedures on anus and perianal tissue

49.21 Anoscopy

49.22 Biopsy of perianal tissue

49.23 Biopsy of anus

49.29 Other diagnostic procedures on anus and perianal tissue

Excludes *microscopic examination of specimen from anus (90.91–90.99)*

● 49.3 Local excision or destruction of other lesion or tissue of anus
Anal cryptotomy
Cauterization of lesion of anus

Excludes *biopsy of anus (49.23)*
control of (postoperative) hemorrhage of anus (49.95)
hemorrhoidectomy (49.46)

49.31 Endoscopic excision or destruction of lesion or tissue of anus

✖49.39 Other local excision or destruction of lesion or tissue of anus

Excludes *that by endoscopic approach (49.31)*

● 49.4 Procedures on hemorrhoids

49.41 Reduction of hemorrhoids

49.42 Injection of hemorrhoids

49.43 Cauterization of hemorrhoids
Clamp and cautery of hemorrhoids

✖49.44 Destruction of hemorrhoids by cryotherapy

✖49.45 Ligation of hemorrhoids

✖49.46 Excision of hemorrhoids
Hemorrhoidectomy NOS

49.47 Evacuation of thrombosed hemorrhoids

✖49.49 Other procedures on hemorrhoids
Lord procedure

● 49.5 Division of anal sphincter

✖49.51 Left lateral anal sphincterotomy

✖49.52 Posterior anal sphincterotomy

✖49.59 Other anal sphincterotomy
Division of sphincter NOS

✖49.6 Excision of anus

● 49.7 Repair of anus

Excludes *repair of current obstetric laceration (75.62)*

✖49.71 Suture of laceration of anus

✖49.72 Anal cerclage

✖49.73 Closure of anal fistula

Excludes *excision of anal fistula (49.12)*

✖49.74 Gracilis muscle transplant for anal incontinence

✖49.75 Implantation or revision of artificial anal sphincter
Removal with subsequent replacement
Replacement during same or subsequent operative episode

✖49.76 Removal of artificial anal sphincter
Explanation or removal without replacement

Excludes *revision with implantation during same operative episode (49.75)*

✖49.79 Other repair of anal sphincter
Repair of old obstetric laceration of anus

Excludes *anoplasty with synchronous hemorrhoidectomy (49.46)*
repair of current obstetric laceration (75.62)

● 49.9 Other operations on anus

Excludes *dilation of anus (sphincter) (96.23)*

✖49.91 Incision of anal septum

✖49.92 Insertion of subcutaneous electrical anal stimulator

✖49.93 Other incision of anus
Removal of:
foreign body from anus with incision
seton from anus

Excludes *anal fistulotomy (49.11)*
removal of intraluminal foreign body without incision (98.05)

✖49.94 Reduction of anal prolapse

Excludes *manual reduction of rectal prolapse (96.26)*

✖49.95 Control of (postoperative) hemorrhage of anus

✖49.99 Other

● 50 Operations on liver

Code also any application or administration of an adhesion barrier substance (99.77)

✖50.0 Hepatotomy
Incision of abscess of liver
Removal of gallstones from liver
Stromeyer-Little operation

● 50.1 Diagnostic procedures on liver

50.11 Closed (percutaneous) [needle] biopsy of liver
Diagnostic aspiration of liver

✖50.12 Open biopsy of liver
Wedge biopsy

✖50.19 Other diagnostic procedures on liver

Excludes *liver scan and radioisotope function study (92.02)*
microscopic examination of specimen from liver (91.01–91.09)

● 50.2 Local excision or destruction of liver tissue or lesion

✖50.21 Marsupialization of lesion of liver

✖50.22 Partial hepatectomy
Wedge resection of liver

Excludes *biopsy of liver (50.11–50.12)*
hepatic lobectomy (50.3)

✖50.29 Other destruction of lesion of liver
Cauterization of hepatic lesion
Enucleation of hepatic lesion
Evacuation of hepatic lesion

Excludes *percutaneous aspiration of lesion (50.91)*

✖50.3 Lobectomy of liver
Total hepatic lobectomy with partial excision of other lobe

✖ **50.4 Total hepatectomy**

● **50.5 Liver transplant**

✖ **50.51 Auxiliary liver transplant**
Auxiliary hepatic transplantation leaving patient's own liver in situ

✖ **50.59 Other transplant of liver**

● **50.6 Repair of liver**

✖ **50.61 Closure of laceration of liver**

✖ **50.69 Other repair of liver**
Hepatopexy

● **50.9 Other operations on liver**
Excludes *lysis of adhesions (54.5)*

50.91 Percutaneous aspiration of liver
Excludes *percutaneous biopsy (50.11)*

50.92 Extracorporeal hepatic assistance
Includes: Liver dialysis

50.93 Localized perfusion of liver

50.94 Other injection of therapeutic substance into liver

50.99 Other

● **51 Operations on gallbladder and biliary tract**
Code also any application or administration of an adhesion barrier substance (99.77)

Includes: operations on:
ampulla of Vater
common bile duct
cystic duct
hepatic duct
intrahepatic bile duct
sphincter of Oddi

● **51.0 Cholecystotomy and cholecystostomy**

51.01 Percutaneous aspiration of gallbladder
Percutaneous cholecystotomy for drainage
That by: needle or catheter
Excludes *needle biopsy (51.12)*

✖ **51.02 Trocar cholecystostomy**

✖ **51.03 Other cholecystostomy**

✖ **51.04 Other cholecystotomy**
Cholelithotomy NOS

● **51.1 Diagnostic procedures on biliary tract**
Excludes *that for endoscopic procedures classifiable to 51.64, 51.84–51.88, 52.14, 52.21, 52.93–52.94, 52.97–52.98*

51.10 Endoscopic retrograde cholangiopancreatography [ERCP]
Excludes *endoscopic retrograde:*
cholangiography [ERC] (51.11)
pancreatography [ERP] (52.13)

51.11 Endoscopic retrograde cholangiography [ERC]
Includes: Laparoscopic exploration of common bile duct
Excludes *endoscopic retrograde:*
cholangiopancreatography [ERCP] (51.10)
pancreatography [ERP] (52.13)

51.12 Percutaneous biopsy of gallbladder or bile ducts
Needle biopsy of gallbladder

✖ **51.13 Open biopsy of gallbladder or bile ducts**

51.14 Other closed [endoscopic] biopsy of biliary duct or sphincter of Oddi
Brushing or washing for specimen collection
Closed biopsy of biliary duct or sphincter of Oddi by procedures classifiable to 51.10–51.11, 52.13

51.15 Pressure measurement of sphincter of Oddi
Pressure measurement of sphincter by procedures classifiable to 51.10–51.11, 52.13

✖ **51.19 Other diagnostic procedures on biliary tract**
Excludes *biliary tract x-ray (87.51–87.59)*
microscopic examination of specimen from biliary tract (91.01–91.09)

● **51.2 Cholecystectomy**

✖ **51.21 Other partial cholecystectomy**
Revision of prior cholecystectomy
Excludes *that by laparoscope (51.24)*

✖ **51.22 Cholecystectomy**
Excludes *laparoscopic cholecystectomy (51.23)*

✖ **51.23 Laparoscopic cholecystectomy**
That by laser

✖ **51.24 Laparoscopic partial cholecystectomy**

● **51.3 Anastomosis of gallbladder or bile duct**
Excludes *resection with end-to-end anastomosis (51.61–51.69)*

✖ **51.31 Anastomosis of gallbladder to hepatic ducts**

✖ **51.32 Anastomosis of gallbladder to intestine**

✖ **51.33 Anastomosis of gallbladder to pancreas**

✖ **51.34 Anastomosis of gallbladder to stomach**

✖ **51.35 Other gallbladder anastomosis**
Gallbladder anastomosis NOS

✖ **51.36 Choledochoenterostomy**

✖ **51.37 Anastomosis of hepatic duct to gastrointestinal tract**
Kasai portoenterostomy

✖ **51.39 Other bile duct anastomosis**
Anastomosis of bile duct NOS
Anastomosis of unspecified bile duct to:
intestine
liver
pancreas
stomach

● **51.4 Incision of bile duct for relief of obstruction**

✖ **51.41 Common duct exploration for removal of calculus**
Excludes *percutaneous extraction (51.96)*

✖ **51.42 Common duct exploration for relief of other obstruction**

✖ **51.43 Insertion of choledochohepatic tube for decompression**
Hepatocholedochostomy

✖ **51.49 Incision of other bile ducts for relief of obstruction**

● **51.5 Other incision of bile duct**
Excludes *that for relief of obstruction (51.41–51.49)*

✖ **51.51 Exploration of common duct**
Incision of common bile duct

✖ **51.59 Incision of other bile duct**

● **51.6 Local excision or destruction of lesion or tissue of biliary ducts and sphincter of Oddi**

Code also anastomosis other than end-to-end (51.31, 51.36–51.39)

Excludes *biopsy of bile duct (51.12–51.13)*

✖ **51.61 Excision of cystic duct remnant**

✖ **51.62 Excision of ampulla of Vater (with reimplantation of common duct)**

✖ **51.63 Other excision of common duct**
Choledochectomy

Excludes *fistulectomy (51.72)*

51.64 Endoscopic excision or destruction of lesion of biliary ducts or sphincter of Oddi
Excision or destruction of lesion of biliary duct by procedures classifiable to 51.10–51.11, 52.13

✖ **51.69 Excision of other bile duct**
Excision of lesion of bile duct NOS

Excludes *fistulectomy (51.79)*

● **51.7 Repair of bile ducts**

✖ **51.71 Simple suture of common bile duct**

✖ **51.72 Choledochoplasty**
Repair of fistula of common bile duct

✖ **51.79 Repair of other bile ducts**
Closure of artificial opening of bile duct NOS
Suture of bile duct NOS

Excludes *operative removal of prosthetic device (51.95)*

● **51.8 Other operations on biliary ducts and sphincter of Oddi**

✖ **51.81 Dilation of sphincter of Oddi**
Dilation of ampulla of Vater

Excludes *that by endoscopic approach (51.84)*

✖ **51.82 Pancreatic sphincterotomy**
Incision of pancreatic sphincter
Transduodenal ampullary sphincterotomy

Excludes *that by endoscopic approach (51.85)*

✖ **51.83 Pancreatic sphincteroplasty**

51.84 Endoscopic dilation of ampulla and biliary duct
Dilation of ampulla and biliary duct by procedures classifiable to 51.10–51.11, 52.13

51.85 Endoscopic sphincterotomy and papillotomy
Sphincterotomy and papillotomy by procedures classifiable to 51.10–51.11, 52.13

51.86 Endoscopic insertion of nasobiliary drainage tube
Insertion of nasobiliary tube by procedures classifiable to 51.10–51.11, 52.13

51.87 Endoscopic insertion of stent (tube) into bile duct
Endoprosthesis of bile duct
Insertion of stent into bile duct by procedures classifiable to 51.10–51.11, 52.13

Excludes *nasobiliary drainage tube (51.86)*
replacement of stent (tube) (97.05)

51.88 Endoscopic removal of stone(s) from biliary tract
Laparoscopic removal of stone(s) from biliary tract
Removal of biliary tract stone(s) by procedures classifiable to 51.10–51.11, 52.13

Excludes *percutaneous extraction of common duct stones (51.96)*

✖ **51.89 Other operations on sphincter of Oddi**

● **51.9 Other operations on biliary tract**

✖ **51.91 Repair of laceration of gallbladder**

✖ **51.92 Closure of cholecystostomy**

✖ **51.93 Closure of other biliary fistula**
Cholecystogastroenteric fistulectomy

✖ **51.94 Revision of anastomosis of biliary tract**

✖ **51.95 Removal of prosthetic device from bile duct**

Excludes *nonoperative removal (97.55)*

51.96 Percutaneous extraction of common duct stones

51.98 Other percutaneous procedures on biliary tract
Percutaneous biliary endoscopy via existing T-tube or other tract for:
dilation of biliary duct stricture
removal of stone(s) except common duct stone
exploration (postoperative)
Percutaneous transhepatic biliary drainage

Excludes *percutaneous aspiration of gallbladder (51.01)*
percutaneous biopsy and/or collection of specimen by brushing or washing (51.12)
percutaneous removal of common duct stone(s) (51.96)

✖ **51.99 Other**
Insertion or replacement of biliary tract prosthesis

Excludes *biopsy of gallbladder (51.12–51.13)*
irrigation of cholecystostomy and other biliary tube (96.41)
lysis of peritoneal adhesions (54.5)
nonoperative removal of:
cholecystostomy tube (97.54)
tube from biliary tract or liver (97.55)

● **52 Operations on pancreas**

Code also any application or administration of an adhesion barrier substance (99.77)

Includes: operations on pancreatic duct

● **52.0 Pancreatotomy**

✖ **52.01 Drainage of pancreatic cyst by catheter**

✖ **52.09 Other pancreatotomy**
Pancreatolithotomy

Excludes *drainage by anastomosis (52.4, 52.96)*
incision of pancreatic sphincter (51.82)
marsupialization of cyst (52.3)

● **52.1 Diagnostic procedures on pancreas**

52.11 Closed [aspiration] [needle] [percutaneous] biopsy of pancreas

✖ **52.12 Open biopsy of pancreas**

52.13 Endoscopic retrograde pancreatography [ERP]

Excludes *endoscopic retrograde:*
cholangiography [ERC] (51.11)
cholangiopancreatography [ERCP] (51.10)
that for procedures classifiable to 51.14–51.15, 51.64, 51.84–51.88, 52.14, 52.21, 52.92–52.94, 52.97–52.98

52.14 Closed [endoscopic] biopsy of pancreatic duct
Closed biopsy of pancreatic duct by procedures classifiable to 51.10–51.11, 52.13

✖ **52.19 Other diagnostic procedures on pancreas**

Excludes *contrast pancreatogram (87.66)*
endoscopic retrograde pancreatography [ERP] (52.13)
microscopic examination of specimen from pancreas (91.01–91.09)

● 52.2 **Local excision or destruction of pancreas and pancreatic duct**

Excludes *biopsy of pancreas (52.11–52.12, 52.14)*
pancreatic fistulectomy (52.95)

52.21 **Endoscopic excision or destruction of lesion or tissue of pancreatic duct**
Excision or destruction of lesion or tissue of pancreatic duct by procedures classifiable to 51.10–51.11, 52.13

✖ 52.22 **Other excision or destruction of lesion or tissue of pancreas or pancreatic duct**

✖ 52.3 **Marsupialization of pancreatic cyst**

Excludes *drainage of cyst by catheter (52.01)*

✖ 52.4 **Internal drainage of pancreatic cyst**
Pancreaticocystoduodenostomy
Pancreaticocystogastrostomy
Pancreaticocystojejunostomy

● 52.5 **Partial pancreatectomy**

Excludes *pancreatic fistulectomy (52.95)*

✖ 52.51 **Proximal pancreatectomy**
Excision of head of pancreas (with part of body)
Proximal pancreatectomy with synchronous duodenectomy

✖ 52.52 **Distal pancreatectomy**
Excision of tail of pancreas (with part of body)

✖ 52.53 **Radical subtotal pancreatectomy**

✖ 52.59 **Other partial pancreatectomy**

✖ 52.6 **Total pancreatectomy**
Pancreatectomy with synchronous duodenectomy

✖ 52.7 **Radical pancreaticoduodenectomy**
One-stage pancreaticoduodenal resection with choledochojejunal anastomosis, pancreaticojejunal anastomosis, and gastrojejunostomy
Two-stage pancreaticoduodenal resection (first stage) (second stage)
Radical resection of the pancreas
Whipple procedure

Excludes *radical subtotal pancreatectomy (52.53)*

● 52.8 **Transplant of pancreas**

✖ 52.80 **Pancreatic transplant, not otherwise specified**

✖ 52.81 **Reimplantation of pancreatic tissue**

✖ 52.82 **Homotransplant of pancreas**

✖ 52.83 **Heterotransplant of pancreas**

52.84 **Autotransplantation of cells of Islets of Langerhans**
Homotransplantation of islet cells of pancreas

52.85 **Allotransplantation of cells of Islets of Langerhans**
Heterotransplantation of islet cells of pancreas

✖ 52.86 **Transplantation of cells of Islets of Langerhans, not otherwise specified**

● 52.9 **Other operations on pancreas**

✖ 52.92 **Cannulation of pancreatic duct**

Excludes *that by endoscopic approach (52.93)*

52.93 **Endoscopic insertion of stent (tube) into pancreatic duct**
Insertion of cannula or stent into pancreatic duct by procedures classifiable to 51.10–51.11, 52.13

Excludes *endoscopic insertion of nasopancreatic drainage tube (52.97)*
replacement of stent (tube) (97.05)

52.94 **Endoscopic removal of stone(s) from pancreatic duct**
Removal of stone(s) from pancreatic duct by procedures classifiable to 51.10–51.11, 52.13

✖ 52.95 **Other repair of pancreas**
Fistulectomy of pancreas
Simple suture of pancreas

✖ 52.96 **Anastomosis of pancreas**
Anastomosis of pancreas (duct) to:
intestine
jejunum
stomach

Excludes *anastomosis to:*
bile duct (51.39)
gallbladder (51.33)

52.97 **Endoscopic insertion of nasopancreatic drainage tube**
Insertion of nasopancreatic drainage tube by procedures classifiable to 51.10–51.11, 52.13

Excludes *drainage of pancreatic cyst by catheter (52.01)*
replacement of stent (tube) (97.05)

52.98 **Endoscopic dilation of pancreatic duct**
Dilation of Wirsung's duct by procedures classifiable to 51.10–51.11, 52.13

✖ 52.99 **Other**
Dilation of pancreatic [Wirsung's] duct by open approach
Repair of pancreatic [Wirsung's] duct by open approach

Excludes *irrigation of pancreatic tube (96.42)*
removal of pancreatic tube (97.56)

● 53 **Repair of hernia**

Code also any application or administration of an adhesion barrier substance (99.77)

Includes: hernioplasty
herniorrhaphy

Excludes *manual reduction of hernia (96.27)*

● 53.0 **Unilateral repair of inguinal hernia**

✖ 53.00 **Unilateral repair of inguinal hernia, not otherwise specified**
Inguinal herniorrhaphy NOS

✖ 53.01 **Repair of direct inguinal hernia**

✖ 53.02 **Repair of indirect inguinal hernia**

✖ 53.03 **Repair of direct inguinal hernia with graft or prosthesis**

✖ 53.04 **Repair of indirect inguinal hernia with graft or prosthesis**

✖ 53.05 **Repair of inguinal hernia with graft or prosthesis, not otherwise specified**

● 53.1 **Bilateral repair of inguinal hernia**

✖ 53.10 **Bilateral repair of inguinal hernia, not otherwise specified**

✖ 53.11 **Bilateral repair of direct inguinal hernia**

✖ 53.12 **Bilateral repair of indirect inguinal hernia**

✖ 53.13 **Bilateral repair of inguinal hernia, one direct and one indirect**

✖ 53.14 **Bilateral repair of direct inguinal hernia with graft or prosthesis**

✖ 53.15 **Bilateral repair of indirect inguinal hernia with graft or prosthesis**

✖ 53.16 **Bilateral repair of inguinal hernia, one direct and one indirect, with graft or prosthesis**

✖ 53.17 **Bilateral inguinal hernia repair with graft or prosthesis, not otherwise specified**

● 53.2 **Unilateral repair of femoral hernia**

✖ 53.21 **Unilateral repair of femoral hernia with graft or prosthesis**

✖ 53.29 **Other unilateral femoral herniorrhaphy**

● 53.3 **Bilateral repair of femoral hernia**

✖ 53.31 **Bilateral repair of femoral hernia with graft or prosthesis**

✖ 53.39 **Other bilateral femoral herniorrhaphy**

● 53.4 **Repair of umbilical hernia**

Excludes *repair of gastroschisis (54.71)*

✖ 53.41 **Repair of umbilical hernia with prosthesis**

✖ 53.49 **Other umbilical herniorrhaphy**

● 53.5 **Repair of other hernia of anterior abdominal wall (without graft or prosthesis)**

✖ 53.51 **Incisional hernia repair**

✖ 53.59 **Repair of other hernia of anterior abdominal wall**

Repair of hernia:
- epigastric
- hypogastric
- spigelian
- ventral

● 53.6 **Repair of other hernia of anterior abdominal wall with graft or prosthesis**

✖ 53.61 **Incisional hernia repair with prosthesis**

✖ 53.69 **Repair of other hernia of anterior abdominal wall with prosthesis**

✖ 53.7 **Repair of diaphragmatic hernia, abdominal approach**

● 53.8 **Repair of diaphragmatic hernia, thoracic approach**

✖ 53.80 **Repair of diaphragmatic hernia with thoracic approach, not otherwise specified**

Thoracoabdominal repair of diaphragmatic hernia

✖ 53.81 **Plication of the diaphragm**

✖ 53.82 **Repair of parasternal hernia**

✖ 53.9 **Other hernia repair**

Repair of hernia:
- ischiatic
- ischiorectal
- lumbar
- obturator
- omental
- retroperitoneal
- sciatic

Excludes *relief of strangulated hernia with exteriorization of intestine (46.01, 46.03)*
repair of pericolostomy hernia (46.42)
repair of vaginal enterocele (70.92)

● 54 **Other operations on abdominal region**

Code also any application or administration of an adhesion barrier substance (99.77)

Includes: operations on:
- epigastric region
- flank
- groin region
- hypochondrium
- inguinal region
- loin region
- male pelvic cavity
- mesentery
- omentum
- peritoneum
- retroperitoneal tissue space

Excludes *female pelvic cavity (69.01–70.92)*
hernia repair (53.00–53.9)
obliteration of cul-de-sac (70.92)
retroperitoneal tissue dissection (59.00–59.09)
skin and subcutaneous tissue of abdominal wall (86.01–86.99)

✖ 54.0 **Incision of abdominal wall**

Drainage of:
- abdominal wall
- extraperitoneal abscess
- retroperitoneal abscess

Excludes *incision of peritoneum (54.95)*
laparotomy (54.11–54.19)

● 54.1 **Laparotomy**

✖ 54.11 **Exploratory laparotomy**

Excludes *exploration incidental to intra- abdominal surgery—omit code*

✖ 54.12 **Reopening of recent laparotomy site**

Reopening of recent laparotomy site for:
- control of hemorrhage
- exploration
- incision of hematoma

✖ 54.19 **Other laparotomy**

Drainage of intraperitoneal abscess or hematoma

Excludes *culdocentesis (70.0)*
drainage of appendiceal abscess (47.2)
exploration incidental to intra-abdominal surgery—omit code
Ladd operation (54.95)
percutaneous drainage of abdomen (54.91)
removal of foreign body (54.92)

● 54.2 **Diagnostic procedures of abdominal region**

✖ 54.21 **Laparoscopy**

Peritoneoscopy

Excludes *laparoscopic cholecystectomy (51.23)*
that incidental to destruction of fallopian tubes (66.21–66.29)

✖ 54.22 **Biopsy of abdominal wall or umbilicus**

✖ 54.23 **Biopsy of peritoneum**

Biopsy of:
- mesentery
- omentum
- peritoneal implant

Excludes *closed biopsy of:*
omentum (54.24)
peritoneum (54.24)

54.24 **Closed [percutaneous] [needle] biopsy of intra-abdominal mass**

Closed biopsy of:
- omentum
- peritoneal implant
- peritoneum

Excludes *that of:*
fallopian tube (66.11)
ovary (65.11)
uterine ligaments (68.15)
uterus (68.16)

54.25 Peritoneal lavage
Diagnostic peritoneal lavage

Excludes *peritoneal dialysis (54.98)*

✖ **54.29 Other diagnostic procedures on abdominal region**

Excludes *abdominal lymphangiogram (88.04)*
abdominal x-ray NEC (88.19)
angiocardiography of venae cava (88.51)
C.A.T. scan of abdomen (88.01)
contrast x-ray of abdominal cavity (88.11–88.15)
intra-abdominal arteriography NEC (88.47)
microscopic examination of peritoneal and retroperitoneal specimen (91.11–91.19)
phlebography of:
intra-abdominal vessels NEC (88.65)
portal venous system (88.64)
sinogram of abdominal wall (88.03)
soft tissue x-ray of abdominal wall NEC (88.09)
tomography of abdomen NEC (88.02)
ultrasonography of abdomen and retroperitoneum (88.76)

✖ **54.3 Excision or destruction of lesion or tissue of abdominal wall or umbilicus**
Debridement of abdominal wall
Omphalectomy

Excludes *biopsy of abdominal wall or umbilicus (54.22)*
size reduction operation (86.83)
that of skin of abdominal wall (86.22, 86.26, 86.3)

✖ **54.4 Excision or destruction of peritoneal tissue**
Excision of:
appendices epiploicae
falciform ligament
gastrocolic ligament
lesion of:
mesentery
omentum
peritoneum
presacral lesion NOS
retroperitoneal lesion NOS

Excludes *biopsy of peritoneum (54.23)*
endometrectomy of cul-de-sac (70.32)

54.5 Lysis of peritoneal adhesions
Freeing of adhesions of:
biliary tract
intestines
liver
pelvic peritoneum
peritoneum
spleen
uterus

Excludes *lysis of adhesions of:*
bladder (59.11)
fallopian tube and ovary
laparoscopic (65.81)
other (65.89)
kidney (59.02)
ureter (59.02)

✖ **54.51 Laparoscopic lysis of peritoneal adhesions**

✖ **54.59 Other lysis of peritoneal adhesions**

● **54.6 Suture of abdominal wall and peritoneum**

✖ **54.61 Reclosure of postoperative disruption of abdominal wall**

✖ **54.62 Delayed closure of granulating abdominal wound**
Tertiary subcutaneous wound closure

✖ **54.63 Other suture of abdominal wall**
Suture of laceration of abdominal wall

Excludes *closure of operative wound—omit code*

✖ **54.64 Suture of peritoneum**
Secondary suture of peritoneum

Excludes *closure of operative wound—omit code*

● **54.7 Other repair of abdominal wall and peritoneum**

✖ **54.71 Repair of gastroschisis**

✖ **54.72 Other repair of abdominal wall**

✖ **54.73 Other repair of peritoneum**
Suture of gastrocolic ligament

✖ **54.74 Other repair of omentum**
Epiplorrhaphy
Graft of omentum
Omentopexy
Reduction of torsion of omentum

Excludes *cardio-omentopexy (36.39)*

✖ **54.75 Other repair of mesentery**
Mesenteric plication
Mesenteropexy

● **54.9 Other operations of abdominal region**

Excludes *removal of ectopic pregnancy (74.3)*

54.91 Percutaneous abdominal drainage
Paracentesis

Excludes *creation of cutaneoperitoneal fistula (54.93)*

✖ **54.92 Removal of foreign body from peritoneal cavity**

✖ **54.93 Creation of cutaneoperitoneal fistula**

✖ **54.94 Creation of peritoneovascular shunt**
Peritoneovenous shunt

✖ **54.95 Incision of peritoneum**
Exploration of ventriculoperitoneal shunt at peritoneal site
Ladd operation
Revision of distal catheter of ventricular shunt
Revision of ventriculoperitoneal shunt at peritoneal site

Excludes *that incidental to laparotomy (54.11–54.19)*

54.96 Injection of air into peritoneal cavity
Pneumoperitoneum

Excludes *that for:*
collapse of lung (33.33)
radiography (88.12–88.13, 88.15)

54.97 Injection of locally-acting therapeutic substance into peritoneal cavity

Excludes *peritoneal dialysis (54.98)*

54.98 Peritoneal dialysis

Excludes *peritoneal lavage (diagnostic) (54.25)*

54.99 Other

Excludes *removal of:*
abdominal wall suture (97.83)
peritoneal drainage device (97.82)
retroperitoneal drainage device (97.81)

10. OPERATIONS ON THE URINARY SYSTEM (55–59)

● 55 **Operations on kidney**

Code also any application or administration of an adhesion barrier substance (99.77)

Includes: operations on renal pelvis

Excludes *perirenal tissue (59.00–59.09, 59.21–59.29, 59.91–59.92)*

● 55.0 **Nephrotomy and nephrostomy**

Excludes *drainage by:*
anastomosis (55.86)
aspiration (55.92)
incision of kidney pelvis (55.11–55.12)

✖ 55.01 **Nephrotomy**
Evacuation of renal cyst
Exploration of kidney
Nephrolithotomy

✖ 55.02 **Nephrostomy**

✖ 55.03 **Percutaneous nephrostomy without fragmentation**
Nephrostolithotomy, percutaneous (nephroscopic)
Percutaneous removal of kidney stone(s) by:
basket extraction
forceps extraction (nephroscopic)
Pyelostolithotomy, percutaneous (nephroscopic)
With placement of catheter down ureter

Excludes *percutaneous removal by fragmentation (55.04)*
repeat nephroscopic removal during current episode (55.92)

✖ 55.04 **Percutaneous nephrostomy with fragmentation**
Percutaneous nephrostomy with disruption of kidney stone by ultrasonic energy and extraction (suction) through endoscope
With placement of catheter down ureter
With fluoroscopic guidance

Excludes *repeat fragmentation during current episode (59.95)*

● 55.1 **Pyelotomy and pyelostomy**

Excludes *drainage by anastomosis (55.86)*
percutaneous pyelostolithotomy (55.03)
removal of calculus without incision (56.0)

✖ 55.11 **Pyelotomy**
Exploration of renal pelvis
Pyelolithotomy

✖ 55.12 **Pyelostomy**
Insertion of drainage tube into renal pelvis

● 55.2 **Diagnostic procedures on kidney**

55.21 **Nephroscopy**

55.22 **Pyeloscopy**

55.23 **Closed [percutaneous] [needle] biopsy of kidney**
Endoscopic biopsy via existing nephrostomy, nephrotomy, pyelostomy, or pyelotomy

✖ 55.24 **Open biopsy of kidney**

✖ 55.29 **Other diagnostic procedures on kidney**

Excludes *microscopic examination of specimen from kidney (91.21–91.29)*
pyelogram:
intravenous (87.73)
percutaneous (87.75)
retrograde (87.74)
radioisotope scan (92.03)
renal arteriography (88.45)
tomography:
C.A.T. scan (87.71)
other (87.72)

● 55.3 **Local excision or destruction of lesion or tissue of kidney**

✖ 55.31 **Marsupialization of kidney lesion**

✖ 55.39 **Other local destruction or excision of renal lesion or tissue**
Obliteration of calyceal diverticulum

Excludes *biopsy of kidney (55.23–55.24)*
partial nephrectomy (55.4)
percutaneous aspiration of kidney (55.92)
wedge resection of kidney (55.4)

✖ 55.4 **Partial nephrectomy**
Calycectomy
Wedge resection of kidney

Code also any synchronous resection of ureter (56.40–56.42)

● 55.5 **Complete nephrectomy**

Code also any synchronous excision of:
bladder segment (57.6)
lymph nodes (40.3, 40.52–40.59)

✖ 55.51 **Nephroureterectomy**
Nephroureterectomy with bladder cuff
Total nephrectomy (unilateral)

Excludes *removal of transplanted kidney (55.53)*

✖ 55.52 **Nephrectomy of remaining kidney**
Removal of solitary kidney

Excludes *removal of transplanted kidney (55.53)*

✖ 55.53 **Removal of transplanted or rejected kidney**

✖ 55.54 **Bilateral nephrectomy**

Excludes *complete nephrectomy NOS (55.51)*

● 55.6 **Transplant of kidney**

✖ 55.61 **Renal autotransplantation**

✖ 55.69 **Other kidney transplantation**

✖ 55.7 **Nephropexy**
Fixation or suspension of movable [floating] kidney

● 55.8 **Other repair of kidney**

✖ 55.81 **Suture of laceration of kidney**

✖ 55.82 **Closure of nephrostomy and pyelostomy**

✖ 55.83 **Closure of other fistula of kidney**

✖ 55.84 **Reduction of torsion of renal pedicle**

✖ 55.85 **Symphysiotomy for horseshoe kidney**

✖ 55.86 **Anastomosis of kidney**
Nephropyeloureterostomy
Pyeloureterovesical anastomosis
Ureterocalyceal anastomosis

Excludes *nephrocystanastomosis NOS (56.73)*

✖ 55.87 **Correction of ureteropelvic junction**

✖ 55.89 **Other**

● 55.9 **Other operations on kidney**

Excludes *lysis of perirenal adhesions (59.02)*

✖ 55.91 **Decapsulation of kidney**
Capsulectomy of kidney
Decortication of kidney

55.92 **Percutaneous aspiration of kidney (pelvis)**
Aspiration of renal cyst
Renipuncture

Excludes *percutaneous biopsy of kidney (55.23)*

55.93 **Replacement of nephrostomy tube**

55.94 **Replacement of pyelostomy tube**

55.95 **Local perfusion of kidney**

55.96 Other injection of therapeutic substance into kidney
Injection into renal cyst

✖**55.97 Implantation or replacement of mechanical kidney**

✖**55.98 Removal of mechanical kidney**

✖**55.99 Other**
Excludes *removal of pyelostomy or nephrostomy tube (97.61)*

● **56 Operations on ureter**

Code also any application or administration of an adhesion barrier substance (99.77)

✖**56.0 Transurethral removal of obstruction from ureter and renal pelvis**
Removal of:
blood clot from ureter or renal pelvis without incision
calculus from ureter or renal pelvis without incision
foreign body from ureter or renal pelvis without incision
Excludes *manipulation without removal of obstruction (59.8)*
that by incision (55.11, 56.2)
transurethral insertion of ureteral stent for passage of calculus (59.8)

✖**56.1 Ureteral meatotomy**

✖**56.2 Ureterotomy**
Incision of ureter for:
drainage
exploration
removal of calculus
Excludes *cutting of ureterovesical orifice (56.1)*
removal of calculus without incision (56.0)
transurethral insertion of ureteral stent for passage of calculus (59.8)
urinary diversion (56.51–56.79)

● **56.3 Diagnostic procedures on ureter**

56.31 Ureteroscopy

56.32 Closed percutaneous biopsy of ureter
Excludes *endoscopic biopsy of ureter (56.33)*

56.33 Closed endoscopic biopsy of ureter
Cystourethroscopy with ureteral biopsy
Transurethral biopsy of ureter
Ureteral endoscopy with biopsy through ureterotomy
Ureteroscopy with biopsy
Excludes *percutaneous biopsy of ureter (56.32)*

✖**56.34 Open biopsy of ureter**

56.35 Endoscopy (cystoscopy) (looposcopy) of ileal conduit

✖**56.39 Other diagnostic procedures on ureter**
Excludes *microscopic examination of specimen from ureter (91.21–91.29)*

● **56.4 Ureterectomy**

Code also anastomosis other than end-to-end (56.51–56.79)

Excludes *fistulectomy (56.84)*
nephroureterectomy (55.51–55.54)

✖**56.40 Ureterectomy, not otherwise specified**

✖**56.41 Partial ureterectomy**
Excision of lesion of ureter
Shortening of ureter with reimplantation
Excludes *biopsy of ureter (56.32–56.34)*

✖**56.42 Total ureterectomy**

● **56.5 Cutaneous uretero-ileostomy**

✖**56.51 Formation of cutaneous uretero-ileostomy**
Construction of ileal conduit
External ureteral ileostomy
Formation of open ileal bladder
Ileal loop operation
Ileoureterostomy (Bricker's) (ileal bladder)
Transplantation of ureter into ileum with external diversion
Excludes *closed ileal bladder (57.87)*
replacement of ureteral defect by ileal segment (56.89)

✖**56.52 Revision of cutaneous uretero-ileostomy**

● **56.6 Other external urinary diversion**

✖**56.61 Formation of other cutaneous ureterostomy**
Anastomosis of ureter to skin
Ureterostomy NOS

✖**56.62 Revision of other cutaneous ureterostomy**
Revision of ureterostomy stoma
Excludes *nonoperative removal of ureterostomy tube (97.62)*

● **56.7 Other anastomosis or bypass of ureter**
Excludes *ureteropyelostomy (55.86)*

✖**56.71 Urinary diversion to intestine**
Anastomosis of ureter to intestine
Internal urinary diversion NOS

Code also any synchronous colostomy (46.10–46.13)

Excludes *external ureteral ileostomy (56.51)*

✖**56.72 Revision of ureterointestinal anastomosis**
Excludes *revision of external ureteral ileostomy (56.52)*

✖**56.73 Nephrocystanastomosis, not otherwise specified**

✖**56.74 Ureteroneocystostomy**
Replacement of ureter with bladder flap
Ureterovesical anastomosis

✖**56.75 Transureteroureterostomy**
Excludes *ureteroureterostomy associated with partial resection (56.41)*

✖**56.79 Other**

● **56.8 Repair of ureter**

✖**56.81 Lysis of intraluminal adhesions of ureter**
Excludes *lysis of periureteral adhesions (59.01–59.02)*
ureterolysis (59.01–59.02)

✖**56.82 Suture of laceration of ureter**

✖**56.83 Closure of ureterostomy**

✖**56.84 Closure of other fistula of ureter**

✖**56.85 Ureteropexy**

✖**56.86 Removal of ligature from ureter**

✖**56.89 Other repair of ureter**
Graft of ureter
Replacement of ureter with ileal segment implanted into bladder
Ureteroplication

● **56.9 Other operations on ureter**

56.91 Dilation of ureteral meatus

✖**56.92 Implantation of electronic ureteral stimulator**

✖**56.93 Replacement of electronic ureteral stimulator**

✖ **56.94 Removal of electronic ureteral stimulator**

Excludes *that with synchronous replacement (56.93)*

✖ **56.95 Ligation of ureter**

✖ **56.99 Other**

Excludes *removal of ureterostomy tube and ureteral catheter (97.62)*
ureteral catheterization (59.8)

● **57 Operations on urinary bladder**

Code also any application or administration of an adhesion barrier substance (99.77)

Excludes *perivesical tissue (59.11–59.29, 59.91–59.92)*
ureterovesical orifice (56.0–56.99)

57.0 Transurethral clearance of bladder
Drainage of bladder without incision
Removal of:
blood clots from bladder without incision
calculus from bladder without incision
foreign body from bladder without incision

Excludes *that by incision (57.19)*

● **57.1 Cystotomy and cystostomy**

Excludes *cystotomy and cystostomy as operative approach—omit code*

57.11 Percutaneous aspiration of bladder

✖ **57.12 Lysis of intraluminal adhesions with incision into bladder**

Excludes *transurethral lysis of intraluminal adhesions (57.41)*

57.17 Percutaneous cystostomy
Closed cystostomy
Percutaneous suprapubic cystostomy

Excludes *removal of cystostomy tube (97.63)*
replacement of cystostomy tube (59.94)

✖ **57.18 Other suprapubic cystostomy**

Excludes *percutaneous cystostomy (57.17)*
removal of cystostomy tube (97.63)
replacement of cystostomy tube (59.94)

✖ **57.19 Other cystotomy**
Cystolithotomy

Excludes *percutaneous cystostomy (57.17)*
suprapubic cystostomy (57.18)

● **57.2 Vesicostomy**

Excludes *percutaneous cystostomy (57.17)*
suprapubic cystostomy (57.18)

✖ **57.21 Vesicostomy**
Creation of permanent opening from bladder to skin using a bladder flap

✖ **57.22 Revision or closure of vesicostomy**

Excludes *closure of cystostomy (57.82)*

● **57.3 Diagnostic procedures on bladder**

57.31 Cystoscopy through artificial stoma

57.32 Other cystoscopy
Transurethral cystoscopy

Excludes *cystourethroscopy with ureteral biopsy (56.33)*
retrograde pyelogram (87.74)
that for control of hemorrhage (postoperative):
bladder (57.93)
prostate (60.94)

✖ **57.33 Closed [transurethral] biopsy of bladder**

✖ **57.34 Open biopsy of bladder**

✖ **57.39 Other diagnostic procedures on bladder**

Excludes *cystogram NEC (87.77)*
microscopic examination of specimen from bladder (91.31–91.39)
retrograde cystourethrogram (87.76)
therapeutic distention of bladder (96.25)

● **57.4 Transurethral excision or destruction of bladder tissue**

✖ **57.41 Transurethral lysis of intraluminal adhesions**

✖ **57.49 Other transurethral excision or destruction of lesion or tissue of bladder**
Endoscopic resection of bladder lesion

Excludes *transurethral biopsy of bladder (57.33)*
transurethral fistulectomy (57.83–57.84)

● **57.5 Other excision or destruction of bladder tissue**

Excludes *that with transurethral approach (57.41–57.49)*

✖ **57.51 Excision of urachus**
Excision of urachal sinus of bladder

Excludes *excision of urachal cyst of abdominal wall (54.3)*

✖ **57.59 Open excision or destruction of other lesion or tissue of bladder**
Endometrectomy of bladder
Suprapubic excision of bladder lesion

Excludes *biopsy of bladder (57.33–57.34)*
fistulectomy of bladder (57.83–57.84)

✖ **57.6 Partial cystectomy**
Excision of bladder dome
Trigonectomy
Wedge resection of bladder

● **57.7 Total cystectomy**

Includes: total cystectomy with urethrectomy

✖ **57.71 Radical cystectomy**
Pelvic exenteration in male
Removal of bladder, prostate, seminal vesicles, and fat
Removal of bladder, urethra, and fat in a female

Code also any:
lymph node dissection (40.3, 40.5)
urinary diversion (56.51–56.79)

Excludes *that as part of pelvic exenteration in female (68.8)*

✖ **57.79 Other total cystectomy**

● **57.8 Other repair of urinary bladder**

Excludes *repair of:*
current obstetric laceration (75.61)
cystocele (70.50–70.51)
that for stress incontinence (59.3–59.79)

✖ **57.81 Suture of laceration of bladder**

✖ **57.82 Closure of cystostomy**

✖ **57.83 Repair of fistula involving bladder and intestine**
Rectovesicovaginal fistulectomy
Vesicosigmoidovaginal fistulectomy

✖ **57.84 Repair of other fistula of bladder**
Cervicovesical fistulectomy
Urethroperineovesical fistulectomy
Uterovesical fistulectomy
Vaginovesical fistulectomy

Excludes *vesicoureterovaginal fistulectomy (56.84)*

✖ **57.85 Cystourethroplasty and plastic repair of bladder neck**
Plication of sphincter of urinary bladder
V-Y plasty of bladder neck

✖ **57.86 Repair of bladder exstrophy**

57.87 Reconstruction of urinary bladder
Anastomosis of bladder with isolated segment of ileum
Augmentation of bladder
Replacement of bladder with ileum or sigmoid [closed ileal bladder]

Code also resection of intestine (45.50–45.52)

57.88 Other anastomosis of bladder
Anastomosis of bladder to intestine NOS
Cystocolic anastomosis

Excludes *formation of closed ileal bladder (57.87)*

57.89 Other repair of bladder
Bladder suspension, not elsewhere classified
Cystopexy NOS
Repair of old obstetric laceration of bladder

Excludes *repair of current obstetric laceration (75.61)*

57.9 Other operations on bladder

57.91 Sphincterotomy of bladder
Division of bladder neck

57.92 Dilation of bladder neck

57.93 Control of (postoperative) hemorrhage of bladder

57.94 Insertion of indwelling urinary catheter

57.95 Replacement of indwelling urinary catheter

57.96 Implantation of electronic bladder stimulator

57.97 Replacement of electronic bladder stimulator

57.98 Removal of electronic bladder stimulator

Excludes *that with synchronous replacement (57.97)*

57.99 Other

Excludes *irrigation of:*
cystostomy (96.47)
other indwelling urinary catheter (96.48)
lysis of external adhesions (59.11)
removal of:
cystostomy tube (97.63)
other urinary drainage device (97.64)
therapeutic distention of bladder (96.25)

58 Operations on urethra

Code also any application or administration of an adhesion barrier substance (99.77)

Includes: operations on:
bulbourethral gland [Cowper's gland]
periurethral tissue

58.0 Urethrotomy
Excision of urethral septum
Formation of urethrovaginal fistula
Perineal urethrostomy
Removal of calculus from urethra by incision

Excludes *drainage of bulbourethral gland or periurethral tissue (58.91)*
internal urethral meatotomy (58.5)
removal of urethral calculus without incision (58.6)

58.1 Urethral meatotomy

Excludes *internal urethral meatotomy (58.5)*

58.2 Diagnostic procedures on urethra

58.21 Perineal urethroscopy

58.22 Other urethroscopy

58.23 Biopsy of urethra

58.24 Biopsy of periurethral tissue

58.29 Other diagnostic procedures on urethra and periurethral tissue

Excludes *microscopic examination of specimen from urethra (91.31–91.39)*
retrograde cystourethrogram (87.76)
urethral pressure profile (89.25)
urethral sphincter electromyogram (89.23)

58.3 Excision or destruction of lesion or tissue of urethra

Excludes *biopsy of urethra (58.23)*
excision of bulbourethral gland (58.92)
fistulectomy (58.43)
urethrectomy as part of:
complete cystectomy (57.79)
pelvic evisceration (68.8)
radical cystectomy (57.71)

58.31 Endoscopic excision or destruction of lesion or tissue of urethra
Fulguration of urethral lesion

58.39 Other local excision or destruction of lesion or tissue of urethra
Excision of:
congenital valve of urethra
lesion of urethra
stricture of urethra
Urethrectomy

Excludes *that by endoscopic approach (58.31)*

58.4 Repair of urethra

Excludes *repair of current obstetric laceration (75.61)*

58.41 Suture of laceration of urethra

58.42 Closure of urethrostomy

58.43 Closure of other fistula of urethra

Excludes *repair of urethroperineovesical fistula (57.84)*

58.44 Reanastomosis of urethra
Anastomosis of urethra

58.45 Repair of hypospadias or epispadias

58.46 Other reconstruction of urethra
Urethral construction

58.47 Urethral meatoplasty

58.49 Other repair of urethra
Benenenti rotation of bulbous urethra
Repair of old obstetric laceration of urethra
Urethral plication

Excludes *repair of:*
current obstetric laceration (75.61)
urethrocele (70.50–70.51)

58.5 Release of urethral stricture
Cutting of urethral sphincter
Internal urethral meatotomy
Urethrolysis

58.6 Dilation of urethra
Dilation of urethrovesical junction
Passage of sounds through urethra
Removal of calculus from urethra without incision

Excludes *urethral calibration (89.29)*

58.9 Other operations on urethra and periurethral tissue

58.91 Incision of periurethral tissue
Drainage of bulbourethral gland

58.92 Excision of periurethral tissue

Excludes *biopsy of periurethral tissue (58.24)*
lysis of periurethral adhesions
laparoscopic (59.12)
other (59.11)

✖58.93 **Implantation of artificial urinary sphincter [AUS]**
Placement of inflatable:
bladder sphincter
urethral sphincter
Removal with replacement of sphincter device [AUS]
With pump and/or reservoir

✖58.99 **Other**
Removal of inflatable urinary sphincter without replacement
Repair of inflatable sphincter pump and/or reservoir
Surgical correction of hydraulic pressure of inflatable sphincter device

Excludes *removal of:*
intraluminal foreign body from urethra without incision (98.19)
urethral stent (97.65)

● 59 **Other operations on urinary tract**

Code also any application or administration of an adhesion barrier substance (99.77)

● 59.0 **Dissection of retroperitoneal tissue**

✖59.00 **Retroperitoneal dissection, not otherwise specified**

✖59.02 **Other lysis of perirenal or periureteral adhesions**

Excludes *that by laparoscope (59.03)*

✖59.03 **Laparoscopic lysis of perirenal or periureteral adhesions**

✖59.09 **Other incision of perirenal or periureteral tissue**
Exploration of perinephric area
Incision of perirenal abscess

● 59.1 **Incision of perivesical tissue**

✖59.11 **Other lysis of perivesical adhesions**

✖59.12 **Laparoscopic lysis of perivesical adhesions**

✖59.19 **Other incision of perivesical tissue**
Exploration of perivesical tissue
Incision of hematoma of space of Retzius
Retropubic exploration

● 59.2 **Diagnostic procedures on perirenal and perivesical tissue**

✖59.21 **Biopsy of perirenal or perivesical tissue**

✖59.29 **Other diagnostic procedures on perirenal tissue, perivesical tissue, and retroperitoneum**

Excludes *microscopic examination of specimen from:*
perirenal tissue (91.21–91.29)
perivesical tissue (91.31–91.39)
retroperitoneum NEC (91.11–91.19)
retroperitoneal x-ray (88.14–88.16)

✖59.3 **Plication of urethrovesical junction**
Kelly-Kennedy operation on urethra
Kelly-Stoeckel urethral plication

✖59.4 **Suprapubic sling operation**
Goebel-Frangenheim-Stoeckel urethrovesical suspension
Millin-Read urethrovesical suspension
Oxford operation for urinary incontinence
Urethrocystopexy by suprapubic suspension

✖59.5 **Retropubic urethral suspension**
Burch procedure
Marshall-Marchetti-Krantz operation
Suture of periurethral tissue to symphysis pubis
Urethral suspension NOS

✖59.6 **Paraurethral suspension**
Pereyra paraurethral suspension
Periurethral suspension

● 59.7 **Other repair of urinary stress incontinence**

✖59.71 **Levator muscle operation for urethrovesical suspension**
Cystourethropexy with levator muscle sling
Gracilis muscle transplant for urethrovesical suspension
Pubococcygeal sling

59.72 **Injection of implant into urethra and/or bladder neck**
Collagen implant
Endoscopic injection of implant
Fat implant
Polytef implant

✖59.79 **Other**
Anterior urethropexy
Repair of stress incontinence NOS
Tudor "rabbit ear" urethropexy

59.8 **Ureteral catheterization**
Drainage of kidney by catheter
Insertion of ureteral stent
Ureterovesical orifice dilation

Code also any ureterotomy (56.2)

Excludes *that for:*
retrograde pyelogram (87.74)
transurethral removal of calculus or clot from ureter and renal pelvis (56.0)

● 59.9 **Other operations on urinary system**

Excludes *nonoperative removal of therapeutic device (97.61–97.69)*

✖59.91 **Excision of perirenal or perivesical tissue**

Excludes *biopsy of perirenal or perivesical tissue (59.21)*

✖59.92 **Other operations on perirenal or perivesical tissue**

59.93 **Replacement of ureterostomy tube**
Change of ureterostomy tube
Reinsertion of ureterostomy tube

Excludes *nonoperative removal of ureterostomy tube (97.62)*

59.94 **Replacement of cystostomy tube**

Excludes *nonoperative removal of cystostomy tube (97.63)*

59.95 **Ultrasonic fragmentation of urinary stones**
Shattered urinary stones

Excludes *percutaneous nephrostomy with fragmentation (55.04)*
shock-wave disintegration (98.51)

59.99 **Other**

Excludes *instillation of medication into urinary tract (96.49)*
irrigation of urinary tract (96.45–96.48)

11. OPERATIONS ON THE MALE GENITAL ORGANS (60–64)

● 60 Operations on prostate and seminal vesicles

Code also any application or administration of an adhesion barrier substance (99.77)

Includes: operations on periprostatic tissue

Excludes *that associated with radical cystectomy (57.71)*

✖ 60.0 Incision of prostate
Drainage of prostatic abscess
Prostatolithotomy

Excludes *drainage of periprostatic tissue only (60.81)*

● 60.1 Diagnostic procedures on prostate and seminal vesicles

60.11 Closed [percutaneous] [needle] biopsy of prostate
Approach:
transrectal
transurethral
Punch biopsy

✖ 60.12 Open biopsy of prostate

60.13 Closed [percutaneous] biopsy of seminal vesicles
Needle biopsy of seminal vesicles

✖ 60.14 Open biopsy of seminal vesicles

✖ 60.15 Biopsy of periprostatic tissue

✖ 60.18 Other diagnostic procedures on prostate and periprostatic tissue

Excludes *microscopic examination of specimen from prostate (91.31–91.39)*
x-ray of prostate (87.92)

✖ 60.19 Other diagnostic procedures on seminal vesicles

Excludes *microscopic examination of specimen from seminal vesicles (91.31–91.39)*
x-ray:
contrast seminal vesiculogram (87.91)
other (87.92)

● 60.2 Transurethral prostatectomy

Excludes *local excision of lesion of prostate (60.61)*

✖ 60.21 Transurethral (ultrasound) guided laser induced prostatectomy (TULIP)
Ablation (contact) (noncontact) by laser

✖ 60.29 Other transurethral prostatectomy
Excision of median bar by transurethral approach
Transurethral electrovaporization of prostrate (TEVAP)
Transurethral enucleative procedure
Transurethral prostatectomy NOS
Transurethral resection of prostate (TURP)

✖ 60.3 Suprapubic prostatectomy
Transvesical prostatectomy

Excludes *local excision of lesion of prostate (60.61)*
radical prostatectomy (60.5)

✖ 60.4 Retropubic prostatectomy

Excludes *local excision of lesion of prostate (60.61)*
radical prostatectomy (60.5)

✖ 60.5 Radical prostatectomy
Prostatovesiculectomy
Radical prostatectomy by any approach

Excludes *cystoprostatectomy (57.71)*

● 60.6 Other prostatectomy

✖ 60.61 Local excision of lesion of prostate
Excision of prostatic lesion by any approach

Excludes *biopsy of prostate (60.11–60.12)*

✖ 60.62 Perineal prostatectomy
Cryoablation of prostate
Cryoprostatectomy
Cryosurgery of prostate
Radical cryosurgical ablation of prostate (RCSA)

Excludes *local excision of lesion of prostate (60.61)*

✖ 60.69 Other

● 60.7 Operations on seminal vesicles

60.71 Percutaneous aspiration of seminal vesicle

Excludes *needle biopsy of seminal vesicle (60.13)*

✖ 60.72 Incision of seminal vesicle

✖ 60.73 Excision of seminal vesicle
Excision of Müllerian duct cyst
Spermatocystectomy

Excludes *biopsy of seminal vesicle (60.13–60.14)*
prostatovesiculectomy (60.5)

✖ 60.79 Other operations on seminal vesicles

● 60.8 Incision or excision of periprostatic tissue

✖ 60.81 Incision of periprostatic tissue
Drainage of periprostatic abscess

✖ 60.82 Excision of periprostatic tissue
Excision of lesion of periprostatic tissue

Excludes *biopsy of periprostatic tissue (60.15)*

● 60.9 Other operations on prostate

60.91 Percutaneous aspiration of prostate

Excludes *needle biopsy of prostate (60.11)*

60.92 Injection into prostate

✖ 60.93 Repair of prostate

✖ 60.94 Control of (postoperative) hemorrhage of prostate
Coagulation of prostatic bed
Cystoscopy for control of prostatic hemorrhage

✖ 60.95 Transurethral balloon dilation of the prostatic urethra

60.96 Transurethral destruction of prostate tissue by microwave thermotherapy
Transurethral microwave thermotherapy (TUMT) of prostate

Excludes *prostatectomy:*
other (60.61–60.69)
radical (60.5)
retropubic (60.4)
suprapubic (60.3)
transurethral (60.21–60.29)

60.97 Other transurethral destruction of prostate tissue by other thermotherapy
Radiofrequency thermotherapy
Transurethral needle ablation (TUNA) of prostate

Excludes *prostatectomy:*
other (60.61–60.69)
radical (60.5)
retropubic (60.4)
suprapubic (60.3)
transurethral (60.21–60.29)

✖ 60.99 Other

Excludes *prostatic massage (99.94)*

● 61 **Operations on scrotum and tunica vaginalis**

61.0 **Incision and drainage of scrotum and tunica vaginalis**

Excludes *percutaneous aspiration of hydrocele (61.91)*

● 61.1 **Diagnostic procedures on scrotum and tunica vaginalis**

61.11 **Biopsy of scrotum or tunica vaginalis**

61.19 **Other diagnostic procedures on scrotum and tunica vaginalis**

✖ 61.2 **Excision of hydrocele (of tunica vaginalis)**
Bottle repair of hydrocele of tunica vaginalis

Excludes *percutaneous aspiration of hydrocele (61.91)*

61.3 **Excision or destruction of lesion or tissue of scrotum**
Fulguration of lesion of scrotum
Reduction of elephantiasis of scrotum
Partial scrotectomy of scrotum

Excludes *biopsy of scrotum (61.11)*
scrotal fistulectomy (61.42)

● 61.4 **Repair of scrotum and tunica vaginalis**

61.41 **Suture of laceration of scrotum and tunica vaginalis**

✖ 61.42 **Repair of scrotal fistula**

✖ 61.49 **Other repair of scrotum and tunica vaginalis**
Reconstruction with rotational or pedicle flaps

● 61.9 **Other operations on scrotum and tunica vaginalis**

61.91 **Percutaneous aspiration of tunica vaginalis**
Aspiration of hydrocele of tunica vaginalis

✖ 61.92 **Excision of lesion of tunica vaginalis other than hydrocele**
Excision of hematocele of tunica vaginalis

✖ 61.99 **Other**

Excludes *removal of foreign body from scrotum without incision (98.24)*

● 62 **Operations on testes**

✖ 62.0 **Incision of testis**

● 62.1 **Diagnostic procedures on testes**

62.11 **Closed [percutaneous] [needle] biopsy of testis**

✖ 62.12 **Open biopsy of testis**

✖ 62.19 **Other diagnostic procedures on testes**

✖ 62.2 **Excision or destruction of testicular lesion**
Excision of appendix testis
Excision of cyst of Morgagni in the male

Excludes *biopsy of testis (62.11–62.12)*

✖ 62.3 **Unilateral orchiectomy**
Orchidectomy (with epididymectomy) NOS

● 62.4 **Bilateral orchiectomy**
Male castration
Radical bilateral orchiectomy (with epididymectomy)

Code also any synchronous lymph node dissection (40.3, 40.5)

✖ 62.41 **Removal of both testes at same operative episode**
Bilateral orchidectomy NOS

✖ 62.42 **Removal of remaining testis**
Removal of solitary testis

✖ 62.5 **Orchiopexy**
Mobilization and replacement of testis in scrotum
Orchiopexy with detorsion of testis
Torek (-Bevan) operation (orchidopexy) (first stage) (second stage)
Transplantation to and fixation of testis in scrotum

● 62.6 **Repair of testes**

Excludes *reduction of torsion (63.52)*

✖ 62.61 **Suture of laceration of testis**

✖ 62.69 **Other repair of testis**
Testicular graft

✖ 62.7 **Insertion of testicular prosthesis**

● 62.9 **Other operations on testes**

62.91 **Aspiration of testis**

Excludes *percutaneous biopsy of testis (62.11)*

62.92 **Injection of therapeutic substance into testis**

✖ 62.99 **Other**

● 63 **Operations on spermatic cord, epididymis, and vas deferens**

● 63.0 **Diagnostic procedures on spermatic cord, epididymis, and vas deferens**

63.01 **Biopsy of spermatic cord, epididymis, or vas deferens**

✖ 63.09 **Other diagnostic procedures on spermatic cord, epididymis, and vas deferens**

Excludes *contrast epididymogram (87.93)*
contrast vasogram (87.94)
other x-ray of epididymis and vas deferens (87.95)

✖ 63.1 **Excision of varicocele and hydrocele of spermatic cord**
High ligation of spermatic vein
Hydrocelectomy of canal of Nuck

✖ 63.2 **Excision of cyst of epididymis**
Spermatocelectomy

✖ 63.3 **Excision of other lesion or tissue of spermatic cord and epididymis**
Excision of appendix epididymis

Excludes *biopsy of spermatic cord or epididymis (63.01)*

✖ 63.4 **Epididymectomy**

Excludes *that synchronous with orchiectomy (62.3–62.42)*

● 63.5 **Repair of spermatic cord and epididymis**

✖ 63.51 **Suture of laceration of spermatic cord and epididymis**

63.52 **Reduction of torsion of testis or spermatic cord**

Excludes *that associated with orchiopexy (62.5)*

✖ 63.53 **Transplantation of spermatic cord**

✖ 63.59 **Other repair of spermatic cord and epididymis**

63.6 **Vasotomy**
Vasostomy

● 63.7 **Vasectomy and ligation of vas deferens**

63.70 **Male sterilization procedure, not otherwise specified**

63.71 **Ligation of vas deferens**
Crushing of vas deferens
Division of vas deferens

63.72 **Ligation of spermatic cord**

63.73 **Vasectomy**

● 63.8 **Repair of vas deferens and epididymis**

✖63.81 **Suture of laceration of vas deferens and epididymis**

✖63.82 **Reconstruction of surgically divided vas deferens**

✖63.83 **Epididymovasostomy**

63.84 **Removal of ligature from vas deferens**

✖63.85 **Removal of valve from vas deferens**

✖63.89 **Other repair of vas deferens and epididymis**

● 63.9 **Other operations on spermatic cord, epididymis, and vas deferens**

63.91 **Aspiration of spermatocele**

✖63.92 **Epididymotomy**

✖63.93 **Incision of spermatic cord**

✖63.94 **Lysis of adhesions of spermatic cord**

✖63.95 **Insertion of valve in vas deferens**

✖63.99 **Other**

● 64 **Operations on penis**

Includes: operations on:
corpora cavernosa
glans penis
prepuce

✖64.0 **Circumcision**

● 64.1 **Diagnostic procedures on the penis**

✖64.11 **Biopsy of penis**

64.19 **Other diagnostic procedures on penis**

✖64.2 **Local excision or destruction of lesion of penis**

Excludes *biopsy of penis (64.11)*

✖64.3 **Amputation of penis**

● 64.4 **Repair and plastic operation on penis**

✖64.41 **Suture of laceration of penis**

✖64.42 **Release of chordee**

✖64.43 **Construction of penis**

✖64.44 **Reconstruction of penis**

✖64.45 **Replantation of penis**
Reattachment of amputated penis

✖64.49 **Other repair of penis**

Excludes *repair of epispadias and hypospadias (58.45)*

✖64.5 **Operations for sex transformation, not elsewhere classified**

● 64.9 **Other operations on male genital organs**

64.91 **Dorsal or lateral slit of prepuce**

✖64.92 **Incision of penis**

✖64.93 **Division of penile adhesions**

64.94 **Fitting of external prosthesis of penis**
Penile prosthesis NOS

✖64.95 **Insertion or replacement of non-inflatable penile prosthesis**
Insertion of semi-rigid rod prosthesis into shaft of penis

Excludes *external penile prosthesis (64.94)*
inflatable penile prosthesis (64.97)
plastic repair, penis (64.43–64.49)
that associated with:
construction (64.43)
reconstruction (64.44)

✖64.96 **Removal of internal prosthesis of penis**
Removal without replacement of non-inflatable or inflatable penile prosthesis

✖64.97 **Insertion or replacement of inflatable penile prosthesis**
Insertion of cylinders into shaft of penis and placement of pump and reservoir

Excludes *external penile prosthesis (64.94)*
non-inflatable penile prosthesis (64.95)
plastic repair, penis (64.43–64.49)

✖64.98 **Other operations on penis**
Corpora cavernosa-corpus spongiosum shunt
Corpora-saphenous shunt
Irrigation of corpus cavernosum

Excludes *removal of foreign body:*
intraluminal (98.19)
without incision (98.24)
stretching of foreskin (99.95)

✖64.99 **Other**

Excludes *collection of sperm for artificial insemination (99.96)*

12. OPERATIONS ON THE FEMALE GENITAL ORGANS (65–71)

● **65 Operations on ovary**

Code also any application or administration of an adhesion barrier substance (99.77)

● **65.0 Oophorotomy**
Salpingo-oophorotomy

✖ **65.01 Laparoscopic oophorotomy**

✖ **65.09 Other oophorotomy**

● **65.1 Diagnostic procedures on ovaries**

✖ **65.11 Aspiration biopsy of ovary**

✖ **65.12 Other biopsy of ovary**

✖ **65.13 Laparoscopic biopsy of ovary**

✖ **65.14 Other laparoscopic diagnostic procedures on ovaries**

✖ **65.19 Other diagnostic procedures on ovaries**

Excludes *microscopic examination of specimen from ovary (91.41–91.49)*

● **65.2 Local excision or destruction of ovarian lesion or tissue**

✖ **65.21 Marsupialization of ovarian cyst**

Excludes *that by laparoscope (65.23)*

✖ **65.22 Wedge resection of ovary**

Excludes *that by laparoscope (65.24)*

✖ **65.23 Laparoscopic marsupialization of ovarian cyst**

✖ **65.24 Laparoscopic wedge resection of ovary**

✖ **65.25 Other laparoscopic local excision or destruction of ovary**

✖ **65.29 Other local excision or destruction of ovary**
Bisection of ovary
Cauterization of ovary
Partial excision of ovary

Excludes *biopsy of ovary (65.11–65.13)*
that by laparoscope (65.25)

● **65.3 Unilateral oophorectomy**

✖ **65.31 Laparoscopic unilateral oophorectomy**

✖ **65.39 Other unilateral oophorectomy**

Excludes *that by laparoscope (65.31)*

● **65.4 Unilateral salpingo-oophorectomy**

✖ **65.41 Laparoscopic unilateral salpingo-oophorectomy**

✖ **65.49 Other unilateral salpingo-oophorectomy**

● **65.5 Bilateral oophorectomy**

✖ **65.51 Other removal of both ovaries at same operative episode**
Female castration

Excludes *that by laparoscope (65.53)*

✖ **65.52 Other removal of remaining ovary**
Removal of solitary ovary

Excludes *that by laparoscope (65.54)*

✖ **65.53 Laparoscopic removal of both ovaries at same operative episode**

✖ **65.54 Laparoscopic removal of remaining ovary**

● **65.6 Bilateral salpingo-oophorectomy**

✖ **65.61 Other removal of both ovaries and tubes at same operative episode**

Excludes *that by laparoscope (65.63)*

✖ **65.62 Other removal of remaining ovary and tube**
Removal of solitary ovary and tube

Excludes *that by laparoscope (65.64)*

✖ **65.63 Laparoscopic removal of both ovaries and tubes at same operative episode**

✖ **65.64 Laparoscopic removal of remaining ovary and tube**

● **65.7 Repair of ovary**

Excludes *salpingo-oophorostomy (66.72)*

✖ **65.71 Other simple suture of ovary**

Excludes *that by laparoscope (65.74)*

✖ **65.72 Other reimplantation of ovary**

Excludes *that by laparoscope (65.75)*

✖ **65.73 Other salpingo-oophoroplasty**

Excludes *that by laparoscope (65.76)*

✖ **65.74 Laparoscopic simple suture of ovary**

✖ **65.75 Laparoscopic reimplantation of ovary**

✖ **65.76 Laparoscopic salpingo-oophoroplasty**

✖ **65.79 Other repair of ovary**
Oophoropexy

● **65.8 Lysis of adhesions of ovary and fallopian tube**

✖ **65.81 Laparoscopic lysis of adhesions of ovary and fallopian tube**

✖ **65.89 Other lysis of adhesions of ovary and fallopian tube**

Excludes *that by laparoscope (65.81)*

● **65.9 Other operations on ovary**

✖ **65.91 Aspiration of ovary**

Excludes *aspiration biopsy of ovary (65.11)*

✖ **65.92 Transplantation of ovary**

Excludes *reimplantation of ovary*
laparoscopic (65.75))
other (65.72)

✖ **65.93 Manual rupture of ovarian cyst**

✖ **65.94 Ovarian denervation**

✖ **65.95 Release of torsion of ovary**

✖ **65.99 Other**

● **66 Operations on fallopian tubes**

Code also any application or administration of an adhesion barrier substance (99.77)

● **66.0 Salpingotomy and salpingostomy**

✖ **66.01 Salpingotomy**

✖ **66.02 Salpingostomy**

● **66.1 Diagnostic procedures on fallopian tubes**

✖ **66.11 Biopsy of fallopian tube**

✖ **66.19 Other diagnostic procedures on fallopian tubes**

Excludes *microscopic examination of specimen from fallopian tubes (91.41–91.49)*
radiography of fallopian tubes (87.82–87.83, 87.85)
Rubin's test (66.8)

● **66.2 Bilateral endoscopic destruction or occlusion of fallopian tubes**

Includes: bilateral endoscopic destruction or occlusion of fallopian tubes by:
culdoscopy
endoscopy
hysteroscopy
laparoscopy
peritoneoscopy
endoscopic destruction of solitary fallopian tube

✖ **66.21 Bilateral endoscopic ligation and crushing of fallopian tubes**

✖ **66.22 Bilateral endoscopic ligation and division of fallopian tubes**

✖ **66.29 Other bilateral endoscopic destruction or occlusion of fallopian tubes**

● **66.3 Other bilateral destruction or occlusion of fallopian tubes**

Includes: destruction of solitary fallopian tube

Excludes *endoscopic destruction or occlusion of fallopian tubes (66.21–66.29)*

✖ **66.31 Other bilateral ligation and crushing of fallopian tubes**

✖ **66.32 Other bilateral ligation and division of fallopian tubes**
Pomeroy operation

✖ **66.39 Other bilateral destruction or occlusion of fallopian tubes**
Female sterilization operation NOS

✖ **66.4 Total unilateral salpingectomy**

● **66.5 Total bilateral salpingectomy**

Excludes *bilateral partial salpingectomy for sterilization (66.39)*
that with oophorectomy (65.61–65.64)

✖ **66.51 Removal of both fallopian tubes at same operative episode**

✖ **66.52 Removal of remaining fallopian tube**
Removal of solitary fallopian tube

● **66.6 Other salpingectomy**

Includes: salpingectomy by:
cauterization
coagulation
electrocoagulation
excision

Excludes *fistulectomy (66.73)*

✖ **66.61 Excision or destruction of lesion of fallopian tube**

Excludes *biopsy of fallopian tube (66.11)*

✖ **66.62 Salpingectomy with removal of tubal pregnancy**

Code also any synchronous oophorectomy (65.31, 65.39)

✖ **66.63 Bilateral partial salpingectomy, not otherwise specified**

✖ **66.69 Other partial salpingectomy**

● **66.7 Repair of fallopian tube**

✖ **66.71 Simple suture of fallopian tube**

✖ **66.72 Salpingo-oophorostomy**

✖ **66.73 Salpingo-salpingostomy**

✖ **66.74 Salpingo-uterostomy**

✖ **66.79 Other repair of fallopian tube**
Graft of fallopian tube
Reopening of divided fallopian tube
Salpingoplasty

66.8 Insufflation of fallopian tube
Insufflation of fallopian tube with:
air
dye
gas
saline
Rubin's test

Excludes *insufflation of therapeutic agent (66.95)*
that for hysterosalpingography (87.82–87.83)

● **66.9 Other operations on fallopian tubes**

66.91 Aspiration of fallopian tube

✖ **66.92 Unilateral destruction or occlusion of fallopian tube**

Excludes *that of solitary tube (66.21–66.39)*

✖ **66.93 Implantation or replacement of prosthesis of fallopian tube**

✖ **66.94 Removal of prosthesis of fallopian tube**

✖ **66.95 Insufflation of therapeutic agent into fallopian tubes**

✖ **66.96 Dilation of fallopian tube**

✖ **66.97 Burying of fimbriae in uterine wall**

✖ **66.99 Other**

Excludes *lysis of adhesions of ovary and tube*
laparoscopic (65.81)
other (65.89)

● **67 Operations on cervix**

Code also any application or administration of an adhesion barrier substance (99.77)

67.0 Dilation of cervical canal

Excludes *dilation and curettage (69.01–69.09)*
that for induction of labor (73.1)

● **67.1 Diagnostic procedures on cervix**

✖ **67.11 Endocervical biopsy**

Excludes *conization of cervix (67.2)*

✖ **67.12 Other cervical biopsy**
Punch biopsy of cervix NOS

Excludes *conization of cervix (67.2)*

✖ **67.19 Other diagnostic procedures on cervix**

Excludes *microscopic examination of specimen from cervix (91.41–91.49)*

✖ **67.2 Conization of cervix**

Excludes *that by:*
cryosurgery (67.33)
electrosurgery (67.32)

● **67.3 Other excision or destruction of lesion or tissue of cervix**

✖ **67.31 Marsupialization of cervical cyst**

✖ **67.32 Destruction of lesion of cervix by cauterization**
Electroconization of cervix
LEEP (loop electrosurgical excision procedure)
LLETZ (large loop excision of the transformation zone)

✖ **67.33 Destruction of lesion of cervix by cryosurgery**
Cryoconization of cervix

✖ **67.39 Other excision or destruction of lesion or tissue of cervix**

Excludes *biopsy of cervix (67.11–67.12)*
cervical fistulectomy (67.62)
conization of cervix (67.2)

✖ **67.4 Amputation of cervix**
Cervicectomy with synchronous colporrhaphy

● 67.5 Repair of internal cervical os

✖ 67.51 Transabdominal cerclage of cervix

✖ 67.59 Other repair of internal cervical os
Cerclage of isthmus uteri
McDonald operation
Shirodkar operation
Transvaginal cerclage

Excludes *transabdominal cerclage of cervix (67.51)*
laparoscopically assisted supracervical hysterectomy (LASH) (68.31) ◀

● 67.6 Other repair of cervix

Excludes *repair of current obstetric laceration (75.51)*

✖ 67.61 Suture of laceration of cervix

✖ 67.62 Repair of fistula of cervix
Cervicosigmoidal fistulectomy

Excludes *fistulectomy:*
cervicovesical (57.84)
ureterocervical (56.84)
vesicocervicovaginal (57.84)

✖ 67.69 Other repair of cervix
Repair of old obstetric laceration of cervix

● 68 Other incision and excision of uterus

Code also any application or administration of an adhesion barrier substance (99.77)

✖ 68.0 Hysterotomy
Hysterotomy with removal of hydatidiform mole

Excludes *hysterotomy for termination of pregnancy (74.91)*

● 68.1 Diagnostic procedures on uterus and supporting structures

68.11 Digital examination of uterus

Excludes *pelvic examination, so described (89.26)*
postpartal manual exploration of uterine cavity (75.7)

68.12 Hysteroscopy

Excludes *that with biopsy (68.16)*

✖ 68.13 Open biopsy of uterus

Excludes *closed biopsy of uterus(68.16)*

✖ 68.14 Open biopsy of uterine ligaments

Excludes *closed biopsy of uterine ligaments (68.15)*

✖ 68.15 Closed biopsy of uterine ligaments
Endoscopic (laparoscopy) biopsy of uterine adnexa, except ovary and fallopian tube

✖ 68.16 Closed biopsy of uterus
Endoscopic (laparoscopy) (hysteroscopy) biopsy of uterus

Excludes *open biopsy of uterus (68.13)*

✖ 68.19 Other diagnostic procedures on uterus and supporting structures

Excludes *diagnostic:*
aspiration curettage (69.59)
dilation and curettage (69.09)
microscopic examination of specimen from uterus (91.41–91.49)
pelvic examination (89.26)
radioisotope scan of:
placenta (92.17)
uterus (92.19)
ultrasonography of uterus (88.78–88.79)
x-ray of uterus (87.81–87.89)

● 68.2 Excision or destruction of lesion or tissue of uterus

✖ 68.21 Division of endometrial synechiae
Lysis of intraluminal uterine adhesions

✖ 68.22 Incision or excision of congenital septum of uterus

✖ 68.23 Endometrial ablation
Dilation and curettage
Hysteroscopic endometrial ablation

✖ 68.29 Other excision or destruction of lesion of uterus
Uterine myomectomy

Excludes *biopsy of uterus (68.13)*
uterine fistulectomy (69.42)

● 68.3 Subtotal abdominal hysterectomy ⬅

✖ 68.31 Laparoscopic supracervical hysterectomy [LSH] ◀
Classic infrafascial SEMM hysterectomy [CISH] ◀
Laparoscopically assisted supracervical hysterectomy [LASH] ◀

✖ 68.39 Other subtotal abdominal hysterectomy, NOS ◀
Supracervical hysterectomy ◀

Excludes *classic infrafascial SEMM hysterectomy [CISH] (68.31)* ◀
laparoscopic supracervical hysterectomy [LSH] (68.31) ◀

✖ 68.4 Total abdominal hysterectomy
Hysterectomy:
extended

Code also any synchronous removal of tubes and ovaries (65.3–65.6)

● 68.5 Vaginal hysterectomy

Code also any synchronous:
removal of tubes and ovaries (65.31–65.64)
repair of cystocele or rectocele (70.50–70.52)
repair of pelvic floor (70.79)

✖ 68.51 Laparoscopically assisted vaginal hysterectomy (LAVH)

✖ 68.59 Other vaginal hysterectomy

Excludes *laparoscopically assisted vaginal hysterectomy (LAVH) (68.51)*
radical vaginal hysterectomy (68.7)

✖ 68.6 Radical abdominal hysterectomy
Modified radical hysterectomy
Wertheim's operation

Code also any synchronous:
lymph gland dissection (40.3, 40.5)
removal of tubes and ovaries (65.61–65.64)

Excludes *pelvic evisceration (68.8)*

✖ 68.7 Radical vaginal hysterectomy
Schauta operation

Code also any synchronous:
lymph gland dissection (40.3, 40.5)
removal of tubes and ovaries (65.61–65.64)

✖ 68.8 Pelvic evisceration
Removal of ovaries, tubes, uterus, vagina, bladder, and urethra (with removal of sigmoid colon and rectum)

Code also any synchronous:
colostomy (46.12–46.13)
lymph gland dissection (40.3, 40.5)
urinary diversion (56.51–56.79)

✖ 68.9 Other and unspecified hysterectomy
Hysterectomy NOS

Excludes *abdominal hysterectomy, any approach (68.31-68.39, 68.4, 68.6)* ⬅
vaginal hysterectomy, any approach (68.51, 68.59, 68.7)

● **69 Other operations on uterus and supporting structures**

Code also any application or administration of an adhesion barrier substance (99.77)

● **69.0 Dilation and curettage of uterus**

Excludes *aspiration curettage of uterus (69.51–69.59)*

✖ **69.01 Dilation and curettage for termination of pregnancy**

✖ **69.02 Dilation and curettage following delivery or abortion**

✖ **69.09 Other dilation and curettage**
Diagnostic D and C

● **69.1 Excision or destruction of lesion or tissue of uterus and supporting structures**

✖ **69.19 Other excision or destruction of uterus and supporting structures**

Excludes *biopsy of uterine ligament (68.14)*

● **69.2 Repair of uterine supporting structures**

✖ **69.21 Interposition operation**
Watkins procedure

✖ **69.22 Other uterine suspension**
Hysteropexy
Manchester operation
Plication of uterine ligament

✖ **69.23 Vaginal repair of chronic inversion of uterus**

✖ **69.29 Other repair of uterus and supporting structures**

✖ **69.3 Paracervical uterine denervation**

● **69.4 Uterine repair**

Excludes *repair of current obstetric laceration (75.50–75.52)*

✖ **69.41 Suture of laceration of uterus**

✖ **69.42 Closure of fistula of uterus**

Excludes *uterovesical fistulectomy (57.84)*

✖ **69.49 Other repair of uterus**
Repair of old obstetric laceration of uterus

● **69.5 Aspiration curettage of uterus**

Excludes *menstrual extraction (69.6)*

✖ **69.51 Aspiration curettage of uterus for termination of pregnancy**
Therapeutic abortion NOS

✖ **69.52 Aspiration curettage following delivery or abortion**

69.59 Other aspiration curettage of uterus

69.6 Menstrual extraction or regulation

69.7 Insertion of intrauterine contraceptive device

● **69.9 Other operations on uterus, cervix, and supporting structures**

Excludes *obstetric dilation or incision of cervix (73.1, 73.93)*

69.91 Insertion of therapeutic device into uterus

Excludes *insertion of:*
intrauterine contraceptive device (69.7)
laminaria (69.93)
obstetric insertion of bag, bougie, or pack (73.1)

69.92 Artificial insemination

69.93 Insertion of laminaria

69.94 Manual replacement of inverted uterus

Excludes *that in immediate postpartal period (75.94)*

✖ **69.95 Incision of cervix**

Excludes *that to assist delivery (73.93)*

69.96 Removal of cerclage material from cervix

✖ **69.97 Removal of other penetrating foreign body from cervix**

Excludes *removal of intraluminal foreign body from cervix (98.16)*

✖ **69.98 Other operations on supporting structures of uterus**

Excludes *biopsy of uterine ligament (68.14)*

✖ **69.99 Other operations on cervix and uterus**

Excludes *removal of:*
foreign body (98.16)
intrauterine contraceptive device (97.71)
obstetric bag, bougie, or pack (97.72)
packing (97.72)

● **70 Operations on vagina and cul-de-sac**

Code also any application or administration of an adhesion barrier substance (99.77)

70.0 Culdocentesis

● **70.1 Incision of vagina and cul-de-sac**

70.11 Hymenotomy

✖ **70.12 Culdotomy**

✖ **70.13 Lysis of intraluminal adhesions of vagina**

✖ **70.14 Other vaginotomy**
Division of vaginal septum
Drainage of hematoma of vaginal cuff

● **70.2 Diagnostic procedures on vagina and cul-de-sac**

70.21 Vaginoscopy

70.22 Culdoscopy

✖ **70.23 Biopsy of cul-de-sac**

✖ **70.24 Vaginal biopsy**

✖ **70.29 Other diagnostic procedures on vagina and cul-de-sac**

● **70.3 Local excision or destruction of vagina and cul-de-sac**

✖ **70.31 Hymenectomy**

✖ **70.32 Excision or destruction of lesion of cul-de-sac**
Endometrectomy of cul-de-sac

Excludes *biopsy of cul-de-sac (70.23)*

✖ **70.33 Excision or destruction of lesion of vagina**

Excludes *biopsy of vagina (70.24)*
vaginal fistulectomy (70.72–70.75)

✖ **70.4 Obliteration and total excision of vagina**
Vaginectomy

Excludes *obliteration of vaginal vault (70.8)*

● **70.5 Repair of cystocele and rectocele**

✖ **70.50 Repair of cystocele and rectocele**

✖ **70.51 Repair of cystocele**
Anterior colporrhaphy (with urethrocele repair)

✖ **70.52 Repair of rectocele**
Posterior colporrhaphy

● **70.6 Vaginal construction and reconstruction**

✖ **70.61 Vaginal construction**

✖ **70.62 Vaginal reconstruction**

● **70.7 Other repair of vagina**

Excludes *lysis of intraluminal adhesions (70.13)*
repair of current obstetric laceration (75.69)
that associated with cervical amputation (67.4)

✖ **70.71 Suture of laceration of vagina**

✖ **70.72 Repair of colovaginal fistula**

✖ **70.73 Repair of rectovaginal fistula**

✖ **70.74 Repair of other vaginoenteric fistula**

✖ **70.75 Repair of other fistula of vagina**

Excludes *repair of fistula:*
rectovesicovaginal (57.83)
ureterovaginal (56.84)
urethrovaginal (58.43)
uterovaginal (69.42)
vesicocervicovaginal (57.84)
vesicosigmoidovaginal (57.83)
vesicoureterovaginal (56.84)
vesicovaginal (57.84)

✖ **70.76 Hymenorrhaphy**

✖ **70.77 Vaginal suspension and fixation**

✖ **70.79 Other repair of vagina**
Colpoperineoplasty
Repair of old obstetric laceration of vagina

✖ **70.8 Obliteration of vaginal vault**
LeFort operation

● **70.9 Other operations on vagina and cul-de-sac**

✖ **70.91 Other operations on vagina**

Excludes *insertion of:*
diaphragm (96.17)
mold (96.15)
pack (96.14)
pessary (96.18)
suppository (96.49)
removal of:
diaphragm (97.73)
foreign body (98.17)
pack (97.75)
pessary (97.74)
replacement of:
diaphragm (97.24)
pack (97.26)
pessary (97.25)
vaginal dilation (96.16)
vaginal douche (96.44)

✖ **70.92 Other operations on cul-de-sac**
Obliteration of cul-de-sac
Repair of vaginal enterocele

● **71 Operations on vulva and perineum**

Code also any application or administration of an adhesion barrier substance (99.77)

● **71.0 Incision of vulva and perineum**

✖ **71.01 Lysis of vulvar adhesions**

✖ **71.09 Other incision of vulva and perineum**
Enlargement of introitus NOS

Excludes *removal of foreign body without incision (98.23)*

● **71.1 Diagnostic procedures on vulva**

✖ **71.11 Biopsy of vulva**

✖ **71.19 Other diagnostic procedures on vulva**

● **71.2 Operations on Bartholin's gland**

71.21 Percutaneous aspiration of Bartholin's gland (cyst)

✖ **71.22 Incision of Bartholin's gland (cyst)**

✖ **71.23 Marsupialization of Bartholin's gland (cyst)**

✖ **71.24 Excision or other destruction of Bartholin's gland (cyst)**

✖ **71.29 Other operations on Bartholin's gland**

✖ **71.3 Other local excision or destruction of vulva and perineum**
Division of Skene's gland

Excludes *biopsy of vulva (71.11)*
vulvar fistulectomy (71.72)

✖ **71.4 Operations on clitoris**
Amputation of clitoris
Clitoridotomy
Female circumcision

✖ **71.5 Radical vulvectomy**

Code also any synchronous lymph gland dissection (40.3, 40.5)

● **71.6 Other vulvectomy**

✖ **71.61 Unilateral vulvectomy**

✖ **71.62 Bilateral vulvectomy**
Vulvectomy NOS

● **71.7 Repair of vulva and perineum**

Excludes *repair of current obstetric laceration (75.69)*

✖ **71.71 Suture of laceration of vulva or perineum**

✖ **71.72 Repair of fistula of vulva or perineum**

Excludes *repair of fistula:*
urethroperineal (58.43)
urethroperineovesical (57.84)
vaginoperineal (70.75)

✖ **71.79 Other repair of vulva and perineum**
Repair of old obstetric laceration of vulva or perineum

✖ **71.8 Other operations on vulva**

Excludes *removal of:*
foreign body without incision (98.23)
packing (97.75)
replacement of packing (97.26)

✖ **71.9 Other operations on female genital organs**

13. OBSTETRICAL PROCEDURES (72–75)

● 72 Forceps, vacuum, and breech delivery

72.0 Low forceps operation
Outlet forceps operation

72.1 Low forceps operation with episiotomy
Outlet forceps operation with episiotomy

● 72.2 Mid forceps operation

72.21 Mid forceps operation with episiotomy

72.29 Other mid forceps operation

● 72.3 High forceps operation

72.31 High forceps operation with episiotomy

72.39 Other high forceps operation

72.4 Forceps rotation of fetal head
De Lee maneuver
Key-in-lock rotation
Kielland rotation
Scanzoni's maneuver

Code also any associated forceps extraction (72.0–72.39)

● 72.5 Breech extraction

72.51 Partial breech extraction with forceps to aftercoming head

72.52 Other partial breech extraction

72.53 Total breech extraction with forceps to aftercoming head

72.54 Other total breech extraction

72.6 Forceps application to aftercoming head
Piper forceps operation

Excludes *partial breech extraction with forceps to aftercoming head (72.51)*
total breech extraction with forceps to aftercoming head (72.53)

● 72.7 Vacuum extraction

Includes: Malström's extraction

72.71 Vacuum extraction with episiotomy

72.79 Other vacuum extraction

72.8 Other specified instrumental delivery

72.9 Unspecified instrumental delivery

● 73 Other procedures inducing or assisting delivery

● 73.0 Artificial rupture of membranes

73.01 Induction of labor by artificial rupture of membranes
Surgical induction NOS

Excludes *artificial rupture of membranes after onset of labor (73.09)*

73.09 Other artificial rupture of membranes
Artificial rupture of membranes at time of delivery

73.1 Other surgical induction of labor
Induction by cervical dilation

Excludes *injection for abortion (75.0)*
insertion of suppository for abortion (96.49)

● 73.2 Internal and combined version and extraction

73.21 Internal and combined version without extraction
Version NOS

73.22 Internal and combined version with extraction

73.3 Failed forceps
Application of forceps without delivery
Trial forceps

73.4 Medical induction of labor

Excludes *medication to augment active labor— omit code*

● 73.5 Manually assisted delivery

73.51 Manual rotation of fetal head

73.59 Other manually assisted delivery
Assisted spontaneous delivery
Credé maneuver

73.6 Episiotomy
Episioproctotomy
Episiotomy with subsequent episiorrhaphy

Excludes *that with:*
high forceps (72.31)
low forceps (72.1)
mid forceps (72.21)
outlet forceps (72.1)
vacuum extraction (72.71)

73.8 Operations on fetus to facilitate delivery
Clavicotomy on fetus
Destruction of fetus
Needling of hydrocephalic head

● 73.9 Other operations assisting delivery

73.91 External version

73.92 Replacement of prolapsed umbilical cord

73.93 Incision of cervix to assist delivery
Dührssen's incisions

✖ 73.94 Pubiotomy to assist delivery
Obstetric symphysiotomy

✖ 73.99 Other

Excludes *dilation of cervix, obstetrical to induce labor (73.1)*
insertion of bag or bougie to induce labor (73.1)
removal of cerclage material (69.96)

● 74 Cesarean section and removal of fetus

Code also any synchronous:
hysterectomy (68.3–68.4, 68.6, 68.8)
myomectomy (68.29)
sterilization (66.31–66.39, 66.63)

✖ 74.0 Classical cesarean section
Transperitoneal classical cesarean section

✖ 74.1 Low cervical cesarean section
Lower uterine segment cesarean section

✖ 74.2 Extraperitoneal cesarean section
Supravesical cesarean section

✖ 74.3 Removal of extratubal ectopic pregnancy
Removal of:
ectopic abdominal pregnancy
fetus from peritoneal or extraperitoneal cavity following uterine or tubal rupture

Excludes *that by salpingostomy (66.02)*
that by salpingotomy (66.01)
that with synchronous salpingectomy (66.62)

✖ 74.4 Cesarean section of other specified type
Peritoneal exclusion cesarean section
Transperitoneal cesarean section NOS
Vaginal cesarean section

● 74.9 Cesarean section of unspecified type

✖ 74.91 Hysterotomy to terminate pregnancy
Therapeutic abortion by hysterotomy

✖ 74.99 Other cesarean section of unspecified type
Cesarean section NOS
Obstetrical abdominouterotomy
Obstetrical hysterotomy

● **75 Other obstetric operations**

75.0 Intra-amniotic injection for abortion
Injection of:
prostaglandin for induction of abortion
saline for induction of abortion
Termination of pregnancy by intrauterine injection

Excludes *insertion of prostaglandin suppository for abortion (96.49)*

75.1 Diagnostic amniocentesis

75.2 Intrauterine transfusion
Exchange transfusion in utero
Insertion of catheter into abdomen of fetus for transfusion

Code also any hysterotomy approach (68.0)

● **75.3 Other intrauterine operations on fetus and amnion**

Code also any hysterotomy approach (68.0)

75.31 Amnioscopy
Fetoscopy
Laparoamnioscopy

75.32 Fetal EKG (scalp)

75.33 Fetal blood sampling and biopsy

75.34 Other fetal monitoring

Includes: Fetal monitoring, not otherwise specified

Excludes *fetal pulse oximetry (75.38)*

75.35 Other diagnostic procedures on fetus and amnion
Intrauterine pressure determination

Excludes *amniocentesis (75.1)*
diagnostic procedures on gravid uterus and placenta (87.81, 88.46, 88.78, 92.17)

✖ **75.36 Correction of fetal defect**

75.37 Amnioinfusion
Code also injection of antibiotic (99.21)

75.38 Fetal pulse oximetry
Transcervical fetal oxygen saturation monitoring
Transcervical fetal SpO_2 monitoring

75.4 Manual removal of retained placenta

Excludes *aspiration curettage (69.52)*
dilation and curettage (69.02)

● **75.5 Repair of current obstetric laceration of uterus**

✖ **75.50 Repair of current obstetric laceration of uterus, not otherwise specified**

✖ **75.51 Repair of current obstetric laceration of cervix**

✖ **75.52 Repair of current obstetric laceration of corpus uteri**

● **75.6 Repair of other current obstetric laceration**

✖ **75.61 Repair of current obstetric laceration of bladder and urethra**

75.62 Repair of current obstetric laceration of rectum and sphincter ani

75.69 Repair of other current obstetric laceration
Episioperineorrhaphy
Repair of:
pelvic floor
perineum
vagina
vulva
Secondary repair of episiotomy

Excludes *repair of routine episiotomy (73.6)*

75.7 Manual exploration of uterine cavity, postpartum

75.8 Obstetric tamponade of uterus or vagina

Excludes *antepartum tamponade (73.1)*

● **75.9 Other obstetric operations**

75.91 Evacuation of obstetric incisional hematoma of perineum
Evacuation of hematoma of:
episiotomy
perineorrhaphy

75.92 Evacuation of other hematoma of vulva or vagina

✖ **75.93 Surgical correction of inverted uterus**
Spintelli operation

Excludes *vaginal repair of chronic inversion of uterus (69.23)*

75.94 Manual replacement of inverted uterus

✖ **75.99 Other**

14. OPERATIONS ON THE MUSCULOSKELETAL SYSTEM (76–84)

● 76 Operations on facial bones and joints

Excludes *accessory sinuses (22.00–22.9)*
nasal bones (21.00–21.99)
skull (01.01–02.99)

● **76.0 Incision of facial bone without division**

✖ **76.01 Sequestrectomy of facial bone**
Removal of necrotic bone chip from facial bone

✖ **76.09 Other incision of facial bone**
Reopening of osteotomy site of facial bone

Excludes *osteotomy associated with orthognathic surgery (76.61–76.69)*
removal of internal fixation device (76.97)

● **76.1 Diagnostic procedures on facial bones and joints**

✖ **76.11 Biopsy of facial bone**

✖ **76.19 Other diagnostic procedures on facial bones and joints**

Excludes *contrast arthrogram of temporomandibular joint (87.13)*
other x-ray (87.11–87.12, 87.14–87.16)

✖ **76.2 Local excision or destruction of lesion of facial bone**

Excludes *biopsy of facial bone (76.11)*
excision of odontogenic lesion (24.4)

● **76.3 Partial ostectomy of facial bone**

✖ **76.31 Partial mandibulectomy**
Hemimandibulectomy

Excludes *that associated with temporomandibular arthroplasty (76.5)*

✖ **76.39 Partial ostectomy of other facial bone**
Hemimaxillectomy (with bone graft or prosthesis)

● **76.4 Excision and reconstruction of facial bones**

✖ **76.41 Total mandibulectomy with synchronous reconstruction**

✖ **76.42 Other total mandibulectomy**

✖ **76.43 Other reconstruction of mandible**

Excludes *genioplasty (76.67–76.68)*
that with synchronous total mandibulectomy (76.41)

✖ **76.44 Total ostectomy of other facial bone with synchronous reconstruction**

✖ **76.45 Other total ostectomy of other facial bone**

✖ **76.46 Other reconstruction of other facial bone**

Excludes *that with synchronous total ostectomy (76.44)*

✖ **76.5 Temporomandibular arthroplasty**

● **76.6 Other facial bone repair and orthognathic surgery**

Code also any synchronous:
bone graft (76.91)
synthetic implant (76.92)

Excludes *reconstruction of facial bones (76.41–76.46)*

✖ **76.61 Closed osteoplasty [osteotomy] of mandibular ramus**
Gigli saw osteotomy

✖ **76.62 Open osteoplasty [osteotomy] of mandibular ramus**

✖ **76.63 Osteoplasty [osteotomy] of body of mandible**

✖ **76.64 Other orthognathic surgery on mandible**
Mandibular osteoplasty NOS
Segmental or subapical osteotomy

✖ **76.65 Segmental osteoplasty [osteotomy] of maxilla**
Maxillary osteoplasty NOS

✖ **76.66 Total osteoplasty [osteotomy] of maxilla**

✖ **76.67 Reduction genioplasty**
Reduction mentoplasty

✖ **76.68 Augmentation genioplasty**
Mentoplasty:
NOS
with graft or implant

✖ **76.69 Other facial bone repair**
Osteoplasty of facial bone NOS

● **76.7 Reduction of facial fracture**

Includes: internal fixation

Code also any synchronous:
bone graft (76.91)
synthetic implant (76.92)

Excludes *that of nasal bones (21.71–21.72)*

✖ **76.70 Reduction of facial fracture, not otherwise specified**

76.71 Closed reduction of malar and zygomatic fracture

✖ **76.72 Open reduction of malar and zygomatic fracture**

76.73 Closed reduction of maxillary fracture

✖ **76.74 Open reduction of maxillary fracture**

76.75 Closed reduction of mandibular fracture

✖ **76.76 Open reduction of mandibular fracture**

✖ **76.77 Open reduction of alveolar fracture**
Reduction of alveolar fracture with stabilization of teeth

76.78 Other closed reduction of facial fracture
Closed reduction of orbital fracture

Excludes *nasal bone (21.71)*

✖ **76.79 Other open reduction of facial fracture**
Open reduction of orbit rim or wall

Excludes *nasal bone (21.72)*

● **76.9 Other operations on facial bones and joints**

✖ **76.91 Bone graft to facial bone**
Autogenous graft to facial bone
Bone bank graft to facial bone
Heterogenous graft to facial bone

✖ **76.92 Insertion of synthetic implant in facial bone**
Alloplastic implant to facial bone

76.93 Closed reduction of temporomandibular dislocation

✖ **76.94 Open reduction of temporomandibular dislocation**

76.95 Other manipulation of temporomandibular joint

76.96 Injection of therapeutic substance into temporomandibular joint

✖ **76.97 Removal of internal fixation device from facial bone**

Excludes *removal of:*
dental wiring (97.33)
external mandibular fixation device NEC (97.36)

✖ **76.99 Other**

● 77 **Incision, excision, and division of other bones**

Excludes *laminectomy for decompression (03.09)*
operations on:
accessory sinuses (22.00–22.9)
ear ossicles (19.0–19.55)
facial bones (76.01–76.99)
joint structures (80.00–81.99)
mastoid (19.9–20.99)
nasal bones (21.00–21.99)
skull (01.01–02.99)

The following fourth-digit subclassification is for use with appropriate categories in section 77 to identify the site. Valid fourth-digit categories are in brackets under each code.

0 unspecified site
1 scapula, clavicle, and thorax [ribs and sternum]
2 humerus
3 radius and ulna
4 carpals and metacarpals
5 femur
6 patella
7 tibia and fibula
8 tarsals and metatarsals
9 other
Pelvic bones
Phalanges (of foot) (of hand)
Vertebrae

✖● **77.0 Sequestrectomy**
[0–9]

✖● **77.1 Other incision of bone without division**
[0–9] Reopening of osteotomy site

Excludes *aspiration of bone marrow (41.31, 41.91)*
removal of internal fixation device (78.60–78.69)

✖● **77.2 Wedge osteotomy**
[0–9]

Excludes *that for hallux valgus (77.51)*

✖● **77.3 Other division of bone**
[0–9] Osteoarthrotomy

Excludes *clavicotomy of fetus (73.8)*
laminotomy or incision of vertebra (03.01–03.09)
pubiotomy to assist delivery (73.94)
sternotomy incidental to thoracic operation—omit code

✖● **77.4 Biopsy of bone**
[0–9]

● **77.5 Excision and repair of bunion and other toe deformities**

✖ **77.51 Bunionectomy with soft tissue correction and osteotomy of the first metatarsal**

✖ **77.52 Bunionectomy with soft tissue correction and arthrodesis**

✖ **77.53 Other bunionectomy with soft tissue correction**

✖ **77.54 Excision or correction of bunionette**
That with osteotomy

✖ **77.56 Repair of hammer toe**
Filleting of hammer toe
Fusion of hammer toe
Phalangectomy (partial) of hammer toe

✖ **77.57 Repair of claw toe**
Capsulotomy of claw toe
Fusion of claw toe
Phalangectomy (partial) of claw toe
Tendon lengthening of claw toe

✖ **77.58 Other excision, fusion and repair of toes**
Cockup toe repair
Overlapping toe repair
That with use of prosthetic materials

✖ **77.59 Other bunionectomy**
Resection of hallux valgus joint with insertion of prosthesis

✖● **77.6 Local excision of lesion or tissue of bone**
[0–9]

Excludes *biopsy of bone (77.40–77.49)*
debridement of compound fracture (79.60–79.69)

✖● **77.7 Excision of bone for graft**
[0–9]

✖● **77.8 Other partial ostectomy**
[0–9] Condylectomy

Excludes *amputation (84.00–84.19, 84.91)*
arthrectomy (80.90–80.99)
excision of bone ends associated with:
arthrodesis (81.00–81.29)
arthroplasty (81.31–81.87)
excision of cartilage (80.5–80.6, 80.80–80.99)
excision of head of femur with synchronous replacement (81.51–81.53)
hemilaminectomy (03.01–03.09)
laminectomy (03.01–03.09)
ostectomy for hallux valgus (77.51–77.59)
partial amputation:
finger (84.01)
thumb (84.02)
toe (84.11)
resection of ribs incidental to thoracic operation—omit code
that incidental to other operation—omit code

✖● **77.9 Total ostectomy**
[0–9]

Excludes *amputation of limb (84.00–84.19, 84.91)*
that incidental to other operation—omit code

● 78 **Other operations on bones, except facial bones**

Excludes *operations on:*
accessory sinuses (22.00–22.9)
facial bones (76.01–76.99)
joint structures (80.00–81.99)
nasal bones (21.00–21.99)
skull (01.01–02.99)

The following fourth-digit subclassification is for use with categories in section 78 to identify the site. Valid fourth-digit categories are in [brackets] under each code.

0 unspecified site
1 scapula, clavicle, and thorax [ribs and sternum]
2 humerus
3 radius and ulna
4 carpals and metacarpals
5 femur
6 patella
7 tibia and fibula
8 tarsals and metatarsals
9 other
Pelvic bones
Phalanges (of foot) (of hand)
Vertebrae

✖● **78.0 Bone graft**
[0–9] Bone:
bank graft
graft (autogenous) (heterogenous)
That with debridement of bone graft site (removal of sclerosed, fibrous or necrotic bone or tissue)
Transplantation of bone

Code also any excision of bone for graft (77.70–77.79)

Excludes *that for bone lengthening (78.30–78.39)*

✖● 78.1 **Application of external fixation device**
[0–9] Minifixator with insertion of pins/wires/screws into bone

Excludes *other immobilization, pressure, and attention to wound (93.51–93.59)*

✖● 78.2 **Limb shortening procedures**
[0, 2–5, 7–9] Epiphyseal stapling
Open epiphysiodesis
Percutaneous epiphysiodesis
Resection/osteotomy

✖● 78.3 **Limb lengthening procedures**
[0, 2–5, 7–9] Bone graft with or without internal fixation devices or osteotomy
Distraction technique with or without corticotomy/osteotomy

Code also any application of an external fixation device (78.10–78.19)

✖● 78.4 **Other repair or plastic operations on bone**
[0–9] Other operation on bone NEC
Repair of malunion or nonunion fracture NEC

Excludes *application of external fixation device (78.10–78.19)*
limb lengthening procedures (78.30–78.39)
limb shortening procedures (78.20–78.29)
osteotomy (77.3)
reconstruction of thumb (82.61–82.69)
repair of pectus deformity (34.74)
repair with bone graft (78.00–78.09)

✖● 78.5 **Internal fixation of bone without fracture reduction**
[0–9] Internal fixation of bone (prophylactic)
Reinsertion of internal fixation device
Revision of displaced or broken fixation device

Excludes *arthroplasty and arthrodesis (81.00–81.85)*
bone graft (78.00–78.09)
limb shortening procedures (78.20–78.29)
that for fracture reduction (79.10–79.19, 79.30–79.59)

✖● 78.6 **Removal of implanted devices from bone**
[0–9] External fixator device (invasive)
Internal fixation device
Removal of bone growth stimulator (invasive)

Excludes *removal of cast, splint, and traction device (Kirschner wire) (Steinmann pin) (97.88)*
removal of skull tongs or halo traction device (02.95)

✖● 78.7 **Osteoclasis**
[0–9]

✖● 78.8 **Diagnostic procedures on bone, not elsewhere classified**
[0–9]

Excludes *biopsy of bone (77.40–77.49)*
magnetic resonance imaging (88.94)
microscopic examination of specimen from bone (91.51–91.59)
radioisotope scan (92.14)
skeletal x-ray (87.21–87.29, 87.43, 88.21–88.33)
thermography (88.83)

✖● 78.9 **Insertion of bone growth stimulator**
[0–9] Insertion of:
bone stimulator (electrical) to aid bone healing
osteogenic electrodes for bone growth stimulation
totally implanted device (invasive)

Excludes *non-invasive (transcutaneous) (surface) stimulator (99.86)*

● 79 **Reduction of fracture and dislocation**

Includes: application of cast or splint
Reduction with insertion of traction device (Kirschner wire) (Steinmann pin)

Code also any application of external fixation device (78.10–78.19)

Excludes *external fixation alone for immobilization of fracture (93.51–93.56, 93.59)*
internal fixation without reduction of fracture (78.50–78.59)
operations on:
facial bones (76.70–76.79)
nasal bones (21.71–21.72)
orbit (76.78–76.79)
skull (02.02)
vertebrae (03.53)
removal of cast or splint (97.88)
replacement of cast or splint (97.11–97.14)
traction alone for reduction of fracture (93.41–93.46)

The following fourth-digit subclassification is for use with appropriate categories in section 79 to identify the site. Valid fourth-digit categories are in [brackets] under each code.

0 unspecified site
1 humerus
2 radius and ulna
Arm NOS
3 carpals and metacarpals
Hand NOS
4 phalanges of hand
5 femur
6 tibia and fibula
Leg NOS
7 tarsals and metatarsals
Foot NOS
8 phalanges of foot
9 other specified bone

● 79.0 **Closed reduction of fracture without internal fixation**

Excludes *that for separation of epiphysis (79.40–79.49)*

✖● 79.1 **Closed reduction of fracture with internal fixation**

Excludes *that for separation of epiphysis (79.40–79.49)*

✖● 79.2 **Open reduction of fracture without internal fixation**
[0–9]

Excludes *that for separation of epiphysis (79.50–79.59)*

✖● 79.3 **Open reduction of fracture with internal fixation**
[0–9]

Excludes *that for separation of epiphysis (79.50–79.59)*

✖● 79.4 **Closed reduction of separated epiphysis**
[0–2, 5, 6, 9] Reduction with or without internal fixation

✖● 79.5 **Open reduction of separated epiphysis**
[0–2, 5, 6, 9] Reduction with or without internal fixation

✖● 79.6 **Debridement of open fracture site**
[0–9] Debridement of compound fracture

● 79.7 **Closed reduction of dislocation**

Includes: closed reduction (with external traction device)

Excludes *closed reduction of dislocation of temporomandibular joint (76.93)*

79.70 **Closed reduction of dislocation of unspecified site**

79.71 **Closed reduction of dislocation of shoulder**

79.72 **Closed reduction of dislocation of elbow**

79.73 **Closed reduction of dislocation of wrist**

79.74 **Closed reduction of dislocation of hand and finger**

79.75 **Closed reduction of dislocation of hip**

79.76 **Closed reduction of dislocation of knee**

79.77 **Closed reduction of dislocation of ankle**

79.78 **Closed reduction of dislocation of foot and toe**

79.79 **Closed reduction of dislocation of other specified sites**

● 79.8 **Open reduction of dislocation**

Includes: open reduction (with internal and external fixation devices)

Excludes *open reduction of dislocation of temporomandibular joint (76.94)*

✖79.80 **Open reduction of dislocation of unspecified site**

✖79.81 **Open reduction of dislocation of shoulder**

✖79.82 **Open reduction of dislocation of elbow**

✖79.83 **Open reduction of dislocation of wrist**

✖79.84 **Open reduction of dislocation of hand and finger**

✖79.85 **Open reduction of dislocation of hip**

✖79.86 **Open reduction of dislocation of knee**

✖79.87 **Open reduction of dislocation of ankle**

✖79.88 **Open reduction of dislocation of foot and toe**

✖79.89 **Open reduction of dislocation of other specified sites**

✖● 79.9 **Unspecified operation on bone injury**
[0–9]

● 80 **Incision and excision of joint structures**

Includes: operations on:
capsule of joint
cartilage
condyle
ligament
meniscus
synovial membrane

Excludes *cartilage of:*
ear (18.01–18.9)
nose (21.00–21.99)
temporomandibular joint (76.01–76.99)

The following fourth-digit subclassification is for use with appropriate categories in section 80 to identify the site:

- 0 **unspecified site**
- 1 **shoulder**
- 2 **elbow**
- 3 **wrist**
- 4 **hand and finger**
- 5 **hip**
- 6 **knee**
- 7 **ankle**
- 8 **foot and toe**
- 9 **other specified sites**
  Spine

✖● 80.0 **Arthrotomy for removal of prosthesis**
Cement spacer

✖● 80.1 **Other arthrotomy**
Arthrostomy

Excludes *that for:*
arthrography (88.32)
arthroscopy (80.20–80.29)
injection of drug (81.92)
operative approach—omit code

✖● 80.2 **Arthroscopy**

● 80.3 **Biopsy of joint structure**
Aspiration biopsy

✖● 80.4 **Division of joint capsule, ligament, or cartilage**
Goldner clubfoot release
Heyman-Herndon(-Strong) correction of metatarsus varus
Release of:
adherent or constrictive joint capsule
joint
ligament

Excludes *symphysiotomy to assist delivery (73.94)*
that for:
carpal tunnel syndrome (04.43)
tarsal tunnel syndrome (04.44)

● 80.5 **Excision or destruction of intervertebral disc**

✖80.50 **Excision or destruction of intervertebral disc, unspecified**
Unspecified as to excision or destruction

✖80.51 **Excision of intervertebral disc**
Diskectomy
Removal of herniated nucleus pulposus
Level:
cervical
thoracic
lumbar (lumbosacral)
That by laminotomy or hemilaminectomy
That with decompression of spinal nerve root at same level
Requires additional code for any concomitant decompression of spinal nerve root at different level from excision site
Code also any concurrent spinal fusion (81.00–81.09)

Excludes *intervertebral chemonucleolysis (80.52)*
laminectomy for exploration of intraspinal canal (03.09)
laminotomy for decompression of spinal nerve root only (03.09)

80.52 **Intervertebral chemonucleolysis**
With aspiration of disc fragments
With diskography
Injection of proteolytic enzyme into intervertebral space (chymopapain)

Excludes *injection of anesthetic substance (03.91)*
injection of other substances (03.92)

✖80.59 **Other destruction of intervertebral disc**
Destruction NEC
That by laser

✖80.6 **Excision of semilunar cartilage of knee**
Excision of meniscus of knee

✖● 80.7 **Synovectomy**
Complete or partial resection of synovial membrane

Excludes *excision of Baker's cyst (83.39)*

✖● 80.8 **Other local excision or destruction of lesion of joint**

✖● 80.9 **Other excision of joint**

Excludes *cheilectomy of joint (77.80–77.89)*
excision of bone ends (77.80–77.89)

● 81 **Repair and plastic operations on joint structures**

● 81.0 **Spinal fusion**
Code also the total number of vertebrae fused (81.62–81.64) ◀
Code also any 360 degree spinal fusion by a single incision (81.61)
Code also any insertion of interbody spinal fusion device (84.51)
Code also any insertion of recombinant bone morphogenetic protein (84.52)

Includes: arthrodesis of spine with:
bone graft
internal fixation

Excludes *correction of pseudarthrosis of spine (81.30–81.39)*
refusion of spine (81.30–81.39)

✖**81.00 Spinal fusion, not otherwise specified**

✖**81.01 Atlas-axis spinal fusion**
Craniocervical fusion by anterior, transoral, or posterior technique
C1-C2 fusion by anterior, transoral, or posterior technique
Occiput C2 fusion by anterior, transoral, or posterior technique

✖**81.02 Other cervical fusion, anterior technique**
Arthrodesis of C2 level or below:
anterior (interbody) technique
anterolateral technique

✖**81.03 Other cervical fusion, posterior technique**
Arthrodesis of C2 level or below:
posterior (interbody) technique
posterolateral technique

✖**81.04 Dorsal and dorsolumbar fusion, anterior technique**
Arthrodesis of thoracic or thoracolumbar region:
anterior (interbody) technique
anterolateral technique

✖**81.05 Dorsal and dorsolumbar fusion, posterior technique**
Arthrodesis of thoracic or thoracolumbar region:
posterior (interbody) technique
posterolateral technique

✖**81.06 Lumbar and lumbosacral fusion, anterior technique**
Arthrodesis of lumbar or lumbosacral region:
anterior (interbody) technique
anterolateral technique

✖**81.07 Lumbar and lumbosacral fusion, lateral transverse process technique**

✖**81.08 Lumbar and lumbosacral fusion, posterior technique**
Arthrodesis of lumbar or lumbosacral region:
posterior (interbody) technique
posterolateral technique

● **81.1 Arthrodesis of foot and ankle**

Includes: arthrodesis of foot and ankle with:
bone graft
external fixation device

✖**81.11 Ankle fusion**
Tibiotalar fusion

✖**81.12 Triple arthrodesis**
Talus to calcaneus and calcaneus to cuboid and navicular

✖**81.13 Subtalar fusion**

✖**81.14 Midtarsal fusion**

✖**81.15 Tarsometatarsal fusion**

✖**81.16 Metatarsophalangeal fusion**

✖**81.17 Other fusion of foot**

● **81.2 Arthrodesis of other joint**

Includes: arthrodesis with:
bone graft
external fixation device
excision of bone ends and compression

✖**81.20 Arthrodesis of unspecified joint**

✖**81.21 Arthrodesis of hip**

✖**81.22 Arthrodesis of knee**

✖**81.23 Arthrodesis of shoulder**

✖**81.24 Arthrodesis of elbow**

✖**81.25 Carporadial fusion**

✖**81.26 Metacarpocarpal fusion**

✖**81.27 Metacarpophalangeal fusion**

✖**81.28 Interphalangeal fusion**

✖**81.29 Arthrodesis of other specified joints**

● **81.3 Refusion of spine**

Includes: arthrodesis of spine with:
bone graft
internal fixation
correction of pseudarthrosis of spine

Code also the total number of vertebra fused (81.62–81.64) ◀

Code also any 360 degree spinal fusion by a single incision (81.61)

Code also any insertion of interbody spinal fusion device (84.51)

Code also any insertion of recombinant bone morphogenetic protein (84.52)

✖**81.30 Refusion of spine, not otherwise specified**

✖**81.31 Refusion of atlas-axis spine**
Craniocervical fusion by anterior, transoral or posterior technique
C1-C2 fusion by anterior, transoral or posterior technique
Occiput C2 fusion by anterior, transoral or posterior technique

✖**81.32 Refusion of other cervical spine, anterior technique**
Arthrodesis of C2 level or below:
anterior (interbody) technique
anterolateral technique

✖**81.33 Refusion of other cervical spine, posterior technique**
Arthrodesis of C2 level or below:
posterior (interbody) technique
posterolateral technique

✖**81.34 Refusion of dorsal and dorsolumbar spine, anterior technique**
Arthrodesis of thoracic or thoracolumbar region:
anterior (interbody) technique
anterolateral technique

✖**81.35 Refusion of dorsal and dorsolumbar spine, posterior technique**
Arthrodesis of thoracic or thoracolumbar region:
posterior (interbody) technique
posterolateral technique

✖**81.36 Refusion of lumbar and lumbosacral spine, anterior technique**
Arthrodesis of lumbar or lumbosacral region:
anterior (interbody) technique
anterolateral technique

✖**81.37 Refusion of lumbar and lumbosacral spine, lateral transverse process technique**

✖**81.38 Refusion of lumbar and lumbosacral spine, posterior technique**
Arthrodesis of lumbar or lumbosacral region:
posterior (interbody) technique
posterolateral technique

✖**81.39 Refusion of spine, not elsewhere classified**

● **81.4 Other repair of joint of lower extremity**

Includes: arthroplasty of lower extremity with:
external traction or fixation
graft of bone (chips) or cartilage
internal fixation device

✖ **81.40 Repair of hip, not elsewhere classified**

✖ **81.42 Five-in-one repair of knee**
Medial meniscectomy, medial collateral ligament repair, vastus medialis advancement, semitendinosus advancement, and pes anserinus transfer

✖ **81.43 Triad knee repair**
Medial meniscectomy with repair of the anterior cruciate ligament and the medial collateral ligament
O'Donoghue procedure

✖ **81.44 Patellar stabilization**
Roux-Goldthwait operation for recurrent dislocation of patella

✖ **81.45 Other repair of the cruciate ligaments**

✖ **81.46 Other repair of the collateral ligaments**

✖ **81.47 Other repair of knee**

✖ **81.49 Other repair of ankle**

● **81.5 Joint replacement of lower extremity**

Includes: arthroplasty of lower extremity with:
external traction or fixation
graft of bone (chips) or cartilage
internal fixation device or prosthesis
removal of cement spacer

✖ **81.51 Total hip replacement**
Replacement of both femoral head and acetabulum by prosthesis
Total reconstruction of hip

✖ **81.52 Partial hip replacement**
Bipolar endoprosthesis

✖ **81.53 Revision of hip replacement**
Partial
Total

✖ **81.54 Total knee replacement**
Bicompartmental
Tricompartmental
Unicompartmental (hemijoint)

✖ **81.55 Revision of knee replacement**

Excludes *arthrodesis of knee (81.22)*

✖ **81.56 Total ankle replacement**

✖ **81.57 Replacement of joint of foot and toe**

✖ **81.59 Revision of joint replacement of lower extremity, not elsewhere classified**

● **81.6 Other procedures on spine**

Note: Number of vertebrae ◀

The vertebral spine consists of 25 vertebrae in the following order and number: ◀

Cervical: C1 (atlas), C2 (axis), C3, C4, C5, C6, C7 ◀

Thoracic or Dorsal: T1, T2, T3, T4, T5, T6, T7, T8, T9, T10, T11. T12 ◀

Lumbar and Sacral: L1, L2, L3, L4, L5, S1 ◀

Coders should report only one code from the series 81.62 or 81.63 or 81.64 to show the total number of vertebrae fused on the patient. ◀

Code also the level and approach of the fusion or refusion (81.00–81.08, 81.30–81.39) ◀

● **81.61 360 degree spinal fusion, single incision approach**
That by a single incision but fusing or refusion both anterior and posterior spine

Code also refusion of spine (81.30–81.39)

Code also spinal fusion (81.00–81.08)

Code also the total number of vertebrae fused (81.62–81.64) ◀

✖ **81.62 Fusion or refusion of 2–3 vertebrae** ◀

✖ **81.63 Fusion or refusion of 4–8 vertebrae** ◀

✖ **81.64 Fusion or refusion of 9 or more vertebrae** ◀

● **81.7 Arthroplasty and repair of hand, fingers and wrist**

Includes: arthroplasty of hand and finger with:
external traction or fixation
graft of bone (chips) or cartilage
internal fixation device or prosthesis

Excludes *operations on muscle, tendon and fascia of hand (82.01–82.99)*

✖ **81.71 Arthroplasty of metacarpophalangeal and interphalangeal joint with implant**

✖ **81.72 Arthroplasty of metacarpophalangeal and interphalangeal joint without implant**

✖ **81.73 Total wrist replacement**

✖ **81.74 Arthroplasty of carpocarpal or carpometacarpal joint with implant**

✖ **81.75 Arthroplasty of carpocarpal or carpometacarpal joint without implant**

✖ **81.79 Other repair of hand, fingers and wrist**

● **81.8 Arthroplasty and repair of shoulder and elbow**

Includes: arthroplasty of upper limb NEC with:
external traction or fixation
graft of bone (chips) or cartilage
internal fixation device or prosthesis

✖ **81.80 Total shoulder replacement**

✖ **81.81 Partial shoulder replacement**

✖ **81.82 Repair of recurrent dislocation of shoulder**

✖ **81.83 Other repair of shoulder**
Revision of arthroplasty of shoulder

✖ **81.84 Total elbow replacement**

✖ **81.85 Other repair of elbow**

● **81.9 Other operations on joint structures**

81.91 Arthrocentesis
Joint aspiration

Excludes *that for:*
arthrography (88.32)
biopsy of joint structure (80.30–80.39)
injection of drug (81.92)

81.92 Injection of therapeutic substance into joint or ligament

✖ **81.93 Suture of capsule or ligament of upper extremity**

Excludes *that associated with arthroplasty (81.71–81.75, 81.80–81.81, 81.84)*

✖ **81.94 Suture of capsule or ligament of ankle and foot**

Excludes *that associated with arthroplasty (81.56–81.59)*

✖ **81.95 Suture of capsule or ligament of other lower extremity**

Excludes *that associated with arthroplasty (81.51–81.55, 81.59)*

✖ **81.96 Other repair of joint**

✖ **81.97 Revision of joint replacement of upper extremity**
Partial
Removal of cement spacer
Total

✖81.98 Other diagnostic procedures on joint structures
Excludes *arthroscopy (80.20–80.29)*
biopsy of joint structure (80.30–80.39)
microscopic examination of specimen from joint (91.51–91.59)
thermography (88.83)
x-ray (87.21–87.29, 88.21–88.33)

✖81.99 Other

● 82 Operations on muscle, tendon, and fascia of hand

Includes: operations on:
aponeurosis
synovial membrane (tendon sheath)
tendon sheath

● 82.0 Incision of muscle, tendon, fascia, and bursa of hand

✖82.01 Exploration of tendon sheath of hand
Incision of tendon sheath of hand
Removal of rice bodies in tendon sheath of hand
Excludes *division of tendon (82.11)*

✖82.02 Myotomy of hand
Excludes *myotomy for division (82.19)*

✖82.03 Bursotomy of hand

82.04 Incision and drainage of palmar or thenar space

✖82.09 Other incision of soft tissue of hand
Excludes *incision of skin and subcutaneous tissue alone (86.01–86.09)*

● 82.1 Division of muscle, tendon, and fascia of hand

✖82.11 Tenotomy of hand
Division of tendon of hand

✖82.12 Fasciotomy of hand
Division of fascia of hand

✖82.19 Other division of soft tissue of hand
Division of muscle of hand

● 82.2 Excision of lesion of muscle, tendon, and fascia of hand

✖82.21 Excision of lesion of tendon sheath of hand
Ganglionectomy of tendon sheath (wrist)

✖82.22 Excision of lesion of muscle of hand

✖82.29 Excision of other lesion of soft tissue of hand
Excludes *excision of lesion of skin and subcutaneous tissue (86.21–86.3)*

● 82.3 Other excision of soft tissue of hand

Code also any skin graft (86.61–86.62, 86.73)
Excludes *excision of skin and subcutaneous tissue (86.21–86.3)*

✖82.31 Bursectomy of hand

✖82.32 Excision of tendon of hand for graft

✖82.33 Other tenonectomy of hand
Tenosynovectomy of hand
Excludes *excision of lesion of:*
tendon (82.29)
sheath (82.21)

✖82.34 Excision of muscle or fascia of hand for graft

✖82.35 Other fasciectomy of hand
Release of Dupuytren's contracture
Excludes *excision of lesion of fascia (82.29)*

✖82.36 Other myectomy of hand
Excludes *excision of lesion of muscle (82.22)*

✖82.39 Other excision of soft tissue of hand
Excludes *excision of skin (86.21–86.3)*
excision of soft tissue lesion (82.29)

● 82.4 Suture of muscle, tendon, and fascia of hand

✖82.41 Suture of tendon sheath of hand

✖82.42 Delayed suture of flexor tendon of hand

✖82.43 Delayed suture of other tendon of hand

✖82.44 Other suture of flexor tendon of hand
Excludes *delayed suture of flexor tendon of hand (82.42)*

✖82.45 Other suture of other tendon of hand
Excludes *delayed suture of other tendon of hand (82.43)*

✖82.46 Suture of muscle or fascia of hand

● 82.5 Transplantation of muscle and tendon of hand

✖82.51 Advancement of tendon of hand

✖82.52 Recession of tendon of hand

✖82.53 Reattachment of tendon of hand

✖82.54 Reattachment of muscle of hand

✖82.55 Other change in hand muscle or tendon length

✖82.56 Other hand tendon transfer or transplantation
Excludes *pollicization of thumb (82.61)*
transfer of finger, except thumb (82.81)

✖82.57 Other hand tendon transposition

✖82.58 Other hand muscle transfer or transplantation

✖82.59 Other hand muscle transposition

● 82.6 Reconstruction of thumb

Includes: digital transfer to act as thumb

Code also any amputation for digital transfer (84.01, 84.11)

✖82.61 Pollicization operation carrying over nerves and blood supply

✖82.69 Other reconstruction of thumb
"Cocked-hat" procedure [skin flap and bone]
Grafts:
bone to thumb skin (pedicle) to thumb

● 82.7 Plastic operation on hand with graft or implant

✖82.71 Tendon pulley reconstruction
Reconstruction for opponensplasty

✖82.72 Plastic operation on hand with graft of muscle or fascia

✖82.79 Plastic operation on hand with other graft or implant
Tendon graft to hand

● 82.8 Other plastic operations on hand

✖82.81 Transfer of finger, except thumb
Excludes *pollicization of thumb (82.61)*

✖82.82 Repair of cleft hand

✖82.83 Repair of macrodactyly

✖82.84 Repair of mallet finger

✖82.85 Other tenodesis of hand
Tendon fixation of hand NOS

✖82.86 Other tenoplasty of hand
Myotenoplasty of hand

✖82.89 Other plastic operations on hand
Plication of fascia
Repair of fascial hernia
Excludes *that with graft or implant (82.71–82.79)*

● 82.9 **Other operations on muscle, tendon, and fascia of hand**

Excludes *diagnostic procedures on soft tissue of hand (83.21–83.29)*

✖ 82.91 **Lysis of adhesions of hand**
Freeing of adhesions of fascia, muscle, and tendon of hand

Excludes *decompression of carpal tunnel (04.43)*
that by stretching or manipulation only (93.26)

82.92 **Aspiration of bursa of hand**

82.93 **Aspiration of other soft tissue of hand**

Excludes *skin and subcutaneous tissue (86.01)*

82.94 **Injection of therapeutic substance into bursa of hand**

82.95 **Injection of therapeutic substance into tendon of hand**

82.96 **Other injection of locally-acting therapeutic substance into soft tissue of hand**

Excludes *subcutaneous or intramuscular injection (99.11–99.29)*

✖ 82.99 **Other operations on muscle, tendon, and fascia of hand**

● 83 **Operations on muscle, tendon, fascia, and bursa, except hand**

Includes: operations on:
aponeurosis
synovial membrane of bursa and tendon sheaths
tendon sheaths

Excludes *diaphragm (34.81–34.89)*
hand (82.01–82.99)
muscles of eye (15.01–15.9)

● 83.0 **Incision of muscle, tendon, fascia, and bursa**

✖ 83.01 **Exploration of tendon sheath**
Incision of tendon sheath
Removal of rice bodies from tendon sheath

✖ 83.02 **Myotomy**

Excludes *cricopharyngeal myotomy (29.31)*

✖ 83.03 **Bursotomy**
Removal of calcareous deposit of bursa

Excludes *aspiration of bursa (percutaneous) (83.94)*

✖ 83.09 **Other incision of soft tissue**
Incision of fascia

Excludes *incision of skin and subcutaneous tissue alone (86.01–86.09)*

● 83.1 **Division of muscle, tendon, and fascia**

✖ 83.11 **Achillotenotomy**

✖ 83.12 **Adductor tenotomy of hip**

✖ 83.13 **Other tenotomy**
Aponeurotomy
Division of tendon
Tendon release
Tendon transection
Tenotomy for thoracic outlet decompression

✖ 83.14 **Fasciotomy**
Division of fascia
Division of iliotibial band
Fascia stripping
Release of Volkmann's contracture by fasciotomy

✖ 83.19 **Other division of soft tissue**
Division of muscle
Muscle release
Myotomy for thoracic outlet decompression
Myotomy with division
Scalenotomy
Transection of muscle

● 83.2 **Diagnostic procedures on muscle, tendon, fascia, and bursa, including that of hand**

✖ 83.21 **Biopsy of soft tissue**

Excludes *biopsy of chest wall (34.23)*
biopsy of skin and subcutaneous tissue (86.11)

✖ 83.29 **Other diagnostic procedures on muscle, tendon, fascia, and bursa, including that of hand**

Excludes *microscopic examination of specimen (91.51–91.59)*
soft tissue x-ray (87.09, 87.38–87.39, 88.09, 88.35, 88.37)
thermography of muscle (88.84)

● 83.3 **Excision of lesion of muscle, tendon, fascia, and bursa**

Excludes *biopsy of soft tissue (83.21)*

✖ 83.31 **Excision of lesion of tendon sheath**
Excision of ganglion of tendon sheath, except of hand

✖ 83.32 **Excision of lesion of muscle**
Excision of:
heterotopic bone
muscle scar for release of Volkmann's contracture
myositis ossificans

✖ 83.39 **Excision of lesion of other soft tissue**
Excision of Baker's cyst

Excludes *bursectomy (83.5)*
excision of lesion of skin and subcutaneous tissue (86.3)
synovectomy (80.70–80.79)

● 83.4 **Other excision of muscle, tendon, and fascia**

✖ 83.41 **Excision of tendon for graft**

✖ 83.42 **Other tenonectomy**
Excision of:
aponeurosis
tendon sheath
Tenosynovectomy

✖ 83.43 **Excision of muscle or fascia for graft**

✖ 83.44 **Other fasciectomy**

✖ 83.45 **Other myectomy**
Debridement of muscle NOS
Scalenectomy

✖ 83.49 **Other excision of soft tissue**

✖ 83.5 **Bursectomy**

● 83.6 **Suture of muscle, tendon, and fascia**

✖ 83.61 **Suture of tendon sheath**

✖ 83.62 **Delayed suture of tendon**

✖ 83.63 **Rotator cuff repair**

✖ 83.64 **Other suture of tendon**
Achillorrhaphy
Aponeurorrhaphy

Excludes *delayed suture of tendon (83.62)*

✖ 83.65 **Other suture of muscle or fascia**
Repair of diastasis recti

● 83.7 **Reconstruction of muscle and tendon**

Excludes *reconstruction of muscle and tendon associated with arthroplasty*

✖ 83.71 **Advancement of tendon**

✖ 83.72 **Recession of tendon**

✖ 83.73 **Reattachment of tendon**

✖ 83.74 **Reattachment of muscle**

✖ 83.75 **Tendon transfer or transplantation**

✖ 83.76 **Other tendon transposition**

✖ 83.77 **Muscle transfer or transplantation**
Release of Volkmann's contracture by muscle transplantation

✖ 83.79 **Other muscle transposition**

● 83.8 **Other plastic operations on muscle, tendon, and fascia**

Excludes *plastic operations on muscle, tendon, and fascia associated with arthroplasty*

✖ 83.81 **Tendon graft**

✖ 83.82 **Graft of muscle or fascia**

✖ 83.83 **Tendon pulley reconstruction**

✖ 83.84 **Release of clubfoot, not elsewhere classified**
Evans operation on clubfoot

✖ 83.85 **Other change in muscle or tendon length**
Hamstring lengthening
Heel cord shortening
Plastic achillotenotomy
Tendon plication

✖ 83.86 **Quadricepsplasty**

✖ 83.87 **Other plastic operations on muscle**
Musculoplasty
Myoplasty

✖ 83.88 **Other plastic operations on tendon**
Myotenoplasty
Tendon fixation
Tenodesis
Tenoplasty

✖ 83.89 **Other plastic operations on fascia**
Fascia lengthening
Fascioplasty
Plication of fascia

● 83.9 **Other operations on muscle, tendon, fascia, and bursa**

Excludes *nonoperative:*
manipulation (93.25–93.29)
stretching (93.27–93.29)

✖ 83.91 **Lysis of adhesions of muscle, tendon, fascia, and bursa**

Excludes *that for tarsal tunnel syndrome (04.44)*

✖ 83.92 **Insertion or replacement of skeletal muscle stimulator**
Implantation, insertion, placement, or replacement of skeletal muscle:
electrodes
stimulator

✖ 83.93 **Removal of skeletal muscle stimulator**

83.94 **Aspiration of bursa**

83.95 **Aspiration of other soft tissue**

Excludes *that of skin and subcutaneous tissue (86.01)*

83.96 **Injection of therapeutic substance into bursa**

83.97 **Injection of therapeutic substance into tendon**

83.98 **Injection of locally-acting therapeutic substance into other soft tissue**

Excludes *subcutaneous or intramuscular injection (99.11–99.29)*

✖ 83.99 **Other operations on muscle, tendon, fascia, and bursa**
Suture of bursa

● 84 **Other procedures on musculoskeletal system**

● 84.0 **Amputation of upper limb**

Excludes *revision of amputation stump (84.3)*

✖ 84.00 **Upper limb amputation, not otherwise specified**
Closed flap amputation of upper limb NOS
Kineplastic amputation of upper limb NOS
Open or guillotine amputation of upper limb NOS
Revision of current traumatic amputation of upper limb NOS

✖ 84.01 **Amputation and disarticulation of finger**

Excludes *ligation of supernumerary finger (86.26)*

✖ 84.02 **Amputation and disarticulation of thumb**

✖ 84.03 **Amputation through hand**
Amputation through carpals

✖ 84.04 **Disarticulation of wrist**

✖ 84.05 **Amputation through forearm**
Forearm amputation

✖ 84.06 **Disarticulation of elbow**

✖ 84.07 **Amputation through humerus**
Upper arm amputation

✖ 84.08 **Disarticulation of shoulder**

✖ 84.09 **Interthoracoscapular amputation**
Forequarter amputation

● 84.1 **Amputation of lower limb**

Excludes *revision of amputation stump (84.3)*

✖ 84.10 **Lower limb amputation, not otherwise specified**
Closed flap amputation of lower limb NOS
Kineplastic amputation of lower limb NOS
Open or guillotine amputation of lower limb NOS
Revision of current traumatic amputation of lower limb NOS

✖ 84.11 **Amputation of toe**
Amputation through metatarsophalangeal joint
Disarticulation of toe
Metatarsal head amputation
Ray amputation of foot (disarticulation of the metatarsal head of the toe extending across the forefoot just proximal to the metatarsophalangeal crease)

Excludes *ligation of supernumerary toe (86.26)*

✖ 84.12 **Amputation through foot**
Amputation of forefoot
Amputation through middle of foot
Chopart's amputation
Midtarsal amputation
Transmetatarsal amputation (amputation of the forefoot, including all the toes)

Excludes *ray amputation of foot (84.11)*

✖ 84.13 **Disarticulation of ankle**

✖ 84.14 **Amputation of ankle through malleoli of tibia and fibula**

✖ 84.15 **Other amputation below knee**
Amputation of leg through tibia and fibula NOS

✖**84.16 Disarticulation of knee**
Batch, Spitler, and McFaddin amputation
Mazet amputation
S.P. Roger's amputation

✖**84.17 Amputation above knee**
Amputation of leg through femur
Amputation of thigh
Conversion of below-knee amputation into above-knee amputation
Supracondylar above-knee amputation

✖**84.18 Disarticulation of hip**

✖**84.19 Abdominopelvic amputation**
Hemipelvectomy
Hindquarter amputation

● **84.2 Reattachment of extremity**

✖**84.21 Thumb reattachment**

✖**84.22 Finger reattachment**

✖**84.23 Forearm, wrist, or hand reattachment**

✖**84.24 Upper arm reattachment**
Reattachment of arm NOS

✖**84.25 Toe reattachment**

✖**84.26 Foot reattachment**

✖**84.27 Lower leg or ankle reattachment**
Reattachment of leg NOS

✖**84.28 Thigh reattachment**

✖**84.29 Other reattachment**

✖**84.3 Revision of amputation stump**
Reamputation of stump
Secondary closure of stump
Trimming of stump

Excludes *revision of current traumatic amputation [revision by further amputation of current injury] (84.00–84.19, 84.91)*

● **84.4 Implantation or fitting of prosthetic limb device**

✖**84.40 Implantation or fitting of prosthetic limb device, not otherwise specified**

84.41 Fitting of prosthesis of upper arm and shoulder

84.42 Fitting of prosthesis of lower arm and hand

84.43 Fitting of prosthesis of arm, not otherwise specified

✖**84.44 Implantation of prosthetic device of arm**

84.45 Fitting of prosthesis above knee

84.46 Fitting of prosthesis below knee

84.47 Fitting of prosthesis of leg, not otherwise specified

✖**84.48 Implantation of prosthetic device of leg**

● **84.5 Implantation of other musculoskeletal devices an substances**

84.51 Insertion of interbody spinal fusion device
Insertion of: cages (carbon, ceramic, metal, plastic or titanium)
interbody fusion cage
synthetic cages or spacers
threaded bone dowels

Code also refusion of spine (81.30–81.39)

Code also spinal fusion (81.00–81.08)

84.52 Insertion of recombinant bone morphogenetic protein rhBMP
That via collagen sponge, coral, ceramic, and other carriers

Code also primary procedure performed:
fracture repair (79.00–79.99)
spinal fusion (81.00–81.08)
spinal refusion (81.30–81.39)

● **84.9 Other operations on musculoskeletal system**

Excludes *nonoperative manipulation (93.25–93.29)*

✖**84.91 Amputation, not otherwise specified**

✖**84.92 Separation of equal conjoined twins**

✖**84.93 Separation of unequal conjoined twins**
Separation of conjoined twins NOS

✖**84.99 Other**

15. OPERATIONS ON THE INTEGUMENTARY SYSTEM (85–86)

● 85 **Operations on the breast**

Includes: operations on the skin and subcutaneous tissue of:
breast female or male
previous mastectomy site female or male
revision of previous mastectomy site

85.0 **Mastotomy**
Incision of breast (skin)
Mammotomy
Excludes *aspiration of breast (85.91)*
removal of implant (85.94)

● 85.1 **Diagnostic procedures on breast**

85.11 **Closed [percutaneous] [needle] biopsy of breast**

✖ 85.12 **Open biopsy of breast**

85.19 **Other diagnostic procedures on breast**
Excludes *mammary ductogram (87.35)*
mammography NEC (87.37)
manual examination (89.36)
microscopic examination of specimen (91.61–91.69)
thermography (88.85)
ultrasonography (88.73)
xerography (87.36)

● 85.2 **Excision or destruction of breast tissue**
Excludes *mastectomy (85.41–85.48)*
reduction mammoplasty (85.31–85.32)

✖ 85.20 **Excision or destruction of breast tissue, not otherwise specified**

✖ 85.21 **Local excision of lesion of breast**
Lumpectomy
Removal of area of fibrosis from breast
Excludes *biopsy of breast (85.11–85.12)*

✖ 85.22 **Resection of quadrant of breast**

✖ 85.23 **Subtotal mastectomy**
Excludes *quadrant resection (85.22)*

✖ 85.24 **Excision of ectopic breast tissue**
Excision of accessory nipple

✖ 85.25 **Excision of nipple**
Excludes *excision of accessory nipple (85.24)*

● 85.3 **Reduction mammoplasty and subcutaneous mammectomy**

✖ 85.31 **Unilateral reduction mammoplasty**
Unilateral:
amputative mammoplasty
size reduction mammoplasty

✖ 85.32 **Bilateral reduction mammoplasty**
Amputative mammoplasty
Reduction mammoplasty (for gynecomastia)

✖ 85.33 **Unilateral subcutaneous mammectomy with synchronous implant**
Excludes *that without synchronous implant (85.34)*

✖ 85.34 **Other unilateral subcutaneous mammectomy**
Removal of breast tissue with preservation of skin and nipple
Subcutaneous mammectomy NOS

✖ 85.35 **Bilateral subcutaneous mammectomy with synchronous implant**
Excludes *that without synchronous implant (85.36)*

✖ 85.36 **Other bilateral subcutaneous mammectomy**

● 85.4 **Mastectomy**

✖ 85.41 **Unilateral simple mastectomy**
Mastectomy:
NOS
complete

✖ 85.42 **Bilateral simple mastectomy**
Bilateral complete mastectomy

✖ 85.43 **Unilateral extended simple mastectomy**
Extended simple mastectomy NOS
Modified radical mastectomy
Simple mastectomy with excision of regional lymph nodes

✖ 85.44 **Bilateral extended simple mastectomy**

✖ 85.45 **Unilateral radical mastectomy**
Excision of breast, pectoral muscles, and regional lymph nodes [axillary, clavicular, supraclavicular]
Radical mastectomy NOS

✖ 85.46 **Bilateral radical mastectomy**

✖ 85.47 **Unilateral extended radical mastectomy**
Excision of breast, muscles, and lymph nodes [axillary, clavicular, supraclavicular, internal mammary, and mediastinal]
Extended radical mastectomy NOS

✖ 85.48 **Bilateral extended radical mastectomy**

● 85.5 **Augmentation mammoplasty**
Excludes *that associated with subcutaneous mammectomy (85.33, 85.35)*

✖ 85.50 **Augmentation mammoplasty, not otherwise specified**

85.51 **Unilateral injection into breast for augmentation**

85.52 **Bilateral injection into breast for augmentation**
Injection into breast for augmentation NOS

✖ 85.53 **Unilateral breast implant**

✖ 85.54 **Bilateral breast implant**
Breast implant NOS

✖ 85.6 **Mastopexy**

✖ 85.7 **Total reconstruction of breast**

● 85.8 **Other repair and plastic operations on breast**
Excludes *that for:*
augmentation (85.50–85.54)
reconstruction (85.7)
reduction (85.31–85.32)

85.81 **Suture of laceration of breast**

✖ 85.82 **Split-thickness graft to breast**

✖ 85.83 **Full-thickness graft to breast**

✖ 85.84 **Pedicle graft to breast**

✖ 85.85 **Muscle flap graft to breast**

✖ 85.86 **Transposition of nipple**

✖ 85.87 **Other repair or reconstruction of nipple**

✖ 85.89 **Other mammoplasty**

● 85.9 **Other operations on the breast**

85.91 **Aspiration of breast**
Excludes *percutaneous biopsy of breast (85.11)*

85.92 **Injection of therapeutic agent into breast**
Excludes *that for augmentation of breast (85.51–85.52)*

✖ 85.93 **Revision of implant of breast**

✖ 85.94 **Removal of implant of breast**

✖ 85.95 **Insertion of breast tissue expander**
Insertion (soft tissue) of tissue expander (one or more) under muscle or platysma to develop skin flaps for donor use

✖ **85.96 Removal of breast tissue expander(s)**

✖ **85.99 Other**

● **86 Operations on skin and subcutaneous tissue**

Includes: operations on:
- hair follicles
- male perineum
- nails
- sebaceous glands
- subcutaneous fat pads
- sudoriferous glands
- superficial fossae

Excludes *those on skin of:*
- *anus (49.01–49.99)*
- *breast (mastectomy site) (85.0–85.99)*
- *ear (18.01–18.9)*
- *eyebrow (08.01–08.99)*
- *eyelid (08.01–08.99)*
- *female perineum (71.01–71.9)*
- *lips (27.0–27.99)*
- *nose (21.00–21.99)*
- *penis (64.0–64.99)*
- *scrotum (61.0–61.99)*
- *vulva (71.01–71.9)*

● **86.0 Incision of skin and subcutaneous tissue**

86.01 Aspiration of skin and subcutaneous tissue

Aspiration of:
- abscess of nail, skin, or subcutaneous tissue
- hematoma of nail, skin, or subcutaneous tissue
- seroma of nail, skin, or subcutaneous tissue

86.02 Injection or tattooing of skin lesion or defect

Injection of filling material
Insertion of filling material
Pigmenting of skin of filling material

86.03 Incision of pilonidal sinus or cyst

Excludes *marsupialization (86.21)*

86.04 Other incision with drainage of skin and subcutaneous tissue

Excludes *drainage of:*
- *fascial compartments of face and mouth (27.0)*
- *palmar or thenar space 82.04)*
- *pilonidal sinus or cyst 86.03)*

86.05 Incision with removal of foreign body from skin and subcutaneous tissue

Removal of loop recorder
Removal of tissue expander(s) from skin or soft tissue other than breast tissue

Excludes *removal of foreign body without incision (98.20–98.29)*

✖ **86.06 Insertion of totally implantable infusion pump**

Code also any associated catheterization

Excludes *insertion of totally implantable vascular access device (86.07)*

86.07 Insertion of totally implantable vascular access device [VAD]

Totally implanted port

Excludes *insertion of totally implantable infusion pump (86.06)*

86.09 Other incision of skin and subcutaneous tissue

Creation of loop recorder pocket, new site and insertion/relocation of device
Creation of pocket for implantable, patient-activated cardiac event recorder and insertion/relocation of device
Creation of thalamic stimulator pulse generator pocket, new site
Escharotomy
Exploration:
- sinus tract, skin
- superficial fossa

Undercutting of hair follicle

Excludes *that of:*
- *cardiac pacemaker pocket, new site (37.79)*
- *fascial compartments of face and mouth (27.0)*

● **86.1 Diagnostic procedures on skin and subcutaneous tissue**

86.11 Biopsy of skin and subcutaneous tissue

86.19 Other diagnostic procedures on skin and subcutaneous tissue

Excludes *microscopic examination of specimen from skin and subcutaneous tissue (91.61–91.79)*

● **86.2 Excision or destruction of lesion or tissue of skin and subcutaneous tissue**

✖ **86.21 Excision of pilonidal cyst or sinus**

Marsupialization of cyst

Excludes *incision of pilonidal cyst or sinus (86.03)*

✖ **86.22 Excisional debridement of wound, infection, or burn**

Removal by excision of:
- devitalized tissue
- necrosis
- slough

Excludes *debridement of:*
- *abdominal wall (wound) (54.3)*
- *bone (77.60–77.69)*
- *muscle (83.45)*
- *of hand (82.36)*
- *nail (bed) (fold) (86.27)*
- *nonexcisional debridement of wound, infection, or burn (86.28)*
- *open fracture site (79.60–79.69)*
- *pedicle or flap graft (86.75)*

86.23 Removal of nail, nail bed, or nail fold

86.24 Chemosurgery of skin

Chemical peel of skin

✖ **86.25 Dermabrasion**

That with laser

Excludes *dermabrasion of wound to remove embedded debris (86.28)*

86.26 Ligation of dermal appendage

Excludes *excision of preauricular appendage (18.29)*

86.27 Debridement of nail, nail bed, or nail fold

Removal of:
- necrosis
- slough

Excludes *removal of nail, nail bed, or nail fold (86.23)*

86.28 Nonexcisional debridement of wound, infection or burn

Debridement NOS
Maggot therapy
Removal of devitalized tissue, necrosis and slough by such methods as:
- brushing
- irrigation (under pressure)
- scrubbing
- washing

86.3 Other local excision or destruction of lesion or tissue of skin and subcutaneous tissue

Destruction of skin by:
- cauterization cryosurgery
- fulguration
- laser beam

That with Z-plasty

Excludes *adipectomy (86.83)*
biopsy of skin (86.11)
wide or radical excision of skin (86.4)
Z-plasty without excision (86.84)

✖**86.4 Radical excision of skin lesion**
Wide excision of skin lesion involving underlying or adjacent structure

Code also any lymph node dissection (40.3–40.5)

● **86.5 Suture or other closure of skin and subcutaneous tissue**

86.51 **Replantation of scalp**

86.59 **Closure of skin and subcutaneous tissue of other sites**
Adhesives (surgical) (tissue)
Staples
Sutures

Excludes *application of adhesive strips (butterfly)—omit code*

● **86.6 Free skin graft**

Includes: excision of skin for autogenous graft

Excludes *construction or reconstruction of:*
penis (64.43–64.44)
trachea (31.75)
vagina (70.61–70.62)

✖86.60 **Free skin graft, not otherwise specified**

✖86.61 **Full-thickness skin graft to hand**

Excludes *heterograft (86.65)*
homograft (86.66)

✖86.62 **Other skin graft to hand**

Excludes *heterograft (86.65)*
homograft (86.66)

✖86.63 **Full-thickness skin graft to other sites**

Excludes *heterograft (86.65)*
homograft (86.66)

86.64 **Hair transplant**

Excludes *hair follicle transplant to eyebrow or eyelash (08.63)*

✖86.65 **Heterograft to skin**
Pigskin graft
Porcine graft

Excludes *application of dressing only (93.57)*

✖86.66 **Homograft to skin**
Graft to skin of:
amnionic membrane from donor skin from donor

86.67 **Dermal regenerative graft**
Artificial skin, NOS
Creation of "neodermis"
Decellularized allodermis
Integumentary matrix implants
Prosthetic implant of dermal layer of skin
Regenerate dermal layer of skin

Excludes *heterograft to skin (86.65)*
homograft to skin (86.66)

✖86.69 **Other skin graft to other sites**

Excludes *heterograft (86.65)*
homograft (86.66)

● **86.7 Pedicle grafts or flaps**

Excludes *construction or reconstruction of:*
penis (64.43–64.44)
trachea (31.75)
vagina (70.61–70.62)

✖86.70 **Pedicle or flap graft, not otherwise specified**

✖86.71 **Cutting and preparation of pedicle grafts or flaps**
Elevation of pedicle from its bed
Flap design and raising
Partial cutting of pedicle or tube
Pedicle delay

Excludes *pollicization or digital transfer (82.61, 82.81)*
revision of pedicle (86.75)

✖86.72 **Advancement of pedicle graft**

✖86.73 **Attachment of pedicle or flap graft to hand**

Excludes *pollicization or digital transfer (82.61, 82.81)*

✖86.74 **Attachment of pedicle or flap graft to other sites**
Attachment by:
advanced flap
double pedicled flap
pedicle graft
rotating flap
sliding flap
tube graft

✖86.75 **Revision of pedicle or flap graft**
Debridement of pedicle or flap graft
Defatting of pedicle or flap graft

● **86.8 Other repair and reconstruction of skin and subcutaneous tissue**

✖86.81 **Repair for facial weakness**

✖86.82 **Facial rhytidectomy**
Face lift

Excludes *rhytidectomy of eyelid (08.86–08.87)*

✖86.83 **Size reduction plastic operation**
Reduction of adipose tissue of:
abdominal wall (pendulous)
arms (batwing)
buttock
liposuction
thighs (trochanteric lipomatosis)

Excludes *breast (85.31–85.32)*

✖86.84 **Relaxation of scar or web contracture of skin**
Z-plasty of skin

Excludes *Z-plasty with excision of lesion (86.3)*

✖86.85 **Correction of syndactyly**

✖86.86 **Onychoplasty**

✖86.89 **Other repair and reconstruction of skin and subcutaneous tissue**

Excludes *mentoplasty (76.67–76.68)*

● **86.9 Other operations on skin and subcutaneous tissue**

✖86.91 **Excision of skin for graft**
Excision of skin with closure of donor site

Excludes *that with graft at same operative episode (86.60–86.69)*

86.92 **Electrolysis and other epilation of skin**

Excludes *epilation of eyelid (08.91–08.93)*

✖86.93 **Insertion of tissue expander**
Insertion (subcutaneous) (soft tissue) of expander (one or more) in scalp (subgaleal space), face, neck, trunk except breast, and upper and lower extremities for development of skin flaps for donor use

Excludes *flap graft preparation (86.71)*
tissue expander, breast (85.95)

86.99 **Other**

Excludes *removal of sutures from:*
abdomen (97.83)
head and neck (97.38)
thorax (97.43)
trunk NEC (97.84)
wound catheter:
irrigation (96.58)
replacement (97.15)

16. MISCELLANEOUS DIAGNOSTIC AND THERAPEUTIC PROCEDURES (87–99)

● 87 Diagnostic Radiology

● 87.0 Soft tissue x-ray of face, head, and neck

Excludes *angiography (88.40–88.68)*

87.01 **Pneumoencephalogram**

87.02 **Other contrast radiogram of brain and skull**
Pneumocisternogram
Pneumoventriculogram
Posterior fossa myelogram

87.03 **Computerized axial tomography of head**
C.A.T. scan of head

87.04 **Other tomography of head**

87.05 **Contrast dacryocystogram**

87.06 **Contrast radiogram of nasopharynx**

87.07 **Contrast laryngogram**

87.08 **Cervical lymphangiogram**

87.09 **Other soft tissue x-ray of face, head, and neck**
Noncontrast x-ray of:
adenoid
larynx
nasolacrimal duct
nasopharynx
salivary gland
thyroid region
uvula

Excludes *x-ray study of eye (95.14)*

● 87.1 Other x-ray of face, head, and neck

Excludes *angiography (88.40–88.68)*

87.11 **Full-mouth x-ray of teeth**

87.12 **Other dental x-ray**
Orthodontic cephalogram or cephalometrics
Panorex examination of mandible
Root canal x-ray

87.13 **Temporomandibular contrast arthrogram**

87.14 **Contrast radiogram of orbit**

87.15 **Contrast radiogram of sinus**

87.16 **Other x-ray of facial bones**
X-ray of:
frontal area
mandible
maxilla
nasal sinuses
nose
orbit
supraorbital area
symphysis menti
zygomaticomaxillary complex

87.17 **Other x-ray of skull**
Lateral projection of skull
Sagittal projection of skull
Tangential projection of skull

● 87.2 X-ray of spine

87.21 **Contrast myelogram**

87.22 **Other x-ray of cervical spine**

87.23 **Other x-ray of thoracic spine**

87.24 **Other x-ray of lumbosacral spine**
Sacrococcygeal x-ray

87.29 **Other x-ray of spine**
Spinal x-ray NOS

● 87.3 Soft tissue x-ray of thorax

Excludes *angiocardiography (88.50–88.58)*
angiography (88.40–88.68)

87.31 **Endotracheal bronchogram**

87.32 **Other contrast bronchogram**
Transcricoid bronchogram

87.33 **Mediastinal pneumogram**

87.34 **Intrathoracic lymphangiogram**

87.35 **Contrast radiogram of mammary ducts**

87.36 **Xerography of breast**

87.37 **Other mammography**

87.38 **Sinogram of chest wall**
Fistulogram of chest wall

87.39 **Other soft tissue x-ray of chest wall**

● 87.4 Other x-ray of thorax

Excludes *angiocardiography (88.50–88.58)*
angiography (88.40–88.68)

87.41 **Computerized axial tomography of thorax**
C.A.T. scan of thorax
Crystal linear scan of x-ray beam of thorax
Electronic subtraction of thorax
Photoelectric response of thorax
Tomography with use of computer, x-rays, and camera of thorax

87.42 **Other tomography of thorax**
Cardiac tomogram

87.43 **X-ray of ribs, sternum, and clavicle**
Examination for:
cervical rib
fracture

87.44 **Routine chest x-ray, so described**
X-ray of chest NOS

87.49 **Other chest x-ray**
X-ray of:
bronchus NOS
diaphragm NOS
heart NOS
lung NOS
mediastinum NOS
trachea NOS

● 87.5 Biliary tract x-ray

87.51 **Percutaneous hepatic cholangiogram**

87.52 **Intravenous cholangiogram**

✖ 87.53 **Intraoperative cholangiogram**

87.54 **Other cholangiogram**

87.59 **Other biliary tract x-ray**
Cholecystogram

● 87.6 Other x-ray of digestive system

87.61 **Barium swallow**

87.62 **Upper GI series**

87.63 **Small bowel series**

87.64 **Lower GI series**

87.65 **Other x-ray of intestine**

87.66 **Contrast pancreatogram**

87.69 **Other digestive tract x-ray**

● 87.7 X-ray of urinary system

Excludes *angiography of renal vessels (88.45, 88.65)*

87.71 **Computerized axial tomography of kidney**
C.A.T. scan of kidney

87.72 **Other nephrotomogram**

87.73 **Intravenous pyelogram**
Diuretic infusion pyelogram

87.74 **Retrograde pyelogram**

87.75 **Percutaneous pyelogram**

87.76 **Retrograde cystourethrogram**

87.77 **Other cystogram**

87.78 **Ileal conduitogram**

87.79 **Other x-ray of the urinary system**
KUB x-ray

● **87.8** **X-ray of female genital organs**

87.81 **X-ray of gravid uterus**
Intrauterine cephalometry by x-ray

87.82 **Gas contrast hysterosalpingogram**

87.83 **Opaque dye contrast hysterosalpingogram**

87.84 **Percutaneous hysterogram**

87.85 **Other x-ray of fallopian tubes and uterus**

87.89 **Other x-ray of female genital organs**

● **87.9** **X-ray of male genital organs**

87.91 **Contrast seminal vesiculogram**

87.92 **Other x-ray of prostate and seminal vesicles**

87.93 **Contrast epididymogram**

87.94 **Contrast vasogram**

87.95 **Other x-ray of epididymis and vas deferens**

87.99 **Other x-ray of male genital organs**

● **88** **Other diagnostic radiology and related techniques**

● **88.0** **Soft tissue x-ray of abdomen**

Excludes *angiography (88.40–88.68)*

88.01 **Computerized axial tomography of abdomen**
C.A.T. scan of abdomen

Excludes *C.A.T. scan of kidney (87.71)*

88.02 **Other abdomen tomography**

Excludes *nephrotomogram (87.72)*

88.03 **Sinogram of abdominal wall**
Fistulogram of abdominal wall

88.04 **Abdominal lymphangiogram**

88.09 **Other soft tissue x-ray of abdominal wall**

● **88.1** **Other x-ray of abdomen**

88.11 **Pelvic opaque dye contrast radiography**

88.12 **Pelvic gas contrast radiography**
Pelvic pneumoperitoneum

88.13 **Other peritoneal pneumogram**

88.14 **Retroperitoneal fistulogram**

88.15 **Retroperitoneal pneumogram**

88.16 **Other retroperitoneal x-ray**

88.19 **Other x-ray of abdomen**
Flat plate of abdomen

● **88.2** **Skeletal x-ray of extremities and pelvis**

Excludes *contrast radiogram of joint (88.32)*

88.21 **Skeletal x-ray of shoulder and upper arm**

88.22 **Skeletal x-ray of elbow and forearm**

88.23 **Skeletal x-ray of wrist and hand**

88.24 **Skeletal x-ray of upper limb, not otherwise specified**

88.25 **Pelvimetry**

88.26 **Other skeletal x-ray of pelvis and hip**

88.27 **Skeletal x-ray of thigh, knee, and lower leg**

88.28 **Skeletal x-ray of ankle and foot**

88.29 **Skeletal x-ray of lower limb, not otherwise specified**

● **88.3** **Other x-ray**

88.31 **Skeletal series**
X-ray of whole skeleton

88.32 **Contrast arthrogram**

Excludes *that of temporomandibular joint (87.13)*

88.33 **Other skeletal x-ray**

Excludes *skeletal x-ray of:*
extremities and pelvis 88.21–88.29)
face, head, and neck (87.11–87.17)
spine (87.21–87.29)
thorax (87.43)

88.34 **Lymphangiogram of upper limb**

88.35 **Other soft tissue x-ray of upper limb**

88.36 **Lymphangiogram of lower limb**

88.37 **Other soft tissue x-ray of lower limb**

Excludes *femoral angiography (88.48, 88.66)*

88.38 **Other computerized axial tomography**
C.A.T. scan NOS

Excludes *C.A.T. scan of:*
abdomen (88.01)
head (87.03)
kidney (87.71)
thorax (87.41)

88.39 **X-ray, other and unspecified**

● **88.4** **Arteriography using contrast material**

Includes: angiography of arteries
arterial puncture for injection of contrast material
radiography of arteries (by fluoroscopy)
retrograde arteriography

Note: The fourth-digit subclassification identifies the site to be viewed, not the site of injection.

Excludes *arteriography using:*
radioisotopes or radionuclides (92.01–92.19)
ultrasound (88.71–88.79)
fluorescein angiography of eye (95.12)

88.40 **Arteriography using contrast material, unspecified site**

88.41 **Arteriography of cerebral arteries**
Angiography of:
basilar artery
carotid (internal)
posterior cerebral circulation
vertebral artery

88.42 **Aortography**
Arteriography of aorta and aortic arch

88.43 **Arteriography of pulmonary arteries**

88.44 **Arteriography of other intrathoracic vessels**

Excludes *angiocardiography (88.50–88.58)*
arteriography of coronary arteries (88.55–88.57)

88.45 **Arteriography of renal arteries**

88.46 **Arteriography of placenta**
Placentogram using contrast material

88.47 **Arteriography of other intra-abdominal arteries**

88.48 **Arteriography of femoral and other lower extremity arteries**

88.49 **Arteriography of other specified sites**

● **88.5 Angiocardiography using contrast material**

Includes: arterial puncture and insertion of arterial catheter for injection of contrast material
cineangiocardiography
selective angiocardiography

Code also synchronous cardiac catheterization (37.21–37.23)

Excludes *angiography of pulmonary vessels (88.43, 88.62)*

88.50 Angiocardiography, not otherwise specified

88.51 Angiocardiography of venae cavae
Inferior vena cavography
Phlebography of vena cava (inferior) (superior)

88.52 Angiocardiography of right heart structures
Angiocardiography of:
pulmonary valve
right atrium
right ventricle (outflow tract)

Excludes *that combined with left heart angiocardiography (88.54)*

88.53 Angiocardiography of left heart structures
Angiocardiography of:
aortic valve
left atrium
left ventricle (outflow tract)

Excludes *that combined with right heart angiocardiography (88.54)*

88.54 Combined right and left heart angiocardiography

88.55 Coronary arteriography using a single catheter
Coronary arteriography by Sones technique
Direct selective coronary arteriography using a single catheter

88.56 Coronary arteriography using two catheters
Coronary arteriography by:
Judkins technique
Ricketts and Abrams technique
Direct selective coronary arteriography using two catheters

88.57 Other and unspecified coronary arteriography
Coronary arteriography NOS

88.58 Negative-contrast cardiac roentgenography
Cardiac roentgenography with injection of carbon dioxide

● **88.6 Phlebography**

Includes: angiography of veins
radiography of veins (by fluoroscopy)
retrograde phlebography
venipuncture for injection of contrast material
venography using contrast material

Note: The fourth-digit subclassification (88.60–88.67) identifies the site to be viewed, not the site of injection.

Excludes *angiography using:*
radioisotopes or radionuclides (92.01–92.19)
ultrasound (88.71–88.79)
fluorescein angiography of eye (95.12)

88.60 Phlebography using contrast material, unspecified site

88.61 Phlebography of veins of head and neck using contrast material

88.62 Phlebography of pulmonary veins using contrast material

88.63 Phlebography of other intrathoracic veins using contrast material

88.64 Phlebography of the portal venous system using contrast material
Splenoportogram (by splenic arteriography)

88.65 Phlebography of other intra-abdominal veins using contrast material

88.66 Phlebography of femoral and other lower extremity veins using contrast material

88.67 Phlebography of other specified sites using contrast material

88.68 Impedance phlebography

● **88.7 Diagnostic ultrasound**

Includes: echography
ultrasonic angiography
ultrasonography

Excludes *therapeutic ultrasound (00.01–00.09)*

88.71 Diagnostic ultrasound of head and neck
Determination of midline shift of brain
Echoencephalography

Excludes *eye (95.13)*

88.72 Diagnostic ultrasound of heart
Echocardiography
Intravascular ultrasound of heart

88.73 Diagnostic ultrasound of other sites of thorax
Aortic arch ultrasonography
Breast ultrasonography
Lung ultrasonography

88.74 Diagnostic ultrasound of digestive system

88.75 Diagnostic ultrasound of urinary system

88.76 Diagnostic ultrasound of abdomen and retroperitoneum

88.77 Diagnostic ultrasound of peripheral vascular system
Deep vein thrombosis ultrasonic scanning

88.78 Diagnostic ultrasound of gravid uterus
Intrauterine cephalometry:
echo
ultrasonic
Placental localization by ultrasound

88.79 Other diagnostic ultrasound
Ultrasonography of:
multiple sites
nongravid uterus
total body

● **88.8 Thermography**

88.81 Cerebral thermography

88.82 Ocular thermography

88.83 Bone thermography
Osteoarticular thermography

88.84 Muscle thermography

88.85 Breast thermography

88.86 Blood vessel thermography
Deep vein thermography

88.89 Thermography of other sites
Lymph gland thermography
Thermography NOS

● **88.9 Other diagnostic imaging**

88.90 Diagnostic imaging, not elsewhere classified

88.91 Magnetic resonance imaging of brain and brain stem

Excludes *intraoperative magnetic resonance imaging (88.96)*
real-time magnetic resonance imaging (88.96)

88.92 Magnetic resonance imaging of chest and myocardium
For evaluation of hilar and mediastinal lymphadenopathy

88.93 Magnetic resonance imaging of spinal canal
Spinal cord levels:
cervical
thoracic
lumbar (lumbosacral)
Spinal cord
Spine

88.94 Magnetic resonance imaging of musculoskeletal
Bone marrow blood supply
Extremities (upper) (lower)

88.95 Magnetic resonance imaging of pelvis, prostate, and bladder

88.96 Other intraoperative magnetic resonance imaging
iMRI
Real-time magnetic resonance imaging

88.97 Magnetic resonance imaging of other and unspecified sites
Abdomen
Eye orbit
Face
Neck

88.98 Bone mineral density studies
Dual photon absorptiometry
Quantitative computed tomography (CT) studies
Radiographic densitometry
Single photon absorptiometry

● **89 Interview, evaluation, consultation, and examination**

● **89.0 Diagnostic interview, consultation, and evaluation**

Excludes *psychiatric diagnostic interview (94.11–94.19)*

89.01 Interview and evaluation, described as brief
Abbreviated history and evaluation

89.02 Interview and evaluation, described as limited
Interval history and evaluation

89.03 Interview and evaluation, described as comprehensive
History and evaluation of new problem

89.04 Other interview and evaluation

89.05 Diagnostic interview and evaluation, not otherwise specified

89.06 Consultation, described as limited
Consultation on a single organ system

89.07 Consultation, described as comprehensive

89.08 Other consultation

89.09 Consultation, not otherwise specified

● **89.1 Anatomic and physiologic measurements and manual examinations—nervous system and sense organs**

Excludes *ear examination (95.41–95.49)*
eye examination (95.01–95.26)
the listed procedures when done as part of a general physical examination (89.7)

89.10 Intracarotid amobarbital test
Wada test

89.11 Tonometry

89.12 Nasal function study
Rhinomanometry

89.13 Neurologic examination

89.14 Electroencephalogram

Excludes *that with polysomnogram (89.17)*

89.15 Other nonoperative neurologic function tests

89.16 Transillumination of newborn skull

89.17 Polysomnogram
Sleep recording

89.18 Other sleep disorder function tests
Multiple sleep latency test [MSLT]

89.19 Video and radio-telemetered electroencephalographic monitoring
Radiographic EEG monitoring
Video EEG monitoring

● **89.2 Anatomic and physiologic measurements and manual examinations—genitourinary system**

Excludes *the listed procedures when done as part of a general physical examination (89.7)*

89.21 Urinary manometry
Manometry through:
indwelling ureteral catheter
nephrostomy
pyelostomy
ureterostomy

89.22 Cystometrogram

89.23 Urethral sphincter electromyogram

89.24 Uroflowmetry [UFR]

89.25 Urethral pressure profile [UPP]

89.26 Gynecological examination
Pelvic examination

89.29 Other nonoperative genitourinary system measurements
Bioassay of urine
Renal clearance
Urine chemistry

● **89.3 Other anatomic and physiologic measurements and manual examinations**

Excludes *the listed procedures when done as part of a general physical examination (89.7)*

89.31 Dental examination
Oral mucosal survey
Periodontal survey

89.32 Esophageal manometry

89.33 Digital examination of enterostomy stoma
Digital examination of colostomy stoma

89.34 Digital examination of rectum

89.35 Transillumination of nasal sinuses

89.36 Manual examination of breast

89.37 Vital capacity determination

89.38 Other nonoperative respiratory measurements
Plethysmography for measurement of respiratory function
Thoracic impedance plethysmography

89.39 Other nonoperative measurements and examinations
14 C-Urea breath test
Basal metabolic rate [BMR]
Gastric:
analysis
function NEC

Excludes *body measurement (93.07)*
cardiac tests (89.41–89.69)
fundus photography (95.11)
limb length measurement (93.06)

● 89.4 Cardiac stress tests and pacemaker checks

89.41 **Cardiovascular stress test using treadmill**

89.42 **Masters' two-step stress test**

89.43 **Cardiovascular stress test using bicycle ergometer**

89.44 **Other cardiovascular stress test**
Thallium stress test with or without transesophageal pacing

89.45 **Artificial pacemaker rate check**
Artificial pacemaker function check NOS

89.46 **Artificial pacemaker artifact wave form check**

89.47 **Artificial pacemaker electrode impedance check**

89.48 **Artificial pacemaker voltage or amperage threshold check**

● 89.5 **Other nonoperative cardiac and vascular diagnostic procedures**

Excludes *fetal EKG (75.32)*

89.50 **Ambulatory cardiac monitoring**
Analog devices [Holter-type]

89.51 **Rhythm electrocardiogram**
Rhythm EKG (with one to three leads)

89.52 **Electrocardiogram**
ECG NOS
EKG (with 12 or more leads)

89.53 **Vectorcardiogram (with ECG)**

89.54 **Electrographic monitoring**
Telemetry

Excludes *ambulatory cardiac monitoring (89.50)*
electrographic monitoring during surgery—omit code

89.55 **Phonocardiogram with ECG lead**

89.56 **Carotid pulse tracing with ECG lead**

Excludes *oculoplethysmography (89.58)*

89.57 **Apexcardiogram (with ECG lead)**

89.58 **Plethysmogram**

Includes: Penile plethysmography with nerve stimulation

Excludes *plethysmography (for):*
measurement of respiratory function (89.38)
thoracic impedance (89.38)

89.59 **Other nonoperative cardiac and vascular measurements**

89.60 **Continuous intra-arterial blood gas monitoring**
Insertion of blood gas monitoring system and continuous monitoring of blood gases through an intra-arterial sensor

● 89.6 **Circulatory monitoring**

Excludes *electrocardiographic monitoring during surgery—omit code*

89.61 **Systemic arterial pressure monitoring**

89.62 **Central venous pressure monitoring**

89.63 **Pulmonary artery pressure monitoring**

Excludes *pulmonary artery wedge monitoring (89.64)*

89.64 **Pulmonary artery wedge monitoring**
Pulmonary capillary wedge [PCW] monitoring
Swan-Ganz catheterization

89.65 **Measurement of systemic arterial blood gases**

Excludes *continuous intra-arterial blood gas monitoring (89.60)*

89.66 **Measurement of mixed venous blood gases**

89.67 **Monitoring of cardiac output by oxygen consumption technique**
Fick method

89.68 **Monitoring of cardiac output by other technique**
Cardiac output monitor by thermodilution indicator

89.69 **Monitoring of coronary blood flow**
Coronary blood flow monitoring by coincidence counting technique

89.7 **General physical examination**

89.8 **Autopsy**

● 90 **Microscopic examination-I**

The following fourth-digit subclassification is for use with categories in section 90 to identify type of examination:
1 **bacterial smear**
2 **culture**
3 **culture and sensitivity**
4 **parasitology**
5 **toxicology**
6 **cell block and Papanicolaou smear**
9 **other microscopic examination**

● 90.0 **Microscopic examination of specimen from nervous system and of spinal fluid**

● 90.1 **Microscopic examination of specimen from endocrine gland, not elsewhere classified**

● 90.2 **Microscopic examination of specimen from eye**

● 90.3 **Microscopic examination of specimen from ear, nose, throat, and larynx**

● 90.4 **Microscopic examination of specimen from trachea, bronchus, pleura, lung, and other thoracic specimen, and of sputum**

● 90.5 **Microscopic examination of blood**

● 90.6 **Microscopic examination of specimen from spleen and of bone marrow**

● 90.7 **Microscopic examination of specimen from lymph node and of lymph**

● 90.8 **Microscopic examination of specimen from upper gastrointestinal tract and of vomitus**

● 90.9 **Microscopic examination of specimen from lower gastrointestinal tract and of stool**

● 91 **Microscopic examination-II**

The following fourth-digit subclassification is for use with categories in section 91 to identify type of examination
1 **bacterial smear**
2 **culture**
3 **culture and sensitivity**
4 **parasitology**
5 **toxicology**
6 **cell block and Papanicolaou smear**
9 **other microscopic examination**

● 91.0 **Microscopic examination of specimen from liver, biliary tract, and pancreas**

● 91.1 **Microscopic examination of peritoneal and retroperitoneal specimen**

● 91.2 **Microscopic examination of specimen from kidney, ureter, perirenal and periureteral tissue**

● 91.3 **Microscopic examination of specimen from bladder, urethra, prostate, seminal vesicle, perivesical tissue, and of urine and semen**

● 91.4 **Microscopic examination of specimen from female genital tract**
Amnionic sac
Fetus

● 91.5 **Microscopic examination of specimen from musculoskeletal system and of joint fluid**
Microscopic examination of:
bone
bursa
cartilage
fascia
ligament
muscle
synovial membrane
tendon

● 91.6 **Microscopic examination of specimen from skin and other integument**
Microscopic examination of:
hair
nails
skin

Excludes *mucous membrane—code to organ site that of operative wound (91.70–91.79)*

● 91.7 **Microscopic examination of specimen from operative wound**

● 91.8 **Microscopic examination of specimen from other site**

● 91.9 **Microscopic examination of specimen from unspecified site**

● 92 **Nuclear medicine**

● 92.0 **Radioisotope scan and function study**

92.01 **Thyroid scan and radioisotope function studies**
Iodine-131 uptake
Protein-bound iodine
Radio-iodine uptake

92.02 **Liver scan and radioisotope function study**

92.03 **Renal scan and radioisotope function study**
Renal clearance study

92.04 **Gastrointestinal scan and radioisotope function study**
Radio-cobalt B12 Schilling test
Radio-iodinated triolein study

92.05 **Cardiovascular and hematopoietic scan and radioisotope function study**
Bone marrow scan or function study
Cardiac output scan or function study
Circulation time scan or function study
Radionuclide cardiac ventriculogram scan or function study
Spleen scan or function study

92.09 **Other radioisotope function studies**

● 92.1 **Other radioisotope scan**

92.11 **Cerebral scan**
Pituitary

92.12 **Scan of other sites of head**

Excludes *eye (95.16)*

92.13 **Parathyroid scan**

92.14 **Bone scan**

92.15 **Pulmonary scan**

92.16 **Scan of lymphatic system**

92.17 **Placental scan**

92.18 **Total body scan**

92.19 **Scan of other sites**

● 92.2 **Therapeutic radiology and nuclear medicine**

Excludes *that for:*
ablation of pituitary gland (07.64–07.69)
destruction of chorioretinal lesion (14.26–14.27)

92.21 **Superficial radiation**
Contact radiation [up to 150 KVP]

92.22 **Orthovoltage radiation**
Deep radiation [200–300 KVP]

92.23 **Radioisotopic teleradiotherapy**
Teleradiotherapy using:
Cobalt-60
Iodine-125
radioactive cesium

92.24 **Teleradiotherapy using photons**
Megavoltage NOS
Supervoltage NOS
Use of:
Betatron
linear accelerator

92.25 **Teleradiotherapy using electrons**
Beta particles

92.26 **Teleradiotherapy of other particulate radiation**
Neutrons
Protons NOS

✖ 92.27 **Implantation or insertion of radioactive elements**
Code also incision of site

Includes: Intravascular brachytherapy

92.28 **Injection or instillation of radioisotopes**
Injection or infusion of radioimmunoconjugate ◀
Intracavitary injection or instillation
Intravenous injection or instillation
Iodine-131 [I-131] tositumomab ◀
Radioimmunotherapy ◀
Ytrium-90 [Y-90] ibritumomab tiuxetan ◀

92.29 **Other radiotherapeutic procedure**

● 92.3 **Stereotactic radiosurgery**

Excludes *stereotactic biopsy*

Code also stereotactic head frame application (93.59)

92.30 **Stereotactic radiosurgery, not otherwise specified**

92.31 **Single source photon radiosurgery**
High energy x-rays
Linear accelerator (LINAC)

92.32 **Multi-source photon radiosurgery**
Cobalt 60 radiation
Gamma irradiation

92.33 **Particulate radiosurgery**
Particle beam radiation (cyclotron)
Proton accelerator

92.39 **Stereotactic radiosurgery, not elsewhere classified**

● 93 **Physical therapy, respiratory therapy, rehabilitation, and related procedures**

● 93.0 **Diagnostic physical therapy**

93.01 **Functional evaluation**

93.02 **Orthotic evaluation**

93.03 **Prosthetic evaluation**

93.04 **Manual testing of muscle function**

93.05 Range of motion testing

93.06 Measurement of limb length

93.07 Body measurement
Girth measurement
Measurement of skull circumference

93.08 Electromyography
Excludes *eye EMG (95.25)*
that with polysomnogram (89.17)
urethral sphincter EMG (89.23)

93.09 Other diagnostic physical therapy procedure

● **93.1 Physical therapy exercises**

93.11 Assisting exercise
Excludes *assisted exercise in pool (93.31)*

93.12 Other active musculoskeletal exercise

93.13 Resistive exercise

93.14 Training in joint movements

93.15 Mobilization of spine

93.16 Mobilization of other joints
Excludes *manipulation of temporomandibular joint (76.95)*

93.17 Other passive musculoskeletal exercise

93.18 Breathing exercise

93.19 Exercise, not elsewhere classified

● **93.2 Other physical therapy musculoskeletal manipulation**

93.21 Manual and mechanical traction
Excludes *skeletal traction (93.43–93.44)*
skin traction (93.45–93.46)
spinal traction (93.41–93.42)

93.22 Ambulation and gait training

93.23 Fitting of orthotic device

93.24 Training in use of prosthetic or orthotic device
Training in crutch walking

93.25 Forced extension of limb

93.26 Manual rupture of joint adhesions

93.27 Stretching of muscle or tendon

93.28 Stretching of fascia

93.29 Other forcible correction of deformity

● **93.3 Other physical therapy therapeutic procedures**

93.31 Assisted exercise in pool

93.32 Whirlpool treatment

93.33 Other hydrotherapy

93.34 Diathermy

93.35 Other heat therapy
Acupuncture with smoldering moxa
Hot packs
Hyperthermia NEC
Infrared irradiation
Moxibustion
Paraffin bath
Excludes *hyperthermia for treatment of cancer (99.85)*

93.36 Cardiac retraining

93.37 Prenatal training
Training for natural childbirth

93.38 Combined physical therapy without mention of the components

93.39 Other physical therapy

● **93.4 Skeletal traction and other traction**

93.41 Spinal traction using skull device
Traction using:
caliper tongs
Crutchfield tongs
halo device
Vinke tongs
Excludes *insertion of tongs or halo traction device (02.94)*

93.42 Other spinal traction
Cotrel's traction
Excludes *cervical collar (93.52)*

93.43 Intermittent skeletal traction

93.44 Other skeletal traction
Bryant's traction
Dunlop's traction
Lyman Smith traction
Russell's traction

93.45 Thomas' splint traction

93.46 Other skin traction of limbs
Adhesive tape traction
Boot traction
Buck's traction
Gallows traction

● **93.5 Other immobilization, pressure, and attention to wound**
Excludes *wound cleansing (96.58–96.59)*

93.51 Application of plaster jacket
Excludes *Minerva jacket (93.52)*

93.52 Application of neck support
Application of:
cervical collar
Minerva jacket
molded neck support

93.53 Application of other cast

93.54 Application of splint
Plaster splint
Tray splint
Excludes *periodontal splint (24.7)*

93.55 Dental wiring
Excludes *that for orthodontia (24.7)*

93.56 Application of pressure dressing
Application of:
Gibney bandage
Robert Jones' bandage
Shanz dressing

93.57 Application of other wound dressing
Porcine wound dressing

93.58 Application of pressure trousers
Application of:
anti-shock trousers
MAST trousers
vasopneumatic device

93.59 Other immobilization, pressure, and attention to wound
Elastic stockings
Electronic gaiter
Intermittent pressure device
Oxygenation of wound (hyperbaric)
Stereotactic head frame application
Velpeau dressing

● **93.6 Osteopathic manipulative treatment**

93.61 Osteopathic manipulative treatment for general mobilization
General articulatory treatment

93.62 Osteopathic manipulative treatment using high- velocity, low-amplitude forces
Thrusting forces

93.63 Osteopathic manipulative treatment using low-velocity, high-amplitude forces
Springing forces

93.64 Osteopathic manipulative treatment using isotonic, isometric forces

93.65 Osteopathic manipulative treatment using indirect forces

93.66 Osteopathic manipulative treatment to move tissue fluids
Lymphatic pump

93.67 Other specified osteopathic manipulative treatment

● **93.7 Speech and reading rehabilitation and rehabilitation of the blind**

93.71 Dyslexia training

93.72 Dysphasia training

93.73 Esophageal speech training

93.74 Speech defect training

93.75 Other speech training and therapy

93.76 Training in use of lead dog for the blind

93.77 Training in braille or Moon

93.78 Other rehabilitation for the blind

● **93.8 Other rehabilitation therapy**

93.81 Recreation therapy
Diversional therapy
Play therapy

Excludes *play psychotherapy (94.36)*

93.82 Educational therapy
Education of bed-bound children
Special schooling for the handicapped

93.83 Occupational therapy
Daily living activities therapy

Excludes *training in activities of daily living for the blind (93.78)*

93.84 Music therapy

93.85 Vocational rehabilitation
Sheltered employment
Vocational:
assessment
retraining
training

93.89 Rehabilitation, not elsewhere classified

● **93.9 Respiratory therapy**

Excludes *insertion of airway (96.01–96.05)*
other continuous mechanical ventilation (96.70–96.72)

93.90 Continuous positive airway pressure [CPAP]

93.91 Intermittent positive pressure breathing [IPPB]

93.93 Nonmechanical methods of resuscitation
Artificial respiration
Manual resuscitation
Mouth-to-mouth resuscitation

93.94 Respiratory medication administered by nebulizer
Mist therapy

93.95 Hyperbaric oxygenation

Excludes *oxygenation of wound (93.59)*

93.96 Other oxygen enrichment
Catalytic oxygen therapy
Cytoreductive effect
Oxygenators
Oxygen therapy

Excludes *oxygenation of wound (93.59)*

93.97 Decompression chamber

93.98 Other control of atmospheric pressure and composition
Antigen-free air conditioning
Helium therapy

Excludes *inhaled nitric oxide therapy (INO) (00.12)*

93.99 Other respiratory procedures
Continuous negative pressure ventilation [CNP]
Postural drainage

● **94 Procedures related to the psyche**

● **94.0 Psychologic evaluation and testing**

94.01 Administration of intelligence test
Administration of:
Stanford-Binet
Wechsler Adult Intelligence Scale
Wechsler Intelligence Scale for Children

94.02 Administration of psychologic test
Administration of:
Bender Visual-Motor Gestalt Test
Benton Visual Retention Test
Minnesota Multiphasic Personality Inventory
Wechsler Memory Scale

94.03 Character analysis

94.08 Other psychologic evaluation and testing

94.09 Psychologic mental status determination, not otherwise specified

● **94.1 Psychiatric interviews, consultations, and evaluations**

94.11 Psychiatric mental status determination
Clinical psychiatric mental status determination
Evaluation for criminal responsibility
Evaluation for testimentary capacity
Medicolegal mental status determination
Mental status determination NOS

94.12 Routine psychiatric visit, not otherwise specified

94.13 Psychiatric commitment evaluation
Pre-commitment interview

94.19 Other psychiatric interview and evaluation
Follow-up psychiatric interview NOS

● **94.2 Psychiatric somatotherapy**

94.21 Narcoanalysis
Narcosynthesis

94.22 Lithium therapy

94.23 Neuroleptic therapy

94.24 Chemical shock therapy

94.25 Other psychiatric drug therapy

94.26 Subconvulsive electroshock therapy

94.27 Other electroshock therapy
Electroconvulsive therapy (ECT)
EST

94.29 Other psychiatric somatotherapy

● **94.3 Individual psychotherapy**

94.31 Psychoanalysis

94.32 Hypnotherapy
Hypnodrome
Hypnosis

94.33 Behavior therapy
Aversion therapy
Behavior modification
Desensitization therapy
Extinction therapy
Relaxation training
Token economy

94.34 Individual therapy for psychosexual dysfunction
Excludes *that performed in group setting (94.41)*

94.35 Crisis intervention

94.36 Play psychotherapy

94.37 Exploratory verbal psychotherapy

94.38 Supportive verbal psychotherapy

94.39 Other individual psychotherapy
Biofeedback

● **94.4 Other psychotherapy and counselling**

94.41 Group therapy for psychosexual dysfunction

94.42 Family therapy

94.43 Psychodrama

94.44 Other group therapy

94.45 Drug addiction counselling

94.46 Alcoholism counselling

94.49 Other counselling

● **94.5 Referral for psychologic rehabilitation**

94.51 Referral for psychotherapy

94.52 Referral for psychiatric aftercare:
That in:
halfway house
outpatient (clinic) facility

94.53 Referral for alcoholism rehabilitation

94.54 Referral for drug addiction rehabilitation

94.55 Referral for vocational rehabilitation

94.59 Referral for other psychologic rehabilitation

● **94.6 Alcohol and drug rehabilitation and detoxification**

94.61 Alcohol rehabilitation

94.62 Alcohol detoxification

94.63 Alcohol rehabilitation and detoxification

94.64 Drug rehabilitation

94.65 Drug detoxification

94.66 Drug rehabilitation and detoxification

94.67 Combined alcohol and drug rehabilitation

94.68 Combined alcohol and drug detoxification

94.69 Combined alcohol and drug rehabilitation and detoxification

● **95 Ophthalmologic and otologic diagnosis and treatment**

● **95.0 General and subjective eye examination**

95.01 Limited eye examination
Eye examination with prescription of spectacles

95.02 Comprehensive eye examination
Eye examination covering all aspects of the visual system

95.03 Extended ophthalmologic work-up
Examination (for):
glaucoma
neuro-ophthalmology
retinal disease

✖ **95.04 Eye examination under anesthesia**
Code also type of examination

95.05 Visual field study

95.06 Color vision study

95.07 Dark adaptation study

95.09 Eye examination, not otherwise specified
Vision check NOS

● **95.1 Examinations of form and structure of eye**

95.11 Fundus photography

95.12 Fluorescein angiography or angioscopy of eye

95.13 Ultrasound study of eye

95.14 X-ray study of eye

95.15 Ocular motility study

95.16 P32 and other tracer studies of eye

● **95.2 Objective functional tests of eye**
Excludes *that with polysomnogram (89.17)*

95.21 Electroretinogram [ERG]

95.22 Electro-oculogram [EOG]

95.23 Visual evoked potential [VEP]

95.24 Electronystagmogram [ENG]

95.25 Electromyogram of eye [EMG]

95.26 Tonography, provocative tests, and other glaucoma testing

● **95.3 Special vision services**

95.31 Fitting and dispensing of spectacles

95.32 Prescription, fitting, and dispensing of contact lens

95.33 Dispensing of other low vision aids

95.34 Ocular prosthetics

95.35 Orthoptic training

95.36 Ophthalmologic counselling and instruction
Counselling in:
adaptation to visual loss
use of low vision aids

● **95.4 Nonoperative procedures related to hearing**

95.41 Audiometry
Békésy 5-tone audiometry
Impedance audiometry
Stapedial reflex response
Subjective audiometry
Tympanogram

95.42 Clinical test of hearing
Tuning fork test
Whispered speech test

95.43 Audiological evaluation
Audiological evaluation by:
Bárány noise machine
blindfold test
delayed feedback
masking
Weber lateralization

95.44 Clinical vestibular function tests
Thermal test of vestibular function

95.45 Rotation tests
Bárány chair

95.46 Other auditory and vestibular function tests

95.47 Hearing examination, not otherwise specified

95.48 Fitting of hearing aid
Excludes *implantation of electromagnetic hearing device (20.95)*

95.49 Other nonoperative procedures related to hearing
Adjustment (external components) of cochlear prosthetic device

● **96 Nonoperative intubation and irrigation**

● **96.0 Nonoperative intubation of gastrointestinal and respiratory tracts**

96.01 Insertion of nasopharyngeal airway

96.02 Insertion of oropharyngeal airway

96.03 Insertion of esophageal obturator airway

96.04 Insertion of endotracheal tube

96.05 Other intubation of respiratory tract

96.06 Insertion of Sengstaken tube
Esophageal tamponade

96.07 Insertion of other (naso-)gastric tube
Intubation for decompression

Excludes *that for enteral infusion of nutritional substance (96.6)*

96.08 Insertion of (naso-)intestinal tube
Miller-Abbott tube (for decompression)

96.09 Insertion of rectal tube
Replacement of rectal tube

● 96.1 Other nonoperative insertion

Excludes *nasolacrimal intubation (09.44)*

96.11 Packing of external auditory canal

96.14 Vaginal packing

96.15 Insertion of vaginal mold

96.16 Other vaginal dilation

96.17 Insertion of vaginal diaphragm

96.18 Insertion of other vaginal pessary

96.19 Rectal packing

● 96.2 Nonoperative dilation and manipulation

96.21 Dilation of frontonasal duct

96.22 Dilation of rectum

96.23 Dilation of anal sphincter

96.24 Dilation and manipulation of enterostomy stoma

96.25 Therapeutic distention of bladder
Intermittent distention of bladder

96.26 Manual reduction of rectal prolapse

96.27 Manual reduction of hernia

96.28 Manual reduction of enterostomy prolapse

96.29 Reduction of intussusception of alimentary tract
With:
Fluoroscopy
Ionizing radiation enema
Ultrasonography guidance
Hydrostatic reduction
Pneumatic reduction

Excludes *intra-abdominal manipulation of intestine, not otherwise specified (46.80)*

● 96.3 Nonoperative alimentary tract irrigation, cleaning, and local instillation

96.31 Gastric cooling
Gastric hypothermia

96.32 Gastric freezing

96.33 Gastric lavage

96.34 Other irrigation of (naso-)gastric tube

96.35 Gastric gavage

96.36 Irrigation of gastrostomy or enterostomy

96.37 Proctoclysis

96.38 Removal of impacted feces
Removal of impaction:
by flushing
manually

96.39 Other transanal enema
Rectal irrigation

Excludes *reduction of intussusception of alimentary tract by ionizing radiation enema (96.29)*

● 96.4 Nonoperative irrigation, cleaning, and local instillation of other digestive and genitourinary organs

96.41 Irrigation of cholecystostomy and other biliary tube

96.42 Irrigation of pancreatic tube

96.43 Digestive tract instillation, except gastric gavage

96.44 Vaginal douche

96.45 Irrigation of nephrostomy and pyelostomy

96.46 Irrigation of ureterostomy and ureteral catheter

96.47 Irrigation of cystostomy

96.48 Irrigation of other indwelling urinary catheter

96.49 Other genitourinary instillation
Insertion of prostaglandin suppository

● 96.5 Other nonoperative irrigation and cleaning

96.51 Irrigation of eye
Irrigation of cornea

Excludes *irrigation with removal of foreign body (98.21)*

96.52 Irrigation of ear
Irrigation with removal of cerumen

96.53 Irrigation of nasal passages

96.54 Dental scaling, polishing, and debridement
Dental prophylaxis
Plaque removal

96.55 Tracheostomy toilette

96.56 Other lavage of bronchus and trachea

Excludes *diagnostic bronchoalveolar lavage (BAL) (33.24)*
whole lung lavage (33.99)

96.57 Irrigation of vascular catheter

96.58 Irrigation of wound catheter

96.59 Other irrigation of wound
Wound cleaning NOS

Excludes *debridement (86.22, 86.27–86.28)*

96.6 Enteral infusion of concentrated nutritional substances

● 96.7 Other continuous mechanical ventilation

Includes: Endotracheal respiratory assistance
Intermittent mandatory ventilation [IMV]
Positive end expiratory pressure [PEEP]
Pressure support ventilation [PSV]
That by tracheostomy
Weaning of an intubated (endotracheal tube) patient

Excludes *bi-level airway pressure (93.90)*
continuous negative pressure ventilation [CNP] (iron lung) (cuirass) (93.99)
continuous positive airway pressure [CPAP] (93.90)
intermittent positive pressure breathing [IPPB] (93.91)
that by face mask (93.90–93.99)
that by nasal cannula (93.90–93.99)
that by nasal catheter (93.90–93.99)

Code also any associated:
endotracheal tube insertion (96.04)
tracheostomy (31.1–31.29)

Note: Endotracheal Intubation

To calculate the number of hours (duration) of continuous mechanical ventilation during a hospitalization, begin the count from the start of the (endotracheal) intubation. The duration ends with (endotracheal) extubation.

If a patient is intubated prior to admission, begin counting the duration from the time of the admission. If a patient is transferred (discharged) while intubated, the duration would end at the time of transfer (discharge).

For patients who begin on (endotracheal) intubation and subsequently have a tracheostomy performed for mechanical ventilation, the duration begins with the (endotracheal) intubation and ends when the mechanical ventilation is turned off (after the weaning period).

Tracheostomy

To calculate the number of hours of continuous mechanical ventilation during a hospitalization, begin counting the duration when mechanical ventilation is started. The duration ends when the mechanical ventilator is turned off (after the weaning period).

If a patient has received a tracheostomy prior to admission and is on mechanical ventilation at the time of admission, begin counting the duration from the time of admission. If a patient is transferred (discharged) while still on mechanical ventilation via tracheostomy, the duration would end at the time of the transfer (discharge).

96.70 Continuous mechanical ventilation of unspecified duration
Mechanical ventilation NOS

96.71 Continuous mechanical ventilation for less than 96 consecutive hours

96.72 Continuous mechanical ventilation for 96 consecutive hours or more

● **97 Replacement and removal of therapeutic appliances**

● **97.0 Nonoperative replacement of gastrointestinal appliance**

97.01 Replacement of (naso-)gastric or esophagostomy tube

97.02 Replacement of gastrostomy tube

97.03 Replacement of tube or enterostomy device of small intestine

97.04 Replacement of tube or enterostomy device of large intestine

97.05 Replacement of stent (tube) in biliary or pancreatic duct

● **97.1 Nonoperative replacement of musculoskeletal and integumentary system appliance**

97.11 Replacement of cast on upper limb

97.12 Replacement of cast on lower limb

97.13 Replacement of other cast

97.14 Replacement of other device for musculoskeletal immobilization

97.15 Replacement of wound catheter

97.16 Replacement of wound packing or drain

Excludes *repacking of:*
dental wound (97.22)
vulvar wound (97.26)

● **97.2 Other nonoperative replacement**

97.21 Replacement of nasal packing

97.22 Replacement of dental packing

97.23 Replacement of tracheostomy tube

97.24 Replacement and refitting of vaginal diaphragm

97.25 Replacement of other vaginal pessary

97.26 Replacement of vaginal or vulvar packing or drain

97.29 Other nonoperative replacements

● **97.3 Nonoperative removal of therapeutic device from head and neck**

97.31 Removal of eye prosthesis

Excludes *removal of ocular implant (16.71)*
removal of orbital implant (16.72)

97.32 Removal of nasal packing

97.33 Removal of dental wiring

97.34 Removal of dental packing

97.35 Removal of dental prosthesis

97.36 Removal of other external mandibular fixation device

97.37 Removal of tracheostomy tube

97.38 Removal of sutures from head and neck

97.39 Removal of other therapeutic device from head and neck

Excludes *removal of skull tongs (02.94)*

● **97.4 Nonoperative removal of therapeutic device from thorax**

97.41 Removal of thoracotomy tube or pleural cavity drain

97.42 Removal of mediastinal drain

97.43 Removal of sutures from thorax

97.44 Nonoperative removal of heart assist system
Intra-aortic balloon pump [IABP]

97.49 Removal of other device from thorax

● **97.5 Nonoperative removal of therapeutic device from digestive system**

97.51 Removal of gastrostomy tube

97.52 Removal of tube from small intestine

97.53 Removal of tube from large intestine or appendix

97.54 Removal of cholecystostomy tube

97.55 Removal of T-tube, other bile duct tube, or liver tube

Includes: Removal of bile duct stent

97.56 Removal of pancreatic tube or drain

97.59 Removal of other device from digestive system
Removal of rectal packing

● **97.6 Nonoperative removal of therapeutic device from urinary system**

97.61 Removal of pyelostomy and nephrostomy tube

97.62 Removal of ureterostomy tube and ureteral catheter

97.63 **Removal of cystostomy tube**

97.64 **Removal of other urinary drainage device**
Removal of indwelling urinary catheter

97.65 **Removal of urethral stent**

97.69 **Removal of other device from urinary system**

● 97.7 **Nonoperative removal of therapeutic device from genital system**

97.71 **Removal of intrauterine contraceptive device**

97.72 **Removal of intrauterine pack**

97.73 **Removal of vaginal diaphragm**

97.74 **Removal of other vaginal pessary**

97.75 **Removal of vaginal or vulvar packing**

97.79 **Removal of other device from genital tract**
Removal of sutures

● 97.8 **Other nonoperative removal of therapeutic device**

97.81 **Removal of retroperitoneal drainage device**

97.82 **Removal of peritoneal drainage device**

97.83 **Removal of abdominal wall sutures**

97.84 **Removal of sutures from trunk, not elsewhere classified**

97.85 **Removal of packing from trunk, not elsewhere classified**

97.86 **Removal of other device from abdomen**

97.87 **Removal of other device from trunk**

97.88 **Removal of external immobilization device**
Removal of:
brace
cast
splint

97.89 **Removal of other therapeutic device**

● 98 **Nonoperative removal of foreign body or calculus**

● 98.0 **Removal of intraluminal foreign body from digestive system without incision**

Excludes *removal of therapeutic device (97.51–97.59)*

98.01 **Removal of intraluminal foreign body from mouth without incision**

98.02 **Removal of intraluminal foreign body from esophagus without incision**

98.03 **Removal of intraluminal foreign body from stomach and small intestine without incision**

98.04 **Removal of intraluminal foreign body from large intestine without incision**

98.05 **Removal of intraluminal foreign body from rectum and anus without incision**

● 98.1 **Removal of intraluminal foreign body from other sites without incision**

Excludes *removal of therapeutic device (97.31–97.49, 97.61–97.89)*

98.11 **Removal of intraluminal foreign body from ear without incision**

98.12 **Removal of intraluminal foreign body from nose without incision**

98.13 **Removal of intraluminal foreign body from pharynx without incision**

98.14 **Removal of intraluminal foreign body from larynx without incision**

98.15 **Removal of intraluminal foreign body from trachea and bronchus without incision**

98.16 **Removal of intraluminal foreign body from uterus without incision**

Excludes *removal of intrauterine contraceptive device (97.71)*

98.17 **Removal of intraluminal foreign body from vagina without incision**

98.18 **Removal of intraluminal foreign body from artificial stoma without incision**

98.19 **Removal of intraluminal foreign body from urethra without incision**

● 98.2 **Removal of other foreign body without incision**

Excludes *removal of intraluminal foreign body (98.01–98.19)*

98.20 **Removal of foreign body, not otherwise specified**

98.21 **Removal of superficial foreign body from eye without incision**

98.22 **Removal of other foreign body without incision from head and neck**
Removal of embedded foreign body from eyelid or conjunctiva without incision

98.23 **Removal of foreign body from vulva without incision**

98.24 **Removal of foreign body from scrotum or penis without incision**

98.25 **Removal of other foreign body without incision from trunk except scrotum, penis, or vulva**

98.26 **Removal of foreign body from hand without incision**

98.27 **Removal of foreign body without incision from upper limb, except hand**

98.28 **Removal of foreign body from foot without incision**

98.29 **Removal of foreign body without incision from lower limb, except foot**

● 98.5 **Extracorporeal shockwave lithotripsy [ESWL]**
Lithotriptor tank procedure
Disintegration of stones by extracorporeal induced shockwaves
That with insertion of stent

98.51 **Extracorporeal shockwave lithotripsy [ESWL] of the kidney, ureter and/or bladder**

98.52 **Extracorporeal shockwave lithotripsy [ESWL] of the gallbladder and/or bile duct**

98.59 **Extracorporeal shockwave lithotripsy of other sites**

● 99 **Other nonoperative procedures**

● 99.0 **Transfusion of blood and blood components**
Use additional code for that done via catheter or cutdown (38.92–38.94)

99.00 **Perioperative autologous transfusion of whole blood or blood components**
Intraoperative blood collection
Postoperative blood collection
Salvage

99.01 **Exchange transfusion**
Transfusion:
exsanguination
replacement

99.02 **Transfusion of previously collected autologous blood**
Blood component

99.03 Other transfusion of whole blood
Transfusion:
blood NOS
hemodilution
NOS

99.04 Transfusion of packed cells

99.05 Transfusion of platelets
Transfusion of thrombocytes

99.06 Transfusion of coagulation factors
Transfusion of antihemophilic factor

99.07 Transfusion of other serum
Transfusion of plasma

Excludes *injection [transfusion] of:*
antivenin (99.16)
gamma globulin (99.14)

99.08 Transfusion of blood expander
Transfusion of Dextran

99.09 Transfusion of other substance
Transfusion of:
blood surrogate
granulocytes

Excludes *transplantation [transfusion] of bone marrow (41.0)*

● **99.1 Injection or infusion of therapeutic or prophylactic substance**

Includes: injection or infusion given:
hypodermically acting locally or systemically
intramuscularly acting locally or systemically
intravenously acting locally or systemically

99.10 Injection or infusion of thrombolytic agent
Streptokinase
Tissue plasminogen activator (TPA)
Urokinase

Excludes *aspirin—omit code*
GP IIB/IIIa platelet inhibitors (99.20)
heparin (99.19)
single vessel percutaneous transluminal coronary angioplasty [PTCA] or coronary atherectomy with mention of thrombolytic agent (36.02)
warfarin—omit code

99.11 Injection of Rh immune globulin
Injection of:
Anti-D (Rhesus) globulin
RhoGAM

99.12 Immunization for allergy
Desensitization

99.13 Immunization for autoimmune disease

99.14 Injection of gamma globulin
Injection of immune sera

99.15 Parenteral infusion of concentrated nutritional substances
Hyperalimentation
Total parenteral nutrition [TPN]
Peripheral parenteral nutrition [PPN]

99.16 Injection of antidote
Injection of:
antivenin
heavy metal antagonist

99.17 Injection of insulin

99.18 Injection or infusion of electrolytes

99.19 Injection of anticoagulant

Excludes *infusion of drotrecogin alfa (activated) (00.11)*

● **99.2 Injection or infusion of other therapeutic or prophylactic substance**

Includes: injection or infusion given:
hypodermically acting locally or systemically
intramuscularly acting locally or systemically
intravenously acting locally or systemically

Use additional code for:
injection (into):
breast (85.92)
bursa (82.94, 83.96)
intraperitoneal (cavity) (54.97)
intrathecal (03.92)
joint (76.96, 81.92)
kidney (55.96)
liver (50.94)
orbit (16.91)
other sites—see Alphabetic Index
perfusion:
NOS (39.97)
intestine (46.95, 46.96)
kidney (55.95)
liver (50.93)
total body (39.96)

99.20 Injection or infusion of platelet inhibitor
Glycoprotein IIB/IIIa inhibitor
GP IIB/IIIa inhibitor
GP IIB/IIa inhibitor

Excludes *infusion of heparin (99.19)*
injection or infusion of thrombolytic agent (99.10)

99.21 Injection of antibiotic

Excludes *injection or infusion of oxazolidinones class of antibiotics (00.14)*

99.22 Injection of other anti-infective

Excludes *injection or infusion of oxazolidinones class of antibiotics (00.14)*

99.23 Injection of steroid
Injection of cortisone
Subdermal implantation of progesterone

99.24 Injection of other hormone

99.25 Injection or infusion of cancer chemotherapeutic substance
Chemoembolization
Injection or infusion of antineoplastic agent

Excludes *immunotherapy, antineoplastic (00.15, 99.28)* ⬅
implantation of chemotherapeutic agent (00.10)
injection of radioisotope (92.28)
injection or infusion of biological response modifier [BRM] as an antineoplastic agent (99.28)

99.26 Injection of tranquilizer

99.27 Iontophoresis

99.28 Injection or infusion of biological response modifier [BRM] as an antineoplastic agent
Low-dose interleukin-2 (IL-2) therapy ⬅
Immunotherapy, antineoplastic
Interleukin therapy
Tumor vaccine

Excludes *high-dose infusion interleukin-2 [IL-2] (00.15)* ◀

99.29 Injection or infusion of other therapeutic or prophylactic substance

Excludes *administration of neuroprotective agent (99.75)*
immunization (99.31–99.59)
injection of sclerosing agent into:
esophageal varices (42.33)
hemorrhoids (49.42)
veins (39.92)
injection or infusion of human B-type natriuretic peptide (hBNP) (00.13)
injection or infusion of nesiritide (00.13)
injection or infusion of platelet inhibitor (99.20)
injection or infusion of thrombolytic agent (99.10)

● **99.3 Prophylactic vaccination and inoculation against certain bacterial diseases**

99.31 Vaccination against cholera

99.32 Vaccination against typhoid and paratyphoid fever
Administration of TAB vaccine

99.33 Vaccination against tuberculosis
Administration of BCG vaccine

99.34 Vaccination against plague

99.35 Vaccination against tularemia

99.36 Administration of diphtheria toxoid

Excludes *administration of:*
diphtheria antitoxin (99.58)
diphtheria-tetanus-pertussis, combined (99.39)

99.37 Vaccination against pertussis

Excludes *administration of diphtheria-tetanus-pertussis, combined (99.39)*

99.38 Administration of tetanus toxoid

Excludes *administration of:*
diphtheria-tetanus-pertussis, combined (99.39)
tetanus antitoxin (99.56)

99.39 Administration of diphtheria-tetanus-pertussis, combined

● **99.4 Prophylactic vaccination and inoculation against certain viral diseases**

99.41 Administration of poliomyelitis vaccine

99.42 Vaccination against smallpox

99.43 Vaccination against yellow fever

99.44 Vaccination against rabies

99.45 Vaccination against measles

Excludes *administration of measles-mumps-rubella vaccine (99.48)*

99.46 Vaccination against mumps

Excludes *administration of measles-mumps-rubella vaccine (99.48)*

99.47 Vaccination against rubella

Excludes *administration of measles-mumps-rubella vaccine (99.48)*

99.48 Administration of measles-mumps-rubella vaccine

● **99.5 Other vaccination and inoculation**

99.51 Prophylactic vaccination against the common cold

99.52 Prophylactic vaccination against influenza

99.53 Prophylactic vaccination against arthropod-borne viral encephalitis

99.54 Prophylactic vaccination against other arthropod-borne viral diseases

99.55 Prophylactic administration of vaccine against other diseases
Vaccination against:
anthrax
brucellosis
Rocky Mountain spotted fever
Staphylococcus
Streptococcus
typhus

99.56 Administration of tetanus antitoxin

99.57 Administration of botulism antitoxin

99.58 Administration of other antitoxins
Administration of:
diphtheria antitoxin
gas gangrene antitoxin
scarlet fever antitoxin

99.59 Other vaccination and inoculation
Vaccination NOS

Excludes *injection of:*
gamma globulin (99.14)
Rh immune globulin (99.11)
immunization for:
allergy (99.12)
autoimmune disease (99.13)

● **99.6 Conversion of cardiac rhythm**

Excludes *open chest cardiac:*
electric stimulation (37.91)
massage (37.91)

99.60 Cardiopulmonary resuscitation, not otherwise specified

99.61 Atrial cardioversion

99.62 Other electric countershock of heart
Cardioversion:
NOS
external
Conversion to sinus rhythm
Defibrillation
External electrode stimulation

99.63 Closed chest cardiac massage
Cardiac massage NOS
Manual external cardiac massage

99.64 Carotid sinus stimulation

99.69 Other conversion of cardiac rhythm

● **99.7 Therapeutic apheresis or other injection, administration, or infusion of other therapeutic or prophylactic substance**

99.71 Therapeutic plasmapheresis

Excludes *extracorporeal immunoadsorption [ECI] 99.76*

99.72 Therapeutic leukopheresis
Therapeutic leukocytapheresis

99.73 Therapeutic erythrocytapheresis
Therapeutic erythropheresis

99.74 Therapeutic plateletpheresis

99.75 Administration of neuroprotective agent

99.76 Extracorporeal immunoadsorption
Removal of antibodies from plasma with protein A columns

99.77 Application or administration of adhesion barrier substance

99.79 Other
Apheresis (harvest) of stem cells

● **99.8 Miscellaneous physical procedures**

99.81 Hypothermia (central) (local)

Excludes *gastric cooling (96.31)*
gastric freezing (96.32)
that incidental to open heart surgery (39.62)

99.82 Ultraviolet light therapy
Actinotherapy

99.83 Other phototherapy
Phototherapy of the newborn

Excludes *extracorporeal photochemotherapy (99.88)*
photocoagulation of retinal lesion (14.23–14.25, 14.33–14.35, 14.53–14.55)

99.84 Isolation
Isolation after contact with infectious disease
Protection of individual from his surroundings
Protection of surroundings from individual

99.85 Hyperthermia for treatment of cancer
Hyperthermia (adjunct therapy) induced by microwave, ultrasound, low energy radio frequency, probes (interstitial), or other means in the treatment of cancer

Code also any concurrent chemotherapy or radiation therapy

99.86 Non-invasive placement of bone growth stimulator
Transcutaneous (surface) placement of pads or patches for stimulation to aid bone healing

Excludes *insertion of invasive or semi-invasive bone growth stimulators (device) (percutaneous electrodes) (78.90–78.99)*

99.88 Therapeutic photopheresis
Extracorporeal photochemotherapy
Extracorporeal photopheresis

Excludes *other phototherapy (99.83)*
ultraviolet light therapy (99.82)

● **99.9 Other miscellaneous procedures**

99.91 Acupuncture for anesthesia

99.92 Other acupuncture

Excludes *that with smoldering moxa (93.35)*

99.93 Rectal massage (for levator spasm)

99.94 Prostatic massage

99.95 Stretching of foreskin

99.96 Collection of sperm for artificial insemination

99.97 Fitting of denture

99.98 Extraction of milk from lactating breast

99.99 Other
Leech therapy

UNIT TWO

HCPCS 2003: LEVEL II NATIONAL CODES

2004 HCPCS Updates available on the companion website at:
http://evolve.elsevier.com/Buck/icd

DISCLAIMER

Every effort has been made to make this text complete and accurate, but no guarantee, warranty, or representation is made for its accuracy or completeness. It is based on the Centers for Medicare and Medicaid Services Healthcare Common Procedure Coding System (HCPCS).

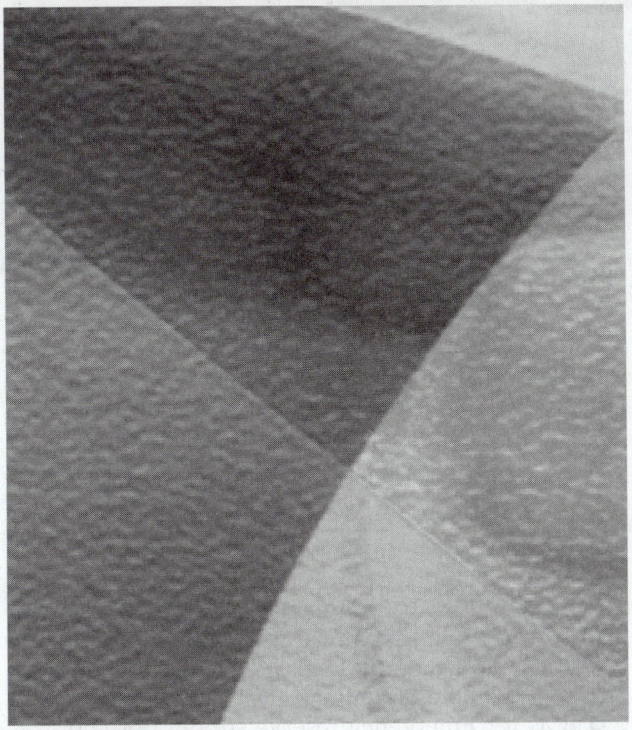

PART I

Introduction

2004 HCPCS Updates available on the companion website at: http://evolve.elsevier.com/Buck/icd

The Centers for Medicare and Medicaid Services (CMS) (formerly Health Care Financing Administration [HCFA]) Healthcare Common Procedure Coding System (HCPCS) is a collection of codes and descriptors that represent procedures, supplies, products, and services that may be provided to Medicare beneficiaries and to individuals enrolled in private health insurance programs. The codes are divided into three levels, or groups, as follows:

Level I: Codes and descriptors copyrighted by the American Medical Association's (AMA's) Current Procedural Terminology, ed. 4 (CPT-4). Five-position numeric codes primarily represent physician services.

Level II: Five-position alpha-numeric codes representing primarily items and nonphysician services that are not represented in the Level I codes. Codes and descriptors copyrighted by the American Dental Association's (ADA's) Current Dental Terminology, ed. 2 (CDT-2), are five-position alpha-numeric codes comprising the D series. **This book does not contain codes D0100 through D9999.** They can be purchased from the ADA. All other Level II codes and descriptors are approved and maintained jointly by the Alpha-Numeric Editorial Panel (consisting of CMS, the Health Insurance Association of America, and the Blue Cross and Blue Shield Association).

Level III: The CMS has eliminated Level III local codes. Select temporary national codes are included in the annual HCPCS update (see Program Memorandum AB-02-113).

Headings are provided as a means of grouping similar or closely related items. The placement of a code under a heading does not indicate additional means of classification, nor does it relate to any health insurance coverage categories.

HCPCS also contains modifiers, which are two-position codes and descriptors used to indicate that a service or procedure that has been performed has been altered by some specific circumstance but not changed in its definition or code. Modifiers are grouped by the three levels. Level I modifiers and descriptors are copyrighted by the AMA. Modifiers in the D series are copyrighted by the ADA. **This book does not contain D series modifiers.** They are available directly from the ADA.

HCPCS is designed to promote uniform reporting and statistical data collection of medical procedures, supplies, products, and services.

HCPCS Disclaimer

Inclusion or exclusion of a procedure, supply, product, or service does not imply any health insurance coverage or reimbursement policy.

HCPCS makes as much use as possible of generic descriptions, but the inclusion of brand names to describe devices or drugs is intended only for indexing purposes; it is not meant to convey endorsement of any particular product or drug.

Updating HCPCS

The primary updates are made annually.

Legend

❂ Special coverage instructions
◆ Not covered by or valid for Medicare
✻ Carrier discretion
◀▶ New
⬅➡ Revised code

LEVEL II NATIONAL MODIFIERS

▶✻ A1	Dressing for one wound
▶✻ A2	Dressing for two wounds
▶✻ A3	Dressing for three wounds
▶✻ A4	Dressing for four wounds
▶✻ A5	Dressing for five wounds
▶✻ A6	Dressing for six wounds
▶✻ A7	Dressing for seven wounds
▶✻ A8	Dressing for eight wounds
▶✻ A9	Dressing for nine or more wounds
✪ AA	Anesthesia services performed personally by anesthesiologist
✪ AD	Medical supervision by a physician: more than four concurrent anesthesia procedures MCM 3350.5
✪ AH	Clinical psychologist MCM 2150, MCM 5112
✪ AJ	Clinical social worker MCM 2152, MCM 5113
✪ AM	Physician, team member service MCM 4105.7, Cross Reference QM
✻ AP	Determination of refractive state was not performed in the course of diagnostic ophthalmological examination
✻ AS	Physician assistant, nurse practitioner, or clinical nurse specialist services for assistant at surgery
✻ AT	Acute treatment (this modifier should be used when reporting service 98940, 98941, 98942*)
▶✻ AU	Item furnished in conjunction with a urological, ostomy, or tracheostomy supply
▶✻ AV	Item furnished in conjunction with a prosthetic device, prosthetic or orthotic
▶✻ AW	Item furnished in conjunction with a surgical dressing
▶✻ AX	Item furnished in conjunction with dialysis services
▶✻ BA	Item furnished in conjunction with parenteral enteral nutrition (PEN) services
▶✻ BO	Orally administered nutrition, not by feeding tube
✻ BP	The beneficiary has been informed of the purchase and rental options and has elected to purchase the item.
✻ BR	The beneficiary has been informed of the purchase and rental options and has elected to rent the item.
✻ BU	The beneficiary has been informed of the purchase and rental options and after 30 days has not informed the supplier of his/her decision.
▶✻ CA	Procedure payable only in inpatient setting when performed emergently on an outpatient who expires prior to admission
▶◆ CB	Service ordered by a renal dialysis facility (RDF) physician as part of the beneficiary's benefit, is not part of the composite rate, and is separately reimbursable
✻ CC	Procedure code change. (Use CC when the procedure code submitted was changed either for administrative reasons or because an incorrect code was filed.)
✻ E1	Upper left eyelid
✻ E2	Lower left eyelid
✻ E3	Upper right eyelid
✻ E4	Lower right eyelid
✪ EJ	Subsequent claim for a defined course of therapy (e.g., EPO, sodium hyaluronate, infliximab
✪ EM	Emergency reserve supply (for end state renal disease [ESRD] benefit only)
✻ EP	Service provided as part of Medicaid early periodic screening diagnosis and treatment (EPSDT) program
✻ ET	Emergency services
▶✻ EY	No physician or other licensed health care provider order for this item or service
✻ F1	Left hand, second digit
✻ F2	Left hand, third digit
✻ F3	Left hand, fourth digit
✻ F4	Left hand, fifth digit
✻ F5	Right hand, thumb
✻ F6	Right hand, second digit
✻ F7	Right hand, third digit
✻ F8	Right hand, fourth digit
✻ F9	Right hand, fifth digit
✻ FA	Left hand, thumb
✻ FP	Service provided as part of Medicaid Family Planning Program
✻ G1	Most recent URR reading of less than 60
✻ G2	Most recent URR reading of 60 to 64.9
✻ G3	Most recent URR reading of 65 to 69.9
✻ G4	Most recent URR reading of 70 to 74.9
✻ G5	Most recent URR reading of 75 or greater
✻ G6	ESRD patient for whom less than six dialysis sessions have been provided in a month
✪ G7	Pregnancy resulting from rape or incest or pregnancy certified by physician as life threatening MCM 2005.1, CIM 35-99
✻ G8	Monitored anesthesia care (MAC) for deep complex, complicated, or markedly invasive surgical procedure
✻ G9	Monitored anesthesia care patient who has history of severe cardio-pulmonary condition

*CPT only ©*Current Procedural Terminology 2002, Professional Edition*. American Medical Association.

✻	GA	Waiver of liability statement on file
✻	GB	Claims being resubmitted for payment because it is no longer covered under a global payment demonstration
❂	GC	This service has been performed in part by a resident under the direction of a teaching physician. MCM 3350.5, MCM 4116
❂	GE	This service has been performed by a resident without the presence of a teaching physician under the primary care exception. MCM 4116
✻	GG	Performance and payment of a screening mammogram and diagnostic mammogram on the same patient, same day
✻	GH	Diagnostic mammogram converted from screening mammogram on same day
✻	GJ	"Opt out" physician or practitioner emergency or urgent service
✻	GK	Actual item/service ordered by physician, item associated with GA or GZ modifier
✻	GL	Medically unnecessary upgrade provided instead of standard item, no charge, no Advance Beneficiary Notice (ABN)
✻	GM	Multiple patients on one ambulance trip
➠ ✻	GN	Services delivered under an outpatient speech-language pathology plan of care
➠ ✻	GO	Services delivered under an outpatient occupational therapy plan of care
➠ ✻	GP	Services delivered under an outpatient physical therapy plan of care
✻	GQ	Via asynchronous telecommunications system
❂	GT	Via interactive audio and video telecommunication systems
	GU	Deleted 01/01/02
❂	GV	Attending physician not employed or paid under arrangement by the patient's hospice provider MCM 4175-5
❂	GW	Service not related to the hospice patient's terminal condition MCM 4175-5
	GX	Deleted 01/01/02
◆	GY	Item or service statutorily excluded or does not meet the definition of any Medicare benefit
◆	GZ	Item or service expected to be denied as not reasonable or necessary MCM 2000
▶ ◆	H9	Court-ordered
▶ ◆	HA	Child/adolescent program
▶ ◆	HB	Adult program, non geriatric
▶ ◆	HC	Adult program, geriatric
▶ ◆	HD	Pregnant/parenting women's program
▶ ◆	HE	Mental health program
▶ ◆	HF	Substance abuse program
▶ ◆	HG	Opioid addiction treatment program
▶ ◆	HH	Integrated mental health/substance abuse program
▶ ◆	HI	Integrated mental health and mental retardation/developmental disabilities program
▶ ◆	HJ	Employee assistance program
▶ ◆	HK	Specialized mental health programs for high-risk populations
▶ ◆	HL	Intern
▶ ◆	HM	Less than bachelor degree level
▶ ◆	HN	Bachelor's degree level
▶ ◆	HO	Master's degree level
▶ ◆	HP	Doctoral level
▶ ◆	HQ	Group setting
▶ ◆	HR	Family/couple with client present
▶ ◆	HS	Family/couple without client present
▶ ◆	HT	Multi-disciplinary team
▶ ◆	HU	Funded by child welfare agency
▶ ◆	HV	Funded state addictions agency
▶ ◆	HW	Funded by state mental health agency
▶ ◆	HX	Funded by county/local agency
▶ ◆	HY	Funded by juvenile justice agency
▶ ◆	HZ	Funded by criminal justice agency
▶ ✻	JW	Drug amount discarded/not administered to any patient
➠ ✻	K0	Lower extremity prosthesis functional Level 0 does not have the ability or potential to ambulate or transfer safely with or without assistance and a prosthesis does not enhance their quality of life or mobility
✻	K1	Lower extremity prosthesis functional Level 1 has the ability or potential to use a prosthesis for transfers or ambulation on level surfaces at fixed cadence. Typical of the limited and unlimited household ambulator.
✻	K2	Lower extremity prosthesis functional Level 2 has the ability or potential for ambulation with the ability to traverse low level environmental barriers such as curbs, stairs or uneven surfaces. Typical of the limited community ambulator.
✻	K3	Lower extremity prosthesis functional Level 3 has the ability or potential for ambulation with variable cadence. Typical of the community ambulator who has the ability to traverse most environmental barriers and may have vocational, therapeutic, or exercise activity that demands prosthetic utilization beyond simple locomotion.
✻	K4	Lower extremity prosthesis functional Level 4 has the ability or potential for prosthetic ambulation that exceeds the basic ambulation skills, exhibiting high impact, stress, or energy levels, typical of the prosthetic demands of the child, active adult, or athlete.

✻ KA Add on option/accessory for wheelchair

▶✻ KB Beneficiary requested upgrade for ABN, more than 4 modifiers identified on claim

✻ KH Durable medical equipment prosthetics and orthotics supplies (DMEPOS) item, initial claim, purchase or first month rental

✻ KI DMEPOS item, second or third month rental

✻ KJ DMEPOS item, parenteral enteral nutrition (PEN) pump or capped rental, months four to fifteen

✻ KM Replacement of facial prosthesis including new impression/moulage

✻ KN Replacement of facial prosthesis using previous master model

✻ KO Single drug unit dose formulation

✻ KP First drug of a multiple drug unit dose formulation

✻ KQ Second or subsequent drug of a multiple drug unit dose formulation

✻ KR Rental item, billing for partial month

✪ KS Glucose monitor supply for diabetic beneficiary not treated with insulin

▶✻ KX Specific required documentation on file

✻ LC Left circumflex coronary artery

✻ LD Left anterior descending coronary artery

✻ LL Lease/rental (use the LL modifier when durable medical equipment [DME] rental is to be applied against the purchase price)

✻ LR Laboratory round trip
CIM 65-7

✪ LS Food and Drug Administration (FDA)–monitored intraocular lens implant

✻ LT Left side (used to identify procedures performed on the left side of the body)

✻ MS Six-month maintenance and servicing fee for reasonable and necessary parts and labor, which are not covered under any manufacturer or supplier warranty

✻ NR New when rented (use the NR modifier when DME which was new at the time of rental is subsequently purchased)

✻ NU New equipment

✻ PL Progressive addition lenses

✻ Q2 HCFA/ORD demonstration project procedure/service

➡✻ Q3 Live kidney donor surgery and related services

✻ Q4 Service for ordering/referring physician qualifies as a service exemption

✪ Q5 Service furnished by a substitute physician under a reciprocal billing arrangement
MCM 3060.6

✪ Q6 Service furnished by a locum tenens physician
MCM 3060.7

✻ Q7 One Class A finding

✻ Q8 Two Class B findings

✻ Q9 One Class B and two Class C findings

✻ QA FDA investigational device exemption

✪ QB Physician providing service in a rural health professional shortage area (HPSA)
MCM 3050.3

✻ QC Single channel monitoring

✻ QD Recording and storage in solid state memory by a digital recorder

✻ QE Prescribed amount of oxygen is less than 1 liter per minute (LPM)

✻ QF Prescribed amount of oxygen exceeds 4 LPM and portable oxygen is prescribed

✻ QG Prescribed amount of oxygen is greater than 4 LPM

✻ QH Oxygen-conserving device is being used with an oxygen delivery system

▶✪ QJ Services/items provided to a prisoner or patient in state or local custody, however the state or local government, as applicable, meets the requirements in 42 CFR 411.4 (B)

✪ QK Medical direction of two, three, or four concurrent anesthesia procedures involving qualified individuals
MCM 3350.5

✻ QL Patient pronounced dead after ambulance called

✻ QM Ambulance service provided under arrangement by a provider of services

✻ QN Ambulance service furnished directly by a provider of services

✪ QP Documentation is on file showing that the laboratory test(s) was ordered individually or ordered as a CPT-recognized panel other than automated profile codes 80002 to 80019,* G0058, G0059, and G0060
MCM 7517.1

✻ QQ Claim submitted with a written statement of intent

✪ QS Monitored anesthesia care service
MCM 150181

✻ QT Recording and storage on tape by an analog tape recorder

✪ QU Physician providing service in an urban HPSA
MCM 3350.3

✪ QV Item or service provided as routine care in a Medicare qualifying clinical trial
CIM 30-1

✻ QW CLIA-waived test

✻ QX Certified registered nurse anesthetist (CRNA) service: with medical direction by a physician

---

*CPT only ©*Current Procedural Terminology 2002, Professional Edition*. American Medical Association.

✪ QY Medical direction of one CRNA by an anesthesiologist MCM 3350.5
✻ QZ CRNA service: without medical direction by a physician
✻ RC Right coronary artery
✻ RP Replacement and repair (RP may be used to indicate replacement of DME or orthotic and prosthetic devices that have been in use for sometime.) The claim shows the code for the part, followed by the *RP* modifier and the charge for the part.
✻ RR Rental (use the RR modifier when DME is to be rented)
✻ RT Right side (used to identify procedures performed on the right side of the body
◆ SA Nurse practitioner rendering service in collaboration with a physician
◆ SB Nurse midwife
◆ SC Medically necessary service or supply
◆ SD Services provided by registered nurse with specialized, highly technical home infusion training
◆ SE State and/or federally funded programs/services
✻ SF Second opinion ordered by a professional review organization (PRO) per Section 9401, P.L. 99-272 (100% reimbursement/no Medicare deductible or coinsurance)
✻ SG Ambulatory surgical center (ASC) facility service
◆ SH Second concurrently administered infusion therapy
◆ SJ Third or more concurrently administered infusion therapy
▶◆ SK Member of high risk population (use only with codes for immunization)
▶◆ SL State supplied vaccine
▶◆ SM Second surgical opinion
▶◆ SN Third surgical opinion
▶◆ SQ Item ordered by home health
▶◆ ST Related to trauma or injury
▶◆ SU Procedure performed in physician's office (to denote use of facility and equipment)
▶◆ SV Pharmaceuticals delivered to patient's home but not utilized
✻ T1 Left foot, second digit
✻ T2 Left foot, third digit
✻ T3 Left foot, fourth digit
✻ T4 Left foot, fifth digit
✻ T5 Right foot, great toe
✻ T6 Right foot, second digit
✻ T7 Right foot, third digit
✻ T8 Right foot, fourth digit
✻ T9 Right foot, fifth digit
✻ TA Left foot, great toe
✻ TC Technical component (Under certain circumstances, a charge may be made for the technical component alone. Under those circumstances the technical component charge is identified by adding modifier TC to the usual procedure number. Technical component charges are institutional charges and not billed separately by physicians. However, portable x-ray suppliers only bill for technical component and should utilize modifier TC. The charge data from portable x-ray suppliers will then be used to build customary and prevailing profiles.)
◆ TD RN
◆ TE LPN/LVN
◆ TF Intermediate level of care
◆ TG Complex/high-tech level of care
◆ TH Obstetrical treatment/services, prenatal or postpartum
◆ TJ Program group, child, and/or adolescent
▶◆ TK Extra patient or passenger, non-ambulance
▶◆ TL Early intervention/individualized family services plan (IFSP)
▶◆ TM Individualized education program (IEP)
▶◆ TN Rural/outside providers customary service area
▶◆ TP Medical transport, unloaded vehicle
▶◆ TQ Basic life support (BLS) transport by a volunteer ambulance provider
▶◆ TR School-based IEP services provided outside the public school district responsible for the student
▶◆ TS Follow-up service
▶◆ TT Individualized service provided to more than one patient in same setting
▶◆ TU Special payment rate, overtime
▶◆ TV Special payment rates, holidays/weekends
▶◆ TW Back-up equipment
▶◆ U1 Medicaid Level of Care 1, as defined by each State
▶◆ U2 Medicaid Level of Care 2, as defined by each State
▶◆ U3 Medicaid Level of Care 3, as defined by each State
▶◆ U4 Medicaid Level of Care 4, as defined by each State
▶◆ U5 Medicaid Level of Care 5, as defined by each State
▶◆ U6 Medicaid Level of Care 6, as defined by each State
▶◆ U7 Medicaid Level of Care 7, as defined by each State
▶◆ U8 Medicaid Level of Care 8, as defined by each State
▶◆ U9 Medicaid Level of Care 9, as defined by each State
▶◆ UA Medicaid Level of Care 10, as defined by each State

▶◆ UB Medicaid Level of Care 11, as defined by each State
▶◆ UC Medicaid Level of Care 12, as defined by each State
▶◆ UD Medicaid Level of Care 13, as defined by each State
✻ UE Used DME
✻ VP Aphakic patient

Ambulance Modifiers

Modifiers that are used on claims for ambulance services are created by combining two alpha characters. Each alpha character, with the exception of X, represents an origin (source) code or a destination code. The pair of alpha codes creates one modifier. The first position alpha-code = origin; the second position alpha-code = destination. On form HCFA-1491, used to report ambulance services, Item 12 should contain the origin code and Item 13 should contain the destination code. Origin and destination codes and their descriptions are listed below:

D Diagnostic or therapeutic site other than *P* or *H* when these are used as origin codes
E Residential, domiciliary, custodial facility (other than an 1819 facility)
G Hospital-based dialysis facility (hospital or hospital related)
H Hospital
I Site of transfer (e.g., airport or helicopter pad) between modes of ambulance transport
J Non–hospital-based dialysis facility
N Skilled nursing facility (SNF) (1819 facility)
P Physician's office (includes HMO non-hospital facility, clinic, etc.)
R Residence
S Scene of accident or acute event
X Destination code only. Intermediate stop at physician's office en route to the hospital (includes non-hospital facility, clinic, etc.)

TRANSPORT SERVICES INCLUDING AMBULANCE (A0000-A0999)

◆ A0021 Ambulance service, outside state per mile, transport (Medicaid only)
Cross Reference A0030
➠◆ A0080 Non-emergency transportation: per mile—vehicle provided by volunteer (individual or organization), with no vested interest
➠◆ A0090 Non-emergency transportation, per mile—vehicle provided by volunteer (individual or organization), with no vested interest
➠◆ A0100 Non-emergency transportation: taxi
◆ A0110 Non-emergency transportation and bus, intra or inter state carrier
➠◆ A0120 Non-emergency transportation: mini-bus, mountain area transports, or other transportation systems
◆ A0130 Non-emergency transportation: wheel-chair van
◆ A0140 Non-emergency transportation and air travel (private or commercial), intra or inter state
◆ A0160 Non-emergency transportation: per mile—caseworker or social worker
➠◆ A0170 Transportation: ancillary: parking fees, tolls, other
◆ A0180 Non-emergency transportation: ancillary: lodging—recipient
◆ A0190 Non-emergency transportation: ancillary: meals—recipient
◆ A0200 Non-emergency transportation: ancillary: lodging—escort
◆ A0210 Non-emergency transportation: ancillary: meals—escort
✻ A0225 Ambulance service, neonatal transport, base rate, emergency transport, one way
✻ A0380 BLS mileage (per mile)
Cross Reference A0425
✻ A0382 BLS routine disposable supplies
✻ A0384 BLS specialized service disposable supplies; defibrillation (used by advanced life support [ALS] ambulances and BLS ambulances in jurisdictions where defibrillation is permitted in BLS ambulances)
✻ A0390 ALS mileage (per mile)
Cross Reference A0425
✻ A0392 ALS specialized service disposable supplies; defibrillation (to be used only in jurisdictions where defibrillation cannot be performed in BLS ambulances)
✻ A0394 ALS specialized service disposable supplies; intravenous (IV) drug therapy
✻ A0396 ALS specialized service disposable supplies; esophageal intubation
✻ A0398 ALS routine disposable supplies
✻ A0420 Ambulance waiting time (ALS or BLS), one half (½) hour increments

Waiting Time Table

Units	Time	Units	Time
1	½ to 1 hrs.	6	3 to 3½ hrs.
2	1 to 1½ hrs.	7	3½ to 4 hrs.
3	1½ to 2 hrs	8	4 to 4½ hrs.
4	2 to 2½ hrs.	9	4½ to 5 hrs.
5	2½ to 3 hrs.	10	5 to 5½ hrs.

✻ A0422 Ambulance (ALS or BLS) oxygen and oxygen supplies, life-sustaining situation
➠✻ A0424 Extra ambulance attendant, ALS or BLS or air (fixed or rotary winged); (requires medical review)
✻ A0425 Ground mileage, per statute mile

✻ A0426 Ambulance service, advanced life support, non-emergency transport, Level 1 (ALS1)

✻ A0427 Ambulance service, advanced life support, emergency transport, Level 1 (ALS1-Emergency)

✻ A0428 Ambulance service, BLS, non-emergency transport

✻ A0429 Ambulance service, basic life support, emergency transport (BLS-Emergency)

✻ A0430 Ambulance service, conventional air services, transport, one way (fixed wing)

✻ A0431 Ambulance service, conventional air services, transport, one way (rotary wing)

✻ A0432 Paramedic intercept (PI), rural area, transport furnished by a volunteer ambulance company, which is prohibited by state law from billing third-party payers

✻ A0433 Advanced life support, Level 2 (ALS2)

✻ A0434 Specialty care transport (SCT)

✻ A0435 Fixed wing air mileage, per statute mile

✻ A0436 Rotary wing air mileage, per statute mile

◆ A0888 Noncovered ambulance mileage, per mile (e.g., for miles traveled beyond closest appropriate facility)
MCM 2125

✪ A0999 Unlisted ambulance service
MCM 2120.1, MCM 2125

MEDICAL AND SURGICAL SUPPLIES (A4000-A8999)

◆ A4206 Syringe with needle, sterile 1 cc, each

◆ A4207 Syringe with needle, sterile 2 cc, each

◆ A4208 Syringe with needle, sterile 3 cc, each

◆ A4209 Syringe with needle, sterile 5 cc or greater, each

◆ A4210 Needle-free injection device, each
CIM 60-9

✪ A4211 Supplies for self-administered injections
MCM 2049

✻ A4212 Non-coring needle or stylet with or without catheter

◆ A4213 Syringe, sterile, 20 cc or greater, each

✻ A4214 Sterile saline or water, 30 cc vial

◆ A4215 Needles only, sterile, any size, each

✪ A4220 Refill kit for implantable infusion pump
CIM 60-14

✻ A4221 Supplies for maintenance of drug infusion catheter, per week (list drug separately)

✻ A4222 Supplies for external drug infusion pump, per cassette or bag (list drug separately)

✪ A4230 Infusion set for external insulin pump, non-needle cannula type
CIM 60-14

✪ A4231 Infusion set for external insulin pump, needle type
CIM 60-14

✪ A4232 Syringe with needle for external insulin pump, sterile, 3 cc
CIM 60-14

◆ A4244 Alcohol or peroxide, per pint

◆ A4245 Alcohol wipes, per box

◆ A4246 Betadine or pHisoHex solution, per pint

◆ A4247 Betadine or iodine swabs/wipes, per box

◆ A4250 Urine test or reagent strips or tablets (100 tablets or strips)
MCM 2100

✪ A4253 Blood glucose test or reagent strips for home blood glucose monitor, per 50 strips
CIM 60-11

✪ A4254 Replacement battery, any type, for use with medically necessary home blood glucose monitor owned by patient, each
CIM 60-11

✪ A4255 Platforms for home blood glucose monitor, 50 per box
CIM 60-11

✪ A4256 Normal, low and high calibrator solution/chips
CIM 60-11

✻ A4257 Replacement lens shield cartridge for use with laser skin piercing device, each

✪ A4258 Spring-powered device for lancet, each
CIM 60-11

✪ A4259 Lancets, per box of 100
CIM 60-11

◆ A4260 Levonorgestrel (contraceptive) implants system, including implants and supplies
Medicare Statute 1862a1A

◆ A4261 Cervical cap for contraceptive use
Medicare Statute 1862a1

✪ A4262 Temporary, absorbable lacrimal duct implant, each

✪ A4263 Permanent, long-term, non-dissolvable lacrimal duct implant, each
MCM 15030

✪ A4265 Paraffin, per pound
CIM 60-9

▶◆ A4266 Diaphragm for contraceptive use

▶◆ A4267 Contraceptive supply, condom, male, each

▶◆ A4268 Contraceptive supply, condom, female, each

▶◆ A4269 Contraceptive supply, spermicide (e.g., foam, gel), each

✻ A4270 Disposable endoscope sheath, each

✻ A4280 Adhesive skin support attachment for use with external breast prosthesis, each

▶◆ A4281 Tubing for breast pump, replacement

▶◆ A4282 Adapter for breast pump, replacement

▶◆ A4283 Cap for breast pump bottle, replacement

▶◆ A4284 Breast shield and splash protector for use with breast pump, replacement

▶◆ A4285 Polycarbonate bottle for use with breast pump, replacement

▶◆ A4286 Locking ring for breast pump, replacement

✻ A4290 Sacral nerve stimulation test lead, each

Vascular Catheters

✪ A4300 Implantable access catheter, (e.g., venous, arterial, epidural subarachnoid, or peritoneal, etc.) external access
MCM 2130

➠✻ A4301 Implantable access total; catheter, port/reservoir (e.g., venous, arterial, epidural, or subarachnoid, peritoneal etc.)

✻ A4305 Disposable drug delivery system, flow rate of 50 cc or greater per hour

✻ A4306 Disposable drug delivery system, flow rate of 5 cc or less per hour

Incontinence Appliances and Care Supplies

✪ A4310 Insertion tray without drainage bag and without catheter (accessories only)
MCM 2130

✪ A4311 Insertion tray without drainage bag with indwelling catheter, Foley type, two-way latex with coating (Teflon, silicone, silicone elastomer or hydrophilic, etc.)
MCM 2130

✪ A4312 Insertion tray without drainage bag with indwelling catheter, Foley type, two-way, all silicone
MCM 2130

✪ A4313 Insertion tray without drainage bag with indwelling catheter, Foley type, three-way, for continuous irrigation
MCM 2130

✪ A4314 Insertion tray with drainage bag with indwelling catheter, Foley type, two-way latex with coating (Teflon, silicone, silicone elastomer or hydrophilic, etc.)
MCM 2130

✪ A4315 Insertion tray with drainage bag with indwelling catheter, Foley type, two-way, all silicone
MCM 2130

✪ A4316 Insertion tray with drainage bag with indwelling catheter, Foley type, three-way, for continuous irrigation
MCM 2130

✻ A4319 Sterile water irrigation solution, 1000 cc

✪ A4320 Irrigation tray with bulb or piston syringe, any purpose
MCM 2130

✻ A4321 Therapeutic agent for urinary catheter irrigation

✪ A4322 Irrigation syringe, bulb or piston, each
MCM 2130

✪ A4323 Sterile saline irrigation solution, 1000 cc
MCM 2130

✻ A4324 Male external catheter, with adhesive coating, each

✻ A4325 Male external catheter, with adhesive strip, each

✪ A4326 Male external catheter specialty type (e.g., inflatable, faceplate, etc.), each
MCM 2130

✪ A4327 Female external urinary collection device; metal cup, each
MCM 2130

✪ A4328 Female external urinary collection device; pouch, each
MCM 2130

A4329 Deleted 01/01/02

✪ A4330 Perianal fecal collection pouch with adhesive, each
MCM 2130

✻ A4331 Extension drainage tubing, any type, any length, with connector/adaptor, for use with urinary leg bag or urostomy pouch, each

✻ A4332 Lubricant, individual sterile packet, for insertion of urinary catheter, each

✻ A4333 Urinary catheter anchoring device, adhesive skin attachment, each

✻ A4334 Urinary catheter anchoring device, leg strap, each

✪ A4335 Incontinence supply; miscellaneous
MCM 2130

✪ A4338 Indwelling catheter; Foley type, two-way latex with coating (Teflon, silicone, silicone elastomer, or hydrophilic, etc.), each
MCM 2130

✪ A4340 Indwelling catheter; specialty type (e.g., coudé, mushroom, wing, etc.), each
MCM 2130

✪ A4344 Indwelling catheter, Foley type, two-way, all silicone, each
MCM 2130A

✪ A4346 Indwelling catheter; Foley type, three-way for continuous irrigation, each
MCM 2130

✪ A4347 Male external catheter with or without adhesive, with or without anti-reflux device; per dozen
MCM 2130

✻ A4348 Male external catheter with integral collection compartment, extended wear, (e.g., two per month)

✪ A4351 Intermittent urinary catheter; straight tip, with or without coating (Teflon, silicone, silicone elastomer, or hydrophilic, etc.), each
MCM 2130

✪ A4352 Intermittent urinary catheter; coudé (curved) tip, with or without coating (Teflon, silicone, silicone elastomeric, or hydrophilic, etc.), each
MCM 2130

✻ A4353 Intermittent urinary catheter, with insertion supplies

✪ A4354 Insertion tray with drainage bag but without catheter
MCM 2130

✪ A4355 Irrigation tubing set for continuous bladder irrigation through a three-way indwelling Foley catheter, each
MCM 2130

External Urinary Supplies

✪ A4356 External urethral clamp or compression device (not to be used for catheter clamp), each
MCM 2130

✪ A4357 Bedside drainage bag, day or night, with or without anti-reflux device, with or without tube, each
MCM 2130

✪ A4358 Urinary drainage bag, leg or abdomen, vinyl, with or without tube, with straps, each
MCM 2130

✪ A4359 Urinary suspensory without leg bag, each
MCM 2130

4360 Deleted 12/31/02

Ostomy Supplies

✪ A4361 Ostomy faceplate, each
MCM 2130A

✪ A4362 Skin barrier; solid, 4 × 4 or equivalent; each
MCM 2130

A4363 Deleted 01/01/00; Cross Reference A4369, A4370, A4371

✻ A4364 Adhesive, liquid or equal, any type, per ounce (oz)

✻ A4365 Adhesive remover wipes, any type, per 50

✪ A4367 Ostomy belt, each
MCM 2130A

✻ A4368 Ostomy filter, any type, each

✻ A4369 Ostomy skin barrier, liquid (spray, brush, etc.), per oz

A4370 Deleted 12/31/02

✻ A4371 Ostomy skin barrier, powder, per oz

➠✻ A4372 Ostomy skin barrier, solid 4 × 4 or with built-in convexity, each
MCM 2130

➠✻ A4373 Ostomy skin barrier, with flange (solid, flexible, or accordion), with built-in convexity, any size, each
MCM 2130

A4374 Deleted 12/31/02

✻ A4375 Ostomy pouch, drainable, with faceplate attached, plastic, each

✻ A4376 Ostomy pouch, drainable, with faceplate attached, rubber, each

✻ A4377 Ostomy pouch, drainable, for use on faceplate, plastic, each

✻ A4378 Ostomy pouch, drainable, for use on faceplate, rubber, each

✻ A4379 Ostomy pouch, urinary, with faceplate attached, plastic, each

✻ A4380 Ostomy pouch, urinary, with faceplate attached, rubber, each

✻ A4381 Ostomy pouch, urinary, with faceplate attached, plastic, each

✻ A4382 Ostomy pouch, urinary, for use on faceplate, heavy plastic, each

✻ A4383 Ostomy pouch, urinary, for use on faceplate, rubber, each

✻ A4384 Ostomy faceplate equivalent, silicone ring, each

✻ A4385 Ostomy skin barrier, solid 4 × 4 or equivalent, extended wear, without built-in convexity, each

A4386 Deleted 12/31/02

➠✻ A4387 Ostomy pouch closed, with barrier attached, with built-in convexity (1 piece), each
MCM 2130

➠✻ A4388 Ostomy pouch, drainable, with extended wear barrier attached (1 piece), each
MCM 2130

➠✻ A4389 Ostomy pouch, drainable, with barrier attached, with built-in convexity (1 piece), each
MCM 2130

✻ A4390 Ostomy pouch, drainable, with extended wear barrier attached, with built-in convexity (1 piece), each

➠✻ A4391 Ostomy pouch, urinary, with extended wear barrier attached (1 piece), each
MCM 2130

✻ A4392 Ostomy pouch, urinary, with standard wear barrier attached, with built-in convexity (1 piece), each

✻ A4393 Ostomy pouch, urinary, with extended wear barrier attached, with built-in convexity (1 piece), each

✻ A4394 Ostomy deodorant for use in ostomy pouch, liquid, per fluid ounce

✻ A4395 Ostomy deodorant for use in ostomy pouch, solid, per tablet

✻ A4396 Ostomy belt with peristomal hernia support

⊕ A4397 Irrigation supply; sleeve, each
MCM 2130

⊕ A4398 Ostomy irrigation supply; bag, each
MCM 2130A

⊕ A4399 Ostomy irrigation supply; cone/catheter, including brush
MCM 2130A

⊕ A4400 Ostomy irrigation set
MCM 2130

⊕ A4402 Lubricant, per ounce
MCM 2130

⊕ A4404 Ostomy ring, each
MCM 2130

▶⊕ A4405 Ostomy skin barrier, non-pectin based, paste, per ounce
MCM 2130

▶⊕ A4406 Ostomy skin barrier, pectin-based, paste, per ounce
MCM 2130

▶⊕ A4407 Ostomy skin barrier, with flange (solid, flexible, or accordion), extended wear, with built-in convexity, 4 x 4 inches or smaller, each
MCM 2130

▶⊕ A4408 Ostomy skin barrier, with flange (solid, flexible or accordion), extended wear, with built-in convexity, larger than 4 x 4 inches, each
MCM 2130

▶⊕ A4409 Ostomy skin barrier, with flange (solid, flexible or accordion), extended wear, without built-in convexity, 4 x 4 inches or smaller, each
MCM 2130

▶⊕ A4410 Ostomy skin barrier, with flange (solid, flexible or accordion), extended wear, without built-in convexity, larger than 4 × 4 inches, each
MCM 2130

▶⊕ A4413 Ostomy pouch, drainable, high output, for use on a barrier with flange (2 piece system), with filter, each
MCM 2130

▶⊕ A4414 Ostomy skin barrier, with flange (solid, flexible or accordion), without built-in convexity, 4 × 4 inches or smaller, each
MCM 2130

▶⊕ A4415 Ostomy skin barrier, with flange (solid, flexible or accordion), without built-in convexity, larger than 4 × 4 inches, each
MCM 2130

⊕ A4421 Ostomy supply; miscellaneous
MCM 2130

▶⊕ A4422 Ostomy absorbent material (sheet/pad/crystal packet) for use in ostomy pouch to thicken liquid stomal output, each
MCM 2130

▶⊕ A4450 Tape, non-waterproof, per 18 square inches
MCM 2130

▶⊕ A4452 Tape, waterproof, per 18 square inches
MCM 2130

Miscellaneous Supplies

A4454 Deleted 12/31/02

⊕ A4455 Adhesive remover or solvent (for tape, cement or other adhesive), per ounce
MCM 2130

▶◆ A4458 Enema bag with tubing, reusable

A4460 Deleted 12/31/02

➠✻ A4462 Abdominal dressing holder, each
MCM 2130

A4464 Deleted 12/31/02

✻ A4465 Non-elastic binder for extremity

⊕ A4470 Gravlee jet washer
MCM 2320, CIM 50-4

⊕ A4480 VABRA aspirator
MCM 2320, CIM 50-4

✻ A4481 Tracheostoma filter, any type, any size, each

✻ A4483 Moisture exchanger, disposable, for use with invasive mechanical ventilation

◆ A4490 Surgical stockings above knee length, each
MCM 2079, MCM 2133, CIM 60-9

◆ A4495 Surgical stockings thigh length, each
MCM 2079, MCM 2133, CIM 60-9

◆ A4500 Surgical stockings below knee length, each
MCM 2079, MCM 2133, CIM 60-9

◆ A4510 Surgical stockings full length, each
MCM 2079, MCM 2133, CIM 60-9

▶◆ A4521 Adult-sized incontinence product, diaper, small size, each
CIM 60-9

▶◆ A4522 Adult-sized incontinence product, diaper, medium size, each
CIM 60-9

▶◆ A4523 Adult-sized incontinence product, diaper, large size, each
CIM 60-9

▶◆ A4524 Adult-sized incontinence product, diaper, extra large size, each
CIM 60-9

▶◆ A4525 Adult-sized incontinence product, brief, small size, each
CIM 60-9

▶◆ A4526 Adult-sized incontinence product, brief, medium size, each
CIM 60-9

▶◆ A4527 Adult-sized incontinence product, brief, large size, each
CIM 60-9

▶◆ A4528 Adult-sized incontinence product, brief, extra-large size, each
CIM 60-9

▶◆ A4529 Child-sized incontinence product, diaper, small/medium size, each
CIM 60-9

▶◆ A4530 Child-sized incontinence product, diaper, large size, each
CIM 60-9

▶◆ A4531 Child-sized incontinence product, brief, small/medium size, each
CIM 60-9

▶◆ A4532 Child-sized incontinence product, brief, large size, each
CIM 60-9

▶◆ A4533 Youth-sized incontinence product, diaper, each
CIM 60-9

▶◆ A4534 Youth-sized incontinence product, brief, each
CIM 60-9

▶◆ A4535 Disposable liner/shield for incontinence, each
CIM 60-9

▶◆ A4536 Protective underwear, washable, any size, each
CIM 60-9

▶◆ A4537 Under pad, reusable/washable, any size, each
CIM 60-9

▶◆ A4538 Diaper service, reusable diaper, each diaper
CIM 60-9

✪ A4550 Surgical trays
MCM 15030

◆ A4554 Disposable underpads, all sizes, (e.g., Chux's)
MCM 2130, CIM 60-9

✱ A4556 Electrodes, (e.g., apnea monitor), per pair

✱ A4557 Lead wires, (e.g., apnea monitor), per pair

✱ A4558 Conductive paste or gel

✱ A4561 Pessary, rubber, any type

✱ A4562 Pessary, non-rubber, any type

✱ A4565 Slings

◆ A4570 Splint
MCM 2079

A4572 Deleted 12/31/02, Cross Reference L0210

◆ A4575 Topical hyperbaric oxygen chamber, disposable
CIM 35-10

◆ A4580 Cast supplies (e.g., plaster)
MCM 2079

◆ A4590 Special casting material (e.g., fiberglass)

➠✱ A4595 Electrical stimulators supplies, 2-lead, per month (e.g. tens, NMES)
CIM 45-25

Supplies for Respiratory and Oxygen Equipment

▶✱ A4606 Oxygen probe for use with oximeter device, replacement

✱ A4608 Transtracheal oxygen catheter, each

▶✱ A4609 Tracheal suction catheter, closed system, for less than 72 hours of use, each

▶✱ A4610 Tracheal suction catheter, closed system, for 72 or more hours of use, each

✱ A4611 Battery, heavy duty; replacement for patient-owned ventilator

✱ A4612 Battery cables; replacement for patient-owned ventilator

✱ A4613 Battery charger; replacement for patient-owned ventilator

✱ A4614 Peak expiratory flow rate meter, hand-held

✪ A4615 Cannula, nasal
MCM 3312, CIM 60-4

✪ A4616 Tubing (oxygen), per foot
MCM 3312, CIM 60-4

✪ A4617 Mouth piece
MCM 3312, CIM 60-4

✪ A4618 Breathing circuits
MCM 3312, CIM 60-4

✪ A4619 Face tent
MCM 3312, CIM 60-4

✪ A4620 Variable concentration mask
MCM 3312, CIM 60-4

✱ A4621 Tracheotomy mask or collar

✪ A4622 Tracheostomy or laryngectomy tube
CIM 65-16

✪ A4623 Tracheostomy, inner cannula (replacement only)
CIM 65-16

➠✱ A4624 Tracheal suction catheter, any type, other than closed system, each

✱ A4625 Tracheostomy care kit for new tracheostomy

✱ A4626 Tracheostomy cleaning brush, each

◆ A4627 Spacer, bag or reservoir, with or without mask, for use with metered dose inhaler
MCM 2100

✱ A4628 Oropharyngeal suction catheter, each

✱ A4629 Tracheostomy care kit for established tracheostomy

Supplies for Other Durable Medical Equipment

✪ A4630 Replacement batteries; medically necessary TENS owned by patient
CIM 65-8

⊙ A4631 Replacement batteries for medically necessary electronic wheelchair owned by patient
CIM 60-9

▶✻ A4632 Replacement battery for external infusion pump, any type, each

▶✻ A4633 Replacement bulb/lamp for ultraviolet light therapy system, each

▶✻ A4634 Replacement bulb for therapeutic light box, tabletop model

⊙ A4635 Underarm pad, crutch, replacement, each
CIM 60-9

⊙ A4636 Replacement, handgrip, cane, crutch, or walker, each
CIM 60-9

⊙ A4637 Replacement, tip, cane, crutch, walker, each
CIM 60-9

▶✻ A4639 Replacement pad for infrared heating pad system, each

⊙ A4640 Replacement pad for use with medically necessary alternating pressure pad owned by patient
MCM 4107.6, CIM 60-9

Supplies for Radiological Procedures

✻ A4641 Supply of radiopharmaceutical diagnostic imaging agent, not otherwise classified
MCM 15030

✻ A4642 Supply of satumomab pendetide, radiopharmaceutical diagnostic imaging agent, per dose
MCM 15030

✻ A4643 Supply of additional high dose contrast material(s) during magnetic resonance imaging (e.g., gadoteridol injection)
MCM 15030

⊙ A4644 Supply of low osmolar contrast material (100 to 199 milligram [mg] of iodine)
MCM 15022, MCM 15030

⊙ A4645 Supply of low osmolar contrast material (200 to 299 mg of iodine)
MCM 15022, MCM 15030

⊙ A4646 Supply of low osmolar contrast material (300 to 399 mg of iodine)
MCM 15022, MCM 15030

⊙ A4647 Supply of paramagnetic contrast material (e.g., gadolinium)
MCM 15022, MCM 15030

✻ A4649 Surgical supply, miscellaneous

Supplies for End State Renal Disease

NOTE: For DME items for ESRD see procedures codes E1550 to E1699.

A4650 Deleted 01/01/02

⊙ A4651 Calibrated microcapillary tube, each
MCM 4270

⊙ A4652 Microcapillary tube sealant
MCM 4270

▶✻ A4653 Peritoneal dialysis catheter anchoring device, belt, each

⊙ A4655 Deleted 01/01/02

➠ ⊙ A4656 Needle, any size, each
MCM 4270

➠ ⊙ A4657 Syringe, with or without needle, each
MCM 4270

➠ ⊙ A4660 Sphygmomanometer/blood pressure apparatus with cuff and stethoscope
MCM 4270

➠ ⊙ A4663 Blood pressure cuff only
MCM 4270

➠ ◆ A4670 Automatic blood pressure monitor
MCM 4270, CIM 50-42

⊙ A4680 Activated carbon filters for hemodialysis, each
MCM 4270, CIM 55-1

⊙ A4690 Dialyzers (artificial kidneys) all types, all sizes, for hemodialysis, each
MCM 4270

A4700 Deleted 01/01/02

A4705 Deleted 01/01/02

⊙ A4706 Bicarbonate concentrate, solution, for hemodialysis, per gallon
MCM 4270

⊙ A4707 Bicarbonate concentrate, powder, for hemodialysis, per packet
MCM 4270

⊙ A4708 Acetate concentrate solution, for hemodialysis, per gallon
MCM 4270

⊙ A4709 Acid concentrate, solution, for hemodialysis, per gallon
MCM 4270

➠ ⊙ A4712 Water, sterile, for injection for dialysis, per 10 ml
MCM 4270

⊙ A4714 Treated water (deionized, distilled, reverse osmosis) for peritoneal dialysis, per gallon
MCM 4270, CIM 55-1

⊙ A4719 "Y set" tubing for peritoneal dialysis
MCM 4270

⊙ A4720 Dialysate solution, any concentrate of dextrose, fluid volume greater than 249 cc, but less than or equal to 999 cc, for peritoneal dialysis
MCM 4270

⊛ A4721 Dialysate solution, any concentrate of dextrose, fluid volume greater than 999 cc, but less than or equal to 1999 cc, for peritoneal dialysis
MCM 4270

⊛ A4722 Dialysate solution, any concentrate of dextrose, fluid volume greater than 1999 cc, but less than or equal to 2999 cc, for peritoneal dialysis
MCM 4270

⊛ A4723 Dialysate solution, any concentrate of dextrose, fluid volume greater than 2999 cc, but less than or equal to 3999 cc, for peritoneal dialysis
MCM 4270

⊛ A4724 Dialysate solution, any concentrate of dextrose, fluid volume greater than 3999 cc, but less than or equal to 4999 cc, for peritoneal dialysis
MCM 4270

⊛ A4725 Dialysate solution, any concentrate of dextrose, fluid volume greater than 4999 cc, but less than or equal to 5999 cc, for peritoneal dialysis
MCM 4270

⊛ A4726 Dialysate solution, any concentrate of dextrose, fluid volume greater than 5999 cc, for peritoneal dialysis
MCM 4270

⊛ A4730 Fistula cannulation set for hemodialysis, each
MCM 4270

A4735 Deleted 01/01/02

⊛ A4736 Topical anesthetic, for dialysis, per gram
MCM 4270

⊛ A4737 Injectable anesthetic, for dialysis, per 10 cc
MCM 4270

⊛ A4740 Shunt accessories for hemodialysis, any type, each
MCM 4270

⊛ A4750 Blood tubing, arterial or venous for hemodialysis, each
MCM 4270

⊛ A4755 Blood tubing, arterial and venous combined, for hemodialysis, each
MCM 4270

⊛ A4760 Dialysate solution test kit, for peritoneal dialysis, any type, each
MCM 4270

⊛ A4765 Dialysate concentrate, powder, additive for peritoneal dialysis, per packet
MCM 4270

⊛ A4766 Dialysate concentrate, solution, additive for peritoneal dialysis, per 10 cc
MCM 4270

⊛ A4770 Blood collection tube, vacuum, for dialysis, per 50
MCM 4270

⊛ A4771 Serum clotting time tube, for dialysis, per 50
MCM 4270

⊛ A4772 Blood glucose test strips, for dialysis, per 50
MCM 4270

⊛ A4773 Occult blood test strips, for dialysis, per 50
MCM 4270

⊛ A4774 Ammonia test strips, for dialysis, per 50
MCM 4270

A4780 Deleted 01/01/02

A4790 Deleted 01/01/02

A4800 Deleted 01/01/02, Cross Reference A4801

A4801 Deleted 12/31/02, Cross Reference J1644

⊛ A4802 Protamine sulfate, for hemodialysis, per 50 mg
MCM 4270

A4820 Deleted 01/01/02

A4850 Deleted 01/01/02, Cross Reference E1637

⊛ A4860 Disposable catheter tips for peritoneal dialysis, per 10

⊛ A4870 Plumbing and/or electrical work for home dialysis equipment

A4880 Deleted 12/31/01

⊛ A4890 Contracts, repair and maintenance, for hemodialysis equipment
MCM 2100.4

A4900 Deleted 01/01/02

A4901 Deleted 01/01/02

A4905 Deleted 01/01/02

A4910 Deleted 01/01/02

⊛ A4911 Drain bag/bottle, for dialysis, each

A4912 Deleted 01/01/02, Cross Reference A4911

⊛ A4913 Miscellaneous dialysis supplies, not otherwise specified

A4914 Deleted 01/01/02

⊛ A4918 Venous pressure clamp, for hemodialysis, each

A4919 Deleted 01/01/02

A4920 Deleted 01/01/02

A4921 Deleted 01/01/02

➠ ⊛ A4927 Gloves, non-sterile, per 100

➠ ⊛ A4928 Surgical mask, per 20

⊛ A4929 Tourniquet for dialysis, each

▶ ⊛ A4930 Gloves, sterile, per pair

▶ ✻ A4931 Oral thermometer, reusable, any type, each

▶ ◆ A4932 Rectal thermometer, reusable, any type, each

Additional Ostomy Supplies

➠ ⊛ A5051 Ostomy pouch, closed; with barrier attached (1 piece), each
MCM 2130

➠ ✪ A5052 Ostomy pouch, closed; without barrier attached (1 piece), each
MCM 2130

➠ ✪ A5053 Ostomy pouch, closed; for use on faceplate, each
MCM 2130

➠ ✪ A5054 Ostomy pouch, closed; for use on barrier with flange (2 piece), each
MCM 2130

✪ A5055 Stoma cap
MCM 2130

➠ ✪ A5061 Ostomy pouch, drainable; with barrier attached (1 piece), each
MCM 2130

➠ ✪ A5062 Ostomy pouch, drainable; without barrier attached (1 piece), each
MCM 2130

➠ ✪ A5063 Ostomy pouch, drainable; for use on barrier with flange (2 piece), each
MCM 2130

A5064 Deleted 01/01/02

➠ ✪ A5071 Ostomy pouch, urinary; with barrier attached (1 piece), each
MCM 2130

➠ ✪ A5072 Ostomy pouch, urinary; without barrier attached (1 piece), each
MCM 2130

➠ ✪ A5073 Ostomy pouch, urinary; for use on barrier with flange (2 piece), each
MCM 2130

A5074 Deleted 01/01/02

A5075 Deleted 01/01/02

✪ A5081 Continent device; plug for continent stoma
MCM 2130

✪ A5082 Continent device; catheter for continent stoma
MCM 2130

✪ A5093 Ostomy accessory; convex insert
MCM 2130

Additional Incontinence Appliances/Supplies

✪ A5102 Bedside drainage bottle with or without tubing, rigid or expandable, each
MCM 2130

✪ A5105 Urinary suspensory; with leg bag, with or without tube
MCM 2130

✪ A5112 Urinary leg bag; latex
MCM 2130

✪ A5113 Leg strap; latex, replacement only, per set
MCM 2130

✪ A5114 Leg strap; foam or fabric, replacement only, per set
MCM 2130

Supplies for Either Incontinence or Ostomy Appliances

✪ A5119 Skin barrier; wipes, box per 50
MCM 2130

✪ A5121 Skin barrier; solid, 6 × 6 or equivalent, each
MCM 2130

✪ A5122 Skin barrier; solid, 8 × 8 or equivalent, each
MCM 2130

A5123 Deleted 12/31/02

✪ A5126 Adhesive or non-adhesive; disc or foam pad
MCM 2130

✪ A5131 Appliance cleaner, incontinence and ostomy appliances, per 16 oz
MCM 2130

* A5200 Percutaneous catheter/tube anchoring device, adhesive skin attachment

Diabetic Shoes, Fitting and Modifications

✪ A5500 For diabetics only, fitting (including follow-up), custom preparation and supply of off-the-shelf depth-inlay shoe manufactured to accommodate multidensity insert(s), per shoe
MCM 2134

✪ A5501 For diabetics only, fitting (including follow-up), custom preparation and supply of shoe molded from cast(s) of patient's foot (custom molded shoe), per shoe
MCM 2134

A5502 Deleted 01/01/02

✪ A5503 For diabetics only, modification (including fitting) of off-the-shelf depth-inlay shoe or custommolded shoe with roller or rigid rocker bottom, per shoe
MCM 2134

✪ A5504 For diabetics only, modification (including fitting) of off-the-shelf depth-inlay shoe or custom-molded shoe with wedge(s), per shoe
MCM 2134

✪ A5505 For diabetics only, modification (including fitting) of off-the-shelf depth-inlay shoe or custom-molded shoe with metatarsal bar, per shoe
MCM 2134

✪ A5506 For diabetics only, modification (including fitting) of off-the-shelf depth-inlay shoe or custom-molded shoe with offset heel(s), per shoe
MCM 2134

✪ A5507 For diabetics only, not otherwise specified modification (including fitting) of off-the-shelf depth-inlay shoe or custom-molded shoe, per shoe
MCM 2134

* A5508 For diabetics only, deluxe feature of off-the-shelf depth-inlay shoe or custom-molded shoe, per shoe

✪ A5509 For diabetics only, direct formed, molded to foot with external heat source (e.g., heat gun) multiple density insert(s), prefabricated, per shoe
MCM 2134

✪ A5510 For diabetics only, direct formed, compression molded to patient's foot without external heat source, multiple-density insert(s) prefabricated, per shoe
MCM 2134

✪ A5511 For diabetics only, custom-molded from model of patient's foot, multiple density insert(s), custom-fabricated, per shoe
MCM 2134

Dressings

* A6000 Non-contact wound warming wound cover for use with the non-contact wound warming device and warming card

* A6010 Collagen based wound filler, dry form, per gram of collagen

▶✪ A6011 Collagen based wound filler, gel/paste, per gram of collagen
MCM 2079

* A6021 Collagen dressing, pad size 16 square inch (in^2) or less, each

* A6022 Collagen dressing, pad size more than 16 in^2 but less than or equal to 48 in^2, each

* A6023 Collagen dressing, pad size more than 48 in^2, each

* A6024 Collagen dressing wound filler, per 6 in

◆ A6025 Silicone gel sheet, each

* A6154 Wound pouch, each

* A6196 Alginate or other fiber gelling dressing, wound cover, pad size 16 in^2 or less, each dressing

* A6197 Alginate or other fiber gelling dressing, wound cover, pad size more than 16 in^2, but less than or equal to 48 in^2, each dressing

* A6198 Alginate or other fiber gelling dressing, wound cover, pad size more than 48 in^2, each dressing

* A6199 Alginate or other fiber gelling dressing, wound filler, per 6 in

* A6200 Composite dressing, pad size 16 in^2 or less, without adhesive border, each dressing

* A6201 Composite dressing, pad size more than 16 in^2 but less than or equal to 48 in^2, without adhesive border, each dressing

* A6202 Composite dressing, pad size more than 48 in^2, without adhesive border, each dressing

* A6203 Composite dressing, pad size 16 in^2 or less, with any size adhesive border, each dressing

* A6204 Composite dressing, pad size more than 16 in^2 but less than or equal to 48 in, with any size adhesive border, each dressing

* A6205 Composite dressing, pad size more than 48 in^2, with any size adhesive, each dressing

* A6206 Contact layer, 16 in^2 or less, each dressing

* A6207 Contact layer, more than 16 in^2 but less than or equal to 48 in^2, each dressing

* A6208 Contact layer, more than 48 in^2, each dressing

* A6209 Foam dressing, wound cover, pad size 16 in^2 or less, without adhesive border, each dressing

* A6210 Foam dressing, wound cover, pad size more than 16 in^2 but less than or equal to 48 in^2, without adhesive border, each dressing

* A6211 Foam dressing, wound cover, pad size more than 48 in^2, without adhesive border, each dressing

* A6212 Foam dressing, wound cover, pad size 16 in^2 or less, with any size adhesive border, each dressing

* A6213 Foam dressing, wound cover, pad size more than 16 in^2 but less than or equal to 48 in^2, with any size adhesive border, each dressing

* A6214 Foam dressing, wound cover, pad size more than 48 in^2, with any size adhesive border, each dressing

* A6215 Foam dressing, wound filler, per gram

* A6216 Gauze, non-impregnated, non-sterile, pad size 16 in^2 or less, without adhesive border, each dressing

* A6217 Gauze, non-impregnated, non-sterile, pad size more than 16 in^2 but less than or equal to 48 in^2, without adhesive border, each dressing

* A6218 Gauze, non-impregnated, non-sterile, pad size more than 48 in^2, without adhesive border, each dressing

* A6219 Gauze, non-impregnated, pad size 16 in^2 or less, with any size adhesive border, each dressing

✻ A6220 Gauze, non-impregnated, pad size more than 16 in^2 but less than or equal to 48 in^2, with any size adhesive border, each dressing

✻ A6221 Gauze, non-impregnated, pad size more than 48 in^2, with any size adhesive border, each dressing

✻ A6222 Gauze, impregnated, other than water, normal saline or hydrogel, pad size 16 in^2 or less, without adhesive border, each dressing

✻ A6223 Gauze, impregnated, with other than water, normal saline or hydrogel, pad size more than 16 in^2 but less than or equal to 48 in^2, without adhesive border, each dressing

✻ A6224 Gauze, impregnated, other than water or normal saline or hydrogel, pad size more than 48 in^2, without adhesive border, each dressing

✻ A6228 Gauze, impregnated, water or normal saline, pad size 16 in^2 or less, without adhesive border, each dressing

✻ A6229 Gauze, impregnated, water or normal saline, pad size more than 16 in^2 but less than or equal to 48 in^2, without adhesive border, each dressing

✻ A6230 Gauze, impregnated, water or normal saline, pad size more than 48 in^2, without adhesive border, each dressing

✻ A6231 Gauze, impregnated, hydrogel, for direct wound contact, pad size 16 in^2 or less, each dressing

✻ A6232 Gauze, impregnated, hydrogel, for direct wound contact, pad size greater than 16 in^2, but less than or equal to 48 in^2, each dressing

✻ A6233 Gauze, impregnated, hydrogel, for direct wound contact, pad size more than 48 in^2, each dressing

✻ A6234 Hydrocolloid dressing, wound cover, pad size 16 in^2 or less, without adhesive border, each dressing

✻ A6235 Hydrocolloid dressing, wound cover, pad size more than 16 in^2 but less than or equal to 48 in^2, without adhesive border, each dressing

✻ A6236 Hydrocolloid dressing, wound cover, pad size more than 48 in^2, without adhesive border, each dressing

✻ A6237 Hydrocolloid dressing, wound cover, pad size 16 in^2 or less, with any size adhesive border, each dressing

✻ A6238 Hydrocolloid dressing, wound cover, pad size more than 16 in^2 but less than or equal to 48 in^2, with any size adhesive border, each dressing

✻ A6239 Hydrocolloid dressing, wound cover, pad size more than 48 in^2, with any size adhesive border, each dressing

✻ A6240 Hydrocolloid dressing, wound filler, paste, per fluid ounce

✻ A6241 Hydrocolloid dressing, wound filler, dry form, per gram

✻ A6242 Hydrogel dressing, wound cover, pad size 16 in^2 or less, without adhesive border, each dressing

✻ A6243 Hydrogel dressing, wound cover, pad size more than 16 in^2 but less than or equal to 48 in^2, without adhesive border, each dressing

✻ A6244 Hydrogel dressing, wound cover, pad size more than 48 in^2, without adhesive border, each dressing

✻ A6245 Hydrogel dressing, wound cover, pad size 16 in^2 or less, with any size adhesive border, each dressing

✻ A6246 Hydrogel dressing, wound cover, pad size more than 16 in^2 but less than or equal to 48 in^2, with any size adhesive border, each dressing

✻ A6247 Hydrogel dressing, wound cover, pad size more than 48 in^2, with any size adhesive border, each dressing

✻ A6248 Hydrogel dressing, wound filler, gel, per fluid ounce

✻ A6250 Skin sealants, protectants, moisturizers, ointments, any type, any size

✻ A6251 Specialty absorptive dressing, wound cover, pad size 16 in^2 or less, without adhesive border, each dressing

✻ A6252 Specialty absorptive dressing, wound cover, pad size more than 16 in^2 but less than or equal to 48 in^2, without adhesive border, each dressing

✻ A6253 Specialty absorptive dressing, wound cover, pad size more than 48 in^2, without adhesive border, each dressing

✻ A6254 Specialty absorptive dressing, wound cover, pad size 16 in^2 or less, with any size adhesive border, each dressing

✻ A6255 Specialty absorptive dressing, wound cover, pad size more than 16 in^2 but less than or equal to 48 in^2, with any size adhesive border, each dressing

✻ A6256 Specialty absorptive dressing, wound cover, pad size more than 48 in^2, with any size adhesive border, each dressing

✻ A6257 Transparent film, 16 in^2 or less, each dressing

✻ A6258 Transparent film, more than 16 in^2 but less than or equal to 48 in^2, each dressing

✻ A6259 Transparent film, more than 48 in^2, each dressing

✻ A6260 Wound cleansers, any type, any size

✻ A6261 Wound filler, not elsewhere classified, gel/paste, per fluid ounce

✻ A6262 Wound filler, not elsewhere classified, dry form, per gram

A6263 Deleted 12/31/02
A6264 Deleted 12/31/02
A6265 Deleted 12/31/02
➡ * A6266 Gauze, impregnated, other than water normal saline, or zinc paste, any width, per linear yard
MCM 2079
* A6402 Gauze, non-impregnated, sterile, pad size 16 in^2 or less, without adhesive border, each dressing
* A6403 Gauze, non-impregnated, sterile, pad size more than 16 in^2, less than or equal to 48 in^2, without adhesive border, each dressing
* A6404 Gauze, non-impregnated, sterile, pad size more than 48 in^2, without adhesive border, each dressing
A6405 Deleted 12/31/02
A6406 Deleted 12/31/02
▶ ✪ A6410 Eye pad, sterile, each
MCM 2079
▶ ✪ A6411 Eye pad, non-sterile, each
MCM 2079
▶ ◆ A6412 Eye patch, occlusive, each
▶ * A6421 Padding bandage, non-elastic, non-woven/non-knitted, width greater than or equal to 3 inches and less than 5 inches, per roll (at least 3 yards, unstretched)
▶ * A6422 Conforming bandage, non-elastic, knitted/woven, non-sterile, width greater than or equal to 3 inches and less than 5 inches per roll (at least 3 yards, unstretched)
▶ * A6424 Conforming bandage, non-elastic, knitted/woven, non-sterile, width greater than or equal to 5 inches, per roll (at least 3 yards, unstretched)
▶ * A6426 Conforming bandage, non-elastic, knitted/woven, sterile width greater than or equal to 3 inches and less than 5 inches, per roll (at least 3 yards, unstretched)
▶ * A6428 Conforming bandage, non-elastic, knitted/woven, sterile, width greater than or equal to 5 inches, per roll (at least 3 yards, unstretched)
▶ * A6430 Light compression bandage, elastic, knitted/woven, load resistance less than 1.25 foot pounds at 50% maximum stretch, width greater than or equal to 3 inches and less than 5 inches, per roll (at least 3 yards, unstretched)
▶ * A6432 Light compression bandage, elastic, knitted/woven, load resistance less than 1.25 foot pounds at 50% maximum stretch, width greater than or equal to 5 inches, per roll (at least 3 yards, unstretched)
▶ * A6434 Moderate compression bandage, elastic, knitted/woven, load resistance of 1.25 to 1.34 foot pounds at 50% maximum stretch, width greater than or equal to 3 inches or less than 5 inches, per roll (at least 3 yards, unstretched)
▶ * A6436 High compression bandage, elastic, knitted/woven, load resistance greater than or equal to 1.35 foot pounds at 50% maximum stretch, width greater than or equal to 3 inches and less than 5 inches, per roll (at least 3 yards, unstretched)
▶ * A6438 Self-adherent bandage, elastic, non-knitted/non-woven, load resistance greater than or equal to 0.55 foot pounds at 50% maximum stretch, width greater than or equal to 3 inches and less than 5 inches, per roll (at least 3 yards, unstretched)
▶ * A6440 Zinc paste impregnated bandage, non-elastic, knitted/woven, width greater than or equal to 3 inches and less than 5 inches, per roll (at least 10 yards, unstretched)
▶ ✪ A6501 Compression burn garment, bodysuit (head to foot), custom fabricated
MCM 2079
▶ ✪ A6502 Compression burn garment, chin strap, custom fabricated
MCM 2079
▶ ✪ A6503 Compression burn garment, facial hood, custom fabricated
MCM 2079
▶ ✪ A6504 Compression burn garment, glove to wrist, custom fabricated
MCM 2079
▶ ✪ A6505 Compression burn garment, glove to elbow, custom fabricated
MCM 2079
▶ ✪ A6506 Compression burn garment, glove to axilla, custom fabricated
MCM 2079
▶ ✪ A6507 Compression burn garment, foot to knee length, custom fabricated
MCM 2079
▶ ✪ A6508 Compression burn garment, foot to thigh length, custom fabricated
MCM 2079
▶ ✪ A6509 Compression burn garment, upper trunk to waist including arm openings (vest), custom fabricated
MCM 2079
▶ ✪ A6510 Compression burn garment, trunk, including arms down to leg openings (leotard), custom fabricated
MCM 2079
▶ ✪ A6511 Compression burn garment, lower trunk including leg openings (panty), custom fabricated
MCM 2079

▶✪ A6512 Compression burn garment, not otherwise classified
MCM 2079

RESPIRATORY DURABLE MEDICAL EQUIPMENT, INEXPENSIVE AND ROUTINELY PURCHASED (A7700-A7509)

* A7700 Canister, disposable, used with suction pump, each
* A7001 Canister, non-disposable, used with suction pump, each
* A7002 Tubing, used with suction pump, each
* A7003 Administration set, with small volume nonfiltered pneumatic nebulizer, disposable
* A7004 Small volume nonfiltered pneumatic nebulizer, disposable
* A7005 Administration set, with small volume nonfiltered pneumatic nebulizer, non-disposable
* A7006 Administration set, with small volume filtered pneumatic nebulizer
* A7007 Large volume nebulizer, disposable, unfilled, used with aerosol compressor
* A7008 Large volume nebulizer, disposable, prefilled, used with aerosol compressor
* A7009 Reservoir bottle, nondisposable, used with large volume ultrasonic nebulizer
* A7010 Corrugated tubing, disposable, used with large volume nebulizer, 100 feet
* A7011 Corrugated tubing, non-disposable, used with large volume nebulizer, 10 feet
* A7012 Water collection device, used with large volume nebulizer
* A7013 Filter, disposable, used with aerosol compressor
* A7014 Filter, non-disposable, used with aerosol compressor or ultrasonic generator
* A7015 Aerosol mask, used with DME nebulizer
* A7016 Dome and mouthpiece, used with small volume ultrasonic nebulizer

✪ A7017 Nebulizer, durable, glass or autoclavable plastic, bottle type, not used with oxygen
CIM 60-9

* A7018 Water, distilled, used with large volume nebulizer, 1000 cc
* A7019 Saline solution, per 10 cc, metered dose dispenser, for use with inhalation drugs
* A7020 Sterile water or sterile saline, 1000 cc, used with large volume nebulizer

▶* A7025 High frequency chest wall oscillation system vest, replacement for use with patient-owned equipment, each
▶* A7026 High frequency chest wall oscillation system hose, replacement for use with patient-owned equipment, each
▶* A7030 Full face mask used with positive airway pressure device, each
▶* A7031 Face mask interface, replacement for full-face mask, each
▶* A7032 Replacement cushion for nasal application device, each
▶* A7033 Replacement pillows for nasal application device, pair
▶* A7034 Nasal interface (mask or cannula type) used with positive airway pressure device, with or without head strap
▶* A7035 Headgear used with positive airway pressure device
▶* A7036 Chinstrap used with positive airway pressure device
▶* A7037 Tubing used with positive airway pressure device
▶* A7038 Filter, disposable, used with positive airway pressure device
▶* A7039 Filter, non disposable, used with positive airway pressure device
▶* A7042 Implanted pleural catheter, each
▶* A7043 Vacuum drainage bottle and tubing for use with implanted catheter
▶* A7044 Oral interface used with positive airway pressure device, each

✪ A7501 Tracheostoma valve, including diaphragm, each
MCM 2130

✪ A7502 Replacement diaphragm/faceplate for tracheostoma valve, each
MCM 2130

✪ A7503 Filter holder or filter cap, reusable, for use in a tracheostoma heat and moisture exchange system, each
MCM 2130

✪ A7504 Filter for use in a tracheostoma heat and moisture exchange system, each
MCM 2130

✪ A7505 Housing, reusable without adhesive, for use in a heat and moisture exchange system and/or with a tracheostoma valve, each
MCM 2130

✪ A7506 Adhesive disc for use in a heat and moisture exchange system and/or with tracheostoma valve, any type, each
MCM 2130

✪ A7507 Filter holder and integrated filter without adhesive, for use in a tracheostoma heat and moisture exchange system, each
MCM 2130

✪ A7508 Housing and integrated adhesive, for use in a tracheostoma heat and moisture exchange system and/or with a tracheostoma valve, each
MCM 2130

- ⊙ A7509 Filter holder and integrated filter housing, and adhesive, for use as a tracheostoma heat and moisture exchange system, each
  MCM 2130

ADMINISTRATIVE, MISCELLANEOUS AND INVESTIGATIONAL (A9000-A9999)

NOTE: The following codes do not imply that codes in other sections are necessarily covered.

- ⊙ A9150 Non-prescription drugs
  MCM 2050.5
- A9160 Deleted 01/01/02
- A9170 Deleted 12/31/01
- A9190 Deleted 12/31/01
- ◆ A9270 Non-covered item or service
  MCM 2303
- ◆ A9300 Exercise equipment
  MCM 2100.1, CIM 60-9

Supplies for Radiology Procedures

- ⊙ A9500 Supply of radiopharmaceutical diagnostic imaging agent, technetium Tc99m sestamibi, per dose
  MCM 15022
- ⊙ A9502 Supply of radiopharmaceutical diagnostic imaging agent, technetium Tc99m tetrofosmin, per unit dose
  MCM 15022
- ⊙ A9503 Supply of radiopharmaceutical diagnostic imaging agent, technetium Tc99m, medronate, up to 30 mCi
  MCM 15022
- ✻ A9504 Supply of radiopharmaceutical diagnostic imaging agent, technetium Tc99m apcitide
  MCM 15022
- ⊙ A9505 Supply of radiopharmaceutical diagnostic imaging agent, thallous chloride Tl-201, per mCi
  MCM 15022
- ✻ A9507 Supply of radiopharmaceutical diagnostic imaging agent, indium In 111-capromab pendetide, per dose
  MCM 15022
- ⊙ A9508 Supply of radiopharmaceutical diagnostic imaging agent, iobenguane sulfate I-131, per 0.5 mCi
  MCM 15030
- ⊙ A9510 Supply of radiopharmaceutical diagnostic imaging agent, technetium Tc99m disofenin, per vial
  MCM 15030
- ✻ A9511 Supply of radiopharmaceutical diagnostic imaging agent, technetium Tc99m, depreotide, per mCi
- ▶✻ A9512 Supply of radiopharmaceutical diagnostic imaging agent, technetium Tc-99m pertechnetate, per mCi
- ▶✻ A9513 Supply of radiopharmaceutical diagnostic imaging agent, technetium Tc-99m mebrofenin, per mCi
- ▶✻ A9514 Supply of radiopharmaceutical diagnostic imaging agent, technetium Tc-99m pyrophosphate, per mCi
- ▶✻ A9515 Supply of radiopharmaceutical diagnostic imaging agent, technetium Tc-99m pentetate, per mCi
- ▶✻ A9516 Supply of radiopharmaceutical diagnostic imaging agent, i-123 sodium iodide capsule, per 100 uCi
- ▶✻ A9517 Supply of radiopharmaceutical therapeutic imaging agent, I-131 sodium iodide capsule, per mCi
- ▶✻ A9518 Supply of radiopharmaceutical therapeutic imaging agent, I-131 sodium iodide solution, per uCi
- ▶✻ A9519 Supply of radiopharmaceutical diagnostic imaging agent, technetium Tc-99m macroaggregated albumin, per mCi
- ▶✻ A9520 Supply of radiopharmaceutical diagnostic imaging agent, technetium Tc-99m sulfur colloid, per mCi
- ▶✻ A9521 Supply of radiopharmaceutical diagnostic imaging agent, technetium Tc-99m exametazime, per dose
- ▶⊙ A9522 Supply of radiopharmaceutical diagnostic imaging agent, indium-111 ibritumomab tiuxetan, per mCi
  MCM 15022
- ▶⊙ A9523 Supply of radiopharmaceutical therapeutic imaging agent, yttrium 90 ibritumomab tiuxetan, per mCi
  MCM 15022
- ▶⊙ A9524 Supply of radiopharmaceutical diagnostic imaging agent, iodinated I-131 serum albumin, 5 uCi
  MCM 15022
- ✻ A9600 Supply of therapeutic radiopharmaceutical, strontium-89 chloride, per mCi
- ✻ A9605 Supply of therapeutic radiopharmaceutical, samarium Sm-153 lexidronamm, 50 mCi
- ▶✻ A9699 Supply of radiopharmaceutical therapeutic imaging agent, not otherwise classified
- ⊙ A9700 Supply of injectable contrast material for use in echocardiography, per study
  MCM 15360

Miscellaneous Service Component

✻ A9900 Miscellaneous DME supply, accessory, and/or service component of another HCPCS code

✻ A9901 DME delivery, set up, and/or dispensing service component of another HCPCS code

ENTERAL AND PARENTERAL THERAPY (B4000-B9999)

Enteral Formulae and Enteral Medical Supplies

✪ B4034 Enteral feeding supply kit; syringe, per day
MCM 2130, MCM 4450, CIM 65-10

✪ B4035 Enteral feeding supply kit; pump fed, per day
MCM 2130, MCM 4450, CIM 65-10

✪ B4036 Enteral feeding supply kit; gravity fed, per day
MCM 2130, MCM 4450, CIM 65-10

✪ B4081 Nasogastric tubing with stylet
MCM 2130, MCM 4450, CIM 65-10

✪ B4082 Nasogastric tubing without stylet
MCM 2130, MCM 4450, CIM 65-10

✪ B4083 Stomach tube, Levine type
MCM 2130, MCM 4450, CIM

B4084 Deleted 01/01/02

B4085 Deleted 01/01/02

✻ B4086 Gastrostomy/jejunostomy tube, any material, any type, (standard or low profile), each

▶◆ B4100 Food thickener, administered orally, per ounce

✪ B4150 Enteral formulae; category I; semi-synthetic intact protein/protein isolates, administered through an enteral feeding tube at 100 calories = 1 unit
MCM 2130, MCM 4450, CIM 65-10

✪ B4151 Enteral formulae; category I: natural intact protein/protein isolates, administered through an enteral feeding tube at 100 calories = 1 unit
MCM 2130, MCM 4450, CIM 65-10

✪ B4152 Enteral formulae; category II: intact protein/protein isolates (calorically dense), administered through an enteral feeding tube at 100 calories = 1 unit
MCM 2130, MCM 4450, CIM 65-10

✪ B4153 Enteral formulae; category III: hydrolized protein/amino acids, administered through an enteral feeding tube at 100 calories = 1 unit
MCM 2130, MCM 4450, CIM 65-10

✪ B4154 Enteral formulae; category IV: defined formula for special metabolic need, administered through an enteral feeding tube at 100 calories = 1 unit
MCM 2130, MCM 4450, CIM 65-10

✪ B4155 Enteral formulae; category V: modular components, administered through an enteral feeding tube at 100 calories = 1 unit
MCM 2130, MCM 4450, CIM 65-10

✪ B4156 Enteral formulae; category VI: standardized nutrients, administered through an enteral feeding tube at 100 calories = 1 unit
MCM 2130, MCM 4450, CIM 65-10

Parenteral Nutritional Solutions and Supplies

✪ B4164 Parenteral nutrition solution: carbohydrates (dextrose), 50% or less (500 cc = 1 unit)—home mix
MCM 2130, MCM 4450, CIM 65-10

✪ B4168 Parenteral nutrition solution; amino acid, 3.5% (500 cc = 1 unit)—home mix
MCM 2130, MCM 4450, CIM 65-10

✪ B4172 Parenteral nutrition solution; amino acid, 5.5% through 7% (500 cc = 1 unit)—home mix
MCM 2130, MCM 4450, CIM 65-10

✪ B4176 Parenteral nutrition solution; amino acid, 7% through 8.5% (500 cc = 1 unit)—home mix
MCM 2130, MCM 4450, CIM 65-10

✪ B4178 Parenteral nutrition solution: amino acid, greater than 8.5% (500 cc = 1 unit)—home mix
MCM 2130, MCM 4450, CIM 65-10

✪ B4180 Parenteral nutrition solution; carbohydrates (dextrose), greater than 50% (500 cc = 1 unit)—home mix
MCM 2130, MCM 4450, CIM 65-10

✪ B4184 Parenteral nutrition solution; lipids, 10% with administration set (500 cc = 1 unit)
MCM 2130, MCM 4450, CIM 65-10

✪ B4186 Parenteral nutrition solution, lipids, 20% with administration set (500 cc = 1 unit)
MCM 2130, MCM 4450, CIM 65-10

✪ B4189 Parenteral nutrition solution; compounded amino acid and carbohydrates with electrolytes, trace elements, and vitamins, including preparation, any strength, 10 to 51 gram (gm) of protein—premix
MCM 2130, MCM 4450, CIM 65-10

B4193 Parenteral nutrition solution; compounded amino acid and carbohydrates with electrolytes, trace elements, and vitamins, including preparation, any strength, 52 to 73 gm of protein—premix
MCM 2130, MCM 4450, CIM 65-10

B4197 Parenteral nutrition solution; compounded amino acid and carbohydrates with electrolytes, trace elements and vitamins, including preparation, any strength, 74 to 100 gm of protein—premix
MCM 2130, MCM 4450, CIM 65-10

B4199 Parenteral nutrition solution; compounded amino acid and carbohydrates with electrolytes, trace elements and vitamins, including preparation, any strength, over 100 gm of protein—premix

B4216 Parenteral nutrition additives (vitamins, trace elements, heparin, electrolytes) home mix, per day
MCM 2130, MCM 4450, CIM 65-10

B4220 Parenteral nutrition supply kit; premix, per day
MCM 2130, MCM 4450, CIM 65-10

B4222 Parenteral nutrition supply kit; home mix, per day
MCM 2130, MCM 4450, CIM 65-10

B4224 Parenteral nutrition administration kit, per day
MCM 2130, MCM 4450, CIM 65-10

B5000 Parenteral nutrition solution; compounded amino acid and carbohydrates with electrolytes, trace elements, and vitamins, including preparation, any strength, renal—Amirosyn-RF, NephrAmine, RenAmine—premix
MCM 2130, MCM 4450, CIM 65-10

B5100 Parenteral nutrition solution; compounded amino acid and carbohydrates with electrolytes, trace elements, and vitamins, including preparation, any strength, hepatic—FreAmine HBC, HepatAmine—premix
MCM 2130, MCM 4450, CIM 65-10

B5200 Parenteral nutrition solution; compounded amino acid and carbohydrates with electrolytes, trace elements, and vitamins, including preparation, any strength, stress—branch chain amino acids—premix
MCM 2130, MCM 4450, CIM 65-10

Enteral and Parenteral Pumps

B9000 Enteral nutrition infusion pump, without alarm
MCM 2130, MCM 4450, CIM 65-10

B9002 Enteral nutrition infusion pump, with alarm
MCM 2130, MCM 4450, CIM 65-10

B9004 Parenteral nutrition infusion pump, portable
MCM 2130, MCM 4450, CIM 65-10

B9006 Parenteral nutrition infusion pump, stationary
MCM 2130, MCM 4450, CIM 65-10

B9998 NOC for enteral supplies
MCM 2130, MCM 4450, CIM 65-10

B9999 NOC for parenteral supplies
MCM 2130, MCM 4450, CIM 65-10

C CODES FOR USE ONLY UNDER THE HOSPITAL OUTPATIENT PROSPECTIVE PAYMENT SYSTEM (C1000-C9999)

Note: C-codes are used ONLY as a part of Hospital Outpatient Prospective Payment System (OPPS) and are not to be used to report other services. C-codes are updated quarterly by the Centers for Medicare and Medicaid Services.

C1010 Whole blood or red blood cells, leukoreduced, CMV negative, each unit
Medicare Statute 1833(t)

C1011 Platelet, HLA-matched leukoreduced, apheresis/pheresis, each unit
Medicare Statute 1833(t)

C1012 Deleted 12/31/02, Cross Reference P9003

C1013 Deleted 12/31/02, Cross Reference P9031

C1014 Deleted 12/31/02, Cross Reference P9035

C1015 Platelets, pheresis, leukocyte-reduced, CMV negative, irradiated, each unit
Medicare Statute 1833(t)

C1016 Whole blood or red blood cells, leukoreduced, frozen/deglycerol/washed, each unit
Medicare Statute 1833(t)

C1017 Platelet, leukoreduced, CMV-negative, apheresis/pheresis, each unit
Medicare Statute 1833(t)

C1018 Whole blood, leukoreduced, irradiated, each unit
Medicare Statute 1833(t)

C1019 Deleted 01/01/02

▶ ✪ C1020 Red blood cells, frozen/deglycerolized/washed, leukocyte-reduced, irradiated, each unit
Medicare Statute 1833(t)

▶ ✪ C1021 Red blood cells, leukocyte-reduced, CMV negative, irradiated, each unit
Medicare Statute 1833(t)

▶ ✪ C1022 Plasma, frozen within 24 hours of collection, each unit
Medicare Statute 1833(t)

C1058 Deleted 12/31/02, Cross Reference Q3009

C1064 Deleted 12/31/02

C1065 Deleted 12/31/02

C1066 Deleted 12/31/02, Cross Reference A4642

✪ C1079 Supply of radiopharmaceutical diagnostic imaging agent, cyanocobalamin Co-58/57, per 0.5 mCi
Medicare Statute 1833(t)

C1087 Deleted 12/31/02

✪ C1088 Laser optic treatment system, Indigo LaserOptic Treatment System
Medicare Statute 1833(t)

C1090 Deleted 01/01/02

✪ C1091 Supply of radiopharmaceutical diagnostic imaging agent, indium-111 oxyquinoline, per 0.5 mCi
Medicare Statute 1833(t)

✪ C1092 Supply of radiopharmaceutical diagnostic imaging agent, indium-111 pentetate, per 0.5 mCi
Medicare Statute 1833(t)

C1094 Deleted 12/31/02

C1095 Deleted 01/01/02

C1096 Deleted 12/31/02

C1097 Deleted 12/31/02

C1098 Deleted 12/31/02

C1099 Deleted 12/31/02

✪ C1122 Supply of radiopharmaceutical diagnostic imaging agent, technetium Tc99m arcitumomab, per vial
Medicare Statute 1833(t)

➡ ✪ C1166 Injection, cytarabine liposome, per 10 mg
Medicare Statute 1833(t)

✪ C1167 Injection, epirubicin hydrochloride (HCl), 2 mg
Medicare Statute 1833(t)

➡ ✪ C1178 Injection, bisulfan, per 6 mg
Medicare Statute 1833(t)

C1188 Deleted 12/31/02

✪ C1200 Supply of radiopharmaceutical diagnostic imaging agent, technetium Tc99m sodium glucoheptonate, per vial
Medicare Statute 1833(t)

✪ C1201 Supply of radiopharmaceutical diagnostic imaging agent, technetium Tc99m succimer, per vial
Medicare Statute 1833(t)

C1202 Deleted 12/31/02

C1207 Deleted 12/31/02, Cross Reference J2352

✪ C1300 Hyperbaric oxygen under pressure, full body chamber, per 30-minute interval lead defibrillator, TVL SQ01
Medicare Statute 1833(t)

✪ C1305 Apligraf, per 44 sqare centimeter (cm^2)
Medicare Statute 1833(t)

C1348 Deleted 12/31/02

C1713-C1715 Deleted 12/31/02

✪ C1716 Brachytherapy seed, gold-198
Medicare Statute 1833 (t)

C1717 Deleted 12/31/02

✪ C1718 Brachytherapy seed, Iodine 125
Medicare Statute 1833 (t)

✪ C1719 Brachytherapy seed, non-high dose rate iridium-192
Medicare Statute 1833 (t)

C1720 Brachytherapy seed, Palladium 103
Medicare Statute 1833 (t)

C1721-C1764 Deleted 12/31/02

✪ C1765 Adhesion barrier
Medicare Statute 1833 (t)

C1766-C1773 Deleted 12/31/02

➡ ✪ C1774 Injection, darbepoetin alfa (for non ESRD use), per 1 mcg
Medicare Status 1833(t)

▶ ✪ C1775 Supply of radiopharmaceutical diagnostic imaging agent, fluorodeoxyglucose f18 (2-deoxy-2-[18f] fluoro-d-glucose), per dose (4-40 mCi/ml)
Medicare Statute 1833(t)

C1776-C1782 Deleted 12/31/02

▶ C1783 Ocular implant, aqueous drainage assist device
Medicare Statute 1833(t)

C1784-C1789 Deleted 12/31/02

C1813-C1817 Deleted 12/31/02

C1874-C1887 Deleted 12/31/02

▶ ✪ C1888 Catheter, ablation, non-cardiac, endovascular (implantable)
Medicare Statute 1833(t)

C1891-C1899 Deleted 12/31/02

▶ ✪ C1900 Lead, left ventricular coronary venous system
Medicare Statute 1833(t)

▶ ✪ C2614 Probe, percutaneous lumbar disectomy
Medicare Statute 1833(t)

✪ C2615 Deleted 12/31/02

✪ C2616 Brachytherapy seed, yttrium-90
Medicare Statute 1833(T)

C2617-C2631 Deleted 12/31/02

▶ ✪ C2632 Brachytherapy solution, iodine-125, per mCi
Medicare Statute 1833(t)

✪ C8900 Magnetic resonance angiography (MRA) with contrast, abdomen
Medicare Statute 1833(t)(2)

✪ C8901 MRA without contrast, abdomen
Medicare Statute 1833(t)(2)

- ⚙ C8902 MRA without contrast followed by with contrast, abdomen Medicare Statute 1833(t)(2)
- ⚙ C8903 Magnetic resonance imaging (MRI) with contrast, breast; unilateral Medicare Statute 1833(t)(2)
- ⚙ C8904 MRI without contrast, breast; unilateral Medicare Statute 1833(t)(2)
- ⚙ C8905 MRI without contrast followed by with contrast, breast; unilateral Medicare Statute 1833(t)(2)
- ⚙ C8906 MRI with contrast, breast; bilateral Medicare Statute 1833(t)(2)
- ⚙ C8907 MRI without contrast, breast; bilateral Medicare Statute 1833(t)(2)
- ⚙ C8908 MRI without contrast followed by with contrast, breast; bilateral Medicare Statute 1833(t)(2)
- ⚙ C8909 MRA with contrast, chest (excluding myocardium) Medicare Statute 1833(t)(2)
- ⚙ C8910 MRA without contrast, chest (excluding myocardium) Medicare Statute 1833(t)(2)
- ⚙ C8911 MRA without contrast followed by with contrast, chest (excluding myocardium) Medicare Statute 1833(t)(2)
- ⚙ C8912 MRA with contrast, lower extremity Medicare Statute 1833(t)(2)
- ⚙ C8913 MRA without contrast, lower extremity Medicare Statute 1833(t)(2)
- ⚙ C8914 MRA without contrast followed by with contrast, lower extremity Medicare Statute 1833(t)(2)
- ⚙ C9000 Injection, sodium chromate Cr51, per 0.25 mCi Medicare Statute 1833(t)
- ⚙ C9003 Palivizumab-RSV-IGM, per 50 mg Medicare Statute 1833(t)
- ⚙ C9007 Baclofen intrathecal screening kit (1 amp) Medicare Statute 1833(t)
- ⚙ C9008 Baclofen intrathecal refill kit, per 500 micrograms (mcg) Medicare Statute 1833(t)
- ⚙ C9009 Baclofen intrathecal refill kit, per 2000 mcg Medicare Statute 1833(t)
- ⚙ C9010 Baclofen intrathecal refill kit, per 4000 mcg Medicare Statute 1833(t)
- ⚙ C9013 Supply of cobaltous chloride CO-57, radiopharmaceutical diagnostic imaging agent Medicare Statute 1833(t)(2)
- C9018 Deleted 01/01/02
- C9019 Deleted 12/31/02, Cross Reference J0637
- C9020 Deleted 01/01/02, Cross Reference J7520
- C9100 Deleted 12/31/02
- ⚙ C9102 Supply of radiopharmaceutical diagnostic imaging agent, 51-sodium chromate, per 50 mCi Medicare Statute 1833(t)
- ⚙ C9103 Supply of radiopharmaceutical diagnostic imaging agent, sodium iothalamate I-125 injection, per 10 mCi Medicare Statute 1833(t)
- C9104 Deleted 01/01/02
- ⚙ C9105 Injection, hepatitis B immune globulin, per 1 cc Medicare Statute 1833(t)
- C9108 Deleted 12/31/02, Cross Reference J3240
- ⚙ C9109 Injection, tirofiban HCl, 6.25 mg Medicare Statute 1833(t)
- C9110 Deleted 12/31/02, Cross Reference J9010
- ⚙ C9111 Injection, bivalirudin, 250 mg per vial Medicare Statute 1833(t)
- ⚙ C9112 Injection, perflutren lipid microsphere, per 2 cc vial Medicare Statute 1833(t)
- ⚙ C9113 Injection, pantoprazole sodium, per vial Medicare Statute 1833(t)
- C9114 Deleted 12/31/02, Cross Reference J2324
- C9115 Deleted 12/31/02 Cross Reference J3487
- ▶⚙ C9116 Injection, ertapenem sodium, per 1 gram vial Medicare Statute 1833(t)
- C9117 Deleted 12/31/02, Cross Reference A9523
- C9118 Deleted 12/31/02, Cross Reference A9522
- ▶⚙ C9119 Injection, pegfilgrastim, per 6 mg single dose vial Medicare Statute 1833(t)
- ▶⚙ C9120 Injection, fulvestrant, per 50 mg Medicare Statute 1833(t)
- ▶⚙ C9121 Injection, argatroban, per 5 mg Medicare Statute 1833(t)
- ⚙ C9200 Orcel, per 36 cm^2 Medicare Statute 1833(t)
- ⚙ C9201 Dermagraft, per 37.5 cm^2 Medicare Statute 1833(t)
- ⚙ C9503 Fresh frozen plasma, donor retested, each unit Medicare Statute 1833(t)
- ⚙ C9701 STRETTA system Medicare Statute 1833(t)
- ⚙ C9703 Bard endoscopic suturing system Medicare Statute 1833(t)
- C9708 Deleted 12/31/02
- ⚙ C9711 H.E.L.P. apheresis system Medicare Statute 1833(t)

DENTAL PROCEDURES (D0000-D9999)

Codes D0100-D9999 are dental codes copyrighted to the ADA. A copy of the Current Dental Terminology (CDT), which contains all of the dental codes, can be purchased from the ADA.

DURABLE MEDICAL EQUIPMENT (E0100-E9999)

Canes

- ✪ E0100 Cane, includes canes of all materials, adjustable or fixed, with tip
  MCM 2100.1, CIM 60-3, CIM 60-9
- ✪ E0105 Cane, quad or three prong, includes canes of all materials, adjustable or fixed, with tips
  MCM 2100.1, CIM 60-9, CIM 60-15

Crutches

- ✪ E0110 Crutches, forearm, includes crutches of various materials, adjustable or fixed, pair, complete with tips and handgrips
  MCM 2100.1, CIM 60-9
- ✪ E0111 Crutches, forearm, includes crutches of various materials, adjustable or fixed, each, with tips and handgrips
  MCM 2100.1, CIM 60-9
- ✪ E0112 Crutches, underarm, wood, adjustable or fixed, pair, with pads, tips and handgrips
  MCM 2100.1, CIM 60-9
- ✪ E0113 Crutches, underarm, wood, adjustable or fixed, each, with pads, tips and handgrip
  MCM 2100.1, CIM 60-9
- ✪ E0114 Crutches, underarm, other than wood, adjustable or fixed, pair, with pads, tips and handgrips
  MCM 2100.1, CIM 60-9
- ✪ E0116 Crutches, underarm, other than wood, adjustable or fixed, each, with pads, tips and handgrips
  MCM 2100.1, CIM 60-9
- ▶✪ E0117 Crutch, underarm, articulating, spring assisted, each
  MCM 2100.1

Walkers

- ✪ E0130 Walker, rigid (pickup), adjustable or fixed height
  MCM 2100.1, CIM 60-9
- ✪ E0135 Walker, folding (pickup), adjustable or fixed height
  MCM 2100.1, CIM 60-9
- ✪ E0141 Rigid walker, wheeled, without seat
  MCM 2100.1, CIM 60-9
- ✪ E0142 Rigid walker, wheeled, with seat
  MCM 2100.1, CIM 60-9
- ✪ E0143 Folding walker, wheeled, without seat
  MCM 2100.1, CIM 60-9
- ✪ E0144 Enclosed, framed folding walker, wheeled, with posterior seat
  MCM 2100.1, CIM 60-9
- ✪ E0145 Walker, wheeled, with seat and crutch attachments
  MCM 2100.1, CIM 60-9
- ✪ E0146 Folding walker, wheeled, with seat
  MCM 2100.1, CIM 60-9
- ✪ E0147 Heavy-duty, multiple breaking system, variable wheel resistance walker
  MCM 2100.1, CIM 60-15
- ✻ E0148 Walker, heavy-duty, without wheels, rigid or folding, any type, each
- ✻ E0149 Walker, heavy-duty, wheeled, rigid or folding, any type, each
- ✻ E0153 Platform attachment, forearm crutch, each
- ✻ E0154 Platform attachment, walker, each
- ✻ E0155 Wheel attachment, rigid pick-up walker, per pair

Attachments

- ✻ E0156 Seat attachment, walker
- ✻ E0157 Crutch attachment, walker, each
- ✻ E0158 Leg extensions for a walker, per set of four (4)
- ✻ E0159 Brake attachment for wheeled walker, replacement, each

Commodes

- ✪ E0160 Sitz type bath or equipment, portable, used with or without commode
  CIM 60-9
- ✪ E0161 Sitz type bath or equipment, portable, used with or without commode, with faucet attachment/s
  CIM 60-9
- ✪ E0162 Sitz bath chair
  CIM 60-9
- ✪ E0163 Commode chair, stationary, with fixed arms
  MCM 2100.1, CIM 60-9
- ✪ E0164 Commode chair, mobile, with fixed arms
  MCM 2100.1, CIM 60-9

- ❂ E0165 Commode chair, stationary, with detachable arms
  MCM 2100.1, CIM 60-9
- ❂ E0166 Commode chair, mobile, with detachable arms
  MCM 2100.1, CIM 60-9
- ❂ E0167 Pail or pan for use with commode chair
  CIM 60-9
- ✻ E0168 Commode chair, extra wide and/or heavy duty, stationary or mobile, with or without arms, any type, each
- ✻ E0169 Commode chair with seat lift mechanism
- ✻ E0175 Foot rest, for use with commode chair, each

Decubitus Care Equipment

- ❂ E0176 Air pressure pad or cushion, nonpositioning
  CIM 60-9
- ❂ E0177 Water pressure pad or cushion, nonpositioning
  CIM 60-9
- ❂ E0178 Gel or gel-like pressure pad or cushion, nonpositioning
  CIM 60-9
- ❂ E0179 Dry pressure pad or cushion, nonpositioning
  CIM 60-9
- ❂ E0180 Pressure pad, alternating with pump
  MCM 4107.6, CIM 60-9
- ❂ E0181 Pressure pad, alternating with pump, heavy duty
  MCM 4107.6, CIM 60-9
- ❂ E0182 Pump for alternating pressure pad
  MCM 4107.6, CIM 60-9
- ❂ E0184 Dry pressure mattress
  MCM 4107.6, CIM 60-9
- ❂ E0185 Gel or gel-like pressure pad for mattress, standard mattress length and width
  MCM 4107.6, CIM 60-9
- ❂ E0186 Air pressure mattress
  CIM 60-9
- ❂ E0187 Water pressure mattress
  CIM 60-9
- ❂ E0188 Synthetic sheepskin pad
  MCM 4107.6, CIM 60-9
- ❂ E0189 Lambswool sheepskin pad, any size
  MCM 4107.6, CIM 60-9
- ✻ E0191 Heel or elbow protector, each
- ❂ E0192 Low pressure and positioning equalization pad, for wheelchair
  MCM 4107.6, CIM 60-9
- ✻ E0193 Powered air flotation bed (low air loss therapy)
- ❂ E0194 Air fluidized bed
  CIM 60-19, Cross Reference Q0049
- ❂ E0196 Gel pressure mattress
  CIM 60-9
- ❂ E0197 Air pressure pad for mattress, standard mattress length and width
  CIM 60-9
- ❂ E0198 Water pressure pad for mattress, standard mattress length and width
  CIM 60-9
- ❂ E0199 Dry pressure pad for mattress, standard mattress length and width
  CIM 60-9

Heat/Cold Application

- ❂ E0200 Heat lamp, without stand (table model), includes bulb, or infrared element
  MCM 2100.1, CIM 60-9
- ✻ E0202 Phototherapy (bilirubin) light with photometer
- ▶ ◆ E0203 Therapeutic lightbox, minimum 10,000 lux, table top model
- ❂ E0205 Heat lamp, with stand, includes bulb, or infrared element
  MCM 2100.1, CIM 60-9
- ❂ E0210 Electric heat pad, standard
  CIM 60-9
- ❂ E0215 Electric heat pad, moist
  CIM 60-9
- ❂ E0217 Water circulating heat pad with pump
  CIM 60-9
- ❂ E0218 Water circulating cold pad with pump
  CIM 60-9
- ✻ E0220 Hot water bottle
- ✻ E0221 Infrared heating pad system
- ❂ E0225 Hydrocollator unit, includes pads
  MCM 2210.3, CIM 60-9
- ✻ E0230 Ice cap or collar
- ✻ E0231 Non-contact wound warming device (temperature control unit, AC adapter and power cord) for use with warming card and wound cover
- ✻ E0232 Warming card for use with the non-contact wound warming device and non-contact wound warming wound cover
- ❂ E0235 Paraffin bath unit, portable (see medical supply code A4265 for paraffin)
  MCM 2210.3, CIM 60-9
- ❂ E0236 Pump for water circulating pad
  CIM 60-9
- ❂ E0238 Non-electric heat pad, moist
  CIM 60-9
- ❂ E0239 Hydrocollator unit, portable
  MCM 2210.3, CIM 60-9

Bath and Toilet Aids

◆ E0241 Bath tub wall rail, each
MCM 2100.1, CIM 60-9

◆ E0242 Bath tub rail, floor base
MCM 2100.1, CIM 60-9

◆ E0243 Toilet rail, each
MCM 2100.1, CIM 60-9

◆ E0244 Raised toilet seat
CIM 60-9

◆ E0245 Tub stool or bench
CIM 60-9

✻ E0246 Transfer tub rail attachment

✪ E0249 Pad for water circulating heat unit
CIM 60-9

Hospital Beds and Accessories

✪ E0250 Hospital bed, fixed height, with any type side rails, with mattress
MCM 2100.1, CIM 60-18

✪ E0251 Hospital bed, fixed height, with any type side rails, without mattress
MCM 2100.1, CIM 60-18

✪ E0255 Hospital bed, variable height, high-low (hi-lo), with any type side rails, with mattress
MCM 2100.1, CIM 60-18

✪ E0256 Hospital bed, variable height, hi-lo, with any type side rails, without mattress
MCM 2100.1, CIM 60-18

✪ E0260 Hospital bed, semi-electric (head and foot adjustment), with any type side rails, with mattress
MCM 2100.1, CIM 60-18

✪ E0261 Hospital bed, semi-electric (head and foot adjustment), with any type side rails, without mattress
MCM 2100.1, CIM 60-18

✪ E0265 Hospital bed, total electric (head, foot and height adjustments), with any type side rails, with mattress
MCM 2100.1, CIM 60-18

✪ E0266 Hospital bed, total electric (head, foot and height adjustments), with any type side rails, without mattress
MCM 2100.1, CIM 60-18

◆ E0270 Hospital bed, institutional type includes: oscillating, circulating and Stryker frame, with mattress
CIM 60-9

✪ E0271 Mattress, innerspring
CIM 60-9, CIM 60-18

✪ E0272 Mattress, foam rubber
CIM 60-9, CIM 60-18

◆ E0273 Bed board
CIM 60-9

◆ E0274 Over-bed table
CIM 60-9

✪ E0275 Bed pan, standard, metal or plastic
CIM 60-9

✪ E0276 Bed pan, fracture, metal or plastic
CIM 60-9

✪ E0277 Powered pressure-reducing air mattress
CIM 60-9

✻ E0280 Bed cradle, any type

✪ E0290 Hospital bed, fixed height, without side rails, with mattress
MCM 2100.1, CIM 60-18

✪ E0291 Hospital bed, fixed height, without side rails, without mattress
MCM 2100.1, CIM 60-18

✪ E0292 Hospital bed, variable height, hi-lo, without side rails, with mattress
MCM 2100.1, CIM 60-18

✪ E0293 Hospital bed, variable height, hi-lo, without side rails, without mattress
MCM 2100.1, CIM 60-18

✪ E0294 Hospital bed, semi-electric (head and foot adjustment), without side rails, with mattress
MCM 2100.1, CIM 60-18

✪ E0295 Hospital bed, semi-electric (head and foot adjustment), without side rails, without mattress
MCM 2100.1, CIM 60-18

✪ E0296 Hospital bed, total electric (head, foot and height adjustments), without side rails, with mattress
MCM 2100.1, CIM 60-18

✪ E0297 Hospital bed, total electric (head, foot and height adjustments), without side rails, without mattress
MCM 2100.1, CIM 60-18

E0298 Deleted 01/01/02, Cross Reference K0549

Bed Accessories

✪ E0305 Bed side rails, half length
CIM 60-18

✪ E0310 Bed side rails, full length
CIM 60-18

◆ E0315 Bed accessory: board, table, or support device, any type
CIM 60-9

✻ E0316 Safety enclosure frame/canopy for use with hospital bed, any type

✪ E0325 Urinal; male, jug-type, any material
CIM 60-9

✪ E0326 Urinal; female, jug-type, any material
CIM 60-9

✻ E0350 Control unit for electronic bowel irrigation/evacuation system

∗ E0352 Disposable pack (water reservoir bag, speculum, valving mechanism and collection bag/box) for use with the electronic bowel irrigation/evacuation system
∗ E0370 Air pressure elevator for heel
∗ E0371 Non-powered advanced pressure-reducing overlay for mattress, standard mattress length and width
∗ E0372 Powered air overlay for mattress, standard mattress length and width
∗ E0373 Non-powered advanced pressure-reducing mattress

Oxygen and Related Respiratory Equipment

✪ E0424 Stationary compressed gaseous oxygen system, rental; includes container, contents, regulator, flowmeter, humidifier, nebulizer, cannula or mask, and tubing
MCM 4107.9, CIM 60-4
✪ E0425 Stationary compressed gas system, purchase; includes regulator, flowmeter, humidifier, nebulizer, cannula or mask, and tubing
MCM 4107.9, CIM 60-4
✪ E0430 Portable gaseous oxygen system, purchase; includes regulator, flowmeter, humidifier, cannula or mask, and tubing
MCM 4107.9, CIM 60-4
✪ E0431 Portable gaseous oxygen system, rental; includes portable container, regulator, flowmeter, humidifier, cannula or mask, and tubing
MCM 4107.9, CIM 60-4
✪ E0434 Portable liquid oxygen system, rental; includes portable container, supply reservoir, humidifier, flowmeter, refill adaptor, contents gauge, cannula or mask, and tubing
MCM 4107.9, CIM 60-4
✪ E0435 Portable liquid oxygen system, purchase; includes portable container, supply reservoir, flowmeter, humidifier, contents gauge, cannula or mask, tubing and refill adaptor
MCM 4107.9, CIM 60-4
✪ E0439 Stationary liquid oxygen system, rental; includes container, contents, regulator, flowmeter, humidifier, nebulizer, cannula or mask, and tubing
MCM 4107.9, CIM 60-4
✪ E0440 Stationary liquid oxygen system, purchase; includes use of reservoir, contents indicator, regulator, flowmeter, humidifier, nebulizer, cannula or mask, and tubing
MCM 4107.9, CIM 60-4
➠ ✪ E0441 Oxygen contents, gaseous (for use with owned gaseous stationary systems or when both a stationary and portable gaseous system are owned), 1 month's supply = 1 unit
MCM 4107.9, CIM 60-4
➠ ✪ E0442 Oxygen contents, liquid, (for use with owned liquid stationary systems or when both a stationary and portable liquid system are owned), 1 month's supply = 1 unit
MCM 4107.9, CIM 60-4
➠ ✪ E0443 Portable oxygen contents, gaseous, (for use only with portable gaseous systems when no stationary gas or liquid system is used), 1 month's supply = 1 unit
MCM 4107.9, CIM 60-4
➠ ✪ E0444 Portable oxygen contents, liquid (for use only with portable liquid systems when no stationary gas or liquid system is used), 1 month's supply = 1 unit
MCM 4107.9, CIM 60-4
▶ ∗ E0445 Oximeter device for measuring blood oxygen levels non-invasively
✪ E0450 Volume ventilator, stationary or portable, with backup rate feature, used with invasive interface (e.g., tracheostomy tube)
CIM 60-9
▶ ✪ E0454 Pressure ventilator with pressure control, pressure support and flow triggering features
CIM 60-9
✪ E0455 Oxygen tent, excluding croup or pediatric tents
MCM 4107.9, CIM 60-4
∗ E0457 Chest shell (cuirass)
∗ E0459 Chest wrap
✪ E0460 Negative pressure ventilator, portable or stationary
CIM 60-9
▶ ✪ E0461 Volume ventilator, stationary or portable, with backup rate feature, used with non-invasive interface
CIM 60-9
∗ E0462 Rocking bed, with or without side rails
CIM 60-9
✪ E0480 Percussor, electric or pneumatic, home model
CIM 60-9
◆ E0481 Intrapulmonary percussive ventilation system and related accessories
CIM 60-21
∗ E0482 Cough stimulating device, alternating positive and negative airway pressure
▶ ∗ E0483 High frequency chest wall oscillation air-pulse generator system, (includes hoses and vest), each

▶✻ E0484 Oscillatory positive expiratory pressure device, non-electric, any type, each

IPPB Machines

✪ E0500 IPPB machine, all types, with built-in nebulization; manual or automatic valves; internal or external power source
CIM 60-9

Humidifiers/Nebulizers/Compressors for Use with Oxygen IPPB Equipment

✪ E0550 Humidifier, durable for extensive supplemental humidification during IPPB treatments or oxygen delivery
CIM 60-9

✪ E0555 Humidifier, durable, glass or autoclavable plastic bottle type, for use with regulator or flowmeter
MCM 4107.9, CIM 60-9

✪ E0560 Humidifier, durable for supplemental humidification during IPPB treatment or oxygen delivery
CIM 60-9

✻ E0565 Compressor, air power source for equipment which is not self-contained or cylinder driven

✪ E0570 Nebulizer, with compressor
MCM 4107.9, CIM 60-9

✪ E0571 Aerosol compressor, battery powered, for use with small volume nebulizer
CIM 60-9

✻ E0572 Aerosol compressor, adjustable pressure, light duty for intermittent use

➠✻ E0574 Ultrasonic electronic aerosol generator with small volume nebulizer

✪ E0575 Nebulizer, ultrasonic, large volume
CIM 60-9

✪ E0580 Nebulizer, durable, glass or autoclavable plastic, bottle type, for use with regulator or flowmeter
MCM 4107.9, CIM 60-9

✪ E0585 Nebulizer, with compressor and heater
MCM 4107.9, CIM 60-9

✻ E0590 Dispensing fee for covered drug administered through DME nebulizer

Suction Pump/Room Vaporizers

✪ E0600 Respiratory such pump, home model, portable or stationary, electric
CIM 60-9

✪ E0601 Continuous airway pressure (CPAP) device
CIM 60-17

✻ E0602 Breast pump, manual, any type

✻ E0603 Breast pump, electric (AC and/or DC), any type

✻ E0604 Breast pump, heavy duty, hospital grade, piston operated, pulsatile, vacuum suction/release cycles, vacuum regulator, supplies, transformer, electric (AC and/or DC)

✪ E0605 Vaporizer, room type
CIM 60-9

✪ E0606 Postural drainage board
CIM 60-9

Monitoring Equipment

✪ E0607 Home blood glucose monitor
CIM 60-11

E0608 Deleted 12/31/02, Cross Reference E0618

E0609 Deleted 01/01/02

Pacemaker Monitor

✪ E0610 Pacemaker monitor, self-contained (checks battery depletion, includes audible and visible check systems)
CIM 50-1, CIM 60-7

✪ E0615 Pacemaker monitor, self-contained (checks battery depletion and other pacemaker components, includes digital/visible check systems)
CIM 50-1, CIM 60-7

✻ E0616 Implantable cardiac event recorder with memory, activator, and programmer

✻ E0617 External defibrillator with integrated electrocardiogram analysis

▶✻ E0618 Apnea monitor, without recording feature

▶✻ E0619 Apnea monitor, with recording feature

✻ E0620 Skin piercing device for collection of capillary blood, laser, each

Patient Lifts

✪ E0621 Sling or seat, patient lift, canvas or nylon
CIM 60-9

◆ E0625 Patient lift, Kartop, bathroom or toilet
CIM 60-9

✪ E0627 Seat lift mechanism incorporated into a combination lift-chair mechanism
MCM 4107.8, CIM 60-8, Cross Reference Q0080

- E0628 Separate seat lift mechanism for use with patient owned furniture—electric MCM 4107.8, CIM 60-8, Cross Reference Q0078
- E0629 Separate seat lift mechanism for use with patient owned furniture—non-electric MCM 4107.8, Cross Reference Q0079
- E0630 Patient lift, hydraulic, with seat or sling CIM 60-9
- E0635 Patient lift, electric, with seat or sling CIM 60-9
- ▶* E0636 Multipositional patient support system, with integrated lift, patient accessible controls

Pneumatic Compressor and Appliances

- E0650 Pneumatic compressor, non-segmental home model CIM 60-16
- E0651 Pneumatic compressor, segmental home model without calibrated gradient pressure CIM 60-16
- E0652 Pneumatic compressor, segmental home model with calibrated gradient pressure CIM 60-16
- E0655 Non-segmental pneumatic appliance for use with pneumatic compressor, half arm CIM 60-16
- E0660 Non-segmental pneumatic appliance for use with pneumatic compressor, full leg CIM 60-16
- E0665 Non-segmental pneumatic appliance for use with pneumatic compressor, full arm CIM 60-16
- E0666 Non-segmental pneumatic appliance for use with pneumatic compressor, half leg CIM 60-16
- E0667 Segmental pneumatic appliance for use with pneumatic compressor, full leg CIM 60-16
- E0668 Segmental pneumatic appliance for use with pneumatic compressor, full arm CIM 60-16
- E0669 Segmental pneumatic appliance for use with pneumatic compressor, half leg CIM 60-16
- E0671 Segmental gradient pressure pneumatic appliance, full leg CIM 60-16
- E0672 Segmental gradient pressure pneumatic appliance, full arm CIM 60-16
- E0673 Segmental gradient pressure pneumatic appliance, half leg CIM 60-16

Ultraviolet Cabinet

- E0690 Deleted 12/31/02
- ▶* E0691 Ultraviolet light therapy system panel, includes bulbs/lamps, timer and eye protection; treatment area 2 square feet or less
- ▶* E0692 Ultraviolet light therapy system panel, includes bulbs/lamps, timer and eye protection, 4 foot panel
- ▶* E0693 Ultraviolet light therapy system panel, includes bulbs/lamps, timer and eye protection, 6 foot panel
- ▶* E0694 Ultraviolet multidirectional light therapy system in 6 foot cabinet, includes bulbs/lamps, timer and eye protection

Safety Equipment

- * E0700 Safety equipment (e.g., belt, harness or vest)
- ▶* E0701 Helmet with face guard and soft interface material, prefabricated

Restraints

- * E0710 Restraints, any type (body, chest, wrist or ankle)

Transcutaneous and/or Neuromuscular Electrical Nerve Stimulators

- E0720 TENS, two lead, localized stimulation MCM 4107.6, CIM 35-20, CIM 35-46
- E0730 Transcutaneous electrical nerve stimulation device, four or more leads, for multiple nerve stimulation MCM 4107.6, CIM 35-20, CIM 35-46
- E0731 Form fitting conductive garment for delivery of TENS or NMES (with conductive fibers separated from the patient's skin by layers of fabric) CIM 45-25
- E0740 Incontinence treatment system, pelvic floor stimulator, monitor, sensor and/or trainer CIM 65-24
- * E0744 Neuromuscular stimulator for scoliosis

✪ E0745 Neuromuscular stimulator, electronic shock unit
CIM 35-77

✪ E0746 Electromyography (EMG), biofeedback device
CIM 35-27

✪ E0747 Osteogenesis stimulator, electrical, non-invasive, other than spinal applications
CIM 35-48

✪ E0748 Osteogensis stimulator, electrical, non-invasive, spinal applications
CIM 35-48

✪ E0749 Osteogenesis stimulator, electrical, surgically implanted
CIM 35-48

✪ E0752 Implantable neurostimulator electrode, each
CIM 65-8

E0753 Deleted 01/01/02

✪ E0754 Patient programmer (external) for use with implantable programmable neurostimulator pulse generator
CIM 65-8

* E0755 Electronic salivary reflex stimulator (intra-oral/non-invasive)

✪ E0756 Implantable neurostimulator pulse generator
CIM 65-8

✪ E0757 Implantable neurostimulator radiofrequency receiver
CIM 65-8

✪ E0758 Radiofrequency transmitter (external) for use with implantable neurostimulator radiofrequency receiver
CIM 65-8

* E0759 Radiofrequency transmitter (external) for use with implantable sacral root neurostimulator receiver for bowel and bladder management, replacement
CIM 65-8

✪ E0760 Osteogenesis stimulator, low intensity ultrasound, non-invasive
CIM 35-48

▶◆ E0761 Non-thermal pulsed high frequency radio waves, high peak power electromagnetic energy treatment device

* E0765 FDA-approved nerve stimulator, with replaceable batteries, for treatment of nausea and vomiting

Infusion Supplies

* E0776 IV pole

* E0779 Ambulatory infusion pump, mechanical, reusable, for infusion 8 hours or greater

* E0780 Ambulatory infusion pump, mechanical, reusable, for infusion less than 8 hours

✪ E0781 Ambulatory infusion pump, single or multiple channels, electric or battery operated with administrative equipment, worn by patient
CIM 60-14

➠✪ E0782 Infusion pump, implantable, non-programmable (includes all components, e.g., pump, cathether, connectors, etc.)
CIM 60-14

✪ E0783 Infusion pump system, implantable, programmable (includes all components, e.g., pump, catheter, connectors, etc.)
CIM 60-14

✪ E0784 External ambulatory infusion pump, insulin
CIM 60-14

✪ E0785 Implantable intraspinal (epidural/intrathecal) catheter used with implantable infusion pump, replacement
CIM 60-14

✪ E0786 Implantable programmable infusion pump, replacement (excludes implantable intraspinal catheter
CIM 60-14

✪ E0791 Parenteral infusion pump, stationary, single or multi-channel
MCM 2130, MCM 4450, CIM 65-10

Traction Equipment: Cervical

✪ E0830 Ambulatory tract device, all types, each
CIM 60-9

✪ E0840 Traction frame, attached to headboard, cervical traction
CIM 60-9

✪ E0850 Traction stand, free-standing, cervical traction
CIM 60-9

* E0855 Cervical traction equipment not requiring additional stand or frame

Traction: Overdoor

✪ E0860 Traction equipment, overdoor, cervical
CIM 60-9

Traction: Extremity

✪ E0870 Traction frame, attached to footboard, extremity traction (e.g., Buck's)
CIM 60-9

✪ E0880 Traction stand, free-standing, extremity traction (e.g., Buck's)
CIM 60-9

Traction: Pelvic

- ✪ E0890 Traction frame, attached to footboard, pelvic traction
  CIM 60-9
- ✪ E0900 Traction stand, free-standing, pelvic traction (e.g., Buck's)
  CIM 60-9

Trapeze Equipment, Fracture Frame and Other Orthopedic Devices

- ✪ E0910 Trapeze bars, also known as patient helper, attached to bed, with grab bar
  CIM 60-9
- ✪ E0920 Fracture frame, attached to bed, includes weights
  CIM 60-9
- ✪ E0930 Fracture frame, free-standing, includes weights
  CIM 60-9
- ✪ E0935 Passive motion exercise device
  CIM 60-9
- ✪ E0940 Trapeze bar, free-standing, complete with grab bar
  CIM 60-9
- ✪ E0941 Gravity assisted traction device, any type
  CIM 60-9
- ✻ E0942 Cervical head harness/halter
- ✻ E0943 Cervical pillow
- ✻ E0944 Pelvic belt/harness/boot
- ✻ E0945 Extremity belt/harness
- ✪ E0946 Fracture, frame, dual with cross bars, attached to bed, (e.g., Balken, Four Poster)
  CIM 60-9
- ✪ E0947 Fracture frame, attachments for complex pelvic traction
  CIM 60-9
- ✪ E0948 Fracture frame, attachments for complex cervical traction
  CIM 60-9

Wheelchairs

- ◆ E0950 Tray, Cross Reference K0107
- ◆ E0951 Loop heel, each; Cross Reference K0034
- ◆ E0952 Loop toe, each; Cross Reference K0036
- ◆ E0953 Pneumatic tire, each
  CIM 60-9, Cross Reference K0067
- ◆ E0954 Semi-pneumatic caster, each
  CIM 60-9, Cross Reference K0075

Wheelchair Accessories

- ◆ E0958 Wheelchair attachment to convert any wheelchair to one arm drive
  CIM 60-9, Cross Reference K0101
- ◆ E0959 Amputee adapter (device used to compensate for transfer of weight due to lost limbs to maintain proper balance)
  CIM 60-9, Cross Reference K0100
- ◆ E0961 Brake extension, for wheelchair
  CIM 60-9, Cross Reference K0079
- ✪ E0962 1" cushion, for wheelchair
  CIM 60-9
- ✪ E0963 2" cushion, for wheelchair
  CIM 60-9
- ✪ E0964 3" cushion, for wheelchair
  CIM 60-9
- ✪ E0965 4" cushion, for wheelchair
  CIM 60-9
- ◆ E0966 Hook-on head rest extension
  CIM 60-9, Cross Reference K0025
- ✪ E0967 Wheelchair hand rims with eight vertical rubber-tipped projections, pair
  CIM 60-9
- ✪ E0968 Commode seat, wheelchair
  CIM 60-9
- ✪ E0969 Narrowing device, wheelchair
  CIM 60-9
- ◆ E0970 No. 2 footplates, except for elevating leg rest
  CIM 60-9; Cross Reference K0037, K0042
- ◆ E0971 Anti-tipping device wheelchair
  CIM 60-9, Cross Reference K0021
- ◆ E0972 Transfer board or device, Cross Reference K0103
- ◆ E0973 Adjustable-height detachable arms, desk or full length, wheelchair
  CIM 60-9, Cross Reference K0016
- ◆ E0974 "Grade-aid" (device to prevent rolling back on an incline) for wheelchair
  Cross Reference K0080
- ◆ E0975 Reinforced seat upholstery, wheelchair
  CIM 60-9, Cross Reference K0029
- ◆ E0976 Reinforced back, wheelchair, upholstery or other material
  CIM 60-9, Cross Reference K0022
- ✻ E0977 Wedge cushion, wheelchair
- ◆ E0978 Belt, safety with airplane buckle, wheelchair; Cross Reference K0031
- ◆ E0979 Belt, safety with velcro closure, wheelchair; Cross Reference K0031
- ✻ E0980 Safety vest, wheelchair
- ◆ E0990 Elevating leg rest, each
  CIM 60-9, Cross Reference K0048
- ◆ E0991 Upholstery seat
  CIM 60-9, Cross Reference K0032, K0033
- ◆ E0992 Solid seat insert
  CIM 60-9, Cross Reference K0030

◆ E0993 Back, upholstery
CIM 60-9, Cross Reference K0027

⊛ E0994 Arm rest, each
CIM 60-9

◆ E0995 Calf rest, each
CIM 60-9, Cross Reference K0049

◆ E0996 Tire, solid, each
CIM 60-9, Cross Reference K0066

⊛ E0997 Caster with a fork
CIM 60-9

⊛ E0998 Caster without fork
CIM 60-9

⊛ E0999 Pneumatic tire with wheel
CIM 60-9

◆ E1000 Tire, pneumatic caster
CIM 60-9, Cross Reference K0074

⊛ E1001 Wheel, single
CIM 60-9

▶⊛ E1011 Modification to pediatric wheelchair, width adjustment package (not to be dispensed with initial chair)
CIM 60-9

▶⊛ E1012 Integrated seating system, planar, for pediatric wheelchair
CIM 60-9

▶⊛ E1013 Integrated seating system, contoured, for pediatric wheelchair
CIM 60-9

▶⊛ E1014 Reclining back, addition to pediatric wheelchair
CIM 60-9

▶⊛ E1015 Shock absorber for manual wheelchair, each
CIM 60-9

▶⊛ E1016 Shock absorber for power wheelchair, each
CIM 60-9

▶⊛ E1017 Heavy duty shock absorber for heavy duty or extra heavy duty manual wheelchair, each
CIM 60-9

▶⊛ E1018 Heavy duty shock absorber for heavy duty or extra heavy duty power wheelchair, each
CIM 60-9

▶⊛ E1020 Residual limb support system for wheelchair
CIM 60-6

▶⊛ E1025 Lateral thoracic support, non-contoured, for pediatric wheelchair, each (includes hardware)
CIM 60-9

▶⊛ E1026 Lateral thoracic support, contoured, for pediatric wheelchair, each (includes hardware)
CIM 60-9

▶⊛ E1027 Lateral/anterior support, for pediatric wheelchair, each (includes hardware)
CIM 60-9

Rollabout Chair and Transfer System

⊛ E1031 Rollabout chair, any and all types with castors 5 inches or greater
CIM 60-9

⊛ E1035 Multi-positional patient transfer system, with integrated seat, operated by care giver
MCM 2100

▶⊛ E1037 Transport chair, pediatric size
CIM 60-9

▶⊛ E1038 Transport chair, adult size
CIM 60-9

Wheelchair: Fully Reclining

⊛ E1050 Fully reclining wheelchair, fixed full-length arms, swing-away detachable elevating leg rests
CIM 60-9

⊛ E1060 Fully reclining wheelchair, detachable arms, desk or full-length, swing-away detachable elevating leg rests
CIM 60-9

⊛ E1065 Power attachment (to convert any wheelchair to motorized wheelchair, e.g., Solo)
CIM 60-9

◆ E1066 Battery charger
CIM 60-9, Cross Reference K0088

◆ E1069 Deep cycle battery
CIM 60-9, Cross Reference K0082, K0086

⊛ E1070 Fully reclining wheelchair, detachable arms (desk or full-length), swing-away detachable foot rests
CIM 60-9

⊛ E1083 Hemi-wheelchair, fixed full-length arms, swing-away detachable elevating leg rests
CIM 60-9

⊛ E1084 Hemi-wheelchair, detachable arms (desk or full-length) arms, swing-away detachable elevating leg rests
CIM 60-9

◆ E1085 Hemi-wheelchair, fixed full-length arms, swing-away detachable foot rests
CIM 60-9, Cross Reference K0002

◆ E1086 Hemi-wheelchair, detachable arms (desk or full-length), swing-away detachable foot rests
CIM 60-9, Cross Reference K0002

⊛ E1087 High-strength lightweight wheelchair, fixed full-length arms, swing-away detachable elevating leg rests
CIM 60-9

- ❂ E1088 High-strength lightweight wheelchair, detachable arms (desk or full-length), swing-away detachable elevating leg rests
  CIM 60-9
- ◆ E1089 High-strength lightweight wheelchair, fixed-length arms, swing-away detachable foot rests
  CIM 60-9, Cross Reference K0004
- ◆ E1090 High-strength lightweight wheelchair, detachable arms (desk or full-length), swing-away detachable foot rests
  CIM 60-9, Cross Reference K0004
- E1091 Deleted 12/31/02
- ❂ E1092 Wide, heavy duty wheelchair, detachable arms (desk or full-length), swing-away detachable elevating leg rests
  CIM 60-9
- ❂ E1093 Wide, heavy duty wheelchair, detachable arms (desk or full-length) swing-away detachable foot rests
  CIM 60-9

Wheelchair: Semi-reclining

- ❂ E1100 Semi-reclining wheelchair, fixed full-length arms, swing-away detachable elevating leg rests
  CIM 60-9
- ❂ E1110 Semi-reclining wheelchair, detachable arms (desk or full-length), elevating leg rests
  CIM 60-9

Wheelchair: Standard

- ◆ E1130 Standard wheelchair, fixed full-length arms, fixed or swing-away detachable foot rests
  CIM 60-9, Cross Reference K0001
- ◆ E1140 Wheelchair, detachable arms (desk or full-length), swing-away detachable foot rests
  CIM 60-9, Cross Reference K0001
- ❂ E1150 Wheelchair, detachable arms (desk or full-length), swing-away detachable elevating leg rests
  CIM 60-9
- ❂ E1160 Wheelchair, fixed full-length arms, swing-away detachable elevating leg rests
  CIM 60-9
- ▶✻ E1161 Manual adult size wheelchair, includes tilt in space

Wheelchair: Amputee

- ❂ E1170 Amputee wheelchair, fixed full-length arms, swing-away detachable elevating leg rests
  CIM 60-9
- ❂ E1171 Amputee wheelchair, fixed full-length arms, without foot rests or leg rests
  CIM 60-9
- ❂ E1172 Amputee wheelchair, detachable arms (desk or full-length), without foot rests or leg rests
  CIM 60-9
- ❂ E1180 Amputee wheelchair, detachable arms (desk or full-length) swing-away detachable foot rests
  CIM 60-9
- ❂ E1190 Amputee wheelchair, detachable arms (desk or full-length), swing-away detachable elevating leg rests
  CIM 60-9
- ❂ E1195 Heavy duty wheelchair, fixed full-length arms, swing-away detachable elevating leg rests
  CIM 60-9
- ❂ E1200 Amputee wheelchair, fixed full-length arms, swing-away detachable foot rests
  CIM 60-9

Wheelchair: Power

- ❂ E1210 Motorized wheelchair, fixed full-length arms, swing-away detachable elevating leg rests
  CIM 60-5, CIM 60-9
- ❂ E1211 Motorized wheelchair, detachable arms (desk or full-length) swing-away, detachable elevating leg rests
  CIM 60-5, CIM 60-9
- ◆ E1212 Motorized wheelchair, fixed full-length arms, swing-away detachable foot rests
  CIM 60-5, CIM 60-9, Cross Reference K0010
- ◆ E1213 Motorized wheelchair, detachable arms (desk or full-length), swing-away detachable foot rests
  CIM 60-5, CIM 60-9, Cross Reference K0010

Wheelchair: Special Size

- ❂ E1220 Wheelchair; specially sized or constructed (indicate brand name, model number, if any) and justification
  CIM 60-6
- ❂ E1221 Wheelchair with fixed arm, foot rests
  CIM 60-6

⊙ E1222 Wheelchair with fixed arm, elevating leg rests
CIM 60-6

⊙ E1223 Wheelchair with detachable arms, foot rests
CIM 60-6

⊙ E1224 Wheelchair with detachable arms, elevating leg rests
CIM 60-6

⊙ E1225 Semi-reclining back for customized wheelchair
CIM 60-6

◆ E1226 Full-reclining back for customized wheelchair
CIM 60-6, Cross Reference K0028

⊙ E1227 Special height arms for wheelchair
CIM 60-6

⊙ E1228 Special back height for wheelchair
CIM 60-6

⊙ E1230 Power operated vehicle (three- or four-wheel non-highway); specify brand name and model number
MCM 4107.6, CIM 60-5

▶⊙ E1231 Wheelchair, pediatric size, tilt-in-space, rigid, adjustable, with seating system
CIM 60-9

▶⊙ E1232 Wheelchair, pediatric size, tilt-in-space, folding, adjustable, with seating system
CIM 60-9

▶⊙ E1233 Wheelchair, pediatric size, tilt-in-space, rigid, adjustable, without seating system
CIM 60-9

▶⊙ E1234 Wheelchair, pediatric size, tilt-in-space, folding, adjustable, without seating system
CIM 60-9

▶⊙ E1235 Wheelchair, pediatric size, rigid, adjustable, with seating system
CIM 60-9

▶⊙ E1236 Wheelchair, pediatric size, folding, adjustable, with seating system
CIM 60-9

▶⊙ E1237 Wheelchair, pediatric size, rigid, adjustable, without seating system
CIM 60-9

▶⊙ E1238 Wheelchair, pediatric size, folding, adjustable, without seating system
CIM 60-9

Wheelchair: Lightweight

⊙ E1240 Lightweight wheelchair, detachable arms (desk or full-length), swing-away detachable, elevating leg rests
CIM 60-9

◆ E1250 Lightweight wheelchair, fixed full-length arms, swing-away detachable foot rests
CIM 60-9, Cross Reference K0003

◆ E1260 Lightweight wheelchair, detachable arms (desk or full-length), swing-away detachable foot rests
CIM 60-9, Cross Reference K0003

⊙ E1270 Lightweight wheelchair, fixed full-length arms, swing-away detachable elevating leg rests
CIM 60-9

Wheelchair: Heavy Duty

⊙ E1280 Heavy duty wheelchair, detachable arms (desk or full-length), elevating leg rests
CIM 60-9

◆ E1285 Heavy duty wheelchair, fixed full-length arms, swing-away detachable foot rests
CIM 60-9, Cross Reference K0006

◆ E1290 Heavy duty wheelchair, detachable arms (desk or full-length), swing-away detachable foot rests
CIM 60-9, Cross Reference K0006

⊙ E1295 Heavy duty wheelchair, fixed full-length arms, elevating leg rests
CIM 60-9

⊙ E1296 Special wheelchair seat, height from floor
CIM 60-6

⊙ E1297 Special wheelchair seat depth, by upholstery
CIM 60-6

⊙ E1298 Special wheelchair seat depth and/or width, by construction
CIM 60-6

Whirlpool Equipment

◆ E1300 Whirlpool, portable (overtub type)
CIM 60-9

⊙ E1310 Whirlpool, non-portable (built-in type)
CIM 60-9

Repairs and Replacement Parts

⊙ E1340 Repair or nonroutine service for durable medical equipment requiring the skill of a technician, labor component, per 15 minutes
MCM 2100.4

Additional Oxygen Related Equipment

- ✪ E1353 Regulator
  MCM 4107.9, CIM 60-4
- ✪ E1355 Stand/rack
  CIM 60-4
- ✪ E1372 Immersion external heater for nebulizer
  CIM 60-4
- ✪ E1390 Oxygen concentrator, capable of delivering 85 percent or greater oxygen concentration at the prescribed flow rate
  CIM 60-4
- * E1399 Durable medical equipment, miscellaneous
- ✪ E1405 Oxygen and water vapor enriching system with heated delivery
  MCM 4107, CIM 60-4
- ✪ E1406 Oxygen and water vapor enriching system without heated delivery
  MCM 4107, CIM 60-4
- ✪ E1500 Centrifuge, for dialysis

Artificial Kidney Machines and Accessories

- ✪ E1510 Kidney, dialysate delivery system, kidney machine, pump recirculating, air removal system, flow rate meter, power off, heater and temperature control with alarm, IV poles, pressure gauge, concentrate container
- ✪ E1520 Heparin infusion pump for hemodialysis
- ✪ E1530 Air bubble detector for hemodialysis, each, replacement
- ✪ E1540 Pressure alarm for hemodialysis, each
- ✪ E1550 Bath conductivity meter for hemodialysis, each
- ✪ E1560 Blood leak detector for hemodialysis, each, replacement
- ✪ E1570 Adjustable chair, for ESRD patients
- ✪ E1575 Transducer protectors/fluid barriers for hemohemodialysis, any size, per 10
- ✪ E1580 Unipuncture control system for hemodialysis
- ✪ E1590 Hemodialysis machine
- ✪ E1592 Automatic intermittent peritoneal dialysis system
- ✪ E1594 Cycler dialysis machine for peritoneal dialysis
- ✪ E1600 Delivery and/or installation charges for hemodialysis equipment
- ✪ E1610 Reverse osmosis water purification system, for hemodialysis
  CIM 55-1A
- ✪ E1615 Deionizer water purification system, for hemodialysis
  CIM 55-1A
- ✪ E1620 Blood pump for hemodialysis replacement
- ✪ E1625 Water softening system, for hemodialysis
  CIM 55-1B
- * E1630 Reciprocating peritoneal dialysis system
- ✪ E1632 Wearable artificial kidney, each
- ✪ E1635 Compact (portable) travel hemodialyzer system
- ✪ E1636 Sorbent cartridges, per case, for hemodialysis, per 10
- ➠ ✪ E1637 Hemostats, each
- E1638 Deleted 12/31/02, Cross Reference E0210
- ➠ ✪ E1639 Scale, each
- E1640 Deleted 01/01/02
- ✪ E1699 Dialysis equipment, not otherwise specified

Jaw Motion Rehabilitation System and Accessories

- * E1700 Jaw motion rehabilitation system
- * E1701 Replacement cushions for jaw motion rehabilitation system, package of 6
- * E1702 Replacement measuring scales for jaw motion rehabilitation system, package of 200

Other Orthopedic Devices

- * E1800 Dynamic adjustable elbow extension/flexion device, includes soft interface material
- * E1801 Bi-directional static progressive stretch elbow device with range of motion adjustment, includes cuffs
- ▶ * E1802 Dynamic adjustable forearm pronation/supination device, includes soft interface material
- * E1805 Dynamic adjustable wrist extension/flexion device, includes soft interface material
- * E1806 Bi-directional static progressive stretch wrist device with range of motion adjustment, includes cuffs
- * E1810 Dynamic adjustable knee extension/flexion device, includes soft interface material
- * E1811 Bi-directional static progressive stretch knee device with range of motion adjustment, includes cuffs
- * E1815 Dynamic adjustable ankle extension/flexion device, includes soft interface material
- * E1816 Bi-directional static progressive stretch ankle device with range of motion adjustment, includes cuffs

✻ E1818 Bi-directional static progressive stretch forearm pronation/supination device with range of motion adjustment, includes cuffs

✻ E1820 Replacement of soft interface material, dynamic adjustable extension/flexion device

✻ E1821 Replacement of soft interface material/cuffs for bi-directional static progressive stretch device

✻ E1825 Dynamic adjustable finger extension/flexion device, includes soft interface material

✻ E1830 Dynamic adjustable toe extension/flexion device, includes soft interface material

✻ E1840 Dynamic adjustable shoulder flexion/abduction/rotation device, includes soft interface material

E1900 Deleted 01/01/02

✻ E1902 Communication board, non-electronic augmentative or alternative communication device

✻ E2000 Gastric suction pump, home model, portable or stationary, electric

✪ E2100 Blood glucose monitor with integrated voice synthesizer
CIM 60-11

✪ E2101 Blood glucose monitor with integrated lancing/blood sample
CIM 60-11

PROCEDURES/PROFESSIONAL SERVICES (TEMPORARY) (G0000-G9999)

NOTE: This section contains national codes assigned by CMS on a temporary basis to identify procedures/professional services.

Positron Emission Tomography Scan Code Modifiers

Modifiers that are used on claims for positron emission tomography (PET) myocardial perfusion imaging are created by combining two alpha characters. Each alpha character represents the results of the PET scan and the previous test, with the first letter indicating the results of the PET scan, while the second letter indicates the test done prior to the PET scan.The test result codes and their descriptions are listed below:

Code	
N	Negative
E	Equivocal
P	Positive, but not suggestive of extensive ischemia
S	Positive and suggestive of extensive ischemia (greater than 20% of the left ventricle)

✻ G0001 Routine venipuncture for collection of specimen(s)

G0002 Deleted 12/31/02, Cross Reference 51702*, 51703*

G0004 Deleted 12/31/02, Cross Reference 93268

G0005 Deleted 12/31/02, Cross Reference 93270

G0006 Deleted 12/31/02, Cross Reference 93271

G0007 Deleted 12/31/02, Cross Reference 93272

✻ G0008 Administration of influenza virus vaccine

✻ G0009 Administration of pneumococcal vaccine

✻ G0010 Administration of hepatitis B vaccine

G0015 Deleted 12/31/02, Cross Reference 93012

G0016 Deleted 01/01/02

✪ G0025 Collagen skin test kit
CIM 65-9

G0026 Deleted 12/31/02

G0027 Deleted 12/31/02, Cross Reference 89310

✪ G0030 PET myocardial perfusion imaging (following previous PET, G0030-G0047); single study, rest or stress (exercise and/or pharmacologic)
CIM 50-36

✪ G0031 PET myocardial perfusion imaging (following previous PET, G0030-G0047); multiple studies, rest or stress (exercise and/or pharmacologic)
CIM 50-36

✪ G0032 PET myocardial perfusion imaging (following rest SPECT, 78464); single study, rest or stress (exercise and/or pharmacologic)
CIM 50-36

✪ G0033 PET myocardial perfusion imaging (following rest SPECT, 78464*); multiple studies, rest or stress (exercise and/or pharmacologic)
CIM 50-36

✪ G0034 PET myocardial perfusion imaging (following stress SPECT, 78465*); single study, rest or stress (exercise and/or pharmacologic)
CIM 50-36

✪ G0035 PET myocardial perfusion imaging (following stress SPECT, 78465*); multiple studies, rest or stress (exercise and/or pharmacologic)
CIM 50-36

⊙ G0036 PET myocardial perfusion imaging (following coronary angiography, 93510-93529*); single study, rest or stress (exercise and/or pharmacologic)
CIM 50-36

⊙ G0037 PET myocardial perfusion imaging (following coronary angiography, 93510-93529*); multiple studies, rest or stress (exercise and/or pharmacologic)
CIM 50-36

⊙ G0038 PET myocardial perfusion imaging, (following stress planar myocardial perfusion, 78460*); single study, rest or stress (exercise and/or pharmacologic)
CIM 50-36

⊙ G0039 PET myocardial perfusion imaging (following stress planar myocardial perfusion, 78460*); multiple studies, rest or stress (exercise and/or pharmacologic)
CIM 50-36

⊙ G0040 PET myocardial perfusion imaging (following stress echocardiogram, 93350*); single study, rest or stress (exercise and/or pharmacologic)
CIM 50-36

⊙ G0041 PET myocardial perfusion imaging (following stress echocardiogram, 93350*); multiple studies, rest or stress (exercise and/or pharmacologic)
CIM 50-36

⊙ G0042 PET myocardial perfusion imaging (following stress nuclear ventriculogram, 78481 or 78483*); single study, rest or stress (exercise and/or pharmacologic)
CIM 50-36

⊙ G0043 PET myocardial perfusion imaging, (following stress nuclear ventriculogram, 78488 or 78483*); multiple studies, rest or stress (exercise and/or pharmacologic)
CIM 50-36

⊙ G0044 PET myocardial perfusion imaging (following rest electrocardiogram [ECG], 93000*); single study, rest or stress (exercise and/or pharmacologic)
CIM 50-36

⊙ G0045 PET myocardial perfusion imaging (following rest ECG, 93000*); multiple studies, rest or stress (exercise and/or pharmacologic)
CIM 50-36

⊙ G0046 PET myocardial perfusion imaging (following stress ECG, 93015*); single study, rest or stress (exercise and/or pharmacologic)
CIM 50-36

*CPT only ©*Current Procedural Terminology 2002, Professional Edition*. American Medical Association.

⊙ G0047 PET myocardial perfusion imaging, (following stress ECG, 93015*); multiple studies, rest or stress (exercise and/or pharmacologic)
CIM 50-36

G0050 Deleted 12/31/02, Cross Reference 51798*

⊙ G0101 Cervical or vaginal cancer screening; pelvic and clinical breast examination

⊙ G0102 Prostate cancer screening; digital rectal examination
MCM 4182, CIM 50-55

⊙ G0103 Prostate cancer screening; prostate specific antigen test (PSA), total
MCM 4182, CIM 50-55

⊙ G0104 Colorectal cancer screening; flexible sigmoidoscopy

⊙ G0105 Colorectal cancer screening; colonoscopy on individual at high risk

⊙ G0106 Colorectal cancer screening; alternative to G0104, screening sigmoidoscopy, barium enema

⊙ G0107 Colorectal cancer screening; fecal-occult blood test, 1-3 simultaneous determinations

✻ G0108 Diabetes outpatient self-management training services, individual, per 30 minute

✻ G0109 Diabetes outpatient self-management training services, group session, two or more, per 30 minutes

⊙ G0110 NETT pulmonary-rehabilitation; education/skills training, individual
CIM 35-93

⊙ G0111 NETT pulmonary-rehabilitation; education/skills training, group
CIM 35-93

⊙ G0112 NETT pulmonary-rehabilitation; nutritional guidance, initial
CIM 35-93

⊙ G0113 NETT pulmonary-rehabilitation; nutritional guidance, subsequent
CIM 35-93

⊙ G0114 NETT pulmonary-rehabilitation; psychosocial consultation
CIM 35-93

⊙ G0115 NETT pulmonary-rehabilitation; psychological testing
CIM 35-93

⊙ G0116 NETT pulmonary-rehabilitation; psychosocial counseling
CIM 35-93

✻ G0117 Glaucoma screening for high risk patients furnished by optometrist or ophthalmologist

✻ G0118 Glaucoma screening for high risk patient furnished under direct supervision by optometrist or ophthalmologist

⊙ G0120 Colorectal cancer screening; alternative to G0105, screening colonoscopy, barium enema

✪ G0121 Colorectal cancer screening; colonoscopy on individual not meeting criteria for high risk

◆ G0122 Colorectal cancer screening; barium enema

✪ G0123 Screening cytopathology, cervical or vaginal (any reporting system); collected in preservative fluid, automated thin layer preparation, screening by cytotechnologist under physician supervision
CIM 50-20, Laboratory Certification: cytology

✪ G0124 Screening cytopathology, cervical or vaginal (any reporting system); collected in preservative fluid, automated thin layer preparation, requiring interpretation by physician
CIM 50-20, Laboratory Certification: cytology

➡ ✪ G0125 PET imaging regional or whole body; single pulmonary nodule
MCM 4173, CIM 50-36

✪ G0127 Trimming of dystrophic nails, any number
MCM 2323, MCM 4120

✪ G0128 Direct (face-to-face with patient) skilled nursing services of a registered nurse provided in a comprehensive outpatient rehabilitation facility, each 10 minutes beyond the first 5 minutes
Medicare Statute 1833a

G0129 Occupational therapy requiring the skills of a qualified occupational therapist, furnished as a component of a partial hospitalization treatment program, per day

✪ G0130 Single energy x-ray absorptiometry (SEXA) bone density study, one or more sites; appendicular skeleton (peripheral) (e.g., radius, wrist, heel)
CIM 50-44

G0131 Deleted 12/31/02, Cross Reference 76070*

G0132 Deleted 12/31/02, Cross Reference 76071*

✻ G0141 Screening cytopathology smears, cervical or vaginal, performed by automated system, with manual rescreening requiring interpretation by physician; Laboratory Certification: cytology

✻ G0143 Screening cytopathology, cervical or vaginal (any reporting system); collected in preservative fluid, automated thin layer preparation, with manual screening and rescreening by cytotechnologist under physician supervision; Laboratory Certification: cytology

*CPT only ©*Current Procedural Terminology 2002, Professional Edition*. American Medical Association. All rights reserved.

➡ ✻ G0144 Screening cytopathology, cervical or vaginal (any reporting system); collected in preservative fluid, automated thin layer preparation, with screening by automated system, under physician supervision; Laboratory Certification: cytology

➡ ✻ G0145 Screening cytopathology, cervical or vaginal (any reporting system); collected in preservative fluid, automated thin layer preparation, with screening by automated system and manual rescreening under physician supervision; Laboratory Certification: cytology

✻ G0147 Screening cytopathology smears, cervical or vaginal; performed by automated system under physician supervision; Laboratory Certification: cytology

✻ G0148 Screening cytopathology smears, cervical or vaginal; performed by automated system with manual rescreening; Laboratory Certification: cytology

✻ G0151 Services of physical therapist in home health setting, each 15 minutes

✻ G0152 Services of occupational therapist in home health setting, each 15 minutes

✻ G0153 Services of speech and language pathologist in home health setting, each 15 minutes

✻ G0154 Services of skilled nurse in home health setting, each 15 minutes

✻ G0155 Services of clinical social worker in home health setting, each 15 minutes

✻ G0156 Services of home health aide in home health setting, each 15 minutes

✪ G0166 External counterpulsation, per treatment session
CIM 35-74

✪ G0167 Hyperbaric oxygen treatment not requiring physician attendance, per treatment session
CIM 35-10

✻ G0168 Wound closure utilizing tissue adhesive(s) only

✪ G0173 Stereotactic radiosurgery, complete course of therapy in one session

✪ G0174 Deleted 01/01/02

✻ G0175 Scheduled interdisciplinary team conference (minimum of three exclusive of patient care nursing staff) with patient present

✪ G0176 Activity therapy, such as music, dance, art or play therapies not for recreation, related to the care and treatment of patient's disabling mental health problems, per session (45 minutes or more)

✪ G0177 Training and educational services related to the care and treatment of patient's disabling mental health problems per session (45 minutes or more)

G0178 Deleted 01/01/02

➠ ✻ G0179 Physician re-certification for Medicare-covered home health services under a home health plan of care (patient not present), including contacts with home health agency and review of reports of patient status required by physicians to affirm the initial implementation of the plan of care that meets patient's needs, per re-certification period

➠ ✻ G0180 Physician certification for Medicare-covered home health services under a home health plan of care (patient not present), including contacts with home health agency and review of reports of patient status required by physicians to affirm the initial implementation of the plan of care that meets patient's needs, per certification period

✻ G0181 Physician supervision of a patient receiving Medicare-covered services provided by a participating home health agency (patient not present) requiring complex and multidisciplinary care modalities involving regular physician development and/or revision of care plans, review of subsequent reports of patient status, review of laboratory and other studies, communication (including telephone calls) with other health care professionals involved in the patient's care, integration of new information into the medical treatment plan, and/or adjustment of medical therapy, within a calendar month, 30 minutes or more

✻ G0182 Physician supervision of a patient under a Medicare-approved hospice (patient not present) requiring complex and multidisciplinary care modalities involving regular physician development and/or revision of care plans, review of subsequent reports of patient status, review of laboratory and other studies, communication (including telephone calls) with other health care professionals involved in the patient's care, integration of new information into the medical treatment plan, and/or adjustment of medical therapy, within a calendar month, 30 minutes or more

G0184 Deleted 01/01/02

G0185 Deleted 12/31/02, Cross Reference 0016T

✻ G0186 Destruction of localized lesion of choroid (for example, choroidal neovascularization); photocoagulation, feeder vessel technique (one or more sessions)

G0187 Deleted 12/31/02

G0188 Deleted 01/01/02

G0190 Deleted 01/01/02

G0191 Deleted 01/01/02

G0192 Deleted 12/31/02

G0193 Deleted 12/31/02, Cross Reference 92612

G0194 Deleted 12/31/02, Cross Reference 92614

G0195 Deleted 12/31/02, Cross Reference 92610

G0196 Deleted 12/31/02, Cross Reference 92611

G0197 Deleted 12/31/02, Cross Reference 92607

G0198 Deleted 12/31/02, Cross Reference 92609

G0199 Deleted 12/31/02, Cross Reference 92607 and 92608

G0200 Deleted 12/31/02, Cross Reference 92506

G0201 Deleted 12/31/02, Cross Reference 92507

✻ G0202 Screening mammography, producing direct digital image, bilateral, all views

G0203 Deleted 01/01/02

✻ G0204 Diagnostic mammography, producing direct digital image, bilateral, all views

G0205 Deleted 01/01/02

✻ G0206 Diagnostic mammography, producing direct digital image, unilateral, all views

G0207 Deleted 01/01/02

➠ ✪ G0210 PET imaging whole body; diagnosis; lung cancer, non-small cell
MCM 4173 CIM 50-36

➠ ✪ G0211 PET imaging whole body; initial staging; lung cancer; non-small cell (replaces G0126)
MCM 4173 CIM 50-36

➠ ✪ G0212 PET imaging whole body; restaging; lung cancer; non-small cell
MCM 4173 CIM 50-36

➠ ✪ G0213 PET imaging whole body; diagnosis; colorectal cancer
MCM 4173 CIM 50-36

➠ ✪ G0214 PET imaging whole body; initial staging; colorectal cancer
MCM 4173 CIM 50-36

➠ ✪ G0215 PET imaging whole body; restaging; colorectal cancer (replaces G0163)
MCM 4173 CIM 50-36

➠ ✪ G0216 PET imaging whole body; diagnosis; melanoma
MCM 4173 CIM 50-36

➠ ✪ G0217 PET imaging whole body; initial staging; melanoma
MCM 4173 CIM 50-36

➠ ✪ G0218 PET imaging whole body; restaging; melanoma (replaces G0165)
MCM 4173 CIM 50-36

➠ ✪ G0219 PET imaging whole body melanoma; for non-covered indications
MCM 4173 CIM 50-36

➡✪ G0220 PET imaging whole body; diagnosis; lymphoma
MCM 4173 CIM 50-36

➡✪ G0221 PET imaging whole body; initial staging; lymphoma (replaces G0164)
MCM 4173 CIM 50-36

➡✪ G0222 PET imaging whole body; restaging; lymphoma (replaces G0164)
MCM 4173 CIM 50-36

➡✪ G0223 PET imaging whole body or regional; diagnosis; head and neck cancer; excluding thyroid and CNS cancers
MCM 4173 CIM 50-36

➡✪ G0224 PET imaging whole body or regional; initial staging; head and neck cancer; excluding thyroid and CNS cancers
MCM 4173 CIM 50-36

➡✪ G0225 PET imaging whole body or regional; restaging; head and neck cancer, excluding thyroid and CNS cancers
MCM 4173 CIM 50-36

➡✪ G0226 PET imaging whole body; diagnosis; esophageal cancer
MCM 4173 CIM 50-36

➡✪ G0227 PET imaging whole body; initial staging; esophageal cancer
MCM 4173 CIM 50-36

➡✪ G0228 PET imaging whole body; restaging; esophageal cancer
MCM 4173 CIM 50-36

➡✪ G0229 PET imaging; metabolic brain imaging for pre-surgical evaluation of refractory seizures
MCM 4173 CIM 50-36

➡✪ G0230 PET imaging; metabolic assessment for myocardial viability following inconclusive SPECT study
MCM 4173 CIM 50-36

✪ G0231 PET, whole body, for recurrence of colorectal or colorectal metastatic cancer; gamma cameras only
CIM 50-36

✪ G0232 PET, whole body, staging and characterization of lymphoma; gamma cameras only
CIM 50-36

✪ G0233 PET, whole body, for recurrence of melanoma or melanoma metastatic cancer; gamma cameras only
CIM 50-36

✪ G0234 PET, regional or whole body, for solitary pulmonary nodule following CT or for initial staging of pathologically diagnosed non-small cell lung cancer; gamma cameras only
CIM 50-36

➡* G0236 Digitization of film radiographic images with computer analysis for lesion detection, or computer analysis of digital mammogram for lesion detection, and further physician review for interpretation, diagnostic mammography (list separately in addition to code for primary procedure)

* G0237 Therapeutic procedures to increase strength or endurance of respiratory muscles, face to face, one on one, each 15 minutes

* G0238 Therapeutic procedures to improve respiratory function, other than described by G0237, one on one, face to face, per 15 minutes

* G0239 Therapeutic procedures to improve respiratory function or increase strength or endurance of respiratory muscles, two or more individuals (includes monitoring)

G0240 Deleted 12/31/02

G0241 Deleted 12/31/02

✪ G0242 Multi-source photon stereotactic radiosurgery (cobalt-60 multi-source converging beams) plan, including dose volume histograms for target and critical structure tolerances, plan optimization performed for highly conformal distributions, plan positional accuracy and dose verification, all lesions treated, per course of treatment

✪ G0243 Multi-source photon stereotactic radiosurgery, delivery including collimator changes and custom plugging, complete course of treatment, all lesions

✪ G0244 Observation care provided by a facility to a patient with congestive heart failure, chest pain, or asthma, minimum 8 hours, maximum 48 hours

LOSS OF PROTECTIVE SENSATION

▶✪ G0245 Initial physician evaluation of a diabetic patient with diabetic sensory neuropathy resulting in a loss of protective sensation (LOPS) which must include (1) the diagnosis of LOPS; (2) a patient history; (3) a physical examination that consist of *at least* the following elements:

a. Visual inspection of the forefoot, hindfoot and toeweb spaces
b. Evaluation of a protective sensation
c. Evaluation of foot structure and biomechanics
d. Evaluation of vascular status and skin integrity
e. Evaluation and recommendation of footwear
4. Patient education
CIM 50-81

▶✪ G0246 Follow-up physician evaluation and management of a diabetic patient with diabetic sensory neuropathy resulting in a loss of protective sensation (LOPS) to include at least the following, (1) a patient history (2) a physical examination that includes:
a. Visual inspection of the forefoot, hindfoot and toe web spaces
b. Evaluation of protective sensation
c. Evaluation of foot structure and biomechanics
d. Evaluation of vascular status and skin integrity
e. Evaluation and recommendation of footwear
3. Patient education

▶✪ G0247 Routine foot care by a physician of a diabetic patient with diabetic sensory neuropathy resulting in a LOPS to include if present, at least the following:
1. Local care of superficial wounds
2. Débridement of corns and calluses, trimming and débridement of nails
3. Trimming and débridement of nails

"G" Codes for International Normalized Ratio Monitoring

Codes established for CIM 50.55 effective for services furnished on or after July 1, 2002. Use of the International Normalized Ratio (INR) allows physician to determine the level of anti-coagulation in a patient independent of the laboratory reagents used. Home prothrombin monitoring with the use of INR devices is only covered for patients with mechanical heart valves.

CIM reference 50-36 details coverage indications. FDG Positron Emission Tomography is a minimally invasive diagnostic procedure using positron camera (tomograph) to measure the decay of radioisotopes such as FDG, CMS determined that the benefit category for the requested indications fell under 1861(s)(3) of the Social Security Act diagnostic service.

▶✪ G0248 Demonstration, at initial use, of home INR monitoring for patient with mechanical heart valve(s) who meets Medicare coverage criteria, under the direction of a physician; includes: demonstrating use and care of the INR monitor, obtaining at least one blood sample, provision of instructions for reporting home INR test results, and documentation of patient ability to perform testing.
CIM 50-55

▶✪ G0249 Provision of test materials and equipment for home INR monitoring to patient with mechanical heart valve(s) who meets Medicare coverage criteria; includes provision of materials for use in the home and reporting of test results to physician; per 4 tests.
CIM 50-55

▶✪ G0250 Physician review, interpretation and patient management of home INR testing for a patient with mechanical heart valve(s) who meets other coverage criteria; per 4 tests (does not require face-to-face service)
CIM 50-55

▶✪ G0251 Linear accelerator based stereotactic radiosurgery, delivery including collimator changes and custom plugging, fractionated treatment, all lesions, per session, maximum five sessions per course of treatment

▶✪ G0252 PET imaging, full and partial-ring PET scanners only, for initial diagnosis of breast cancer and/or surgical planning for breast cancer (e.g. initial staging of axillary lymph nodes)
CIM 50-36

▶✻ G0253 Pet imaging for breast cancer, full and partial-ring PET scanners only, staging/restaging of local regional recurrence or distant metastases (i.e., staging/restaging after or prior to course of treatment)
CIM 50-36

▶✻ G0254 PET imaging for breast cancer, full and partial ring PET scanners only, evaluation of response to treatment, performed during course of treatment
CIM 50-36

▶◆ G0255 Current perception threshold/sensory nerve conduction test, (SNCT) per limb, any nerve
CIM 50-57

▶✪ G0256 Prostate brachytherapy using permanently implanted palladium seeds, including transperitoneal placement of needles or catheters into the prostate, cystoscopy and application of permanent interstitial radiation source

▶❂ G0257 Unscheduled or emergency dialysis treatment for an ESRD patient in a hospital outpatient department that is not certified as an ESRD facility

G0258 Deleted

▶❂ G0259 Injection procedure for sacroiliac joint; arthrography

▶❂ G0260 Injection procedure for sacroiliac joint; provision of anesthetic, steroid and/or other therapeutic agent and arthrography

▶❂ G0261 Prostate brachytherapy using permanently implanted iodine seeds, including transperineal placement of needles or catheters into the prostate, cystoscopy and application of permanent interstitial radiation source

▶* G0262 Small intestinal imaging; intraluminal, from ligament of Treitz to the ileo cecal valve, includes physician interpretation and report

▶❂ G0263 Direct admission of patient with diagnosis of congestive heart failure, chest pain or asthma for observation services that meet all criteria from G0244

▶❂ G0264 Initial nursing assessment of patient directly admitted to observation with diagnosis other than congestive heart failure, chest pain or asthma or patient directly admitted to observation with diagnosis of CHF, chest pain or asthma when the observation stay does not qualify for G0244

▶* G0265 Cryopreservation, freezing and storage of cells for therapeutic use, each cell line

▶* G0266 Thawing and expansion of frozen cells for therapeutic use, each aliquot

▶* G0267 Bone marrow or peripheral stem cell harvest, modification or treatment to eliminate cell type(s) (e.g. t-cells, metastatic carcinoma)

▶* G0268 Removal of impacted cerumen (one or both ears) by physician on same date of service as audiologic function testing

▶❂ G0269 Placement of occlusive device into either a venous or arterial access site, post surgical or interventional procedure (e.g. angioseal plug, vascular plug)

▶* G0270 Medical nutrition therapy; reassessment and subsequent intervention(s) following second referral in same year for change in diagnosis, medical condition or treatment regimen (including additional hours needed for renal disease), individual, face to face with the patient, each 15 minutes

▶* G0271 Medical nutrition therapy, reassessment and subsequent intervention(s) following second referral in same year for change in diagnosis, medical condition, or treatment regimen (including additional hours needed for renal disease), group (2 or more individuals), each 30 minutes

▶* G0272 Naso/oro gastric tube placement, requiring physician's skill and fluoroscopic guidance (includes fluoroscopy, image documentation and report)

▶* G0273 Radiopharmaceutical biodistribution, single or multiple scans on one or more days, pre-treatment planning for radiopharmaceutical therapy of non-Hodgkin's lymphoma, includes administration of radiopharmaceutical (e.g., radiolabeled antibodies)

▶* G0274 Radiopharmaceutical therapy, non-Hodgkin's lymphoma, includes administration of radiopharmaceutical (.e.g. radiolabeled antibodies)

▶* G0275 Renal artery angiography (unilateral or bilateral) performed at the time of cardiac catheterization, includes catheter placement, injection of dye, flush aortogram and radiologic supervision and interpretation and production of images (list separately in addition to primary procedure)

▶* G0278 Iliac artery angiography performed at the same time of cardiac catheterization, includes catheter placement, injection of dye, radiologic supervision and interpretation and production of images (list separately in addition to primary procedure)

▶* G0279 Extracorporeal shock wave therapy; involving elbow epicondylitis

▶* G0280 Extracorporeal shock wave therapy; involving other than elbow epicondylitis or plantar fascitis

▶* G0281 Electrical stimulation, (unattended), to one or more areas, for chronic stage iii and stage iv pressure ulcers, arterial ulcers, diabetic ulcers, and venous stasis ulcers not demonstrating measurable signs of healing after 30 days of conventional care, as part of a therapy plan of care

▶* G0282 Electrical stimulation, (unattended), to one or more areas, for wound care other than described in G0281
CIM 35-98

▶* G0283 Electrical stimulation (unattended), to one or more areas for indication(s) other than wound care, as part of a therapy plan of care

▶✻ G0288 Reconstruction, computed tomographic angiography of aorta for surgical planning for vascular surgery

▶✻ G0289 Arthroscopy, knee, surgical, for removal of loose body, foreign body, debridement/shaving of articular cartilage (chondroplasty) at the time of other surgical knee arthroscopy in a different compartment of the same knee

▶✪ G0290 Transcatheter placement of a drug eluting intracoronary stent(s), percutaneous, with or without other therapeutic intervention, any method; single vessel

▶✪ G0291 Transcatheter placement of a drug eluting intracoronary stent(s), percutaneous, with or without other therapeutic intervention, any method; each additional vessel

▶✪ G0292 Administration(s) of experimental drug(s) only in a Medicare qualifying clinical trial (includes administration for chemotherapy and other types of therapy via infusion and/or other than infusion), per day

▶✪ G0293 Noncovered surgical procedure(s) using conscious sedation, regional, general or spinal anesthesia in a Medicare qualifying clinical trial, per day

▶✪ G0294 Noncovered procedure(s) using either no anesthesia or local anesthesia only, in a Medicare qualifying clinical trial, per day

▶◆ G0295 Electromagnetic stimulation, to one or more areas
CIM 35-98

✪ G9001 Coordination fee, initial rate

✪ G9002 Coordinated care fee, maintenance rate

✪ G9003 Coordinated care fee, risk adjusted high, initial

✪ G9004 Coordinated care fee, risk adjusted low, initial

✪ G9005 Coordinated care fee, risk adjusted maintenance

✪ G9006 Coordinated care fee, home monitoring

✪ G9007 Coordinated care fee, scheduled team conference

✪ G9008 Coordinated care fee, physician coordinated care oversight services

✪ G9009 Coordination care fee, risk adjustment maintenance, level 3

✪ G9010 Coordination care fee, risk adjustment maintenance, level 4

✪ G9011 Coordination care fee, risk adjustment maintenance, level 5

✪ G9012 Other specified care management services not elsewhere classified

◆ G9016 Smoking cessation counseling, individual, in the absence of or in addition to any other evaluation and management service, per session (6-10 minutes) (demo project code only)

ALCOHOL AND/OR DRUG SERVICES (H0001-H1005)

◆ H0001 Alcohol and/or drug assessment

➠◆ H0002 Behavioral health screening to determine eligibility for admission to treatment program

◆ H0003 Alcohol and/or drug screening; laboratory analysis of specimens for presence of alcohol and/or drugs

➠◆ H0004 Behavioral health counseling and therapy, per 15 minutes

◆ H0005 Alcohol and/or drug services; group counseling by a clinician

◆ H0006 Alcohol and/or drug services; case management

◆ H0007 Alcohol and/or drug services; crisis intervention (outpatient)

◆ H0008 Alcohol and/or drug services; subacute detoxification (hospital inpatient)

◆ H0009 Alcohol and/or drug services; acute detoxification (hospital inpatient)

◆ H0010 Alcohol and/or drug services; subacute detoxification (residential addiction program inpatient)

◆ H0011 Alcohol and/or drug services; acute detoxification (residential addiction program inpatient)

◆ H0012 Alcohol and/or drug services; subacute detoxification (residential addiction program outpatient)

◆ H0013 Alcohol and/or drug services; acute detoxification (residential addiction program outpatient)

◆ H0014 Alcohol and/or drug services; ambulatory detoxification

◆ H0015 Alcohol and/or drug services; intensive outpatient (treatment program that operates at least 3 hours per day and at least 3 days per week and is based on an individualized treatment plan), including assessment, counseling; crisis intervention, and activity therapies or education

◆ H0016 Alcohol and/or drug services; medical/somatic (medical intervention in ambulatory setting)

➠◆ H0017 Behavioral health; residential (hospital residential treatment program), without room and board, per diem

➠◆ H0018 Behavioral health; short-term residential (non-hospital residential treatment program), without room and board, per diem

➠◆ H0019 Behavioral health; long-term residential (non-medial, non-acute care in a residential treatment program where stay is typically longer than 30 days), without room and board, per diem

◆ H0020 Alcohol and/or drug services; methadone administration and/or service (provision of the drug by a licensed program)

◆ H0021 Alcohol and/or drug training service (for staff and personnel not employed by providers)

◆ H0022 Alcohol and/or drug intervention service (planned facilitation)

➡ ◆ H0023 Behavioral health outreach service (planned approach to reach a target population)

➡ ◆ H0024 Behavioral health prevention information dissemination service (one-way direct or non-direct contact with service audiences to affect knowledge or attitude)

➡ ◆ H0025 Behavioral health prevention education service (delivery of services with target population to affect knowledge, attitude, and/or behavior)

◆ H0026 Alcohol and/or drug prevention process service, community-based (delivery of services to develop skills of impactors)

◆ H0027 Alcohol and/or drug prevention environmental service (broad range of external activities geared toward modifying systems in order to mainstream prevention through policy and law)

◆ H0028 Alcohol and/or drug prevention problem identification and referral service (e.g., student assistance and employee assistance programs), does not include assessment

◆ H0029 Alcohol and/or drug prevention alternatives service (services for populations that exclude alcohol and other drug use [e.g., alcohol-free social events])

➡ ◆ H0030 Behavioral health hotline service

▶ ◆ H0031 Mental health assessment, by non-physician

▶ ◆ H0032 Mental health service plan development by non-physician

▶ ◆ H0033 Oral medication administration, direct observation

▶ ◆ H0034 Medication training and support, per 15 minutes

▶ ◆ H0035 Mental health partial hospitalization, treatment, less than 24 hours

▶ ◆ H0036 Community psychiatric supportive treatment, face-to-face, per 15 minutes

▶ ◆ H0037 Community psychiatric supportive treatment program, per diem

▶ ◆ H0038 Self-help/peer services, per 15 minutes

▶ ◆ H0039 Assertive community treatment, face-to-face, per 15 minutes

▶ ◆ H0040 Assertive community treatment program, per diem

▶ ◆ H0041 Foster care, child, non-therapeutic, per diem

▶ ◆ H0042 Foster care, child, non-therapeutic, per month?

▶ ◆ H0043 Supported housing, per diem

▶ ◆ H0044 Supported housing, per month

▶ ◆ H0045 Respite care services, not in the home, per diem

▶ ◆ H0046 Mental health services, not otherwise specified

▶ ◆ H0047 Alcohol and/or other drug abuse services, not otherwise specified

▶ ◆ H0048 Alcohol and/or other drug testing: collection and handling only, specimens other than blood

◆ H1000 Prenatal care, at-risk assessment

◆ H1001 Prenatal care, at-risk enhanced service; antepartum management

◆ H1002 Prenatal care, at-risk enhanced service; care coordination

◆ H1003 Prenatal care, at-risk enhanced service; education

◆ H1004 Prenatal care, at-risk enhanced service; follow-up home visit

◆ H1005 Prenatal care, at-risk enhanced service package (includes H1001-H1004)

▶ ◆ H1010 Non-medical family planning education, per session

▶ ◆ H1011 Family assessment by licensed behavioral health professional for state defined purposes

▶ ◆ H2000 Comprehensive multidisciplinary evaluation

▶ ◆ H2001 Rehabilitation program, per 1/2 day

DRUGS OTHER THAN CHEMOTHERAPY (J0100-J8999)

✪ J0120 Injection, tetracycline, up to 250 mg
MCM 2049

✪ J0130 Injection abciximab, 10 mg
MCM 2049

✪ J0150 Injection, adenosine, 6 mg (not to be used to report any adenosine phosphate compounds; instead use A9270)
MCM 2049

✪ J0151 Injection, adenosine, 90 mg (not to be used to report any adenosine phosphate compounds; instead use A9270)
MCM 2049

✪ J0170 Injection, adrenalin, epinephrine, up to 1 cc ampule
MCM 2049

✪ J0190 Injection, biperiden lactate, per 5 mg
MCM 2049

✪ J0200 Injection, alatrofloxacin mesylate, 100 mg
MCM 2049.5

✪ J0205 Injection, alglucerase, per 10 units
MCM 2049

- ✪ J0207 Injection, amifostine, 500 mg
  MCM 2049
- ✪ J0210 Injection, methyldopate HCl, up to 250 mg
  MCM 2049
- ✪ J0256 Injection, alpha-1-proteinase inhibitor (human), 10 mg
  MCM 2049
- ✪ J0270 Injection, alprostadil, per 1.25 mcg (Code may be used for Medicare when drug administered under the direct supervision of a physician, not for use when drug is self-administered.)
  MCM 2049
- ✪ J0275 Alprostadil urethral suppository (Code may be used for Medicare when drug administered under the direct supervision of a physician, not for use when drug is self-administered.)
  MCM 2049
- ✪ J0280 Injection, aminophylline, up to 250 mg
  MCM 2049
- ✪ J0282 Injection, amiodarone HCl, 30 mg
  MCM 2049
- ✪ J0285 Injection, amphotericin B, 50 mg
  MCM 2049
- J0286 Deleted 12/31/02
- ▶✪ J0287 Injection, amphotericin B lipid complex, 10 mg
  MCM 2049
- ▶✪ J0288 Injection, amphotericin B cholesteryl sulfate complex, 10 mg
  MCM 2049
- ▶✪ J0289 Injection, amphotericin B liposome, 10 mg
  MCM 2049
- ✪ J0290 Injection, ampicillin sodium, 500 mg
  MCM 2049
- ✪ J0295 Injection, ampicillin sodium/sulbactam sodium, per 1.5 gm
  MCM 2049
- ✪ J0300 Injection, amobarbital, up to 125 mg
  MCM 2049
- ✪ J0330 Injection, succinylcholine chloride, up to 20 mg
  MCM 2049
- J0340 Deleted 01/01/02
- ✪ J0350 Injection, anistreplase, per 30 units
  MCM 2049
- ✪ J0360 Injection, hydralazine HCl, up to 20 mg
  MCM 2049
- ✪ J0380 Injection, metaraminol bitartrate, per 10 mg
  MCM 2049
- ✪ J0390 Injection, chloroquine HCl, up to 250 mg
  MCM 2049
- ✪ J0395 Injection, arbutamine HCl, 1 mg
  MCM 2049
- J0400 Deleted 01/01/02
- ✪ J0456 Injection, azithromycin, 500 mg
  MCM 2049.5
- ✪ J0460 Injection, atropine sulfate, up to 0.3 mg
  MCM 2049
- ✪ J0470 Injection, dimercaprol, per 100 mg
  MCM 2049
- ✪ J0475 Injection, baclofen, 10 mg
  MCM 2049
- ✪ J0476 Injection, baclofen 50 mcg for intrathecal trial
  MCM 2049
- ✪ J0500 Injection, dicyclomine HCl, up to 20 mg
  MCM 2049
- J0510 Deleted 01/01/02
- ✪ J0515 Injection, benztropine mesylate, per 1 mg
  MCM 2049
- ✪ J0520 Injection, bethanechol chloride, myotonachol or urecholine, up to 5 mg
  MCM 2049
- ✪ J0530 Injection, penicillin G benzathine and penicillin G procaine, up to 600,000 units
  MCM 2049
- ✪ J0540 Injection, penicillin G benzathine and penicillin G procaine, up to 1,200,000 units
  MCM 2049
- ✪ J0550 Injection, penicillin G benzathine and penicillin G procaine, up to 2,400,000 units
  MCM 2049
- ✪ J0560 Injection, penicillin G benzathine, up to 600,000 units
  MCM 2049
- ✪ J0570 Injection, penicillin G benzathine, up to 1,200,000 units
  MCM 2049
- ✪ J0580 Injection, penicillin G benzathine, up to 2,400,000 units
  MCM 2049
- ✪ J0585 Botulinum toxin type A, per unit
  MCM 2049
- ✪ J0587 Botulinum toxin type B, per 100 units
- J0590 Deleted 01/01/02
- ▶✪ J0592 Injection, buprenorphine hydrochloride, 0.1 mg
  MCM 2049
- ✪ J0600 Injection, edetate calcium disodium, up to 1000 mg
  MCM 2049
- ✪ J0610 Injection, calcium gluconate, per 10 cc
  MCM 2049
- ✪ J0620 Injection, calcium glycerophosphate and calcium lactate, per 10 cc
  MCM 2049
- ✪ J0630 Injection, calcitonin (salmon), up to 400 units
  MCM 2049
- J0635 Deleted 12/31/02

▶✪ J0636 Injection, calcitriol, 0.1 mcg
MCM 2049

▶* J0637 Injection, caspofungin acetate, 5 mg

✪ J0640 Injection, leucovorin calcium, per 50 mg
MCM 2049

✪ J0670 Injection, mepivacaine HCl, per 10 cc
MCM 2049

✪ J0690 Injection, cefazolin sodium, 500 mg
MCM 2049

J0690 Injection, cefepime HCl, 500 mg

* J0692 Injection, cefepime HCl, 500 mg

✪ J0694 Injection, cefoxitin sodium, 1 gm
MCM 2049, Cross Reference Q0090

J0695 Deleted 01/01/02

✪ J0696 Injection, ceftriaxone sodium, per 250 mg
MCM 2049

✪ J0697 Injection, sterile cefuroxime sodium, per 750 mg
MCM 2049

✪ J0698 Injection, cefotaxime sodium, per gm
MCM 2049

✪ J0702 Injection, betamethasone acetate and betamethasone sodium phosphate, per 3 mg
MCM 2049

✪ J0704 Injection, betamethasone sodium phosphate, per 4 mg
MCM 2049

* J0706 Injection, caffeine citrate, 5 mg

✪ J0710 Injection, cephapirin sodium, up to 1 gm
MCM 2049

✪ J0713 Injection, ceftazidime, per 500 mg
MCM 2049

✪ J0715 Injection, ceftizoxime sodium, per 500 mg
MCM 2049

✪ J0720 Injection, chloramphenicol sodium succinate, up to 1 gm
MCM 2049

✪ J0725 Injection, chorionic gonadotropin, per 1,000 USP units
MCM 2049

J0730 Deleted 01/01/02

✪ J0735 Injection, clonidine HCl, 1 mg
MCM 2049

✪ J0740 Injection, cidofovir, 375 mg
MCM 2049

✪ J0743 Injection, cilastatin sodium; imipenem, per 250 mg
MCM 2049

* J0744 Injection, ciprofloxacin for IV infusion, 200 mg

✪ J0745 Injection, codeine phosphate, per 30 mg
MCM 2049

✪ J0760 Injection, colchicine, per 1 mg
MCM 2049

✪ J0770 Injection, colistimethate sodium, up to 150 mg
MCM 2049

✪ J0780 Injection, prochlorperazine, up to 10 mg
MCM 2049

✪ J0800 Injection, corticotropin, up to 40 units
MCM 2049

J0810 Deleted 01/01/02

✪ J0835 Injection, cosyntropin, per 0.25 mg
MCM 2049

✪ J0850 Injection, cytomegalovirus immune globulin IV (human), per vial
MCM 2049

▶* J0880 Injection, darbepoetin alfa, 5 mcg

✪ J0895 Injection, deferoxamine mesylate, 500 mg
MCM 2049, Cross Reference Q0087

✪ J0900 Injection, testosterone enanthate and estradiol valerate, up to 1 cc
MCM 2049

✪ J0945 Injection, brompheniramine maleate, per 10 mg
MCM 2049

✪ J0970 Injection, estradiol valerate, up to 40 mg
MCM 2049

✪ J1000 Injection, depo-estradiol cypionate, up to 5 mg
MCM 2049

✪ J1020 Injection, methylprednisolone acetate, 20 mg
MCM 2049

✪ J1030 Injection, methylprednisolone acetate, 40 mg
MCM 2049

✪ J1040 Injection, methylprednisolone acetate, 80 mg
MCM 2049

J1050 Deleted 12/31/02

▶✪ J1051 Injection, medroxyprogesterone acetate, 50 mg
MCM 2049

◆ J1055 Injection, medroxyprogesterone acetate for contraceptive use, 150 mg
Medicare Statute 1862A1

* J1056 Injection, medroxyprogesterone acetate/estradiol cypionate, 5 mg/ 25 mg

✪ J1060 Injection, testosterone cypionate and estradiol cypionate, up to 1 cc
MCM 2049

✪ J1070 Injection, testosterone cypionate, up to 100 mg
MCM 2049

✪ J1080 Injection, testosterone cypionate, 1 cc, 200 mg
MCM 2049

J1090 Deleted 01/01/02

▶✪ J1094 Injection, dexamethasone acetate, 1 mg
MCM 2049

J1095 Deleted 12/31/02

✪ J1100 Injection, dexamethasone sodium phosphate, 1 mg
MCM 2049

✪	J1110	Injection, dihydroergotamine mesylate, per 1 mg MCM 2049
✪	J1120	Injection, acetazolamide sodium, up to 500 mg MCM 2049
✪	J1160	Injection, digoxin, up to 0.5 mg MCM 2049
✪	J1165	Injection, phenytoin sodium, per 50 mg MCM 2049
✪	J1170	Injection, hydromorphone, up to 4 mg MCM 2049
✪	J1180	Injection, dyphylline, up to 500 mg MCM 2049
✪	J1190	Injection, dexrazoxane HCl, per 250 mg MCM 2049
✪	J1200	Injection, diphenhydramine HCl, up to 50 mg MCM 2049
✪	J1205	Injection, chlorothiazide sodium, per 500 mg MCM 2049
✪	J1212	Injection, dimethyl sulfoxide, DMSO, 50%, 50 cc MCM 2049, CIM 45-23
✪	J1230	Injection, methadone HCl, up to 10 mg MCM 2049
✪	J1240	Injection, dimenhydrinate, up to 50 mg MCM 2049
✪	J1245	Injection, dipyridamole, per 10 mg MCM 2049, MCM 15030
✪	J1250	Injection, dobutamine HCl, per 250 mg MCM 2049
✪	J1260	Injection, dolasetron mesylate, 10 mg MCM 2049
*	J1270	Injection, doxercalciferol, 1 mcg
✪	J1320	Injection, amitriptyline HCl, up to 20 mg MCM 2049
✪	J1325	Injection, epoprostenol, 0.5 mg MCM 2049
✪	J1327	Injection, eptifibatide, 5 mg MCM 2049
✪	J1330	Injection, ergonovine maleate, up to 0.2 mg MCM 2049
	J1362	Deleted 01/01/02
✪	J1364	Injection, erythromycin lactobionate, per 500 mg MCM 2049
✪	J1380	Injection, estradiol valerate, up to 10 mg MCM 2049
✪	J1390	Injection, estradiol valerate, up to 20 mg MCM 2049
✪	J1410	Injection, estrogen conjugated, per 25 mg MCM 2049
✪	J1435	Injection, estrone, per 1 mg MCM 2049
✪	J1436	Injection, etidronate disodium, per 300 mg MCM 2049
✪	J1438	Injection, etanercept, 25 mg (Code may be used for Medicare when drug administered under the direct supervision of a physician, not for use when drug is self-administered.)
✪	J1440	Injection, filgrastim (G-CSF), 300 mcg MCM 2049
✪	J1441	Injection, filgrastim (G-CSF), 480 mcg MCM 2049
✪	J1450	Injection, fluconazole, 200 mg MCM 2049.5
✪	J1452	Injection, fomivirsen sodium, intraocular, 1.65 mg MCM 2049.3
✪	J1455	Injection, foscarnet sodium, per 1000 mg MCM 2049
✪	J1460	Injection, gamma globulin, intramuscular, 1 cc MCM 2049
✪	J1470	Injection, gamma globulin, intramuscular, 2 cc MCM 2049
✪	J1480	Injection, gamma globulin, intramuscular, 3 cc MCM 2049
✪	J1490	Injection, gamma globulin, intramuscular, 4 cc MCM 2049
✪	J1500	Injection, gamma globulin, intramuscular, 5 cc MCM 2049
✪	J1510	Injection, gamma globulin, intramuscular, 6 cc MCM 2049
✪	J1520	Injection, gamma globulin, intramuscular, 7 cc MCM 2049
✪	J1530	Injection, gamma globulin, intramuscular, 8 cc MCM 2049
✪	J1540	Injection, gamma globulin, intramuscular, 9 cc MCM 2049
✪	J1550	Injection, gamma globulin, intramuscular, 10 cc MCM 2049
✪	J1560	Injection, gamma globulin, intramuscular, over 10 cc MCM 2049
	J1561	Deleted 12/31/02
	J1562	Deleted 01/01/01
✪	J1563	Injection, immune globulin, IV, 1 gm MCM 2049
▶ ✪	J1564	Injection, immune globulin, 10 mg MCM 2049

✪ J1565 Injection, respiratory syncytial virus immune globulin, IV, 50 mg
MCM 2049

✪ J1570 Injection, ganciclovir sodium, 500 mg
MCM 2049

✪ J1580 Injection, Garamycin, gentamicin, up to 80 mg
MCM 2049

✻ J1590 Injection, gatifloxacin, 10 mg

✪ J1600 Injection, gold sodium thiomalate, up to 50 mg
MCM 2049

✪ J1610 Injection, glucagon HCl, per 1 mg
MCM 2049

✪ J1620 Injection, gonadorelin HCl, per 100 mcg
MCM 2049

✪ J1626 Injection, granisetron HCl, 100 mcg
MCM 2049

✪ J1630 Injection, haloperidol, up to 5 mg
MCM 2049

✪ J1631 Injection, haloperidol decanoate, per 50 mg
MCM 2049

✪ J1642 Injection, heparin sodium, (heparin lock flush), per 10 units
MCM 2049

✪ J1644 Injection, heparin sodium, per 1000 units
MCM 2049

✪ J1645 Injection, dalteparin sodium, per 2500 IU
MCM 2049

✪ J1650 Injection, enoxaparin sodium, 10 mg
MCM 2049

✪ J1652 Injection, fondaparinux sodium, 0.5 mg
MCM 2049

✻ J1655 Injection, tinzaparin sodium 1000 IU

✪ J1670 Injection, tetanus immune globulin (human), up to 250 units
MCM 2049

J1690 Deleted 01/01/02

✪ J1700 Injection, hydrocortisone acetate, up to 25 mg
MCM 2049

✪ J1710 Injection, hydrocortisone sodium phosphate, up to 50 mg
MCM 2049

✪ J1720 Injection, hydrocortisone sodium succinate, up to 100 mg
MCM 2049

✪ J1730 Injection, diazoxide, up to 300 mg
MCM 2049

J1739 Deleted 01/01/02

J1741 Deleted 01/01/02

✪ J1742 Injection, ibutilide fumarate, 1 mg
MCM 2049

✪ J1745 Injection, infliximab, 10 mg
MCM 2049

✪ J1750 Injection, iron dextran, 50 mg
MCM 2049.5

J1755 Deleted 12/31/02

▶✻ J1756 Injection, iron sucrose, 1 mg

✪ J1785 Injection, imiglucerase, per unit
MCM 2049

✪ J1790 Injection, droperidol, up to 5 mg
MCM 2049

✪ J1800 Injection, propranolol HCl, up to 1 mg
MCM 2049

✪ J1810 Injection, droperidol and fentanyl citrate, up to 2 cc ampule
MCM 2049

▶✪ J1815 Injection, insulin, per 5 units
MCM 2049, CIM 60-14

▶✻ J1817 Insulin for administration through DME (i.e., insulin pump) per 50 units

J1820 Deleted 12/31/02, Cross Reference J1815

➠✪ J1825 Injection, interferon beta-1a, 33 mcg
MCM 2049

✪ J1830 Injection interferon beta-1b, per 0.25 mg (Code may be used for Medicare when drug administered under the direct supervision of a physician, not for use when drug is self-administered.)
MCM 2049

✻ J1835 Injection, itraconazole

✪ J1840 Injection, kanamycin sulfate, up to 500 mg
MCM 2049

✪ J1850 Injection, kanamycin sulfate, up to 75 mg
MCM 2049

✪ J1885 Injection, ketorolac tromethamine, per 15 mg
MCM 2049

✪ J1890 Injection, cephalothin sodium, up to 1 gm
MCM 2049

✪ J1910 Injection, Kutapressin, up to 2 cc
MCM 2049

J1930 Deleted 01/01/02

✪ J1940 Injection, furosemide, up to 20 mg
MCM 2049

✪ J1950 Injection, leuprolide acetate (for depot suspension), per 3.75 mg
MCM 2049

✪ J1955 Injection, levocarnitine, per 1 gm
MCM 2049

✪ J1956 Injection, levofloxacin, 250 mg
MCM 2049

✪ J1960 Injection, levorphanol tartrate, up to 2 mg
MCM 2049

J1970 Deleted 01/01/02

✪ J1980 Injection, hyoscyamine sulfate, up to 0.25 mg
MCM 2049

✪ J1990 Injection, chlordiazepoxide HCl, up to 100 mg
MCM 2049

✪ J2000 Injection, lidocaine HCl, 50 cc
MCM 2049

✪ J2010 Injection, lincomycin HCl, up to 300 mg
MCM 2049
✻ J2020 Injection, linezolid, 200 mg
✪ J2060 Injection, lorazepam, 2 mg
MCM 2049
✪ J2150 Injection, mannitol, 25% in 50 cc
MCM 2049
✪ J2175 Injection, meperidine HCl, per 100 mg
MCM 2049
✪ J2180 Injection, meperidine and promethazine HCl, up to 50 mg
MCM 2049
✪ J2210 Injection, methylergonovine maleate, up to 0.2 mg
MCM 2049
J2240 Deleted 01/01/02
✪ J2250 Injection, midazolam HCl, per 1 mg
MCM 2049
✪ J2260 Injection milrinone lactate, 5 mg
MCM 2049
✪ J2270 Injection, morphine sulfate, up to 10 mg
MCM 2049
✪ J2271 Injection, morphine sulfate, 100 mg
MCM 2049, CIM 60-14a
✪ J2275 Injection, morphine sulfate (preservative-free sterile solution), per 10 mg
MCM 2049, CIM 60-14b
✪ J2300 Injection, nalbuphine HCl, per 10 mg
MCM 2049
✪ J2310 Injection, naloxone HCl, per 1 mg
MCM 2049
✪ J2320 Injection, nandrolone decanoate, up to 50 mg
MCM 2049
✪ J2321 Injection, nandrolone decanoate, up to 100 mg
MCM 2049
✪ J2322 Injection, nandrolone decanoate, up to 200 mg
MCM 2049
▶✪ J2324 Injection, nesiritide, 0.5 mg
MCM 2049
J2330 Deleted 01/01/02
J2350 Deleted 01/01/02
✪ J2352 Injection, octreotide acetate, 1 mg
MCM 2049
✪ J2355 Injection, oprelvekin, 5 mg
MCM 2049
✪ J2360 Injection, orphenadrine citrate, up to 60 mg
MCM 2049
✪ J2370 Injection, phenylephrine HCl, up to 1 cc
MCM 2049
✪ J2400 Injection, chloroprocaine HCl, per 30 cc
MCM 2049
✪ J2405 Injection, ondansetron HCl, per 1 mg
MCM 2049
✪ J2410 Injection, oxymorphone HCl, up to 1 mg
MCM 2049

✪ J2430 Injection, pamidronate disodium, per 30 mg
MCM 2049
✪ J2440 Injection, papaverine HCl, up to 60 mg
MCM 2049
✪ J2460 Injection, oxytetracycline HCl, up to 50 mg
MCM 2049
J2480 Deleted 01/01/02
J2500 Deleted 12/31/02
▶✪ J2501 Injection, paricalcitol, 1 mcg
MCM 2049
✪ J2510 Injection, penicillin G procaine, aqueous, up to 600,000 units
MCM 2049
J2512 Deleted 01/01/02
✪ J2515 Injection, pentobarbital sodium, per 50 mg
MCM 2049
✪ J2540 Injection, penicillin G potassium, up to 600,000 units
MCM 2049
✪ J2543 Injection, piperacillin sodium/tazobactam sodium, 1/0.125 gm (1.125 gm)
MCM 2049
✪ J2545 Pentamidine isethionate, inhalation solution, per 300 mg, administered through a DME
MCM 2049, Cross Reference Q0077
✪ J2550 Injection, promethazine HCl, up to 50 mg
MCM 2049
✪ J2560 Injection, phenobarbital sodium, up to 120 mg
MCM 2049
✪ J2590 Injection, oxytocin, up to 10 units
MCM 2049
✪ J2597 Injection, desmopressin acetate, per 1 mcg
MCM 2049
J2640 Deleted 01/01/02
✪ J2650 Injection, prednisolone acetate, up to 1 cc
MCM 2049
✪ J2670 Injection, tolazoline HCl, up to 25 mg
MCM 2049
▶✪ J2675 Injection, progesterone, per 50 mg
MCM 2049
✪ J2680 Injection, fluphenazine decanoate, up to 25 mg
MCM 2049
✪ J2690 Injection, procainamide HCl, up to 1 gm
MCM 2049
✪ J2700 Injection, oxacillin sodium, up to 250 mg
MCM 2049
✪ J2710 Injection, neostigmine methylsulfate, up to 0.5 mg
MCM 2049

⊕ J2720 Injection, protamine sulfate, per 10 mg
MCM 2049

⊕ J2725 Injection, protirelin, per 250 mcg
MCM 2049

⊕ J2730 Injection, pralidoxime chloride, up to 1 gm
MCM 2049

⊕ J2760 Injection, phentolamine mesylate, up to 5 mg
MCM 2049

⊕ J2765 Injection, metoclopramide HCl, up to 10 mg
MCM 2049

J2770 Injection quinupristin/dalfopristin, 500 mg (150/350)
MCM 2049

⊕ J2780 Injection, ranitidine HCl, 25 mg
MCM 2049

▶⊕ J2788 Injection, Rho (d) immune globulin, human, minidose, 50 mcg
MCM 2049

➡⊕ J2790 Injection, Rho (D) immune globulin, human, full dose, 300 mcg
MCM 2049

⊕ J2792 Injection, Rho (D) immune globulin (human), IV, solvent detergent, 100 IU
MDC 2049

✻ J2795 Injection, ropivacaine HCl, 1 mg

⊕ J2800 Injection, methocarbamol, up to 10 cc
MCM 2049

⊕ J2810 Injection, theophylline, per 40 mg
MCM 2049

⊕ J2820 Injection, sargramostim (GM-CSF), 50 mcg
MCM 2049

J2860 Deleted 01/01/02

⊕ J2910 Injection, aurothioglucose, up to 50 mg
MCM 2049

⊕ J2912 Injection, sodium chloride, 0.9%, per 2 cc
MCM 2049

J2915 Deleted 12/31/02

▶⊕ J2916 Injection, sodium ferric gluconate complex in sucrose injection, 12.5 mg
MCM 2049.2, MCM 2049.4

⊕ J2920 Injection, methylprednisolone sodium succinate, up to 40 mg
MCM 2049

⊕ J2930 Injection, methylprednisolone sodium succinate, up to 125 mg
MCM 2049

⊕ J2940 Injection, somatrem, 1 mg
MCM 2049, Medicare Statute 1861s2b

⊕ J2941 Injection, somatropin, 1 mg
MCM 2049, Medicare Statute 1861s2b

⊕ J2950 Injection, promazine HCl, up to 25 mg
MCM 2049

J2970 Deleted 01/01/02

⊕ J2993 Injection, reteplase, 18.1 mg
MCM 2049

⊕ J2995 Injection, streptokinase, per 250,000 IU
MCM 2049

⊕ J2997 Injection, alteplase recombinant, 1 mg
MCM 2049

⊕ J3000 Injection, streptomycin, up to 1 gm
MCM 2049

⊕ J3010 Injection, fentanyl citrate, 0.1 mg
MCM 2049

⊕ J3030 Injection, sumatriptan succinate, 6 mg (Code may be used for Medicare when drug administered under the direct supervision of a physician, not for use when drug is self-administered.)
MCM 2049

➡⊕ J3070 Injection, pentazocine 30 mg
MCM 2049

J3080 Deleted 01/01/02

✻ J3100 Injection, tenecteplase, 50 mg

⊕ J3105 Injection, terbutaline sulfate, up to 1 mg
MCM 2049

⊕ J3120 Injection, testosterone enanthate, up to 100 mg
MCM 2049

⊕ J3130 Injection, testosterone enanthate, up to 200 mg
MCM 2049

➡⊕ J3140 Injection, testosterone suspension, up to 50 mg provided in 1.1 mg vial
MCM 2049

⊕ J3150 Injection, testosterone propionate, up to 100 mg
MCM 2049

⊕ J3230 Injection, chlorpromazine HCl, up to 50 mg
MCM 2049

➡⊕ J3240 Injection, thyrotropin alfa, 0.9 mg provided in 1.1 mg vial
MCM 2049

⊕ J3245 Injection, tirofiban HCl, 12.5 mg
MCM 2049

⊕ J3250 Injection, trimethobenzamide HCl, up to 200 mg
MCM 2049

⊕ J3260 Injection, tobramycin sulfate, up to 80 mg
MCM 2049

⊕ J3265 Injection, torsemide, 10 mg/cc
MCM 2049

J3270 Deleted 01/01/02

⊕ J3280 Injection, thiethylperazine maleate, up to 10 mg
MCM 2049

⊕ J3301 Injection triamcinolone acetonide, per 10 mg
MCM 2049

⊕ J3302 Injection triamcinolone diacetate, per 5 mg
MCM 2049

⊕ J3303 Injection triamcinolone hexacetonide, per 5 mg
MCM 2049

- ✪ J3305 Injection, trimetrexate glucuronate, per 25 mg
  MCM 2049
- ✪ J3310 Injection, perphenazine, up to 5 mg
  MCM 2049
- ▶✪ J3315 Injection, triptorelin pamoate, 3.75 mg
  MCM 2049
- ✪ J3320 Injection, spectinomycin dihydrochloride, up to 2 gm
  MCM 2049
- ✪ J3350 Injection, urea, up to 40 gm
  MCM 2049
- ✪ J3360 Injection, diazepam, up to 5 mg
  MCM 2049
- ✪ J3364 Injection, urokinase, 5000 international units (IU) vial
  MCM 2049
- ✪ J3365 Injection, IV, urokinase, 250,000 IU vial
  MCM 2049, Cross Reference Q0089
- ✪ J3370 Injection, vancomycin HCl, 500 mg
  MCM 2049, CIM 60-14
- J3390 Deleted 01/01/02
- ✪ J3395 Injection, verteporfin, 15 mg
  CIM 35-100, CIM 45-30
- ✪ J3400 Injection, triflupromazine HCl, up to 20 mg
  MCM 2049
- ✪ J3410 Injection, hydroxyzine HCl, up to 25 mg
  MCM 2049
- ✪ J3420 Injection, vitamin B-12 cyanocobalamin, up to 1000 mcg
  MCM 2049, CIM 45-4
- ✪ J3430 Injection, phytonadione (vitamin K), per 1 mg
  MCM 2049
- ✪ J3450 Deleted 01/01/02
- ✪ J3470 Injection, hyaluronidase, up to 150 units
  MCM 2049
- ✪ J3475 Injection, magnesium sulfate, per 500 mg
  MCM 2049
- ✪ J3480 Injection, potassium chloride, per 2 milliequivalents (mEq)
  MCM 2049
- ✪ J3485 Injection, zidovudine, 10 mg
  MCM 2049
- ▶✻ J3487 Injection, zoledronic acid, 1 mg
- ✪ J3490 Unclassified drugs
  MCM 2049
- ◆ J3520 Edetate disodium, per 150 mg
  CIM 35-64, CIM 45-20
- ✪ J3530 Nasal vaccine inhalation
  MCM 2049
- ◆ J3535 Drug administered through a metered dose inhaler
  MCM 2050.5
- ◆ J3570 Laetrile, amygdalin, vitamin B-17
  CIM 45-10
- ▶✻ J3590 Unclassified biologics

Miscellaneous Drugs and Solutions

- ✪ J7030 Infusion, normal saline solution, 1000 cc
  MCM 2049
- ✪ J7040 Infusion, normal saline solution, sterile (500 cc = 1 unit)
  MCM 2049
- ✪ J7042 5% dextrose/normal saline (500 cc = 1 unit)
  MCM 2049
- ✪ J7050 Infusion, normal saline solution, 250 cc
  MCM 2049
- ✪ J7051 Sterile saline or water, up to 5 cc
  MCM 2049
- ✪ J7060 5% dextrose/water (500 cc = 1 unit)
  MCM 2049
- ✪ J7070 Infusion, D-5-W, 1000 cc
  MCM 2049
- ✪ J7100 Infusion, dextran 40, 500 cc
  MCM 2049
- ✪ J7110 Infusion, dextran 75, 500 cc
  MCM 2049
- ✪ J7120 Ringer's lactate infusion, up to 1000 cc
  MCM 2049
- ✪ J7130 Hypertonic saline solution, 50 or 100 mEq, 20 cc vial
  MCM 2049
- ✪ J7190 Factor VIII, anti-hemophilic factor (human), per IU
  MCM 2049
- ✪ J7191 Factor VIII, anti-hemophilic factor (porcine), per IU
  MCM 2049
- ✪ J7192 Factor VIII (anti-hemophilic factor recombinant), per IU
  MCM 2049
- ✪ J7193 Factor IX (anti-hemophilic factor, purified, non-recombinant) per IU
  MCM 2049
- ✪ J7194 Factor IX, complex, per IU
  MCM 2049
- ✪ J7195 Factor IX (anti-hemophilic factor, recombinant) per IU
  MCM 2049
- J7196 Deleted 01/01/00
- ✪ J7197 Anti-thrombin III (human), per IU
  MCM 2049
- ✪ J7198 Anti-inhibitor, per IU
  MCM 2049, CIM 45-24
- ✪ J7199 Hemophilia clotting factor, not otherwise classified
  MCM 2049, CIM 45-24
- ◆ J7300 Intrauterine copper contraceptive
  Medicare Statute 1862A1
- ◆ J7302 Levonorgestrel-releasing intrauterine contraceptive system, 52 mg
  Medicare Statute 1862a1

✻ J7308 Aminolevulinic acid HCL for topical administration, 20%, single unit dosage form (354 mg)

⊕ J7310 Ganciclovir, 4.5 mg, long-acting implant
MCM 2049

J7315 Deleted 01/01/02

J7316 Deleted 12/31/02, Cross Reference J7317

▶✻ J7317 Sodium hyaluronate, per 20 to 25 mg dose for intra-articular injection

✻ J7320 Hylan G-F 20, 16 mg, for intra-articular injection

✻ J7330 Autologous cultured chondrocytes, implant

➠✻ J7340 Dermal and epidermal, tissue of human origin, with or without bioengineered of processed elements, with metabolically active elements, per square centimeter

▶✻ J7342 Dermal tissue, of human origin, with or without other bioengineered or processed elements, with metabolically active elements, per square centimeter

▶✻ J7350 Dermal tissue of human origin, injectable, with or without other bioengineered or processed elements, but without metabolized active elements, per 10 mg

Immunosuppressive Drugs (Includes Non-injectibles)

⊕ J7500 Azathioprine, oral, 50 mg
MCM 2049.5

⊕ J7501 Azathioprine, parenteral, 100 mg
MCM 2049

⊕ J7502 Cyclosporine, oral, 100 mg
MCM 2049.5

⊕ J7504 Lymphocyte immune globulin, anti-thymocyte globulin, equine, parenteral 250 mg
MCM 2049, CIM 45-22

⊕ J7505 Muromonab-CD3, parenteral, 5 mg
MCM 2049

⊕ J7506 Prednisone, oral, per 5 mg
MCM 2049.5

⊕ J7507 Tacrolimus, oral, per 1 mg
MCM 2049.5

⊕ J7508 Tacrolimus, oral, per 5 mg
MCM 2049.5

⊕ J7509 Methylprednisolone oral, per 4 mg
MCM 2049.5

⊕ J7510 Prednisolone oral, per 5 mg
MCM 2049.5

✻ J7511 Lymphocyte immune globulin, anti-thymocyte globulin, rabbit, parenteral, 25 mg

⊕ J7513 Daclizumab, parenteral, 25 mg
MCM 2049.5

✻ J7515 Cyclosporine, oral, 25 mg

✻ J7516 Cyclosporin, parenteral, 250 mg

✻ J7517 Mycophenolate mofetil, oral, 250 mg

⊕ J7520 Sirolimus, oral, 1 mg
MCM 2049.5

⊕ J7525 Tacrolimus, parenteral, 5 mg
MCM 2049.5

⊕ J7599 Immunosuppressive drug, not otherwise classified
MCM 2049.5

Inhalation Solutions

⊕ J7608 Acetylcysteine, inhalation solution administered through DME, unit dose form, per gm
MCM 2100.5

⊕ J7618 Albuterol, all formulations including separated isomers, inhalation solution administered through DME, concentrated form, per 1 mg (albuterol) or per 0.5 mg (levalbuterol)
MCM 2100.5

⊕ J7619 Albuterol, all formulations including separated isomers, inhalation solution administered through DME, unit dose form, per 1 mg (albuterol) or per 0.5 mg (levalbuterol)
MCM 2100.5

✻ J7622 Beclomethasone, inhalation solution administered through DME, unit dose form, per mg

✻ J7624 Betamethasone, inhalation solution administered through DME, unit dose form, per mg

➠✻ J7626 Budesonide inhalation solution, administered through DME, unit dose form, 0.25 to 0.50 mg

⊕ J7628 Bitolterol mesylate, inhalation solution administered through DME, concentrated form, per mg
MCM 2100.5

⊕ J7629 Bitolterol mesylate, inhalation solution administered through DME, unit dose form, per mg
MCM 2100.5

⊕ J7631 Cromolyn sodium, inhalation solution administered through DME, unit dose form, per 10 mg
MCM 2100.5

▶✻ J7633 Budesonide, inhalation solution administered through DME, concentrated form, per 0.25 milligram

⊕ J7635 Atropine, inhalation solution administered through DME, concentrated form, per mg
MCM 2100.5

- ❂ J7636 Atropine, inhalation solution administered through DME, unit dose form, per mg
  MCM 2100.5
- ❂ J7637 Dexamethasone, inhalation solution administered through DME, concentrated form, per mg
  MCM 2100.5
- ❂ J7638 Dexamethasone, inhalation solution administered through DME, unit dose form, per mg
  MCM 2100.5
- ❂ J7639 Dornase alpha, inhalation solution administered through DME, unit dose form, per mg
  MCM 2100.5
- * J7641 Flunisolide, inhalation solution administered through DME, unit dose, per mg
- ❂ J7642 Glycopyrrolate, inhalation solution administered through DME, concentrated form, per mg
  MCM 2100.5
- ❂ J7643 Glycopyrrolate, inhalation solution administered through DME, unit dose form, per mg
  MCM 2100.5
- ❂ J7644 Ipratropium bromide, inhalation solution administered through DME, unit dose form, per mg
  MCM 2100.5
- ❂ J7648 Isoetharine HCl, inhalation solution administered through DME, concentrated form, per mg
  MCM 2100.5
- ❂ J7649 Isoetharine HCl, inhalation solution administered through DME, unit dose form, per mg
  MCM 2100.5
- ❂ J7658 Isoproterenol HCl, inhalation solution administered through DME, concentrated form, per mg
  MCM 2100.5
- ❂ J7659 Isoproterenol HCl, inhalation solution administered through DME, unit dose form, per mg
  MCM 2100.5
- ❂ J7668 Metaproterenol sulfate, inhalation solution administered through DME, concentrated form, per 10 mg
  MCM 2100.5
- ❂ J7669 Metaproterenol sulfate, inhalation solution administered through DME, unit dose form, per 10 mg
  MCM 2100.5
- ❂ J7680 Terbutaline sulfate, inhalation solution administered through DME, concentrated form, per mg
  MCM 2100.5
- ❂ J7681 Terbutaline sulfate, inhalation solution administered through DME, unit dose form, per mg
  MCM 2100.5
- ❂ J7682 Tobramycin, unit dose form, 300 mg, inhalation solution, administered through DME
  MCM 2100.5
- ❂ J7683 Triamcinolone, inhalation solution administered through DME, concentrated form, per mg
  MCM 2100.5
- ❂ J7684 Triamcinolone, inhalation solution administered through DME, unit dose form, per mg
  MCM 2100.5
- ❂ J7699 NOC drugs, inhalation solution administered through DME
  MCM 2100.5
- ❂ J7799 NOC drugs, other than inhalation drugs, administered through DME
  MCM 2100.5
- ◆ J8499 Prescription drug, oral, non-chemotherapeutic, NOS
  MCM 2049
- ❂ J8510 Busulfan; oral, 2 mg
  MCM 2049.5
- ❂ J8520 Capecitabine, oral, 150 mg
  MCM 2049.5
- ❂ J8521 Capecitabine, oral, 500 mg
  MCM 2049.5
- ❂ J8530 Cyclophosphamide, oral, 25 mg
  MCM 2049.5
- ❂ J8560 Etoposide, oral, 50 mg
  MCM 2049.5
- ❂ J8600 Melphalan, oral, 2 mg
  MCM 2049.5
- ❂ J8610 Methotrexate, oral, 2.5 mg
  MCM 2049.5
- ❂ J8700 Temozolomide, oral, 5 mg
  MCM 2049.5c
- ❂ J8999 Prescription drug, oral, chemotherapeutic, NOS
  MCM 2049.5

CHEMOTHERAPY DRUGS (J9000-J9999)

NOTE: The cost of the chemotherapy drug only, not to include the administration

- ❂ J9000 Doxorubicin HCl, 10 mg
  MCM 2049
- ❂ J9001 Doxorubicin HCl, all lipid formulations, 10 mg
  MCM 2049
- ▶❂ J9010 Alemtuzumab, 10 mg
  Medicare Statute 1833(t)
- ❂ J9015 Aldesleukin, per single use vial
  MCM 2049
- * J9017 Arsenic trioxide, 1 mg

⊕ J9020 Asparaginase, 10,000 units
MCM 2049

⊕ J9031 BCG (intravesical), per instillation
MCM 2049

⊕ J9040 Bleomycin sulfate, 15 units
MCM 2049

⊕ J9045 Carboplatin, 50 mg
MCM 2049

⊕ J9050 Carmustine, 100 mg
MCM 2049

⊕ J9060 Cisplatin, powder or solution, per 10 mg
MCM 2049

⊕ J9062 Cisplatin, 50 mg
MCM 2049

⊕ J9065 Injection, cladribine, per 1 mg
MCM 2049

⊕ J9070 Cyclophosphamide, 100 mg
MCM 2049

⊕ J9080 Cyclophosphamide, 200 mg
MCM 2049

⊕ J9090 Cyclophosphamide, 500 mg
MCM 2049

⊕ J9091 Cyclophosphamide, 1.0 gm
MCM 2049

⊕ J9092 Cyclophosphamide, 2.0 gm
MCM 2049

⊕ J9093 Cyclophosphamide, lyophilized, 100 mg
MCM 2049

⊕ J9094 Cyclophosphamide, lyophilized, 200 mg
MCM 2049

⊕ J9095 Cyclophosphamide, lyophilized, 500 mg
MCM 2049

⊕ J9096 Cyclophosphamide, lyophilized, 1.0 gm
MCM 2049

⊕ J9097 Cyclophosphamide, lyophilized, 2.0 gm
MCM 2049

⊕ J9100 Cytarabine 100 mg
MCM 2049

⊕ J9110 Cytarabine, 500 mg
MCM 2049

⊕ J9120 Dactinomycin, 0.5 mg
MCM 2049

⊕ J9130 Dacarbazine, 100 mg
MCM 2049

⊕ J9140 Dacarbazine, 200 mg
MCM 2049

⊕ J9150 Daunorubicin, HCl, 10 mg
MCM 2049

⊕ J9151 Daunorubicin citrate liposomal formulation, 10 mg
MCM 2049

* J9160 Denileukin diftitox, 300 mcg

⊕ J9165 Diethylstilbestrol diphosphate, 250 mg
MCM 2049

⊕ J9170 Docetaxel, 20 mg
MCM 2049

⊕ J9180 Epirubicin HCl, 50 mg
MCM 2049

⊕ J9181 Etoposide, 10 mg
MCM 2049

⊕ J9182 Etoposide, 100 mg
MCM 2049

⊕ J9185 Fludarabine phosphate, 50 mg
MCM 2049

⊕ J9190 Fluorouracil, 500 mg
MCM 2049

⊕ J9200 Floxuridine, 500 mg
MCM 2049

⊕ J9201 Gemcitabine HCl, 200 mg
MCM 2049

⊕ J9202 Goserelin acetate implant, per 3.6 mg
MCM 2049

⊕ J9206 Irinotecan, 20 mg
MCM 2049

⊕ J9208 Ifosfamide, 1 gm
MCM 2049

⊕ J9209 Mesna, 200 mg
MCM 2049

⊕ J9211 Idarubicin HCl, 5 mg
MCM 2049

⊕ J9212 Injection, interferon alfacon-1, recombinant, 1 mcg
MCM 2049

⊕ J9213 Interferon, alfa-2a, recombinant, 3 million units
MCM 2049

⊕ J9214 Interferon, alfa-2b, recombinant, 1 million units
MCM 2049

⊕ J9215 Interferon, alfa-n3 (human leukocyte derived), 250,000 IU
MCM 2049

⊕ J9216 Interferon, gamma-1B, 3 million units
MCM 2049

⊕ J9217 Leuprolide acetate (for depot suspension), 7.5 mg
MCM 2049

⊕ J9218 Leuprolide acetate, per 1 mg
MCM 2049

⊕ J9219 Leuprolide acetate implant, 65 mg
MCM 2049

⊕ J9230 Mechlorethamine HCl (nitrogen mustard), 10 mg
MCM 2049

⊕ J9245 Injection, melphalan HCl, 50 mg
MCM 2049

⊕ J9250 Methotrexate sodium, 5 mg
MCM 2049

⊕ J9260 Methotrexate sodium, 50 mg
MCM 2049

⊕ J9265 Paclitaxel, 30 mg
MCM 2049

⊕ J9266 Pegaspargase, per single dose vial
MCM 2049

⊕ J9268 Pentostatin, per 10 mg
MCM 2049

⊕ J9270 Plicamycin, 2.5 mg
MCM 2049

⊕ J9280 Mitomycin, 5 mg
MCM 2049

⊕ J9290 Mitomycin, 20 mg
MCM 2049

⊕ J9291 Mitomycin, 40 mg
MCM 2049

⊕ J9293 Injection, mitoxantrone HCl, per 5 mg
MCM 2049

* J9300 Gemtuzumab ozogamicin, 5 mg, not for use for Gemzer

⊕ J9310 Rituximab, 100 mg
MCM 2049

⊕ J9320 Streptozocin, 1 gm
MCM 2049

⊕ J9340 Thiotepa, 15 mg
MCM 2049

⊕ J9350 Topotecan, 4 mg
MCM 2049

* J9355 Trastuzumab, 10 mg

⊕ J9357 Valrubicin, intravesical, 200 mg
MCM 2049

⊕ J9360 Vinblastine sulfate, 1 mg
MCM 2049

⊕ J9370 Vincristine sulfate, 1 mg
MCM 2049

⊕ J9375 Vincristine sulfate, 2 mg
MCM 2049

⊕ J9380 Vincristine sulfate, 5 mg
MCM 2049

⊕ J9390 Vinorelbine tartrate, per 10 mg
MCM 2049

⊕ J9600 Porfimer sodium, 75 mg
MCM 2049

⊕ J9999 Not otherwise classified, anti-neoplastic drugs
MCM 2049, CIM 45-16

K CODES FOR DURABLE MEDICAL EQUIPMENT: TEMPORARY CODES (K0000-K9999)

Wheelchairs

NOTE: This section contains national codes assigned by CMS on a temporary basis and for the exclusive use of the durable medical equipment regional carriers (DMERC).

* K0001 Standard wheelchair
* K0002 Standard hemi (low seat) wheelchair
* K0003 Lightweight wheelchair
* K0004 High-strength, lightweight wheelchair
* K0005 Ultra lightweight wheelchair
* K0006 Heavy-duty wheelchair
* K0007 Extra heavy-duty wheelchair
* K0009 Other manual wheelchair/base
* K0010 Standard-weight frame motorized/power wheelchair
* K0011 Standard-weight frame motorized/power wheelchair, with programmable control parameters for speed adjustment, tremor dampening, acceleration control and braking
* K0012 Lightweight portable motorized/power wheelchair
* K0014 Other motorized/power wheelchair base
* K0015 Detachable, non-adjustable height arm rest, each
* K0016 Detachable, adjustable height arm rest, complete assembly, each
* K0017 Detachable, adjustable height arm rest, base, each
* K0018 Detachable, adjustable height arm rest, upper portion, each
* K0019 Arm pad, each
* K0020 Fixed, adjustable height arm rest, pair

K0021 Deleted 12/31/02, Cross Reference E0971

* K0022 Reinforced back upholstery
* K0023 Solid back insert, planar back, single density foam, attached with straps
* K0024 Solid back insert, planar back, single density form, with adjustable hook-on hardware
* K0025 Hook-on headrest extension
* K0026 Back upholstery for ultra lightweight or high-strength lightweight wheelchair
* K0027 Back upholstery for wheelchair type other than ultra lightweight or high-strength lightweight wheelchair
* K0028 Manual, fully reclining back
* K0029 Reinforced seat upholstery
* K0030 Solid seat insert, planar seat, single density foam
* K0031 Safety belt/pelvic strap, each
* K0032 Seat upholstery for ultra lightweight or high-strength lightweight wheelchair
* K0033 Seat upholstery for wheelchair type other than ultra lightweight or high-strength lightweight wheelchair

K0034 Deleted 12/31/02, Cross Reference E0951

* K0035 Heel loop with ankle strap, each
* K0036 Toe loop, each
* K0037 High mount flip-up footrest, each
* K0038 Leg strap, each
* K0039 Leg strap, H-style, each
* K0040 Adjustable angle footplate, each
* K0041 Large size footplate, each
* K0042 Standard size footplate, each
* K0043 Foot rest, lower extension tube, each
* K0044 Foot rest, upper hanger bracket, each
* K0045 Foot rest, complete assembly
* K0046 Elevating leg rests, lower extension tube, each
* K0047 Elevating leg rests, upper hanger bracket, each
* K0048 Elevating leg rests, complete assembly

∗ K0049 Calf pad, each
∗ K0050 Ratchet assembly
∗ K0051 Cam release assembly, footrest or leg rests, each
∗ K0052 Swing-away, detachable foot rests, each
∗ K0053 Elevating foot rests, articulating (telescoping), each
∗ K0054 Seat width of 10″, 11″, 12″, 15″, 17″, or 20″ for a high-strength, lightweight or ultra lightweight wheelchair
∗ K0055 Seat depth of 15″, 17″, or 18″ for a high-strength, lightweight or ultra lightweight wheelchair
∗ K0056 Seat height less than 17″ or equal to or greater than 21″ for a high-strength, lightweight, or ultra lightweight wheelchair
∗ K0057 Seat width 19″ or 20″ for heavy duty or extra heavy duty chair
∗ K0058 Seat depth 17″ or 18″ for motorized/power wheelchair
∗ K0059 Plastic coated hand rim, each
∗ K0060 Steel hand rim, each
∗ K0061 Aluminum hand rim, each
∗ K0062 Hand rim with 8 to 10 vertical or oblique projections, each
∗ K0063 Hand rim with 12 to 16 vertical or oblique projections, each
∗ K0064 Zero pressure tube (flat-free inserts), any size, each
∗ K0065 Spoke protectors, each
∗ K0066 Solid tire, any size, each
∗ K0067 Pneumatic tire, any size, each
∗ K0068 Pneumatic tire tube, each
∗ K0069 Rear wheel assembly, complete, with solid tire, spokes or molded, each
∗ K0070 Rear wheel assembly, complete, with pneumatic tire, spokes or molded, each
∗ K0071 Front caster assembly, complete, with pneumatic tire, each
∗ K0072 Front caster assembly, complete, with semi-pneumatic tire, each
∗ K0073 Caster pin lock, each
∗ K0074 Pneumatic caster tire, any size, each
∗ K0075 Semi-pneumatic caster tire, any size, each
∗ K0076 Solid caster tire, any size, each
∗ K0077 Front caster assembly, complete, with solid tire, each
∗ K0078 Pneumatic caster tire tube, each
∗ K0079 Wheel lock extension, pair
∗ K0080 Anti-rollback device, pair
∗ K0081 Wheel lock assembly, complete, each
➡ ∗ K0082 22NF non-sealed lead acid battery, each
➡ ∗ K0083 22NF sealed lead acid battery, each (e.g., gel cell, absorbed glass mat)
➡ ∗ K0084 Group 24 non-sealed lead acid battery, each
➡ ∗ K0085 Group 24 sealed lead acid battery, each (e.g., gel cell, absorbed glass mat)
➡ ∗ K0086 U-1 non-sealed lead acid battery, each
➡ ∗ K0087 U-1 sealed lead acid battery, each (e.g., gel cell, absorbed glass mat)
➡ ∗ K0088 Battery charger, single mode, for use with only one battery type, sealed or non-sealed
➡ ∗ K0089 Battery charger, dual mode, for use with either battery type, sealed or non-sealed
∗ K0090 Rear wheel tire for power wheelchair, any size, each
∗ K0091 Rear wheel tire tube other than zero pressure for power wheelchair, any size, each
∗ K0092 Rear wheel assembly for power wheelchair, complete each
∗ K0093 Rear wheel, zero pressure tire tube (flat-free insert) for power wheelchair, any size, each
∗ K0094 Wheel tire for power base, any size, each
∗ K0095 Wheel tire tube other than zero pressure for each base, any size, each
∗ K0096 Wheel assembly for power base, complete, each
∗ K0097 Wheel zero pressure tire tube (flat-free insert) for power base, any size, each
∗ K0098 Drive belt for power wheelchair
∗ K0099 Front caster for power wheelchair, each
∗ K0100 Wheelchair adapter for amputee, pair (device used to compensate for transfer of weight due to lost limbs to maintain proper balance)
K0101 Deleted 12/31/02, Cross Reference E0958
∗ K0102 Crutch and cane holder, each
∗ K0103 Transfer board, less than 25″
∗ K0104 Cylinder tank carrier, each
∗ K0105 IV hanger, each
∗ K0106 Arm trough, each
∗ K0107 Wheelchair tray
∗ K0108 Wheelchair component or accessory, not otherwise specified

Spinal Orthotics

∗ K0112 Trunk support device, vest type, with inner frame, prefabricated
∗ K0113 Trunk support device, vest type, without inner frame, prefabricated
∗ K0114 Back support system for use with a wheelchair, with inner frame, prefabricated
∗ K0115 Seating system, back module, posterior-lateral control, with or without lateral supports, custom fabricated for attachment to wheelchair base
∗ K0116 Seating system, combined back and seat module, custom fabricated for attachment to wheelchair base

Other

K0183 Deleted 12/31/02, Cross Reference A7034
K0184 Deleted 12/31/02, Cross Reference A7032, A7033
K0185 Deleted 12/31/02, Cross Reference A7035
K0186 Deleted 12/31/02, Cross Reference A7036
K0187 Deleted 12/31/02, Cross Reference A7037
K0188 Deleted 12/31/02, Cross Reference A7038
K0189 Deleted 12/31/02, Cross Reference A7039
✪ K0195 Elevating leg rests, pair (for use with capped rental wheelchair base)
CIM 60-9
* K0268 Humidifier, non-heated, used with positive airway pressure device
✪ K0415 Prescription antiemetic drug, oral, per 1 mg, for use in conjunction with oral anti-cancer drug, not otherwise specified
MCM 2049.5C
✪ K0416 Prescription antiemetic drug, rectal, per 1 mg, for use in conjunction with oral anti-cancer drug, not otherwise specified
MCM 2049.5C
* K0452 Wheelchair bearings, any type
✪ K0455 Infusion pump used for uninterrupted administration of epoprostenol
CIM 60-14
* K0460 Power add-on, to convert manual wheelchair to motorized wheelchair, joystick control
* K0461 Power add-on, to convert manual wheelchair to power-operated vehicle, tiller control
✪ K0462 Temporary replacement for patient owned equipment being repaired, any type
MCM 5102.3
✪ K0531 Humidifier, heated, used with positive airway pressure device
CIM 60-9
✪ K0532 Respiratory assist device, bi-level pressure capability, without backup rate feature, used with noninvasive interface such as nasal or facial mask (intermittent assist device with continuous positive airway pressure device)
CIM 60-9
✪ K0533 Respiratory assist device, bi-level pressure capability, with backup rate feature, used with noninvasive interface such as a nasal or facial mask (intermittent assist device with continuous positive airway pressure device)
CIM 60-9
✪ K0534 Respiratory assist device, bi-level pressure capability, with backup rate feature, used with invasive interface such as a tracheostomy tube (intermittent assist device with continuous positive airway pressure device)
CIM 60-9
* K0538 Negative pressure wound therapy electrical pump, stationary or portable
* K0539 Dressing set for negative pressure wound therapy electrical pump, stationary or portable, each
* K0540 Canister set for negative pressure wound therapy electrical pump, stationary or portable, each
✪ K0541 Speech generating device, digitized speech using pre-recorded messages, less than or equal to 8 minutes recording time
CIM 60-23
✪ K0542 Speech generating device, digitized speech, using pre-recorded messages, greater than 8 minutes recording time
CIM 60-23
✪ K0543 Speech generating device, synthesized speech, requiring message formulation by spelling and access by physical contact with the device
CIM 60-23
✪ K0544 Speech generating device, synthesized speech, permitting multiple methods of message formulation and multiple methods of device access
CIM 60-23
✪ K0545 Speech generating software program, for personal computer or personal digital assistant
CIM 60-23
✪ K0546 Accessory for speech generating device, mounting system
CIM 60-23
✪ K0547 Accessory for speech generating device, not otherwise classified
CIM 60-23
* K0548 Deleted 12/31/02, Cross Reference J1817
✪ K0549 Hospital bed, heavy duty, extra wide, with weight capacity greater than 350 pounds (lb), but less than or equal to 600 lb, with any type side rails, with mattress
CIM 60-18

❂ K0550 Hospital bed, extra heavy duty, extra wide, with weight capacity greater than 600 lb, with any type side rails, with mattress
CIM 60-18

K0551 Deleted 12/31/02, Cross Reference E1020

▶✻ K0556 Addition to lower extremity, below knee/above knee, custom fabricated from existing mold or prefabricated, socket insert, silicone gel, elastomeric or equal, for use with locking mechanism

▶✻ K0557 Addition to lower extremity, below knee/above knee, custom fabricated from existing mold or prefabricated, socket insert, silicone gel, elastomeric or equal, not for use with locking mechanism

▶✻ K0558 Addition to lower extremity, below knee/above knee, custom fabricated socket insert for congenital or atypical traumatic amputee, silicone gel, elastomeric or equal, for use with or without locking mechanism, initial only (for other than initial, use code K0556 or K0557)

▶✻ K0559 Addition to lower extremity, below knee/above knee, custom fabricated socket insert for other than congenital or atypical traumatic amputee, silicone gel, elastomeric or equal, for use with or without locking mechanism, initial only (for other than initial, use code K0556 or K0557)

Ostomy Supplies

K0561 Deleted 12/31/02, Cross Reference A4405

K0562 Deleted 12/31/02, Cross Reference A4406

K0563 Deleted 12/31/02, Cross Reference A4407

K0564 Deleted 12/31/02, Cross Reference A4408

K0565 Deleted 12/31/02, Cross Reference A4409

K0566 Deleted 12/31/02, Cross Reference A4410

K0567 Deleted 12/31/02

K0568 Deleted 12/31/02

K0569 Deleted 12/31/02, Cross Reference A4413

K0570 Deleted 12/31/02, Cross Reference A4414

K0571 Deleted 12/31/02, Cross Reference A4415

K0572 Deleted 12/31/02, Cross Reference A4450

K0573 Deleted 12/31/02, Cross Reference A4452

K0574 Deleted 12/31/02

K0575 Deleted 12/31/02

K0576 Deleted 12/31/02

K0577 Deleted 12/31/02

K0578 Deleted 12/31/02

K0579 Deleted 12/31/02, Cross Reference A4422

K0580 Deleted 12/31/02

▶✻ K0581 Ostomy pouch, closed, with barrier attached, with filter (1 piece), each

▶✻ K0582 Ostomy pouch, closed, with barrier attached, with built-in convexity, with filter (1 piece), each

▶✻ K0583 Ostomy pouch, closed; without barrier attached, with filter (1 piece), each

▶✻ K0584 Ostomy pouch, closed; for use on barrier with flange, with filter (2 piece), each

▶✻ K0585 Ostomy pouch, closed; for use on barrier with locking flange (2 piece), each

▶✻ K0586 Ostomy pouch, closed; for use on barrier with locking flange, with filter (2 piece), each

▶✻ K0587 Ostomy pouch, drainable, with barrier attached, with filter (1 piece), each

▶✻ K0588 Ostomy pouch, drainable; for use on barrier with flange, with filter (2 piece system), each

▶✻ K0589 Ostomy pouch, drainable; for use on barrier with locking flange (2 piece system), each

▶✻ K0590 Ostomy pouch, drainable; for use on barrier with locking flange, with filter (2 piece system), each

▶✻ K0591 Ostomy pouch, urinary, with extended wear barrier attached, with faucet-type tap with valve (1 piece), each

▶✻ K0592 Ostomy pouch, urinary, with barrier attached, with built-in convexity, with faucet-type tap with valve (1 piece), each

▶✻ K0593 Ostomy pouch, urinary, with extended wear barrier attached, with built-in convexity, with faucet-type tap with valve (1 piece), each

▶✻ K0594 Ostomy pouch, urinary; with barrier attached, with faucet-type tap with valve (1 piece), each

▶✻ K0595 Ostomy pouch, urinary; for use on barrier with flange, with faucet-type tap with valve (2 piece), each

▶✻ K0596 Ostomy pouch, urinary; for use on barrier with locking flange (2 piece), each

▶✻ K0597 Ostomy pouch, urinary; for use on barrier with locking flange, with faucet-type tap with valve (2 piece), each

ORTHOTIC PROCEDURES (L0100-L4999)

Orthotic Devices: Spinal

Cervical

* ∗ L0100 Cranial orthosis (helmet,), with or without soft interface, molded to patient model
* ∗ L0110 Cranial orthosis (helmet), with or without soft-interface, non-molded
* ∗ L0120 Cervical, flexible, non-adjustable (foam collar)
* ∗ L0130 Cervical, flexible, thermoplastic collar, molded to patient
* ∗ L0140 Cervical, semi-rigid, adjustable (plastic collar)
* ∗ L0150 Cervical, semi-rigid, adjustable molded chin cup (plastic collar with mandibular/occipital piece)
* ∗ L0160 Cervical, semi-rigid, wire frame occipital/mandibular support
* ∗ L0170 Cervical, collar, molded to patient model
* ∗ L0172 Cervical, collar, semi-rigid thermoplastic foam, two piece
* ∗ L0174 Cervical, collar, semi-rigid, thermoplastic foam, two piece with thoracic extension

Multiple Post Collar

* ∗ L0180 Cervical, multiple post collar, occipital/mandibular supports, adjustable
* ∗ L0190 Cervical, multiple post collar, occipital/mandibular supports, adjustable cervical bars (SOMI, Guilford, Taylor types)
* ∗ L0200 Cervical, multiple post collar, occipital/mandibular supports, adjustable cervical bars, and thoracic extension

Thoracic

* ∗ L0210 Thoracic, rib belt
* ∗ L0220 Thoracic, rib belt, custom fabricated

Thoracic-Lumbar-Sacral

Flexible

L0300 Deleted 12/31/02
L0310 Deleted 12/31/02
L0315 Deleted 12/31/02
L0317 Deleted 12/31/02

Anterior-Posterior Control

L0320 Deleted 12/31/02
L0321 Deleted 12/31/02
L0330 Deleted 12/31/02
L0331 Deleted 12/31/02

Anterior-Posterior-Lateral Rotary-Control

L0340 Deleted 12/31/02
L0350 Deleted 12/31/02
L0360 Deleted 12/31/02
L0370 Deleted 12/31/02
L0380 Deleted 12/31/02
L0390 Deleted 12/31/02
L0391 Deleted 12/31/02
L0400 Deleted 12/31/02
L0410 Deleted 12/31/02
L0420 Deleted 12/31/02
L0430 Deleted 12/31/02
L0440 Deleted 12/31/02

* ▶∗ L0450 TLSO, flexible, provides trunk support, upper thoracic region, produces intracavitary pressure to reduce load on the intevertebral disks with rigid stays or panel(s), includes shoulder straps and closures, prefabricated, includes fitting and adjustment
* ▶∗ L0452 TLSO TLSO, flexible, provides trunk support, upper thoracic region, produces intracavitary pressure to reduce load on the intervertebral disks with rigid stays or panel(s), includes shoulder straps and closures, custom fabricated
* ▶∗ L0454 TLSO flexible, provides trunk support, extends from sacrococcygeal junction to above t-9 vertebra, restricts gross trunk motion in the sagittal plane, produces intracavitary pressure to reduce load on the intervertebral disks with rigid stays or panel(s), includes shoulder straps and closures, prefabricated, includes fitting and adjustment
* ▶∗ L0456 TLSO, flexible, provides trunk support, thoracic region, rigid posterior panel and soft anterior apron, extends from the sacrococcygeal junction and terminates just inferior to the scapular spine, restricts gross trunk motion in the sagittal plane, produces intracavitary pressure to reduce load on the intervertebral disks, includes straps and closures, prefabricated, includes fitting and adjustment

▶✻ L0458 TLSO, triplanar control, modular segmented spinal system, two rigid plastic shells, posterior extends from the sacrococcygeal junction and terminates just inferior to the scapular spine, anterior extends from the symphysis pubis to the xiphoid, soft liner, restricts gross trunk motion in the sagittal, coronal, and transverse planes, lateral strength is provided by overlapping plastic and stabilizing closures, includes straps and closures, prefabricated, includes fitting and adjustment

▶✻ L0460 TLSO, triplanar control, modular segmented spinal system, two rigid plastic shells, posterior extends from the sacrococcygeal junction and terminates just inferior to the scapular spine, anterior extends from the symphysis pubis to the sternal notch, soft liner, restricts gross trunk motion in the sagittal, coronal, and transverse planes, lateral strength is provided by overlapping plastic and stabilizing closures, includes straps and closures, prefabricated, includes fitting and adjustment

▶✻ L0462 TLSO, triplanar control, modular segmented spinal system, three rigid plastic shells, posterior extends from the sacrococcygeal junction and terminates just inferior to the scapular spine, anterior extends from the symphysis pubis to the sternal notch, soft liner, restricts gross trunk motion in the sagittal, coronal, and transverse planes, lateral strength is provided by overlapping plastic and stabilizing closures, includes straps and closures, prefabricated, includes fitting and adjustment

▶✻ L0464 TLSO, triplanar control, modular segmented spinal system, four rigid plastic shells, posterior extends from sacrococcygeal junction and terminates just inferior to scapular spine, anterior extends from symphysis pubis to the sternal notch, soft liner, restricts gross trunk motion in sagittal, coronal, and transverse planes, lateral strength is provided by overlapping plastic and stabilizing closures, includes straps and closures, prefabricated, includes fitting and adjustment

▶✻ L0466 TLSO, sagittal control, rigid posterior frame and flexible soft anterior apron with straps, closures and padding, restricts gross trunk motion in sagittal plane, produces intracavitary pressure to reduce load on intervertebral disks, includes fitting and shaping the frame, prefabricated, includes fitting and adjustment

▶✻ L0468 TLSO, sagittal-coronal control, rigid posterior frame and flexible soft anterior apron with straps, closures and padding, extends from sacrococcygeal junction over scapulae, lateral strength provided by pelvic, thoracic, and lateral frame pieces, restricts gross trunk motion in sagittal, and coronal planes, produces intracavitary pressure to reduce load on intervertebral disks, includes fitting and shaping the frame, prefabricated, includes fitting and adjustment

▶✻ L0470 TLSO, triplanar control, rigid posterior frame and flexible soft anterior apron with straps, closures and padding, extends from sacrococcygeal junction to scapula, lateral strength provided by pelvic, thoracic, and lateral frame pieces, rotational strength provided by subclavicular extensions, restricts gross trunk motion in sagittal, coronal, and transverse planes, produces intracavitary pressure to reduce load on the intervertebral disks, includes fitting and shaping the frame, prefabricated, includes fitting and adjustment

▶✻ L0472 TLSO, triplanar control, hyperextension, rigid anterior and lateral frame extends from symphysis pubis to sternal notch with two anterior components (one pubic and one sternal), posterior and lateral pads with straps and closures, limits spinal flexion, restricts gross trunk motion in sagittal, coronal, and transverse planes, includes fitting and shaping the frame, prefabricated, includes fitting and adjustment

▶✻ L0476 TLSO, sagittal-coronal control, flexion compression jacket, two rigid plastic shells with soft liner, posterior extends from sacrococcygeal junction and terminates at or before the T-9 vertebra, anterior extends from symphysis pubis to xiphoid, usually laced together on one side, restricts gross trunk motion in sagittal and coronal planes, allows free flexion and compression of the LS region, includes straps and closures, prefabricated, includes fitting and adjustment

▶✻ L0478 TLSO, sagittal-coronal control, flexion compression jacket, two rigid plastic shells with soft liner, posterior extends from sacrococcygeal junction and terminates at or before the T-9 vertebra, anterior extends from symphysis pubis to xiphoid, usually laced together on one side, restricts gross trunk motion in sagittal and coronal planes, allows free flexion and compression of LS region, includes straps and closures, custom fabricated

▶✻ L0480 TLSO, triplanar control, one piece rigid plastic shell without interface liner, with multiple straps and closures, posterior extends from sacrococcygeal junction and terminates just inferior to scapular spine, anterior extends from symphysis pubis to sternal notch, anterior or posterior opening, restricts gross trunk motion in sagittal, coronal, and transverse planes, includes a carved plaster or Cad-Cam model, custom fabricated

▶✻ L0482 TLSO, triplanar control, one piece rigid plastic shell with interface liner, multiple straps and closures, posterior extends from sacrococcygeal junction and terminates just inferior to scapular spine, anterior extends from symphysis pubis to sternal notch, anterior or posterior opening, restricts gross trunk motion in sagittal, coronal, and transverse planes, includes a carved plaster or Cad-Cam model, custom fabricated

▶✻ L0484 TLSO, triplanar control, two piece rigid plastic shell without interface liner, with multiple straps and closures, posterior extends from sacrococcygeal junction and terminates just inferior to scapular spine, anterior extends from symphysis pubis to sternal notch, lateral strength is enhanced by overlapping plastic, restricts gross trunk motion in the sagittal, coronal, and transverse planes, includes a carved plaster or Cad-Cam model, custom fabricated

▶✻ L0486 TLSO, triplanar control, two piece rigid plastic shell with interface liner, multiple straps and closures, posterior extends from sacrococcygeal junction and terminates just inferior to scapular spine, anterior extends from symphysis pubis to sternal notch, lateral strength is enhanced by overlapping plastic, restricts gross trunk motion in the sagittal, coronal, and transverse planes, includes a carved plaster or Cad-Cam model, custom fabricated

▶✻ L0488 TLSO, triplanar control, one piece rigid plastic shell with interface liner, multiple straps and closures, posterior extends from sacrococcygeal junction and terminates just inferior to scapular spine, anterior extends from symphysis pubis to sternal notch, anterior or posterior opening, restricts gross trunk motion in sagittal, coronal, and transverse planes, prefabricated, includes fitting and adjustment

▶✻ L0490 TLSO, sagittal-coronal control, one piece rigid plastic shell, with overlapping reinforced anterior, with multiple straps and closures, posterior extends from sacrococcygeal junction and terminates at or before the T-9 vertebra, anterior extends from symphysis pubis to xiphoid, anterior opening, restricts gross trunk motion in sagittal and coronal planes, prefabricated, includes fitting and adjustment

Lumbar-Sacral

Flexible

➡✻ L0500 Lumbar-sacral orthosis (LSO), flexible, (lumbar-sacral support)

➡✻ L0510 LSO, flexible (lumbar-sacral support), custom fabricated

✻ L0515 LSO, anterior-posterior control, with rigid or semi-rigid posterior panel, prefabricated

Anterior-Posterior-Lateral Control

✻ L0520 LSO, anterior-posterior-lateral control (Knight, Wilcox types), with apron front

Anterior-Posterior Control

✻ L0530 LSO, anterior-posterior control (Macausland type), with apron front

Lumbar-Flexion

✻ L0540 LSO, lumbar flexion (Williams flexion type)

Anterior-Posterior-Lateral Control (Body Jacket)

✻ L0550 LSO, anterior-posterior-lateral control, molded to patient model

✻ L0560 LSO, anterior-posterior lateral control, molded to patient model, with interface material

✻ L0561 LSO, anterior-posterior-lateral control, with rigid or semi-rigid posterior panel, prefabricated

✻ L0565 LSO, anterior-posterior-lateral control, custom fitted

Sacroiliac

Flexible

*	L0600	Sacroiliac, flexible (sacroiliac surgical support)
*	L0610	Sacroiliac, flexible (sacroiliac surgical support), custom fabricated

Semi-rigid

*	L0620	Sacroiliac, semi-rigid (Goldthwaite, Osgood types), with apron front

Cervical-Thoracic-Lumbar-Sacral

Anterior-Posterior-Lateral Control

*	L0700	Cervical-thoracic-lumbar-sacral orthosis (CTLSO), anterior-posterior-lateral control, molded to patient model (Minerva type)
*	L0710	CTLSO, anterior-posterior-lateral control, molded to patient model, with interface material (Minerva type)

HALO Procedure

*	L0810	HALO procedure, cervical halo incorporated into jacket vest
*	L0820	HALO procedure, cervical halo incorporated into plaster body jacket
*	L0830	HALO procedure, cervical halo incorporated into Milwaukee type orthosis
*	L0860	Addition to HALO procedures, magnetic resonance image compatible system

Torso Supports

	L0900	Deleted 12/31/02, Cross Reference L0500
	L0910	Deleted 12/31/02, Cross Reference L0510
	L0920	Deleted 12/31/02, Cross Reference L0500
	L0930	Deleted 12/31/02, Cross Reference L0510
	L0940	Deleted 12/31/02, Cross Reference L0500
	L0950	Deleted 12/31/02, Cross Reference L0510
*	L0960	Torso support, postsurgical support, pads for postsurgical support

Additions to Spinal Orthoses

*	L0970	TLSO, corset front
*	L0972	LSO, corset front
*	L0974	TLSO, full corset
*	L0976	LSO, full corset
*	L0978	Axillary crutch extension
*	L0980	Peroneal straps, pair
*	L0982	Stocking supporter grips, set of four (4)
*	L0984	Protective body sock, each
	L0986	Deleted 12/31/02
*	L0999	Addition to spinal orthosis, not otherwise specified

Orthotic Devices: Scoliosis Procedures (L1000-L1499)

NOTE: Orthotic care of scoliosis differs from other orthotic care in that the treatment is more dynamic in nature and uses ongoing continual modification of the orthosis to the patient's changing condition. This coding structure uses the proper names, or eponyms, of the procedures because they have historic and universal acceptance in the profession. It should be recognized that variations to the basic procedures described by the founders/developers are accepted in various medical and orthotic practices throughout the country. All procedures include a model of patient when indicated.

Scoliosis: Cervical-Thoracic-Lumbar-Sacral (Milwaukee)

*	L1000	CTLSO (Milwaukee), inclusive of furnishing initial orthosis, including model
*	L1005	Tension-based scoliosis orthosis and accessory pads, includes fitting and adjustment
*	L1010	Addition to CTLSO or scoliosis orthosis, axilla sling

Correction Pads

*	L1020	Addition to CTLSO or scoliosis orthosis, kyphosis pad
*	L1025	Addition to CTLSO or scoliosis orthosis, kyphosis pad, floating
*	L1030	Addition to CTLSO or scoliosis orthosis, lumbar bolster pad
*	L1040	Addition to CTLSO or scoliosis orthosis, lumbar or lumbar rib pad
*	L1050	Addition to CTLSO or scoliosis orthosis, sternal pad
*	L1060	Addition to CTLSO or scoliosis orthosis, thoracic pad
*	L1070	Addition to CTLSO or scoliosis orthosis, trapezius sling

- ✱ L1080 Addition to CTLSO or scoliosis orthosis, outrigger
- ✱ L1085 Addition to CTLSO or scoliosis orthosis, outrigger, bilateral with vertical extensions
- ✱ L1090 Addition to CTLSO or scoliosis orthosis, lumbar sling
- ✱ L1100 Addition to CTLSO or scoliosis orthosis, ring flange, plastic or leather
- ✱ L1110 Addition to CTLSO or scoliosis orthosis, ring flange, plastic or leather, molded to patient model
- ✱ L1120 Addition to CTLSO, scoliosis orthosis, cover for upright, each

Scoliosis: Cervical-Thoracic-Lumbar-Sacral (Low Profile)

- ✱ L1200 TLSO, inclusive of furnishing initial orthosis only
- ✱ L1210 Addition to TLSO, (low profile), lateral thoracic extension
- ✱ L1220 Addition to TLSO (low profile), anterior thoracic extension
- ✱ L1230 Addition to TLSO (low profile), Milwaukee type superstructure
- ✱ L1240 Addition to TLSO (low profile), lumbar derotation pad
- ✱ L1250 Addition to TLSO (low profile), anterior ASIS pad
- ✱ L1260 Addition to TLSO (low profile), anterior thoracic derotation pad
- ✱ L1270 Addition to TLSO (low profile), abdominal pad
- ✱ L1280 Addition to TLSO (low profile), rib gusset (elastic), each
- ✱ L1290 Addition to TLSO (low profile), lateral trochanteric pad

Other Scoliosis Procedures

- ✱ L1300 Other scoliosis procedure, body jacket molded to patient model
- ✱ L1310 Other scoliosis procedure, postoperative body jacket
- ✱ L1499 Spinal orthosis, NOS

Scoliosis: Thoracic-Hip-Knee-Ankle

- ✱ L1500 Thoracic-hip-knee-ankle orthosis (THKAO), mobility frame (Newington, Parapodium types)
- ✱ L1510 THKAO, standing frame, with or without tray and accessories
- ✱ L1520 THKAO, swivel walker

Orthotic Devices: Lower Limb

NOTE: the procedures in L1600-L2999 are considered as *base* or *basic procedures* and may be modified by listing procedure from the Additions Sections and adding them to the base procedure.

Hip: Flexible

- ✱ L1600 Hip orthosis (HO), abduction control of hip joints, flexible, Frejka type with cover, prefabricated, includes fitting and adjustment
- ✱ L1610 HO, abduction control of hip joints, flexible, Frejka cover only, prefabricated, includes fitting and adjustment
- ✱ L1620 HO, abduction control of hip joints, flexible, Pavlik harness, prefabricated, includes fitting and adjustment
- ✱ L1630 HO, abduction control of hip joints, semi-flexible (Von Rosen type), custom fabrication
- ✱ L1640 HO, abduction control of hip joints, static, pelvic band or spreader bar, thigh cuffs, custom fabrication
- ✱ L1650 HO, abduction control of hip joints, static, adjustable, (Ilfeld type), prefabricated, includes fitting and adjustment
- ▶✱ L1652 Hip orthosis, bilateral thigh cuffs with adjustable abductor spreader bar, adult size, prefabricated, includes fitting and adjustment, any type
- ✱ L1660 HO, abduction control of hip joints, static, plastic, prefabricated, includes fitting and adjustment
- ✱ L1680 HO, abduction control of hip joints, dynamic, pelvic control, adjustable hip motion control, thigh cuffs (Rancho hip action type), custom fabrication
- ✱ L1685 HO, abduction control of hip joint, postoperative hip abduction type, custom fabricated
- ✱ L1686 HO, abduction control of hip joint, postoperative hip abduction type, prefabricated, includes fitting and adjustment
- ✱ L1690 Combination, bilateral, lumbar sacral, hip, femur orthosis providing adduction and internal rotation control, prefabricated, includes fitting and adjustment

Legg-Perthes

- ✱ L1700 Legg-Perthes orthosis (Toronto type), custom fabrication
- ✱ L1710 Legg-Perthes orthosis (Newington type), custom fabrication

✻ L1720 Legg-Perthes orthosis, trilateral (Tachdjian type), custom fabrication

✻ L1730 Legg-Perthes orthosis (Scottish Rite type), custom fabrication

✻ L1750 Legg-Perthes orthosis, Legg Perthes sling (Sam Browne type), prefabricated, includes fitting and adjustment

✻ L1755 Legg-Perthes orthosis (Patten bottom type), custom fabrication

Knee

✻ L1800 Knee orthosis (KO), elastic with stays, prefabricated, includes fitting and adjustment

✻ L1810 KO, elastic with joints, prefabricated, includes fitting and adjustment

✻ L1815 KO, elastic or other elastic type material with condylar pads, prefabricated, includes fitting and adjustment

✻ L1820 KO, elastic with condylar pads and joints, prefabricated, includes fitting and adjustment

✻ L1825 KO, elastic kneecap, prefabricated, includes fitting and adjustment

✻ L1830 KO, immobilizer, canvas longitudinal, prefabricated, includes fitting and adjustment

✻ L1832 KO, adjustable knee joints, positional orthosis, rigid support, prefabricated, includes fitting and adjustment

✻ L1834 KO, without knee joint, rigid, custom fabrication

▶✻ L1836 Knee orthosis, rigid, without joint(s), includes soft interface material, prefabricated, includes fitting and adjustment

✻ L1840 KO, derotation, medial-lateral, anterior cruciate ligament, custom fabricated

➡✻ L1843 KO, single upright, thigh and calf, with adjustable flexion and extension joint, medial-lateral and rotation control, includes varus/valgus adjustment; prefabricated, includes fitting and adjustment

➡✻ L1844 KO, single upright, thigh and calf, with adjustable flexion and extension joint, medial-lateral and rotation control, includes varus/valgus adjustment custom fabrication

✻ L1845 KO, double upright, thigh and calf, with adjustable flexion and extension joint, medial-lateral and rotation control; prefabricated, includes fitting and adjustment

✻ L1846 KO, double upright, thigh and calf, with adjustable flexion and extension joint, medial-lateral and rotation control, custom fabrication

✻ L1847 Knee orthosis, double upright with adjustable joint, with inflatable air support chambers, prefabricated, includes fitting and adjustment

✻ L1850 KO, Swedish type, prefabricated, includes fitting and adjustment

✻ L1855 KO, molded plastic, thigh and calf sections, with double upright knee joints, custom fabrication

✻ L1858 KO, molded plastic, polycentric knee joints, pneumatic knee pads (CTI), custom fabrication

✻ L1860 KO, modification of supracondylar prosthetic socket, custom fabrication (SK)

✻ L1870 KO, double upright, thigh and calf lacers, with knee joints, custom fabrication

✻ L1880 KO, double upright, non-molded thigh and calf cuffs/lacers with knee joints, custom fabrication

✻ L1885 KO, single or double upright, thigh and calf, with functional active resistance control, prefabricated, includes fitting and adjustment

Ankle-Foot

✻ L1900 Ankle-foot orthosis (AFO), spring wire, dorsiflexion assist calf band, custom fabrication

▶✻ L1901 Ankle orthosis, elastic, prefabricated, includes fitting and adjustment (e.g. neoprene, Lycra)

✻ L1902 AFO, ankle gauntlet, prefabricated, includes fitting and adjustment

✻ L1904 AFO, molded ankle gauntlet, custom fabrication

✻ L1906 AFO, multiligamentus ankle support, prefabricated, includes fitting and adjustment

✻ L1910 AFO, posterior, single bar, clasp attachment to shoe counter, prefabricated, includes fitting and adjustment

✻ L1920 AFO, single upright with static or adjustable stop (Phelps or Perlstein type), custom fabrication

✻ L1930 AFO, plastic or other material, prefabricated, includes fitting and adjustment

✻ L1940 AFO, plastic or other material, custom fabrication

✻ L1945 AFO, plastic, rigid anterior tibial section (floor reaction), custom fabrication

✻ L1950 AFO, spiral, (IRM type), plastic, custom fabrication

✻ L1960 AFO, posterior solid ankle, plastic, custom fabrication

✻ L1970 AFO, plastic, with ankle joint, custom fabrication

∗ L1980 AFO, single upright free plantar dorsiflexion, solid stirrup, calf band/cuff (single bar BK orthosis), custom fabrication

∗ L1990 AFO, double upright free plantar dorsiflexion, solid stirrup, calf band/cuff (double bar BK orthosis), custom fabrication

Hip-Knee-Ankle-Foot (or Any Combination)

NOTE: L2000, L2020, and L2036 are base procedures to be used with any knee joint. L2010 and L2030 are to be used only with no knee joint.

∗ L2000 Knee-ankle-foot orthosis (KAFO), single upright, free knee, free ankle, solid stirrup, thigh and calf bands/cuffs (single bar 'AK' orthosis), custom fabrication

∗ L2010 KAFO, single upright, free ankle, solid stirrup, thigh and calf bands/cuffs (single bar AK orthosis), without knee joint, custom fabrication

∗ L2020 KAFO, double upright, free knee, free ankle, solid stirrup, thigh and calf bands/cuffs (double bar AK orthosis), custom fabrication

∗ L2030 KAFO, double upright, free ankle, solid stirrup, thigh and calf bands/cuffs (double bar AK orthosis), without knee joint, custom fabrication

∗ L2035 KAFO, full plastic, static, prefabricated (pediatric size), prefabricated, includes fitting and adjustment

∗ L2036 KAFO, full plastic, double upright, free knee, custom fabrication

∗ L2037 KAFO, full plastic, single upright, free knee, custom fabrication

∗ L2038 KAFO, full plastic, without knee joint, multi-axis ankle, (lively orthosis or equal), custom fabrication

∗ L2039 KAFO, full plastic, single upright, polyaxial hinge, medial-lateral rotation control, custom fabrication

Torsion Control

∗ L2040 Hip-knee-ankle-foot orthosis (HKAFO), torsion control, bilateral rotation straps, pelvic band/belt, custom fabrication

∗ L2050 HKAFO, torsion control, bilateral torsion cables, hip joint, pelvic band/belt, custom fabrication

∗ L2060 HKAFO, torsion control, bilateral torsion cables, ball bearing hip joint, pelvic band/belt, custom fabrication

∗ L2070 HKAFO, torsion control, unilateral rotation straps, pelvic band/belt, custom fabrication

∗ L2080 HKAFO, torsion control, unilateral torsion cable, hip joint, pelvic band/belt, custom fabrication

∗ L2090 HKAFO, torsion control, unilateral torsion cable, ball bearing hip joint, pelvic band/belt, custom fabrication

Fracture Orthoses

◆ L2102 AFO, fracture orthosis, tibial fracture cast orthosis, plaster type casting material, custom fabrication

◆ L2104 AFO, fracture orthosis, tibial fracture cast orthosis, synthetic type casting material, custom fabrication

∗ L2106 AFO, fracture orthosis, tibial fracture cast orthosis, thermoplastic type casting material, custom fabrication

∗ L2108 AFO, fracture orthosis, tibial fracture cast orthosis, custom fabrication

∗ L2112 AFO, fracture orthosis, tibial fracture orthosis, soft, prefabricated, includes fitting and adjustment

∗ L2114 AFO, fracture orthosis, tibial fracture orthosis, semi-rigid, prefabricated, includes fitting and adjustment

∗ L2116 AFO, fracture orthosis, tibial fracture orthosis, rigid, prefabricated, includes fitting and adjustment

◆ L2122 KAFO, fracture orthosis, femoral fracture cast orthosis, plaster type casting material, custom fabrication

◆ L2124 KAFO, fracture orthosis, femoral fracture cast orthosis, synthetic type casting material, custom fabrication

∗ L2126 KAFO, fracture orthosis, femoral fracture cast orthosis, thermoplastic type casting material, custom fabrication

∗ L2128 KAFO, fracture orthosis, femoral fracture cast orthosis, custom fabrication

∗ L2132 KAFO, fracture orthosis, femoral fracture cast orthosis, soft, prefabricated, includes fitting and adjustment

∗ L2134 KAFO, fracture orthosis, femoral fracture cast orthosis, semi-rigid, prefabricated, includes fitting and adjustment

∗ L2136 KAFO, fracture orthosis, femoral fracture cast orthosis, rigid, prefabricated, includes fitting and adjustment

Additions to Fracture Orthosis

∗ L2180 Addition to lower extremity fracture orthosis, plastic shoe insert with ankle joints

∗ L2182 Addition to lower extremity fracture orthosis, drop lock knee joint

∗ L2184 Addition to lower extremity fracture orthosis, limited motion knee joint

* L2186 Addition to lower extremity fracture orthosis, adjustable motion knee joint (Lerman type)
* L2188 Addition to lower extremity fracture orthosis, quadrilateral brim
* L2190 Addition to lower extremity fracture orthosis, waist belt
* L2192 Addition to lower extremity fracture orthosis, hip joint, pelvic band, thigh flange, and pelvic belt

Additions to Lower Extremity Orthosis

Shoe-Ankle-Shin-Knee

* L2200 Addition to lower extremity, limited ankle motion, each joint
* L2210 Addition to lower extremity, dorsiflexion assist (plantar flexion resist), each joint
* L2220 Addition to lower extremity, dorsiflexion and plantar flexion assist/resist, each joint
* L2230 Addition to lower extremity, split flat caliper stirrups and plate attachment
* L2240 Addition to lower extremity, round caliper and plate attachment
* L2250 Addition to lower extremity, footplate, molded to patient model, stirrup attachment
* L2260 Addition to lower extremity, reinforced solid stirrup (Scott-Craig type)
* L2265 Addition to lower extremity, long tongue stirrup
* L2270 Addition to lower extremity, varus/valgus correction (T) strap, padded/lined or malleolus pad
* L2275 Addition to lower extremity, varus/valgus correction, plastic modification, padded/lined
* L2280 Addition to lower extremity, molded inner boot
* L2300 Addition to lower extremity, abduction bar (bilateral hip involvement), jointed, adjustable
* L2310 Addition to lower extremity, abduction bar, straight
* L2320 Addition to lower extremity, non-molded lacer
* L2330 Addition to lower extremity, lacer molded to patient model
* L2335 Addition to lower extremity, anterior swing band
* L2340 Addition to lower extremity, pre-tibial shell, molded to patient model
* L2350 Addition to lower extremity, prosthetic type, (BK) socket, molded to patient model, (used for PTB and AFO orthoses)
* L2360 Addition to lower extremity, extended steel shank
* L2370 Addition to lower extremity, Patten bottom
* L2375 Addition to lower extremity, torsion control, ankle joint and half solid stirrup
* L2380 Addition to lower extremity, torsion control, straight knee joint, each joint
* L2385 Addition to lower extremity, straight knee joint, heavy duty, each joint
* L2390 Addition to lower extremity, offset knee joint, each joint
* L2395 Addition to lower extremity, offset knee joint, heavy duty, each joint
* L2397 Addition to lower extremity orthosis, suspension sleeve

Straight Knee or Offset Knee Joints

* L2405 Addition to knee joint, drop lock, each joint
* L2415 Addition to knee lock with integrated release mechanism (bail, cable, or equal), any material, each joint
* L2425 Addition to knee joint, disc or dial lock for adjustable knee flexion, each joint
* L2430 Addition to knee joint, ratchet lock for active and progressive knee extension, each joint
* L2435 Addition to knee joint, polycentric joint, each joint
* L2492 Addition to knee joint, lift loop for drop lock ring

Additions to Thigh/Weight Bearing

Gluteal/Ischial Weight

* L2500 Addition to lower extremity, thigh/weight bearing, gluteal/ischial weight bearing, ring
* L2510 Addition to lower extremity, thigh/weight bearing, quadri-lateral brim, molded to patient model
* L2520 Addition to lower extremity, thigh/weight bearing, quadri-lateral brim, custom fitted
* L2525 Addition to lower extremity, thigh/weight bearing, ischial containment/narrow M-L brim molded to patient model
* L2526 Addition to lower extremity, thigh/weight bearing, ischial containment/narrow M-L brim, custom fitted
* L2530 Addition to lower extremity, thigh-weight bearing, lacer, non-molded
* L2540 Addition to lower extremity, thigh/weight bearing, lacer, molded to patient model
* L2550 Addition to lower extremity, thigh/weight bearing, high roll cuff

Additions to Pelvic and Thoracic Control

* ✻ L2570 Addition to lower extremity, pelvic control, hip joint, Clevis type two position joint, each
* ✻ L2580 Addition to lower extremity, pelvic control, pelvic sling
* ✻ L2600 Addition to lower extremity, pelvic control, hip joint, Clevis type, or thrust bearing, free, each
* ✻ L2610 Addition to lower extremity, pelvic control, hip joint, Clevis or thrust bearing, lock, each
* ✻ L2620 Addition to lower extremity, pelvic control, hip joint, heavy duty, each
* ✻ L2622 Addition to lower extremity, pelvic control, hip joint, adjustable flexion, each
* ✻ L2624 Addition to lower extremity, pelvic control, hip joint, adjustable flexion, extension, abduction control, each
* ✻ L2627 Addition to lower extremity, pelvic control, plastic, molded to patient model, reciprocating hip joint and cables
* ✻ L2628 Addition to lower extremity, pelvic control, metal frame, reciprocating hip joint and cables
* ✻ L2630 Addition to lower extremity, pelvic control, band and belt, unilateral
* ✻ L2640 Addition to lower extremity, pelvic control, band and belt, bilateral
* ✻ L2650 Addition to lower extremity, pelvic and thoracic control, gluteal pad, each
* ✻ L2660 Addition to lower extremity, thoracic control, thoracic band
* ✻ L2670 Addition to lower extremity, thoracic control, paraspinal uprights
* ✻ L2680 Addition to lower extremity, thoracic control, lateral support uprights

General Additions

* ✻ L2750 Addition to lower extremity orthosis, plating chrome or nickel, per bar
* ✻ L2755 Addition to lower extremity orthosis, high strength, lightweight material, all hybrid lamination/prepreg composite, per segment
* ✻ L2760 Addition to lower extremity orthosis, extension, per extension, per bar (for lineal adjustment for growth)
* ✻ L2768 Orthotic side bar disconnect device, per bar
* ✻ L2770 Addition to lower extremity orthosis, any material—per bar or joint
* ✻ L2780 Addition to lower extremity orthosis, non-corrosive finish, per bar
* ✻ L2785 Addition to lower extremity orthosis, drop lock retainer, each
* ✻ L2795 Addition to lower extremity orthosis, knee control, full kneecap
* ✻ L2800 Addition to lower extremity orthosis, knee control, knee cap, medial or lateral pull
* ✻ L2810 Addition to lower extremity orthosis, knee control, condylar pad
* ✻ L2820 Addition to lower extremity orthosis, soft interface for molded plastic, below knee section
* ✻ L2830 Addition to lower extremity orthosis, soft interface for molded plastic, above knee section
* ✻ L2840 Addition to lower extremity orthosis, tibial length sock, fracture or equal, each
* ✻ L2850 Addition to lower extremity orthosis, femoral length sock, fracture or equal, each
* ✻ L2860 Addition to lower extremity joint, knee or ankle, concentric adjustable torsion style mechanism, each
* ✻ L2999 Lower extremity orthoses, not otherwise specified

Foot (Orthopedic Shoes)

Insert, Removable, Molded to Patient Model

* ✪ L3000 Foot, insert, removable, molded to patient model, UCB type, Berkeley shell, each
  MCM 2323
* ✪ L3001 Foot, insert, removable, molded to patient model, Spenco, each
  MCM 2323
* ✪ L3002 Foot, insert, removable, molded to patient model, Plastazote or equal, each
  MCM 2323
* ✪ L3003 Foot, insert, removable, molded to patient model, silicone gel, each
  MCM 2323
* ✪ L3010 Foot, insert, removable, molded to patient model, longitudinal arch support, each
  MCM 2323
* ✪ L3020 Foot, insert, removable, molded to patient model, longitudinal/metatarsal support, each
  MCM 2323
* ✪ L3030 Foot, insert, removable, formed to patient foot, each
  MCM 2323

Arch Support, Removable, Premolded

* ✪ L3040 Foot, arch support, removable, premolded, longitudinal, each
  MCM 2323

✪ L3050 Foot, arch support, removable, premolded, metatarsal, each
MCM 2323

✪ L3060 Foot, arch support, removable, premolded, longitudinal/metatarsal, each
MCM 2323

Arch Support, Non-removable, Attached to Shoe

✪ L3070 Foot, arch support, non-removable attached to shoe, longitudinal, each
MCM 2323

✪ L3080 Foot, arch support, non-removable attached to shoe, metatarsal, each
MCM 2323

✪ L3090 Foot, arch support, non-removable attached to shoe, longitudinal/metatarsal, each
MCM 2323

✪ L3100 Hallus-valgus night dynamic splint
MCM 2323

Abduction and Rotation Bars

✪ L3140 Foot, abduction rotation bar, including shoes
MCM 2323

✪ L3150 Foot, abduction rotation bar, without shoes
MCM 2323

* L3160 Foot, adjustable shoe-styled positioning device

✪ L3170 Foot, plastic heel stabilizer
MCM 2323

Orthopedic Footwear

✪ L3201 Orthopedic shoe, oxford with supinator or pronator, infant
MCM 2323

✪ L3202 Orthopedic shoe, oxford with supinator or pronator, child
MCM 2323

✪ L3203 Orthopedic shoe, oxford with supinator or pronator, junior
MCM 2323

✪ L3204 Orthopedic shoe, hightop with supinator or pronator, infant
MCM 2323

✪ L3206 Orthopedic shoe, hightop with supinator or pronator, child
MCM 2323

✪ L3207 Orthopedic shoe, hightop with supinator or pronator, junior
MCM 2323

✪ L3208 Surgical boot, infant, each
MCM 2079

✪ L3209 Surgical boot, each, child
MCM 2079

✪ L3211 Surgical boot, each, junior
MCM 2079

✪ L3212 Benesch boot, pair, infant
MCM 2079

✪ L3213 Benesch boot, pair, child
MCM 2079

✪ L3214 Benesch boot, pair, junior
MCM 2079

◆ L3215 Orthopedic footwear, ladies' shoes, oxford
Medicare Statute 1862A8

◆ L3216 Orthopedic footwear, ladies' shoes, depth inlay
Medicare Statute 1862A8

◆ L3217 Orthopedic footwear, ladies' shoes, hightop, depth inlay
Medicare Statute 1862A8

L3218 Deleted 12/31/02, Cross Reference L3260

◆ L3219 Orthopedic footwear, men's shoes, oxford
Medicare Statute 1862A8

◆ L3221 Orthopedic footwear, men's shoes, depth inlay
Medicare Statute 1862A8

◆ L3222 Orthopedic footwear, men's shoes, high-top, depth inlay
Medicare Statute 1862A8

L3223 Deleted 12/31/02, Cross Reference L3260

✪ L3224 Orthopedic footwear, ladies' shoe, oxford, used as an integral part of a brace (orthosis)
MCM 2323D

✪ L3225 Orthopedic footwear, men's shoe, oxford, used as an integral part of a brace (orthosis)
MCM 2323D

✪ L3230 Orthopedic footwear, custom shoes, depth inlay
MCM 2323

✪ L3250 Orthopedic footwear, custom molded shoe, removable inner mold, prosthetic shoe, each
MCM 2323

✪ L3251 Foot, shoe molded to patient model, silicone shoe, each
MCM 2323

✪ L3252 Foot, shoe molded to patient model, Plastazote (or similar), custom fabricated, each
MCM 2323

✪ L3253 Foot, molded shoe Plastazote (or similar), custom fitted, each
MCM 2323

✪ L3254 Non-standard size or width
MCM 2323

✪ L3255 Non-standard size or length
MCM 2323

✪ L3257 Orthopedic footwear, additional charge for split size
MCM 2323

➡✪ L3260 Surgical boot/shoe, each
MCM 2079

∗ L3265 Plastazote sandal, each

Shoe Modifications

Lifts

✪ L3300 Lift, elevation, heel, tapered to metatarsals, per inch
MCM 2323

✪ L3310 Lift, elevation, heel and sole, Neoprene, per inch
MCM 2323

✪ L3320 Lift, elevation, heel and sole, cork, per inch
MCM 2323

✪ L3330 Lift, elevation, metal extension (skate)
MCM 2323

✪ L3332 Lift, elevation, inside shoe, tapered, up to 0.5 in
MCM 2323

✪ L3334 Lift, elevation, heel, per inch
MCM 2323

Wedges

✪ L3340 Heel wedge, SACH
MCM 2323

✪ L3350 Heel wedge
MCM 2323

✪ L3360 Sole wedge, outside sole
MCM 2323

✪ L3370 Sole wedge, between sole
MCM 2323

✪ L3380 Clubfoot wedge
MCM 2323

✪ L3390 Outflare wedge
MCM 2323

✪ L3400 Metatarsal bar wedge, rocker
MCM 2323

✪ L3410 Metatarsal bar wedge, between sole
MCM 2323

✪ L3420 Full sole and heel wedge, between sole
MCM 2323

Heels

✪ L3430 Heel, counter, plastic reinforced
MCM 2323

✪ L3440 Heel, counter, leather reinforced
MCM 2323

✪ L3450 Heel, SACH cushion type
MCM 2323

✪ L3455 Heel, new leather, standard
MCM 2323

✪ L3460 Heel, new rubber, standard
MCM 2323

✪ L3465 Heel, Thomas with wedge
MCM 2323

✪ L3470 Heel, Thomas extended to ball
MCM 2323

✪ L3480 Heel, pad and depression for spur
MCM 2323

✪ L3485 Heel, pad, removable for spur
MCM 2323

Additions to Orthopedic Shoes

✪ L3500 shoe addition, insole, leather
MCM 2323

✪ L3510 Orthopedic shoe addition, insole, rubber
MCM 2323

✪ L3520 Orthopedic shoe addition, insole, felt covered with leather
MCM 2323

✪ L3530 Orthopedic shoe addition, sole, half
MCM 2323

✪ L3540 Orthopedic shoe addition, sole, full
MCM 2323

✪ L3550 Orthopedic shoe addition, toe tap, standard
MCM 2323

✪ L3560 Orthopedic shoe addition, toe tap, horseshoe
MCM 2323

✪ L3570 Orthopedic shoe addition, special extension to instep (leather with eyelets)
MCM 2323

✪ L3580 Orthopedic shoe addition, convert instep to Velcro closure
MCM 2323

✪ L3590 Orthopedic shoe addition, convert firm shoe counter to soft counter
MCM 2323

✪ L3595 Orthopedic shoe addition, March bar
MCM 2323

Transfer or Replacement

✪ L3600 Transfer of an orthosis from one shoe to another, caliper plate, existing
MCM 2323

✪ L3610 Transfer of an orthosis from one shoe to another, caliper plate, new
MCM 2323

✪ L3620 Transfer of an orthosis from one shoe to another, solid stirrup, existing
MCM 2323

✪ L3630 Transfer of an orthosis from one shoe to another, solid stirrup, new
MCM 2323

✪ L3640 Transfer of an orthosis from one shoe to another, Dennis Browne splint (Riveton), both shoes
MCM 2323

✪ L3649 Orthopedic shoe, modification, addition or transfer, not otherwise specified
MCM 2323

Orthotic Devices: Upper Limb

NOTE: The procedures in this section are considered as *base* or *basic procedures* and may be modified by listing procedures from the Additions section and adding them to the base procedure.

Shoulder

* L3650 Shoulder orthosis, (SO), figure of eight (8) design abduction restrainer, prefabricated, includes fitting and adjustment

▶* L3651 Shoulder orthosis, single shoulder, elastic, prefabricated, includes fitting and adjustment (e.g. neoprene, Lycra)

▶* L3652 Shoulder orthosis, double shoulder, elastic, prefabricated, includes fitting and adjustment (e.g. neoprene, Lycra)

* L3660 SO, figure of eight (8) design abduction restrainer, canvas and webbing, prefabricated, includes fitting and adjustment

* L3670 SO, acromio/clavicular (canvas and webbing type), prefabricated, includes fitting and adjustment

* L3675 SO, vest type abduction restrainer, canvas webbing type, or equal, prefabricated, includes fitting and adjustment

✪ L3677 SO, hard plastic, shoulder stabilizer, pre-fabricated, includes fitting and adjustment
MCM 2130

Elbow

* L3700 Elbow orthosis (EO), elastic with stays, prefabricated, includes fitting and adjustment

▶* L3701 Elbow orthosis, elastic, prefabricated, includes fitting and adjustment (e.g. neoprene, Lycra)

* L3710 EO, elastic with metal joints, prefabricated, includes fitting and adjustment

* L3720 EO, double upright with forearm/arm cuffs, free motion, custom fabrication

* L3730 EO, double upright with forearm/arm cuffs, extension/flexion assist, custom fabrication

* L3740 EO, double upright with forearm/arm cuffs, adjustable position lock with active control, custom fabrication

* L3760 Elbow orthosis, with adjustable position locking joint(s), prefabricated, includes fitting and adjustments, any type

▶* L3762 Elbow orthosis, rigid, without joints, includes soft interface material, prefabricated, includes fitting and adjustment

Wrist-Hand-Finger

* L3800 Wrist-hand-finger orthosis (WHFO), short opponens, no attachments, custom fabrication

* L3805 WHFO, long opponens, no attachment, custom fabrication

* L3807 WHFO, without joint(s), prefabricated, includes fitting and adjustments, any type

Additions and Extensions

* L3810 WHFO, addition to short and long opponens, thumb abduction (C) bar

* L3815 WHFO, addition to short and long opponens, second MP abduction assist

* L3820 WHFO, addition to short and long opponens, IP extension assist, with MP extension stop

* L3825 WHFO, addition to short and long opponens, MP extension stop

* L3830 WHFO, addition to short and long opponens, MP extension assist

* L3835 WHFO, addition to short and long opponens, MP spring extension assist

* L3840 WHFO, addition to short and long opponens, spring swivel thumb

* L3845 WHFO, addition to short and long opponens, thumb IP extension assist, with MP stop

* L3850 WHO, addition to short and long opponens, action wrist, with dorsiflexion assist

* L3855 WHFO, addition to short and long opponens, adjustable MP flexion control

* L3860 WHFO, addition to short and long opponens, adjustable MP flexion control and IP

* L3890 Addition to upper extremity joint, wrist or elbow, concentric adjustable torsion style mechanism, each

* L3900 WHFO, dynamic flexor hinge, reciprocal wrist extension/flexion, finger flexion/extension, wrist or finger driven, custom fabrication

* L3901 WHFO, dynamic flexor hinge, reciprocal wrist extension/flexion, finger flexion/extension, cable driven, custom fabrication

External Power

✻ L3902 WHFO, external powered, compressed gas, custom fabrication

✻ L3904 WHFO, external powered, electric, custom fabrication

Other Wrist-Hand-Finger Orthoses: Custom Fitted

✻ L3906 WHO, wrist gauntlet, molded to patient model, custom fabrication

✻ L3907 WHFO, wrist gauntlet with thumb spica, molded to patient model, custom fabrication

✻ L3908 WHO, wrist extension control cock-up, non-molded, prefabricated, includes fitting and adjustment

▶✻ L3909 Wrist orthosis, elastic, prefabricated, includes fitting and adjustment (e.g. neoprene, Lycra)

✻ L3910 WHFO, Swanson design, prefabricated, includes fitting and adjustment

▶✻ L3911 Wrist hand finger orthosis, elastic, prefabricated, includes fitting and adjustment (e.g. neoprene, Lycra)

✻ L3912 HFO, flexion glove with elastic finger control, prefabricated, includes fitting and adjustment

✻ L3914 WHO, wrist extension cock-up, prefabricated, includes fitting and adjustment

✻ L3916 WHFO, wrist extension cock-up, with outrigger, prefabricated, includes fitting and adjustment

✻ L3918 HFO, knuckle bender, prefabricated, includes fitting and adjustment

✻ L3920 HFO, knuckle bender, with outrigger, prefabricated, includes fitting and adjustment

✻ L3922 HFO, knuckle bender, two segment to flex joints, prefabricated, includes fitting and adjustment

✻ L3923 HFO, without joint(s), prefabricated, includes fitting and adjustments, any type

✻ L3924 WHFO, Oppenheimer, prefabricated, includes fitting and adjustment

✻ L3926 WHFO, Thomas suspension, prefabricated, includes fitting and adjustment

✻ L3928 HFO, finger extension, with clock spring, prefabricated, includes fitting and adjustment

✻ L3930 WHFO, finger extension, with wrist support, prefabricated, includes fitting and adjustment

✻ L3932 FO, safety pin, spring wire, prefabricated, includes fitting and adjustment

✻ L3934 FO, safety pin, modified, prefabricated, includes fitting and adjustment

✻ L3936 WHFO, palmar, prefabricated, includes fitting and adjustment

✻ L3938 WHFO, dorsal wrist, prefabricated, includes fitting and adjustment

✻ L3940 WHFO, dorsal wrist, with outrigger attachment, prefabricated, includes fitting and adjustment

✻ L3942 HFO, reverse knuckle bender, prefabricated, includes fitting and adjustment

✻ L3944 HFO, reverse knuckle bender, with outrigger, prefabricated, includes fitting and adjustment

✻ L3946 HFO, composite elastic, prefabricated, includes fitting and adjustment

✻ L3948 FO, finger knuckle bender, prefabricated, includes fitting and adjustment

✻ L3950 WHFO, combination Oppenheimer, with knuckle bender and two attachments, prefabricated, includes fitting and adjustment

✻ L3952 WHFO, combination Oppenheimer, with reverse knuckle and two attachments, prefabricated, includes fitting and adjustment

✻ L3954 HFO, spreading hand, prefabricated, includes fitting and adjustment

✻ L3956 Addition of joint to upper extremity orthosis, any material, per joint

Shoulder-Elbow-Wrist-Hand

Abduction Positioning: Custom Fitted

✻ L3960 Shoulder-elbow-wrist-hand orthosis, (SEWHO), abduction positioning, airplane design, prefabricated, includes fitting and adjustment

✻ L3962 SEWHO, abduction positioning, Erb's palsy design, prefabricated, includes fitting and adjustment

✻ L3963 SEWHO, molded shoulder, arm, forearm, and wrist, with articulating elbow joint, custom fabrication

✻ L3964 SEO, mobile arm support attached to wheelchair, balanced, adjustable, prefabricated, includes fitting and adjustment

✻ L3965 SEO, mobile arm support attached to wheelchair, balanced, adjustable Rancho type, prefabricated, includes fitting and adjustment

✻ L3966 SEO, mobile arm support attached to wheelchair, balanced, reclining, prefabricated, includes fitting and adjustment

✻ L3968 SEO, mobile arm support attached to wheelchair, balanced, friction arm support (friction dampening to proximal and distal joints), prefabricated, includes fitting and adjustment

✻ L3969 SEO, mobile arm support, monosuspension arm and hand support, overhead elbow forearm hand sling support, yoke type arm suspension support, prefabricated, includes fitting and adjustment

Additions to Mobile Arm Supports

✻ L3970 SEO, addition to mobile arm support, elevating proximal arm

✻ L3972 SEO, addition to mobile arm support, offset or lateral rocker arm with elastic balance control

✻ L3974 SEO, addition to mobile arm support, supinator

Fracture Orthoses

✻ L3980 Upper extremity fracture orthosis, humeral, prefabricated, includes fitting and adjustment

✻ L3982 Upper extremity fracture orthosis, radius/ulnar, prefabricated, includes fitting and adjustment

✻ L3984 Upper extremity fracture orthosis, wrist, prefabricated, includes fitting and adjustment

✻ L3985 Upper extremity fracture orthosis, forearm, hand with wrist hinge, custom fabrication

✻ L3986 Upper extremity fracture orthosis, combination of humeral, radius/ulnar, wrist, (e.g., Colles' fracture), custom fabrication

✻ L3995 Addition to upper extremity orthosis, sock, fracture or equal, each

✻ L3999 Upper limb orthosis, not otherwise specified

Specific Repair

✻ L4000 Replace girdle for spinal orthosis (CTLSO or SO)

✻ L4010 Replace trilateral socket brim

✻ L4020 Replace quadrilateral socket brim, molded to patient model

✻ L4030 Replace quadrilateral socket brim, custom fitted

✻ L4040 Replace molded thigh lacer

✻ L4045 Replace non-molded thigh lacer

✻ L4050 Replace molded calf lacer

✻ L4055 Replace non-molded calf lacer

✻ L4060 Replace high roll cuff

✻ L4070 Replace proximal and distal upright for KAFO

✻ L4080 Replace metal bands, KAFO, proximal thigh

✻ L4090 Replace metal bands, KAFO-AFO, calf or distal thigh

✻ L4100 Replace leather cuff, KAFO, proximal thigh

✻ L4110 Replace leather cuff, KAFO-AFO, calf or distal thigh

✻ L4130 Replace pretibial shell

Repairs

✪ L4205 Repair of orthotic device, labor component, per 15 minutes
MCM 2100.4

✪ L4210 Repair of orthotic device, repair or replace minor parts
MCM 2100.4, MCM 2130D, MCM 2133

Ancillary Orthotic Services

➡✻ L4350 Pneumatic ankle control splint prefabricated, includes fitting and adjustment

➡✻ L4360 Pneumatic ankle foot orthosis, with or without joints, prefabricated, includes fitting and adjustment

➡✻ L4370 Pneumatic full leg splint, prefabricated, includes fitting and adjustment

➡✻ L4380 Pneumatic knee splint, prefabricated, includes fitting and adjustment

▶✻ L4386 Non-pneumatic walking splint, with or without joints, prefabricated, includes fitting and adjustment

✻ L4392 Replace soft interface material, static AFO

✻ L4394 Replace soft interface material, foot drop splint

✻ L4396 Static AFO, including soft interface material, adjustable for fit, for positioning, pressure reduction, may be used for minimal ambulation, prefabricated, includes fitting and adjustment

✻ L4398 Foot drop splint, recumbent positioning device, prefabricated, includes fitting and adjustment

PROSTHETIC PROCEDURES (L5000-L9999)

Lower Limb (L5000-L5999)

NOTE: The procedures in this sections are considered as *base* or *basic procedures* and may be modified by listing items/procedures or special materials from the Additions section and adding them to the base procedure.

Partial Foot

- ❂ L5000 Partial foot, shoe insert with longitudinal arch, toe filler MCM 2323
- ❂ L5010 Partial foot, molded socket, ankle height, with toe filler MCM 2323
- ❂ L5020 Partial foot, molded socket, tibial tubercle height, with toe filler MCM 2323

Ankle

- * L5050 Ankle, Symes, molded socket, SACH foot
- * L5060 Ankle, Symes, metal frame, molded leather socket, articulated ankle/foot

Below Knee

- * L5100 Below knee, molded socket, shin, SACH foot
- * L5105 Below knee, plastic socket, joints and thigh lacer, SACH foot

Knee Disarticulation

- * L5150 Knee disarticulation (or through knee), molded socket, external knee joints, shin, SACH foot
- * L5160 Knee disarticulation (or through knee), molded socket, bent knee configuration, external knee joints, shin, SACH foot

Above Knee

- * L5200 Above knee, molded socket, single axis constant friction knee, shin, SACH foot
- * L5210 Above knee, short prosthesis, no knee joint ('stubbies'), with foot blocks, no ankle joints, each
- * L5220 Above knee, short prosthesis, no knee joint ('stubbies'), with articulated ankle/foot, dynamically aligned, each
- * L5230 Above knee, for proximal femoral focal deficiency, constant friction knee, shin, SACH foot

Hip Disarticulation

- * L5250 Hip disarticulation, Canadian type; molded socket, hip joint, single axis constant friction knee, shin, SACH foot
- * L5270 Hip disarticulation, tilt table type; molded socket, locking hip joint, single axis constant friction knee, shin, SACH foot

Hemipelvectomy

- * L5280 Hemipelvectomy, Canadian type; molded socket, hip joint, single axis constant friction knee, shin, SACH foot

Endoskeleton: Below Knee

- * L5301 Below knee, molded socket, shin, SACH foot, endoskeletal system

Endoskeletal: Knee Disarticulation

- * L5311 Knee disarticulation (or through knee), molded socket, external knee joints, shin, SACH foot, endoskeletal system

Endoskeletal: Above Knee

- * L5321 Above knee, molded socket, open end, SACH foot, endoskeletal system, single axis knee

Endoskeletal: Hip Disarticulation

- * L5331 Hip disarticulation, Canadian type, molded socket, endoskeletal system, hip joint, single axis knee, SACH foot

Endoskeletal: Hemipelvectomy

- L5340 Deleted 01/01/02, Cross Reference L5341
- * L5341 Hemipelvectomy, Canadian type, molded socket, endoskeletal system, hip joint, single axis knee, SACH foot

Immediate Postsurgical or Early Fitting Procedures

- * L540 Immediate postsurgical or early fitting, application of initial rigid dressing, including fitting, alignment, suspension, and one cast change, below knee
- * L5410 Immediate post surgical or early fitting, application of initial rigid dressing, including fitting, alignment and suspension, below knee, each additional cast change and realignment
- * L5420 Immediate postsurgical or early fitting, application of initial rigid dressing, including fitting, alignment and suspension and one cast change AK or knee disarticulation
- * L5430 Immediate postsurgical or early fitting, application of initial rigid dressing, including fitting, alignment and suspension, AK or knee disarticulation, each additional cast change and realignment

* L5450 Immediate postsurgical or early fitting, application of non-weight bearing rigid dressing, below knee
* L5460 Immediate postsurgical or early fitting, application of non-weight bearing rigid dressing, above knee

Initial Prosthesis

* L5500 Initial, below knee PTB type socket, non-alignable system, pylon, no cover, SACH foot, plaster socket, direct formed
* L5505 Initial, above knee–knee disarticulation, ischial level socket, non-alignable system, pylon, no cover, SACH foot, plaster socket, direct formed

Preparatory Prosthesis

* L5510 Preparatory, below knee PTB type socket, non-alignable system, pylon, no cover, SACH foot, plaster socket, molded to model
* L5520 Preparatory, below knee PTB type socket, non-alignable system, pylon, no cover, SACH foot, thermoplastic or equal, direct formed
* L5530 Preparatory, below knee PTB type socket, non-alignable system, pylon, no cover, SACH foot, thermoplastic or equal, molded to model
* L5535 Preparatory, below knee PTB type socket, non-alignable system, no cover, SACH foot, prefabricated, adjustable open end socket
* L5540 Preparatory, below knee PTB type socket, non-alignable system, pylon, no cover, SACH foot, laminated socket, molded to model
* L5560 Preparatory, above knee-knee disarticulation, ischial level socket, non-alignable system, pylon, no cover, SACH foot, plaster socket, molded to model
* L5570 Preparatory, above knee-knee disarticulation, ischial level socket, non-alignable system, pylon, no cover, SACH foot, thermoplastic or equal, direct formed
* L5580 Preparatory, above knee-knee disarticulation, ischial level socket, non-alignable system, pylon, no cover, SACH foot, thermoplastic or equal, molded to model
* L5585 Preparatory, above knee-knee disarticulation, ischial level socket, non-alignable system, pylon, no cover, SACH foot, prefabricated adjustable open end socket
* L5590 Preparatory, above knee-knee disarticulation, ischial level socket, non-alignable system, pylon, no cover, SACH foot, laminated socket, molded to model
* L5595 Preparatory, hip disarticulation-hemipelvectomy, pylon, no cover, SACH foot, thermoplastic or equal, molded to patient model

Additions to Lower Extremity

* L5600 Preparatory, hip disarticulation-hemipelvectomy, pylon, no cover, SACH foot, laminated socket, molded to patient model
* L5610 Addition to lower extremity, endoskeletal system, above knee, hydracadence system
* L5611 Addition to lower extremity, endoskeletal system, above knee-knee disarticulation, 4-bar link-age, with friction wing phase control
* L5613 Addition to lower extremity, endoskeletal system, above knee-knee disarticulation, 4-bar linkage, with hydraulic swing phase control
* L5614 Addition to lower extremity, exoskeletal system, above knee-knee disarticulation, 4-bar linkage, with pneumatic swing phase control
* L5616 Addition to lower extremity, endoskeletal system, above knee, universal multiplex system, friction swing phase control
* L5617 Addition to lower extremity, quick change self-aligning unit, above knee or below knee, each

Additions to Test Sockets

* L5618 Addition to lower extremity, test socket, Symes
* L5620 Addition to lower extremity, test socket, below knee
* L5622 Addition to lower extremity, test socket, knee disarticulation
* L5624 Addition to lower extremity, test socket, above knee
* L5626 Addition to lower extremity, test socket, hip disarticulation
* L5628 Addition to lower extremity, test socket, hemipelvectomy
* L5629 Addition to lower extremity, below knee, acrylic socket

Additions to Socket Variations

* L5630 Addition to lower extremity, Symes type, expandable wall socket
* L5631 Addition to lower extremity, above knee or knee disarticulation, acrylic socket
* L5632 Addition to lower extremity, Symes type, PTB brim design socket
* L5634 Addition to lower extremity, Symes type, posterior opening (Canadian) socket
* L5636 Addition to lower extremity, Symes type, medial opening socket
* L5637 Addition to lower extremity, below knee, total contact
* L5638 Addition to lower extremity, below knee, leather socket
* L5639 Addition to lower extremity, below knee, wood socket
* L5640 Addition to lower extremity, knee disarticulation, leather socket
* L5642 Addition to lower extremity, above knee, leather socket
* L5643 Addition to lower extremity, hip disarticulation, flexible inner socket, external frame
* L5644 Addition to lower extremity, above knee, wood socket
* L5645 Addition to lower extremity, below knee, flexible inner socket, external frame
* L5646 Addition to lower extremity, below knee, air cushion socket
* L5647 Addition to lower extremity, below knee, suction socket
* L5648 Addition to lower extremity, above knee, air cushion socket
* L5649 Addition to lower extremity, ischial containment/narrow M-L socket
* L5650 Additions to lower extremity, total contact, above knee or knee disarticulation socket
* L5651 Addition to lower extremity, above knee, flexible inner socket, external frame
* L5652 Addition to lower extremity, suction suspension, above knee or knee disarticulation socket
* L5653 Addition to lower extremity, knee disarticulation, expandable wall socket

Additions to Socket Insert and Suspension

* L5654 Addition to lower extremity, socket insert, Symes, (Kemblo, Pelite, Aliplast, Plastazote or equal)
* L5655 Addition to lower extremity, socket insert, below knee (Kemblo, Pelite, Aliplast, Plastazote or equal)
* L5656 Addition to lower extremity, socket insert, knee disarticulation (Kemblo, Pelite, Aliplast, Plastazote or equal)
* L5658 Addition to lower extremity, socket insert, above knee (Kemblo, Pelite, Aliplast, Plastazote or equal)

L5660 Deleted 12/31/02

* L5661 Addition to lower extremity, socket insert, multi-durometer Symes

L5662 Deleted 12/31/02
L5663 Deleted 12/31/02
L5664 Deleted 12/31/02

* L5665 Addition to lower extremity, socket insert, multi-durometer, below knee
* L5666 Addition to lower extremity, below knee, cuff suspension

L5667 Deleted 01/01/02

* L5668 Addition to lower extremity, below knee, molded distal cushion

L5669 Deleted 01/01/02; Cross Reference L5660, L5662, L5663, L5664

* L5670 Addition to lower extremity, below knee, molded supracondylar suspension (PTS or similar)
* L5671 Addition to lower extremity, below knee/above knee suspension locking mechanism (shuttle, lanyard or equal), excludes socket insert
* L5672 Addition to lower extremity, below knee, removable medial brim suspension
* L5674 Addition to lower extremity, below knee, suspension sleeve, any material, each
* L5675 Addition to lower extremity, below knee, suspension sleeve, heavy duty, any material, each
* L5676 Addition to lower extremity, below knee, knee joints, single axis, pair
* L5677 Addition to lower extremity, below knee, knee joints, polycentric, pair
* L5678 Addition to lower extremity, below knee, joint covers, pair
* L5680 Addition to lower extremity, below knee, thigh lacer, non-molded
* L5682 Addition to lower extremity, below knee, thigh lacer, gluteal/ischial, molded
* L5684 Addition to lower extremity, below knee, fork strap
* L5686 Addition to lower extremity, below knee, back check (extension control)
* L5688 Addition to lower extremity, below knee, waist belt, webbing
* L5690 Addition to lower extremity, below knee, waist belt, padded and lined
* L5692 Addition to lower extremity, above knee, pelvic control belt, light
* L5694 Addition to lower extremity, above knee, pelvic control belt, padded and lined

✻ L5695 Addition to lower extremity, above knee, pelvic control, sleeve suspension, neoprene or equal, each

✻ L5696 Addition to lower extremity, above knee or knee disarticulation, pelvic joint

✻ L5697 Addition to lower extremity, above knee or knee disarticulation, pelvic band

✻ L5698 Addition to lower extremity, above knee or knee disarticulation, Silesian bandage

✻ L5699 All lower extremity prostheses, shoulder harness

Additions to Feet-Ankle Units

✻ L5700 Replacement, socket, below knee, molded to patient model

✻ L5701 Replacement, socket, above knee-knee disarticulation, including attachment plate, molded to patient model

✻ L5702 Replacement, socket, hip disarticulation, including hip joint, molded to patient model

✻ L5704 Custom shaped protective cover, below knee

✻ L5705 Custom shaped protective cover, above knee

✻ L5706 Custom shaped protective cover, knee disarticulation

✻ L5707 Custom shaped protective cover, hip disarticulation

Additions to Exoskeletal—Knee-Shin System

✻ L5710 Addition, exoskeletal knee-shin system, single axis, manual lock

✻ L5711 Addition, exoskeletal knee-shin system, single axis, manual lock, ultralight material

✻ L5712 Addition, exoskeletal knee-shin system, single axis, friction swing and stance phase control (safety knee)

✻ L5714 Addition, exoskeletal knee-shin system, single axis, variable friction swing phase control

✻ L5716 Addition, exoskeletal knee-shin system, polycentric, mechanical stance phase lock

✻ L5718 Addition, exoskeletal knee-shin system, polycentric, friction swing and stance phase control

✻ L5722 Addition, exoskeletal knee-shin system, single axis, pneumatic swing, friction stance phase control

✻ L5724 Addition, exoskeletal knee-shin system, single axis, fluid swing phase control

✻ L5726 Addition, exoskeletal knee-shin system, single axis, external joints, fluid swing phase control

✻ L5728 Addition, exoskeletal knee-shin system, single axis, fluid swing and stance phase control

✻ L5780 Addition, exoskeletal knee-shin system, single axis, pneumatic/hydra pneumatic swing phase control

▶✻ L5781 Addition to lower limb prosthesis, vacuum pump, residual limb volume management and moisture evacuation system

▶✻ L5782 Addition to lower limb prosthesis, vacuum pump, residual limb volume management and moisture evacuation system, heavy duty

Component Modification

✻ L5785 Addition, exoskeletal system, below knee, ultra-light material (titanium, carbon fiber or equal)

✻ L5790 Addition, exoskeletal system, above knee, ultra-light material (titanium, carbon fiber or equal)

✻ L5795 Addition, exoskeletal system, hip disarticulation, ultra-light material (titanium, carbon fiber or equal)

Endoskeletal

✻ L5810 Addition, endoskeletal knee-shin system, single axis, manual lock

✻ L5811 Addition, endoskeletal knee-shin system, single axis, manual lock, ultra light material

✻ L5812 Addition, endoskeletal knee-shin system, single axis, friction swing and stance phase control (safety knee)

✻ L5814 Addition, endoskeletal knee-shin system, polycentric, hydraulic swing phase control, mechanical stance phase lock

✻ L5816 Addition, endoskeletal knee-shin system, polycentric, mechanical stance phase lock

✻ L5818 Addition, endoskeletal knee-shin system, polycentric, friction swing, and stance phase control

✻ L5822 Addition, endoskeletal knee-shin system, single axis, pneumatic swing, friction stance phase control

✻ L5824 Addition, endoskeletal knee-shin system, single axis, fluid swing phase control

✻ L5826 Addition, endoskeletal knee-shin system, single axis, hydraulic swing phase control, with miniature high activity frame

✻ L5828 Addition, endoskeletal knee-shin system, single axis, fluid swing and stance phase control

✻ L5830 Addition, endoskeletal knee-shin system, single axis, pneumatic/ swing phase control
✻ L5840 Addition, endoskeletal knee-shin system, four-bar linkage or multiaxial, pneumatic swing phase control
✻ L5845 Addition, endoskeletal, knee-shin system, stance flexion feature, adjustable
✻ L5846 Addition, endoskeletal, knee-shin system, microprocessor control feature, swing phase only
✻ L5847 Addition, endoskeletal knee-shin system, microprocessor control feature, stance phase
▶✻ L5848 Addition to endoskeletal, knee-shin system, hydraulic stance extension, dampening feature, adjustable
✻ L5850 Addition, endoskeletal system, above knee or hip disarticulation, knee extension assist
✻ L5855 Addition, endoskeletal system, hip disarticulation, mechanical hip extension assist
✻ L5910 Addition, endoskeletal system, below knee, alignable system
✻ L5920 Addition, endoskeletal system, above knee or hip disarticulation, alignable system
✻ L5925 Addition, endoskeletal system, above knee, knee disarticulation or hip disarticulation, manual lock
✻ L5930 Addition, endoskeletal system, high activity knee control frame
✻ L5940 Addition, endoskeletal system, below knee, ultra light material (titanium, carbon fiber or equal)
✻ L5950 Addition, endoskeletal system, above knee, ultra light material (titanium, carbon fiber or equal)
✻ L5960 Addition, endoskeletal system, hip disarticulation, ultra light material (titanium, carbon fiber or equal)
✻ L5962 Addition, endoskeletal system, below knee, flexible protective outer surface covering system
✻ L5964 Addition, endoskeletal system, above knee, flexible protective outer surface covering system
✻ L5966 Addition, endoskeletal system, hip disarticulation, flexible protective outer surface covering system
✻ L5968 Addition to lower limb prosthesis, multiaxial ankle with swing phase active dorsiflexion feature
✻ L5970 All lower extremity prostheses, foot, external heel, SACH foot
✻ L5972 All lower extremity prostheses, flexible heel foot (Safe, Sten, Bock Dynamic or equal)
✻ L5974 All lower extremity prostheses, foot, single axis ankle/foot
✻ L5975 All lower extremity prostheses, combination single axis ankle and flexible heel foot
✻ L5976 All lower extremity prostheses, energy storing foot (Seattle Carbon Copy II or equal)
✻ L5978 All lower extremity prostheses, foot, multiaxial ankle/foot
✻ L5979 All lower extremity prostheses, multiaxial ankle, dynamic response foot, one piece system
✻ L5980 All lower extremity prostheses, flex foot system
✻ L5981 All lower extremity prostheses, flexwalk system or equal
✻ L5982 All exoskeletal lower extremity prostheses, axial rotation unit
✻ L5984 All endoskeletal lower extremity prostheses, axial rotation unit
✻ L5985 All endoskeletal lower extremity prostheses, dynamic prosthetic pylon
✻ L5986 All lower extremity prostheses, multiaxial rotation unit (MCP or equal)
✻ L5987 All lower extremity prostheses, shank foot system with vertical loading pylon
✻ L5988 Addition to lower limb prosthesis, vertical shock reducing pylon feature
✻ L5989 Addition to lower extremity prosthesis, endoskeletal system, pylon with integrated electronic force sensors
✻ L5990 Addition to lower extremity prosthesis, user adjustable heel height
▶✻ L5995 Addition to lower extremity prosthesis, heavy duty feature (for patient weight > 300 lbs)
✻ L5999 Lower extremity prosthesis, not otherwise specified

Upper Limb

NOTE: The procedures in L6000-L6599 are considered as base or basic procedures and may be modified by listing procedures from the additions sections. The base procedures include only standard friction wrist and control cable system unless otherwise specified.

Partial Hand

✻ L6000 Partial hand, Robin-Aids, thumb remaining (or equal)
✻ L6010 Partial hand, Robin-Aids, little and/or ring finger remaining (or equal)
✻ L6020 Partial hand, Robin-Aids, no finger remaining (or equal)

▶✻ L6025 Transcarpal/metacarpal or partial hand disarticulation prosthesis, external power, self-suspended, inner socket with removable forearm section, electrodes and cables, two batteries, charger, myoelectric control of terminal device

Wrist Disarticulation

✻ L6050 Wrist disarticulation, molded socket, flexible elbow hinges, triceps pad

✻ L6055 Wrist disarticulation, molded socket with expandable interface, flexible elbow hinges, triceps pad

Below Elbow

✻ L6100 Below elbow, molded socket, flexible elbow hinge, triceps pad

✻ L6110 Below elbow, molded socket, (Muenster or Northwestern suspension types)

✻ L6120 Below elbow, molded double wall split socket, step-up hinges, half cuff

✻ L6130 Below elbow, molded double wall split socket, stump activated locking hinge, half cuff

Elbow Disarticulation

✻ L6200 Elbow disarticulation, molded socket, outside locking hinge, forearm

✻ L6205 Elbow disarticulation, molded socket with expandable interface, outside locking hinges, forearm

Above Elbow

✻ L6250 Above elbow, molded double wall socket, internal locking elbow, forearm

Shoulder Disarticulation

✻ L6300 Shoulder disarticulation, molded socket, shoulder bulkhead, humeral section, internal locking elbow, forearm

✻ L6310 Shoulder disarticulation, passive restoration (complete prosthesis)

✻ L6320 Shoulder disarticulation, passive restoration (shoulder cap only)

Interscapular Thoracic

✻ L6350 Interscapular thoracic, molded socket, shoulder bulkhead, humeral section, internal locking elbow, forearm

✻ L6360 Interscapular thoracic, passive restoration (complete prosthesis)

✻ L6370 Interscapular thoracic, passive restoration (shoulder cap only)

Immediate and Early Postsurgical Procedures

✻ L6380 Immediate postsurgical or early fitting, application of initial rigid dressing, including fitting alignment and suspension of components, and one cast change, wrist disarticulation or below elbow

✻ L6382 Immediate postsurgical or early fitting, application of initial rigid dressing including fitting alignment and suspension of components, and one cast change, elbow disarticulation or above elbow

✻ L6384 Immediate postsurgical or early fitting, application of initial rigid dressing including fitting alignment and suspension of components, and one cast change, shoulder disarticulation or interscapular thoracic

✻ L6386 Immediate postsurgical or early fitting, each additional cast change and realignment

✻ L6388 Immediate postsurgical or early fitting, application of rigid dressing only

Endoskeletal: Below Elbow

✻ L6400 Below elbow, molded socket, endoskeletal system, including soft prosthetic tissue shaping

Endoskeletal: Elbow Disarticulation

✻ L6450 Elbow disarticulation, molded socket, endoskeletal system, including soft prosthetic tissue shaping

Endoskeletal: Above Elbow

✻ L6500 Above elbow, molded socket, endoskeletal system, including soft prosthetic tissue shaping

Endoskeletal: Shoulder Disarticulation

✻ L6550 Shoulder disarticulation, molded socket, endoskeletal system, including soft prosthetic tissue shaping

Endoskeletal: Interscapular Thoracic

✻ L6570 Interscapular thoracic, molded socket, endoskeletal system, including soft prosthetic tissue shaping

✻ L6580 Preparatory, wrist disarticulation or below elbow, single wall plastic socket, friction wrist, flexible elbow hinges, figure of eight harness, humeral cuff, Bowden cable control, USMC or equal pylon, no cover, molded to patient model

✻ L6582 Preparatory, wrist disarticulation or below elbow, single wall socket, friction wrist, flexible elbow hinges, figure of eight harness, humeral cuff, Bowden cable control, USMC or equal pylon, no cover, direct formed

✻ L6584 Preparatory, elbow disarticulation or above elbow, single wall plastic socket, friction wrist, locking elbow, figure of eight harness, fair lead cable control, USMC or equal pylon, no cover, molded to patient model

✻ L6586 Preparatory, elbow disarticulation or above elbow, single wall socket, friction wrist, locking elbow, figure of eight harness, fair lead cable control, USMC or equal pylon, no cover, direct formed

✻ L6588 Preparatory, shoulder disarticulation or interscapular thoracic, single wall plastic socket, shoulder joint, locking elbow, friction wrist, chest strap, fair lead cable control, USMC or equal pylon, no cover, molded to patient model

✻ L6590 Preparatory, shoulder disarticulation or interscapular thoracic, single wall socket, shoulder joint, locking elbow, friction wrist, chest strap, fair lead cable control, USMC or equal pylon, no cover, direct formed

Additions to Upper Limb

NOTE: The following procedures/modifications/components may be added to other base procedures. The items in this section should reflect the additional complexity of each modification procedure, in addition to base procedure, at the time of the original order.

✻ L6600 Upper extremity addition, polycentric hinge, pair

✻ L6605 Upper extremity addition, single pivot hinge, pair

✻ L6610 Upper extremity addition, flexible metal hinge, pair

✻ L6615 Upper extremity addition, disconnect locking wrist unit

✻ L6616 Upper extremity addition, additional disconnect insert for locking wrist unit, each

✻ L6620 Upper extremity addition, flexion-friction wrist unit

✻ L6623 Upper extremity addition, spring assisted rotational wrist unit with latch release

✻ L6625 Upper extremity addition, rotation wrist unit with cable lock

✻ L6628 Upper extremity addition, quick disconnect hook adapter, Otto Bock or equal

✻ L6629 Upper extremity addition, quick disconnect lamination collar with coupling piece, Otto Bock or equal

✻ L6630 Upper extremity addition, stainless steel, any wrist

✻ L6632 Upper extremity addition, latex suspension sleeve, each

✻ L6635 Upper extremity addition, lift assist for elbow

✻ L6637 Upper extremity addition, nudge control elbow lock

▶✻ L6638 Upper extremity addition to prosthesis, electric locking feature, only for use with manually powered elbow

✻ L6640 Upper extremity additions, shoulder abduction joint, pair

✻ L6641 Upper extremity addition, excursion amplifier, pulley type

✻ L6642 Upper extremity addition, excursion amplifier, lever type

✻ L6645 Upper extremity addition, shoulder flexion-abduction joint, each

▶✻ L6646 Upper extremity addition, shoulder joint, multipositional locking, flexion, adjustable abduction friction control, for use with body powered or external powered system

▶✻ L6647 Upper extremity addition, shoulder lock mechanism, body powered actuator

▶✻ L6648 Upper extremity addition, shoulder lock mechanism, external powered actuator

✻ L6650 Upper extremity addition, shoulder universal joint, each

✻ L6655 Upper extremity addition, standard control cable, extra

✻ L6660 Upper extremity addition, heavy duty control cable

✻ L6665 Upper extremity addition, Teflon, or equal, cable lining

✻ L6670 Upper extremity addition, hook to hand, cable adapter

✻ L6672 Upper extremity addition, harness, chest or shoulder, saddle type

✻ L6675 Upper extremity addition, harness, figure of eight (8) type, for single control

✻ L6676 Upper extremity addition, harness, figure of eight (8) type, for dual control

* L6680 Upper extremity addition, test socket, wrist disarticulation or below elbow
* L6682 Upper extremity addition, test socket, elbow disarticulation or above elbow
* L6684 Upper extremity addition, test socket, shoulder disarticulation or interscapular thoracic
* L6686 Upper extremity addition, suction socket
* L6687 Upper extremity addition, frame type socket, below elbow or wrist disarticulation
* L6688 Upper extremity addition, frame type socket, above elbow or elbow disarticulation
* L6689 Upper extremity addition, frame type socket, shoulder disarticulation
* L6690 Upper extremity addition, frame type socket, interscapular-thoracic
* L6691 Upper extremity addition, removable insert, each
* L6692 Upper extremity addition, silicone gel insert or equal, each
* L6693 Upper extremity addition, locking elbow, forearm counterbalance

Terminal Devices

Hooks

⊕ L6700 Terminal device, hook, Dorrance, or equal, model #3
MCM 2133

⊕ L6705 Terminal device, hook, Dorrance, or equal, model #5
MCM 2133

⊕ L6710 Terminal device, hook, Dorrance, or equal, model #5X
MCM 2133

⊕ L6715 Terminal device, hook, Dorrance, or equal, model #5XA
MCM 2133

⊕ L6720 Terminal device, hook, Dorrance, or equal, model #6
MCM 2133

⊕ L6725 Terminal device, hook, Dorrance, or equal, model #7
MCM 2133

⊕ L6730 Terminal device, hook, Dorrance, or equal, model #7LO
MCM 2133

⊕ L6735 Terminal device, hook, Dorrance, or equal, model #8
MCM 2133

⊕ L6740 Terminal device, hook, Dorrance, or equal, model #8X
MCM 2133

⊕ L6745 Terminal device, hook, Dorrance, or equal, model #88X
MCM 2133

⊕ L6750 Terminal device, hook, Dorrance, or equal, model #10P
MCM 2133

⊕ L6755 Terminal device, hook, Dorrance, or equal, model #10X
MCM 2133

⊕ L6765 Terminal device, hook, Dorrance, or equal, model #12P
MCM 2133

⊕ L6770 Terminal device, hook, Dorrance, or equal, model #99X
MCM 2133

⊕ L6775 Terminal device, hook, Dorrance, or equal, model #555
MCM 2133

⊕ L6780 Terminal device, hook, Dorrance, or equal, model #SS555
MCM 2133

⊕ L6790 Terminal device, hook, Accu hook, or equal
MCM 2133

⊕ L6795 Terminal device, hook, 2 load, or equal
MCM 2133

⊕ L6800 Terminal device, hook, APRL VC, or equal
MCM 2133

⊕ L6805 Terminal device, modifier wrist flexion unit
MCM 2133

⊕ L6806 Terminal device, hook, TRS Grip, Grip III, VC, or equal
MCM 2133

⊕ L6807 Terminal device, hook, Grip I, Grip II, VC, or equal
MCM 2133

⊕ L6808 Terminal device, hook, TRS Adept, infant or child, VC, or equal
MCM 2133

⊕ L6809 Terminal device, hook, TRS Super Sport, passive
MCM 2133

⊕ L6810 Terminal device, pincher tool, Otto Bock or equal
MCM 2133

Hands

⊕ L6825 Terminal device, hand, Dorrance, VO
MCM 2133

⊕ L6830 Terminal device, hand, APRL, VC
MCM 2133

⊕ L6835 Terminal device, hand, Sierra, VO
MCM 2133

⊕ L6840 Terminal device, hand, Becker Imperial
MCM 2133

⊕ L6845 Terminal device, hand, Becker Lock Grip
MCM 2133

⊕ L6850 Terminal device, hand, Becker Plylite
MCM 2133

✪ L6855 Terminal device, hand, Robin-Aids, VO
MCM 2133

✪ L6860 Terminal device, hand, Robin-Aids, VO soft
MCM 2133

✪ L6865 Terminal device, hand, passive hand
MCM 2133

✪ L6867 Terminal device, hand, Detroit infant hand (mechanical)
MCM 2133

✪ L6868 Terminal device, hand, passive infant hand, (Steeper, Hosmer or equal)
MCM 2133

✪ L6870 Terminal device, hand, child MITT
MCM 2133

✪ L6872 Terminal device, hand, NYU child hand
MCM 2133

✪ L6873 Terminal device, hand, mechanical infant hand, Steeper or equal
MCM 2133

✪ L6875 Terminal device, hand, Bock, VC
MCM 2133

✪ L6880 Terminal device, hand, Bock, VO
MCM 2133

✻ L6881 Automatic grasp feature, addition to upper limb prosthetic terminal device

✪ L6882 Microprocessor control feature, addition to upper limb prosthetic terminal device
MCM 2133

Gloves for Above Hands

✻ L6890 Terminal device, glove for above hands, production glove

✻ L6895 Terminal device, glove for above hands, custom glove

Hand Restoration

✻ L6900 Hand restoration (casts, shading and measurements included), partial hand, with glove, thumb or one finger remaining

✻ L6905 Hand restoration (casts, shading and measurements included), partial hand, with glove, multiple fingers remaining

✻ L6910 Hand restoration (casts, shading and measurements included), partial hand, with glove, no fingers remaining

✻ L6915 Hand restoration (shading, and measurements included), replacement glove for above

External Power

Base Devices

✻ L6920 Wrist disarticulation, external power, self-suspended inner socket, removable forearm shell, Otto Bock or equal, switch, cables, two batteries and one charger, switch control of terminal device

✻ L6925 Wrist disarticulation, external power, self-suspended inner socket, removable forearm shell, Otto Bock or equal, electrodes, cables, two batteries and one charger, myoelectronic control of terminal device

✻ L6930 Below elbow, external power, self-suspended inner socket, removable forearm shell, Otto Bock or equal, switch, cables, two batteries and one charger, switch control of terminal device

✻ L6935 Below elbow, external power, self-suspended inner socket, removable forearm shell, Otto Bock or equal, electrodes, cables, two batteries and one charger, myoelectronic control of terminal device

✻ L6940 Elbow disarticulation, external power, molded inner socket, removable humeral shell, outside locking hinges, forearm, Otto Bock or equal, switch, cables, two batteries and one charger, switch control of terminal device

✻ L6945 Elbow disarticulation, external power, molded inner socket, removable humeral shell, outside locking hinges, forearm, Otto Bock or equal, electrodes, cables, two batteries and one charger, myoelectronic control of terminal device

✻ L6950 Above elbow, external power, molded inner socket, removable humeral shell, internal locking elbow, forearm, Otto Bock or equal, switch, cables, two batteries and one charger, switch control of terminal device

✻ L6955 Above elbow, external power, molded inner socket, removable humeral shell, internal locking elbow, forearm, Otto Bock or equal, electrodes, cables, two batteries and one charger, myoelectronic control of terminal device

✻ L6960 Shoulder disarticulation, external power, molded inner socket, removable shoulder shell, shoulder bulkhead, humeral section, mechanical elbow, forearm, Otto Bock or equal, switch, cables, two batteries and one charger, switch control of terminal device

✻ L6965 Shoulder disarticulation, external power, molded inner socket, removable shoulder shell, shoulder bulkhead, humeral section, mechanical elbow, forearm, Otto Bock or equal, electrodes, cables, two batteries and one charger, myoelectronic control of terminal device

✻ L6970 Interscapular-thoracic, external power, molded inner socket, removable shoulder shell, shoulder bulkhead, humeral section, mechanical elbow, forearm, Otto Bock or equal, switch, cables, two batteries and one charger, switch control of terminal device

✻ L6975 Interscapular-thoracic, external power, molded inner socket, removable shoulder shell, shoulder bulkhead, humeral section, mechanical elbow, forearm, Otto Bock or equal, electrodes, cables, two batteries and one charger, myoelectronic control of terminal device

Terminal Devices

✻ L7010 Electronic hand, Otto Bock, Steeper or equal, switch controlled

✻ L7015 Electronic hand, System Teknik, Variety Village or equal, switch controlled

✻ L7020 Electronic greifer, Otto Bock or equal, switch controlled

✻ L7025 Electronic hand, Otto Bock or equal, myoelectronically controlled

✻ L7030 Electronic hand, System Teknik, Variety Village or equal, myoelectronically controlled

✻ L7035 Electronic greifer, Otto Bock or equal, myoelectronically controlled

✻ L7040 Prehensile actuator, Hosmer or equal, switch controlled

✻ L7045 Electronic hook, child, Michigan or equal, switch controlled

Elbow

✻ L7170 Electronic elbow, Hosmer or equal, switch controlled

✻ L7180 Electronic elbow, Boston, Utah or equal, myoelectronically controlled

✻ L7185 Electronic elbow, adolescent, Variety Village or equal, switch controlled

✻ L7186 Electronic elbow, child, Variety Village or equal, switch controlled

✻ L7190 Electronic elbow, adolescent, Variety Village or equal, myoelectronically controlled

✻ L7191 Electronic elbow, child, Variety Village or equal, myoelectronically controlled

✻ L7260 Electronic wrist rotator, Otto Bock or equal

✻ L7261 Electronic wrist rotator, for Utah arm

✻ L7266 Servo control, Steeper or equal

✻ L7272 Analogue control, UNB or equal

✻ L7274 Proportional control, 6-12 volt, Liberty, Utah or equal

Battery Components

✻ L7360 Six-volt battery, Otto Bock or equal, each

✻ L7362 Battery charger, 6 volt, Otto Bock or equal

✻ L7364 Twelve volt battery, Utah or equal, each

✻ L7366 Battery charger, 12 volt, Utah or equal

▶✻ L7367 Lithium ion battery, replacement

▶✻ L7368 Lithium ion battery charger

✻ L7499 Upper extremity prosthesis, not otherwise specified

Repairs

✪ L7500 Repair of prosthetic device, hourly rate (excludes V5335 repair of oral or laryngeal prosthesis or artificial larynx)
MCM 2100.4, MCM 2130D, MCM 2133

➡✪ L7510 Repair of prosthetic device, repair or replace minor parts
MCM 2100.4, MCM 2130D, MCM 2133

✻ L7520 Repair prosthetic device, labor component, per 15 minutes

➡✻ L7900 Male vacuum erection system

Breast Prostheses

✪ L8000 Breast prosthesis, mastectomy bra
MCM 2130A

✪ L8001 Breast prosthesis, mastectomy bra, with integrated breast prosthesis form, unilateral
MCM 2130A

✪ L8002 Breast prosthesis, mastectomy bra, with integrated breast prosthesis form, bilateral
MCM 2130A

✪ L8010 Breast prosthesis, mastectomy sleeve
MCM 2130A

✪ L8015 External breast prosthesis garment, with mastectomy form, post mastectomy
MCM 2130

✪ L8020 Breast prosthesis, mastectomy form
MCM 2130A

✪ L8030 Breast prosthesis, silicone or equal
MCM 2130A

✪ L8035 Custom breast prosthesis, post mastectomy, molded to patient mode
IMCM 2130

✻ L8039 Breast prosthesis, not otherwise specified

Nasal, Orbital, Auricular Prosthesis

✻ L8040 Nasal prosthesis, provided by a non-physician
✻ L8041 Midfacial prosthesis, provided by a non-physician
✻ L8042 Orbital prosthesis, provided by a non-physician
✻ L8043 Upper facial prosthesis, provided by a non-physician
✻ L8044 Hemi-facial prosthesis, provided by a non-physician
✻ L8045 Auricular prosthesis, provided by a non-physician
✻ L8046 Partial facial prosthesis, provided by a non-physician
✻ L8047 Nasal septal prosthesis, provided by a non-physician
✻ L8048 Unspecified maxillofacial prosthesis, by report, provided by a non-physician
✻ L8049 Repair or modification of maxillofacial prosthesis, labor component, 15-minute increments, provided by a non-physician

Elastic Supports

◆ L8100 Gradient compression stocking, below knee, 18-30 mm Hg, each
MCM 2133, CIM 60-9
◆ L8110 Gradient compression stocking, below knee, 30-40 mm Hg, each
MCM 2133, CIM 60-9
◆ L8120 Gradient compression stocking, below knee, 40-50 mm Hg, each
MCM 2133, CIM 60-9
◆ L8130 Gradient compression stocking, thigh length, 18-30 mm Hg, each
MCM 2133, CIM 60-9
◆ L8140 Gradient compression stocking, thigh length, 30-40 mm Hg, each
MCM 2133, CIM 60-9
◆ L8150 Gradient compression stocking, thigh length, 40-50 mm Hg, each
MCM 2133, CIM 60-9
◆ L8160 Gradient compression stocking, full length/chap style, 18-30 mm Hg, each
MCM 2133, CIM 60-9
◆ L8170 Gradient compression stocking, full length/chap style, 30-40 mm Hg, each
MCM 2133, CIM 60-9
◆ L8180 Gradient compression stocking, full length/chap style, 40-50 mm Hg, each
MCM 2133, CIM 60-9
◆ L8190 Gradient compression stocking, waist length, 18-30 mm Hg, each
MCM 2133, CIM 60-9
◆ L8195 Gradient compression stocking, waist length, 30-40 mm Hg, each
MCM 2133, CIM 60-9
◆ L8200 Gradient compression stocking, waist length, 40-50 mm Hg, each
MCM 2133, CIM 60-9
◆ L8210 Gradient compression stocking, custom made
MCM 2133, CIM 60-9
◆ L8220 Gradient compression stocking, lymphedema
MCM 2133, CIM 60-9
◆ L8230 Gradient compression stocking, garter belt
MCM 2133, CIM 60-9
✻ L8239 Gradient compression stocking, not otherwise specified

Trusses

✪ L8300 Truss, single with standard pad
MCM 2133, CIM 70-1, CIM 70-2
✪ L8310 Truss, double with standard pads
MCM 2133, CIM 70-1, CIM 70-2
✪ L8320 Truss, addition to standard pad, water pad
MCM 2133, CIM 70-1, CIM 70-2
✪ L8330 Truss, addition to standard pad, scrotal pad
MCM 2133, CIM 70-1, CIM 70-2

Prosthetic Socks

✪ L8400 Prosthetic sheath, below knee, each
MCM 2133
✪ L8410 Prosthetic sheath, above knee, each
MCM 2133
✪ L8415 Prosthetic sheath, upper limb, each
MCM 2133
✻ L8417 Prosthetic sheath/sock, including a gel cushion layer, below knee or above knee, each
✪ L8420 Prosthetic sock, multiple ply, below knee, each
MCM 2133
✪ L8430 Prosthetic sock, multiple ply, above knee, each
MCM 2133
✪ L8435 Prosthetic sock, multiple ply, upper limb, each
MCM 2133
✪ L8440 Prosthetic shrinker, below knee, each
MCM 2133
✪ L8460 Prosthetic shrinker, above knee, each
MCM 2133
✪ L8465 Prosthetic shrinker, upper limb, each
MCM 2133
✪ L8470 Prosthetic sock, single ply, fitting, below knee, each
MCM 2133

⊕ L8480 Prosthetic sock, single ply, fitting, above knee, each
MCM 2133

⊕ L8485 Prosthetic sock, single ply, fitting, upper limb, each
MCM 2133

* L8490 Addition to prosthetic sheath/sock, air seal suction retention system

* L8499 Unlisted procedure for miscellaneous prosthetic services

Prosthetic Implants

Integumentary System

⊕ L8500 Artificial larynx, any type
MCM 2130, CIM 65-5

⊕ L8501 Tracheostomy speaking valve
CIM 65-16

* L8505 Artificial larynx replacement battery/accessory, any type

* L8507 Tracheo-esophageal voice prosthesis, patient inserted, any type, each

* L8509 Tracheo-esophageal voice prosthesis, inserted by licensed health car provider, any type

⊕ L8510 Voice amplifier
CIM 65-5

⊕ L8600 Implantable breast prosthesis, silicone or equal
MCM 2130, CIM 35-47

⊕ L8603 Injectable bulking agent, collagen implant, urinary tract, per 2.5 cc syringe, includes shipping and necessary supplies
CIM 65-9

Urinary System

⊕ L8606 Injectable bulking agent, synthetic implant, urinary tract, 1 cc syringe, includes shipping and necessary supplies
CIM 65.9

Head (Skull, Facial Bones, and Temporomandibular Joint)

⊕ L8610 Ocular implant
MCM 2130

⊕ L8612 Aqueous shunt
MCM 2130, Cross Reference Q0074

⊕ L8613 Ossicula implant
MCM 2130

⊕ L8614 Cochlear device/system
MCM 2130, CIM 65-14

⊕ L8619 Cochlear implant external speech processor, replacement
CIM 65-14

Upper Extremity

⊕ L8630 Metacarpophalangeal joint implant
MCM 2130

Lower Extremity (Joint: Knee, Ankle, Toe)

⊕ L8641 Metatarsal joint implant
MCM 2130

⊕ L8642 Hallux implant
MCM 2130, Cross Reference Q0073

Miscellaneous Muscular-Skeletal

⊕ L8658 Interphalangeal joint implant
MCM 2130

Cardiovascular System

⊕ L8670 Vascular graft material, synthetic, implant
MCM 2130

Genital

* L8699 Prosthetic implant, not otherwise specified

* L9900 Orthotic and prosthetic supply, accessory, and/or service component of another HCPCS L code

MEDICAL SERVICES (M0000-M0399)

Other Medical Services

⊕ M0064 Brief office visit for the sole purpose of monitoring or changing drug prescriptions used in the treatment of mental psychoneurotic and personality disorders
MCM 2476.3

◆ M0075 Cellular therapy
CIM 35-5

◆ M0076 Prolotherapy
CIM 35-13

◆ M0100 Intragastric hypothermia using gastric freezing (MNP)
CIM 35-65

◆ M0300 IV chelation therapy (chemical endarterectomy)
CIM 35-64

◆ M0301 Fabric wrapping of abdominal aneurysm (MNP)
CIM 35-34

M0302 Deleted 01/01/02, Cross Reference CPT

PATHOLOGY AND LABORATORY TESTS (P2000-P2999)

Chemistry and Toxicology Tests

- ✪ P2028 Cephalin flocculation, blood
  CIM 50-34
- ✪ P2029 Congo red, blood
  CIM 50-34
- ◆ P2031 Hair analysis (excluding arsenic)
  CIM 50-24
- ✪ P2033 Thymol turbidity, blood
  CIM 50-34
- ✪ P2038 Mucoprotein, blood (seromucoid) (medical necessity procedure)
  CIM 50-34

Pathology Screening Tests

- ✪ P3000 Screening Papanicolaou smear, cervical or vaginal, up to three smears, by technician under physician supervision
  CIM 50-20, Laboratory Certification: cytology
- ✪ P3001 Screening Papanicolaou smear, cervical or vaginal, up to three smears, requiring interpretation by physician
  CIM 50-20, Laboratory Certification: cytology

Microbiology Tests

- ◆ P7001 Culture, bacterial, urine; quantitative, sensitivity study
  Cross Reference CPT, Laboratory Certification: bacteriology

Miscellaneous Pathology

- ✪ P9010 Blood (whole), for transfusion, per unit
  MCM 2455A
- ✪ P9011 Blood (split unit), specify amount
  MCM 2455A
- ✪ P9012 Cryoprecipitate, each unit
  MCM 2455B
- ✪ P9016 Red blood cells, leukocytes reduced, each unit
  MCM 2455B
- ✪ P9017 Fresh frozen plasma (single donor), each unit
  MCM 2455B
- P9018 Deleted 01/01/01
- ✪ P9019 Platelets, each unit
  MCM 2455B
- ✪ P9020 Platelet rich plasma, each unit
  MCM 2455B
- ✪ P9021 Red blood cells, each unit
  MCM 2455A
- ✪ P9022 Red blood cells, washed, each unit
  MCM 2455A
- ✪ P9023 Plasma, pooled multiple donor, solvent/detergent treated, frozen, each unit
  MCM 2455B
- ✪ P9031 Platelets, leukocytes reduced, each unit
  MCM 2455
- ✪ P9032 Platelets, irradiated, each unit
  MCM 2455
- ✪ P9033 Platelets, leukocytes reduced, irradiated, each unit
  MCM 2455
- ✪ P9034 Platelets, pheresis, each unit
  MCM 2455
- ✪ P9035 Platelets, pheresis, leukocytes reduced, each unit
  MCM 2455
- ✪ P9036 Platelets, pheresis, irradiated, each unit
  MCM 2455
- ✪ P9037 Platelets, pheresis, leukocytes reduced, irradiated, each unit
  MCM 2455
- ✪ P9038 Red blood cells, irradiated, each unit
  MCM 2455
- ✪ P9039 Red blood cells, deglycerolized, each unit
  MCM 2455
- ✪ P9040 Red blood cells, leukocytes reduced, irradiated, each unit
  MCM 2455
- ✻ P9041 Infusion, albumin (human), 5%, 50 cc
- P9042 Deleted 01/01/02, Cross Reference P9046
- ✪ P9043 Infusion, plasma protein fraction (human), 5%, 50 cc
  MCM 2455B
- ✪ P9044 Plasma, cryoprecipitate reduced, each unit
  MCM 2455B
- ✻ P9045 Infusion, albumin (human), 5%, 250 cc
- ✻ P9046 Infusion, albumin (human), 25%, 20 cc
- ✻ P9047 Infusion, albumin (human), 25%, 50 cc
- ✻ P9048 Infusion, plasma protein fraction (human), 5%, 250 cc
- ✻ P9050 Granulocytes, pheresis, each unit
- ✪ P9603 Travel allowance one way in connection with medically necessary laboratory specimen collection drawn from home bound or nursing home bound patient; prorated miles actually traveled.
  MCM 5114.1K

⊙ P9604 Travel allowance one way in connection with medically necessary laboratory specimen collection drawn from home bound or nursing home bound patient; prorated trip charge
MCM 5114.1K

⊙ P9612 Catheterization for collection of specimen, single patient, all places of service
MCM 5114.1D

⊙ P9615 Catheterization for collection of specimen(s) (multiple patients)
MCM 5114.1D

Q CODES: TEMPORARY CODES (Q0000-Q9999)

⊙ Q0035 Cardiokymography
CIM 50-50

⊙ Q0081 Infusion therapy, using other than chemotherapy drugs, per visit
CIM 60-14

* Q0083 Chemotherapy administration by other than infusion technique only (e.g., subcutaneous, intramuscular, push), per visit

⊙ Q0084 Chemotherapy administration by infusion technique only, per visit
CIM 60-14

* Q0085 Chemotherapy administration by both infusion technique and other technique(s) (e.g., subcutaneous, intramuscular, push), per visit

* Q0086 Physical therapy evaluation/treatment, per visit
MCI 2210

⊙ Q0091 Screening Papanicolaou smear; obtaining, preparing and conveyance of cervical or vaginal smear to laboratory
CIM 50-20

⊙ Q0092 Setup portable x-ray equipment
MCM 2070.4

* Q0111 Wet mounts, including preparations of vaginal, cervical or skin specimens; Laboratory Certification: bacteriology, mycology, parasitology

* Q0112 All potassium hydroxide (KOH) preparations; Laboratory Certification: mycology

* Q0113 Pinworm examinations; Laboratory Certification: parasitology

* Q0114 Fern test; Laboratory certification: routine chemistry

* Q0115 Post-coital direct, qualitative examinations of vaginal or cervical mucus; Laboratory Certification: hematology

⊙ Q0136 Injection, epoetin alfa, (for non-ESRD use), per 1000 units
MCM 2049

▶◆ Q0144 Azithromycin dihydrate, oral, capsules/powder, 1 gm

Q0160 Deleted 01/01/02, Cross Reference J7193

Q0161 Deleted 01/01/02, Cross Reference J7195

⊙ Q0163 Diphenhydramine HCl, 50 mg, oral, FDA-approved prescription antiemetic, for use as a complete therapeutic substitute for an IV antiemetic at time of chemotherapy treatment not to exceed a 48-hour dosage regimen
Medicare Statute 4557

⊙ Q0164 Prochlorperazine maleate, 5 mg, oral, FDA-approved prescription antiemetic, for use as a complete therapeutic substitute for an IV antiemetic at the time of chemotherapy treatment, not to exceed a 48-hour dosage regimen
Medicare Statute 4557

⊙ Q0165 Prochlorperazine maleate, 10 mg, oral, FDA-approved prescription antiemetic, for use as a complete therapeutic substitute for an IV antiemetic at the time of chemotherapy treatment, not to exceed a 48-hour dosage regimen
Medicare Statute 4557

⊙ Q0166 Granisetron HCl, 1 mg, oral, FDA-approved prescription antiemetic, for use as a complete therapeutic substitute for an IV antiemetic at the time of chemotherapy treatment, not to exceed a 24-hour dosage regimen
Medicare Statute 4557

⊙ Q0167 Dronabinol, 2.5 mg, oral, FDA-approved prescription antiemetic, for use as a complete therapeutic substitute for an IV antiemetic at the time of chemotherapy treatment, not to exceed a 48-hour dosage regimen
Medicare Statute 4557

⊙ Q0168 Dronabinol, 5 mg, oral, FDA-approved prescription antiemetic, for use as a complete therapeutic substitute for an IV antiemetic at the time of chemotherapy treatment, not to exceed a 48-hour dosage regimen
Medicare Statute 4557

⊙ Q0169 Promethazine HCl, 12.5 mg, oral, FDA-approved prescription antiemetic, for use as a complete therapeutic substitute for an IV antiemetic at the time of chemotherapy treatment, not to exceed a 48-hour dosage regimen
Medicare Statute 4557

⊙ Q0170 Promethazine HCl, 25 mg, oral, FDA-approved prescription antiemetic, for use as a complete therapeutic substitute for an IV antiemetic at the time of chemotherapy treatment, not to exceed a 48-hour dosage regimen
Medicare Statute 4557

❂	Q0171	Chlorpromazine HCl, 10 mg, oral, FDA-approved prescription antiemetic, for use as a complete therapeutic substitute for an IV antiemetic at the time of chemotherapy treatment, not to exceed a 48-hour dosage regimen Medicare Statute 4557
❂	Q0172	Chlorpromazine HCl, 25 mg, oral, FDA-approved prescription antiemetic, for use as a complete therapeutic substitute for an IV antiemetic at the time of chemotherapy treatment, not to exceed a 48-hour dosage regimen Medicare Statute 4557
❂	Q0173	Trimethobenzamide HCl, 250 mg, oral, FDA-approved prescription antiemetic, for use as a complete therapeutic substitute for an IV antiemetic at the time of chemotherapy treatment, not to exceed a 48-hour dosage regimen Medicare Statute 4557
❂	Q0174	Thiethylperazine maleate, 10 mg, oral, FDA-approved prescription antiemetic, for use as a complete therapeutic substitute for an IV antiemetic at the time of chemotherapy treatment, not to exceed a 48-hour dosage regimen Medicare Statute 4557
❂	Q0175	Perphenazine, 4 mg, oral, FDA-approved prescription antiemetic, for use as a complete therapeutic substitute for an IV antiemetic at the time of chemotherapy treatment, not to exceed a 48-hour dosage regimen Medicare Statute 4557
❂	Q0176	Perphenazine, 8 mg, oral, FDA-approved prescription antiemetic, for use as a complete therapeutic substitute for an IV antiemetic at the time of chemotherapy treatment, not to exceed a 48-hour dosage regimen Medicare Statute 4557
❂	Q0177	Hydroxyzine pamoate, 25 mg, oral, FDA-approved prescription antiemetic, for use as a complete therapeutic substitute for an IV antiemetic at the time of chemotherapy treatment, not to exceed a 48-hour dosage regimen Medicare Statute 4557
❂	Q0178	Hydroxyzine pamoate, 50 mg, oral, FDA-approved prescription antiemetic, for use as a complete therapeutic substitute for an IV antiemetic at the time of chemotherapy treatment, not to exceed a 48-hour dosage regimen Medicare Statute 4557
❂	Q0179	Ondansetron HCl, 8 mg, oral, FDA-approved prescription antiemetic, for use as a complete therapeutic substitute for an IV antiemetic at the time of chemotherapy treatment, not to exceed a 48-hour dosage regimen Medicare Statute 4557
❂	Q0180	Dolasetron mesylate, 100 mg, oral, FDA-approved prescription antiemetic, for use as a complete therapeutic substitute for an IV antiemetic at the time of chemotherapy treatment, not to exceed a 24-hour dosage regimen Medicare Statute 4557
❂	Q0181	Unspecified oral dosage form, FDA-approved prescription antiemetic, for use as a complete therapeutic substitute for a IV antiemetic at the time of chemotherapy treatment, not to exceed a 48-hour dosage regimen Medicare Statute 4557
*	Q0183	Dermal tissue, of human origin, with and without other bioengineered or processed elements, but without metabolically active elements, per square centimeter
	Q0184	Deleted 12/31/02
	Q0185	Deleted 01/01/02, Cross Reference J7340
❂	Q0187	Factor VIIA (coagulation factor, recombinant) per 1.2 mg MCM 2049
❂	Q1001	New technology intraocular lens category 1 as defined in Federal Register notice, Vol 65, dated May 3, 2000
❂	Q1002	New technology intraocular lens category 2 as defined in Federal Register notice, Vol 65, dated May 3, 2000
❂	Q1003	New technology intraocular lens category 3 as defined in Federal Register notice
❂	Q1004	New technology intraocular lens category 4 as defined in Federal Register notice
❂	Q1005	New technology intraocular lens category 5 as defined in Federal Register notice
◆	Q2001	Oral, cabergoline, 0.5 mg MCM 2049.5
❂	Q2002	Injection, Elliott's B solution, per milliliter MCM 2049, Medicare Statute 1861S2B
❂	Q2003	Injection, aprotinin, 10,000 KIU MCM 2049, Medicare Statute 1861S2B
❂	Q2004	Irrigation solution for treatment of bladder calculi, for example Renacidin, per 500 cc MCM 2049, Medicare Statute 1861S2B
❂	Q2005	Injection, corticorelin ovine triflutate, per dose MCM 2049, Medicare Statute 1861S2B

⊕ Q2006 Injection, digoxin immune FAB (ovine), per vial
MCM 2049, Medicare Statute 1861S2B

⊕ Q2007 Injection, ethanolamine oleate, 100 mg
MCM 2049, Medicare Statute 1861S2B

⊕ Q2008 Injection, fomepizole, 15 mg
MCM 2049, Medicare Statute 1861S2B

⊕ Q2009 Injection, fosphenytoin, 50 mg
MCM 2049, Medicare Statute 1861S2B

⊕ Q2010 Injection, glatiramer acetate, per dose
MCM 2049, Medicare Statute 1861S2B

⊕ Q2011 Injection, hemin, per 1 mg
MCM 2049, Medicare Statute 1861S2B

⊕ Q2012 Injection, pegademase bovine, 25 IU
MCM 2049, Medicare Statute 1861S2B

⊕ Q2013 Injection, pentastarch, 10% solution, per 100 cc
MCM 2049, Medicare Statute 1861S2B

⊕ Q2014 Injection, sermorelin acetate, 0.5 mg
Medicare Statute 1861S2B MCM 2049

Q2015 Deleted 01/01/02

Q2016 Deleted 01/01/02

⊕ Q2017 Injection, teniposide, 50 mg
MCM 2049, Medicare Statute 1861S2B

⊕ Q2018 Injection, urofollitropin, 75 IU
MCM 2049, Medicare Statute 1861S2B

⊕ Q2019 Injection, basiliximab, 20 mg
MCM 2049, Medicare Statute 1861S2B

⊕ Q2020 Injection, histrelin acetate, 10 mcg
MCM 2049, Medicare Statute 1861S2B

⊕ Q2021 Injection, lepirudin, 50 mg
MCM 2049, Medicare Statute 1861S2B

⊕ Q2022 Von Willebrand factor complex, human, per IU
MCM 2049.5, CIM 35-30

▶⊕ Q3000 Supply of radiopharmaceutical diagnostic imaging agent, rubidium RB-82, per dose

⊕ Q3001 Radioelements for brachytherapy, any type, each
MCM 15022

⊕ Q3002 Supply of radiopharmaceutical diagnostic imaging agent, gallium GA-67, per millicurie
MCM 15022

⊕ Q3003 Supply of radiopharmaceutical diagnostic imaging agent, technetium Tc99m bicisate, per unit dose
MCM 15022

⊕ Q3004 Supply of radiopharmaceutical diagnostic imaging agent, xenon XE-133, per 10 mCi
MCM 15022

⊕ Q3005 Supply of radiopharmaceutical diagnostic imaging agent, technetium Tc99m mertiatide, per mCi
MCM 15022

⊕ Q3006 Supply of radiopharmaceutical diagnostic imaging agent, technetium Tc99m gluceptate, per 5 mCi
MCM 15022

⊕ Q3007 Supply of radiopharmaceutical diagnostic imaging agent, sodium phosphate P-32, per mCi
MCM 15022

⊕ Q3008 Supply of radiopharmaceutical diagnostic imaging agent, indium In-111 pentetreotide, per 3 mCi
MCM 15022

⊕ Q3009 Supply of radiopharmaceutical diagnostic imaging agent, technetium Tc99m oxidronate, per millicurie
MCM 15022

⊕ Q3010 Supply of radiopharmaceutical diagnostic imaging agent, technetium Tc99m–labeled red blood cells, per millicurie
MCM 15022

⊕ Q3011 Supply of radiopharmaceutical diagnostic imaging agent, chromic phosphate P-32 suspension, per millicurie
MCM 15022

⊕ Q3012 Supply of oral radiopharmaceutical diagnostic imaging agent, cyanocobalamin cobalt Co-57, per 0.5 mCi
MCM 15022

Q3013 Deleted 01/01/02, Cross Reference J3395

* Q3014 Telehealth originating site facility fee

Q3017 Deleted 03/31/02

▶* Q3019 ALS vehicle used, emergency transport, no ALS level services furnished.

▶* Q3020 ALS vehicle used, non-emergency transport, no ALS level service furnished

▶◆ Q3021 Injection, hepatitis B vaccine, pediatric or adolescent, per dose

▶◆ Q3022 Injection, hepatitis B vaccine, adult, per dose

▶◆ Q3023 Injection, hepatitis B vaccine, immunosuppressed patients (including renal dialysis patients), per dose

▶⊕ Q3025 Injection, interferon beta-1a, 11 mcg for intramuscular use
MCM 2049

▶◆ Q3026 Injection, interferon beta-1a, 11 mcg for subcutaneous use

Q3030 Deleted 12/31/02, Cross Reference J7317

* Q4001 Casting supplies, body cast adult, with or without head, plaster

* Q4002 Cast supplies, body cast adult, with or without head, fiberglass

* Q4003 Cast supplies, shoulder cast, adult (11 years +), plaster

* Q4004 Cast supplies, shoulder cast, adult (11 years +), fiberglass

* Q4005 Cast supplies, long arm cast, adult (11 years +), plaster

* Q4006 Cast supplies, long arm cast, adult (11 years +), fiberglass

* Q4007 Cast supplies, long arm cast, pediatric (0-10 years), plaster

✱ Q4008 Cast supplies, long arm cast, pediatric (0-10 years), fiberglass
✱ Q4009 Cast supplies, short arm cast, adult (11 years +), plaster
✱ Q4010 Cast supplies, short arm cast, adult (11 years +), fiberglass
✱ Q4011 Cast supplies, short arm cast, pediatric (0-10 years), plaster
✱ Q4012 Cast supplies, short arm cast, pediatric (0-10 years), fiberglass
✱ Q4013 Cast supplies, gauntlet cast (includes lower forearm and hand), adult (11 years +), plaster
✱ Q4014 Cast supplies, gauntlet cast (includes lower forearm and hand), adult (11 years +), fiberglass
✱ Q4015 Cast supplies, gauntlet cast (includes lower forearm and hand), pediatric (0-10 years), plaster
✱ Q4016 Cast supplies, gauntlet cast (includes lower forearm and hand), pediatric (0-10 years), fiberglass
✱ Q4017 Cast supplies, long arm splint, adult (11 years +), plaster
✱ Q4018 Cast supplies, long arm splint, adult (11 years +), fiberglass
✱ Q4019 Cast supplies, long arm splint, pediatric (0-10 years), plaster
✱ Q4020 Cast supplies, long arm splint, pediatric (0-10 years), fiberglass
✱ Q4021 Cast supplies, short arm splint, adult (11 years +), plaster
✱ Q4022 Cast supplies, short arm splint, adult (11 years +), fiberglass
✱ Q4023 Cast supplies, short arm splint, pediatric (0-10 years), plaster
✱ Q4024 Cast supplies, short arm splint, pediatric (0-10 years), fiberglass
✱ Q4025 Cast supplies, hip spica (one or both legs), adult (11 years +), plaster
✱ Q4026 Cast supplies, hip spica (one or both legs), adult (11 years +), fiberglass
✱ Q4027 Cast supplies, hip spica (one or both legs), pediatric (0-10 years), plaster
✱ Q4028 Cast supplies, hip spica (one or both legs), pediatric (0-10 years), fiberglass
✱ Q4029 Cast supplies, long leg cast, adult (11 years +), plaster
✱ Q4030 Cast supplies, long leg cast, adult (11 years +), fiberglass
✱ Q4031 Cast supplies, long leg cast, pediatric (0-10 years), plaster
✱ Q4032 Cast supplies, long leg cast, pediatric (0-10 years), fiberglass
✱ Q4033 Cast supplies, long leg cylinder cast, adult (11 years +), plaster
✱ Q4034 Cast supplies, long leg cylinder cast, adult (11 years +), fiberglass
✱ Q4035 Cast supplies, long leg cylinder cast, pediatric (0-10 years), plaster
✱ Q4036 Cast supplies, long leg cylinder cast, pediatric (0-10 years), fiberglass
✱ Q4037 Cast supplies, short leg cast, adult (11 years +), plaster
✱ Q4038 Cast supplies, short leg cast, adult (11 years +), fiberglass
✱ Q4039 Cast supplies, short leg cast, pediatric (0-10 years), plaster
✱ Q4040 Cast supplies, short leg cast, pediatric (0-10 years), fiberglass
✱ Q4041 Cast supplies, long leg splint, adult (11 years +), plaster
✱ Q4042 Cast supplies, long leg splint, adult (11 years +), fiberglass
✱ Q4043 Cast supplies, long leg splint, pediatric (0-10 years), plaster
✱ Q4044 Cast supplies, long leg splint, pediatric (0-10 years), fiberglass
✱ Q4045 Cast supplies, short leg splint, adult (11 years +), plaster
✱ Q4046 Cast supplies, short leg splint, adult (11 years +), fiberglass
✱ Q4047 Cast supplies, short leg splint, pediatric (0-10 years), plaster
✱ Q4048 Cast supplies, short leg splint, pediatric (0-10 years), fiberglass
✱ Q4049 Finger splint, static
✱ Q4050 Cast supplies, for unlisted types and materials of casts
✱ Q4051 Splint supplies, miscellaneous (includes thermoplastics, strapping, fasteners, padding and other supplies)

Injection Codes for Epoetin Alfa

✪ Q9920 Injection of epoetin alfa (EPO), per 1000 units, at patient HCT of 20 or less
MCM 4273.1
✪ Q9921 Injection of EPO, per 1000 units, at patient HCT of 21
MCM 4273.1
✪ Q9922 Injection of EPO, per 1000 units, at patient HCT of 22
MCM 4273.1
✪ Q9923 Injection of EPO, per 1000 units, at patient HCT of 23
MCM 4273.1
✪ Q9924 Injection of EPO, per 1000 units, at patient HCT of 24
MCM 4273.1
✪ Q9925 Injection of EPO, per 1000 units, at patient HCT of 25
MCM 4273.1
✪ Q9926 Injection of EPO, per 1000 units, at patient HCT of 26
MCM 4273.1
✪ Q9927 Injection of EPO, per 1000 units, at patient HCT of 27
MCM 4273.1

✪ Q9928 Injection of EPO, per 1000 units, at patient HCT of 28
MCM 4273.1

✪ Q99[illegible] Injection of EPO, per 1000 units, at patient HCT of 29
MCM 4273.1

[illegible]930 Injection of EPO, per 1000 units, at patient HCT of 30
MCM 4273.1

✪ Q9931 Injection of EPO, per 1000 units, at patient HCT of 31
MCM 4273.1

✪ Q9932 Injection of EPO, per 1000 units, at patient HCT of 32
MCM 4273.1

✪ Q9933 Injection of EPO, per 1000 units, at patient HCT of 33
MCM 4273.1

✪ Q9934 Injection of EPO, per 1000 units, at patient HCT of 34
MCM 4273.1

✪ Q9935 Injection of EPO, per 1000 units, at patient HCT of 35
MCM 4273.1

✪ Q9936 Injection of EPO, per 1000 units, at patient HCT of 36
MCM 4273.1

✪ Q9937 Injection of EPO, per 1000 units, at patient HCT of 37
MCM 4273.1

✪ Q9938 Injection of EPO, per 1000 units, at patient HCT of 38
MCM 4273.1

✪ Q9939 Injection of EPO, per 1000 units, at patient HCT of 39
MCM 4273.1

✪ Q9940 Injection of EPO, per 1000 units, at patient HCT of 40 or above
MCM 4273.1

DOMESTIC RADIOLOGY SERVICES (R0000-R5999)

Transportation/Setup of Portable X-Ray Equipment

✪ R0070 Transportation of portable x-ray equipment and personnel to home or nursing home, per trip to facility or location, one patient seen
MCM 2070.4, MCM 5244B

✪ R0075 Transportation of portable x-ray equipment and personnel to home or nursing home, per trip to facility or location, more than one patient seen, per patient
MCM 2070.4, MCM 5244B

✪ R0076 Transportation of portable ECG to facility or location, per patient
MCM 2070.1, MCM 2070.4, CIM 50-15

TEMPORARY NATIONAL CODES (S0009-S9999)

▶ SK Member of high risk population (use only with codes for immunization)

▶ SL State supplied vaccine

▶ SM Second surgical opinion

▶ SN Third surgical opinion

◆ S0009 Injection, butorphanol tartrate, 1 mg

◆ S0012 Butorphanol tartrate, nasal spray, 25 mg

◆ S0014 Tacrine HCl, 10 mg

◆ S0016 Injection, amikacin sulfate, 500 mg

◆ S0017 Injection, aminocaproic acid, 5 gm

◆ S0020 Injection, bupivacaine HCl, 30 cc

◆ S0021 Injection, cefoperazone sodium, 1 gm

◆ S0023 Injection, cimetidine HCl, 300 mg

S0024 Deleted 01/01/02

◆ S0028 Injection, famotidine, 20 mg

S0029 Deleted 01/01/02, Cross Reference J1450

◆ S0030 Injection, metronidazole, 500 mg

◆ S0032 Injection, nafcillin sodium, 2 gm

◆ S0034 Injection, ofloxacin, 400 mg

◆ S0039 Injection, sulfamethoxazole and trimethoprim, 10 cc

◆ S0040 Injection, ticarcillin disodium and clavulanate potassium, 3.1 gm

◆ S0071 Injection, acyclovir sodium, 50 mg

◆ S0072 Injection, amikacin sulfate, 100 mg

◆ S0073 Injection, aztreonam, 500 mg

◆ S0074 Injection, cefotetan disodium, 500 mg

◆ S0077 Injection, clindamycin phosphate, 300 mg

◆ S0078 Injection, fosphenytoin sodium, 750 mg

◆ S0079 Injection, octreotide acetate, 100 mcg (for doses over 1 mg use J2352 or C1207)

◆ S0080 Injection, pentamidine isethionate, 300 mg

◆ S0081 Injection, piperacillin sodium, 500 mg

S0085 Deleted 12/31/02, Cross Reference J1590

S0086 Deleted 01/01/02, Cross Reference J3395

S0087 Deleted 12/31/02, Cross Reference J9010

➡◆ S0088 Imatinib, 100 mg

◆ S0090 Sildenafil citrate, 25 mg

➡◆ S0091 Granisetron hydrochloride, 1 mg (for circumstances falling under the Medicare statute, use Q0166)

➡◆ S0092 Injection, hydromorphone hydrochloride, 250 mg (loading dose for infusion pump)

➡◆ S0093 Injection, morphine sulfate, 500 mg (loading dose for infusion pump)

S0096 Deleted 01/01/02

▶◆ S0104 Zidovudine, oral, 100 mg

▶◆ S0106 Bupropion HCl sustained release tablet, 150 mg, per bottle of 60 tablets

▶◆ S0108 Mercaptopurine, oral, 50 mg

S0112 Deleted 12/31/02, Cross Reference J0880

▶◆ S0114 Injection, treprostinil sodium, 0.5 mg

▶◆ S0122 Injection, menotropins, 75 IU

▶◆ S0124 Injection, urofollitropin, purified, 75 IU

▶◆ S0126 Injection, follitropin alfa, 75 IU

▶◆ S0128 Injection, follitropin beta, 75 IU

▶◆ S0130 Injection, chorionic gonadotropin, 5000 units

▶◆ S0132 Injection, ganirelix acetate, 250 mcg

▶◆ S0135 Injection, pegfilgrastim, 6 mg

◆ S0155 Sterile dilatant for epoprostenol, 50 cc

◆ S0156 Exemestane, 25 mg

◆ S0157 Becaplermin gel 0.01%, 0.5 gm

◆ S0170 Anastrozole, oral, 1mg

◆ S0171 Injection, bumetanide, 0.5mg

◆ S0172 Chlorambucil, oral, 2mg

◆ S0173 Dexamethasone, oral, 4mg

◆ S0174 Dolasetron mesylate, oral 50mg (for circumstances falling under the Medicare statute, use Q0180)

◆ S0175 Flutamide, oral, 125mg

◆ S0176 Hydroxyurea, oral, 500mg

◆ S0177 Levamisole HCl, oral, 50mg

◆ S0178 Lomustine, oral, 10mg

◆ S0179 Megestrol acetate, oral, 20mg

◆ S0181 Ondansetron HCl, oral, 4mg (for circumstances falling under the Medicare statute, use Q0179)

◆ S0182 Procarbazine HCl, oral, 50mg

◆ S0183 Prochlorperazine maleate, oral, 5mg (for circumstances falling under the Medicare statute, use Q0164-Q0165)

◆ S0187 Tamoxifen citrate, oral, 10mg

◆ S0189 Testosterone pellet, 75mg

◆ S0190 Mifepristone, oral, 200 mg

◆ S0191 Misoprostol, oral 200 mcg

▶◆ S0195 Pneumococcal conjugate vaccine, polyvalent, intramuscular, for children from five years to nine years of age who have not previously received the vaccine

◆ S0199 Medically induced abortion by oral ingestion of medication including all associated services and supplies (e.g., patient counseling, office visits, confirmation of pregnancy by HCG, ultrasound to confirm duration of pregnancy, ultrasound to confirm completion of abortion), except drugs

▶◆ S0201 Partial hospitalization services, less than 24 hours, per diem

S0206 Deleted 12/31/02, Cross Reference modifier SU

▶◆ S0207 Paramedic intercept, non-hospital based ALS service (non-voluntary), non-transport

◆ S0208 Paramedic intercept, hospital-based ALS service (non-voluntary), non-transport

◆ S0209 Wheelchair van, mileage, per mile

➡◆ S0215 Non-emergency transportation; mileage per mile

◆ S0220 Medical conference by a physician with interdisciplinary team of health professionals or representatives of community agencies to coordinate activities of patient care (patient is present); approximately 30 minutes

◆ S0221 Medical conference by a physician with interdisciplinary team of health professionals or representatives of community agencies to coordinate activities of patient care (patient is present); approximately 60 minutes

◆ S0250 Comprehensive geriatric assessment and treatment planning performed by assessment team

◆ SO255 Hospice referral visit (advising patient and family of care options) performed by nurse, social worker, or other designated staff

◆ S0260 History and physical (outpatient or office) related to surgical procedure (list separately in addition to code for appropriate evaluation and management service)

◆ S0302 Completed EPSDT service (list in addition to code for appropriate evaluation and management service)

◆ S0310 Hospitalist services (list separately in addition to code for appropriate evaluation and management service)

▶◆ S0315 Disease management program; initial assessment and initiation of the program

▶◆ S0316 Follow-up/assessment

▶◆ S0320 Telephone calls by a registered nurse to a disease management program member for monitoring purposes; per month

◆ S0340 Lifestyle modification program for management of coronary artery disease, including all supportive services; first quarter/stage

◆ S0341 Lifestyle modification program for management of coronary artery disease, including all supportive services; second or third quarter/stage

◆ S0342 Lifestyle modification program for management of coronary artery disease, including all supportive services; fourth quarter/stage

▶◆ S0390 Routine foot care; removal and/or trimming of corns, calluses and/or nails and preventive maintenance in specific medical conditions (e.g., diabetes), per visit

◆ S0395 Impression casting of a foot performed by a practitioner other than the manufacturer of the orthotic

- ◆ S0400 Global fee for extracorporeal shock wave lithotripsy treatment of kidney stone(s)
- ◆ S0500 Disposable contact lens, per lens
- ◆ S050[illegible] Single vision prescription lens (safety, athletic, or sunglass), per lens
- ◆ S0506 Bifocal vision prescription lens (safety, athletic, or sunglass), per lens
- ◆ S0508 Trifocal vision prescription lens (safety, athletic, or sunglass), per lens
- ◆ S0510 Non-prescription lens (safety, athletic, or sunglass), per lens
- ◆ S0512 Daily wear specialty contact lens, per lens
- ◆ S0514 Color contact lens, per lens
- ◆ S0516 Safety eyeglass frames
- ◆ S0518 Sunglasses frames
- ◆ S0580 Polycarbonate lens (list this code in addition to the basic code for the lens)
- ◆ S0581 Nonstandard lens (list this code in addition to the basic code for the lens)
- ◆ S0590 Integral lens service, miscellaneous services reported separately
- ◆ S0592 Comprehensive contact lens evaluation
- ◆ S0601 Screening proctoscopy
- ◆ S0605 Digital rectal examination, annual
- ◆ S0610 Annual gynecological examination, new patient
- ◆ S0612 Annual gynecological examination, established patient
- ◆ S0620 Routine ophthalmological examination including refraction; new patient
- ◆ S0621 Routine ophthalmological examination including refraction; established patient
- ◆ S0622 Physical exam for college, new or established patient (list separately) in addition to appropriate evaluation and management code)
- ◆ S0630 Removal of sutures; by a physician other than the physician who originally closed the wound
- ◆ S0800 Laser in situ keratomileusis (lasik)
- ◆ S0810 Photorefractive keratectomy (PRK)
- ◆ S0812 Phototherapeutic keratectomy (PTK)
- ◆ S0820 Computerized corneal topography, unilateral
- ◆ S0830 Ultrasound pachymetry to determine corneal thickness, with interpretation and report, unilateral
- ◆ S1001 Deluxe item, patient aware (list in addition to code for basic item)
- ◆ S1002 Customized item (list in addition to code for basic item)
- ◆ S1015 IV tubing extension set
- ◆ S1016 Non–polyvinyl chloride (PVC) IV administration set, for use with drugs that are not stable in PVC (e.g., paclitaxel)
- ◆ S1025 Inhaled nitric oxide for the treatment of hypoxic respiratory failure in the neonate; per diem
- ◆ S1030 Continuous noninvasive glucose monitoring device, purchase (for physician interpretation of data, use CPT code
- ◆ S1031 Continuous noninvasive glucose monitoring device, rental, including sensor, sensor replacement, and download to monitor (for physician interpretation of data, use CPT code
- ▶◆ S1040 Cranial remolding orthosis, rigid, with soft interface material, custom fabricated, includes fitting and adjustment(s)
- S2052 Deleted 01/01/02
- ◆ S2053 Transplantation of small intestine and liver allografts
- ◆ S2054 Transplantation of multivisceral organs
- ◆ S2055 Harvesting of donor multivisceral organs, with preparation and maintenance of allografts; from cadaver donor
- ◆ S2060 Lobar lung transplantation
- ◆ S2061 Donor lobectomy (lung) for transplantation, living donor
- ◆ S2065 Simultaneous pancreas kidney transplantation
- ◆ S2080 Laser-assisted uvulopalatoplasty (LAUP)
- ◆ S2102 Islet cell tissue transplant from pancreas allogeneic
- ◆ S2103 Adrenal tissue transplant to brain
- ▶◆ S2107 Adoptive immunotherapy i.e. development of specific anti-tumor reactivity (e.g. tumor-infiltrating lymphocyte therapy) per course of treatment
- ◆ S2112 Arthroscopy, knee, surgical for harvesting of cartilage (chondrocyte cells)
- ◆ S2115 Osteotomy, periacetabular, with internal fixation
- ◆ S2120 Low-density lipoprotein (LDL) apheresis using heparin-induced extracorporeal LDL precipitation
- ▶◆ S2130 Endoluminal radiofrequency ablation of refluxing saphenous vein
- ◆ S2140 Cord blood harvesting for transplantation, allogeneic
- ◆ S2142 Cord blood–derived stem cell transplantation, allogeneic
- ◆ S2150 Bone marrow or blood-derived peripheral stem cell harvesting and transplantation, allogenic or autologous, including pheresis, high-dose chemotherapy, and 28 days of post-transplant care (including drugs; hospitalization; medical, surgical, diagnostic and emergency services
- S2180 Deleted 12/31/02, Cross Reference 38242
- ◆ S2202 Echosclerotherapy

◆ S2205 Minimally invasive direct coronary artery bypass surgery involving mini-thoracotomy or mini-sternotomy surgery, performed under direct vision; using arterial graft(s), single coronary arterial graft

◆ S2206 Minimally invasive direct coronary artery bypass surgery involving mini-thoracotomy or mini-sternotomy surgery, performed under direct vision; using arterial graft(s), two coronary arterial grafts

◆ S2207 Minimally invasive direct coronary artery bypass surgery involving mini-thoracotomy or mini-sternotomy surgery, performed under direct vision; using venous graft only, single coronary venous graft

◆ S2208 Minimally invasive direct coronary artery bypass surgery involving mini-thoracotomy or mini-sternotomy surgery, performed under direct vision; using single arterial and venous graft(s), single venous graft

◆ S2209 Minimally invasive direct coronary artery bypass surgery involving mini-thoracotomy or mini-sternotomy surgery, performed under direct vision; using two arterial grafts and single venous graft

▶◆ S2211 Transcatheter placement of intravascular stent(s), carotid artery, percutaneous, unilateral (if performed bilaterally, use −50 modifier)

S2220 Deleted 01/01/02

◆ S2250 Uterine artery embolization for uterine fibroids

◆ S2260 Induced abortion, 17-24 weeks, any surgical method

▶◆ S2262 Abortion for maternal indications, 25 weeks or greater

▶◆ S2265 Abortion for fetal indications, 25-28 weeks

▶◆ S2266 Abortion for fetal indication, 29-31 weeks

▶◆ S2267 Abortion for fetal indication, 32 weeks or greater

◆ S2300 Arthroscopy, shoulder, surgical; with thermally induced capsulorrhaphy

◆ S2340 Chemodenervation of abductor muscle(s) of vocal cord

◆ S2341 Chemodenervation of adductor muscle(s) of vocal cord

◆ S2342 Nasal endoscopy for post-operative debridement following functional endoscopic sinus surgery, nasal and/or sinus cavity(s), unilateral or bilateral

◆ S2350 Diskectomy, anterior, with decompression of spinal cord and/or nerve root(s) including osteophytectomy; lumbar, single interspace

◆ S2351 Diskectomy, anterior, with decompression of spinal cord and/or nerve root(s) including osteophytectomy; lumbar, each additional interspace (list separately in addition to code for primary procedure)

◆ S2360 Percutaneous vertebroplasty, one vertebral body, unilateral or bilateral injection; cervical

◆ S2361 Each additional cervical vertebral body (list separately in addition to code for primary procedure)

◆ S2370 Intradiscal electrothermal therapy, single interspace

◆ S2371 Each additional interspace (list separately in addition to code for primary procedure)

➡◆ S2400 Repair, congenital diaphragmatic hernia in the fetus using temporary tracheal occlusion, procedure performed in utero

◆ S2401 Repair, urinary tract obstruction in the fetus, procedure performed in utero

◆ S2402 Repair, congenital cystic adenomatoid malformation in the fetus, procedure performed in utero

◆ S2403 Repair, extralobar pulmonary sequestration in the fetus, procedure performed in utero

◆ S2404 Repair, myelomeningocele in the fetus, procedure performed in utero

▶◆ S2405 Repair of sacrococcygeal teratoma in the fetus, procedure performed in utero

◆ S2409 Repair, congenital malformation of fetus, procedure performed in utero, not otherwise classified

◆ S2411 Fetoscopic laser therapy for treatment of twin-to-twin transfusion syndrome (TTTS)

◆ S3600 Stat laboratory request (situations other than S3601)

◆ S3601 Emergency stat laboratory charge for patient who is homebound or residing in a nursing facility

✪ S3620 Newborn metabolic screening panel, includes test kit, postage, and the laboratory tests specified by the sate for inclusion in this panel (e.g., galactose, hemoglobin; electrophoresis; hydroxyprogesterone; 17-D; phenylalanine (PKU); and thyroxine, total)

◆ S3630 Eosinophil count, blood, direct

◆ S3645 Human immunodeficiency virus-1 (HIV-1) antibody testing of oral mucosal transudate

◆ S3650 Saliva test, hormone level; during menopause

◆ S3652 Saliva test, hormone level; to assess preterm labor risk

▶◆ S3655 Antisperm antibodies test (immunobead)

◆ S3701 Imm[illegible]oassay for nuclear matrix protei[illegible]22 (NMP-22), quantitative

◆ S3708 [illegible]strointestinal fat absorption study

◆ S3818 [illegible]omplete gene sequence analysis; *BRCA1* gene

◆ S38[illegible] Complete gene sequence analysis; *BRCA2* gene

◆ [illegible]330 Complete *CCHI* and *CCH2* gene sequence analysis for hereditary nonpolyposis colorectal cancer (HNPCC) genetic testing

◆ S3831 Single-mutation analysis (in individual with a known *CCH1* and *CCH2* mutation in the family) for hereditary nonpolyposis colorectal cancer (HNPCC) genetic testing

◆ S3835 Complete gene sequence analysis for cystic fibrosis genetic testing

◆ S3837 Complete gene sequence analysis for hemochromatosis genetic testing

◆ S3900 Surface electromyography (EMG)

◆ S3902 Ballistrocardiogram

◆ S3904 Masters two step

S3906 Deleted 01/01/02

▶◆ S4005 Interim labor facility global (labor occurring but not resulting in delivery)

◆ S4011 In vitro fertilization (IVF); including but not limited to identification and incubation of mature oocytes, fertilization with sperm, incubation of embryo(s), and subsequent visualization for determination of development

▶◆ S4013 Complete cycle, gamete intrafallopian transfer (GIFT), case rate

▶◆ S4014 Complete cycle, zygote intrafallopian transfer (ZIFT), case rate

➠◆ S4015 Complete in vitro fertilization cycle, not otherwise specified, case rate

◆ S4016 Frozen in vitro fertilization cycle, case rate

▶◆ S4017 Incomplete cycle, treatment canceled prior to stimulation, case rate

◆ S4018 Frozen embryo transfer procedure cancelled before transfer, case rate

◆ S4020 In vitro fertilization procedure cancelled before aspiration, case rate

◆ S4021 In vitro fertilization procedure cancelled after aspiration, case rate

◆ S4022 Assisted oocyte fertilization, case rate

▶◆ S4023 Donor egg cycle, incomplete, case rate

◆ S4025 Donor services for in vitro fertilization (sperm or embryo), case rate

◆ S4026 Procurement of donor sperm from sperm bank

◆ S4027 Storage of previously frozen embryos

◆ S4028 Microsurgical epididymal sperm aspiration (MESA)

◆ S4030 Sperm procurement and cryopreservation services; initial visit

◆ S4031 Sperm procurement and cryopreservation services; subsequent visit

▶◆ S4035 Stimulated intrauterine insemination (IUI), case rate

▶◆ S4036 Intravaginal culture (IVC), case rate

▶◆ S4037 Cryopreserved embryo transfer, case rate

▶◆ S4040 Monitoring and storage of cryopreserved embryos, per 30 days

◆ S4981 Insertion of levonorgestrel-releasing intrauterine system

◆ S4989 Contraceptive intrauterine device (IUD) (e.g. Progestasert), including implants and supplies

◆ S4990 Nicotine patches, legend

◆ S4991 Nicotine patches, non-legend

▶◆ S4993 Contraceptive pills for birth control

▶◆ S4995 Smoking cessation gum

◆ S5000 Prescription drug, generic

◆ S5001 Prescription drug, brand name

S5002 Deleted 01/01/02

S5003 Deleted 01/01/02

◆ S5010 5% dextrose and 0.45% normal saline, 1000 cc

◆ S5011 5% dextrose in lactated Ringer's, 1000 cc

◆ S5012 5% dextrose with potassium chloride, 1000 cc

◆ S5013 5% dextrose/0.45% normal saline with potassium chloride and magnesium sulfate, 1000 cc

◆ S5014 5% dextrose/0.45% normal saline with potassium chloride and magnesium sulfate, 1500 cc

S5016 Deleted 01/01/02

S5017 Deleted 01/01/02

S5018 Deleted 01/01/02

S5019 Deleted 01/01/02

S5020 Deleted 01/01/02

S5021 Deleted 01/01/02

S5022 Deleted 01/01/02

S5025 Deleted 01/01/02

◆ S5035 Home infusion therapy, routine service of infusion device (e.g., pump maintenance)

◆ S5036 Home infusion therapy, repair of infusion device (e.g., pump repair)

▶◆ S5100 Day care services, adult; per 15 minutes

▶◆ S5101 Day care services, adult; per half day

▶◆ S5102 Day care services, adult; per diem

▶◆ S5105 Day care services, center-based; services not included in program fee, per diem

▶◆ S5110 Home care training, family; per 15 minutes

▶◆ S5111 Home care training, family; per session

▶◆ S5115 Home care training, non-family; per 15 minutes

▶◆ S5116 Home care training, non-family; per session

▶◆ S5120 Chore services; per 15 minutes

▶◆ S5121 Chore services; per diem

▶◆ S5125 Attendant care services; per 15 minutes

▶◆ S5126 Attendant care services; per diem

▶◆ S5130 Homemaker service, NOS; per 15 minutes
▶◆ S5131 Homemaker service, NOS; per diem
▶◆ S5135 Companion care, adult (e.g., IADL/ADL); per 15 minutes
▶◆ S5136 Companion care, adult (e.g., IADL/ADL); per diem
▶◆ S5140 Foster care, adult; per diem
▶◆ S5141 Foster care, adult; per month
▶◆ S5145 Foster care, therapeutic, child; per diem
▶◆ S5146 Foster care, therapeutic, child; per month
▶◆ S5150 Unskilled respite care, not hospice; per 15 minutes
▶◆ S5151 Unskilled respite care, not hospice; per diem
▶◆ S5160 Emergency response system; installation and testing
▶◆ S5161 Emergency response system; service fee, per month (excludes installation and testing)
▶◆ S5162 Emergency response system; purchase only
▶◆ S5165 Home modifications; per service
▶◆ S5170 Home delivered meals, including preparation; per meal
▶◆ S5175 Laundry service, external, professional; per order
▶◆ S5180 Home health respiratory therapy, initial evaluation
▶◆ S5181 Home health respiratory therapy, NOS, per diem
▶◆ S5185 Medication reminder service, non-face-to-face; per month
▶◆ S5190 Wellness assessment, performed by non-physician
▶◆ S5199 Personal care item, NOS, each
◆ S5497 Home infusion therapy, catheter care/maintenance, not otherwise classified; includes administration services, professional pharmacy services, care coordination, and all necessary supplies and equipment (drugs and nursing visits coded separately), per diem
◆ S5498 Home infusion therapy, catheter care/maintenance, simple (single lumen), includes administrative services, professional pharmacy services, care coordination and all necessary supplies and equipment, (drugs and nursing visits coded separately), per diem
◆ S5501 Home infusion therapy, catheter care/maintenance, complex (more than one lumen), includes administrative services, professional pharmacy services, care coordination, and all necessary supplies and equipment (drugs and nursing visits coded separately), per diem
◆ S5502 Home infusion therapy, catheter care/maintenance, implanted access device, includes administrative services, professional pharmacy services, care coordination and all necessary supplies and equipment, (drugs and nursing visits coded separately), per diem (use this code for interim maintenance of vascular access not currently in use)
S5503 Deleted 01/01/02
◆ S5517 Home infusion therapy, all supplies necessary for restoration of catheter patency or declotting
◆ S5518 Home infusion therapy, all supplies necessary for catheter repair
◆ S5520 Home infusion therapy, all supplies (including catheter) necessary for a peripherally inserted central venous catheter (PICC) line insertion
◆ S5521 Home infusion therapy, all supplies (including catheter) necessary for a midline catheter insertion
◆ S5522 Home infusion therapy, insertion of PICC, nursing services only (no supplies or catheter included)
◆ S5523 Home infusion therapy, insertion of midline central venous catheter, nursing services only (no supplies or catheter included)
S8001 Deleted 01/01/02
S8002 Deleted 12/31/02, Cross Reference A9522
S8003 Deleted 12/31/02, Cross Reference A9523
▶◆ S8004 Radioimmunopharmaceutical localization of targeted cells; whole body
◆ S8030 Scleral application of tantalum ring(s) for localization of lesions for proton beam therapy
◆ S8035 Magnetic source imaging
◆ S8037 Magnetic resonance cholangiopancreatography (MRCP)
◆ S8040 Topographic brain mapping
▶◆ S8042 Magnetic resonance imaging (MRI), low-field
◆ S8049 Intraoperative radiation therapy (single administration)
◆ S8055 Ultrasound guidance for multifetal pregnancy reduction(s), technical component (only to be used when the physician doing the reduction procedure does not perform the ultrasound, guidance is included in the CPT code for multifetal pregnancy reduction-59866)
◆ S8080 Scintimammography (radioimmunoscintigraphy of the breast), unilateral, including supply of radiopharmaceutical
◆ S8085 Fluorine-18 fluorodeoxyglucose (F-18 FDG) imaging using dual-head coincidence detection system (non-dedicated postiron emissition test [PET] scan)

◆ S8092 Electron beam computed tomography (also known as *ultrafast CT, cine CT*)
◆ S8095 Wig (for medically or congenitally induced hair loss)
◆ S8096 Portable peak flow meter
◆ S8097 Asthma kit (including but not limited to portable peak expiratory flow meter, instructional video, brochure, and/or spacer)
◆ S8100 Holding chamber or spacer for use with an inhaler or nebulizer; without mask
◆ S8101 Holding chamber or spacer for use with an inhaler or nebulizer; with mask
S8105 Deleted 12/31/02
◆ S8110 Peak expiratory flow rate (physician services)
◆ S8180 Tracheostomy shower protector
◆ S8181 Tracheostomy tube holder
◆ S8182 Humidifier, heated, used with ventilator, non-servo-controlled
◆ S8183 Humidifier, heated, used with ventilator, dual servo-controlled with temperature monitoring
◆ S8185 Flutter device
◆ S8186 Swivel adaptor
◆ S8189 Tracheostomy supply, not otherwise classified
◆ S8190 Electronic spirometer (or micro spirometer)
S8200 Deleted 12/31/02, Cross Reference E0483
S8205 Deleted 12/31/02, Cross Reference E0483
◆ S8210 Mucus trap
◆ S8260 Oral orthotic for treatment of sleep apnea, includes fitting, fabrication, and materials
▶◆ S8262 Mandibular orthopedic repositioning device, each
▶◆ S8265 Haberman feeder for cleft lip/palate
S8401 Deleted 12/31/02, Cross Reference A4529, A4530
S8402 Deleted 01/01/02
S8403 Deleted 12/31/02
S8404 Deleted 12/31/02, Cross Reference A4531, A4532
S8405 Deleted 12/31/02, Cross Reference A4535
◆ S8415 Supplies for home delivery of infant
◆ S8420 Gradient pressure aid (sleeve and glove combination), custom made
◆ S8421 Gradient pressure aid (sleeve and glove combination), ready made
◆ S8422 Gradient pressure aid (sleeve), custom made, medium weight
◆ S8423 Gradient pressure aid (sleeve), custom made, heavy weight
◆ S8424 Gradient pressure aid (sleeve), ready made
◆ S8425 Gradient pressure aid (glove), custom made, medium weight
◆ S8426 Gradient pressure aid (glove), custom made, heavy weight
◆ S8427 Gradient pressure aid (glove), ready made
◆ S8428 Gradient pressure aid (gauntlet), ready made
◆ S8429 Gradient pressure exterior wrap
◆ S8430 Padding for compression bandage, roll
◆ S8431 Compression bandage, roll
S8433 Deleted 12/31/02, Cross Reference A4280
◆ S8450 Splint, prefabricated, digit (specify digit by use of modifier)
◆ S8451 Splint, prefabricated, wrist or ankle
◆ S8452 Splint, prefabricated, elbow
◆ S8490 Insulin syringes (100 syringes, any size)
▶◆ S8945 Physical medicine treatment (constant attendance by provider) to one area, initial 30 minutes, each visit; phonophoresis
◆ S8950 Complex lymphedema therapy, each 15 minutes
◆ S8999 Resuscitation bag (for use by patient on artificial respiration during power failure or other catastrophic event)
◆ S9001 Home uterine monitor with or without associated nursing services
◆ S9007 Ultrafiltration monitor
◆ S9015 Automated electroencephalogram (EEG) monitoring
◆ S9022 Digital subtraction angiography (use in addition to CPT code for the procedure for further identification)
S9023 Deleted 01/01/02
◆ S9024 Paranasal sinus ultrasound
◆ S9025 Omnicardiogram/cardiointegram
▶◆ S9034 Extracorporeal shockwave lithotripsy for gall stones (if performed with ERCP, use 43265)
S9035 Deleted 01/01/02
◆ S9055 Procuren or other growth factor preparation to promote wound healing
◆ S9056 Coma stimulation per diem
◆ S9061 Home administration of aerosolized drug therapy (e.g., pentamidine); administrative services, professional pharmacy services, care coordination, all necessary supplies and equipment (drugs and nursing visits coded separately), per diem
◆ S9075 Smoking cessation treatment
◆ S9083 Global fee urgent care centers
S9085 Deleted 01/01/02
◆ S9088 Services provided in an urgent care center (list in addition to code for service)
◆ S9090 Vertebral axial decompression, per session

▶◆ S9092 Canolith repositioning, per visit
◆ S9098 Home visit, phototherapy services (e.g. Bili-Lite), including equipment rental, nursing services, blood draw, supplies, and other services, per diem
◆ S9109 Congestive heart failure telemonitoring, equipment rental, including telescale, computer system and software, telephone connections, and maintenance, per month
◆ S9117 Back school, per visit
◆ S9122 Home health aide or certified nurse assistant, providing care in the home; per hour
➠◆ S9123 Nursing care, in the home; by registered nurse, per hour (use for general nursing care only, not to be used when CPT codes 99500-99600 or S codes S9802-S9803 can be used)
◆ S9124 Nursing care, in the home; by licensed practical nurse, per hour
◆ S9125 Respite care, in the home, per diem
◆ S9126 Hospice care, in the home, per diem
◆ S9127 Social work visit, in the home, per diem
◆ S9128 Speech therapy, in the home, per diem
◆ S9129 Occupational therapy, in the home, per diem
◆ S9131 Physical therapy; in the home, per diem
◆ S9140 Diabetic management program, follow-up visit to non-physician provider
◆ S9141 Diabetic management program, follow-up visit to physcian provider
▶◆ S9145 Insulin pump initiation, instruction in initial use of pump (pump not included)
▶◆ S9150 Evaluation by ocularist
S9200 Deleted 01/01/02
◆ S9208 Home management of preterm labor, including administrative services, professional pharmacy services, care coordination, and all necessary supplies or equipment (drugs and nursing visits coded separately), per diem (do not use this code with any home infusion per diem code)
◆ S9209 Home management of preterm premature rupture of membranes (PPROM), including administrative services, professional pharmacy services, care coordination, and all necessary supplies or equipment (drugs and nursing visits coded separately), per diem (do not use this code with any home infusion per diem code)
S9210 Deleted 01/01/02
◆ S9211 Home management of gestational hypertension, includes administrative services, professional pharmacy services, care coordination and all necessary supplies and equipment (drugs and nursing visits coded separately); per diem (do not use this code with any home infusion per diem code)
◆ S9212 Home management of postpartum hypertension, includes administrative services, professional pharmacy services, care coordination, and all necessary supplies and equipment (drugs and nursing visits coded separately), per diem (do not use this code with any home infusion per diem code)
◆ S9213 Home management of preeclampsia, includes administrative services, professional pharmacy services, care coordination, and all necessary supplies and equipment (drugs and nursing services coded separately); per diem (do not use this code with any home infusion per diem code)
◆ S9214 Home management of gestational diabetes, includes administrative services, professional pharmacy services, care coordination, and all necessary supplies and equipment (drugs and nursing visits coded separately); per diem (do not use this code with any home infusion per diem code)
S9216 Deleted 12/31/02, Cross Reference S9211
S9217 Deleted 12/31/02, Cross Reference S9212
S9218 Deleted 12/31/02, Cross Reference S9213
S9220 Deleted 01/01/02
S9225 Deleted 01/01/02
S9230 Deleted 01/01/02
S9300 Deleted 01/01/02
S9308 Deleted 01/01/02
S9310 Deleted 01/01/02
◆ S9325 Home infusion therapy, pain management infusion; administrative services, professional pharmacy services, care coordination, and all necessary supplies and equipment, (drugs and nursing visits coded separately), per diem (do not use this code with S9326, S9327 or S9328)
➠◆ S9326 Home infusion therapy, continuous (twenty-four hours or more) pain management infusion; administrative services, professional pharmacy services, care coordination and all necessary supplies and equipment (drugs and nursing visits coded separately), per diem

➠ ◆ S9327 Home infusion therapy, intermittent (less than twenty-four hours) pain management infusion; administrative services, professional pharmacy services, care coordination, and all necessary supplies and equipment (drugs and nursing visits coded separately), per diem

◆ S9328 Home infusion therapy, implanted pump pain management infusion; administrative services, professional pharmacy services, care coordination, and all necessary supplies and equipment (drugs and nursing visits coded separately), per diem

◆ S9329 Home infusion therapy, chemotherapy infusion; administrative services, professional pharmacy services, care coordination, and all necessary supplies and equipment (drugs and nursing visits coded separately), per diem (do not use this code with S9330 or S9331)

➠ ◆ S9330 Home infusion therapy, continuous (twenty-four hours or more) chemotherapy infusion; administrative services, professional pharmacy services, care coordination, and all necessary supplies and equipment (drugs and nursing visits coded separately), per diem

➠ ◆ S9331 Home infusion therapy, intermittent (less than twenty-four hours) chemotherapy infusion; administrative services, professional pharmacy services, care coordination, and all necessary supplies and equipment (drugs and nursing visits coded separately), per diem

◆ S9336 Home infusion therapy, continuous anticoagulant infusion therapy (e.g. heparin), administrative services, professional pharmacy services, care coordination and all necessary supplies and equipment (drugs and nursing visits coded separately), per diem

➠ ◆ S9338 Home infusion therapy, immunotherapy therapy; (e.g., intravenous immunoglobulin, interferon); administrative services, professional pharmacy services, care coordination, and all necessary supplies and equipment (drug and nursing visits coded separately), per diem

◆ S9339 Home therapy; peritoneal dialysis, administrative services, professional pharmacy services, care coordination and all necessary supplies and equipment (drugs and nursing visits coded separately), per diem

◆ S9340 Home therapy; enteral nutrition; administrative services, professional pharmacy services, care coordination, and all necessary supplies and equipment (enteral formula and nursing visits coded separately), per diem

◆ S9341 Home therapy; enteral nutrition via gravity; administrative services, professional pharmacy services, care coordination, and all necessary supplies and equipment (enteral formula and nursing visits coded separately), per diem

◆ S9342 Home therapy; enteral nutrition via pump; administrative services, professional pharmacy services, care coordination, and all necessary supplies and equipment (enteral formula and nursing visits coded separately), per diem

◆ S9343 Home therapy; enteral nutrition via bolus; administrative services, professional pharmacy services, care coordination, and all necessary supplies and equipment (enteral formula and nursing visits coded separately), per diem

◆ S9345 Home infusion therapy, anti-hemophilic agent infusion therapy (e.g. Factor VIII); administrative services, professional pharmacy services, care coordination, and all necessary supplies and equipment (drugs and nursing visits coded separately), per diem

◆ S9346 Home infusion therapy, alpha-1-proteinase inhibitor (e.g., Prolastin); administrative services, professional pharmacy services, care coordination, and all necessary supplies and equipment (drugs and nursing visits coded separately), per diem

➠ ◆ S9347 Home infusion therapy, uninterrupted, long-term, controlled rate IV or subcutaneous infusion therapy (e.g. Epoprostenol); administrative services, professional pharmacy services, care coordination, and all necessary supplies and equipment (drugs and nursing visits coded separately), per diem

◆ S9348 Home infusion therapy, sympathomimetic/inotropic agent infusion therapy (e.g., Dobutamine); administrative services, professional pharmacy services, care coordination, all necessary supplies and equipment (drugs and nursing visits coded separately), per diem

◆ S9349 Home infusion therapy, tocolytic infusion therapy; administrative services, professional pharmacy services, care coordination, and all necessary supplies and equipment (drugs and nursing visits coded separately), per diem

◆ S9351 Home infusion therapy, continuous antiemetic infusion therapy; administrative services, professional pharmacy services, care coordination, all necessary supplies and equipment (drugs and nursing visits coded separately), per diem

◆ S9353 Home infusion therapy, continuous insulin infusion therapy; administrative services, professional pharmacy services, care coordination, and all necessary supplies and equipment (drugs and nursing visits coded separately), per diem

◆ S9355 Home infusion therapy, chelation therapy; administrative services, professional pharmacy services, care coordination, and all necessary supplies and equipment (drugs and nursing visits coded separately), per diem

◆ S9357 Home infusion therapy, enzyme replacement IV therapy; (e.g. Imiglucerase); administrative services, professional pharmacy services, care coordination, and all necessary supplies and equipment (drugs and nursing visits coded separately), per diem

◆ S9359 Home infusion therapy, anti-tumor necrosis factor IV therapy; (e.g. Infliximab); administrative services, professional pharmacy services, care coordination, and all necessary supplies and equipment (drugs and nursing visits coded separately), per diem

◆ S9361 Home infusion therapy, diuretic IV therapy; administrative services, professional pharmacy services, care coordination, and all necessary supplies and equipment (drugs and nursing visits coded separately), per diem

◆ S9363 Home infusion therapy, anti-spasmotic IV therapy; administrative services, professional pharmacy services, care coordination, and all necessary supplies and equipment (drugs and nursing visits coded separately), per diem

➠ ◆ S9364 Home infusion therapy, total parenteral nutrition (TPN); administrative services, professional pharmacy services, care coordination, and all necessary supplies and equipment including standard TPN formula (lipids, specialty amino acid formulas, drugs other than in standard formula and nursing visits coded separately) per diem (do not use with home infusion codes S9365-S9368 using daily volume scales)

➠ ◆ S9365 Home infusion therapy, total parenteral nutrition (TPN); one liter per day, administrative services, professional pharmacy services, care coordination, and all necessary supplies and equipment including standard TPN formula (lipids, specialty amino acid formulas, drugs other than in standard formula and nursing visits coded separately), per diem

➠ ◆ S9366 Home infusion therapy, total parenteral nutrition (TPN); more than one liter but no more than two liters per day, administrative services, professional pharmacy services, care coordination, and all necessary supplies and equipment including standard TPN formula; (lipids, specialty amino acid formulas, drugs other than in standard formula and nursing visits coded separately), per diem

➠ ◆ S9367 Home infusion therapy, total parenteral nutrition (TPN); more than two liters but no more than three liters per day, administrative services, professional pharmacy services, care coordination, and all necessary supplies and equipment including standard TPN formula; (lipids, specialty amino acid formulas, drugs other than in standard formula and nursing visits coded separately), per diem

➠ ◆ S9368 Home infusion therapy, total parenteral nutrition (TPN); more than three liters per day, administrative services, professional pharmacy services, care coordination, and all necessary supplies and equipment (includes standard TPN formula; (lipids, specialty amino acid formulas, drugs other than in standard formula and nursing visits coded separately), per diem

◆ S9370 Home therapy, intermittent antiemetic injection therapy; administrative services, professional pharmacy services, care coordination, and all necessary supplies and equipment (drugs and nursing visits coded separately), per diem

◆ S9372 Home therapy; intermittent anti-coagulant injection therapy (e.g. heparin); administrative services, professional pharmacy services, care coordination, and all necessary supplies and equipment (drugs and nursing visits coded separately), per diem (do not use this code for flushing of infusion devices with heparin to maintain patency)

◆ S9373 Home infusion therapy, hydration therapy; administrative services, professional pharmacy services, care coordination, and all necessary supplies and equipment (drugs and nursing visits coded separately), per diem (do not use with hydration therapy codes S9374-S9377 using daily volume scales)

◆ S9374 Home infusion therapy, hydration therapy; one liter per day, administrative services, professional pharmacy services, care coordination, and all necessary supplies and equipment (drugs and nursing visits coded separately), per diem

◆ S9375 Home infusion therapy, hydration therapy; more than one liter but no more than two liters per day, administrative services, professional pharmacy services, care coordination, and all necessary supplies and equipment (drugs and nursing visits coded separately), per diem

◆ S9376 Home infusion therapy, hydration therapy; more than two liters but no more than three liters per day, administrative services, professional pharmacy services, care coordination, and all necessary supplies and equipment (drugs and nursing visits coded separately), per diem

◆ S9377 Home infusion therapy, hydration therapy; more than three liters per day, administrative services, professional pharmacy services, care coordination, and all necessary supplies (drugs and nursing visits coded separately), per diem

◆ S9379 Home infusion therapy, infusion therapy, not otherwise classified; administrative services, professional pharmacy services, care coordination, and all necessary supplies and equipment (drugs and nursing visits coded separately), per diem

◆ S9381 Delivery or service to high risk areas requiring escort or extra protection, per visit

S9395 Deleted 01/01/02

▶◆ S9401 Anti-coagulation clinic, inclusive of all services except laboratory tests, per session

S9420 Deleted 01/01/02

S9423 Deleted 01/01/02

S9425 Deleted 01/01/02

▶◆ S9430 Pharmacy compounding and dispensing services

◆ S9435 Medical foods for inborn errors of metabolism

▶◆ S9436 Childbirth preparation/Lamaze classes, non-physician provider, per session

▶◆ S9437 Childbirth refresher classes, non-physician provider, per session

▶◆ S9438 Cesarean birth classes, non-physician provider, per session

▶◆ S9439 Vaginal birth after cesarean (VBAC) classes, non-physician provider, per session

◆ S9441 Asthma education, non-physician provider, per session

◆ S9442 Birthing classes, non-physician provider, per session

◆ S9443 Lactation classes, non-physician provider, per session

▶◆ S9444 Parenting classes, non-physician provider, per session

◆ S9445 Patient education, not otherwise classified, non-physician provider, individual, per session

◆ S9446 Patient education, not otherwise classified, non-physician provider, group, per session

▶◆ S9447 Infant safety (including cardiopulmonary resuscitation [CPR]) classes, non-physician provider, per session

▶◆ S9449 Weight management classes, non-physician provider, per session

▶◆ S9451 Exercise classes, non-physician provider, per session

▶◆ S9452 Nutrition classes, non-physician provider, per session

▶◆ S9453 Smoking cessation classes, non-physician provider, per session

▶◆ S9454 Stress management classes, non-physician provider, per session

◆ S9455 Diabetic management program, group session

◆ S9460 Diabetic management program, nurse visit

◆ S9465 Diabetic management program, dietitian visit

◆ S9470 Nutritional counseling, dietitian visit

◆ S9472 Cardiac rehabilitation program, non-physician provider, per diem

◆ S9473 Pulmonary rehabilitation program, non-physician provider, per diem

◆ S9474 Enterostomal therapy by a registered nurse certified in enterostomal therapy, per diem

◆ S9475 Ambulatory setting substance abuse treatment or detoxification services, per diem

◆ S9480 Intensive outpatient psychiatric services, per diem

▶◆ S9484 Crisis intervention mental health services, per hour

◆ S9485 Crisis intervention mental health services, per diem

▶◆ S9490 Home infusion therapy, corticosteroid infusion; administrative services, professional pharmacy services, care coordination, and all necessary supplies and equipment (drugs and nursing visits coded separately), per diem

▶◆ S9494 Home infusion therapy, antibiotic, antiviral, or anti-fungal therapy; administrative services, professional pharmacy services, care coordination, and all necessary supplies and equipment (drug and nursing visits coded separately, per diem), (do not use with home infusion codes for hourly dosing schedules S9497-S9504)

◆ S9497 Home infusion therapy, antibiotic, antiviral, or anti-fungal therapy; once every 3 hours; administrative services, professional pharmacy services, care coordination, and all necessary supplies and equipment (drugs and nursing visits coded separately), per diem

◆ S9500 Home infusion therapy, antibiotic, antiviral, or anti-fungal therapy; once every 24 hours; administrative services, professional pharmacy services, care coordination, and all necessary supplies and equipment (drugs and nursing visits coded separately), per diem

◆ S9501 Home infusion therapy, antibiotic, antiviral, or anti-fungal therapy; once every 12 hours; administrative services, professional pharmacy services, care coordination, and all necessary supplies and equipment (drugs and nursing visits coded separately), per diem

◆ S9502 Home infusion therapy, antibiotic, antiviral, or anti-fungal therapy; once every 8 hours, administrative services, professional pharmacy services, care coordination, and all necessary supplies and equipment (drugs and nursing visits coded separately), per diem

◆ S9503 Home infusion therapy, antibiotic, antiviral, or anti-fungal; once every 6 hours; administrative services, professional pharmacy services, care coordination, and all necessary supplies and equipment (drugs and nursing visits coded separately), per diem

◆ S9504 Home infusion therapy, antibiotic, antiviral, or anti-fungal; once every 4 hours; administrative services, professional pharmacy services, care coordination, and all necessary supplies and equipment (drugs and nursing visits coded separately), per diem

◆ S9524 Nursing services related to home iv therapy, per diem

S9526 Deleted 01/01/02

S9527 Deleted 01/01/02

S9528 Deleted 01/01/02

◆ S9529 Routine venipuncture for collection of specimen(s), single home bound, nursing home, or skilled nursing facility patient

S9533 Deleted 01/01/02

S9535 Deleted 01/01/02

➠◆ S9537 Home therapy; hematopoietic hormone injection therapy (e.g. erythropoietin, G-CSF, GM-CSF); administrative services, professional pharmacy services, care coordination, and all necessary supplies and equipment (drugs and nursing visits coded separately), per diem

◆ S9538 Home transfusion of blood product(s); administrative services, professional pharmacy services, care coordination and all necessary supplies and equipment (blood products, drugs, and nursing visits coded separately), per diem

S9539 Deleted 01/01/02

➠◆ S9542 Home injectable therapy; not otherwise classified, including administrative services, professional pharmacy services, care coordination, and all necessary supplies and equipment (drugs and nursing visits coded separately), per diem

S9543 Deleted 04/01/02

S9545 Deleted 01/01/02

▶◆ S9546 Home infusion of blood products, nursing services, per visit

S9550 Deleted 01/01/02

S9555 Deleted 01/01/02

➠◆ S9558 Home infusion therapy; growth hormone, including administrative services, professional pharmacy services, care coordination, and all necessary supplies and equipment (drugs and nursing visits coded separately), per diem

➠◆ S9559 Home infusion therapy; interferon, including administrative services, professional pharmacy services, care coordination, and all necessary supplies and equipment (drugs and nursing visits coded separately), per diem

◆ S9560 Home injectable therapy; hormonal therapy (e.g.; Leuprolide, Goserelin), including administrative services, professional pharmacy services, care coordination, and all necessary supplies and equipment (drugs and nursing visits coded separately), per diem

▶◆ S9562 Home injectable therapy, palivizumab, including administrative services, professional pharmacy services, care coordination, and all necessary supplies and equipment (drugs and nursing visits coded separately), per diem

▶◆ S9590 Home therapy, irrigation therapy (e.g. sterile irrigation of an organ or anatomical cavity); including administrative services, professional pharmacy services, care coordination, and all necessary supplies and equipment (drugs and nursing visits coded separately), per diem

S9800 Deleted 12/31/02, Cross Reference S9802, S9803

▶◆ S9802 Home infusion/specialty drug administration, nursing services; per visit (up to 2 hours)

▶◆ S9803 Each additional hour (list separately in addition to code S9802)

▶◆ S9806 RN services in the infusion suite of the IV therapy provider, per visit

◆ S9810 Home therapy; professional pharmacy services for provision of infusion, specialty drug administration, and/or disease state management, not otherwise classified, per hour (do not use this code with any per diem code)

▶◆ S9900 Services by authorized Christian Science Practitioner for the process of healing, per diem; not to be used for rest or study; excludes in-patient services

▶◆ S9970 Health club membership, annual

▶◆ S9975 Transplant related lodging, meals and transportation, per diem

◆ S9981 Medical records copying fee, administrative

◆ S9982 Medical records copying fee, per page

◆ S9986 Not medically necessary service (patient is aware that service not medically necessary)

◆ S9989 Services provided outside of the United States of America (list in addition to code[s] for services[s])

◆ S9990 Services provided as part of a phase II clinical trial

◆ S9991 Services provided as part of a phase III clinical trial

◆ S9992 Transportation costs to and from trial location and local transportation costs (e.g., fares for taxicab or bus) for clinical trial participant and one caregiver/companion

◆ S9994 Lodging costs (e.g., hotel charges) for clinical trial participant and one caregiver/companion

◆ S9996 Meals for clinical trial participant and one caregiver/companion

◆ S9999 Sales tax

NATIONAL T CODES FOR STATE MEDICAID AGENCIES (T1000-T1015)

Not Valid For Medicare

◆ T1000 Private duty/independent nursing service(s), licensed, up to 15 minutes

◆ T1001 Nursing assessment/evaluation

◆ T1002 RN services, up to 15 minutes

◆ T1003 Licensed practical nurse/licensed nurse (LPN/LVN) services, up to 15 minutes

◆ T1004 Services of a qualified nursing aide, up to 15 minutes

◆ T1005 Respite care services, up to 15 minutes

◆ T1006 Alcohol and/or substance abuse services, family/couple counseling

◆ T1007 Alcohol and/or substance abuse services, treatment plan development and/or modification

◆ T1008 Day treatment for individual alcohol and/or substance abuse services

◆ T1009 Child sitting services for children of the individual receiving alcohol and/or substance abuse services

◆ T1010 Meals for individuals receiving alcohol and/or substance abuse services (when meals not included in the program)

◆ T1011 Alcohol and/or substance abuse services, not otherwise classified

◆ T1012 Alcohol and/or substance abuse services, skills development

➠◆ T1013 Sign language or oral interpreter services, per 15 minutes

◆ T1014 TEL health transmission, per minute, professional services bill separately

◆ T1015 Clinic visit/encounter, all-inclusive

▶◆ T1016 Case Management, each 15 minutes

▶◆ T1017 Targeted Case Management, each 15 minutes

▶◆ T1018 School-based IEP services, bundled

▶◆ T1019 Personal care services, per 15 minutes, not for an in-patient or resident of a hospital, nursing facility, ICF/MR or IMD, part of the individualized plan of treatment (code may not be used to identify services provided by home health aide or certified nurse assistant)

▶◆ T1020 Personal care services, per diem, not for an inpatient or resident of a hospital, nursing facility, ICF/MR or IMD, part of the individualized plan of treatment (code may not be used to identify services provided by home health aide or certified nurse assistant)

▶◆ T1021 Home health aide or certified nurse assistant, per visit

▶◆ T1022 Contracted home health agency services, all services provided under contract, per day

▶◆ T1023 Screening to determine the appropriateness of consideration of an individual for participation in a specified program, project or treatment protocol, per encounter

▶◆ T1024 Evaluation and treatment by an integrated, specialty team contracted to provide coordinated care to multiple or severely handicapped children, per encounter

▶◆ T1025 Intensive, extended multidisciplinary services provided in a clinic setting to children with complex medical, physical, mental and psychosocial impairments, per diem

▶◆ T1026 Intensive, extended multidisciplinary services provided in a clinic setting to children with complex medical, physical, medical and psychosocial impairments, per hour

▶◆ T1027 Family training and counseling for child development, per 15 minutes

▶◆ T1028 Assessment of home, physical and family environment, to determine suitability to meet patient's medical needs

▶◆ T1029 Comprehensive environmental lead investigation, not including laboratory analysis, per dwelling

▶◆ T1030 Nursing care, in the home, by registered nurse, per diem

▶◆ T1031 Nursing care, in the home, by licensed practical nurse, per diem

▶◆ T1500 Diaper/incontinent pant, reusable/washable, any size, each

▶◆ T1502 Administration of oral, intramuscular and/or subcutaneous medication by health care agency/professional, per visit

▶◆ T1999 Miscellaneous therapeutic items and supplies, retail purchases, not otherwise classified; identify product in "remarks"

▶◆ T2001 Non-emergency transportation; patient attendant/escort

▶◆ T2002 Non-emergency transportation; per diem

▶◆ T2003 Non-emergency transportation; encounter/trip

▶◆ T2004 Non-emergency transport; commercial carrier, multi-pass

▶◆ T2005 Non-emergency transportation: non-ambulatory stretcher van

▶◆ T2006 Ambulance response and treatment, no transport

▶◆ T2007 Transportation waiting time, air ambulance and non-emergency vehicle, one-half (1/2) hour increments

VISION SERVICES (V0000-V2799)

Frames

❂ V2020 Frames, purchases
MCM 2130

◆ V2025 Deluxe frame
MCM 3045.4

Spectacle Lenses

NOTE: If a CPT procedure code for supply of spectacles or a permanent prosthesis is reported, recode with the specific lens type listed below. For aphakic temporary spectacle correction, see CPT.

Single Vision, Glass or Plastic

∗ V2100 Sphere, single vision, plano to plus or minus 4.00, per lens

∗ V2101 Sphere, single vision, plus or minus 4.12 to plus or minus 7.00d, per lens

∗ V2102 Sphere, single vision, plus or minus 7.12 to plus or minus 20.00d, per lens

∗ V2103 Spherocylinder, single vision, plano to plus or minus 4.00d sphere, 0.12 to 2.00d cylinder, per lens

∗ V2104 Spherocylinder, single vision, plano to plus or minus 4.00d sphere, 2.12 to 4.00d cylinder, per lens

∗ V2105 Spherocylinder, single vision, plano to plus or minus 4.00d sphere, 4.25 to 6.00d cylinder, per lens

∗ V2106 Spherocylinder, single vision, plano to plus or minus 4.00d sphere, over 6.00d cylinder, per lens

∗ V2107 Spherocylinder, single vision, plus or minus 4.25 to plus or minus 7.00 sphere, 0.12 to 2.00d cylinder, per lens

∗ V2108 Spherocylinder, single vision, plus or minus 4.25d to plus or minus 7.00d sphere, 2.12 to 4.00d cylinder, per lens

∗ V2109 Spherocylinder, single vision, plus or minus 4.25 to plus or minus 7.00d sphere, 4.25 to 6.00d cylinder, per lens

∗ V2110 Sperocylinder, single vision, plus or minus 4.25 to 7.00d sphere, over 6.00d cylinder, per lens

∗ V2111 Spherocylinder, single vision, plus or minus 7.25 to plus or minus 12.00d sphere, 0.25 to 2.25d cylinder, per lens

∗ V2112 Spherocylinder, single vision, plus or minus 7.25 to plus or minus 12.00d sphere, 2.25d to 4.00d cylinder, per lens

∗ V2113 Spherocylinder, single vision, plus or minus 7.25 to plus or minus 12.00d sphere, 4.25 to 6.00d cylinder, per lens

* V2114 Spherocylinder, single vision, sphere over plus or minus 12.00d, per lens
* V2115 Lenticular (myodisc), per lens, single vision
* V2116 Lenticular lens, nonaspheric, per lens, single vision
* V2117 Lenticular, aspheric, per lens, single vision
* V2118 Aniseikonic lens, single vision
* V2199 Not otherwise classified, single vision lens

Bifocal, Glass or Plastic

* V2200 Sphere, bifocal, plano to plus or minus 4.00d, per lens
* V2201 Sphere, bifocal, plus or minus 4.12 to plus or minus 7.00d, per lens
* V2202 Sphere, bifocal, plus or minus 7.12 to plus or minus 20.00d, per lens
* V2203 Spherocylinder, bifocal, plano to plus or minus 4.00d sphere, 0.12 to 2.00d cylinder, per lens
* V2204 Spherocylinder, bifocal, plano to plus or minus 4.00d sphere, 2.12 to 4.00d cylinder, per lens
* V2205 Spherocylinder, bifocal, plano to plus or minus 4.00d sphere, 4.25 to 6.00d cylinder, per lens
* V2206 Spherocylinder, bifocal, plano to plus or minus 4.00d sphere, over 6.00d cylinder, per lens
* V2207 Spherocylinder, bifocal, plus or minus 4.25 to plus or minus 7.00d sphere, 0.12 to 2.00d cylinder, per lens
* V2208 Spherocylinder, bifocal, plus or minus 4.25 to plus or minus 7.00d sphere, 2.12 to 4.00d cylinder, per lens
* V2209 Spherocylinder, bifocal, plus or minus 4.25 to plus or minus 7.00d sphere, 4.25 to 6.00d cylinder, per lens
* V2210 Spherocylinder, bifocal, plus or minus 4.25 to plus or minus 7.00d sphere, over 6.00d cylinder, per lens
* V2211 Spherocylinder, bifocal, plus or minus 7.25 to plus or minus 12.00d sphere, 0.25 to 2.25d cylinder, per lens
* V2212 Spherocylinder, bifocal, plus or minus 7.25 to plus or minus 12.00d sphere, 2.25 to 4.00d cylinder, per lens
* V2213 Spherocylinder, bifocal, plus or minus 7.25 to plus or minus 12.00d sphere, 4.25 to 6.00d cylinder, per lens
* V2214 Spherocylinder, bifocal, sphere over plus or minus 12.00d, per lens
* V2215 Lenticular (myodisc), per lens, bifocal
* V2216 Lenticular, nonaspheric, per lens, bifocal
* V2217 Lenticular, aspheric lens, bifocal
* V2218 Aniseikonic, per lens, bifocal
* V2219 Bifocal seg width over 28 mm
* V2220 Bifocal add over 3.25d
* V2299 Specialty bifocal (by report)

Trifocal, Glass or Plastic

* V2300 Sphere, trifocal, plano to plus or minus 4.00d, per lens
* V2301 Sphere, trifocal, plus or minus 4.12 to plus or minus 7.00d per lens
* V2302 Sphere, trifocal, plus or minus 7.12 to plus or minus 20.00, per lens
* V2303 Spherocylinder, trifocal, plano to plus or minus 4.00d sphere, 0.12 to 2.00d cylinder, per lens
* V2304 Spherocylinder, trifocal, plano to plus or minus 4.00d sphere, 2.25 to 4.00d cylinder, per lens
* V2305 Spherocylinder, trifocal, plano to plus or minus 4.00d sphere, 4.25 to 6.00 cylinder, per lens
* V2306 Spherocylinder, trifocal, plano to plus or minus 4.00d sphere, over 6.00d cylinder, per lens
* V2307 Spherocylinder, trifocal, plus or minus 4.25 to plus or minus 7.00d sphere, 0.12 to 2.00d cylinder, per lens
* V2308 Spherocylinder, trifocal, plus or minus 4.25 to plus or minus 7.00d sphere, 2.12 to 4.00d cylinder, per lens
* V2309 Spherocylinder, trifocal, plus or minus 4.25 to plus or minus 7.00d sphere, 4.25 to 6.00d cylinder, per lens
* V2310 Spherocylinder, trifocal, plus or minus 4.25 to plus or minus 7.00d sphere, over 6.00d cylinder, per lens
* V2311 Spherocylinder, trifocal, plus or minus 7.25 to plus or minus 12.00d sphere, 0.25 to 2.25d cylinder, per lens
* V2312 Spherocylinder, trifocal, plus or minus 7.25 to plus or minus 12.00d sphere, 2.25 to 4.00d cylinder, per lens
* V2313 Spherocylinder, trifocal, plus or minus 7.25 to plus or minus 12.00d sphere, 4.25 to 6.00d cylinder, per lens
* V2314 Spherocylinder, trifocal, sphere over plus or minus 12.00d, per lens
* V2315 Lenticular (myodisc), per lens, trifocal
* V2316 Lenticular nonaspheric, per lens, trifocal
* V2317 Lenticular, aspheric lens, trifocal
* V2318 Aniseikonic lens, trifocal
* V2319 Trifocal seg width over 28 mm
* V2320 Trifocal add over 3.25d
* V2399 Specialty trifocal (by report)

Variable Asphericity

* V2410 Variable asphericity lens, single vision, full field, glass or plastic, per lens

✻ V2430 Variable asphericity lens, bifocal, full field, glass or plastic, per lens
✻ V2499 Variable sphericity lens, other type

Contact Lenses

If a CPT procedure code for supply of contact lens is reported, recode with specific lens type listed below (per lens).

✻ V2500 Contact lens, PMMA, spherical, per lens
✻ V2501 Contact lens, PMMA, toric or prism ballast, per lens
✻ V2502 Contact lens PMMA, bifocal, per lens
✻ V2503 Contact lens PMMA, color vision deficiency, per lens
✻ V2510 Contact lens, gas permeable, spherical, per lens
✻ V2511 Contact lens, gas permeable, toric, prism ballast, per lens
✻ V2512 Contact lens, gas permeable, bifocal, per lens
✻ V2513 Contact lens, gas permeable, extended wear, per lens
✪ V2520 Contact lens, hydrophilic, spherical, per lens
CIM 45-7, CIM 65-1
✪ V2521 Contact lens, hydrophilic, toric, or prism ballast, per lens
CIM 45-7, CIM 65-1
✪ V2522 Contact lens, hydrophilic, bifocal, per lens
CIM 45-7, CIM 65-1
✪ V2523 Contact lens, hydrophilic, extended wear, per lens
CIM 45-7, CIM 65-1
✻ V2530 Contact lens, scleral, gas impermeable, per lens (for modification, see contact lens, 92325*)
✪ V2531 Contact lens, scleral, gas permeable, per lens (for contact lens modification, see 92325*)
CIM 65-3
✻ V2599 Contact lens, other type

Low Vision Aids

If a CPT procedure code for supply of low vision aid is reported, recode with specific systems listed below.

✻ V2600 Hand-held low vision aids and other nonspectacle mounted aids
✻ V2610 Single lens spectacle mounted low vision aids

*CPT only ©*Current Procedural Terminology 2002, Professional Edition*. American Medical Association.

✻ V2615 Telescopic and other compound lens system, including distance vision telescopic, near vision telescopes and compound microscopic lens system

Prosthetic Eye

✪ V2623 Prosthetic eye, plastic, custom
MCM 2133
✻ V2624 Polishing/resurfacing of ocular prosthesis
✻ V2625 Enlargement of ocular prosthesis
✻ V2626 Reduction of ocular prosthesis
✪ V2627 Scleral cover shell
CIM 65-3
✻ V2628 Fabrication and fitting of ocular conformer
✻ V2629 Prosthetic eye, other type

Intraocular Lenses

✪ V2630 Anterior chamber intraocular lens
MCM 2130
✪ V2631 Iris supported intraocular lens
MCM 2130
✪ V2632 Posterior chamber intraocular lens
MCM 2130

Miscellaneous

✻ V2700 Balance lens, per lens
✻ V2710 Slab off prism, glass or plastic, per lens
✻ V2715 Prism, per lens
✻ V2718 Press-on lens, Fresnel prism, per lens
✻ V2730 Special base curve, glass or plastic, per lens
✪ V2740 Tint, plastic, rose 1 or 2 per lens
MCM 2130B
✪ V2741 Tint, plastic, other than rose 1-2, per lens
MCM 2130B
✪ V2742 Tint, glass, rose, 1 or 2, per lens
MCM 2130B
✪ V2743 Tint, glass, other than rose, 1 or 2 per lens
MCM 2130B
✪ V2744 Tint, photochromatic, per lens
MCM 2130B
✪ V2750 Anti-reflective coating, per lens
MCM 2130B
✪ V2755 U-V lens, per lens
MCM 2130B
✻ V2760 Scratch resistant coating, per lens
✻ V2770 Occluder lens, per lens
✻ V2780 Oversize lens, per lens
✻ V2781 Progressive lens, per lens
✻ V2785 Processing, preserving and transporting corneal tissue

✻ V2790 Amniotic membrane for surgical reconstruction, per procedure
✻ V2799 Vision service, miscellaneous

HEARING SERVICES (V5000-V5299)

NOTE: These codes are for non-physician services.

◆ V5008 Hearing screening
MCM 2320
◆ V5010 Assessment for hearing aid
Medicare Statute 1862A7
◆ V5011 Fitting/orientation/checking of hearing aid
Medicare Statute 1862A7
◆ V5014 Repair/modification of a hearing aid
Medicare Statute 1862A7
◆ V5020 Conformity evaluation
Medicare Statute 1862A7
◆ V5030 Hearing aid, monaural, body worn, air conduction
Medicare Statute 1862A7
◆ V5040 Hearing aid, monaural, body worn, bone conduction
Medicare Statute 1862A7
◆ V5050 Hearing aid, monaural, in the ear
Medicare Statute 1862A7
◆ V5060 Hearing aid, monaural, behind the ear
Medicare Statute 1862A7
◆ V5070 Glasses, air conduction
Medicare Statute 1862A7
◆ V5080 Glasses, bone conduction
Medicare Statute 1862A7
◆ V5090 Dispensing fee, unspecified hearing aid
Medicare Statute 1862A7
▶ ◆ V5095 Semi-implantable middle ear hearing prosthesis
Medicare Statute 1862a7
◆ V5100 Hearing aid, bilateral, body worn
Medicare Statute 1862A7
◆ V5110 Dispensing fee, bilateral
Medicare Statute 1862A7
◆ V5120 Binaural, body
Medicare Statute 1862A7
◆ V5130 Binaural, in the ear
Medicare Statute 1862A7
◆ V5140 Binaural, behind the ear
Medicare Statute 1862A7
◆ V5150 Binaural, glasses
Medicare Statute 1862A7
◆ V5160 Dispensing fee, binaural
Medicare Statute 1862A7
◆ V5170 Hearing aid, CROS, in the ear
Medicare Statute 1862A7
◆ V5180 Hearing aid, CROS, behind the ear
Medicare Statute 1862A7
◆ V5190 Hearing aid, CROS, glasses
Medicare Statute 1862A7
◆ V5200 Dispensing fee, CROS
Medicare Statute 1862A7
◆ V5210 Hearing aid, BICROS, in the ear
Medicare Statute 1862A7
◆ V5220 Hearing aid, BICROS, behind the ear
Medicare Statute 1862A7
◆ V5230 Hearing aid, BICROS, glasses
Medicare Statute 1862A7
◆ V5240 Dispensing fee, BICROS
Medicare Statute 1862A7
◆ V5241 Dispensing fee, monaural hearing aid, any type
Medicare Statute 1862A7
◆ V5242 Hearing aid, analog, monaural, completely in the ear canal (CIC)
Medicare Statute 1862A7
◆ V5243 Hearing aid, analog, monaural, in the canal (ITC)
Medicare Statute 1862A9
◆ V5244 Hearing aid, digitally programmable analog, monaural, CIC
Medicare Statute 1862A7
◆ V5245 Hearing aid, digitally programmable, analog, monaural, ITC
Medicare Statute 1862A7
◆ V5246 Hearing aid, digitally programmable analog, monaural, in the ear (ITE)
Medicare Statute 1862A7
◆ V5247 Hearing aid, digitally programmable analog, monaural, behind the ear (BTE)
Medicare Statute 1862A7
◆ V5248 Hearing aid, analog, binaural, CIC
Medicare Statute 1862A7
◆ V5249 Hearing aid, analog, binaural, ITC
Medicare Statute 1862A7
◆ V5250 Hearing aid, digitally programmable analog, binaural, CIC
Medicare Statute 1862A7
◆ V5251 Hearing aid, digitally programmable analog, binaural, ITC
Medicare Statute 1862A7
◆ V5252 Hearing aid, digitally programmable, binaural, ITE
Medicare Statute 1862A7
◆ V5253 Hearing aid, digitally programmable, binaural, BTE
Medicare Statute 1862A7
◆ V5254 Hearing aid, digital, monaural, CIC
Medicare Statute 1862A7
◆ V5255 Hearing aid, digital, monaural, ITC
Medicare Statute 1862A7
◆ V5256 Hearing aid, digital, monaural, ITE
Medicare Statute 1862A7
◆ V5257 Hearing aid, digital, monaural, BTE
Medicare Statute 1862A7
◆ V5258 Hearing aid, digital, binaural, CIC
Medicare Statute 1862A7
◆ V5259 Hearing aid, digital, binaural, ITC
Medicare Statute 1862A7
◆ V5260 Hearing aid, digital, binaural, ITE
Medicare Statute 1862A7
◆ V5261 Hearing aid, digital, binaural, BTE
Medicare Statute 1862A7

◆ V5262 Hearing aid, disposable, any type, monaural
Medicare Statute 1862A7

◆ V5263 Hearing aid, disposable, any type, binaural
Medicare Statute 1862A7

◆ V5264 Ear mold/insert, not disposable, any type
Medicare Statute 1862A7

◆ V5265 Ear mold/insert, disposable, any type
Medicare Statute 1862A7

◆ V5266 Battery for use in hearing device
Medicare Statute 1862A7

◆ V5267 Hearing aid supplies/accessories
Medicare Statute 1862A7

◆ V5268 Assistive listening device, telephone amplifier, any type
Medicare Statute 1862A7

◆ V5269 Assistive listening device, alerting, any type
Medicare Statute 1862A7

◆ V5270 Assistive listening device, television amplifier, any type
Medicare Statute 1862A7

◆ V5271 Assistive listening device, television caption decoder
Medicare Statute 1862A7

◆ V5272 Assistive listening device, TDD
Medicare Statute 1862A7

◆ V5273 Assistive listening device, for use with cochlear implant
Medicare Statute 1862A7

◆ V5274 Assistive listening device, not otherwise specified
Medicare Statute 1862A7

◆ V5275 Ear impression, each
Medicare Statute 1862A7

▶◆ V5298 Hearing aid, not otherwise classified
Medicare Statute 1862a7

✪ V5299 Hearing service, miscellaneous
MCM 2320

Speech-Language Pathology Services

NOTE: These codes are for non-physician services.

◆ V5336 Repair/modification of augmentative communicative system or device (excludes adaptive hearing aid)
Medicare Statute 1862A7

✪ V5362 Speech screening
MCM 2320

✪ V5363 Language screening
MCM 2320

✪ V5364 Dysphagia screening
MCM 2320

2003 TABLE OF DRUGS

IA—Intra-arterial administration
IV—Intravenous administration
IM—Intramuscular administration
IT—Intrathecal
SC—Subcutaneous administration
INH—Administration by inhaled solution
VAR—Various routes of administration
OTH—Other routes of administration
ORAL—Administered orally

Intravenous administration includes all methods, such as gravity infusion, injections, and timed pushes. The "VAR" posting denotes various routes of administration and is used for drugs that are commonly administered into joints, cavities, tissues, or topical applications, in addition to other parenteral administrations. Listings posted with "OTH" indicate other administration methods, such as suppositories or catheter injections.

A			
Abbokinase, *see* Urokinase			
Abbokinase, Open Cath, *see* Urokinase			
Abciximab	10 mg	IV	J0130
Abelcet, *see* Amphotericin B lipid complex			
ABLC, *see* Amphotericin B			
Acetazolamide sodium	up to 500 mg	IM, IV	J1120
Acetylcysteine, unit dose form	per gram	INH	J7608
Achromycin, *see* Tetracycline			
ACTH, *see* Corticotropin			
Acthar, *see* Corticotropin			
Actimmune, *see* Interferon gamma 1-B			
Activase, *see* Alteplase recombinant			
Adenocard, *see* Adenosine			
Adenoscan, *see* Adenosine			
Adenosine	6 mg	IV	J0150
Adenosine	90 mg	IV	J0151
Adrenalin Chloride, *see* Adrenalin, epinephrine			
Adrenalin, epinephrine	up to 1 ml ampule	SC, IM	J0170
Adriamycin PFS, *see* Doxorubicin HCl			
Adriamycin RDF, *see* Doxorubicin HCl			
Adrucil, *see* Fluorouracil			
Aggrastat, *see* Tirofiban hydrochloride			
A-hydroCort, *see* Hydrocortisone sodium phosphate			
Akineton, *see* Biperiden			
Alatrofloxacin mesylate, injection 100 mg		IV	J0200
Albuterol, concentrated form	per mg	INH	J7618
Albuterol, unit dose form	per mg	INH	J7619
Aldesleukin	per single use vial	IM, IV	J9015
Aldomet, *see* Methyldopate HCl			
Alemtuzumab	10 mg		J9010
Alferon N, *see* Interferon alfa-n3			
Alglucerase	per 10 units	IV	J0205
Alkaban-AQ, *see* Vinblastine sulfate			
Alkeran, *see* Melphalan, oral			
Alpha-1-proteinase inhibitor (human)	per 10 mg	IV	J0256
Alprostadil, injection	1.25 mcg	OTH	J0270
		injection	J0275
Alprostadil, urethral suppository		OTH	
Alteplase recombinant	per 1 mg	IV	J2997
Alupent, *see* Metaproterenol sulfate or Metaproterenol, compounded			
Amcort, *see* Triamcinolone diacetate			
A-Methapred, *see* Methylprednisolone sodium succinate			
Amgen, *see* Interferon alphacon-1			
Amifostine	500 mg	IV	J0207
Aminolevalinic acid HCl	unit dose (354 mg)	OTH	J7308
Aminophylline/Aminophyllin	up to 250 mg	IV	J0280
Amiodarone HCl	30 mg	IV	J0282
Amitriptyline HCl	up to 20 mg	IM	J1320
Amobarbital	up to 125 mg	IM, IV	J0300
Amphocin, *see* Amphotericin B			
Amphotericin B	50 mg	IV	J0285
Amphotericin B lipid complex	10 mg	IV	J0287-J0289
Ampicillin sodium	up to 500 mg	IM, IV	J0290
Ampicillin sodium/sulbactam sodium	per 1.5 gm	IM, IV	J0295
Amygdalin, *see* Laetrile, Amygdalin, vitamin B-17			
Amytal, *see* Amobarbital			
Anabolin LA 100, *see* Nandrolone decanoate			
Ancef, *see* Cefazolin sodium			
Andrest 90-4, *see* Testosterone enanthate and estradiol valerate			
Andro-Cyp, *see* Testosterone cypionate			
Andro-Cyp 200, *see* Testosterone cypionate			
Andro L.A. 200, *see* Testosterone enanthate			
Andro-Estro 90-4, *see* Testosterone enanthate and estradiol valerate			
Andro/Fem, *see* Testosterone cypionate and estradiol cypionate			
Androgyn L.A., *see* Testosterone enanthate and estradiol valerate			
Androlone-50, *see* Nandrolone phenpropionate			
Androlone-D 100, *see* Nandrolone decanoate			
Andronaq-50, *see* Testosterone suspension			
Andronaq-LA, *see* Testosterone cypionate			
Andronate-200, *see* Testosterone cypionate			
Andronate-100, *see* Testosterone cypionate			
Andropository 100, *see* Testosterone enanthate			
Andryl 200, *see* Testosterone enanthate			

Anectine, *see* Succinylcholine chloride			
Anergan 25, *see* Promethazine HCl			
Anergan 50, *see* Promethazine HCl			
Anistreplase	30 units	IV	J0350
Anti-Inhibitor	per IU	IV	J7198
Antispas, *see* Dicyclomine HCl			
Antithrombin III (human)	per IU	IV	J7197
Anzemet, *see* Dolasetron mesylate injection			
A.P.L., *see* Chorionic gonadotropin			
Apresoline, *see* Hydralazine HCl			
Aprotinin	10,000 KIU		Q2003
AquaMEPHYTON, *see* Vitamin K			
Aralen, *see* Chloroquine HCl			
Aramine, *see* Metaraminol			
Aranesp, *see* Darbepoietin Alfa			
Arbutamine	1 mg	IV	J0395
Aredia, *see* Pamidronate disodium			
Arfonad, *see* Trimethaphan camsylate			
Aristocort Forte, *see* Triamcinolone diacetate			
Aristocort Intralesional, *see* Triamcinolone diacetate			
Aristospan Intra-Articular, *see* Triamcinolone hexacetonide			
Aristospan Intralesional, *see* Triamcinolone hexacetonide			
Arrestin, *see* Trimethobenzamide HCl			
Arsenic trioxide	1 mg	IV	J9017
Asparaginase	10,000 units	IV, IM	J9020
Astramorph PF, *see* Morphine sulfate			
Atgam, *see* Lymphocyte immune globulin			
Ativan, *see* Lorazepam			
Atropine, concentrated form	per mg	INH	J7635
Atropine, unit dose form	per mg	INH	J7636
Atropine sulfate	up to 0.3 mg	IV, IM, SC	J0460
Atrovent, *see* Ipratropium bromide			
Aurothioglucose	up to 50 mg	IM	J2910
Autologous cultured chondrocytes implant			J7330
Autoplex T, *see* Hemophilia clotting factors			
Avonex, *see* Interferon beta-1a			
Azathioprine	50 mg	ORAL	J7500
Azathioprine, parenteral	100 mg	IV	J7501
Azithromycin, dihydrate	1 gm	ORAL	Q0144
Azithromycin, injection	500 mg	IV	J0456
B			
Baclofen	10 mg	IT	J0475
Baclofen for intrathecal trial	50 mcg	OTH	J0476
Bactocill, *see* Oxacillin sodium			
BAL in oil, *see* Dimercaprol			
Banflex, *see* Orphenadrine citrate			
Basiliximab	20 mg		Q2019
BCG (Bacillus Calmette and Guérin), live	per vial instillation	IV	J9031
Beclomethasone inhalation solution, unit dose form	per mg	INH	J7622
Bena-D 10, *see* Diphenhydramine HCl			
Bena-D 50, *see* Diphenhydramine HCl			
Benadryl, *see* Diphenhydramine HCl			
Benahist 10, *see* Diphenhydramine HCl			
Benahist 50, *see* Diphenhydramine HCl			
Ben-Allergin-50, *see* Diphenhydramine HCl			
Benefix, *see* Factor IX, recombinant			
Benoject-10, *see* Diphenhydramine HCl			
Benoject-50, *see* Diphenhydramine HCl			
Bentyl, *see* Dicyclomine			
Benztropine mesylate	per 1 mg	IM, IV	J0515
Berubigen, *see* Vitamin B-12, cyanocobalamin			
Betalin 12, *see* Vitamin B-12, cyanocobalamin			
Betameth, *see* Betamethasone sodium phosphate			
Betamethasone acetate & betamethasone sodium phosphate	3 mg of ea	IM	J0702
Betamethasone inhalation solution, unit dose form	per mg	INH	J7624
Betamethasone sodium phosphate	4 mg	IM, IV	J0704
Betaseron, *see* Interferon beta-1b			
Bethanechol chloride	up to 5 mg	SC	J0520
Bicillin L-A, *see* Penicillin G benzathine			
Bicillin C-R 900/300, *see* Penicillin G procaine and penicillin G benzathine			
Bicillin C-R, *see* Penicillin G benzathine and penicillin G procaine			
BiCNU, *see* Carmustine			
Biperiden lactate	per 5 mg	IM, IV	J0190
Bitolterol mesylate, concentrated form	per mg	INH	J7628
Bitolterol mesylate, unit dose form	per mg	INH	J7629
Blenoxane, *see* Bleomycin sulfate			
Bleomycin sulfate	15 units	IM, IV, SC	J9040
Botulinum toxin type A	per unit	IM	J0585
Botulinum toxin type B	per 100 units	IM	J0587
Brethine, *see* Terbutaline sulfate or Terbutaline, compounded			
Bricanyl Subcutaneous, *see* Terbutaline sulfate			
Brompheniramine maleate	per 10 mg	IM, SC, IV	J0945
Bronkephrine, *see* Ethylnorepinephrine HCl			
Bronkosol, *see* Isoetharine HCl			
Budesonide inhalation solution, concentrated form	0.25 mg	INH	J7633
Budesonide inhalation solution, unit dose form	0.25 mg	INH	J7626
Buprenorphine Hydrochloride	0.1 mg		J0592
Busulfan	2 mg	ORAL	J8510

C			
Cabergoline	0.5 mg	ORAL	Q2001
Cafcit, *see* Caffeine citrate			
Caffeine citrate	5 mg	IV	J0706
Caine-1, *see* Lidocaine HCl			
Caine-2, *see* Lidocaine HCl			
Calcijex, *see* Calcitriol			
Calcimar, *see* Calcitonin-salmon			
Calcitonin-salmon	up to 400 units	SC, IM	J0630
Calcitriol	0.1 mcg	IM	J0636
Calcium Disodium Versenate, *see* Edetate calcium disodium			
Calcium gluconate	per 10 ml	IV	J0610
Calcium glycerophosphate & calcium lactate	per 10 ml	IM, SC	J0620
Calphosan, *see* Calcium glycerophosphate & calcium lactate			
Camptosar, *see* Irinotecan			
Capecitabine	150 mg	ORAL	J8520
	500 mg	ORAL	J8521
Carbocaine with Neo-Cobefrin, *see* Mepivacaine			
Carbocaine, *see* Mepivacaine			
Carboplatin	50 mg	IV	J9045
Carmustine	100 mg	IV	J9050
Carnitor, *see* Levocarnitine			
Carticel, *see* Autologous cultured chondrocytes			
Caspofungin Acetate	5 mg	IV	J0637
Cefadyl, *see* Cephapirin sodium			
Cefazolin sodium	up to 500 mg	IV, IM	J0690
Cefepime hydrochloride	500 mg	IV	J0692
Cefizox, *see* Ceftizoxime sodium			
Cefotaxime sodium	per 1 g	IV, IM	J0698
Cefoxitin sodium	1 g	IV, IM	J0694
Ceftazidime	per 500 mg	IM, IV	J0713
Ceftizoxime sodium	per 500 mg	IV, IM	J0715
Ceftriaxone sodium	per 250 mg	IV, IM	J0696
Cefuroxime sodium, sterile	per 750 mg	IM, IV	J0697
Celestone Phosphate, *see* Betamethasone sodium phosphate			
Celestone Soluspan, *see* Betamethasone acetate and betamethasone sodium phosphate			
CellCept, *see* Mycophenolate mofetil			
Cel-U-Jec, *see* Betamethasone sodium phosphate			
Cenacort Forte, *see* Triamcinolone diacetate			
Cenacort A-40, *see* Triamcinolone acetonide			
Cephalothin sodium	up to 1 g	IM, IV	J1890
Cephapirin sodium	up to 1 g	IV, IM	J0710
Ceredase, *see* Alglucerase			
Cerezyme, *see* Imiglucerase			
Cerubidine, *see* Daunorubicin HCl			
Chealamide, *see* Endrate ethylenediamine-tetra-/acetic acid			
Chloramphenicol sodium succinate	up to 1 g	IV	J0720
Chlordiazepoxide HCl	up to 100 mg	IM, IV	J1990
Chloromycetin Sodium Succinate, *see* Chloramphenicol sodium succinate			
Chloroprocaine HCl	per 30 ml	VAR	J2400
Chlorpromazine HCl, oral	10 mg	ORAL	Q0171
	25 mg	ORAL	Q0172
Chloroquine HCl	up to 250 mg	IM	J0390
Chlorothiazide sodium	per 500 mg	IV	J1205
Chlorpromazine HCl	10 mg	ORAL	Q0171
	25 mg	ORAL	Q0172
	up to 50 mg	IM, IV	J3230
Chorex-5, *see* Chorionic gonadotropin			
Chorex-10, *see* Chorionic gonadotropin			
Chorignon, *see* Chorionic gonadotropin			
Chorionic gonadotropin	per 1,000 USP units	IM	J0725
Choron-10, *see* Chorionic gonadotropin			
Cidofovir	375 mg	IV	J0740
Cilastatin sodium, imipenem	per 250 mg	IV, IM	J0743
Cipro IV, *see* Ciprofloxacin			
Ciprofloxacin	200 mg	IV	J0706
Cisplatin, powder or solution	per 10 mg	IV	J9060
Cisplatin	50 mg	IV	J9062
Cladribine	per mg	IV	J9065
Claforan, *see* Cefotaxime sodium			
Clonidine HCl	1 mg	epidural	J0735
Cobex, *see* Vitamin B-12, cyanocobalamin			
Codeine phosphate	per 30 mg	IM, IV, SC	J0745
Codimal-A, *see* Brompheniramine maleate			
Cogentin, *see* Benztropine mesylate			
Colchicine	per 1 mg	IV	J0760
Colistimethate sodium	up to 150 mg	IM, IV	J0770
Coly-Mycin M, *see* Colistimethate sodium			
Compa-Z, *see* Prochlorperazine			
Compazine, *see* Prochlorperazine			
Cophene-B, *see* Brompheniramine maleate			
Copper contraceptive, intrauterine	—	OTH	J7300
Cordarone, *see* Amiodarone HCl			
Corgonject-5, *see* Chorionic gonadotropin			
Corticorelin ovine triflutate	per dose		Q2005
Corticotropin	up to 40 units	IV, IM, SC	J0800
Cortrosyn, *see* Cosyntropin			
Cosmegen, *see* Dactinomycin			
Cosyntropin	per 0.25 mg	IM, IV	J0835
Cotranzine, *see* Prochlorperazine			
Cromolyn sodium, unit dose form	per 10 mg	INH	J7631
Crysticillin 300 A.S., *see* Penicillin G procaine			
Crysticillin 600 A.S., *see* Penicillin G procaine			
Cyclophosphamide	100 mg	IV	J9070
	200 mg	IV	J9080
	500 mg	IV	J9090
	1 g	IV	J9091
	2 g	IV	J9092

Cyclophosphamide, lyophilized	100 mg	IV	J9070
	200 mg	IV	J9080
	500 mg	IV	J9090
	1 g	OV	J9091
	2g	IV	J9092
Cyclophosphamide, oral	25 mg	ORAL	J8530
Cyclosporine, oral	25 mg	ORAL	J7515
	100 mg	ORAL	J7502
Cyclosporine, parenteral	250 mg	IV	J7516
Cytarabine	100 mg	SC, IV	J9100
	500 mg	SC, IV	J9110
Cytomegalovirus immune globulin intravenous (human)	per vial	IV	J0850
Cytosar-U, *see* Cytarabine			
Cytovene, *see* Ganciclovir sodium			
Cytoxan, *see* Cyclophosphamide; cyclophosphamide, lyophilized; and cyclophosphamide, oral			
D			
D-5-W, infusion	1000 cc	IV	J7070
Dacarbazine	100 mg	IV	J9130
	200 mg	IV	J9140
Daclizumab	25 mg	IV	J7513
Dactinomycin	0.5 mg	IV	J9120
Dalalone, *see* Dexamethasone sodium phosphate			
Dalalone L.A., *see* Dexamethasone acetate			
Dalteparin sodium	per 2500 IU	SC	J1645
Darbepoetin Alfa	5 mcg		J0880
Daunorubicin citrate, liposomal formulation	10 mg	IV	J9151
Daunorubicin HCl	10 mg	IV	J9150
DaunoXome, (*see* Daunorubicin citrate)			
DDAVP, *see* Desmopressin acetate			
Decadron Phosphate, *see* Dexamethasone sodium phosphate			
Decadron, *see* Dexamethasone sodium phosphate			
Decadron-LA, *see* Dexamethasone acetate			
Deca-Durabolin, *see* Nandrolone decanoate			
Decaject, *see* Dexamethasone sodium phosphate			
Decaject-L.A., *see* Dexamethasone acetate			
Decolone-50, *see* Nandrolone decanoate			
Decolone-100, *see* Nandrolone decanoate			
De-Comberol, *see* Testosterone cypionate and estradiol cypionate			
Deferoxamine mesylate	500 mg	IM, SC, IV	J0895
Dehist, *see* Brompheniramine maleate			
Deladumone, *see* Testosterone enanthate and estradiol valerate			
Deladumone OB, *see* Testosterone enanthate and estradiol valerate			
Delatest, *see* Testosterone enanthate			
Delatestadiol, *see* Testosterone enanthate and estradiol valerate			
Delatestryl, *see* Testosterone enanthate			
Delta-Cortef, *see* Prednisolone, oral			
Delestrogen, *see* Estradiol valerate			
Demadex, *see* Torsemide			
Demerol HCl, *see* Meperidine HCl			
Denileukin diftitox	300 mcg		J9160
DepAndro 100, *see* Testosterone cypionate			
DepAndro 200, *see* Testosterone cypionate			
DepAndrogyn, *see* Testosterone cypionate and estradiol cypionate			
DepGynogen, *see* Depo-estradiol cypionate			
DepMedalone 40, *see* Methylprednisolone acetate			
DepMedalone 80, *see* Methylprednisolone acetate			
Depo-estradiol cypionate	up to 5 mg	IM	J1000
Depogen, *see* Depo-estradiol cypionate			
Depoject, *see* Methylprednisolone acetate			
Depo-Medrol, *see* Methylprednisolone acetate			
Depopred-40, *see* Methylprednisolone acetate			
Depopred-80, *see* Methylprednisolone acetate			
Depo-Provera, *see* Medroxyprogesterone acetate			
Depotest, *see* Testosterone cypionate			
Depo-Testadiol, *see* Testosterone cypionate and estradiol cypionate			
Depotestogen, *see* Testosterone cypionate and estradiol cypionate			
Depo-Testosterone, *see* Testosterone cypionate			
Desferal Mesylate, *see* Deferoxamine mesylate			
Desmopressin acetate	1 mcg	IV, SC	J2597
Dexacen LA-8, *see* Dexamethasone acetate			
Dexacen-4, *see* Dexamethasone sodium phosphate			
Dexamethasone, concentrated form	per mg	INH	J7637
Dexamethasone, unit form	per mg	INH	J7638
Dexamethasone acetate	1 mg	IM	J1094
Dexamethasone sodium phosphate	1 mg	IM, IV, OTH	J1100
Dexasone, *see* Dexamethasone sodium phosphate			
Dexasone L.A., *see* Dexamethasone acetate			
Dexferrum, *see* Iron dextran			
Dexone, *see* Dexamethasone sodium phosphate			
Dexone LA, *see* Dexamethasone acetate			
Dexrazoxane HCl	250 mg	IV	J1190
Dextran 40	500 ml	IV	J7100
Dextran 75	500 ml	IV	J7110
Dextrose 5%/normal saline solution	500 ml = 1 unit	IV	J7042
Dextrose/water (5%)	500 ml = 1 unit	IV	J7060

D.H.E. 45, *see* Dihydroergotamine			
Diamox, *see* Acetazolamide sodium			
Diazepam	up to 5 mg	IM, IV	J3360
Diazoxide	up to 300 mg	IV	J1730
Dibent, *see* Dicyclomine HCl			
Dicyclomine HCl	up to 20 mg	IM	J0500
Didronel, *see* Etidronate disodium			
Diethylstilbestrol diphosphate	250 mg	IV	J9165
Diflucan, see Fluconazole			
Digoxin	up to 0.5 mg	IM, IV	J1160
Digoxin immune Fab (ovine)	per vial		Q2006
Dihydrex, *see* Diphenhydramine HCl			
Dihydroergotamine mesylate	per 1 mg	IM, IV	J1110
Dilantin, *see* Phenytoin sodium			
Dilaudid, *see* Hydromorphone HCl			
Dilocaine, *see* Lidocaine HCl			
Dilomine, *see* Dicyclomine HCl			
Dilor, *see* Dyphylline			
Dimenhydrinate	up to 50 mg	IM, IV	J1240
Dimercaprol	per 100 mg	IM	J0470
Dimethyl sulfoxide, *see* DMSO, Dimethyl sulfoxide			
Dinate, *see* Dimenhydrinate			
Dioval, *see* Estradiol valerate			
Dioval 40, *see* Estradiol valerate			
Dioval XX, *see* Estradiol valerate			
Diphenacen-50, *see* Diphenhydramine HCl			
Diphenhydramine HCl, injection	up to 50 mg	IV, IM	J1200
Diphenhydramine HCl, oral	50 mg	ORAL	Q0163
Dipyridamole	per 10 mg	IV	J1245
Disotate, *see* Endrate ethylenediamine-tetra-acetic acid			
Di-Spaz, *see* Dicyclomine HCl			
Ditate-DS, *see* Testosterone enanthate and estradiol valerate			
Diuril Sodium, *see* Chlorothiazide sodium			
D-Med 80, *see* Methylprednisolone acetate			
DMSO, Dimethyl sulfoxide	50%, 50 ml	OTH	J1212
Dobutamine HCl	per 250 mg	IV	J1250
Dobutrex, *see* Dobutamine HCl			
Docetaxel	20 mg	IV	J9170
Dolasetron mesylate, injection	10 mg	IV	J1260
Dolasetron mesylate, tablets	100 mg	ORAL	Q0180
Dolophine HCl, *see* Methadone HCl			
Dommanate, *see* Dimenhydrinate			
Dornase alpha, unit dose form	per mg	INH	J7639
Doxercalciferol	1 mcg	IV	J1270
Doxil, *see* Doxorubicin HCl, lipid			
Doxorubicin HCl	10 mg	IV	J9000
Doxorubicin HCl, all lipid	10 mg	IV	J9001
Dramamine, *see* Dimenhydrinate			
Dramanate, *see* Dimenhydrinate			
Dramilin, *see* Dimenhydrinate			
Dramocen, *see* Dimenhydrinate			
Dramoject, *see* Dimenhydrinate			
Dronabinol, oral	2.5 mg	ORAL	Q0167
Dronabinol, oral	5 mg	ORAL	Q0168
Droperidol	up to 5 mg	IM, IV	J1790
Drug administered through a metered dose inhaler		INH	J3535
Droperidol and fentanyl citrate	up to 2 ml ampule	IM, IV	J1810
DTIC-Dome, *see* Dacarbazine			
Dua-Gen L.A., *see* Testosterone enanthate and estradiol valerate cypionate			
Duoval P.A., *see* Testosterone enanthate and estradiol valerate			
Durabolin, *see* Nandrolone phenpropionate			
Duraclon, *see* Clonidine HCl			
Dura-Estrin, *see* Depo-estradiol cypionate			
Duracillin A.S., *see* Penicillin G procaine			
Duragen-10, *see* Estradiol valerate			
Duragen-20, *see* Estradiol valerate			
Duragen-40, *see* Estradiol valerate			
Duralone-40, *see* Methylprednisolone acetate			
Duralone-80, *see* Methylprednisolone acetate			
Duralutin, *see* Hydroxyprogesterone caproate			
Duramorph, *see* Morphine sulfate			
Duratest-100, *see* Testosterone cypionate			
Duratest-200, *see* Testosterone cypionate			
Duratestrin, *see* Testosterone cypionate and estradiol cypionate			
Durathate-200, *see* Testosterone enanthate			
Dymenate, *see* Dimenhydrinate			
Dyphylline	up to 500 mg	IM	J1180

E

Edetate calcium disodium	up to 1000 mg	IV, SC, IM	J0600
Edetate disodium	per 150 mg	IV	J3520
Elavil, *see* Amitriptyline HCl			
Ellence, *see* Epirubicin HCl			
Elliott's B solution	per ml	OTH	Q2002
Elspar, *see* Asparaginase			
Emete-Con, *see* Benzquinamide			
Eminase, *see* Anistreplase			
Enbrel, *see* Etanercept			
Endrate ethylenediamine-tetra-acetic acid, *see* Edetate disodium			
Enovil, *see* Amitriptyline HCl			
Enoxaparin sodium	10 mg	SC	J1650

Drug	Dosage	Route	Code
Epinephrine, adrenalin	up to 1 ml ampule	SC, IM	J0170
Epirubicin hydrochloride	50 mg		J9180
Epoprostenol	0.5 mg	IV	J1325
Eptifibatide, injection	5 mg	IM, IV	J1327
Ergonovine maleate	up to 0.2 mg	IM, IV	J1330
Erythromycin lactobionate	500 mg	IV	J1364
Estra-D, *see* Depo-estradiol cypionate			
Estra-L 20, *see* Estradiol valerate			
Estra-L 40, *see* Estradiol valerate			
Estra-Testrin, *see* Testosterone enanthate and estradiol valerate			
Estradiol Cypionate, *see* Depo-estradiol cypionate			
Estradiol L.A., *see* Estradiol valerate			
Estradiol L.A. 20, *see* Estradiol valerate			
Estradiol L.A. 40, *see* Estradiol valerate			
Estradiol valerate	up to 10 mg	IM	J1380
	up to 20 mg	IM	J1390
	up to 40 mg	IM	J0970
Estro-Cyp, *see* Depo-estradiol cypionate			
Estrogen, conjugated	per 25 mg	IV, IM	J1410
Estroject L.A., *see* Depo-estradiol cypionate			
Estrone	per 1 mg	IM	J1435
Estrone 5, *see* Estrone			
Estrone Aqueous, *see* Estrone			
Estronol, *see* Estrone			
Estronol-L.A., *see* Depo-estradiol cypionate			
Etanercept, injection	25 mg	IM, IV	J1438
Ethanolamine	100 mg		Q2007
Ethyol, *see* Amifostine			
Etidronate disodium	per 300 mg	IV	J1436
Etopophos, *see* Etoposide			
Etoposide	10 mg	IV	J9181
	100 mg	IV	J9182
Etoposide, oral	50 mg	ORAL	J8560
Everone, *see* Testosterone enanthate			
F			
Factor VIIa (coagulation factor, recombinant)	per mg	IV	Q0187
Factor VIII (anti-hemophilic factor, human)	per IU	IV	J7190
Factor VIII (anti-hemophilic factor, porcine)	per IU	IV	J7191
Factor VIII, (anti-hemophilic factor, recombinant)	per IU	IV	J7192
Factor IX (anti-hemophilic factor, purified, non-recombinant)	per IU	IV	Q0160
Factor IX (anti-hemophilic factor, recombinant)	per IU	IV	Q0161
Factor IX, complex	per IU	IV	J7194
Factors, other hemophilia clotting	per IU	IV	J7196
Factrel, *see* Gonadorelin HCl			
Feiba VH Immuno, *see* Factors, other hemophilia clotting			
Fentanyl citrate	0.1 mg	IM, IV	J3010
Ferrlecit, *see* Sodium ferricgluconate complex in sucrose injection			
Filgrastim (G-CSF)	300 mcg	SC, IV	J1440
	480 mcg	SC, IV	J1441
Flexoject, *see* Orphenadrine citrate			
Flexon, *see* Orphenadrine citrate			
Flolan, *see* Epoprostenol			
Floxuridine	500 mg	IV	J9200
Fluconazole	200 mg	IV	J1450
Fludara, *see* Fludarabine phosphate			
Fludarabine phosphate	50 mg	IV	J9185
Flunisolide inhalation solution, unit dose form	per mg	INH	J7641
Fluorouracil	500 mg	IV	J9190
Folex, *see* Methotrexate sodium			
Folex PFS, *see* Methotrexate sodium			
Follutein, *see* Chorionic gonadotropin			
Fomepizole	1.5 mg		Q2008
Fomivirsen sodium	1.65 mg	Intraocular	J1452
Fondaparinux sodium	0.5 mg		J1652
Fortaz, *see* Ceftazidime			
Foscarnet sodium	per 1,000 mg	IV	J1455
Foscavir, *see* Foscarnet sodium			
Fosphenytoin	50 mg		Q2009
FUDR, *see* Floxuridine			
Fungizone Intravenous, *see* Amphotericin B			
Furomide M.D., *see* Furosemide			
Furosemide	up to 20 mg	IM, IV	J1940
G			
Gamastan, *see* Gamma globulin and Immune globulin			
Gamma globulin	1 cc	IM	J1460
	2 cc	IM	J1470
	3 cc	IM	J1480
	4 cc	IM	J1490
	5 cc	IM	J1500
	6 cc	IM	J1510
	7 cc	IM	J1520
	8 cc	IM	J1530
	9 cc	IM	J1540
	10 cc	IM	J1550
	over 10 cc	IM	J1560
Gammar, *see* Gamma globulin and immune globulin			
Gammar-IV, *see* Immune globulin intravenous (human)			
Gamulin RH, *see* Rho(D) immune globulin			
Ganciclovir, implant	4.5 mg	OTH	J7310
Ganciclovir sodium	500 mg	IV	J1570
Garamycin, gentamicin	up to 80 mg	IM, IV	J1580
Gatifloxacin	10 mg	IV	J1590
Gemcitabine HCl	200 mg	IV	J9201
Gemtuzumab ozogamicin	5 mg	IV	J9300
Gemzar, *see* Gemcitabine HCl			
Gentamicin Sulfate, *see* Garamycin, gentamicin			
Gentran, *see* Dextran 40			
Gentran 75, *see* Dextran 75			
Gesterol 50, *see* Progesterone			
Glatiramer acetate	per dose		Q2010
Glucagon HCl	per 1 mg	SC, IM, IV	J1610
Glukor, *see* Chorionic gonadotropin			
Glycopyrrolate, concentrated form	per 1 mg	INH	J7642

Glycopyrrolate, unit dose form	per 1 mg	INH	J7643
Gold sodium thiomalate	up to 50 mg	IM	J1600
Gonadorelin HCl	per 100 mcg	SC, IV	J1620
Gonic, *see* Chorionic gonadotropin			
Goserelin acetate implant	per 3.6 mg	SC	J9202
Granisetron HCl, injection	100 mcg	IV	J1626
Granisetron HCl, oral	1 mg	ORAL	Q0166
Gynogen L.A. "A10," *see* Estradiol valerate			
Gynogen L.A. "A20," *see* Estradiol valerate			
Gynogen L.A. "A40," *see* Estradiol valerate			
H			
Haldol, *see* Haloperidol			
Haloperidol	up to 5 mg	IM, IV	J1630
Haloperidol decanoate	per 50 mg	IM	J1631
Hectorol, *see* Doxercalciferol			
Hemin	per 1 mg		Q2011
Hemofil M, *see* Factor VIII			
Hemophilia clotting factors (e.g., anti-inhibitors)	per IU	IV	J7198
Hemophilia clotting factors, NOC	per IU	IV	J7199
Hepatitis B vaccine			Q3021-Q3023
Hep-Lock, *see* Heparin sodium (heparin lock flush)			
Heparin sodium	1,000 units	IV, SC	J1644
Heparin sodium (heparin lock flush)	10 units	IV	J1642
Herceptin, *see* Trastuzumab			
Hexadrol Phosphate, *see* Dexamethasone sodium phosphate			
Histaject, *see* Brompheniramine maleate			
Histerone 50, *see* Testosterone suspension			
Histerone 100, *see* Testosterone suspension			
Histrelin acetate	10 mg		Q2020
Hyalgan, *see* Sodium hyaluronate			
Hyaluronidase	up to 150 units	SC, IV	J3470
Hyate:C, *see* Factor VIII (anti-hemophilic factor, porcine)			
Hybolin Improved, *see* Nandrolone phenpropionate			
Hybolin Decanoate, *see* Nandrolone decanoate			
Hycamtin, *see* Topotecan			
Hydralazine HCl	up to 20 mg	IV, IM	J0360
Hydrate, *see* Dimenhydrinate			
Hydrochlorides of opium alkaloids	up to 20 mg	IM, SC	J2480
Hydrocortisone acetate	up to 25 mg	IV, IM, SC	J1700
Hydrocortisone sodium phosphate	up to 50 mg	IV, IM, SC	J1710
Hydrocortisone succinate sodium	up to 100 mg	IV, IM, SC	J1720
Hydrocortone Acetate, *see* Hydrocortisone acetate			
Hydrocortone Phosphate, *see* Hydrocortisone sodium phosphate			
Hydromorphone HCl	up to 4 mg	SC, IM, IV	J1170
Hydroxyzine HCl	up to 25 mg	IM	J3410
Hydroxyzine pamoate	25 mg	ORAL	Q0177
	50 mg	ORAL	Q0178
Hylan G-F 20	16 mg	OTH	J7320
Hyoscyamine sulfate	up to 0.25 mg	SC, IM, IV	J1980
Hyperstat IV, *see* Diazoxide			
Hyper-Tet, *see* Tetanus immune globulin, human			
HypRho-D, *see* Rho(D) immune globulin			
Hyrexin-50, *see* Diphenhydramine HCl			
Hyzine-50, *see* Hydroxyzine HCl			
I			
Ibutilide fumarate	1 mg	IV	J1742
Idamycin, *see* Idarubicin HCl			
Idarubicin HCl	5 mg	IV	J9211
Ifex, *see* Ifosfamide			
Ifosfamide	per 1 g	IV	J9208
Ilotycin, *see* Erythromycin gluceptate			
Imferon, *see* Iron dextran			
Imiglucerase	per unit	IV	J1785
Imitrex, *see* Sumatriptan succinate			
Immune globulin	per 500 mg	IV	J1561
Immune globulin, anti-thymocyte globulin	25 mg	IV	J7504
Immune globulin intravenous	1 gm	IV	J1563
	10 mg	IV	J1564
Immunosuppressive drug, not otherwise classified			J7599
Imuran, *see* Azathioprine			
Inapsine, *see* Droperidol			
Inderal, *see* Propranolol HCl			
Infed, *see* Iron dextran-			
Infergen, *see* Interferon alfa-1			
Infliximab, injection	10 mg	IM, IV	J1745
Innohep, *see* Tinzarparin			
Innovar, *see* Droperidol with fentanyl citrate			
Insulin	5 units	SC	J1815
	50 units	SC	J1817
Insulin lispro	up to 50 units	SC	K0548
Intal, *see* Cromolyn sodium or Cromolyn sodium, compounded			
Integrilin, injection, *see* Eptifibatide			
Interferon alphacon-1, recombinant	1 mcg	SC	J9212
Interferon alfa-2a, recombinant	3 million units	SC, IM	J9213
Interferon alfa-2b, recombinant	1 million units	SC, IM	J9214
Interferon alfa-n3 (human leukocyte derived)	250,000 IU	IM	J9215
Interferon beta-1a	33 mcg	IM	J1825
	11 mcg	IM	Q3025
	11 mcg	SC	Q3026
Interferon beta-1b	0.25 mg	SC	J1830
Interferon gamma-1b	3 million units	SC	J9216
Intrauterine copper contraceptive, *see* Copper contraceptive, intrauterine			
Ipratropium bromide, unit dose form	per mg	INH	J7644
Irinotecan	20 mg	IV	J9206

Drug	Dosage	Route	Code
Iron dextran	50 mg	IV, IM	J1750
Iron sucrose	1 mg	IV	J1756
Irrigation solution for Tx of bladder calculi	per 50 ml	OTH	Q2004
Isocaine HCl, *see* Mepivacaine			
Isoetharine HCl, concentrated form	per mg	INH	J7648
Isoetharine HCl, unit dose form	per mg	INH	J7649
Isoproterenol HCl, concentrated form	per mg	INH	J7658
Isoproterenol HCl, unit dose form	per mg	INH	J7659
Isuprel, *see* Isoproterenol HCl			
Itraconazole	50 mg	IV	J1835
J			
Jenamicin, *see* Garamycin, gentamicin			
K			
Kabikinase, *see* Streptokinase			
Kaleinate, *see* Calcium gluconate			
Kanamycin sulfate	up to 75 mg	IM, IV	J1850
Kanamycin sulfate	up to 500 mg	IM, IV	J1840
Kantrex, *see* Kanamycin sulfate			
Keflin, *see* Cephalothin sodium			
Kefurox, *see* Cufuroxime sodium			
Kefzol, *see* Cefazolin sodium			
Kenaject-40, *see* Triamcinolone acetonide			
Kenalog-10, *see* Triamcinolone acetonide			
Kenalog-40, *see* Triamcinolone acetonide			
Kestrone 5, *see* Estrone			
Ketorolac tromethamine	per 15 mg	IM, IV	J1885
Key-Pred 25, *see* Prednisolone acetate			
Key-Pred 50, *see* Prednisolone acetate			
Key-Pred-SP, *see* Prednisolone sodium phosphate			
K-Flex, *see* Orphenadrine citrate			
Klebcil, *see* Kanamycin sulfate			
Konate-HP, *see* Factor VIII			
Kogenate, *see* Factor VIII			
Konakion, *see* Vitamin K, phytonadione, etc.			
Konyne 80, *see* Factor IX, complex			
Kutapressin	up to 2 ml	SC, IM	J1910
Kytril, *see* Granisetron HCl			
L			
L.A.E. 20, *see* Estradiol valerate			
Laetrile, Amygdalin, vitamin B-17			J3570
Lanoxin, *see* Digoxin			
Largon, *see* Propiomazine HCl			
Lasix, *see* Furosemide			
L-Caine, *see* Lidocaine HCl			
Lepirudin	50 mg		Q2021
Leucovorin calcium	per 50 mg	IM, IV	J0640
Leukine, *see* Sargramostim (GM-CSF)			
Leuprolide acetate (for depot suspension)	3.75 mg	IM	J1950
	7.5 mg	IM	J9217
Leuprolide acetate	per 1 mg	IM	J9218
Leuprolide acetate implant	65 mg		J9219
Leustatin, *see* Cladribine			
Levalbuterol HCl, concentrated form	0.5 mg	INH	J7618
Levalbuterol HC1, unit form	0.5 mg	INH	J7619
Levaquin I.U., *see* Levofloxacin			
Levocarnitine	per 1 gm	IV	J1955
Levo-Dromoran, *see* Levorphanol tartrate			
Levofloxacin	250 mg	IV	J1956
Levonorgestrel releasing intrauterine contraceptive	52 mg	OTH	J7302
Levorphanol tartrate	up to 2 mg	SC, IV	J1960
Levsin, *see* Hyoscyamine sulfate			
Levulan Kerastick, *see* Aminolevulinic acid HC1			
Librium, *see* Chlordiazepoxide HCl			
Lidocaine HCl	50 cc	VAR	J2000
Lidoject-1, *see* Lidocaine HCl			
Lidoject-2, *see* Lidocaine HCl			
Lincocin, *see* Lincomycin HCl			
Lincomycin HCl	up to 300 mg	IV	J2010
Linezolid	200 mg	IV	J2020
Liquaemin Sodium, *see* Heparin sodium			
Lioresal, *see* Baclofen			
LMD (10%), *see* Dextran 40			
Lovenox, *see* Enoxaparin sodium			
Lorazepam	2 mg	IM, IV	J2060
Lufyllin, *see* Dyphylline			
Luminal Sodium, *see* Phenobarbital sodium			
Lunelle, *see* Medroxyprogesterone acetate/estradiol cypionate			
Lupron, *see* Leuprolide acetate			
Lymphocyte immune globulin			
anti-thymocyte globulin, equine	250 mg	IV	J7504
anti-thymocyte, globulin, rabbit	25 mg	IV	J7511
Lyophilized, *see* Cyclophosphamide, lyophilized			
M			
Magnesium sulfate	500 mg		J3475
Mannitol	25% in 50 ml	IV	J2150
Marmine, *see* Dimenhydrinate			
Maxipime, *see* Cefepime hydrochloride			
Mechlorethamine HCl (nitrogen mustard), HN2	10 mg	IV	J9230
Medralone 40, *see* Methylprednisolone acetate			
Medralone 80, *see* Methylprednisolone acetate			
Medrol, *see* Methylprednisolone			
Medroxyprogesterone acetate	50 mg	IM	J1051
	150 mg	IM	J1055
Medroxyprogesterone acetate/estradiol cypionate	5 mg/25 mg	IV	J1056
Mefoxin, *see* Cefoxitin sodium			

Drug Name	Dosage	Route	Code
Melphalan HCl	50 mg	IV	J9245
Melphalan, oral	2 mg	ORAL	J8600
Menoject LA, *see* Testosterone cypionate and estradiol cypionate			
Mepergan Injection, *see* Meperidine and promethazine HCl			
Meperidine HCl	per 100 mg	IM, IV, SC	J2175
Meperidine and promethazine HCl	up to 50 mg	IM, IV	J2180
Mepivacaine HCL	per 10 ml	VAR	J0670
Mesna	200 mg	IV	J9209
Mesnex, *see* Mesna			
Metaprel, *see* Metaproterenol sulfate			
Metaproterenol sulfate, concentrated form	per 10 mg	INH	J7668
Metaproterenol sulfate, unit dose form	per 10 mg	INH	J7669
Metaraminol bitartrate	per 10 mg	IV, IM, SC	J0380
Metastron, *see* Strontium-89 chloride			
Methadone HCl	up to 10 mg	IM, SC	J1230
Methergine, *see* Methylergonovine maleate			
Methocarbamol	up to 10 ml	IV, IM	J2800
Methotrexate, oral	2.5 mg	ORAL	J8610
Methotrexate sodium	5 mg	IV, IM, IT, IA	J9250
	50 mg	IV, IM, IT, IA	J9260
Methotrexate LPF, *see* Methotrexate sodium			
Methylergonovine maleate	up to 0.2 mg	IM, IV	J2210
Methyldopate HCl	up to 250 mg	IV	J0210
Methylergonovine maleate	up to 0.2 mg		J2210
Methylprednisolone, oral	per 4 mg	ORAL	J7509
Methylprednisolone acetate	20 mg	IM	J1020
	40 mg	IM	J1030
	80 mg	IM	J1040
Methylprednisolone sodium succinate	up to 40 mg	IM, IV	J2920
	up to 125 mg	IM, IV	J2930
Metoclopramide HCl	up to 10 mg	IV	J2765
Miacalcin, *see* Calcitonin-salmon			
Midazolam HCl	per 1 mg	IM, IV	J2250
Milrinone lactate	per 5 mg	IV	J2260
Mirena, *see* Levonorgestrel releasing intrauterine contraceptive			
Mithracin, *see* Plicamycin			
Mitomycin	5 mg	IV	J9280
	20 mg	IV	J9290
	40 mg	IV	J9291
Mitoxantrone HCl	per 5 mg	IV	J9293
Monocid, *see* Cefonicid sodium			
Monoclate-P, *see* Factor VIII			
Monoclonal antibodies, parenteral	5 mg	IV	J7505
Mononine, *see* Factor IX, purified, non-recombinant			
Morphine sulfate	up to 10 mg	IM, IV, SC	J2270
	100 mg	IM, IV, SC	J2271
Morphine sulfate, preservative-free	per 10 mg	IM, IV, SC	J2275
M-Prednisol-40, *see* Methylprednisolone acetate			
M-Prednisol-80, *see* Methylprednisolone acetate			
Mucomyst, *see* Acetylcysteine or Acetylcysteine, compounded			
Mucosol, *see* Acetylcysteine			
Muromonab-CD3	5 mg	IV	J7505
Muse, *see* Alprostadil			
Mustargen, *see* Mechlorethamine HCl			
Mutamycin, *see* Mitomycin			
Mycophenolate mofetil	250 mg	ORAL	J7517
Myleran, *see* Busulfan			
Mylotarg, *see* Gemtuzumab ozogamicin			
Myobloc, *see* Botulinum toxin type B			
Myochrysine, *see* Gold sodium thiomalate			
Myolin, *see* Orphenadrine citrate			
N			
Nalbuphine HCl	per 10 mg	IM, IV, SC	J2300
Naloxone HCl	per 1 mg	IM, IV, SC	J2310
Nandrobolic L.A., *see* Nandrolone decanoate			
Nandrolone decanoate	up to 50 mg	IM	J2320
	up to 100 mg	IM	J2321
	up to 200 mg	IM	J2322
Narcan, *see* Naloxone HCl			
Naropin, *see* Ropivacaine HCl			
Nasahist B, *see* Brompheniramine maleate			
Nasal vaccine inhalation		INH	J3530
Navane, *see* Thiothixene			
Navelbine, *see* Vinorelbine tartrate			
ND Stat, *see* Brompheniramine maleate			
Nebcin, *see* Tobramycin sulfate			
NebuPent, *see* Pentamidine isethionate			
Nembutal Sodium Solution, *see* Pentobarbital sodium			
Neocyten, *see* Orphenadrine citrate			
Neo-Durabolic, *see* Nandrolone decanoate			
Neoquess, *see* Dicyclomine HCl			
Neosar, *see* Cyclophosphamide			
Neostigmine methylsulfate	up to 0.5 mg	IM, IV, SC	J2710
Neo-Synephrine, *see* Phenylephrine HCl			
Nervocaine 1%, *see* Lidocaine HCl			
Nervocaine 2%, *see* Lidocaine HCl			
Nesacaine, *see* Chloroprocaine HCl			
Nesacaine-MPF, *see* Chloroprocaine HCl			
Nesiritide	0.5 mg		J2324
Neumega, *see* Oprelvekin			
Neupogen, *see* Filgrastim (G-CSF)			
Neutrexin, *see* Trimetrexate glucuronate			
Nipent, *see* Pentostatin			
Nordryl, *see* Diphenhydramine HCl			
Norflex, *see* Orphenadrine citrate			
Norzine, *see* Thiethylperazine maleate			
Not otherwise classified drugs			J3490

Drug Name	Unit Per	Route	Code
Not otherwise classified drugs	other than INH, administered thru DME		J7799
Not otherwise classified drugs	INH, administered thru DME		J7699
Not otherwise classified drugs, anti-neoplastic		—	J9999
Not otherwise classified drugs, chemotherapeutic		ORAL	J8999
Not otherwise classified drugs, immunosuppressive		—	J7599
Not otherwise classified drugs, nonchemotherapeutic		ORAL	J8499
Novantrone, *see* Mitoxantrone HCl			
Novo Seven, *see* Factor VIIa			
NPH, *see* Insulin			
Nubain, *see* Nalbuphine HCl			
Nulicaine, *see* Lidocaine HCl			
Numorphan, *see* Oxymorphone HCl			
Numorphan H.P., *see* Oxymorphone HCl			
O			
Octreotide Acetate, injection	1 mg	IM, IV	J2352
Oculinum, *see* Botulinum toxin type A			
Odansetron HCl	1 mg	IV	J2405
O-Flex, *see* Orphenadrine citrate			
Omnipen-N, *see* Ampicillin			
Oncaspar, *see* Pegaspargase			
Oncovin, *see* Vincristine sulfate			
Ondansetron HCl, oral	8 mg	ORAL	Q0179
Oprelvekin	5 mg	SC	J2355
Oraminic II, *see* Brompheniramine maleate			
Ormazine, *see* Chlorpromazine HCl			
Orphenadrine citrate	up to 60 mg	IV, IM	J2360
Orphenate, *see* Orphenadrine citrate			
Or-Tyl, *see* Dicyclomine			
Oxacillin sodium	up to 250 mg	IM, IV	J2700
Oxymorphone HCl	up to 1 mg	IV, SC, IM	J2410
Oxytetracycline HCl	up to 50 mg	IM	J2460
Oxytocin	up to 10 units	IV, IM	J2590
P			
Paclitaxel	30 mg	IV	J9265
Pamidronate disodium	per 30 mg	IV	J2430
Papaverine HCl	up to 60 mg	IV, IM	J2440
Paragard T 380 A, *see* Copper contraceptive, intrauterine			
Paraplatin, *see* Carboplatin			
Paricalcitol, injection	1 mcg	IV, IM	J2501
Pegademase bovine	25 IU		Q2012
Pegaspargase	per single dose vial	IM, IV	J9266
Penicillin G benzathine	up to 600,000 units	IM	J0560
	up to 1,200,000 units	IM	J0570
	up to 2,400,000 units	IM	J0580
Penicillin G benzathine and penicillin G procaine	up to 600,000 units	IM	J0530
	up to 1,200,000 units	IM	J0540
	up to 2,400,000 units	IM	J0550
Penicillin G potassium	up to 600,000 units	IM, IV	J2540
Penicillin G procaine, aqueous	up to 600,000 units	IM, IV	J2510
Pentamidine isethionate	per 300 mg	INH	J2545
Pentastarch, 10%	per 100 ml		Q2013
Pentazocine HCl	up to 30 mg	IM, SC, IV	J3070
Pentobarbital sodium	per 50 mg	IM, IV, OTH	J2515
Pentostatin	per 10 mg	IV	J9268
Permapen, *see* Penicillin G benzathine			
Perphenazine, injection	up to 5 mg	IM, IV	J3310
Perphenazine, tablets	4 mg	ORAL	Q0175
	8 mg	ORAL	Q0176
Persantine IV, *see* Dipyridamole			
Pfizerpen, *see* Penicillin G potassium			
Pfizerpen A.S., *see* Penicillin G procaine			
Phenazine 25, *see* Promethazine HCl			
Phenazine 50, *see* Promethazine HCl			
Phenergan, *see* Promethazine HCl			
Phenobarbital sodium	up to 120 mg	IM, IV	J2560
Phentolamine mesylate	up to 5 mg	IM, IV	J2760
Phenylephrine HCl	up to 1 ml	SC, IM, IV	J2370
Phenytoin sodium	per 50 mg	IM, IV	J1165
Photofrin, *see* Porfimer sodium			
Phytonadione (Vitamin K)	per 1 mg	IM, SC, IV	J3430
Piperacillin/Tazobactam Sodium, injection	1.125 g	IV	J2543
Pitocin, *see* Oxytocin			
Plantinol AQ, *see* Cisplatin			
Plas + SD, *see* Plasma, pooled multiple donor			
Plasma, cryoprecipitate reduced	each unit		P9044
Plasma, pooled multiple donor, frozen, each unit		IV	P9023
Platinol, *see* Cisplatin			
Plicamycin	2,500 mcg	IV	J9270
Polocaine, *see* Mepivacaine			
Polycillin-N, *see* Ampicillin			
Porfimer Sodium	75 mg	IV	J9600
Potassium chloride	per 2 mEq	IV	J3480
Pralidoxime chloride	up to 1 g	IV, IM, SC	J2730
Predalone-50, *see* Prednisolone acetate			
Predcor-25, *see* Prednisolone acetate			
Predcor-50, *see* Prednisolone acetate			
Predicort-50, *see* Prednisolone acetate			
Prednisone	per 5 mg	ORAL	J7506
Prednisolone, oral	5 mg	ORAL	J7510
Prednisolone acetate	up to 1 ml	IM	J2650
Predoject-50, *see* Prednisolone acetate			
Pregnyl, *see* Chorionic gonadotropin			

Drug	Dosage	Route	Code
Premarin Intravenous, *see* Estrogen, conjugated			
Prescription, chemotherapeutic, not otherwise specified		ORAL	J8999
Prescription, nonchemotherapeutic, not otherwise specified		ORAL	J8499
Primacor, *see* Milrinone lactate			
Primaxin I.M., *see* Cilastatin sodium, imipenem			
Primaxin I.V., *see* Cilastatin sodium, imipenem			
Priscoline HCl, *see* Tolazoline HCl			
Pro-Depo, *see* Hydroxyprogesterone Caproate			
Procainamide HCl	up to 1 g	IM, IV	J2690
Prochlorperazine	up to 10 mg	IM, IV	J0780
Prochlorperazine maleate, oral	5 mg	ORAL	Q0164
	10 mg	ORAL	Q0165
Profasi HP, *see* Chorionic gonadotropin			
Profilnine Heat-Treated, *see* Factor IX			
Progestaject, *see* Progesterone			
Progesterone	per 50 mg		J2675
Prograf, *see* Tacrolimus, oral or parenteral			
Prokine, *see* Sargramostim (GM-CSF)			
Prolastin, *see* Alpha 1-proteinase inhibitor (human)			
Proleukin, *see* Aldesleukin			
Prolixin Decanoate, *see* Fluphenazine decanoate			
Promazine HCl	up to 25 mg	IM	J2950
Promethazine HCl, injection	up to 50 mg	IM, IV	J2550
Promethazine HCl, oral	12.5 mg	ORAL	Q0169
	25 mg	ORAL	Q0170
Pronestyl, *see* Procainamide HCl			
Proplex T, *see* Factor IX			
Proplex SX-T, *see* Factor IX			
Propranolol HCl	up to 1 mg	IV	J1800
Prorex-25, *see* Promethazine HCl			
Prorex-50, *see* Promethazine HCl			
Prostaphlin, *see* Procainamide HCl			
Prostigmin, *see* Neostigmine methylsulfate			
Protamine sulfate	per 10 mg	IV	J2720
Protirelin	per 250 mcg	IV	J2725
Prothazine, *see* Promethazine HCl			
Protopam Chloride, *see* Pralidoxime chloride			
Proventil, *see* Albuterol sulfate, compounded			
Prozine-50, *see* Promazine HCl			
Pulmicort Respules, *see* Budesonide			

Q

Drug	Dosage	Route	Code
Quelicin, *see* Succinylcholine chloride			
Quinupristin/dalfopristin	500 mg (150/350)	IV	J2770

R

Drug	Dosage	Route	Code
Ranitidine HCl, injection	25 mg	IV, IM	J2780
Rapamune, *see* Sirolimus			
Recombinate, *see* Factor VIII			
Redisol, *see* Vitamin B-12 cyanocobalamin			
Regitine, *see* Phentolamine mesylate			
Reglan, *see* Metoclopramide HCl			
Regular, *see* Insulin			
Relefact TRH, *see* Protirelin			
Remicade, *see* Infliximab, injection			
Reo Pro, *see* Abciximab			
Rep-Pred 40, *see* Methylprednisolone acetate			
Rep-Pred 80, *see* Methylprednisolone acetate			
RespiGam, *see* Respiratory Syncytial Virus			
Respiratory Syncytial Virus Immune-globulin	50 mg	IV	J1565
Retavase, *see* Reteplase			
Reteplase	18.8 mg	IV	J2993
Retrovir, *see* Zidovudine			
Rheomacrodex, *see* Dextran 40			
Rhesonativ, *see* Rho(D) immune globulin, human			
Rheumatrex Dose Pack, *see* Methotrexate, oral			
Rho(D) immune globulin, human	1 dose package, 300 mcg	IM	J2790
	1 dose package, 50 mcg	IM	J2798
Rho(D)immune globulin (human), solvent detergent	100 IU	IV	J2792
RhoGAM, *see* Rho(D) immune globulin, human			
Ringer's lactate infusion	up to 1,000 cc	IV	J7120
Rituxan, *see* Rituximab			
Rituximab	100 mg	IV	J9310
Robaxin, *see* Methocarbamol			
Rocephin, *see* Ceftriaxone sodium			
Roferon-A, *see* Interferon alfa-2A, recombinant			
Ropivacaine HCl	1 mg		J2795
Rubex, *see* Doxorubicin HCl			
Rubramin PC, *see* Vitamin B-12 cyanocobalamin			

S

Drug	Dosage	Route	Code
Saline solution	5% dextrose, 500 ml	IV	J7042
	infusion, 250 cc	IV	J7050
	infusion, 1,000 cc	IV	J7030
Saline solution, sterile	500 ml = 1 unit	IV, OTH	J7040
	up to 5 cc	IV, OTH	J7051
Sandimmune, *see* Cyclosporine			
Sandoglobulin, *see* Immune globulin intravenous (human)			
Sandostatin Lar Depot, *see* Octreotide			
Sargramostim (GM-CSF)	50 mcg	IV	J2820

Drug	Dosage	Route	Code
Secobarbital sodium	up to 250 mg	IM, IV	J2860
Seconal, *see* Secobarbital sodium			
Selestoject, *see* Betamethasone sodium phosphate			
Sermorelin acetate	0.5 mg		Q2014
Sinusol-B, *see* Brompheniramine maleate	per 2 ml	IV	J2912
Sirolimus	1 mg	ORAL	J7520
Sodium chloride, 0.9%	per 2 ml		J2912
Sodium ferricgluconate in sucrose	12.5 mg		J2916
Sodium hyaluronate	5 mg	OTH	J7316
Solganal, *see* Aurothioglucose			
Solu-Cortef, *see* Hydrocortisone sodium phosphate			J1710
Solu-Medrol, *see* Methylprednisolone sodium succinate			
Solurex, *see* Dexamethasone sodium phosphate			
Solurex LA, *see* Dexamethasone acetate			
Somatrem	1 mg		J2940
Somatropin	1 mg		J2941
Sparine, *see* Promazine HCl			
Spasmoject, *see* Dicyclomine HCl			
Spectinomycin HCl	up to 2 g	IM	J3320
Sporanox, *see* Itraconazole			
Staphcillin, *see* Methicillin sodium			
Stilphostrol, *see* Diethylstilbestrol diphosphate			
Streptase, *see* Streptokinase			
Streptokinase	per 250,000 IU	IV	J2995
Streptomycin Sulfate, *see* Streptomycin			
Streptomycin	up to 1 g	IM	J3000
Streptozocin	1 gm	IV	J9320
Strontium-89 chloride	per 10 ml	IV	J3005
Sublimaze, *see* Fentanyl citrate			
Succinylcholine chloride	up to 20 mg	IV, IM	J0330
Sumatriptan succinate	6 mg	SC	J3030
Supartz *see* Sodium hyaluronate			
Surostrin, *see* Succinycholine chloride			
Sus-Phrine, *see* Adrenalin, epinephrine			
Synercid, *see* Quinupristin/dalfopristin			
Synkavite, *see* Vitamin K, phytonadione, etc.			
Syntocinon, *see* Oxytocin			
Synvisc, *see* Hylan G-F 20			
Sytobex, *see* Vitamin B-12 cyanocobalamin			
T			
Tacrolimus, oral	per 1 mg	ORAL	J7507
	per 5 mg	ORAL	J7508
Tacrolimus, parenteral	5 mg		J7515
Talwin, *see* Pentazocine HCl			
Taractan, *see* Chlorprothixene			
Taxol, *see* Paclitaxel			
Taxotere, *see* Docetaxel			
Tazidime, *see* Ceftazidime			
Technetium TC Sestamibi	per dose		A9500
TEEV, *see* Testosterone enanthate and estradiol valerate			
Temozolomide	5 mg	ORAL	J8700
Tenecteplase	50 mg		J3100
Teniposide	50 mg		Q2017
Tequin, *see* Gatifloxacin			
Terbutaline sulfate	up to 1 mg	SC, IV	J3105
Terbutaline sulfate, concentrated form	per 1 mg	INH	J7680
Terbutaline sulfate, unit dose form	per 1 mg	INH	J7681
Terramycin IM, *see* Oxytetracycline HCl			
Testa-C, *see* Testosterone cypionate			
Testadiate, *see* Testosterone enanthate and estradiol valerate			
Testadiate-Depo, *see* Testosterone cypionate			
Testaject-LA, *see* Testosterone cypionate			
Testaqua, *see* Testosterone suspension			
Test-Estro Cypionates, *see* Testosterone cypionate and estradiol cypionate			
Test-Estro-C, *see* Testosterone cypionate and estradiol cypionate			
Testex, *see* Testosterone propionate			
Testoject-50, *see* Testosterone suspension			
Testoject-LA, *see* Testosterone cypionate			
Testone LA 200, *see* Testosterone enanthate			
Testone LA 100, *see* Testosterone enanthate			
Testosterone Aqueous, *see* Testosterone suspension			
Testosterone enanthate and estradiol valerate	up to 1 cc	IM	J0900
Testosterone enanthate	up to 100 mg	IM	J3120
	up to 200 mg	IM	J3130
Testosterone cypionate	up to 100 mg	IM	J1070
	1 cc, 200 mg	IM	J1080
Testosterone cypionate and estradiol cypionate	up to 1 ml	IM	J1060
Testosterone propionate	up to 100 mg	IM	J3150
Testosterone suspension	up to 50 mg	IM	J3140
Testradiol 90/4, *see* Testosterone enanthate and estradiol valerate			
Testrin PA, *see* Testosterone enanthate			
Tetanus immune globulin, human	up to 250 units	IM	J1670
Tetracycline	up to 250 mg	IM, IV	J0120
Thallous Chloride TL 201	per MCI		A9505
Theelin Aqueous, *see* Estrone			
Theophylline	per 40 mg	IV	J2810
TheraCys, *see* BCG live			
Thiethylperazine maleate, injection	up to 10 mg	IM	J3280
Thiethylperazine maleate, oral	10 mg	ORAL	Q0174

Drug	Dosage	Route	Code
Thiotepa	15 mg	IV	J9340
Thorazine, *see* Chlorpromazine HCl			
Thymoglobulin, *see* Immune globulin, anti-thymocyte			
Thypinone, *see* Protirelin			
Thyrogen, *see* Thyrotropin Alfa			
Thyrotropin Alpha, injection	0.9 mg	IM, SC	J3240
Tice BCG, *see* BCG live			
Ticon, *see* Trimethobenzamide HCl			
Tigan, *see* Trimethobenzamide HCl			
Tiject-20, *see* Trimethobenzamide HCl			
Tinzarparin	1000 IU	SC	J1655
Tirofiban hydrochloride, injection	12.5 mg	IM, IV	J3245
TNKase, *see*, Tenecteplase			
Tobi, *see* Tobramycin, inhalation solution			
Tobramycin, inhalation solution	300 mg	INH	J7682
Tobramycin sulfate	up to 80 mg	IM, IV	J3260
Tofranil, *see* Imipramine HCl			
Tolazoline HCl	up to 25 mg	IV	J2670
Topotecan	4 mg	IV	J9350
Toradol, *see* Ketorolac tromethamine			
Torecan, *see* Thiethylperazine maleate			
Tornalate, *see* Bitolterol mesylate			
Torsemide	10 mg/ml	IV	J3265
Totacillin-N, *see* Ampicillin			
Trastuzumab	10 mg	ORAL	J9355
Tri-Kort, *see* Triamcinolone acetonide			
Triam-A, *see* Triamcinolone acetonide			
Triamcinolone, concentrated form	per 1 mg	INH	J7683
Triamcinolone, unit dose	per 1 mg	INH	J7684
Triamcinolone acetonide	per 10 mg	IM	J3301
Triamcinolone diacetate	per 5 mg	IM	J3302
Triamcinolone hexacetonide	per 5 mg	VAR	J3303
Triflupromazine HCl	up to 20 mg	IM, IV	J3400
Trilafon, *see* Perphenazine			
Trilog, *see* Triamcinolone acetonide			
Trilone, *see* Triamcinolone diacetate			
Trimethobenzamide HCl, injection	up to 200 mg	IM	J3250
Trimethobenzamide HCl, oral	250 mg	ORAL	Q0173
Trimetrexate glucuronate	per 25 mg	IV	J3305
Triptorelin Pamoate	3.75 mg		J3315
Trisenox, *see* Arsenic trioxide			
Trobicin, *see* Spectinomycin HCl			
Trovan, *see* Alatrofloxacin mesylate			
U			
Ultrazine-10, *see* Prochlorperazine			
Unasyn, *see* Ampicillin sodium/sulbactam sodium			
Unclassified drugs (*see also* Not otherwise classified)			J3490
Unspecified oral antiemetic			Q0181
Urea	up to 40 gm	IV	J3350
Ureaphil, *see* Urea			
Urecholine, *see* Bethanechol chloride			
Urofollitropin	75 IU		Q2018
Urokinase	5,000 IU vial	IV	J3364
	250,000 IU vial	IV	J3365
V			
V-Gan 25, *see* Promethazine HCl			
V-Gan 50, *see* Promethazine HCl			
Valergen 10, *see* Estradiol valerate			
Valergen 20, *see* Estradiol valerate			
Valergen 40, *see* Estradiol valerate			
Valertest No. 1, *see* Testosterone enanthate and estradiol valerate			
Valertest No. 2, *see* Testosterone enanthate and estradiol valerate			
Valium, *see* Diazepam			
Valrubicin, intravesical	200 mg	OTH	J9357
Valstar, *see* Valrubicin			
Vancocin, *see* Vancomycin HCl			
Vancoled, *see* Vancomycin HCl			
Vancomycin HCl	up to 500 mg	IV, IM	J3370
Vasoxyl, *see* Methoxamine HCl			
Velban, *see* Vinblastine sulfate			
Velsar, *see* Vinblastine sulfate			
Venofer, *see* Iron sucrose			
Ventolin, *see* Albuterol sulfate			
VePesid, *see* Etoposide and Etoposide, oral			
Versed, *see* Midazolam HCl			
Verteporfin	15 mg	IV	J3395
Vesprin, *see* Triflupromazine HCl			
Viadur, *see* Leuprolide acetate implant			
Vinblastine sulfate	1 mg	IV	J9360
Vincasar PFS, *see* Vincristine sulfate			
Vincristine sulfate	1 mg	IV	J9370
	2 mg	IV	J9375
	5 mg	IV	J9380
Vinorelbine tartrate	per 10 mg	IV	J9390
Vistaject-25, *see* Hydroxyzine HCl			
Vistaril, *see* Hydroxyzine HCl			
Vistide, *see* Cidofovir			
Visudyne, *see* Verteporfin			
Vitamin K, phytonadione, menadione, menadiol sodium diphosphate	per 1 mg	IM, SC, IV	J3430
Vitamin B-12 cyanocobalamin	up to 1,000 mcg	IM, SC	J3420
Von Willebrand factor complex, human	per IU	IV	Q2022
W			
Wehamine, *see* Dimenhydrinate			

HCPCS 2003 INDEX

B

C

D

E

F

G

H

I

J

K

L

M

N

O

P

Q

R

S

T

U

APPENDIX A

MEDICARE CARRIERS MANUAL (MCM), SELECT

2005 WHEN PART B EXPENSES ARE INCURRED

2005.1 Physicians' Expense for Surgery, Childbirth, and Treatment for Infertility

A. Surgery and Childbirth.—Skilled medical management is appropriate throughout the events of pregnancy, beginning with diagnosis, continuing through delivery, and ending after the necessary postnatal care. Similarly, in the event of termination of pregnancy, regardless of whether terminated spontaneously or for therapeutic reasons (i.e., where the life of the mother would be endangered if the fetus were brought to term), the need for skilled medical management and/or medical services is equally important as in those cases carried to full term. After the infant is delivered and is a separate individual, items and services furnished to the infant are not covered on the basis of the mother's eligibility.

Most surgeons and obstetricians bill patients an all-inclusive package charge intended to cover all services associated with the surgical procedure or delivery of the child. All expenses for surgical and obstetrical care, including preoperative/prenatal examinations and tests and postoperative/postnatal services are considered incurred on the date of surgery or delivery, as appropriate. This policy applies whether the physician bills on a package charge basis, or itemizes his/her bill separately for these items.

Occasionally, a physician's bill may include charges for additional services not directly related to the surgical procedure or the delivery. Such charges are considered incurred on the date the additional services are furnished.

The above policy applies only where the charges are imposed by one physician or by a clinic on behalf of a group of physicians. Where charges are imposed by more than one physician for surgical or obstetrical services, all preoperative/prenatal and postoperative/postnatal services performed by the physician who performed the surgery or delivery are considered incurred on the date of the surgery or delivery. Expenses for services rendered by other physicians are considered incurred on the date they were performed.

B. Treatment for Infertility.—Reasonable and necessary services associated with treatment for infertility are covered under Medicare. Infertility is a condition sufficiently at variance with the usual state of health to make it appropriate for a person who normally is expected to be fertile to seek medical consultation and treatment. Coordinate with PROs to see that utilization guidelines are established for this treatment if inappropriate utilization or abuse is suspected.

2049 DRUGS AND BIOLOGICALS

Generally, drugs and biologicals are covered only if all of the following requirements are met:

- They meet the definition of drugs or biologicals (see section 2049.1);
- They are of the type that cannot be self-administered (see section 2049.2);
- They meet all the general requirements for coverage of items as incident to a physician's services (see sections 2050.1 and 2050.3);
- They are reasonable and necessary for the diagnosis or treatment of the illness or injury for which they are administered according to accepted standards of medical practice (see section 2049.4);
- They are not excluded as immunizations (see section 2049.4.B); and
- They have not been determined by the FDA to be less than effective. (See section 2049.4D.)

Drugs that can be self-administered, such as those in pill form, or that are used for self-injection are generally not covered by Part B. However, the statute provides for the coverage of some self-administered drugs. Examples of self-administered drugs that are covered include blood clotting factors, drugs used in immunosuppressive therapy, erythropoietin for dialysis patients, osteoporosis drugs for certain homebound patients, and certain oral cancer drugs. (See sections 2100.5 and 2130D for coverage of drugs that are necessary to the effective use of DME or prosthetic devices.)

2049.1 Definition of Drug or Biological.—Drugs and biologicals must be determined to meet the statutory definition. Under the statute, payment may be made for a drug or biological only where it is included, or approved for inclusion, in the latest official edition of the United States Pharmacopoeia-National Formulary (USP-NF), the United States Pharmacopoeia Drug Information (USPDI), or the American Dental Association (ADA) Guide to Dental Therapeutics, except for those drugs and biologicals unfavorably evaluated in the ADA Guide to Dental Therapeutics. Combination drugs are also included in the definition of drugs if the combination itself or all of the therapeutic ingredients of the combination are included, or approved for inclusion, in any of the above drug compendia.

Drugs and biologicals are considered approved for inclusion in a compendium if approved under the established procedure by the professional organization responsible for revision of the compendium.

2049.2 Determining Self-Administration of Drug or Biological.—Whether a drug or biological is of a type that cannot be self-administered is based on the usual method of administration of the form of that drug or biological as furnished by the physician. Thus, where a physician gives a patient pills or other oral medication, these are excluded from coverage since the form of the drug given to the patient is usually self-administered. Similarly, if a physician gives a patient an injection that is usually self-injected (e.g., insulin or calcitonin), this drug is excluded from coverage, unless administered to the patient in an emergency situation (e.g., diabetic coma). Where, however, a physician injects a drug that is not usually self-injected, this drug is not subject to the self-administrable drug exclusion (regardless of whether the drug may also be available in oral form) since it is not self-administrable in the form in which it was furnished to the patient.

Whole blood is a biological that cannot be self-administered and is covered when furnished incident to a physician's services. Payment may also be made for blood fractions if all coverage requirements are satisfied. (See section 2455 on Part B blood deductible.)

2049.3 Incident-to Requirements.—In order to meet all the general requirements for coverage under the incident-to provision, an FDA-approved drug or biological must be of a form that cannot be self-administered and must be furnished by a physician and administered by him/her or by auxiliary personnel employed by him/her under his/her personal supervision. The charge, if any, for the drug or biological must be included in the physician's bill, and the cost of the drug or biological must represent an expense to the physician. Drugs and biologicals furnished by other health professionals may also meet these requirements. (See sections 2154, 2156, 2158 and 2160 for specific instructions.)

2049.4 Reasonableness and Necessity.—Use of the drug or biological must be safe and effective and otherwise reasonable and necessary. (See section 2303.) Drugs or biologicals approved for marketing by the Food and Drug Administration (FDA) are considered safe and effective for purposes of this requirement when used for indications specified on the labeling. Therefore you may pay for the use of an FDA approved drug or biological, if:

- It was injected on or after the date of the FDA's approval;
- It is reasonable and necessary for the individual patient; and
- All other applicable coverage requirements are met.

Deny coverage for drugs and biologicals that have not received final marketing approval by the FDA unless you receive instructions from HCFA to the contrary. For specific guidelines on coverage of Group C cancer drugs, see the Coverage Issues Manual.

If there is reason to question whether the FDA has approved a drug or biological for marketing, obtain satisfactory evidence of FDA approval. Acceptable evidence includes a copy of the FDA's letter to the drug's manufacturer approving the new drug application (NDA); or listing of the drug or biological in the FDA's Approved Drug Products or FDA Drug and Device Product Approvals; or a copy of the manufacturer's package insert, approved by the FDA as part of the labeling of the drug, containing its recommended uses and dosage, as well as possible adverse reactions and recommended precautions in using it. When necessary, the RO may be able to help in obtaining information.

An unlabeled use of a drug is a use that is not included as an indication on the drug's label as approved by the FDA. FDA-approved drugs used for indications other than what is indicated on the official label may be covered under Medicare if the carrier determines the use to be medically accepted, taking into consideration the major drug compendia, authoritative medical literature, and/or accepted standards of medical practice. In the case of drugs used in an anti-cancer chemotherapeutic regimen, unlabeled uses are covered for a medically accepted indication as defined in section 2049.4.C.

Determinations as to whether medication is reasonable and necessary for an individual patient should be made on the same basis as all other such determinations (i.e., with the advice of medical consultants and with reference to accepted standards of medical practice and the medical circumstances of the individual case). The following guidelines identify three categories with specific examples of situations in which medications would not be reasonable and necessary according to accepted standards of medical practice.

1. Not for Particular Illness.—Medications given for a purpose other than the treatment of a particular condition, illness, or injury are not covered (except for certain immunizations). Exclude the charge for medications, e.g., vitamins, given simply for the general good and welfare of the patient and not as accepted therapy for a particular illness.

2. Injection Method Not Indicated.—Medication given by injection (parenterally) is not covered if standard medical practice indicates that the administration of the medication by mouth (orally) is effective and is an accepted or preferred method of administration. For example, the accepted standards of medical practice for the treatment of certain diseases is to initiate therapy with parenteral penicillin and to complete therapy with oral penicillin. Exclude the entire charge for penicillin injections given after the initiation of therapy if oral penicillin is indicated unless there are special medical circumstances that justify additional injections.

3. Excessive Medications.—Medications administered for treatment of a disease that exceed the frequency or duration of injections indicated by accepted standards of medical practice are not covered. For example, the accepted standard of medical practice in the maintenance treatment of pernicious anemia is one vitamin B-12 injection per month. Exclude the entire charge for injections given in excess of this frequency unless there are special medical circumstances that justify additional injections.

Supplement the guidelines as necessary with guidelines concerning appropriate use of specific injections in other situations. Use the guidelines to screen out questionable cases for special review, further development, or denial when the injection billed for would not be reasonable and necessary. Coordinate any type of drug treatment review with the PRO.

If a medication is determined not to be reasonable and necessary for diagnosis or treatment of an illness or injury according to these guidelines, exclude the entire charge (i.e., for both the drug and its administration). Also exclude from payment any charges for other services (such as office visits) that were primarily for the purpose of administering a noncovered injection (i.e., an injection that is not reasonable and necessary for the diagnosis or treatment of an illness or injury).

A. Antigens.—Payment may be made for a reasonable supply of antigens that have been prepared for a particular patient if: (1) the antigens are prepared by a physician who is a doctor of medicine or osteopathy, and (2) the physician who prepared the antigens has examined the patient and has determined a plan of treatment and a dosage regimen. Antigens must be administered in accordance with the plan of treatment and by a doctor of medicine or osteopathy or by a properly instructed person (who could be the patient) under the supervision of the doctor. The associations of allergists that HCFA consulted advised that a reasonable supply of antigens is considered to be not more than a 12-week supply of antigens that has been prepared for a particular patient at any one time. The purpose of the reasonable supply limitation is to assure that the antigens retain their potency and effectiveness over the period in which they are to be administered to the patient. (See sections 2005.2 and 2050.2.)

B. Immunizations.—Vaccinations or inoculations are excluded as immunizations unless they are directly related to the treatment of an injury or direct exposure to a disease or condition, such as antirabies treatment, tetanus antitoxin or booster vaccine, botulin antitoxin, antivenin sera, or immune globulin. In the absence of injury or direct exposure, preventive immunization (vaccination or inoculation) against such diseases as smallpox, polio, diphtheria, etc., is not covered. However, pneumococcal, hepatitis B, and influenza virus vaccines are exceptions to this rule. (See items 1, 2 and 3.) In cases where a vaccination or inoculation is excluded from coverage, deny the entire charge.

1. Pneumococcal Pneumonia Vaccinations.—Effective for services furnished on or after May 1, 1981, the Medicare Part B program covers pneumococcal pneumonia vaccine and its administration when furnished in compliance with any applicable State law by any provider of services or any entity or individual with a supplier number. This includes revaccination of patients at highest risk of pneumococcal infection. Typically, these vaccines are administered once in a lifetime except for persons at highest risk. Effective July 1, 2000, Medicare does not require for coverage purposes that the vaccine must be ordered by a doctor of medicine or osteopathy. Therefore, the beneficiary may receive the vaccine upon request without a physician's order and without physician supervision. An initial vaccine may be administered only to persons at high risk (see below) of pneumococcal disease. Revaccination may be administered only to persons at highest risk of serious pneumococcal infection and those likely to have a rapid decline in pneumococcal antibody levels, provided that at least 5 years have passed since receipt of a previous dose of pneumococcal vaccine.

Persons at high risk for whom an initial vaccine may be administered include all people age 65 and older; immunocompetent adults who are at increased risk of pneumococcal disease or its complications because of chronic illness (e.g., cardiovascular disease, pulmonary disease, diabetes mellitus, alcoholism, cirrhosis, or cerebrospinal fluid leaks); and individuals with compromised immune systems (e.g., splenic dysfunction or anatomic asplenia, Hodgkin's disease, lymphoma, multiple myeloma, chronic renal failure, HIV infection, nephrotic syndrome, sickle cell disease, or organ transplantation).

Persons at highest risk and those most likely to have rapid declines in antibody levels are those for whom revaccination may be appropriate. This group includes persons with functional or anatomic asplenia (e.g., sickle cell disease, splenectomy), HIV infection, leukemia, lymphoma, Hodgkin's disease, multiple myeloma, generalized malignancy, chronic renal failure, nephrotic syndrome, or other conditions associated with immunosuppression such as organ or bone marrow transplantation, and those receiving immunosuppressive chemotherapy. Routine revaccination of people age 65 or older who are not at highest risk is not appropriate.

Those administering the vaccine should not require the patient to present an immunization record prior to administering the pneumococcal vaccine, nor should they feel compelled to review the patient's complete medical record if it is not available. Instead, provided that the patient is competent, it is acceptable for them to rely on the patient's verbal history to determine prior vaccination status. If the patient is uncertain about his/her vaccination history in the past 5 years, the vaccine should be given. However, if the patient is certain he/she was vaccinated in the last 5 years, the vaccine should not be given. If the patient is certain that the vaccine was given and that more than 5 years have passed since receipt of the previous dose, revaccination is not appropriate unless the patient is at highest risk.

2. Hepatitis B Vaccine.—With the enactment of P.L. 98-369, coverage under Part B was extended to hepatitis B vaccine and its administration, furnished to a Medicare beneficiary who is at high or intermediate risk of contracting hepatitis B. This coverage is effective for services furnished on or after September 1, 1984.

High-risk groups currently identified include (see exception below):

- End stage renal disease (ESRD) patients;
- Hemophiliacs who receive Factor VIII or IX concentrates;
- Clients of institutions for the mentally retarded;
- Persons who live in the same household as a hepatitis B virus (HBV) carrier;
- Homosexual men; and
- Illicit injectable drug abusers.

Intermediate risk groups currently identified include:

- Staff in institutions for the mentally retarded; and
- Workers in health care professions who have frequent contact with blood or blood-derived body fluids during routine work.

EXCEPTION: Persons in the above-listed groups would not be considered at high or intermediate risk of contracting hepatitis B, however, if there is laboratory evidence positive for antibodies to hepatitis B. (ESRD patients are routinely tested for hepatitis B antibodies as part of their continuing monitoring and therapy.)

For Medicare program purposes, the vaccine may be administered upon the order of a doctor of medicine or osteopathy by home health agencies, skilled nursing facilities, ESRD facilities, hospital outpatient departments, persons recognized under the incident to physicians' services provision of law, and doctors of medicine and osteopathy.

A charge separate from the ESRD composite rate will be recognized and paid for administration of the vaccine to ESRD patients.

For ESRD laboratory tests, see Coverage Issues Manual, section 50-17.

3. Influenza Virus Vaccine.—Effective for services furnished on or after May 1, 1993, the Medicare Part B program covers influenza virus vaccine and its administration when furnished in compliance with any applicable State law by any provider of services or any entity or individual with a supplier number. Typically, these vaccines are administered once a year in the fall or winter. Medicare does not require for coverage purposes that the vaccine must be ordered by a doctor of medicine or osteopathy. Therefore the beneficiary may receive the vaccine upon request without a physician's order and without physician supervision.

C. Unlabeled Use For Anti-Cancer Drugs.—Effective January 1, 1994, unlabeled uses of FDA-approved drugs and biologicals used in an anti-cancer chemotherapeutic regimen for a medically accepted indication are evaluated under the conditions described in this paragraph. A regimen is a combination of anti-cancer agents that has been clinically recognized for the treatment of a specific type of cancer. An example of a drug regimen is: Cyclophosphamide + vincristine + prednisone (CVP) for non-Hodgkin's lymphoma.

In addition to listing the combination of drugs for a type of cancer, there may be a different regimen or combinations that are used at different times in the history of the cancer (induction, prophylaxis of CNS involvement, post remission, and relapsed or refractory disease). A protocol may specify the combination of drugs, doses, and schedules for administration of the drugs. For purposes of this provision, a cancer treatment regimen includes drugs used to treat toxicities or side effects of the cancer treatment regimen when the drug is administered incident to a chemotherapy treatment. Contractors must not deny coverage based solely on the absence of FDA-approved labeling for the use, if the use is supported by one of the following and the use is not listed as "not indicated" in any of the three compendia. (See note at the end of this subsection.)

1. American Hospital Formulary Service Drug Information.—Drug monographs are arranged in alphabetical order within therapeutic classifications. Within the text of the monograph, information concerning indications is provided, including both labeled and unlabeled uses. Unlabeled uses are identified with daggers. The text must be analyzed to make a determination whether a particular use is supported.

2. American Medical Association Drug Evaluations.—Drug evaluations are organized into sections and chapters that are based on therapeutic classifications. The evaluation of a drug provides information concerning indications, including both labeled and unlabeled uses. Unlabeled uses are not specifically identified as such. The text must be analyzed to make a determination whether a particular use is supported. In making these determinations, also refer to the AMA Drug Evaluations Subscription, Volume III, section 17 (Oncolytic Drugs), chapter 1 (Principles of Cancer Chemotherapy), tables 1 and 2.

Table 1, Specific Agents Used in Cancer Chemotherapy, lists the anti-neoplastic agents that are currently available for use in various cancers. The indications presented in this table for a particular anti-cancer drug include labeled and unlabeled uses (although they are not identified as such). Any indication appearing in this table is considered to be a medically accepted use.

Table 2, Clinical Responses to Chemotherapy, lists some of the currently preferred regimens for various cancers. The table headings include (1) type of cancer, (2) drugs or regimens currently preferred, (3) alternative or secondary drugs or regimens, and (4) other drugs or regimens with reported activity.

A regimen appearing under the preferred or alternative/secondary headings is considered to be a medically accepted use.

A regimen appearing under the heading "Other Drugs or Regimens with Reported Activity" is considered to be for a medically accepted use provided:

- The preferred and alternative/secondary drugs or regimens are contraindicated; or
- A preferred and/or alternative/secondary drug or regimen was used but was not tolerated or was ineffective; or
- There was tumor progression or recurrence after an initial response.

3. United States Pharmacopoeia Drug Information (USPDI).—Monographs are arranged in alphabetical order by generic or family name. Indications for use appear as accepted, unaccepted, or insufficient data. An indication is considered to be a medically accepted use only if the indication is listed as accepted. Unlabeled uses are identified with brackets. A separate indications index lists all indications included in USPDI along with the medically accepted drugs used in treatment or diagnosis.

4. A Use Supported by Clinical Research that Appears in Peer Reviewed Medical Literature.—This applies only when an unlabeled use does not appear in any of the compendia or is listed as insufficient data or investigational. If an unlabeled use of a drug meets these criteria, contact the compendia to see if a report regarding this use is forthcoming. If a report is forthcoming, use this information as a basis for your decision making. The compendium process for making decisions concerning unlabeled uses is very thorough and continuously updated. Peer-reviewed medical literature includes scientific, medical, and pharmaceutical publications in which original manuscripts are published, only after having been critically reviewed for scientific accuracy, validity, and reliability by unbiased independent experts. This does

not include in-house publications of pharmaceutical manufacturing companies or abstracts (including meeting abstracts).

In determining whether there is supportive clinical evidence for a particular use of a drug, your medical staff (in consultation with local medical specialty groups) must evaluate the quality of the evidence in published, peer-reviewed medical literature. When evaluating this literature, consider (among other things) the following:

- The prevalence and life history of the disease when evaluating the adequacy of the number of subjects and the response rate. While a 20% response rate may be adequate for highly prevalent disease states, a lower rate may be adequate for rare diseases or highly unresponsive conditions.
- The effect on the patient's well-being and other responses to therapy that indicate effectiveness, e.g., a significant increase in survival rate or life expectancy or an objective and significant decrease in the size of the tumor or a reduction in symptoms related to the tumor. Stabilization is not considered a response to therapy.
- The appropriateness of the study design. Consider:

1. Whether the experimental design in light of the drugs and conditions under investigation is appropriate to address the investigative question. (For example, in some clinical studies, it may be unnecessary or not feasible to use randomization, double blind trials, placebos, or crossover.);

2. That nonrandomized clinical trials with a significant number of subjects may be a basis for supportive clinical evidence for determining accepted uses of drugs; and

3. That case reports are generally considered uncontrolled and anecdotal information and do not provide adequate supportive clinical evidence for determining accepted uses of drugs.

Use peer reviewed medical literature appearing in the following publications:

- American Journal of Medicine;
- Annals of Internal Medicine;
- The Journal of the American Medical Association;
- Journal of Clinical Oncology;
- Blood;
- Journal of the National Cancer Institute;
- The New England Journal of Medicine;
- British Journal of Cancer;
- British Journal of Hematology;
- British Medical Journal;
- Cancer;
- Drugs;
- European Journal of Cancer (formerly the European Journal of Cancer and Clinical Oncology);
- Lancet; or
- Leukemia.

You are not required to maintain copies of these publications. If a claim raises a question about the use of a drug for a purpose not included in the FDA-approved labeling or the compendia, ask the physician to submit copies of relevant supporting literature.

4. Unlabeled uses may also be considered medically accepted if determined by you to be medically accepted generally as safe and effective for the particular use.

NOTE: If a use is identified as not indicated by HCFA or the FDA, or if a use is specifically identified as not indicated in one or more of the three compendia mentioned, or if you determine based on peer-reviewed medical literature that a particular use of a drug is not safe and effective, the off-label usage is not supported and therefore the drug is not covered.

5. Less Than Effective Drug.—This is a drug that has been determined by the Food and Drug Administration (FDA) to lack substantial evidence of effectiveness for all labeled indications. Also, a drug that has been the subject of a Notice of an Opportunity for a Hearing (NOOH) published in the Federal Register before being withdrawn from the market, and for which the Secretary has not determined there is a compelling justification for its medical need, is considered less than effective. This includes any other drug product that is identical, similar, or related. Payment may not be made for a less than effective drug.

Because the FDA has not yet completed its identification of drug products that are still on the market, existing FDA efficacy decisions must be applied to all similar products once they are identified.

6. Denial of Medicare Payment for Compounded Drugs Produced in Violation of Federal Food, Drug, and Cosmetic Act.—The Food and Drug Administration (FDA) has found that, from time to time, firms established as retail pharmacies engage in mass production of compounded drugs, beyond the normal scope of pharmaceutical practice, in violation of the Federal Food, Drug, and Cosmetic Act (FFDCA). By compounding drugs on a large scale, a company may be operating as a drug manufacturer within the meaning of the FFDCA, without complying with requirements of that law. Such companies may be manufacturing drugs that are subject to the new drug application (NDA) requirements of the FFDCA, but for which FDA has not approved an NDA or which are misbranded or adulterated. If the manufacturing and processing procedures used by these facilities have not been approved by the FDA, the FDA has no assurance that the drugs these companies are producing are safe and effective. The safety and effectiveness issues pertain to such factors as chemical stability, purity, strength, bioequivalency, and biovailability.

Section 1862(a)(1)(A) of the Act requires that drugs must be reasonable and necessary in order to be covered under Medicare. This means, in the case of drugs, they must have been approved for marketing by the FDA. Section 2049.4 instructs carriers to deny coverage for drugs that have not received final marketing approval by the FDA, unless instructed otherwise by HCFA. Section 2300.1 instructs carriers to deny coverage of services related to the use of noncovered drugs as well. Hence, if DME or a prosthetic device is used to administer a noncovered drug, coverage is denied for both the nonapproved drug and the DME or prosthetic device.

In those cases in which the FDA has determined that a company is producing compounded drugs in violation of the FFDCA, Medicare does not pay for the drugs because they do not meet the FDA approval requirements of the Medicare program. In addition, Medicare does not pay for the DME or prosthetic device used to administer such a drug if the FDA determines that a required NDA has not been approved or that the drug is misbranded or adulterated.

HCFA will notify you when the FDA has determined that compounded drugs are being produced in violation of the FFDCA. Do not stop Medicare payment for such a drug unless you are notified that it is appropriate to do so through a subsequent instruction. In addition, if you or ROs become aware that other companies are possibly operating in violation of the FFDCA, notify:

Health Care Financing Administration
Bureau of Policy Development
Office of Physician and Ambulatory Care Policy
7500 Security Blvd.
Baltimore, MD 21244-1850

2049.5 Self-Administered Drugs and Biologicals.—Drugs that are self-administered are not covered by Medicare Part B unless the statute provides for such coverage. This includes blood clotting factors, drugs used in immunosuppressive therapy, erythropoietin for dialysis patients, certain oral anti-cancer drugs, and oral anti-nausea drugs when used in certain situations.

A. Immunosuppressive Drugs.—Until January 1, 1995, immunosuppressive drugs are covered under Part B for a period of 1 year following discharge from a hospital for a Medicare-covered organ transplant. HCFA interprets the 1-year period after the date of the transplant procedure to mean 365 days from the day on which an inpatient is discharged from the hospital. Beneficiaries are eligible to receive additional Part B coverage within 18 months after the discharge date for drugs furnished in 1995; within 24 months for drugs furnished in 1996; within 30 months for drugs furnished in 1997; and within 36 months for drugs furnished after 1997.

Covered drugs include those immunosuppressive drugs that have been specifically labeled as such and approved for marketing by the FDA, as well as those prescription drugs, such as prednisone, that are used in conjunction with immunosuppressive drugs as part of a therapeutic regimen reflected in FDA-approved labeling for immunosuppressive drugs. Therefore, antibiotics, hypertensives, and other drugs that are not directly related to rejection are not covered. The FDA has identified and approved for marketing five specifically labeled immunosuppressive drugs. They are Sandimmune (cyclosporine), Sandoz Pharmaceutical; Imuran (azathioprine), Burroughs Wellcome; Atgam (antithymocyte globulin), Upjohn; and Orthoclone OKT3 (Muromonab-CD3), Ortho Pharmaceutical, and Prograf (tacrolimus), Fujisawa USA, Inc. You are expected to keep informed of FDA additions to the list of the immunosuppressive drugs.

B. Erythropoietin (EPO).—The statute provides that EPO is covered for the treatment of anemia for patients with chronic renal failure who are on dialysis. Coverage is available regardless of whether the drug is administered by the patient or the patient's caregiver. EPO is a biologically engineered protein that stimulates the bone marrow to make new red blood cells.

NOTE: Non-ESRD patients who are receiving EPO to treat anemia induced by other conditions such as chemotherapy or the drug zidovudine (commonly called AZT) must meet the coverage requirements in section 2049.

EPO is covered for the treatment of anemia for patients with chronic renal failure who are on dialysis when:

- It is administered in the renal dialysis facility; or
- It is self-administered in the home by any dialysis patient (or patient caregiver) who is determined competent to use the drug and meets the other conditions detailed below.

NOTE: Payment may not be made for EPO under the incident to provision when EPO is administered in the renal dialysis facility. (See section 5202.4.)

Medicare covers EPO and items related to its administration for dialysis patients who use EPO in the home when the following conditions are met.

1. Patient Care Plan.—A dialysis patient who uses EPO in the home must have a current care plan (a copy of which must be maintained by the designated back-up facility for Method II patients) for monitoring home use of EPO that includes the following:

a. Review of diet and fluid intake for aberrations as indicated by hyperkalemia and elevated blood pressure secondary to volume overload;

b. Review of medications to ensure adequate provision of supplemental iron;

c. Ongoing evaluations of hematocrit and iron stores;

d. Reevaluation of the dialysis prescription taking into account the patient's increased appetite and red blood cell volume;

e. Method for physician and facility (including back-up facility for Method II patients) follow-up on blood tests and a mechanism (such as a patient log) for keeping the physician informed of the results;

f. Training of the patient to identify the signs and symptoms of hypotension and hypertension; and

g. The decrease or discontinuance of EPO if hypertension is uncontrollable.

2. Patient Selection.—The dialysis facility, or the physician responsible for all dialysis-related services furnished to the patient, must make a comprehensive assessment that includes the following:

a. Pre-selection monitoring. The patient's hematocrit (or hemoglobin), serum iron, transferrin saturation, serum ferritin, and blood pressure must be measured.

b. Conditions the patient must meet. The assessment must find that the patient meets the following conditions:

(1) Is a dialysis patient;

(2) Has a hematocrit (or comparable hemoglobin level) that is as follows:

(a) For a patient who is initiating EPO treatment, no higher than 30 percent unless there is medical documentation showing the need for EPO despite a hematocrit (or comparable hemoglobin level) higher than 30 percent. Patients with severe angina, severe pulmonary distress, or severe hypotension may require EPO to prevent adverse symptoms even if they have higher hematocrit or hemoglobin levels.

(b) For a patient who has been receiving EPO from the facility or the physician, between 30 and 36 percent; and

(3) Is under the care of:

(a) A physician who is responsible for all dialysis-related services and who prescribes the EPO and follows the drug labeling instructions when monitoring the EPO home therapy; and

(b) A renal dialysis facility that establishes the plan of care and monitors the progress of the home EPO therapy.

c. The assessment must find that the patient or a caregiver meets the following conditions:

(1) Is trained by the facility to inject EPO and is capable of carrying out the procedure;

(2) Is capable of reading and understanding the drug labeling; and

(3) Is trained in, and capable of observing, aseptic techniques.

d. Care and storage of drug. The assessment must find that EPO can be stored in the patient's residence under refrigeration and that the patient is aware of the potential hazard of a child's having access to the drug and syringes.

3. Responsibilities of Physician or Dialysis Facility.—The patient's physician or dialysis facility must:

a. Develop a protocol that follows the drug label instructions;

b. Make the protocol available to the patient to ensure safe and effective home use of EPO;

c. Through the amounts prescribed, ensure that the drug on hand at any time does not exceed a 2-month supply; and

d. Maintain adequate records to allow quality assurance for review by the network and State survey agencies. For Method II patients, current records must be provided to and maintained by the designated back-up facility.

See section 5202.4 for information on EPO payment.

Submit claims for EPO in accordance with section 4273.1 and 4273.2.

C. Oral Anti-Cancer Drugs.—Effective January 1, 1994, Medicare Part B coverage is extended to include oral anti-cancer drugs that are prescribed as anti-cancer chemotherapeutic agents providing they have the same active ingredients and are used for the same indications as anti-cancer chemotherapeutic agents that would be covered if they were not self-administered and they were furnished incident to a physician's service as drugs and biologicals.

This provision applies only to the coverage of anti-neoplastic chemotherapeutic agents. It does not apply to oral drugs and/or biologicals used to treat toxicity or side effects such as nausea or bone marrow depression. Medicare will cover anti-neoplastic chemotherapeutic agents, the primary drugs that directly fight the cancer, and self-administered antiemetics that are necessary for the administration and absorption of the anti-neoplastic chemotherapeutic agents when a high likelihood of vomiting exists. The substitution of an oral form of an anti-neoplastic drug requires that the drug be retained for absorption. The antiemetic drug is covered as a necessary means for administration of the oral drug (similar to a syringe and needle necessary for injectable administration). Oral drugs prescribed for use with the primary drug that enhance the anti-neoplastic effect of the primary drug or permit the patient to tolerate the primary anti-neoplastic drug in higher doses for longer periods are not covered. Self-administered antiemetics to reduce the side effects of nausea and vomiting brought on by the primary drug are not included beyond the administration necessary to achieve drug absorption.

In order to assure uniform coverage policy, regional carriers and FIs must be apprised of local carriers' anti-cancer drug medical review policies that may impact on future medical review policy development. Local carriers' current and proposed anti-cancer drug medical review polices should be provided by local carrier medical directors to regional carrier or FI medical directors, upon request.

For an oral anti-cancer drug to be covered under Part B, it must:

- Be prescribed by a physician or other practitioner licensed under State law to prescribe such drugs as anti-cancer chemotherapeutic agents;
- Be a drug or biological that has been approved by the Food and Drug Administration (FDA);
- Have the same active ingredients as a non-self-administrable anti-cancer chemotherapeutic drug or biological that is covered when furnished incident to a physician's service. The oral anti-cancer drug and the non-self-administrable drug must have the same chemical/generic name as indicated by the FDA's Approved Drug Products (Orange Book), Physician's Desk Reference (PDR), or an authoritative drug compendium; or, effective January 1, 1999, be a prodrug—an oral drug ingested into the body that metabolizes into the same active ingredient that is found in the non-self-administrable form of the drug;
- Be used for the same indications, including unlabeled uses, as the non-self-administrable version of the drug; and
- Be reasonable and necessary for the individual patient.

D. *Oral Anti-Nausea Drugs*.—Section 4557 of the Balanced Budget Act of 1997 amends section 1861(s)(2) by extending the coverage of oral anti-emetic drugs under the following conditions:

- Coverage is provided only for oral drugs approved by the Food and Drug Administration (FDA) for use as anti-emetics;
- The oral anti-emetics must either be administered by the treating physician or in accordance with a written order from the physician as part of a cancer chemotherapy regimen;
- Oral anti-emetics drugs administered with a particular chemotherapy treatment must be initiated within 2 hours of the administration of the chemotherapeutic agent and may be continued for a period not to exceed 48 hours from that time; and
- The oral anti-emetic drugs provided must be used as a full therapeutic replacement for the intravenous anti-emetic drugs that would have otherwise been administered at the time of the chemotherapy treatment.

Only drugs pursuant to a physician's order at the time of the chemotherapy treatment qualify for this benefit. The dispensed number of dosage units may not exceed a loading dose administered within 2 hours of that treatment, plus a supply of additional dosage units not to exceed 48 hours of therapy. However, more than one oral anti-emetic drug may be prescribed and will be covered for concurrent usage within these parameters if more than one oral drug is needed to fully replace the intravenous drugs that would otherwise have been given.

Oral drugs that are not approved by the FDA for use as anti-emetics and that are used by treating physicians adjunctively in a manner incidental to cancer chemotherapy are not covered by this benefit and are not reimbursable within the scope of this benefit.

It is recognized that a limited number of patients will fail on oral anti-emetic drugs. Intravenous anti-emetics may be covered (subject to the rules of medical necessity) when furnished to patients who fail on oral anti-emetic therapy.

This coverage, effective for services on or after January 1, 1998, is subject to regular Medicare Part B coinsurance and deductible provisions.

NOTE: Existing coverage policies authorizing the administration of suppositories to prevent vomiting when oral cancer drugs are used are unchanged by this new coverage.

E. Hemophilia Clotting Factors.—Section 1861(s)(2)(I) of the Act provides Medicare coverage of blood clotting factors for hemophilia patients competent to use such factors to control bleeding without medical supervision, and items related to the administration of such factors. Hemophilia, a blood disorder characterized by prolonged coagulation time, is caused by deficiency of a factor in plasma necessary for blood to clot. (The discovery in 1964 of a cryoprecipitate rich in antihemophilic factor activity facilitated management of acute bleeding episodes.) For purposes of Medicare Part B coverage, hemophilia encompasses the following conditions:

- Factor VIII deficiency (classic hemophilia);
- Factor IX deficiency (also termed plasma thromboplastin component (PTC) or Christmas factor deficiency); and
- Von Willebrand's disease.

Claims for blood clotting factors for hemophilia patients with these diagnoses may be covered if the patient is competent to use such factors without medical supervision.

The amount of clotting factors determined to be necessary to have on hand and thus covered under this provision is based on the historical utilization pattern or profile developed by the carrier for each patient. It is expected that the treating source (e.g., a family physician or comprehensive hemophilia diagnostic and treatment center) has such information. From this data, the contractor is able to make reasonable projections concerning the quantity of clotting factors anticipated to be needed by the patient over a specific period of time. Unanticipated occurrences involving extraordinary events, such as automobile accidents of inpatient hospital stays, will change this base line data and should be appropriately considered. In addition, changes in a patient's medical needs over a period of time require adjustments in the profile. (See section 5245 for payment policies.)

2070 DIAGNOSTIC X-RAY, DIAGNOSTIC LABORATORY, AND OTHER DIAGNOSTIC TESTS

2070.1 Independent Laboratories.—Diagnostic laboratory services furnished by an independent laboratory are covered under medical insurance if the laboratory is an approved Independent Clinical Laboratory. (However, as is the case of all diagnostic services, in order to be covered these services must be related to a patient's illness or injury (or symptom or complaint) and ordered by a physician. See section 2020.1 for the definition of a "physician".)

A. Definition of Independent.—An independent laboratory is one that is independent both of an attending or consulting physician's office and of a hospital that meets at least the requirements to qualify as an emergency hospital as defined in section 1861(e) of the Act. (A consulting physician is one whose services include history taking, examination of the patient, and, in each case, furnishing to the attending physician an opinion regarding diagnosis or treatment. A physician providing clinical laboratory services for patients of other physicians is not considered to be a consulting physician.)

A laboratory that is operated by or under the supervision of a hospital (or the organized medical staff of the hospital) which does not meet at least the definition of an emergency hospital is considered to be an independent laboratory. However, a laboratory serving hospital patients and operated on the premises of a hospital that meets the definition of an emergency hospital is presumed to be subject to the supervision of the hospital or its organized medical staff and is not an independent laboratory. A laboratory that a physician or group of physicians maintains for performing diagnostic tests in connection with his own or the group practice is also not considered to be an independent laboratory.

An out-of-hospital laboratory is ordinarily presumed to be independent unless there is written evidence establishing that it is operated by or under the supervision of a hospital that meets at least the definition of an emergency hospital or of the organized medical staff of such a hospital.

Where a laboratory operated on hospital premises is claimed to be independent or where an out-of-hospital facility is designated as a hospital laboratory, the RO makes the determination concerning the laboratory's status.

B. Clinical Defined.—A clinical laboratory is a laboratory where microbiological, serological, chemical, hematological, radiobioassay, cytological, immunohematological, or pathological examinations are performed on materials derived from the human body, to provide information for the diagnosis, prevention, or treatment of a disease or assessment of a medical condition.

C. Approval of Laboratories.—An approved independent clinical laboratory is one that is approved by the Secretary of Health, Education, and Welfare as meeting the specific conditions for coverage under the program. These require that: (l) where State or applicable local law provides for licensing of independent clinical laboratories, the laboratory is either licensed under such law or it is approved as meeting the requirements for licensing laboratories; and (2) such laboratories also meet the health and safety requirements prescribed by the Secretary of Health, Education, and Welfare. See "Conditions for Coverage of Services of Independent Laboratories" (HIRM l Subpart M).

Diagnostic laboratory tests performed by a laboratory of a nonparticipating hospital that meet the statutory definition of an emergency hospital are covered only if the laboratory meets the requirements set forth in the regulations for hospital laboratories.

Services rendered by an independent clinical laboratory are covered under medical insurance only if the laboratory has been approved under the program. Carriers are furnished lists of approved laboratories and their approved specialties by HCFA. If you have any reason to question the lists concerning additions or deletions of particular laboratories or specialties, clarifying information should be requested from the RO.

Laboratory Certification and Decertification

You must notify your physicians of the initial certification of the laboratories in your service areas and also furnished certification information about laboratories outside your service area upon request from individual physicians or clinics. This information is available from the RO (see section 2070.1D below). Where there are any changes in the certification of a laboratory, i.e., addition or deletion of tests for which the laboratory is certified, notify the physicians in your service areas of these changes.

When some or all of the services of an independent laboratory no longer meet the conditions for coverage, inform all physicians having an interest in the laboratory's certification status of the effective date of decertification, reasons for the decertification, and the applicability of the determination to the various categories of diagnostic tests performed by the independent laboratory. Notification to the physicians must be made prior to the termination date since you cannot honor any bill for services performed after the termination date.

If you issue a monthly bulletin or newsletter to physicians in your service area, you may wish to use this vehicle to inform the physicians involved. If, in a particular instance, timely notification cannot be made by use of the regular monthly bulletin or newsletter, a special bulletin will be necessary. In cases where there are a limited number of physicians in a remote area, a notification to all physicians in your service area may not be necessary. In these situations, you may wish to limit the scope of the notification and use means other than the monthly newsletter. You must secure the prior approval of the regional office for limited notification.

For notices of decertification, you will receive a copy of the decertification letter to the laboratory from the RO. Language suitable for use in the carrier notices to physicians concerning the reasons for the decertification will also be supplied. The following information will be included in the notification:

1. Name and address of laboratory;
2. Effective date of decertification;
3. Which services are not covered (all or particular specialty(ies); and
4. Reason for decertification.

Your notification to the physicians should contain a statement that no payment can be made under title XVIII on behalf of Medicare patients receiving these services from the laboratory on or after the effective decertification dates.

A copy of all notifications to physicians concerning laboratory decertifications, whether by regular monthly newsletter or by a special bulletin, should be sent to the RO Contractor Operations Staff on the date of issuance.

NOTE: The notification to physicians also applies to services performed by suppliers of portable x-ray services (see section 2070.4B).

D. The Specialty Provision.—One of the conditions for coverage of services of independent laboratories is that the laboratory agrees to perform tests for Medicare beneficiaries only in the specialties for which it is certified. Clinical laboratory services rendered in a specialty for which an independent laboratory is not certified are not covered and claims for payment of benefits for these services must be denied.

HCFA furnishes lists to the carriers showing specialties and subspecialties in which each laboratory has been certified. The lists are updated quarterly. Each carrier receives two lists showing the independent laboratories located in its service area: one list by provider number and the other list alphabetical. For information on laboratories not located within a carrier's service area, the RO maintains national lists showing all approved laboratories. A key is furnished for interpreting the codes on the lists. See section 4110ff. for additional information.

2130 PROSTHETIC DEVICES

A. General.—Prosthetic devices (other than dental) that replace all or part of an internal body organ (including contiguous tissue), or replace all or part of the function of a permanently inoperative or malfunctioning internal body organ are covered when furnished on a physician's order. This does not require a determination that there is no possibility that the patient's condition may improve sometime in the future. If the medical record, including the judgment of the attending physician, indicates the condition is of long and indefinite duration, the test of permanence is considered met. (Such a device may also be covered under section 2050.1 as a supply when furnished incident to a physician's service.)

Examples of prosthetic devices include cardiac pacemakers, prosthetic lenses (see subsection B), breast prostheses (including a surgical brassiere) for postmastectomy patients, maxillofacial devices, and devices that replace all or part of the ear or nose. A urinary collection and retention system with or without a tube is a prosthetic device replacing bladder function in case of permanent urinary incontinence. The Foley catheter is also considered a prosthetic device when ordered for a patient with permanent urinary incontinence. However, Chux, diapers, rubber sheets, etc., are supplies that are not covered under this provision. (Although hemodialysis equipment is a prosthetic device, payment for the rental or purchase of such equipment for use in the home is made only under the provisions for payment applicable to durable medical equipment [see section 4105ff] or the special rules that apply to the ESRD program.)

NOTE: Medicare does not cover a prosthetic device dispensed to a patient prior to the time at which the patient undergoes the procedure that makes necessary the use of the device. For example, do not make a separate Part B payment for an intraocular lens (IOL) or pacemaker that a physician, during an office visit prior to the actual surgery, dispenses to the patient for his/her use. Dispensing a prosthetic device in this manner raises health and safety issues. Moreover, the need for the device cannot be clearly established until the procedure that makes its use possible is successfully performed. Therefore, dispensing a prosthetic device in this manner is not considered reasonable and necessary for the treatment of the patient's condition.

Colostomy (and other ostomy) bags and necessary accouterments required for attachment are covered as prosthetic devices. This coverage also includes irrigation and flushing equipment and other items and supplies directly related to ostomy care, whether the attachment of a bag is required.

Accessories and/or supplies that are used directly with an enteral or parenteral device to achieve the therapeutic benefit of the prosthesis or to assure the proper functioning of the device are covered under the prosthetic device benefit subject to the additional guidelines in the Coverage Issues Manual section 65-10 to 65-10.3.

Covered items include catheters, filters, extension tubing, infusion bottles, pumps (either food or infusion), intravenous (IV) pole, needles, syringes, dressings, tape, heparin sodium (parenteral only), volumetric monitors (parenteral only), and parenteral and enteral nutrient solutions. Baby food and other regular grocery products that can be blenderized and used with the enteral system are not covered. Note that some of these items, e.g., a food pump and an IV pole, qualify as DME. Although coverage of the enteral and parenteral nutritional therapy systems is provided on the basis of the prosthetic device benefit, the payment rules relating to rental or purchase of DME apply to such items. (See section 4105.3.) Code claims in accordance with the Healthcare Common Procedure Coding System (HCPCS).

The coverage of prosthetic devices includes replacement of and repairs to such devices as explained in subsection D.

B. Prosthetic Lenses.—The term "internal body organ" includes the lens of an eye. Prostheses replacing the lens of an eye include postsurgical lenses customarily used during convalescence from eye surgery in which the lens of the eye was removed. In addition, permanent lenses are also covered when required by an individual lacking the organic lens of the eye because of surgical removal or congenital absence. Prosthetic lenses obtained on or after the beneficiary's date of entitlement to supplementary medical insurance benefits may be covered even though the surgical removal of the crystalline lens occurred before entitlement.

1. Prosthetic Cataract Lenses.—Make payment for one of the following prosthetic lenses or combinations of prosthetic lenses when determined to be medically necessary by a physician (see section 2020.25 for coverage of prosthetic lenses prescribed by a doctor of optometry) to restore essentially the vision provided by the crystalline lens of the eye:

- Prosthetic bifocal lenses in frames;
- Prosthetic lenses in frames for far vision, and prosthetic lenses in frames for near vision; or
- When a prosthetic contact lens(es) for far vision is prescribed (including cases of binocular and monocular aphakia), make payment for the contact lens(es) and prosthetic lenses in frames for near vision to be worn at the same time as the contact lens(es), and prosthetic lenses in frames to be worn when the contacts have been removed.

Make payment for lenses that have ultraviolet absorbing or reflecting properties, in lieu of payment for regular (untinted) lenses, if it has been determined that such lenses are medically reasonable and necessary for the individual patient.

Do not make payment for cataract sunglasses obtained in addition to the regular (untinted) prosthetic lenses since the sunglasses duplicate the restoration of vision function performed by the regular prosthetic lenses.

2. Payment for IOLs Furnished in Ambulatory Surgical Centers (ASCs). Effective for services furnished on or after March 12, 1990, payment for IOLs inserted during or subsequent to cataract surgery in a Medicare certified ASC is included with the payment for facility services that are furnished in connection with the covered surgery. Section 5243.3 explains payment procedures for ASC facility services and the IOL allowance.

3. Limitation on Coverage of Conventional Lenses.—Make payment for no more than one pair of conventional eyeglasses or conventional contact lenses furnished after each cataract surgery with insertion of an IOL.

C. Dentures.—Dentures are excluded from coverage. However, when a denture or a portion thereof is an integral part (built-in) of a covered prosthesis (e.g., an obturator to fill an opening in the palate), it is covered as part of that prosthesis.

D. Supplies, Repairs, Adjustments, and Replacement.—Make payment for supplies that are necessary for the effective use of a prosthetic device (e.g., the batteries needed to operate an artificial larynx). Adjustment of prosthetic devices required by wear or by a change in the patient's condition is covered when ordered by a physician. To the extent applicable, follow the provisions relating to the repair and replacement of durable medical equipment in section 2100.4 for the repair and replacement of prosthetic devices. (See section 2306.D in regard to payment for devices replaced under a warranty.) Regardless of the date that the original eyewear was furnished (i.e., whether before, on, or after January 1, 1991), do not pay for replacement of conventional eyeglasses or contact lenses covered under subsection B.3.

Necessary supplies, adjustments, repairs, and replacements are covered even when the device had been in use before the user enrolled in Part B of the program, so long as the device continues to be medically required.

2133 LEG, ARM, BACK, AND NECK BRACES, TRUSSES, AND ARTIFICIAL LEGS, ARMS, AND EYES

These appliances are covered when furnished incident to physicians' services or on a physician's order. A brace includes rigid and semi-rigid devices that are used for the purpose of supporting a weak or deformed body member or restricting or eliminating motion in a diseased or injured part of the body. Elastic stockings, garter belts, and similar devices do not come within the scope of the definition of a brace. Back braces include, but are not limited to, special corsets, e.g., sacroiliac, sacrolumbar, dorsolumbar corsets and belts. A terminal device (e.g., hand or hook) is covered under this provision whether an artificial limb is required by the patient. (See section 2323.) Stump stockings and harnesses (including replacements) are also covered when these appliances are essential to the effective use of the artificial limb.

Adjustments to an artificial limb or other appliance required by wear or by a change in the patient's condition are covered when ordered by a physician. To the extent applicable, follow the provisions in section 2100.4 relating to the repair and replacement of durable medical equipment for the repair and replacement of artificial limbs, braces, etc. Adjustments, repairs and replacements are covered even when the item had been in use before the user enrolled in Part B of the program so long as the device continues to be medically required.

2150. CLINICAL PSYCHOLOGIST SERVICES

Section 6113(a) of OBRA 1989 (P. L. 101-239) eliminates the restriction on clinical psychologist (CP) services imposed by prior law, which required that, to be paid for directly, the services be furnished at community mental health centers (CMHCs) or offsite at a CMHC for those who are institutionalized or are physically or mentally impaired.

A CMHC is an institution that provides the mental health services required by §1916(c)(4) of the PHS Act and is certified by the appropriate State authorities as meeting such requirements.

Services furnished by a CP and services furnished incident to the services of a CP to hospital patients during the period July 1, 1990, through December 31, 1990, were bundled. Therefore, Medicare made payment to the hospital for these services. However, as a result of the enactment of §4157 of OBRA 1990, effective January 1, 1991, professional CP services furnished to hospital patients are no longer bundled under 42 CFR 411.15(m). Section 4157 amended §1862(a)(14) of the Act to permit direct payment to CPs under Medicare Part B for such services. However, services furnished incident to the professional services of CPs to hospital patients remain bundled. Therefore, payment must continue to be made to the hospital for such "incident to" services.

The diagnostic services of psychologists who are not clinical psychologists, and who are practicing independently, are discussed in §2070.2.

A. Clinical Psychologist Defined.—To qualify as a CP, a practitioner must meet the following requirements:

- Hold a doctoral degree in psychology;
- Be licensed or certified, on the basis of the doctoral degree in psychology, by the State in which he or she practices, at the independent practice level of psychology to furnish diagnostic, assessment, preventive, and therapeutic services directly to individuals.

B. Qualified Clinical Psychologist Services Defined.—Effective July 1, 1990, the diagnostic and therapeutic services of CPs and services and supplies furnished incident to such services are covered as the services furnished by a physician or as incident to physician's services are covered. However, the CP must be legally authorized to perform the services under applicable licensure laws of the State in which they are furnished.

C. Types of Clinical Psychologist Services That May Be Covered.—CPs may provide the following services:

- Diagnostic and therapeutic services that the CP is legally authorized to perform in accordance with State law and/or regulation. Pay all qualified CPs based on the fee schedule for their diagnostic and therapeutic services. Also, pay those practitioners who do not meet the requirements for a CP on the basis of the physician fee schedule for the provision of diagnostic services under §2070.2.
- Services and supplies furnished incident to a CP's services are covered if the requirements that apply to services incident to a physician's services, as described in §2050.1 are met. These services must be:

1. Mental health services that are commonly furnished in CPs' offices;

2. An integral, although incidental, part of professional services performed by the CP;

3. Performed under the direct personal supervision of the CP, i.e., the CP must be physically present and immediately available; and

4. Furnished without charge or included in the CP's bill.

Any person involved in performing the service must be an employee of the CP (or an employee of the legal entity that employs the supervising CP) under the common law control test of the Act, as set forth in 20 CFR 404.1007 and §RS 2101.020 of the Retirement and Survivors Insurance part of the Social Security Program Operations Manual System.

Be familiar with appropriate State laws and/or regulations governing a CP's scope of practice. The development of lists of appropriate services may prove useful.

D. Noncovered Services.—The services of CPs are not covered if they are otherwise excluded from Medicare coverage even though a clinical psychologist is authorized by State law to perform them. For example, §1862(a)(1)(A) of the Act excludes from coverage services that are not "reasonable and necessary for the diagnosis or treatment of an illness or injury or to improve the functioning of a malformed body member." Therefore, even though the services are authorized by State law, the services of a CP that are determined to be not reasonable and necessary are not covered. Additionally, any therapeutic services that are billed by CPs under CPT psychotherapy codes that include medical evaluation and management services are not covered.

E. Requirement for Consultation.—When applying for a Medicare provider number, a CP must submit to the carrier a signed Medicare provider/supplier enrollment form that indicates an agreement to the effect that, contingent upon the patient's consent, he or she will attempt to consult with the patient's attending or primary care physician in accordance with accepted professional ethical norms, taking into consideration patient confidentiality.

If the patient assents to the consultation, the CP must attempt to consult with the patient's physician within a reasonable time after receiving the consent. If the CP's attempts to consult directly with the physician are not successful, the CP must notify the physician within a reasonable time that he or she is furnishing services to the patient. Additionally, the CP must document, in the patient's medical record, the date the patient consented or declined consent to consultations, the date of consultation, or, if attempts to consult did not succeed, that date and manner of notification to the physician.

The only exception to the consultation requirement for CPs is in cases where the patient's primary care or attending physician refers the patient to the CP. Also, neither a CP nor a primary care or attending physician may bill Medicare or the patient for this required consultation.

See H.R. Conf. Rep. No. 386, 101st Cong., 1st Sess. 789 (1989).

F. Payment Methodology Limitation.—Payment for the services of CPs is made on the basis of a fee schedule or the actual charge, whichever is less, and only on the basis of assignment.

G. Outpatient Mental Health Services Limitation.—All covered therapeutic services furnished by qualified CPs are subject to the outpatient mental health services limitation in §2470ff (i.e., only 62.5 percent of expenses for these services are considered incurred expenses for Medicare purposes). The limitation does not apply to diagnostic services. (See §2472.4.C.)

H. Assignment Requirement.—Make all claims for covered services rendered by CPs on an assignment basis.

2152 CLINICAL SOCIAL WORKER SERVICES

Medical and other health services include the services provided by a clinical social worker (CSW). Payment is made only under assignment. The amount payable cannot exceed 80 percent of the lesser of the actual charge for the services or 75 percent of the amount paid to a psychologist for the same service. See section 5112 for the payment guidelines and subsection F for application of the mental health payment limitation.

A. Clinical Social Worker Defined.—Section 1861(hh) of the Act defines a "clinical social worker" as an individual who:

- Possesses a master's or doctor's degree in social work;
- Has performed at least 2 years of supervised clinical social work; and either:
- Is licensed or certified as a clinical social worker by the State in which the services are performed; or
- In the case of an individual in a State that does not provide for licensure or certification, has completed at least 2 years or 3,000 hours of post master's degree supervised clinical social work practice under the supervision of a master's level social worker in an appropriate setting such as a hospital, SNF, or clinic.

B. Clinical Social Worker Services Defined.—Section 1861(hh)(2) of the Act defines "clinical social worker services" as those services that the CSW is legally authorized to perform under State law (or the State regulatory mechanism provided by State law) of the State in which such services are performed for the diagnosis and treatment of mental illnesses. Services furnished to an inpatient of a hospital or an inpatient of an SNF that the SNF is required to provide as a requirement for participation are not included. The services that are covered are those that are otherwise covered if furnished by a physician or as incident to a physician's professional service.

C. Covered Services.—Coverage is limited to the services a CSW is legally authorized to perform in accordance with State law (or State regulatory mechanism established by State law). The services of a CSW may be covered under Part B if they are:

- The type of services that are otherwise covered if furnished by a physician, or as incident to a physician's service. (See section 2020 for a description of physicians' services and section 2020.2 for the definition of a physician.);
- Performed by a person who meets the definition of a CSW (see subsection A.); and
- Not otherwise excluded from coverage.

Become familiar with the State law or regulatory mechanism governing a CSW's scope of practice in your service area. The development of a list of services within the scope of practice may prove useful.

D. Noncovered Services.—Services of a CSW are not covered when furnished to inpatients of a hospital or to inpatients of a SNF if the services furnished in the SNF are those that the SNF is required to furnish as a condition of participation in Medicare. In addition, CSW services are not covered if they are otherwise excluded from Medicare coverage even though a CSW is authorized by State law to perform them. For example, the Medicare law excludes from coverage services that are not "reasonable and necessary for the diagnosis or treatment of an illness or injury or to improve the functioning of a malformed body member."

E. Outpatient Mental Health Services Limitation.—All covered therapeutic services furnished by qualified CSWs are subject to the outpatient psychiatric services limitation in section 2470ff. (i.e., only 62.5 percent of expenses for these services are considered incurred expenses for Medicare purposes). The limitation does not apply to diagnostic services. (See section 2476.5.)

2210 PAYABLE PHYSICAL THERAPY (PT)

A. General.—To be covered PT services, the services must relate directly and specifically to an active written treatment regimen established by the physician after any needed consultation with the qualified physical therapist and must be reasonable and necessary to the treatment of the individual's illness or injury. Effective July 18, 1984, a plan of treatment for OPT services may be established by either the physician or the qualified physical therapist providing such services. Services related to activities for the general good and welfare of patients, e.g., general exercises to promote overall fitness and flexibility and activities to provide diversion or general motivation, do not constitute PT services for Medicare purposes.

Services furnished beneficiaries must constitute PT where entitlement to benefits is at issue. Since the OPT benefit under Part B provides coverage only of PT services, payment can be made only for those services that constitute PT.

B. Reasonable and Necessary.—To be considered reasonable and necessary, the following conditions must be met:

- The services must be considered under accepted standards of medical practice to be a specific and effective treatment for the patient's condition.
- The services must be of such a level of complexity and sophistication or the condition of the patient must be such that the services required can be safely and effectively performed only by a qualified physical therapist or under his supervision. Services that do not require the performance or supervision of a physical therapist are not considered reasonable or necessary PT services, even if they are performed or supervised by a physical therapist. (When you determine the services furnished were of a type that could have been safely and effectively performed only by a qualified physical therapist or under his/her supervision, presume that such services were properly supervised. However, this assumption is rebuttable, and, if in the course of processing claims you find that PT services are not being furnished under proper supervision, deny the claim and bring this matter to the attention of the Division of Survey and Certification of the RO.)
- The development, implementation, management, and evaluation of a patient care plan constitute skilled physical therapy services when, because of the beneficiary's condition, those activities require the skills of a physical therapist to meet the beneficiary's needs, promote recovery, and ensure medical safety. Where the skills of a physical therapist are needed to manage and periodically reevaluate the appropriateness of a maintenance program because of an identified danger to the patient, those reasonable and necessary management and evaluation services could be covered, even if the skills of a therapist are not needed to carry out the activities performed as part of the maintenance program.
- While a beneficiary's particular medical condition is a valid factor in deciding if skilled physical therapy services are needed, a beneficiary's diagnosis or prognosis should never be the sole factor in deciding that a service is or is not skilled. The key issue is whether the skills of a physical therapist are needed to treat the illness or injury, or whether the services can be carried out by nonskilled personnel.
- A service that ordinarily would be performed by nonskilled personnel could be considered a skilled physical therapy service in cases in which there is clear documentation that, because of special medical complications, a skilled physical therapist is required to perform or supervise the service. However, the importance of a particular service to a beneficiary or the frequency with which it must be performed does not, by itself, make a nonskilled service into a skilled service.
- There must be an expectation that the patient's condition will improve significantly in a reasonable (and generally predictable) period of time, or the services must be necessary for the establishment of a safe and effective maintenance program required in connection with a specific disease state.
- The amount, frequency, and duration of the services must be reasonable.

NOTE: Claims for PT services denied because they are not considered reasonable and necessary are excluded by section 1862(a)(1) of the Act and are thus subject to consideration under the waiver of liability provision in section 1879 of the Act. (See section 7300.10.)

2210.3 Application of Guidelines.—The following discussion illustrates the application of the above guidelines to some of the more common physical therapy modalities and procedures utilized in the treatment of patients:

1. Hot Pack, Hydrocollator, Infra-Red Treatments, Paraffin Baths and Whirlpool Baths.—Heat treatments of this type and whirlpool baths do not ordinarily require the skills of a qualified physical therapist. However, in a particular case the skills, knowledge, and judgment of a qualified physical therapist might be required in such treatments or baths, e.g., where the patient's condition is complicated by circulatory deficiency, areas of desensitization, open wounds, or other complications. Also, if such treatments are given prior to but as an integral part of a skilled physical therapy procedure, they would be considered part of the physical therapy service.

2. Gait Training.—Gait evaluation and training furnished a patient whose ability to walk has been impaired by neurological, muscular, or skeletal abnormality require the skills of a qualified physical therapist. However, if gait evaluation and training cannot reasonably be expected to improve significantly the patient's ability to walk, such services would not be considered reasonable and necessary. Repetitive exercises to improve gait or maintain strength and endurance, and assistive walking, such as provided in support for feeble or unstable patients, are appropriately provided by supportive personnel, e.g., aides or nursing personnel and do not require the skills of a qualified physical therapist.

3. Ultrasound, Shortwave, and Microwave Diathermy Treatments.—These modalities must always be performed by or under the supervision of a qualified physical therapist, and therefore, such treatments constitute physical therapy.

4. Range of Motion Tests.—Only the qualified physical therapist may perform range of motion tests and, therefore, such tests would constitute physical therapy.

5. Therapeutic Exercises.—Therapeutic exercises that must be performed by or under the supervision of a qualified physical therapist due either to the type of exercise employed or to the condition of the patient would constitute physical therapy. Range of motion exercises require the skills of a qualified physical therapist only when they are part of the active treatment of a specific disease that has resulted in a loss or restriction of mobility (as evidenced by physical therapy notes showing the degree of motion lost and the degree to be restored) and such exercises, either because of their nature or the condition of the patient, may only be performed safely and effectively by or under the supervision of a qualified physical therapist. Generally, range of motion exercises that are not related to the restoration of a specific loss of function but rather are related to the maintenance of function (see section 2210.2) do not require the skills of a qualified physical therapist.

2303 SERVICES NOT REASONABLE AND NECESSARY

Items and services that are not reasonable and necessary for the diagnosis or treatment of illness or injury, or to improve the functioning of a malformed body member; e.g., payment *cannot* be made for the rental of a special hospital bed to be used by the patient in his home unless it was a reasonable and necessary part of the patient's treatment. See also section 2318.

2323 FOOT CARE AND SUPPORTIVE DEVICES FOR FEET

A. Exclusion of Coverage.—The following foot care services are generally excluded from coverage under both Part A and Part B. Exceptions to this general exclusion for limited treatment of routine foot care services are described in subsections A.2 and B. (See section 4120 for procedural instructions in applying foot care exclusions.)

1. Treatment of Flat Foot.—The term "flat foot" is defined as a condition in which one or more arches of the foot have flattened out. Services or devices directed toward the care or correction of such conditions, including the prescription of supportive devices, are not covered.

2. Treatment of Subluxation of Foot.—Subluxations of the foot are defined as partial dislocations or displacements of joint surfaces, tendons, ligaments, or muscles of the foot. Surgical or nonsurgical treatments undertaken for the sole purpose of correcting a subluxated structure in the foot as an isolated entity are not covered.

This exclusion does not apply to medical or surgical treatment of subluxation of the ankle joint (talo-crural joint). In addition, reasonable and necessary medical or surgical services, diagnosis, or treatment for medical conditions that have resulted from or are associated with partial displacement of structures is covered. For example, if a patient has osteoarthritis that has resulted in a partial displacement of joints in the foot, and the primary treatment is for the osteoarthritis, coverage is provided.

3. Routine Foot Care.—Except as provided in subsection B, routine foot care is excluded from coverage. Services that normally are considered routine and not covered by Medicare include the following:

- The cutting or removal of corns and calluses;
- The trimming, cutting, clipping, or debriding of nails; and
- Other hygienic and preventive maintenance care, such as cleaning and soaking the feet, the use of skin creams to maintain skin tone of either ambulatory or bedfast patients, and any other service performed in the absence of localized illness, injury, or symptoms involving the foot.

B. Exceptions to Routine Foot Care Exclusion

1. Necessary and Integral Part of Otherwise Covered Services.—In certain circumstances, services ordinarily considered to be routine may be covered if they are performed as a necessary and integral part of otherwise covered services, such as diagnosis and treatment of ulcers, wounds, or infections.

2. Treatment of Warts on Foot.—The treatment of warts (including plantar warts) on the foot is covered to the same extent as services provided for the treatment of warts located elsewhere on the body.

3. Presence of Systemic Condition.—The presence of a systemic condition such as metabolic, neurologic, or peripheral vascular disease may require scrupulous foot care by a professional that in the absence of such condition(s) would be considered routine (and, therefore, excluded from coverage). Accordingly, foot care that would otherwise be considered routine may be covered when systemic condition(s) result in severe circulatory embarrassment or areas of diminished sensation in the individual's legs or feet. (See subsection C.)

In these instances, certain foot care procedures that otherwise are considered routine (e.g., cutting or removing corns and calluses, or trimming, cutting, clipping, or debriding nails) may pose a hazard when performed by a nonprofessional person on patients with such systemic conditions. (See section 4120 for procedural instructions.)

4. Mycotic Nails.—In the absence of a systemic condition, treatment of mycotic nails may be covered.

The treatment of mycotic nails for an ambulatory patient is covered only when the physician attending the patient's mycotic condition documents that (1) there is clinical evidence of mycosis of the toenail, and (2) the patient has marked limitation of ambulation, pain, or secondary infection resulting from the thickening and dystrophy of the infected toenail plate.

The treatment of mycotic nails for a nonambulatory patient is covered only when the physician attending the patient's mycotic condition documents that (1) there is clinical evidence of mycosis of the toenail, and (2) the patient suffers from pain or secondary infection resulting from the thickening and dystrophy of the infected toenail plate.

For the purpose of these requirements, documentation means any written information that is required by the carrier in order for services to be covered. Thus, the information submitted with claims must be substantiated by information found in the patient's medical record. Any information, including that contained in a form letter, used for documentation purposes is subject to carrier verification in order to ensure that the information adequately justifies coverage of the treatment of mycotic nails. (See section 4120 for claims processing criteria.)

C. Systemic Conditions.—Although not intended as a comprehensive list, the following metabolic, neurologic, and peripheral vascular diseases (with synonyms in parentheses) most commonly represent the underlying conditions that might justify coverage for routine foot care.

*Diabetes mellitus
*Arteriosclerosis obliterans (ASO, arteriosclerosis of the extremities, occlusive peripheral arteriosclerosis)
*Buerger's disease (thromboangiitis obliterans)
*Chronic thrombophlebitis
*Peripheral neuropathies involving the feet
*Associated with malnutrition and vitamin deficiency
  Malnutrition (general, pellagra)
  Alcoholism
  Malabsorption (celiac disease, tropical sprue)
  Pernicious anemia
*Associated with carcinoma
*Associated with diabetes mellitus
*Associated with drugs and toxins
*Associated with multiple sclerosis
*Associated with uremia (chronic renal disease)
*Associated with traumatic injury
*Associated with leprosy or neurosyphilis
*Associated with hereditary disorders
*Hereditary sensory radicular neuropathy
*Angiokeratoma corporis diffusum (Fabry's)
*Amyloid neuropathy

When the patient's condition is one of those designated by an asterisk (*), routine procedures are covered only if the patient is under the active care of a doctor of medicine or osteopathy who documents the condition.

D. Supportive Devices for Feet.—Orthopedic shoes and other supportive devices for the feet generally are not covered. However, this exclusion does not apply to such a shoe if it is an integral part of a leg brace (see section 2133), and its expense is included as part of the cost of the brace. Also, this exclusion does not apply to therapeutic shoes furnished to diabetics. (See section 2134.)

E. Coding.—You are responsible for informing all medical specialties that codes and policies for routine foot care and supportive devices for the feet are not exclusively for the use of podiatrists. These codes must be used to report foot care services regardless of the specialty of the physician who furnishes the services. Instruct physicians to use the most appropriate code available when billing for routine foot care.

2455 MEDICAL INSURANCE BLOOD DEDUCTIBLE

A. General.—Program payment under Part B may not be made for the first three units of whole blood, or packed red cells, received by a beneficiary in a calendar year. For purpose of the blood deductible, a unit of whole blood means a pint of whole blood. The term "whole blood" means human blood from which none of the liquid or cellular components has been removed. Where packed red cells are furnished, a unit of packed red cells is considered equivalent to a pint of whole blood. After the three unit deductible has been satisfied, payment may be made for all blood charges, subject to the normal coverage and reasonable charge criteria.

NOTE: Blood is a biological and can be covered under Part B only when furnished incident to a physician's services. (See sections 2050.1ff. for a more complete explanation of services rendered "incident to a physician's services.")

B. Application of the Blood Deductible.—The blood deductible applies only to whole blood or packed red cells. Other components of blood such as platelets, fibrinogen, plasma, gamma globulin, and serum albumin are not subject to the blood deductible. These components of blood are covered biologicals.

The blood deductible involves only the charges for the blood (or packed red cells). Charges for the administration of blood or packed cells are not subject to the blood deductible. Accordingly, although payment may not be made for the first three pints of blood and/or units of packed red cells furnished to a beneficiary in a calendar year, payment may be made (subject to the cash deductible) for the administration charges for all covered pints or units including the first three furnished in a calendar year.

The blood deductible applies only to the first three pints and/or units furnished in a calendar year, even though more than one physician or clinic furnished blood. Furthermore, to count toward the deductible, the blood must be covered with respect to all applicable criteria (i.e., it must be medically necessary, it must be furnished incident to a physician's services, etc.). (See section 2050.5.)

C. Physician or Supplier Right to Charge for Deductible Blood.—A physician or other supplier who accepts assignment may bill a beneficiary the reasonable charge for unreplaced deductible blood (i.e., any of the first three units in a calendar year) but may not charge for blood that has been replaced.

Once a physician or supplier accepts a replacement unit of whole blood or packed red cells from a beneficiary or another individual acting on his behalf, the beneficiary may not be charged for the blood.

When a supplier accepts blood donated in advance, in anticipation of need by a specific beneficiary, whether the beneficiary's own blood, that is, an autologous donation, or blood furnished by another individual or blood assurance group, such donations are considered replacement for units subsequently furnished the beneficiary.

D. Distinction Between Blood Charges and Blood Administration Charges.—Since the blood deductible applies only to charges for blood and does not apply to charges for blood administration, these two charges must be considered separately. Where a bill for unreplaced blood shows only a single blood charge, break down the charge between blood and blood administration in accordance with the supplier's customary charges for these items. If the supplier does not customarily bill separately for blood and for blood administration, the portion of the single charge that is considered to be a charge for blood is determined by reference to the established reasonable charge in the locality as it applies to blood. The remainder of the charge is considered a blood administration charge.

E. Relationship to Other Deductibles.—Part B payment for all blood administration charges and for blood charges after the beneficiary has received three pints and/or units in a calendar year is subject to the annual cash deductible and coinsurance provisions. Expenses incurred in meeting the Part B blood deductible do not count as incurred expenses under Part B for purposes of meeting the cash deductible or for purposes of payment.

There is also a Part A blood deductible applicable to the first three pints of whole blood or equivalent units of packed red cells received by a beneficiary in a benefit period. The Part A and Part B blood deductibles are applied separately.

F. Example of Application of the Part B Blood Deductible.—In 1991, a beneficiary received three pints of blood from a physician for which the total charge is $100 per pint. (The physician does not specify how much of the charge is for blood, and how much is for blood administration.) The physician accepted assignment and submitted a claim for Part B payment.

Determine that the beneficiary has not met any part of the Part B blood deductible and has met only $40 of the cash deductible. You determine that the physician's customary charge for blood administration is $50 per unit and that it is reasonable. Consequently, charges for blood administration are $50 per unit or a total of $150 for the three units furnished, and charges for blood are $50 per unit or a total of $150 for the three units furnished. The beneficiary replaces one pint of blood. Since the beneficiary had not met any of the Part B blood deductible, none of the $150 in blood charges are payable, nor may any of such charges be applied to satisfy the annual cash deductible ($100). Of the $150 in blood administration charges, $60 is applied to satisfy the beneficiary's unmet cash deductible, and a payment of $72 is made on the remaining $90 in charges ($90 x 80%). Since the physician accepted assignment and since the beneficiary replaced one pint of blood, the physician may charge the beneficiary the reasonable charge only for the two remaining deductible pints.

2470 OUTPATIENT MENTAL HEALTH TREATMENT LIMITATION

Regardless of the actual expenses a beneficiary incurs for treatment of mental, psychoneurotic, and personality disorders while the beneficiary is not an inpatient of a hospital at the time such expenses are incurred, the amount of those expenses that may be recognized for Part B deductible and payment purposes is limited to 62.5 percent of the Medicare allowed amount for those services. This limitation is called the outpatient mental health treatment limitation. Expenses for diagnostic services (e.g., psychiatric testing and evaluation to diagnose the patient's illness) are not subject to this limitation. This limitation applies only to therapeutic services and to services performed to evaluate the progress of a course of treatment for a diagnosed condition, as described in section 2472.3.

3045 FILING THE REQUEST - ASSIGNMENTS

3045.4 Effect of Assignment Upon Purchase of Cataract Glasses from Participating Physician or Supplier.—A pair of cataract glasses is composed of two distinct products: a professional product (the prescribed lenses) and a retail commercial product (the frames). The frames serve not only as a holder of lenses but also as an article of personal apparel. As such, they are usually selected on the basis of personal taste and style. Although Medicare will pay only for standard frames, most patients want deluxe frames. Participating physicians and suppliers cannot profitably furnish such deluxe frames unless they can make an extra (noncovered) charge for the frames even though they accept assignment.

Therefore a participating physician or supplier (whether an ophthalmologist, optometrist, or optician) who accepts assignment on cataract glasses with deluxe frames may charge the Medicare patient the difference between his usual charge to private pay patients for glasses with standard frames and his usual charge to such patients for glasses with deluxe frames, in addition to the applicable deductible and coinsurance on glasses with standard frames, if all of the following requirements are met:

A. The participating physician or supplier has standard frames available, offers them for sale to the patient, and explains to the patient the price and other differences between standard and deluxe frames.

B. The participating physician or supplier obtains from the patient (or his representative) and keeps on file the following signed and dated statement:

Name of Patient Medicare Claim Number

Having been informed that an extra charge is being made by the physician or supplier for deluxe frames, that this extra charge is not covered by Medicare, and that standard frames are available for purchase from the physician or supplier at no extra charge, I have chosen to purchase deluxe frames.

Signature Date

C. The participating physician or supplier itemizes on his claim his actual charge for the lenses, his actual charge for the standard frames, and his actual extra charge for the deluxe frames (charge differential).

Once the assigned claim for deluxe frames has been processed, the carrier will explain the extra charge for the deluxe frames on the EOMB, as indicated in the following example.

		BILLED	APPROVED
CATARACT LENSES	JULY 20, 1985	$200.00	$175.00
APPROVED AMOUNT LIMITED BY ITEM 5C ON BACK			
STANDARD FRAMES	JULY 20, 1985	$ 20.00	$ 15.00
APPROVED AMOUNT LIMITED BY ITEM 5C ON BACK			
DR. JONES AGREED TO CHARGE NO MORE FOR THE ABOVE SERVICES THAN THE AMOUNT APPROVED BY MEDICARE.			
EXTRA CHARGE DELUXE	JULY 20, 1985	$ 35.00	$ 00.00
MEDICARE DOES NOT PAY THE EXTRA CHARGE FOR DELUXE FRAMES.			
TOTAL APPROVED AMOUNT			$190.00
MEDICARE PAYMENT (80% OF THE APPROVED AMOUNT)			$152.00

WE ARE PAYING A TOTAL OF $152.00 TO DR. JONES FOR THE ABOVE SERVICES. YOU ARE RESPONSIBLE FOR THE DIFFERENCE OF $38.00 BETWEEN THE APPROVED AMOUNT AND THE MEDICARE PAYMENT, PLUS THE EXTRA CHARGE OF $35.00 FOR DELUXE FRAMES.

3045.7 Mandatory Assignment and Other Requirements for Home Dialysis Supplies and Equipment Paid Under Method II.

A. General.—Effective for services furnished on or after February 1, 1990, pay only on an assignment basis for home dialysis supplies and equipment furnished a beneficiary who has selected Method II. There is also a monthly payment limitation: $2,080 for continuous cycling peritoneal dialysis (CCPD) and $1,600 for all other methods of dialysis. (Note, however, that beneficiaries are permitted to have on hand one month's emergency reserve supplies.) This payment may be made to only one supplier per beneficiary. (See sections 4270-4271.)

B. Billing Instructions.—Claims for these supplies must be completed as follows:

- You may allow suppliers to bill for more than one month's supplies at a time. However, the date of service field must identify the month for which the supplies are purchased, so that you can apply the monthly payment limit. This may be accomplished by using a separate line for each month's supplies or by using inclusive service dates and the units field.

Example: In July 1990, a supplier bills for 2 CCPD supply kits. The first kit was supplied for the patient's use in June, and the second for use in July.

If the supplier lists both kits on the same line, that item must include the following information:

- Date of service: From: 060190 To 073190
- Procedure Code: A4900
- Units: 2

If the supplier lists each month's supplies on a separate line, the inclusive dates of service for each month are the first to the last date of each month (e.g., 060190 to 063090).

- Modifier "QR" must be used to designate the one month's emergency reserve supplies. This allows you to identify situations in which the payment limit for a given month may be exceeded if an emergency reserve is billed for in addition to regular monthly supplies. It also allows you to ensure that emergency supplies are not purchased more frequently than required.
- HCPCS code A4901 identifies CCPD supplies.

3060 CLAIMS, FILING, JURISDICTION AND DEVELOPMENT PROCEDURES

3060.6 Payment Under Reciprocal Billing Arrangements

A. General.—The patient's regular physician may submit the claim, and (if assignment is accepted) receive the Part B payment, for covered visit services (including emergency visits and related services) that the regular physician arranges to be provided by a substitute physician on an occasional reciprocal basis, if:

- The regular physician is unavailable to provide the visit services;
- The Medicare patient has arranged or seeks to receive the visit services from the regular physician;
- The substitute physician does not provide the visit services to Medicare patients over a continuous period of longer than 60 days; and
- The regular physician identifies the services as substitute physician services meeting the requirements of this section by entering in item 24d of Form HCFA-1500 HCPCS Q5 modifier (service furnished by a substitute physician under a reciprocal billing arrangement) after the procedure code. When Form HCFA-1500 is next revised, provision will be made to identify the substitute physician by entering his/her unique physician identification number (UPIN) on the form and cross-referring the entry to the appropriate service line item(s) by number(s). Until further notice, the regular physician must keep in file a record of each service provided by the substitute physician, associated with the substitute physician's UPIN, and make this record available to you upon request.

If the only substitution services a physician performs in connection with an operation are postoperative services furnished during the period covered by the global fee, these services need not be identified on the claim as substitution services.

A physician may have reciprocal arrangements with more than one physician. The arrangements need not be in writing.

B. Definitions

1. Covered Visit Service.—The term "covered visit service" includes not only those services ordinarily characterized as a covered physician visit, but also any other covered items and services furnished by the substitute physician or by others as incident to his/her services.

Items and services furnished by the staff of the substitute physician covered as incident to his/her services if billed by him/her are still covered if billed by the regular physician under this section.

Items and services furnished by the staff of the regular physician covered as incident to his/her services if furnished under his/her supervision are still covered if furnished under the supervision of the substitute physician.

2. Continuous Period of Covered Visit Services.—A continuous period of covered visit services begins with the first day on which the substitute physician provides covered visit services to Medicare Part B patients of the regular physician, and it ends with the last day on which the substitute physician provides these services to these patients before the regular physician returns to work. This period continues without interruption on days on which no covered visit services are provided to patients on behalf of the regular physician or are furnished by some other substitute physician on behalf of the regular physician. A new period of covered visit services can begin after the regular physician has returned to work.

Example: The regular physician goes on vacation on June 30, 1992, and returns to work on September 4, 1992. A substitute physician provides services to Medicare Part B patients of the regular physician on July 2, 1992, and at various times thereafter, including August 30th and September 2, 1992. The continuous period of covered visit services begins on July 2nd and runs through September 2nd, a period of 63 days. Since the September 2nd services are furnished after the expiration of 60 days of the period, the regular physician is not entitled to bill and receive direct payment for them. The substitute physician must bill for these services in his/her own name. The regular physician may, however, bill and receive payment for the services that the substitute physician provides on his/her behalf in the period July 2nd through August 30th.

C. Unassigned Claims Under Reciprocal Billing Arrangements.—The requirements for the submission of claims under reciprocal billing arrangements are the same for assigned and unassigned claims.

D. Medical Group Claims Under Reciprocal Billing Arrangements.—The requirements of this section do not apply to the substitution arrangements among physicians in the same medical group where claims are submitted in the name of the group. On claims submitted by the group, the group physician who actually performed the service must be identified in the manner described in section 3060.9.

For a medical group to submit assigned and unassigned claims for the covered visit services of a substitute physician who is not a member of the group, the requirements of subsection A must be met. The medical group must enter in item 24d of Form HCFA-1500 the HCPCS modifier Q5 after the procedure code. Until further notice, the medical group must keep in file a record of each service provided by the substitute physician, associated with the substitute physician's UPIN, and make this record available to you upon request. In addition, the medical group physician for whom the substitution services are furnished must be identified by his/her provider identification number (PIN) in block 24k of the appropriate line item.

For an independent physician to submit assigned and unassigned claims for the substitution services of a physician who is a member of a medical group, the requirements of subsection A must be met. The independent physician must enter in item 24 of Form HCFA-1500 HCPCS modifier Q5 after the procedure code. Until further notice, the independent physician must keep in file a record of each service provided by the substitute medical group physician, associated with the substitute physician's UPIN, and make this record available to you upon request.

Physicians who are members of a group but who bill in their own names are treated as independent physicians for purposes of applying the requirements of this section.

E. Guidance to Physicians.—Inform physicians of the requirements of this section. Advise physicians and, if necessary, remind them that, in entering the code Q5 modifier, the regular physician (or the medical group, where applicable) is certifying that the services are covered visit services furnished by the substitute physician identified in a record of the regular physician that is available for inspection, and are services for which the regular physician (or group) is entitled under this section to submit the claim. Mention the possible penalties under subsection F for false certifications.

F. Penalties.—A physician or other person who falsely certifies that the requirements of this section are met may be subject to possible civil and criminal penalties for fraud. Also, the physician's right to receive payment or to submit claims under this section or even to accept any assignments may be revoked. The revocation procedures are set forth in section 14025.

G. Claims Review.—If a line item includes the code Q5 certification, assume that the claim meets the requirements of this section in the absence of evidence to the contrary. You need not track the 60-day period or validate the billing arrangement on a prepayment basis, absent postpayment findings that indicate that the certifications by a particular physician may not be valid.

H. Payment Amount.—When you make Part B payment under this section, you determine the payment amount as though the regular physician or his/her staff provided the services. The identification of the substitute physician is primarily for purposes of providing an audit trail to verify that the services were furnished, not for purposes of the payment or the limiting charge. Also, notices of noncoverage under section 7300ff. and 7330ff. are to be given in the name of the regular physician.

3060.7 Payment Under Locum Tenens Arrangements

A. Background.—It is a longstanding and widespread practice for physicians to retain substitute physicians to take over their professional practices when the regular physicians are absent for reasons such as illness, pregnancy, vacation, or continuing medical education, and for the regular physician to bill and receive payment for the substitute physician's services as though he/she performed them himself/herself. The substitute physician generally has no practice of his/her own and moves from area to area as needed. The regular physician generally pays the substitute physician a fixed amount per diem, with the substitute physician having the status of an independent contractor rather than of an employee. These substitute physicians are generally called "locum tenens" physicians.

Section 125(b) of the Social Security Act Amendments of 1994 makes this procedure available on a permanent basis. Thus, beginning January 1, 1995, a regular physician may bill for the services of "locum tenens" physicians. A regular physician is the physician who is normally scheduled to see a patient. Thus, a regular physician may include physician specialists (such as a cardiologist, oncologist, urologist, etc.).

B. Payment Procedure.—A patient's regular physician may submit the claim, and (if assignment is accepted) receive the Part B payment, for covered visit services (including emergency visits and related services) of a locum tenens physician who is not an employee of the regular physician and whose services for patients of the regular physician are not restricted to the regular physician's offices, if:

- The regular physician is unavailable to provide the visit services;
- The Medicare beneficiary has arranged or seeks to receive the visit services from the regular physician;
- The regular physician pays the locum tenens for his/her services on a per diem or similar fee-for-time basis;
- The substitute physician does not provide the visit services to Medicare patients over a continuous period of longer than 60 days; and
- The regular physician identifies the services as substitute physician services meeting the requirements of this section by entering HCPCS Q6 modifier (service furnished by a locum tenens physician) after the procedure code. When Form HCFA-1500 is next revised, provision will be made to identify the substitute physician by entering his/her unique physician identification number (UPIN).

See section 3060.6B for definitions of covered visit services and continuous period of covered visit services.

If the only substitution services a physician performs in connection with an operation are postoperative services furnished during the period covered by the global fee, these services need not be identified on the claim as substitution services.

C. Unassigned Claims Under Locum Tenens Arrangements.—The requirements for the submission of claims under reciprocal billing arrangements are the same for assigned and unassigned claims.

D. Medical Group Claims Under Locum Tenens Arrangements.—For a medical group to submit assigned and unassigned claims for the services a locum tenens physician provides for patients of the regular physician who is a member of the group, the requirements of subsection B must be met. For purposes of these requirements, per diem or similar fee-for-time compensation that the group pays the locum tenens physician is considered paid by the regular physician. Also, a physician who has left the group and for whom the group has engaged a locum tenens physician as a temporary replacement may still be considered a member of the group until a permanent replacement is obtained. The group must enter in item 24d of Form HCFA-1500 the HCPCS Q6 modifier after the procedure code. Until further notice, the group must keep in file a record of each service provided by the substitute physician, associated with the substitute physician's UPIN, and make this record available to you upon request. In addition, the medical group physician for whom the substitution services are furnished must be identified by his/her provider identification number (PIN) on block 24k of the appropriate line item.

Physicians who are members of a group but who bill in their own names are generally treated as independent physicians for purposes of applying the requirements of subsection A for payment for locum tenens physician services. Compensation paid by the group to the locum tenens physician is considered paid by the regular physician for purposes of those requirements. The term "regular physician" includes a physician who has left the group and for whom the group has hired the locum tenens physician as a replacement.

E. Guidance to Physicians, Penalties, Claims Review and Payment Amount.—In regard to guidance for physicians, possible penalties, claims review, and payment amounts, proceed as in §3060.6.

3312 EVIDENCE OF MEDICAL NECESSITY FOR DURABLE MEDICAL EQUIPMENT

Section 3312 has been moved to Chapter 5 of the Program Integrity Manual, which can be found at http://www.hcfa.gov/pubforms/83_pim/pim83toc.htm.

3350.3 Claims Coding Requirements.—Physicians must indicate that their services were provided in an incentive-eligible rural or urban HPSA by using one of the following modifiers:

- QB—physician providing a service in a rural HPSA; or
- QU—physician providing a service in an urban HPSA.

3350.4 Payment.—The incentive payment is 10 percent of the amount actually paid, not the approved amount. Pay the incentive payment for services identified on either assigned or unassigned claims.

Do not include the incentive payment with each claim payment. Establish a quarterly schedule for issuing incentive payments. These payments are taxable and must be reported to the IRS.

Prepare a list to accompany each payment. Include a line item for each assigned claim represented in the incentive check and a "summary" item showing the number of unassigned claims represented. The sum of the line items and the "summary" items should equal the amount of the check.

3350.5 Services Eligible for HPSA Bonus Payments

A. Information in the professional Component/Technical Component (PC/TC) Indicator Field of the Medicare Physician Fee Schedule Database.—Use the information in the Professional Component/Technical Component (PC/TC) indicator field of the Medicare Physician Fee Schedule Database to identify professional services eligible for HPSA bonus payments. The following are the rules to apply in determining whether to pay the bonus on services furnished within a geographic HPSA and billed with a QB or QU modifier, as appropriate.

PC/TC Indicator	HPSA Payment Policy
0	Pay the HPSA bonus.
1	Globally billed. Only the professional component of this service qualifies for the HPSA bonus payment. The HPSA bonus cannot be paid on the technical component of globally billed services.

ACTION: Return the service as unprocessable. Instruct the provider to re-bill the service as two components with separate charges for the professional component (billed with the "26" and "HPSA" modifiers) and the technical component (billed with the "TC" modifier but not the "HPSA" modifier). (See §3350.6(A).)

PC/TC Indicator	HPSA Payment Policy
1	Professional Component (modifier 26). Pay the bonus.
1	Technical Component (modifier TC). Do not pay the bonus. (See §3350.6(B).)
2	Professional Component only. Pay the bonus.
3	Technical Component only. Do not pay the bonus. (See §3350.6(B).)
4	Global test only. Only the professional component of this service qualifies for the HPSA bonus payment.

ACTION: Return the service as unprocessable. Instruct the provider to re-bill the service as separate professional and technical component procedure codes. The HPSA modifier should only be used with the professional component code. (See §3350.6(A).)

PC/TC Indicator	HPSA Payment Policy
5	Incident to codes. Do not pay the bonus. (See §3350.6(B).)
6	Laboratory physician interpretation codes. Pay the bonus.
7	Physical therapy service. Do not pay the bonus. (See §3350.6(B).)
8	Physician interpretation codes. Pay the bonus.
9	Concept of PC/TC does not apply. Do not pay the bonus. (See §3350.6(B).)

NOTE: Codes that have a status of "X" on the Medicare Physician Fee Schedule Database (MFSDB) have been assigned PC/TC indicator 9 and are not considered physician services for MFSDB payment purposes. Therefore, the HPSA bonus payment will not be paid for these codes.

B. Anesthesia Codes (CPT Codes 00100 through 01999*) that Do Not Appear on the MFSDB.—Anesthesia codes (CPT codes 00100 through 01999*) do not appear on the MFSDB. However, when a medically necessary anesthesia service is furnished within a HPSA area by a physician, a HPSA bonus is payable. In addition to using the MFSDB PC/TC indicator to identify HPSA services, pay physicians the HPSA bonus when CPT codes 00100 through 01999* are billed with the following modifiers: QY, QK, AD, AA, or GC. These modifiers signify that the anesthesia service was performed by a physician.

4105 DURABLE MEDICAL EQUIPMENT, PROSTHETIC, AND ORTHOTIC SUPPLIES

Sections 4105–4105.7 have been deleted and moved to the Program Integrity Manual (PIM), which can be found at the following Internet address: www.hcfa.gov/pubforms/83pim/pimtoc.htm.

4107 DURABLE MEDICAL EQUIPMENT BILLING AND PAYMENT CONSIDERATIONS UNDER THE FEE SCHEDULE

The Omnibus Budget Reconciliation Act of 1987 requires that payment for DME, prosthetics and orthotics be made under fee schedules effective January 1, 1989. The allowable charge is limited to the lower of the actual charge for the equipment, or the fee schedule amount. The equipment is categorized into one of six classes:

- Inexpensive or other routinely purchased DME;
- Items requiring frequent and substantial servicing;
- Customized items;
- Prosthetic and orthotic devices;
- Capped rental items; or
- Oxygen and oxygen equipment.

The fee schedule allowances for each class are determined in accord with section 5102ff.

4107.1 General Billing and Claims Processing.—Subject to some of the specific billing and processing requirements, bills are to be submitted, processed and paid in accordance with section 4105ff. and 5102ff.

You are responsible for processing outpatient and noninstitutional claims for DME and oxygen previously paid by fiscal intermediaries to hospitals, CORFs, SNFs, and OPT providers. Prosthetic, orthotic, and inpatient DME and oxygen claims, however, continue to be billed by these providers to their FIs. You will not receive any claims from HHAs that have transferred to regional home health intermediaries (RHHIs). Issue billing numbers as necessary and pay the appropriate fee schedule amounts. If the item billed is in the capped rental category, develop with the beneficiary or assignee, as appropriate, to determine the length of time the beneficiary has continuously rented the item. Process in accordance with section 4107.4.

Payable bills or claims must specify whether equipment is rented or purchased. For purchased equipment, the itemized bill or claim must also indicate whether equipment is new or used. If the supplier fails to indicate on an assigned claim whether equipment was new or used, assume purchased equipment is used and process the claim accordingly, i.e., pay on the basis of the used purchase fee. If an unassigned purchase claim does not specify whether the item was new or used, develop the claim in accordance with section 3311.

4107.2 Rent/Purchase Decisions.—For services provided on or after October 1, 1988, discontinue making rent/purchase decisions on rental claims. (See section 5101.2.) For purchase claims with dates of service before January 1, 1989, continue to make rent/purchase decisions. Discontinue making rent/purchase decisions for purchase claims with dates of service on or after January 1, 1989. Do not pay for oxygen delivery systems, items requiring frequent and substantial servicing or capped rental items that were purchased on or after June 1, 1989.

4107.3 Comparability and Inherent Reasonableness Limitations.—For services provided on or after January 1, 1989, do not apply the comparable circumstances provision in section 5026. Also, for services provided between January 1, 1989 and December 31, 1990, do not apply the special payment limitation provisions in section 5246 to DME and orthotics/prosthetics subject to the fee schedules in section 5102ff.

4107.4 15-Month Ceiling on Capped Rental Items.—Ensure that your system accurately computes the 15 month period for capped rental items. (See section 5102.1E3 and 5102.3C1 and 2.)

4107.5 Transcutaneous Electrical Nerve Stimulator (TENS).—To permit an attending physician time to determine whether purchase of a TENS unit is medically appropriate, ensure that your system allows no more than 10 percent of the fee schedule purchase amount for up to 2 months of rental prior to purchase. Do not apply the rentals toward the purchase allowance.

4107.6 Written Order Prior to Delivery.—Ensure that your system will pay for the equipment listed below only when the supplier has a written order in hand prior to delivery. Otherwise, do not pay for that item even if a written order is subsequently furnished. However, you can pay for a similar item if it is subsequently provided by an unrelated supplier that has a written order in hand prior to delivery. The HCPCS codes for the equipment requiring a written order are:

- E0180
- E0181
- E0182
- E0183
- E0184
- E0185
- E0188
- E0189
- E0190
- E0192
- E0195
- E0620
- E0720
- E0730
- E1230

4107.7 Special Requirements for Oxygen Claims.—There are a number of billing considerations for oxygen claims. The chart in section 4107.9 indicates what is payable under which situation.

A. Monthly Billing.—Fee schedule payments for stationary oxygen system rentals are all inclusive and represent a monthly allowance per beneficiary. Accordingly, a supplier must bill on a monthly basis for stationary oxygen equipment and contents furnished during a rental month.

A portable equipment add-on is also payable when portable oxygen is prescribed and you determine it to be medically necessary in accordance with Medicare coverage requirements. The portable add-on must be claimed in order to be paid. (See section 4107.10.)

Claims may be submitted when expenses are incurred for initial rentals of oxygen systems, or no sooner than the monthly anniversary date in the case of an established oxygen patient. In the latter situation, suppliers must indicate the monthly volume of oxygen contents delivered, rounded in accordance with subsection D3.

Where the beneficiary has purchased a stationary system (other than a concentrator and/or a portable delivery system), oxygen contents must be billed and paid on a monthly basis, except for unassigned oxygen contents claims submitted by a beneficiary. For beneficiary filed claims, allow, on a claim-by-claim basis, the submitted charge until the applicable monthly fee for oxygen contents has been met.

B. Reduced Number of HCPCS Codes.—The number of HCPCS codes for billing of oxygen claims have been reduced. See section 4107.9 for the codes and their definitions.

C. Use of Payment Modifiers.—The monthly payment amount for stationary oxygen is subject to adjustment depending on the amount of oxygen prescribed (liters per minute (LPM)), and whether or not portable oxygen is also prescribed. (See section 5102.1.) To make proper payment adjustments, supplier claims must indicate the appropriate HCPCS modifier described below, if applicable. On unassigned claims, suppliers should indicate this information on the itemized bill.

If the prescribed amount of oxygen is less than 1 LPM, the modifier is "QE". Reduce the monthly payment amount for stationary oxygen by 50 percent.

If the prescribed amount of oxygen is greater than 4 LPM, the modifier is "QG". Increase the monthly payment amount for stationary oxygen by 50 percent. Conduct prepayment medical review of these claims.

If the prescribed amount of oxygen exceeds 4 LPM and portable oxygen is prescribed, the modifier is "QF". Increase the monthly payment for stationary oxygen by the higher of 50 percent of the monthly stationary oxygen payment amount, or the fee schedule amount for the portable oxygen add-on. (See section 5102.1.F2j.) Conduct a prepayment medical review of these claims.

D. Units Required.—Excluding concentrators, suppliers must furnish units of oxygen contents in Item 24F of their HCFA-1500 claims, or the itemized bill furnished to the beneficiary for unassigned claims.

1. Initial Oxygen Claims.—When submitting an initial claim for rental of a gaseous or liquid oxygen delivery system, units of oxygen contents furnished for the first month need not be indicated. Base your payment upon the lower of the actual charge for the initial rental month or the monthly payment amount.

2. Subsequent Oxygen Claims.—For dates of service subsequent to the initial rental month, suppliers should indicate actual content usage for the month billed or, if billed prospectively, the actual content usage during the previous rental month, rounded in accordance with subsection D3. Base your payment determination on the lower of the actual charge submitted or the monthly payment amount.

For applying these instructions, treat claims submitted under recertifications of continuing and uninterrupted need for oxygen therapy as subsequent claims if a change in suppliers is not involved.

If a change in suppliers has occurred, apply the initial rule in subsection D.1 above for specifying oxygen contents delivered for the initial rental month by the new supplier.

Develop subsequent rental claims for gaseous or liquid oxygen delivery systems that do not include "unit" information. (See section 3311.)

3. Rounding of Oxygen Contents.—For stationary gas system rentals, suppliers should indicate, in item 24F of the HCFA-1500, oxygen contents in unit multiples of 50 cubic feet, rounded to the nearest increment of 50. For example, if 73 cubic feet of oxygen was delivered during the rental month, the item 24F unit entry "01" indicates the nearest 50 cubic foot increment. For stationary liquid systems, units of contents should be specified in multiples of 10 pounds of liquid contents delivered, rounded to the nearest 10 pound increment. For example, if 63 pounds of liquid oxygen were delivered during the applicable rental month billed, the unit entry "06" is made in Item 24F. For units of portable contents only (i.e., no stationary gas or liquid system used), round to the nearest five cubic feet or one liquid pound, respectively.

Periodically audit supplier records to verify that gaseous and liquid content usage is reported correctly.

E. Conserving Device Modifier.—Suppliers must indicate if an oxygen conserving device is being used with an oxygen delivery system by using HCPCS modifier "QH".

4107.8 EOMB Messages.—The following EOMB messages are suggested: (See section 7012ff. for other applicable messages.)

A. General

- "This is the maximum approved amount for this item." (Use when payment is reduced for a line item.)

B. Inexpensive/Frequently Purchased Equipment

- "The total approved amount for this item is whether this item is purchased or rented." (Use in first month.)
- "This is your next to last rental payment."
- "This is your last rental payment."
- "This item has been rented up to the Medicare payment limit."
- "The approved amount has been reduced by the previously approved rental amounts."

C. Items Requiring Frequent and Substantial Servicing.—Use the general rental messages in section 4107.8A, if applicable. If the beneficiary has purchased the item prior to June 1, 1989, follow section 7014.6. If the beneficiary purchased an item in this category on or after June 1, 1989, use the following message:

- "This equipment can only be paid for on a rental basis."

D. Customized Items and Other Prosthetic and Orthotic Devices

- "The total approved amount for this item is ________."

E. Capped Rental Items

- "Under a provision of Medicare law, monthly rental payments for this item can continue for up to 15 months from the first rental month or until the equipment is no longer needed, whichever comes first."
- "If you no longer are using this equipment or have recently moved and will rent this item from a different supplier, please contact our office." (Use on beneficiary's EOMB.)
- "This is your next to last rental payment."
- "This is your last rental payment."
- "This item has been rented up to the 15 month Medicare payment limit."
- "Your equipment supplier must supply and service this item for as long as you continue to need it."
- "Medicare cannot pay for maintenance and/or servicing of this item until 6 months have elapsed since the end of the 15th paid rental month."

If the beneficiary purchased a capped rental item prior to June 1, 1989, follow section 7014.6. If the beneficiary purchased a capped rental item on or after June 1, 1989, use the following denial message:

- "This equipment can only be paid for on a rental basis."

F. Oxygen and Oxygen Equipment

- "The monthly allowance includes payment for all covered oxygen contents and supplies."
- "Payment for the amount of oxygen supplied has been reduced or denied based on the patient's medical condition." (To supplier after medical review.)
- "The approved amount has been reduced to the amount allowable for medically necessary oxygen therapy." (To beneficiary.)
- "Payment denied because the allowance for this item is included in the monthly payment amount."
- "Payment denied because Medicare oxygen coverage requirements are not met."

If the beneficiary purchased an oxygen system prior to June 1, 1989, follow section 7014.6. If the beneficiary purchased an oxygen system on or after June 1, 1989, use the following denial message:

- "This item can only be paid for on a rental basis."

G. Items Requiring a Written Order Prior to Delivery

- "Payment is denied because the supplier did not obtain a written order from your doctor prior to the delivery of this item."

4107.9 Oxygen HCPCS Codes Effective 1/1/89

NEW	OLD	DEFINITION
Q0036 See notes (1) and (8)	E1377-E1385, E1387	Oxygen concentrator, high humidity
Q0038 See note (2)	E0400, E0405	Oxygen contents, gaseous, per unit (for use with owned gaseous stationary systems or when both a stationary and portable gaseous system are owned; 1 unit = 50 cu ft)
Q0039 See note (2)	E0410, E04150	Oxygen contents, liquid, per unit (for use with owned stationary liquid systems or when both a stationary and portable liquid system are owned; 1 unit = 10 lb)
Q0040 See note (2)	E0416	Portable oxygen contents, per unit (for use only with portable gaseous systems when no stationary gas system is used; 1 unit = 5 cu ft)

NEW	OLD	DEFINITION
Q0041 See note (2)	None	Portable oxygen contents, liquid, per unit (for use only with portable liquid systems when no stationary liquid system is used; 1 unit = 1 lb)
Q0042 See note (3)	E0425	Stationary compressed, gas system rental, includes contents (per unit), regulator with flow gauge, humidifier, nebulizer, cannula or mask and tubing; 1 unit = 50 cu ft
E0425 See notes (4) and (8)	Same	No change
E0430 See notes (8) and (9)	Same	No change
E0435 See notes (7) and (8)	Same	No change in terminology, but see note (7).
Q0043 See note (3)	E0440	Stationary liquid oxygen system rental, includes contents (per unit), use of reservoir, contents indicator, flowmeter, humidifier, nebulizer, cannula or mask and tubing; 1 unit of contents = 10 lb
E0440 See note (4)	Same	No change
E0455 See note (6)	Same	No change
E0555 See note (6)	Same	No change
E0580 See note (6)	Same	No change
E1351 See note (6)	Same	No change
E1352 See note (6)	Same	No change
E1353 See notes (6) and (8)	Same	No change
E1354 See note (6)	Same	No change
E1371 See note (6)	Same	No change
E1374 See note (6)	Same	No change
E1400 See notes (1) and (8)	E1388–E1396	Same as Q0014
E1401 See notes (1) and (8)	E1388–E1396	Same as Q0015
E1402	Same	No change
E1403	Same	No change
E1404	Same	No change
E1405 See note (10)	Q0037	Combine the fee schedule amounts for the stationary oxygen system and the nebulizer with a compressor and heater (code E0585) to determine the fee schedule amount to apply to oxygen enrichers with a heater (code E1405)
E1406	Q0037	Combine the fee schedule amounts for the stationary oxygen system and the nebulizer with only a compressor (i.e., without a heater, code E0570) to determine the fee schedule amount to apply to oxygen enrichers without a heater (code E1406)

NOTES:
(1) For billing concentrator rentals or purchases
(2) For monthly billing of contents used with purchased gas or liquid oxygen delivery systems (i.e., no stationary system is being rented)
(3) For billing gas or liquid system rentals only
(4) For billing of purchased stationary gas or liquid systems
(5) For billing the portable add-on for liquid systems
(6) For billing of replacement items for oxygen delivery systems purchased prior to 6/1/89
(7) For services furnished on or after 6/1/89, use E0435 when only portable liquid is prescribed (i.e., no stationary liquid system prescribed) or both stationary and portable oxygen were prescribed but the patient uses a stationary system other than a liquid system (e.g., stationary system is concentrator)
(8) Do not pay for oxygen systems purchased on or after 6/1/89
(9) For billing the portable add-on for gas systems
(10) For billing of rental oxygen and water vapor enriching systems only.

4120 FOOT CARE

4120.1 Application of Foot Care Exclusions to Physicians' Services.—The exclusion of foot care is determined by the nature of the service (section 2323). Thus, reimbursement for an excluded service should be denied whether performed by a podiatrist, osteopath, or a doctor of medicine, and without regard to the difficulty or complexity of the procedure.

When an itemized bill shows both covered services and noncovered services not integrally related to the covered service, the portion of charges attributable to the noncovered services should be denied. (For example, if an itemized bill shows surgery for an ingrown toenail and also removal of calluses not necessary for the performance of toe surgery, any additional charge attributable to removal of the calluses should be denied.)

In reviewing claims involving foot care, the carrier should be alert to the following exceptional situations:

1. Payment may be made for incidental noncovered services performed as a necessary and integral part of, and secondary to, a covered procedure. For example, if trimming of toenails is required for application of a cast to a fractured foot, the carrier need not allocate and deny a portion of the charge for the trimming of the nails. However, a separately itemized charge for such excluded service should be disallowed. When the primary procedure is covered the administration of anesthesia necessary for the performance of such procedure is also covered.

2. Payment may be made for initial diagnostic services performed in connection with a specific symptom or complaint if it seems likely that its treatment would be covered even though the resulting diagnosis may be one requiring only noncovered care.

3. Payment may be made for routine-type foot care such as cutting or removal of corns, calluses, or nails when the patient has a systemic disease of sufficient severity that unskilled performance of such procedure would be hazardous (section 2323C).

a. Claims for such routine services would show in item 7D of the SSA-1490 the complicating systemic disease. Where these services were rendered by a podiatrist this item should also include the name of the MD or DO who diagnosed the complicating condition. In those cases where active care is required, the approximate date the beneficiary was last seen by such physician must also be indicated.

NOTE: Section 939 of P.L. 96-499 removed "warts" from the routine foot care exclusion effective July 1, 1981.

b. Relatively few claims for routine-type care are anticipated considering the severity of conditions contemplated as the basis for this exception. Claims for this type of foot care should not be paid in the absence of convincing evidence that nonprofessional performance of the service would have been hazardous for the beneficiary because of an underlying systemic disease. The mere statement of a diagnosis such as those mentioned in section 2323C does not of itself indicate the severity of the condition. Where development is indicated to verify diagnosis and/or severity the carrier should follow existing claims processing practices that may include review of carrier's history and medical consultation as well as physician contacts.

c. A presumption of coverage may be made by the carrier where the claim or other evidence available discloses certain physical and/or clinical findings consistent with the diagnosis and indicative of severe peripheral involvement. For purposes of applying this presumption, the following findings are pertinent:

- Class A Findings
  —Nontraumatic amputation of foot or integral skeletal portion thereof
- Class B Findings
  —Absent posterior tibial pulse
  —Advanced trophic changes as (three required): hair growth (decrease or absence); nail changes (thickening); pigmentary changes (discoloration); skin texture (thin, shiny); skin color (rubor or redness)
  —Absent dorsalis pedis pulse
- Class C Findings
  —Claudication
  —Temperature changes (e.g., cold feet)
  —Edema
  —Paresthesia (abnormal spontaneous sensations in the feet)
  —Burning

The presumption of coverage may be applied when the physician rendering the routine foot care has identified: (1) a Class A finding; (2) two of the Class B findings; or (3) one Class B and two Class C findings. Case evidencing findings falling short of these alternatives may involve podiatric treatment that may constitute covered care and should be reviewed by the carrier's medical staff and developed as necessary.

For purposes of applying the coverage presumption where the routine services have been rendered by a podiatrist, the carrier may deem the active care requirement met if the claim or other evidence available discloses that the patient has seen an MD or DO for treatment and/or evaluation of the complicating disease process during the 6-month period prior to the rendition of the routine-type service or had come under such care shortly after the services were furnished usually as a result of a referral.

4120.2 Application of the "Reasonable and Necessary" Limitation to Foot Care Services.—In evaluating claims for foot care services, in addition to determining whether any of the other statutory limitations apply, carriers should assure that payment is made only for services that are "reasonable and necessary" for diagnosis or treatment of an illness or injury or to improve the functioning of a malformed body member. (See section 2303.) Determinations as to whether a foot care service is reasonable and necessary should be made on the same basis as all other such determinations—that is, with the advice of medical consultants and with reference to accepted standards of medical practice and the circumstances of the individual case. With appropriate professional consultation, guidelines should be established concerning the scope, frequency, and duration of services that would constitute reasonable and necessary utilization of services for various foot conditions; these guidelines should be used to screen out for denial, claims in which the services billed would clearly not be reasonable and necessary and to screen out questionable cases for special review or further development.

For example, infections of the feet and toenails that cause pain or deformity of sufficient degree to markedly limit ambulation may require a variety of medical services such as physical examination, and laboratory tests for the purpose of diagnosing the existence and type of infectious condition (and differentiating it from other types of dermatoses), prescription of a regimen of treatment, periodic examinations throughout the course of treatment to evaluate the status of the lesion and watch for complicating factors, and active treatment by one or a combination of the following modalities:

(1) Surgical excision (avulsion) of the affected nail(s);
(2) Mechanical debridement of the lesion;
(3) Topical treatment; or
(4) Systemic treatment.

With the appropriate advice from physicians who treat foot infections (e.g., dermatologists, podiatrists and surgeons), guidelines should be developed concerning accepted standards of medical practice with respect to appropriate utilization of the above types of services for different types of infectious conditions, taking into account such factors as the indications for various modalities of treatment, the required duration of different courses of therapy, and the required frequency of follow-up evaluation examinations. For example, when a physician prescribes a topical medication for an infection, patients are usually expected to perform most of the treatment by themselves at home (or if residing in nursing homes or skilled nursing facilities, etc., the staff of the facility is expected to perform most of the treatment), with perhaps occasional follow-up visits to (or by) the physician for evaluation of the status of the lesion. As part of the initial diagnostic and follow-up evaluation visits, the physician may cleanse the lesion and apply medication and these services would, of course, be covered where they are an accepted integral component of such visits; however, if the patient regularly comes to the physician to receive the care that he is expected to perform himself at home and there are no special medical circumstances relating to the infection warranting such special care, this would represent excessive utilization of physicians' services and should be excluded.

Carriers' utilization guidelines should enable them to identify where a course of therapy involves more frequent follow-up visits than are the accepted standards of physician care for that modality of therapy and to deny payment for such excessive visits unless there is documentation of special medical circumstances relating to the infection justifying the extra visits. For instance, in the case of claims for patients whose initial course of treatment includes a medically necessary visit to the physician for mechanical debridement of a mycotic lesion of the toenail, carriers must use a 60-day claims processing screen for identifying excessive follow-up services for the patient (i.e., the presumption would be that only one follow-up visit is covered every 60 days following the end of the initial treatment period unless medical documentation is submitted that supports more frequent visits). Similarly, utilization guidelines should identify when visits extend beyond the period of follow-up evaluation that is the accepted standard for a particular course of treatment for an infection and to deny payment for visits beyond the period unless development reveals complications in the infectious condition necessitating more prolonged treatment.

4173 POSITRON EMISSION TOMOGRAPHY (PET) SCANS BACKGROUND

For dates of service on or after March 14, 1995, Medicare covers one use of PET scans, imaging of the perfusion of the heart using Rubidium 82 (Rb 82).

For dates of service on or after January 1, 1998, Medicare expanded coverage of PET scans for the characterization of solitary pulmonary nodules and for the initial staging of lung cancer, conditioned upon its ability to effect the management and treatment of patients with either suspected or demonstrated lung cancer. All other uses of PET scans remain not covered by Medicare.

Beginning for dates of service on or after July 1, 1999, Medicare will cover PET scans for evaluation of recurrent colorectal cancer in patients with levels of carcinoembryonic antigen (CEA), staging lymphoma (both Hodgkin's and non-Hodgkin's) in place of a gallium study or lymphangiogram, and for the staging of recurrent melanoma prior to surgery.

See Coverage Issues Manual §50-36 for specific coverage criteria for PET scans.

Regardless of any other terms or conditions, all uses of PET scans, in order to be covered by the Medicare program, must meet the following conditions:

- Scans must be performed using PET scanners that have either been approved or cleared for marketing by the FDA as PET scanners;
- Submission of claims for payment must include any information Medicare requires to assure that the PET scans performed were: (a) reasonable and necessary; (b) did not unnecessarily duplicate other covered diagnostic tests; and (c) did not involve investigational drugs or procedures using investigational drugs, as determined by the Food and Drug Administration (FDA); and
- The PET scan entity submitting claims for payment must keep such patient records as Medicare requires on file for each patient for whom a PET scan claim is made.

4173.1 Conditions for Medicare Coverage of Pet Scans for Noninvasive Imaging of the Perfusion of the Heart.—PET scans done at rest or with pharmacological stress used for noninvasive imaging of the perfusion of the heart for the diagnosis and management of patients with known or suspected coronary artery disease using the FDA-approved radiopharmaceutical Rubidium 82 (Rb 82) are covered for the services performed on or after March 15, 1995, provided such scans meet either of the two following conditions:

- The PET scan, whether rest alone or rest with stress, is used in place of, but not in addition to, a single photon emission computed tomography (SPECT); or
- The PET scan, whether rest alone or rest with stress, is used following a SPECT that was found inconclusive. In these cases, the PET scan must have been considered necessary in order to determine what medical or surgical intervention is required to treat the patient. (For purposes of this requirement, an inconclusive test is a test whose results are equivocal, technically uninterpretable, or discordant with a patient's other clinical data.)

NOTE: PET scans using Rubidium 82, whether rest or stress, are not covered by Medicare for routine screening of asymptomatic patients, regardless of the level of risk factors applicable to such patients.

4173.2 Conditions of Coverage of PET Scans for Characterization of Solitary Pulmonary Nodules (SPNs) and PET Scans Using FDG to Initially Stage Lung Cancer.—PET scans using the glucose analog 2-[fluorine-18]-fluoro-2-deoxy-D-glucose (FDG) are covered for services on or after January 1, 1998, subject to the condition and limitations described in CIM 50-36.

NOTE: A tissue sampling procedure (TSP) should not be routinely covered in the case of a negative PET scan for characterization of SPNs, since the patient is presumed not to have a malignant lesion, based upon the PET scan results. Claims for a TSP after a negative PET must be submitted with documentation in order to determine whether the TSP is reasonable and necessary in spite of a negative PET. Claims submitted for a TSP after a negative PET without documentation should be denied. Physicians should discuss with their patients the implications of this decision, both with respect to the patient's responsibility for payment for such a biopsy, if desired, as well as the confidence the physician has in the results of such PET scans, prior to ordering such scans for this purpose. This physician-patient decision should occur with a clear discussion and understanding of the sensitivity and specificity of trade-offs between a computerized tomography (CT) and PET scan. In cases where a TSP is performed, it is the responsibility of the physician ordering the TSP to provide sufficient documentation of the reasonableness and necessity for such procedure or procedures. Such documentation should include, but is not necessarily limited to, a description of the features of the PET scan that call into question whether it is an accurate representation of the patient's condition, the existence of other factors in the patient's condition that call into question the accuracy of the PET scan, and such other information as the contractor deems necessary to determine whether the claim for the TSP should be covered and paid.

In cases of serial evaluation of SPNs using both CT and regional PET chest scanning, such PET scans will not be covered if repeated within 90 days following a negative PET scan.

4173.3 Conditions of Coverage of PET Scans for Recurrence of Colorectal Cancer, Staging and Characterization of Lymphoma, and Recurrence of Melanoma.—Medicare adds coverage for these three new indications for PET, one for evaluation of recurrent colorectal cancer in patients with rising levels of carcinoembryonic antigen (CEA), one for staging of lymphoma (both Hodgkin's and non-Hodgkin's) when the PET scan substitutes for a gallium scan, and one for the detection of recurrent melanoma, provided certain conditions are met. All three indications are covered only when using the radiopharmaceutical FDA (2-[fluorine-18]-fluoro-2-deoxy-D-glucose), and are further predicated on the legal availability of FDG for use in such scans.

4173.4 Billing Requirements for PET Scans

A. Effective for Services on or After January 1, 1998, Claims for Characterizing SPNs Should Include:

- Evidence of the initial detection of a primary lung tumor, usually by CT. This should include an indication of the results of such CT or other detection method, indicating an indeterminate or possibly malignant lesion, not exceeding four centimeters (cm) in diameter. This indication should be included with the claim, along with the result of the PET scan, using the appropriate modifiers. For example, you should not get a claim showing G0125 with modifier N; if you do, deny the claim.
- In order to ensure that the PET scan is properly coordinated with other diagnostic modalities, PET scan claims must include the results of concurrent thoracic CT, which is necessary for anatomic information.
- In view of the limitations on this coverage, you may consider conducting pre- or post-payment reviews to determine that the use of PET scans is consistent with Medicare instructions. Providers must keep patient record information on file for each Medicare patient for whom a PET scan claim is made. These medical records may be used in any review and must include information necessary to substantiate the need for the PET scan.

NOTE: PET scans are not covered by Medicare for routine screening of asymptomatic patients, regardless of the level of risk factors applicable to such patients.

B. Effective for Services on or After January 1, 1998, Claims for Staging Metastatic Non-Small-Cell Lung Carcinoma (NSCLC) Must Include:

- Since this service is covered only in those cases in which a primary cancerous lung tumor has been confirmed, claims for PET must show evidence of the detection of such primary lung tumor. For example, a diagnosis code indicating the existence of a primary tumor or any other evidence you deem appropriate. A surgical pathology report that documents the presence of an NSCLC must be kept on file with the provider. If you deem it necessary, contact the provider for a copy of this documentation.
- Whole body PET scan results and results of concurrent CT and follow-up lymph node biopsy. In order to ensure that the PET scan is properly coordinated with other diagnostic modalities, claims must include both (1) the results of concurrent thoracic CT, which is necessary for anatomic information, and (2) the results of any lymph node biopsy performed to finalize whether the patient will be a surgical candidate.

NOTE: A lymph node biopsy is not covered in the case of a negative CT and negative PET where the patient is considered a surgical candidate, given the presumed absence of metastatic NSCLC.

C. Effective for Dates of Service on or After July 1, 1999, PET Claims For the Following Conditions Must Include:

- Recurring colorectal cancer with rising CEA:
  - —A statement or other evidence of previous colorectal tumor;
  - —The results of the concurrent CT, which is necessary for anatomic information; and
  - —The necessary procedure codes and/or modifiers.
- Staging or restaging of lymphoma in place of a gallium study or lymphangiogram:
  - —A statement or other evidence of previously made diagnosis of lymphoma;
  - —The results of the concurrent CT, which is necessary for anatomic information; and
  - —The date of the last gallium scan or lymphangiogram when done in the same facility as the PET scan.
- Recurrent melanoma prior to surgery:
  - —A statement or other evidence of previous melanoma;
  - —The results of the concurrent CT, which is necessary for anatomic information; and
  - —The date of the last gallium scan when done in the same facility as the PET scan.

As with any claim, but particularly in view of the limitations on this coverage, you may decide to conduct post-payment reviews to determine that the use of PET scans is consistent with this instruction. PET scan facilities must keep patient record information on file for each Medicare patient for whom a PET scan claim is made. These medical records will be used in any post-payment reviews and must include the information necessary to substantiate the need for the PET scan.

4173.5 HCPCS and Modifiers for PET Scans.—Providers should use HCPCS codes G0030 through G0047 to indicate the conditions under which a PET scan was done for imaging of the perfusion of the heart. These codes represent the global service, so providers performing just the technical or professional component of the test should use modifier TC or 26, respectively. The following codes should be reported for PET scans used for the imaging of the lungs:

- G0125—PET lung imaging of solitary pulmonary nodules using 2-[fluorine-18]-fluoro-2-deoxy-D-glucose (FDG), following CT (71250/71260* or 1270*); or
- G0126—PET lung imaging of solitary pulmonary nodules using 2-[fluorine-18]-fluoro-2-deoxy-D-glucose (FDG), following CT (71250/71260* or 71270*); for initial staging of pathologically diagnosed NSCLC.
- G0163—PET, whole body for recurrence of colorectal or colorectal metastatic cancer; or
- G0164—PET, whole body, for staging and characterization of lymphoma; or
- G0165—PET, whole body, for recurrence of melanoma or melanoma metastatic cancer.

NOTE: The payment for the radiotracer or radiopharmaceutical is included in the relative value units of the technical components of the above procedure codes. Do not make any separate payments for these agents for PET scans.

In addition, providers must indicate the results of the PET scan and the previous test using a two-digit modifier. (The modifier is not required for technical component-only billings or billings to the intermediary.) The first character should indicate the result of the PET scan; the second character should indicate the results of the prior test. Depending on the procedure codes with which the modifiers are used, the meaning of the modifier will be apparent. The test result modifiers and their descriptions are as follows:

*CPT only © *Current Procedural Terminology, 2002 Professional Edition*, American Medical Association. All rights reserved.

Modifier	Description
N	Negative;
E	Equivocal;
P	Positive, but not suggestive of, extensive ischemia or not suggestive of malignant single pulmonary nodule; and
S	Positive and suggestive of extensive ischemia (greater than 20 percent of the left ventricle) or malignant single pulmonary nodule.

These modifiers may be used in any combination.

4173.6 Claims Processing Instructions for PET Scan Claims

A. FDA Approval.—PET scans are covered only when performed at a PET imaging center with a PET scanner that has been approved or cleared by the FDA. When submitting the claim, the provider is certifying this and must be able to produce a copy of this approval upon request. An official approval letter need not be submitted with the claim.

You may consider conducting a review on a post-payment basis to verify, based on a sample of PET scan claims, that the PET scan was performed at a center with a PET scanner that was / Penta/.default/.import ascii/42404 appa approved or cleared for marketing.

B. EOMB and Remittance Messages.—Providers must indicate the results of the PET scan and the previous test using a two-digit modifier as specified in §4173.4. Deny assigned claims received prior to April 1, 1996 without such modifier, using the following EOMB message:

> "Your service was denied because information required to make payment was missing. We have asked your provider to resubmit a claim with the missing information so that it may be reprocessed." (Message 9.33)

Deny unassigned claims received prior to April 1, 1996, without the two-digit modifier using the following EOMB message:

> "Medicare cannot pay for this service because the claim is missing information/documentation. Please ask your provider to submit a new, complete claim to us." (Messages 9.8 and 9.15)

Claims received on or after April 1, 1996, without the two-digit modifier must be returned as unprocessable. (See §3005.)

Use the following remittance message for assigned claims:

> "The procedure code is inconsistent with the modifier used, or a required modifier is missing." (Reason Code 4)

Assigned claims for dates of service on or after January 1, 1998 without the proper documentation must be denied using the following EOMB message:

> "Your service was denied because information required to make payment was missing. We have asked your provider to resubmit a claim with the missing information so that it may be reprocessed." (Message 9.33)

C. Type of Service.—The type of service for the PET scan codes in the "G" range is 4, Diagnostic Radiology.

NOTE: Advise providers of this payment requirement and recommend that they coordinate the billing of their claims to avoid delays resulting from a claim for G0161 preceding the corresponding claim for G0160.

4182 PROSTATE CANCER SCREENING TESTS AND PROCEDURES

The following sections summarize coverage requirements and detail claims processing procedures for prostate cancer screening tests and procedures.

4182.1 Coverage Summary.—Sections 1861(s)(2)(P) and 1861(oo) of the Social Security Act (as added by section 4103 of the Balanced Budget Act of 1997), provide for coverage of certain prostate cancer screening tests and procedures subject to certain coverage, frequency, and payment limitations. Effective for services furnished on or after January 1, 2000, Medicare will cover prostate cancer screening tests and procedures for the early detection of prostate cancer. Coverage currently consists of the following tests and procedures furnished to an individual for the early detection of prostate cancer:

A. Screening Digital Rectal Examination.—This test is a clinical examination of an individual's prostate for nodules or other abnormalities of the prostate; and

B. Screening Prostate Specific Antigen (PSA) Blood Test.—This test detects the marker for adenocarcinoma of the prostate.

For more information regarding coverage of prostate cancer screening tests and procedures, refer to section 50-55 of the *Coverage Issues Manual.*

4182.2 Requirements for Submitting Claims.—Submit claims for prostate cancer screening tests on Health Insurance Claim Form HCFA-1500 or electronic equivalent. Follow the general instructions in section 2010, Purpose of Health Insurance Claim Form HCFA-1500, *Medicare Carriers Manual,* Part 4, Chapter 2.

4182.3 HCPCS Codes and Payment Requirements.—The following table lists coverable codes and services for prostate cancer screening tests and procedures. Pay for these services according to the appropriate fee schedule when all of the requirements noted are met.

4182.4 Calculating the Frequency.—Once a beneficiary has received any (or all) of the covered prostate cancer screening test/procedures, he may receive another (or all) of such test/procedures after 11 full months have passed. To determine the 11-month period, start your count beginning with the month after the month in which any (or all) of the previous covered screening test/procedures was performed.

Example: The beneficiary received a screening PSA test on February 25, 2000. Start your count beginning March 2000. The beneficiary is eligible to receive another screening PSA test on February 1, 2001 (the month after 11 months have passed.)

4182.5 CWF Edits—CWF will edit prostate cancer screening tests and procedures for age, frequency, sex, and valid HCPCS code.

4182.6 Correct Coding Requirements.—Billing and payment for a Digital Rectal Exam (DRE) (G0102) is to be bundled into the payment for a covered E/M service (CPT codes 99201-99456* and 99499*) when the two services are furnished to a patient on the same day. If the DRE is the only service or is provided as part of an otherwise noncovered service, HCPCS code G0102 would be payable separately if all other coverage requirements are met.

4182.7 Diagnosis Coding Requirements.—There are no specific diagnosis requirements for prostate screening tests and procedures. However, prostate cancer screening digital rectal examina-

HCPCS Code; Type of Service (TOS)	Description	Payment	
		Requirements	Methodology/Fee Schedule
G0102; TOS = 1	Prostate cancer screening; digital rectal examination	1. Performed on a male Medicare beneficiary over 50 years of age (i.e., for services starting at least one day after the beneficiary attained age 50). 2. Performed by one of the following, who is authorized under State law to perform the examination, is fully knowledgeable about the beneficiary, and is responsible for explaining the results of the examination to the beneficiary: a. Doctor of medicine or osteopathy b. Qualified physician assistant c. Qualified nurse practitioner d. Qualified clinical nurse specialist e. Qualified certified nurse midwife 3. Performed at a frequency no greater than once every 12 months (See §4182.4).	1. Refer to the physician's fee schedule. 2. Apply deductible and coinsurance. 3. Claims from physicians for these examinations where assignment was not taken are subject to the Medicare limiting charge. (See §7555). 4. Correct Coding Initiative requirements apply. See §4182.6
G0103; TOS = 5	Prostate cancer screening; PSA test	1. Performed on a male Medicare beneficiary over 50 years of age (i.e., for services starting at least one day after the beneficiary attained age 50) 2. Ordered by one of the following, who is authorized under State law to perform the examination, is fully knowledgeable about the beneficiary, and is responsible for explaining the results of the examination to the beneficiary: a. Physician (doctor of medicine or osteopathy) b. Qualified physician assistant c. Qualified nurse practitioner d. Qualified clinical nurse specialist e. Qualified certified nurse midwife 3. Performed at a frequency no greater than once every 12 months. (See §4182.4.)	1. Refer to the clinical laboratory fee schedule; payment for this test is the same as for code "84153*, PSA; total." 2. Do not apply deductible and coinsurance.

tions and screening Prostate Specific Antigen (PSA) blood tests must be billed using screening ("V") code V76.44 (Special Screening for Malignant Neoplasms, Prostate).

4182.8 Denial Messages.

A. Remittance Advice Notices.—If the claim for a screening prostate antigen test or screening digital rectal examination is being denied because the patient is not over 50 years of age, use existing American National Standard Institute (ANSI) X12-835 claim adjustment reason code 6 "the procedure code is inconsistent with the patient's age" , at the line level along with line level Remark Code M140 "Service not covered until after the patient's 50th birthday, i.e., no coverage prior to the day after the patient's 50th birthday"

If the claim for a screening prostate antigen test or screening digital rectal examination is being denied because the time period between the test/procedure has not passed, use existing ANSI X12-835 claim adjustment reason code 119 "Benefit maximum for this time period has been reached" at the line level.

If the claim for a screening prostate antigen test or screening digital rectal examination is being denied due to the absence of diagnosis code V76.44 on the claim, use existing ANSI X-12-835 claim adjustment reason code 47, "This (these) diagnosis (es) is (are) not covered, missing, or invalid."

B. Medicare Summary Notice (MSN) and Explanation of Your Medicare Benefits (EOMB) Messages.—If the claim for a screening prostate specific antigen test or screening digital rectal examination is being denied because the patient is not over 50 years of age, the following new line (May 2000) MSN or EOMB message:

- "This service is not covered until after the beneficiary's 50th birthday." (MSN Message 18.19, EOMB Message 18.27)

The Spanish version of this MSN or EOMB message should read:

- "Este servicio no está cubierto hasta después de que el beneficiario cumpla 50 años."

If a claim for screening prostate specific antigen test or screening digital rectal examination is being denied because the minimum time period between the same test or procedure has not elapsed, use the following MSN or EOMB message:

- "Service is being denied because it has not been [12/24/48] months since your last [test/procedure] of this kind." (MSN Message 18.14, EOMB Message 18.23)

The Spanish version of this MSN or EOMB message should read:

- "Este servicio está siendo denegado ya que no han transcurrido [12, 24, 48] meses desde el último [examen/procedimiento] de esta clase."

4270. ESRD BILL PROCESSING PROCEDURES

Physicians, independent laboratories, and beneficiaries must submit claims (Form CMS-1500 and Form CMS-1490S) to their local carrier for services furnished to end stage renal disease (ESRD) beneficiaries. Suppliers of Method II dialysis equipment and supplies will submit their claims (Form CMS-1500 or electronic equivalent) to the appropriate Durable Medical Equipment Regional Carriers (DMERCs). All ESRD facilities must submit their claims to their appropriate fiscal intermediary (FI).

4270.1 Home Dialysis Supplies and Equipment.—Only a supplier that is not a dialysis facility may submit a claim to a DMERC for home dialysis supplies and equipment. Suppliers will submit these claims on Form CMS-1500. Under Method II, beneficiaries may not submit any claims and cannot be directly paid any benefits for home dialysis equipment and supplies. DMERCs must deny unassigned claims.

Use the following messages for beneficiary submitted or unassigned claims."

MSN # 16.6: "This item or service cannot be paid unless the provider accepts assignment.

Spanish: "Este article servicio no se pagará a menos de que el proveedor acepte asignación."

MSN # 16.7: "Your provider must complete and submit your claim."

Spanish: "Su proveedor debe completar y someter su reclamación."

MSN # 16.36: "If you have already paid it, you are entitled to a refund from this provider."

Spanish: "Si usted ya lo ha pagado, tiene derecho a un reebolso de su proveedor."

In accordance with the Code of Federal Regulations (CFR), Method II patients who self-administer erythropoietin (EPO) may only obtain EPO from either their Method II supplier, or a Medicare certified ESRD facility. (See 42 CFR 414.335)

For purposes of home dialysis, a skilled nursing facility (SNF) may qualify as a beneficiary's home.

A. Requirements for Payment.—DMERCS may make payment to home dialysis suppliers only if all of the following conditions are met:

- The beneficiary has elected Method II (see §4271);
- The supplier accepts assignment for all Method II equipment and supplies;
- The supplier agrees to be the beneficiary's sole supplier for all home dialysis equipment and supplies;
- The supplier agrees to bill on a monthly basis for the quantity of supplies used during that period. (However, there is one exception to this rule. Beneficiaries are permitted to retain 1 month's worth of supplies in reserve in case of emergency);
- The supplier maintains a written certification in its files that it has a written agreement with a Medicare approved dialysis facility under which the facility will furnish all necessary support, backup, and emergency dialysis services, for each beneficiary the supplier services. (For Medicare beneficiaries who are also entitled to military or veterans benefits, a military or Veteran's Administration (VA) hospital satisfies this requirement.) The supplier may not provide supplies or services to the beneficiary, or submit a claim to the DMERC, until they have a valid written support service facility agreement for that beneficiary. The dialysis facility must be a reasonable distance from the beneficiary's home in order to furnish these services. Determine a reasonable distance by considering such variables as terrain, whether the patient's home is located in a rural or urban area, and the usual distances traveled and time in transit by patients in the area in obtaining health care services.

In cases where a supplier cannot establish an agreement with a support service facility that is within a reasonable distance from the patient's home, the supplier must establish a written agreement with a support service facility outside of the geographic area of the patient's home. However, in this situation, the support service facility must establish a written agreement with a dialysis facility within the beneficiary's geographic region to provide any required in-facility dialysis treatments. In this situation, the support service facility will be responsible for providing all other necessary services for the patient, and must provide for the coordination of the patient's care and monitor the patient through frequent visits to the patient's home. The signed agreement with the Method II supplier must stipulate how the support services facility will provide each of the required support services. The written agreement must include documentation to support the arrangement with the local facility for any needed in-facility services.

Home dialysis support services include, but are not limited to:

- Surveillance of the patient's home adaptation, including provisions for visits to the home in accordance with a written plan prepared and periodically reviewed by a team that includes the patient's physician and other professionals familiar with the patient's condition;
- Furnishing dialysis-related emergency services;
- Consultation for the patient with a qualified social worker and a qualified dietician;
- Maintaining a recordkeeping system which assures continuity of care;

- Maintaining and submitting all required documentation to the ESRD network;
- Assuring that the water supply is of the appropriate quality;
- Assuring that the appropriate supplies are ordered on an ongoing basis;
- Arranging for the provision of all ESRD related laboratory tests;
- Testing and appropriate treatment of water used in dialysis;
- Monitoring the functioning of dialysis equipment;
- All other necessary dialysis services as required under the ESRD conditions for coverage; and
- Since home dialysis support services include maintaining a medical record for each home dialysis patient, the Method II supplier must report to the support service dialysis facility within 30 days all items and services that it furnished to the patient so that the facility can record this information in the patient's medical record.

Method II suppliers must maintain documentation to support the existence of a written agreement with a Medicare certified support service facility within a reasonable distance from the beneficiary's home. Effective July 1, 2002, suppliers must use the "ZX" modifier on the line item level for all home. Effective July 1, 2002, suppliers must use the "KX" modifier on the line item level for all Method II home dialysis claims to indicate that they have this documentation on file, and must provide it to the DMERC upon request. As of July 1, 2002, DMERCs must front end reject any Method II claims that do not have the "KX" modifier at the line item level. The supplier may correct and resubmit the claim with the appropriate modifier. DMERCs and the standard systems must make all systems changes necessary to reject Method II claims that do not have the "KX" modifier. DMERCs must publish this new requirement on their websites and in their next regularly scheduled supplier bulletins.

B. Amount of Payment.—If the supplier bills a package or kit of supplies, the DMERC must request a list of the items in the kit in order to price it initially. The allowance per month under Method II for home dialysis equipment and supplies may not exceed $1,490.85 per month for all forms of dialysis except continuous cycling peritoneal dialysis (CCPD). For CCPD, the allowance may not exceed $1,974.45 per month. The actual amount paid is based on this limit or any lower limit that you have set (e.g., by applying the usual reasonable charge rules or the inherent reasonableness instructions in §5246.7) less the Part B coinsurance and any unmet Part B deductible amounts.

C. Sample Letter to Method II Supplier.—DMERCs must explain the Medicare requirements to every Method II supplier that they service. Below is a sample letter for DMERC use.

Dear Method II Supplier:

Our records show that you supply home dialysis equipment and/or supplies to Medicare home dialysis beneficiaries who have chosen payment Method II. The Medicare law was recently changed for Method II. Effective February 1, 1990, there will be a limit on the amount that a dialysis supplier may be paid under Method II.

The payment limit for Method II benefits for all forms of dialysis except CCPD cannot exceed the median composite rate for hospital-based dialysis facilities. The portion of this amount that applies to supplies and equipment is $1,490.85 per month. The limit for CCPD supplies and equipment is based on 130 percent of the composite rate and is $1,974.45 per month. These limits are subject to the usual Medicare Part B deductible and coinsurance amounts.

There are additional requirements for Method II benefits. Each Method II beneficiary must certify in writing that he or she deals with a single supplier for all home dialysis equipment and supplies. Beneficiaries who have chosen Method II before February 1, 1990, are presumed to meet this requirement and need not submit this certification. If a beneficiary chooses Method II on or after February 1, 1990, the beneficiary (or the dialysis facility or the supplier on the beneficiary's behalf) writes the following in Block 8 of the Form HCFA-382:

"I certify that I have only one Method II supplier."

As a Method II home dialysis supplier, in order to be paid Medicare benefits, you must:

- Be the beneficiary's sole supplier for all home dialysis equipment and supplies needed by the beneficiary;
- Accept assignment of Medicare benefits for all home dialysis equipment and supplies you supply to Medicare beneficiaries. If you do not accept assignment, inform your Medicare beneficiaries that you do not accept assignment and that, therefore, Medicare CANNOT pay for his/her home dialysis equipment or supplies;
- Certify in writing to each beneficiary's DMERC that, on behalf of each of your Medicare beneficiaries, you have a written agreement with a Medicare approved dialysis facility under which the facility will furnish all necessary support, backup, and emergency dialysis services. Support services inlcude maintaining the patient's medical record and providing information required by the ESRD network. For each of your Medicare beneficiaries, you must have this agreement with a dialysis facility that is a reasonable distance from the beneficiary's home. A reasonable distance is determined by taking into account variables such as terrain, whether the patient's home is located in an urban or rural area, and the usual distances traveled and time in transit by patients in the area when obtaining health care services. You need not identify the individual beneficiaries;
- Report to the back-up dialysis facility within 30 days all items and services that you furnish to the patient so that his information can be recorded by the facility in the medical record; and
- Agree to generally bill once a month and for only 1 month's quantity of supplies at a time. In the event that a beneficiary becomes a hospital inpatient for at least 3 days (not counting the day of admission or discharge), you must prorate the following month's supply bills to account for supplies the beneficiary did not use while an inpatient.

4270.2 Bill Review of Laboratory Services.—See §5114.1 for a detailed description of payment for outpatient clinical diagnostic laboratory tests using fee schedules and for specimen collection fees.

All laboratory tests not included under the ESRD composite rate payment and performed by an independent laboratory for dialysis patients of independent dialysis facilities must be billed by the independent laboratory to carriers. The fee schedule applies to all clinical diagnostic tests except for tests already included under the ESRD composite rate payment. These tests are reimbursed only through the composite rate paid by the intermediary.

Laboratory tests not included under the ESRD composite rate payment, including all laboratory tests furnished to home dialysis patients who have selected payment Method II (see §4271), are billed to and paid by you at the fee schedule, if the tests are performed by an independent laboratory for an independent dialysis facility patient.

For purposes of the fee schedule, clinical diagnostic laboratory services include all laboratory tests listed in codes 80002-89399* of the Current Procedural Terminology Fourth Edition (CPT-4) with the following exceptions:

85095-85109*	Codes dealing with bone marrow smears and biopsies
85120*	Bone marrow transplant
88000-88130*	Certain cytopathology services
88160-88199*	Certain cytopathology services
88260-88299*	Cytogenetic studies
88300-88399*	Surgical pathology services

Services excluded from the fee schedule when billed by an independent laboratory are payable under existing reasonable charge rules.

Where tests not included in the composite rate are performed, the lab includes all tests (both those included in the composite rate and those that meet the frequency guidelines) on the bill. The tests listed below are included in the composite rate if their frequency does not exceed that which is indicated. Do not pay for tests up to the frequency described as they are paid under the composite rate. Tests in excess of the frequency may be paid unless you determine they are not medically necessary. Medical documentation is required to substantiate the frequency. A diagnosis of renal disease is not sufficient. The nature of the illness or injury (diagnosis, complaint, or symptom) requiring the performance of the test(s) must be present on the claim. A diagnosis from the ICD-9-CM coding system may be shown in lieu of a narrative description.

Laboratory Tests For Hemodialysis, Peritoneal Dialysis, and CCPD Included in the Composite Rate

1. Per Treatment
   - All hematocrit or hemoglobin and clotting time tests furnished incident to dialysis treatments.
2. Weekly
   - Prothrombin time for patients on anti-coagulant therapy
   - Serum creatinine
   - Weekly or thirteen per quarter
   - BUN
3. Monthly

• Serum calcium	• Serum bicarbonate	• Alkaline phosphatase
• Serum chloride	• Serum phosphorous	• AST, SGOT
• Total protein	• Serum potassium	• LDH
• CBC	• Serum albumin	

Laboratory Tests For CAPD Included in the Composite Rate

Monthly

BUN	Magnesium	Alkaline Phosphatase
Creatinine	Phosphate	LDH
Sodium	Potassium	AST, SGOT
CO2	Total Protein	HCT
Calcium	Albumin	Hgb
		Dialysate Protein

A. Automated Profile Tests.—Clinical laboratory tests can be performed individually or in groups on automated profile equipment. If a clinical laboratory test is performed individually, it is paid in accordance with §§5114ff. If clinical laboratory tests are performed as part of an automated profile, then the following procedure applies:

1. Determine which of the laboratory tests in the automated profile are included under the composite rate and which are separately billable ESRD laboratory tests.

2. Determine the payment allowance of the automated profile by comparing it to the total payment allowances of the covered laboratory tests in the automated profile when the medically necessary tests in the profile are performed individually. The payment allowance of the automated profile is the lower of these two amounts. (See §5114.1.L.) If the payment allowance for the automated profile containing only the medically necessary tests is lower, you must determine the percentage of covered tests included under the composite rate payment. If 50 percent or more of the covered tests are included under the composite rate payment, then the entire profile is included within the composite payment. In this case, no separate payment in addition to the composite rate is made for any of the separately billable tests. If more than 50 percent of the covered tests are separately billable, the entire automated profile is considered separately billable. In this case, the entire automated profile is paid for in addition to the ESRD composite rate.

If the lower payment allowance is the payment allowance of the laboratory tests taken individually, the tests may be billed individually. In this case, the tests included under the composite rate are not billed or paid separately, and the tests that are not included under the composite rate are billed and paid separately.

B. Separately Billable Tests Furnished by Hospital-Based Facilities.—Hospital-based facilities are paid for the separately billable ESRD laboratory tests furnished to their outpatients following the same rules that apply to all other Medicare covered outpatient laboratory services furnished by a hospital.

C. Separately Billable Tests Furnished to Patients of Independent Dialysis Facilities.—All separately billable ESRD clinical laboratory services furnished to patients of independent dialysis facilities must be billed by and reimbursed to the person or entity that performs the laboratory test in accordance with usual Medicare program rules. Independent dialysis facilities with the appropriate clinical laboratory certification may perform and bill their intermediary for separately billable laboratory services. Independent dialysis facilities are paid for separately billable clinical laboratory tests according to the Medicare laboratory fee schedule for independent laboratories.

Following are tests not included in the composite rate that may be paid at the frequency shown without medical documentation. Tests in excess of that frequency require medical documentation. A diagnosis of ESRD alone is not sufficient medical documentation. The nature of the illness or injury (diagnosis, complaint, or symptom) requiring the performance of the test(s) must be present on the claim. A diagnosis from the ICD-9-CM coding system may be shown in lieu of a narrative description.

- Guidelines for Separately Billable Tests for Hemodialysis, IPD, and CCPD
  - Serum aluminum—one every 3 months
  - Serum ferritin—one every 3 months
- Guidelines for CAPD
  - Every 3 months
    - WBC
    - RBC
    - Platelet count
  - Every 6 months
    - Residual renal function
    - 24 hour urine volume

Specimen Collection Fee.—(See §5114.6D for additional information concerning the specimen collection fee.) Allow separate charges made by independent laboratories for drawing or collecting specimens up to $3. Do not pay this fee to anyone who has not actually extracted the specimen from the patient. Only one collection fee is allowed for each patient encounter, regardless of the number of specimens drawn. When a series of specimens is required to complete single tests, treat the series as a single encounter. Allow a specimen collection fee in circumstances such as drawing a blood sample through venipuncture or collecting a urine sample by catheterization.

A specimen collection fee is not allowed when the specimen is taken to perform a laboratory test reimbursed under the composite rate. However, if a home dialysis patient selects reimbursement Method II and all other criteria for payment are met, pay an independent laboratory the specimen collection fee for specimens collected from the patient.

4273 CLAIMS FOR PAYMENT FOR EPOETIN ALFA (EPO)

4273.1 Completion of Initial Claim for EPO.—The following information is required. Due to space limitations, some items must be documented on a separate form. Therefore, initial claims are generally submitted on paper unless your electronic billers are able to submit supplemental documentation with EMC claims. Return incomplete assigned claims in accordance with §3311. Develop incomplete unassigned claims.

A. Diagnoses.—The diagnoses must be submitted according to ICD-9-CM and correlated to the procedure. This information is in Items 23A and 24D of the Form HCFA-1500.

B. Hematocrit (HCT)/Hemoglobin (Hgb).—There are special HCPCS codes for reporting the injection of EPO. These allow the simultaneous reporting of the patient's latest HCT or Hgb reading before administration of EPO.

Instruct the physician and/or staff to enter a separate line item for injections of EPO at different HCT/Hgb levels. The Q code for each line item is entered in Item 24C.

1. Code Q9920—Injection of EPO, per 1,000 units, at patient HCT of 20 or less/Hgb of 6.8 or less.

2. Codes Q9921 through Q9939—Injection of EPO, per 1,000 units, at patient HCT of 21 to 39/Hgb of 6.9 to 13.1. For HCT levels of 21 or more, up to a HCT of 39/Hgb of 6.9 to 13.1, a Q code that includes the actual HCT levels is used. To convert actual Hgb to corresponding HCT values for Q code reporting, multiply the Hgb value by 3 and round to the nearest whole number. Use the whole number to determine the appropriate Q code.

EXAMPLES: If the patient's HCT is 25/Hgb is 8.2–8.4, Q9925 must be entered on the claim. If the patient's HCT is 39/Hgb is 12.9–13.1, Q9939 is entered.

3. Code Q9940—Injection of EPO, per 1,000 units at patient HCT of 40 or above.

A single line item may include multiple doses of EPO administered while the patient's HCT level remained the same.

C. Units Administered.—The standard unit of EPO is 1,000. The number of 1,000 units administered per line item is included on the claim. The physician's office enters 1 in the units field for each multiple of 1,000 units. For example, if 12,000 units are administered, 12 is entered. This information is shown in Item 24F (Days/Units) on Form HCFA-1500.

In some cases, the dosage for a single line item does not total an even multiple of 1,000. If this occurs, the physician's office rounds down supplemental dosages of 0 to 499 units to the prior 1,000 units. Supplemental dosages of 500 to 999 are rounded up to the next 1,000 units.

EXAMPLES: A patient's HCT reading on August 6 was 22/Hgb was 7.3. The patient received 5,000 units of EPO on August 7, August 9, and August 11, for a total of 15,000 units. The first line of Item 24 of Form HCFA-1500 shows:

Dates of Service	Procedure Code	Days or Units
8/7–8/11	Q9922	15

On September 13, the patient's HCT reading increased to 27/Hgb increased to 9. The patient received 5,100 units of EPO on September 13, September 15, and September 17, for a total of 15,300 units. Since less than 15,500 units were given, the figure is rounded down to 15,000. This line on the claim form shows:

Dates of Service	Procedure Code	Days or Units
9/13–9/17	Q9927	15

On October 16, the HCT level increased to 33/Hgb increased to 11. The patient received doses of 4,850 units on October 16, October 18, and October 20 for a total of 14,500 units. Since more than 14,500 units were administered, the figure is rounded up to 15,000. Form HCFA-1500 shows:

Dates of Service	Procedure Code	Days or Units
10/16–10/20	Q9933	15

D. Date of the patient's most recent HCT or Hgb.

E. Most recent HCT or Hgb level prior to initiation of EPO therapy.

F. Date of most recent HCT or Hgb level prior to initiation of EPO therapy.

G. Patient's most recent serum creatinine, within the last month, prior to initiation of EPO therapy.

H. Date of most recent serum creatinine prior to initiation of EPO therapy.

I. Patient's weight in kilograms.

J. Patient's starting dose per kilogram. (The usual starting dose is 50–100 units per kilogram.)

When a claim is submitted on Form HCFA-1500, these items are submitted on a separate document. It is not necessary to enter them into your claims processing system. This information is used in utilization review.

4450 PARENTERAL AND ENTERAL NUTRITION (PEN)

PEN coverage is determined by information provided by the attending physician and the PEN supplier. A certification of medical necessity (CMN) contains pertinent information needed to ensure consistent coverage and payment determinations nationally. A completed CMN must accompany and support the claims for PEN to establish whether coverage criteria are met and to ensure that the PEN provided is consistent with the attending physician's prescription.

The medical and prescription information on a PEN CMN can be completed most appropriately by the attending physician, or from information in the patient's records by an employee of the physician for the physician's review and signature. Although PEN suppliers may assist in providing PEN items, they cannot complete the CMN since they do not have the same access to patient information needed to properly enter medical or prescription information.

A. Scheduling and Documenting Certifications and Recertifications of Medical Necessity for PEN.—A PEN CMN must accompany the initial claim submitted. The initial certification is valid for three months. Establish the schedule on a case-by-case basis for recertifying the need for PEN therapy. A change in prescription for a beneficiary past the initial certification period does not restart the certification process. A period of medical necessity ends when PEN is not medically required for two consecutive months. The entire certification process, if required, begins after the period of two consecutive months has elapsed.

B. Initial Certifications.—In reviewing the claim and the supporting data on the CMN, compare certain items, especially pertinent dates of treatment. For example, the start date of PEN coverage cannot precede the date of physician certification. The estimated duration of therapy must be contained on the CMN. Use this information to verify that the test of permanence is met. Once coverage is established, the estimated length of need at the start of PEN services will determine the recertification schedule. (See §4450 A.)

Verify that the information shown on the certification supports the need for PEN supplies as billed. A diagnosis must show a functional impairment that precludes the enteral patient from swallowing and the parenteral patient from absorbing nutrients.

The attending physician and/or his/her designated employee are in a position to accurately complete the patient's medical information, including:

- The patient's general condition, estimated duration of therapy, and other treatments or therapies (see §3329 B.2.);
- The patient's clinical assessment relating to the need for PEN therapy (see §3329 B.3.); and
- The nutritional support therapy (i.e., the enteral or parenteral formulation). (See §3329 B.4.)

Initial assigned claims with the following conditions can be denied without development:

- Inappropriate or missing diagnosis or functional impairment;
- Estimated duration of therapy is less than 90 consecutive days;
- Duration of therapy is not listed;
- Supplies have not been provided;
- Supplies were provided prior to onset date of therapy; and
- Stamped physician's signature.

Develop unassigned claims for missing or incomplete information. (See §3329 C.)

Review all claims with initial certifications and recertifications before payment is authorized.

C. Revised Certifications/Change in Prescription.—Remind suppliers to submit revised certifications if the attending physician changes the PEN prescription. A revised certification is appropriate when:

- There is a change in the attending physician's orders in the category of nutrients and/or calories prescribed;
- There is a change by more than one liter in the daily volume of parenteral solutions;

- There is a change from home-mix to pre-mix to home-mix parenteral solutions;
- There is a change from enteral to parenteral or parenteral to enteral therapy; or
- There is a change in the method of infusion (e.g., from gravity-fed to pump-fed).

Do not adjust payments on PEN claims unless a revised or renewed certification documents the necessity for the change. Adjust payments timely, if necessary, for supplies since the PEN prescription was changed.

Do not exceed payment levels for the most current certification or recertification if a prescription change is not documented by a new recertification.

Adjust your diary for scheduled recertifications. When the revised certification has been considered, reschedule the next recertification according to the recertification schedule. (See §4450 A.)

D. Items Requiring Special Attention

1. Nutrients.—Category IB of enteral nutrients contains products that are natural intact protein/protein isolates commonly known as blenderized nutrients. Additional documentation is required to justify the necessity of Category IB nutrients. The attending physician must provide sufficient information to indicate that the patient:

- Has an intolerance to nutritionally equivalent (semi-synthetic) products;
- Had a severe allergic reaction to a nutritionally equivalent (semi-synthetic) product; or
- Was changed to a blenderized nutrient to alleviate adverse symptoms expected to be of permanent duration with continued use of semi-synthetic products.

Also, enteral nutrient categories III through VI require additional medical justification for coverage.

Parenteral nutrition may be either "self-mixed" (i.e., the patient is taught to prepare the nutrient solution aseptically) or "pre-mixed" (i.e., the nutrient solution is prepared by trained professionals employed or contracted by the PEN supplier). The attending physician must provide information to justify the reason for "pre-mixed" parenteral nutrient solutions.

2. Prospective Billing.—Pay for no more than a one-month supply of parenteral or enteral nutrients for any one prospective billing period. Claims submitted retroactively may include multiple months.

3. Pumps.—Enteral nutrition may be administered by syringe, gravity, or pump. The attending physician must specify the reason that necessitates the use of an enteral feeding pump. Ensure that the equipment for which payment is claimed is consistent with that prescribed (e.g., expect a claim for an I.V. pole, if a pump is used).

Effective April 1, 1990, claims for parenteral and enteral pumps are limited to rental payments for a total of 15 months during a period of medical need. A period of medical need ends when enteral or parenteral nutrients are not medically necessary for two consecutive months.

Do not allow additional rental payments once the 15-month limit is reached, unless the attending physician changes the prescription between parenteral and enteral nutrients.

Do not continue rental payments after a pump is purchased unless the attending physician changes the prescription between parenteral and enteral nutrients.

Do not begin a new 15-month rental period when a patient changes suppliers. The new supplier is entitled to the balance remaining on the 15-month rental period.

Effective October 1, 1990, necessary maintenance and servicing of pumps after the 15-month rental limit is reached includes repairs and extensive maintenance that involves the breaking down of sealed components or performing tests that require specialized testing equipment not available to the beneficiary or nursing home.

4. Supplies.—Enteral care kits contain all the necessary supplies for the enteral patient using the syringe, gravity, or pump method of nutrient administration. Parenteral nutrition care kits and their components are considered all-inclusive items necessary to administer therapy during a monthly period.

Compare the enteral feeding care kits on the claim with the method of administration indicated on the CMN.

Reduce the allowance to the amount paid for a gravity-fed care kit when billed for a pump feeding kit in the absence of documentation or unacceptable documentation for a pump.

Limit payment to a one-month supply.

Deny payment for additional components included as part of the PEN supply kit.

5. Attending Physician Identification.—A CMN must contain the attending physician's Unique Physician Identification Number (UPIN) and be signed and dated by the attending physician. A stamped signature is unacceptable.

Deny certifications and recertifications altered by "whiting out" or "pasting over" and entering new data. Consider suppliers that show a pattern of altering CMNs for educational contact and/or audit.

Be alert to certifications from suppliers who have questionable utilization or billing practices or who are under sanction. Consider an audit of any such situations.

5102.3 Transition to Fee Schedule-Relationship to Prior Rules.

A. Comparability and Inherent Reasonableness Limitations.—Effective January 1, 1989, until further notice, you may no longer apply the comparable circumstances provision contained in section 5026. Between January 1, 1989 and December 31, 1990, you may not apply the special limitations provision contained in section 5246.

B. Purchase of Items Requiring Frequent and Substantial Servicing or Capped Rental Items

1. Purchase Prior to January 1, 1989.—If the beneficiary purchased an item of equipment in either of these two categories (see section 5102.1.B or E) prior to January 1, 1989, pay the reasonable and necessary charges for maintenance and servicing of this equipment. In the event the item of equipment needs to be replaced on or after June 1, 1989, pay on a rental basis according to the instructions in section 5102.1.B. or E.

If the beneficiary purchased the equipment even though you determined that rental was more economical under the rent/purchase guidelines, or if the beneficiary made an approved purchase on an installment plan, make payment on an installment basis until the purchase price has been reached or medical necessity terminated. If the purchase price has not been reached by January 1, 1989, continue paying on an installment basis but at the monthly fee schedule amount until the purchase price is reached, the purchase price fee schedule calculated under prior instructions is reached, or the medical necessity ends, whichever occurs first. The limitation on total payments to 15 months rental (as described in section 5102.1.E) does not apply.

2. Purchase on or After June 1, 1989.—If a beneficiary purchased an item of equipment that requires frequent and substantial servicing on or after June 1, 1989, do not make payment. Also, do not make payment for maintenance and servicing or for replacement of items in either category that are purchased on or after June 1, 1989. If a beneficiary purchased an item of equipment in the capped rental category between June 1, 1989 and April 30, 1991, do not make payment. Also, do not make payment for maintenance and servicing. However, see section 5102.1.E.5 or 6 for payment of purchase options after April 30, 1991 and for payment of replacement of items purchased between June 1, 1989 and April 30, 1991.

3. Purchase Between January 1, 1989 and June 1, 1989.—If a beneficiary purchased an item of equipment in either category after December 31, 1988, but before June 1, 1989, pay monthly

installments equivalent to the rental fee schedule amounts until the medical necessity ends, the purchase price fee schedule calculated under prior instructions is reached, or the actual purchase charge has been reached, whichever occurs first. Pay the reasonable and necessary charges for maintenance and servicing of this equipment. In the event the item of equipment needs to be replaced on or after June 1, 1989, pay on a rental basis according to the instructions in section 5102.1.B. or E. Payment may be made for purchase even if the purchase was preceded by a period of rental. However, total payments for rental plus purchase of capped rental items may not exceed the amount that would have been paid had the equipment been continuously rented for 15 months. (Therefore, if a purchase occurs during a period of continuous use after 15 months of rentals have been paid, no payment may be made other than the reasonable and necessary charges for servicing as described in section 5102.1.E.4.)

C. Purchase of Oxygen Equipment

1. Purchase Prior to June 1, 1989.—If the beneficiary purchased stationary or portable oxygen equipment (see section 5102.1.F) prior to June 1, 1989, pay the reasonable and necessary charges for maintenance and servicing of this equipment. In the event the item of equipment needs to be replaced on or after June 1, 1989, pay on a rental basis according to the instructions in section 5102.1.F.

If the beneficiary purchased the equipment even though you determined that rental was more economical under the rent/purchase guidelines, or if the beneficiary made an approved purchase on an installment plan, make payment on an installment basis until the purchase price had been reached or medical necessity terminated. If the purchase price has not been reached by June 1, 1989, continue paying on an installment basis (see section 5102.1.F.9) but at the monthly fee schedule amount until the purchase price is reached or the medical necessity ends, whichever occurs first.

2. Purchase on or After June 1, 1989.—If a beneficiary purchased stationary or portable oxygen equipment on or after June 1, 1989, do not make payment for the equipment. However, make payment for the contents in accordance with section 5102.1.F.4 or 5. Also, do not make payment for maintenance and servicing or for replacement of oxygen equipment that is purchased on or after June 1, 1989.

D. 15-Month Ceiling.—For purposes of computing the 10-month purchase option or the 15-month period for capped rental items, begin counting the first month that the beneficiary continuously rented the equipment. For example, if the beneficiary began renting the equipment in July 1988, the rental month that begins in January 1989 is counted as the beneficiary's 7th month of rental. Therefore, if the equipment has been continuously rented prior to October 2, 1987, no further rental payments are made since the 15-month period is terminated before January 1, 1989. The maintenance and service provision in section 5102.1.E.4 begins July 1, 1989.

If the beneficiary has reached (on a date of service prior to January 1989) the purchase price limitation on a rental claim, do not make any further purchase or rental payments until the useful life has elapsed according to the instructions in section 5102.1.E.7. However, for capped rental items previously rented that have reached the purchase cap under the rent/purchase rules, pay claims for maintenance and servicing fees in accordance with section 5102.1.E.4 effective July 1, 1989.

E. Oxygen.—Claims for oxygen contents provided after May 31, 1989, but prior to the start of the June equipment rental month, may be paid in either of the following two ways. Either continue paying the reasonable charge payment amount for contents through the end of the May monthly rental period; or pay the reasonable charge payment amount for contents through the end of May and pay the actual charge for contents up to the fee schedule allowance for oxygen contents only as prorated for the period June 1 through the end of the May rental period. Begin paying the appropriate full fee schedule amount at the beginning of the new rental period. For example, a beneficiary's rental period began May 15, 1989. Pay on a reasonable charge basis from May 15 through June 14; or pay on a reasonable charge basis from May 15 through May 31, 1989 and pay the actual charge up to 14/31 of the oxygen contents fee (established in section 5102.1.F.4) from June 1 through June 14, 1989. Pay the lesser of the full fee schedule amount or actual charge beginning June 15, 1989.

F. Purchase Options for Capped Rental Items.

1. Electric Wheelchairs.—If the beneficiary purchases an electric wheelchair prior to May 1, 1991, pay for the wheelchair as a routinely purchased item in accordance with section 5102.1.A. If the beneficiary elects to rent an electric wheelchair prior to May 1, 1991, pay the rental fee schedule amount not to exceed the purchase price in accordance with section 5102.1.A. If, on May 1, 1991, the purchase price has not been reached, convert the monthly fee schedule amount from routinely purchased to capped rental. As such, each month's rental before and after conversion must be counted toward the 10 month purchase option in section 5102.1.E.6 and the 15 month rental cap in section 5102.1.E.2.

2. All Other Capped Rental Items.—If the beneficiary purchased a capped rental item prior to May 1, 1991, do not make payment. If the beneficiary rented a capped rental item prior to May 1, 1991, pay the rental fee schedule amount not to exceed the 15 month rental cap in accordance with section 5102.1.E.2. Each month's rental must be counted toward the 10 month purchase option in section 5102.1.E.6 and the 15 month rental cap in section 5102.1.E.2.

5112 PAYMENT TO PSYCHOLOGISTS

The methodology used for determining payment to psychologists varies according to the professional classification of the psychologist: clinical psychologist (CP) or a psychologist other than a clinical psychologist. (See §2150 and §2070.2.)

5113 PAYMENT TO CLINICAL SOCIAL WORKERS

Effective July 1, 1990, direct payment may be made to clinical social workers (CSW) for covered diagnostic and therapeutic services. (See §2152 for coverage guidelines.) Payment for all covered services is based on the lower of the actual charge or a fee schedule.

A. Fee Schedule to Be Used for Payment of Clinical Social Worker Services.—The fee schedule for clinical social worker services is set at 75 percent of the fee schedule for comparable services furnished by clinical psychologists.

B. Payment Limitation.—Clinical social worker services are subject to the outpatient mental health services limitation in §1833(c) of the Act and in §2470ff. Apply the limitation of 62.5 percent (see §2472) to the lesser of the actual charge or fee schedule amount. Diagnostic services are not subject to the limitation. (See §2476.5.)

C. Assignment Requirement.—All claims for clinical social worker services must be made on an assignment-related basis, i.e., the social worker must accept assignment, claim direct Medicare payment after the death of the beneficiary, or submit the claim under the indirect payment procedure in §7065.

D. Coinsurance and Deductible.—The annual deductible and the 20 percent Part B coinsurance apply to clinical social worker services.

E. Coding.—Use professional specialty code 80 for clinical social workers. Use HCPCS procedure codes M0601 for diagnostic services and H5010–H5030 for therapeutic services billed by clinical social workers in independent practice. Where the social worker is not practicing independently and is employed by a provider, physician, or supplier who bills for the social worker, claims for services M0601 and H5010–H5030 must be submitted with modifier QS.

See §4162 for billing instructions for CSW services in outpatient settings.

5114. PAYMENT FOR DIAGNOSTIC LABORATORY SERVICES

This section sets out payment rules for diagnostic laboratory services, i.e., (1) outpatient clinical diagnostic laboratory tests subject to the fee schedule, and (2) other diagnostic laboratory tests.

Regardless of whether a diagnostic laboratory test is performed in a physician's office, by an independent laboratory, or by a hospital laboratory for its outpatients or nonpatients, it is considered a laboratory service. When a hospital laboratory performs diagnostic laboratory tests for nonhospital patients, the laboratory is functioning as an independent laboratory. Also, when physicians and laboratories perform the same test, whether manually or with automated equipment, the services are deemed similar.

The laboratory services for which this instruction applies are those listed in §2070.1.D. The tests are not subject to the economic index under the guidelines in §5020.3.A. Any test not listed in §2070.1.D is considered a physicians' service, is subject to the economic index as described in §5020.3.A, and is not considered in implementing this instruction. The only exceptions are as specified in §5020.3.A. For example, the taking of an EKG is a laboratory service when billed separately; but an EKG interpretation alone, as well as the taking of an EKG billed with interpretation, is a physician service subject to the economic index. Similarly, clinical laboratory services not subject to the fee schedule (see '5114.1) included in office visits for which a single prevailing charge screen is maintained are subject to the economic index.

Clinical diagnostic laboratory tests subject to the fee schedule are specifically delineated in §5114.1.B.

Other diagnostic laboratory tests are laboratory tests other than clinical diagnostic laboratory tests subject to fee schedule reimbursement. Such tests include EKGs and physiological testing.

Payment for clinical diagnostic laboratory tests subject to the fee schedule is made in accordance with the instructions in §5114.1.

Generally, payment for other diagnostic laboratory tests is made in accordance with the reasonable charge methodology. Special payment rules for physicians who do not personally perform or supervise other diagnostic laboratory tests but who bill for such tests are referenced in §5258. In accordance with '5262, payment for diagnostic radiology tests is made on a fee schedule basis.

5114.1 Payment for Outpatient Clinical Diagnostic Laboratory Tests Using Fee Schedules and for Specimen Collection.—Under Part B, for services rendered on or after July 1, 1984, clinical diagnostic laboratory tests performed in a physician's office, by an independent laboratory, or by a hospital laboratory for its outpatients are reimbursed on the basis of fee schedules.

The fee schedules are established on a carrierwide basis (not to exceed a statewide basis). National fee schedules may be established beginning January 1, 1990.

The lowest charge level provisions no longer apply to clinical diagnostic laboratory tests. In addition, §5100.2.C no longer applies. This section provides that laboratory tests furnished to CAPD End Stage Renal Disease (ESRD) patients dialyzing at home are billed in the same way as any other test furnished home patients. The reasonable charge criteria were used for tests performed by an independent laboratory for the home patient. Since clinical diagnostic laboratory tests are no longer paid in accordance with the reasonable charge criteria, the fee schedule now applies to laboratory tests performed for the home ESRD dialysis patient described in §4270.2 when the tests are not covered under the ESRD composite rate.

A. Application of Fee Schedule.—The fee schedule applies to all clinical diagnostic laboratory tests except:

- Laboratory tests furnished to a hospital inpatient whose stay is covered under Part A. Laboratory tests provided by a hospital for an inpatient of such hospital that are payable under Part B (due to lack of Part A coverage) continue to be reimbursed on a reasonable cost basis.
- Laboratory tests performed by a Skilled Nursing Facility (SNF) for its own SNF inpatients and reimbursed under Part A or Part B and any laboratory tests furnished under arrangements to an SNF inpatient with Part A coverage. (The only covered source for laboratory services furnished under Part A is the SNF itself or a hospital with which the facility has a transfer agreement in effect.) Continue to reimburse such tests on a reasonable cost basis. All Part B tests, furnished by a laboratory other than the SNF's own are reimbursable only to the laboratory under the fee schedule; and
- Laboratory tests furnished by hospital-based or independent ESRD dialysis facilities that are included under the ESRD composite rate payment. (See §4270.2 for discussion of laboratory tests included in composite rate payment.) These tests are reimbursed only through this payment. Never pay anyone else for these tests. Laboratory tests that are not included under the ESRD composite rate payment and are performed by an independent laboratory for dialysis patients of independent dialysis facilities are billed to you and paid at the fee schedule. This procedure applies to all laboratory tests furnished to home dialysis patients who have selected payment Method II. (See §4271.)
- Laboratory tests furnished by hospitals in States or areas which have been granted demonstration waivers of Medicare reimbursement principles for outpatient services. The State of Maryland has been granted such demonstration waivers. This also may apply to hospitals in States granted approval for alternative payment methods for paying for hospital outpatient services under §1886(c) of the Act.
- Laboratory tests furnished to inpatients of a hospital with a waiver under §602(k) of the 1983 Amendments to the Act. (See '2255.) This section of the Act provides that an outside supplier may bill under Part B for laboratory and other nonphysician services furnished to inpatients that are otherwise paid only through the hospital. Part B payment to the outside supplier for laboratory tests furnished to inpatients under the 602(k) waiver is made at 80 percent of the reasonable charge if the claim is unassigned or at 100 percent of the reasonable charge if the claim is assigned. The fee schedule does apply to any tests furnished by the outside supplier to hospital outpatients and to nonhospital patients.
- Laboratory tests furnished to patients of rural health clinics under an all inclusive rate.
- Laboratory tests provided by a participating health maintenance organization (HMO) or health care prepayment plan (HCPP) to an enrolled member of the plan.
- Laboratory test furnished by a hospice.

B. Clinical Diagnostic Laboratory Services Subject to Fee Schedule.—For purposes of the fee schedule, clinical diagnostic laboratory services include laboratory tests listed in codes 80002-89399 of the Current Procedural Terminology, Fourth Edition (CPT-4), 1991 printing. Certain tests, however, are required to be performed by a physician and are therefore exempt from the fee schedule. These tests include:

80500-80502	Clinical pathology consultation
85095-85109	Codes dealing with bone marrow smears and biopsies
86077-86079	Blood bank services
88000-88125	Certain cytopathology services
88160-88199	Certain cytopathology services
88300-88399	Surgical pathology services

Some CPT-4 codes in the 8000 series are not clinical diagnostic laboratory tests. Such codes include codes for procedures, services, blood products and autotransfusions. Other codes for tests primarily associated with the provision of blood products are also not considered clinical diagnostic tests.

These codes include the various blood crossmatching techniques. The following codes are never subject to fee schedule limitations:

85060	86070	86595
86012	86100	89100-89105
86013	86120	89130-89141
86016-86019	86128	89350

86024 86130 89360
86034 86265-86267
86068 86455-86585

The following codes are not subject to fee schedule limitations when they are submitted for payment on the same bill with charges for blood products:

86011 86080
86014 86082-86095
86031-86033 86015

If no blood product is provided and billed on the same claim, these codes are subject to the fee schedule.

The following codes that delineate allergy, organ or disease oriented panels/profiles are not currently subject to the national limitation amounts because laboratories do not always utilize the same array or number of tests in a particular panel. However, the national limitation amount applies to each test included in the panel/profile. (See §§5114.1.F and 5114.1.G.)

80050-80099
86421-86422

Know which individual tests have been performed when claims are received using panel/profile codes. This does not need to be reported on each bill as long as you are confident that every laboratory reporting a panel or profile uses a consistent set of tests. If there is variation in content of the panel or profile, establish a uniform definition and require laboratories that do not comply with this definition to identify the individual tests when billing the panel or profile.

The following codes for unlisted or not otherwise classified clinical diagnostic laboratory tests are not subject to the national limitation amounts.

81099 87999
84999 88299
85999 89399
86999

Please note that for purposes of the fee schedule, clinical diagnostic laboratory tests include some services described as anatomic pathology services in CPT-4 (i.e., certain cervical, vaginal, or peripheral blood smears). Use the CPT-4 code 85060 only when a physician interprets an abnormal peripheral blood smear for a hospital inpatient or a hospital outpatient, and the hospital is responsible for the technical component. When a physician interpretation of an abnormal peripheral blood smear is billed by an independent laboratory, it is considered a complete or global service, and the service is not billed under the CPT-4 code 85060. A physician interpretation of an abnormal peripheral blood smear performed by an independent laboratory is considered a routine part of the ordered hematology service (i.e., those tests that include a different white blood count).

HCPCS code 88150 (cervical or vaginal smears) included both screening and interpretation in CPT-4 1986 terminology while the CPT-4 1987 terminology includes only screening. A new code, 88151, was added for those smears which require physician interpretation. Code 88151 is treated and priced in the same manner as you previously treated code 88150. Code 88151 with a "26" modifier is paid when a physician performs an interpretation of an abnormal smear for a hospital inpatient or outpatient, and the hospital is responsible for the technical component. No longer recognize the "26" modifier for code 88150. Price code 88151(26) as you would have priced code 88150(26) if the coding terminology had not been revised. Independent laboratories bill under code 88150 for normal smears and under code 88151 for abnormal smears. However, the fee schedule amount is equivalent.

Certain blood gas levels are determined either by invasive means through use of a blood specimen for a clinical diagnostic laboratory tests or by noninvasive means through ear or pulse oximetry which is not considered a clinical diagnostic laboratory test. Use CPT-4 code 82792 for invasive oximetry. Use HCPCS code M0592 for ear and pulse oximetry. Code M0592 is not subject to fee schedules. (See Coverage Issues Manual, §60-4C, for coverage requirements and Medicare Carriers Manual §5246.6 for pricing consideration.)

Services excluded from the fee schedule when billed by an independent laboratory are reimbursable under existing reasonable charge rules and assignment may be taken on a case-by-case basis unless the laboratory enrolls as a participating supplier in which event assignment is mandatory. Where a service is performed by a physician for a hospital inpatient or outpatient and meets the definition of a physician service under §8318-B, the service is subject to the Medicare Economic Index and the limitation on physician fees under §9331 of the Omnibus Budget Reconciliation Act of 1986. Such service, however, when billed by an independent laboratory as a laboratory service for a nonhospital patient (e.g., surgical pathology) is not considered a physician service for purposes of the Medicare Economic Index or the limitation on physician fees.

C. Calculation of Fee Schedule Amounts.—Set the fee schedule amounts at 60 percent of the prevailing charges for laboratory tests performed in physicians' offices by independent laboratories and for laboratory tests performed by hospital laboratories for nonhospital patients for the fee screen year beginning July 1, 1984. For hospital outpatient laboratory tests, the fee schedule amount is established at 62 percent of the prevailing charges. Beginning January 1, 1987, the fee schedule amount of 62 percent is paid for outpatient laboratory services only if provided by a qualified hospital laboratory, as described below. Beginning April 1, 1988, the fee schedule amount of 62 percent is payable only in a qualified hospital laboratory located in a sole community hospital. For this purpose, a qualified hospital laboratory is one which provides some clinical diagnostic laboratory tests 24 hours a day, 7 days a week, in order to serve a hospital's emergency room which is available to provide services 24 hours a day, 7 days week. To meet this requirement, a hospital must have physicians physically present or available within 30 minutes through a medical staff call roster to handle emergencies 24 hour a day, 7 days a week. Hospital laboratory personnel must be on duty or on call at all times to provide testing for the emergency room.

The prevailing charge is calculated as the 75th percentile of the customary charges, weighted by frequency, that were determined for the fee screen year beginning on July 1, 1984, for both physicians and independent laboratories (including hospital laboratories acting as independent laboratories) in (1) your existing service area or (2) no more than one State where your service area includes more than one entire State. In several instances, e.g., Kansas City and Washington, D.C. metropolitan areas, the area of a carrier includes portions of more than one State and that area is used in determining the prevailing charge.

Effective April 1, 1988, the fee schedules for certain automated tests, and for tests (with the exception of cytopathology) that were subject to the lowest charge level (LCL) provision prior to July 1, 1984, are adjusted in accordance with §5114.1.F.

Any rounding of initial fee schedule amounts is handled in the same manner as rounding for the application of the Medicare Economic Index. (See §5021.)

Where a hospital laboratory acts as an independent laboratory, i.e., performs tests for persons who are nonhospital patients or, where, commencing January 1, 1987, the hospital laboratory is not a qualified hospital laboratory, the services are reimbursed using the 60 percent of prevailing charge fee schedule or the adjusted fee schedule (see §5114.1.F), as appropriate. A hospital outpatient is a person who has not been admitted by the hospital as an inpatient but is registered on the hospital records as an outpatient and receives services (rather than supplies alone) from the hospital. Where a tissue sample, blood sample, or specimen is taken by personnel who are not employed by the hospital and is sent to the hospital for performance of tests, the tests are not outpatient hospital services since the patient does not directly receive services from the hospital. Where the hospital uses the category "day patient," i.e., an individual who receives hospital services during the day and is not expected to be lodged in the hospital at midnight, the individual is classified as an outpatient.

The fee schedule amounts are adjusted annually to reflect changes in the Consumer Price Index (CPI) for all Urban Consumers (U.S. city average). For laboratory tests performed on or after July 1, 1985 through December 31, 1986, the fee schedules are increased 4.1 percent. Beginning January 1, 1987, CPI adjustments are made January 1 of each year instead of July 1. The annualized index changes are as follows:

FSY	Annual Adjustment by Percent
1986	4.1
1987	5.4
1988	.0
1989	4.0
1990	4.7
1991	2.0
1992	2.0
1993	2.0

Information regarding the index changes for subsequent periods is furnished to you in time to make the necessary adjustments. In applying the annual adjustment, round calculations to the nearest penny.

The provisions in §5020.3.A provide for using the economic index to limit the prevailing charges for office visits combined with clinical laboratory tests for which you maintained a single prevailing charge screen. Since clinical diagnostic laboratory tests are no longer paid on the basis of the customary and prevailing charge criteria, do not allow the combination of laboratory tests with the physician's office visit in one prevailing charge. The fee schedule is used in determining the payment amount allowed for the laboratory tests, and the regular reasonable charge criteria and economic index are used for the office visit.

The codes and terminology in HCPCS are used in the fee schedule to identify and describe the laboratory tests. If you have not yet converted your coding systems to HCPCS, identify the equivalent tests in your own systems and use HCPCS codes for those services in establishing the fee schedules.

D. Specimen Collection Fee.—Separate charges made by physicians (except for services furnished to dialysis patients as indicated below), independent laboratories (except for services furnished to dialysis patients as indicated below), or hospital laboratories for drawing or collecting specimens are allowed up to $3 whether the specimens are referred to physicians or other laboratories for testing. This fee is not paid to anyone who has not actually extracted the specimen from the patient. Only one collection fee is allowed for each patient encounter, regardless of the number of specimens drawn. When a series of specimens is required to complete a single text (e.g., glucose tolerance test), the series is treated as a single encounter. A specimen collection fee is allowed in circumstances such as drawing a blood sample through venipuncture (i.e., inserting into a vein a needle with syringe or Vacutainer to draw the specimen) or collecting a urine sample by catheterization.

A specimen collection fee for physicians is allowed *only* when (1) it is the accepted and prevailing practice among physicians in the locality to make separate charges for drawing or collecting a specimen, *and* (2) it is the customary practice of the physician performing such services to bill separate charges for them.

A specimen collection fee is not allowed when the cost of collecting the specimen is minimal, such as a throat culture or a routine capillary puncture for clotting or bleeding time. Stool specimen collection for an occult blood test is usually done by the patient at home, and a fee for such collection is not allowed. When a stool specimen is collected during a rectal examination, the collection is an incidental byproduct of that examination. Costs such as gloves are related to the rectal examination and compensated for in the payment for the visit. Payment for performing the test is separate from the specimen collection fee. Costs such as media (e.g., the slides) and labor are included in the payment for the test.

You no longer have authority to make payment for routine handling charges where a specimen is referred by one laboratory to another. Preparatory services, e.g., where a referring laboratory prepares a specimen before transfer to a reference laboratory, are considered an integral part of the testing process, and the costs of such services are included in the charge for the total testing service.

A specimen collection fee is allowed when it is medically necessary for a laboratory technician to draw a specimen from either a nursing home patient or homebound patient. The technician must personally draw the specimen, e.g., venipuncture or urine sample by catheterization. A specimen collection fee is not allowed in situations where a patient is not in a nursing facility or confined to his home. When a laboratory performs the specimen collection, it may receive payment both for the draw and for the associated travel to obtain the specimen(s) for testing. Payment may be made to the laboratory even if the nursing facility has on-duty personnel qualified to perform the specimen collection. When the nursing home performs the specimen collection, it may only receive payment for the draw. Specimen collection performed by nursing home personnel for patients covered under Part A is paid for as part of the facility's payment for its reasonable costs, not on the basis of the specimen collection fee.

Special rules apply when services are furnished to dialysis patients. ESRD facilities are only paid by intermediaries. Therefore, never pay a specimen collection fee to an ESRD facility. The specimen collection fee is not allowed when a physician or one of the physician's employees draws the specimen from the dialysis patient because it is included in the Monthly Capitation Payment (MCP). (See section 5037.) Independent laboratories are not paid the specimen collection fee for specimens collected that are used in performing a laboratory test reimbursed under the composite rate. If a home dialysis patient selects reimbursement Method II (see section 4271) and all other criteria for payment are met, pay an independent laboratory the specimen collection fee for specimens collected from the patient.

The coinsurance and deductible provisions do not apply to the specimen collection fee where 100 percent of the fee schedule amount is payable on the basis of an assignment to the persons or entities drawing the specimen. For services (including specimen collection) rendered on or after January 1, 1987, payment to laboratories or physicians is only made on the basis of an assignment. For services rendered prior to January 1, 1987, acceptance of an assignment is optional for physicians. However, the coinsurance and deductible is applied to the specimen collection fee where a physician collects the specimen and does not accept assignment.

Complex vascular injection procedures, such as arterial punctures and venesections, are not subject either to this specimen collection policy or to the assignment provisions.

E. Who Can Bill and Receive Payment for Clinical Laboratory Tests.—

1. General

It is your responsibility to determine whether the laboratory services were performed in the office of the physician or by another laboratory. If they were performed by another laboratory, payment may be made only if the laboratory performed tests in the specialties for which it is certified under the program. (See §2070.1.D.)

When Part B payment for clinical laboratory tests is subject to the fee schedule, payment is only made to the person or entity which performed or supervised the performance of the tests, except as follows:

- Payment may be made to an independent laboratory (if it meets the special conditions below) or hospital laboratory for tests performed by another laboratory on specimens referred to it by the first laboratory. Section 3102.F describes the guidelines regarding jurisdiction for payment of independent laboratory services.
- Payment may be made to one physician for tests performed or supervised by another physician with whom he shares his practice, i.e., where the two physicians are members of a medical

group whose physicians bill in their own names rather than in the name of the group. Where the medical group bills in the name of the group for the services of the physician who performed or supervised the performance of these tests, payment is made to the group if the claim is assigned or, for services rendered on or before December 31, 1986, to the beneficiary if the claim is not assigned. See §2070.1 regarding the determination of when a laboratory is considered independent.

- Payment may only be made to the beneficiary, including home dialysis patients under Method II (see §4271), when:
  - — For services rendered on or before December 31, 1986, on the basis of an itemized bill of a physician or medical group for tests performed or supervised by that physician or group, where the physician or group is not required to meet the conditions of coverage of an independent laboratory because during any calendar year the physician or medical group performs the tests on less than 100 specimens in any particular category on referral from other physicians not in the same practice; *and* neither the physician or group has entered into an agreement to be a participating physician or supplier; or
  - — On the basis of an itemized bill of a rural health clinic for tests performed for a nonpatient of the clinic where the rural health clinic is not required to meet the conditions of coverage of an independent laboratory because, during any calendar year, the clinic performs tests on less than 100 specimens in a particular category on referral from outside physicians.

Except as noted above, unless a laboratory, physician or medical group accepts assignment, no Part B payment may be made for laboratory tests. Laboratories, physicians or medical groups that have entered into a participation agreement must accept assignment. Effective January 1, 1988, sanctions of double the violative charges, civil money penalties (up to $2,000 per violation) and/or disbarment from the program for a period of up to 5 years may be imposed on physicians and laboratories with the exception of rural health clinic laboratories that knowingly, willfully, and repeatedly bill patients on an unassigned basis. However, sole community physicians and physicians who are the sole source of an essential specialty in a community are not excluded from the program. Whenever you are notified of a sanction action, follow the procedures contained in §4165 regarding processing of claims after the imposition of a sanction. (See §§3040.3 and 3040.4 for processing instructions for claims which have been inadvertently submitted as unassigned.)

For purposes of this section, the term assignment includes assignment in the strict sense of the term as well as the procedure under which payment is made, after the death of the beneficiary, to the person or entity which furnished the service, on the basis of that person's or entity's agreement to accept the approved charge or fee you determine as the full charge or fee for the service.

When payment is made under the above rules to the beneficiary but the beneficiary is deceased, follow §7201 and §A7201. If the beneficiary has a legal guardian or representative payee, follow §7050. If an approved health benefits plan pays for the test on behalf of the beneficiary, follow §7065.

Ordinarily a physician or laboratory does not bill the Medicare program for noncovered tests. However, if the beneficiary (or his representative) contends that a clinical diagnostic laboratory test which a physician or laboratory believes is noncovered may be covered, the physician or laboratory must file a claim that includes the test, to effectuate the beneficiary's right to a determination. The physician or laboratory notes on the claim that he or it believes that the test is noncovered and is including it at the beneficiary's insistence.

Before furnishing a beneficiary a test which the physician or laboratory believes is excluded from coverage as not reasonable and necessary (rather than excluded from coverage as part of a routine physical checkup), the physician or laboratory obtains a statement from the beneficiary (or his representative) that the physician or laboratory has informed him of the noncoverage of the test and that there is a charge for the test. This is needed to protect the physician or laboratory against possible liability for the test under the limitation of liability provision.

2. Special Conditions for Referring Laboratories—In accordance with §6111(b) of OBRA of 1989 as amended by §4154 of OBRA of 1990, a referring laboratory may bill for tests for Medicare beneficiaries performed on or after May 1, 1990, by a reference laboratory only if it meets any one of the following three exceptions:

- The rural hospital exception. The referring laboratory is located in, or is part of, a rural hospital;
- The ownership related exception (formerly, the subsidiary related exception). The referring laboratory and reference laboratory are ownership related. That is:
  - — The referring laboratory is wholly-owned by the reference laboratory; or
  - — The referring laboratory wholly owns the reference laboratory; or
  - — Both the referring laboratory and the reference laboratory are wholly-owned subsidiaries of the same entity; or
- The 30 percent exception
  - — For services rendered from May 1, 1990 through April 30, 1991, no more than 30 percent of the clinical diagnostic laboratory tests *billed* annually by the referring laboratory may be performed by another laboratory other than an ownership related laboratory.
  - — For services rendered on or after January 1, 1991, no more than 30 percent of the clinical diagnostic laboratory tests for which the referring laboratory *receives requests* annually may be performed by another laboratory, other than an ownership related laboratory described above.

EXAMPLE: A laboratory receives requests for 200 tests, performs 70 tests, and refers 130 tests to a non-related laboratory. The laboratory bills Medicare for the 70 tests it performed and 30 of the tests it referred. Before January 1, 1991, the laboratory would have met the 30 percent exception. Since only the referred tests that the laboratory billed itself would have been counted, no more than 30 percent of the tests (30/100) are counted, and the laboratory may receive Medicare payment for the tests for which it bills. However, under the amended rule, all referred tests are counted. Thus, 65 percent (130/200) of the tests are considered referred tests and, since this exceeds the 30 percent standard, the laboratory may not bill for any referred tests for Medicare beneficiaries.

Effective with services rendered on or after January 1, 1991, deny bills from a referring laboratory for tests performed by a reference laboratory unless you are informed in writing by the referring laboratory that it meets one of the exceptions.

If it is later found that a referring laboratory does not, in fact, meet an exception criterion recoup payment for the referred tests improperly billed. For services rendered between January 1, 1991 and April 30, 1991, there is a date overlap in the criteria for a referring laboratory to meet the 30 percent exception. Therefore, payments made to referring laboratories for referred tests performed between January 1, 1991 and April 30, 1991 are subject to recoupment if the referring laboratory fails to meet either of the 30 percent criteria.

NOTE: This provision of §6111(b) of OBRA of 1989 has no effect on hospitals that are paid under §1833(h)(5)(A)(iii).

F. Adjusted Fee Schedule.—Beginning April 1, 1988, the 987 fee schedules for automated tests, and for tests (with the exception of cytopathology) that were subject to the LCL provision prior to July 1, 1984, are reduced by 8.3 percent. To determine the adjusted fee schedules, multiply the 1987 fee schedules by .9170 (100 percent of the 1987 fee schedule minus 8.3 percent).

The automated tests subject to the adjusted fee schedules tests are listed in codes 80002-80019 of the 1990 printing of the CPT-4.

The adjusted fee schedules also apply to the following tests that were subject to the LCL provision prior to the establishment of the fee schedule methodology. The current CPT-4 codes are provided.

Test	1989 CPT-4 Code
Cholesterol, Serum	82465
Complete Blood Count	85022
	85031
Hemoglobin	85018
Hematocrit	85014
Prothrombin Time	85610
Sedimentation Rate (ESR)	85650
	85651
Glucose	82947
	82948
Urinalysis	81000*
Blood Uric Acid	84550
Blood Urea Nitrogen	84520
White Blood Cell Count	85048

* If 81002 and 81015 are both billed, pay as though the combined service (81000) has been billed.

Where these adjusted fee schedule tests are part of allergy, disease or organ panels/profiles, you must assure that your fee for the panel/profile does not exceed the sum of the fees for the individual components after accounting for the reductions due to the adjustment.

G. National Limitation Amount.—The Consolidated Omnibus Budget Reconciliation Act (COBRA) requires national limitation amounts to be applied to the payments for outpatient clinical diagnostic laboratory services. For services rendered on or after July 1, 1986 and before April 1, 1988, the national limitation amount is 115 percent of the median of all the fee schedules established for a test for each laboratory code (separately calculated for 60 and 62 percent fee schedules). HCFA furnished you a tape file of these initial national limitation amounts for each HCPCS code for both the 60 and 62 percent fee schedules. For laboratory tests performed on or after January 1, 1987 through March 31, 1988, the initial national limitation amounts are increased by 5.4 percent and the result is the 1987 national limitation amount.

For laboratory tests performed on or after April 1, 1988 and before January 1, 1990, the national limitation amount is 100 percent of the median of all the fee schedules established for a test for each laboratory code (separately calculated for 60 and 62 percent fee schedules). The 100 percent national limitation amount for automated tests and tests formerly subject to the LCL limit, is determined by reducing the current national limitation amount by 8.3 percent (i.e., by multiplying the national limitation by .9170) and multiplying this result by .8696 (100 percent divided by 115 percent). In a single step computation, the 1987 national limitation amount is multiplied by .7974 (.9170 × .8696). For all other tests, the 100 percent national limitation amount is determined by multiplying the 1987 national limitation amount by .8696 (100 percent divided by 115 percent). Each HCFA regional office has a listing of the computed 1988 national limitation amounts which is available to you.

For laboratory tests performed on or after January 1, 1990 and before January 1, 1991, the national limitation amount is 93 percent of the median of all the fee schedules established for a test for each laboratory code (separately calculated for 60 and 62 percent fee schedules).

For laboratory tests performed on or after January 1, 1991, the national limitation amount is 88 percent of the median of all the fee schedules established for a test for each laboratory code (separately calculated for 60 and 62 percent fee schedules).

Currently, no specific national limitation amounts apply to allergy, organ, or disease oriented panels/profiles. However, the individual tests that comprise such panels are subject to the national limitation and where applicable, to the adjusted fee schedule. Ensure that the payment allowance for the panel/profile, therefore, does not exceed the lower of (1) the sum of the applicable fee schedule amounts (or national limitation amounts, if lower) for the individual tests included in the panel/profile, or (2) the sum of the fee schedule amount you have established for the panel/profile.

You are responsible for applying the national limitations in calculating your payment allowances. The national limitation amounts are computed to the nearest cent. Do not round in applying these limits. Do not use the national limitation amounts to fill gaps in your prevailing charge screens for clinical laboratory tests. Establish a fee schedule for each HCPCS code that requires gap filling and then apply the national limitation amount.

H. Summary of Payment Rules for Clinical Diagnostic Laboratory Tests.—The following rules apply in determining the amount of Part B payment for clinical laboratory tests:

- For tests performed by an independent laboratory, by a hospital or SNF laboratory (for a nonpatient of the hospital or SNF), or by a physician or medical group, the payment is the lesser of the actual charge, the fee schedule amount or the national limitation amount and the Part B deductible and coinsurance do not apply.
- If payment is made to a hospital for tests furnished for an outpatient of that hospital, the payment is the lesser of the actual charge, the fee schedule amount, or the national limitation amount and Part B deductible and coinsurance do not apply.
- For tests performed by a reference laboratory, the payment is the lesser of the actual charge by the billing laboratory, the fee schedule amount or the national limitation amount. Existing carrier jurisdiction rules apply. Part B deductible and coinsurance do not apply.
- If payment is made to a beneficiary for services prior to January 1, 1987 (see §5114.1.E.3) on the basis of an unassigned itemized bill from a physician, medical group or rural health clinic, the payment is 80 percent of the lesser of the fee schedule, the actual charge or the national limitation amount and Part B deductible and coinsurance applies.
- If payment is made to a participating hospital for tests performed for an inpatient of that hospital without Part A coverage, payment is made on a cost basis and is subject to Part B deductible and coinsurance.
- If payment is made to a participating SNF for tests performed by that SNF for an inpatient of the SNF, payment is made on a cost basis and is subject to Part B deductible and coinsurance.
- If payment is made to a hospital-based or independent dialysis facility for laboratory tests included under the composite rate payment and performed for a patient of that facility, the facility's composite rate payment includes payment for these tests and is subject to the Part B deductible and coinsurance.
- If payment is made to a rural health clinic for laboratory tests performed for a patient of that clinic, payment is made as part of the all-inclusive rate and is subject to Part B deductible and coinsurance.
- If payment is made to a hospital which has been granted a waiver of Medicare reimbursement principles for outpatient services, Part B deductible and coinsurance apply unless otherwise waived as part of an approved waiver.
- If payment is made to a participating HMO or HCPP for laboratory tests performed for a patient who is not a member, payment is the lesser of the actual charge, the national limitation amount or the fee schedule amount and the Part B deductible and coinsurance do not apply.

I. Coordination Between Intermediaries, Carriers, and the Railroad Retirement Board (RRB).—Furnish copies of fee schedules and updates (including national limitation amounts where applicable) to Medicare fiscal intermediaries and to the appropriate Travelers RRB office. (See §4540.) Provide updates at least 30 days prior to the Scheduled implementation. The fiscal intermediaries and the RRB use the fee schedules in paying for hospital laboratory tests performed for outpatients of the hospital and for persons who are not patients of the hospital. The Travelers RRB offices use the fee schedules in paying for outpatient clinical diagnostic laboratory tests. Fiscal intermediaries and the Travelers RRB consult with carriers on filling gaps in fee schedules for certain tests. If intermediaries or the Travelers RRB offices have bills for payment on laboratory tests that are not in the fee schedule, they consult with the carriers that gave them the fee schedules. If those carriers are unable to help the intermediaries, the carriers consult with other nearby carriers. HCPCS contains the American Medical Association's CPT-4 (Physician's Current Procedural Terminology). For those entities which are not familiar with HCPCS but have used the CPT-4, the coding and terminology for laboratory tests are the same in both HCPCS and the CPT-4. The CPT-4 may be used before receipt of the HCPCS.

J. Application of Fee Schedules to Medicaid.—Furnish copies of the fee schedules and the annual update (including national limitation amounts where applicable) to State agencies. Provide updates at least 30 days prior to the scheduled implementation. To obtain Federal matching funds for clinical diagnostic laboratory services, State Medicaid agencies may not pay more for the services and specimen collections than are paid for them under Medicare. This applies to payments for calendar quarters beginning on or after October 1, 1984.

Since the fee schedule provisions have been implemented on a carrierwide basis, a State may have more than one carrier servicing Medicare beneficiaries residing there. A Medicaid agency for such a State may, if it deems necessary, use the fee schedules of either one or both of the carriers to meet the Federal fund matching requirement. State Medicaid agencies may consult with ROs concerning the fee schedule, the national limitation amounts and specimen collection provisions.

K. Travel Allowance.—In addition to a specimen collection fee allowed under section 5114.1D, a travel allowance can also be made to cover the costs of travel to collect a specimen from a nursing home or homebound patient. The additional allowance can be made only where a specimen collection fee is also payable, i.e., no travel allowance is made where the technician merely performs a messenger service to pick up a specimen drawn by a physician or nursing home personnel. The travel allowance may not be paid to a physician unless the trip to the home or nursing home was solely for the purpose of drawing a specimen. Otherwise travel costs are considered to be associated with the other purposes of the trip. Since a travel allowance can now be paid routinely, the differential specimen collection amount formerly allowed when a specimen is collected from a single patient rather than multiple patients (i.e., $5 rather than $3) is discontinued.

The allowance is intended to cover the estimated travel costs of collecting a specimen and is an allowance reflecting the technician's salary and travel costs. The following HCPCS codes are used for travel allowances:

P9603—Travel allowance-one way, in connection with medically necessary laboratory specimen collection drawn from homebound or nursing home bound patient; prorated miles actually traveled (carrier allowance on per mile basis); or

P9604—Travel allowance-one way, in connection with medically necessary laboratory specimen collection drawn from homebound or nursing home bound patient; prorated trip charge (carrier allowance on flat fee basis).

Identify round trip travel by use of modifier LR.

If you determine that it results in equitable payment, you may extend your former payment allowances for additional travel (such as to a distant rural nursing home) to all circumstances where travel is required. This might be appropriate, for example, if your former payment allowance was on a per mile basis. Otherwise you must establish an appropriate allowance. If you decide to establish a new allowance, one method is to consider developing a travel allowance consisting of:

- The current Federal mileage allowance for operating personal automobiles, plus
- A personnel allowance per mile to cover personnel costs based on an estimate of average hourly wages and average driving speed.

Four your convenience, a chronology of mileage rates from July 1, 1984 to date is listed below:

Mileage Rate	From	To
20.5 cents	July 1, 1984	July 31, 1987
21 cents	August 1, 1987	August 13, 1988
22.5 cents	August 14, 1988	September 16, 1989
24 cents	September 17, 1989	June 29, 1991
25 cents	June 30, 1991	

Travel allowance amounts claimed by suppliers are prorated by the total number of patients (including Medicare and non-Medicare patients) from whom specimens are drawn or picked up on a given trip.

Example 1: On October 1, 1989, a carrier determines that the average technician is paid $9 per hour and estimates 45 miles per hour as the average speed driven or $.20 per mile. This amount plus the Federal mileage allowance of $0.24 per mile results in a total allowance of $0.44 per mile. A laboratory technician makes a trip to two nursing homes involving a total mileage of 20 miles and draws specimens from three patients, Medicare as well as non-Medicare patients. In addition, specimens that were not drawn by the technician are picked up from two patients. A travel allowance per Medicare claim of $1.76 can be made (20 miles round trip / $0.44 per mile divided by 5). The supplier bills 4 miles (20 miles / 5) under code P9603LR.

Example 2: The carrier, through a review of the laboratory records, estimates that on average four specimens are drawn or picked up each trip, and that the average trip is 30 miles including both round trips and one way trips. Assuming the same facts as Example 1 (i.e., $9 per hour and 45 miles per hour), the carrier establishes a flat travel allowance of $3.30. Suppliers bill code P9604 and are paid 3.30 regardless of actual distance or number of patients served.

In keeping with the principles of section 5024 and section 5200, a payment in addition to the routine travel allowance determined under this section may be allowed to cover the additional costs of travel to collect a specimen from a nursing home or homebound patient when clinical diagnostic laboratory tests are needed on an emergency basis outside the general business hours of the laboratory making the collection.

L. Laboratory Tests Utilizing Automated Equipment.—Because of the numerous technological advances and innovations in the clinical laboratory field and the increased availability of automated testing equipment to all entities that perform clinical diagnostic laboratory tests, no distinction is generally made in determining payment allowances (i.e., the lower of the respective fee schedules or the national limitations) for such tests between (1) the sites where the service is performed, i.e., physician's office or other laboratory, or (2) the method of the testing process used, whether manual or automated.

When physicians and laboratories perform the same test, whether manually or with automated equipment, the services are considered similar.

1. Determining Payment for Automated Tests.—The common automated tests comprise specific groupings of blood chemistries which enable physicians to more accurately diagnose their patients' medical problems.

The following list contains some of the tests which can be and are frequently done as groups and combinations on automated profile equipment.

Alanine Aminotransferase (ALT, SGPT)	Albumin
Alkaline phosphatase	Aspartate aminotransferase
Bilirubin, direct (AST, SGOT)	
Bilirubin, total	Carbon dioxide content
Calcium	Chloride
Creatinine	Cholesterol
Glucose (sugar)	Creatine kinase (CK, CPK)

GammaGlutamylTransferase (GGT)	Lactate dehydrogenase (LDH, LD)
Phosphorus	Potassium
Protein, total	Sodium
Triglyceride	Urea nitrogen (BUN)
Uric Acid	

While the component tests in automated profiles may vary somewhat from one laboratory to another, or from one physician's office or clinic to another, group together those profile tests which can be performed at the same time on the same equipment for purposes of developing appropriate payment allowances. For Medicare payment purposes, the tests on this list must be grouped together when billed separately and considered automated profile tests. While laboratory entities may bill additional tests using automated profile codes and be paid according to §5114.1, the above listed 22 tests are the only tests that you may group into automated profiles if they are billed separately. Future revisions to this list will be made through manual revisions.

Payment is made only for those tests in an automated profile that meet Medicare coverage rules. Where only some of the tests in a profile of tests are covered, payment cannot exceed the amount that would have been paid if only the covered tests had been ordered. For example, the use of the 12-channel serum chemistry test to determine the blood sugar level in a proven case of diabetes is unreasonable because the results of a blood sugar test performed separately provides the essential information. Normally, the payment allowance for a blood sugar test is lower than the payment allowance for the automated profile of tests. In no event, however, may payment for the covered tests exceed the payment allowance for the profile.

Periodically, at least annually, remind physicians and suppliers that you will review claims for patterns of high utilization of automated profiles with large number of tests and if your review shows that the documentation does not support Medicare coverage that you will pursue recoupment. Encourage physicians to target their test ordering to only those tests that are related to specific symptoms or disease conditions. Remind physicians of Medicare coverage rules that require that payment may be made only for medically necessary tests and that payment is not made for routine screening tests. As a general rule, you may assume that where a physician orders automated profile tests on a test-by-test basis (i.e., not as part of a profile or custom panel), each of the tests is covered. (See §7517.1.) If, after analysis, you find that a pattern of overutilization exists, even if tests were individually ordered, follow the procedures of §7517.2 to aid you in ameliorating the problems.

2. Separately Billed Tests That Are Commonly Part of Automated Test Profiles.—If you receive claims for laboratory services in which the physician or laboratory has separately billed for tests that are available as part of an automated profile test, make the following determinations:

- If the sum of the payment allowance for the separately billed tests exceeds the payment allowance for the profile that includes these tests, make payment at the lesser amount for the profile. Conversely, the payment allowance for a profile cannot exceed the payment allowances for the individual tests.
- The limitation that payment for individual tests not exceed the payment allowance for an automated profile is applied whether or not a particular laboratory has the automated equipment. A higher amount may be paid in unusual circumstances where justified or where individual tests are unavailable on automated equipment. (See §5024.) Suppliers are to provide a detailed explanation to you of the justification for a higher level of payment. Review to determine if unusual circumstances exist and warrant a higher payment amount.
- When one or more automated profile tests are performed for a patient on the same day, determine whether to base payment on an automated profile that includes such tests rather than to base payment on the individual or separately billed tests. For example, compare the allowance for code 80002 of the Current Procedural Terminology - Fourth Edition (CPT-4) for the above determination when one or two tests from the commonly performed automated tests are included on a claim.

M. Organ or Disease Oriented Panels.—The American Medical Association (AMA) is responsible for the nomenclature of codes in the Current Procedural Terminology (CPT). The AMA has developed codes for panels of tests commonly ordered together and related through their use to diagnose a disease state or to evaluate an organ system. The tests listed in the CPT with each panel code are the defined components of that code for Medicare purposes.

Payment for panels is the same as found in subsection L. Payment for the total panel cannot exceed the allowance for individual tests. All Medicare coverage rules apply.

7517.1 Laboratory Claims.—7517.1 Sections 7500–7536.4 have been deleted and moved to the Program Integrity Manual (PIM).

15030 SUPPLIES

Make a separate payment for supplies furnished in connection with a procedure only when one of the two following conditions exists:

A. HCPCS codes A4550, A4200, and A4263 are billed in conjunction with the appropriate procedure in the Medical Physician Fee Schedule Data Base (place of service is physician's office); or

B. The supply is a pharmaceutical or radiopharmaceutical diagnostic imaging agent (including codes A4641 through A4647); pharmacologic stressing agent (code J1245); or therapeutic radionuclide (CPT code 79900*). The procedures performed are:

- Diagnostic radiologic procedures (including diagnostic nuclear medicine) requiring pharmaceutical or radiopharmaceutical contrast media and/or pharmocological stressing agent,
- Other diagnostic tests requiring a pharmacological stressing agent,
- Clinical brachytherapy procedures (other than remote afterloading high intensity brachytherapy procedures (CPT codes 77781 through 77784*), for which the expendable source is included in the TC RVUs), or Therapeutic nuclear medicine procedures.

APPENDIX B

COVERAGE ISSUES MANUAL (CIM), SELECT

30-1 ROUTINE COSTS IN CLINICAL TRIALS

Effective for items and services furnished on or after September 19, 2000, Medicare covers the routine costs of qualifying clinical trials, as such costs are defined below, as well as reasonable and necessary items and services used to diagnose and treat complications arising from participation in all clinical trials. All other Medicare rules apply.

Routine costs of a clinical trial include all items and services that are otherwise generally available to Medicare beneficiaries (i.e., there exists a benefit category, it is not statutorily excluded, and there is not a national noncoverage decision) that are provided in either the experimental or the control arms of a clinical trial **except**:

- The investigational item or service, itself;
- Items and services provided solely to satisfy data collection and analysis needs and that are not used in the direct clinical management of the patient (e.g., monthly CT scans for a condition usually requiring only a single scan); and
- Items and services customarily provided by the research sponsors free of charge for any enrollee in the trial.

Routine costs in clinical trials include:

- Items or services that are typically provided absent a clinical trial (e.g., conventional care);
- Items or services required solely for the provision of the investigational item or service (e.g., administration of a noncovered chemotherapeutic agent), the clinically appropriate monitoring of the effects of the item or service, or the prevention of complications; and
- Items or services needed for reasonable and necessary care arising from the provision of an investigational item or service—in particular, for the diagnosis or treatment of complications.

This policy does not withdraw Medicare coverage for items and services that may be covered according to local medical review policies or the regulations on category B investigational device exemptions (IDE) found in 42 CFR 405.201-405.215, 411.15, and 411.406. For information about LMRPs, refer to www.lmrp.net, a searchable database of Medicare contractors' local policies.

For noncovered items and services, including items and services for which Medicare payment is statutorily prohibited, Medicare only covers the treatment of complications arising from the delivery of the noncovered item or service and unrelated reasonable and necessary care. (Refer to MCM §§2300.1 and MIM 3101.) However, if the item or service is not covered by virtue of a national noncoverage policy in the Coverage Issues Manual and is the focus of a qualifying clinical trial, the routine costs of the clinical trial (as defined above) will be covered by Medicare but the noncovered item or service, itself, will not.

A. Requirements for Medicare Coverage of Routine Costs.—Any clinical trial receiving Medicare coverage of routine costs must meet the following three requirements:

1. The subject or purpose of the trial must be the evaluation of an item or service that falls within a Medicare benefit category (e.g., physicians' service, durable medical equipment, diagnostic test) and is not statutorily excluded from coverage (e.g., cosmetic surgery, hearing aids).

2. The trial must not be designed exclusively to test toxicity or disease pathophysiology. It must have therapeutic intent.

3. Trials of therapeutic interventions must enroll patients with diagnosed disease rather than healthy volunteers. Trials of diagnostic interventions may enroll healthy patients in order to have a proper control group.

The three requirements above are insufficient by themselves to qualify a clinical trial for Medicare coverage of routine costs. Clinical trials also should have the following desirable characteristics; however, some trials, as described below, are presumed to meet these characteristics and are automatically qualified to receive Medicare coverage:

1. The principal purpose of the trial is to test whether the intervention potentially improves the participants' health outcomes;

2. The trial is well-supported by available scientific and medical information or it is intended to clarify or establish the health outcomes of interventions already in common clinical use;

3. The trial does not unjustifiably duplicate existing studies;

4. The trial design is appropriate to answer the research question being asked in the trial;

5. The trial is sponsored by a credible organization or individual capable of executing the proposed trial successfully;

6. The trial is in compliance with Federal regulations relating to the protection of human subjects; and

7. All aspects of the trial are conducted according to the appropriate standards of scientific integrity.

B. Qualification Process for Clinical Trials.—Using the authority found in §1142 of the Act (cross-referenced in §1862(a)(1)(E) of the Act), the Agency for Healthcare Research and Quality (AHRQ) will convene a multi-agency Federal panel (the "panel") composed of representatives of the Department of Health and Human Services research agencies (National Institutes of Health (NIH), Centers for Disease Control and Prevention (CDC), the Food and Drug Administration (FDA), AHRQ, and the Office of Human Research Protection), and the research arms of the Department of Defense (DOD) and the Department of Veterans Affairs (VA) to develop qualifying criteria that will indicate a strong probability that a trial exhibits the desirable characteristics listed above. These criteria will be easily verifiable, and where possible, dichotomous. Trials that meet these qualifying criteria will receive Medicare coverage of their associated routine costs. This panel is not reviewing or approving individual trials. The multi-agency panel will meet periodically to review and evaluate the program and recommend any necessary refinements to HCFA.

Clinical trials that meet the qualifying criteria will receive Medicare coverage of routine costs after the trial's lead principal investigator certifies that the trial meets the criteria. This process will require the principal investigator to enroll the trial in a Medicare clinical trials registry, currently under development.

Some clinical trials are automatically qualified to receive Medicare coverage of their routine costs because they have been deemed by AHRQ, in consultation with the other agencies represented on the multi-agency panel to be highly likely to have the above-listed seven desirable characteristics of clinical trials. The principal investigators of these automatically qualified trials do not need to certify that the trials meet the qualifying criteria, but must enroll the trials in the Medicare clinical trials registry for administrative purposes, once the registry is established.

Effective September 19, 2000, clinical trials that are deemed to be automatically qualified are:

1. Trials funded by NIH, CDC, AHRQ, HCFA, DOD, and VA;

2. Trials supported by centers or cooperative groups that are funded by the NIH, CDC, AHRQ, HCFA, DOD and VA;

3. Trials conducted under an investigational new drug application (IND) reviewed by the FDA; and

4. Drug trials that are exempt from having an IND under 21 CFR 312.2(b)(1) will be deemed automatically qualified until the qualifying criteria are developed and the certification process is in place. At that time the principal investigators of these trials must certify that the trials meet the qualifying criteria in order to main-

tain Medicare coverage of routine costs. This certification process will only affect the future status of the trial and will not be used to retroactively change the earlier deemed status.

Medicare will cover the routine costs of qualifying trials that either have been deemed to be automatically qualified or have certified that they meet the qualifying criteria unless HCFA's Chief Clinical Officer subsequently finds that a clinical trial does not meet the qualifying criteria or jeopardizes the safety or welfare of Medicare beneficiaries.

Should HCFA find that a trial's principal investigator misrepresented that the trial met the necessary qualifying criteria in order to gain Medicare coverage of routine costs, Medicare coverage of the routine costs would be denied under §1862(a)(1)(E) of the Act. In the case of such a denial, the Medicare beneficiaries enrolled in the trial would not be held liable (i.e., would be held harmless from collection) for the costs consistent with the provisions of §§1879, 1842(l), or 1834(j)(4) of the Act, as applicable.Where appropriate, the billing providers would be held liable for the costs and fraud investigations of the billing providers and the trial's principal investigator may be pursued.

Medicare regulations require Medicare+Choice (M+C) organizations to follow HCFA's national coverage decisions. This NCD raises special issues that require some modification of most M+C organizations' rules governing provision of items and services in and out of network. The items and services covered under this NCD are inextricably linked to the clinical trials with which they are associated and cannot be covered outside of the context of those clinical trials. M+C organizations therefore must cover these services regardless of whether they are available through in-network providers. M+C organizations may have reporting requirements when enrollees participate in clinical trials, in order to track and coordinate their members' care, but cannot require prior authorization or approval.

35-3 HEAT TREATMENT, INCLUDING THE USE OF DIATHERMY AND ULTRASOUND FOR PULMONARY CONDITIONS—NOT COVERED

There is no physiological rationale or valid scientific documentation of effectiveness of diathermy or ultrasound heat treatments for asthma, bronchitis, or any other pulmonary condition, and for such purpose this treatment cannot be considered reasonable and necessary within the meaning of section 1862(a)(1) of the law.

35-5 CELLULAR THERAPY—NOT COVERED

Cellular therapy involves the practice of injecting humans with foreign proteins like the placenta or lungs of unborn lambs. Cellular therapy is without scientific or statistical evidence to document its therapeutic efficacy and, in fact, is considered a potentially dangerous practice. Accordingly, cellular therapy is not considered reasonable and necessary within the meaning of section 1862(a)(1) of the law.

35-10 HYPERBARIC OXYGEN THERAPY

For purposes of coverage under Medicare, hyperbaric oxygen (HBO) therapy is a modality in which the entire body is exposed to oxygen under increased atmospheric pressure.

A. Covered Conditions.—Program reimbursement for HBO therapy will be limited to that which is administered in a chamber (including the one man unit) and is limited to the following conditions:

1. Acute carbon monoxide intoxication.
2. Decompression illness.
3. Gas embolism.
4. Gas gangrene.
5. Acute traumatic peripheral ischemia. HBO therapy is a valuable adjunctive treatment to be used in combination with accepted standard therapeutic measures when loss of function, limb, or life is threatened.
6. Crush injuries and suturing of severed limbs. As in the previous conditions, HBO therapy would be an adjunctive treatment when loss of function, limb, or life is threatened.
7. Progressive necrotizing infections (necrotizing fasciitis, Meleney ulcer).
8. Acute peripheral arterial insufficiency.
9. Preparation and preservation of compromised skin grafts (not for primary management of wounds), (ICD-9-CM diagnosis 996.52, excludes artifical skin grafts).
10. Chronic refractory osteomyelitis, unresponsive to conventional medical and surgical management.
11. Osteoradionecrosis as an adjunct to conventional treatment.
12. Soft tissue radionecrosis as an adjunct to conventional treatment.
13. Cyanide poisoning.

The following use of HBO is covered for services rendered on or after 2/22/84.

14. Actinomycosis, only as an adjunct to conventional therapy when the disease process is refractory to antibiotics and surgical treatment.
15. Diabetic wounds of the lower extremities in patients who meet the following three criteria:
    a. Patient has type I or type II diabetes and has a lower extremity wound that is due to diabetes;
    b. Patient has a wound classified as Wagner grade III or higher; and
    c. Patient has failed an adequate course of standard wound therapy.

The use of HBO therapy is covered as adjunctive therapy only after there are no measurable signs of healing for at least 30 days of treatment with standard wound therapy and must be used in addition to standard wound care. Standard wound care in patients with diabetic wounds includes: assessment of a patient's vascular status and correction of any vascular problems in the affected limb if possible, optimization of nutritional status, optimization of glucose control, debridement by any means to remove devitalized tissue, maintenance of a clean, moist bed of granulation tissue with appropriate moist dressings, appropriate off-loading, and necessary treatment to resolve any infection that might be present. Failure to respond to standard wound care occurs when there are not measurable signs of healing for at least 30 consecutive days. Wounds must be evaluated at least every 30 days during administration of HBO therapy. Continued treatment with HBO therapy is not covered if measurable signs of healing have not been demonstrated within any 30-day period of treatment.

B. Noncovered Conditions.—All other indications not specified under section 35-10 (A) are not covered under the Medicare program. No program payment may be made for any conditions other than those listed in section 35-10 (A).

No program payment may be made for HBO in the treatment of the following conditions:

1. Cutaneous, decubitus, and stasis ulcers.
2. Chronic peripheral vascular insufficiency.
3. Anaerobic septicemia and infection other than clostridial.
4. Skin burns (thermal).
5. Senility.
6. Myocardial infarction.
7. Cardiogenic shock.
8. Sickle cell anemia.
9. Acute thermal and chemical pulmonary damage, i.e., smoke inhalation with pulmonary insufficiency.

10. Acute or chronic cerebral vascular insufficiency.
11. Hepatic necrosis.
12. Aerobic septicemia.
13. Nonvascular causes of chronic brain syndrome (Pick's disease, Alzheimer's disease, Korsakoff's disease).
14. Tetanus.
15. Systemic aerobic infection.
16. Organ transplantation.
17. Organ storage.
18. Pulmonary emphysema.
19. Exceptional blood loss anemia.
20. Multiple Sclerosis.
21. Arthritic Diseases.
22. Acute cerebral edema.

C. Topical Application of Oxygen.—This method of administering oxygen does not meet the definition of HBO therapy as stated above. Also, its clinical efficacy has not been established. Therefore, no Medicare reimbursement may be made for the topical application of oxygen. (Cross refer: section 35-31.)

35-13 PROLOTHERAPY, JOINT SCLEROTHERAPY, AND LIGAMENTOUS INJECTIONS WITH SCLEROSING AGENTS—NOT COVERED

The medical effectiveness of the above therapies has not been verified by scientifically controlled studies. Accordingly, reimbursement for these modalities should be denied on the ground that they are not reasonable and necessary as required by section 1862(a)(1) of the law.

35-20 TREATMENT OF MOTOR FUNCTION DISORDERS WITH ELECTRIC NERVE STIMULATION—NOT COVERED

While electric nerve stimulation has been employed to control chronic intractable pain for some time, its use in the treatment of motor function disorders, such as multiple sclerosis, is a recent innovation, and the medical effectiveness of such therapy has not been verified by scientifically controlled studies. Therefore, where electric nerve stimulation is employed to treat motor function disorders, no reimbursement may be made for the stimulator or for the services related to its implantation since this treatment cannot be considered reasonable and necessary.

See sections 35-27 and 65-8.

NOTE: Medicare coverage of deep brain stimulation by implantation of a stimulator device is not prohibited. Therefore, coverage of deep brain stimulation provided by an implanted deep brain stimulator is at the carrier's discretion.

35-27 BIOFEEDBACK THERAPY

Biofeedback therapy provides visual, auditory or other evidence of the status of certain body functions so that a person can exert voluntary control over the functions, and thereby alleviate an abnormal bodily condition. Biofeedback therapy often uses electrical devices to transform bodily signals indicative of such functions as heart rate, blood pressure, skin temperature, salivation, peripheral vasomotor activity, and gross muscle tone into a tone or light, the loudness or brightness of which shows the extent of activity in the function being measured.

Biofeedback therapy differs from electromyography, which is a diagnostic procedure used to record and study the electrical properties of skeletal muscle. An electromyography device may be used to provide feedback with certain types of biofeedback.

Biofeedback therapy is covered under Medicare only when it is reasonable and necessary for the individual patient for muscle re-education of specific muscle groups or for treating pathological muscle abnormalities of spasticity, incapacitating muscle spasm, or weakness, and more conventional treatments (heat, cold, massage, exercise, support) have not been successful. This therapy is not covered for treatment of ordinary muscle tension states or for psychosomatic conditions.

(See HCFA-Pub. 14-3, sections 2200ff., 2215, and 4161; HCFA-Pub. 13-3, section 3133.3, 3148, and 3149; HCFA-Pub. 10, section 242 and 242.5 for special physical therapy requirements. See also sections 35-20 and 65-8.)

35-27.1 BIOFEEDBACK THERAPY FOR THE TREATMENT OF URINARY INCONTINENCE

Biofeedback therapy for the treatment of urinary incontinence (Effective for services performed on or after July 1, 2001.) This policy applies to biofeedback therapy rendered by a practitioner in an office or other facility setting.

Biofeedback is covered for the treatment of stress and/or urge incontinence in cognitively intact patients who have failed a documented trial of pelvic muscle exercise (PME) training. Biofeedback is not a treatment, per se, but a tool to help patients learn how to perform PME. Biofeedback-assisted PME incorporates the use of an electronic or mechanical device to relay visual and/or auditory evidence of pelvic floor muscle tone, in order to improve awareness of pelvic floor musculature and to assist patients in the performance of PME.

A failed trial of PME training is defined as no clinically significant improvement in urinary incontinence after completing 4 weeks of an ordered plan of pelvic muscle exercises to increase periurethral muscle strength.

Contractors may decide whether or not to cover biofeedback as an initial treatment modality.

Home use of biofeedback therapy is not covered.

35-31 TREATMENT OF DECUBITUS ULCERS

An accepted procedure for healing decubitus ulcers is to remove dead tissue from the lesions and to keep them clean to promote the growth of new tissue. This may be accomplished by hydrotherapy (whirlpool) treatments. Hydrotherapy (whirlpool) treatment for decubitus ulcers is a covered service under Medicare for patients when treatment is reasonable and necessary. Some other methods of treating decubitus ulcers, the safety and effectiveness of which have not been established, are not covered under the Medicare program. Some examples of these types of treatments are: ultraviolet light, low intensity direct current, topical application of oxygen, and topical dressings with Balsam of Peru in castor oil.

35-34 FABRIC WRAPPING OF ABDOMINAL ANEURYSMS—NOT COVERED

Fabric wrapping of abdominal aneurysms is not a covered Medicare procedure. This is a treatment for abdominal aneurysms which involves wrapping aneurysms with cellophane or fascia lata. This procedure has not been shown to prevent eventual rupture. In extremely rare instances, external wall reinforcement may be indicated when the current accepted treatment (excision of the aneurysm and reconstruction with synthetic materials) is not a viable alternative, but external wall reinforcement is not fabric wrapping. Accordingly, fabric wrapping of abdominal aneurysms is not considered reasonable and necessary within the meaning of section 1862(a)(1) of the Act.

35-41 DIATHERMY TREATMENT

High-energy pulsed-wave diathermy machines have been found to produce some degree of therapeutic benefit for essentially the same conditions and to the same extent as standard diathermy. Accordingly, when the contractor's medical staff has determined that the pulsed-wave diathermy apparatus used is one which is considered therapeutically effective, the treatments are considered a covered service, but only for those conditions for which standard diathermy is medically indicated and only when rendered by a physician or incident to a physician's professional services.

Further, when the charge for covered pulsed-wave diathermy treatment is substantially in excess of that which is reasonable for standard diathermy, payment is based on the reasonable charge for standard diathermy (CPT-4 code 97024,* ICD-9-CM code 93.34).

Cross-refer: §35-3.

35-46 ASSESSING PATIENT'S SUITABILITY FOR ELECTRICAL NERVE STIMULATION THERAPY

Electrical nerve stimulation is an accepted modality for assessing a patient's suitability for ongoing treatment with a transcutaneous or an implanted nerve stimulator. Accordingly, program payment may be made for the following techniques when used to determine the potential therapeutic usefulness of an electrical nerve stimulator:

A. Transcutaneous Electrical Nerve Stimulation (TENS).—This technique involves attachment of a transcutaneous nerve stimulator to the surface of the skin over the peripheral nerve to be stimulated. It is used by the patient on a trial basis and its effectiveness in modulating pain is monitored by the physician, or physical therapist. Generally, the physician or physical therapist is able to determine whether the patient is likely to derive a significant therapeutic benefit from continuous use of a transcutaneous stimulator within a trial period of 1 month; in a few cases this determination may take longer to make. Document the medical necessity for such services which are furnished beyond the first month. (See section 45-25 for an explanation of coverage of medically necessary supplies for the effective use of TENS.)

If TENS significantly alleviates pain, it may be considered as primary treatment; if it produces no relief or greater discomfort than the original pain, electrical nerve stimulation therapy is ruled out. However, where TENS produces incomplete relief, further evaluation with percutaneous electrical nerve stimulation may be considered to determine whether an implanted peripheral nerve stimulator would provide significant relief from pain. (See section 35-46B.)

Usually, the physician or physical therapist providing the services will furnish the equipment necessary for assessment. Where the physician or physical therapist advises the patient to rent the TENS from a supplier during the trial period rather than supplying it himself/herself, program payment may be made for rental of the TENS as well as for the services of the physician or physical therapist who is evaluating its use. However, the combined program payment which is made for the physician's or physical therapist's services and the rental of the stimulator from a supplier should not exceed the amount which would be payable for the total service, including the stimulator, furnished by the physician or physical therapist alone.

B. Percutaneous Electrical Nerve Stimulation (PENS).—This diagnostic procedure which involves stimulation of peripheral nerves by a needle electrode inserted through the skin is performed only in a physician's office, clinic, or hospital outpatient department. Therefore, it is covered only when performed by a physician or incident to physician's service. If pain is effectively controlled by percutaneous stimulation, implantation of electrodes is warranted.

As in the case of TENS (described in subsection A), generally the physician should be able to determine whether the patient is likely to derive a significant therapeutic benefit from continuing use of an implanted nerve stimulator within a trial period of 1 month. In a few cases, this determination may take longer to make. The medical necessity for such diagnostic services which are furnished beyond the first month must be documented.

NOTE: Electrical nerve stimulators do not prevent pain but only alleviate pain as it occurs. A patient can be taught how to employ the stimulator, and once this is done, can use it safely and effectively without direct physician supervision. Consequently, it is inappropriate for a patient to visit his physician, physical therapist or an outpatient clinic on a continuing basis for treatment of pain with electrical nerve stimulation. Once it is determined that electrical nerve stimulation should be continued as therapy and the patient has been trained to use the stimulator, it is expected that a stimulator will be implanted or the patient will employ the TENS on a continual basis in his home. Electrical nerve stimulation treatments furnished by a physician in his office, by a physical therapist or outpatient clinic are excluded from coverage by section 1862(a)(1) of the law. (See section 65-8 for an explanation of coverage of the therapeutic use of implanted peripheral nerve stimulators under the prosthetic devices benefit. See section 60-20 for an explanation of coverage of the therapeutic use of TENS under the durable medical equipment benefit.)

35-47 BREAST RECONSTRUCTION FOLLOWING MASTECTOMY

During recent years there has been a considerable change in the treatment of diseases of the breast such as fibrocystic disease, and cancer. While extirpation of the disease remains of primary importance, the quality of life following initial treatment is increasingly recognized as of great concern. The increased use of breast reconstruction procedures is due to several factors:

- A change in epidemiology of breast cancer, including an apparent increase in incidence;
- Improved surgical skills and techniques;
- The continuing development of better prostheses; and
- Increasing awareness by physicians of the importance of post-surgical psychological adjustment.

Reconstruction of the affected and the contralateral unaffected breast following a medically necessary mastectomy is considered a relatively safe and effective noncosmetic procedure. Accordingly, program payment may be made for breast reconstruction surgery following removal of a breast for any medical reason.

Program payment may not be made for breast reconstruction for cosmetic reasons. (Cosmetic surgery is excluded from coverage under section 1862(a)(10) of the Social Security Act.)

35-48 OSTEOGENIC STIMULATION

Electrical stimulation to augment bone repair can be attained either invasively or noninvasively. Invasive devices provide electrical stimulation directly at the fracture site either through percutaneously placed cathodes or by implantation of a coiled cathode wire into the fracture site. The power pack for the latter device is implanted into soft tissue near the fracture site and subcutaneously connected to the cathode, creating a self-contained system with no external components. The power supply for the former device is externally placed and the leads connected to the inserted cathodes. With the noninvasive device, opposing pads, wired to an external power supply, are placed over the cast. An electromagnetic field is created between the pads at the fracture site.

1. Noninvasive Stimulator.—The noninvasive stimulator device is covered only for the following indications:

- Nonunion of long bone fractures;
- Failed fusion, where a minimum of 9 months has elapsed since the last surgery;
- Congenital pseudarthroses; and
- As an adjunct to spinal fusion surgery for patients at high risk of pseudarthrosis due to previously failed spinal fusion at the same site or for those undergoing multiple level fusion. A multiple level fusion involves 3 or more vertebrae (e.g., L3-L5, L4-S1, etc).

2. Invasive (Implantable) Stimulator.—The invasive stimulator device is covered only for the following indications:

- Nonunion of long bone fractures;
- As an adjunct to spinal fusion surgery for patients at high risk of pseudarthrosis due to previously failed spinal fusion at the

---

*CPT only © *Current Procedural Terminology, 2002 Professional Edition*, American Medical Association. All rights reserved.

same site or for those undergoing muliple level fusion. A multiple level fusion involves 3 or more vertebrae (e.g., L3-L5, L4-S1, etc).

Effective for services performed on or after September 15, 1980, nonunion of long bone fractures, for both noninvasive and invasive devices, is considered to exist only after six or more months have elapsed without healing of the fracture.

Effective for services performed on or after April 1, 2000, nonunion of long bone fractures, for both noninvasive and invasive devices, is considered to exist only when serial radiographs have confirmed that fracture healing has ceased for three or more months prior to starting treatment with the electrical osteogenic stimulator. Serial radiographs must include a minimum of two sets of radiographs, each including multiple views of the fracture site, separated by a minimum of 90 days.

B. Ultrasonic Osteogenic Stimulators.—An ultrasonic osteogenic stimulator is a non-invasive device that emits low intensity, pulsed ultrasound. The ultrasound signal is applied to the skin surface at the fracture location via ultrasound conductive gel in order to stimulate fracture healing.

Effective for services performed on or after January 1, 2001, ultrasonic osteogenic stimulators are covered as medically reasonable and necessary for the treatment of non-union fractures. In demonstrating nonunion of fractures, we would expect:

1. A minimum of two sets of radiographs obtained prior to starting treatment with the osteogenic stimulator, separated by a minimum of 90 days. Each radiograph must include multiple views of the fracture site accompanied with a written interpretation by a physician stating that there has been no clinically significant evidence of fracture healing between the two sets of radiographs.

2. Indications that the patient failed at least one surgical intervention for the treatment of the fracture.

Non-unions of the skull, vertebrae, and those that are tumor-related are excluded from coverage. The ultrasonic osteogenic stimulator may not be used concurrently with other non-invasive osteogenic devices. The national non-coverage policy related to ultrasonic osteogenic stimulators for fresh fractures and delayed unions remains in place. This policy relates only to non-union as defined above.

35-61 TRANSSEXUAL SURGERY

Transsexual surgery, also known as sex reassignment surgery or intersex surgery, is the culmination of a series of procedures designed to change the anatomy of transsexuals to conform to their gender identity. Transsexuals are persons with an overwhelming desire to change anatomic sex because of their fixed conviction that they are members of the opposite sex. For the male-to-female, transsexual surgery entails castration, penectomy and vulva-vaginal construction. Surgery for the female-to-male transsexual consists of bilateral mammectomy, hysterectomy and salpingo-oophorectomy, which may be followed by phalloplasty and the insertion of testicular prostheses.

Transsexual surgery for sex reassignment of transsexuals is controversial. Because of the lack of well-controlled, long-term studies of the safety and effectiveness of the surgical procedures and attendant therapies for transsexualism, the treatment is considered experimental. Moreover, there is a high rate of serious complications for these surgical procedures. For these reasons, transsexual surgery is not covered.

35-64 CHELATION THERAPY FOR TREATMENT OF ATHEROSCLEROSIS

Chelation therapy is the application of chelation techniques for the therapeutic or preventive effects of removing unwanted metal ions from the body. The application of chelation therapy using ethylenediamine-tetra-acetic acid (EDTA) for the treatment and prevention of atherosclerosis is controversial. There is no widely accepted rationale to explain the beneficial effects attributed to this therapy. Its safety is questioned and its clinical effectiveness has never been established by well designed, controlled clinical trials. It is not widely accepted and practiced by American physicians. EDTA chelation therapy for atherosclerosis is considered experimental. For these reasons, EDTA chelation therapy for the treatment or prevention of atherosclerosis is not covered.

Some practitioners refer to this therapy as chemoendarterectomy and may also show a diagnosis other than atherosclerosis, such as arteriosclerosis or calcinosis. Claims employing such variant terms should also be denied under this section.

Cross-refer: section 45-20

35-65 GASTRIC FREEZING

Gastric freezing for chronic peptic ulcer disease is a non-surgical treatment which was popular about 20 years ago but now is seldom done. It has been abandoned due to a high complication rate, only temporary improvement experienced by patients, and lack of effectiveness when tested by double-blind, controlled clinical trials. Since the procedure is now considered obsolete, it is not covered.

35-74 EXTERNAL COUNTERPULSATION (ECP) FOR SEVERE ANGINA—COVERED

External counterpulsation (ECP), commonly referred to as enhanced external counterpulsation, is a non-invasive outpatient treatment for coronary artery disease refractory to medical and/or surgical therapy. Although ECP devices are cleared by the Food and Drug Administration (FDA) for use in treating a variety of cardiac conditions, including stable or unstable angina pectoris, acute myocardial infarction, and cardiogenic shock. The use of this device to treat cardiac conditions other than stable angina pectoris is not covered, since only that use has developed sufficient evidence to demonstrate its medical effectiveness.

Coverage is provided for the use of ECP for patients who have been diagnosed with disabling angina (Class III or Class IV, Canadian Cardiovascular Society Classification or equivalent classification) who, in the opinion of a cardiologist or cardiothoracic surgeon, are not readily amenable to surgical intervention, such as PTCA or cardiac bypass because: (1) their condition is inoperable, or at high risk of operative complications or post-operative failure; (2) their coronary anatomy is not readily amenable to such procedures; or (3) they have co-morbid states which create excessive risk.

A full course of therapy usually consists of 35 one-hour treatments which may be offered once or twice daily, usually 5 days per week. The patient is placed on a treatment table where the lower trunk and lower extremities are wrapped in a series of three compressive air cuffs which inflate and deflate in synchronization with the patient's cardiac cycle.

During diastole the three sets of air cuffs are inflated sequentially (distal to proximal) compressing the vascular beds within the muscles of the calves, lower thighs, and upper thighs. This action results in an increase in diastolic pressure, generation of retrograde arterial blood flow, and an increase in venous return. The cuffs are deflated simultaneously just prior to systole, which produces a rapid drop in vascular impedance, a decrease in ventricular workload, and an increase in cardiac output.

The augmented diastolic pressure and retrograde aortic flow appear to improve myocardial perfusion, while systolic unloading appears to reduce cardiac workload and oxygen requirements. The increased venous return coupled with enhanced systolic flow appears to increase cardiac output. As a result of this treatment, most patients experience increased time until onset of ischemia, increased exercise tolerance, and a reduction in the number and severity of anginal episodes. Evidence was presented that this effect lasted well beyond the immediate post-treatment phase, with patients symptom-free for several months to two years.

This procedure must be done under direct supervision of a physician.

35-77 NEUROMUSCULAR ELECTRICAL STIMULATION (NMES)

Neuromuscular electrical stimulation (NMES) involves the use of a device which transmits an electrical impulse to activate muscle groups by way of electrodes. There are two broad categories of NMES. One type of device stimulates the muscle when the patient is in a resting state to treat muscle atrophy. The second type is used to enhance functional activity of neurologically impaired patients.

Treatment of Muscle Atrophy

Coverage of NMES to treat muscle atrophy is limited to the treatment of patients with disuse atrophy where the nerve supply to the muscle is intact, including brain, spinal cord and peripheral nerves and other nonneurological reasons for disuse atrophy. Examples include casting or splinting of a limb, contracture due to scarring of soft tissue as in burn lesions, and hip replacement surgery (until orthotic training begins). (See CIM 45-25 for an explanation of coverage of medically necessary supplies for the effective use of NMES).

Use for Walking in Patients with Spinal Cord Injury (SCI)

The type of NMES that is used to enhance the ability to walk of SCI patients is commonly referred to as functional electrical stimulation (FES). These devices are surface units that use electrical impulses to activate paralyzed or weak muscles in precise sequence. Coverage for the use of NMES/FES is limited to SCI patients, for walking, who have completed a training program, which consists of at least 32 physical therapy sessions with the device over a period of 3 months. The trial period of physical therapy will enable the physician treating the patient for his or her spinal cord injury to properly evaluate the person's ability to use these devices frequently and for the long term. Physical therapy sessions are only covered in the inpatient hospital, outpatient hospital, comprehensive outpatient rehabilitation facilities, and outpatient rehabilitation facilities. The physical therapy necessary to perform this training must be directly performed by the physical therapist as part of a one-on-one training program; this service cannot be done unattended.

The goal of physical therapy must be to train SCI pateints on the use of NMES/FES devices to achieve walking, not to reverse or retard muscle atrophy.

Coverage for NMES/FES for walking will be limited to SCI patients with all of the following characteristics:

1. Persons with intact lower motor units (L1 and below) (both muscle and peripheral nerve);
2. Persons with muscle and joint stability for weight bearing at upper and lower extremitities that can demonstrate balance and control to maintain an upright support posture independently;
3. Persons that demonstrate brisk muscle contraction to NMES and have sensory perception of electrical stimulation sufficient for muscle contraction;
4. Persons that possess high motivation, commitment and cognitive ability to use such devices for walking;
5. Persons that can transfer independently and can demonstrate independent standing tolerance for at least 3 minutes;
6. Persons that can demonstrate hand and finger function to manipulate controls;
7. Persons with at least 6-month post recovery spinal cord injury and restorative surgery;
8. Persons without hip and knee degenerative disease and no history of long bone fracture secondary to osteoporosis; and
9. Persons who have demonstrated a willingness to use the device long-term.

NMES/FES for walking will not be covered in SCI patients with any of the following:

1. Persons with cardiac pacemakers;
2. Severe scoliosis or severe osteoporosis;
3. Skin disease or cancer at area of stimulation;
4. Irreversible contracture; or
5. Autonomic dysreflexia.

The only settings where therapists with the sufficient skills to provide these services are employed, are inpatient hospitals, outpatient hospitals, comprehensive outpatient rehabilitation facilities and outpatient rehabilitation facilities. The physical therapy necessary to perform this training must be part of a one-on-one training program.

Additional therapy after the purchase of the DME would be limited by our general policies on coverage of skilled physical therapy.

All other uses of NMES remain non-covered.

(Also reference Medicare Carriers Manual, Part 3, Claims-§2210 and Medicare Intermediary Manual, Part 3, Claims-§3653—See—Maintenance Program 271.1)

35-90 EXTRACORPOREAL IMMUNOADSORPTION (ECI) USING PROTEIN A COLUMNS

Extracorporeal immunoadsorption (ECI), using protein A columns, has been developed for the purpose of selectively removing circulating immune complexes (CIC) and immunoglobulins (IgG) from patients in whom these substances are associated with their diseases. The technique involves pumping the patient's anticoagulated venous blood through a cell separator from which 1 to 3 liters of plasma are collected and perfused over adsorbent columns, after which the plasma rejoins the separated, unprocessed cells and is retransfused to the patient.

For claims with dates of service on or after January 1, 2001, Medicare covers the use of Protein A columns for the treatment of ITP. In addition, Medicare will cover Protein A columns for the treatment of rheumatoid arthritis (RA) under the following conditions:

1. Patient has severe RA. Patient disease is active, having > 5 swollen joints, > 20 tender joints, and morning stiffness > 60 minutes.

2. Patient has failed an adequate course of a minimum of 3 Disease Modifying Anti-Rheumatic Drugs (DMARDs). Failure does not include intolerance.

Other uses of these columns are currently considered to be investigational and, therefore, not reasonable and necessary under the Medicare law. (See '1862(a)(1)(A) of the Act.)

35-93 LUNG VOLUME REDUCTION SURGERY (REDUCTION PNEUMOPLASTY, ALSO CALLED LUNG SHAVING OR LUNG CONTOURING) UNILATERAL OR BILATERAL BY OPEN OR THORACOSCOPIC APPROACH FOR TREATMENT OF EMPHYSEMA OR CHRONIC OBSTRUCTIVE PULMONARY DISEASE—NOT GENERALLY COVERED

Lung volume reduction surgery (LVRS) or reduction pneumoplasty, also referred to as lung shaving or lung contouring, is performed on patients with emphysema and chronic obstructive pulmonary disease (COPD) in order to allow the underlying compressed lung to expand, and thus, establish improved respiratory function. The goal of this procedure is to offer a better quality of life for patients with emphysema and COPD. In addition, LVRS may be offered as a "bridge to transplant" for patients who otherwise may not have been considered candidates for lung transplantation.

Unilateral or bilateral LVRS by open or thoracoscopic approach is not generally covered, because there is insufficient medical evidence available to base a determination that this procedure is generally safe and effective. Therefore, LVRS generally cannot be considered reasonable and necessary under section 1862(a)(1)(A) of the Act in most cases.

When this policy was first established in December 1995, HCFA committed Medicare to reviewing the scientific literature as it was published in order to modify coverage policy as clinical data were developed. HCFA has reviewed data that suggest the need for a randomized clinical trial regarding the safety and effectiveness of LVRS. On April 24, 1996, the Health Care Financing Administration (HCFA) and the National Heart, Lung and Blood Institute (NHLBI) of the National Institutes of Health announced their intention to collaborate on a multi-center, randomized clinical study evaluating the effectiveness of LVRS. On December 20, 1996, HCFA and NHLBI announced the clinical centers and the data coordinating center that will be participating in the study. HCFA has determined that LVRS is reasonable and necessary when it is provided under the conditions detailed by the protocol of the HCFA/NHLBI clinical study. Therefore, Medicare will cover LVRS in those limited circumstances when it is provided to a Medicare beneficiary under the protocols established for the study. Coverage will be provided where the care is furnished in facilities that are approved as meeting the criteria established by HCFA and NHLBI for this study.

This study will consist of a registry of all patients referred to the participating clinical centers for LVRS. In addition, a subset of patients from the registry who meet specific inclusion criteria will be invited to participate in the randomized trial. All randomized patients will receive intensive medical therapy and pulmonary rehabilitation. Half will be selected randomly to undergo LVRS, which will be performed via median sternotomy or video-assisted thoracoscopy.

Medicare will provide coverage to those beneficiaries who may participate in the randomized trial for all services integral to the study and for which the Medicare statute does not prohibit. This includes tests performed to determine whether a beneficiary qualifies for randomization, LVRS, and follow-up tests that are necessary during participation in the randomized study. However, Medicare will not provide coverage for those services that are prohibited by the Act. For example, Medicare will provide coverage for pulmonary rehabilitation and pulmonary function testing, but will not provide coverage for oral steroids provided as part of a physician's service under section 1862(S)(2) of the Act because they are self-administrable and thus statutorily excluded from coverage.

Payment for these services will be provided under the usual payment systems. For example, Part A services will be paid for according to the DRG system, and Part B physician services will be paid for according to the physician fee schedule.

The data from the randomized phase of the study will be analyzed and monitored continuously in order to determine any appropriate changes in Medicare coverage. These determinations will include if and how coverage will be continued.

35-96 CRYOSURGERY OF PROSTATE (Effective for services performed on or after July 1, 1999)

Cryosurgery of the prostate gland, also known as cryosurgical ablation of the prostate (CSAP), destroys prostate tissue by applying extremely cold temperatures in order to reduce the size of the prostate gland. It is safe and effective, as well as medically necessary and appropriate, as primary treatment for patients with clinically localized prostate cancer, Stages T1–T3.

Cryosurgery of the prostate as a salvage therapy is not covered for any services performed prior to June 30, 2001.

35-103 MULTIPLE ELECTROCONVULSIVE THERAPY (MECT) (Effective for services provided on or after April 1, 2003)

The clinical effectiveness of the multiple-seizure electroconvulsive therapy has not been verified by scientifically controlled studies. In addition, studies have demonstrated an increased risk of adverse effects with multiple seizures. Accordingly, MECT cannot be considered reasonable and necessary and is not covered by the Medicare program.

45-4 VITAMIN B12 INJECTIONS TO STRENGTHEN TENDONS, LIGAMENTS, ETC., OF THE FOOT—NOT COVERED

Vitamin B12 injections to strengthen tendons, ligaments, etc., of the foot are not covered under Medicare because (1) there is no evidence that vitamin B12 injections are effective for the purpose of strengthening weakened tendons and ligaments, and (2) this is nonsurgical treatment under the subluxation exclusion. Accordingly, vitamin B12 injections are not considered reasonable and necessary within the meaning of section 1862(a)(1) of the Act.

See Intermediary Manual sections 3101.3 and 3158, and Carriers Manual, sections 2050.5 and 2323.

45-7 HYDROPHILIC CONTACT LENS FOR CORNEAL BANDAGE

Some hydrophilic contact lenses are used as moist corneal bandages for the treatment of acute or chronic corneal pathology, such as bullous keratopathy, dry eyes, corneal ulcers and erosion, keratitis, corneal edema, descemetocele, corneal ectasis, Mooren's ulcer, anterior corneal dystrophy, neurotrophic keratoconjunctivitis, and for other therapeutic reasons.

Payment may be made under section 1861(s)(2) of the Act for a hydrophilic contact lens approved by the Food and Drug Administration (FDA) and used as a supply incident to a physician's service. Payment for the lens is included in the payment for the physician's service to which the lens is incident. Contractors are authorized to accept an FDA letter of approval or other FDA published material as evidence of FDA approval. (See section 65-1 for coverage of a hydrophilic contact lens as a prosthetic device.)

See Intermediary Manual, section 3112.4 and Carriers Manual, sections 2050.1 and 15010.

45-10 LAETRILE AND RELATED SUBSTANCES—NOT COVERED

Laetrile (and the other drugs called by the various terms mentioned below) have been used primarily in the treatment or control of cancer. Although the terms "Laetrile," "laetrile," "amygdalin," "Sarcarcinase," "vitamin B-17," and "nitriloside" have been used interchangeably, the chemical identity of the substances to which these terms refer has varied.

The FDA has determined that neither Laetrile nor any other drug called by the various terms mentioned above, nor any other product which might be characterized as a "nitriloside" is generally recognized (by experts qualified by scientific training and experience to evaluate the safety and effectiveness of drugs) to be safe and effective for any therapeutic use. Therefore, use of this drug cannot be considered to be reasonable and necessary within the meaning of section 1862(a)(1) of the Act and program payment may not be made for its use or any services furnished in connection with its administration.

A hospital stay only for the purpose of having laetrile (or any other drug called by the terms mentioned above) administered is not covered. Also, program payment may not be made for laetrile (or other drug noted above) when it is used during the course of an otherwise covered hospital stay, since the FDA has found such drugs to not be safe and effective for any therapeutic purpose.

45-15 PHYSICIAN'S OFFICE WITHIN AN INSTITUTION—COVERAGE OF SERVICES AND SUPPLIES INCIDENT TO A PHYSICIAN'S SERVICES

When a physician establishes an office within a nursing home or other institution, coverage of services and supplies furnished in the office must be determined in accordance with the "incident to a physician's professional service" provision (see Intermediary Manual, §3112.4A or Carriers Manual, §2050.1), as in any physician's office. A physician's office within an institution must be confined to a separately identified part of the facility that is used solely as the physician's office and cannot be construed to extend throughout the entire institution. Thus, services performed outside the "office" area would be subject to the coverage rules applicable to services furnished outside the office setting.

In order to accurately apply the criteria in §3112.4 or §2050.1, give consideration to the physical proximity of the institution and physician's office. When his office is located within a facility, a physician may not be reimbursed for services, supplies, and use of equipment which fall outside the scope of services "commonly furnished" in physicians' offices generally, even though such services may be furnished in his institutional office. Additionally, make a distinction between the physician's office practice and the institution, especially when the physician is administrator or owner of the facility. Thus, for their services to be covered under the criteria in §3112.4A or §2050.1, the auxiliary medical personnel must be members of the office staff rather than of the institution's staff, and the cost of supplies must represent an expense to the physician's office practice. Finally, services performed by the employees of the physician outside the "office" area must be directly supervised by the physician; his presence in the facility as a whole would not suffice to meet this requirement. (In any setting, of course, supervision of auxiliary personnel in and of itself is not considered a "physician's professional service" to which the services of the auxiliary personnel could be an incidental part—i.e., in addition to supervision, the physician must perform or have performed a personal professional service to the patient to which the services of the auxiliary personnel could be considered an incidental part.) Denials for failure to meet any of these requirements would be based on §1861(s)(2)(A) of the Act.

Establishment of an office within an institution would not modify rules otherwise applicable for determining coverage of the physician's personal professional services within the institution. However, in view of the opportunity afforded to a physician who maintains such an office for rendering services to a sizable number of patients in a short period of time or for performing frequent services for the same patient, claims for physicians' services rendered under such circumstances would require careful evaluation by the carrier to assure that payment is made only for services that are reasonable and necessary.

Cross-refer: Intermediary Manual, §3112.4A; Carriers Manual, §2050.1.

45-16 CERTAIN DRUGS DISTRIBUTED BY THE NATIONAL CANCER INSTITUTE

Under its Cancer Therapy Evaluation, the Division of Cancer Treatment of the National Cancer Institute (NCI), in cooperation with the Food and Drug Administration, approves and distributes certain drugs for use in treating terminally ill cancer patients. One group of these drugs, designated as Group C drugs, unlike other drugs distributed by the NCI, are not limited to use in clinical trials for the purpose of testing their efficacy. Drugs are classified as Group C drugs only if there is sufficient evidence demonstrating their efficacy within a tumor type and that they can be safely administered.

A physician is eligible to receive Group C drugs from the Divison of Cancer Treatment only if the following requirements are met:

- A physician must be registered with the NCI as an investigator by having completed an FD-Form 1573;
- A written request for the drug, indicating the disease to be treated, must be submitted to the NCI;
- The use of the drug must be limited to indications outlined in the NCI's guidelines; and
- All adverse reactions must be reported to the Investigational Drug Branch of the Division of Cancer Treatment.

In view of these NCI controls on distribution and use of Group C drugs, intermediaries may assume, in the absence of evidence to the contrary, that a Group C drug and the related hospital stay are covered if all other applicable coverage requirements are satisfied.

If there is reason to question coverage in a particular case, the matter should be resolved with the assistance of the local PSRO, or if there is none, the assistance of your medical consultants.

Information regarding those drugs which are classified as Group C drugs may be obtained from:

Office of the Chief, Investigational Drug Branch
Division of Cancer Treatment, CTEP, Landow Building
Room 4C09, National Cancer Institute
Bethesda, Maryland 20205

45-20 ETHYLENEDIAMINE-TETRA-ACETIC (EDTA) CHELATION THERAPY FOR TREATMENT OF ATHEROSCLEROSIS

The use of EDTA as a chelating agent to treat atherosclerosis, arteriosclerosis, calcinosis, or similar generalized condition not listed by the FDA as an approved use is not covered. Any such use of EDTA is considered experimental.

See section 35-64 for an explanation of this conclusion.

45-22 LYMPHOCYTE IMMUNE GLOBULIN, ANTI-THYMOCYTE GLOBULIN (EQUINE)

The lymphocyte immune globulin preparations are biologic drugs not previously approved or licensed for use in the management of renal allograft rejection. A number of other lymphocyte immune globulin products of equine, lapine, and murine origin are currently under investigation for their potential usefulness in controlling allograft rejections in human transplantation. These biologic drugs are viewed as adjunctive to traditional immunosuppressive products such as steroids and anti-metabolic drugs. At present, lymphocyte immune globulin preparations are not recommended to replace conventional immunosuppressive drugs, but to supplement them and to be used as alternatives to elevated or accelerated dosing with conventional immunosuppressive agents.

The FDA has approved one lymphocyte immune globulin preparation for marketing, lymphocyte immune globulin, anti-thymocyte globulin (equine). This drug is indicated for the management of allograft rejection episodes in renal transplantation. It is covered under Medicare when used for this purpose. Other forms of lymphocyte globulin preparation which the FDA approves for this indication in the future may be covered under Medicare.

45-23 DIMETHYL SULFOXIDE (DMSO)

DMSO is an industrial solvent produced as a chemical byproduct of paper production from wood pulp. The Food and Drug Administration has determined that the only purpose for which DMSO is safe and effective for humans is in the treatment of the bladder condition, interstitial cystitis. Therefore, the use of DMSO for all other indications is not considered to be reasonable and necessary. Payment may be made for its use only when reasonable and necessary for a patient in the treatment of interstitial cystitis.

45-24 ANTI-INHIBITOR COAGULANT COMPLEX (AICC)

Anti-inhibitor coagulant complex, AICC, is a drug used to treat hemophilia in patients with factor VIII inhibitor antibodies. AICC has been shown to be safe and effective and has Medicare coverage when furnished to patients with hemophilia A and inhibitor antibodies to factor VIII who have major bleeding episodes and who fail to respond to other, less expensive therapies.

45-25 SUPPLIES USED IN THE DELIVERY OF TRANSCUTANEOUS ELECTRICAL NERVE STIMULATION (TENS) AND NEUROMUSCULAR ELECTRICAL STIMULATION (NMES)

Transcutaneous Electrical Nerve Stimulation (TENS) and/or Neuromuscular Electrical Stimulation (NMES) can ordinarily be delivered to patients through the use of conventional electrodes, adhesive tapes and lead wires. There may be times, however, where it might be medically necessary for certain patients receiving TENS or NMES treatment to use, as an alternative to conventional electrodes, adhesive tapes and lead wires, a form-fitting conductive garment (i.e., a garment with conductive fibers which are separated from the patients' skin by layers of fabric).

A form-fitting conductive garment (and medically necessary related supplies) may be covered under the program only when:

1. It has received permission or approval for marketing by the Food and Drug Administration;

2. It has been prescribed by a physician for use in delivering covered TENS or NMES treatment; and

3. One of the medical indications outlined below is met:

- The patient cannot manage without the conductive garment because there is such a large area or so many sites to be stimulated and the stimulation would have to be delivered so frequently that it is not feasible to use conventional electrodes, adhesive tapes and lead wires;
- The patient cannot manage without the conductive garment for the treatment of chronic intractable pain because the areas or sites to be stimulated are inaccessible with the use of conventional electrodes, adhesive tapes and lead wires;
- The patient has a documented medical condition such as skin problems that preclude the application of conventional electrodes, adhesive tapes and lead wires;
- The patient requires electrical stimulation beneath a cast either to treat disuse atrophy, where the nerve supply to the muscle is intact, or to treat chronic intractable pain; or
- The patient has a medical need for rehabilitation strengthening (pursuant to a written plan of rehabilitation) following an injury where the nerve supply to the muscle is intact.

A conductive garment is not covered for use with a TENS device during the trial period specified in section 35-46 unless:

4. The patient has a documented skin problem prior to the start of the trial period; and

5. The carrier's medical consultants are satisfied that use of such an item is medically necessary for the patient.

(See conditions for coverage of the use of TENS in the diagnosis and treatment of chronic intractable pain in sections 35-46 and 60-20 and the use of NMES in the treatment of disuse atrophy in section 35-77.)

45-30 PHOTOSENSITIVE DRUGS

Photosensitive drugs are the light-sensitive agents used in photodynamic therapy. Once introduced into the body, these drugs selectively identify and adhere to diseased tissue. The drugs remain inactive until they are exposed to a specific wavelength of light, by means of a laser, that corresponds to their absorption peak. The activation of a photosensitive drug results in a photochemical reaction which treats the diseased tissue without affecting surrounding normal tissue.

Verteporfin

Verteporfin, a benzoporphyrin derivative, is an intravenous lipophilic photosensitive drug with an absorption peak of 690 nm. This drug was first approved by the Food and Drug Administration (FDA) on April 12, 2000, and subsequently, approved for inclusion in the United States Pharmacopoeia on July 18, 2000, meeting Medicare's definition of a drug as defined under §1861(t)(1) of the Social Security Act. Effective July 1, 2001, Verteporfin (Q3013 – Injection, Verteporfin) is only covered when used in conjunction with ocular photodynamic therapy (see §35-100 PHOTODYNAMIC THERAPY) when furnished intravenously incident to a physician's service. For patients with age-related macular degeneration, Verteporfin is only covered with a diagnosis of neovascular age-related macular degeneration (ICD-9-CM 362.52) with predominately classic subfoveal choroidal neovascular (CNV) lesions (where the area of classic CNV occupies ≥ 50% of the area of the entire lesion) at the initial visit as determined by a fluorescein angiogram (CPT code 92235*). Subsequent follow-up visits will require a fluorescein angiogram prior to treatment. There are no requirements regarding visual acuity, lesion size, and number of retreatments.

50 DIAGNOSTIC SERVICES

50-1 Cardiac Pacemaker Evaluation Services—Medicare covers a variety of services for the post-implant follow-up and evaluation of implanted cardiac pacemakers. The following guidelines are designed to assist contractors in identifying and processing claims for such services.

NOTE: These new guidelines are limited to lithium battery-powered pacemakers, because mercury-zinc battery-powered pacemakers are no longer being manufactured and virtually all have been replaced by lithium units. Contractors still receiving claims for monitoring such units should continue to apply the guidelines published in 1980 to those units until they are replaced.

There are two general types of pacemakers in current use—single-chamber pacemakers, which sense and pace the ventricles of the heart, and dual-chamber pacemakers which sense and pace both the atria and the ventricles. These differences require different monitoring patterns over the expected life of the units involved. One fact of which contractors should be aware is that many dual-chamber units may be programmed to pace only the ventricles; this may be done either at the time the pacemaker is implanted or at some time afterward. In such cases, a dual-chamber unit, when programmed or reprogrammed for ventricular pacing, should be treated as a single-chamber pacemaker in applying screening guidelines.

The decision as to how often any patient's pacemaker should be monitored is the responsibility of the patient's physician who is best able to take into account the condition and circumstances of the individual patient. These may vary over time, requiring modifications of the frequency with which the patient should be monitored. In cases where monitoring is done by some entity other than the patient's physician, such as a commercial monitoring service or hospital outpatient department, the physician's prescription for monitoring is required and should be periodically renewed (at least annually) to assure that the frequency of monitoring is proper for the patient. Where a patient is monitored both during clinic visits and transtelephonically, the contractor should be sure to include frequency data on both types of monitoring in evaluating the reasonableness of the frequency of monitoring services received by the patient.

Since there are over 200 pacemaker models in service at any given point, and a variety of patient conditions that give rise to the need for pacemakers, the question of the appropriate frequency of monitorings is a complex one. Nevertheless, it is possible to develop guidelines within which the vast majority of pacemaker monitorings will fall and contractors should do this, using their own data and experience, as well as the frequency guidelines which follow, in order to limit extensive claims development to those cases requiring special attention.

Guidelines for Transtelephonic Monitoring of Cardiac Pacemakers

A. General.—Transtelephonic monitoring of pacemakers is coming into increasingly widespread use, with the services being furnished by commercial suppliers, hospital outpatient departments and physicians' offices.

Telephone monitoring of cardiac pacemakers as described below is medically efficacious in identifying early signs of possible pacemaker failure, thus reducing the number of sudden pacemaker failures requiring emergency replacement. All systems which monitor the pacemaker rate (bpm) in both the free-running and/or magnetic mode are effective in detecting subclinical pacemaker failure due to battery depletion. More sophisticated systems are also capable of detecting internal electronic problems within the pulse generator itself and other potential problems. In the case of dual chamber pacemakers in particular, such monitoring may detect failure of synchronization of the atria and ventricles, and the need for adjustment and reprogramming of the device.

*CPT only © *Current Procedural Terminology, 2002 Professional Edition*, American Medical Association.

NOTE: The transmitting device furnished to the patient is simply one component of the diagnostic system, and is not covered as durable medical equipment. Those engaged in trans-telephonic pacemaker monitoring should reflect the costs of the transmitters in setting their charges for monitoring.

B. Definition of Transtelephonic Monitoring.—In order for transtelephonic monitoring services to be covered, the services must consist of the following elements:

1. A minimum 30-second readable strip of the pacemaker in the free-running mode;

2. Unless contraindicated, a minimum 30-second readable strip of the pacemaker in the magnetic mode; and

3. A minimum 30 seconds of readable ECG strip.

C. Frequency Guidelines for Transtelephonic Monitoring.—The guidelines below constitute a system which contractors should use, in conjunction with their knowledge of local medical practices, to screen claims for transtelephonic monitoring prior to payment. It is important to note that they are not recommendations with respect to a minimum frequency for such monitorings, but rather a maximum frequency (within which payment may be made without further claims development). As with previous guidelines, more frequent monitorings may be covered in cases where contractors are satisfied that such monitorings are medically necessary; e.g., based on the condition of the patient, or with respect to pacemakers exhibiting unexpected defects or premature failure. Contractors should seek written justification for more frequent monitorings from the patient's physician and/or any monitoring service involved.

These guidelines are divided into two broad categories—Guideline I, which will apply to the majority of pacemakers now in use, and Guideline II, which will apply only to pacemaker systems (pacemaker and leads) for which sufficient long-term clinical information exists to assure that they meet the standards of the Inter-Society Commission for Heart Disease Resources (ICHD) for longevity and end-of-life decay. (The ICHD standards are: (1) 90 percent cumulative survival at 5 years following implant; and (2) an end-of-life decay of less than a 50 percent drop of output voltage and less than 20 percent deviation of magnet rate, or a drop of 5 beats per minute or less, over a period of 3 months or more.) Contractors should consult with their medical advisers and other appropriate individuals and organizations (such as the North American Society of Pacing and Electrophysiology, which publishes product reliability information) should questions arise over whether a pacemaker system meets the ICHD standards.

The two groups of guidelines are then further broken down into two general categories—single chamber and dual-chamber pacemakers. Contractors should be aware that the frequency with which a patient is monitored may be changed from time to time for a number of reasons, such as a change in the patient's overall condition, a reprogramming of the patient's pacemaker, the development of better information on the pacemaker's longevity or failure mode, etc. Consequently, changes in the proper set of guidelines may be required. Contractors should inform physicians and monitoring services to alert contractors to any changes in the patient's monitoring prescription that might necessitate changes in the screening guidelines applied to that patient. (Of particular importance is the reprogramming of a dual-chamber pacemaker to a single-chamber mode of operation. Such reprogramming would shift the patient from the appropriate dual-chamber guideline to the appropriate single-chamber guideline.)

Guideline I

1. Single-chamber pacemakers:
   1st month—every 2 weeks.
   2nd through 36th month—every 8 weeks.
   37th month to failure—every 4 weeks.
2. Dual-chamber pacemaker:
   1st month—every 2 weeks.
   2nd through 6th month—every 4 weeks.
   7th through 36th month—every 8 weeks.
   37th month to failure—every 4 weeks.

Guideline II

1. Single-chamber pacemakers:
   1st month—every 2 weeks.
   2nd through 48th month—every 12 weeks.
   49th through 72nd month—every 8 weeks.
   Thereafter—every 4 weeks.
2. Dual-chamber pacemaker:
   1st month—every 2 weeks.
   2nd through 30th month—every 12 weeks.
   31st through 48th month—every 8 weeks.
   Thereafter—every 4 weeks.

D. Pacemaker Clinic Services

1. General—Pacemaker monitoring is also covered when done by pacemaker clinics. Clinic visits may be done in conjunction with transtelephonic monitoring or as a separate service; however, the services rendered by a pacemaker clinic are more extensive than those currently possible by telephone. They include, for example, physical examination of patients and reprogramming of pacemakers. Thus, the use of one of these types of monitoring does not preclude concurrent use of the other.

2. Frequency Guidelines—As with transtelephonic pacemaker monitoring, the frequency of clinic visits is the decision of the patient's physician, taking into account, among other things, the medical condition of the patient. However, contractors can develop monitoring guidelines that will prove useful in screening claims. The following are recommendations for monitoring guidelines on lithium-battery pacemakers:

a. For single-chamber pacemakers—twice in the first 6 months following implant, then once every 12 months.

b. For dual-chamber pacemakers—twice in the first 6 months, then once every 6 months.

50-15 ELECTROCARDIOGRAPHIC SERVICES

Reimbursement may be made under Part B for electrocardiographic (EKG) services rendered by a physician or incident to his/her services or by an approved laboratory or an approved supplier of portable X-ray services. Since there is no coverage for EKG services of any type rendered on a screening basis or as part of a routine examination, the claim must indicate the signs and symptoms or other clinical reason necessitating the services.

A separate charge by an attending or consulting physician for EKG interpretation is allowed only when it is the normal practice to make such charge in addition to the regular office visit charge. No payment is made for EKG interpretations by individuals other than physicians.

On a claim involving EKG services furnished by a laboratory or a portable X-ray supplier, identify the physician ordering the service and, when the charge includes both the taking of the tracing and its interpretation, include the identity of the physician making the interpretation. No separate bill for the services of a physician is paid unless it is clear that he/she was the patient's attending physician or was acting as a consulting physician. The taking of an EKG in an emergency, i.e., when the patient is or may be experiencing what is commonly referred to as a heart attack, is covered as a laboratory service or a diagnostic service by a portable X-ray supplier only when the evidence shows that a physician was in attendance at the time the service was performed or immediately thereafter.

Where EKG services are rendered in the patient's home and the laboratory's or portable X-ray supplier's charge is higher than that imposed for the same service when performed in the laboratory or portable X-ray supplier's office, the medical need for home service should be documented. In the absence of such justification, reimbursement for the service if otherwise medically necessary should be based on the reasonable charge applicable when performed in the laboratory or X-ray supplier's office.

The documentation required in the various situations mentioned above must be furnished not only when the laboratory or portable X-ray supplier bills the patient or carrier for its service, but also when such a facility bills the attending physician who, in turn, bills the patient or carrier for the EKG services. (In addition to the evidence required to document the claim, the laboratory or portable X-ray supplier must maintain in its records the referring physician's written order and the identity of the employee taking the tracing.)

Long-term EKG monitoring, also referred to as long-term EKG recording, Holter recording, or dynamic electrocardiography, is a diagnostic procedure which provides a continuous record of the electrocardiographic activity of a patient's heart while he is engaged in his daily activities.

The basic components of the long-term EKG monitoring systems are a sensing element, the design of which may provide either for the recording of electrocardiographic information on magnetic tape or for detecting significant variations in rate or rhythm as they occur, and a component for either graphically recording the electrocardiographic data or for visual or computer assisted analysis of the information recorded on magnetic tape. The long-term EKG permits the examination in the ambulant or potentially ambulant patient of as many as 70,000 heartbeats in a 12-hour recording while the standard EKG which is obtained in the recumbent position, yields information on only 50 to 60 cardiac cycles and provides only a limited data base on which diagnostic judgments may be made.

Many patients with cardiac arrhythmias are unaware of the presence of an irregularity in heart rhythm. Due to the transient nature of many arrhythmias and the short intervals in which the rhythm of the heart is observed by conventional standard EKG techniques, the offending arrhythmias can go undetected. With the extended examination provided by the long-term EKG, the physician is able not only to detect but also to classify various types of rhythm disturbances and waveform abnormalities and note the frequency of their occurrence. The knowledge of the reaction of the heart to daily activities with respect to rhythm, rate, conduction disturbances, and ischemic changes are of great assistance in directing proper therapy and rehabilitation.

This modality is valuable in both inpatient and outpatient diagnosis and therapy. Long-term monitoring of ambulant or potentially ambulant inpatients provides significant potential for reducing the length of stay for post-coronary infarct patients in the intensive care setting and may result in earlier discharge from the hospital with greater assurance of safety to the patients. The indications for the use of this technique, noted below, are similar for both inpatients and outpatients.

The long-term EKG has proven effective in detecting transient episodes of cardiac dysrhythmia and in permitting the correlation of these episodes with cardiovascular symptomatology. It is also useful for patients who have symptoms of obscure etiology suggestive of cardiac arrhythmia. Examples of such symptoms include palpitations, chest pain, dizziness, light-headedness, near syncope, syncope, transient ischemic episodes, dyspnea, and shortness of breath.

This technique would also be appropriate at the time of institution of any arrhythmic drug therapy and may be performed during the course of therapy to evaluate response. It is also appropriate for evaluating a change of dosage and may be indicated shortly before and after the discontinuation of anti-arrhythemic medication. The therapeutic response to a drug whose duration of action and peak of effectiveness is defined in hours cannot be properly assessed by examining 30 to 40 cycles on a standard EKG rhythm strip. The knowledge that all patients placed on anti-arrhythmic medication do not respond to therapy and the known toxicity of anti-arrhythmic agents clearly indicate that proper assessment should be made on an individual basis to determine whether medication should be continued and at what dosage level.

The long-term EKG is also valuable in the assessment of patients with coronary artery disease. It enables the documentation of etiology of such symptoms as chest pain and shortness of breath. Since the standard EKG is often normal during the intervals between the episodes of precordial pain, it is essential to obtain EKG information while the symptoms are occurring. The long-term EKG has enabled the correlation of chest symptoms with the objective evidence of ST-segment abnormalities. It is appropriate for patients who are recovering from an acute mycardial infarction or coronary insufficiency before and after discharge from the hospital, since it is impossible to predict which of these patients is subject to ventricular arrhythmias on the basis of the presence or absence of rhythm disturbances during the period of initial coronary care. The long-term EKG enables the physician to identify patients who are at a higher risk of dying suddenly in the period following an acute myocardial infarction. It may also be reasonable and necessary where the high-risk patient with known cardiovascular disease advances to a substantially higher level of activity which might trigger increased or new types of arrhythmias necessitating treatment. Such a high-risk case would be one in which there is documentation that acute phase arrhythmias have not totally disappeared during the period of convalesence.

In view of recent developments in cardiac pacemaker monitoring techniques (see CIA 50-1), the use of the long-term EKG for routine assessment of pacemaker function can no longer be justified. Its use for the patient with an internal pacemaker would be covered only when he has symptoms suggestive of arrhythmia not revealed by the standard EKG or rhythm strip.

These guidelines are intended as a general outline of the circumstances under which the use of this diagnostic procedure would be warranted. Each patient receiving a long-term EKG should be evaluated completely, prior to performance of this diagnostic study. A complete history and physical examination should be obtained and the indications for use of the long-term EKG should be reviewed by the referring physician.

The performance of a long-term EKG does not necessarily require the prior performance of a standard EKG. Nor does the demonstration of a normal standard EKG preclude the need for a long-term EKG. Finally, the demonstration of an abnormal standard EKG does not obviate the need for a long-term EKG if there is suspicion that the dysrhythmia is transient in nature.

A period of recording of up to 24 hours would normally be adequate to detect most transient arrhythmias and provide essential diagnostic information. The medical necessity for longer periods of monitoring must be documented.

Medical documentation for adjudicating claims for the use of the long-term EKG should be similar to other EKG services, X-ray services, and laboratory procedures. Generally, a statement of the diagnostic impression of the referring physician with an indication of the patient's relevant signs and symptoms should be sufficient for purposes of making a determination regarding the reasonableness and medical necessity for the use of this procedure. However, the intermediaries or carriers should require whatever additional documentation their medical consultants deem necessary to properly adjudicate the individual claim where the information submitted is not adequate.

It should be noted that the recording device furnished to the patient is simply one component of the diagnostic system and a separate charge for it will not be recognized under the durable medical equipment benefit.

Patient-Activated EKG Recorders, distributed under a variety of brand names, permit the patient to record an EKG upon manifestation of symptoms, or in response to a physician's order (e.g., immediately following strong exertion). Most such devices also permit the patient to simultaneously voice-record in order to describe symptoms and/or activity. In addition, some of these devices permit transtelephonic transmission of the recording to a physician's office, clinic, hospital, etc., having a decoder/recorder for review and analysis, thus eliminating the need to physically transport the tape. Some of these devices also permit a "time sampling" mode of operation. However, the "time sampling" mode is not covered—only the patient-activated mode of operation, when used for the indications described below, is covered at this time.

Services in connection with patient-activated EKG recorders are covered when used as an alternative to the long-term EKG monitoring (described above) for similar indications—detecting and characterizing symptomatic arrhythmias, regulation of anti-arrhythmic drug therapy, etc. Like long-term EKG monitoring, use of these devices is covered for evaluating patients with symptoms of obscure etiology suggestive of cardiac arrhythmia such as palpitations, chest pain, dizziness, lightheadedness, near syncope, syncope, transient ischemic episodes, dyspnea and shortness of breath.

As with long-term EKG monitors, patient-activated EKG recorders may be useful for both inpatient and outpatient diagnosis and therapy. While useful for assessing some post-coronary infarct patients in the hospital setting, these devices should not, however, be covered for outpatient monitoring of recently discharged post-infarct patients.

Computer Analyzed Electrocardiograms.—Computer interpretation of EKGs is recognized as a valid and effective technique which will improve the quality and availability of cardiology services. Reimbursement may be made for such computer service when furnished in the setting and under the circumstances required for coverage of other electrocardiographic services. Where either a laboratory's or a portable x-ray supplier's charge for EKG services includes the physician review and certification of the printout as well as the computer interpretation, the certifying physician must be identified on the HCFA-1490 before the entire charge can be considered a reimbursable charge. Where the laboratory's (or portable x-ray supplier's) reviewing physician is not identified, the carrier should conclude that no professional component is involved and make its charge determination accordingly. If the supplying laboratory (or portable x-ray supplier when supplied by such a facility) does not include professional review and certification of the hard copy, a charge by the patient's physician may be recognized for the service. In any case the charge for the physician component should be substantially less than that for physician interpretation of the conventional EKG tracing in view of markedly reduced demand on the physician's time where computer interpretation is involved. Considering the unit cost reduction expected of this innovation, the total charge for the complete EKG service (taking of tracing and interpretation) when computer interpretation is employed should never exceed that considered reasonable for the service when physician interpretation is involved.

Transtelephonic Electrocardiographic Transmissions (Formerly Referred to as EKG Telephone Reporter Systems).—Effective for services furnished on and after March 1, 1980, coverage is extended to include the use of transtelephonic electrocardiographic (EKG) transmissions as a diagnostic service for the indications described below, when performed with equipment meeting the standards described below, subject to the limitations and conditions specified below. Coverage is further limited to the amounts payable with respect to the physician's service in interpreting the results of such transmissions, including charges for rental of the equipment. The device used by the beneficiary is part of a total diagnostic system and is not considered durable medical equipment.

1. Covered Uses.—The use of transtelephonic EKGs is covered for the following uses:

a. To detect, characterize, and document symptomatic transient arrhythmias;

b. To overcome problems in regulating antiarrhythmic drug dosage;

c. To carry out early posthospital monitoring of patients discharged after myocardial infarction; (only if 24-hour coverage is provided, see 4. below).

Since cardiology is a rapidly changing field, some uses other than those specified above may be covered if, in the judgment of the contractor's medical consultants, such a use was justifiable in the particular case. The enumerated uses above represent uses for which a firm coverage determination has been made, and for which contractors may make payment without extensive claims development or review.

2. Specifications for Devices.—The devices used by the patient are highly portable (usually pocket-sized) and detect and convert the normal EKG signal so that it can be transmitted via ordinary telephone apparatus to a receiving station. At the receiving end, the signal is decoded and transcribed into a conventional EKG. There are numerous devices available which transmit EKG readings in this fashion. For purposes of Medicare coverage, however, the transmitting devices must meet at least the following criteria:

a. They must be capable of transmitting EKG Leads, I, II, or III;

b. These lead transmissions must be sufficiently comparable to readings obtained by a conventional EKG to permit proper interpretation of abnormal cardiac rhythms.

3. Potential for Abuse—Need for Screening Guidelines.—While the use of these devices may often compare favorably with more costly alternatives, this is the case only where the information they contribute is actively utilized by a knowledgeable practitioner as part of overall medical management of the patient. Consequently, it is vital that contractors be aware of the potential for abuse of these devices, and adopt necessary screening and physician education policies to detect and halt potentially abusive situations. For example, use of these devices to diagnose and treat suspected arrhythmias as a routine substitute for more conventional methods of diagnosis, such as a careful history, physical examination, and standard EKG and rhythm strip would not be appropriate. Moreover, contractors should require written justification for use of such devices in excess of 30 consecutive days in cases involving detection of transient arrhythmias.

Contractors may find it useful to review claims for these devices with a view toward detecting patterns of practice which may be useful in developing schedules which may be adopted for screening such claims in the future.

4. Twenty-Four Hour Coverage.—No payment may be made for the use of these devices to carry out early posthospital monitoring of patients discharged after myocardial infarction unless provision is made for 24 hour coverage in the manner described below.

Twenty-four hour coverage means that there must be, at the monitoring site (or sites) an experienced EKG technician receiving calls; tape recording devices do not meet this requirement. Further, such technicians should have immediate access to a physician, and have been instructed in when and how to contact available facilities to assist the patient in case of emergencies.

Cross-refer: HCFA-Pub. 13-3, sections 3101.5, 3110, 3112.3, HCFA-Pub. 14-3, sections 2070, 2255, 2050.1

50-17 LABORATORY TESTS—CRD PATIENTS

A. Laboratory tests are essential to monitor the progress of CRD patients. The following list and frequencies of tests constitute the level and types of routine laboratory tests that are covered. Bills for other types of tests are considered non-routine. Routine tests at greater frequencies must include medical justification. Non-routine tests generally are justified by the diagnosis. The routinely covered regimen includes the following tests:

Per Dialysis

All hematocrit or hemoglobin and clotting time tests furnished incident to dialysis treatments.

Per Week

Prothrombin time for patients on anticoagulant therapy
Serum creatinine

Per Week or Thirteen Per Quarter

BUN

Monthly

CBC	Serum calcium
Serum potassium	Serum chloride
Serum bicarbonate	Serum phosphorous
Total protein	Serum albumin
Alkaline phosphatase	AST, SGOT
LDH	

Guidelines for tests other than those routinely performed include:
Serum aluminum—one every 3 months
Serum ferritin—one every 3 months

The following tests for hepatitis B are covered when patients first enter a dialysis facility: hepatitis B surface antigen (HBsAg) and Anti-HBs. Coverage of future testing in these patients depends on their serologic status and on whether they have been successfully immunized against hepatitis B virus. The following table summarizes the frequency of serologic surveillance for hepatitis B. Tests furnished according to this table do not require additional documentation and are paid separately because payment for maintenance dialysis treatments does not take them into account.

Vaccination and Serologic Status	Frequency of Screening	
	HBsAg Patients	Anti-HBs Patients
UNVACCINATED		
Susceptible	Monthly	Semiannually
HBsAg carrier	Annually	None
Anti-HBs-positive*	None	Annually
VACCINATED		
Anti-HBs-positive*	None	Annually
Low level or no anti-HBs	Monthly	Semiannually

*At least 10 sample ration units by radioimmunoassay or positive by enzyme immunoassay.

Patients who are in the process of receiving hepatitis B vaccines, but have not received the complete series, should continue to be routinely screened as susceptible. Between one and six months after the third dose, all vaccines should be tested for anti-HBs to confirm their response to the vaccine. Patients who have a level of anti-HBs of at least 10 sample ratio units (SRUs) by radioimmunoassay (RIA) or who are positive by enzyme immunoassay (EIA) are considered adequate responders to vaccine and need be tested only for anti-HBs annually to verify their immune status. If anti-HBs drops below 10 SRUs by RIA or is negative by EIA, a booster dose of hepatitis B vaccine should be given.

B. Laboratory tests are subject to the normal coverage requirements. If the laboratory services are performed by a free-standing facility, be sure it meets the conditions of coverage for independent laboratories.

50-20 DIAGNOSTIC PAP SMEARS

A diagnostic Pap smear and related medically necessary services are covered under Medicare Part B when ordered by a physician under one of the following conditions:

- Previous cancer of the cervix, uterus, or vagina that has been or is presently being treated;
- Previous abnormal Pap smear;
- Any abnormal findings of the vagina, cervix, uterus, ovaries, or adnexa;
- Any significant complaint by the patient referrable to the female reproductive system; or
- Any signs or symptoms that might in the physician's judgment reasonably be related to a gynecologic disorder.

In respect to the last bullet, the contractor's medical staff must determine whether in a particular case a previous malignancy at another site is an indication for a diagnostic Pap smear or whether the test must be considered a screening Pap smear as described in section 50-20.1. Use the following CPT codes for indicating diagnostic Pap smears:

- 88150* Cytopathology, smears, cervical or vaginal (e.g., Papanicolaou), up to three smears; screening by technician under physician supervision; *or*
- 88151* Cytopathology, smears, cervical or vaginal (e.g., Papanicolaou), up to three smears; requiring interpretation by physician.

*CPT only © *Current Procedural Terminology, 2002 Professional Edition*, American Medical Association. All rights reserved.

50-20.1 Screening PAP Smears and Pelvic Examinations for Early Detection of Cervical or Vaginal Cancer—(For screening Pap smears, effective for services performed on or after July 1, 1990. For pelvic examinations including clinical breast examination, effective for services furnished on or after January 1, 1998.)

A screening Pap smear (use HCPCS code P3000 Screening Papanicolaou smear, cervical or vaginal, up to three smears; by technician under physician supervision *or* P3001 Screening Papanicolaou smear, cervical or vaginal, up to three smears requiring interpretation by physician). (Use HCPCS codes G0123 Screening Cytopathology, cervical or vaginal (any reporting system), collected in preservative fluid, automated thin layer preparation, screening by cytotechnologist under physician supervision *or* G0124 Screening Cytopathology, cervical or vaginal (any reporting system) collected in preservative fluid, automated thin layer preparation, requiring interpretation by physician) and related medically necessary services provided to a woman for the early detection of cervical cancer (including collection of the sample of cells and a physician's interpretation of the test results) and pelvic examination (including clinical breast examination) (use HCPCS code G0101 cervical or vaginal cancer screening; pelvic and clinical breast examination) are covered under Medicare Part B when ordered by a physician (or authorized practitioner) under one of the following conditions:

- She has not had such a test during the preceding 3 years or is a woman of childbearing age (section 1861(nn) of the Act).
- There is evidence (on the basis of her medical history or other findings) that she is at high risk of developing cervical cancer and her physician (or authorized practitioner) recommends that she have the test performed more frequently than every 3 years.

High risk factors for cervical and vaginal cancer are:

- Early onset of sexual activity (under 16 years of age)
- Multiple sexual partners (five or more in a lifetime)
- History of sexually transmitted disease (including HIV infection)
- Fewer than three negative or any Pap smears within the previous 7 years; and
- DES (diethylstilbestrol)-exposed daughters of women who took DES during pregnancy.

NOTE: Claims for Pap smears must indicate the beneficiary's low or high risk status by including the appropriate ICD-9-CM on the line item (Item 24E of the HCFA-1500).

- V76.2, special screening for malignant neoplasms of the cervix, **indicates low risk**; and
- V15.89, other specified personal history presenting hazards to health, **indicates high risk.**

If Pap smear or pelvic exam claims do not point to one of these diagnosis codes, the claim will reject in the Common Working File. Claims can contain up to four diagnosis codes, but the one pointed to on the line item must be either V76.2 or V15.89.

Definitions:

A woman as described in section 1861(nn) of the Act is a woman who is of childbearing age and has had a Pap smear test during any of the preceding 3 years that indicated the presence of cervical or vaginal cancer or other abnormality, or is at high risk of developing cervical or vaginal cancer.

A woman of childbearing age is one who is premenopausal and has been determined by a physician or other qualified practitioner to be of childbearing age, based upon the medical history or other findings.

"Other qualified practitioner," as defined in 42 CFR 410.56(a) includes a certified nurse midwife (as defined in section 1861(gg) of the Act), or a physician assistant, nurse practitioner, or clinical nurse specialist (as defined in section 1861(aa) of the Act) who is authorized under State law to perform the examination.

Screening Pelvic Examination:

Section 4102 of the Balanced Budget Act of 1997 provides for coverage of screening pelvic examinations (including a clinical breast examination) for all female beneficiaries, effective January 1, 1998, subject to certain frequency and other limitations. A screening pelvic examination (including a clinical breast examination) should include at least seven of the following eleven elements:

- Inspection and palpation of breasts for masses or lumps, tenderness, symmetry, or nipple discharge.
- Digital rectal examination including sphincter tone, presence of hemorrhoids, and rectal masses. Pelvic examination (with or without specimen collection for smears and cultures) including:
- External genitalia (e.g., general appearance, hair distribution, or lesions).
- Urethral meatus (e.g., size, location, lesions, or prolapse).
- Urethra (e.g., masses, tenderness, or scarring).
- Bladder (e.g., fullness, masses, or tenderness).
- Vagina (e.g., general appearance, estrogen effect, discharge lesions, pelvic support, cystocele, or rectocele).
- Cervix (e.g., general appearance, lesions, or discharge).
- Uterus (e.g., size, contour, position, mobility, tenderness, consistency, descent, or support).
- Adnexa/parametria (e.g., masses, tenderness, organomegaly, or nodularity).
- Anus and perineum.

This description is from Documentation Guidelines for Evaluation and Management Services, published in May 1997 and was developed by the Health Care Financing Administration and the American Medical Association.

50-24 HAIR ANALYSIS—NOT COVERED

Hair analysis to detect mineral traces as an aid in diagnosing human disease is not a covered service under Medicare.

The correlation of hair analysis to the chemical state of the whole body is not possible at this time, and therefore this diagnostic procedure cannot be considered to be reasonable and necessary under section 1862(a)(1) of the law.

50-36 POSITRON EMISSION TOMOGRAPHY (PET) SCANS

I. General Description

Positron emission tomography (PET) is a noninvasive diagnostic imaging procedure that assesses the level of metabolic activity and perfusion in various organ systems of the [human] body. A positron camera (tomograph) is used to produce cross-sectional tomographic images, which are obtained from positron emitting radioactive tracer substances (radiopharmaceuticals) such as 2-[F-18] Fluoro-D-Glucose (FDG), that are administered intravenously to the patient.

The following indications may be covered for PET under certain circumstances. Details of Medicare PET coverage are discussed later in this section. Unless otherwise indicated, the clinical conditions below are covered when PET utilizes FDG as a tracer.

NOTE: All other uses of PET scans not listed in this manual are NOT covered.

Clinical Condition	Effective Date	Coverage
Solitary Pulmonary Nodules (SPNs)	January 1, 1998	Characterization
Lung Cancer (Non Small Cell)	January 1, 1998	Initial staging
Lung Cancer (Non Small Cell)	July 1, 2001	Diagnosis, staging and restaging
Esophageal Cancer	July 1, 2001	Diagnosis, staging and restaging
Colorectal Cancer	July 1, 1999	Determining location of tumors if rising CEA level suggests recurrence
Colorectal Cancer	July 1, 2001	Diagnosis, staging and restaging
Lymphoma	July 1, 1999	Staging and restaging only when used as an alternative to Gallium scan
Lymphoma	July 1, 2001	Diagnosis, staging and restaging
Melanoma	July 1, 1999	Evaluating recurrence prior to surgery as an alternative to a Gallium scan
Melanoma	July 1, 2001	Diagnosis, staging and restaging; Non-covered for evaluating regional nodes
Breast Cancer	October 1, 2002	As an adjunct to standard imaging modalities for staging patients with distant metastasis or restaging patients with locoregional recurrence or metastasis; as an adjunct to standard imaging modalities for monitoring tumor response to treatment for women with locally advanced and metastatic breast cancer when a change in therapy is anticipated.
Head and Neck Cancers (excluding CNS and thyroid)	July 1, 2001	Diagnosis, staging and restaging
Myocardial Viability	July 1, 2001 to September 30, 2002	Covered only following inconclusive SPECT
Myocardial Viability	October 1, 2002	Primary or initial diagnosis, or following an inconclusive SPECT prior to revascularization. SPECT may not be used following an inconclusive PET scan.
Refractory Seizures	July 1, 2001	Covered for pre-surgical evaluation only
Perfusion of the heart using Rubidium 82* tracer	March 14, 1995	Covered for noninvasive imaging of the perfusion of the heart

* Not FDG-PET.

II. General Conditions of Coverage

A. Allowable FDG PET Systems

1. Definitions: For purposes of this section,

a. "Any FDA approved" means all systems approved or cleared for marketing by the FDA to image radionuclides in the body.

b. "FDA approved" means that the system indicated has been approved for cleared for marketing by the FDA to image radionuclides in the body.

c. "Certain coincidence sytems" refers to the systems that have all the following features:

- crystal at least 5/8-inch thick

• techniques to minimize or correct for scatter and/or randoms, and

• digital detectors and iterative reconstruction.

Scans performed with gamma camera PET systems with crystals thinner than 5/8-inch will not be covered by Medicare. In addition, scans performed with systems with crystals greater than or equal to 5/8-inch in thickness, but that do not meet the other listed design characteristics are not covered by Medicare.

2. Allowable PET systems by covered clinical indication:

Covered Clinical Condition	Allowable Type of FDG PET System		
	Prior to July 1, 2001	July 1, 2001 through December 31, 2001	On or after January 1, 2002
Characterization of single pulmonary nodules	Effective 1/1/1998, any FDA approved	Any FDA approved	FDA approved: Full ring Partial ring Certain coincidence systems
Initial staging of lung cancer (non small cell)	Effective 1/1/1998, any FDA approved	Any FDA approved	FDA approved: Full ring Partial ring Certain coincidence systems
Evaluating recurrence of melanoma prior to surgery as an alternative to a gallium scan	Effective 7/1/1999, any FDA approved	Any FDA approved	FDA approved: Full ring Partial ring Certain coincidence systems
Diagnosis, staging, and restaging of colorectal cancer	Not covered by Medicare	Full ring	FDA approved: Full ring Partial ring
Diagnosis, staging, and restaging of esophageal cancer	Not covered by Medicare	Full ring	FDA approved: Full ring Partial ring
Diagnosis, staging, and restaging of head and neck cancers (exclusing CNS and thyroid)	Not covered by Medicare	Full ring	FDA approved: Full ring Partial ring
Diagnosis, staging, and restaging of lung cancer (non small cell)	Not covered by Medicare	Full ring	FDA approved: Full ring Partial ring
Diagnosis, staging, and restaging of lymphoma	Not covered by Medicare	Full ring	FDA approved: Full ring Partial ring
Diagnosis, staging, and restaging of melanoma (noncovered for evaluating regional nodes)	Not covered by Medicare	Full ring	FDA approved: Full ring Partial ring
Determination of myocardial viability only following an inconclusive SPECT	Not covered by Medicare	Full ring	FDA approved: Full ring Partial ring
Presurgical evaluation of refractory seizures	Not covered by Medicare	Full ring	FDA approved: Full ring Partial ring
Breast Cancer	Not covered	Not covered	Effective October 1, 2002, Full and partial ring
Myocardial Viability Primary or initial diagnosis prior to revascularization	Not covered	Not covered	Effective October 1, 2002, Full and partial ring

B. Regardless of any other terms or conditions, all uses of FDG PET scans, in order to be covered by the Medicare program, must meet the following general conditions as of July 1, 2001:

1. PET scans are covered for those indications otherwise listed in this document. For indications covered beginning July 1, 2001, scans performed with dedicated full-ring scanners will be covered. In the decision memorandum of December 15, 2000, HCFA had indicated that gamma camera systems with at least a 1 inch thick crystal would be eligible for coverage. However, coverage of PET using camera-based systems is now under further review as a separate national coverage determination. A final decision on what systems other than dedicated PET will be eligible for coverage, if any, will be announced prior to July 1, 2001. For those indications covered prior to July 1, 2001, all PET scanners approved or cleared for marketing by the FDA remain covered.

2. The provider of the PET scan should maintain on file the doctor's referral and documentation that the procedure involved only FDA approved drugs and devices, as is normal business practice.

3. The ordering physician is responsible for documenting the medical necessity of the study and that it meets the conditions specified in the instructions. The physician should have documentation in the beneficiary's medical record to support the referral to the PET scan provider.

4. Medicare coverage is predicated upon the use of PET scans with FDG for the purpose of development of appropriate treatment plans for patients. HCFA will evaluate both the data produced by claims for these services, and data obtained from other sources, to determine whether, and to what extent, this coverage policy may need additional modification in order to assure that the services covered are medically effective for the treatment of Medicare beneficiaries.

III. Covered Indications for PET Scans and Limitations/Requirements for Usage

For all uses of PET relating to malignancies the following conditions apply:

1. Diagnosis: PET is covered only in clinical situations in which the PET results may assist in avoiding an invasive diagnostic procedure, or in which the PET results may assist in determining the optimal anatomical location to perform an invasive diagnostic procedure. In general, for most solid tumors, a tissue diagnosis is made prior to the performance of PET scanning. PET scans following a tissue diagnosis are performed for the purpose of staging, not diagnosis. Therefore, the use of PET in the diagnosis of lymphoma, esophageal, and colorectal cancers as well as in melanoma should be rare.

PET is not covered for other diagnostic uses, and is not covered for screening (testing of patients without specific signs and symptoms of disease).

2. Staging and or Restaging: PET is covered in clinical situations in which 1) (a) the stage of the cancer remains in doubt after completion of a standard diagnostic workup, including conventional imaging (computed tomography, magnetic resonance imaging, or ultrasound) or (b) the use of PET would also be considered reasonable and necessary if it could potentially replace one or more conventional imaging studies when it is expected that conventional study information is insufficient for the clinical management of the patient and 2) clinical management of the patient would differ depending on the stage of the cancer identified. PET will be covered for restaging after the completion of treatment for the purpose of detecting residual disease, for detecting suspected recurrence or to determine the extent of a known recurrence. Use of PET would also be considered reasonable and necessary if it could potentially replace one or more conventional imaging studies when it is expected that conventional study information is insufficient for the clinical management of the patient.

3. Monitoring: Use of PET to monitor tumor response during the planned course of therapy (i.e. when no change in therapy is being contemplated) is not covered, except for breast cancer. Restaging only occurs after a course of treatment is completed, and this is covered, subject to the conditions above.

NOTE: In the absence of national frequency limitations, contractors may, if necessary, develop frequency requirements on any or all of the indications covered on and after July 1, 2001.

IV. Coverage of PET for Perfusion of the Heart Using Rubidium 82

Effective for services performed on or after March 14, 1995, PET scans performed at rest or with pharmacological stress used for noninvasive imaging of the perfusion of the heart for the diagnosis and management of patients with known or suspected coronary artery disease using the FDA-approved radiopharmaceutical Rubidium 82 (Rb 82) are covered, provided the requirements below are met.

Requirements:

- The PET scan, whether at rest alone, or rest with stress, is performed in place of, but not in addition to, a single photon emission computed tomography (SPECT); or
- The PET scan, whether at rest alone or rest with stress, is used following a SPECT that was found to be inconclusive. In these cases, the PET scan must have been considered necessary in order to determine what medical or surgical intervention is required to treat the patient. (For purposes of this requirement, an inconclusive test is a test(s) whose results are equivocal, technically uninterpretable, or discordant with a patient's other clinical data and must be documented in the beneficiary's file.)
- For any PET scan for which Medicare payment is claimed for dates of services prior to July 1, 2001, the claimant must submit additional specified information on the claim form (including proper codes and/or modifiers), to indicate the results of the PET scan. The claimant must also include information on whether the PET scan was done after an inconclusive noninvasive cardiac test. The information submitted with respect to the previous noninvasive cardiac test must specify the type of test done prior to the PET scan and whether it was inconclusive or unsatisfactory. These explanations are in the form of special G codes used for billing PET scans using Rb 82. Beginning July 1, 2001 claims should be submitted with the appropriate codes.

V. Coverage of FDG PET for Lung Cancer

The coverage for FDG PET for lung cancer, effective January 1, 1998, has been expanded. Beginning July 1, 2001 usage of FDG PET for lung cancer has been expanded to include diagnosis, staging, and restaging (see section III) of the disease.

A. Effective for services performed on or after January 1, 1998, Medicare covers regional FDG PET chest scans, on any FDA approved scanner, for the characterization of single pulmonary nodules (SPNs). The primary purpose of such characterization should be to determine the likelihood of malignancy in order to plan future management and treatment for the patient.

Beginning July 1, 2001, documentation should be maintained in the beneficiary's medical file at the referring physician's office to support the medical necessity of the procedure, as is normal business practice.

Requirements:

- There must be evidence of primary tumor. Claims for regional PET chest scans for characterizing SPNs should include evidence of the initial detection of a primary lung tumor, usually by computed tomography (CT). This should include, but is not restricted to, a report on the results of such CT or other detection method, indicating an indeterminate or possibly malignant lesion, not exceeding four centimeters (cm) in diameter.
- PET scan claims must include the results of concurrent thoracic CT (as noted above), which is necessary for anatomic information, in order to ensure that the PET scan is properly coordinated with other diagnostic modalities.
- In cases of serial evaluation of SPNs using both CT and regional PET chest scanning, such PET scans will not be covered if repeated within 90 days following a negative PET scan.

NOTE: A tissue sampling procedure (TSP) is not routinely covered in the case of a negative PET scan for characterization of SPNs, since the patient is presumed not to have a malignant lesion, based upon the PET scan results. When there has been a negative PET, the provider must submit additional information with the claim to support the necessity of a TSP, for review by the Medicare contractor.

B. Effective for services performed from January 1, 1998 through June 30, 2001, Medicare approved coverage of FDG PET for initial staging of non-small-cell lung carcinoma (NSCLC).

Limitations: This service is covered only when the primary cancerous lung tumor has been pathologically confirmed; claims for PET must include a statement or other evidence of the detection of such primary lung tumor. The evidence should include, but is not restricted to, a surgical pathology report, which documents the presence of an NSCLC. Whole body PET scan results and results of concurrent computed tomography (CT) and follow-up lymph node biopsy must be properly coordinated with other diagnostic modalities. Claims must include both:

- The results of concurrent thoracic CT, necessary for anatomic information, and
- The results of any lymph node biopsy performed to finalize whether the patient will be a surgical candidate. The ordering physician is responsible for providing this biopsy result to the PET facility.

NOTE: Where the patient is considered a surgical candidate, (given the presumed absence of metastatic NSCLC unless medical review supports a determination of medical necessity of a biopsy) a lymph node biopsy will not be covered in the case of a negative CT and negative PET. A lymph node biopsy will be covered in all other cases, i.e., positive CT + positive PET; negative CT + positive PET; positive CT + negative PET.

C. Beginning July 1, 2001, Medicare covers FDG PET for diagnosis, staging, and restaging of NSCLC. Documentation should be maintained in the beneficiary's medical file to support the medical necessity of the procedure, as is normal business practice.

Requirements: PET is covered in either/or both of the following circumstances:

- Diagnosis—PET is covered only in clinical situations in which the PET results may assist in avoiding an invasive diagnostic procedure, or in which the PET results may assist in determining the optimal anatomical location to perform an invasive diagnostic procedure. In general, for most solid tumors, a tissue diagnosis is made prior to the performance of PET scanning. PET scans following a tissue diagnosis are performed for the purpose of staging, not diagnosis. Therefore, the use of PET in the diagnosis of lymphoma, esophageal, and colorectal cancers as well as in melanoma should be rare.
- Staging and/or Restaging—PET is covered in clinical situations in which 1) (a) the stage of the cancer remains in doubt after completion of a standard diagnostic workup, including conventional imaging (computed tomography, magnetic resonance imaging, or ultrasound) or (b) the use of PET would also be considered reasonable and necessary if it could potentially replace one or more conventional imaging studies when it is expected that conventional study information is insufficient for the clinical management of the patient and 2) clinical management of the patient would differ depending on the stage of the cancer identified. PET will be covered for restaging after the completion of treatment for the purpose of detecting residual disease, for detecting suspected recurrence or to determine the extent of a known recurrence. Use of PET would also be considered reasonable and necessary if it could potentially replace one or more conventional imaging studies when it is expected that conventional study information is insufficient for the clinical management of the patient.

Documentation should be maintained in the beneficiary's medical record at the referring physician's office to support the medical necessity of the procedure, as is normal business practice.

VI. Coverage of FDG PET for Esophageal Cancer

A. Beginning July 1, 2001, Medicare covers FDG PET for the diagnosis, staging, and restaging of esophageal cancer. Medical evidence is present to support the use of FDG PET in pre-surgical staging of esophageal cancer.

Requirements: PET is covered in either/or both of the following circumstances:

- Diagnosis - PET is covered only in clinical situations in which the PET results may assist in avoiding an invasive diagnostic procedure, or in which the PET results may assist in determining the optimal anatomical location to perform an invasive diagnostic procedure. In general, for most solid tumors, a tissue diagnosis is made prior to the performance of PET scanning. PET scans following a tissue diagnosis are performed for the purpose of staging, not diagnosis. Therefore, the use of PET in the diagnosis of lymphoma, esophageal and colorectal cancers as well as in melanoma should be rare.
- Staging and/or Restaging - PET is covered in clinical situations in which 1) (a) the stage of the cancer remains in doubt after completion of a standard diagnostic workup, including conventional imaging (computed tomography, magnetic resonance imaging, or ultrasound) or (b) the use of PET would also be considered reasonable and necessary if it could potentially replace one or more conventional imaging studies when it is expected that conventional study information is insufficient for the clinical management of the patient, and 2) clinical management of the patient would differ depending on the stage of the cancer identified. PET will be covered for restaging after the completion of treatment for the purpose of detecting residual disease, for detecting suspected recurrence, or to determine the extent of a known recurrence. Use of PET would also be considered reasonable and necessary if it could potentially replace one or more conventional imaging studies when it is expected that conventional study information is insufficient for the clinical management of the patient.

Documentation should be maintained in the beneficiary's medical record at the referring physician's office to support the medical necessity of the procedure, as is normal business practice.

VII. Coverage of FDG PET for Colorectal Cancer

Medicare coverage of FDG PET for colorectal cancer where there is a rising level of carcinoembryonic antigen (CEA) was effective July 1, 1999 through June 30, 2001. Beginning July 1, 2001, usage of FDG PET for colorectal cancer has been expanded to include diagnosis, staging, and restaging of the disease(see part III).

A. Effective July 1, 1999, Medicare covers FDG PET for patients with recurrent colorectal carcinomas, which are suggested by rising levels of the biochemical tumor marker CEA.

1. Frequency Limitations: Whole body PET scans for assessment of recurrence of colorectal cancer cannot be ordered more frequently than once every 12 months unless medical necessity documentation supports a separate re-elevation of CEA within this period.

2. Limitations: Because this service is covered only in those cases in which there has been a recurrence of colorectal tumor, claims for PET should include a statement or other evidence of previous colorectal tumor, through June 30, 2001.

B. Beginning July 1, 2001, Medicare coverage has been expanded for colorectal carcinomas for diagnosis, staging and restaging. New medical evidence supports the use of FDG PET as a useful tool in determining the presence of hepatic/extrahepatic metastases in the primary staging of colorectal carcinoma, prior to selecting a treatment regimen. Use of FDG PET is also supported in evaluating recurrent colorectal cancer beyond the limited presentation of a rising CEA level where the patient presents clinical signs or symptoms of recurrence.

Requirements: PET is covered in either/both of the following circumstances:

- Diagnosis - PET is covered only in clinical situations in which the PET results may assist in avoiding an invasive diagnostic procedure, or in which the PET results may assist in determining the optimal anatomical location to perform an invasive diagnostic procedure. In general, for most solid tumors, a tissue diagnosis is made prior to the performance of PET scanning. PET scans following a tissue diagnosis are performed for the purpose of staging, not diagnosis. Therefore, the use of PET in the diagnosis of lymphoma, esophageal, and colorectal cancers as well as in melanoma should be rare.
- Staging and/or Restaging - PET is covered in clinical situations in which 1) (a) the stage of the cancer remains in doubt after completion of a standard diagnostic workup, including conventional imaging (computed tomography, magnetic resonance imaging, or ultrasound) or (b) the use of PET would also be considered reasonable and necessary if it could potentially replace one or more conventional imaging studies when it is expected that conventional study information is insufficient for the clinical management of the patient, and 2) clinical management of the patient would differ depending on the stage of the cancer identified. PET will be covered for restaging after the completion of treatment for the purpose of detecting residual disease, for detecting suspected recurrence, or to determine the extent of a known recurrence. Use of PET would also be considered reasonable and necessary if it could potentially replace one or more conventional imaging studies when it is expected that conventional study information is insufficient for the clinical management of the patient.

Documentation that these conditions are met should be maintained by the referring physician in the beneficiary's medical record, as is normal business practice.

VIII. Coverage of FDG PET for Lymphoma

Medicare coverage of FDG PET to stage and re-stage lymphoma as alternative to a Gallium scan, was effective July 1, 1999. Beginning July 1, 2001 usage of FDG PET for lymphoma has been expanded to include diagnosis, staging and restaging (see section III) of the disease.

A. Effective July 1, 1999, FDG PET is covered for the staging and restaging of lymphoma.

Requirements:

- FDG PET is covered only for staging or follow-up restaging of lymphoma. Claims must include a statement or other evidence of previous diagnosis of lymphoma when used as an alternative to a Gallium scan.
- To ensure that the PET scan is properly coordinated with other diagnostic modalities, claims must include the results of concurrent computed tomography (CT) and/or other diagnostic modalities when they are necessary for additional anatomic information.
- In order to ensure that the PET scan is covered only as an alternative to a Gallium scan, no PET scan may be covered in cases where it is done within 50 days of a Gallium scan done by the same facility where the patient has remained during the 50-day period. Gallium scans done by another facility less than 50 days prior to the PET scan will not be counted against this screen. The purpose of this screen is to assure that PET scans are covered only when done as an alternative to a Gallium scan within the same facility. We are aware that, in order to assure proper patient care, the treating physician may conclude that previously performed Gallium scans are either inconclusive or not sufficiently reliable.

Frequency Limitation for Restaging: PET scans will be allowed for restaging no sooner than 50 days following the last staging PET scan or Gallium scan, unless sufficient evidence is presented to convince the Medicare contractor that the restaging at an earlier date is medically necessary. Since PET scans for restaging are generally done following cycles of chemotherapy, and since such cycles usually take at least 8 weeks, we believe this screen will adequately prevent medically unnecessary scans while allowing some adjustments for unusual cases. In all cases, the determination of the medical necessity for a PET scan for re-staging lymphoma is the responsibility of the local Medicare contractor.

Beginning July 1, 2001, documentation should be maintained in the beneficiary's medical record at the referring physician's office to support the medical necessity of the procedure, as is normal business practice.

B. Effective for services performed on or after July 1, 2001, the Medicare program has broadened coverage of FDG PET for the diagnosis, staging and restaging of lymphoma.

Requirements: PET is covered in either/both of the following circumstances:

- Diagnosis - PET is covered only in clinical situations in which the PET results may assist in avoiding an invasive diagnostic procedure, or in which the PET results may assist in determining the optimal anatomical location to perform an invasive diagnostic procedure. In general, for most solid tumors, a tissue diagnosis is made prior to the performance of PET scanning. PET scans following a tissue diagnosis are performed for the purpose of staging, not diagnosis. Therefore, the use of PET in the diagnosis of lymphoma, esophageal, and colorectal cancers as well as in melanoma should be rare.
- Staging and/or Restaging - PET is covered in clinical situations in which 1) (a) the stage of the cancer remains in doubt after completion of a standard diagnostic workup, including conventional imaging (computed tomography, magnetic resonance imaging, or ultrasound) or (b) the use of PET would also be considered reasonable and necessary if it could potentially replace one or more conventional imaging studies when it is expected that conventional study information is insufficient for the clinical management of the patient, and 2) clinical management of the patient would differ depending on the stage of the cancer identified. PET will be covered for restaging after the completion of treatment for the purpose of detecting residual disease, for detecting suspected recurrence, or to determine the extent of a known recurrence. Use of PET would also be considered reasonable and necessary if it could potentially replace one or more conventional imaging studies when it is expected that conventional study information is insufficient for the clinical management of the patient.

Documentation that these conditions are met should be maintained by the referring physician in the beneficiary's medical record, as is normal business practice.

IX. Coverage of FDG PET for Melanoma

Medicare covered the evaluation of recurrent melanoma prior to surgery when used as an alternative to a Gallium scan, effective July 1, 1999. For services furnished on or after July 1, 2001 FDG PET is covered for the diagnosis, staging, and restaging of malignant melanoma (see part III). FDG PET is not covered for the use of evaluating regional nodes in melanoma patients.

A. Effective for services furnished July 1, 1999 through June 30, 2001, in the case of patients with recurrent melanoma prior to surgery, FDG PET (when used as an alternative to a Gallium scan) is covered for tumor evaluation.

Frequency Limitations: Whole body PET scans cannot be ordered more frequently than once every 12 months, unless medical necessity documentation, maintained in the beneficiaries medical record, supports the specific need for anatomic localization of possible recurrent tumor within this period.

Limitations: The FDG PET scan is covered only as an alternative to a Gallium scan. PET scans can not be covered in cases where it is done within 50 days of a Gallium scan done by the same PET facility where the patient has remained under the care of the same facility during the 50-day period. Gallium scans done by another facility less than 50 days prior to the PET scan will not be counted against this screen. The purpose of this screen is to assure that PET scans are covered only when done as an alternative to a Gallium scan within the same facility. We are aware that, in order to assure proper patient care, the treating physician may conclude that previously performed Gallium scans are either inconclusive or not sufficiently reliable to make the determination covered by this provision. Therefore, we will apply this 50-day rule only to PET scans done by the same facility that performed the Gallium scan.

Beginning July 1, 2001, documentation should be maintained in the beneficiary's medical file at the referring physician's office to support the medical necessity of the procedure, as is normal business practice.

B. Effective for services performed on or after July 1, 2001 FDG PET scan coverage for the diagnosis, staging and restaging of melanoma (not the evaluation regional nodes) has been broadened.

Limitations: PET scans are not covered for the evaluation of regional nodes.

Requirements: PET is covered in either/both of the following circumstances:

- Diagnosis—PET is covered only in clinical situations in which the PET results may assist in avoiding an invasive diagnostic procedure, or in which the PET results may assist in determining the optimal anatomical location to perform an invasive diagnostic procedure. In general, for most solid tumors, a tissue diagnosis is made prior to the performance of PET scanning. PET scans following a tissue diagnosis are performed for the purpose of staging, not diagnosis. Therefore, the use of PET in the diagnosis of lymphoma, esophageal, and colorectal cancers as well as in melanoma should be rare.
- Staging and/or Restaging—PET is covered in clinical situations in which 1) (a) the stage of the cancer remains in doubt after completion of a standard diagnostic workup, including conventional imaging (computed tomography, magnetic resonance imaging, or ultrasound) or (b) the use of PET would also be considered reasonable and necessary if it could potentially replace one or more conventional imaging studies when it is expected that conventional study information is insufficient for the clinical management of the patient, and 2) clinical management of the patient would differ depending on the stage of the cancer identified. PET will be covered for restaging after the completion of treatment for the purpose of detecting residual disease, for detecting suspected recurrence, or to determine the extent of a known recurrence. Use of PET would also be consid-

ered reasonable and necessary if it could potentially replace one or more conventional imaging studies when it is expected that conventional study information is insufficient for the clinical management of the patient.

Documentation that these conditions are met should be maintained by the referring physician in the beneficiary's medical file, as is normal business practice.

X. Coverage of FDG PET for Head and Neck Cancers (Cancers of the central nervous system (CNS) and thyroid are not covered)

Effective for services performed on or after July 1, 2001, Medicare will provide coverage for cancer of the head and neck, excluding the central nervous system (CNS) and thyroid. The head and neck cancers encompass a diverse set of malignancies of which the majority is squamous cell carcinomas. Patients may present with metastases to cervical lymph nodes but conventional forms of diagnostic imaging fail to identify the primary tumor. Patients that present with cancer of the head and neck are left with two options either to have a neck dissection or to have radiation of both sides of the neck with random biopsies. PET scanning attempts to reveal the site of primary tumor to prevent the adverse effects of random biopsies or unneeded radiation.

Limitations: PET scans for head and neck cancers are not covered for CNS or thyroid cancers.

Requirements: PET is covered in either/or both of the following circumstances:

- Diagnosis—PET is covered only in clinical situations in which the PET results may assist in avoiding an invasive diagnostic procedure, or in which the PET results may assist in determining the optimal anatomical location to perform an invasive diagnostic procedure. In general, for most solid tumors, a tissue diagnosis is made prior to the performance of PET scanning. PET scans following a tissue diagnosis are performed for the purpose of staging, not diagnosis. Therefore, the use of PET in the diagnosis of lymphoma, esophageal, and colorectal cancers as well as in melanoma should be rare.
- Staging and/or Restaging—PET is covered in clinical situations in which 1) (a) the stage of the cancer remains in doubt after completion of a standard diagnostic workup, including conventional imaging (computed tomography, magnetic resonance imaging, or ultrasound) or (b) the use of PET would also be considered reasonable and necessary if it could potentially replace one or more conventional imaging studies when it is expected that conventional study information is insufficient for the clinical management of the patient, and 2) clinical management of the patient would differ depending on the stage of the cancer identified. PET will be covered for restaging after the completion of treatment for the purpose of detecting residual disease, for detecting suspected recurrence, or to determine the extent of a known recurrence. Use of PET would also be considered reasonable and necessary if it could potentially replace one or more conventional imaging studies when it is expected that conventional study information is insufficient for the clinical management of the patient.

Documentation that these conditions are met should be maintained by the referring physician in the beneficiary's medical record, as is normal business practice.

XI. Coverage of FDG PET for Myocardial Viability

The identification of patients with partial loss of heart muscle movement or hibernating myocardium is important in selecting candidates with compromised ventricular function to determine appropriateness for revascularization. Diagnostic tests such as FDG PET distinguish between dysfunctional but viable myocardial tissue and scar tissue in order to affect management decisions in patients with ischemic cardiomyopathy and left ventricular dysfunction.

FDG PET is covered for the determination of myocardial viability following an inconclusive SPECT from July 1, 2001 through September 30, 2002. Only fully ring PET scanners are covered from July 1, 2001 through December 31, 2001. However, as of January 1, 2002, full and partial ring scanners are covered.

Beginning October 1, 2002, Medicare covers FDG PET for the determination of myocardial viability as a primary or initial diagnostic study prior to revascularization, or following an inconclusive SPECT. Studies performed by full and partial ring scanners are covered.

Limitations: In the event that a patient has received a single photon computed tomography test (SPECT) with inconclusive results, a PET scan may be covered. However, if a patient received a FDG PET study with inconclusive results, a follow up SPECT is not covererd.

Documentation that these conditions are met should be maintained by the referring physician in the beneficiary's medical record, as is normal business practice.

(See §50-58 of the CIM for SPECT coverage.)

XII. Coverage of FDG-PET for Refractory Seizures

Beginning July 1, 2001, Medicare will cover FDG-PET for pre-surgical evaluation for the purpose of localization of a focus of refractory seizure activity.

Limitations: Covered only for pre-surgical evaluation.

Documentation that these conditions are met should be maintained by the referring physician in the beneficiary's medical record, as is normal business practice.

XIII. Breast Cancer

Beginning October 1, 2002, Medicare covers FDG PET as an adjunct to other imaging modalities for staging patients with distant metastasis, or restaging patients with locoregional recurrence or metastasis. Monitoring treatment of a breast cancer tumor when a change in therapy is contemplated is also covered as an adjunct to other imaging modalities.

Limitations: Effective October 1, 2002, Medicare continues to have a national non-coverage determination for initial diagnosis of breast cancer and staging of axillary lymph nodes. Medicare coverage for staging patients with distant metastasis or restaging patients with locoregional recurrence or metastasis; and for monitoring tumor response to treatment for women with locally advanced and metastatic breast cancer when a change in therapy is anticipated, is only covered as an adjunct to other imaging modalities.

Documentation that these conditions are met should be maintained by the referring physician in the beneficiary's medical record, as is normal business practice.

50-44 BONE (MINERAL) DENSITY STUDIES

Bone (mineral) density studies are used to evaluate diseases of bone and/or the responses of bone diseases to treatment. The studies assess bone mass or density associated with such diseases as osteoporosis, osteomalacia, and renal osteodystrophy. Various single or combined methods of measurement may be required to: (a) diagnose bone disease, (b) monitor the course of bone changes with disease progression, or (c) monitor the course of bone changes with therapy. Bone density is usually studied by using photodensitometry, single or dual photon absorptiometry, or bone biopsy. The following bone (mineral) density studies are covered under Medicare:

A. Single Photon Absorptiometry.—A non-invasive radiological technique that measures absorption of a monochromatic photon beam by bone material. The device is placed directly on the patient, uses a low dose of radionuclide, and measures the mass absorption efficiency of the energy used. It provides a quantitative measurement of the bone mineral of cortical and trabecular bone, and is used in assessing an individual's treatment response at appropriate intervals.

Single photon absorptiometry is covered under Medicare when used in assessing changes in bone density of patients with osteodystrophy or osteoporosis when performed on the same individual at intervals of 6 to 12 months.

B. Bone Biopsy.—A physiologic test which is a surgical, invasive procedure. A small sample of bone (usually from the ilium) is removed, generally by a biopsy needle. The biopsy sample is then examined histologically, and provides a qualitative measurement of the bone mineral of trabecular bone. This procedure is used in ascertaining a differential diagnosis of bone disorders and is used primarily to differentiate osteomalacia from osteoporosis.

Bone biopsy is covered under Medicare when used for the qualitative evaluation of bone no more than four times per patient, unless there is special justification given. When used more than four times on a patient, bone biopsy leaves a defect in the pelvis and may produce some patient discomfort.

C. Photodensitometry (Radiographic Absorptiometry).—A noninvasive radiological procedure that attempts to assess bone mass by measuring the optical density of extremity radiographs with a photodensitometer, usually with a reference to a standard density wedge placed on the film at the time of exposure. This procedure provides a quantitative measurement of the bone mineral of cortical bone, and is used for monitoring gross bone change.

The following bone (mineral) density study is not covered under Medicare: dual photon absorptiometry. A noninvasive radiological technique that measures absorption of a dichromatic beam by bone material. This procedure is not covered under Medicare because it is still considered to be in the investigational stage.

50-50 DISPLACEMENT CARDIOGRAPHY

Displacement cardiography, including cardiokymography and photokymography, is a noninvasive diagnostic test used in evaluating coronary artery disease.

A. Cardiokymography.—(Effective for Services Rendered on or after October 12, 1988).—Cardiokymography is a covered service only when it is used as an adjunct to electrocardiographic stress testing in evaluating coronary artery disease and only when the following clinical indications are present:

- For male patients, atypical angina pectoris or nonischemic chest pain; or
- For female patients, angina, either typical or atypical.

B. Photokymography.—not covered. Photokymography remains excluded from coverage.

50-54 CARDIAC OUTPUT MONITORING BY ELECTRICAL BIOIMPEDANCE—NOT COVERED (Effective for services performed on or after July 1, 1999)

Cardiac monitoring using electrical bioimpedance, a form of plethysmography, is covered, effective for services furnished on or after July 1, 1999, for the uses and conditions described below. Contractors should be aware that this technology is in the process of being proven for additional uses. Therefore, the uses below represent the current situation. Contractors may cover additional uses when they believe there is sufficient evidence of the medical effectiveness of such uses.

These devices utilize electrical bioimpedance to noninvasively produce hemodynamic measurements of cardiac output, specifically, stroke volume, contractility, systemic vascular resistance, and thoracic fluid content. These devices are covered for the following uses:

1. Noninvasive diagnosis or monitoring of hemodynamics in patients with suspected or known cardiovascular disease;

2. Differentiation of cardiogenic from pulmonary causes of acute dyspnea;

3. Optimization of atrioventricular interval for patient with A/V sequential cardiac pacemakers;

4. Patients with need of determination for intravenous inotropic therapy;

5. Post heart transplant myocardial biopsy patients; and,

6. Patients with a need for fluid management.

Not covered at this time are the use of such devices for any monitoring of patients with proven or suspected disease involving severe regurgitation of the aorta, or for patients with minute ventilation (MV) sensor function pacemakers, since the device may adversely affect the functioning of that type of pacemaker. Also, these devices do not render accurate measurements in cardiac bypass patients while on a cardiopulmonary bypass machine, but do provide accurate measurements prior to and post bypass pump.

Covered uses of cardiac output monitoring by electrical bioimpedance should be billed using HCPCS code M0302.

50-55 PROSTATE CANCER SCREENING TESTS—COVERED (Effective for services furnished on or after January 1, 2000)

A. General—Section 4103 of the Balanced Budget Act of 1997 provides for coverage of certain prostate cancer screening tests subject to certain coverage, frequency, and payment limitations. Effective for services furnished on or after January 1, 2000. Medicare will cover prostate cancer screening tests/procedures for the early detection of prostate cancer.

Coverage of prostate cancer screening tests includes the following procedures furnished to an individual for the early detection of prostate cancer:

- Screening digital rectal examination; and
- Screening prostate specific antigen blood test.

B. Screening Digital Rectal Examinations—Screening digital rectal examinations (HCPCS code G0102) are covered at a frequency of once every 12 months for men who have attained age 50 (at least 11 months have passed following the month in which the last Medicare-covered screening digital rectal examination was performed). Screening digital rectal examination means a clinical examination of an individual's prostate for nodules or other abnormalities of the prostate. This screening must be performed by a doctor of medicine or osteopathy (as defined in section 1861(r)(1) of the Act), or by a physician assistant, nurse practitioner, clinical nurse specialist, or certified nurse midwife (as defined in section 1861(aa) and section 1861(gg) of the Act) who is authorized under State law to perform the examination, fully knowledgeable about the beneficiary's medical condition, and would be responsible for using the results of any examination performed in the overall management of the beneficiary's specific medical problem.

C. Screening Prostate Specific Antigen Tests.—Screening prostate specific antigen tests (code G0103) are covered at a frequency of once every 12 months for men who have attained age 50 (at least 11 months have passed following the month in which the last Medicare-covered screening prostate specific antigen test was performed). Screening prostate specific antigen tests (PSA) means a test to detect the marker for adenocarcinoma of prostate. PSA is a reliable immunocytochemical marker for primary and metastatic adenocarcinoma of prostate. This screening must be ordered by the beneficiary's physician or by the beneficiary's physician assistant, nurse practitioner, clinical nurse specialist, or certified nurse midwife (the term "attending physician" is defined in section 1861(r)(1) of the Act to mean a doctor of medicine or osteopathy and the terms "physician assistant, nurse practitioner, clinical nurse specialist, or certified nurse midwife" are defined in section 1861(aa) and section 1861(gg) of the Act) who is fully knowledgeable about the beneficiary's medical condition, and who would be responsible for using the results of any examination (test) performed in the overall management of the beneficiary's specific medical problem.

55 DIALYSIS EQUIPMENT

55-1 WATER PURIFICATION AND SOFTENING SYSTEMS USED IN CONJUNCTION WITH HOME DIALYSIS

A. Water Purification Systems.—Water used for home dialysis should be chemically free of heavy trace metals and/or organic contaminants which could be hazardous to the patient. It should also be as free of bacteria as possible but need not be biologically sterile. Since the characteristics of natural water supplies in most areas of the country are such that some type of water purification system is needed, such a system used in conjunction with a home dialysis (either peritoneal or hemodialysis) unit is covered under Medicare.

There are two types of water purification systems which will satisfy these requirements:

- Deionization—The removal of organic substances, mineral salts of magnesium and calcium (causing hardness), compounds of fluoride and chloride from tap water using the process of filtration and ion exchange; or
- Reverse Osmosis—The process used to remove impurities from tap water utilizing pressure to force water through a porous membrane.

Use of both a deionization unit and reverse osmosis unit in series, theoretically to provide the advantages of both systems, has been determined medically unnecessary since either system can provide water which is both chemically and bacteriologically pure enough for acceptable use in home dialysis. In addition, spare deionization tanks are not covered since they are essentially a precautionary supply rather than a current requirement for treatment of the patient.

Activated carbon filters used as a component of water purification systems to remove unsafe concentrations of chlorine and chloramines are covered when prescribed by a physician.

B. Water Softening System.—Except as indicated below, a water softening system used in conjunction with home dialysis is excluded from coverage under Medicare as not being reasonable and necessary within the meaning of section 1862(a)(1) of the law. Such a system, in conjunction with a home dialysis unit, does not adequately remove the hazardous heavy metal contaminants (such as arsenic) which may be present in trace amounts.

A water softening system may be covered when used to pretreat water to be purified by a reverse osmosis (RO) unit for home dialysis where:

- The manufacturer of the RO unit has set standards for the quality of water entering the RO (e.g., the water to be purified by the RO must be of a certain quality if the unit is to perform as intended);
- The patient's water is demonstrated to be of a lesser quality than required; and
- The softener is used only to soften water entering the RO unit, and thus, used only for dialysis. (The softener need not actually be built into the RO unit, but must be an integral part of the dialysis system.)

C. Developing Need When a Water Softening System Is Replaced with a Water Purification Unit in an Existing Home Dialysis System.—The medical necessity of water purification units must be carefully developed when they replace water softening systems in existing home dialysis systems. A purification system may be ordered under these circumstances for a number of reasons. For example, changes in the medical community's opinions regarding the quality of water necessary for safe dialysis may lead the physician to decide the quality of water previously used should be improved, or the water quality itself may have deteriorated. Patients may have dialyzed using only an existing water softener previous to Medicare ESRD coverage because of inability to pay for a purification system. On the other hand, in some cases, the installation of a purification system is not medically necessary. Thus, when such a case comes to your attention, ask the physician to furnish the reason for the changes. Supporting documentation, such as the supplier's recommendations or water analysis, may be required. All such cases should be reviewed by your medical consultants.

Cross-refer: Intermediary Manual, sections 3113, 3643 (item 1c); Carriers Manual, sections 2100, 2100.2 2130, 2105 (item 1c); Hospital Manual, section 235.

55-2 PERIDEX CAPD FILTER SET—NOT COVERED

The Peridex Filter Set is used by home continuous ambulatory peritoneal dialysis (CAPD) patients. The Peridex Filter Set is designed to provide sterile filtration during infusion of the dialysis solution in a beneficiary's peritoneal cavity; included in the filter set is a bacterial filter designed to block peritonitis-causing organisms and thus reduce the incidence of peritonitis.

Based upon advice of our medical consultants, we have determined that the Peridex CAPD Filter Set cannot be covered at this time by Medicare because it has not yet been shown to be safe and effective in preventing peritonitis.

55-3 ULTRAFILTRATION MONITOR (Effective for services performed on and after July 11, 1983.)

The Ultrafiltration Monitor is designed to reduce the clinical risks of overfiltration and underfiltration during hemodialysis. Overfiltration is the removal of too much fluid from body tissues and underfiltration is removal of too little fluid.

Covered: Ultrafiltration and ultrafiltration monitoring as a component of hemodialysis has an established and critical role in maintaining the well-being of ESRD patients and is a covered service. The Ultrafiltration Monitor is covered under the Medicare program when it is used to calculate fluid rates for those recipients who present difficult fluid management problems. Determine the medical necessity of this device on a case-by-case basis.

Not Covered: Ultrafiltration, independent of conventional dialysis, is considered experimental, and technology exclusively designed for this purpose is not covered under Medicare.

60 DURABLE MEDICAL EQUIPMENT

60-3 WHITE CANE FOR USE BY A BLIND PERSON—NOT COVERED

A white cane for use by a blind person is more an identifying and self-help device rather than an item which makes a meaningful contribution in the treatment of an illness or injury.

60-4 HOME USE OF OXYGEN

A. General.—Medicare coverage of home oxygen and oxygen equipment under the durable medical equipment (DME) benefit (see section 1861(s)(6) of the Act) is considered reasonable and necessary only for patients with significant hypoxemia who meet the medical documentation, laboratory evidence, and health conditions specified in subsections B, C, and D. This section also includes special coverage criteria for portable oxygen systems. Finally, a statement on the absence of coverage of the professional services of a respiratory therapist under the DME benefit is included in subsection F.

B. Medical Documentation.—Initial claims for oxygen services must include a completed Form HCFA-484 (Certificate of Medical Necessity: Oxygen Therapy) to establish whether coverage criteria are met and to ensure that the oxygen services provided are consistent with the physician's prescription or other medical documentation. The treating physician's prescription or other medical documentation must indicate that the other forms of treatment (e.g., medical and physical therapy directed at secretions, bronchospasm and infection) have been tried, have not been sufficiently successful, and oxygen therapy is still required. While there is no substitute for oxygen therapy, each patient must receive optimum therapy before long-term home oxygen therapy is ordered. Use Form HCFA-484 for recertifications. (See Medicare Carriers Manual section 3312 for completion of Form HCFA-484.)

The medical and prescription information in section B of Form HCFA-484 can be completed only by the treating physician, the physician's employee, or another clinician (e.g., nurse, respiratory therapist, etc.) as long as that person is not the DME supplier. Although hospital discharge coordinators and medical social workers may assist in arranging for physician-prescribed home oxygen, they do not have the authority to prescribe the services. Suppliers may not enter this information. While this section may be completed by a nonphysician clinician or a physician employee, it must be reviewed and the form HCFA-484 signed by the attending physician.

A physician's certification of medical necessity for oxygen equipment must include the results of specific testing before coverage can be determined.

Claims for oxygen must also be supported by medical documentation in the patient's record. Separate documentation is used with electronic billing. (See Medicare Carriers Manual, Part 3, section 4105.5.) This documentation may be in the form of a prescription written by the patient's attending physician who has recently examined the patient (normally within a month of the start of therapy) and must specify:

- A diagnosis of the disease requiring home use of oxygen;
- The oxygen flow rate; and
- An estimate of the frequency, duration of use (e.g., 2 liters per minute, 10 minutes per hour, 12 hours per day), and duration of need (e.g., 6 months or lifetime).

NOTE: A prescription for "Oxygen PRN" or "Oxygen as needed" does not meet this last requirement. Neither provides any basis for determining if the amount of oxygen is reasonable and necessary for the patient.

A member of the carrier's medical staff should review all claims with oxygen flow rates of more than 4 liters per minute before payment can be made.

The attending physician specifies the type of oxygen delivery system to be used (i.e., gas, liquid, or concentrator) by signing the completed form HCFA-484. In addition the supplier or physician may use the space in section C for written confirmation of additional details of the physician's order. The additional order information contained in section C may include the means of oxygen delivery (mask, nasal, cannula, etc.), the specifics of varying flow rates, and/or the noncontinuous use of oxygen as appropriate. The physician confirms this order information with his or her signature in section D.

New medical documentation written by the patient's attending physician must be submitted to the carrier in support of revised oxygen requirements when there has been a change in the patient's condition and need for oxygen therapy.

Carriers are required to conduct periodic, continuing medical necessity reviews on patients whose conditions warrant these reviews and on patients with indefinite or extended periods of necessity as described in Medicare Carriers Manual, Part 3, section 4105.5. When indicated, carriers may also request documentation of the results of a repeat arterial blood gas or oximetry study.

NOTE: Section 4152 of OBRA 1990 requires earlier recertification and retesting of oxygen patients who begin coverage with an arterial blood gas result at or above a partial pressure of 55 or an arterial oxygen saturation percentage at or above 89. (See Medicare Carriers Manual, section 4105.5 for certifications and retesting schedules.)

C. Laboratory Evidence.—Initial claims for oxygen therapy must also include the results of a blood gas study that has been ordered and evaluated by the attending physician. This is usually in the form of a measurement of the partial pressure of oxygen (PO2) in arterial blood. (See Medicare Carriers Manual, Part 3, section 2070.1 for instructions on clinical laboratory tests.) A measurement of arterial oxygen saturation obtained by ear or pulse oximetry, however, is also acceptable when ordered and evaluated by the attending physician and performed under his or her supervision or when performed by a qualified provider or supplier of laboratory services. When the arterial blood gas and the oximetry studies are both used to document the need for home oxygen therapy and the results are conflicting, the arterial blood gas study is the preferred source of documenting medical need. A DME supplier is not considered a qualified provider or supplier of laboratory services for purposes of these guidelines. This prohibition does not extend to the results of a blood gas test conducted by a hospital certified to do such tests. The conditions under which the laboratory tests are performed must be specified in writing and submitted with the initial claim, i.e., at rest, during exercise, or during sleep.

The preferred sources of laboratory evidence are existing physician and/or hospital records that reflect the patient's medical condition. Since it is expected that virtually all patients who qualify for home oxygen coverage for the first time under these guidelines have recently been discharged from a hospital where they submitted to arterial blood gas tests, the carrier needs to request that such test results be submitted in support of their initial claims for home oxygen. If more than one arterial blood gas test is performed during the patient's hospital stay, the test result obtained closest to, but no earlier than 2 days prior to, the hospital discharge date is required as evidence of the need for home oxygen therapy.

For those patients whose initial oxygen prescription did not originate during a hospital stay, blood gas studies should be done while the patient is in the chronic stable state, i.e., not during a period of an acute illness or an exacerbation of their underlying disease.

Carriers may accept an attending physician's statement of recent hospital test results for a particular patient, when appropriate, in lieu of copies of actual hospital records.

A repeat arterial blood gas study is appropriate when evidence indicates that an oxygen recipient has undergone a major change in their condition relevant to home use of oxygen. If the carrier has reason to believe that there has been a major change in the patient's physical condition, it may ask for documentation of the results of another blood gas or oximetry study.

D. Health Conditions.—Coverage is available for patients with significant hypoxemia in the chronic stable state if: (1) the attending physician has determined that the patient has a health condition outlined in subsection D1, (2) the patient meets the blood gas evidence requirements specified in subsection D3, and (3) the patient has appropriately tried other alternative treatment measures without complete success. (See subsection B.)

1. Conditions for Which Oxygen Therapy May Be Covered:

- A severe lung disease, such as chronic obstructive pulmonary disease, diffuse interstitial lung disease, whether of known or unknown etiology; cystic fibrosis bronchiectasis; widespread pulmonary neoplasm; or
- Hypoxia-related symptoms or findings that might be expected to improve with oxygen therapy. Examples of these symptoms and findings are pulmonary hypertension, recurring congestive heart failure due to chronic cor pulmonale, erythrocytosis, impairment of the cognitive process, nocturnal restlessness, and morning headache.

2. Conditions for Which Oxygen Therapy Is Not Covered:

- Angina pectoris in the absence of hypoxemia. This condition is generally not the result of a low oxygen level in the blood, and there are other preferred treatments;
- Breathlessness without cor pulmonale or evidence of hypoxemia. Although intermittent oxygen use is sometimes prescribed to relieve this condition, it is potentially harmful and psychologically addicting;
- Severe peripheral vascular disease resulting in clinically evident desaturation in one or more extremities. There is no evidence that increased PO2 improves the oxygenation of tissues with impaired circulation; or
- Terminal illnesses that do not affect the lungs.

3. Covered Blood Gas Values.—If the patient has a condition specified in subsection D1, the carrier must review the medical documentation and laboratory evidence that has been submitted for a particular patient (see subsections B and C) and determine if coverage is available under one of the three group categories outlined below.

a. Group I.—Except as modified in subsection D, coverage is provided for patients with significant hypoxemia evidenced by any of the following:

(1) An arterial PO_2 at or below 55 mm Hg, or an arterial oxygen saturation at or below 88 percent, taken at rest, breathing room air.

(2) An arterial PO_2 at or below 55 mm Hg, or an arterial

oxygen saturation at or below 88 percent, taken during sleep for a patient who demonstrates an arterial PO_2 at or above 56 mm Hg, or an arterial oxygen saturation at or above 89 percent, while awake; or a greater than normal fall in oxygen level during sleep (a decrease in arterial PO_2 more than 10 mm Hg, or decrease in arterial oxygen saturation more than 5 percent) associated with symptoms or signs reasonably attributable to hypoxemia (e.g., impairment of cognitive processes and nocturnal restlessness or insomnia). In either of these cases, coverage is provided only for use of oxygen during sleep, and then only one type of unit will be covered. Portable oxygen, therefore, would not be covered in this situation.

(3) An arterial PO_2 at or below 55 mm Hg or an arterial oxygen saturation at or below 88 percent, taken during exercise for a patient who demonstrates an arterial PO_2 at or above 56 mm Hg, or an arterial oxygen saturation at or above 89 percent, during the day while at rest. In this case, supplemental oxygen is provided for during exercise if there is evidence the use of oxygen improves the hypoxemia that was demonstrated during exercise when the patient was breathing room air.

b. Group II.—Except as modified in subsection D, coverage is available for patients whose arterial PO_2 is 56 to 59 mm Hg or whose arterial blood oxygen saturation is 89 percent, if there is evidence of:

(1) Dependent edema suggesting congestive heart failure;

(2) Pulmonary hypertension or cor pulmonale, determined by measurement of pulmonary artery pressure, gated blood pool scan, echocardiogram, or "P" pulmonale on EKG (P wave greater than 3 mm in standard leads II, III, or AVF); or

(3) Erythrocythemia with a hematocrit greater than 56 percent.

c. Group III.—Except as modified in subsection D, carriers must apply a rebuttable presumption that a home program of oxygen use is not medically necessary for patients with arterial PO_2 levels at or above 60 mm Hg, or arterial blood oxygen saturation at or above 90 percent. In order for claims in this category to be reimbursed, the carrier's reviewing physician needs to review any documentation submitted in rebuttal of this presumption and grant specific approval of the claims. HCFA expects few claims to be approved for coverage in this category.

d. Variable Factors That May Affect Blood Gas Values.—In reviewing the arterial PO_2 levels and the arterial oxygen saturation percentages specified in subsections D3A, B and C, the carrier's medical staff must take into account variations in oxygen measurements that may result from such factors as the patient's age, the altitude level, or the patient's decreased oxygen carrying capacity.

E. Portable Oxygen Systems.—A patient meeting the requirements specified below may qualify for coverage of a portable oxygen system either (1) by itself or (2) to use in addition to a stationary oxygen system. Portable oxygen is not covered when it is provided only as a backup to a stationary oxygen system. A portable oxygen system is covered for a particular patient if:

- The claim meets the requirements specified in subsections A-D, as appropriate; and
- The medical documentation indicates that the patient is mobile in the home and would benefit from the use of a portable oxygen system in the home. Portable oxygen systems are not covered for patients who qualify for oxygen solely based on blood gas studies obtained during sleep.

F. Respiratory Therapists.—Respiratory therapists' services are not covered under the provisions for coverage of oxygen services under the Part B durable medical equipment benefit as outlined above. This benefit provides for coverage of home use of oxygen and oxygen equipment, but does not include a professional component in the delivery of such services.

(See section 60-9; Intermediary Manual, Part 3, section 3113ff; and Medicare Carriers Manual, Part 3, section 2100ff.)

60-5 POWER-OPERATED VEHICLES THAT MAY BE USED AS WHEELCHAIRS

Power-operated vehicles that may be appropriately used as wheelchairs are covered under the durable medical equipment provision.

These vehicles have been appropriately used in the home setting for vocational rehabilitation and to improve the ability of chronically disabled persons to cope with normal domestic, vocational and social activities. They may be covered if a wheelchair is medically necessary and the patient is unable to operate a wheelchair manually.

A specialist in physical medicine, orthopedic surgery, neurology, or rheumatology must provide an evaluation of the patient's medical and physical condition and a prescription for the vehicle to assure that the patient requires the vehicle and is capable of using it safely. When an intermediary determines that such a specialist is not reasonably accessible, e.g., more than 1 day's round trip from the beneficiary's home, or the patient's condition precludes such travel, a prescription from the beneficiary's physician is acceptable.

The intermediary's medical staff reviews all claims for a power-operated vehicle, including the specialists' or other physicians' prescriptions and evaluations of the patient's medical and physical conditions, to insure that all coverage requirements are met. (See section 60-9 and Intermediary Manual, Part 3, section 3629.)

60-6 SPECIALLY SIZED WHEELCHAIRS

Payment may be made for a specially sized wheelchair even though it is more expensive than a standard wheelchair. For example, a narrow wheelchair may be required because of the narrow doorways of a patient's home or because of a patient's slender build. Such difference in the size of the wheelchair from the standard model is not considered a deluxe feature.

A physician's certification or prescription that a special size is needed is not required where you can determine from the information in file or other sources that a specially sized wheelchair (rather than a standard one) is needed to accommodate the wheelchair to the place of use or the physical size of the patient.

To determine the reasonable charge in these cases, use the criteria set out in Carriers Manual, sections 5022, 5022.1, 5200, and 5205, as necessary.

Cross-refer: Intermediary Manual, sections 3113.2C, 3642.1, 3643 (item 3); Carriers Manual, sections 2100.2c, 2105, 4105.2, 5107; Hospital Manual, sections 235.2c, 420.1 (item 13).

60-7 SELF-CONTAINED PACEMAKER MONITORS

Self-contained pacemaker monitors are accepted devices for monitoring cardiac pacemakers. Accordingly, program payment may be made for the rental or purchase of either of the following pacemaker monitors when it is prescribed by a physician for a patient with a cardiac pacemaker:

A. Digital Electronic Pacemaker Monitor.—This device provides the patient with an instantaneous digital readout of his pacemaker pulse rate. Use of this device does not involve professional services until there has been a change of five pulses (or more) per minute above or below the initial rate of the pacemaker; when such change occurs, the patient contacts his physician.

B. Audible/Visible Signal Pacemaker Monitor.—This device produces an audible and visible signal which indicates the pacemaker rate. Use of this device does not involve professional services until a change occurs in these signals; at such time, the patient contacts his physician.

NOTE: The design of the self-contained pacemaker monitor makes it possible for the patient to monitor his pacemaker periodically and minimizes the need for regular visits to the outpatient department of the provider.

Therefore, documentation of the medical necessity for pacemaker evaluation in the outpatient department of the provider should be obtained where such evaluation is employed in addition to the self-contained pacemaker monitor used by the patient in his home.

Cross-refer: section 50-1

60-8 SEAT LIFT

Reimbursement may be made for the rental or purchase of a medically necessary seat lift when prescribed by a physician for a patient with severe arthritis of the hip or knee and patients with muscular dystrophy or other neuromuscular diseases when it has been determined the patient can benefit therapeutically from use of the device. In establishing medical necessity for the seat lift, the evidence must show that the item is included in the physician's course of treatment, that it is likely to effect improvement, or arrest or retard deterioration in the patient's condition, and that the severity of the condition is such that the alternative would be chair or bed confinement.

Coverage of seat lifts is limited to those types which operate smoothly, can be controlled by the patient, and effectively assist a patient in standing up and sitting down without other assistance. Excluded from coverage is the type of lift which operates by a spring release mechanism with a sudden, catapult-like motion and jolts the patient from a seated to a standing position. Limit the payment for units which incorporate a recliner feature along with the seat lift to the amount payable for a seat lift without this feature.

Cross-refer: Carriers Manual, section 5107

60-9 DURABLE MEDICAL EQUIPMENT REFERENCE LIST

The durable medical equipment (DME) list which follows is designed to facilitate your processing of DME claims. This section is designed to be used as a quick reference tool for determining the coverage status of certain pieces of DME and especially for those items which are commonly referred to by both brand and generic names. The information contained herein is applicable (where appropriate) to all DME coverage determinations discussed in the DME portion of this manual. The list is organized into two columns. The first column lists alphabetically various generic categories of equipment on which national coverage decisions have been made by HCFA; and the second column notes the coverage status of each equipment category.

In the case of equipment categories that have been determined by HCFA to be covered under the DME benefit, the list outlines the conditions of coverage that must be met if payment is to be allowed for the rental or purchase of the DME by a particular patient, or cross-refers to another section of the manual where the applicable coverage criteria are described in more detail. With respect to equipment categories that cannot be covered as DME, the list includes a brief explanation of why the equipment is not covered. This DME list will be updated periodically to reflect any additional national coverage decisions that HCFA may make with regard to other categories of equipment.

When you receive a claim for an item of equipment which does not appear to fall logically into any of the generic categories listed, you have the authority and responsibility for deciding whether those items are covered under the DME benefit. These decisions must be made by each contractor based on the advice of its medical consultants, taking into account:

- The general DME coverage instructions in the Carriers Manual, section 2100ff and Intermediary Manual, section 3113ff (see below for brief summary);
- Whether the item has been approved for marketing by the Food and Drug Administration (FDA) (see Carriers Manual, section 2303.1 and Intermediary Manual, section 3151.1) and is otherwise generally considered to be safe and effective for the purpose intended; and
- Whether the item is reasonable and necessary for the individual patient.

As provided in the Carriers Manual, section 2100.1, and Intermediary Manual, section 3113.1, the term DME is defined as equipment which:

- Can withstand repeated use; i.e., could normally be rented, and used by successive patients;
- Is primarily and customarily used to serve a medical purpose;
- Generally is not useful to a person in the absence of illness or injury; and
- Is appropriate for use in a patient's home.

Durable Medical Equipment Reference List

Air Cleaners—deny—environmental control equipment; not primarily medical in nature (section 1861(n) of the Act)

Air Conditioners—deny—environmental control equipment; not primarily medical in nature (section 1861(n) of the Act)

Air-Fluidized Bed—(*See* section 60-19.)

Alternating Pressure Pads—covered if patient has, or is highly susceptible to, and matresses and decubitus ulcers and patient's physician has Lambs Wool Pads specified that he will be supervising its use in connection with his course of treatment.

Audible/Visible Signal—(*See* Self-Contained Pacemaker Monitor.) Pacemaker Monitor

Augmentative Communication Device—(*See* speech Generating Devices. Section 60-23.)

Bathtub Lifts—deny—convenience item; not primarily medical in nature (section 1861(n) of the Act)

Bathtub Seats—deny—comfort or convenience item; hygienic equipment; not primarily medical in nature (section 1861(n) of the Act)

Bead Bed—(*See* section 60-19.)

Bed Baths (home type)—deny—hygienic equipment; not primarily medical in nature (section 1861(n) of the Act)

Bed Lifter (bed elevator)—deny—not primarily medical in nature (section 1861(n) of the Act).

Bedboards—deny—not primarily medical in nature (section 1861(n) of the Act)

Bed Pans (autoclavable hospital type)—covered if patient is bed confined

Bed Side Rails—(*See* Hospital Beds, section 60-18.)

Beds—Lounge (power or manual)—deny—not a hospital bed; comfort or convenience item; not primarily medical in nature (section 1861(n) of the Act)

Beds—Oscillating—deny—institutional equipment; inappropriate for home use

Bidet Toilet Seat—(*See* Toilet Seats.)

Blood Glucose Analyzer—deny—unsuitable for home use (*See* section 60-11.)

Blood Glucose Monitor—covered if patient meets certain conditions (*See* section 60-11.)

Braille Teaching Texts—deny—educational equipment; not primarily medical in nature (section 1861(n) of the Act)

Canes—covered if patient's condition impairs ambulation (*See* section 1861(m).)

Carafes—deny—convenience item; not primarily medical in nature (section 1861(n) of the Act)

Catheters—deny—nonreusable disposable supply (section l861(n) of the Act)

Commodes—covered if patient is confined to bed or room

NOTE: The term "room confined" means that the patient's condition is such that leaving the room is medically contraindicated. The accessibility of bathroom facilities generally would not be a factor in this determination. However, confinement of a patient to his home in a case where there are no toilet facilities in the home may be equated to room confinement. Moreover, payment may also be made if a patient's medical condition confines him to a floor of his home and there is no bathroom located on that floor (*See* Hospital Beds in section 60-18 for definition of "bed confinement".)

Communicator—deny—convenience item; not primarily medical in nature (See section 60-23. Speech Generating Devices)

Continuous Passive Motion—Continuous Passive Motion (CPM) devices are covered for patients who have received a total knee replacement. To qualify for coverage, use of the device must commence within two days following surgery. In addition, coverage is limited to that portion of the three week period following surgery during which the device is used in the patient's home.

There is insufficient evidence to justify coverage of these devices for longer periods of time or for other applications.

Continuous Positive Airway Pressure (CPAP)—(*See* section 60-17.)

Crutches—covered if patient's condition impairs ambulation

Cushion Lift Power Seat—(*See* Seat Lifts.)

Dehumidifiers (room or central heating system type)—deny—environmental control equipment; not primarily medical in nature (section 1861(n) of the Act)

Diathermy Machines (standard wave types)—deny—inappropriate for home use (*See* section 35-41.)

Digital Electronic Pacemaker Monitor—(*See* Self-Contained Pacemaker Monitor.)

Disposable Sheets and Bags—deny—nonreusable disposable supplies (section 1861(n) of the Act)

Elastic Stockings—deny—nonreusable supply; not rental-type items (section 1861(n) of the Act)

Electric Air Cleaners—deny—(See Air Cleaners.) (section 1861(n) of the Act)

Electric Hospital Beds—(*See* Hospital Beds section 60-18.)

Electrical Stimulation for Wounds—deny—inappropriate for home use

Electrostatic Machines—deny—(*See* Air Cleaners and Air Conditioners.) (section 1861(n) of the Act)

Elevators—deny—convenience item; not primarily medical in nature (section 1861(n) of the Act)

Emesis Basins—deny—convenience item; not primarily medical in nature (section 1861(n) of the Act)

Esophageal Dilator—deny—physician instrument; inappropriate for patient use

Exercise Equipment—deny—not primarily medical in nature (section 1861(n) of the Act)

Fabric Supports—deny—nonreusable supplies; not rental-type item (section 1861(n) of the Act)

Face Masks (oxygen)—covered if oxygen is covered (*See* section 60-4.)

Face Masks (surgical)—deny—nonreusable disposable items (section 1861(n) of the Act)

Flowmeter—(*See* Medical Oxygen Regulators)

Fluidic Breathing Assister—(*See* IPPB Machines.)

Fomentation Device—(*See* Heating Pads.)

Gel Flotation Pads and Mattresses—(*See* Alternating Pressure Pads.)

Grab Bars—deny—self-help device; not primarily medical in nature (section 1861(n) of the Act)

Heat and Massage Foam Cushion Pad—deny—not primarily medical in nature; personal comfort item (section 1861(n) and 1862(a)(6) of the Act)

Heating and Cooling Plants—deny—environmental control equipment; not primarily medical in nature (section 1861(n) of the Act)

Heating Pads—covered if the contractor's medical staff determines patient's medical condition is one for which the application of heat in the form of a heating pad is therapeutically effective.

Heat Lamps—covered if the contractor's medical staff determines patient's medical condition is one for which the application of heat in the form of a heat lamp is therapeutically effective.

Hospital Beds—(*See* section 60-18.)

Hot Packs—(*See* Heating Pads.)

Humidifiers (oxygen)—(*See* Oxygen Humidifiers.)

Humidifiers (room or central heating system types)—deny—environmental control equipment; not medical in nature (section 1861(n) of the Act)

Hydraulic Lift—(*See* Patient Lifts.)

Incontinent Pads—deny—non-reusable supply; hygienic item (section 1861(n) of the Act.)

Infusion Pumps—For external and implantable pumps, see section 60-14. If the pump is used with an enteral or parenteral malnutritional therapy system, *see* section 65-10 to 65.10.2 0.2 for special coverage rules.

Injectors (hypodermic jet devices for injection of insulin)—deny—noncovered self-administered drug supply; pressure powered devices (section 1861(s)(2)(A) of the Act)

IPPB Machines—covered if patient's ability to breathe is severely impaired

Iron Lungs—(*See* Ventilators.)

Irrigating Kit—deny—nonreusable supply; hygienic equipment (section 1861(n) of the Act)

Lambs Wool Pads—covered under same conditions as alternating pressure pads and mattresses

Leotards—deny—(*See* Pressure Leotards.) (section 1861(n) of the Act)

Lymphedema Pumps (segmental and non-segmental therapy types)—covered (*See* section 60-16.)

Massage Devices—deny—personal comfort items; not primarily medical in nature (section 1861(n) and 1862(a)(6) of the Act)

Mattress—covered only where hospital bed is medically necessary (Separate charge for replacement mattress should not be allowed where a hospital bed with mattress is rented.) (*See* section 60-18.)

Medical Oxygen Regulators—covered if patient's ability to breathe is severely impaired (*See* section 60-4.)

Mobile Geriatric Chair—(*See* Rolling Chairs.)

Motorized Wheelchairs—(*See* Wheelchairs (power operated).)

Muscle Stimulators—Covered for certain conditions (*See* section 35-77.)

Nebulizers—covered if patient's ability to breathe is severely impaired

Oscillating Beds—deny—institutional equipment—inappropriate for home use

Overbed Tables—deny—convenience item; not primarily medical in nature (section 1861(n) of the Act)

Oxygen—covered if the oxygen has been prescribed for use in connection with medically necessary durable medical equipment (*See* section 60-4.)

Oxygen Humidifiers—covered if a medical humidifier has been prescribed for use in connection with medically necessary durable medical equipment for purposes of moisturizing oxygen (*See* section 60-4.)

Oxygen Regulators (Medical)—(*See* Medical Oxygen Regulators.)

Oxygen Tents—(*See* section 60-4.)

Paraffin Bath Units (Portable)—(*See* Paraffin Bath Units [Portable].)

Paraffin Bath Units (Standard)—deny—institutional equipment; inappropriate for home use

Parallel Bars—deny—support exercise equipment; primarily for institutional use; in the home setting other devices (e.g., a walker) satisfy the patient's need

Patient Lifts—covered if contractor's medical staff determines patient's condition is such that periodic movement is necessary to effect improvement or to arrest or retard deterioration in his condition.

Percussors—covered for mobilizing respiratory tract secretions in patients with chronic obstructive lung disease, chronic bronchitis, or emphysema, when patient or operator of powered percussor has received appropriate training by a physician or therapist, and no one competent to administer manual therapy is available.

Portable Oxygen Systems:

1. Regulated (adjustable—covered under conditions specified in flow rate) section 60-4. Refer all claims to medical staff for this determination.

2. Preset (flow rate—deny—emergency, first-aid, or not adjustable) precautionary equipment; essentially not therapeutic in nature.

Portable Paraffin Bath Units—covered when the patient has undergone a successful trial period of paraffin therapy ordered by a physician and the patient's condition is expected to be relieved by long term use of this modality.

Portable Room Heaters—deny—environmental control equipment; not primarily medical in nature (section 1861(n) of the Act)

Portable Whirlpool Pumps—deny—not primarily medical in nature; personal comfort items (section 1861(n) and 1862(a)(6) of the Act)

Postural Drainage Boards—covered if patient has a chronic pulmonary condition

Preset Portable Oxygen Units—deny—emergency, first-aid, or precautionary equipment; essentially not therapeutic in nature

Pressure Leotards—deny—nonreusable supply, not rental-type item (section 1861(n) of the Act)

Pulse Tachometer—deny—not reasonable or necessary for monitoring pulse of homebound patient with or without a cardiac pacemaker

Quad-Canes—(*See* Walkers.)

Raised Toilet Seats—deny—convenience item; hygienic equipment; not primarily medical in nature (section 1861(n) of the Act)

Reflectance Colorimeters—(*See* Blood Glucose Analyzer.)

Respirators—(*See* Ventilators.)

Rolling Chairs—covered if the contractor's medical staff determines that the patient's condition is such that there is a medical need for this item and it has been prescribed by the patient's physician in lieu of a wheelchair. Coverage is limited to those roll about chairs having casters of at least 5 inches in diameter and specifically designed to meet the needs of ill, injured, or otherwise impaired individuals. Coverage is denied for the wide range of chairs with smaller casters as are found in general use in homes, offices, and institutions for many purposes not related to the care or treatment of ill or injured persons. This type is not primarily medical in nature. (section 1861(n) of the Act)

Safety Roller—(*See* section 60-15.)

Sauna Baths—deny—not primarily medical in nature; personal comfort items (section 1861(n) and (1862(a)(6) of the Act)

Seat Lift—covered under the conditions specified in section 60-8. Refer all to medical staff for this determination.

Self-Contained Pacemaker—covered when prescribed by a physician. Monitor for a patient with a cardiac pacemaker (*See* section 50-1C and 60-7.)

Sitz Bath—covered if the contractor's medical staff determines patient has an infection or injury of the perineal area and the item has been prescribed by the patient's physician as a part of his planned regimen of treatment in the patient's home.

Spare Tanks of Oxygen—deny—convenience or precautionary supply

Speech Teaching Machine—deny—education equipment; not primarily medical in nature (section 1861(n) of the Act)

Stairway Elevators—deny—(*See* Elevators.) (section l861(n) of the Act)

Standing Table—deny—convenience item; not primarily medical in nature (section 1861(n) of the Act)

Steam Packs—these packs are covered under the same condition as a heating pad (*See* Heating Pads.)

Suction Machine—covered if the contractor's medical staff determines that the machine specified in the claim is medically required and appropriate for home use without technical or professional supervision.

Support Hose—deny (*See* Fabric Supports.) (section 1861(n) of the Act)

Surgical Leggings—deny—nonreusable supply; not rental-type item (section 1861(n) of the Act)

Telephone Alert Systems—deny—these are emergency communications systems and do not serve a diagnostic or therapeutic purpose

Telephone Arms—deny—convenience item; not medical in nature (section 1861(n) of the Act)

Toilet Seats—deny—not medical equipment (section 1861(n) of the Act)

Traction Equipment—covered if patient has orthopedic impairment requiring traction equipment which prevents ambulation during the period of use. (Consider covering devices usable during ambulation; e.g., cervical traction collar, under the brace provision.)

Trapeze Bars—covered if patient is bed confined and the patient needs a trapeze bar to sit up because of respiratory condition, to change body position for other medical reasons, or to get in and out of bed.

Treadmill Exerciser—deny—exercise equipment; not primarily medical in nature (section 1861(n) of the Act)

Ultraviolet Cabinet—covered for selected patients with generalized intractable psoriasis. Using appropriate consultation, the contractor should determine whether medical and other factors justify treatment at home rather than at alternative sites, e.g., outpatient department of a hospital.

Urinals (autoclavable hospital type)—covered if patient is bed confined

Vaporizers—covered if patient has a respiratory illness

Ventilators—covered for treatment of neuromuscular diseases, thoracic restrictive diseases, and chronic respiratory failure consequent to chronic obstructive pulmonary disease. Includes both positive and negative pressure types.

Walkers—covered if patient's condition impairs ambulation (*See* also section 60-15.)

Water and Pressure Pads and Mattresses—(*See* Alternating Pressure Pads and Mattresses.)

Wheelchairs—covered if patient's condition is such that without the use of a wheelchair he would otherwise be bed or chair confined. An individual may qualify for a wheelchair and still be considered bed confined.

Wheelchairs (power operated) and wheelchairs with other spe-

cial features—covered if patient's condition is such that a wheelchair is medically necessary and the patient is unable to operate the wheelchair manually. Any claim involving a power wheelchair or a wheelchair with other special features should be referred for medical consultation since payment for the special features is limited to those which are medically required because of the patient's condition. (See section 60-5 for power operated and section 60-6 for specially sized wheelchairs.)

NOTE: A power-operated vehicle that may appropriately be used as a wheelchair can be covered. (*See* section 60-5 for coverage details.)

Whirlpool Bath Equipment—covered if patient is homebound and has a (standard) condition for which the whirlpool bath can be expected to provide substantial therapeutic benefit justifying its cost. Where patient is not homebound but has such a condition, payment is restricted to the cost of providing the services elsewhere; e.g., an outpatient department of a participating hospital, if that alternative is less costly. In all cases, refer claim to medical staff for a determination.

Whirlpool Pumps—deny—(*See* Portable Whirlpool Pumps.) (section 1861(n) of the Act)

White Cane—deny—(*See* section 60-3.)

60-11 HOME BLOOD GLUCOSE MONITORS

There are several different types of blood glucose monitors which use reflectance meters to determine blood glucose levels. Medicare coverage of these devices varies, both with respect to the type of device and the medical condition of the patient for whom the device is prescribed.

Reflectance colorimeter devices used for measuring blood glucose levels in clinical settings are not covered as durable medical equipment for use in the home because their need for frequent professional recalibration makes them unsuitable for home use. However, some types of blood glucose monitors which use a reflectance meter specifically designed for home use by diabetic patients may be covered as durable medical equipment, subject to the conditions and limitations described below.

Blood glucose monitors are meter devices which read color changes produced on specially treated reagent strips by glucose concentrations in the patient's blood. The patient, using a disposable sterile lancet, draws a drop of blood, places it on a reagent strip and, following instructions which may vary with the device used, inserts it into the device to obtain a reading. Lancets, reagent strips, and other supplies necessary for the proper functioning of the device are also covered for patients for whom the device is indicated. Home blood glucose monitors enable certain patients to better control their blood glucose levels by frequently checking and appropriately contacting their attending physician for advice and treatment. Studies indicate that the patient's ability to carefully follow proper procedures is critical to obtaining satisfactory results with these devices. In addition, the cost of the devices, with their supplies, limits economical use to patients who must make frequent checks of their blood glucose levels. Accordingly, coverage of home blood glucose monitors is limited to patients meeting the following conditions:

- The patient must be an insulin-treated diabetic;
- The patient's physician states that the patient is capable of being trained to use the particular device prescribed in an appropriate manner. In some cases, the patient may not be able to perform this function, but a responsible individual can be trained to use the equipment and monitor the patient to assure that the intended effect is achieved. This is permissible if the record is properly documented by the patient's physician; and
- The device is designed for home rather than clinical use.

There is also a blood glucose monitoring system designed especially for use by those with visual impairments. The monitors used in such systems are identical in terms of reliability and sensitivity to the standard blood glucose monitors described above. They differ by having such features as voice synthesizers, automatic timers, and specially designed arrangements of supplies and materials to enable the visually impaired to use the equipment without assistance.

These special blood glucose monitoring systems are covered under Medicare if the following conditions are met:

- The patient and device meet the four conditions listed above for coverage of standard home blood glucose monitors; and
- The patient's physician certifies that he or she has a visual impairment severe enough to require use of this special monitoring system.

The additional features and equipment of these special systems justify a higher reimbursement amount than allowed for standard blood glucose monitors. Separately identify claims for such devices and establish a separate reimbursement amount for them. For those carriers using HCPCS, the procedure code and definition is: EO609—Blood Glucose Monitor—with special features (e.g., voice synthesizers, automatic timer).

60-14 INFUSION PUMPS

The following indications for treatment using infusion pumps are covered under medicare:

A. External Infusion Pumps.—

1. Iron Poisoning (Effective for Services Performed On or After 9/26/84).—When used in the administration of deferoxamine for the treatment of acute iron poisoning and iron overload, only external infusion pumps are covered.

2. Thromboembolic Disease (Effective for Services Performed On or After 9/26/84).—When used in the administration of heparin for the treatment of thromboembolic disease and/or pulmonary embolism, only external infusion pumps used in an institutional setting are covered.

3. Chemotherapy for Liver Cancer (Effective for Services Performed On or After 1/29/85).—The external chemotherapy infusion pump is covered when used in the treatment of primary hepatocellular carcinoma or colorectal cancer where this disease is unresectable or where the patient refuses surgical excision of the tumor.

4. Morphine for Intractable Cancer Pain (Effective for Services Performed On or After 4/22/85).—Morphine infusion via an external infusion pump is covered when used in the treatment of intractable pain caused by cancer (in either an inpatient or outpatient setting, including a hospice).

5. Continuous Subcutaneous Insulin Infusion Pumps (CSII) (Effective for Services Performed On or After 4/1/2000).—An external infusion pump and related drugs/supplies are covered as medically necessary in the home setting in the following situation: Treatment of diabetes.

In order to be covered, patients must meet criterion A or B:

(A) The patient has completed a comprehensive diabetes education program and has been on a program of multiple daily injections of insulin (i.e., at least 3 injections per day), with frequent self-adjustments of insulin dose, for at least 6 months prior to initiation of the insulin pump and has documented frequency of glucose self-testing an average of at least four times per day during the 2 months prior to initiation of the insulin pump, and meets one or more of the following criteria while on the multiple daily injection regimen:

(1) Glycosylated hemoglobin level (HbAlc) > 7.0%

(2) History of recurring hypoglycemia

(3) Wide fluctuations in blood glucose before mealtime

(4) Dawn phenomenon, with fasting blood sugars frequently exceeding 200 mg/dl

(5) History of severe glycemic excursions

(B) The patient with diabetes has been on a pump prior to enrollment in Medicare and has documented frequency of glucose self-testing an average of at least four times per day during the month prior to Medicare enrollment. Diabetes needs to be documented by a fasting C-peptide level that is less than or equal to 110 percent of the lower limit of normal of the laboratory's measurement method. (Effective for Services Performed on or after January 1, 2002)

Continued coverage of the insulin pump would require that the patient has been seen and evaluated by the treating physician at least every 3 months. The pump must be ordered by and follow-up care of the patient must be managed by a physician who manages multiple patients with CSII and who works closely with a team including nurses, diabetes educators, and dietitians who are knowledgeable in the use of CSII.

Subcutaneous insulin infusion pumps will continue to be denied as not medically necessary and reasonable for all Type II diabetics, including insulin-requiring Type II diabetics.

6. Other uses of external infusion pumps are covered if the contractor's medical staff verifies the appropriateness of the therapy and of the prescribed pump for the individual patient.

NOTE: Payment may also be made for drugs necessary for the effective use of an external infusion pump as long as the drug being used with the pump is itself reasonable and necessary for the patient's treatment.

B. Implantable Infusion Pumps.—

1. Chemotherapy for Liver Cancer (Effective for Services Performed On or After 9/26/84).—The implantable infusion pump is covered for intra-arterial infusion of 5-FUdR for the treatment of liver cancer for patients with primary hepatocellular carcinoma or Duke's Class D colorectal cancer, in whom the metastases are limited to the liver, and where (1) the disease is unresectable or (2) where the patient refuses surgical excision of the tumor.

2. Anti-Spasmodic Drugs for Severe Spasticity.—An implantable infusion pump is covered when used to administer anti-spasmodic drugs intrathecally (e.g., baclofen) to treat chronic intractable spasticity in patients who have proven unresponsive to less invasive medical therapy as determined by the following criteria:

- As indicated by at least a 6-week trial, the patient cannot be maintained on noninvasive methods of spasm control, such as oral anti-spasmodic drugs, either because these methods fail to control adequately the spasticity or produce intolerable side effects, and
- Prior to pump implantation, the patient must have responded favorably to a trial intrathecal dose of the anti-spasmodic drug.

3. Opioid Drugs for Treatment of Chronic Intractable Pain.—An implantable infusion pump is covered when used to administer opioid drugs (e.g., morphine) intrathecally or epidurally for treatment of severe chronic intractable pain of malignant or non-malignant origin in patients who have a life expectancy of at least 3 months and who have proven unresponsive to less invasive medical therapy as determined by the following criteria:

- The patient's history must indicate that he/she would not respond adequately to noninvasive methods of pain control, such as systemic opioids (including attempts to eliminate physical and behavioral abnormalities which may cause an exaggerated reaction to pain); and
- A preliminary trial of intraspinal opioid drug administration must be undertaken with a temporary intrathecal/epidural catheter to substantiate adequately acceptable pain relief and degree of side effects (including effects on the activities of daily living) and patient acceptance.

4. Coverage of Other Uses of Implanted Infusion Pumps.—Determinations may be made on coverage of other uses of implanted infusion pumps if the contractor's medical staff verifies that:

- The drug is reasonable and necessary for the treatment of the individual patient;
- It is medically necessary that the drug be administered by an implanted infusion pump; and
- The FDA approved labeling for the pump must specify that the drug being administered and the purpose for which it is administered is an indicated use for the pump.

5. Implantation of Infusion Pump Is Contraindicated.—The implantation of an infusion pump is contraindicated in the following patients:

- Patients with a known allergy or hypersensitivity to the drug being used (e.g., oral baclofen, morphine, etc.);
- Patients who have an infection;
- Patients whose body size is insufficient to support the weight and bulk of the device; and
- Patients with other implanted programmable devices since crosstalk between devices may inadvertently change the prescription.

NOTE: Payment may also be made for drugs necessary for the effective use of an implantable infusion pump as long as the drug being used with the pump is itself reasonable and necessary for the patient's treatment.

The following indications for treatment using infusion pumps are not covered under Medicare:

A. External Infusion Pumps.—

1. Vancomycin (Effective for Services Beginning On or After September 1, 1996).—Medicare coverage of vancomycin as a durable medical equipment infusion pump benefit is not covered. There is insufficient evidence to support the necessity of using an external infusion pump, instead of a disposable elastomeric pump or the gravity drip method, to administer vancomycin in a safe and appropriate manner.

B. Implantable Infusion Pump.—

1. Thromboembolic Disease (Effective for Services Performed On or After 9/26/84).—According to the Public Health Service, there is insufficient published clinical data to support the safety and effectiveness of the heparin implantable pump. Therefore, the use of an implantable infusion pump for infusion of heparin in the treatment of recurrent thromboembolic disease is not covered.

2. Diabetes—Implanted infusion pumps for the infusion of insulin to treat diabetes is not covered. The data do not demonstrate that the pump provides effective administration of insulin.

60-15 SAFETY ROLLER

"Safety roller" is the generic name applied to devices for patients who cannot use standard wheeled walkers. They may be appropriate, and therefore covered, for some patients who are obese, have severe neurological disorders, or restricted use of one hand, which makes it impossible to use a wheeled walker that does not have the sophisticated braking system found on safety rollers.

In order to assure that payment is not made for a safety roller when a less expensive standard wheeled walker would satisfy the patient's medical needs, carriers refer safety roller claims to their medical consultants. The medical consultant determines whether some or all of the features provided in a safety roller are necessary, and therefore covered and reimbursable. If it is determined that the patient could use a standard wheeled walker, the charge for the safety roller is reduced to the charge of a standard wheeled walker.

Some obese patients who could use a standard wheeled walker if their weight did not exceed the walker's strength and stability limits can have it reinforced and its wheel base expanded. Such modifications are routine mechanical adjustments and justify a moderate surcharge. In these cases the carrier reduces the charge for the safety roller to the charge for the standard wheeled walker plus the surcharge for modifications.

In the case of patients with medical documentation showing severe neurological disorders or restricted use of one hand which makes it impossible for them to use a wheeled walker that does not have a sophisticated braking system, a reasonable charge for the safety roller may be determined without relating it to the reasonable charge for a standard wheeled walker. (Such reasonable charge should be developed in accordance with the instructions in Medicare Carriers Manual, sections 5010 and 5205.)

Cross Refer: Carriers Manual, sections 2100ff., section 60-9.

60-16 PNEUMATIC COMPRESSION DEVICES

Lymphedema

Lymphedema is the swelling of subcutaneous tissues due to the accumulation of excessive lymph fluid. The accumulation of lymph fluid results from an impairment to the normal clearing function of the lymphatic system and/or from an excessive production of lymph. Lymphedema is divided into two broad classes according to etiology. Primary lymphedema is a relatively uncommon, chronic condition which may be due to such causes as Milroy's Disease or congenital anomalies. Secondary lymphedema, which is much more common, results from the destruction of or damage to formerly functioning lymphatic channels, such as surgical removal of lymph nodes or post radiation fibrosis, among other causes.

Pneumatic compression devices are covered in the home setting for the treatment of lymphedema if the patient has undergone a four-week trial of conservative therapy and the treating physician determines that there has been no significant improvement or if significant symptoms remain after the trial. The trial of conservative therapy must include use of an appropriate compression bandage system or compression garment, exercise, and elevation of the limb. The garment may be prefabricated or custom-fabricated but must provide adequate graduated compression.

Chronic Venous Insufficiency With Venous Statis Ulcers

Chronic venous insufficiency (CVI) of the lower extremities is a condition caused by abnormalities of the venous wall and valves, leading to obstruction or reflux of blood flow in the veins. Sings of CVI include hyperpigmentation, statis dermatitis, chronic edema, and venous ulcers.

Pneumatic compression devices are covered in the home setting for the treatment of CVI of the lower extremities only if the patient has one or more venous statis ulcer(s) which have failed to heal after a 6 month trial of conservative therapy directed by the treating physician. The trial of conservative therapy must include a compression bandage system or compression garment, appropriate dressings for the wound, exercise, and elevation of the limb.

General Coverage Criteria

Pneumatic compression devices are covered only when prescribed by a physician and when they are used with appropriate physician oversight, i.e., physician evaluation of the patient's condition to determine medical necessity of the device, assuring suitable instruction in the operation of the machine, a treatment plan defining the pressure to be used and the frequency and duration of use, and ongoing monitoring of use and response to treatment.

The determination by the physician of the medical necessity of a pneumatic compression device must include (1) the patient's diagnosis and prognosis; (2) symptoms and objective findings, including measurements which establish the severity of the condition; (3) the reason the device is required, including the treatments which have been tried and failed, and (4) the clinical response to an initial treatment with the device. The clinical response includes the change in pre-treatment measurements, ability to tolerate the treatment session and parameters, and ability of the patient (or caregiver) to apply the device for continued use in the home.

The only time that a segmented, calibrated gradient pneumatic compression device (HCPCs code E0652) would be covered is when the individual has unique characteristics that prevent them from receiving satisfactory pneumatic compression treatment using a nonsegmented device in conjunction with a segmented appliance or a segmented compression device without manual control of pressure in each chamber.

Cross Refer: §60-9.

60-17 CONTINUOUS POSITIVE AIRWAY PRESSURE (CPAP)

CPAP is a noninvasive technique for providing low levels of air pressure from a flow generator, via a nose mask, through the nares. The purpose is to prevent the collapse of the oropharyngeal walls and the obstruction of airflow during sleep, which occurs in obstructive sleep apnea (OSA). Effective for services furnished between and including January 12, 1987 and March 31, 2002: The diagnosis of OSA requires documentation of at least 30 episodes of apnea, each lasting a minimum of 10 seconds, during 6 to 7 hours of recorded sleep. The use of CPAP is covered under Medicare when used in adult patients with moderate or severe OSA for whom surgery is a likely alternative to CPAP.

Initial claims must be supported by medical documentation (separate documentation where electronic billing is used), such as a prescription written by the patient's attending physician, that specifies:

- a diagnosis of moderate or severe obstructive sleep apnea, and
- surgery is a likely alternative.

The claim must also certify that the documentation supporting a diagnosis of OSA (described above) is available.

Effective for services furnished on or after April 1, 2002:

The use of CPAP devices are covered under Medicare when ordered and prescribed by the licensed treating physician to be used in adult patients with OSA if either of the following criteria using the Apnea-Hypopnea Index (AHI) are met:

AHI $\geq$ 15 events per hour, or

AHI $\geq$ 5 and $\leq$ 14 events per hour with documented symptoms of excessive daytime sleepiness, impaired cognition, mood disorders or insomnia, or documented hypertension, ischemic heart disease or history of stroke.

The AHI is equal to the average number of episodes of apnea and hypopnea per hour and must be based on a minimum of 2 hours of sleep recorded by polysomnography using actual recorded hours or sleep (i.e., the AHI may not be extrapolated or projected).

Apnea is defined as a cessation of airflow for at least 10 seconds. Hypopnea is defined as an abnormal respiratory event lasting at least 10 seconds with at least 30% reduction in thoracoabdominal movement or airflow as compared to baseline, and with at least a 4% oxygen desaturation.

The polysomnography must be performed in a facility-based sleep study laboratory, and not in the home or in a mobile facility.

Initial claims for CPAP devices must be supported by information contained in the medical record indicating that the patient meets Medicare's stated coverage criteria.

Cross Refer: section 60-9.

60-18 HOSPITAL BEDS

A. General Requirements for Coverage of Hospital Beds.—A physician's prescription, and such additional documentation as the contractors' medical staffs may consider necessary, including medical records and physicians' reports, must establish the medical necessity for a hospital bed due to one of the following reasons:

- The patient's condition requires positioning of the body; e.g., to alleviate pain, promote good body alignment, prevent contractures, avoid respiratory infections, in ways not feasible in an ordinary bed; or
- The patient's condition requires special attachments that cannot be fixed and used on an ordinary bed.

B. Physician's Prescription.—The physician's prescription, which must accompany the initial claim, and supplementing documentation when required, must establish that a hospital bed is medically necessary. If the stated reason for the need for a hospital bed is the patient's condition requires positioning, the prescription or other documentation must describe the medical condition, e.g., cardiac disease, chronic obstructive pulmonary disease, quadriplegia or paraplegia, and also the severity and frequency of the symptoms of the condition, that necessitates a hospital bed for positioning.

If the stated reason for requiring a hospital bed is the patient's condition requires special attachments, the prescription must describe the patient's condition and specify the attachments that require a hospital bed.

C. Variable Height Feature.—In well documented cases, the contractors' medical staffs may determine that a variable height feature of a hospital bed, approved for coverage under subsection A above, is medically necessary and, therefore, covered, for one of the following conditions:

- Severe arthritis and other injuries to lower extremities; e.g., fractured hip. The condition requires the variable height feature to assist the patient to ambulate by enabling the patient to place his or her feet on the floor while sitting on the edge of the bed;
- Severe cardiac conditions. For those cardiac patients who are able to leave bed, but who must avoid the strain of "jumping" up or down;
- Spinal cord injuries, including quadriplegic and paraplegic patients, multiple limb amputee and stroke patients. For those patients who are able to transfer from bed to a wheelchair, with or without help; or
- Other severely debilitating diseases and conditions, if the variable height feature is required to assist the patient to ambulate.

D. Electric Powered Hospital Bed Adjustments.—Electric powered adjustments to lower and raise head and foot may be covered when the contractor's medical staff determines that the patient's condition requires frequent change in body position and/or there may be an immediate need for a change in body position (i.e., no delay can be tolerated) and the patient can operate the controls and cause the adjustments. Exceptions may be made to this last requirement in cases of spinal cord injury and brain damaged patients.

E. Side Rails.—If the patient's condition requires bed side rails, they can be covered when an integral part of, or an accessory to, a hospital bed.

Cross refer: Carriers Manual, section 5015.4

60-19 AIR-FLUIDIZED BED

An air-fluidized bed uses warm air under pressure to set small ceramic beads in motion which simulate the movement of fluid. When the patient is placed in the bed, his body weight is evenly distributed over a large surface area which creates a sensation of "floating." Medicare payment for home use of the air-fluidized bed for treatment of pressure sores can be made if such use is reasonable and necessary for the individual patient.

A decision that use of an air-fluidized bed is reasonable and necessary requires that:

- The patient has a stage 3 (full thickness tissue loss) or stage 4 (deep tissue destruction) pressure sore;
- The patient is bedridden or chair bound as a result of severely limited mobility;
- In the absence of an air-fluidized bed, the patient would require institutionalization;
- The air-fluidized bed is ordered in writing by the patient's attending physician based upon a comprehensive assessment and evaluation of the patient after completion of a course of conservative treatment designed to optimize conditions that promote wound healing. This course of treatment must have been at least one month in duration without progression toward wound healing. This month of prerequisite conservative treatment may include some period in an institution as long as there is documentation available to verify that the necessary conservative treatment has been rendered.
- Use of wet-to-dry dressings for wound debridement, begun during the period of conservative treatment and which continue beyond 30 days, will not preclude coverage of air-fluidized bed. Should additional debridement again become necessary, while a patient is using an air-fluidized bed (after the first 30-day course of conservative treatment) that will not cause the air-fluidized bed to become non-covered. In all instances documentation verifying the continued need for the bed must be available.
- Conservative treatment must include:
  - Frequent repositioning of the patient with particular attention to relief of pressure over bony prominences (usually every 2 hours);
  - Use of a specialized support surface (Group II) designed to reduce pressure and shear forces on healing ulcers and to prevent new ulcer formation;
  - Necessary treatment to resolve any wound infection;
  - Optimization of nutrition status to promote wound healing;
  - Debridement by any means (including wet to dry dressings-which does not require an occulsive covering) to remove devitalized tissue from the wound bed;
  - Maintenance of a clean, moist bed of granulation tissue with appropriate moist dressings protected by an occlusive covering, while the wound heals.
- A trained adult caregiver is available to assist the patient with activities of daily living, fluid balance, dry skin care, repositioning, recognition and management of altered mental status, dietary needs, prescribed treatments, and management and support of the air-fluidized bed system and its problems such as leakage;
- A physician directs the home treatment regimen, and reevaluates and recertifies the need for the air-fluidized bed on a monthly basis; and
- All other alternative equipment has been considered and ruled out.

Home use of the air-fluidized bed is not covered under any of the following circumstances:

- The patient has coexisting pulmonary disease (the lack of firm back support makes coughing ineffective and dry air inhalation thickens pulmonary secretions);
- The patient requires treatment with wet soaks or moist wound dressings that are not protected with an impervious covering such as plastic wrap or other occlusive material;
- The caregiver is unwilling or unable to provide the type of care required by the patient on an air-fluidized bed;
- Structural support is inadequate to support the weight of the air-fluidized bed system (it generally weighs 1600 pounds or more);
- Electrical system is insufficient for the anticipated increase in energy consumption; or
- Other known contraindications exist.

Coverage of an air-fluidized bed is limited to the equipment itself. Payment for this covered item may only be made if the written order from the attending physician is furnished to the supplier prior to the delivery of the equipment. Payment is not included for the caregiver or for architectural adjustments such as electrical or structural improvement.

Cross refer: Carriers Manual, section 5102.2

60-23 SPEECH GENERATING DEVICES

Effective January 1, 2001, augmentative and alternative communication devices or communicators, which are hereafter referred to as "speech generating devices" are now considered to fall within the DME benefit category established by §1861(n) of the Social Security Act. They may be covered if the contractor's medical staff determines that the patient suffers from a severe speech impairment and that the medical condition warrants the use of a device based on the following definitions.

Definition of Speech Generating Devices.—Speech generating devices are defined as speech aids that provide an individual who has a severe speech impairment with the ability to meet his functional speaking needs. Speech generating are characterized by:

- Being a dedicated speech device, used solely by the individual who has a severe speech impairment;
- May have digitized speech output, using pre-recorded messages, less than or equal to 8 minutes recording time;
- May have digitized speech output, using pre-recorded messages, greater than 8 minutes recording time;
- May have synthesized speech output, which requires message formulation by spelling and device access by physical contact with the device-direct selection techniques;
- May have synthesized speech output, which permits multiple methods of message formulation and multiple methods of device access; or
- May be software that allows a laptop computer, desktop computer or personal digital assistant (PDA) to function as a speech generating device.
- Devices that are not dedicated speech devices, but are devices that are capable of running software for purposes other than for speech generation, e.g., devices that can also run a word processing package, an accounting program, or perform other non-medical function.
- Laptop computers, desktop computers, or PDAs, which may be programmed to perform the same function as a speech generating device, are non-covered since they are not primarily medical in nature and do not meet the definition of DME. For this reason, they cannot be considered speech generating devices for Amedicare coverage purposes.
- A devices that is useful to someone without severe speech impairment is not considered a speech generating devices for Medicare coverage purposes.

60-24 NON-IMPLANTABLE PELVIC FLOOR ELECTRICAL STIMULATOR

Non-implantable pelvic floor electrical stimulators provide neuromuscular electrical stimulation through the pelvic floor with the intent of strengthening and exercising pelvic floor musculature. Stimulation is generally delivered by vaginal or anal probes connected to an external pulse generator.

The methods of pelvic floor electrical stimulation vary in location, stimulus frequency (Hz), stimulus intensity or amplitude (mA), pulse duration (duty cycle), treatments per day, number of treatment days per week, length of time for each treatment session, overall time period for device use and between clinic and home settings. In general, the stimulus frequency and other parameters are chosen based on the patient's clinical diagnosis.

Pelvic floor electrical stimulation with a non-implantable stimulator is covered for the treatment of stress and/or urge urinary incontinence in cognitively intact patients who have failed a documented trial of pelvic muscle exercise (PME) training.

A failed trial of PME training is defined as no clinically significant improvement in urinary continence after completing 4 weeks of an ordered plan of pelvic muscle exercises designed to increase periurethral muscle strength.

65 PROSTHETIC DEVICES

65-1 HYDROPHILIC CONTACT LENSES

Hydrophilic contact lenses are eyeglasses within the meaning of the exclusion in section 1862(a)(7) of the law and are not covered when used in the treatment of nondiseased eyes with spherical ametrophia, refractive astigmatism, and/or corneal astigmatism. Payment may be made under the prosthetic device benefit, however, for hydrophilic contact lenses when prescribed for an aphakic patient.

Contractors are authorized to accept an FDA letter of approval or other FDA published material as evidence of FDA approval.

(*See* section 45-7 for coverage of a hydrophilic lens as a corneal bandage.)

Cross-refer: Intermediary Manual, sections 3110.3, 3110.4, 3151, and 3157; Carriers Manual, sections 2130, 2320; Hospital Manual, sections 228.3, 228.4, 260.1 and 260.7.

65-3 SCLERAL SHELL

Scleral shell (or shield) is a catch-all term for different types of hard scleral contact lenses.

A scleral shell fits over the entire exposed surface of the eye as opposed to a corneal contact lens which covers only the central non-white area encompassing the pupil and iris. Where an eye has been rendered sightless and shrunken by inflammatory disease, a scleral shell may, among other things, obviate the need for surgical enucleation and prosthetic implant and act to support the surrounding orbital tissue.

In such a case, the device serves essentially as an artificial eye. In this situation, payment may be made for a scleral shell under section 1861(s)(8) of the law.

Scleral shells are occasionally used in combination with artificial tears in the treatment of "dry eye" of diverse etiology. Tears ordinarily dry at a rapid rate, and are continually replaced by the lacrimal gland. When the lacrimal gland fails, the half-life of artificial tears may be greatly prolonged by the use of the scleral contact lens as a protective barrier against the drying action of the atmosphere. Thus, the difficult and sometimes hazardous process of frequent instillation of artificial tears may be avoided. The lens acts in this instance to substitute, in part, for the functioning of the diseased lacrimal gland and would be covered as a prosthetic device in the rare case when it is used in the treatment of "dry eye."

Cross-refer: HCFA-Pub. 13-3, sections 3110.4, 3110.5; HCFA-Pub. 14-3, sections 2130, 2133; HCFA-Pub. 10, sections 210.4, 211

65-5 ELECTRONIC SPEECH AIDS

Electronic speech aids are covered under Part B as prosthetic devices when the patient has had a laryngectomy or his larynx is permanently inoperative. There are two types of speech aids. One operates by placing a vibrating head against the throat; the other amplifies sound waves through a tube which is inserted into the user's mouth. A patient who has had radical neck surgery and/or extensive radiation to the anterior part of the neck would generally be able to use only the "oral tube" model or one of the more sensitive and more expensive "throat contact" devices.

Cross-refer: HCFA-Pub. 13-3, section 3110.4; HCFA-Pub. 14-3, section 2130; HCFA-Pub. 10, section 228.4

65-7 INTRAOCULAR LENSES (IOLs)

An intraocular lens, or pseudophakos, is an artificial lens which may be implanted to replace the natural lens after cataract surgery. Intraocular lens implantation services, as well as the lens itself, may be covered if reasonable and necessary for the individual. Implantation services may include hospital, surgical, and other medical services, including pre-implantation ultrasound (A-scan) eye measurement of one or both eyes.

Cross-refer: HCFA Pub. 13-3, §§3110.4, 3151, and 3157; HCFA Pub.14-3, §2130; HCFA Pub.10, §228.4

65-8 ELECTRICAL NERVE STIMULATORS

Two general classifications of electrical nerve stimulators are employed to treat chronic intractable pain: peripheral nerve stimulators and central nervous system stimulators.

A. Implanted Peripheral Nerve Stimulators.—Payment may be made under the prosthetic device benefit for implanted peripheral nerve stimulators. Use of this stimulator involves implantation of electrodes around a selected peripheral nerve. The stimulating electrode is connected by an insulated lead to a receiver unit which is implanted under the skin at a depth not greater than 1/2 inch. Stimulation is induced by a generator connected to an antenna unit which is attached to the skin surface over the receiver unit. Implantation of electrodes requires surgery and usually necessitates an operating room.

NOTE: Peripheral nerve stimulators may also be employed to assess a patient's suitability for continued treatment with an electric nerve stimulator. As explained in section 35-46, such use of the stimulator is covered as part of the total diagnostic service furnished to the beneficiary rather than as a prosthesis.

B. Central Nervous System Stimulators (Dorsal Column and Depth Brain Stimulators).—The implantation of central nervous system stimulators may be covered as therapies for the relief of chronic intractable pain, subject to the following conditions:

1. Types of Implantations.—There are two types of implantations covered by this instruction:

a. Dorsal Column (Spinal Cord) Neurostimulation.—The surgical implantation of neurostimulator electrodes within the dura mater (endodural) or the percutaneous insertion of electrodes in the epidural space is covered.

b. Depth Brain Neurostimulation.—The stereotactic implantation of electrodes in the deep brain (e.g., thalamus and periaqueductal gray matter) is covered.

2. Conditions for Coverage.—No payment may be made for the implantation of dorsal column or depth brain stimulators or services and supplies related to such implantation, unless all of the conditions listed below have been met:

a. The implantation of the stimulator is used only as a late resort (if not a last resort) for patients with chronic intractable pain;

b. With respect to item a, other treatment modalities (pharmacological, surgical, physical, or psychological therapies) have been tried and did not prove satisfactory, or are judged to be unsuitable or contraindicated for the given patient;

c. Patients have undergone careful screening, evaluation and diagnosis by a multidisciplinary team prior to implantation. (Such screening must include psychological, as well as physical evaluation);

d. All the facilities, equipment, and professional and support personnel required for the proper diagnosis, treatment training, and followup of the patient (including that required to satisfy item c must be available; and

e. Demonstration of pain relief with a temporarily implanted electrode precedes permanent implantation.

Contractors may find it helpful to work with PROs to obtain the information needed to apply these conditions to claims.

See Intermediary Manual, section 3110.4 and section 35-20 and 35-27.

65-9 INCONTINENCE CONTROL DEVICES

A. Mechanical/Hydraulic Incontinence Control Devices.—Mechanical/hydraulic incontinence control devices are accepted as safe and effective in the management of urinary incontinence in patients with permanent anatomic and neurologic dysfunctions of the bladder. This class of devices achieves control of urination by compression of the urethra. The materials used and the success rate may vary somewhat from device to device. Such a device is covered when its use is reasonable and necessary for the individual patient.

B. Collagen Implant.—A collagen implant, which is injected into the submucosal tissues of the urethra and/or the bladder neck and into tissues adjacent to the urethra, is a prosthetic device used in the treatment of stress urinary incontinence resulting from intrinsic sphincter deficiency (ISD). ISD is a cause of stress urinary incontinence in which the urethral sphincter is unable to contract and generate sufficient resistance in the bladder, especially during stress maneuvers.

Prior to collagen implant therapy, a skin test for collagen sensitivity must be administered and evaluated over a 4 week period.

In male patients, the evaluation must include a complete history and physical examination and a simple cystometrogram to determine that the bladder fills and stores properly. The patient then is asked to stand upright with a full bladder and to cough or otherwise exert abdominal pressure on his bladder. If the patient leaks, the diagnosis of ISD is established.

In female patients, the evaluation must include a complete history and physical examination (including a pelvic exam) and a simple cystometrogram to rule out abnormalities of bladder compliance and abnormalities of urethral support. Following that determination, an abdominal leak point pressure (ALLP) test is performed. Leak point pressure, stated in cm H2O, is defined as the intra-abdominal pressure at which leakage occurs from the bladder (around a catheter) when the bladder has been filled with a minimum of 150 cc fluid. If the patient has an ALLP of less than 100 cm H2O, the diagnosis of ISD is established.

To use a collagen implant, physicians must have urology training in the use of a cystoscope and must complete a collagen implant training program.

Coverage of a collagen implant, and the procedure to inject it, is limited to the following types of patients with stress urinary incontinence due to ISD:

- Male or female patients with congenital sphincter weakness secondary to conditions such as myelomeningocele or epispadias;
- Male or female patients with acquired sphincter weakness secondary to spinal cord lesions;
- Male patients following trauma, including prostatectomy and/or radiation; and
- Female patients without urethral hypermobility and with abdominal leak point pressures of 100 cm H2O or less.

Patients whose incontinence does not improve with 5 injection procedures (5 separate treatment sessions) are considered treatment failures, and no further treatment of urinary incontinence by collagen implant is covered. Patients who have a reoccurrence of incontinence following successful treatment with collagen implants in the past (e.g., 6 to 12 months previously) may benefit from additional treatment sessions. Coverage of additional sessions may be allowed but must be supported by medical justification.

See Intermediary Manual, §3110.4.

C. Non-Implantable Pelvic Floor Electrical Stimulator.—(See section 60-24)

65-10 ENTERAL AND PARENTERAL NUTRITIONAL THERAPY COVERED AS PROSTHETIC DEVICE

There are patients who, because of chronic illness or trauma, cannot be sustained through oral feeding. These people must rely on either enteral or parenteral nutritional therapy, depending upon the particular nature of their medical condition.

Coverage of nutritional therapy as a Part B benefit is provided under the prosthetic device benefit provision, which requires that the patient must have a permanently inoperative internal body organ or function thereof. (See Intermediary Manual, section 3110.4.) Therefore, enteral and parenteral nutritional therapy are not covered under Part B in situations involving temporary impairments. Coverage of such therapy, however, does not require a medical judgment that the impairment giving rise to the therapy will persist throughout the patient's remaining years. If the medical record, including the judgment of the attending physician, indicates that the impairment will be of long and indefinite duration, the test of permanence is considered met.

If the coverage requirements for enteral or parenteral nutritional therapy are met under the prosthetic device benefit provision, related supplies, equipment and nutrients are also covered under the conditions in the following paragraphs and Intermediary Manual, section 3110.4.

65-10.1 Parenteral Nutrition Therapy.—Daily parenteral nutrition is considered reasonable and necessary for a patient with severe pathology of the alimentary tract which does not allow absorption of sufficient nutrients to maintain weight and strength commensurate with the patient's general condition.

Since the alimentary tract of such a patient does not function adequately, an indwelling catheter is placed percutaneously in the subclavian vein and then advanced into the superior vena cava where intravenous infusion of nutrients is given for part of the day. The catheter is then plugged by the patient until the next infusion. Following a period of hospitalization, which is required to initiate parenteral nutrition and to train the patient in catheter care, solution preparation, and infusion technique, the parenteral nutrition can be provided safely and effectively in the patient's home by nonprofessional persons who have undergone special training. However, such persons cannot be paid for their services, nor is payment available for any services furnished by nonphysician professionals except as services furnished incident to a physician's service.

For parenteral nutrition therapy to be covered under Part B, the claim must contain a physician's written order or prescription and sufficient medical documentation to permit an independent conclusion that the requirements of the prosthetic device benefit are met and that parenteral nutrition therapy is medically necessary. An example of a condition that typically qualifies for coverage is a massive small bowel resection resulting in severe nutritional deficiency in spite of adequate oral intake. However, coverage of parenteral nutrition therapy for this and any other condition must be approved on an individual, case-by-case basis initially and at periodic intervals of no more than 3 months by the carrier's medical consultant or specially trained staff, relying on such medical and other documentation as the carrier may require. If the claim involves an infusion pump, sufficient evidence must be provided to support a determination of medical necessity for the pump. Program payment for the pump is based on the reasonable charge for the simplest model that meets the medical needs of the patient as established by medical documentation.

Nutrient solutions for parenteral therapy are routinely covered. However, Medicare pays for no more than one month's supply of nutrients at any one time. Payment for the nutrients is based on the reasonable charge for the solution components unless the medical record, including a signed statement from the attending physician, establishes that the beneficiary, due to his/her physical or mental state, is unable to safely or effectively mix the solution and there is no family member or other person who can do so. Payment will be on the basis of the reasonable charge for more expensive pre-mixed solutions only under the latter circumstances.

65-10.2 Enteral Nutrition Therapy.—Enteral nutrition is considered reasonable and necessary for a patient with a functioning gastrointestinal tract who, due to pathology to or nonfunction of the structures that normally permit food to reach the digestive tract, cannot maintain weight and strength commensurate with his or her general condition. Enteral therapy may be given by nasogastric, jejunostomy, or gastrostomy tubes and can be provided safely and effectively in the home by nonprofessional persons who have undergone special training. However, such persons cannot be paid for their services, nor is payment available for any services furnished by nonphysician professionals except as services furnished incident to a physician's service.

Typical examples of conditions that qualify for coverage are head and neck cancer with reconstructive surgery and central nervous system disease leading to interference with the neuromuscular mechanisms of ingestion of such severity that the beneficiary cannot be maintained with oral feeding. However, claims for Part B coverage of enteral nutrition therapy for these and any other conditions must be approved on an individual, case-by-case basis. Each claim must contain a physician's written order or prescription and sufficient medical documentation (e.g., hospital records, clinical findings from the attending physician) to permit an independent conclusion that the patient's condition meets the requirements of the prosthetic device benefit and that enteral nutrition therapy is medically necessary. Allowed claims are to be reviewed at periodic intervals of no more than 3 months by the contractor's medical consultant or specially trained staff, and additional medical documentation considered necessary is to be obtained as part of this review.

Medicare pays for no more than one month's supply of enteral nutrients at any one time.

If the claim involves a pump, it must be supported by sufficient medical documentation to establish that the pump is medically necessary, i.e., gravity feeding is not satisfactory due to aspiration, diarrhea, dumping syndrome. Program payment for the pump is based on the reasonable charge for the simplest model that meets the medical needs of the patient as established by medical documentation.

65-10.3 Nutritional Supplementation—Some patients require supplementation of their daily protein and caloric intake. Nutritional supplements are often given as a medicine between meals to boost protein-caloric intake or the mainstay of a daily nutritional plan. Nutritional supplementation is not covered under Medicare Part B.

65-11 BLADDER STIMULATORS (PACEMAKERS)—NOT COVERED

There are a number of devices available to induce emptying of the urinary bladder by using electrical current which forces the muscles of the bladder to contract. These devices (commonly known as bladder stimulators or pacemakers) are characterized by the implantation of electrodes in the wall of the bladder, the rectal cones, or the spinal cord. While these treatments may effectively empty the bladder, the issue of safety involving the initiation of infection, erosion, placement, and material selection has not been resolved. Further, some facilities previously using electronic emptying have stopped using this method due to the pain experienced by the patient.

The use of spinal cord electrical stimulators, rectal electrical stimulators, and bladder wall stimulators is not considered reasonable and necessary. Therefore, no program payment may be made for these devices or for their implantation.

65-14 COCHLEAR IMPLANTATION

A cochlear implant device is an electronic instrument, part of which is implanted surgically to stimulate auditory nerve fibers, and part of which is worn or carried by the individual to capture, analyze, and code sound. Cochlear implant devices are available in single channel and multi-channel models. The purpose of implanting the device is to provide an awareness and identification of sounds and to facilitate communication for persons who are profoundly hearing impaired.

Medicare coverage is provided only for those patients who meet all of the following selection guidelines.

A. General.—

- Diagnosis of bilateral severe-to-profound sensorineural hearing impairment with limited benefit from appropriate hearing (or vibrotactile) aids;
- Cognitive ability to use auditory clues and a willingness to undergo an extended program of rehabilitation;
- Freedom from middle ear infection, an accessible cochlear lumen that is structurally suited to implantation, and freedom from lesions in the auditory nerve and acoustic areas of the central nervous system;
- No contraindications to surgery; and
- The device must be used in accordance with the FDA-approved labeling.

B. Adults.—Cochlear implants may be covered for adults (over age 18) for prelinguistically, perilinguistically, and postlinguistically deafened adults. Postlinguistically deafened adults must demonstrate test scores of 30 percent or less on sentence recognition scores from tape recorded tests in the patient's best listening condition.

C. Children.—Cochlear implants may be covered for prelinguistically and postlinguistically deafened children aged 2 through 17. Bilateral profound sensorineural deafness must be demonstrated by the inability to improve on age appropriate closed-set word identification tasks with amplification.

65-16 TRACHEOSTOMY SPEAKING VALVE

A trachea tube has been determined to satisfy the definition of a prosthetic device, and the tracheostomy speaking valve is an add-on to the trachea tube which may be considered a medically necessary accessory that enhances the function of the tube. In other words, it makes the system a better prosthesis. As such, a tracheostomy speaking valve is covered as an element of the trachea tube which makes the tube more effective.

65-18 SACRAL NERVE STIMULATION FOR URINARY INCONTINENCE

Effective January 1, 2002, sacral nerve stimulation is covered for the treatment of urinary urge incontinence, urgency-frequency syndrome, and urinary retention. Sacral nerve stimulation involves both a temporary test stimulation to determine if an implantable stimulator would be effective and a permanent implantation in appropriate candidates. Both the test and the permanent implantation are covered.

The following limitations for coverage apply to all three indications:

(1) Patient must be refractory to conventional therapy (documented behavioral, pharmacologic and/or surgical corrective therapy) and be an appropriate surgical candidate such that implantation with anesthesia can occur.

(2) Patients with stress incontinence, urinary obstruction, and specific neurologic diseases (e.g., diabetes with peripheral nerve involvement) which are associated with secondary manifestation of the above three indications are excluded.

(3) Patient must have had a successful test stimulation in order to support subsequent implantation. Before a patient is eligibile for permanent implantation, he/she must demonstrate a 50% or greater improvement through test stimulation. Improvement is measured through voiding diaries.

(4) Patient must be able to demonstrate adequate ability to record voiding diary data such that clinical results of the implant procedure can be properly evaluated.

70 BRACES—TRUSSES—ARTIFICIAL LIMBS AND EYES

70-1 CORSET USED AS HERNIA SUPPORT

A hernia support (whether in the form of a corset or truss) which meets the definition of a brace is covered under Part B under section 1861(s)(9) of the Act.

See Intermediary Manual, section 3110.5; Medicare Carriers Manual, section 2133; and Hospital Manual, section 228.5.

70-2 SYKES HERNIA CONTROL

Based on professional advice, it has been determined that the Sykes hernia control (a spring-type, U-shaped, strapless truss) is not functionally more beneficial than a conventional truss. Make program reimbursement for this device only when an ordinary truss would be covered. (Like all trusses, it is only of benefit when dealing with a reducible hernia). Thus, when a charge for this item is substantially in excess of that which would be reasonable for a conventional truss used for the same condition, base reimbursement on the reasonable charges for the conventional truss.

See Intermediary Manual, section 3110.5; Medicare Carriers Manual, section 2133; and Hospital Manual, section 228.5.

UNIT THREE

HCPCS 2004 UPDATES

2004 HCPCS Updates are also available on the companion website at: http://evolve.elsevier.com/Buck/icd

DISCLAIMER

Every effort has been made to make this text complete and accurate, but no guarantee, warranty, or representation is made for its accuracy or completeness. It is based on the Centers for Medicare and Medicaid Services Healthcare Common Procedure Coding System (HCPCS).

2004 HCPCS NEW CODES

▶✻ KZ New coverage not implemented by managed care
▶◆ UF Services provided in the morning
▶◆ UG Services provided in the afternoon
▶◆ UH Services provided in the evening
▶◆ UJ Services provided at night
▶◆ UK Services provided on behalf of the client to someone other than the client (collateral relationship)
▶✻ UN Two patients served
▶✻ UP Three patients served
▶✻ UQ Four patients served
▶✻ UR Five patients served
▶✻ US Six or more patients served
▶✻ A0800 Ambulance transport provided between the hours of 7 pm and 7 am
▶❂ A4216 Sterile water/saline, 10 ml
MCM 2049
▶❂ A4217 Sterile water/saline, 500 ml
MCM 2049
▶✻ A4248 Chlorhexidine containing antiseptic, 1 ml
▶✻ A4366 Ostomy vent, any type, each
▶✻ A4416 Ostomy pouch, closed, with barrier attached, with filter (1 piece), each
▶✻ A4417 Ostomy pouch, closed, with barrier attached, with built-in convexity, with filter (1 piece), each
▶✻ A4418 Ostomy pouch, closed; without barrier attached, with filter (1 piece), each
▶✻ A4419 Ostomy pouch, closed; for use on barrier with non-locking flange, with filter (2 piece), each
▶✻ A4420 Ostomy pouch, closed; for use on barrier with locking flange (2 piece), each
▶✻ A4423 Ostomy pouch, closed; for use on barrier with locking flange, with filter (2 piece), each
▶✻ A4424 Ostomy pouch, drainable, with barrier attached, with filter (1 piece), each
▶✻ A4425 Ostomy pouch, drainable; for use on barrier with non-locking flange, with filter (2 piece system), each
▶✻ A4426 Ostomy pouch, drainable; for use on barrier with locking flange (2 piece system), each
▶✻ A4427 Ostomy pouch, drainable; for use on barrier with locking flange, with filter (2 piece system), each
▶✻ A4428 Ostomy pouch, urinary, with extended wear barrier attached, with faucet-type tap with valve (1 piece), each
▶✻ A4429 Ostomy pouch, urinary, with barrier attached, with built-in convexity, with faucet-type tap with valve (1 piece), each
▶✻ A4430 Ostomy pouch, urinary, with extended wear barrier attached, with built-in convexity, with faucet-type tap with valve (1 piece), each
▶✻ A4431 Ostomy pouch, urinary; with barrier attached, with faucet-type tap with valve (1 piece), each
▶✻ A4432 Ostomy pouch, urinary; for use on barrier with non-locking flange, with faucet-type tap with valve (2 piece), each
▶✻ A4433 Ostomy pouch, urinary; for use on barrier with locking flange (2 piece), each
▶✻ A4434 Ostomy pouch, urinary; for use on barrier with locking flange, with faucet-type tap with valve (2 piece), each
▶✻ A4638 Replacement battery for patient-owned ear pulse generator, each
▶❂ A4671 Disposable cycler set used with cycler dialysis machine, each
MCM 4270
▶❂ A4672 Drainage extension line, sterile, for dialysis, each
MCM 4270
▶❂ A4673 Extension line with easy lock connectors, used with dialysis
MCM 4270
▶❂ A4674 Chemicals/antiseptics solution used to clean/sterilize dialysis equipment, per 8 oz
MCM 4270
▶✻ A4728 Dialysate solution, non-dextrose containing, 500 ml
▶✻ A6407 Packing strips, non-impregnated, up to 2 inches in width, per linear yard
▶✻ A6441 Padding bandage, non-elastic, non-woven/non-knitted, width greater than or equal to three inches and less than five inches, per yard
▶✻ A6442 Conforming bandage, non-elastic, knitted/woven, non-sterile, width less than three inches, per yard
▶✻ A6443 Conforming bandage, non-elastic, knitted/woven, non-sterile, width greater than or equal to three inches and less than five inches, per yard
▶✻ A6444 Conforming bandage, non-elastic, knitted/woven, non-sterile, width greater than or equal to 5 inches, per yard
▶✻ A6445 Conforming bandage, non-elastic, knitted/woven, sterile, width less than three inches, per yard
▶✻ A6446 Conforming bandage, non-elastic, knitted/woven, sterile, width greater than or equal to three inches and less than five inches, per yard
▶✻ A6447 Conforming bandage, non-elastic, knitted/woven, sterile, width greater than or equal to five inches, per yard
▶✻ A6448 Light compression bandage, elastic, knitted/woven, width less than three inches, per yard

▶✻ A6449 Light compression bandage, elastic, knitted/woven, width greater than or equal to three inches and less than five inches, per yard

▶✻ A6450 Light compression bandage, elastic, knitted/woven, width greater than or equal to five inches, per yard

▶✻ A6451 Moderate compression bandage, elastic, knitted/woven, load resistance of 1.25 to 1.34 foot pounds at 50% maximum stretch, width greater than or equal to three inches and less than five inches, per yard

▶ A6452 High compression bandage, elastic, knitted/woven, load resistance greater than or equal to 1.35 foot pounds at 50% maximum stretch, width greater than or equal to three inches and less than five inches, per yard

▶✻ A6453 Self-adherent bandage, elastic, non-knitted/non-woven, width less than three inches, per yard

▶✻ A6454 Self-adherent bandage, elastic, non-knitted/non-woven, width greater than or equal to three inches and less than five inches, per yard

▶✻ A6455 Self-adherent bandage, elastic, non-knitted/non-woven, width greater than or equal to five inches, per yard

▶✻ A6456 Zinc paste impregnated bandage, non-elastic, knitted/woven, width greater than or equal to three inches and less than five inches, per yard

▶✻ A6550 Dressing set for negative pressure wound therapy electrical pump, stationary or portable, each

▶✻ A6551 Canister set for negative pressure wound therapy electrical pump, stationary or portable, each

▶✪ A7046 Water chamber for humidifier, used with positive airway pressure device, replacement, each
CIM 60-17

▶✻ A7520 Tracheostomy/laryngectomy tube, non-cuffed, polyvinylchloride (PVC), silicone or equal, each

▶✻ A7521 Tracheostomy/laryngectomy tube, cuffed, polyvinylchloride (PVC), silicone or equal, each

▶✻ A7522 Tracheostomy/laryngectomy tube, stainless steel or equal (sterilizable and reusable), each

▶✻ A7523 Tracheostomy shower protector, each

▶✻ A7524 Tracheostoma stent/stud/button, each

▶✻ A7525 Tracheostomy mask, each

▶✻ A7526 Tracheostomy tube collar/holder, each

▶◆ A9280 Alert or alarm device, not otherwise classified
Medicare Statute 1861

▶✪ A9525 Supply of low or ISO-osmolar contrast material, 10 mg of iodine
MCM 15022, MCM 15-30

▶✪ A9526 Supply of radiopharmaceutical diagnostic imaging agent, ammonia N-13, per dose
CIM 50-36

▶✻ A9528 Supply of radiopharmaceutical diagnostic agent, I-131 sodium iodide capsule, per millicurie

▶✻ A9529 Supply of radiopharmaceutical diagnostic agent, I-131 sodium iodide solution, per millicurie

▶✻ A9530 Supply of radiopharmaceutical therapeutic agent, I-131 sodium iodide solution, per millicurie

▶✻ A9531 Supply of radiopharmaceutical diagnostic agent, I-131 sodium iodide, per microcurie (up to 100 microcuries)

▶✻ A9532 Supply of radiopharmaceutical therapeutic agent, iodinated I-125, serum albumin, 5 microcuries

▶✻ A9533 Supply of radiopharmaceutical diagnostic imaging agent, I-131 tositumomab, per millicurie

▶✻ A9534 Supply of radiopharmaceutical therapeutic imaging agent, I-131 tositumomab, per millicurie

▶✻ A9999 Miscellaneous DME supply or accessory, not otherwise specified

▶✪ C1814 Retinal tamponade device, silicone oil
Medicare Statute 1833(t)

▶✪ C1818 Integrated keratoprosthesis
Medicare Statute 1833(t)

▶✪ C1884 Embolization protective system
Medicare Statute 1833(t)

▶✪ C8918 Magnetic resonance angiography with contrast, pelvis
Medicare Statute 430 BIPA

▶✪ C8919 Magnetic resonance angiography without contrast, pelvis
Medicare Statute 430 BIPA

▶✪ C8920 Magnetic resonance angiography without contrast followed by with contrast, pelvis
Medicare Statute 430 BIPA

▶✪ C9123 Transcyte, per 247 square centimeters
Medicare Statute 1833(t)

▶✪ C9202 Injection, suspension of microspheres of human serum albumin with octafluoropropane, per 3 ml
Medicare Statute 1833(t)

▶✪ C9203 Injection, perflexane lipid microspheres, per 10 ml vial
Medicare Statute 1833(t)

▶✪ C9208 Injection, agalsidase beta, per 1 mg
Medicare Statute 1833(t)

▶✪ C9209 Injection, laronidase, per 2.9 mg
Medicare Statute 1833(t)

▶◆ E0118 Crutch substitute, lower leg platform, with or without wheels, each

▶✪ E0140 Walker, with trunk support, adjustable or fixed height, any type
MCM 2100.1, CIM 60-9

▶◆ E0190 Positioning cushion/pillow/wedge, any shape or size

▶◆ E0240 Bath/shower chair, with or without wheels, any size
CIM 60-9

▶◆ E0247 Transfer bench for tub or toilet with or without commode opening

▶◆ E0248 Transfer bench, heavy duty, for tub or toilet with or without commode opening

▶* E0300 Pediatric crib, hospital grade, fully enclosed

▶✪ E0301 Hospital bed, heavy duty, extra wide, with weight capacity greater than 350 pounds, but less than or equal to 600 pounds, with any type side rails, without mattress
CIM 60-18

▶✪ E0302 Hospital bed, extra heavy duty, extra wide, with weight capacity greater than 600 pounds, with any type side rails, without mattress
CIM 60-18

▶✪ E0303 Hospital bed, heavy duty, extra wide, with weight capacity greater than 350 pounds, but less than or equal to 600 pounds, with any type side rails, with mattress
CIM 60-18

▶✪ E0304 Hospital bed, extra heavy duty, extra wide, with weight capacity greater than 600 pounds, with any type side rails, with mattress
CIM 60-18

▶✪ E0470 Respiratory assist device, bi-level pressure capability, without backup rate feature, used with noninvasive interface, e.g., nasal or facial mask (intermittent assist device with continuous positive airway pressure device)
CIM 60-9

▶✪ E0471 Respiratory assist device, bi-level pressure capability, with back-up rate feature, used with noninvasive interface, e.g., nasal or facial mask (intermittent assist device with continuous positive airway pressure device)
CIM 60-9

▶✪ E0472 Respiratory assist device, bi-level pressure capability, with backup rate feature, used with invasive interface, e.g., tracheostomy tube (intermittent assist device with continuous positive airway pressure device)
CIM 60-9

▶* E0561 Humidifier, non-heated, used with positive airway pressure device

▶* E0562 Humidifier, heated, used with positive airway pressure device

▶* E0637 Combination sit to stand system, any size, with seat lift feature, with or without wheels

▶* E0638 Standing frame system, any size, with or without wheels

▶* E0675 Pneumatic compression device, high pressure, rapid inflation/deflation cycle, for arterial insufficiency (unilateral or bilateral system)

▶* E0955 Wheelchair accessory, headrest, cushioned, prefabricated, including fixed mounting hardware, each

▶* E0956 Wheelchair accessory, lateral trunk or hip support, prefabricated, including fixed mounting hardware, each

▶* E0957 Wheelchair accessory, medial thigh support, prefabricated, including fixed mounting hardware, each

▶* E0960 Wheelchair accessory, shoulder harness/straps or chest strap, including any type mounting hardware

▶* E0981 Wheelchair accessory, seat upholstery, replacement only, each

▶* E0982 Wheelchair accessory, back upholstery, replacement only, each

▶* E0983 Manual wheelchair accessory, power add-on to convert manual wheelchair to motorized wheelchair, joystick control

▶* E0984 Manual wheelchair accessory, power add-on to convert manual wheelchair to motorized wheelchair, tiller control

▶* E0985 Wheelchair accessory, seat lift mechanism

▶* E0986 Manual wheelchair accessory, push-rim activated power assist, each

▶* E1002 Wheelchair accessory, power seating system, tilt only

▶* E1003 Wheelchair accessory, power seating system, recline only, without shear reduction

▶* E1004 Wheelchair accessory, power seating system, recline only, with mechanical shear reduction

▶* E1005 Wheelchair accessory, power seating system, recline only, with power shear reduction

▶* E1006 Wheelchair accessory, power seating system, combination tilt and recline, without shear reduction

▶* E1007 Wheelchair accessory, power seating system, combination tilt and recline, with mechanical shear reduction

▶* E1008 Wheelchair accessory, power seating system, combination tilt and recline, with power shear reduction

▶* E1009 Wheelchair accessory, addition to power seating system, mechanically linked leg elevation system, including pushrod and leg rest, each

▶✻ E1010 Wheelchair accessory, addition to power seating system, power leg elevation system, including leg rest, each

▶✻ E1019 Wheelchair accessory, power seating system, heavy duty feature, patient weight capacity greater than 250 pounds and less than or equal to 400 pounds

▶✻ E1021 Wheelchair accessory, power seating system, extra heavy duty feature, weight capacity greater than 400 pounds

▶✻ E1028 Wheelchair accessory, manual swing away, retractable or removable mounting hardware for joystick, other control interface or positioning accessory

▶✻ E1029 Wheelchair accessory, ventilator tray, fixed

▶✻ E1030 Wheelchair accessory, ventilator tray, gimbaled

▶✪ E1391 Oxygen concentrator, dual delivery port, capable of delivering 85 percent or greater oxygen concentration at the prescribed flow rate, each
CIM 60-4

▶✪ E1634 Peritoneal dialysis clamps, each
MCM 4270

▶✻ E2120 Pulse generator system for tympanic treatment of inner ear endolymphatic fluid

▶✻ E2201 Manual wheelchair accessory, nonstandard seat frame, width greater than or equal to 20 inches and less than 24 inches

▶✻ E2202 Manual wheelchair accessory, nonstandard seat frame width, 24-27 inches

▶✻ E2203 Manual wheelchair accessory, nonstandard seat frame depth, 20 to less than 22 inches

▶✻ E2204 Manual wheelchair accessory, nonstandard seat frame depth, 22 to 25 inches

▶✻ E2300 Power wheelchair accessory, power seat elevation system

▶✻ E2301 Power wheelchair accessory, power standing system

▶✻ E2310 Power wheelchair accessory, electronic connection between wheelchair controller and one power seating system motor, including all related electronics, indicator feature, mechanical function selection switch, and fixed mounting hardware

▶✻ E2311 Power wheelchair accessory, electronic connection between wheelchair controller and two or more power seating system motors, including all related electronics, indicator feature, mechanical function selection switch, and fixed mounting hardware

▶✻ E2320 Power wheelchair accessory, hand or chin control interface, remote joystick or touchpad, proportional, including all related electronics, and fixed mounting hardware

▶✻ E2321 Power wheelchair accessory, hand control interface, remote joystick, nonproportional, including all related electronics, mechanical stop switch, and fixed mounting hardware

▶✻ E2322 Power wheelchair accessory, hand control interface, multiple mechanical switches, nonproportional, including all related electronics, mechanical stop switch, and fixed mounting hardware

▶✻ E2323 Power wheelchair accessory, specialty joystick handle for hand control interface, prefabricated

▶✻ E2324 Power wheelchair accessory, chin cup for chin control interface

▶✻ E2325 Power wheelchair accessory, sip and puff interface, nonproportional, including all related electronics, mechanical stop switch, and manual swingaway mounting hardware

▶✻ E2326 Power wheelchair accessory, breath tube kit for sip and puff interface

▶✻ E2327 Power wheelchair accessory, head control interface, mechanical, proportional, including all related electronics, mechanical direction change switch, and fixed mounting hardware

▶✻ E2328 Power wheelchair accessory, head control or extremity control interface, electronic, proportional, including all related electronics and fixed mounting hardware

▶✻ E2329 Power wheelchair accessory, head control interface, contact switch mechanism, nonproportional, including all related electronics, mechanical stop switch, mechanical direction change switch, head array, and fixed mounting hardware

▶✻ E2330 Power wheelchair accessory, head control interface, proximity switch mechanism, nonproportional, including all related electronics, mechanical stop switch, mechanical direction change switch, head array, and fixed mounting hardware

▶✻ E2331 Power wheelchair accessory, attendant control, proportional, including all related electronics and fixed mounting hardware

▶✻ E2340 Power wheelchair accessory, nonstandard seat frame width, 20-23 inches

▶✻ E2341 Power wheelchair accessory, nonstandard seat frame width, 24-27 inches

▶✻ E2342 Power wheelchair accessory, nonstandard seat frame depth, 20 or 21 inches

▶✻ E2343 Power wheelchair accessory, nonstandard seat frame depth, 22-25 inches

▶✻ E2351 Power wheelchair accessory, electronic interface to operate speech generating device using power wheelchair control interface

▶✻ E2360 Power wheelchair accessory, 22 NF non-sealed lead acid battery, each

▶✻ E2361 Power wheelchair accessory, 22 NF sealed lead acid battery, each, (e.g., gel cell, absorbed glassmat)

▶✻ E2362 Power wheelchair accessory, Group 24 non-sealed lead acid battery, each

▶✻ E2363 Power wheelchair accessory, Group 24 sealed lead acid battery, each (e.g., gel cell, absorbed glassmat)

▶✻ E2364 Power wheelchair accessory, U-1 non-sealed lead acid battery, each

▶✻ E2365 Power wheelchair accessory, U-1 sealed lead acid battery, each (e.g. gel cell, absorbed glassmat)

▶✻ E2366 Power wheelchair accessory, battery charger, single mode, for use with only one battery type, sealed or non-sealed, each

▶✻ E2367 Power wheelchair accessory, battery charger, dual mode, for use with either battery type, sealed or non-sealed, each

▶✻ E2399 Power wheelchair accessory, not otherwise classified interface, including all related electronics and any type mounting hardware

▶✻ E2402 Negative pressure wound therapy electrical pump, stationary or portable

▶❂ E2500 Speech generating device, digitized speech, using pre-recorded messages, less than or equal to 8 minutes recording time
CIM 60-23

▶❂ E2502 Speech generating device, digitized speech, using pre-recorded messages, greater than 8 minutes but less than or equal to 20 minutes recording time
CIM 60-23

▶❂ E2504 Speech generating device, digitized speech, using pre-recorded messages, greater than 20 minutes but less than or equal to 40 minutes recording time
CIM 60-23

▶❂ E2506 Speech generating device, digitized speech, using pre-recorded messages, greater than 40 minutes recording time
CIM 60-23

▶❂ E2508 Speech generating device, synthesized speech, requiring message formulation by spelling and access by physical contact with the device
CIM 60-23

▶❂ E2510 Speech generating device, synthesized speech, permitting multiple methods of message formulation and multiple methods of device access
CIM 60-23

▶❂ E2511 Speech generating software program, for personal computer or personal digital assistant
CIM 60-23

▶❂ E2512 Accessory for speech generating device, mounting system
CIM 60-23

▶❂ E2599 Accessory for speech generating device, not otherwise classified
CIM 60-23

▶✻ G0296 Pet imaging, full and partial ring pet scanner only, for restaging of previously treated thyroid cancer of follicular cell origin following negative I-131 whole body scan

▶✻ G0297 Insertion of single chamber pacing cardioverter defibrillator pulse generator

▶✻ G0298 Insertion of dual chamber pacing cardioverter defibrillator pulse generator

▶✻ G0299 Insertion or repositioning of electrode lead for single chamber pacing cardioverter defibrillator and insertion of pulse generator

▶✻ G0300 Insertion or repositioning of electrode lead(s) for dual chamber pacing cardioverter defibrillator and insertion of pulse generator

▶✻ G0302 Pre-operative pulmonary surgery services for preparation for LVRS, complete course of services, to include a minimum of 16 days of services

▶✻ G0303 Pre-operative pulmonary surgery services for preparation for LVRS, 10 to 15 days of services

▶✻ G0304 Pre-operative pulmonary surgery services for preparation for LVRS, 1 to 9 days of services

▶✻ G0305 Post-discharge pulmonary surgery services after LVRS, minimum of 6 days of services

▶✻ G0306 Complete CBC, automated (HGB, HCT, RBC, WBC, without platelet count) and automated WBC differential count
Laboratory Certification 400

▶✻ G0307 Complete (CBC), automated (HGB, HCT, RBC, WBC; without platelet count)
Laboratory Certification 400

▶✻ G3001 Administration and supply of TO situmomab, 450 mg

▶◆ H2010 Comprehensive medication services, per 15 minutes

▶◆ H2011 Crisis intervention service, per 15 minutes

▶◆ H2012 Behavioral health day treatment, per hour
▶◆ H2013 Psychiatric health facility service, per diem
▶◆ H2014 Skills training and development, per 15 minutes
▶◆ H2015 Comprehensive community support services, per 15 minutes
▶◆ H2016 Comprehensive community support services, per diem
▶◆ H2017 Psychosocial rehabilitation services, per 15 minutes
▶◆ H2018 Psychosocial rehabilitation services, per diem
▶◆ H2019 Therapeutic behavioral services, per 15 minutes
▶◆ H2020 Therapeutic behavioral services, per diem
▶◆ H2021 Community-based wrap-around services, per 15 minutes
▶◆ H2022 Community-based wrap-around services, per diem
▶◆ H2023 Supported employment, per 15 minutes
▶◆ H2024 Supported employment, per diem
▶◆ H2025 Ongoing support to maintain employment, per 15 minutes
▶◆ H2026 Ongoing support to maintain employment, per diem
▶◆ H2027 Psychoeducational service, per 15 minutes
▶◆ H2028 Sexual offender treatment service, per 15 minutes
▶◆ H2029 Sexual offender treatment service, per diem
▶◆ H2030 Mental health clubhouse services, per 15 minutes
▶◆ H2031 Mental health clubhouse services, per diem
▶◆ H2032 Activity therapy, per 15 minutes
▶◆ H2033 Multisystemic therapy for juveniles, per 15 minutes
▶◆ H2034 Alcohol and/or drug abuse halfway house services, per diem
▶◆ H2035 Alcohol and/or other drug treatment program, per hour
▶◆ H2036 Alcohol and/or other drug treatment program, per diem
▶◆ H2037 Developmental delay prevention activities, dependent child of client, per 15 minutes
▶✻ J0152 Injection, adenosine, 30 mg (not to be used to report any adenosine phosphate compounds; instead use A9270)
▶✻ J0215 Injection, alefacept, 0.5 mg
▶✻ J0583 Injection, bivalirudin, 1 mg
▶✻ J0595 Injection, butorphanol tartrate, 1 mg
▶✻ J1335 Injection, ertapenem sodium, 500 mg
▶✪ J1595 Injection, glatiramer acetate, 20 mg
MCM 2049
▶✪ J2001 Injection, lidocaine hcl for intravenous infusion, 10 mg
MCM 2049
▶✻ J2185 Injection, meropenem, 100 mg
▶✻ J2280 Injection, moxifloxacin, 100 mg
▶✻ J2353 Injection, octreotide, depot form for intramuscular injection, 1 mg
▶✻ J2354 Injection, octreotide, non-depot form for subcutaneous or intravenous injection, 25 mcg
▶✻ J2505 Injection, pegfilgrastim, 6 mg
▶✻ J2783 Injection, rasburicase, 0.5 mg
▶✻ J3411 Injection, thiamine HCL, 100 mg
▶✻ J3415 Injection, pyridoxine HCL, 100 mg
▶✪ J3465 Injection, voriconazole, 10 mg
MCM 2049
▶✻ J3486 Injection, ziprasidone mesylate, 10 mg
▶◆ J7303 Contraceptive supply, hormone containing vaginal ring, each
Medicare Statute 1862.1
▶✻ J7621 Albuterol, all formulations, including separated isomers, up to 5 mg (albuterol) or 2.5 mg (levoalbuterol), and ipratropium bromide, up to 1 mg, compounded inhalation solution, administered through DME
▶✻ J9098 Cytarabine liposome, 10 mg
▶✻ J9178 Injection, epirubicin HCL, 2 mg
▶✻ J9263 Injection, oxaliplatin, 0.5 mg
▶✻ J9395 Injection, fulvestrant, 25 mg
▶✪ K0552 Supplies for external drug infusion pump, syringe type cartridge, sterile, each
CIM 60-14
▶✻ K0601 Replacement battery for external infusion pump owned by patient, silver oxide, 1.5 volt, each
▶✻ K0602 Replacement battery for external infusion pump owned by patient, silver oxide, 3 volt, each
▶✻ K0603 Replacement battery for external infusion pump owned by patient, alkaline, 1.5 volt, each
▶✻ K0604 Replacement battery for external infusion pump owned by patient, lithium, 3.6 volt, each
▶✻ K0605 Replacement battery for external infusion pump owned by patient, lithium, 4.5 volt, each
▶✻ K0606 Automatic external defibrillator, with integrated electrocardiogram analysis, garment type
▶✻ K0607 Replacement battery for automated external defibrillator, garment type only, each
▶✻ K0608 Replacement garment for use with automated external defibrillator, each
▶✻ K0609 Replacement electrodes for use with automated external defibrillator, garment type only, each

▶✻ K0618 TLSO, sagittal-coronal control, modular segmented spinal system, two rigid plastic shells, posterior extends from the sacrococcygeal junction and terminates just inferior to the scapular spine, anterior extends from the symphysis pubis to the xiphoid, soft liner, restricts gross trunk motion in the sagittal and coronal planes, lateral strength is provided by overlapping plastic and stabilizing closures, includes straps and closures, prefabricated, includes fitting and adjustment

▶✻ K0619 TLSO, sagittal-coronal control, modular segmented spinal system, three rigid plastic shells, posterior extends from the sacrococcygeal junction and terminates just inferior to the scapular spine, anterior extends from the symphysis pubis to the xiphoid, soft liner, restricts gross trunk motion in the sagittal and coronal planes, lateral strength is provided by overlapping plastic and stabilizing closures, includes straps and closures, prefabricated, includes fitting and adjustment

▶✻ K0620 Tubular elastic dressing, any width, per linear yard

▶✻ L0112 Cranial cervical orthosis, congenital torticollis type, with or without soft interface material, adjustable range of motion joint, custom fabricated

▶✻ L0861 Addition to halo procedure, replacement liner/interface material

▶✻ L1831 Knee orthosis, locking knee joint(s), positional orthosis, prefabricated, includes fitting and adjustment

▶✻ L1907 AFO, supramalleolar with straps, with or without interface/pads, custom fabricated

▶✻ L1951 Ankle foot orthosis, spiral, (institute of rehabilitative medicine type), plastic or other material, prefabricated, includes fitting and adjustment

▶✻ L1971 Ankle foot orthosis, plastic or other material with ankle joint, prefabricated, includes fitting and adjustment

▶◆ L3031 Foot, insert/plate, removable, addition to lower extremity orthosis, high strength, lightweight material, all hybrid lamination/prepreg composite, each

▶✻ L3917 Hand orthosis, metacarpal fracture orthosis, prefabricated, includes fitting and adjustment

▶✻ L5673 Addition to lower extremity, below knee/above knee, custom fabricated from existing mold or prefabricated, socket insert, silicone gel, elastomeric or equal, for use with locking mechanism

▶✻ L5679 Addition to lower extremity, below knee/above knee, custom fabricated from existing mold or prefabricated, socket insert, silicone gel, elastomeric or equal, not for use with locking mechanism

▶✻ L5681 Addition to lower extremity, below knee/above knee, custom fabricated socket insert for congenital or atypical traumatic amputee, silicone gel, elastomeric or equal, for use with or without locking mechanism, initial only (for other than initial, use code l5673 or l5679)

▶✻ L5683 Addition to lower extremity, below knee/above knee, custom fabricated socket insert for other than congenital or atypical traumatic amputee, silicone gel, elastomeric or equal, for use with or without locking mechanism, initial only (for other than initial, use code l5673 or l5679)

▶✻ L8511 Insert for indwelling tracheoesophageal prosthesis, with or without valve, replacement only, each

▶✻ L8512 Gelatin capsules or equivalent, for use with tracheoesophageal voice prosthesis, replacement only, per 10

▶✻ L8513 Cleaning device used with tracheoesophageal voice prosthesis, pipet, brush, or equal, replacement only, each

▶✻ L8514 Tracheoesophageal puncture dilator, replacement only, each

▶✪ L8631 Metacarpal phalangeal joint replacement, two or more pieces, metal (e.g., stainless steel or cobalt chrome), ceramic-like material (e.g., pyrocarbon), for surgical implantation (all sizes, includes entire system)
MCM 2130

▶✪ L8659 Interphalangeal finger joint replacement, 2 or more pieces, metal (e.g., stainless steel or cobalt chrome), ceramic-like material (e.g., pyrocarbon) for surgical implantation, any size
MCM 2130

▶✪ P9051 Whole blood or red blood cells, leukocytes reduced, CMV-negative, each unit
Medicare Statute 1833(t)

▶✪ P9052 Platelets, HLA-matched leukocytes reduced, apheresis/pheresis, each unit
Medicare Statute 1833(t)

▶✪ P9053 Platelets, pheresis, leukocytes reduced, CMV-negative, irradiated, each unit
Medicare Statute 1833(t)

▶✪ P9054 Whole blood or red blood cells, leukocytes reduced, frozen, deglycerol, washed, each unit
Medicare Statute 1833(t)

▶⚙ P9055 Platelets, leukocytes reduced, CMV-negative, apheresis/pheresis, each unit
Medicare Statute 1833(t)

▶⚙ P9056 Whole blood, leukocytes reduced, irradiated, each unit
Medicare Statute 1833(t)

▶⚙ P9057 Red blood cells, frozen/deglycerolized/washed, leukocytes reduced, irradiated, each unit
Medicare Statute 1833(t)

▶⚙ P9058 Red blood cells, leukocytes reduced, CMV-negative, irradiated, each unit
Medicare Statute 1833(t)

▶⚙ P9059 Fresh frozen plasma between 8-24 hours of collection, each unit
Medicare Statute 1833(t)

▶⚙ P9060 Fresh frozen plasma, donor retested, each unit
Medicare Statute 1833(t)

▶⚙ Q0137 Injection, darbepoetin alfa, 1 mcg (non-ESRD use)
MCM 4273.1

▶* Q0182 Dermal and epidermal, tissue of non-human origin, with or without other bioengineered or processed elements, without metabolically active elements, per square centimeter

▶⚙ Q3031 Collagen skin test
CIM 65-9

▶⚙ Q4054 Injection, darbepoetin alfa, 1 mcg (for ESRD on dialysis)
MCM 4273.1

▶⚙ Q4055 Injection, epoetin alfa, 1000 units (for ESRD on dialysis)
MCM 4273.1

▶* Q4075 Injection, acyclovir, 5 mg

▶* Q4076 Injection, dopamine HCL, 40 mg

▶* Q4077 Injection, treprostinil, 1 mg

▶◆ S0107 Injection, omalizumab, 25 mg

▶◆ S0115 Bortezomib, 3.5 mg

▶◆ S0136 Clozapine, 25 mg

▶◆ S0137 Didanosine (DDI), 25 mg

▶◆ S0138 Finasteride, 5 mg

▶◆ S0139 Minoxidil, 10 mg

▶◆ S0140 Saquinavir, 200 mg

▶◆ S0141 Zalcitabine (DDC), 0.375 mg

▶◆ S0317 Disease management program; per diem

▶◆ S2070 Cystourethroscopy, with ureteroscopy and/or pyeloscopy; with endoscopic laser treatment of ureteral calculi (includes ureteral catheterization)

▶◆ S2085 Laparoscopy, gastric restrictive procedure, with gastric bypass for morbid obesity, with short limb (less than 100 cm) roux-en-y gastroenterostomy

▶◆ S2090 Ablation, open, one or more renal tumor(s); cryosurgical

▶◆ S2091 Ablation, percutaneous, one or more renal tumor(s); cryosurgical

▶◆ S2095 Transcatheter occlusion or embolization for tumor destruction, percutaneous, any method, using yttrium-90 microspheres

▶◆ S2113 Arthroscopy, knee, surgical for implantation of cultured analogous chondrocytes

▶◆ S2135 Neurolysis, by injection, of metatarsal neuroma/interdigital neuritis, any interspace of the foot

▶◆ S2213 Implantation of gastric electrical stimulation device

▶◆ S2225 Myringotomy, laser-assisted

▶◆ S2230 Implantation of magnetic component of semi-implantable hearing device on ossicles in middle ear

▶◆ S2235 Implantation of auditory brain stem implant

▶◆ S2362 Kyphoplasty, one vertebral body, unilateral or bilateral injection

▶◆ S2363 Kyphoplasty, one vertebral body, unilateral or bilateral injection; each additional vertebral body (list separately in addition to code for primary procedure)

▶◆ S3000 Diabetic indicator; retinal eye exam, dilated, bilateral

▶◆ S3625 Maternal serum triple marker screen including alpha-fetoprotein (AFP), estriol, and human chorionic gonadotropin (HCG)

▶◆ S3820 Complete BRAL1 and BRCA2 gene sequence analysis for susceptibility to breast and ovarian cancer

▶◆ S3822 Single mutation analysis (in individual with a known BRCA1 or BRCA2 mutation in the family) for susceptibility to breast and ovarian cancer

▶◆ S3823 Three-mutation BRCA1 and BRCA2 analysis for susceptibility to breast and ovarian cancer in Ashkenazi individuals

▶◆ S3828 Complete gene sequence analysis; MLH1 gene

▶◆ S3829 Complete gene sequence analysis; MLH2 gene

▶◆ S3833 Complete APC gene sequence analysis for susceptibility to familial adenomatous polyposis (FAP) and attenuated FAP

▶◆ S3834 Single-mutation analysis (in individual with a known APC mutation in the family) for susceptibility to familial adenomatous polyposis (FAP) and attenuated FAP

▶◆ S3840 DNA analysis for germline mutations of the ret proto-oncogene for susceptibility to multiple endocrine neoplasia type 2

▶◆ S3841 Genetic testing for retinoblastoma

▶◆ S3842 Genetic testing for von Hippel-Lindau disease
▶◆ S3843 DNA analysis of the F5 gene for susceptibility to Factor V leiden thrombophilia
▶◆ S3844 DNA analysis of the connexin 26 gene (GJB2) for susceptibility to congenital, profound deafness
▶◆ S3845 Genetic testing for alpha-thalassemia
▶◆ S3846 Genetic testing for hemoglobin e beta-thalassemia
▶◆ S3847 Genetic testing for Tay-Sachs disease
▶◆ S3848 Genetic testing for Gaucher disease
▶◆ S3849 Genetic testing for Niemann-Pick disease
▶◆ S3850 Genetic testing for sickle cell anemia
▶◆ S3851 Genetic testing for Canavan disease
▶◆ S3852 DNA analysis for apoe epilson 4 Allele for susceptibility to Alzheimer's disease
▶◆ S3853 Genetic testing for myotonic muscular dystrophy
▶◆ S5108 Home care training to home care client, per 15 minutes
▶◆ S5109 Home care training to home care client, per session
▶◆ S5550 Insulin, rapid onset, 5 units
▶◆ S5551 Insulin, most rapid onset (LISPRO or ASPART); 5 units
▶◆ S5552 Insulin, intermediate acting (NPH or LENTE); 5 units
▶◆ S5553 Insulin, long acting; 5 units
▶◆ S5560 Insulin delivery device, reusable pen; 1.5 ml size
▶◆ S5561 Insulin delivery device, reusable pen; 3 ml size
▶◆ S5565 Insulin cartridge for use in insulin delivery device other than pump; 150 units
▶◆ S5566 Insulin cartridge for use in insulin delivery device other than pump; 300 units
▶◆ S5570 Insulin delivery device, disposable pen (including insulin); 1.5 ml size
▶◆ S5571 Insulin delivery device, disposable pen (including insulin); 3 ml size
▶◆ S8075 Computer analysis of full-field digital mammogram and further physician review for interpretation, mammography (list separately in addition to code for primary procedure)
▶◆ S8120 Oxygen contents, gaseous, 1 unit equals 1 cubic foot
▶◆ S8121 Oxygen contents, liquid, 1 unit equals 1 pound
▶◆ S8460 Camisole, post-mastectomy
▶◆ S8948 Application of a modality (requiring constant provider attendance) to one or more areas; low-level laser; each 15 minutes
▶◆ S8990 Physical or manipulative therapy performed for maintenance rather than restoration
▶◆ S9335 Home therapy, hemodialysis; administrative services, professional pharmacy services, care coordination, and all necessary supplies and equipment (drugs and nursing services coded separately), per diem
▶◆ S9434 Modified solid food supplements for inborn errors of metabolism
▶◆ S9476 Vestibular rehabilitation program, non-physician provider, per diem
▶◆ T2010 Preadmission screening and resident review (PASRR) level I identification screening, per screen
▶◆ T2011 Preadmission screening and resident review (PASRR) level II evaluation, per evaluation
▶◆ T2012 Habilitation, educational; waiver, per diem
▶◆ T2013 Habilitation, educational, waiver; per hour
▶◆ T2014 Habilitation, prevocational, waiver; per diem
▶◆ T2015 Habilitation, prevocational, waiver; per hour
▶◆ T2016 Habilitation, residential, waiver; per diem
▶◆ T2017 Habilitation, residential, waiver; 15 minutes
▶◆ T2018 Habilitation, supported employment, waiver; per diem
▶◆ T2019 Habilitation, supported employment, waiver; per 15 minutes
▶◆ T2020 Day habilitation, waiver; per diem
▶◆ T2021 Day habilitation, waiver; per 15 minutes
▶◆ T2022 Case management, per month
▶◆ T2023 Targeted case management; per month
▶◆ T2024 Service assessment/plan of care development, waiver
▶◆ T2025 Waiver services; not otherwise specified (NOS)
▶◆ T2026 Specialized childcare, waiver; per diem
▶◆ T2027 Specialized childcare, waiver; per 15 minutes
▶◆ T2028 Specialized supply, not otherwise specified, waiver
▶◆ T2029 Specialized medical equipment, not otherwise specified, waiver
▶◆ T2030 Assisted living, waiver; per month
▶◆ T2031 Assisted living; waiver, per diem
▶◆ T2032 Residential care, not otherwise specified (NOS), waiver; per month
▶◆ T2033 Residential care, not otherwise specified (NOS), waiver; per diem
▶◆ T2034 Crisis intervention, waiver; per diem

▶◆ T2035 Utility services to support medical equipment and assistive technology/devices, waiver

▶◆ T2036 Therapeutic camping, overnight, waiver; each session

▶◆ T2037 Therapeutic camping, day, waiver; each session

▶◆ T2038 Community transition, waiver; per service

▶◆ T2039 Vehicle modifications, waiver; per service

▶◆ T2040 Financial management, self-directed, waiver; per 15 minutes

▶◆ T2041 Supports brokerage, self-directed, waiver; per 15 minutes

▶◆ T2042 Hospice routine home care; per diem

▶◆ T2043 Hospice continuous home care; per hour

▶◆ T2044 Hospice inpatient respite care; per diem

▶◆ T2045 Hospice general inpatient care; per diem

▶◆ T2046 Hospice long term care, room and board only; per diem

▶◆ T2048 Behavioral health; long-term care residential (non-acute care in a residential treatment program where stay is typically longer than 30 days), with room and board, per diem

▶◆ T2101 Human breast milk processing, storage and distribution only

▶◆ T5001 Positioning seat for persons with special orthopedic needs, for use in vehicles

▶◆ T5999 Supply, not otherwise specified

▶❂ V2121 Lenticular lens, per lens, single
MCM 2130B

▶❂ V2221 Lenticular lens, per lens, bifocal
MCM 2130B

▶❂ V2321 Lenticular lens, per lens, trifocal
MCM 2130B

▶❂ V2745 Addition to lens, tint, any color, solid, gradient or equal, excludes photochroatic, any lens material, per lens
MCM 2130B

▶◆ V2756 Eye glass case

▶❂ V2761 Mirror coating, any type, solid, gradient or equal, any lens material, per lens
MCM 2130B

▶❂ V2762 Polarization, any lens material, per lens
MCM 2130B

▶❂ V2782 Lens, index 1.54 to 1.65 plastic or 1.60 to 1.79 glass, excludes polycarbonate, per lens
MCM 2130B

▶❂ V2783 Lens, index greater than or equal to 1.66 plastic or greater than or equal to 1.80 glass, excludes polycarbonate, per lens
MCM 2130B

▶❂ V2784 Lens, polycarbonate or equal, any index, per lens
MCM 2130B

▶❂ V2786 Specialty occupational multifocal lens, per lens
MCM 2130B

▶✻ V2797 Vision supply, accessory and/or service component of another HCPCS vision code

2004 HCPCS REVISED CODES

➠ ✪ A4326 Male external catheter specialty type ~~(e.g., inflatable, faceplate, etc.)~~ with integral collection chamber, each
MCM 2130

➠ ◆ A4538 Diaper, ~~service~~ reusable ~~diaper~~, provided by a diaper service, each diaper
CIM 60-9

➠ ✪ A4623 Tracheostomy, inner cannula ~~(replacement only)~~
MCM 2130, CIM 65-16

➠ ◆ A6025 ~~Silicone~~ Gel sheet for dermal or epidermal application, (e.g., silicone, hydrogel, other), each

➠ ✪ C1716 Brachytherapy ~~seed~~ source, gold-198
Medicare Statute 1833(t)

➠ ✪ C1718 Brachytherapy ~~seed~~ source, iodine 125
Medicare Statute 1833(t)

➠ ✪ C1719 Brachytherapy ~~seed~~ source, non-high dose rate iridium-192
Medicare Statute 1833(t)

➠ ✪ C1720 Brachytherapy ~~seed~~ source, palladium 103
Medicare Statute 1833(t)

➠ ✪ C2616 Brachytherapy ~~seed~~ source, yttrium-90
Medicare Statute 1833(t)

➠ ✪ E0141 ~~Rigid walker~~ Walker, rigid, wheeled, adjustable or fixed height ~~without seat~~
MCM 2100.1, CIM 60-9

➠ ✪ E0143 ~~Folding~~ Walker, folding, wheeled, ~~without seat~~ adjustable or fixed height
MCM 2100.1, CIM 60-9

➠ ✪ E0144 ~~Enclosed, framed folding walker~~ Walker, enclosed, four-sided framed, rigid or folding, wheeled with posterior seat
MCM 2100.1, CIM 60-9

➠ ✪ E0147 ~~Heavy-duty~~, Walker, heavy duty, multiple ~~breaking~~ braking system, variable wheel resistance ~~walker~~
MCM 2100.1, CIM 60-9

➠ ✻ E0149 Walker, heavy duty, wheeled, rigid or folding, any type, ~~each~~

➠ ◆ E0950 Wheelchair accessory, tray, each
Cross Reference K0107

➠ ✻ E0951 ~~Loop heal~~ Heel loop/holder, with or without ankle strap, each
Cross Reference K0034

➠ ◆ E0952 ~~Loop toe~~ Toe loop/holder, each

➠ ✻ E0958 Manual wheelchair accessory ~~attachment~~, ~~to convert any wheelchair to~~ one-arm drive attachment, each
Cross Reference K0101

➠ ◆ E0959 ~~Amputee adapter (device used to compensate for transfer of weight due to lost limbs to maintain proper balance)~~ Manual wheelchair accessory, adapter for amputee, each
Cross Reference K0100

➠ ◆ E0961 ~~Brake extension, for wheelchair~~ Manual wheelchair accessory, wheel lock brake extension (handle), each
CIM 60-9, Cross Reference K0079

➠ ◆ E0966 ~~Hook-on head rest extension~~ Manual wheelchair accessory, headrest extension, each
CIM 60-9, Cross Reference K0025

➠ ✪ E0967 Manual wheelchair accessory, ~~with eight vertical rubber-tipped projections, pair~~ hand rim with projections, ~~pair~~ each
CIM 60-9

➠ ◆ E0972 Wheelchair accessory, transfer board or device, each
Cross Reference K0103

➠ ◆ E0973 Wheelchair accessory, adjustable height, detachable armrests ~~desk or full length, wheelchair~~, complete assembly, each
CIM 60-9 ~~Cross Reference K0016~~

➠ ◆ E0974 ~~"Grade-aid" (device to prevent rolling back on incline) for wheelchair~~ Manual wheelchair accessory, anti-rollback device, each

➠ ◆ E0978 ~~Belt, safety with airplane buckle~~ Wheelchair accessory, safety belt/pelvic strap, each
~~Cross Reference K0031~~

➠ ◆ E0990 ~~Elevating leg rest, each~~ Wheelchair accessory, elevating leg rest, complete assembly, each
CIM 60-9, Cross Reference K0048

➠ ✻ E0992 Manual wheelchair accessory, solid seat insert
~~CIM 60-9~~, Cross Reference K0030

➠ ◆ E0995 Wheelchair accessory, calf rest/pad, each
Cross Reference K0049

➠ ✪ E1225 Manual wheelchair accessory, semi-reclining back ~~for customized wheelchair~~, (recline greater than 15 degrees, but less than 80 degrees), each
CIM 60-6

➠ ◆ E1226 Manual wheelchair accessory, ~~Full-reclining back for customized wheelchair fully~~ reclining back, each
CIM 60-6 ~~Cross Reference K0028~~

➠ ✪ E1390 Oxygen concentrator, single delivery port, capable of delivering 85 percent or greater oxygen concentration at the prescribed flow rate
CIM 60-4

➠ ✪ G0247 Routine foot care by a physician of a diabetic patient with diabetic sensory neuropathy resulting in a loss of protective sensation (LOPS) to include the local care of superficial wounds (i.e.

superficial to muscle and fascia) and at least the following if present: (1) local care of superficial wounds, (2) debridement of corns and calluses, and (3) trimming and debridement of nails.

➠ ✪ K0455 Infusion pump used for uninterrupted parenteral administration of ~~epoprostenol~~ medication, (e.g., epoprostenol or treprostinol)
CIM 60-14

➠ ✻ L1843 ~~KO~~ Knee orthosis, single upright, thigh and calf, with adjustable flexion and extension joint, medial-lateral and rotation control, ~~includes~~ with or without varus/valgus adjustment, prefabricated, includes fitting and adjustment

➠ ✻ L1844 ~~KO~~ Knee orthosis, single upright, thigh and calf, with adjustable flexion and extension joint, medial-lateral and rotation control, ~~includes~~ with or without varus/valgus adjustment, custom fabricated

➠ ✻ L1950 ~~AFO~~ Ankle foot orthosis, spiral, (~~IRM~~ institute of rehabilitative medicine type), plastic, custom-fabricated

➠ ✻ L2405 Addition to knee joint, lock; drop, stance or swing phase, each joint

➠ ✻ L4350 ~~Pneumatic~~ Ankle control orthosis, ~~splint~~ stirrup style, rigid, includes any type interface (e.g., pneumatic, gel), prefabricated, includes fitting and adjustment

➠ ✻ L4360 ~~Pneumatic ankle foot orthosis,~~ Walking boot, pneumatic, with or without joints, with or without interface material, prefabricated, includes fitting and adjustment

➠ ✻ L4386 Walking boot, non-pneumatic, ~~walking splint~~ with or without joints, with or without interface material, prefabricated, includes fitting and adjustment

➠ ✻ L5648 Addition to lower extremity, above knee, air, fluid, gel or equal, cushion socket

➠ ✻ L5848 Addition to endoskeletal, knee-shin system, hydraulic stance extension, dampening feature, ~~adjustable~~ with or without adjustability

➠ ✻ L5984 All endoskeletal lower extremity prosthesis, axial rotation unit, with or without adjustability

➠ ✻ L6620 Upper extremity addition, flexion/extension wrist unit, with or without friction

➠ ✻ L6675 Upper extremity addition, harness, ~~figure of eight (8) type~~ (e.g. figure of eight type), ~~for single control~~ single cable design

➠ ✻ L6676 Upper extremity addition, harness, ~~figure of eight (8) type~~ (e.g. figure of eight type), dual cable design

➠ ✪ L8658 Interphalangeal joint ~~implant~~ spacer, silicone or equal, each
MCM 2130

➠ ◆ M0100 Intragastric hypothermia using gastric freezing ~~(MNP)~~
CIM 35-65

➠ ◆ M0301 Fabric wrapping of abdominal aneurysm ~~(MNP)~~
CIM 35-64

➠ ✪ P9017 Fresh frozen plasma (single donor), frozen within 8 hours of collection, each unit
MCM 2455B

➠ ◆ S2150 Bone marrow or blood-derived peripheral stem cell harvesting and transplantation, allogenic or autologous, including pheresis, high-dose chemotherapy, and ~~28~~ the number of days of post-transplant care in the global definition (including drugs; hospitalization; medical, surgical, diagnostic and emergency services)

➠ ◆ S9123 Nursing care, in the home; by registered nurse, per hour (use for general nursing care only, not to be used when CPT codes 99500-99602 ~~or S codes S9802-S9803~~ can be used)

2004 HCPCS DELETED CODES

A4214
A4319
A4323
A4621
A4622
A4631
A4644
A4645
A4646
A4712
A6421
A6422
A6424
A6426
A6428
A6430
A6432
A6434
A6436
A6438
A6440
A7019
A7020
A9518
C1010
C1011
C1015
C1016
C1017
C1018
C1020
C1021
C1022
C1166
C1167
C1774
C9010
C9111
C9116
C9119
C9120
C9503
E0142
E0145
E0146
E0165
E0943
E0975
E0976
E0979
E0991
E0993
E1066
E1069
G0025
G0110
G0111
G0112
G0113
G0114
G0115
G0116
G0167
G0236
G0262
G0272
G0273
G0274
J0151
J1910
J2000
J2352
J7508
J9180
K0016
K0022
K0025
K0026
K0027
K0028
K0029
K0030
K0031
K0032
K0033
K0035
K0036
K0048
K0049
K0054
K0055
K0057
K0058
K0062
K0063
K0079
K0080
K0082
K0083
K0084
K0085
K0086
K0087
K0088
K0089
K0100
K0103
K0107
K0112
K0113
K0268
K0460
K0461
K0531
K0532
K0533
K0534
K0538
K0539
K0540
K0541
K0542
K0543
K0544
K0545
K0546
K0547
K0549
K0550
K0556
K0557
K0558
K0559
K0581
K0582
K0583
K0584
K0585
K0586
K0587
K0588
K0589
K0590
K0591
K0592
K0593
K0594
K0595
K0596
K0597
K0610
L1885
L2102
L2104
L2122
L2124
Q0086
Q2010
Q9920
Q9921
Q9922
Q9923
Q9924
Q9925
Q9926
Q9927
Q9928
Q9929
Q9930
Q9931
Q9932
Q9933
Q9934
Q9935
Q9936
Q9937
Q9938
Q9939
Q9940
S0009
S0079
S0124
S0130
S0135
S8180
S8181
S8945
S9524
S9546
S9802
S9803
S9806
T1008
T1011
V2116
V2117
V2216
V2217
V2316
V2317
V2740
V2741
V2742
V2743